Textbook of Dermatopathology

Notice

Medicine is an ever-changing science. As new research and clinical experience broaden our knowledge, changes in treatment and drug therapy are required. The editors and the publisher of this work have checked with sources believed to be reliable in their efforts to provide information that is complete and generally in accord with the standards accepted at the time of publication. However, in view of the possibility of human error or changes in medical sciences, neither the editors, nor the publisher, nor any other party who has been involved in the preparation or publication of this work warrants that the information contained herein is in every respect accurate or complete. Readers are encouraged to confirm the information contained herein with other sources. For example and in particular, readers are advised to check the product information sheet included in the package of each drug they plan to administer to be certain that the information contained in this book is accurate and that changes have not been made in the recommended dose or in the contraindications for administration. This recommendation is of particular importance in connection with new or infrequently used drugs.

Textbook of Dermatopathology

EDITOR

Raymond L. Barnhill, M.D.

Director
Division of Dermatopathology and Oral Pathology
Departments of Dermatology and Pathology
The Johns Hopkins Medical Institutions
Baltimore, Maryland
Formerly Director, Division of Dermatopathology, Brigham
  and Women's Hospital and Children's Hospital
Associate Professor of Pathology
Harvard Medical School
Boston, Massachusetts

ASSOCIATE EDITOR

A. Neil Crowson, M.D.

Director, Central Medical Laboratories
  and Department of Laboratories
Misericordia General Hospital
Winnipeg, Canada

ASSISTANT EDITORS

Klaus J. Busam, M.D.

Assistant Attending Pathologist in the
  Department of Pathology
Memorial Sloan-Kettering Cancer Center
New York, New York

Scott R. Granter, M.D.

Assistant Professor of Pathology
Harvard Medical School
Associate Pathologist
Brigham and Women's Hospital
Consultant in Pathology
Children's Hospital
Boston, Massachusetts

McGraw-Hill

HEALTH PROFESSIONS DIVISION

New York   St. Louis   San Francisco   Auckland   Bogotá   Caracas   Lisbon   London   Madrid
Mexico City   Milan   Montreal   New Delhi   Paris   San Juan   Singapore   Sydney   Tokyo   Toronto

McGraw-Hill

A Division of The McGraw-Hill Companies

Textbook of Dermatopathology

1234567890 QPK QPK 9987

ISBN 0-07-005726-5

This book was set in Times Roman by Better Graphics, Inc.
The editors were Joseph Hefta and Pamela Touboul;
the index was prepared by Irving Condé Tullar;
the production supervisor was Helene G. Landers;
the cover designer was Parallelogram/Marsha Cohen.

Quebecor Printing/Kingsport was printer and binder.

This book is printed on acid-free paper.

Library of Congress Cataloging-in-Publication Data

Textbook of dermatopathology / editor, Raymond L. Barnhill ; associate
    editor, Neil Crowson ; assistant editors, Klaus J. Busam, Scott R.
    Granter.
        p.   cm.
    Includes bibliographical references and index.
    ISBN 0-07-005726-5
    1. Skin—Histopathology.   2. Skin—Diseases.   3. Skin—
Pathophysiology.   I. Barnhill, Raymond L.
    [DNLM: 1. Skin—pathology.   2. Skin Diseases—diagnosis.
3. Diagnosis, Differential.   WR 105 T355 1997]
RL95.T49   1997
616.5′07—dc21
DNLM/DLC
for Library of Congress   97-24101

Dedication

To my father and to others who have had a profound influence on my thinking and writing: Shelby Foote, Walker Percy, and Marcel Proust.

Contents

Part One
INFLAMMATORY REACTIONS IN THE SKIN / 1

Part TWO
PREDOMINANTLY NON-INFLAMMATORY CONDITIONS / 279

Andreas Haeffner
Beatrix Mueller
Reinhard Dummer
Helmut Kerl
Lorenzo Cerroni
Stefan Hoedl
Stanislaw A. Buechner
W.P. Daniel Su

Part Five
DISORDERS OF NAILS AND ORAL MUCOSA / 813

APPENDIX / 843

Contributors

ZSOLT B. ARGENYI, M.D.
Professor of Pathology and Dermatology
Director of Dermatopathology
Departments of Pathology and Dermatology
University of Iowa Hospitals and Clinics
Iowa City, Iowa
(Chapter 33)

SARAH K. BARKSDALE, M.D.
Assistant Professor of Pathology,
Temple University School of Medicine
Philadelphia, Pennsylvania
(Chapter 9)

RAYMOND L. BARNHILL, M.D.
Director
Division of Dermatopathology and Oral Pathology
Professor, Departments of Dermatology and Pathology
The Johns Hopkins Medical Institutions
Baltimore, Maryland
Formerly, Director, Div. of Dermatopathology
Brigham and Women's Hospital
Associate Professor of Pathology
Harvard Medical School
Boston, Massachusetts
(Chapters 1, 7, 9, 11, 15, 16, 18, 20, 21, 27, 28, 29, 31)

ALAN S. BOYD, M.D.
Assistant Professor of Dermatology
Vanderbilt University School of Medicine
Nashville, Tennessee
(Chapter 26)

STANISLAW A. BUECHNER, M.D.
Professor of Dermatology
University of Basel
Basel, Switzerland
(Chapter 34)

GUENTER BURG, M.D.
Professor and Chair
Department of Dermatology
University Hospital
Zurich, Switzerland
(Chapter 34)

KLAUS BUSAM, M.D.
Attending Pathologist
Department of Pathology
Memorial Sloan-Kettering Cancer Center
New York, New York
(Chapters 9, 21, Appendix)

ANDREW CARLSON, M.D.
Associate Professor of Pathology
Albany Medical College
Albany, New York
(Appendix)

LORENZO CERRONI, M.D.
Associate Professor of Dermatology
University of Graz
Graz, Austria
(Chapter 34)

CLAY J. COCKERELL, M.D.
Associate Clinical Professor
Division of Dermatopathology
Departments of Dermatology and Pathology
University of Texas Southwestern Medical Center
Dallas, Texas
(Chapter 22)

A. NEIL CROWSON, M.D.
Director
Central Medical Laboratories and Department of Laboratories
Misericordia General Hospital
Winnipeg, Manitoba, Canada
(Chapters 5, 12, 20)

A. DEL ROSARIO, M.D.
Assistant Professor of Pathology
Department of Pathology
Albany Medical College
Albany, New York
(Appendix)

REINHARD DUMMER, M.D.
Assistant Professor
Department of Dermatology
University Hospital
Zurich, Switzerland
(Chapter 34)

J. STEPHEN DUMLER, M.D.
Director
Division of Medical Microbiology and Associate Professor
Department of Pathology
The Johns Hopkins University School of Medicine
Baltimore, Maryland
(Chapter 20)

PHILIP FLECKMAN, M.D.
Associate Professor of Medicine
University of Washington School of Medicine
Seattle, Washington
(Chapter 14)

CHRISTOPHER D. M. FLETCHER, M.D., M.R.C. PATH.
Professor of Pathology
Harvard Medical School; and Director of Surgical Pathology
Brigham and Women's Hospital
Boston, Massachusetts
(Chapters 30, 32)

PAUL S. GILLUM, M.D.
Assistant Professor of Dermatology
University of Oklahoma
Oklahoma City, Oklahoma
(Chapter 4)

LOREN E. GOLITZ, M.D.
Professor of Dermatology and Pathology
University of Colorado School of Medicine; and Chief of Dermatology
Denver General Hospital
Denver, Colorado
(Chapter 4)

ALDO GONZÁLEZ-SERVA, M.D.
Associate Dermatopathologist
Pathology Services, Inc.; Assistant Professor of Dermatology
Tufts University; Assistant Professor of Pathology
Boston University; and Lecturer in Pathology
Harvard University
Boston, Massachusetts
(Chapter 36)

SCOTT R. GRANTER, M.D.
Assistant Professor of Pathology
Harvard Medical School; and Associate Pathologist,
Brigham and Women's Hospital
Consultant in Pathology
Children's Hospital
Boston, Massachusetts
(Chapter 30)

ANDREAS HAEFFNER, M.D.
Resident, Department of Dermatology
University Hospital
Zurich, Switzerland
(Chapter 34)

VICTORIA HOBBS HAMET, M.D.
Research Fellow, Dermatopathology Laboratory
University of Maryland School of Medicine
Baltimore, Maryland
(Chapter 21)

TERENCE J. HARRIST, M.D.
Assistant Clinical Professor of Pathology
Harvard Medical School
Beth Israel Deaconess Medical Center/Pathology Services, Inc.
Boston, Massachusetts
(Chapter 7)

JEFF D. HARVELL, M.D.
Dermatopathology Fellow, Department of Pathology
Bowman Gray School of Medicine
Winston-Salem, North Carolina
(Chapter 6)

KEN HASHIMOTO, M.D.
Department of Dermatology and Syphilology
Wayne State University School of Medicine
Detroit, Michigan
(Chapters 15, 16)

STEFAN HOEDL, M.D.
Professor of Dermatology
Department of Dermatology
University of Graz
Graz, Austria
(Chapter 34)

THOMAS D. HORN, M.D.
Professor and Chair, Department of Dermatology
University of Arkansas for Medical Sciences
Little Rock, Arkansas
(Chapter 3)

STEVEN J. HUNT, M.D.
Northern Pathology Laboratory
Iron Mountain, Michigan
(Chapter 31)

DANIEL M. JONES, M.D., PH.D.
Clinical Fellow in Pathology
Harvard Medical School; and Resident in Pathology
Brigham and Women's Hospital
Boston, Massachusetts
(Chapter 1)

JACQUELINE JUNKINS-HOPKINS, M.D.
Assistant Professor of Dermatology
Department of Dermatology
University of Pennsylvania School of Medicine
Philadelphia, Pennsylvania
(Chapter 18)

GRACE F. KAO, M.D.
Professor of Dermatology and Pathology
University of Maryland School of Medicine; and
Director, Section of Dermatopathology and Attending Pathologist
University of Maryland Medical Systems Hospital
Consultant Dermatopathologist, VA Medical Center
Baltimore, Maryland
(Chapter 20)

CATHARINE LISA KAUFFMAN, M.D.
Assistant Professor of Dermatology and Pathology; and
Director, Dermatopathology Laboratory
University of Maryland School of Medicine
Baltimore, Maryland
(Chapter 21)

HELMUT KERL, M.D.
Professor and Chair
Department of Dermatology
University of Graz
Graz, Austria
(Chapter 34)

WERNER KEMPF, M.D.
Resident, Department of Dermatology
University Hospital
Zurich, Switzerland
(Chapter 34)

ZAFAR M. KHAN, M.D.
Division of Dermatopathology
University of Texas Southwestern Medical Center
Dallas, Texas
(Chapter 22)

SABINE KOHLER, M.D.
Assistant Professor, Departments of Dermatology and Pathology
Stanford University School of Medicine
Palo Alto, California
(Chapter 8)

THEORDORE H. KWAN, M.D.
Assistant Professor of Pathology
Harvard Medical School; and Associate in Pathology
Beth Israel Deaconess Medical Center
Boston, Massachusetts
(Chapter 2)

JULIA LAGUETTE, M.D.
Instructor in Pathology, Harvard Medical School
Associate Pathologist, Dermatopathology Division
Department of Pathology
Brigham and Women's Hospital
Boston, Massachusetts
(Chapter 13)

FREDDYE LEMONS-ESTES, CDR, MC, USN
Department of Dermatopathology
Armed Forces Institute of Pathology
Washington, D.C.
(Chapter 23)

LISA LERNER, M.D.
Assistant Professor of Pathology and Dermatology
Harvard Medical School
Massachusetts General Hospital
Boston, Massachusetts
(Chapter 7)

FRANZ VON LICHTENBERG, M.D.
Professor of Pathology
Harvard Medical School
Brigham and Women's Hospital
Boston, Massachusetts
(Chapter 24)

CYNTHIA M. MAGRO, M.D.
Assistant Clinical Professor of Pathology
Harvard Medical School
Beth Israel Deaconess Medical Center
Pathology Services, Inc.
Boston, Massachusetts
(Chapters 7, 12, 20)

RANDALL J. MARGOLIS, M.D.
Assistant Clinical Professor of Pathology
Harvard Medical School; Department of Pathology
Harvard Community Health Plan
Brigham and Women's Hospital
Boston, Massachusetts
(Chapter 35)

BEATRIX MUELLER
Technician, Department of Dermatology
University Hospital
Zurich, Switzerland
(Chapter 34)

BERNARD NG, M.D.
Resident in Pathology
Albany Medical College
Albany, New York
(Appendix)

ANN MARIE NELSON, M.D.
Chief,
Division of AIDS Pathology and Emerging Infectious Diseases
Department of Infectious and Parasitic Disease Pathology
Armed Forces Institute of Pathology
Washington, D.C.
(Chapter 23)

NEAL S. PENNEYS, M.D., PH.D.
Professor and Chair, Division of Dermatology
St. Louis University School of Medicine
St. Louis, Missouri
(Chapter 13)

MICHAEL W. PIEPKORN, M.D., PH.D.
Associate Professor of Medicine and Pathology
University of Washington School of Medicine
Seattle, Washington
(Chapter 14)

RONALD P. RAPINI, M.D.
Professor and Chair
Department of Dermatology
Texas Tech University
Lubbock, Texas
(Chapter 19)

ANDREW A. RENSHAW, M.D.
Assistant Professor of Pathology
Harvard Medical School; and Associate Pathologist
Brigham and Women's Hospital
Boston, Massachusetts
(Chapter 32)

DANIEL J. SANTA CRUZ, M.D.
Cutaneous Pathology
St. John's Mercy Medical Center
St. Louis, Missouri
(Chapter 31)

BRIAN SCHAPIRO, M.D.
Fellow in Dermatopathology
Harvard Medical School
Beth Israel Deaconess Medical Center/Pathology Services, Inc.
Boston, Massachusetts
(Chapter 7)

GLYNIS A. SCOTT, M.D.
Associate Professor of Dermatology and Pathology
University of Rochester School of Medicine and Dentistry
Rochester, New York
(Chapter 25)

BRUCE R. SMOLLER, M.D.
Professor of Pathology
University of Arkansas for Medical Sciences
Little Rock, Arkansas
(Chapter 8)

ALVIN R. SOLOMON, M.D.
Professor of Dermatology and Pathology
Emory University School of Medicine
Atlanta, Georgia
(Chapter 10)

KURT S. STENN, M.D.
Director, Skin Biology Research Center
Johnson and Johnson
Skillman, New Jersey
(Appendix)

PAUL E. SWANSON, M.D.
Associate Professor of Pathology
Washington University School of Medicine
St. Louis, Missouri
(Chapters 28, 29)

W. P. DANIEL SU, M.D.
Consultant, Department of Dermatology
Mayo Clinic and Mayo Foundation; and
Professor of Dermatology
Mayo Medical School
Rochester, Minnesota
(Chapter 34)

STEVEN TAHAN, M.D.
Assistant Professor of Pathology
Harvard Medical School
Beth Israel Deaconess Medical Center
Boston, Massachusetts
(Chapter 21)

STEPHEN F. TEMPLETON, M.D.
Assistant Professor of Dermatology and Pathology
Emory University School of Medicine
Atlanta, Georgia
(Chapter 10)

CLIFTON R. WHITE, JR., M.D.
Professor of Dermatology
Oregon Health Sciences University
Portland, Oregon
(Chapter 17)

WAIN L. WHITE, M.D.
Associate Professor of Dermatology and Pathology
Bowman Gray School of Medicine
Wake Forest University
Winston-Salem, North Carolina
(Chapter 6)

DAVID A. WHITING, M.D., FACP, FRCP(ED)
Clinical Professor of Dermatology and Pediatrics
University of Texas Southwestern Medical Center; and
Medical Director, Baylor Hair Research and Treatment Center
Dallas, Texas
(Chapter 10)

MARK R. WICK, M.D.
Professor of Pathology
Director of Surgical Pathology and Co-Director of Dermatopathology
Washington University School of Medicine
St. Louis, Missouri
(Chapters 28, 29)

SOOK-BIN WOO, D.M.D., MMSc
Instructor
Harvard School of Dental Medicine
Attending Dentist
Department of Oral and Maxillofacial Surgery and Consultant in Pathology
Brigham and Women's Hospital; and
Associate Pathologist, Pathology Services, Inc.
Boston, Massachusetts
(Chapter 37)

GARY S. WOOD, M.D.
Professor of Dermatology and Pathology
Department of Dermatology
Case Western Reserve University School of Medicine
Chief, Dermatology Services
VA Medical Center
Cleveland, Ohio
(Appendix)

Preface

The question might be posed, Why another textbook of dermatopathology? since a number of books are currently available and would seem to do justice to the subject. Quite simply, I have perceived the need for another book. Following on the success of a monograph on melanocytic lesions of the skin, *The Pathology of Melanocytic Nevi and Malignant Melanoma*, I believe that there is indeed a need for a general text on dermatopathology emphasizing the same format as the aforementioned monograph: descriptive histopathology and differential diagnosis, critical analysis, balanced perspectives on what is known and what is not, clarity of writing, the use of tables to summarize the key features of major entities, and color photomicrographs.

At the same time it must be acknowledged that the scope of such a book goes well beyond that of a monograph on melanocytic lesions. As a result, I have engaged a scholarly group of individuals to help in writing such a book in a timely fashion. Nonetheless one of my major goals has been to maintain a uniform style in keeping with the philosophy of the book.

In recent years I have been impressed with the need to provide some orientation for beginning the process of learning dermatopathology. Thus the first chapter of this book is devoted to the approach to diagnosis at the microscope. Daniel Jones, M.D., Ph.D. also discusses succinctly the scientific basis of pattern recognition as a prologue to algorithms and the description of the major patterns of inflammation in the skin. Christopher French, M.D. has in addition designed schematic color figures that enhance the recognition of patterns of inflammation in the skin. Another major feature is that Associate Editor Neil Crowson, M.D. has taken high quality photomicrographs for most of the entities in the book. This is another characteristic that provides a uniform style to the book. I am deeply grateful to Dr. Crowson for this enormous undertaking.

Although all major entities have been covered in an erudite fashion in the book, a number of unique features must be mentioned. The chapter on disorders of the skin appendages provides new quantitative information on the alopecias and describes the use of transverse sections in diagnosis of alopecia. Dr. Crowson has written a comprehensive chapter on drug eruptions and included lists of medications implicated in these eruptions. Critical chapters on controversial and difficult topics such as vasculitis, panniculitis, disorders of pigmentation, and melanocytic lesions will provide greater insight and aid to the pathologist dealing with these conditions. Finally, there are more detailed chapters on disorders of the nails and the oral mucosa than are currently available in most other texts. Another modification has been the inclusion of a scholarly section on normal skin histology, laboratory methods, immunohistochemistry, and the molecular biology of cutaneous lymphoid infiltrates in an appendix rather than in the text itself.

It will become evident to the reader that there is occasionally some overlap or duplication of some conditions among the various chapters, since no method of classification is entirely consistent. My intention has been to allow some duplication since this provides different perspectives on a disease process.

Finally and most importantly, I would like to acknowledge the tremendous efforts of many friends and colleagues without whose advice, encouragement, and help this book would not have been possible. First of all I would like to thank Neil Crowson for his enormous contributions in photography, writing, and unflagging encouragement and support throughout the project. I am also indebted to my former fellows Klaus Busam and Scott Granter for their commitment and hard work on the book. I am also most appreciative of my secretaries Robin McCarthy (who has since departed for an undoubtedly easier job!) and Maria Palaima, and the staff at McGraw-Hill for their dedication and efforts in bringing the book to closure. Lastly, I am most grateful to all the contributors who have sacrificed so much of their time and energy to make the book not only possible but a learned work that will have an impact on the field.

Raymond L. Barnhill, M.D.

Foreword

As senior editor of this new Textbook of Dermatopathology, Dr. Raymond Barnhill brings to the task years of experience as a dermatopathologist, clinical dermatologist, clinical investigator, and author. This has given him an unparalleled understanding of inflammatory and neoplastic diseases of the skin and the ability to teach others. As Director of Dermatopathology at the Brigham and Women's Hospital and the Children's Hospital in Boston, he has had contact with both pediatric and adult dermatological conditions, and as a member of the Combined Harvard Dermatopathology Training Program, he has developed the knowledge and skills to interact with pathologists, dermatologists, trainees, and students. The success of his monograph on Melanocytic Lesions of the Skin speaks of the effectiveness of his writing and teaching approaches.

For this book, Dr. Barnhill has assembled a stellar roster of authors from various disciplines, and has appropriately included both established leaders in the field as well as the cream of our younger generation of dermatopathologists. He himself has co-authored one-third of the chapters of the book, and I know first-hand that he has spent a great deal of effort meticulously editing all chapters for consistency, style, and accuracy. His Associate Editor, Dr. Neil Crowson, has been instrumental in providing the high quality micrographs for many of the entities in the book, and two young, energetic Assistant Editors, Drs. Klaus Busam and Scott Granter contributed heavily to the book.

I look forward to the publication of this text and wish it the success it truly deserves.

Ramzi S. Cotran, M.D.

PART ONE

INFLAMMATORY REACTIONS IN THE SKIN

CHAPTER 1

INTRODUCTION TO MICROSCOPIC INTERPRETATION

Raymond L. Barnhill / Daniel M. Jones

Perhaps in no other area of pathology does one encounter such diverse disease processes and bewildering terminology as in dermatopathology. Without a systematic and logical approach to diagnosis, the observer may be hopelessly lost. Unfortunately, the approach to learning dermatopathology, as in many other areas of medicine, has traditionally been disease-oriented, a format not easily mastered by beginners or even more advanced students in the field. However, in recent years there has been greater emphasis on utilizing methods of pattern recognition for diagnosis, particularly for inflammatory conditions in the skin.[1–5]

The objectives of this chapter will be (1) to present new information on visual perception and reaching pathologic diagnoses and (2) to outline a practical step-by-step method for interpreting a microslide and formulating a differential diagnosis, utilizing techniques of pattern recognition and algorithms.

MECHANISMS OF VISUAL PERCEPTION IN DIAGNOSIS

In this section, we will review current understanding of the perceptual principles used in diagnostic dermatopathology. As discussed later in this chapter, a systematic approach to diagnosis of skin lesions stressing an orderly "algorithmic" approach is helpful, especially early in training. However, it is obvious that many lesions are instantly recognized by the experienced dermatopathologist. Indeed, the correct diagnosis of common skin tumors can often be made by inspection of the microslide with the naked eye or at the lowest scanning magnification. This is because the low-power pattern ("tumor silhouette") of a cutaneous proliferation is at least as important as cytologic criteria for diagnosis.[5] Similarly, *low-power* features are the basis for the classification of most inflammatory skin lesions (See Table 1-1). Unfortunately for the beginner, rapid diagnosis involves not only the appreciation of features such as symmetry and shape but also comparison with visual memories of similar lesions seen previously. It is this ability to store and retrieve visual patterns which is the basis of diagnostic pathology.

Certain tumor growth patterns appear to be intrinsically more readily recognizable. This is supported by a large body of perceptual research demonstrating that some simple visual targets (termed *good patterns*) are more rapidly recognized than others. Conversely, there is impaired performance of visual tasks which involve recall of *poor* visual targets. Recent neuroimaging studies have suggested this observation may be explained by inherent differences in the brain's ability to store and/or recall certain images.[6] The same may be true for patterns in histopathology. The easy recognition of some skin tumors (e.g., keratoacanthoma

or cylindroma) in contrast to others (e.g., regressed nevus or fibrous papule) may be an intrinsic function of the visual impact of each tumor's particular growth pattern (Fig. 1-1). Recognition of lesions with poor patterns may take longer or require more expertise.

Although it may appear intuitive and instantaneous, visual pattern and shape recognition is a highly complex process which involves more than simple *wallpaper matching*. For instance, recognition of many patterns occurs independently of the size or orientation of a particular lesion.[7] Basal cell carcinoma is invariably recognized because of its characteristic nests and islands of basaloid cells with peripheral palisading and retraction artifact. This pattern can be extracted even from superficial lesions of small size or those in tangential section (Fig. 1-2). Similarly, schwannomas have such a distinct pattern of alternating hypocellular and hypercellular curvilinear whorled fascicles that recognition is almost instantaneous. This suggests that more than a simple database of tumor images may be stored for comparison. It is not yet clear whether three-dimensional representations of tumor pattern may be constructed and stored by the visual system to hasten their recognition.

Since many diagnoses cannot be made on the overall pattern alone of a biopsy, visual attention must eventually be focused on individual cells or groups of cells (Fig. 1-3). Recent research suggests this is a two-stage process whereby initially all objects in a microscopic field compete for visual attention.[8,9] Once an object of interest (e.g., a subepidermal blister) has been located, the eye moves to place that object at the center of its gaze. This concentrates the enormous processing power of the visual system on a small area, and the surrounding tissue is temporarily (largely) ignored. After a period of close scrutiny, visual attention is once more defocussed, and another microscopic field can be examined for new objects.

During our initial scan of a microscopic field, visual attention can be influenced by specific search targets. Fundamentally, the visual system is most attentive to objects with unusual features (e.g., viral inclusions or foreign-body giant cells) or those that it has not seen recently (e.g., mitoses).[8] However, the specific task and nonvisual information such as clinical history can strongly influence the selection of visual targets. With practice, the visual system becomes increasingly more efficient in its search for specific targets. It appears that the brain is capable of creating an internal image of a search object which it can use for rapid comparison with incoming information. As a result, the search for significant objects in a biopsy (e.g., mitoses or eosinophils) tends to get easier the longer we attend to the task.

Although it also involves pattern recognition, the diagnosis of inflammatory lesions presents a different challenge. Instead of arriving

Examination of microslide with the naked eye
  Size, number, and nature of sections
  Site of pathologic process
    Epidermis
    Dermis
    Subcutis
  Clues from histochemical staining: Basophilic staining suggesting basal cell carcinoma, small round cell tumors, or lymphoid infiltrates
Examination at scanning magnification (2X or 4X objective)
  Determine type of specimen and adequacy for histological evaluation
    Curetting
    Punch biopsy
    Shave
    Skin ellipse
  Determine general anatomic site
    Head and neck
    Trunk and proximal extremities
    Acral and frictional surfaces
  Determine basic nature of the process and stage in development of disease and formulate differential diagnosis
Examination at intermediate magnification (10X and 20X objectives)
  Confirmation of impression at scanning magnification
  Confirmation of particular features, such as parakeratosis, spongiosis, mucin deposition
  Identification of particular cell types, such as lymphocytes, eosinophils, epithelioid histiocytes
  Systematic evaluation of specimen from stratum corneum sequentially to epidermis, dermis, and subcutis for specimens with subtle alterations
  Confirmation of stage in development, if possible
High magnification (40X, 60X, or 100X objectives)
  Careful assessment of cellular and nuclear detail as for cytological atypia
  Identification of infectious organisms
Integration of all information
  Development of histological differential diagnosis without clinical information
  Obtaining clinical information from pathology requisition and speaking directly with clinician if necessary
    Age, gender, site of biopsy
    Detailed information as to distribution, clinical features, and chronology of eruption or individual lesion and clinical differential diagnosis
  Clinicopathological correlation and generation of a differential diagnosis with probability of a diagnosis or a single specific diagnosis if possible

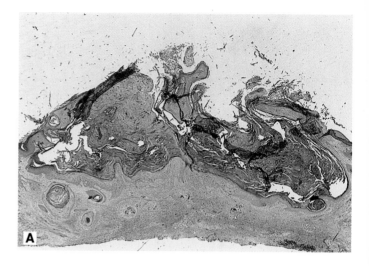

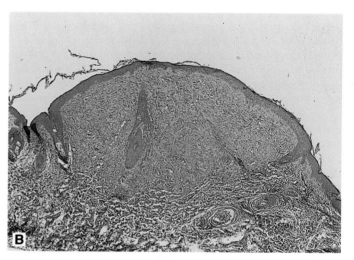

FIGURE 1-1 "Good" pattern versus "poor" pattern. The crateriform appearance of a keratoacanthoma (*A*) is evident at the lowest scanning magnification. This is in contrast with the subtle dermal alteration seen in a sclerosing Spitz tumor (*B*).

at a definite diagnosis, the usual approach is descriptive (i.e., what kinds of inflammatory cells are present and where they are located). In the absence of adequate clinical information, a range of possible diagnoses is usually provided. This is a different perceptual task for which the goal is not to match a stored visual image precisely but to compare the features of a lesion to the entity to which it is (statistically) most similar. Lesions are initially grouped into general categories (see Table 1-2), then specific searches are initiated to narrow (or prioritize) the diagnoses. For instance, once the pattern of interface dermatitis has been

identified, visual search for viral inclusions could support the diagnoses of a viral exanthem.

As discussed later, this stepwise approach depends on a knowledge of the diagnostic differential for each inflammatory pattern. For instance, if a predominantly perivascular inflammatory infiltrate was perceived at low power, recall of an internal visual representation of vasculitis could allow for the subsequent rapid recognition of fibrin thrombi and leukocytoclasia. As a pathologist gains experience with a specialty area, the diagnostic search becomes more efficient. This observation is supported by recent discoveries about learning within the visual system. As visual skill develops, there is increasingly selective use of visual pathways with a decrease in nonspecific brain activity. In the long-term, as with other skill learning, this would also likely be accompanied by an increase in the visual cortical areas devoted to performing the specific visual task of histomorphologic recognition.[10] Full maturation of visual expertise in dermatopathology would require not only a "library" of stored visual images of skin lesions but knowledge of the associated features of particular entities. Using a systematic approach to diagnosis may "teach" the visual system to link discrete diagnostic features with the database of visual images.

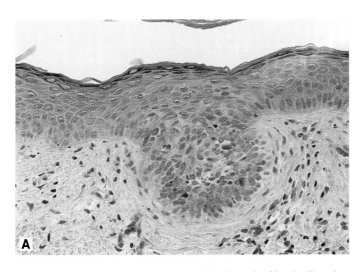
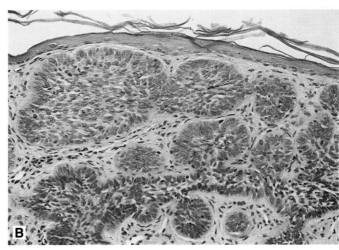

FIGURE 1-2   The power of a good pattern. The diagnosis of basal cell carcinoma can be made even on a small superficial lesion (*A*). The features of basaloid cells with peripheral palisading and retraction artifact are more readily recognizable in a larger well-developed lesion (*B*).

There has been a great interest in designing computer pattern recognition devices capable of automated diagnosis of dermatopathologic material. Most of these systems extract morphometric data (cell size, shape, nuclear contour, shading) and subject it to rules-based algorithms for diagnosis. Although modeled on visual features used by expert pathologists in diagnosis, these systems don't model the holistic property of human pattern recognition. In fact, many trained pathologists will relate that they resort to a systematic approach (e.g., epidermis→dermis→blood vessels→subcutis) only when they can't arrive at the diagnosis by *gestalt* (pattern recognition). The recent use of neural-network circuits that can be trained by test cases to classify lesions without explicit rules may be more successful in imitating the perceptual processes described above. The rest of this chapter outlines a rules-based approach to diagnosis based on pattern recognition.

INTERPRETATION OF THE SLIDE

Initial Examination of the Slide with the Naked Eye

The histopathologist should first inspect the microslide with the naked eye in order to gain some appreciation of the size, number, and nature of the histologic sections on the slide (Table 1-1). Often one can make certain deductions from this gross examination alone. For example, a small specimen is either a curetting, shave, or punch biopsy and connotes particular pathologic processes (see below). In contrast, a large specimen generally indicates an excision. Often it is possible to establish the process as epidermal, dermal, or subcutaneous by this examination. The tinctorial properties (histochemical staining) also may provide clues to diagnosis, e.g., bluish cellular aggregates or nodules suggest

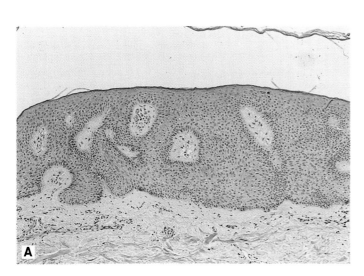
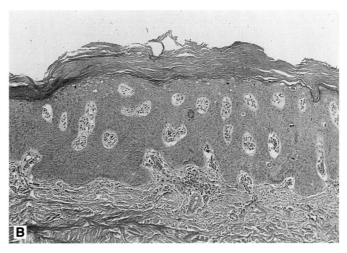

FIGURE 1-3   The limits of pattern recognition. "Low-power" lookalikes. At scanning magnification, both seborrheic keratosis (*A*) and squamous cell carcinoma in situ (*B*) demonstrate epidermal proliferation. Higher magnification is needed to identify the lack of maturation, numerous mitotic figures, and striking nuclear atypia in the carcinoma in situ.

high nuclear-to-cytoplasmic ratios because of basophilic staining of nuclei and, as a result, indicate processes such as basal cell carcinoma, small-cell carcinoma, and infiltrates of small lymphocytes, or calcium deposition.

Examination of the Microslide at Scanning (2X or 4X) Magnification

The microslide should next be viewed at scanning magnification, i.e., with a 2X or 4X objective. Although a 2X objective may prove optimal for the initial examination of many specimens, particularly large specimens, many microscopes are equipped only with 4X objectives. However, the 4X objective is a reasonable alternative, and additional information can generally be obtained at this magnification. If possible, the specimen should always be studied initially without knowledge of age, gender, or other clinical findings in order to gather information and formulate differential diagnosis. Although the experienced pathologist often does not need to resort to such a method unless a diagnosis is not immediately apparent, the beginner should systematically study a slide with specific goals in mind:

1. The pathologist should attempt to identify the *type of specimen* submitted, i.e., is it a curettage, punch, shave, or excisional specimen? Determination of the type of specimen is important, since it often provides clues to the type of disease process suspected by the submitting clinician. For example, curettage specimens are often taken for neoplastic processes such as actinic or seborrheic keratoses or basal cell carcinoma. Shave biopsies are usually obtained for diagnosis of keratoses or basal or squamous cell carcinoma. In general, punch biopsies are submitted for diagnosis of either neoplastic or inflammatory conditions. In some instances, these biopsies are utilized to "excise" a proliferation or tumor, and thus margins may need to be assessed. By and large, skin ellipses (excisions) are submitted for suspected tumors but also on occasion for inflammatory processes such as vasculitis or panniculitis.

2. Next, the pathologist should inspect the specimen with the idea of determining in general terms from what *anatomic site* the tissue was taken. Based on characteristics such as prominence of sebaceous follicles, relative paucity of hair follicles, thickness of the reticular dermis, and thickness of the stratum corneum, one can recognize the following general regions of the integument: (a) head and neck, (b) trunk and proximal extremities, and (c) acral (including frictional) surfaces. Many diseases have characteristic site distributions, and knowledge of the particular localization of the lesion or eruption is useful in formulating one's differential diagnosis.

3. The entire specimen, i.e., epidermis, dermis, subcutis, should be scanned for the principal site of involvement by a disease process, if any, and the nature of the process, whether inflammatory, proliferative, or noninflammatory. Although in most instances the site of involvement is obvious, it is important that the specimen is systematically examined when the process is not so obvious. In general, the specimen should be scrutinized in a sequential fashion, e.g., beginning with the stratum corneum then proceeding to the epidermis, dermis, and subcutis. At scanning magnification, one should be able to appreciate many aspects of the disease process without going to greater magnification. If an inflammatory process is present, one should attempt to recognize the following: the nature of epidermal involvement, e.g., spongiosis, psoriasiform epidermal hyperplasia, or vesicle, blister, or pustule formation; the pattern of the inflammatory infiltrate, whether bandlike (lichenoid), perivascular, interstitial, periadnexal, nodular, or diffuse (pan-dermal); the depth of the infiltrate, e.g., superficial only or superficial and deep; possibly the presence of vascular damage; the essential character of

an infiltrate, i.e., whether it is composed of mononuclear cells, suggesting small lymphocytes, or larger cells; alteration of the dermis as by fibrosis or sclerosis resulting in a "square" punch biopsy versus the typical inverted cone configuration; thickening or atrophy of the dermis; or deposition of material such as calcium. A primary proliferative or neoplastic condition should also be obvious in most instances at scanning magnification.

After the completion of the above exercise, the pathologist often can establish the basic nature and localization of the disease process and begin to develop a preliminary differential diagnosis, if he or she has not already arrived at a specific diagnosis. In some instances, diagnosis may not be possible at scanning magnification because the changes are subtle, or there has been a sampling error. At this point, the pathologist must go to greater magnification to confirm an impression or to gain more information.

Examination at Intermediate Magnification

Again, most information about a pathologic process is obtained at scanning magnification. The tendency to go to higher magnification too soon should be resisted since one will often overlook a crucial feature, in effect missing "the forest for the trees." Closer inspection (with 10x and 20x objectives) of the specimen can confirm particular features of pathologic processes, i.e., parakeratosis, spongiosis, fibrinoid necrosis, mucin deposition, and can allow identification of specific cell types such as lymphocytes or eosinophils. However, in some instances greater magnification may be needed in order to identify a morphological feature not recognizable at low magnification, e.g., hyphal elements in the cornified layer, basal layer vacuolopathy, amyloid deposits in the papillary dermis, or mucinosis in the reticular dermis.

Examination at High Magnification

As mentioned for intermediate magnification, use of the high-power objective should also be reserved for specific indications. Such examination is necessary in order to study the cytologic details of cells, e.g., the nuclear contours of lymphocytes or nuclear atypia in general; to confirm the nature of infectious organisms, and to confirm other findings.

Integration of All Information

During the above exercise of examining the microslide, the histopathologist should consider that he or she is objectively gathering information that can be integrated with other (clinical and laboratory) information to arrive at some conclusion about the disease process and not necessarily to arrive at a single diagnosis. One should, at all times, try to avoid reaching a conclusion too quickly and failing to observe other pertinent findings in the specimen. The pathologist should always try to think expansively of every potential pathologic process that might explain the histologic findings. One should continuously weigh the various points that argue for or against a particular pathologic condition.

After completing the above examination and reaching some tentative impression (or lack of conclusion) about the specimen without knowledge of clinical parameters, it is then necessary consider the clinical context of the specimen. Even if the histopathologic diagnosis appears straightforward, as, e.g., basal cell carcinoma, the pathologist should always have certain clinical information before finalizing the case: age, gender, anatomic site, and clinical diagnosis. Without such information, the pathologist is much more prone to blatant errors, such as mislabeled specimens or misdiagnosis.

However, for many conditions, particularly inflammatory processes, detailed clinical information concerning the onset, evolution, distribution, and specific character of the skin lesions is essential in order to arrive at a diagnosis or to formulate a differential diagnosis. Many inflammatory reaction patterns are not specific and may be secondary to several processes. Thus, an accurate clinical history is needed to establish the most likely condition or group of conditions that might explain the histologic findings.

AN ALGORITHMIC METHOD OF DIAGNOSIS

As outlined in Tables 1-2 to 1-7, the initial decision is whether a process is predominantly inflammatory, predominantly proliferative and neoplastic, both inflammatory and proliferative, or noninflammatory and nonproliferative. This classification is not always possible, but, in general, the vast majority of pathologic processes can be categorized into one of these groups. Thus, one is able proceed along one of the decision trees.

Major Inflammatory Reaction Patterns in the Skin

Since the pathogenesis of most inflammatory dermatitides is unknown, one must of necessity utilize morphologic criteria for classification at present. Although most inflammatory conditions can be categorized into one of the major reaction patterns, some dermatitides show overlapping features, and some defy classification. Some inflammatory conditions may be sampled either too early or late in their evolution to be diagnostic. Inflammatory diseases are dynamic, and knowledge of the point in

---

TABLE 1-2

Algorithmic Approach to Diagnosis

Skin specimen

↓   ↓   ↓   ↓

Principally   Proliferative/   Noninflammatory   "Normal skin"
inflammatory   neoplastic   conditions
conditions   conditions

↓   ↓   ↓

With   Without   ↓   ↓
epidermal   epidermal   Proliferations   Proliferations
alteration   alteration   originating in   localized to
                                the epidermis   dermis and subcutis
↓   ↓

↓

Characterization of
dermal/subcutaneous
inflammatory process

TABLE 1-3

Inflammatory Conditions with Epidermal Alteration

↓   ↓   ↓   ↓

Vesicle/blister/pustule   Spongiotic   Interface   Psoriasiform
                           dermatitis   dermatitis   dermatitis
↓   (Chapter 2)   (Chapter 3)   (Chapter 4)

↓   ↓   ↓

Intraepidermal   Subepidermal   ↓   ↓
(Chapter 7)   (Chapter 8)   Vacuolar   Lichenoid type
                          ↓   type
↓   ↓   ↓

Junctional   Dermolytic

↓   ↓   ↓

Subcorneal/   Intrastratum   Suprabasilar,
substratum   spinosum   intrabasilar
granulosum

↓   ↓   ↓   ↓

Conventional   Eosinophilic   Follicular   Miliarial
spongiosis   spongiosis   spongiosis   spongiosis

TABLE 1-4

Inflammatory Conditions without Epidermal Alterations

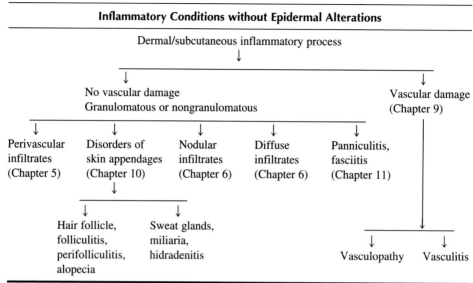

Dermal/subcutaneous inflammatory process
↓

| No vascular damage Granulomatous or nongranulomatous | | | | | Vascular damage (Chapter 9) |

| Perivascular infiltrates (Chapter 5) | Disorders of skin appendages (Chapter 10) | Nodular infiltrates (Chapter 6) | Diffuse infiltrates (Chapter 6) | Panniculitis, fasciitis (Chapter 11) |

Hair follicle, folliculitis, perifolliculitis, alopecia   Sweat glands, miliaria, hidradenitis

Vasculopathy   Vasculitis

TABLE 1-5

Inflammatory Infiltrates with Granulomas/Granulomatous Inflammation

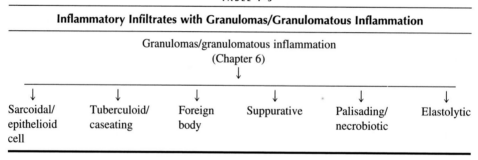

Granulomas/granulomatous inflammation
(Chapter 6)
↓

| Sarcoidal/ epithelioid cell | Tuberculoid/ caseating | Foreign body | Suppurative | Palisading/ necrobiotic | Elastolytic |

TABLE 1-6

Noninflammatory Disorders with Alterations of Stratum Corneum and Epidermis

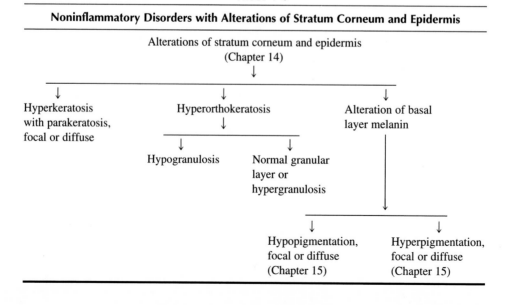

Alterations of stratum corneum and epidermis
(Chapter 14)
↓

| Hyperkeratosis with parakeratosis, focal or diffuse | Hyperorthokeratosis | Alteration of basal layer melanin |

Hypogranulosis   Normal granular layer or hypergranulosis

Hypopigmentation, focal or diffuse (Chapter 15)   Hyperpigmentation, focal or diffuse (Chapter 15)

TABLE 1-7

Noninflammatory Disorders with Dermal Alteration

	Alterations of dermis						
	Papillary dermal alteration			Reticular dermal alteration			
Atrophy	Deposition of material (Chapter 16)	Hypertrophy fibrosis (Chapter 17)	Pigmentary alterations (Chapter 15)	Atrophy (Chapter 17)	Hypertrophy thickening fibrosis ("square biopsy") (Chapter 17)	Deposition of material (Chapter 16)	Pigmentary alterations (Chapter 15)

time when the dermatitis is sampled is critical to optimal microscopic interpretations. The histopathologist should strive to assess specimens with the "fourth dimension," time, always in mind.

As previously mentioned, one initially attempts to ascertain whether the epidermis shows one of the following major reaction patterns or is uninvolved by the inflammatory process.

INFLAMMATORY REACTION PATTERNS OF THE EPIDERMIS

Spongiotic Dermatitis

Spongiotic dermatitis refers specifically to the presence of spongiosis or intercellular edema that stretches apart keratinocytes and sometimes results in the formation of intraepidermal vesicles (Fig. 1-4). Spongiosis is often variable, multifocal, accompanied by intracellular edema and exocytosis of inflammatory cells. The disease process is dynamic and in general has been categorized according to morphologic features correlating with the stages of its life history: (1) acute, (2) subacute, and (3) chronic, and other alterations such as eosinophilic infiltration of the epidermis (eosinophilic spongiosis) or involvement of skin appendages, e.g., follicular spongiosis (Table 1-3).

Spongiosis is a relatively nonspecific morphologic alteration observed in a wide variety of conditions (Table 1-8). It is perhaps most characteristic of the group of conditions referred to as *eczematous dermatitis*. These disorders include endogenous or atopic dermatitis, contact allergic dermatitis, and nummular dermatitis. Other common dermatitides showing spongiosis include seborrheic dermatitis, spongiotic drug eruptions, and some primary bullous conditions.

Interface Dermatitis

Interface dermatitis refers to a morphologic alteration at the junction or interface between the epidermis (or epithelium) and dermis. Specifically, one observes vacuolization (vacuoles or discrete clear spaces) either within basilar keratinocytes or within the basement membrane zone. This reaction pattern is often accompanied by a number of other alterations present to variable extent: individually dyskeratotic keratinocytes (which are probably apoptotic cells), disruption of orderly keratinocytic maturation to the surface, and clefts resulting from coalescence of vacuoles.

Interface dermatitis may be further subclassified according to the density and pattern of the inflammatory cell infiltrate in the papillary dermis: (1) the vacuolar or cell-poor type, based on perivascular or

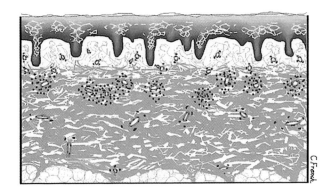

FIGURE 1-4   Spongiotic dermatitis.

patchy infiltrates in the papillary dermis (Fig. 1-5), (2) the lichenoid or cell-rich type, which shows a dense bandlike infiltrate that fills the papillary dermis (Fig. 1-6) (Tables 1-3 and 1-9). As with all inflammatory processes, interface dermatitides also may be characterized according to the stage of their evolution, i.e., acute or early-stage, subacute or developed, and chronic or late-stage. Certain diseases are prototypic of the two patterns of interface dermatitis mentioned above. Erythema multiforme, many drug eruptions, viral exanthems, and connective tissue diseases result in a vacuolar pattern of interface dermatitis. However, lichen planus, lichenoid drug eruption, lichen planus-like keratosis, and "halo" nevus are associated with lichenoid patterns of inflammation.

Psoriasiform Dermatitis

Psoriasiform dermatitis refers to a characteristic pattern of epidermal hyperplasia typified by elongation of the epidermal rete ridges (Fig. 1-7). In general, the topography of the epidermal surface is unaffected, i.e., remains essentially flat-topped. This pattern of epidermal alteration may be further described as either *regular* or *irregular*. Regular psoriasiform hyperplasia, as the name suggests, indicates elongated epidermal rete ridges of fairly uniform length and thickness and is typical of psoriasis in a well-developed stage. This morphologic feature is accompanied by a number of other histologic alterations notable in psoriasis: broad zones of parakeratosis, absence of the granular layer, exocytosis of neutrophils, pallor of keratinocytes (intracellular edema), thinning of the epidermis above the dermal papillae, prominent dilated and tortuous papillary dermal microvessels, and papillary dermal edema.

TABLE 1-8

Spongiotic Dermatitis

Conventional spongiotic dermatitis
  Allergic contact dermatitis
  Irritant contact dermatitis
  Atopic (endogenous) dermatitis
  Nummular dermatitis
  Dyshidrotic eczema (pompholyx)
  Id reaction
  Seborrheic dermatitis
  Stasis dermatitis
  Spongiotic drug eruption
  Erythroderma
  Pityriasis rosea
  Pityriasis alba
  Photoallergic contact dermatitis
  Polymorphous light eruption
  Arthropod bites
  Gyrate/figurate erythemas
  Dermatophyte infection
  Transient acantholytic dermatosis
  Pigmented purpuric dermatitis
  Papular and urticarial eruptions of pregnancy
Eosinophilic spongiosis
  Pemphigus group
  Bullous pemphigoid
  Allergic contact dermatitis
  Spongiotic drug eruptions
  Infestations
  Cutaneous larva migrans
  Arthropod bites
  Incontinentia pigmenti
  Eosinophilic folliculitis
Follicular spongiosis
  Atopic dermatitis
  Pityriasis alba
  Contact dermatitis
  Infundibulofolliculitis
  Eosinophilic folliculitis
  Follicular mucinosis
  Fox-Fordyce disease
Miliarial spongiosis
  Miliaria

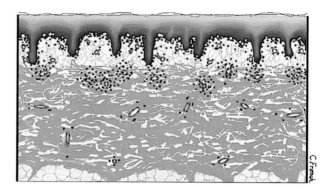

FIGURE 1-5   Vacuolar (cell-poor) interface dermatitis.

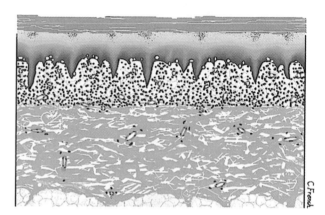

FIGURE 1-6   Lichenoid (cell-rich) interface dermatitis.

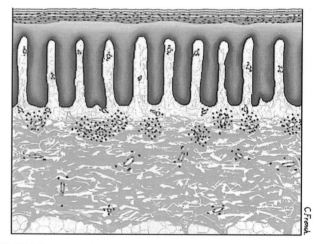

FIGURE 1-7   Psoriasiform dermatitis.

Irregular psoriasiform epidermal hyperplasia may be observed in psoriasis but typifies other processes more commonly, such as chronic eczematous dermatitis, lichen simplex chronicus, or mycosis fungoides (Table 1-10). Other conditions that exhibit this reaction include psoriasiform drug eruptions, lamellar ichthyosis, and secondary syphilis.

Vesicular and Bullous Dermatitis

This reaction pattern refers to the formation of tissue clefts or spaces, which may be accompanied by cellular infiltrates such as eosinophils, neutrophils, or lymphocytes. In general, these disorders are classified according to whether the level of cleavage is: (1) intraepidermal (Fig. 1-8) or (2) subepidermal (Fig. 1-9) (Tables 1-3, 1-11, and 1-12). Intra-

epidermal blisters may include subcorneal or intragranular layer cleavage or cleavage through the superficial layer or suprabasal layer of the epidermis. Subepidermal blisters may be further delineated as cleavage through the lamina lucida of the basement membrane zone or through the superficial dermis.

TABLE 1-9

Interface Dermatitis

Vacuolar interface dermatitis
    Erythema multiforme
    Fixed drug eruption
    Drug eruptions
    Viral exanthems
    HIV interface dermatitis
    Connective tissue disease
    Lupus erythematosus
    Dermatomyositis
    Graft-versus-host reaction
    Pityriasis lichenoides
    Poikiloderma congenitale
    Bloom's syndrome
    Vitiligo
    Pigmented purpuric dermatitis
Lichenoid interface dermatitis
    Lichen planus and variants
    Lichenoid drug eruption
    Lichenoid keratosis
    Lichen striatus
    Lichen nitidus
    Lichenoid purpura
    Porokeratosis
    Histologic regression of many tumors

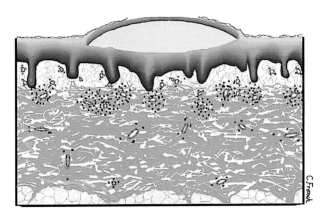

FIGURE 1-8   Intraepidermal vesicular dermatitis.

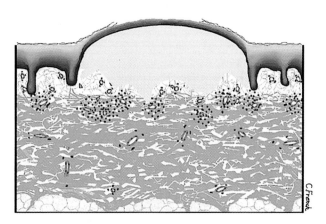

FIGURE 1-9   Subepidermal bullous dermatitis.

TABLE 1-10

Psoriasiform Dermatitis

Psoriasis
Reiter's syndrome
Subacute to chronic eczematous dermatitis
Seborrheic dermatitis
Lichen simplex chronicus
Pityriasis rubra pilaris
Parapsoriasis
Mycosis fungoides
Psoriasiform drug eruption
Erythroderma
Candidiasis
Secondary syphilis
Inflammatory linear verrucous epidermal nevus (ILVEN)
Scabies
Lamellar ichthyosis
Clear cell acanthoma
Pellagra
Acrodermatitis enteropathica
Migratory necrolytic erythema
Bazex syndrome

TABLE 1-11

Intraepidermal Vesicular and Pustular Dermatitis

Intracorneal and subcorneal vesicles and pustules
    Impetigo
    Staphylococcal "scalded skin" syndrome
    Superficial fungal infection
    Pemphigus foliaceus
    Pemphigus erythematosus
    Subcorneal pustular dermatosis
    Infantile acropustulosis
    Erythema toxicum
    Transient neonatal pustular melanosis
    Miliaria crystallina
Intraepidermal vesicles and pustules
    Spongiotic vesicles
    Viral vesicles
    Palmoplantar pustulosis
    Friction blister
    Epidermolysis bullosa

TABLE 1-12

Subepidermal Vesicular Dermatitis

Subepidermal blisters with little inflammation
Epidermolysis bullosa
Porphyria
Pseudoporphyria
Bullous pemphigoid (cell-poor type)
Burns
Toxic epidermal necrolysis
Bullae associated with diabetes
Blisters overlying scars
Bullous amyloidosis
Subepidermal blisters with lymphocytes
Erythema multiforme
Fixed drug eruption
Lichen planus pemphigoides
Polymorphous light eruption
Bullous mycosis fungoides
Bullous fungal infections
Subepidermal blisters with eosinophils
Bullous pemphigoid
Epidermolysis bullosa acquisita
Herpes gestationis
Arthropod bites
Drug reactions
Subepidermal blisters with neutrophils
Dermatitis herpetiformis
Linear IgA bullous dermatosis
Cicatricial pemphigoid and localized cicatricial pemphigoid
Pustular vasculitis
Bullous lupus erythematosus
Sweet's syndrome
Epidermolysis bullosa acquisita
Erysipelas
Bullous urticaria
Subepidermal blisters with mast cells
Bullous mastocytosis
Miscellaneous blistering diseases
Drug-overdose-related bullae
PUVA-induced bulla
Etretinate-induced bullae

Blistering dermatitides may then be characterized as predominantly inflammatory or noninflammatory. If inflammatory, the composition of the infiltrate will further aid classification. Finally, one may be able to recognize the mechanism of vesicle or blister formation as spongiotic, acantholytic, ballooning degeneration, or resulting from prominent basal layer vacuolization or subepidermal edema.

Other Epidermal Reactions and Overlapping Patterns

Inevitably, the procedure of classification is somewhat artificial, and there are always exceptions and entities that defy categorization. Many inflammatory conditions in the skin show two or more of the patterns of epidermal alteration discussed above. The predominant reaction pattern should generally be used as the basis for categorization if possible. The following morphologic reactions represent additional subsets.

Pityriasiform Dermatitis　A small but important group of inflammatory dermatitides shows a constellation of epidermal changes that include focal or spotty parakeratosis, slight epidermal hyperplasia, and variable spongiotic and interface alteration. Depending on which of the above features might predominate, various dermatitides in this group might also be classified as a subacute spongiotic, psoriasiform, or interface dermatitis (see discussion of overlapping patterns below). These conditions generally include pityriasis rosea, pityriasis lichenoides, seborrheic dermatitis, eruptive or guttate psoriasis, pre- or early mycosis fungoides lesions ("parapsoriasis"), some drug eruptions, subacute eczematous dermatitis, pityriasis rubra pilaris, and superficial fungal infections.

Overlapping Reaction Patterns　The four patterns listed below emphasize the prominence of two or more morphologic alterations; particular patterns often correlate with particular disease processes (for example, spongiotic psoriasiform dermatitis is a typical pattern associated with chronic-active eczematous dermatitis):

1. Spongiotic psoriasiform dermatitis
2. Spongiotic interface dermatitis
3. Spongiotic psoriasiform interface dermatitis
4. Psoriasiform interface dermatitis

CHARACTERIZATION OF THE INFLAMMATORY PROCESS IN THE DERMIS

After one has examined the epidermis for morphologic alteration, one proceeds to evaluate the inflammatory process in the dermis (and subcutis and fascia, as the case may be). An immediate concern is whether recognizable vascular injury is present or absent.

Absence of Vascular Injury

In the absence of vascular injury, one proceeds with the assessment of the pattern, depth, density, and composition of the inflammatory cell infiltrate and whether it is granulomatous. The patterns of inflammatory infiltrates in the dermis generally are described as lichenoid, perivascular (Fig. 1-10), periadnexal, interstitial (infiltrating collagen bundles), nodular (Fig. 1-11), and diffuse (Fig. 1-12) (occupying entire dermis) (Table 1-13). The depth of involvement is important to recognize since many dermatitides correlate with depth. For example, drug eruptions and viral exanthems often show superficial perivascular involvement only, whereas conditions such as lupus erythematosus, polymorphous light eruption, and secondary syphilis are prone to involvement of the deep dermal vascular plexus (a so-called superficial and deep perivascular pattern). Depth also may be indicative of likelihood of a systemic disease process, as in lupus or secondary syphilis. Density of an infiltrate is difficult to assess except in rather subjective terms, such as sparse, moderate, or dense. However, recognizing the density of an infiltrate has relevance for particular disease processes, such as acute urticaria (which is sparse), figurate erythema (which is moderately dense), and cutaneous lymphoid hyperplasia or lymphoma (which tend to be dense).

The cellular infiltrates in the dermis are commonly composed of lymphocytes, possibly with varying admixtures of other cell types, including histiocytes (monocyte/macrophages), mast cells, eosinophils, plasma cells, and neutrophils. The particular cellular composition often has diagnostic significance, particularly when integrated with the other features mentioned above, i.e., pattern, depth, and density. Thus, a sparse superficial perivascular infiltrate containing lymphocytes and eosinophils would suggest urticaria. Infiltrates with the same cell types but of greater density (moderate) would suggest the rather broad category of allergic hypersensitivity reactions, and, finally, circumscribed

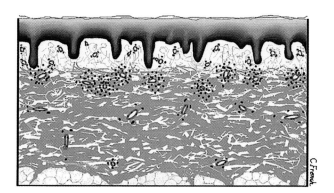

FIGURE 1-10   Superficial perivascular infiltrate.

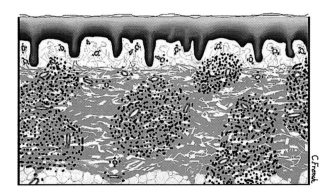

FIGURE 1-11   Nodular dermal infiltrate.

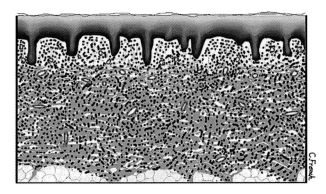

FIGURE 1-12   Diffuse dermal infiltrate.

TABLE 1-13
Dermal Inflammatory Infiltrates without Vascular Injury

Superficial or superficial and deep perivascular infiltrates*
  Urticaria
  Urticarial reactions
  Viral exanthems
  Drug eruptions
  Gyrate/figurate erythemas
  Lupus erythematosus
  Polymorphous light eruption
  Photosensitive eruptions
  Chilblains
  Leprosy (indeterminate)
  Syphilis
  Borreliosis
  Leukemia
  Urticaria pigmentosa
Nodular infiltrates
  Arthropod bite reactions
  Cutaneous lymphoid hyperplasia
  Histiocytic infiltrates
  Neutrophilic dermatoses
  Lymphoma
Diffuse infiltrates*
  Reactive infiltrates
  Leukemia
  Lymphoma
  Histiocytic infiltrates
  Mast cell infiltrates

*Further classified according to cell types present, such as lymphocytes, eosinophils, neutrophils.

TABLE 1-14
Vasculitis and Related Disorders

Vasculopathy
Small-vessel vasculitis
  Neutrophilic/leukocytoclastic vasculitis
  Lymphocytic vasculitis
  Granulomatous vasculitis
Medium-vessel vasculitis

---

superficial and deep perivascular aggregates of epithelioid monocyte/macrophages—the sarcoidal granulomatous reaction pattern. (See below.)

Presence of Vascular Injury

Vascular injury refers to a spectrum of morphologic alteration ranging from endothelial perturbation or activation to frank fibrinoid necrosis. These changes may be primary or secondary (a distinction not always easily made). In assessing vascular injury, a number of parameters must be considered, including caliber and type of vessels involved, degree of vascular injury, as already mentioned, the composition and density of the cellular infiltrate, presence or absence of such factors as antineutrophil cytoplasmic antibodies (Table 1-14).

Granulomatous Reaction Patterns

The essential definition of a *granuloma* is a circumscribed aggregate of monocyte/macrophages. The cytologic characteristics of such cells vary from mononuclear cells with abundant pale, vacuolated, or lipidized cytoplasm to cells with plentiful pink cytoplasm, resembling epithelial cells and hence the term *epithelioid* cells. Multinucleated giant cells are commonly present and are generally one of two types: foreign-body and Langhans' giant cells. Granulomas often contain a variable admixture of other cell types such as lymphocytes, plasma cells, neutrophils, and mast cells. Poorly-defined granulomatous infiltrates are often referred to as granulomatous inflammation. Granulomas may be classified a number of ways, such as infectious or noninfectious, or by morphologic features—there is considerable overlap among many of these entities. A generally accepted scheme is as follows: (1) sarcoidal or epithelioid-cell, (2) tuberculoid or caseating, (3) foreign-body, (4) suppurative, (5) palisading/necrobiotic, and (6) elastolytic granulomas. In general, these reaction patterns are nonspecific and should prompt a differential diagnosis and systematic evaluation, as discussed in more detail in Chapter 6 (Table 1-5).

Disorders of Skin Appendages

The skin appendages, principally the hair follicle and the eccrine sweat apparatus, may show primary inflammatory involvement.

Disorders of the Hair Follicle   In general, *folliculitis* is categorized as to whether it is infectious or noninfectious and according to its depth—superficial only or superficial and deep. Acne is an extremely common form of folliculitis that has a multifactorial basis, for example. The hair follicle also may show a peculiar reaction—follicular mucinosis—which may be associated with a variety of processes that includes mycosis fungoides and inflammatory conditions such as arthropod bites and lupus erythematosus.

Alopecia histologically refers to an overall reduction in the number of terminal anagen hair follicles, which may be reversible or irreversible. Operationally (and perhaps simplistically), alopecia may be classified as nonscarring or scarring. Nonscarring alopecias may result from any number of factors interrupting the hair growth cycle, whether inflammatory, as in the case of alopecia areata, or noninflammatory, as in androgenetic alopecia or telogen effluvium. Scarring alopecia follows a wide variety of processes such as infective follicultis, lupus erythematosus, lichen planus, or traumatic injury.

Disorders of the Sweat Apparatus   The eccrine duct may be primarily involved by an inflammatory reaction termed miliaria and categorized according to depth of involvement as (superficial) miliaria crystallina, miliaria rubra, and miliaria profunda. *Hidradenitis* refers to an inflammatory disorder involving the sweat coil, e.g., neutrophilic eccrine hidradenitis, which may be infectious or noninfectious.

Panniculitis

The primary focus of inflammation may involve the subcutaneous fat. Although traditionally *panniculitis* has been classified as septal or lobular, in fact, in most instances the inflammatory process is both septal (Fig. 1-13) and lobular (Fig. 1-14). Particular factors that should be considered when evaluating panniculitis include presence or absence of infection, vascular injury, cold-related injury, factitial disease, and physical injury. Adequate sampling and the stage of disease when the biopsy is taken will influence the morphologic findings. The reaction pattern of adipose tissue to injury is rather limited. Initially, one observes an influx of neutrophils, followed by mononuclear cells (lymphocytes and macrophages), and finally reparative fibrosis, depending upon the nature and severity of the insult.

Proliferative or Neoplastic Conditions

A large category of conditions encompasses hyperplasias, hamartomas, and benign and malignant neoplasms involving the epidermis, melanocytes, skin appendages, dermis, subcutis, and hematopoietic cells in the skin (Table 1-2).

Noninflammatory Conditions

In the absence of an obvious inflammatory dermatitis or proliferative or neoplastic process, one must proceed along the algorithm for noninflammatory conditions. Histologic alterations may suggest "normal skin" and may include the so-called invisible dermatoses (Table 1-15).

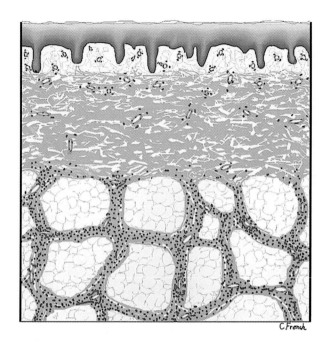

FIGURE 1-13   Septal panniculitis.

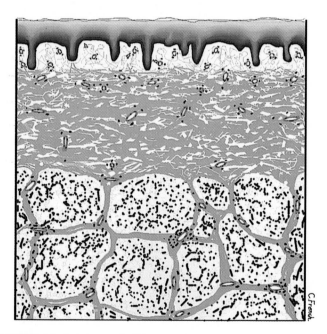

FIGURE 1-14   Lobular panniculitis.

As already outlined above, one must generally resort to systemic study of the specimen beginning with stratum corneum or perhaps with the subcutis in the reverse order. It goes without saying that the histopathologist should have some understanding of the regional microanatomy and age-related variations of skin in order to know what is within normal limits.

Alterations of Stratum Corneum and Epidermis

The stratum corneum is studied for subtle abnormalities such as parakeratosis, hyperkeratosis, and fungal elements. The epidermis is inspected for acanthosis, atrophy, subtle alterations suggesting an inflammatory or vesicular reaction, alterations of the granular layer as in ichthyosiform dermatitides, peculiar processes such as epidermolytic

TABLE 1-15

Differential Diagnosis of "Normal Skin"

Diagnosis	Histopathological Features

Superficial fungal infection
    Dermatophytosis and tinea
    versicolor
	Hyphae and spores in stratum corneum

Porokeratosis	Cornoid lamella
Ichthyosis	Slight hyperkeratosis; diminished or absent granular layer

Hypopigmentation
    Vitiligo
    Piebaldism
    Chemical leukoderma
    Nevus depigmentosus
	Diminished or absent basal layer melanin, melanocytes

Hyperpigmentation
    Café-au-lait macule
    Freckle
    Melasma
    Lentigo
	Increased basilar melanin and possibly melanocytes

Macular amyloidosis	Pink amorphous globules in papillary dermis; pigment incontinence
Onchocerciasis	Microfilaria in superficial dermis
Dermal melanocytosis	Dendritic melanocytes in dermis
Urticaria pigmentosa	Increased numbers of mast cells in dermis
Argyria	Deposition of silver granules in basement membranes, particularly surrounding eccrine sweat coils
Urticaria	Sparse perivascular infiltrate Edema
Anhidrotic ectodermal dysplasia	Absence of eccrine sweat glands
Anetoderma	Focal or diffuse absence of elastic tissue; inflammation present or absent
Cutis laxa	Absence of elastic fibers
Connective tissue nevus	Increased or decreased collagen and/or elastin; abnormal connective tissue

Dermal mucinosis
    Myxedema
    Scleromyxedema
	Increased dermal mucin

Atrophoderma	Decreased thickness of dermis
Lipoatrophy	Fat lobules diminished in size

hyperkeratosis, and finally, pigmentary alterations associated with hypo- and hyperpigmentation.

Alterations of Papillary Dermis
The papillary dermis is then studied for alterations such as deposition of amyloid, hyalinization of vessels as in porphyria, and incontinence of melanin (melanin-laden macrophages in papillary dermis).

Alterations of Reticular Dermis
The reticular dermis is systematically examined for alteration of collagen as in morphea/scleroderma or scleroderma, thickening or atrophy of the reticular dermis, alteration of elastic fibers, and deposition of materials such as mucin or amyloid.

REFERENCES

1. Pinkus H, Mehregan AH: *A Guide to Dermatohistopathology*, 3d ed. New York, Appleton-Century-Crofts, 1981.
2. Ackerman AB: *Histologic Diagnosis of Inflammatory Skin Diseases. A Method of Pattern Analysis.* Philadelphia, Lea & Febiger, 1978.
3. Ackerman AB: An algorithmic method for histologic diagnosis of inflammatory and neoplastic skin diseases by analysis of their patterns. *Am J Dermatopathol* 7:105–107, 1985.
4. Nathwani BN, Burke JS, Winberg CD: Architectural features of normal, neoplastic, and nonneoplastic lymph nodes: A practical diagnostic approach, in Murphy GR, Mihm MC Jr (eds): *Lymphoproliferative Disorders of the Skin.* Boston, Butterworths, 1986.
5. Ackerman AB: Differentiation of benign from malignant neoplasms by silhouette. *Am J Dermatopathol* 1:297–300, 1989.
6. Schacter DL, Reiman E, Uecker A, et al: Brain regions associated with retrieval of structurally coherent visual information. *Nature* 376:587–590, 1995.
7. Bartels PH: The diagnostic pattern in histopathology. *Am J Clin Path* 91:S7–S13, 1989.
8. Desimone R, Duncan J: Neural mechanisms of selective visual attention. *Annu Rev Neurosci* 8:193–222, 1995.
9. Reuter B, Schenck U: Investigation of the visual cytoscreening of conventional gynecologic smears: II. Analysis of eye movements. *Anal Quant Cytol Histol* 8:210–218, 1986.
10. Ungerleider LG: Functional brain imaging studies of cortical mechanisms for memory. *Science* 270:769–775, 1995.
11. Brownstein MH, Rabinowtiz AD: The invisible dermatoses. *J Am Acad Dermatol* 8:579–588, 1983.

SPONGIOTIC DERMATITIS

Theodore H. Kwan

Spongiosis refers to intercellular edema of the epidermis. The histologic appearance of spongiosis is that of expanded spaces between keratinocytes (Fig. 2-1). These spaces are clear on hematoxylin and eosin (H & E) sections, and are traversed by numerous intercellular bridges (the latter are sometimes called *spinous processes*). *Spongiosis* connotes a sponge or spongy quality. Marked spongiosis leads to the formation of intraepidermal multiloculated vesicles. To a lesser extent, intracellular edema (within the keratinocyte) can also be appreciated with spongiosis. The clinical correlate of spongiosis depends on the degree of intercellular edema and varies from mild erythema to weepy, oozing skin with vesicles. Spongiosis is largely associated with the eczematous dermatitides, but it can be seen in many other disorders, as reflected in the algorithm in Tables 2-1 and 2-2 and in Tables 2-3 and 2-4. Hence spongiosis is a useful but not highly specific histologic feature. As with all microscopic interpretation, clinicopathologic correlation is of paramount importance.

Several histologic patterns are sometimes confused with spongiosis. These include epidermolytic hyperkeratosis, reticular degeneration, ballooning degeneration, intracellular glycogen accumulation, intracellular edema, follicular mucinosis, and spongiform pustule. Most of these alterations include some degree of spongiosis, to add some further confusion.

The presumed pathogenesis of spongiosis is passage of fluid from the vascular compartment into the dermis and from there into the epidermis. One would expect therefore to find dermal edema in all cases with spongiosis, and one does, by and large. Spongiosis is almost always accompanied by inflammatory cells in the dermis and/or the epidermis. Some of these inflammatory cells probably elaborate substances which regulate movement of fluid from compartment to compartment. Other inflammatory cells migrate to this location in response to substances elaborated by other cells in the area. The types and distribution of these inflammatory cells are critical to the dermatopathologist in the classification of spongiotic dermatitis.

Spongiosis itself may also be specifically distributed or modified. *Follicular spongiosis* refers to intercellular edema of follicular epithelium. *Miliarial spongiosis* refers to intercellular edema of the acrosyringium. *Eosinophilic spongiosis* refers to migration of eosinophils into the intercellular spaces of the epidermis. These particular types of spongiosis have diseases associated with them (Tables 2-2, 2-5, 2-6, and 12-2).

ECZEMATOUS DERMATITIS

Under the term *eczematous dermatitis* (also referred to as *eczema* or *dermatitis*) are subsumed a number of clinically distinct and indistinct entities including atopic dermatitis, nummular dermatitis, dyshidrotic eczema (pompholyx), asteatotic eczema (eczema crequelé), id reaction (autosensitization), Sulzberger-Garbe syndrome, and others. All these clinical entities share some histologic findings. They also share similarities in the morphology of the individual lesions, namely erythematous macules, papules, plaques, vesicles, scaling, and sometimes lichenification. These many entities achieve clinical distinction in the distribution of their lesions, associations with other disorders, and specific etiologies. The next section provides a brief clinical description of the entities listed above. Other disorders also regarded as eczematous such as follicular eczema, seborrheic dermatitis, contact dermatitis, spongiotic drug reactions, erythroderma, stasis dermatitis, pityriasis alba, and pityriasis rosea are also discussed.

Clinical Features Atopic dermatitis is a common disorder which is associated with asthma and chronic rhinitis (hayfever), a family history of atopy, marked pruritus, and increased serum IgE levels (Table 2-7). In spite of extensive study, the etiology and pathogenesis are not yet understood. The skin lesions of atopic dermatitis can show the entire spectrum of eczematous lesions including erythematous scaly areas, oozing, lichenification, and scaling dry fissured areas (especially palms and soles); secondary changes commonly seen include bacterial infections with crusting and folliculitis and hypo- and/or hyperpigmented areas. Vesicles are not, however, common. The skin of atopics is characterized as dry, lackluster, particularly pruritic, and irritable. The skin lesions of patients with atopic dermatitis are thought to be largely secondary to the scratching and trauma inflicted by the patient in response

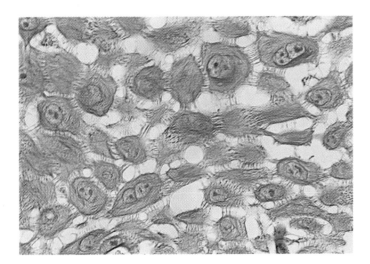

FIGURE 2-1 Spongiosis. Note that keratinocytes are stretched apart by intercellular edema revealing the intercellular bridges.

TABLE 2-1

Algorithm for Spongiosis

↓

↓	↓	↓	↓
Proliferation of the superficial vascular plexus, thickened vessel walls, variable amount of lymphocytic infiltrate, hemorrhage and hemosiderin-laden macrophages: Chronic stasis dermatitis, Angiodermatitis	Superficial perivascular lymphoid infiltrates with hemorrhage and/or hemosiderin-laden macrophages: Pigmentary purpura (eczematid variant of Doucas and Kapetanakis)	Superficial and deep perivascular lymphoid infiltrate, tightly cuffed "coat-sleeve" around vessel: Figurate erythemas ↓ Dyskeratotic cells: Polymorphous light reaction, Photodrug reaction Many dyskeratotic cells, and keratinocytic atypia: Phototoxic reaction	Wedge-shaped superficial and deep perivascular lymphoid infiltrates with eosinophils: Hypersensitivity reaction to arthropod assaults
↓	↓	↓	↓
Superficial perivascular lymphoid infiltrate and intraepidermal or intracorneal neutrophils: Seborrheic dermatitis Early or treated psoriasis Sneddon-Wilkinson disease Contact dermatitis (esp. irritant)	Superficial perivascular lymphoid infiltrate with or without eosinophils and large, well-formed intraepidermal vesicles: Pompholyx Allergic contact dermatitis Dyshidrotic eczema	Superficial perivascular lymphoid infiltrate without eosinophils: Chronic superficial dermatitis Pityriasis lichenoides chronica Pruritic urticarial papules and plaques of pregnancy Gianotti-Crosti syndrome Early mycosis fungoides	Superficial perivascular lymphoid infiltrate with or without eosinophils: Drug hypersensitivity reaction Atopic dermatitis Nummular dermatitis Pityriasis rosea (especially inflammatory variant) Grover's disease (spongiotic variant) Id reaction Hypersensitivity reaction to arthropod assault

↓

With intracorneal hyphal forms:
Dermatophytosis
With intracorneal gram-positive cocci:
Impetigo
With plasma cells and endothelial cell swelling:
Secondary syphilis

TABLE 2-2

Miliarial Spongiosis

Miliarial Spongiosis (spongiosis involving the acrosyringium)

↓	↓	↓	↓
Subcorneal vesicle filled with fluid and less than 50% neutrophils by volume in and around the duct:	Spongiosis involving the upper half of the acrosyringium and lymphocytic infiltrate in and around the duct:	Spongiosis involving the lower half of the acrosyringium and lymphocytic infiltrate:	Inflammatory dermatitis which involves the epidermis and the acrosyringium:
Miliaria crystallina	Miliaria rubra	Miliaria profunda	See relevant pattern

TABLE 2-3

Disorders in which Spongiosis Is Often Seen

Allergic contact dermatitis
Atopic dermatitis
Dermatophytoses
Dyshidrotic eczema
Eczematous drug reactions
Eosinophilic cellulitis
Erythema neonatorum
Erythroderma
Figurate erythemas
Granuloma gluteale infantum
Grover's disease, spongiotic variant
Hyperkeratotic dermatitis of hands
Id reactions
Irritant contact dermatitis
Irritated seborrheic keratosis
Lichen striatus
Mycosis fungoides, early
Next to any erosion or ulcer
Nummular dermatitis
Papular acrodermatitis of childhood

Parapsoriasis
Pigmented purpuras
Pityriasis alba
Pityriasis lichenoides
Pityriasis rosea
Polymorphous light reaction
Pompholyx
Primary syphilis
Prurigo simplex
Pruritic urticarial papules and
    plaques of pregnancy
Psoriasis, early or treated
Pustular psoriasis
Reaction to arthropod assault
Seborrheic dermatitis
Stasis dermatitis
Sulzberger-Garbe
Yaws

TABLE 2-4

Disorders in which Spongiosis Can Be Seen

Acne
Acrodermatitis enteropathica
Acute febrile neutrophilic dermatosis
Acute meningococcemia
Blastomycosislike pyoderma
Erythema multiforme
Inflammatory linear verrucous
    epidermal nevus
Lichen simplex chronicus
Necrolytic migratory erythema

Prurigo nodularis
Pyoderma gangrenosum
Subcorneal pustular dermatosis
Toxic shock syndrome
Vasculitis
Others

TABLE 2-5

Follicular Spongiosis

Apocrine miliaria
Eosinophilic folliculitis
Follicular eczema
Follicular mucinosis
Folliculitis, infectious and others
Impetigo of Bockhart
Infundibulofolliculitis
Pityriasis alba

TABLE 2-6

Eosinophilic Spongiosis

Allergic contact dermatitis
Bullous pemphigoid
Drug eruptions
Herpes gestationis
Idiopathic eosinophilic spongiosis
Incontinentia pigmenti, first stage
Pemphigus, precursor lesions
Pemphigus vegetans
Reactions to arthropod assaults

TABLE 2-7

Atopic Dermatitis

Clinical Features
Common disorder of all ages
Associated with allergic rhinitis and/or asthma
Family history of atopy common
Marked pruritus associated with a variety of lesions
    Erythematous scaling areas
    Edematous, oozing, weepy areas
    Lichenified areas
    Dry fissured scaly areas
Skin of patients generally lackluster, pruritic, and irritable
Abnormalities of vascular and immune responses

Histopathological Features
Acute pattern
    Spongiosis, sometimes spongiotic vesiculation, a usually superfi-
        cial perivascular lymphocytic and eosinophilic infiltrate, epider-
        mis of normal thickness
Subacute pattern
    Thickened epidermis (usually psoriasiform type), spongiosis, a usu-
        ally superficial perivascular lymphocytic and eosinophilic infil-
        trate, variable fibrosis of papillary dermis
Chronic pattern
    Psoriasiform hyperplasia, spongiosis absent, vascular ectasia, a
        usually superficial perivascular lymphocytic infiltrate with
        eosinophils, variable fibrosis of the papillary dermis

Differential Diagnosis
All other types of eczematous dermatitis
Clinicopathologic correlation largely determines the diagnosis
Pathologic diagnosis is usually expressed as acute, subacute, or
    chronic eczematous dermatitis

TABLE 2-8

Nummular (Discoid) Dermatitis

Clinical Features
Coin-shaped, pruritic, erythematous patches on the hands, forearms, and legs
Patches may have tiny vesicles or erosions, which can evolve to form annular plaques or dry scaly areas
Tends to affect men and women 55 years and older as well as women 15–30 years old

Histopathological Features
Varies according to the lesion biopsied: acute, subacute, and chronic eczematous patterns

Differential Diagnosis
All types of eczematous dermatitis
Dermatophytosis
Figurate erythemas
Seborrheic dermatitis

to the pruritus and irritability. Abnormal cutaneous vascular responses (including white dermatographism), abnormal fatty acid metabolism, abnormally decreased delayed hypersensitivity responses, and defects in monocyte and neutrophil function have been reported. Atopic dermatitis can appear as early as 6 months of age. In infants the lesions are usually located on the head, neck, and diaper areas. In children, the flexural areas tend to be particularly involved. In adults, the lesions may be widely distributed.

Nummular (discoid) dermatitis is charactertized by coin-shaped patches on the hands, forearms, and legs (Table 2-8). The patches are usually pruritic and erythematous with tiny vesicles or erosions which can evolve to form larger annular lesions with central clearing or to dry scaly areas. Nummular dermatitis is seen in men and women 55 years and older as well as in young women (15 to 30 years). Sometimes there is a history of atopy or hypersensitivity to nickel.

Dyshidrotic eczema (pompholyx, eczema of palms and soles) affects the digits, palms, and soles (Table 2-9). Typically one sees tense vesicles whose formation may be related to the thick stratum corneum in these areas. The term *dyshidrotic* notwithstanding, the cause of this disorder does not seem to be related to hyperhidrosis, and the cause is not

TABLE 2-9

Dyshidrotic Eczema (Pompholyx)

Clinical Features
Itchy tense vesicles on the digits, palms, and soles

Histopathological Features
Intraepidermal spongiotic vesicles usually on epidermis of normal or increased thickness
Variable amount of superficial perivascular lymphocytic infiltrate

Differential Diagnosis
Atopic dermatitis
Allergic contact dermatitis
Dermatophytosis
Miliaria
Other types of acute vesicular eczematous eruptions

known. Heat, stress, tinea pedis, allergy to nickel, and atopy have been associated from time to time with dyshidrotic eczema.

Asteatotic eczema (eczema craquelé, winter eczema) refers to eczema with dry skin, possibly related to decreased surface lipid. Cold wind, winter weather with its low humidity, exposure to detergents, central heating, and other similar conditions can produce or exacerabate the lesions. The hands, arms, and legs are usually affected by a dry scaly appearance which often has a crisscrossed pattern. Erythema and eczematous changes occur in and around the lesions. Asteatotic eczema is usually seen in elderly adults. The generalized type of asteatotic eczema involves the trunk as well as extremities and may signal the presence of a visceral malignancy.

Id reaction (autosensitization) refers to a poorly understood and somewhat difficult to describe phenomenon of a nonspecific acute eczematous dermatitis arising usually distant to (but sometimes contiguous with) the site of a prior and continuing dermatitis for which there is an etiology. An example is tinea pedis (the dermatitis for which there is an etiology) with the subsequent development of acute eczematous dermatitis on the upper extremity (no dermatophyte is present in the upper extremity lesion, and it is therefore nonspecific). In this situation, the upper extremity rash is sometimes called a *dermatophytid*. Another classic example is a stasis ulcer which develops an extensive contiguous eczematous reaction and a noncontiguous upper extremity acute eczema. In this example, the extensive contiguous rash and upper extremity rash are the id reaction.

Sulzberger-Garbe syndrome (exudative discoid and lichenoid dermatosis) refers to a chronic, very itchy, widespread eruption occurring in male Jews from 40 to 60 years of age. The lesions consist of erythematous, sometimes oozing papules and plaques, as well as discoid and lichenoid lesions which may be present at the same or different times. The lesions may pass through an urticarial phase as they evolve. Persistent penile and scrotal lesions are common and considered to be typical of Sulzberger-Garbe syndrome.

Many other types of eczema have been described largely on the basis of clinical features which are not discussed here.

Histopathological Features   The histopathology of eczematous dermatitis is traditionally divided into acute, subacute, and chronic patterns. Again, these diseases often do not follow the sequence of acute, subacute, and chronic. Some forms of pompholyx show only the acute pattern. Atopic dermatitis, however, may show all the patterns, but the sequence may vary, depending on whether the disease is acute or chronic, stable, waxing, or waning. The histology of each pattern is summarized in Table 2-10. Table 2-11 provides correlation of the clinical disorders described above with the histologic patterns. The *acute pattern* shows an epidermis of normal or slightly increased thickness, marked spongiosis, sometimes with spongiotic vesicle formation (Figs. 2-2 to 2-4), and a deep and/or superficial perivascular infiltrate of lymphocytes, histiocytes, and often eosinophils. If there is secondary impetiginization, the lesions may be surmounted by crust-scale with neutrophils and bacterial colonies. (Fig. 2-5). Dermal edema is often seen with increased dermal mucin. The *chronic form* shows hyperkeratosis, variable parakeratosis, psoriasiform hyperplasia (well described in Chapter 4), a superficial perivascular infiltrate of lymphocytes, histiocytes, and sometimes eosinophils (Fig. 2-6). The chronic pattern merges with that of lichen simplex chronicus (Fig. 2-7), which in addition to the above has hypergranulosis and a distinctive papillary dermal fibrosis which follows the contours of the rete ridges. The *subacute form* merges histologic features of both acute and chronic patterns, showing both psoriasiform hyperplasia and spongiosis with the usually largely perivascular infiltrate of lymphocytes, and variable numbers of eosinophils (Figs. 2-8 and 2-9).

Follicular Eczema

Follicular eczema is part of the spectrum of atopic dermatitis. Some patients show only follicular lesions. Other patients show follicular lesions in addition to lesions typical of atopic dermatitis.

Clinical Features   Follicular-based pruritic papules, flesh-colored or erythematous, are usually seen on the trunk and/or extremities. These primary lesions are usually rapidly transformed by scratching into excoriated, crusted, and lichenified lesions. Young black patients are said to be more often affected by this form of atopic dermatitis; in any case, the lesions are particularly evident when they occur in melanin-rich skin. In some cases follicular eczema appears to be related to an irritant or occlusive phenomenon.

Histopathological Features   The histologic features are not well studied. Spongiosis involves the follicular infundibulum and possibly the isthmus but not the inferior portion of the follicle with variable lymphocytic and eosinophilic infiltrate of the surrounding dermis (Fig. 2-10).

Differential Diagnosis   Table 2-5 indicates the principal differential diagnoses.

Seborrheic Dermatitis

Seborrheic dermatitis is a common disorder affecting the "seborrheic" areas of the body. The etiology is unclear, but many patients have a family history, so a genetic component seems likely. There may be a strong and causative association with Pityrosporum ovale.

Clinical Features   Seborrheic dermatitis can affect the scalp, face, upper chest, back, and to a lesser extent flexural areas (Table 2-12). The morphology of the lesions is greasy, scaly, red to brown demarcated patches. Dandruff is regarded as a type of seborrheic dermatitis. The lesions are sometimes susceptible to bacterial infections. In infancy, seborrheic dermatitis is sometimes called *Leiner's disease*. There is a strong association of seborrheic dermatitis with HIV infection[1] and with Parkinson's disease. Seborrheic dermatitis is less often associated with myocardial ischemia, epilepsy, obesity, malabsorption, and alcoholism.

TABLE 2-10

Eczematous Dermatitis: Acute, Subacute, and Chronic Patterns

	Parakeratosis	*Hyperkeratosis*	*Acanthosis*	*Spongiosis*	*Perivascular dermatitis*
Acute	+/−	+/−	+/−	+, ++, +++	+, ++, +++
Subacute	+	++, +++	++, +++	++, +++	+, ++, +++
Chronic	+, ++	+, ++, +++	++, +++	+/−	+, ++, +++

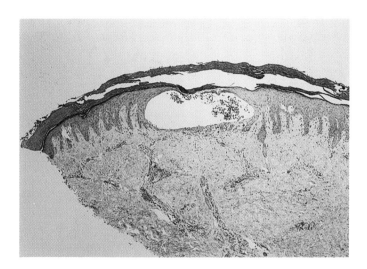

FIGURE 2-2   Dyshidrotic eczema. There is a large spongiotic intraepidermal vesicle.

TABLE 2-11

Histologic Spectrum of Some Eczemas

	Acute	*Subacute*	*Chronic*
Atopic	x	x	x
Nummular	x	x	(x)
Dyshidrotic	x	(x)	
Asteatotic		(x)	x
Id reaction	x	(x)	
Sulzberger-Garbe	x	x	x

x = less commonly observed

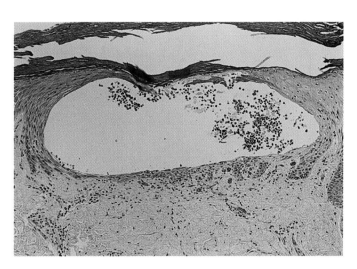

FIGURE 2-3   Dyshidrotic eczema. Higher magnification of Fig. 2-2; shows intraepidermal vesicle containing inflammatory cells.

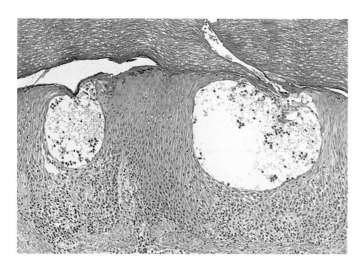

FIGURE 2-4   Acute spongiotic dermatitis with intraepidermal microvesicle formation as seen in this case of acute allergic contact dermatitis.

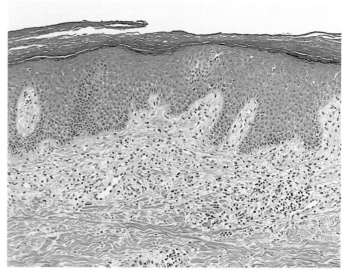

FIGURE 2-6   Chronic spongiotic dermatitis. The epidermis shows irregular psoriasiform hyperplasia with hyperkeratosis, minimal spongiosis, and a superficial perivascular lymphocytic infiltrate.

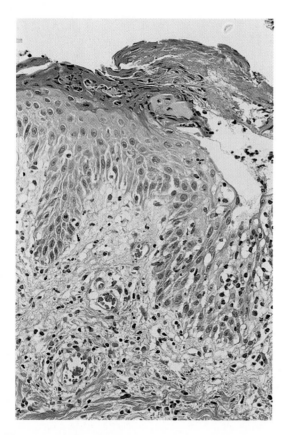

FIGURE 2-5   Id reaction. Note scale-crust containing neutrophils and spongiosis with exocytosis of lymphocytes.

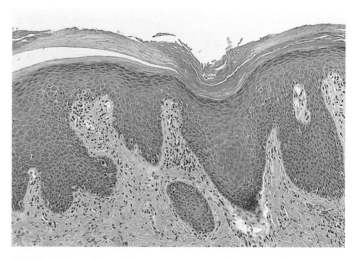

FIGURE 2-7   Lichen simplex chronicus. Note striking hyperkeratosis with some parakeratosis and irregular psoriasiform epidermal hyperplasia. The papillary dermis shows fibroplasia.

Histopathological Features   The microscopic findings show many features in common with eczematous dermatitis and psoriasis (Table 2-12): psoriasiform hyperplasia, parakeratosis (especially around hair follicles), hyperkeratosis, spongiosis, neutrophilic exocytosis, and a superficial perivascular lymphocytic infiltrate (Figs. 2-11 and 2-12); yeast forms may be seen in the stratum corneum. In the early phases, the resemblance to psoriasis may be particularly marked with dilated capillaries in edematous dermal papillae, neutrophils in the suprapapillary epidermis, and a decreased granular layer.

Differential Diagnosis   Seborrheic dermatitis almost always shows more spongiosis than psoriasis, and in many cases seborrheic dermatitis has a subacute eczematous pattern but with neutrophils. Besides psoriasis and subacute eczema, other differential diagnoses include impetigo, dermatophyte infections, secondary syphilis, gyrate erythemas, pityriasis rosea, and irritant contact dermatitis. Impetigo can usually be favored if colonies of gram-positive cocci are identified in the stratum corneum. Yeast and hyphal forms in the stratum corneum seen with a periodic acid–Schiff (PAS) or methenamine silver stain (and sometimes on

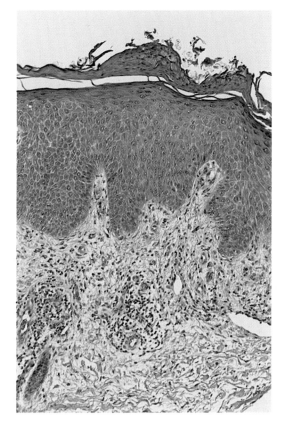

FIGURE 2-8   Subacute spongiotic dermatitis. The parakeratotic scale contains exudate. The epidermis is acanthotic and shows only slight spongiosis.

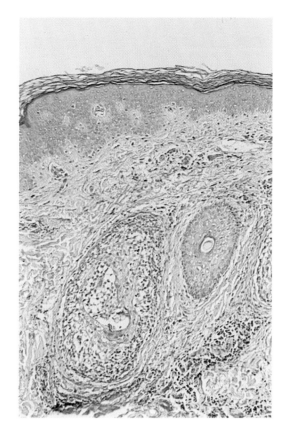

FIGURE 2-10   Follicular eczema. Prominent spongiosis involves the follicular infundibulum.

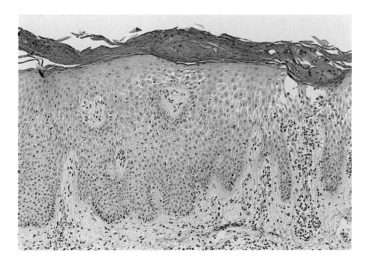

FIGURE 2-9   Nummular eczema. The epidermis shows psoriasiform hyperplasia with foci of spongiosis, including microvesicle formation.

H&E) confirm the diagnosis of dermatophytosis. In cases of secondary syphilis, the neutrophilic aggregates in the corneal layer are often larger than with seborrheic dermatitis, and special stain (modified Steiner or Warthin-Starry) usually shows the characteristic spirochetes in the epidermis and around vessels.

Gyrate erythemas often but not always have a deeper perivascular infiltrate than seborrheic dermatitis. The focal parakeratotic scale of pityriasis rosea is helpful if it is present. The clinical features of gyrate erythemas and pityriasis rosea also distinguish them from seborrheic

---

TABLE 2-12

Seborrheic Dermatitis

Clinical Features
Common disorder affecting the scalp, face, upper chest, and back
Greasy, scaly, red-brown patches
Often pruritic
Dandruff one type of seborrheic dermatitis

Histopathological Features
Psoriasiform hyperplasia
Hyperkeratosis and parakeratosis, especially parafollicular spongiosis
Neutrophilic exocytosis
Superficial perivascular lymphocytic infiltrate

Differential Diagnosis
Psoriasis
Eczematous dermatitis
Impetigo
Dermatophytosis
Secondary syphilis
Gyrate erythemas
Pityriasis rosea
Irritant contact dermatitis
Drug reaction

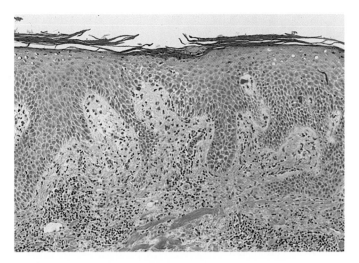

FIGURE 2-11   Seborrheic dermatitis. The epidermis shows a subacute pattern of spongiotic dermatitis with parakeratosis and mild spongiosis. Perivascular lymphoid infiltrates are present in the superficial dermis.

dermatitis. Seborrheic dermatitis in HIV patients tends to show more follicular involvement, more plasma cells in the dermal infiltrate, and more yeast forms in the stratum corneum. Contact dermatitis is discussed in the sections which follow immediately.

Irritant Contact Dermatitis

Irritant contact dermatitis can be caused by almost any substance if it is applied under effective conditions of duration, temperature, and humidity. Physical (heat, cold, light, and other forms of energy) and mechanical agents can also cause an irritant dermatitis. One definition of *irritant contact dermatitis* is cell damage incurred in excess of the skin's ability to repair the damage. Immunologically mediated cell injury is excluded from the category of irritant contact dermatitis. Experimental studies of irritant dermatitis have shown decreased numbers of epidermal Langerhans cells with concurrent increased dermal CD1+ cells, suggesting a net migration of these cells into the dermis.[2] Other studies have also shown gap junction–like structures between Langerhans cells and activated T cells.[3] Some irritants bypass the Langerhans cells and directly induce tumor necrosis factor in keratinocytes.[4]

Clinical Features   Chemical, physical, and mechanical agents can cause a range of clinical appearances from dryness and chapping to all three patterns of eczematous dermatitis to frank burns. Any age and any location of the body can be affected by irritant contact dermatitis. Most human beings have experienced irritant contact dermatitis at least once. Clinical features alone sometimes do not permit differentiation of allergic from irritant contact dermatitis. In one experimental model involucrin expression varies significantly when one compares allergic versus irritant dermatitis.[5]

Histopathological Features   The range of histologic appearances varies with the clinical spectrum: from simple parakeratosis and hyperkeratosis with intracellular edema and a mild infiltrate at the mild end of the spectrum to the three patterns (acute, subacute, and chronic) of eczematous dermatitis with ballooning degeneration and frank necrosis of the epidermis at the other. The above patterns may be complicated by attempts of the skin to regenerate damaged areas. Neutrophils are reported to be common in early phases of irritant contact dermatitis.

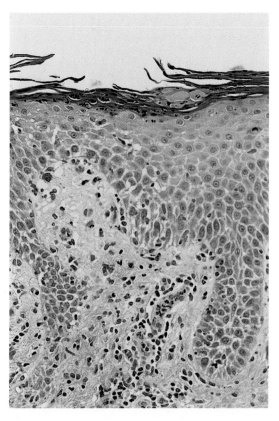

FIGURE 2-12   Seborrheic dermatitis. Higher magnification of Fig. 2-11; shows exocytosis of neutrophils into the superficial epidermis and stratum corneum.

Differential Diagnosis   Allergic contact dermatitis and eczematous dermatitis may be difficult to distinguish from irritant dermatitis. In the early phase, the presence of neutrophils may help to differentiate allergic from irritant dermatitis. When one agent acts as both an irritant and an allergen, the histologic features may be mixed with both eosinophils and neutrophils. Although phototoxic dermatitis may be indistinguishable from irritant dermatitis under the microscope, clinical features, including a good history, will often provide helpful information.

Allergic Contact Dermatitis

This delayed hypersensitivity reaction (type IV immunologic reaction) is a cell-mediated reaction against an antigen. Sensitization occurs when a substance (hapten) applied to the skin binds to Langerhans cells, which in turn interact with T lymphocytes in the skin and in the paracortical area of the lymph node to cause proliferation of helper T cells. The latter cells can recognize the antigen-Langerhans cell complex as they circulate through the blood, skin, and other tissues. This phase of sensitization is a complex interaction, with a host of mediators which up-regulate and down-regulate the response. Suppressor T cells in particular usually prevent sensitization from occurring. The phase of sensitization usually takes 14 to 28 days but can occur in as few as 4 days. Elicitation occurs when the antigen (hapten) binds to the Langerhans cell and is recognized by previously sensitized T cells, which in turn release substances called *lymphokines* which recruit other cells (especially lymphocytes, macrophages, neutrophils, basophils, and to a lesser extent eosinophils) with their attendant cytokines to cause damage to the antigen and surrounding tissues. This phase of elicitation takes 1 to 2 days.

Allergic Contact Dermatitis

Clinical Features
Delayed hypersensitivity reaction (type IV)
All ages affected except below age 5 years and the elderly
Rash occurs at the site of exposure in previously sensitized host
Morphology of rash is eczematous—acute, subacute, or chronic

Histopathological Features
Acute
    Spongiosis often with formation of clinically evident intraepidermal vesicles, superficial perivascular lymphocytic infiltrate usually rich in eosinophils, migration of inflammatory cells into the epidermis
Subacute
    Epidermal hyperplasia with spongiosis, superficial perivascular lymphocytic and eosinophilic infiltrate with variable exocytosis
Chronic
    Psoriasiform hyperplasia with a superficial perivascular lymphocytic and eosinophilic infiltrate; spongiosis absent

Differential Diagnosis
Many forms of eczematous dermatitis
Irritant and photoallergic reactions
Scabetic infestation
Drug reactions
Bullous pemphigoid
Parasitic infestations

Clinical Features   The rash occurs in the area of the skin where the allergen has been applied (but may become generalized if autoeczematization or an id reaction occurs) (Table 2-13). The morphology is basically eczematous, showing acute, subacute, and chronic patterns. The acute is characterized by erythema, edema, oozing, crusting, vesicles, and bullae. The chronic pattern is characterized by erythema, scaling, lichenification, and, not infrequently, hyperpigmentation. Unusual forms of contact dermatitis include follicular contact dermatitis, in which the presumed pathogenesis includes absorption of the antigen preferentially through the pilosebaceous unit. As a rule of thumb, infants and children under the age of 5 years as well as the elderly do not experience allergic contact dermatitis because their immune systems tend not to respond to antigens in this fashion. The reaction of allergic contact dermatitis is generally slower in its formation than that of an irritant contact dermatitis.

Histopathological Features   The microscopic features parallel those described for eczematous dermatitis, again showing acute, subacute, and chronic patterns. The hyperpigmented lesions usually show melanin-laden macrophages in the upper dermis with variable basal pigmentation. Basophils are not seen in routinely prepared sections because their granules are soluble in aqueous solutions. In one experimental model of allergic contact dermatitis, the following time course is observed: spongiosis in the lower epidermis 3 to 4 h after the allergen is applied; increased spongiosis and an infiltrate of lymphocytes and mononuclear cells in the dermis and epidermis at 6 to 12 h; markedly stretched or disrupted desmosomes at 12 to 48 h; keratinocyte necrosis at several days.

Differential Diagnosis   Other forms of eczematous dermatitis can be indistinguishable from allergic contact dermatitis, including scabies, drug reactions, bullous pemphigoid, cutaneous larva migrans, and, espe-

cially, irritant and photoallergic reactions. Clinical features will ultimately arbitrate.

SPONGIOTIC (ECZEMATOUS) DRUG REACTIONS

These delayed hypersensitivity reactions (see Chapter 12) may follow oral or parenteral administration of drugs, foods, or other substances. The sensitizing event may have occurred by the above routes or by cutaneous contact.

Clinical Features   The appearance is that of a spongiotic dermatitis which may be localized or generalized. The rash is often symmetric and may first appear or be more marked at the site of the sensitizing event. Some of the substances reported to cause spongiotic (eczematous) drug reactions are listed in Table 2-14.

Histopathological Features   The microscopic appearance of these reactions is similar to that of eczematous dermatitis with acute, subacute, and chronic patterns. In practice the presence of eosinophils is considered supportive evidence for a hypersensitivity reaction, although it is well understood that these reactions may occur in the absence of eosinophils. The infiltrate is often limited to the superficial plexus.

Differential Diagnosis   Eczematous dermatitis and preeruptive pemphigoid may provide an identical histologic pattern. The latter, however, usually has distinctive findings with direct immunofluorescence studies. Clinical features are usually helpful in differential diagnosis. When the infiltrate involves the deep vascular plexus, it may be difficult to distinguish from a reaction to an arthropod assault.

ERYTHRODERMA AND EXFOLIATIVE DERMATITIS

Erythroderma ("red skin") occurs in association with a variety of disorders, only some of which occur with spongiosis. When scaling predominates as the clinical appearance, the term *exfoliative dermatitis* may be used. Biopsy is often but not always helpful in determining the underlying disorder.[6]

Drugs Associated with Eczematous Reaction

Allopurinol
Bleomycin
Chloramphenicol
Clonidine
Ethylenediamine
Hydroxyquinolines
Indomethacin
Methyldopa
Mitomycin C
Neomycin
Parabens
Penicillin
Quinine
Sulphonamides

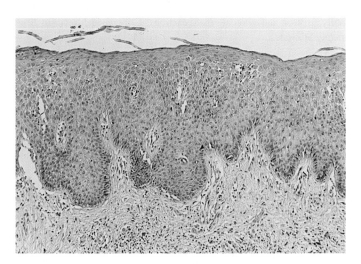

FIGURE 2-13 Erythroderma. The epidermis shows nonspecific psoriasiform dermatitis with slight spongiosis.

TABLE 2-15

Stasis Dermatitis

Clinical Features
Legs, especially inner aspects, are affected
Red, edematous, scaling lesions
Variable oozing
Evidence of stasis such as brown pigmentation, ulcers, varicose veins, and atrophic scars

Histopathological Features
Acute, subacute, or chronic eczematous pattern with lobular proliferation of capillaries, hemorrhage, hemosiderin deposition, and fibrosis

Differential Diagnosis
Granulation tissue next to a leg ulcer
Kaposi's sarcoma

Clinical Features   Large areas of or the entire cutaneous surface are involved. Scaling, erythema, and, in severe cases, oozing are the clinical findings. Severe cases may also be associated with fever and temperature dysregulation, fluid imbalance, and cardiac failure. Pruritus may be a sign of mycosis fungoides. Drug reactions, eczematous dermatitis, and psoriasis are the most common causes of erythroderma. Many disorders have been associated with erythroderma including contact dermatitis, atopic dermatitis, psoriasis, seborrheic dermatitis, stasis dermatitis, scabetic infestation, lichen planus, pityriasis rubra pilaris, pemphigus foliaceus, lamellar ichthyosis, hypereosinophilic syndrome, and Sézary syndrome (mycosis fungoides). Hodgkin's disease and T-cell leukemias are less commonly associated. The history of a prior dermatitis may provide an underlying cause. Cases without a discernable underlying disorder are classified as idiopathic. Up to 25 percent of these idiopathic cases are diagnosed eventually as mycosis fungoides. The erythroderma may precede diagnosable mycosis fungoides by several years.

Histopathological Features   A psoriasiform or eczematous dermatitis (subacute or chronic) is the usual microscopic pattern (Fig. 2-13). An eosinophil-rich infiltrate may indicate a drug reaction or atopic diathesis. Neutrophils forming microabscesses may point to psoriasis or seborrheic dermatitis. Cerebriform cells with formation of Pautrier's microabscesses indicate Sézary syndrome. In many cases the underlying disorder will be evident from the histology. Of course some cases will defy ready analysis. Multiple and/or repeated biopsies may provide more information than a single one.[7] Given that a significant number of cases eventuate in mycosis fungoides, careful examination of lymphocyte morphology merits particular consideration.

STASIS DERMATITIS

Stasis dermatitis (synonyms include *gravitational eczema, venous eczema*) is an eczematous dermatitis involving the lower legs of usually middle-aged to elderly women with increased venous hypertension. The pathogenesis of this disorder is unresolved. Since measurement of venous blood has been found to be faster than expected, stasis as the cause per se has been questioned. However, tissue perfusion appears to be poor.

Clinical Features   The inner legs are often first involved (Table 2-15). The eruption may begin gradually or quite suddenly. Erythema, scaling, edema, and sometimes an exudative appearance are seen as they would be in other types of eczema. Brown pigmentation, ulceration, dilated or varicose veins, and scarring with atrophy are features which are not always present, but when they are seen in this location, they provide evidence of stasis dermatitis. The eczematous features could represent a kind of id reaction (see discussion of autosensitization, above) superimposed upon the background of venous hypertension.

Histopathological Features   The pattern of an acute, subacute, or chronic eczematous dermatitis is seen above dermal changes of chronic venous hypertension, namely, lobular proliferation of capillaries, hemorrhage, variable hemosiderin deposition, and fibrosis (Figs. 2-14 and 2-15). These changes may be confined to the upper dermis in early cases, but advanced cases will show striking changes all through the dermis and sometimes into the subcutaneous fat.

Differential Diagnosis   The histologic changes of stasis dermatitis merge with those of lymphedema. Granulation tissue adjacent to an ulcer may show many of the changes of stasis dermatitis, but it is usually more circumscribed. Kaposi's sarcoma (KS) may share proliferation of vessels in this anatomic location; however, KS usually has more abnormal and poorly formed vessels as well as a characteristic spindle-cell proliferation with slitlike spaces containing erythrocytes. Angiodermatitis (which is a more extreme form of stasis dermatitis) may also be considered part of the differential diagnosis.

PITYRIASIS ALBA

Pityriasis alba is a very common disorder usually seen in children as hypopigmented slightly scaly patches on the face. The cause is unclear, but eczematous dermatitis with postinflammatory hypopigmentation has been proposed as a pathogenetic mechanism, since many of the patients are atopic.

Clinical Features   Children from 3 to 16 years usually present with one or several hypopigmented macules on the face and, less often, on the trunk and extremities. The borders of the lesions are indistinct, and a fine scale (as implied by the term *pityriasis*) can be appreciated. A

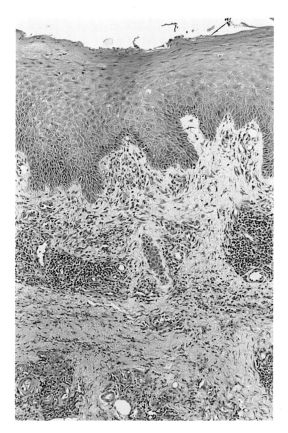

FIGURE 2-14   Stasis dermatitis. The epidermis exhibits irregular psoriasiform epidermal hyperplasia with slight spongiosis and overlying hyperkeratosis. There is some lobular grouping of blood vessels in the dermis with an associated perivascular lymphoid infiltrate.

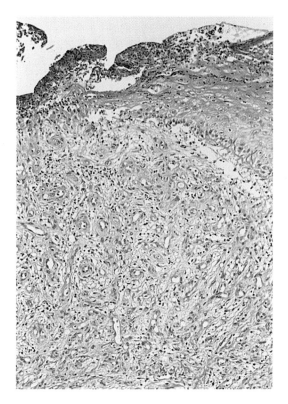

FIGURE 2-15   Stasis dermatitis. There is prominent lobular vascular proliferation in the dermis.

phase of erythematous scaly patches may precede the hypopigmented lesions, providing evidence that pityriasis alba is basically eczematous or atopic in nature. Follicular papules are also sometimes observed. Spontaneous remission with repigmentation usually occurs in 1 to 2 years, but occasionally the lesions persist into adulthood. Clinically, the differential diagnosis includes vitiligo and pityriasis versicolor.

Histopathological Features   Mild eczematous changes are observed including moderate hyperkeratosis, patchy parakeratosis, acanthosis, mild spongiosis, edema of the upper dermis, and a superficial perivascular lymphocytic infiltrate with ectasia of superficial vessels. Follicular spongiosis has been described[8] as well as follicular plugging and atrophic sebaceous glands,[9] if follicular papules are biopsied. The number of melanocytes is not reduced, but decreased melanization is seen with fewer active melanocytes and smaller and few melanosomes in affected skin.

Differential Diagnosis   The histologic features of pityriasis alba are difficult to distinguish from mild eczematous dermatitis and chronic superficial dermatitis. The diagnosis is usually made on the basis of clinical findings—especially the age of the patient and the morphology and distribution of the lesions. Vitiligo is readily distinguished from pityriasis alba, because the former is characterized by loss of melanocytes. Pityriasis versicolor is also separated from pityriasis alba by the presence of yeast and hyphal forms in the former.

PITYRIASIS ROSEA

Pityriasis rosea is a common, self-limited, usually papulosquamous disorder of uncertain but possibly infectious etiology.

Clinical Features   This disorder usually affects children through middle-aged adults (Table 2-16). A mild prodrome of malaise and headache sometimes precedes a herald patch, which is followed some 10 days later by a more generalized eruption which in turn resolves over a period of weeks. The entire disease cycle usually lasts no more than 10 weeks. The herald patch consists of a 2- to 10-cm salmon-colored or erythematous scaly area, usually located on the trunk or extremity. The more generalized eruption is usually located on the trunk and consists of numerous approximately 1-cm oval salmon-rose, erythematous maculopapules with a fine peripheral scale which has been likened to cigarette paper. The distribution of these usually truncal lesions when seen on the back sometimes resembles a fir tree. Oral lesions are seen in a minority (16 percent in one series) of patients.[10]

In contrast to the usual maculopapular lesions, atypical pityriasis rosea may produce vesicular (especially in infants and children), pustular, urticarial, or large hemorrhagic-purpuric lesions. *Inverse pityriasis rosea* refers to the rash when it appears mostly on the extremities rather than on the trunk. Pityriasis rosea–like rash following bone marrow transplantation has also been reported.[11] Pityriasis rosea–like drug rashes have also been seen after treatment with gold, bismuth, barbiturates, and captopril, among others.

Histopathological Features   Similar histologic features are seen for both the herald patch and the generalized eruption and can be summarized as an eczematous pattern with the following caveats. Focal parakeratosis corresponding to the cigarette paper–like scale is seen, and one end of the scale may tilt upward. This upward tilt of focal parakeratosis has been likened to the gesture of tilting open the lid of a teapot. However, a more diffuse mild parakeratosis and hyperkeratosis may also be seen. The epidermis may be of normal or increased thickness.

Pityriasis Rosea

Clinical Features
Duration of disease less than 10 weeks
Herald patch
Generalized eruption, usually on trunk
Multiple salmon-colored macules with fine scale
"Fir-tree" pattern
Atypical pityriasis rosea may exhibit vesicles, pustules, urticarial lesions, purpura
Inverse pityriasis rosea rash distributed on the extremities instead of the trunk
Drug eruptions may resemble pityriasis rosea

Histopathological Features
Mild subacute spongiotic dermatitis often with focal parakeratosis (which may tilt upward)
Perivascular lymphocytic infiltrate with variable exocytosis
Sometimes a microvesicle containing mononuclear cells in the epidermis
Atypical forms tend to show vesicles, dyskeratosis, more parakeratosis and inflammation, hemorrhage, and eosinophils

Differential Diagnosis
Drug reactions
Eczematous dermatitis
Chronic superficial dermatitis (parapsoriasis)
Pityriasis lichenoides
Guttate psoriasis
Dermatophytosis

Patchy loss of the granular layer can be found. Spongiosis is often focal and best seen in areas of exocytosis. An intraepidermal vesicle and mononuclear cell microabscess may be found. Below the epidermis there is a superficial perivascular lymphocytic infiltrate with focal interface involvement and exocytosis. Eosinophils are described in some cases. Dyskeratosis and hemorrhage in the papillary dermis may be seen. The atypical forms of pityriasis rosea often show more inflammation and more hemorrhage and may be so altered from the above histologic picture that the diagnosis devolves heavily upon the clinical aspects.

Differential Diagnosis　A well-oriented biopsy of a well-developed lesion of pityriasis rosea will show all or most of the above features, but clinically obvious cases are rarely biopsied. The differential diagnosis often includes drug reactions, eczematous dermatitis, parapsoriasis, pityriasis lichenoides, guttate psoriasis, dermatophyte infections, and pityriasis alba, among others. The focal parakeratosis with one side tilted upward, if present, is a feature which favors the diagnosis of pityriasis rosea over most of the disorders listed above. Drug reactions and eczematous dermatitis are often more eosinophil-rich than pityriasis rosea. Parapsoriasis may be indistinguishable from pityriasis rosea on biopsy findings alone; clinically parapsoriasis is chronic, whereas pityriasis rosea is usually resolved by 6 to 8 weeks. Eosinophils are usually absent in parapsoriasis and can be absent or present in pityriasis rosea. Compared to pityriasis rosea, pityriasis lichenoides usually has more lymphoid cells at the dermoepidermal interface. Guttate psoriasis usually has more neutrophils in the parakeratotic scale. Dermatophyte infections should be easy to separate from pityriasis rosea once the hyphal forms are identified in the stratum corneum. Pityriasis alba can usually be distinguished from pityriasis rosea on clinical features with its more chronic course leading to decreased pigmentation.

PAPULAR ACRODERMATITIS OF CHILDHOOD (GIANOTTI-CROSTI SYNDROME)

This eruption is considered to be the cutaneous manifestation of a generalized viral infection acquired through the skin or mucous membrane. Hepatitis B is the most common association. Epstein-Barr virus is also described in association with this eruption. Coxsackie viruses, cytomegalovirus, echovirus, poliovirus, respiratory syncytial virus, parainfluenza, and hepatitis A have also been implicated.

Clinical Features　This disorder affects children from age 6 months to 12 years. When hepatitis B is involved, the skin, liver, and lymph nodes are affected. The eruption lasts usually 3 to 4 weeks but may last longer. The eruption consists of an erythematous, nonpruritic, papular eruption which involves the face, buttocks, and extremities. The trunk is usually spared. During the cutaneous phase and for up to 12 months, hepatitis B surface antigen, often of the subtype ayw, is found in the blood, but antibody is undetectable. After about 1 year, well after the rash and acute hepatitis have resolved, antibody to hepatitis B surface antigen may be found. The acute hepatitis lasts about 2 months. Jaundice is usually not seen. Only rarely is there progression to chronic hepatitis. Axillary, inguinal, and sometimes generalized lymphadenopathy may occur. If the infectious agent is other than hepatitis B, the clinical picture will vary—the lesions may be pruritic, and the hepatitis and lymphadenopathy are usually absent.

Histopathological Features　The epidermis may be normal, or it may show slight acanthosis, slight spongiosis, and parakeratosis, sometimes with a mononuclear cell microabscess. An infiltrate of lymphocytes and histiocytes is seen around superficial vessels. All in all, the histologic pattern is not distinctive.

Differential Diagnosis　The differential diagnosis includes viral exanthems, drug reactions, dermatophytosis, and hypersensitivity reactions, among others. Although the histologic picture is not specific, the clinical features and serologic studies are likely to provide the diagnosis.

CHRONIC SUPERFICIAL DERMATITIS

The term *parapsoriasis*, without modifiers, has fallen out of favor, since it refers to several entities and especially since some of these entities eventuate in mycosis fungoides or other cutaneous lymphomas. *Chronic superficial dermatitis* (and synonyms—parapsoriasis—small plaque variant, digitate dermatosis, parapsoriasis en plaques—benign type) refers to a benign type of parapsoriasis which is not associated with mycosis fungoides. This having been said, occasional cases typical of chronic superficial dermatitis have evolved to form lesions of the type associated with mycosis fungoides, so one cannot always be certain of the outcome. Follow-up examinations thus merit particular consideration. Guttate parapsoriasis has been reclassified as pityriasis lichenoides chronica. The pathogenesis of chronic superficial dermatitis is poorly understood. Clonality on the basis of T-cell gene rearrangements has been demonstrated in a few cases,[12] leading to speculation that chronic superficial dermatitis is "an abortive cutaneous T-cell lymphoma."[13]

Clinical Features　This uncommon but not rare disorder usually begins in middle age as one or a few erythematous round to oval scaly patches about 2.5 cm across on the trunk or extremities. With time, the lesions become more numerous. They may be fingerlike, or digitate, on the abdomen. They are often much larger on the lower limb. The face, palms, and soles are usually spared. The well-developed lesions may wrinkle in a way that recalls cigarette paper. Eventually the number and size of patches stabilize. The lesions may be more obvious in the winter and may appear to regress somewhat with sun exposure. Sometimes they are pruritic but almost always mildly so. With treatment, a response can be expected, but the lesions tend to return if treatment is discontinued.

Histopathological Features Variable but usually mild spongiosis, parakeratosis, normal or mildly acanthotic epidermis, mild to moderate superficial perivascular lymphocytic infiltrate, and slight exocytosis define the spectrum. Lymphocytic atypia and fibroplasia are minimal or absent. No Pautrier's microabscesses are seen.

Differential Diagnosis Chronic superficial dermatitis shares many features with mild spongiotic eczematous dermatitis, some drug reactions, and pityriasis lichenoides chronica. Eosinophils are uncommon in chronic superficial dermatitis and are more often seen with eczematous and drug reactions. Pityriasis lichenoides chronica also usually lacks eosinophils and often but not always exhibits more interface and epidermal distribution of lymphocytes. Early mycosis fungoides may be difficult to distinguish from chronic superficial dermatitis. With mycosis fungoides, the following are seen: lymphocytic atypia—notably Sézary cells, a denser lymphocytic infiltrate than with chronic superficial dermatitis, more exocytosis with formation of Pautrier's microabscesses, and relatively little spongiosis. When histologic features are equivocal, the diagnosis will often turn on the response to therapy and clinical observations over time. Several biopsies over the course of several months with close clinical correlation will often provide useful information.

PRURITIC URTICARIAL PAPULES AND PLAQUES OF PREGNANCY (POLYMORPHIC ERUPTION OF PREGNANCY)

Nicknamed *PUPPP*, this disorder is characterized by marked pruritus, periumbilical involvement, and occurrence during the last trimester of pregnancy. The cause and pathogenesis are unknown. This disorder has no association with fetal morbidity or mortality, in possible contrast to herpes gestationis for which the older literature describes these associations.

Clinical Features The eruption usually begins after the thirty-fifth week of gestation, typically in a primigravida, often beginning around the umbilicus and spreading to the rest of the abdomen, buttocks, and thighs. As the name implies, the morphology of the eruption is variable, but commonly urticarial papules coalesce to form plaques. The urtication may be extreme enough to simulate vesicles, but, unlike herpes gestationis, true bullae are absent in PUPPP. Target lesions resembling those seen in erythema multiforme can also form. Pruritus is usually an outstanding complaint, sometimes to the extent that sleep is disturbed. The rash resolves several days after delivery. Infants of mothers with PUPPP are usually unaffected, save for possibly increased birthweight.[14] Increased maternal weight gain and an increased rate of twins was also found in the same series.

Histopathological Features Biopsies of PUPPP usually show slight spongiosis, variable parakeratosis and acanthosis, edema of the papillary dermis, and a superficial perivascular lymphocytic infiltrate with focal exocytosis (usually into the area of spongiosis). Eosinophils may be present within the infiltrate. Erosion with neutrophils may be seen as a secondary finding, not surprisingly, given the marked pruritus. These findings are not specific. Direct immunofluorescence studies are negative, in contrast to herpes gestationis.

Differential Diagnosis Herpes gestationis is usually the main clinical differential consideration, even though it often occurs earlier in pregnancy and has a different morphology. Eosinophils at the dermoepidermal junction are more often seen in herpes gestationis than in PUPPP. Direct immunofluorescence studies are strongly recommended whenever herpes gestationis is a consideration. The histologic pattern of PUPPP is identical to eczematous dermatitis and hypersensitivity reactions, among others. Clinical features may be helpful in separating PUPPP from these other eruptions.

GROVER'S DISEASE (TRANSIENT ACANTHOLYTIC DERMATOSIS)

Grover's disease is a common itchy papular acantholytic dermatosis of unknown etiology. It has often been associated with heat and perspiration. Ultrastructurally there is abnormal keratinization.

Clinical Features Grover's disease usually affects middle-aged to elderly men. The rash consists of red-brown pruritic papules usually located on the chest, back, and thighs. Less commonly there are vesicles and, rarely, bullae, instead of papules. Oral lesions are apparently very rare. The duration of the disorder is usually weeks to months, but there are reported cases lasting over 3 years. Some cases of Grover's disease have been reported in patients with malignant neoplasms[15] and AIDS, but a specific association has not been established. In many of these cases, there is a history of fever, occlusion of the skin, perspiration, or radiation.

Histopathological Features Four patterns have been described, all associated with acantholysis: Darier-like, Hailey-Hailey-like, pemphigus foliaceus–like, and spongiotic. The Darier-like pattern differs from true Darier's disease in that the lesions are smaller and often less well formed (Fig. 2-16). One observes a suprabasal cleft, acantholytic cells, dense keratohyaline granules, and sometimes corps ronds and corps grains. Sometimes "villi" are seen. The Hailey-Hailey-like pattern shows the dilapidated brick-wall appearance, but the lesions are usually smaller than true Hailey-Hailey disease. The pemphigus foliaceus–like pattern shows acantholysis with formation of a cleft within or just below the granular layer. The spongiotic variant shows spongiosis, usually mild, with scattered acantholytic cells. All four patterns have a superficial perivascular lymphocytic infiltrate with spillover into the interstitium. Eosinophils and hemorrhage are sometimes seen.

Differential Diagnosis Darier's disease, warty dyskeratoma, Hailey-Hailey disease, pemphigus foliaceus, spongiotic eczematous dermatitis, and focal acantholytic dyskeratosis may all resemble Grover's disease, but the size and extent of the lesions and clinical morphology usually allow for diagnostic certainty.

ERYTHEMA NEONATORUM (TOXIC ERYTHEMA OF NEWBORN, ERYTHEMA TOXICUM NEONATORUM)

The cause of this common, benign, self-limited process is unknown. High viscosity of the newborn extracellular matrix[16] and mild self-limited acute cutaneous graft-versus-host reaction from maternal-to-fetal lymphocyte transfer[17] are two unusual mechanisms proposed recently. To complicate matters further, others suggest that *erythema neonatorum* and *transient neonatal pustular melanosis* be aggregated under the term *sterile transient neonatal pustulosis*.[18] This disorder is characterized by lack of spongiosis but it appears in this chapter nonetheless so that it can be compared to incontinentia pigmenti.

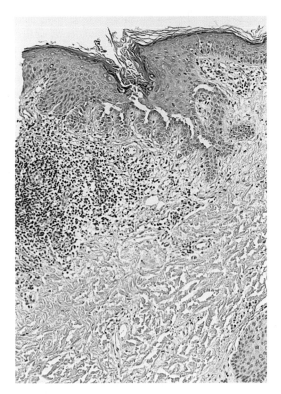

FIGURE 2-16 Transient acantholytic dermatosis (Grover's disease). The epidermis shows focal acantholytic dyskeratosis. The superficial dermis shows a lymphocytic infiltrate with a few eosinophils.

Clinical Features   Erythema neonatorum affects up to 50 percent of all infants. It usually appears within 12 h of birth and resolves without treatment in 2 to 7 days. The asymptomatic lesions may appear as erythematous macules and/or papules. The lesions vary in size and may be few to numerous. About 10 percent of cases have pustules. The trunk is most often involved, followed by the face and proximal thighs. Blood eosinophilia may be noted.

Histopathological Features   The macular lesions may show only dermal edema and a perivascular eosinophilic infiltrate. The papular lesions show, in addition to dermal edema and perivascular eosinophil infiltrates, aggregates of eosinophils and a few neutrophils in the outer root sheath of the follicular infundibulum. The absence of spongiosis is considered to be a key feature in differential diagnosis, favoring erythema neonatorum over incontinentia pigmenti. The pustular lesions show an eosinophil-rich pustule in the subcorneal area of a hair follicle.

Differential Diagnosis   Incontinentia pigmenti shows an eosinophil-rich pustule within the epidermis, but it usually shows spongiosis. Clinically, incontinentia pigmenti may appear as early in life as erythema neonatorum, but, unlike erythema neonatorum, which resolves, incontinentia pigmenti progresses through verrucous to pigmented stages. Miliaria and neonatal pustular melanosis form pustules which are neutrophil-rich.

INFUNDIBULOFOLLICULITIS, DISSEMINATE AND RECURRENT

This uncommon disorder occurs more often in blacks, and the cause is unknown.

Clinical Features   The rash affects the trunk and extremities but spares flexural areas and consists of numerous flesh-colored papules resembling goosebumps. The rash is often but not always pruritic.

Histopathological Features   The follicular infundibulum shows spongiosis. A lymphocytic infiltrate surrounds the follicle, and some lymphocytes are seen within the spongiotic area. There is variable follicular plugging within and parakeratosis above the follicle. The histologic findings are not specific.

Differential Diagnosis   The diagnosis is made largely on the basis of clinical findings. Table 2-5 lists other disorders which may show follicular spongiosis.

INCONTINENTIA PIGMENTI

This uncommon X-linked multisystem disorder is usually seen in females (97 percent of cases). Males with the disorder (3 percent of cases) probably have spontaneous mutations; males who inherit the abnormal gene are thought to die in utero. Females with incontinentia pigmenti are thought to exhibit functional X-chromosome mosaicism.[19] Gene-mapping studies[20] may eventually lead to a better understanding of pathogenesis of the cutaneous and extracutaneous manifestations.

Clinical Features   The cutaneous lesions are of three types which usually follow sequentially, but they may overlap. The first stage usually presents at birth or shortly thereafter and consists of erythematous lesions with vesicles, more prominent on the extremities and arranged in a whorled pattern following Blaschko's lines. Several months later, the second stage consisting of linear verrucous lesions is seen, also mainly on the extremities. The third stage begins several months later and consists of pigmentation in an irregular whorled or spattered pattern, usually widespread on the trunk rather than the extremities, again following Blaschko's lines. The pigmentation often but not always fades to imperceptibility within several years. Blaschko's lines are thought to represent the effects of functional X-chromosome mosaicism, i.e., these are the areas where the abnormal gene which is not inactivated can express its phenotype.[21] The extracutaneous abnormalities involve the teeth, eyes, and central nervous system: widely spaced and/or cone-shaped teeth, hypodontia, strabismus, astigmatism, cataracts, blindness, seizure disorders, spina bifida, and mental retardation. Nail dystrophy and partial scarring alopecia as well as altered immunologic activity are also described. The extracutaneous problems are seen in a significant percentage of patients but are by no means universal.

Histopathological Features   The lesions of the first stage show eosinophilic spongiosis, spongiotic vesicles containing mostly eosinophils (Figs. 2-17 and 2-18) (but also neutrophils), dyskeratotic cells, and whorls of squamous cells. The lesions of the second stage show acanthosis with papillomatosis, dyskeratotic cells, basal cell vacuolar changes, and a mild mononuclear infiltrate with melanin-laden macrophages. The pigmentary changes of the third stage show melanin-laden macrophages in the upper dermis. Changes of different stages may be seen in the same biopsy, just as the clinical features may overlap.

Differential Diagnosis   Erythema neonatorum, which can occur in the same age group, can show eosinophilic spongiosis and eosinophilic vesicles, but spongiosis is usually absent.

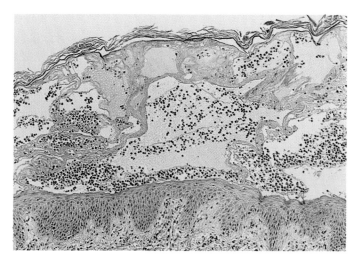

FIGURE 2-17 Incontinentia pigmenti, vesicular stage. There is a large intraepidermal microvesicle containing numerous eosinophils.

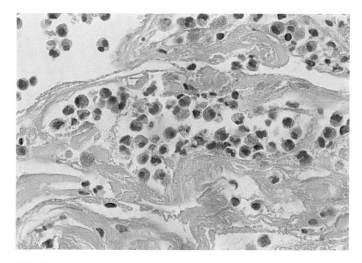

FIGURE 2-18 Incontinentia pigmenti. Higher magnification of Fig. 2-17; shows numerous eosinophils within the intraepidermal vesicle.

MILIARIA

Miliaria refers to rashes caused by blockage of sweat ducts.[22] Eccrine miliaria can be divided into three types based upon where the blockage occurs. From superficial to deep, the types are: miliaria crystallina (sudamina), miliaria rubra, and miliaria profunda. *Miliaria pustulosa* refers to miliaria rubra with a neutrophil-rich infiltrate. Apocrine miliaria is discussed in Chapter 10.

Miliaria Crystallina (Sudamina)

This type of miliaria occurs after superficial damage to the epidermis followed by sweating; sunburn is a commonly cited example of such damage. Miliaria crystallina may also be seen following a fever, particularly in infants and children. The site of the blockage is the intracorneal course of the eccrine duct. Drugs have also been implicated in the etiology of sudamina.

Clinical Features   Numerous 1- to 2-mm droplike vesicles filled with clear fluid are the typical lesions of this type of miliaria. Erythema is notably absent. The lesions often occur on the trunk and are asymptomatic.

Histopathological Features   A subcorneal vesicle filled mostly with fluid but also containing neutrophils is seen. The vesicle is associated with an underlying eccrine duct. This type of miliaria is rarely biopsied, because the lesions are so distinctive and evanescent.

Differential Diagnosis   Subcorneal pustular dermatosis and a pustular drug reaction also show an intracorneal vesicle filled with neutrophils; however, miliaria crystallina has a vesicle with more fluid and fewer neutrophils. Eosinophils are present in erythema toxicum neonatorum and usually absent or inconspicuous in miliaria crystallina.

Miliaria Rubra (Prickly Heat Rash)

This type of miliaria occurs in susceptible individuals under conditions of occlusion and profuse sweating. For example, soldiers sent from temperate zones to the tropics or the desert may develop miliaria rubra. Since gram-positive cocci have been seen in some lesions, an etiologic role for these microorganisms with the following scenario has been proposed: Under conditions of occlusion, resident flora (such as coagulase-negative staphylococci) produce a toxin which damages the ductal epithelial cells from which a PAS&D-positive cast is formed, causing occlusion of the acrosyringium.[22] These investigators also state that microorganisms are necessary for the development of miliaria rubra, since the application of antibacterial solutions appeared to prevent disease. Other investigators have shown that the PAS&D-positive cast is an extracellular polysaccharide substance formed by *Staphylococcus epidermidis*.[23] Miliaria rubra can be produced experimentally if the skin is occluded for several days by an impermeable plastic such as polyethylene. Blockage of the intraepidermal portion of the sweat duct (the acrosyringium), probably near the granular layer, results in miliaria rubra.

Clinical Features   Numerous 1- to 2-mm erythematous papules and, rarely, vesicles often located on the trunk and in the groin area are associated with a distinctive prickly sensation.

Histopathological Features   The acrosyringium shows spongiosis and a largely lymphocytic and mononuclear cell infiltrate. Rarely there is formation of a spongiotic vesicle below the granular layer (Fig. 2-19).

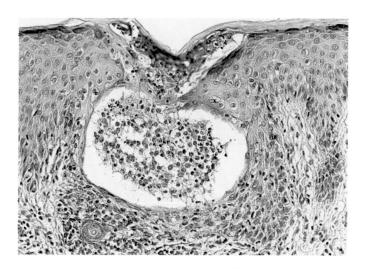

FIGURE 2-19 Miliaria rubra. There is a spongiotic microvesicle associated with the intraepidermal sweat duct. The microvesicle contains both mononuclear and polymorphonuclear leukocytes.

Sometimes gram-positive cocci are seen in the stratum corneum, and a PAS&D-positive plug may occlude the duct lumen. The gram-positive cocci are not seen in the duct lumen.

Differential Diagnosis   If the portions of the epidermis between acrosyringeal units are normal, the histologic features described above speak strongly for miliaria rubra. If the intervening epidermis also shows an interface dermatitis and exocytosis, other differential diagnoses must be considered according to the pattern of inflammation present.

Miliaria Profunda

This type of miliaria often follows repeated or chronic miliaria rubra and is usually seen only in military personnel in the tropics in wartime. It usually occurs after several months of extreme conditions and is often associated with an inability to sweat, causing serious difficulties with thermoregulation and electrolyte imbalances; *tropical anhidrotic asthenia* is the name given to this state. Blockage of the lower portion of the acrosyringium is associated with miliaria profunda.

Clinical Features   Numerous usually asymptomatic 2- to 3-mm papules resembling cutis anserina (but not associated with hair follicles) are present during the attacks of tropical anhidrotic asthenia. During these periods, the patients experience micturation, fatigue, loss of interest in work, and fear of heat. Obesity and rashes due to other causes may also predispose to miliaria profunda. The rash is often absent in periods between attacks of anhidrotic asthenia.

Histopathological Features   Spongiosis and sometimes vesiculation of the lower portion of the acrosyringium and upper dermal part of the sweat duct are associated with a largely lymphocytic infiltrate and dermal edema. Duct rupture may be seen.

Differential Diagnosis   The clinical features and conditions under which miliaria profunda occurs are distinctive.

REFERENCES

1. Lifson AR, Hessol NA, Buchbinder SP, et al: The association of clinical conditions and serologic tests with CD4+ lymphocyte counts in HIV-infected subjects without AIDS. *AIDS* 5:1209, 1991.

2. Mikulowska A, Falck B: Distributional changes of Langerhans cells in human skin during irritant contact dermatitis. *Arch Dermatol Res* 286:429, 1994.

3. Brand CU, Hunziker T, Schaffner T, et al: Activated immunocompetent cells in human skin lymph derived from irritant contact dermatitis: An immunomorphological study. *Br J Dermatol* 132:39, 1995.

4. Lisby S, Muiler KM, Jongeneel CV, et al: Nickel and skin irritants up-regulate tumor necrosis factor alpha-mRNA in keratinocytes by different but potentially synergistic mechanisms. *Int Immunol* 7:343, 1995.

5. Le TK, van der Valk PG, Schalkwijk J, et al: Changes in epidermal proliferation and differentiation in allergic and irritant contact dermatitis reactions. *Br J Dermatol* 133:236, 1995.

6. Walsh NM, Prokopetz R, Tron VA: Histopathology in erythroderma: Review of a series of cases by multiple observers. *J Cutan Pathol* 21:419, 1994.

7. Vasconcellos C, Domingues PP, Aoki V, et al: Erythroderma: Analysis of 247 cases. *Rev Saude Publica* 29:177, 1995.

8. Martin RF, Lugo-Somolinos A, Sanchez JL: Clinicopathological study on pityriasis alba. *Bol Assoc Med P R* 83:463, 1990.

9. Vargas-Ocampo F: Pityriasis alba: A histologic study. *Int J Dermatol* 32:870, 1993.

10. Vidimos AT, Camisa C: Tongue and cheek: Oral lesions in pityriasis rosea. *Cutis* 50:276, 1992.

11. Spelman LJ, Robertson IM, Strutton GM, et al: Pityriasis rosea-like eruption after bone marrow transplantation. *J Am Acad Dermatol* 31:348, 1994.

12. Haeffner AC, Smoller BR, Zepter K: Differentiation and clonality of lesional lymphocytes in small plaque parapsoriasis. *Arch Dermatol* 131:321, 1995.

13. Burg G, Dummer R: Small plaque (digitate) parapsoriasis is an "abortive cutaneous T-cell lymphoma" and is not mycosis fungoides (editorial; comment). *Arch Dermatol* 131:336, 1995.

14. Cohen LM, Capeless EK, Krusinski PA, et al: Pruritic urticarial papules and plaques of pregnancy and its relationship to maternal-fetal weight gain and twin pregnancy. *Arch Dermatol* 125:1534, 1989.

15. Guana AL, Cohen PR: Transient acantholytic dermatosis in oncology patients. *J Clin Oncol* 12:1703, 1994.

16. Stone OJ: High viscosity of newborn extracellular matrix is the etiology of erythema toxicum neonatorum: Neonatal jaundice? Hyaline membrane disease? *Med Hypotheses* 33:15, 1990.

17. Bassukas ID: Is erythema toxicum neonatorum a mild self-limited acute cutaneous graft-versus-host-reaction from maternal-to-fetal lymphocyte transfer? *Med Hypotheses* 38:334, 1992.

18. Ferrandiz C, Corulu W, Ribera M, et al: Sterile transient neonatal pustulosis is a precocious form of erythema toxicum neonatorum. *Dermatology* 185:18, 1992.

19. Curtis AR, Lindsay S, Boye E, et al: A study of X chromosome activity in two incontinentia pigmenti families with probable linkage to Xq28. *Eur J Hum Genet* 2:51, 1994.

20. Smahi A, Hyden-Granskog C, Peterlin B, et al: The gene for the familial form of incontinentia pigmenti (IP2) maps to the distal part of Xq28. *Hum Mol Genet* 3:273, 1994.

21. Happle R: The lines of Blaschko: A developmental pattern visualizing functional X-chromosome mosaicism. *Curr Probl Dermatol* 17:5, 1987.

22. Holze E, Kligman AM: The pathogenesis of miliaria rubra: Role of the microflora. *Br J Dermatol* 99:117, 1978.

23. Mowad CM, McGinley KJ, Foglia A, et al: The role of extracellular polysaccharide substance produced by *Staphylococcus epidermidis* in miliaria. *J Am Acad Dermatol* 33:729, 1995.

CHAPTER 3

INTERFACE DERMATITIS

Thomas D. Horn

A large group of skin diseases is characterized by histologic changes categorized as *interface dermatitis* (Table 3-1). At a minimum, a variable combination of leukocyte infiltration of the dermis, vacuolar change of the basilar epidermis, accumulation of melanophages in the upper dermis, and necrosis of keratinocytes must be observed. The term *interface dermatitis* is, therefore, apt because these findings occur at the interface between the epidermis and dermis. This common thread binds otherwise disparate entities together. Other terms applied to this group of disorders include *vacuolar dermatitis*, *vacuolar interface dermatitis*, and *lichenoid tissue reaction*. Before considering specific diseases, definition and illustration of the common histologic findings is in order.

Leukocyte Infiltration

The term *leukocyte infiltration of the dermis* is cumbersome but more accurate than *inflammation*, since, in the case of mycosis fungoides, some portion of the infiltrating lymphocytes is neoplastic and not inflammatory in nature. In all other disorders considered here, lymphoid infiltration represents inflammation. Some degree of upper dermal perivascular accumulation of leukocytes is observed in interface dermatitides. Extension of cells into surrounding collagen may impart a bandlike appearance (or lichenoid appearance, given the similarity to lichen planus) to the infiltrate. Density, pattern, and composition of the infiltrate are variable elements of interface dermatitis that aid in establishing a more specific diagnosis.

Vacuolar Alteration

Vacuolar alteration of the basilar epidermis is also termed *basal vacuolization*. At the junction between epidermis and dermis, small often contiguous discrete bubbles or vacuoles form in interface dermatitides. The vacuolization imparts a ragged appearance to the basilar epidermis, making the interface indistinct compared with normal skin. As vacuoles coalesce, progressively larger clefts may form until macroscopic vesiculation develops. This phenomenon underlies blister formation in bullous lichen planus and grade 3 or 4 graft-versus-host reaction.

Melanin generally resides mostly in keratinocytes and to a lesser degree in melanocytes. Damage to basilar keratinocytes, as part of an interface dermatitis, results in deposition of melanin granules in the upper dermis. The pigment is phagocytosed by macrophages which become progressively more melanin-laden and are termed *melanophages*. Recognition of melanophages correlates with stage in evolution of the interface dermatitis and consitutive degree of pigmentation. The presence of many melanophages suggests that the process is well-established.

Extension of leukocytes into the epidermis is also termed *exocytosis*. The definition of exocytosis also encompasses extension of erythrocytes into the epidermis. The small round nuclei of lymphocytes are interca-lated between keratinocytes, admixed with variable, but generally little, spongiosis, in the case of interface dermatitis. This infiltration may be subtle or pronounced and may be confined to the basilar epidermis or may extend throughout the thickness of the epidermis. Direct apposition of lymphocytes to necrotic keratinocytes (see below) is termed *satellite cell necrosis*.

A necrotic keratinocyte displays an irregularly shrunken hyperchromatic nucleus positioned adjacent to dense eosinophilic refractile cytoplasm. The nucleus may not be observed. The cytoplasmic change is most apparent and is progressive as the cell dies. The pattern and degree of keratinocyte necrosis help to distinguish among diseases. An unfortunate plethora of terms exists to name a necrotic keratinocyte or the process of keratinocyte necrosis. Based solely on histologic observation there is little validity to the many names, even though important and real differences in pathophysiology may exist. Thus, *dyskeratosis (dyskeratotic keratinocyte)*, *apoptosis*, *(apoptotic keratinocyte)*, *Civatte body*, *colloid body*, and perhaps other terms are historically and possibly mechanistically valid but will not be employed further in this chapter.

Understanding the individual histopathologic elements of interface dermatitis is the framework upon which to build a detailed description of the specific entities discussed in this chapter. Considerable variation exists in histologic expression of specific diseases depending on body site sampled, adequacy of the sample, and, most important, stage of evolution of the lesion sampled. The chapter is organized such that diseases with shared histologic features are considered as a group with the proposed prototype discussed first. The first general categorization to be made lies in the distinction between a lichenoid interface dermatitis, which is heavily inflamed (*cell-rich*), relative to a vacuolar interface dermatitis which contains few inflammatory cells (*cell-poor*) (Table 3-1).

LICHENOID INTERFACE DERMATITIS

Lichen planus serves as the prototype for several disorders (Table 3-2). The main findings in samples from fully evolved lesions include a fairly continuous band of lymphoid cells in the upper dermis, overlying interface changes, and further characteristic epidermal changes consisting of acanthosis, pointed rete ridges, an expanded granular layer, and hyperkeratosis.

Lichen Planus and Variants

Clinical Features   Lichen planus, an inflammatory disorder of uncertain cause, consists of variably distributed erythematous to violaceous polygonal papules and plaques, typically well-defined in contour and often grouped on flexor surfaces, especially the wrists. The genitalia are frequently involved. Scale is generally absent, but surface change consisting of white lines or grooves known as Wickham's striae are often

TABLE 3-1

Interface Dermatitis:
Diagnostic Algorithm

Interface dermatitis

Vacuolar interface dermatitis		Lichenoid interface dermatitis
		Lichen planus and variants
Vacuolar interface dermatitis	**Poikilodermatous interface dermatitis**	Lichenoid drug eruption
Erythema multiforme	Poikiloderma of Civatte	Lichenoid keratosis
Fixed drug eruption	Poikiloderma congenitale	Lichen striatus
Drug eruptions	Bloom's syndrome	Lichen nitidus
Viral xanthems	Dyskeratosis congenita	Lichenoid purpura
HIV interface dermatitis	Dermatomyositis	Porokeratosis
Connective tissue disease	Mycosis fungoides	Histologic regression of many tumors
Lupus erythematosus	Radiation dermatitis	
Dermatomyositis		
Graft-versus-host reaction		
Pityriasis lichenoides		
Vitiligo		

observed. The patient frequently complains of intense pruritus. Oral and nail changes may accompany the cutaneous eruption. Rare cases of esophageal and ocular involvement are reported.[1,2] Lacy white patches commonly involve the buccal mucosa. Dystrophy of the nail plate may develop with ridging and distal splitting. Variants include hypertrophic, atrophic, and bullous forms. Hypertrophic lichen planus commonly occurs on the lower legs and consists of erythematous hyperkeratotic plaques which are quite pruritic. Lichen planus actinicus (actinic lichen planus) is an unusual variant localized to sun-exposed skin. Scarring alopecia in association with lichen planus, known as *lichen planopilaris*, is discussed in Chapter 10. An association between lichen planus and hepatitis C infection is noted.[3]

Histopathological Features   A fully evolved lesion will display a perivascular and interstitial infiltration of the upper dermis by lymphocytes and histiocytes forming a band of cells positioned in the papillary and upper reticular dermis (Figs. 3-1 to 3-3). Interspersed melanophages are usually present, and eosinophils may accompany the mononuclear elements of the infiltrate. The inflammatory cells extend up to and infiltrate the lower epidermis. Significant perivascular inflammation of the middle or deep reticular dermis is uncommon. The density of the infiltrate partially or totally obscures the junction between the epidermis and dermis. Exocytosis of lymphocytes is noted with scattered necrotic keratinocytes generally concentrated in the lower epidermis but possibly arrayed at all epidermal levels (Fig. 3-3). Necrotic keratinocytes may be observed in the upper dermis and the stratum corneum. Direct immunofluorescence studies reveal shaggy deposits of IgM along the basement membrane zone and variable immunoglobulin staining of necrotic keratinocytes. Basilar keratinocytes may be flattened, imparting a "squamatized" appearance. Occasionally, satellite cell necrosis may be observed.

A constellation of additional epidermal changes is also evident. Acanthosis with wedge-shaped hypergranulosis occurs. The rete ridges become pointed with sharply tapering tips, a so-called saw-tooth pattern. Hyperkeratosis is seen, but significant parakeratosis is absent. The combination of a band of mononuclear cells confined to the upper dermis, interface changes, and these characteristic epidermal features represent a theme uniting several entities, as discussed below, but should prompt consideration of lichen planus first. Specimens from early lesions display less inflammation and incompletely evolved epidermal

changes; melanophages may be absent. Old lesions generally show reparative changes in the papillary dermis, vascular ectasia, contain numerous melanophages with little inflammation, and display variable epidermal alteration. Biopsy specimens from mucosa and nail display similar changes.[4]

In hypertrophic lichen planus, irregular acanthosis is pronounced but is accompanied by the elements of interface dermatitis and a band of lymphocytes (Fig. 3-4). This combination of findings represents an element of lichen simplex chronicus in addition to lichen planus. Epidermal atrophy typifies actinic lichen planus.[5,6] Inflammation of the deep vascular plexus and adnexae is absent. In bullous lichen planus the basal vacuolization becomes confluent, leading to separation of the epidermis from the dermis (Fig. 3-5). The clefts, or Max-Joseph spaces, may remain microscopic or become clinically apparent.

As mentioned, the infiltrating lymphocytes express CD3 with a majority of cells in the T helper-inducer phenotype (CD4+). Terminal effector mechanisms are not completely understood. Typical cytokine patterns are found in affected tissue, referable to aberrant keratinocyte and lymphocyte physiology.[7] These cytokines may affect the epidermal keratin expression which tends to resemble keratin expression in wound healing.[8] In addition, the pattern of intercellular adhesion molecule-1 (ICAM-1) expression is restricted to basilar keratinocytes in lichen planus, in contrast to lupus erythematosus and erythema multiforme, where more diffuse staining at upper epidermal levels is attributed to the effects of photosensitivity and herpes simplex virus triggers, respectively.[9] The interface change leads to disruption of the normal integrity of epidermal anchoring mechanisms.[10] Alteration in the structure and distribution of type VII collagen, alpha 6 beta 4 integrin, and kalinin is reported in lichen planus.

Differential Diagnosis   The fully evolved histopathology of lichen planus generally allows confident diagnosis in the correct clinical setting. Specimens of lichenoid keratosis and lichenoid drug eruption (see below) may strongly resemble lichen planus, requiring accompanying clinical information. The lichenoid keratosis is often distinguished from lichen planus by the presence of parakeratosis, delicate laminated hyperkeratosis, a normal granular layer, and in some cases, remnants of a solar lentigo. Most lichenoid keratoses are solitary lesions developing on sun-exposed skin. The lesion is often mistaken clinically for basal cell carcinoma, actinic keratosis, or melanocytic nevus.

Clinical Features

Lichen planus
  Prominent pruritus
  Violaceous polygonal papules
  Flexural surfaces favored
  Oral and genital involvement frequent
Atrophic lichen planus (actinicus)
  Atrophic erythematous patches
  Sun-exposed skin
Hypertrophic lichen planus
  Verrucous plaques
  Extensor surfaces favored
Bullous lichen planus
  Bullae within erythematous patches

Histopathological Features

Lichen planus
  Band of lymphocytes in upper dermis, melanophages
  Acanthosis, hypergranulosis, "sawtoothing" of rete ridges
  Basal vacuolization
Atrophic lichen planus (actinicus)
  Lichenoid interface dermatitis
  Epidermal atrophy
Hypertrophic lichen planus
  Lichenoid interface dermatitis
  Irregular acanthosis
  Hyperkeratosis
Bullous lichen planus
  Lichenoid interface dermatitis
  Subepidermal cleft

Differential Diagnosis

Lichen planus
  Lichenoid drug eruption
  Lichenoid keratosis
  Lichenoid actinic keratosis
  Lupus erythematosus
Atrophic lichen planus (actinicus)
  Lupus erythematosus
  Lichen sclerosus et atrophicus
Hypertrophic lichen planus
  Lichen simplex chronicus
  Verrucous lupus erythematosus
Bullous lichen planus
  Paraneoplastic pemphigus
  Erythema multiforme
  Toxic epidermal necrolysis
  Fixed drug eruption

Lichenoid drug eruptions cannot be reliably distinguished from lichen planus but more commonly display the following features: parakeratosis, a normal granular layer, eosinophils, and plasma cells in the inflammatory infiltrate. Inflammation is also more likely to be perivascular and bandlike in contrast to only bandlike in lichen planus. In general, epidermis involved with lichen planus contains a greater number of Langerhans' cells than seen in lichenoid keratosis and lichenoid actinic keratosis.[11]

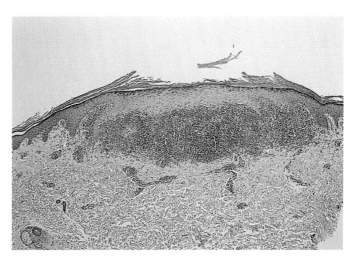

FIGURE 3-1   Lichen planus. The most notable feature is a bandlike infiltrate of lymphocytes that obscures the dermal-epidermal junction.

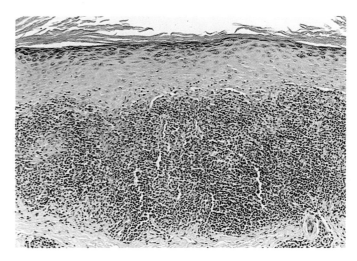

FIGURE 3-2   Lichen planus. This lesion shows hyperkeratosis, hypergranulosis, some acanthosis, and a bandlike infiltrate that fills the papillary dermis and obscures the dermal-epidermal junction.

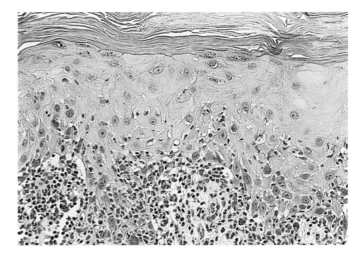

FIGURE 3-3   Lichen planus. There is basal layer vacuolization. The epidermis is slightly acanthotic, and there is a tendency to a sawtooth pattern of the lower epidermis.

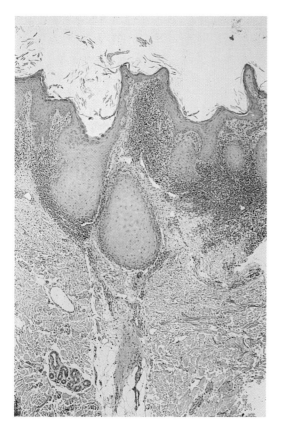

FIGURE 3-4 Hypertrophic lichen planus. The epidermal surface is slightly papillomatous, and there is irregular hyperplasia of the epidermis.

Lichenoid actinic keratosis should possess the diagnostic elements of an actinic keratosis with crowding of keratinocytes and nuclear atypia in addition to the elements of interface dermatitis. As chronic ulcerating lichen planus of mucosal surfaces is rarely associated with the development of squamous cell carcinoma, epithelial dysplasia in these sites must be sought and noted.[12]

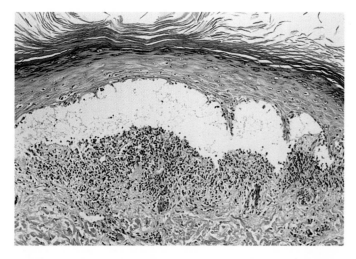

FIGURE 3-5 Bullous lichen planus. There is dermal-epidermal separation leading to formation of a blister cavity. Otherwise features typical of lichen planus are present.

In lupus erythematosus (see below), the pattern of inflammation is quite variable but often extends to involve the deep vascular plexus and adnexal epithelium. In general, the degree of upper dermal inflammation and number of necrotic keratinocytes in lupus erythematosus are less than in lichen planus. Epidermal atrophy suggests the diagnosis of lupus erythematosus, keeping in mind that an atrophic form of lichen planus exists, lacking inflammation of the deep vessels and adnexa. Basement membrane thickening and increased dermal mucin also suggest connective tissue disease rather than lichen planus. Hypertrophic (verrucous) lupus erythematosus may show many of the same features of hypertrophic lichen planus but is discriminated by basement membrane thickening, dermal mucin, and deep extension of the inflammatory infiltrate. Overlap of lupus erythematosus and lichen planus is possible and must be diagnosed based upon clinicopathologic correlation. Erythema multiforme and toxic epidermal necrolysis (see below) are characterized by more keratinocyte necrosis, relative to the degree of inflammation, than in lichen planus. The inflammation in a specimen of fixed drug eruption (see below) often involves the deep vascular plexus and may be polymorphous with occasional eosinophils, neutrophils, and plasma cells. At times, confident discrimination among these disorders requires clinicopathologic correlation.

Any skin biopsy specimen with an upper dermal interstitial infiltrate of lymphocytes should prompt consideration of mycosis fungoides. Interface changes are variably present in mycosis fungoides, although the other epidermal changes of lichen planus are generally absent. Significant nuclear atypia of lymphocytes and aggregation of lymphocytes in epidermal lacunae are absent in lichen planus.

Lichenoid Drug Eruption

Clinical Features   Drug eruptions with clinical and histologic features similar to lichen planus have been described.[13,14] (See also Chapter 12.) Various components of drugs of abuse may also cause lichenoid reactions.[15] Photodistribution is frequently observed. Discontinuation of the offending medication results in resolution of the eruption.

Histopathological Features   Lichenoid drug eruptions may resemble lichen planus. Parakeratosis and inflammation around the middle and deep vascular plexus occur regularly. Eosinophils are variably present. The absence of eosinophils does not preclude the diagnosis of lichenoid drug eruption. Lichenoid drug eruption often displays epidermal atrophy.

Differential Diagnosis   Observation of parakeratosis, epidermal atrophy, eosinophils, and deep dermal inflammation suggests the diagnosis of lichenoid drug eruption when lichen planus is also a consideration. Adequate clinical history is imperative for accurate diagnosis.

Lichenoid Keratosis (Lichen Planus–Like Keratosis) and Lichenoid Actinic Keratosis

Clinical Features   Lichenoid keratoses typically occur as solitary lesions on the chest and arms but may develop elsewhere. Women are more frequently affected than men.[16] The clinical lesion is not specific, consisting of an erythematous papule or plaque. The clinical impression of basal cell carcinoma is common. Lichenoid actinic keratosis occurs mostly in actinically damaged skin as an erythematous scaling patch or plaque.

Histopathological Features   A lichenoid keratosis may greatly resemble lichen planus.[11] As in lichenoid drug eruption, the presence of parakeratosis and middermal inflammation are subtle clues to help in the differentiation. Because solar lentigines may evolve into lichenoid keratoses, the epidermis of a lichenoid keratosis may show changes of solar lentigo with elongated rete ridges. A lichenoid actinic keratosis should possess the epidermal characteristics of the usual actinic keratosis, but with a moderately dense band of lymphocytes in the upper dermis and overlying interface change.

Differential Diagnosis   The distinction of lichenoid keratosis from lichen planus and lichenoid drug eruption often relies in large measure on accompanying clinical history (see differential diagnosis of lichen planus). In lichenoid keratosis, the density of the infiltrate and pattern of epidermal alteration are often not as fully evolved as in lichen planus, but the similarities are often striking. It is important to scan the epidermis and dermis for melanocytic proliferation and features of an inflamed or regressing melanocytic nevus or melanoma in situ, as the inflammation in such nevi or melanoma in situ may assume an interface pattern and may partially obscure the tumor. If clear epidermal features of seborrheic keratosis are observed, yet underlying inflammation is present in an interface pattern, the diagnosis of inflamed seborrheic keratosis is preferable, as a true lichenoid keratosis bears greater resemblance to lichen planus in its epidermal findings.

VACUOLAR INTERFACE DERMATITIS

Compared with lichen planus, the diseases considered under this heading generally display less intense inflammation without the dense band-like pattern. Interface change, especially necrosis of keratinocytes, is prominent relative to the degree of inflammation, and this difference, along with the absence of epidermal changes characteristic of lichen planus, helps to distinguish between diseases in these groups.

Erythema Multiforme

Clinical Features   Clinical and histologic subtypes of eruptions identified as erythema multiforme are likely to exist, and the description of target lesions oversimplifies the range of clinical findings.[17,18] Erythema multiforme exhibits a fairly nonspecific histologic pattern, hence the wide clinical spectrum. The classic target lesion consists of at least three zones of color change: a peripheral rim of erythema, an inner rim of relative pallor, and a central erythematous macule.[19] This concentric pattern imparts a "bull's-eye appearance." Variation from this pattern is described with erythematous patches, some with a dusky, violaceous center but no distinct target appearance. Blisters, when present, form centrally in most cases, but a peripheral pattern also may occur.

The distribution of erythema multiforme is frequently acral with concentration on the palms and soles, but widespread lesions occur commonly. The disease is self-limited, but often recurrent. Involvement of mucosal and conjunctival surfaces occurs and, if extensive, leads to classification of the disease as *major* (possibly synonymous with the term *Stevens-Johnson syndrome*), versus the *minor* form with less severe extracutaneous disease. Universally accepted criteria distinguishing major from minor erythema multiforme and major erythema multiforme from toxic epidermal necrolysis (see below) do not exist. The most common causes of erythema multiforme include herpes simplex virus infection, medications, and other infectious agents, especially *Mycoplasma pneumoniae*.[20] Typical target lesions were more frequently associated with herpes simplex virus infection and "atypical" lesions with drug etiology in one study.[18]

The pathophysiology of erythema multiforme is uncertain. The relative roles of autoimmune triggers, actual presence of virus in clinical lesions,[21] and genetic susceptibility are unclear. Cell-mediated epidermal toxicity and possibly direct drug toxicity are likely factors in the evolution of the eruption.

Histopathological Features   At low magnification, there is a perivascular infiltrate of lymphocytes with some extension between collagen bundles, but a bandlike infiltrate is not observed (Fig. 3-6). Eosinophils in low number are observed in some cases but should not be the predominant infiltrating leukocyte. The papillary dermis is often edematous with dilated capillaries. Subepidermal edema may be marked in some instances, leading to subepidermal blisters. Exocytosis and spongiosis are evident, and variable degrees of epidermal necrosis may be observed. At higher magnification, many elements of interface dermatitis are noted (Fig. 3-7). Necrotic keratinocytes are generally present at all epidermal levels, including the stratum corneum, and may be solitary or grouped. The number of necrotic keratinocytes varies depending upon the age of the lesion and the lesional site selected for sampling. In early lesions, the stratum corneum will retain its basketweave appearance.

Samples from early lesions and from the periphery of established lesions show less keratinocyte necrosis than tissue from the center of fully evolved targets. As the number of necrotic keratinocytes increases, so do the number and size of basal vacuoles. Corresponding to the clinical appearance of blisters are the histologic findings of confluent (or nearly confluent) keratinocyte necrosis and basal vacuolization leading to separation of epidermis from dermis. The relative contribution of lymphocytic infiltrate and interface change to the histopathology in a given specimen is quite variable and may relate to underlying cause. For example, drug etiology may be associated with a less dense infiltrate and eosinophils, as compared to erythema multiforme caused by herpes simplex virus.[17]

Immunophenotypic analysis fails to clearly identify a specific effector lymphocyte population. CD4+ and CD8+ T lymphocytes as well as NK cells are reported. Autoantibodies to desmoplakin I and II may play a role in erythema multiforme major.[22]

Differential Diagnosis   The differential diagnosis of erythema multiforme includes toxic epidermal necrolysis, fixed drug eruption, graft-versus-host reaction, viral exanthem, pityriasis lichenoides, and connective tissue disease (Table 3-3). The relationship between erythema multiforme and toxic epidermal necrolysis is controversial. Some authors consider erythema multiforme and toxic epidermal necrolysis to

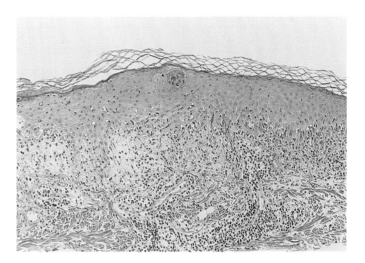

FIGURE 3-6   Erythema multiforme. This lesion exhibits an acute interface dermatitis with basal layer vacuolization, subepidermal edema, and a predominantly lymphocytic infiltrate in the superficial dermis.

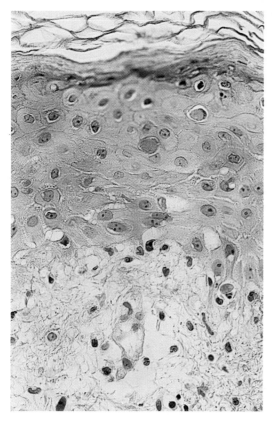

FIGURE 3-7   Erythema multiforme. High magnification shows basal layer vacuolization and scattered necrotic keratinocytes.

be distinct entities, whereas others maintain that they are part of the same disease continuum. In general, typical toxic epidermal necrolysis shows full-thickness necrosis of the epidermis with a scant inflammatory cell infiltrate. In comparison, erythema multiforme shows less epi-

dermal necrosis (except centrally in a given lesion) usually with single and occasionally clumped necrotic keratinocytes and a denser infiltrate. The histologic changes in both disorders constitute a spectrum, and, in some instances, discrimination between the two diseases is exceedingly difficult in the absence of clinical information. Superficial samples from central portions of lesions of fixed drug eruption may also closely resemble erythema multiforme. The presence of a more polymorphous and deep inflammatory cell infiltrate typifies fixed drug eruption. Melanophages progressively accumulate in the upper dermis in both conditions but are somewhat more numerous in a fixed drug eruption.

Histologic differentiation of an acute graft-versus-host reaction from erythema multiforme is generally unnecessary, because these disorders are clinically distinct; the histopathology is quite similar, although a graft-versus-host reaction generally contains fewer lymphocytes and necrotic keratinocytes. Nonspecific viral exanthems may greatly resemble erythema multiforme. The presence of specific viral cytopathic effects, as, for example, multinucleated keratinocytes in herpesvirus infections, allows more specific diagnosis. Erythema multiforme lacks significant inflammation around the deep vascular plexus and around adnexal epithelium, aiding in the differentiation from pityriasis lichenoides et varioliformis acuta and lupus erythematosus. Erythema multiforme also usually does not exhibit parakeratosis containing granulocytes as is typically observed in pityriasis lichenoides. Tissue from pityriasis lichenoides chronica typically displays denser upper dermal inflammation and hemorrhage in the dermal papillae with extension of erythrocytes into the epidermis. Features favoring connective tissue disease over erythema multiforme include hyperkeratosis, follicular plugging, epidermal atrophy, and increased dermal mucin. Correlation with clinical findings is often necessary.

Other miscellaneous conditions requiring differentiation from erythema multiforme include coma bulla, in which variable necrosis of eccrine glandular epithelium occurs in association with overlying epidermal keratinocyte necrosis and sparse inflammation. In addition, many specimens of paraneoplastic pemphigus will only display features of interface dermatitis and will strongly resemble erythema multiforme; tissue from paraneoplastic pemphigus is generally more heavily inflamed.

Toxic Epidermal Necrolysis

Clinical Features   Toxic epidermal necrolysis typically presents as diffuse erythema, becoming dusky over time. The patient often complains of painful skin. Erythema and injection of mucosal surfaces and conjunctivae are common early. As the disease worsens, the eruption becomes generalized, blistering develops, and mucosal surfaces ulcerate. The blisters are occasionally discrete and flaccid, but sheets of sloughing skin, leaving a glistening occasionally bleeding base, is a common presentation. Toxic epidermal necrolysis is reported in patients with the acquired immunodeficiency syndrome, and HIV-1 may be detected in blister fluid.[23] The patient is generally systemically ill. Widespread denudation of the epidermis results in significant risk of sepsis, fluid and electrolyte derangement, and hemodynamic instability. Despite aggressive supportive measures, many patients die.

TABLE 3-3

Erythema Multiforme and Toxic Epidermal Necrolysis

Erythema Multiforme	Toxic Epidermal Necrolysis
Clinical Features	
Erythematous patches with dusky centers	Diffuse erythematous patches with diffuse, full-thickness epidermal denudation
Target lesions	Mucosal and conjunctival involvement
Bullae and erosions	
Mucosal and conjunctival involvement	
Histopathological Features	
Upper dermal interstitial infiltrate of lymphocytes	Little or no inflammation
Basal vacuolization	Vacuolar interface dermatitis
Single and clusters of necrotic keratinocytes	Full-thickness epidermal necrosis typical
Full-thickness epidermal necrosis possible	Scattered necrotic keratinocytes at periphery
Differential Diagnosis	
Toxic epidermal necrolysis	Erythema multiforme
Fixed drug eruption	Fixed drug eruption
Graft-verus-host reaction	
Pityriasis lichenoides	

Most cases of toxic epidermal necrolysis are caused by drugs[24] and there is evidence that an inability to detoxify certain drugs is a predisposing factor in the development of toxic epidermal necrolysis.[25]

Histopathological Features   The essential features include substantial or full-thickness necrosis of the epidermis with little or no inflammation (Figs. 3-8 and 3-9) (Table 3-3). A pattern of single-cell necrosis may occur at the periphery of lesional skin. Mild inflammation around the eccrine apparatus is noted, with necrosis of distal elements of the duct a common finding.[26] Pathologists are often called upon to interpret frozen sections from the blister roof in order to obtain rapid laboratory support for the clinical impression. These sections should reveal full-thickness necrosis of epidermis with occasional evidence of individual keratinocyte necrosis, often in aggregates.

Differential Diagnosis   The final diagnosis of toxic epidermal necrolysis is made based upon clinical examination with consideration given to erythema multiforme and fixed drug eruption based upon histopathology. Specimens from staphylococcal scalded skin syndrome reveal subcorneal or granular layer blister formation with minimal necrosis of keratinocytes.

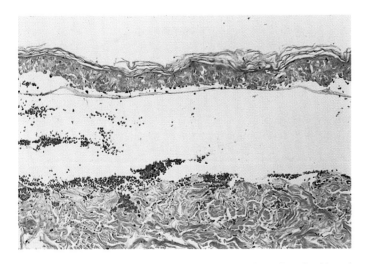

FIGURE 3-8   Toxic epidermal necrolysis. This lesion shows dermal-epidermal separation, necrosis of the overlying epidermis, and almost no inflammation in the dermis.

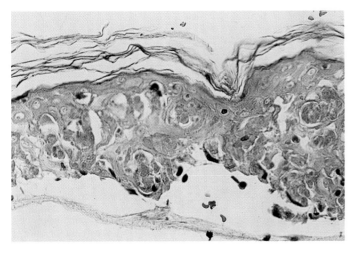

FIGURE 3-9   Toxic epidermal necrolysis. There is full-thickness necrosis of the epidermis.

Other causes of full-thickness epidermal necrosis include environmental trauma, such as excoriation or thermal injury. Thermal injury creates a picture of uniform keratinocyte necrosis without individual cell death. True vasculitis may produce sufficient ischemic damage to the epidermis to cause full-thickness epidermal necrosis. Toxic epidermal necrolysis lacks vessel destruction as an integral part of its histopathology.

Fixed Drug Eruption

Clinical Features (see Chapter 12)   A fixed drug eruption consists of a variable number of well-defined erythematous to violaceous edematous plaques with central duskiness and bulla formation. These plaques often recur in the same anatomic site upon second ingestion of the causative drug. New plaques may develop upon reexposure. As the inflammatory stage resolves, hyperpigmentation, often quite intense, ensues. The plaques may arise at any site but are frequently on the genitalia and other acral locations. Barbiturates, phenolphthalein, tetracyclines, sulfonamides, and nonsteroidal anti-inflammatory agents are most commonly implicated. As many of these medications are compounded in over-the-counter formulations, a detailed history of drug ingestion is necessary.

Histopathological Features   All elements of interface dermatitis are evident in a fixed drug eruption. As with erythema multiforme, the degree of epidermal damage varies with the site of sampling within the individual lesion—full-thickness epidermal necrosis may occur in the central bullous zone. Adequate sampling will allow inspection of the reticular dermis where a moderately intense superficial and deep perivascular and interstitial inflammatory cell infiltrate is generally seen. The composition of this infiltrate is variable. A superficial and deep perivascular lymphocytic infiltrate is common, but inflammation is often polymorphous with lymphocytes, eosinophils, and neutrophils. Neutrophils may predominate, and some karyorrhexis may be evident. No vasculitis is seen.

Samples from early lesions will display few melanophages in the upper dermis. Over time and with continued damage to the basilar epidermis, melanophages progressively accumulate in the papillary and upper reticular dermis. Specimens from late stages of a fixed drug eruption may only contain melanophages.

Differential Diagnosis   In comparison with erythema multiforme and toxic epidermal necrolysis, fixed drug eruption displays heavier and more polymorphous inflammation. Involvement of the deep vascular plexus also helps distinguish these entities. Confident distinctions based upon degree of melanophage accumulation are difficult. Whereas numerous melanophages typify the fixed drug eruption, stage of the lesion sampled and constitutive differences among individuals make this finding a variable component of any interface dermatitis.

Interface Dermatitis of HIV Infection

Clinical Features   Variably distributed but often widespread erythematous patches and plaques characterize this incompletely understood cutaneous eruption associated with HIV-1 infection. The lesions become violaceous over time and result in hyperpigmentation. This hyperpigmentation often involves the face and is of significant cosmetic concern. The eruption is accompanied by pruritus and frequently assumes a photodistribution. The precise cause of the interface dermatitis associated with HIV infection is unknown but may relate to medications, many of which are capable of photosensitization.[27]

Histopathological Features   The principal features include basal layer vacuolization, occasional necrotic keratinocytes, and a superficial perivascular and interstitial predominantly lymphocytic infiltrate. The infiltrate may involve the deeper reticular dermis and often is polymorphous with admixed histiocytes, eosinophils, neutrophils, and plasma cells. Vasculitis is usually absent; melanophages may accumulate progressively in the upper dermis.

Differential Diagnosis   The differential diagnosis includes true lichenoid drug eruption, infectious diseases including viruses, and connective tissue disease. Given adequate clinical information, this combination of findings is reasonably distinct. The occasional presence of plasma cells raises the possibility of syphilis. Cutaneous inflammatory cell infiltrates in the HIV-1 infected person are often polymorphous, making correlation with clinical impression vital for the final diagnosis.

Acute Graft-versus-Host Disease

Clinical Features   Erythematous macules and patches develop usually within the first month after marrow transplant as a manifestation of acute disease. The skin is the earliest and most commonly involved organ in graft-versus-host disease (GVHD), making accurate interpretation of skin biopsy specimens important in patient management. The erythematous patches may remain localized, often acrally, or may generalize to cause erythroderma. Increasing severity is manifested by the formation of blisters and a clinical picture of toxic epidermal necrolysis. Reliable criteria for distinction between a blistering acute cutaneous graft-versus-host reaction (GVHR) and toxic epidermal necrolysis do not exist.

The clinical features of the acute cutaneous GVHR are similar after allogeneic and autologous marrow transplants, although the clinical severity is greater in the former setting. It is imperative that the pathologist be aware of immunologic manipulation of autologous marrow transplants which result in higher incidences and greater severity of cutaneous disease than in unmanipulated scenarios. For example, administration of moderate doses of cyclosporine increases the incidence and severity of cutaneous eruptions, presumably by promoting autoreactive T-cell clones in the peripheral circulation. This autoimmunity can be enhanced by the addition of interferon, resulting in erythroderma after autologous marrow transplantation, an otherwise uncommon event.[28] Accurate identification of histopathologic changes compatible with a GVHR is vital for determining the outcome of clinical trials in the field of autologous marrow transplantation.

Apposition of a lymphocyte to a necrotic keratinocyte may be observed in the epidermis, consistent with satellite cell necrosis. Despite great effort to identify the effector cell responsible for a GVHR, no clear cell population emerges. Epidermal damage mediated by CD8+ T cells is a widely held concept that lacks mechanistic confirmation. To what extent CD4+ T cells and NK cells play a role is unclear. It is unlikely that one specific lymphocyte population acts as the sole effector cell. The mechanism of cytotoxicity is also unclear.[29] Cytokines elaborated by infiltrating lymphocytes may play a role, as may molecules directly damaging cell membranes, such as perforin.

Histopathological Features   A grading scheme exists (Table 3-4) by which all specimens taken for the diagnosis of acute GVHR may be classified.[30] The minimum criteria to establish the diagnosis are codified as *grade 2*; namely, basal vacuolization, keratinocyte necrosis (at least four necrotic keratinocytes per linear millimeter of epidermis), and a lymphocytic infiltrate in the upper dermis with variable exocytosis (Figs. 3-10 and 3-11).[31,32] Confluence of the basal vacuoles and separation of epidermis from dermis define grades 3 and 4, respectively.

TABLE 3-4

Acute Cutaneous Graft-versus-Host Reaction (GVHR)

Grade 0   No pathologic change or diagnosis unrelated to GVHR

Grade 1   Basal vacuolization

Grade 2   Basal vacuolization, necrotic keratinocytes, dermal inflammation

Grade 3   Confluence of basal vacuoles

Grade 4   Separation of epidermis from dermis

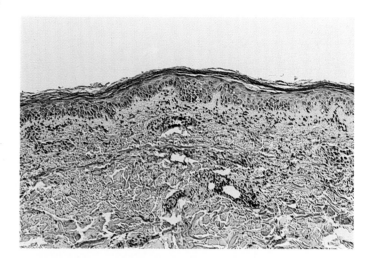

FIGURE 3-10   Acute graft-versus-host reaction. Scanning magnification shows a relatively subtle interface dermatitis. There is a relatively sparse lymphocytic infiltrate in the dermis.

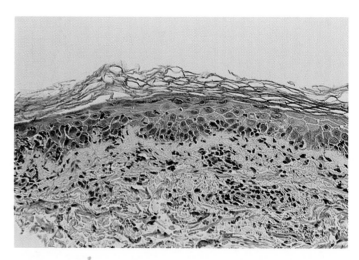

FIGURE 3-11   Acute graft-versus-host reaction. The epidermis shows some disturbance in the maturation of keratinocytes, slight spongiosis, vacuolization of the basal layer, and a relatively scant superficial perivascular lymphocytic infiltrate.

Follicular epithelium is similarly involved. This cytotoxic folliculitis is the earliest manifestation of acute cutaneous GVHR, and it is advisable to study many tissue profiles from a given sample in search of this finding.

Loss of polarity of keratinocytes resulting in disordered maturation of the epidermis from small cuboidal keratinocytes to flattened squames is attributable to antineoplastic chemotherapy effect, as these drugs disrupt the keratinocyte cell cycle. Individual keratinocyte necrosis accompanies this change, and the diagnosis of a GVHR is best made in unaffected portions of the epidermis or not at all, if this change is diffusely present. Similarly, within the first 3 weeks after marrow transplant, increased numbers of necrotic keratinocytes are referable to ionizing radiation, making quantification helpful (see above).[33,34] The matter is made simpler by the requirement for significant dermal inflammation, as neither chemotherapy artifact nor *acute* radiation change is accompanied by large numbers of lymphocytes in the dermis.

Differential Diagnosis   The diagnostic specificity of the interface dermatitis recognized as the acute cutaneous GVHR is debated (Table 3-5). The effect of potentially confounding variables such as prior marrow ablative chemotherapy and ionizing radiation must be considered when interpreting these skin biopsy specimens. Neither preparative regimen induces significant cutaneous inflammation; however, inflammation is necessary for the diagnosis of a GVHR. Similarity to erythema multiforme is great, but clinically, the diffuse erythema of a GVHR is rarely confused with the more discrete patches and plaques of erythema multiforme. The development of blisters makes clinical and histologic distinction of a GVHR from toxic epidermal necrolysis nearly impossible—concomitant development of voluminous watery diarrhea and elevated liver transaminase values typify GVHD and are more helpful than histologic examination of the skin. Samples containing grade-1 changes may require further tissue acquisition over time or may reflect the eruption of lymphocyte recovery, not a true GVHR.

Early after marrow infusion, samples from cutaneous eruptions may display eosinophils in the upper dermis. The presence of eosinophils is generally not compatible with the diagnosis of a GVHR and is often interpreted as drug hypersensitivity. This situation requires caution, as subsequent marrow engraftment may lead to a switch in histologic findings with a clear diagnosis of GVHR and explosive GVHD; meanwhile, the cutaneous eruption has persisted largely unchanged.

Chronic Graft-versus-Host Disease

Clinical Features   Chronic GVHD is divided into lichenoid and sclerodermoid forms. A lichenoid GVHR resembles lichen planus in that the primary lesion is a relatively small discrete erythematous to violaceous flat papule without scale. Oral changes identical to lichen planus also occur and are often the predominant manifestation of the disease. The lichenoid GVHR typically arises after day 60 after a marrow transplant but may occur earlier or later. The development of acute GVHD predisposes to chronic GVHD, but chronic disease may arise *de novo*. Development of lichenoid GVHD is associated with lower incidence of tumor relapse.

A sclerodermoid GVHR typically begins after day 100 after a marrow transplant, but again, the time of onset is variable. Progressive cutaneous sclerosis resembles systemic scleroderma. Fasciitis accompanies the skin changes and is a major cause of morbidity leading to joint contractures. Progressive cutaneous sclerosis leads to ischemia and chronic erosion and ulceration of the skin—particularly the scalp and feet. Alopecia is common. Spontaneous resolution of cutaneous sclerosis with completely normal skin examination may occur. In both forms of chronic GVHD, death is usually due to the accompanying smoldering immunoincompetence which predisposes to frequent infectious complications, including sepsis.

Histopathological Features   The fully evolved picture of a lichenoid GVHR resembles lichen planus (Figs. 3-12 and 3-13) (Table 3-5). The diagnosis rests upon (1) the correct clinical setting, and (2) epidermal changes of lichen planus; namely, acanthosis with pointed rete ridges, hypergranulosis, and hyperkeratosis. The infiltrate in a lichenoid GVHR is sparse compared to the typical case of lichen planus. Oral changes resemble those of oral lichen planus. Samples from the oral mucosa are commonly submitted as this site may be the only manifestation of chronic GVHD.

The sclerodermoid reaction is characterized by progressive thickening of collagen bundles with loss of the normal interstices. This progression reportedly begins in the papillary dermis and extends toward the subcutis, in contrast to progressive systemic sclerosis and morphea, in which the collagen alteration proceeds upward from a superficial panniculitis. Full histologic expression of the sclerodermoid GVHR includes a thickened dermis with loss of pilosebaceous apparatus and loss of adipose tissue around eccrine glands called *entrapment*. Invariably, there is evidence of interface damage as well. Although active inflammation is sparse, the epidermal-dermal junction will display basal vacuolization with occasional necrotic keratinocytes and upper dermal melanophages. This finding raises the interesting possibility that an epidermal cytokine mediates the pathologic collagen alteration during and after chronic damage to the interface.

TABLE 3-5

Acute versus Chronic Graft-versus-Host Reaction (GVHR)

Acute GVHR	*Chronic GVHR*
Clinical Features	
Variably distributed erythematous patches	Discrete erythematous to violaceous
Acral accentuation	papules of variable distribution
Blisters rarely	Lacy white patches on buccal mucosa
Histopathological Features	
Upper dermal perivascular and interstitial infiltrate of lymphocytes, often mild	Denser band of lymphocytes in upper dermis
Basal vacuolization, keratinocyte necrosis	Epidermal features of lichen planus
Subepidermal bullae rarely	Dermal sclerosis, especially involving superficial dermis, in sclerodermoid variant
Differential Diagnosis	
Erythema multiforme	Lichen planus
Toxic epidermal necrolysis	Lichenoid drug eruption
Viral exanthem	Lichenoid keratosis
	Morphea/scleroderma

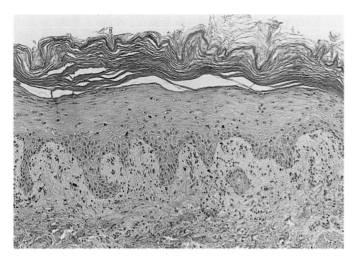

FIGURE 3-12 Chronic graft-versus-host reaction. This lesion shows hyperkeratosis, acanthosis, and a sawtooth pattern reminiscent of lichen planus. However, a bandlike infiltrate typical of lichen planus is not present.

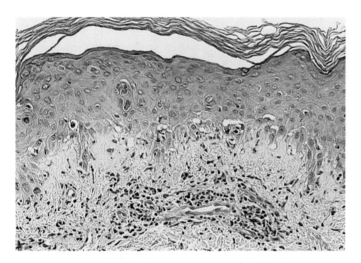

FIGURE 3-13 Lichenoid graft-versus-host reaction. This biopsy shows hypergranulosis, slight acanthosis, a sawtooth pattern of the epidermis, and prominent interface dermatitis with necrotic keratinocytes.

Fasciitis is characterized by lymphocytic inflammation and thickening of collagen bundles.[35] Myositis may also be observed in these samples.

Differential Diagnosis   To what extent the lichenoid chronic GVHR is reliably separable from acute disease is uncertain.[36] Both conditions are interface dermatitides with the main difference residing in the extent to which epidermal change resembles lichen planus. This distinction is important because therapy differs depending upon whether the process is considered acute or chronic. It is the rare biopsy specimen that fulfills all criteria for the diagnosis of a lichenoid chronic GVHR. Therefore, when uncertain, it is advisable to make a diagnosis of "interface dermatitis consistent with graft-versus-host reaction" and allow the clinician to establish the final diagnosis. The differential diagnosis includes lichen planus and lichenoid drug eruption. As noted above, the density of the inflammatory cell infiltrate is relatively less in the lichenoid chronic GVHR.

Provided that an adequate sample was submitted, the diagnosis of sclerodermoid disease is generally not difficult. One pitfall resides in a biopsy of skin which appears normal histologically and which represents normal skin overlying fasciitis. Fascial sampling is rarely necessary (because the diagnosis is clinically evident) but should be requested when appropriate. Other causes of increased fibrosis in the dermis and subcutis should be considered, including morphea, progressive systemic sclerosis, and porphyria.

LUPUS ERYTHEMATOSUS AND RELATED ENTITIES

The entities discussed here share similarities in pattern of inflammation and/or epidermal atrophy, all in association with interface changes, and thus bear resemblance to lupus erythematosus (Table 3-6). The epidermal changes typical of lichen planus combined with the dense band of lymphocytes are not the usual features of this group of disorders. Furthermore, inflammatory infiltrates in the conditions considered in this section tend to display more specific and reproducible distribution within the dermis than erythema multiforme and allied entities. The common theme of interface dermatitis persists.

Lupus Erythematosus

Clinical Features   Cutaneous involvement in lupus erythematosus presents several differing clinical pictures. Whereas photodistribution is common, any form of lupus erythematosus may display generalized distribution of lesions. In acute systemic lupus erythematosus, diffuse erythematous macules and patches are common, often with alopecia. Little surface change is present, and the eruption is evanescent. Photoaccentuation is common, leading to the malar "butterfly" distribution. Fully evolved systemic disease is common, and serologic tests reveal positive antinuclear antibodies in high titer and antibodies to double-stranded DNA. Patients with systemic lupus erythematosus rarely develop a blistering eruption. Bullous lupus erythematosus is discussed in Chapter 8.

Subacute cutaneous lupus erythematosus may bear similarity to psoriasis or may manifest as arcuate and serpiginous plaques. The majority of these patients have positive antinuclear antibodies as well as antibodies to the extractable nuclear antigens Ro and La (SSA and SSB) and may exhibit photosensitivity. Renal disease develops in low frequency.

Discoid (chronic) lupus erythematosus is characterized by varying numbers of lesions, usually erythematous plaques, often with atrophy, scale, and dyspigmentation involving the face and scalp. Systemic disease is rare in patients presenting with discoid lupus erythematosus, although patients with systemic disease may develop discoid lesions. Whereas some patients possess reactive antinuclear antibody titers, no serologic test is reliably positive in this subtype. A hypertrophic (or verrucous) variant exists in which the primary lesions have a verrucous surface. Lupus panniculitis (profundus) is usually associated with discoid lupus erythematosus but may evolve in patients with systemic disease. Lupus panniculitis is discussed in Chapter 11.

In neonatal lupus erythematosus the infant is born with or quickly develops variably distributed erythematous scaling macules and patches. Annular erythema is common. The mother may or may not have an established diagnosis of lupus erythematosus prior to birth, but the large majority will have Ro or La autoantibodies. In most instances, the cutaneous eruption resolves over weeks to months in the child. The major complication of neonatal lupus erythematosus is congenital heart block manifested by bradycardia in about 40 percent of patients. Heart block and the cutaneous eruption occur independently in neonatal lupus erythematosus with only occasional patients exhibiting both clinical manifestations. The risk for subsequent connective tissue disease later in the life of the affected child is uncertain.

TABLE 3-6

Lupus Erythematosus and Variants*

Clinical Features

Systemic lupus erythematosus
    Diffuse erythematous macules, atrophy possible
Subacute lupus erythematosus
    Psoriasiform lesions
    Arcuate or serpiginous plaques
    Ro/La+
Discoid lupus erythematosus
    Erythematous plaques with atrophy, scarring, alopecia, and
        dyspigmentation

Histopathological Features

Systemic lupus erythematosus
    Mild upper dermal perivascular and interstitial infiltrate of
        lymphocytes
    Mild epidermal atrophy
    Dermal mucin
    Thickened basement membrane
Subacute lupus erythematosus
    Denser lymphocytic infiltrate
    Periadnexal inflammation possible
    Dermal mucin
    Moderate regular acanthosis in psoriasiform variant
Discoid lupus erythematosus
    Hyperkeratosis, follicular plugging
    Epidermal atrophy
    Features of vacuolar interface dermatitis (above) with dense
        perivascular, interstitial, and periadnexal inflammation
    Dermal mucinosis
    Loss of adnexae

Differential Diagnosis

Systemic lupus erythematosus
    Dermatomyositis
    Mixed connective tissue disease
    Viral exanthem
    Reticular erythematous mucinosis
Subacute lupus erythematosus
    Dermatomyositis
    Neonatal lupus erythematosus
    PLEVA
    Syphilis
    Photo-drug eruption
    Figurate erythemas
Discoid lupus erythematosus
    Lichen planus
    Lichen sclerosus et atrophicus
    Polymorphous light eruption
    Chilblains
    Deep gyrate erythema
    Pityriasis lichenoides
    Syphilis

*At times, dermatomyositis may resemble any variant of lupus erythematosus.

Deposition of immunoreactants (immunoglobulin and complement) in skin of patients with lupus erythematosus is well described but may be of limited value as a diagnostic aid. A linear array of IgG, C3, and, less reliably, other immunoglobulin subtypes is typically located at the dermal-epidermal junction. This pattern occurs in most lesional skin of all subtypes as well as in nonlesional, sun-protected skin from patients with systemic lupus erythematosus (the *lupus band test*). Improved serologic tests have largely supplanted the diagnostic utility of direct immunofluorescence testing.

Histopathological Features   There is debate whether the clinical subtypes can be reliably distinguished based on histological criteria (Figs. 3-14 to 3-18).[37,38] Although histological features overlap enough to make confident distinction difficult, typical histological patterns are recognized in fully evolved clinical lesions from the various subtypes. The descriptions which follow are intended to characterize these findings according to subtype of disease, with the reminder that in clinical practice specific diagnoses require correlation with the entire clinical picture and with serologic tests. An interface dermatitis is common to all forms of lupus erythematosus.

ACUTE SYSTEMIC LUPUS ERYTHEMATOSUS

Subtle histologic changes often characterize acute disease. A mild upper dermal perivascular and interstitial infiltrate of lymphocytes is present with little or no epidermal change, imparting a nonspecific picture.

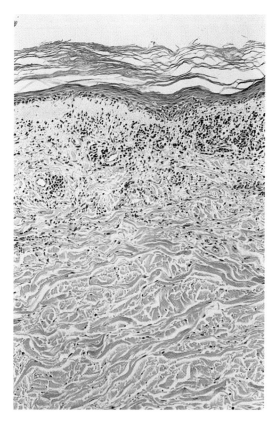

FIGURE 3-14   Acute lupus erythematosus. This lesion exhibits hyperkeratosis, atrophy of the epidermis, homogenization of the papillary dermis near the dermal-epidermal junction, and a mononuclear cell infiltrate in the papillary dermis.

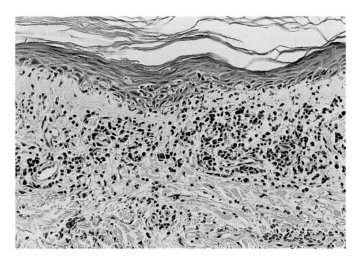

FIGURE 3-15   Acute lupus erythematosus. Higher magnification shows atrophy of the epidermis, basal layer vacuolization, and eosinophilic homogenization of the papillary dermis near the dermal-epidermal junction.

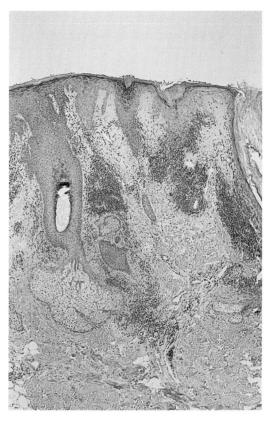

FIGURE 3-17   Discoid lupus erythematosus. This lesion is notable for hyperkeratosis and rather dense lymphoid infiltrates in the dermis.

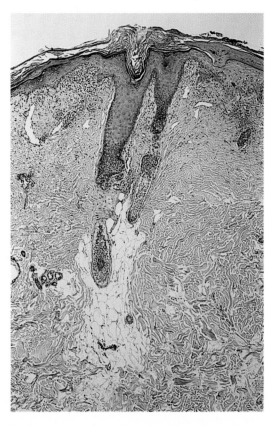

FIGURE 3-16   Subacute lupus erythematosus. The epidermis shows hyperkeratosis and a lymphoid infiltrate that is primarily superficial.

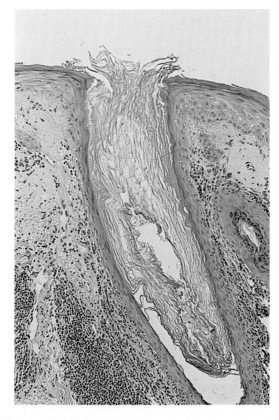

FIGURE 3-18   Discoid lupus erythematosus. There is prominent follicular hyperkeratosis and basement membrane thickening.

Some degree of basal vacuolization and keratinocyte necrosis is present. Atrophy of the epidermis, edema of the upper dermis, and an increase in mucin in the upper reticular dermis may be observed (Figs 3-14 and 3-15). In aggregate these findings allow the diagnosis of lupus erythematosus in the correct clinical setting. The subtle histologic findings often belie the severity of clinical disease; this disparity should be expected. Marked accumulation of mucin throughout the reticular dermis in the absence of significant inflammation may occur in systemic lupus erythematosus (and occasionally skin-limited disease). Mild overlying interface dermatitis is present. This variant is known as *tumid lupus erythematosus*.[39] Systemic lupus erythematosus is also reported to display elements of granulomatous dermatitis with neutrophils accompanying the mononuclear inflammation.[40]

Differential Diagnosis Distinction between acute systemic lupus erythematosus and dermatomyositis is not possible based solely upon histopathology. Mild interface change and scant inflammation may occur in viral exanthems and phototoxic reactions. The observation of increased dermal mucin narrows the focus to connective tissue disease. Tumid forms of lupus erythematosus must be distinguished from reticular erythematous mucinosis, myxedema associated with treatment of hyperthyroidism, and localized mucinosis. Reticular erythematous mucinosis has both mucin and mononuclear infiltrates in common with lupus erythematosus but lacks interface dermatitis and evidence of a systemic disease. The mucin accumulation in papular mucinosis and scleromyxedema is accompanied by a concomitant increase in fibroblasts; this cellular proliferation is absent in lupus erythematosus. These conditions lack significant interface dermatitis.

SUBACUTE CUTANEOUS LUPUS ERYTHEMATOSUS

In contrast to the acute subtype, subacute disease displays more inflammation. A lymphocytic infiltrate is present, primarily surrounding the superficial vascular plexus with possible extension to deeper dermal levels and subcutis (Fig. 3-16). In general, eosinophils are absent. Although lymphocytes extend between collagen bundles in the upper dermis, formation of a dense band of lymphocytes is uncommon. Epidermal interface changes and increased dermal mucin may be observed. The lymphocytic infiltrate extends around pilosebaceous and eccrine epithelium as well but is generally not as dense as in discoid disease (see below). The histopathologic features of neonatal lupus erythematosus resemble those of subacute disease. In the psoriasiform variant, moderate regular acanthosis is present, with a diminished granular layer and parakeratosis, again with interface change at the dermal-epidermal junction. The arcuate form often displays slight epidermal atrophy. Thus, in comparison with acute systemic lupus erythematosus, subacute disease is characterized by a heavier lymphocytic infiltrate with a more distinct superficial perivascular and periadnexal pattern. Subacute cutaneous lupus erythematosus is associated with antibodies directed against Ro/La, SSA/SSB epitopes. Exposure of keratinocytes in tissue culture to UVB results in enhanced expression of these antigens, possibly explaining the photosensitivity in this subtype.[41]

Differential Diagnosis Subacute lupus erythematosus shares histologic features with dermatomyositis. Dermatomyositis is generally less heavily inflamed and lacks significant periadnexal inflammation (Figs 3-17 and 3-18). Interface dermatitis accompanied by a superficial and deep perivascular lymphocytic infiltrate also characterizes pityriasis lichenoides et varioliformis acuta and syphilis. Accumulation of mucin and periadnexal patterning of the infiltrate favor the diagnosis of lupus erythematosus. Rarely, mucin deposition may be observed in pityriasis lichenoides. Furthermore, pityriasis lichenoides et varioliformis acuta and syphilis tend to display heavier exocytosis and more keratinocyte

necrosis than any variant of lupus erythematosus. Plasma cells, although typical of syphilis, may occur in lupus erythematosus.

Lymphocytic infiltrate of Jessner, a condition of uncertain nosology, is best distinguished from subacute lupus erythematosus by the absence of significant epidermal interface change. Otherwise, the pattern of the lymphocytic infiltrate and increase in mucin greatly resemble subacute lupus erythematosus. Polymorphous light eruption and chilblains are distinguished by the presence of upper dermal edema with hemorrhage and lack of significant interface dermatitis. Periadnexal inflammation is also not characteristic of either polymorphous light eruption or chilblains. Certain figurate erythemas may mimic the superficial and deep perivascular nature of the infiltrate in subacute lupus erythematosus, but interface changes are absent, and in the case of erythema chronicum migrans, the infiltrate may contain plasma cells and eosinophils.

Psoriasis is easily distinguished from the psoriasiform variant of subacute lupus erythematosus by the presence of deep perivascular and periadnexal inflammation as well as interface dermatitis in the latter entity.

Occasional photosensitive drug eruptions as, for example, those induced by thiazide diuretics, may closely resemble and possibly induce subacute lupus erythematosus. These drug eruptions are discriminated by clinical history and possibly the presence of eosinophils.

DISCOID LUPUS ERYTHEMATOSUS

Discoid lupus erythematosus is the most common subtype and is thus most frequently sampled. Fully evolved changes include a moderately intense superficial and deep perivascular and interstitial infiltrate of lymphocytes with distinct periadnexal inflammation. The infiltrate extends along the pilosebaceous apparatus, and all elements of interface dermatitis may be found here. Lymphocytes track along eccrine ductal epithelium and surround glandular epithelium as well. Significant keratinocyte necrosis in eccrine ductal and glandular epithelium is generally absent. Aggregates of lymphoid cells may be sufficiently dense to resemble cutaneous lymphoid hyperplasia. Closer inspection reveals the interface nature of the inflammation. Over time, destruction of follicular epithelium ensues, leading to loss of follicles. As a primary manifestation in the scalp, this process leads to the scarring alopecia associated with lupus erythematosus.

The perifollicular inflammation primarily targets sebaceous epithelium and follicular epithelium above the entry of sebaceous glands. It is interesting to note that the same pattern is observed in lichen planopilaris and that both lichen planopilaris and lupus erythematosus result in scarring alopecias primarily due to an inflammation directly against pilosebaceous apparatus. To what extent damage to the follicular bulge and its stem cell population explains this observation is uncertain.

Interface change in lupus erythematosus is characterized by basal vacuolization and exocytosis with necrosis of keratinocytes but at lower levels than lichen planus and erythema multiforme. Additional epidermal changes are variable. Whereas atrophy of the epidermis is typical in combination with the interface change, acanthosis may also develop or the epidermal thickness may be normal. When present, atrophy may be striking, with only two to three layers of keratinocytes evident. Ulceration may develop with crust formation, underlying granulation tissue, and ultimately dermal fibrosis. With atrophy, orthohyperkeratosis is frequently present, forming a sharp contrast to the thinned stratum spinosum. The hypertrophic variant displays irregular acanthosis with papillomatosis and orthohyperkeratosis; interface change is evident. Superficial specimens from the hypertrophic subtype may be mistaken for keratoacanthoma or squamous cell carcinoma.[42] Rarely, squamous cell carcinoma arises in longstanding discoid lupus erythematosus. An additional finding at the dermal-epidermal junction is thickening of the basement membrane, seen as a dense eosinophilic band hugging basal keratinocytes. Periodic acid–Schiff (PAS) stain highlights this finding.

Another variable finding typical of the fully evolved discoid lesion is dilated and keratin-filled epidermal invaginations associated with follicular orifices. These follicular "plugs" are often macroscopically identified. The associated follicular epithelium is usually thinned, and the dilatation generally extends to the level of the sebaceous gland entry in correctly oriented specimens.

Increased dermal mucin is generally present to a variable degree. The dermal vessels may display swelling of endothelium, but true vasculitis is usually absent. If subcutis is included in the specimen, panniculitis is frequently encountered with mixed septal and lobular inflammation composed of lymphocytes, plasma cells, and histiocytes, including lipophages. When panniculitis is the primary histologic manifestation, a specific diagnosis of lupus erythematosus may be difficult to establish without adequate clinical information. Thickened collagen bundles and increased eosinophilia of collagen bundles of the lower reticular dermis often accompany the panniculitis. Dystrophic calcification may ensue.

Differential Diagnosis   The differential diagnosis includes dermatomyositis, lichen planus, lichen sclerosus et atrophicus, polymorphous light eruption, chilblains, deep gyrate erythemas, pityriasis lichenoides, certain viral exanthems, drug eruption, and syphilis. The fully evolved picture of discoid lupus erythematosus is diagnostic. Dermatomyositis lacks heavy inflammation and significant periadnexal patterning but in rare instances may greatly resemble discoid lupus erythematosus. As mentioned, the occasional case of lupus erythematosus may contain sufficient lymphoid aggregation to warrant consideration of lymphocytoma. Hypertrophic lupus erythematosus is distinguished from hypertrophic lichen planus by basement membrane thickening, deep dermal and periadnexal inflammation, and dermal mucin deposition.

Dermatomyositis

Clinical Features   Dermatomyositis is a syndrome consisting of variably distributed erythematous macules and plaques with photoaccentuation,[43] inflammation of skeletal muscle, and malignant neoplasms.[44] Dermatomyositis in association with Lyme disease has been reported.[45] The cutaneous manifestations vary in terms of extent and location, but the typical presentation consists of erythematous infiltrated plaques, usually on the face but possibly generalized. The location of the erythema on the face is often periorbital, assuming a violaceous hue, the so-called heliotrope. Atrophic papules with scale on the knuckles are characteristic and are known as *Gottron's papules*. Poikiloderma as a manifestation of dermatomyositis is considered below.

Myositis may accompany the skin changes, or may precede or follow. Severe proximal muscle weakness may ensue, and determination of serum levels of muscle-derived enzymes and degradation products aids in diagnosis. Muscle biopsy may be necessary to establish the diagnosis. An electromyogram may also be a useful adjunct. On occasion, cutaneous findings or muscle findings may be absent; prompting the terms *polymyositis* and *dermatomyositis sine myositis*, respectively.[46]

A careful search for visceral malignant neoplasms is necessary if not apparent at the time of diagnosis. The neoplasm may predate the onset of the symptoms or may be concomitant or follow the diagnosis of dermatomyositis. A wide range of incidence figures exists for the association between dermatomyositis and malignant neoplasms. The relative risk was 2.4 in men and 3.4 in women in one study.[47] Whereas ovarian cancer is overrepresented in comparison to the general population, the proportion of other malignant neoplasms parallels that of age-matched controls. Dermatomyositis occurs in children, unassociated with malignant neoplasms. Vasculitis and severe calcinosis cutis often accompany the juvenile form.

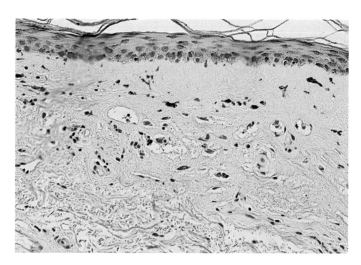

FIGURE 3-19   Dermatomyositis. This lesion exhibits atrophy, eosinophilic homogenization of the papillary dermis, pigment incontinence, and relatively little inflammation.

Histopathological Features   Dermatomyositis is characterized by a variable, but often mild, degree of lymphocytic inflammation in the upper dermis with overlying epidermal atrophy, interface change, and increased mucin deposition in the dermis, largely indistinguishable from lupus erythematosus (Fig. 3-19). This increased ground substance may be more evident than the inflammatory changes. Massive dermal edema may develop in the heliotrope region. Inflammation around the deep vascular plexus and adnexa may occur. The central portion of a Gottron's papule displays atrophy and superficial dermal inflammation with overlying interface change.[48] A septal and lobular panniculitis with lymphoid infiltrates has been described.[49] (See Chapter 11.) Immunoreactants, including complement components, are identified in lesional skin upon direct immunofluorescence testing.[50]

Differential Diagnosis   As discussed above, confident distinction of dermatomyositis from acute lupus erythematosus is not possible.

Mixed Connective Tissue Disease

Although many overlap syndromes are recognized among the connective tissue diseases, mixed connective tissue disease is the most common, consisting of features of systemic lupus erythematosus, scleroderma, polymyositis, and rheumatoid arthritis. Facial erythema, heliotrope, acral telangiectases, and scleroderma are the more common cutaneous manifestations. These patients possess high-titer antinuclear antibodies with antibodies to ribonucleoprotein (RNP) as well.

Histopathological Features   A specific diagnosis of mixed connective tissue disease is not possible based solely on examination of skin biopsy specimens. Erythematous patches display interface dermatitis accompanied by other features of lupus erythematosus to variable degrees.

Lichen Sclerosus et Atrophicus

Clinical Features   Lichen sclerosus et atrophicus (LSA) has protean clinical manifestations ranging from localized disease in the perineum to widespread erythematous plaques. The primary lesion in any site is an erythematous patch or plaque, often with an edematous center. This central zone may display pallor and thus impart a white color.

Over time, dermal fibrosis may ensue, resulting in the clinical impression of sclerosis resembling scleroderma. Rare lesions of LSA blister, often with hemorrhagic contents. Most common, LSA occurs in the genital skin of women, but men and children are affected.[51] On the penis, LSA is termed *balanitis xerotica obliterans*. There is a reported association between squamous cell carcinoma and chronic LSA of the vulva, with the incidence estimated at 3 to 4 percent.[52] Involved vulvar skin displays a higher expression of p53 in association with increased epidermal cell proliferation.[53]

In North America, tissue from LSA lacks evidence of borrelial infection.[54] An association is reported between increased severity of disease and presence of specific interleukin-1 receptor alleles.[55]

Histopathological Features   Histological alterations parallel the age of the lesion. Early, there is an upper dermal perivascular and interstitial lymphocytic infiltrate immediately below the epidermis. Overlying interface change is evident, and the epidermis may be of normal thickness. A fully evolved lesion displays an interstitial band of lymphocytes in the upper to middle reticular dermis (Figs. 3-20 and 3-21). The epidermis is usually atrophic with hyperkeratosis and dilated and keratin-filled acrotrichial and acrosyringeal ostia. Melanophages are present in a variably edematous dermis.

The nature of the collagen alteration in LSA is variable. Initially, the papillary and upper reticular dermis display edema, imparting a light, airy, and indistinct quality to the collagen bundles. This zone of alteration lies above the band of lymphocytes, is of variable thickness, and usually contains ectatic vascular channels. The edema may lead to subepidermal bulla formation, often with hemorrhage in the blister cavity. Over time, this wispy edematous collagen gives place to a more dense homogeneous and deeply eosinophilic collagen that continues to overlie the zone of inflammation.[56]

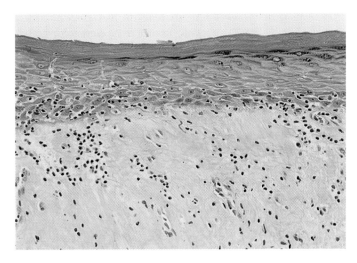

FIGURE 3-21   Lichen sclerosus et atrophicus. Higher magnification shows the homogenous eosinophilic hyalinization of the papillary dermis.

Older lesions of LSA may no longer contain inflammation, or the band of lymphocytes may localize more deeply within the reticular dermis. There is loss of pilosebaceous units and marked atrophy of the epidermis with numerous upper dermal melanophages. The nature of the collagen alteration is often fibrotic rather than edematous. Overlap of histologic features between LSA and morphea occurs but is uncommon and generally consists of a combination of the changes described above as well as collagen alteration consistent with morphea in the deep reticular dermis, including superficial panniculitis and entrapped eccrine coils.[57]

Epidermal atypia should be sought in genital lesions of LSA given the occasional development of squamous cell carcinoma in lichen sclerosus et atrophicus.

Differential Diagnosis   Lupus erythematosus may mimic LSA, but the characteristic collagen alteration is absent and periadnexal inflammation more pronounced in the former disease. Otherwise, the epidermal changes are quite similar. Chronic radiation dermatitis may closely resemble LSA with fibrotic alteration of the upper dermal collagen, vascular ectasia, and interface change. Radiation fibroblasts and the thickened waxy blood vessel walls are absent in LSA. The interstitial pattern of inflammation typical of LSA is absent in radiation dermatitis. Sufficient overlap of histologic features in LSA and morphea make confident distinction difficult on occasion. In general, the predominance of upper dermal collagen alteration in association with interface change and dilated keratin-filled follicular ostia distinguishes LSA from the predominantly deep dermal alterations of morphea. Both diagnoses may be rendered in certain samples, usually as "lichen sclerosus et atrophicus/morphea overlap." The nosology of this entity is unclear.

Acrodermatitis Chronica Atrophicans

Clinical Features   Acrodermatitis chronica atrophicans occurs most commonly in Europe where an association between this disease and borrelial infection (*Borrelia afzellii* subspecies of *B. burgdorferi*) exists.[58,59] Acrodermatitis chronica atrophicans begins as erythematous patches on the arms and legs with progressive atrophy of epidermis, dermis, and adnexal structures. Atrophy is associated with dermal fibrosis leading to linear bands of sclerosis. Severe atrophy leads to ulceration and peripheral neuropathy.[60]

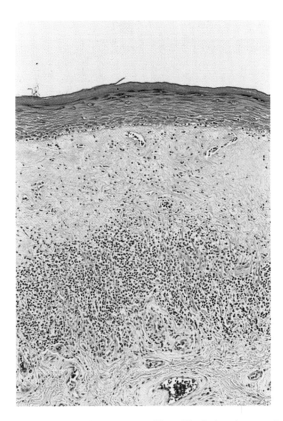

FIGURE 3-20   Lichen sclerosus et atrophicus. The lesion shows typical features of lichen sclerosus: hyperkeratosis, epidermal atrophy, prominent homogenization of the papillary dermis, and a subjacent bandlike lymphoid infiltrate.

Histopathological Features All structures of the skin may appear atrophic. The epidermis is markedly thinned with associated hyperkeratosis. The upper dermis contains an interstitial infiltrate composed largely of plasma cells. Interface change is generally mild and consists mainly of basal vacuolization. Adnexal structures are lost over time. While the upper dermis may be edematous in early stages, samples from the clinically sclerotic areas reveal thickened collagen bundles in the remaining dermis resembling morphea.

During the inflammatory stage of the disease, elastic fibers are progressively lost with retention of the elastic plexus. In the atrophic stage, only fragments of elastic fibers remain with loss of elaunin fibers. Myelin sheaths are abnormal, and axons are absent. In one study, spirochetes were found in 69 percent of specimens with most numerous organisms found in heavily inflamed tissue.[61]

Differential Diagnosis There are histologic similarities between acrodermatitis chronica atrophicans and lupus erythematosus and lichen sclerosus et atrophicus. The combination of cutaneous atrophy with a plasma cell infiltrate should prompt consideration of acrodermatitis chronica atrophicans.

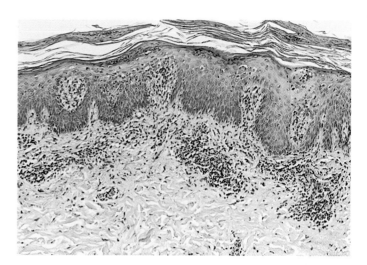

FIGURE 3-22 Pityriasis lichenoides et varioliformis acuta. The lesion displays confluent parakeratosis, basal layer vacuolization, some exocytosis of lymphoid cells, and a perivascular lymphoid infiltrate in the dermis.

PITYRIASIS LICHENOIDES ET VARIOLIFORMIS ACUTA AND RELATED DISEASES

Pityriasis lichenoides et varioliformis acuta (PLEVA) serves as the histologic prototype for several diseases also characterized by interface dermatitis. One distinguishing feature of this group of disorders is marked exocytosis of lymphocytes into the epidermis, as compared to the diseases described thus far. All other elements of interface dermatitis are present in the fully evolved lesion. The pattern of dermal inflammation typically involves the superficial and deep vascular plexuses with interstitial extension in the upper reticular and papillary dermis. Unlike lupus erythematosus, periadnexal inflammation is not a prominent feature, although inflammation involving vessels in the adventitial dermis, especially of the pilosebaceous apparatus, may be noted. Hemorrhage in the papillary dermis accompanies the inflammation in fully evolved lesions.

Pityriasis Lichenoides et Varioliformis Acuta (PLEVA)

Clinical Features The primary lesion of PLEVA is an erythematous papule which undergoes central vesiculation, pustulation, erosion, and ulceration, forming a crust. PLEVA is abrupt in onset with generalized distribution and clustering of lesions in flexural areas. Fever and malaise may accompany the eruption. The papules may enlarge to form nodules, but most lesions remain less than 1 cm in largest diameter. The papules occur in successive crops with individual lesions resolving with hyperpigmentation and scarring over several weeks' time. Systemic symptoms may occur.[62] The pattern of scarring is randomly scattered, as are the active lesions, imparting similarity to varicella. New papules appear as older papules resolve, resulting in an often polymorphous clinical appearance.

PLEVA typically occurs in children and young adults but may develop at any age. The cause is unknown. An infectious agent has been postulated,[63] but no clear pathogen has been clearly implicated, including herpesviruses.[64] If untreated, PLEVA may resolve in several months or persist for years. As the clinical appearance of PLEVA resembles that of lymphomatoid papulosis, periodic skin biopsy specimens are indicated, in persistent cases, to confirm the diagnosis.

Histopathological Features At scanning magnification, a pattern of dermal inflammation is seen which involves the superficial and deep

vascular plexuses and includes extension of lymphocytes between collagen bundles in the upper reticular and papillary dermis (Fig 3-22). The degree of inflammation is variable but usually intense in the fully evolved lesion.[65] Extension of lymphocytes into the overlying epidermis is typically marked, leading to the impression of equal numbers of keratinocyte and lymphocyte nuclei in the epidermis. A characteristic finding in PLEVA is a confluent parakeratotic scale usually containing neutrophils (Fig. 3-23). Basal vacuolization and necrosis of keratino-

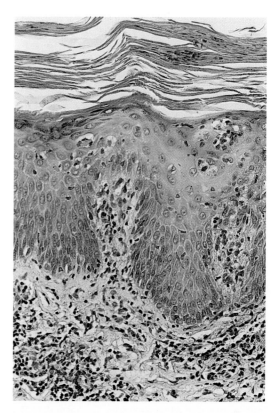

FIGURE 3-23 Pityriasis lichenoides et varioliformis acuta. Higher magnification discloses parakeratosis containing neutrophils, necrotic keratinocytes, and exocytosis of lymphocytes.

cytes are evident. The inflammatory infiltrate is composed of T lymphocytes with a predominant CD3+4+ phenotype. Clonal T-cell populations have been reported.[66] The presence of occasional cells with atypical nuclear forms in PLEVA has led to speculation that this condition is related to lymphomatoid papulosis.[63] In general, significant numbers (greater than 10 percent of total infiltrate, see below) of atypical mononculear cells should not be observed in pityriasis lichenoides et varioliformis acuta. One case of pityriasis lichenoides et varioliformis acuta is noted with enrichment of T cells bearing the γ/δ receptor.[67]

Hemorrhage in the upper dermis is typical of fully evolved lesions. Erythrocytes extend into the epidermis along with lymphocytes. Endothelial cells are plump, partially or entirely occluding vessel lumina. This change has prompted consideration of PLEVA as a lymphocytic vasculitis. True vessel destruction, with fibrin deposition and loss of integrity of the vessel wall, is generally not seen, and thus, categorization of PLEVA in the spectrum of vasculitis is of questionable validity. Rare cases may display histologic changes of vasculitis and are associated with infarction resulting in more epidermal and dermal necrosis typical of the ulceronecrotic type of PLEVA.

As the lesion ages, the keratinocyte necrosis becomes confluent centrally, leading to vesiculation, ulceration with associated crust formation, and granulation tissue. The inflammation becomes progressively less intense. Resolution of the ulceration leaves dermal fibrosis consistent with a scar. The overlying epidermis may be flattened with variable melanin content.

Differential Diagnosis   The differential diagnosis includes drug eruptions, viral exanthems, secondary syphilis, papulonecrotic tuberculid, arthropod bite reactions, polymorphous light eruption, connective tissue disease, and erythema multiforme. Drug eruptions and viral exanthems usually do not exhibit the degree of keratinocyte necrosis, parakeratosis with neutrophils, and inflammation encountered in PLEVA. Drug eruptions generally contain eosinophils. Secondary syphilis may closely mimic the pattern of inflammation seen in PLEVA. The presence of numerous plasma cells suggests the diagnosis of syphilis. Correlation with results of serologic examinations and, possibly, tissue silver stains is indicated. Papulonecrotic tuberculid and occasional necrotic arthropod bite reactions may closely simulate PLEVA. Clinicopathologic correlation is helpful. PLEVA lacks the upper dermal edema characteristic of polymorphous light eruption. Polymorphous light eruption also should not display the degree of interface change typical of PLEVA. Both PLEVA and lupus erythematosus have superficial and deep lymphocytic inifltrates. PLEVA lacks the accompanying changes of follicular plugging, epidermal atrophy, basement membrane thickening, periadnexal inflammation, and increased dermal mucin often seen in lupus erythematosus. In contrast to PLEVA, the inflammatory infiltrate of erythema multiforme is usually restricted to the upper dermis and is less dense. Other features more characteristic of erythema multiforme include upper dermal edema and retention of the basketweave stratum corneum.

Distinction of PLEVA from pityriasis lichenoides chronica (Table 3-7) is generally based upon degree of inflammation with pityriasis lichenoides chronica displaying fewer lymphocytes in general, especially in the deep dermis. The pattern of upper dermal inflammation as well as hemorrhage resembles PLEVA. Vesiculation, confluent epidermal necrosis, and ulceration are uncommon in pityriasis lichenoides chronica.

PLEVA lacks a significant number of atypical lymphocytes. Lymphomatoid papulosis is characterized by numerous atypical lymphocytes expressing the CD30 antigen (Reed-Sternberg-related antigen and a marker of "activated lymphocytes"). The occasional case of PLEVA will contain a subset of activated lymphocytes which possess larger irregular nuclear contours than the typical cell. These cells may express CD30, but should represent a clear minority of the overall lymphocyte population. Examination of multiple samples, especially over time, may be necessary to clearly distinguish PLEVA from lymphomatoid papulosis.

Pityriasis Lichenoides Chronica (PLC)

Clinical Features   PLC is more common than PLEVA. The primary lesion of PLC is an erythematous papule, 3 to 10 mm in diameter, which evolves to form a pinpoint dusky center but rarely displays vesiculation or ulceration. The eruption is widely distributed and chronic. Lesions resolve with dyspigmentation over several weeks, but little or no scarring ensues. The nosology of this entity is uncertain, especially its relationship to PLEVA. Because of the somewhat nonspecific clinical appearance of PLC, diagnosis may be difficult. PLC may evolve from PLEVA but also may arise without antecedent inflammatory condition. PLC may occur at any age and is especially common in children and adolescents. The cause is unknown, but an association with infection is noted.[68]

TABLE 3-7

Pityriasis Lichenoides et Varioliformis Acuta versus Pityriasis Lichenoides Chronica

PLEVA	PLC
Clinical Features	
Abrupt onset of erythematous papules	More gradual onset of erythematous papules with dusky center
Central vesiculation and ulceration	
Scarring	
Histopathological Features	
Superficial and deep perivascular and interstitial infiltrate of lymphocytes; wedge-shaped	Less inflammation, mostly upper dermal
Upper dermal hemorrhage	Interface dermatitis and hemorrhage persist
Features of interface dermatitis with marked exocytosis	
Parakeratotic scale with neutrophils	
Central confluent keratinocyte necrosis	
Differential Diagnosis	
Syphilis	Erythema multiforme
Drug eruption	Syphilis
Viral exanthem	Drug eruption
Papulonecrotic tuberculid	Viral exanthem
Arthropod bite reaction	Lichenoid pigmented purpuric dermatitis
Polymorphous light eruption	Pityriasis rosea
Connective tissue disease	
Erythema multiforme	

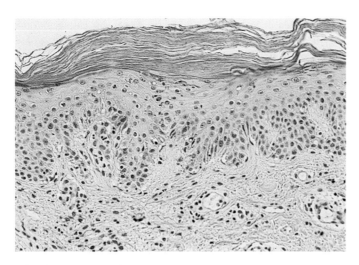

FIGURE 3-24 Pityriasis lichenoides chronica. This lesion exhibits prominent hyperkeratosis, occasional necrotic keratinocytes, and slight basal layer vacuolization.

Histopathological Features   In contrast to PLEVA, the features of an interface dermatitis are more subtle in PLC (Fig. 3-24). One observes parakeratotic scale, occasional or rare necrotic keratinocytes, slight basal layer vacuolization, and a predominantly superficial perivascular infiltrate of lymphocytes. As with PLEVA, the degree of exocytosis of lymphocytes can be striking. Hemorrhage around capillaries and venules of the upper dermis occurs with extension of erythrocytes into the epidermis. In typical PLC, aggregation of keratinocyte necrosis, vesiculation, and ulceration are uncommon. PLEVA and PLC may form part of a disease spectrum termed pityriasis lichenoides. This concept allows for overlapping histologic and clinical features.

Differential Diagnosis   The distinction of PLC from PLEVA is discussed above. Epidermal features of lichen planus are absent in PLC. The degree and pattern of inflammation may resemble erythema multiforme, but significant epidermal necrosis, especially in greater proportion than the degree of inflammation, should not be observed in PLC. As with PLEVA, consideration of secondary syphilis is warranted in the presence of plasma cells.

PLC may be classified among the pityriasiform dermatitides (see Chapter 1), and thus the following entities should be considered in the differential diagnosis: pityriasis rosea, certain drug eruptions, superficial gyrate erythema, subacute spongiotic dermatitis, guttate or eruptive psoriasis, pityriasis rubra pilaris, and early mycosis fungoides. The distinction of PLC from the later stages of pityriasis rosea can be difficult. In general, pityriasis rosea shows greater spongiosis and less interface change with confluent parakeratosis than PLC. This distinction is also true for superficial gyrate erythema and subacute spongiotic dermatitis. The typical drug eruption will contain eosinophils. Pityriasis rubra pilaris may be quite nonspecific but often displays follicular plugging, alternating ortho- and parakeratosis with little inflammation. Guttate and early psoriasis may show parakeratosis, as is the case with PLC, but often exhibit exocytosis of neutrophils, papillary dermal edema, dilated upper dermal vessels, and no significant interface change.

PLC may enter the differential diagnosis of circumscribed hypopigmentation. Consideration of tinea versicolor, vitiligo, leprosy, and mycosis fungoides may be necessary (see Chapters 15, 19, 34).

Secondary Syphilis

Clinical Features   A more comprehensive discussion of syphilis is present in Chapter 20. Secondary syphilis presents with a wide range of clinical findings, but most common is a papulosquamous eruption of variable distribution. Involvement of the palms and soles is typical. Obtaining a skin biopsy specimen in search of the diagnosis of secondary syphilis is less reliable than serologic testing. However, as the diagnosis is occasionally not suspected clinically and often falls within the clinical differential diagnosis of entities that are separable histologically, the pathologist will be asked to identify cutaneous eruptions of secondary syphilis.

Histopathological Features   Any cutaneous infiltrate which contains significant numbers of plasma cells warrants consideration of syphilis. The typical pattern of secondary syphilis is that of an interface dermatitis with a superficial and deep perivascular and to some extent interstitial infiltrate of lymphocytes, including plasma cells.[69,70] The absence of plasma cells does not definitively exclude the diagnosis of syphilis. Psoriasiform epidermal hyperplasia with marked exocytosis of lymphocytes is commonly observed. Endothelial cells are enlarged and partially or totally obliterate vessels.

In older lesions of secondary syphilis, histiocytes accumulate, often leading to the formation of granulomas. These granulomas are generally not well formed when compared to the granulomas of sarcoidosis; rather, they consist of a variable admixture of histiocytes, multinucleated giant cells, lymphocytes, and plasma cells in a loose and somewhat poorly circumscribed aggregate.

Differential Diagnosis   The similarities between secondary syphilis and PLEVA and PLC are noted above. Occasional skin biopsy specimens will contain heavy infiltration by plasma cells. Consideration should be given to plasmacytoma, especially if some degree of atypia is observed. Determination of monoclonality by demonstration of light-chain restriction or immunoglobulin gene rearrangement should be sought.

DISEASES CHARACTERIZED BY POIKILODERMA

The term *poikiloderma* does not imply a specific diagnosis. Poikiloderma is a clinical and histologic finding with many causes. Clinically, poikiloderma consists of patches of skin with variable melanin content, imparting a mottled hyper- and hypopigmented appearance. The epidermis is thin and may be shiny with fine wrinkles. Ectatic papillary dermal vessels are responsible for a faint erythema or distinct telangiectases. The minimum criteria for the histologic diagnosis of poikiloderma include epidermal atrophy with loss of the normal pattern of rete ridges, variable epidermal melanin content, dilated upper dermal vessels, and melanophages with some element of interface change. Determining hyper- and hypopigmentation in a given skin biopsy specimen is generally not possible unless the clinician includes or identifies skin with normal pigmentation for comparison. Mild papillary dermal fibrosis often accompanies these changes. The degree of inflammation is highly variable and depends in part on the stage of evolution of the lesion sampled. This section will discuss entities characterized by poikiloderma. The clinical and pathologic features making these diseases distinctive will be emphasized together, as the histopathology alone is often not specific.

POIKILODERMA OF CIVATTE

Poikiloderma of Civatte occurs as patches of wrinkled skin with mottled pigmentation and telangiectases in sun-exposed sites, frequently on the necks of women. Samples from poikiloderma of Civatte show solar elastosis and lack significant inflammation. This form of poikiloderma is poorly understood but is most likely due to chronic sun exposure.

POIKILODERMA CONGENITALE (ROTHMUND-THOMSON SYNDROME)

Childhood onset of poikiloderma, photosensitivity, mental retardation, short stature, juvenile cataracts, skeletal defects, nail dystrophy, and hypogonadism combine to characterize poikiloderma congenitale. The poikilodermatous changes are typically photodistributed and, viewed histologically, lack significant inflammation.[71]

CONGENITAL TELANGIECTATIC ERYTHEMA (BLOOM'S SYNDROME)

Facial telangiectasia beginning in infancy or early childhood with photosensitivity and progression to a poikilodermatous appearance characterize the cutaneous manifestations of congenital telangiectatic erythema. Skin biopsy specimens reveal interface dermatitis with some features of poikiloderma as noted above. Other features include short stature, genomic instability, development of malignant neoplasms, and variable immunoglobulin deficiencies. Bloom's syndrome is inherited in an autosomal recessive manner and is associated with sister-chromatid-exchange.[72]

DYSKERATOSIS CONGENITA

A retiform erythema with mottled pigmentation is characteristic of dyskeratosis congenita. Recognition of this syndrome is crucial, since there is a high incidence of squamous cell carcinoma arising in dysplastic oral and anal mucosal epithelium. The oral changes consist of white plaques which display variable keratinocyte atypia progressing to full-thickness dysplasia and invasive carcinoma. Skin biopsy specimens of the poikiloderma show the typical findings. Additional features of this syndrome include nail dystrophy and bone marrow failure.[73]

POIKILODERMA ACCOMPANYING DERMATOMYOSITIS

Poikiloderma may represent a prominent clinical finding in patients with dermatomyositis. The poikiloderma generally arises in long-standing plaques of erythema. The histopathology of poikiloderma in the setting of dermatomyositis is often remarkable for other changes typical of the connective tissue disorder, namely, more pronounced interface change and increased dermal mucin deposition.

POIKILODERMA ACCOMPANYING MYCOSIS FUNGOIDES

Poikiloderma as the primary clinical manifestation of cutaneous T-cell lymphoma is rare. Many observers consider this finding to be an involutionary or regressing phase of the disease process. With any clinical description of poikiloderma, the pathologist should consider the diagnosis of cutaneous T-cell lymphoma. In addition to the constellation of findings typical of poikiloderma, the diagnosis rests mainly upon identification of a band of atypical lymphocytes in the upper dermis with variable epidermotropism and possibly formation of Pautrier's microabscesses. The epidermal changes typical of fully evolved cutaneous T-cell lymphoma are generally less pronounced in poikilodermatous forms of the disease, an argument for the resolving lesion theory.

Nonetheless, a diagnosis of cutaneous T-cell lymphoma must rest upon recognition of a neoplastic T-cell population in the skin regardless of specific pattern or density of the infiltrate (see Chapter 34).

MISCELLANEOUS DISEASES WITH FEATURES OF INTERFACE DERMATITIS

Some of the entities considered in this section are covered more extensively elsewhere in the text but display interface change as an integral part of their histopathology. No specific pathophysiology unifies these diseases.

Lichen Nitidus

Clinical Features   Lichen nitidus consists of discrete 1- to 2-mm skin-colored to minimally erythematous papules of variable distribution and extent but often grouped and located on the genital and acral skin. Lichen nitidus occurs commonly in children and is often seen on the penis. The disease is self-limited. Overlap with lichen planus occurs, as both conditions may be recognized in a given patient.

Histopathological Features   A discrete interstitial aggregate of mononuclear cells expands one dermal papilla to form the typical lesion of lichen nitidus (Fig. 3-25). This expansion causes the adjacent epidermal rete ridges to bow outward and give the appearance of extension underneath the inflammatory cell aggregate as a collarette (so-called ball-and-claw effect). This discrete anatomic localization corresponds to the clinical picture of pinpoint papules and is distinct from the histopathology of lichen planus.[74] The infiltrate filling two adjacent dermal papillae may fuse to form a larger lesion on occasion.

Initially, the infiltrate is composed almost entirely of lymphocytes, whereas established lesions exhibit an admixture of lymphocytes and histiocytes with occasional multinucleated giant cells and melanophages. The overlying epidermis is slightly thinned and flattened with basal vacuolization and rare necrotic keratinocytes. Parakeratotic scale often overlies these epidermal changes.

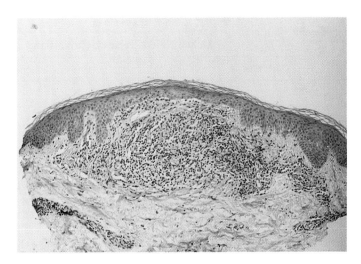

FIGURE 3-25 Lichen nitidus. There is a circumscribed nodular lymphoid infiltrate filling the papillary dermis. The infiltrate contains some multinucleate giant cells.

Differential Diagnosis   The fully evolved lesion is quite characteristic. Serial sectioning of a sample submitted for the diagnosis of lichen nitidus may be necessary, as the diagnostic area may be missed in initial cuts. Some lesions of lichen striatus may resemble lichen nitidus (Table 3-8) but are distinguished by additional features similar to lichen planus; some spongiosis with necrotic keratinocytes and eccrine coil involvement. The clinical appearance of lichen striatus is of a linear patch (see below).

Lichen Striatus

Clinical Features   Lichen striatus may affect individuals of any age but most commonly occurs in children as a linear array of closely set skin-colored to erythematous papules with little or no scale. Almost any skin site may be affected; however, a common presentation is a progressively lengthening collection of erythematous papules beginning on the proximal portion of an extremity with growth over several months to acral skin, commonly a digit. No associated systemic abnormalities occur. As mysteriously as lichen striatus begins, it involutes, leaving variable dyspigmentation.

Histopathological Features   The histopathologic features of lichen striatus are variable. Findings of a lichenoid dermatitis indistinguishable from lichen planus, lichen nitidus, or a combination may occur (Fig. 3-26). Parakeratosis may be seen. Lichen striatus also may present as a spongiotic dermatitis that typically exhibits prominent necrosis of keratinocytes. Another typical feature of lichen striatus is involvement of the eccrine coil by the infiltrate of lymphocytes. Occasional cases are reported with involvement of the deep vascular plexus.[75]

Differential Diagnosis   Although many cutaneous diseases assume a linear patterning, lichen striatus most closely resembles linear lichen planus and inflammatory linear verrucous epidermal nevus (ILVEN). Linear lichen planus displays the same histopathology as conventional lichen planus with its typical epidermal change and band of lymphocytes in the upper dermis. Lichen striatus may show fully evolved features of lichen planus but often also demonstrates parakeratosis, features of lichen nitidus, and deep dermal extension of the infiltrate. Another manifestation of lichen striatus is spongiotic dermatitis, as mentioned above. The epidermal changes in ILVEN usually more closely resemble psoriasis than interface dermatitis. The significant acanthosis and hyperkeratosis which impart the verrucous appearance to ILVEN are absent in lichen striatus.

Lichenoid Pigmented Purpuric Eruption of Gougerot and Blum

As a group, pigmented purpuric dermatitis is discussed in more detail in Chapter 9. The lichenoid variant displays the typical erythematous-hemorrhagic patches and bronze discoloration characteristic of pigmented purpuric dermatitis. Skin samples reveal a perivascular and interstitial infiltrate of lymphocytes in the upper dermis with overlying interface change. This interstitial inflammation and the accompanying epidermal findings separate lichenoid pigmented purpuric eruption from other forms of pigmented purpuric dermatitis. Pericapillary hemorrhage is similar to that in pityriasis lichenoides chronica. In fact, these two entities are best distinguished on clinical grounds. Vasculitis with fibrin deposition and thrombosis are uncommon.

Macular and Lichen Amyloidosis

Macular amyloidosis (see Chapter 16) typically presents as hyperpigmented macules, often on the upper back, whereas the clinical appearance of lichen amyloidosis consists of verrucous plaques which are quite pruritic, usually on the shins. In both entities, there is an accumulation of amorphous eosinophilic material to variable extent in the upper dermis. In general, greater amounts of amyloid are present in lichen amyloidosis than in macular amyloidosis. In both instances, the amyloid is derived from keratin. This fact explains the frequent finding of damage to the epidermal-dermal interface with basal vacuolization, scattered necrotic keratinocytes, and melanophages in the upper dermis admixed with the amyloid. Acanthosis, hyperkeratosis, and papillomatosis further characterize lichen amyloidosis. These changes may reflect the sequela of chronic rubbing of the skin.

Vitiligo

Vitiligo (see Chapter 15) involves progressive hypopigmentation leading to depigmentation of the skin and correlates with the histologic findings of progressive loss of melanin content and melanocytes from the epidermis. Sampling of a chronic lesion reveals minimal inflammation with mild interface changes consisting mainly of basal vacuolization. Samples of the erythematous rim show a mild to moderately dense perivascular and interstitial infiltrate of lymphocytes with more developed interface change, including keratinocyte necrosis, than the central zone.

Morbilliform Drug Eruption

In morbilliform drug eruptions (see Chapter 12), exanthematous drug eruptions present as variably distributed pruritic erythematous macules and papules, often with

TABLE 3-8

Lichen Nitidus versus Lichen Striatus

Lichen nitidus	*Lichen striatus*
Clinical Features	
1- to 2-mm flesh-colored papules, often genital and acral	Grouped erythematous papules in linear array
Histopathological Features	
Discrete aggregate of lymphocytes, histiocytes, and occasional multinucleated giant cells expanding a dermal papilla	Variable findings resembling lichen planus with deep perivascular and perieccrine inflammation at times
Epidermal collarette	May resemble lichen nitidus
	May display spongiosis and dyskeratosis
Differential Diagnosis	
Lichen planus	ILVEN
	Lichen planus

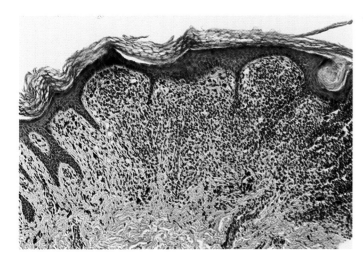

FIGURE 3-26 Lichen striatus. The lesion exhibits a bandlike infiltrate expanding the papillary dermis in a pattern resembling both lichen planus and lichen nitidus.

a generalized distribution. The histopathology is not specific, consisting of an upper dermal perivascular and interstitial infiltrate of lymphocytes and eosinophils. Typically, these eruptions have basal vacuolization as the primary manifestation of interface change. At times, this finding may become pronounced with rare necrotic keratinocytes. Any significant number of necrotic keratinocytes should prompt consideration of erythema multiforme.

Morbilliform Viral Exanthem

Viral exanthems (see Chapter 22) manifest as variably distributed erythematous macules often concentrated on the trunk. Skin biopsy samples display an upper dermal perivascular and interstitial infiltrate of lymphocytes with overlying basal vacuolization and variable numbers of necrotic keratinocytes. Spongiosis and parakeratosis may be present.

Paraneoplastic Pemphigus (PNP)

The clinical and histologic features in PNP (see Chapter 7) are protean. Marked mucositis is a nearly constant finding, and skin lesions range from erythema multiforme–like to overt blisters. The most characteristic skin biopsy specimens will mirror this spectrum with interface dermatitis as well as suprabasal acantholysis. Many, possibly most, specimens will show only interface change. Such lesions exhibit a moderately dense upper dermal infiltrate of lymphocytes and features closely resembling erythema multiforme. Occasional eosinophils may be observed. As a rule, the degree of inflammation is heavier in PNP than in typical erythema multiforme.[76] Acantholysis may be entirely absent or minimal in these specimens. Confirmation of the diagnosis through direct and indirect immunofluorescence is necessary.

MISCELLANEOUS DISEASES WITH SOME FEATURES OF INTERFACE DERMATITIS

Although many diseases of the skin display some elements of interface dermatitis as part of their overall histopathology, as for example, in spongiotic dermatitis, a few entities deserve special mention. The patch and plaques stages of mycosis fungoides are often characterized by basal vacuolization and migration of lymphocytes into the epidermis.

Necrotic keratinocytes may be observed, but not in significant numbers. Ultimately, the atypia and abnormal patterns of lymphocytes in both the epidermis and dermis discriminate mycosis fungoides from other interface dermatitides. Lichenoid contact dermatitis is characterized by a perivascular and interstitial infiltrate composed of lymphocytes and eosinophils with variable overlying spongiosis and features of interface dermatitis. Most cases of contact dermatitis lack the features of interface dermatitis. Occasional immunologic reactions to the foreign materials in a tattoo will exhibit features of interface dermatitis with the moderately heavy inflammatory infiltrate admixed among the exogenous pigments. This pattern is more common in response to mercury implantation.

REFERENCES

1. Kirsch M: Esophageal lichen planus: A forgotten diagnosis. *J Clin Gastroenterol* 20:145, 1995.
2. Hutnik CM, Probst LE, Burt WL, et al: Progressive refractory keratoconjunctivitis associated with lichen planus. *Can J Ophthalmol* 30:211, 1995.
3. Bellman B, Reddy RK, Falanga V: Lichen planus associated with hepatitis C. *Lancet* 346(8984):1234, 1995 (Nov 4).
4. Hanno R, Mathes BM, Krull EA: Longitudinal nail biopsy in evaluation of acquired nail dystrophies. *J Am Acad Dermatol* 14:803, 1986.
5. Dilamy M: Lichen planus subtropicus. *Arch Dermatol* 112:1251, 1976.
6. Albers SE, Glass LF, Fenske NA: Lichen planus subtropicus: Direct immunofluorescence findings and therapeutic response to hydroxychloroquine. *Int J Dermatol* 33:645, 1994.
7. Yamamoto T, Osaki T: Characteristic cytokines generated by keratincoytes and mononuclear infiltrates in oral lichen planus. *J Invest Dermatol* 104:784, 1995.
8. Schofield JK, De Berker D, Milligan A, et al: Keratin expression in cutaneous lichen planus. *Histopathology* 26:153, 1995.
9. Bennion SD, Middleton MH, David-Bajar K, et al: In three types of interface dermatitis, different patterns of expression of intercellular adhesion molecule-1 (ICAM-1) indicate different triggers of disease. *J Invest Dermatol* 105:71s, 1995.
10. Haapalainen T, Oksala O, Kallioinen M, et al: Destruction of the epithelial anchoring system in lichen planus. *J Invest Dermatol* 105:100, 1995.
11. Prieto VG, Casal M, McNutt NS: Immunohistochemistry detects differences between lichen planus–like keratosis, lichen planus, and lichenoid actinic keratosis. *J Cutan Pathol* 20:143,1993.
12. Franck JM, Young AW Jr: Squamous cell carcinoma in situ arising within lichen planus of the vulva. *Dermatol Surg* 21:890, 1995.
13. Beckman KA, Chanes L, Kaufman SR: Lichen planus associated with topical beta-blocker therapy. *Am J Ophthalmol* 120:530, 1995.
14. Halvey S, Sahi A: Lichenoid drug eruptions. *J Am Acad Dermatol* 29:249, 1993.
15. Deloach-Banta LJ: Lichenoid drug eruption: Crystal methamphetamine or adulterant? *Cutis* 53:97, 1994.
16. Prieto VG, Casal M, McNutt NS: Lichen planus–like keratosis: A clinical and histopathological re-examination. *Am J Surg Pathol* 17:259, 1993.
17. Cote B, Wechsler J, Bastuji-Garin S, et al: Clinicopathologic correlation in erythema multiforme and Stevens-Johnson syndrome. *Arch Dermatol* 131:1268, 1995.
18. Assier H, Bastuji-Garin S, Revuz J, Roujeau JC: Erythema multiforme with mucous membrane involvement and Stevens-Johnson syndrome are clinically different disorders with distinct causes. *Arch Dermatol* 131:539, 1995.
19. Howland WW, Golitz LE, Weston WL, Huff JC: Erythema multiforme: Clinical, histopathologic, and immunologic study. *J Am Acad Dermatol* 10:438, 1984.
20. Huff JC, Weston WL, Tonnesen MG: Erythema multiforme: A critical review of characteristics, diagnostic criteria, and causes. *J Am Acad Dematol* 8:763, 1983.
21. Brice SL, Leahy MA, Org L, et al: Examination of non-involved skin, previously involved skin, and peripheral blood for herpes simplex virus DNA in patients with recurrent herpes-associated erythema multiforme. *J Cutan Pathol* 21:408, 1994.
22. Foedinger D, Anhalt GJ, Boecskoer B, et al: Autoantibodies to desmoplakin I and II in patients with erythema multiforme. *J Exp Med* 181:1, 1995.
23. Correia O, Delgado L, Santos C, Miranda AM: HIV-1 in blister fluid of a patient with toxic epidermal necrolysis and AIDS. *Lancet* 344(8934):1432, 1994.
24. Roujeau JC, Kelly JP, Naldi L, et al: Medication use and the risk of Stevens-Johnson syndrome or toxic epidermal necrolysis. *N Engl J Med* 333:1600, 1995.
25. Wolkenstein P, Charue D, Laurent P, et al: Metabolic predisposition to cutaneous adverse drug reactions: Role in toxic epidermal necrolysis caused by sulfonamides and anticonvulsants. *Arch Dermatol* 131:544, 1995.
26. Ukosa AB, Elhaq AM: Toxic epidermal necrolysis: A study of the sweat glands. *J Cutan Pathol* 22:359, 1995.
27. Rico MJ, Kory WP, Gould EW, Penneys NS: Interface dermatitis in patients with the acquired immunodeficiency syndrome. *J Am Acad Dermatol* 16:1209, 1987.
28. Horn TD, Alltomonte V, Vogelsang GB, Kennedy MJ: Erythroderma after autologous

bone marrow transplantation modified by administration of cyclosporine and interferon gamma for breast cancer. *J Am Acad Dermatol* 34:413, 1996.

29. Acevedo A, Aramburu J, Lopez J, et al: Identification of natural killer (NK) cells in lesions of human cutaneous graft-versus-host disease: Expression of a novel NK-associated surface antigen (Kp43) in mononuclear infiltrates. *J Invest Dermatol* 97:659, 1991.

30. Horn TD: Acute cutaneous eruptions after marrow ablation: roses by other names? *J Cutan Pathol* 21:385, 1994.

31. Horn TD, Bauer DJ, Vogelsang GB, Hess AD: Reappraisal of histologic features of the acute cutaneous graft-versus-host reaction based upon an allogeneic rodent model. *J Invest Dermatol* 103:206, 1994.

32. Lerner KG, Kao GF, Storb R, et al: Clinical manifestations of graft-versus-host disease in human recipients of marrow from HLA-matched sibling donors. *Transplantation* 4:376, 1974.

33. Darmstadt GL, Donnenberg AD, Vogelsang GB, et al: Clinical, laboratory, and histopathologic indicators of the development of progressive acute graft-versus-host disease. *J Invest Dermatol* 99:397, 1992.

34. LeBoit PE: Subacute radiation dermatitis: A histologic imitator of acute cutaneous graft-versus-host disease. *J Am Acad Dermatol* 20:236, 1989.

35. Janin A, Socie G, Devergie A, et al: Fasciitis in chronic graft-versus-host disease: A clinicopathologic study of 14 cases. *Ann Intern Med* 120:933, 1994.

36. Horn, TD: unpublished observations.

37. Bielsa I, Herrero C, Collado A, et al: Histopathologic findings in cutaneous lupus erythematosus. *Arch Dermatol* 130:54, 1994.

38. Jerdan MS, Hood AF, Moore GW, et al: Histologic comparisons of subsets of lupus erythematosus. *Arch Dermatol* 126:52, 1990.

39. Pandya AG, Sontheimer RD, Cockerell CJ, et al: Papulonodular mucinosis associated with systemic lupus erythematosus: Possible mechanisms of increased glycosaminoglycan accumulation. *J Am Acad Dermatol* 32:199, 1995.

40. Chu P, Connolly MK, LeBoit PE: The histopathologic spectrum of palisaded neutrophilic and granulomatous dermatitis in patients with collagen vascular disease. *Arch Dermatol* 130:1278, 1994.

41. Kawahima T, Zappi EG, Lieu TS, Sontheimer RD: Impact of ultraviolet radiation on expression of SSA/Ro autoantigenic polypeptides in transformed human epidermal keratinocytes. *Lupus* 3:493, 1994.

42. Perniciaro C, Randle HW, Perry HO: Hypertrophic discoid lupus erythematosus resembling squamous cell carcinoma. *Dermatol Surg* 21:255, 1995.

43. Cheong WK, Hughes GR, Norris PG, Hawk JL: Cutaneous photosensitivity in dermatomyositis. *Br J Dermatol* 131:205, 1994.

44. Whitmore SE, Rosenschein NB, Provost TT: Ovarian cancer in patients with dermatomyositis. *Medicine* 73:153, 1994.

45. Horowitz HW, Sanghera K, Goldberg N, et al: Dermatomyositis associated with Lyme disease: Case report and review of Lyme myositis. *Clin Infec Dis* 18:166, 1994.

46. Cosnes A, Amaudric F, Gherardi R, et al: Dermatomyositis without muscle weakness: Long-term follow-up of 12 patients without systemic corticosteroids. *Arch Dermatol* 131:1458, 1995.

47. Sigurgeirsson B, Lindelof B, Edhag O, et al: Risk of cancer in patients with dermatomyositis or polymyositis: A population-based study. *N Engl J Med* 326:363, 1992.

48. Hanno R, Callen JP: Histopathology of Gottron's papules. *J Cutan Pathol* 12:389, 1985.

49. Fusade T, Belanyi P, Joly P, et al: Subcutaneous changes in dermatomyositis. *Br J Dermatol* 128:451, 1993.

50. Mascaro JM Jr, Hausman G, Herrero C, et al: Membrane attack complex deposits in cutaneous lesions of dermatomyositis. *Arch Dermatol* 131:1386, 1995.

51. Hinchliffe SA, Ciftci AO, Khine MM, et al: Composition of the inflammatory infiltrate in pediatric penile lichen sclerosus et atrophicus (balanitis xerotica obliterans): A prospective, comparative immunophenotyping study. *Pediatr Pathol* 14:223, 1994.

52. Hart WR, Norris HJ, Helwig EB: Relation of lichen sclerosis et atrophicus of the vulva to the development of carcinoma. *Obstet Gynecol* 45:369, 1975.

53. Tan SH, Derrick E, McKee PH, et al: Altered p53 expression and epidermal cell proliferation is seen in vulval lichen sclerosus. *J Cutan Pathol* 21:316, 1994.

54. Dillon WI, Saed GM, Fivenson DP: *Borrelia burgdorferi* DNA is undetectable by polymerase chain reaction in skin lesions of morphea, scleroderma, or lichen sclerosus et atrophicus of patients from North America. *J Am Acad Dermatol* 33:617, 1995.

55. Clay FE, Cork MJ, Tarlow JK, et al: Interleukin-1 receptor antagonist gene polymorphism association with lichen sclerosus. *Hum Genet* 94:407, 1994.

56. Mihara Y, Mihara M, Hagani Y, Shimao S: Lichen sclerosus et atrophicus: A histological, immunohistochemical, and electron microscopic study. *Arch Dermatol Res* 286:434, 1994.

57. Glockenberg A, Cohen-Sobel E, Caselli M, Chico: Rare case of lichen sclerosus et atrophicus associated with morphea. *J Am Podiatr Med Assoc* 84:622, 1994.

58. Lubbe J, Schlupen EM, Fierz W, et al: Identification of *Borrelia afzelli* in a juxta-articular fibroid nodule from a human immunodeficiency virus-positive patient with acrodermatitis chronica atrophicans. *Arch Dermatol* 131:1341, 1995.

59. Balmelli T, Piffaretti J: Association between different clinical manifestations of Lyme disease and different species of Borrelia burgdorferi sensu lato. *Res Microbiol* 146:329, 1995.

60. Kristoferitsch W, Sluga E, Grof M, et al: Neuropathy associated with acrodermatitis chronica atrophicans: Clinical and morphological features. *Ann NY Acad Sci* 539:35, 1988.

61. DeKoning J, Tazelaar DJ, Hoogkamp-Korstanje JA, Elema J: Acrodermatitis chronica atrophicans: A light and electron microscopic study. *J Cutan Pathol* 22:23, 1995.

62. Fink-Puches R, Soyer HP, Kerl H: Febrile ulceronecrotic pityriasis lichenoides et varioliformis acuta. *J Am Acad Dermatol* 30:261, 1994.

63. English JC III, Collins M, Bryant-Bruce C: Pityriasis lichenoides et varioliformis acuta and group A beta hemolytic streptococcal infection. *Int J Dermatol* 34:642, 1995.

64. Brice SL, Jester JD, Friednash M, et al: Examination of cutaneous T cell lymphoma for human herpesviruses by using the polymerase chain reaction. *J Cutan Pathol* 20:304, 1993.

65. Black M: Lymphomatoid papulosis and pityriasis lichenoides: Are they related? *Br J Dermatol* 106:717, 1982.

66. Terhune MH, Cooper K: Gene rearrangements and T-cell lymphomas. *Arch Dermatol* 129:1484, 1993.

67. Alaibac M, Morris J, Yu R, Chu A: T lymphocytes bearing the gamma delta T-cell receptor: A study in normal human skin and pathologic skin conditions. *Br J Dermatol* 127:458, 1992.

68. Takahashi K, Atsumi M: Pityriasis lichenoides chronica resolving after tonsillectomy. *Br J Dermatol* 129:353, 1993.

69. Abell E, Marks R, Wilson-Jones E: Secondary syphilis: A clinicopathological review. *Br J Dermatol* 93:53, 1975.

70. Jeerapaet P, Ackerman A: Histologic patterns of secondary syphilis. *Arch Dermatol* 107:373, 1973.

71. Vennos EN, Collins M, James W: Rothmund-Thomson syndrome: Review of the world literature. *J Am Acad Dermatol* 27:750, 1992.

72. Weksberg R: Low-sister-chromatid-exchange Bloom syndrome cell lines: An important new tool for mapping the basic genetic defect in Bloom syndrome and for unraveling the biology of human tumor development. *Am J Hum Genet* 57:994, 1995.

73. Drachtman RA, Alter B: Dyskeratosis congenita. *Dermatol Clin* 13:33, 1995.

74. Smoller BR, Flynn T: Immunohistochemical examination of lichen nitidus suggests that it is not a localized papular variant of lichen planus. *J Am Acad Dermatol* 27:232, 1992.

75. Gianotti R, Restano L, Grimalt R, et al: Lichen striatus—a chameleon: A histopathological and immunohistological study of forty-one cases. *J Cutan Pathol* 22:18, 1995.

76. Horn TD, Anhalt G: Histologic features of paraneoplastic pemphigus. *Arch Dermatol* 128:1091, 1991.

CHAPTER 4

PSORIASIFORM DERMATITIS

Paul S. Gillum / Loren E. Golitz

Inflammatory dermatoses may be categorized based on the pattern of inflammation[1] and epidermal changes.[2] With psoriasis as the prototype, the psoriasiform dermatitides are characterized by regular elongation of rete ridges.[3] This may result from increased keratinocyte proliferation, due to more rapid turnover of stem cells or an increased pool of proliferating cells. Epidermal thickening may affect any or all of the layers of the epidermis. The stratum corneum may be thickened (hyperkeratosis) and may retain nuclear remnants (parakeratosis). Thickening of the granular layer or spinous layer is termed *hypergranulosis* or *acanthosis*, respectively.

In psoriasis, there is prominent parakeratosis associated with a thin to absent granular layer. Rete are uniformly elongated and expanded at the tips. Neutrophils migrate from dilated capillaries in the papillary dermis and extend into the stratum corneum to form Munro's microabscesses. Many inflammatory dermatoses share these features, including psoriasis, Reiter's syndrome, piytriasis rubra pilaris, and neurodermatitis (lichen simplex chronicus).[4] However, just as there are differences in the clinical appearance and pathogenesis, there are histologic differences which allow these dermatoses to be distinguished from each other.

MAJOR PSORIASIFORM DERMATOSES

Psoriasis

Psoriasis is a chronic papulosquamous disease, affecting about 1 percent of the U.S. population. There is considerable geographic and ethnic variation in incidence. For example, psoriasis is rare in native Americans. The onset is typically in the third decade with a second peak in the sixth.[5] Certain areas of the skin are preferentially involved including the scalp, groin, elbows, knees, umbilicus, and lumbar spine.[6] The disease follows a chronic relapsing course characterized by remission and exacerbation. Psoriasis is characterized by an increased epidermal turnover rate[7] leading to thickening of the epidermis and accumulation of scale.

There is evidence for an inherited component in psoriasis. There is high concordance for disease in monozygotic twins[8] and a linkage disequilibrium with certain human lymphocyte antigen (HLA) types, including HLA-B13 and HLA-Bw17.[9] There is evidence for genomic imprinting in the inheritance of psoriasis, in that children of males with psoriasis are more often affected than children of females with psoriasis. This and other genetic phenomena in psoriasis can be explained by the "allelic instability in mitosis" model of dominantly inherited disease, the subject of recent reviews.[10,11]

An elegant experiment has demonstrated that psoriasis is not a primary defect of keratinocytes: Human psoriatic skin was grafted onto mice with severe combined immunodeficiency. Over time mouse epidermis grew over the human dermis, but the epidermis retained psoriasiform architecture, indicating that the defect more likely lay in the dermis.[12] The pathogenesis of psoriasis involves the interaction between inflammatory cells and keratinocytes. T cell activation and cytokines are involved in epidermal proliferation,[13] and cytokines produced by activated keratinocytes are thought to induce keratinocyte proliferation and lymphocyte migration.[14] One hypothesis is that the inflammatory process may be triggered by activation of T cells by bacterial superantigens.[15,16]

Clinical Features　The most common clinical presentation is chronic stationary psoriasis (psoriasis vulgaris). Individual lesions are sharply demarcated, erythematous, and covered with a thick, silvery scale (Table 4-1). They may show the Auspitz sign, in which forcible removal of scale produces pinpoint areas of bleeding. The tendency to involve the extensors has been attributed to the Koebner (isomorphic) phenomenon, in which typical lesions arise at sites of trauma. Inverse psoriasis is characterized by involvement of the flexures. Here, lesions may show less scale and exhibit a shiny erythema. Fingernails are involved in 50 percent and toenails in 35 percent of patients with psoriasis.[17] Involvement of the proximal nail fold overlying the nail matrix produces pitting of the nail plate. Psoriasis of the nail bed produces yellow-brown discoloration under the nail plate ("oil-spots"). Inflammation of the nail matrix causes a deformed thickened nail plate termed *onychodystrophy*. Mucosal lesions are rare, except on the glans penis.

Abrupt onset of small (guttate) lesions, especially on the trunk and proximal extremities, may follow a streptococcal infection.[18,19] This phenomenon may be related to cross-reactive antibodies between streptococcal M protein and human skin.[20] Psoriasis may be pustular. A generalized form of pustular psoriasis with systemic symptoms is termed *pustular psoriasis of von Zumbusch*, which may be precipitated by systemic corticosteroids.[21] When pustules are localized to the palms and soles, the process is termed *pustular psoriasis of Barber*. Erythrodermic psoriasis is characterized by generalized erythema and shedding of large amounts of scale. In this setting, marked dilatation of cutaneous blood vessels adversely affects temperature regulation.

Histopathological Features　Just as the clinical picture varies with the age of the lesions, so do the histopathologic findings.[22] Biopsies of fully developed plaques show extensive hyperkeratosis and confluent parakeratosis (Figs. 4-1 to 4-6). In areas of parakeratosis, the granular layer is thinned or absent. Parakeratosis may alternate with orthokeratosis, reflecting the episodic nature of the disease. Mitoses are more frequent than in uninvolved skin and may appear one or two layers above the basal layer. There is uniform elongation of rete ridges with thinning of the suprapapillary epidermis. The tips of the rete ridges are often clubbed or fused with adjacent ones. The dermal papillae are edematous and contain dilated, tortuous capillaries. Despite the dermal edema, spongiosis is mild or absent. The granular and spinous layers are

55

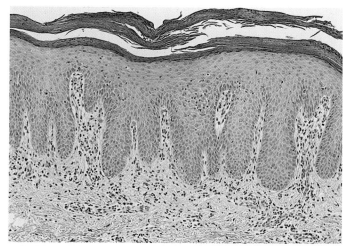

FIGURE 4-2   Psoriasis. The cornified layer shows confluent parakeratosis with exocytosis of neutrophils.

thinned over the edematous dermal papillae, and exocytosis of neutrophils frequently occurs in these areas. It is the thinned suprapapillary plates and the proximity of dilated dermal capillaries to the skin surface that produce the Auspitz sign. Collections of neutrophils with pyknotic nuclei in the stratum corneum, Munro's microabscesses, are found in approximately 75 percent of cases.[23] Neutrophils are also found in the spinous layer, where they may aggregate to form spongiform pustules of Kogoj. The underlying dermis is characterized by a superficial perivascular infiltrate of lymphocytes and neutrophils.

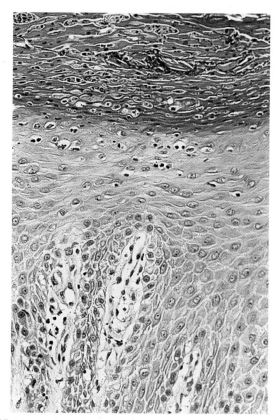

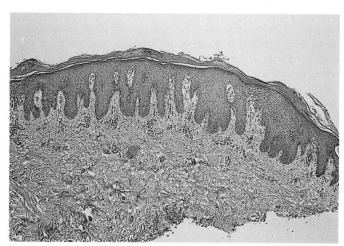

FIGURE 4-1   Psoriasis. The epidermis shows regular elongation of the epidermal rete ridges.

FIGURE 4-3   Psoriasis. The granular layer is absent and there is prominent exocytosis of neutrophils.

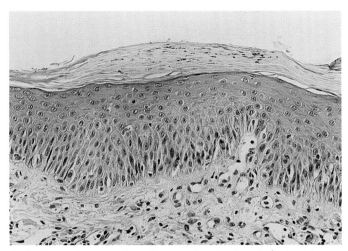

FIGURE 4-4   Guttate psoriasis. Note prominent focal parakeratotic scale.

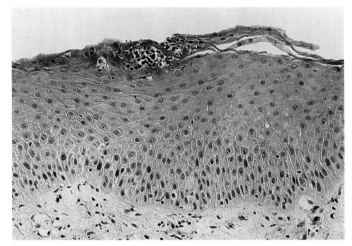

FIGURE 4-5   Guttate psoriasis. There is focal exocytosis of neutrophils.

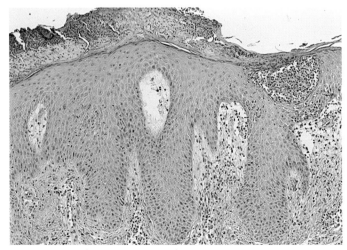

FIGURE 4-6   Pustular psoriasis. This lesion shows prominent parakeratotic scale, an intraepidermal neutrophilic pustule, and prominent subepidermal edema.

This classic picture is seen in only a small percentage of lesions.[24] Earlier or eruptive lesions may show initially a nonspecific pattern of changes confined to the dermis.[25] There is a superficial perivascular lymphocytic infiltrate with extravasation of erythrocytes, associated with papillary dermal edema and vascular dilatation. Only later are the suprapapillary plates thinned in association with elongation of rete ridges. In early lesions parakeratosis is typically mounded or spotty rather than continuous (Fig. 4-4). The migration of neutrophils from dermal papillae into the overlying epidermis has been referred to as *squirting papillae*.[26] Neutrophils are more numerous in eruptive psoriasis than in psoriasis vulgaris (Fig. 4-5).[27]

Differential Diagnosis   The presence of marked spongiosis suggests the diagnosis of a spongiotic dermatitis, such as nummular dermatitis or contact dermatitis. Lichen simplex chronicus shows papillary dermal fibrosis, while psoriasis shows papillary dermal edema and dilated, tortuous capillaries. Neutrophils in the stratum corneum may be seen in candidiasis or dermatophytosis. In these conditions, a fungal stain, such as a periodic acid–Schiff (PAS) stain with diastase predigestion, may reveal hyphae, pseudohyphae, or budding yeast. Secondary syphilis may show psoriasiform epidermal hyperplasia, but may have a deeper dermal infiltrate containing plasma cells.

Pustular Psoriasis

Pustules in psoriasis may occur in several settings. Occasionally pustules may be found at the periphery of typical plaque-type lesions. Pustules may be localized to the palms and soles (Barber) or may be generalized (von Zumbusch). Impetigo herpetiformis is pustular psoriasis in association with pregnancy. Patients with impetigo herpetiformis usually have typical lesions of psoriasis elsewhere.

Clinical Features   Pustular psoriasis of von Zumbusch[28] presents as a sudden eruption of 2- to 3-mm sterile pustules distributed over the trunk and extremities. The pustules may become confluent. The underlying skin shows a fiery red erythema. The face is usually spared, but oral lesions are common.[29] This process is episodic, and may be accompanied by fever, leukocytosis, and arthralgias lasting several days. Nails may be shed. The average age of onset is 50, with males and females affected equally.[30] Hypocalcemia may be present,[21] possibly related to hypoalbuminemia. Pustular psoriasis of von Zumbusch has been precipitated by systemic corticosteroids, iodides, salicylates, and progesterone.[31]

Palmoplantar pustulosis describes psoriasis in which lesions are confined to the palms and soles. Some authors separate clinical variants, such as pustular psoriasis of Barber, acrodermatitis continua of Hallopeau, and pustular bacterid of Andrews. We will consider these entities together since they show identical histopathologic features.

Histopathological Features   The major histologic feature of pustular psoriasis is the spongiform pustule of Kogoj. Neutrophils between residual plasma membranes, accompanied by intercellular edema, produce a spongelike appearance within the Malpighian layer (Figs. 4-6 to 4-8).[32] Epidermal cells in the center of the spongiotic areas degenerate, leaving large unilocular pustules. With time neutrophils arrive in the stratum corneum to form Munro's microabscesses. Other changes are the same as those in psoriasis vulgaris, namely diffuse parakeratosis, hypogranulosis, regular elongation of rete ridges, papillary dermal edema, and capillary dilatation in association with a superficial perivascular infiltrate of lymphocytes and neutrophils. These findings are less well developed in eruptive lesions. On acral skin, as in palmoplantar pustular psoriasis of Barber or acrodermatitis continua of Hallopeau,

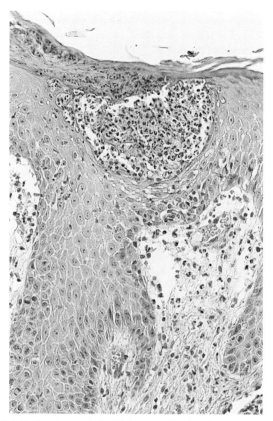

FIGURE 4-7   Pustular psoriasis. Higher magnification showing intraepidermal neutrophilic pustule.

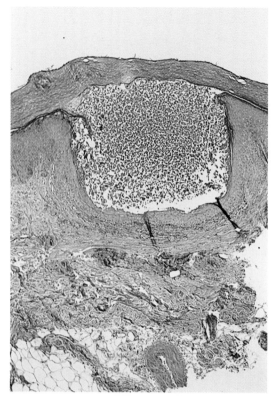

FIGURE 4-9   Palmoplantar pustulosis. Note large intraepidermal pustule.

pustules are large and unilocular, with the typical spongiform pattern seen primarily at the periphery of the pustule (Fig. 4-9).

Differential Diagnosis   Dyshidrotic eczema may show intraepidermal pustules but is more spongiotic and often has eosinophils in the dermal infiltrate. Superficial fungal infections such as candidiasis and dermato-

phytosis may show small pustules in the stratum corneum. Fungal elements cannot be reliably detected without the use of special stains. Impetigo, pustular drug eruptions, and subcorneal pustular dermatosis of Sneddon-Wilkinson may all show subcorneal pustules. In these conditions parakeratosis and epidermal hyperplasia are mild. The presence of eosinophils suggests pustular drug eruption.[33]

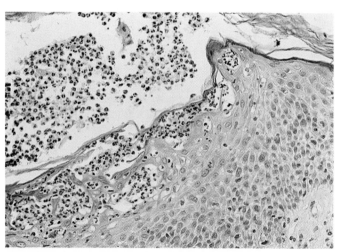

FIGURE 4-8   Pustular psoriasis. There are spongiform pustules in the upper part of the malpighian layer of the epidermis.

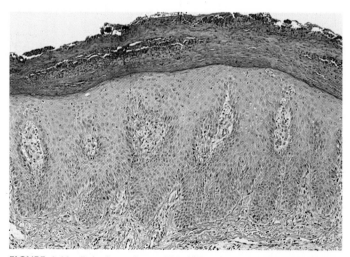

FIGURE 4-10   Reiter's syndrome. This lesion shows a parakeratotic stratum corneum containing neutrophils that overlies psoriasiform epidermal hyperplasia.

Reiter's Syndrome

Reiter's syndrome is characterized by the triad of urethritis, arthritis, and conjunctivitis (Table 4-2). However, only one-third of patients manifest the classic triad. A more recent definition by the American Rheumatism Association requires "an episode of peripheral arthritis of more than one month's duration occurring in association with urethritis and/or cervicitis."[34] Approximately 80 percent of patients have mucocutaneous lesions.[35] There is a well-established genetic component demonstrated by the strong association with human lymphocyte antigen (HLA) B27.[36] In addition to genitourinary infections, enteric infections may trigger the reactive disease in genetically predisposed individuals. There is evidence that microbial antigens persist in patients with Reiter's syndrome.[37] Although organisms are rarely cultured, nucleic acid sequences of *Chlamydia* subspecies have been found in the synovium of affected patients.[38] A comprehensive review of the pathogenesis of Reiter's syndrome is available.[39]

Clinical Features   Patients with Reiter's syndrome tend to be young males in whom arthritis follows urethritis and conjunctivitis by several days or weeks. Urethral cultures are usually negative. One-third of patients manifest the complete triad, and 40 percent have arthritis only.[40] Mucocutaneous lesions include a psoriasiform eruption of the palms and soles (keratoderma blenorrhagicum), a pustular or psoriasiform eruption on the glans penis (balanitis circinata), erosive or ulcerative oral lesions (geographic tongue), and subungual pustules associated with onycholysis.

Histopathological Features   The histopathologic features of keratoderma blenorrhagicum and balanitis circinata are essentially identical to those of pustular psoriasis (Fig. 4-10). Hyperkeratosis and parakeratosis are extensive with thinning of the granular layer. Spongiform pustules are present and may be large, resembling those seen in pustular psoriasis. Rete ridges are elongated and expanded at the tips. Collections of neutrophils with pyknotic nuclei (Munro's microabscesses) are found within the parakeratotic stratum corneum. Geographic tongue shows prominent spongiform pustules with less hyperkeratosis than in cutaneous lesions.[41]

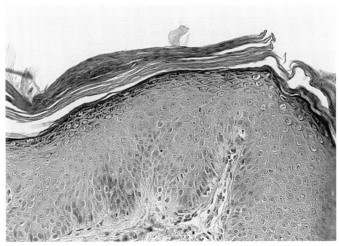

FIGURE 4-11   Pityriasis rubra pilaris. The epidermis shows psoriasiform epidermal hyperplasia with a hyperkeratotic stratum corneum.

Differential Diagnosis   Both the keratoderma of Reiter's syndrome and pustular psoriasis have large, unilocular spongiform pustules. Striking hyperkeratosis favors Reiter's syndrome. Reiter's may show a more prominent superficial dermal inflammatory infiltrate. Mucosal lesions are more common in Reiter's syndrome. Clinical correlation may be necessary to distinguish Reiter's syndrome from pustular psoriasis since the histologic changes may be identical.

Pityriasis Rubra Pilaris

Pitryriasis rubra pilaris (PRP) is a rare, chronic papulosquamous disease with a bimodal age of onset.[42] There is an equal sex ratio. Some cases are familial and are transmitted as an autosomal dominant trait[43] with expression of keratins not normally found in epidermis.[44] In adult onset cases, the etiology is uncertain. As in psoriasis, the epidermal turnover rate is increased.[45]

Clinical Features   PRP usually begins as asymptomatic scaling and erythema of the scalp which resembles seborrheic dermatitis.[43] Later, truncal lesions develop as small, orange-red, accuminate follicular papules with perifollicular erythema (Table 4-3). These coalesce into large plaques with fine scale and distinct borders which expand, leaving islands of normal skin. The disease may progress to generalized erythroderma. There is a yellow-red keratoderma of the palms and soles. Follicular papules on the dorsa of fingers are said to resemble a "nutmeg grater." Nail changes include thickening of the nail plate and subungual hyperkeratosis.[46] Oral lesions are infrequent. In the classic adult form the disease may undergo spontaneous remission, but the childhood form tends to be chronic.

Histopathological Features   In PRP there are discrete foci of lamellar hyperkeratosis and parakeratosis which alternate with orthokeratosis both perpendicularly and parallel to the skin surface (Figs. 4-11 to 4-13). Parakeratotic mounds at the edges of follicular ostia are termed "shoulder parakeratosis." Keratotic plugs fill the follicular ostia and extend above the level of the adjacent epidermis. The epidermis is hyperplastic including the suprapapillary plates.[47] Rete ridges are irregularly elongated and thickened but less so than in psoriasis. There is a mild superficial perivascular lymphocytic infiltrate. The neutrophils and

TABLE 4-2

Reiter's Syndrome

Clinical Features
    Triad of urethritis (negative urethral cultures), arthritis, and
        conjunctivitis
    Predominantly young males, HLA-B27
    Palms and soles (keratoderma blenorrhagicum)
    Penile lesions (balanitis circinata)
Histopathological Features (identical to psoriasis)
    Hyperkeratosis with confluent parakeratosis
    Uniform elongation of rete ridges
    Papillary dermal edema with dilated tortuous capillaries
    Thinned suprapapillary plates
    Neutrophils within the stratum corneum (Munro's microabscesses)
    Neutrophils within the spinous layer (spongiform pustule of Kogoj)
    Superficial perivascular lymphocytic infiltrate
Differential Diagnosis
    Psoriasis
    Chronic dermatitis
    Superficial cutaneous fungal infections
    Secondary syphilis

TABLE 4-3

Pityriasis Rubra Pilaris

Clinical Features
　Inherited (autosomal dominant) and sporadic forms
　Scalp involvement resembling seborrheic dermatitis
　Accuminate follicular papules
　Erythroderma with islands of sparing
　Palmoplantar keratoderma
Histopathological Features
　Vertical and horizontal foci of orthokeratosis alternate with
　　parakeratosis
　Parakeratotic mounds at follicular ostia (shoulder parakeratosis)
　Follicular plugging
　Rete ridges irregularly elongated and thickened
　Thickened suprapapillary plates
　Superficial perivascular lymphocytic inflammation
Differential Diagnosis
　Psoriasis
　Chronic dermatitis
　Keratosis pilaris

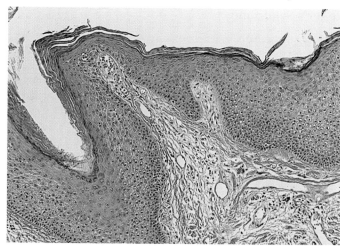

FIGURE 4-13　Pityriasis rubra pilaris. There is follicular hyperkeratosis with parakeratosis involving the shoulders of the follicular infundibulum.

Munro's microabscesses of psoriasis are usually absent. Spongiosis is minimal.

Differential Diagnosis　An objective histologic diagnosis of PRP can be made in about 50 percent of cases. The most distinctive features are follicular hyperkeratosis and shoulder parakeratosis. In psoriasis the hyperkeratosis and parakeratosis tend to be confluent, whereas in PRP the changes are focal. The presence of neutrophils and spongiform pustules in association with dilated, tortuous capillaries argues against the

diagnosis of PRP. Chronic dermatitis usually shows some degree of spongiosis. Follicular plugging may be seen in discoid lupus erythematosus, keratosis pilaris, and lesions of vitamin A deficiency (phrynoderma). In discoid lupus, the pattern of inflammation is lichenoid or deep and periappendageal. Keratosis pilaris and phrynoderma do not show significant epidermal hyperplasia.

Lichen Simplex Chronicus

Lichen simplex chronicus (LSC) is produced by repetitive mechanical trauma to the skin. A variety of stimuli produce pruritus and provoke scratching. Over time the behavior may become unconscious. When the stimuli are localized, papular and nodular lesions are produced (prurigo nodularis, "picker's nodule"). When plaques are produced, the condition is termed LSC or localized neurodermatitis. Psychogenic factors may be involved. Identical lesions can be produced in normal skin by a minimum of 140,000 scratches.[48] The chronic stage of all eczematous dermatitis may be histologically similar.

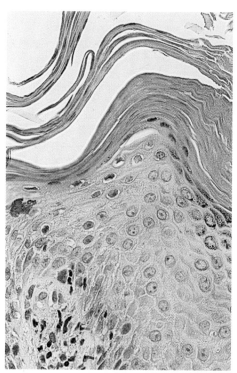

FIGURE 4-12　Pityriasis rubra pilaris. High magnification showing alternating ortho- and parakeratosis.

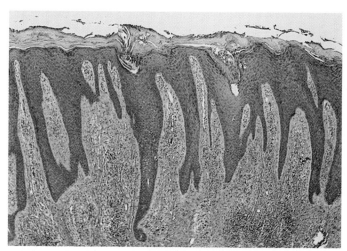

FIGURE 4-14　Lichen simplex chronicus. There is prominent irregular psoriasiform epidermal hyperplasia.

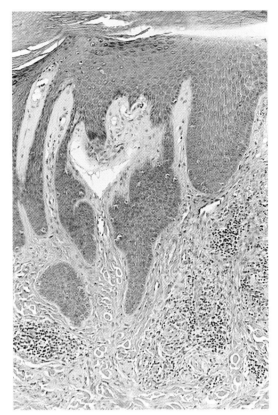

FIGURE 4-15   Prurigo nodularis. Note irregular psoriasiform epidermal hyperplasia as in lichen simplex chronicus.

TABLE 4-4

Lichen Simplex Chronicus

Clinical Features
    Prominent pruritus
    Changes produced by repetitive scratching
    Chronic well-demarcated plaques
    Lichenification/excoriation/hyperpigmentation
    Lateral legs, posterior neck, flexures
Histopathological Features
    Thickening of all layers of the skin above the reticular dermis
        Hyperkeratosis/hypergranulosis/acanthosis
        Papillary dermal fibroplasia
    Stellate/multinucleated fibroblasts
    Superficial perivascular lymphocytic infiltrate
Differential Diagnosis
    Psoriasis
    Chronic dermatitis
    Superficial cutaneous fungal infections

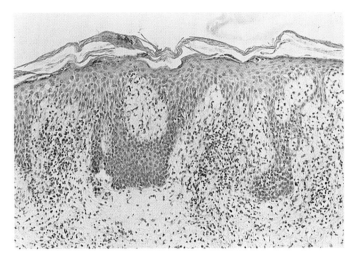

FIGURE 4-16   Pityriasis rosea. The lesion exhibits focal parakeratosis and psoriasiform epidermal hyperplasia.

Clinical Features   Lesions of LSC are always pruritic and often solitary. They are chronic and most commonly involve the lower lateral legs, dorsal feet, extensor forearms, and posterior neck. Lesions of LSC are thickened, well-demarcated, scaly papules, nodules, or plaques which are excoriated and lichenified. Hyperpigmentation is common and persistent. Lesions of prurigo nodularis are usually multiple and symmetrically distributed on the extremities with evidence of chronicity including dyspigmentation and scarring.

Histopathological Features   A biopsy of LSC shows thickening of all layers of the skin above the reticular dermis and a close resemblance to acral skin (Table 4-4) (Figs. 4-14 and 4-15). The epidermis shows hyperkeratosis, hypergranulosis, and acanthosis. Parakeratosis may or may not be present. The rete ridges are irregularly elongated and thickened. The epidermis may be papillomatous, and the superficial Malpighian layer may be pale, as the result of glycogen accumulation.[49] There is usually some spongiosis in the acute stage, but vesicles are rare. The papillary dermis shows thickening of collagen fibers which are oriented perpendicular to the skin surface. There may be stellate or multinucleated fibroblasts in the superficial dermis. The superficial dermis shows vascular ectasia and a perivascular lymphocytic infiltrate with occasional melanophages. Exocytosis of lymphocytes into the epidermis is minimal.

Differential Diagnosis   LSC may show residual intercellular edema and hypergranulosis, which are mild or absent in psoriasis. Both conditions show vascular ectasia, but vessels are more tortuous in psoriasis. Seborrheic dermatitis, psoriasis, and chronic fungal infections are more likely to show neutrophils within the stratum corneum. Psoriasis shows more prominent parakeratosis and papillary dermal edema rather than

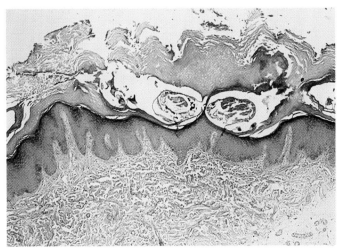

FIGURE 4-17   Crusted scabies. The epidermis shows psoriasiform epidermal hyperplasia. The exoskeleton of two mites can be observed in the lower stratum corneum.

papillary dermal fibrosis. Benign keratoses and other epidermal neoplasms tend to be more sharply circumscribed. Chronic lesions of spongiotic dermatitis may show a superimposed pattern of LSC.

Parapsoriasis En Plaques

Parapsoriasis is not a disease but a group of diseases which includes parapsoriasis en plaques (PeP). This group of diseases was first proposed by Brocq in an attempt to organize the inflammatory dermatoses.[50] The diseases are essentially unrelated, except that all are of unknown etiology, are of long duration, and are relatively unresponsive to therapy. A review of the nosology of these diseases is available.[51]

In addition to a confusing nomenclature, considerable controversy surrounds the relationship between PeP and mycosis fungoides. Many authors consider PeP to be an inflammatory process which may progress to mycosis fungoides.[52] Others consider PeP to be part of the spectrum of cutaneous T-cell lymphoma or mycosis fungoides from the outset[53,54]; a low-grade malignancy which smolders in the majority of cases, and follows a more aggressive course in a few. In support of this view, both processes may show similar abnormalities of T-cell antigen expression,[55] and some cases of PeP may show monoclonal T-cell proliferation.[56,57]

Clinical Features Parapsoriasis en plaques, also known as large plaque parapsoriasis, is a chronic disease of middle age. It is characterized by large, slightly scaly, erythematous patches and plaques with irregular outlines (Table 4-5). Lesions are often larger than 10 cm. The eruption is asymmetric and affects predominantly the buttocks, flexures, and female breasts. Mucosal disease, nail changes, and acral involvement are rare. Lesions are usually asymptomatic but may be pruritic. Plaques often show epidermal atrophy manifested as fine wrinkling of the skin. The skin lesions may resemble poikiloderma atrophicans vasculare, which is characterized by epidermal atrophy, dyspigmentation, and telangiectasia. Progression to mycosis fungoides may be heralded by thickening of the plaques.

Histopathological Features The earliest lesions show only a superficial perivascular lymphocytic infiltrate. The epidermis initially shows mild irregular acanthosis and mounding parakeratosis. Spongiosis is unusual. Later the infiltrate may become more dense and bandlike. Lymphocytes may be seen along the basal layer in association with vacuolar change and pigment incontinence.

TABLE 4-5

Parapsoriasis En Plaques

Clinical Features
   Chronic disease of middle age
   Scaly erythematous patches and plaques
   Predilection for buttocks, flexures, and breasts
   Unresponsive to treatment
Histopathological Features
   Mild irregular acanthosis
   Mounding parakeratosis
   Papillary dermal fibrosis
   Focal vacuolar change
   Superficial perivascular lymphocytic infiltrate
Differential Diagnosis
   Guttate (eruptive) psoriasis
   Mild chronic dermatitis
   Mycosis fungoides (see text)

Differential Diagnosis In early lesions the differential diagnosis includes a mild chronic dermatitis or superficial perivascular dermatitis. Clinically the eruption may be unresponsive to standard therapy. When lymphocytes infiltrate the deeper layers of the epidermis, the histologic features resemble those seen in the earliest or patch stage of mycosis fungoides.[58] Reactive inflammatory dermatoses usually do not show monoclonal T-cell proliferation.[56,57]

OTHER PSORIASIFORM DERMATOSES

Subacute And Chronic Spongiotic Dermatitides

Spongiotic dermatitis is a cutaneous reaction pattern to a variety of endogenous or exogenous stimuli. Acute and subacute lesions are characterized clinically by ill-defined pruritic areas of erythema, vesiculation, and crust formation. The common histologic findings include spongiosis and a superficial perivascular lymphocytic infiltrate. There is exocytosis of lymphocytes into the epidermis. With chronicity, histologic spongiosis and clinical vesiculation diminish and are replaced by lichenification. This pattern of inflammation has been termed *eczema* or *eczematous dermatitis*. However, some authors have argued that the term *eczema* lacks a specific meaning and should be avoided.[59]

Clinical Features Lesions of spongiotic dermatitis have a similar clinical appearance regardless of etiology. This is analogous to the reaction pattern of urticaria, in which different allergens produce similar wheals. Acute lesions show poorly defined pruritic, erythematous, edematous patches studded with vesicles. Subacute lesions show secondary changes of excoriation and crust formation, often with impetiginization. In chronic lesions, the edema and vesiculation are replaced by lichenification, scaling, and pigmentary changes including both hyperpigmentation and hypopigmentation.

The clinical distribution of spongiotic dermatitis may offer clues to the specific etiology. Briefly, allergic contact dermatitis occurs at the site of antigen contact and may be patterned. It is uncommon on the thick skin of the palms and soles but may affect the dorsa of the hands and feet. Atopic dermatitis typically involves the flexures and occurs in people with a personal or family history of asthma or allergic rhinitis. Spongiotic systemic drug eruptions are unusual, but when they do occur, they are typically diffuse. Seborrheic dermatitis involves the central face, scalp, ears, upper chest, axillae, and groin. Lesions of nummular dermatitis are symmetrically distributed on the extremities as small, round plaques. Dyshidrotic dermatitis is characterized by vesicles along the margins of the digits and on the palms and soles.

Histopathological Features The histologic picture of chronic and subacute dermatitis is dominated by the changes produced by chronic rubbing and scratching of the skin, similar to that seen in lichen simplex chronicus. Regardless of the cause there is thickening of the epidermis, corresponding to the clinical finding of lichenification. All layers of the epidermis and papillary dermis are thickened, manifesting as compact hyperkeratosis and parakeratosis, hypergranulosis, acanthosis, and fibrosis of the papillary dermis. Spongiosis and exocytosis of lymphocytes into the epidermis are prominent in acute lesions but are less prominent in chronic ones. Dried serum is present as crust, and there may be superficial ulceration due to excoriation.

Differential Diagnosis Different clinical forms of spongiotic dermatitis may show distinctive histologic features. Stasis dermatitis shows clusters of tortuous vessels and hemosiderin within a fibrotic papillary dermis. Nummular dermatitis shows focal mounding parakeratosis and spongiosis associated with a superficial perivascular infiltrate of lymphocytes and a variable number of eosinophils. In chronic atopic dermatitis one sees a pattern indistinguishable from lichen simplex chronicus except eosinophils are more common in the former. Dyshidrotic dermatitis shows spongiotic vesicles on acral skin. Neutrophils may be present in older vesicles. Allergic contact dermatitis may show intraepidermal spongiotic vesicles which contain Langerhans cells and lymphocytes. Eosinophils are uncommon in allergic contact dermatitis. Seborrheic dermatitis shows follicular plugging, focal spongiosis, hemorrhage, and neutrophils within a parakeratotic scale-crust. Vesicular dermatophyte infections show small collections of neutrophils within the stratum corneum. Hyphae may be recognized in hematoxylin and eosin–stained sections as small holes in the stratum corneum. Fungal stains confirm the diagnosis. Dyshidrotic dermatitis may be pustular, but can be distinguished from pustular psoriasis of the palms and soles by the presence of more extensive spongiosis and the absence of intracorneal collections of neutrophils (Munro's microabscesses).

Erythroderma

Erythroderma is a clinical term referring to generalized redness of the skin. *Exfoliative dermatitis* refers to those cases with extensive scaling. This reaction pattern may result from a number of mechanisms.[60] Generalization of preexisting papulosquamous disease or spongiotic dermatitis accounts for 25 to 62.5 percent of cases. Psoriasis, pityriasis rubra pilaris, atopic dermatitis, and seborrheic dermatitis are common causes. Drugs are another major cause of erythroderma (14 to 42 percent). Lymphoma, especially Sézary syndrome, accounts for 8 to 21 percent of cases. Many cases are idiopathic.

Clinical Features   Erythema, scaling, and desquamation may involve the entire body. High blood flow to the skin may disrupt temperature regulation or lead to high output cardiac failure. Nails or hair may be shed. There may be a history of a drug eruption or a preexisting dermatosis. A careful examination may reveal typical lesions of psoriasis, stigmata of atopy, or "islands of sparing" as seen in pityriasis rubra pilaris. Many cases show no distinguishing features.

Histopathological Features   The histologic pattern varies with the underlying etiology. In those cases resulting from chronic or subacute spongiotic dermatitis the histologic picture is nonspecific. A biopsy may show intercellular and intracellular edema with exocytosis of mononuclear cells. Crusting may be present. The superficial dermis contains a perivascular lymphocytic inflammation and edema. Chronic changes are inversely related to the above. They consist of hyperkeratosis, parakeratosis, acanthosis, and papillary dermal fibrosis. In cases related to a primary inflammatory dermatosis such as psoriasis or pityriasis rubra pilaris, the histologic pattern may still be recognizable[61] but is usually less typical than in the primary disease. Cases of Sézary syndrome may show atypical, cerebriform lymphocytes in the epidermis with minimal associated spongiosis; however, Pautrier's microabscesses are less common than in the plaque stage of mycosis fungoides. Drug eruptions may show atypical lymphocytes along the interface and within the epidermis, leading to confusion with mycosis fungoides. In a blinded retrospective study of erythrodermic patients, histologic impression correlated with final diagnosis in up to 66 percent of cases. The authors suggest that multiple biopsies taken simultaneously may improve diagnostic accuracy.[62]

Pityriasis Rosea

Pityriasis rosea (PR) is a self-limited exanthematous eruption of unknown etiology. However, there is some evidence that it is infectious. There is a seasonal variation with an increased incidence in the fall.[63]

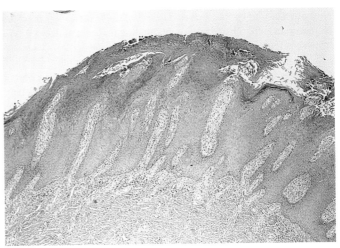

FIGURE 4-18   Inflammatory linear verrucous epidermal nevus. The epidermis shows psoriasiform epidermal hyperplasia with alternating hyperkeratosis and parakeratosis.

Cases are often clustered,[64] recurrence is unusual, and passive transfer of immunity has been demonstrated.[65] Patients are usually in the first to fourth decade of life, and there is a slight female preponderance. Drugs may induce a similar eruption, particularly captopril[66] and gold.[67]

Clinical Features   The classic presentation is that of a single larger initial lesion known as the *herald patch* or *mother patch*. There may be a prodrome consisting of coryza, fever, and malaise. A secondary more diffuse eruption appears 1 to 3 weeks after the initial lesion. Both the primary and the secondary lesions are oval orange-brown- or salmon-colored patches distributed on the upper trunk and proximal extremities. Individual lesions show a collarette of trailing scale. The long axis of lesions follows the lines of skin cleavage, such that the pattern on the back has been compared to a Christmas tree. Less common patterns include flexural (inverse), papular, and purpuric PR. The clinical differential diagnosis includes secondary syphilis, nummular eczema, dermatophytosis, guttate psoriasis, and drug eruptions.

Histopathological Features   Lesional skin shows foci of moundlike parakeratosis, spongiosis, exocytosis of lymphocytes, and extravasation of erythrocytes (Fig. 4-16). There may be small spongiotic microvesicles and slight irregular acanthosis. The superficial dermis contains a patchy, predominantly lymphocytic infiltrate, and the epidermis may contain dyskeratotic cells.[68]

Differential Diagnosis   In PR, dermal papillae are not as elongated as in psoriasis, and neutrophils are not present. Spongiosis and exocytosis are more focal than in chronic spongiotic dermatitis. The eosinophils found in nummular dermatitis are usually absent in PR. Parapsoriasis en plaques shows less spongiosis and a tendency for lymphocytes to line the dermal-epidermal junction. Plasma cells and endothelial swelling are often seen in syphilis. The superficial form of erythema annulare centrifugum may be indistinguishable from PR.

Chronic Candidiasis and Dermatophytosis

Dermatophytosis and candidiasis represent superficial fungal infections of the skin and its appendages. Infection is limited to the nonviable keratinized components including the hair, nails, and stratum corneum. Host factors are important in the development of clinical infection and the subsequent course of disease. Chronic dermatophyte infections are most often caused by *Trichophyton rubrum*. Atopic patients,[69] in whom IgE-mediated type-I hypersensitivity response may inhibit delayed-type hypersensitivity, are susceptible to dermatophytosis.

Clinical Features   Chronic dermatophytosis may involve the glabrous skin (tinea corporis), palms and soles (tinea manuum and pedis), or nails (tinea unguium, onychomycosis). Tinea corporis is characterized by annular, scaly, erythematous plaques with central clearing. Lesions may be psoriasiform with abundant scale. On the feet or hands chronic infection presents as thick hyperkeratotic scale with minimal inflammation. Involvement of the thick stratum corneum of the hands or feet produces a glovelike or moccasinlike pattern. Some patients may have involvement of both feet and one hand. Although candidiasis in otherwise healthy individuals is restricted to the intertriginous areas, chronic mucocutaneous candidiasis may be more extensive, involving the scalp and acral skin. Lesions are often hyperkeratotic or granulomatous rather than the more typical erosive, erythematous, or pustular lesions seen in acute infection. Patients with chronic mucocutaneous candidiasis have an immune deficiency.

Histopathological Features   In acute infections with dermatophytes or *Candida* species, the epidermis is spongiotic with focal parakeratosis. With chronicity the epidermis becomes acanthotic with elongation of rete ridges. There may be aggregates of neutrophils within the parakeratotic scale or in subcorneal pustules resembling the spongiform pustules of Kogoj. Demonstration of organisms within the stratum corneum is diagnostic. The organisms are found only in the nonviable, keratinized components of the epidermis and its appendages, but they are sparse and may not be visible on routinely stained sections. Fungi may be visualized better in sections stained with PAS stain following diastase predigestion or with the methenamine silver stain. Typically, organisms may be found between an orthokeratotic layer and a parakeratotic layer ("sandwich sign").[70]

Mycosis Fungoides (Cutaneous T-Cell Lymphoma)

Mycosis fungoides (MF) is a T-cell lymphoma which primarily affects the skin. It is included here because it may mimic nearly all patterns of inflammatory dermatoses including psoriasiform dermatitis.[71]

Clinical Features   Classically, mycosis fungoides evolves through several stages. The patch stage is characterized by large, erythematous, scaly patches usually located on the trunk and proximal extremities. Lesions tend to be chronic, asymptomatic, and unresponsive to treatment. There may be dyspigmentation, epidermal atrophy, and telangiectasia. The patch stage may persist for years with an average of 6.1 years between the onset of disease and the ultimate diagnosis.[72] Thickened plaques may develop from existing lesions or arise on previously unaffected skin. Plaques may be arcuate or annular as the result of coalescence or central clearing and may have abundant scale resembling psoriasis. The development of cutaneous tumors is correlated with a poor prognosis with a mean survival of 2.5 years.[72] Plaques and tumors have a tendency to ulcerate and may become secondarily infected.

Sézary syndrome represents the leukemic phase of the disease. Clinically patients have generalized erythroderma with red, scaly, pruritic skin. Constitutional symptoms are common, including fever, malaise, and weight loss. Sézary syndrome must be distinguished clinically from other causes of erythroderma, such as pityriasis rubra pilaris, psoriasis, drug eruptions, and widespread spongiotic dermatitis.

Histopathological Features   The histologic findings of mycosis fungoides vary with the clinical stage of the disease. The earliest patches show a nonspecific superficial perivascular or lichenoid infiltrate composed of lymphocytes with occasional plasma cells and eosinophils with little or no epidermal change.[71] Epidermotropism of atypical lymphocytes is highly suggestive of mycosis fungoides.[53] These lymphocytes may show hyperchromatic, cerebriform nuclei, and may be surrounded by clear halos. Similar cells may line the dermal-epidermal junction in association with vacuolar change of the basal layer. The papillary dermis shows random irregular fibrosis. Lymphocytes in the superficial dermis are also surrounded by clear halos.

In biopsies taken from infiltrated plaques, the epidermis is hyperplastic with elongation of the rete ridges, resembling psoriasis. However, there are atypical lymphocytes, both in the epidermis and dermis. The epidermotropic lymphocytes may be single, in small aggregates (Pautrier's microabscesses), or in a diffuse pattern resembling Paget's disease. Adnexal epithelium may be similarly involved,[53] and the pattern of epidermotropism may be limited to follicular epithelium[73] or eccrine glands.[74]

Differential Diagnosis   Because the earliest changes of MF are subtle and may mimic inflammatory dermatoses, multiple specimens taken over time may be necessary to establish the diagnosis. MF may share with psoriasis epidermal hyperplasia and a superficial infiltrate composed of lymphocytes. Features favoring MF include irregular papillary dermal fibrosis and epidermotropism of atypical lymphocytes. Features favoring psoriasis include papillary dermal edema with dilated tortuous capillaries, and neutrophils within the stratum corneum. MF may also resemble chronic dermatitis. Inflammatory dermatoses may show some atypical cells, but the irregularity of nuclear contour, as determined by image analysis, is not as great as in MF.[75] Although spongiosis may be seen in MF, it is mild compared to the number of lymphocytes within the epidermis. Drug eruptions, particularly those due to anticonvulsants, may simulate MF.[76]

Crusted (Norwegian) Scabies

Scabies infestation is a pruritic disease caused by infestation by the human scabies mite, *Sarcoptes scabiei* var. *hominis*. The itch results from sensitization to the mite or its products and subsequent cell-mediated immune response. The mite is usually transmitted by direct contact with infested individuals or, less commonly, by fomites. Mites may survive away from the human host for several days.[77] After mating, the female mite burrows into the superficial layers of the skin and lays her eggs. The female dies after about 5 weeks; the eggs hatch, and the cycle repeats.[78] Typically a patient is infested with only 10 to 15 adult mites,[79] making demonstration and diagnosis occasionally difficult. In crusted scabies, however, mites are much more numerous.[80] This clinical pattern is seen in incapacitated, immunosuppressed, or institutionalized patients.

Clinical Features   Scabies infestation is pruritic, particularly at night. Sites of predilection include the web spaces of fingers and toes, wrists, flexures, elbows, and male genitals. The diagnostic lesion is a linear burrow with a tiny vesicle at the blind end. Although there are typically few mites, intense pruritus and scratching may produce widespread secondary lesions. Areas of excoriation, irritant dermatitis, lichenification, or secondary infection are common.[81] In crusted scabies, one sees hyperkeratotic or psoriasiform papules and plaques. The eruption may be diffuse, presenting as erythroderma. Because mites are numerous, these patients are highly contagious. Testing for human immunodeficiency virus may be appropriate in patients with crusted scabies.[82]

Histopathological Features   The epidermis shows irregular acanthosis and focal spongiosis (Fig. 4-17). There may be a space within or just underneath the stratum corneum, corresponding to the clinical burrow.

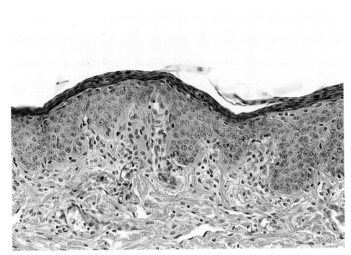

FIGURE 4-19 Acrodermatitis enteropathica. This well-developed lesion displays confluent parakeratosis, absence of the granular layer, and psoriasiform epidermal hyperplasia.

The end of the burrow extends into the superficial stratum malpighii.[83] Step sections may reveal the female mite or its products, including eggs or fecal material. The dermis contains a superficial perivascular or nodular infiltrate composed of lymphocytes and variable numbers of eosinophils. The infiltrate in nodular lesions may have the picture of lymphocytoma cutis, and may contain atypical lymphocytes suggesting lymphoma.[84] In Norwegian (crusted) scabies, mites are usually numerous and easily identified within a greatly thickened stratum corneum.[85] Mites or their products are diagnostic. A nodular dermal infiltrate with eosinophils is not seen in other psoriasiform dermatitides.

Inflammatory Linear Verrucose Epidermal Nevus

Epidermal nevi are hamartomas of the epidermis or its appendages. Some epidermal nevi represent a mosaic state of disorders of cornification. For example, the acantholytic dyskeratotic variant may represent a localized form of Darier's disease (keratosis follicularis), and the epidermolytic variant may represent localized epidermolytic hyperkeratosis, a disorder of keratins 1 or 10.[86] Inflammatory linear verrucose epidermal nevus (ILVEN) was described as a distinct entity in 1971.[87] Most cases are sporadic, but familial cases have been described.[88]

Clinical Features ILVEN consists of grouped or coalescent lichenoid, psoriasiform, or verrucous papules in a linear arrangement, most commonly on the lower extremities. Fifty percent are present by 6 months of age and 75 percent by 5 years of age.[87] Lesions follow the lines of Blaschko,[86] are pruritic, and may wax and wane in intensity. Associated skeletal malformations occur in some cases.[89]

Histopathological Features The characteristic histopathologic features of ILVEN include hyperkeratosis and epidermal hyperplasia. Rete are thickened and elongated with occasional slight spongiosis.[87] Exocytosis of neutrophils as in psoriasis may occur in some instances. A striking pattern consisting of broad columns of parakeratosis without an underlying granular layer alternating with compact hyperkeratosis with underlying hypergranulosis may be seen (Fig. 4-18).[90] The superficial dermis contains a predominantly lymphocytic inflammatory infiltrate arrayed around dilated capillaries.

Differential Diagnosis The clinical differential diagnosis includes other linear papulosquamous lesions, such as linear psoriasis, linear Darier's disease, linear porokeratosis, lichen striatus, and the non-inflammatory form of linear epidermal nevus. Suprapapillary plates are thickened in ILVEN, whereas they are usually thinned in psoriasis. Parakeratosis in psoriasis is diffuse rather than arrayed in broad columns in ILVEN. Linear Darier's disease shows acantholysis and dyskeratosis. Porokeratosis is characterized by cornoid lamellae. Ordinary epidermal nevi show papillomatosis and are not inflammatory.

Bazex Syndrome

Bazex syndrome (acrokeratosis neoplastica) is a paraneoplastic syndrome characterized by psoriasiform skin lesions in association with internal malignancy. A review of 113 cases found the most common neoplasm to be squamous cell carcinoma of the upper aerodigestive tract. Patients had a mean age of 61 years with a striking male predominance (108 of 113 patients).[91] The pathogenesis may be related to a shared antigen between the neoplasm and normal skin or to tumor production of keratinocyte growth factors. An unrelated X-linked disorder showing follicular atrophoderma on the dorsal hands and feet, hypotrichosis, hypohidrosis, and basal cell carcinomas also carries the eponym *Bazex syndrome* (Bazex-Dupre-Christol syndrome).[92]

Clinical Features Acrokeratosis neoplastica is a symmetric psoriasiform eruption, affecting acral areas, including hands and feet, ears, and the nose. Nail involvement is common with periungual and subungual hyperkeratosis and shedding of the nail plate. Lesions are distinctly violaceous and often resistant to treatment. Commonly the skin changes precede the diagnosis of internal malignancy. Treatment of the underlying malignancy reverses the skin changes but not the nail changes. Relapse of skin lesions may herald tumor recurrence.[91]

Histopathologic Features The histopathologic pattern is nonspecific. In addition to psoriasiform epidermal hyperplasia, keratinocytes may show vacuolar change and nuclear pyknosis.[93]

Pellagra

Pellagra results from a dietary deficiency of niacin or its precursor, the essential amino acid tryptophan. The disease is characterized by the three *D*'s—diarrhea, dementia, and dermatitis. The disease was thought to be infectious, until the remarkable work of Joseph Golberger.[94] One hypothesis holds that the clinical manifestations may be caused by increased extracellular matrix viscosity.[95] In this model, cutaneous lesions are localized to areas of sun exposure and trauma because "mediators" cannot diffuse from the site. Increased viscosity in the gastrointestinal tract might limit absorption leading to diarrhea.

A similar rash may occur in the carcinoid syndrome where tryptophan is converted in quantity into serotonin (5-OH tryptophan). Hartnup disease is an autosomal recessive disorder characterized by an impairment of neutral amino acid transport. Tryptophan is not absorbed from the diet and is lost in the urine, leading to a deficiency of niacin.[96] Regardless of the cause of niacin deficiency, the signs and symptoms respond promptly to replacement therapy.

Clinical Features In addition to the gastrointestinal symptoms (diarrhea) and neurologic disease, there is a characteristic skin eruption. Lesions are symmetric and involve sun-exposed skin and areas of pressure. There are first erythema and burning or itching. Early lesions may be bullous. Later the eruption is characterized by hyperpigmentation, scaling, and fissuring. Facial involvement may simulate the "butterfly" eruption of lupus erythematosus. The limitation to sun-exposed sites may be striking, with extremity involvement showing a glove or stocking distribution. Involvement of the neck by a sharply demarcated photoinduced rash has been termed *Casal's necklace*.

Histopathological Features   The histopathologic features of pellagra are essentially identical to those seen in acrodermatitis enteropathica, necrolytic migratory erythema, essential fatty acid deficiency, and various nutritional disorders. They consist of extensive parakeratosis with underlying irregular epidermal hyperplasia. There is a pallor of the upper epidermis, representing diffuse superficial keratinocyte necrosis. There may be a superficial perivascular lymphocytic infiltrate.

Acrodermatitis Enteropathica

Acrodermatitis enteropathica is an autosomal recessive disease caused by a defect in dietary zinc absorption. The defect is not complete, in that the disease may be reversed by zinc supplementation. Identical symptoms may also be produced by a diet deficient in zinc. Causes of noninherited zinc deficiency are numerous, and include chronic diarrhea of any etiology, inadequate dietary content as in alcoholism or crash dieting, or renal loss as in dialysis. Also, chronic diseases with an increased catabolic rate may lead to zinc deficiency. Breast milk may have a low concentration of zinc, leading to zinc deficiency in breast-fed infants.[97] As with the inherited form, dietary deficiency is quickly and completely reversed by supplementation with oral or parenteral zinc salts.

Clinical Features   The hereditary form of zinc deficiency (i.e. acrodermatitis enteropathica) develops earlier in bottle-fed as opposed to breast-fed infants. As the name implies, the eruption typically starts as eczematous, scaly plaques on acral skin, including the scalp, paronychial folds, and perineum. Lesions may be erosive, pustular, or bullous, and secondary infection with candida or bacteria is common. There may be failure to thrive. There may be alopecia or alternating light and dark banding of hair, which may be observed with polarizing light microscopy.[98]

Histopathological Features   The epidermis is verrucous with pallor of the superficial malpighian layer and extensive necrosis of individual keratinocytes. Chronic lesions show psoriasiform epidermal hyperplasia with overlying hyperkeratosis and parakeratosis (Fig. 4-19). The superficial dermis contains a mild perivascular lymphocytic infiltrate. Bullous lesions show intraepidermal vacuolar change and ballooning degeneration associated with extensive epidermal necrosis without acantholysis.[99]

Glucagonoma Syndrome

Glucagon-producing islet cell (alpha cell) tumors of the pancreas are associated with necrolytic migratory erythema.[100] The cutaneous manifestations may be related to a hypoaminoacidemia or to the high levels of glucagon itself. Diagnosis is made by demonstrating increased levels of glucagon in patients with the typical syndrome. Removal of the pancreatic tumor is curative. Necrolytic migratory erythema may also occur without glucagonoma[101] in association with hepatocellular dysfunction and hypoalbuminemia.[102]

Clinical Features   The eruption is periorificial, acral, and flexural, often with severe glossitis. Lesions begin as erythematous papules. Later there are superficial vesicular lesions, erosions, crusting, and fissuring. Older lesions may be psoriasiform.[103] Secondary infection with candida and bacteria is common. Noncutaneous findings include stomatitis, weight loss, glucose intolerance, and diarrhea.

Histopathological Features   Specimens are characterized by psoriasiform epidermal hyperplasia with confluent parakeratosis. There is pallor of the superficial epidermis with dyskeratotic keratinocytes. The pallor may result from intracellular edema.[104] In more acute lesions necrosis may be extensive, producing an intraepidermal bulla. There is a superficial perivascular lymphocytic infiltrate with papillary dermal edema. This condition has also been reported to show extensive suprabasilar acantholysis.[105]

Secondary Syphilis

Syphilis is a venereal disease caused by *Treponema pallidum*. Syphilis is referred to as "the great imitator" because of its protean clinical manifestations. Secondary syphilis may show numerous clinical patterns, including generalized psoriasiform lesions. As in psoriasis, the palms and soles may be involved. Mucosal lesions include condylomata lata which are mamillated or papillomatous whitish papules or plaques. The clinical differential diagnosis of secondary syphilis includes guttate psoriasis, pityriasis rosea, tinea corporis, tinea versicolor, and nummular eczema.

Histopathological Features   The papulosquamous lesions of secondary syphilis may show psoriasiform hyperplasia associated with exocytosis of neutrophils. There are overlying hyperkeratosis and crust. The dermis shows a superficial and deep perivascular[106] infiltrate composed of lymphocytes and plasma cells. Endothelial cells may be swollen, protruding into vascular lumina. A lichenoid pattern is more common than a psoriasiform pattern in secondary syphilis.

Differential Diagnosis   The inflammatory infiltrate of psoriasis, chronic dermatitis, and dermatophytosis is uniformly superficial, rather than deep, and does not contain plasma cells. Mycosis fungoides may have a superficial and deep infiltrate as well as a lichenoid pattern. However, the presence of atypical lymphocytes,[107] Pautrier's microabscesses, and a variable number of eosinophils distinguishes it from syphilis. In difficult cases, serology is useful.

Bowen's Disease

Bowen's disease, originally described in 1912,[108] is a squamous cell carcinoma in situ. Although not a dermatitis, Bowen's disease is included here because it may show psoriasiform epidermal thickening. Lesions arise more commonly on sun exposed than covered skin, usually in patients older than 60 years old.[109] Bowen's disease presents as a long-standing, fairly well circumscribed, scaly erythematous plaque. Lesions are usually solitary but may be multiple. Thus, Bowen's disease may clinically resemble papulosquamous dermatoses.

Histopathological Features   Overall the neoplasm is poorly circumscribed and asymmetric. The epidermis is thickened with elongated rete ridges. The granular layer is absent with broad, thick overlying parakeratosis, which may form a cutaneous horn. Keratinocytes show marked atypia, lack of maturation, and individual cell dyskeratosis. Large atypical cells with ample glycogen-containing cytoplasm may be distributed singly in a pagetoid pattern or in clusters among normal keratinocytes. This pattern may involve adnexal epithelium, particularly follicular infundibula.[110] The superficial dermis often shows extensive solar elastosis and a perivascular lymphocytic infiltrate. At low power, the presence of parakeratosis, a thickened epidermis, and superficial dermal inflammation may suggest psoriasis. However, the presence of full-thickness keratinocyte atypia and lack of maturation defines Bowen's disease as a neoplasm and excludes inflammatory causes of psoriasiform epidermal changes.

Clear Cell Acanthoma

Clear cell acanthoma (CCA, Degos acanthoma, pale cell acanthoma) is included here because it may show psoriasiform epidermal hyperplasia. A study of keratin expression found a pattern similar to that seen in inflammatory dermatoses such as psoriasis, and the authors speculate that CCA is an inflammatory dermatosis rather than a neoplasm.[111] The process is uncommon and most often occurs in adults. The lesion is usually solitary but may be multiple.[112] It is most commonly located on the extensor aspect of the leg. The typical presentation is a red-brown papule with a somewhat eroded surface. Lesions share clinical features with irritated seborrheic keratoses and pyogenic granulomas.[113]

Histopathological Features   CCA resembles a benign epidermal neoplasm in that it is well-circumscribed, symmetric, and sharply demarcated from the surrounding uninvolved skin. The granular layer is absent and the surface may show hyperkeratosis, parakeratosis, or erosion. Rete ridges are elongated and interconnected in an anastomosing pattern. Keratinocytes contain ample pale-staining cytoplasm, except for the basal layer, acrosyringia, and acrotrichia, which are spared. The pale-staining pattern represents accumulation of glycogen, which is PAS positive and diastase labile. Throughout the lesion are numerous neutrophils in association with spongiosis. Neutrophils may extend into the stratum corneum, forming microabscesses[114] resembling psoriasis. The papillary dermis between elongated, interconnected rete is often edematous with dilated capillaries and a perivascular lymphocytic infiltrate.

Lamellar Ichthyosis

Lamellar ichthyosis (LI) is an autosomal recessive disorder of cornification distinct from nonbullous congenital ichthyosiform erythroderma.[115] Affected individuals may be born encased in a colloidion membrane which is shed in the first 2 weeks of life. There is a lifelong thick scale over the entire body. This represents a retention hyperkeratosis, rather than a hyperproliferative process. Palms and soles are hyperkeratotic, and the eyelids and lips are often everted (ectropion and eclabium). The disease has been attributed to a mutation in the gene for transglutaminase 1, leading to defective cross-links required for normal cell envelope production.[116]

Histopathological Features   The histologic pattern of lamellar ichthyosis is nonspecific. In addition to irregular acanthosis, there is striking compact hyperkeratosis without parakeratosis.[117] This pattern reflects the fact that LI is a retention hyperkeratosis, rather than a hyperproliferative disorder. The granular layer may be thickened or thinned.[118] Because LI is a genodermatosis rather than an inflammatory dermatosis, it is usually noninflammatory.

REFERENCES

1. Ackerman AB: *Histologic Diagnosis of Inflammatory Skin Diseases.* Philadelphia, Lea and Febiger, 1978.
2. Farmer ER, Hood AF: *Pathology of the Skin.* East Norwalk, CT, Appleton and Lange; 1990.
3. Pinkus H: Psoriasiform tissue reactions. *Aust J of Dermatol* 3:31–35, 1965.
4. Pinkus H, Mehregan AH: *A Guide to Dermatohistopathology.* East Norwalk, CT, Appleton Lange, 1976.
5. Henseler T, Christophers E: Psoriasis of early and late onset: Characterization of two types of psoriasis vulgaris. *J Acad Dermatol* 13: 450, 1985.
6. Cram DL: Psoriasis: Current advances in etiology and treatment. *J Am Acad Dermatol* 4:1–14, 1981.
7. Weinstein GD: Autoradiographic analysis of turnover times of normal and psoriatic epidermis. *J Invest Dermatol* 45: 257, 1968.
8. Farber EM, Nall ML, Watson W: Natural history of psoriasis in 61 twin pairs. *Arch Dermatol* 109: 207, 1974.
9. Russell TJ: Histocompatibility (HL-A) antigens associated with psoriasis. *N Engl J Med* 287: 738, 1972.
10. Theeuwes M, Morhenn V: Allelic instability in the mitosis model and the inheritance of psoriasis. [Review]. *Am Acad Dermatol* 32: 44–52, 1995.
11. Zheng G, Thomson G, Pen Y: Allelic instability in mitosis can explain "genome imprinting" and other genetic phenomena in psoriasis. *J Med Genet* 51: 163–164, 1994.
12. Boehncke W, Sterry W, Hainzl A, et al: Psoriasiform architecture of murine epidermis overlying human psoriatic dermis transplanted onto SCID mice. *Arch Dermatol Res* 286: 325–330, 1994.
13. Bata-Csorgo Z, Hammerberg C, Voorhees J, Cooper K: Intralesional T-lymphocyte activation as a mediator of psoriatic epidermal hyperplasia. [Review]. *J Invest Dermatol* 105: 89s–94s, 1995.
14. Creamer J, Barker J: Vascular proliferation and angiogenic factors in psoriasis. *Clin Exp Dermatol* 20: 6–9, 1995.
15. Leung D, Walsh P, Giorno R, Norris D: A potential role for superantigens in the pathogenesis of psoriasis. *J Invest Dermatol* 100: 225–228, 1993.
16. Valdimarsson H, Baker B, Jonsdottir I, et al: Psoriasis: A T-cell-mediated autoimmune disease induced by streptococcal superantigens?. [Review]. *Immunol Today* 16: 145–149, 1995.
17. Farber EM, Nall ML: The natural history of psoriasis in 5,600 patients. *Dermatologica* 148: 1, 1974.
18. Whyte HJ, Baughmann RD: Acute guttate psoriasis and streptococcal infection. *Arch Dermatol* 89: 350, 1964.
19. Telfer N, Chalmers R, Whale K, Colman G: The role of streptococcal infection in the initiation of guttate psoriasis. *Arch Dermatol* 128: 39–42, 1992.
20. McFadden J, Valdimarsson H, Fry L: Cross-reactivity between streptococcal M surface antigen and human skin. *Br J Dermatol* 125: 443–447, 1991.
21. Braverman JM, Cohen I, Black MM: Metabolic and ultrastructural studies in a patient with pustular psoriasis. *Br J Dermatol* 105: 189, 1972.
22. Ackerman AB, Ragaz A: *The Lives of Lesions. Chronology in Dermatopathology.* New York, Masson, 1984.
23. Gordon M, Johnson WC: Histopathology and histochemistry of psoriasis: I. The active lesion and clinically normal skin. *Arch Dermatol* 95: 402, 1967.
24. Cox AJ, Watson W: Histologic variation in lesions of psoriasis. *Arch Dermatol* 106: 503, 1972.
25. Ragaz A, Ackerman AB: Evolution, maturation, and regression of lesions of psoriasis. *Am J Dermatopathol* 1: 199–214, 1979.
26. Pinkus H, Mehregan AH: The primary histologic lesion of seborrheic dermatitis and psoriasis. *J Invest Dermatol* 46: 109–116, 1966.
27. Braun-Falco O, Christophers E: Structural aspects of initial psoriatic lesions. *Arch Dermatol Res* 251: 95, 1974.
28. Baker H, Ryan TJ: Generalized pustular psoriasis: A clinical and epidemiological study of 104 cases. *Br J Dermatol* 80: 771, 1968.
29. Wagner G, Luckasen JR, Goltz RW: Mucous membrane involvement in generalized psoriasis. *Arch Dermatol* 112: 1010–1014, 1976.
30. Zelickson B, Muller S: Generalized pustular psoriasis: A review of 63 cases. *Arch Dermatol* 127: 1339–1345, 1991.
31. Shelly WB: *Generalized Pustular Psoriasis: Consultations in Dermatology.* Philadelphia, Saunders, 1972.
32. Rupec M: Zur ultrastruktur der spongiformen pustel. *Arch Klin Exp Dermatol* 239: 30–49, 1970.
33. Spencer J, Silvers D, Grossman M: Pustular eruption after drug exposure: Is it pustular psoriasis or a pustular drug eruption? *Br J Dermatol* 130: 514–519, 1994.
34. Wilkins RF: Reiter's syndrome: Evaluation of preliminary criteria for definite diagnosis. *Arth Rheum* 24: 844, 1981.
35. Engelman EP, Weber HM: Reiter's syndrome. *Clin Orthop* 57: 19, 1968.
36. Brewerton DA: Reiter's disease and HLA 27. *Lancet* 2: 996, 1973.
37. Granfors K: *Yersinia antigens* in synovial fluid cells from patients with reactive arthritis. *N Engl J Med* 320: 216, 1989.
38. Beutler A, Whittum-Hudson J, Nanagara R, et al: Intracellular location of inapparently infecting Chlamydia in synovial tissue from patients with Reiter's syndrome. *Immunologic Res* 13: 163–171, 1994.
39. Hughes R, Keat A: Reiter's syndrome and reactive arthritis: A current view. [Review]. *Sem in Arth Rheum* 24: 190–210, 1994.
40. Arnett FC: Incomplete Reiter's syndrome: Clinical comparison with the classical triad. *Annals Rheumatologic Disease* 38: 73, 1979.
41. Kulka JP: The lesions of Reiter's syndrome. *Arth and Rheum* 5: 195, 1962.
42. Griffiths WAD: Pityriasis rubra pilaris. *Clin and Exp Dermatol* 5: 105, 1980.
43. Gross DA, Landau JW, Newcomer VD: Pityriasis rubra pilaris: Report of a case and analysis of the literature. *Arch Dermatol* 99: 710, 1969.
44. Vanderhooft SL, Francis JS, Holbrook KA, et al: Familial pityriasis rubra pilaris. *Arch Dermatol* 131: 448–453, 1995.
45. Porter D, Shuster S: Epidermal renewal and amino acids in psoriasis and pityriasis rubra pilaris. *Arch Dermatol* 98: 339, 1968.

46. Sonex TS: Nail changes in adult type I pityriasis rubra pilaris. *J Am Acad Dermatol* 15: 956, 1986.

47. Soeprono FF: Histologic criteria for the diagnosis of pityriasis rubra pilaris. *Am J Dermatopathol* 8: 277–283, 1986.

48. Goldblum RW, Piper WN: Artificial lichenification produced by a scratching machine. *J Invest Dermatol* 22: 405–415, 1957.

49. Neumann E, Winter V: The character of cells with "alteration cavitaire" (Leloir). *Acta Dermatol Venereol* 45: 272–274, 1965.

50. Brocq L: Les parapsoriasis. *Ann Dermatol Syphiligr* 3: 433, 1902.

51. Lambert WC, Everett MA: The nosology of parapsoriasis. *J Am Acad Dermatol* 5: 373, 1981.

52. Samman PD: The natural history of parapsoriasis en plaque (chronic superficial dermatitis) and prereticulotic poikiloderma. *Br J Dermatol* 87: 405, 1972.

53. Sanchez JL, Ackerman AB: The patch stage of mycosis fungoides. *Am J Dermatopathol* 1: 5–26, 1979.

54. Wood GS, Haeffner A, Dummer R, Crooks CF: Molecular biology techniques for the diagnosis of cutaneous T-cell lymphoma. [Review]. *Dermatol Clin* 12: 231–241, 1994.

55. Lindae ML: Poikilodermatous mycosis fungoides and atrophic large plaque psoriasis exhibit similar abnormalities of T-cell antigen expression. *Arch Dermatol* 124: 366, 1988.

56. Staib G, Sterry W: Use of polymerase chain reaction in the detection of clones in lymphoproliferative diseases of the skin. *Recent Results Cancer Res* 139: 239–247, 1995.

57. Theodorou I, Delfau-Larue MH, Bigorgne C, et al: Cutaneous T-cell infiltrates: Analysis of T-cell receptor gamma gene rearrangement by polymerase chain reaction and denaturing gradient gel electrophoresis. *Blood* 86: 305–310, 1995.

58. Kikuchi A, Naka W, Harada T, et al: Parapsoriasis en plaques: Its potential for progression to malignant lymphoma. *J Am Acad Dermatol* 29: 419–422, 1993.

59. Ackerman AB, Ragaz A: A plea to expunge the word "eczema" from the lexicon of dermatology and dermatopathology. *Am J Dermatopathol* 4: 315–326, 1982.

60. Botella-Estrada R, Sanmartin O, Oliver V, et al: Erythroderma: A clinicopathological study of 56 cases. *Arch Dermatol* 130: 1503–1507, 1994.

61. Zip C, Murray S, Walsh NM: The specificity of histopathology in erythroderma. *J Cutan Pathol* 20: 393–398, 1993.

62. Walsh N, Prokopetz R, Tron V, et al.: Histopathology in erythroderma: Review of a series of cases by multiple observers. *J Cutan Pathol* 21: 419–423, 1994.

63. Chuang T: Pityriasis rosea in Rochester, Minnesota, 1969 to 1978: A 10-year epidemiologic study. *J Am Acad Dermatol* 7: 80, 1982.

64. Bjornberg A, Hellgren L: Pityriasis rosea: A statistical, clinical, and laboratory investigation of 826 patients and matched healthy controls. *Acta Dermatol Venereol* 42 (suppl 50): 1, 1962.

65. Salin RW: The treatment of pityriasis rosea with convalescent plasma, gamma globulin, and pooled plasma. *Arch Dermatol* 76: 659, 1957.

66. Wilkin JK, Kirkendall WM: Pityriasis rosea-like rash from Captopril. *Arch Dermatol* 118: 186, 1982.

67. Wilkinson SM, Smith AG, Davis MJ, et al: Pityriasis rosea and discoid eczema: Dose related reactions to treatment with gold. *Ann Rheumatol Dis* 51: 881–884, 1992.

68. Okamato H, Imamura S, Aoskima T: Dyskeratotic degeneration of epidermal cells in pityriasis rosea. *Br J Dermatol* 107: 189–194, 1982.

69. Jones HE: The atopic-chronic-dermatophytosis syndrome. *Acta Dermatol Venereol* 92(suppl): 81, 1980.

70. Gottlieb GJ, Ackerman AB: The "sandwich sign" of dermatophytosis. *Am J Dermatopathol* 8: 347–350, 1986.

71. Shapiro P, Pinto F: The histologic spectrum of mycosis fungoides/Sezary syndrome (cutaneous T-cell lymphoma): A review of 222 biopsies, including newly described patterns and the earliest pathologic changes. *Am J Surg Pathol* 18: 645–667, 1994.

72. Epstein EHJ: Mycosis fungoides: Survival, prognostic factors, response to therapy and autopsy findings. *Medicine* (Baltimore) 51: 61, 1972.

73. Goldenhersh M, Zlotogorski A, Rosenmann E: Follicular mycosis fungoides. *Am J Dermatopathol* 16: 52–55, 1994.

74. Zelger B, Sepp N, Weyrer K, et al: Syringotropic cutaneous T-cell lymphoma: A variant of mycosis fungoides? *Br J Dermatol* 130: 756–769, 1994.

75. McNutt NS, Crain WR: Quantitative electron microscopic comparison of lymphocyte nuclear contours in mycosis fungoides and benign infiltrates in the skin. *Cancer* 47: 698, 1981.

76. Rijlaarsdam U, Scheffer E, Meijer CJ, et al: Mycosis fungoides-like lesions associated with phenytoin and carbamazepine therapy. *J Am Acad Dermatol* 24: 216–220, 1991.

77. Arlian LG: Prevalence of Sarcoptes scabiei in the homes and nursing homes of scabietic patients. *J Am Acad Dermatol* 19: 806, 1988.

78. Molinaro MJ, Schwartz RA, Janniger CK: Scabies. *Cutis* 56: 317–321, 1995.

79. Commons CA: We can get rid of scabies: New treatment available soon. *Med J Austral* 160: 317–318, 1994.

80. Sierra G, Ruis F, Romeu J: Hospital outbreak of scabies stemming from two AIDS patients with Norwegian scabies. *Lancet* 335: 1227, 1990.

81. O'Donnell BF, O'Loughlin S, Powell FC: Management of crusted scabies. *Int J Dermatol* 29: 258–266, 1990.

82. Schlesinger I, Oelrich DM, Tyring SK: Crusted (Norwegian) scabies in patients with AIDS: The range of clinical presentations. *South Med J* 87: 352–356, 1994.

83. Hejazi N, Mehregen AH: Histologic study of inflammatory lesions. *Arch Dermatol* 111: 37–39, 1975.

84. Thomson J, Cochrane T, Cochran R: Histology simulating reticulosis in nodular scabies. *Br J Dermatol* 90: 421–429, 1974.

85. Fernandez N, Torres A, Ackerman AB: Pathological findings in human scabies. *Arch Dermatol* 113: 320–324, 1977.

86. Bolognia JL, Orlow SJ, Glick SA: Lines of Blaschko. *J Am Acad Dermatol* 31: 157–190, 1994.

87. Altman L, Mehregan AH: Inflammatory linear verrucose epidermal nevus. *Arch Dermatol* 104: 385–389, 1971.

88. Goldman K, Don PC: Adult onset of inflammatory linear verrucous epidermal nevus in a mother and her daughter. *Dermatol* 189: 170–172, 1994.

89. Golitz LE, Weston WL: Inflammatory linear verrucose epidermal nevus. *Arch Dermatol* 115: 1208–1212, 1979.

90. Dupre A, Christol B: Inflammatory linear verrucose epidermal nevus. *Arch Dermatol* 113: 767–769, 1977.

91. Bolognia JL: Bazex syndrome: Acrokeratosis paraneoplastica. *Sem Dermatol* 14: 84–89, 1995.

92. Plosila M, Kustala R, Niemi KM: Bazex syndrome: Follicular atrophoderma with multiple basal cell carcinomas, hypotrichosis, and hypohidrosis. *Clin Exp Dermatol* 6: 31, 1981.

93. Pecora AL, Landsman L, Imgrund SP: Acrokeratosis neoplastica (Bazex syndrome). *Arch Dermatol* 120: 820–826, 1983.

94. Elmore JG, Feinstein AR: Joseph Goldberger: An unsung hero of American clinical epidemiology. *Ann Intern Med* 121: 372–375, 1994.

95. Stone OJ: Pellagra—increased viscosity of extracellular matrix. *Med Hypotheses* 40: 355–359, 1993.

96. Halvorsen K, Halvorsen S: Hartnup disease. *Pediatrics* 31: 565, 1963.

97. Lee MG: Transient symptomatic zinc deficiency in a full term breast fed infant. *J Am Acad Dermatol* 23:375–379, 1990.

98. Traupe H: Polarizing microscopy of hair in AE. *Pediatr Dermatol* 3: 300, 1986.

99. Borroni G, Brazzelli V, Vignati G, et al: Bullous lesions in acrodermatitis enteropathica: Histopathologic findings regarding two patients. *Am J Dermatopathol* 14: 304–309, 1992.

100. Mallinson: A glucagonoma syndrome. *Ann Intern Med* 108: 64, 1974.

101. Thivolet J: Necrolytic migratory erythema without glucagonoma. *Arch Dermatol* 117: 4, 1981.

102. Marinkovich MP, Botella R, Datloff J, Sangueza OP: Necrolytic migratory erythema without glucagonoma in patients with liver disease. *J Am Acad Dermatol* 32: 604–609, 1995.

103. Kahan RS, Perez-Figaredo RA, Neimanis A: Necrolytic migratory erythema. *Arch Dermatol* 113: 792–797, 1977.

104. Sweet R: A dermatosis specifically associated with a tumor of pancreatic alpha cells. *Br J Dermatol* 90: 301–308, 1974.

105. Long CC, Laidler P, Holt P: Suprabasal acantholysis—an unusual feature of necrolytic migratory erythema. *Clin Exp Dermatol* 18: 464–467, 1993.

106. Jeerapeet P, Ackerman A: Histologic patterns of secondary syphilis. *Arch Dermatol* 107: 373–377, 1973.

107. Cochran R, Thomson J, Flemming K: Histology simulating reticulosis in secondary syphilis. *Br J Dermatol* 95: 251–254, 1976.

108. Bowen JT: Precancerous dermatosis. *J Cutan Dis* 30: 241–255, 1912.

109. Thestrup-Pedersen K, Morbus Bowen: A description of the disease in 617 patients. *Acta Dermatol Venereol* 68: 236, 1988.

110. Brownstein MH, Raboniwitz AD: The precursors of cutaneous squamous cell carcinoma (review). *Int J Dermatol* 18: 1–16, 1979.

111. Ohnishi T, Watanabe S: Immunohistochemical characterization of keratin expression in clear cell acanthoma. *Br J Dermatol* 133: 186–193, 1995.

112. Baden TJ: Multiple clear cell acanthomas. *J Am Acad Dermatol* 16: 1075, 1987.

113. Fine RM, Chernosky ME: Clinical recognition of clear-cell acanthoma (Degos). *Arch Dermatol* 100: 559–563, 1969.

114. Jones EW, Wells GC: Dego's acanthoma (acantome a cellules claires). *Arch Dermatol* 94: 286–294, 1966.

115. Williams ML, Elias PM: Heterogeneity in autosomal recessive ichthyosis: Clinical and biochemical differentiation of lamellar ichthyosis and non-bullous congenital ichthyosiform erythroderma. *Arch Dermatol* 121: 477, 1985.

116. Russell LJ, DiGiovanna JJ, Rogers GR, et al.: Mutations in the gene for transglutaminase 1 in autosomal recessive lamellar ichthyosis. *Nature Genet* 9: 279–283, 1995.

117. Williams ML, Elias PM: Heterogeneity in autosomal recessive ichthyosis. *Arch Dermatol* 121: 477–488, 1985.

118. Vandersteen PR, Muller SA: Lamellar ichthyosis. *Arch Dermatol* 106: 694–701, 1972.

SUPERFICIAL AND DEEP PERIVASCULAR DERMATITIS

A. Neil Crowson

In approaching a skin biopsy showing a dermal inflammatory cell infiltrate, the pathologist must take note of the presence or absence and type of epidermal alteration, vascular changes, the stromal response, and the character of the infiltrate itself. With respect to the former, the presence or absence of parakeratosis and orthohyperkeratosis and concomitant acanthosis or atrophy are clues to the chronicity of the process, and the type of injury pattern, for example, a spongiotic versus a cell-poor vacuolopathic interface dermatitis, point toward a delayed-type hypersensitivity reaction versus a humorally mediated or autoimmune disease, respectively. The infiltrate may be lymphohistiocytic, or may contain an admixture of granulocytes, the former usually a sign of delayed-type hypersensitivity and the latter often a clue to an immune-complex (type III) or an anaphylactic type (type I) hypersensitivity reaction. Histiocyte-predominant infiltrates may be a clue to a drug, viral, or idiopathic granulomatous process. The disposition of the infiltrate, either tightly "cuffed" around the vasculature, or both perivascular and interstitial in distribution, may be a clue to a gyrate erythema on the one hand or to urticaria on the other. The stromal response, either in the context of a fibrosing reaction or of collagen necrobiosis, may be a clue to a chronic process or a systemic disease. Careful attention to the vasculature is essential. The presence or absence of fibrin deposition defining a vasculitis, and the presence or absence of endothelial cell necrosis, telangiectasia, and diminished vascular density of the superficial plexus, features indicative of certain of the connective tissue diseases, must be addressed, as must the type of inflammatory cells in vessel walls and lumina. Although by no means comprehensive, Table 5-1 provides a differential diagnostic approach to the superficial and the superficial and deep perivascular dermatitides. The reader is referred to other sections of this book for an in-depth consideration of many of these entities.

URTICARIA

Clinical Features   The urticarias are common, transient eruptions that affect roughly 15 percent of the population at some time in life.[1] They comprise palpable erythematous papules or wheals that lack surface alteration and wax and wane without a clinical residuum. Confluent plaques may form annular or arcuate lesions. Urticaria may be acute or chronic; in the former, etiologic triggers often are identifiable. Chronic urticarias are those that last longer than 6 weeks and may be either idiopathic or of physical, cholinergic, IgE–, immune complex, or histamine-releasing agent-mediated types (see Table 5-2). There is increasing evidence that delayed-type hypersensitivity mechanisms may play a role in at least some cases of urticaria.[2]

The clinical appearance results from vasodilatation, enhanced vascular permeability, and extravasation of proteins into the dermis. Angioedema represents the same process but extends as well to the subcutis and subjacent soft tissues, and sometimes the upper airways, with potentially fatal consequences; it generally relates to an absolute or relative C1 esterase–inhibitor deficiency that may be familial.

The main mediators include histamine, prostaglandins, and interleukin-1, the liberation of which is provoked by types I and III immune reactions (see Chap. 22) and nonimmunologic mechanisms causing mast cell or basophil degranulation. The latter are exemplified by opiates and foods such as strawberries and shellfish. The IgE-mediated urticarias constitute antigen-specific reactions to certain foods, drugs, pollens, insect bites, and stings. The neutrophilic urticarias usually represent the sequelae of complement activation, causes of which include $C1_q$ esterase deficiency and circulating immune complexes containing antigens of endogenous or exogenous origin, the latter often comprising drug or microbial antigens such as Epstein-Barr or hepatitis viruses.[3] Characteristic endogenous causes include connective tissue diseases, neoplasms, and mixed cryoglobulinemia. Neutrophilic urticaria also may characterize the incipient physical urticarias owing to cold, heat, or pressure.

Chronic urticarias occur mainly in middle age, and relate in some patients to IgG autoantibodies that cross-link alpha subunits of high-affinity IgE receptors on basophils and mast cells,[4] associated with an increased incidence of thyroid autoimmunity.[4] Most other patients with chronic urticaria exhibit allergies to food, acetylsalicylic acid, or other common antigens. Cholinergic urticaria is caused by exercise, heat, or emotional stress, all of which increase body temperature; enhancement of sympathetic activity is postulated to lead to acetylcholine release at nerve endings, triggering degranulation of apposed mast cells. Schnitzler's syndrome is a rare form of chronic urticaria associated with IgM-κ paraproteinemia, bone pain, hyperostosis, and pyrexia.[5]

Histopathological Features   The histology reflects the age of the lesion biopsied and the type of provocative stimulus. One constant is

TABLE 5-1

Perivascular Inflammatory Cell Infiltrates with Minimal or No Epidermal Alteration

Superficial Perivascular Dermatitis	*Superficial and Deep Perivascular Dermatitis*
Urticaria	Urticaria
Perivascular lymphocytic dermatitis	Superficial and deep perivascular lymphocytic dermatitis
Toxic erythema of pregnancy	Toxic erythema of pregnancy
Gyrate erythemas	Gyrate erythemas
Pityriasis lichenoides	Pityriasis lichenoides
Perniosis	Perniosis
Rickettsial and viral infections	Richettsial and viral infections
Polymorphous light eruption (superficial variant)	Polymorphous light eruption (superficial and deep variant)
	Photosensitive eruptions
Connective tissue disease	Connective tissue disease
Systemic lupus erythematosus	Discoid lupus erythematosus
Subacute cutaneous lupus erythematosus	
Mixed connective tissue disease	Leprosy (indeterminate)
	Syphilis
Dermatomyositis	Borreliosis
	Leukemia and leukemids
Urticaria pigmentosa	Urticaria pigmentosa

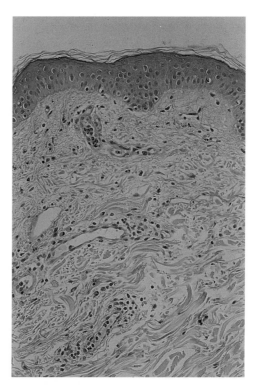

FIGURE 5-1   Urticaria. The reticular dermis shows edema, comprising separation of collagen bundles, accompanied by an interstitial granulocytic infiltrate.

edema, characterized by separation of collagen bundles (Fig. 5-1). Blood vessels and lymphatics usually are dilated and show endothelial swelling. The upper dermis is preferentially involved, except in angioedema, which prominently involves the deep reticular dermis and subcutis. A sparse perivascular inflammatory cell infiltrate composed of a variable admixture of lymphocytes, eosinophils, and neutrophils characterizes the lesions. Mast cells and granulocytes are seen within the interstitium and granulocytes within blood vessels. Degranulated mast cells resemble lymphocytes and, when present, may suggest a mononuclear cell-predominant vascular reaction. The neutrophilic urticarias tend to have a more cellular infiltrate, often with neutrophilic packing of blood vessels (Fig. 5-2). Neutrophilic urticaria may also characterize the incipient physical urticarias caused by cold, heat, or pressure, which are more likely, in their chronic state, to manifest the cell-poor morphology described in the preceding.

Differential Diagnosis   The differential diagnosis of urticaria includes persistent dermal hypersensitivity reactions to drugs, insect bite reactions, dermal contact hypersensitivity, viral exanthems, gyrate erythemas, and small-vessel vasculitides. Most of these can be distinguished from urticaria by epidermal changes such as parakeratosis, acanthosis, spongiosis, and basal layer vacuolization, by lymphocytic infiltrates which usually are heavier and manifest a more pronounced perivascular distribution, and the absence of interstitial granulocytes or prominent reticular dermal edema. With respect to gyrate erythemas, these can either be superficial, associated with the aforementioned epidermal changes, or deep; the latter show striking perivascular "cuffing" of lymphocytes, accompanied in some cases by eosinophils. The absence of vascular fibrin deposition, leukocytoclastic debris, or extravasation of fragmented red blood cells enables distinction from leukocytoclastic vasculitis. More challenging is the distinction from urticarial vasculitis, which characteristically manifests only mild vascular injury, but should be suspected when urticariallike lesions resolve clinically after more than 24 h with a residuum of pigmentation. The histopathology of

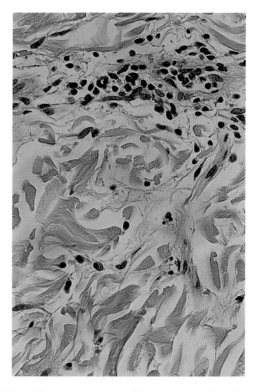

FIGURE 5-2   Urticaria. A sparse superficial and deep perivascular mixed cell infiltrate is seen, including lymphocytes, neutrophils, and eosinophils. Neutrophils are present in blood vessels, and a sparse interstitial infiltrate of granulocytes is present.

TABLE 5-2

The Common Forms of Chronic Urticarias (after Greaves)[1]

Type of Urticaria	Principal Clinical Features	Histopathological Features	Diagnostic Test
Acute and chronic idiopathic	Profuse or sparse edematous papules or wheals, often annular with itching	Absence of epidermal alteration Dermal edema Sparse perivascular infiltrate composed of lymphocytes, eosinophils, neutrophils (variable)	
Symptomatic dermatographism	Itchy, linear wheals with a surrounding bright red flare at sites of scratching or rubbing	As above	Light stroking of skin causes an immediate wheal with itching
Other physical urticarias			
Cold	Itchy pale or red swelling at sites of contact with cold surfaces or fluids	As above but neutrophils may be more prominent	Ten-min application of an ice pack causes a wheal within 5 min of the removal of ice
Pressure	Large painful or itchy red swelling at sites of pressure lasting 24 h or more	As above but neutrophils may be more prominent	Application of pressure produces persistent red swelling after a latent period of 1 to 4 h
Solar	Itchy pale or red swelling at site of exposure to ultraviolet or visible light	As above but neutrophils may be more prominent	Irradiation by a 2.5 kW 290–690 nm source for 30–120 seconds causes wheals in 30 min)
Cholinergic	Itchy wheals on trunk, neck, and limbs	As above but neutrophils may be more prominent	Exercise or a hot shower elicits eruption

urticarial vasculitis is typified by a mild form of leukocytoclastic vasculitis comprising erythrocyte extravasation, slight leukocytoclasia, and neutrophilic infiltration of venular endothelia with minimal fibrin deposition. The same underlying systemic diseases as are implicated in leukocytoclastic vasculitis, such as malignancies or systemic connective tissue diseases, are seen in urticarial vasculitis, extracutaneous manifestations of which include involvement of synovia, kidneys, and ophthalmologic, respiratory, central nervous, and gastrointestinal systems.[2,6]

TOXIC ERYTHEMA OF PREGNANCY

Clinical Features This distinctive eruption, the most common dermatosis of pregnancy, occurs in 1 in 20 pregnancies and is characterized by pruritic papules and urticarial plaques, sometimes with superimposed vesicles, in and near abdominal striae.[7] It usually develops in the last few weeks of pregnancy and may spread to the extremities or become generalized. Periumbilical sparing and spontaneous resolution are characteristic. The association of this eruption with increased fetal weight

and maternal weight gain raises the possibility that it relates somehow to excessive abdominal distention. Alternate appellations include polymorphic eruption of pregnancy and pruritic urticarial papules and plaques of pregnancy (PUPPP) (Table 5-3).

Histopathological Features Superficial perivascular lymphocytic or lymphocytic and eosinophilic infiltrates with a nondescript appearance, accompanied in one-third of cases by exocytosis and spongiosis, are characteristic (Fig. 5-3). Fibroblast proliferation is an infrequent concomitant.[7] Leukocyte debris may be present, but there is no vascular fibrin deposition to suggest a leukocytoclastic vasculitis. Although often nonreactive by direct immunofluorescent testing, lesions of PUPPP may show patchy IgM, C3, and fibrin deposition at the dermoepidermal junction (personal observation) suggesting a delayed-type hypersensitivity reaction as the pathophysiologic basis.[7,8]

Differential Diagnosis The differential diagnosis of PUPPP includes dermal hypersensitivity reactions such as those owing to drugs, atopy, contactants, insect bites, and herpes gestationis. Most of the hypersensi-

TABLE 5-3

Pruritic Urticarial Papules and Plaques of Pregnancy

Clinical Features

Pruritic erythematous urticarial papules, vesicles, and plaques in
  and near abdominal striae
Most common dermatosis of pregnancy
Occurs classically in week 35+

Histopathological Features

Superficial perivascular lymphocytic or lymphocytic and eosinophilic
  dermal infiltrate
Exocytosis and spongiosis in one-third of cases

Differential Diagnosis

Delayed-type hypersensitivity reactions of diverse causes:
  Drugs
  Contactants
  Insect bite reactions (including papular urticaria)
Atopic dermatitis
Herpes gestationis

TABLE 5-4

Erythema Annulare Centrifugum (EAC)

Clinical Features

Erythematous infiltrated papules which slowly enlarge to
  form annular or arciform arrays

Histopathological Features

Superficial EAC
  Superficial perivascular lymphocytic or lymphocytic and
    eosinophilic dermal infiltrate
  Exocytosis and spongiosis with focal parakeratosis
Superficial and deep EAC
  Superficial and deep perivascular lymphocytic or lymphocytic and
    eosinophilic dermal infiltrate with prominent "cuffing" around
    blood vessels

Differential Diagnosis

Superficial EAC
  Delayed-type hypersensitivity reactions including:
    Allergic contact reactions
    Atopy
    Pityriasis rosea
    Pityriasiform and other drug eruptions
    Polymorphous light eruption and other photoallergic conditions
    Insect bite reactions
  Connective tissue diseases including:
    Discoid lupus erythematosus
    Subacute lupus erythematosus
    Relapsing polychondritis
    Sjogren's syndrome
    Mixed connective tissue disease
Superficial and deep EAC
  Jessner's lymphocytic infiltrate
  Connective tissue diseases including:
    Discoid and tumid lupus erythematosus
    Relapsing polychondritis
    Sjogren's syndrome
    Mixed connective tissue disease
  Delayed-type hypersensitivity reactions including:
    Dermal contact hypersensitivity reactions (i.e., to nickel)
    Polymorphous light eruption, deep variant
    Insect bite reactions and papular urticaria

tivity reactions cannot be reliably distinguished from PUPPP because of its nondescript histomorphology. Herpes gestationis can occur at any time during pregnancy, and often is raised as a clinical consideration. Lesions of herpes gestationis often show subepidermal blisters accompanied by eosinophils in the epidermis, at tips of dermal papillae, and in a perivascular disposition, associated with focal necrosis of basal layer keratinocytes and colloid body formation. Circulating anti–basement membrane IgG is demonstrable by indirect immunofluorescence in 25 percent of herpes gestationis patients, associated invariably with linear C3 deposition along the dermoepidermal junction and, in 50 percent of cases, a similar pattern of IgG deposition.[7,9] The distinction between herpes gestationis and PUPPP is an important one, as the former is associated with increased fetal morbidity and may require systemic steroid therapy, whereas PUPPP is a self-limited eruption with no associated fetal morbidity.[7,9] The linear dermoepidermal junction deposition of C3 and IgG that characterizes herpes gestationis is not seen in PUPPP. Direct immunofluorescence testing thus is a valuable adjunct to light microscopy in making the distinction.

GYRATE ERYTHEMAS

Clinical Features   The gyrate erythemas are characterized by annular, polycyclic, often migratory erythematous macular eruptions.

Erythema annulare centrifugum (Table 5-4) comprises one or more annular fixed or migratory erythematous lesions, often with a fine peripheral scale at the advancing edge, involving the trunk and proximal extremities. A number of trigger factors are implicated (see Table 5-5).[10] Although lesions may be seen in the neonatal period, in which they may be a sign of maternal systemic lupus erythematosus, onset is most often in early adulthood or middle age. The initial lesion, a pink infiltrated papule, slowly enlarges to form a ring as its center fades, and in some cases reaches a diameter of 8.0 cm over a 2- to 3-week period. Eccentric expansion may yield an irregular arciform pattern. Lesions may last from days to months and may be associated with purpuric or pigmented residua. The clinical differential diagnosis includes granuloma annulare, which more often has a beaded edge, fungal infections,

parapsoriasis, sarcoidosis, urticaria, urticarial bullous pemphigoid, connective tissue disease, atypical forms of pityriasis rosea (particularly pityriasis marginatum et circinatum of Vidal), and necrolytic migratory erythema associated with pancreatic islet cell neoplasms. The nature of the factors that trigger erythema annulare centrifugum implicate delayed-type hypersensitivity as the pathogenetic basis.

Erythema gyratum repens manifests as broad polycyclic patches that resemble the rings on the cut surface of a tree. This eruption is associated with internal organ malignancies, tuberculosis, ichthyotic states, pityriasis rubra pilaris, and CREST syndrome.[11] Clinical mimics include atypical cases of autoimmune bullous dermatoses, such as bullous pemphigoid or linear IgA disease, and subacute cutaneous lupus erythematosus.[11]

Erythema marginatum is associated with rheumatic fever in less than 10 percent of cases and comprises erythematous macules with a raised edge and a pale center.

TABLE 5-5

Possible Trigger Factors for Erythema Annulare Centrifugum

Infective and Nondrug Hypersensitivity States
Tinea
Candida infection
Ascaris infection
Viral infection
Ingested molds

Autoimmune diseases
Sjogren's syndrome
Hyperthyroidism
Liver disease
Immunologic disturbances

Drug-related
Cimetidine
Salicylates
Diazide
Antimalarials

Neoplastic
Liver disease
Carcinoma
Dysproteinemia
Blood dyscrasias

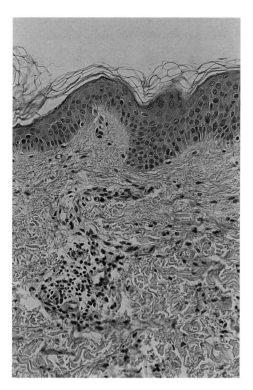

FIGURE 5-3 Pruritic urticarial papules and plaques of pregnancy. A nondescript superficial perivascular infiltrate of lymphocytes and eosinophils is present.

Erythema chronicum migrans, the distinctive cutaneous manifestation of stage I Lyme disease, is discussed elsewhere (Chapter 20).

Histopathological Features There are two discrete forms of erythema annulare centrifugum. The superficial variant shows epidermal spongiosis and parakeratosis with papillary dermal edema, which may be considerable (Fig. 5-4). There are superficial perivascular lymphocytic infiltrates that typically exhibit some degree of "cuffing" about blood vessels in addition to a loose scattering of lymphocytes in the papillary dermis. The second form is a superficial and deep one in which a sharply demarcated perivascular lymphoid infiltrate spares the overlying epidermis (Fig. 5-5).[12] Endothelial swelling may be seen in both types and may be accompanied by hemorrhage, but fibrin deposition is absent. Eosinophils are seen in roughly 10 to 20 percent of cases (Fig. 5-6) (personal observation).

The histopathology of erythema gyratum repens comprises spongiosis with parakeratosis, focal mild perivascular lymphoid infiltrates, and variable edema or eosinophilia of the dermis.

Skin biopsies in erythema marginatum show perivascular neutrophilic, lymphocytic, and eosinophilic infiltrates with perivascular debris but absent vascular fibrin deposition.

Differential Diagnosis The differential diagnosis of the superficial variant of erythema annulare centrifugum includes allergic contact reactions, atopy, pityriasis rosea and pityriasiform drug eruptions, polymorphous light eruption and other photoallergic conditions, insect bite reactions, and occasional cases of lupus erythematosus. With respect to the superficial and deep forms of gyrate erythema, differential diagnostic considerations include Jessner's lymphocytic infiltrate, connective tissue diseases such as discoid and tumid lupus erythematosus, relapsing polychondritis, Sjogren's syndrome, and lesions of mixed connective tissue disease and subacute lupus erythematosus that have been treated

with topical steroids, all of which may manifest perivascular lymphocytic infiltrates without epidermal alterations, and those hypersensitivity reactions whose expression is principally confined to the dermis. With respect to Jessner's lymphocytic infiltrate and the aforementioned connective tissue diseases, eosinophils are most unusual, whereas in tumid lupus erythematosus, massive mucin deposition is characteristic and the lymphocytic infiltrate usually is sparse. The dermal contact hypersensitivity reactions, such as those owing to nickel, manifest perivascular lymphocytic and eosinophilic infiltrates in the absence of epidermal changes.

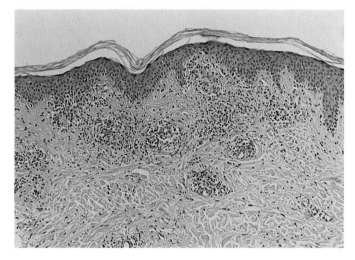

FIGURE 5-4 Erythema annulare centrifugum, superficial type. There is a moderately heavy superficial perivascular infiltrate of lymphocytes and eosinophils, associated with exocytosis of inflammatory cells, concomitant spongiosis, and, often, an adherant plasma-containing scale-crust.

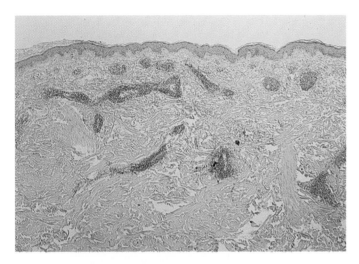

FIGURE 5-5 Erythema annulare centrifugum, superficial and deep type. A moderately heavy superficial and deep perivascular lymphocyte-predominant infiltrate manifests "cuffing" around blood vessel, without exocytosis of inflammatory cells into the epidermis, which shows no appreciable pathology.

With respect to erythema marginatum, other conditions that combine perivascular lymphocytic infiltrates with a neutrophilic and eosinophilic component in the presence of perivascular leukocytoclasia but absent or minimal fibrin deposition include urticaria, urticarial vasculitis, rheumatoid neutrophilic dermatosis, and some cases of Henoch-Schonlein purpura. With respect to the latter, although a mononuclear-cell predominant vascular injury pattern may be seen, most cases manifest a pustular vasculitis, and are easily distinguished from erythema marginatum.[13]

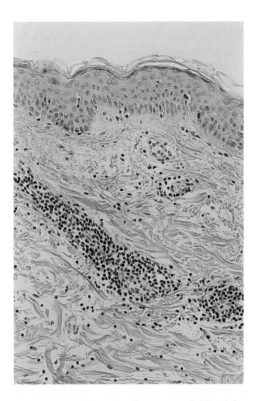

FIGURE 5-6 Erythema annulare centrifugum, superficial and deep type. The dermal lymphocyte-predominant infiltrate is associated with scattered eosinophils and mural and endothelial swelling, but no fibrin deposition within blood vessel walls or lumina.

TABLE 5-6
Pityriasis Lichenoides

Clinical Features

Self-limited dermatosis comprising 10s to 100s of hemorrhagic
  papules, pustules, or vesicles that heal with scars
Onset in first–third decades with male predominance
Spectrum ranging from acute (pityriasis lichenoides et varioliformis
  acuta, or PLEVA) to chronic (pityriasis lichenoides chronica, or
  PLC) eruptions

Histopathological Features

PLEVA
Lymphocytic infiltrate obscures dermoepidermal junction
Erythrocyte extravasation into degenerating epidermis
Papillary dermal edema
Wedge-shaped superficial and deep, purely lymphocytic dermal
  infiltrate
Sometimes atypical transformed lymphocytes

PLC
Confluent parakeratotic scale, often containing neutrophils
More sparse lymphocytic interface injury pattern
Less conspicuous epidermal injury and hemorrhage
Melanophages in papillary dermis

Differential Diagnosis

Pityriasis rosea
Small plaque parapsoriasis
Viral exanthemata
Lymphomatoid papulosis
Secondary syphilis
Connective tissue disease

PITYRIASIS LICHENOIDES

Clinical Features   Pityriasis lichenoides is a self-limited dermatosis which usually presents in the first to third decades of life and shows a predilection for males (Table 5-6).[14] The onset ranges from an acute eruption termed pityriasis lichenoides et varioliformis acuta (PLEVA), comprising hemorrhagic papules (thus "pityriasis lichenoides"), pustules, or vesicles that heal with scars mimicking smallpox (thus "varioliformis"), to a chronic eruption termed pityriasis lichenoides chronica. The latter may heal with postinflammatory hyperpigmention. Lesions number from dozens to hundreds and frequently affect the anterior trunk and flexor aspects of the proximal extremities preferentially. The putative etiology is viral in nature, based in part on the clinical behavior and in part on phenotypic studies that show a characteristic infiltrate comprising CD8+ lymphocytes admixed with a minor populace of Langerhans' cells or indeterminate cells. Epidermal HLA-DR-expressing keratinocytes are common, and IgM and C3 deposition often is seen along the basement membrane zone and in blood vessels.

Histopathological Features   In PLEVA, the dermoepidermal junction often is obscured by a pure population of lymphocytes associated with basal layer vacuolopathy, colloid body formation, and variable, sometimes confluent, epidermal necrosis (see Chap. 3). Intraepidermal hemorrhage, endothelial swelling, papillary dermal edema, bleeding, and wedge-shaped superficial and deep dermal lymphoid infiltrates are characteristic.[14] The parakeratotic scale often contains neutrophils. A rare extreme expression of the disease is the ulceronecrotic variant, in which necrotizing lymphocytic vasculitis produces confluent epidermal necrosis.[15] In pityriasis lichenoides chronica, parakeratosis often is confluent, and epidermal injury less striking.[16] The epidermis may show superficial pallor, and melanophages often are present in the papillary dermis, reflecting basal layer injury. As PLEVA and pityriasis lichenoides chronica represent opposite poles of a spectrum of injury, not all cases can be comfortably classified as one or the other; some authorities sign out most cases simply as pityriasis lichenoides without further qualification.

Differential Diagnosis   The differential diagnosis includes pityriasis rosea, in which discrete mounds of parakeratin overlie foci of epidermal spongiosis, and small-plaque parapsoriasis, where the degree of epithelial injury generally is less and the infiltrate more sparse.[16] The common viral exanthem pattern may mimic PLEVA by virtue of a perivascular and interface lymphocytic infiltrate accompanied by basilar vacuolopathy with scattered cytoid bodies and streak dyskeratosis, but the epidermis usually is surmounted by a basket-weave pattern of orthokeratinization. Similar features also typify evolving lesions of erythema multiforme, which may show scattered eosinophils in the dermal inflammatory populace, enabling distinction. Secondary syphilis merits consideration, but usually has a significant plasma cell component, at variance with the pure lymphoid populace of pityriasis lichenoides. Connective tissue diseases with pronounced keratinocyte degeneration, such as subacute cutaneous lupus erythematosus, can be problematic if a superfical shave biopsy is submitted, and the deep infiltrates of pityriasis lichenoides, which would enable distinction, cannot be assessed (see the following text on connective tissue diseases).

PIGMENTED PURPURIC DERMATOSES

The pigmented purpuric dermatoses, a group of idiopathic disorders having in common a lymphocytic vascular reaction associated with endothelial swelling and perivascular hemorrhage, are discussed in detail elsewhere (see Chap. 9).

PERNIOSIS

Clinical Features   Perniosis, or chilblains, is a form of cold-induced injury that manifests as inflammatory red to purple macules, nodules, papules, or plaques, at times accompanied by overlying blisters, erosions, or ulcers characteristically distributed symmetrically on acral skin, thighs, or buttocks (Table 5-7). It is common in the humid climate of northwest Europe, but is decreasing in frequency with modern home heating methods.[17–20] A vasospastic response to cold with resultant ischemia of vessel walls is the proposed etiology, with humidity playing a role through enhanced air conductivity of temperature. Lesions clear dramatically with warming.[17–21] An association with anorexia nervosa has been reported; it appears that anxiety states and the ingestion of anti-depressant medications such as Prozac (personal observation), which has immune dysregulating properties, may play a role.[22,23]

Histopathological Features   Biopsies show a dense superficial or superficial and deep perivascular lymphocytic infiltrate with exocytosis to retia and acrosyringia (Fig, 5-7). Epithelial necrosis occasionally is observed. Edema of blood vessel walls accompanied by transmural lymphocytic infiltrates is characteristic, and thrombi may be observed in dermal papillae capillaries. Pronounced papillary dermal edema often is present.[19] Mucinosis around the eccrine coil and luminal fibrin thrombi localized to dermal papillae capillaries may be seen, but pan-dermal mucin deposition or reticular dermal vascular thrombosis is unusual.[20,21]

TABLE 5-7

Perniosis (Chilblains)

Clinical Features

Cold-induced purplish macules, papules, and nodules involving acral, thigh, or buttock skin
Occurs in humid climates

Histopathological Features

Dense superficial and deep lymphocytic infiltrates with preferential migration to epidermal retia and acrosyringia
Occasional fibrin thrombi in dermal papillae capillaries
Transmural lymphocytic migration through blood vessel walls
Marked papillary dermal edema
Mucinosis around eccrine coil

Differential Diagnosis

Connective tissue diseases, especially:
    Chilblains lupus erythematosus
    Mixed connective tissue disease
Behçet's disease
Erythema multiforme
Viral exanthems

Differential Diagnosis   Other causes of acral purpuric papulonodular lesions include hyperviscosity and procoagulant states, namely hypergammaglobulinemia, essential cryofibrinogenemia, antiphospholipid antibody syndrome, rheumatoid arthritis, Crohn's disease, Behçet's disease, and systemic lupus erythematosus.[24,25] The latter lesions are termed "chilblains lupus erythematosus," and resemble Behçet's disease by virtue of the distribution of the infiltrate and the presence of a

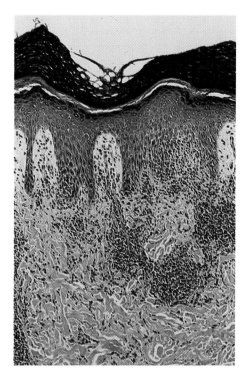

FIGURE 5-7   Perniosis (chilblains). There is a dense superficial and deep perivascular lymphocytic infiltrate associated with marked papillary dermal edema and directed migration of lymphocytes into retia and acrosyringia.

TABLE 5-8

Polymorphous Light Eruption

Clinical Features

Erythematous, pruritic papules or papulovesicles and urticarial plaques

Eruption occurs 30 min to 3 days after sun exposure, and resolves in 7–10 days

Predilection for sun-exposed sites: hands, forearms, head and neck area

Histopathological Features

Perivascular infiltrates of lymphocytes, eosinophils, and neutrophils

Exocytosis, spongiosis, vesiculation, acanthosis, and focal parakeratosis common

Some cases show vacuolopathic interface injury pattern or no epidermal changes

Marked papillary dermal edema classically

Blood vessels show ectasia and endothelial swelling which preferentially affects superficial vasculature

Differential Diagnosis

Delayed-type hypersensitivity reactions including:
    Allergic contact reactions
    Rosacea
    Other photoallergic/phototoxic eruptions
    Insect bite reactions
Connective tissue diseases including:
    Discoid lupus erythematosus
    Subacute lupus erythematosus
Jessner's lymphocytic infiltrate

---

vacuolopathic lymphocytic interface dermatitis.[26] All of the aforementioned differential diagnostic considerations are associated with reticular dermal endovascular thrombi. The perniosislike lesions in Crohn's disease characteristically manifest an interstitial histiocytopathy mimicking granuloma annulare, accompanied at times by granulomatous vasculitis.[27] Pan-dermal mucinosis should prompt consideration of a systemic connective tissue disease.[20,21] Erythema multiforme merits consideration, but rarely shows vasculopathy.

RICKETTSIAL AND VIRAL INFECTION

Rickettsial and viral infections produce a lymphocytic interface injury pattern mimicking the common viral exanthem pattern, often in concert with vascular injury, and are discussed in detail elsewhere (Chapter 20).

POLYMORPHOUS LIGHT ERUPTION

Clinical Features   Polymorphous light eruption is an idiopathic photoinduced eruption. It likely represents the combined effects of phototoxicity and a delayed-type hypersensitivity reaction to ultraviolet light, as early lesions are dominated by CD4+ lymphocytes, whereas late lesions manifest a CD8-predominant populace (Table 5-8). Lesions manifest as pruritic erythematous papules, papulovesicles, or urticarial plaques that erupt 30 min to 3 days after ultraviolet light exposure and characteristically resolve in 7 to 10 days.[28] Lesions may appear eczematous or may resemble pemphigus, prurigo nodularis, erythema multiforme, or insect bite reactions. There is a predilection for the hands, forearms, upper arms, and head and neck region. Females are preferen-

tially affected; onset is classically in the third decade of life. Roughly 50 percent of patients show decreasing photosensitivity over time.

Histopathological Features   Characteristic findings include papillary dermal edema accompanied in early lesions by a superficial perivascular lymphoid infiltrate (Fig. 5-8) and in late lesions by a moderate to intense superficial and deep lymphocytic infiltrate, which often manifests perivascular "cuffing." Eosinophils, neutrophils, hemorrhage, and vesiculation owing to marked papillary dermal edema may be seen (Fig. 5-9). The epidermis may be normal or may show basal layer vacuolization, acanthosis, parakeratosis, spongiosis, vesiculation, and, uncommonly, necrosis.[29] Vascular changes comprising mural and endothelial swelling and edema diminish in the depths of the biopsy. By direct immunofluorescence examination, perivascular IgM and C3 deposition is seen in the setting of a negative lupus band test.

Differential Diagnosis   The differential diagnosis of polymorphous light eruption includes the other photoallergic and phototoxic dermatoses, including those that are drug-related (see Chap. 22); lupus erythematosus; Jessner's lymphocytic infiltrate; the gyrate erythemas, particularly superficial erythema annulare centrifugum; granuloma faciale; and other delayed-type hypersensitivity reactions such as rosacea, atopy, insect bite, and contact reactions. Whereas distinction from photoallergic eruptions may be impossible, epidermal changes tend to be more pronounced than in polymorphous light eruption. Purely phototoxic eruptions show a greater degree of epidermal necrosis. The pattern of epithelial injury in lupus erythematosus is one of vacuolopathic basal layer degeneration usually associated with atrophy, whereas Jessner's lymphocytic infiltrate typically spares the epidermis altogether. The superficial gyrate erythemas show eczematous epithelial changes as may be seen in polymorphous light eruption, accompanied by a similar pattern of dermal inflammation, but generally lack a neutrophilic component. Granuloma faciale manifests a dermal inflammatory infiltrate of a similarly polymorphous composition, but the infiltrate usually is much more dense, is associated with a grenz zone of papillary dermal sparing, and is accompanied by vasculitic alterations and eosinophilic dermal trabeculation, features not seen in polymorphous light eruption. Acne rosacea frequently manifests eczematous alterations, but demodectic mites commonly are present in hair follicles, and the dermal infiltrate usually is folliculocentric. The dermal neutrophilia seen in some examples of polymorphous light eruption would not be a feature of most other types of hypersensitivity reaction.

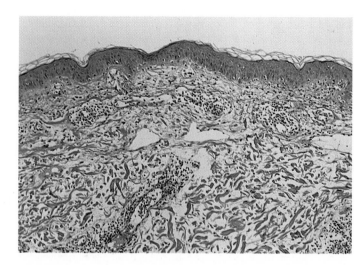

FIGURE 5-8 Polymorphous light eruption. A superficial perivascular lymphocytic infiltrate is associated with papillary dermal edema in the absence of an interface dermatitis or eczematous epithelial alterations.

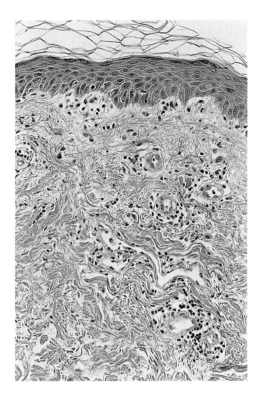

FIGURE 5-9   Polymorphous light eruption. In addition to a superficial perivascular lymphocytic infiltrate and papillary dermal edema, there is an infiltrate of neutrophils approximating the dermoepidermal junction.

CONNECTIVE TISSUE DISEASES

The manifestations of connective tissue disease in the skin encompass vasculopathy and vasculitis of leukocytoclastic, granulomatous, and lymphocytic subtypes; panniculitis; and dermal and epidermal infiltrates. The vasculitides and panniculitides are addressed elsewhere. With respect to the epidermal and dermal findings, the characteristic morphology seen in most skin lesions of lupus erythematosus, dermatomyositis, relapsing polychondritis (personal observation), Sjogren's syndrome, and mixed connective tissue disease comprises a variable superficial or superficial and deep lymphocytic infiltrate in concert with a lymphocytic interface dermatitis ranging from a subtle cell-poor vacuolopathic injury pattern to a lichenoid infiltrate.[30–33] The hallmark of the cell-poor interface dermatitis, the causes of which are listed in Table 5-9, is a sparse number of lymphocytes scattered along the dermoepidermal junction with concomitant degenerative epithelial changes manifested by basilar vacuolopathy and dyskeratosis.

Relatively specific to the connective tissue diseases are hyperkeratosis with follicular and acrosyringeal plugging, epidermal atrophy, basement membrane zone thickening, and prominent dermal mucinosis. In those cases of cell-poor interface dermatitis owing to hypersensitivity reactions, where the insult is acute, no alteration of the stratum corneum or of the basement membrane zone is seen, nor is dermal mucinosis conspicuous.

Lupus Erythematosus

Clinical Features   Lupus erythematosus (LE) is an autoimmune disorder affecting skin, hematopoietic and lymphoreticular organs, joints, kidney, lung, serosa, and cardiovascular structures in concert or in isolation. Lupus erythematosus is subdivided clinically into systemic (SLE), subacute cutaneous (SCLE), and discoid (DLE) forms.[30,34–36] A

TABLE 5-9
Causes of a Cell-Poor Interface Dermatitis

Connective tissue disease syndromes
   Systemic lupus erythematosus
   Subacute cutaneous lupus erythematosus
   Dermatomyositis
   Mixed connective tissue disease
Hypersensitivity reactions
   Erythema multiforme
   Drug reaction
   Viral exanthem
   Graft-versus-host disease

---

diagnosis of SLE is based on the presence of four or more of the criteria of the American Rheumatology Association (see Table 5-10).[34] Patients with SCLE manifest photodistributed, annular papulosquamous eruptions accompanied by extracutaneous manifestations that, if present, are mild in nature, such as microhematuria or arthralgia.[30] In DLE disease is restricted to a cutaneous expression as one or more scaling plaques in photodistributed areas, typically involving the head and neck region.

Histopathological Features   Some authors aver that light microscopy has limitations in the subclassification of LE[36] and that the differences between subtypes reflect lesional age (Table 5-11). However, although it is true that a sparse interface lymphocytic infiltrate in the incipient lesion of DLE may mimic the more ominous systemic form, the pattern of disease progression, seen in a minority of patients, is from DLE to SLE and not vice versa. Certain features prove particularly helpful in subclassification.[30] Lesions of SLE, for example, show a pauci-inflam-

---

TABLE 5-10
Revised Criteria of the American Rheumatology Association for the Classification of Systemic Lupus Erythematosus (SLE) (after Tan et al.)[34]

1. Malar rash
2. Discoid rash
3. Photosensitivity
4. Oral ulcers
5. Arthritis
6. Serositis: (a) pleuritis or (b) pericarditis
7. Renal disorder: (a) proteinuria >0.5 g/24 h or 3+, persistently, or (b) cellular casts
8. Neurological disorder: (a) seizures or (b) psychosis (having excluded other causes, e.g., drugs)
9. Hematologic disorders:
    Hemolytic anemia
    Leukopenia $<4.0 \times 10^9$/L on two or more occasions
    Lymphopenia $<1.5 \times 10^9$/L on two or more occasions
    Thrombocytopenia $<100 \times 10^9$/L
10. Immunologic disorders:
    Positive LE cell
    Raised anti-native DNA antibody binding
    Anti-Sm antibody
    False-positive serologic test for syphilis, present for at least 6 months
11. Antinuclear antibody in raised titer

Sm, Smith antigen

TABLE 5-11

Histopathological Criteria for Subtypes of Lupus Erythematosus (after Magro et al.)[30]

I. *Systemic lupus erythematosus*
   Pauci-inflammatory interface dermatitis
   Slight to absent epidermal atrophy
   Basement membrane zone of normal thickness
   No follicular plugging
   Prominent papillary dermal edema and reticular dermal mucin accumulation

II. *Subacute cutaneous lupus erythematosus*
   Prominent suprabasilar exocytosis of lymphocytes and dyskeratosis extending into upper spinous layers
   Prominent epidermal atrophy
   Follicular plugging or basement membrane zone thickening minimal or absent
   Mild to moderate mononuclear cell infiltrate confined to the superficial dermis

III. *Discoid lupus erythematosus*
   Lymphocyte-rich interface dermatitis
   Less epidermal atrophy than SCLE; sometimes acanthosis
   Prominent basement membrane zone thickening
   Prominent follicular hyperkeratosis
   Dense superficial and deep perivascular and periadnexal infiltrates with prominent follicular degeneration
   Dermal fibrosis

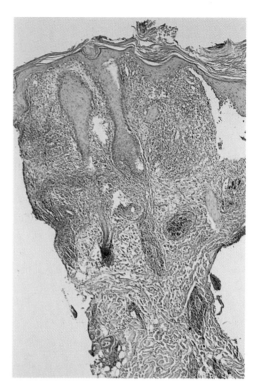

FIGURE 5-10 Discoid lupus erythematosus (DLE). A superficial and deep perivascular and periadnexal lymphocytic interface dermatitis is seen, associated with vacuolar degeneration of basal layer keratinocytes, dermal edema, and mucinosis. There is extension of the lymphocytic infiltrate to the subcutis, a feature that would be unusual in SLE or SCLE.

matory interface dermatitis with subtle basal layer vacuolopathy and none of basement membrane zone thickening, keratotic follicular plugging, or acanthosis. Skin biopsies from patients with SCLE demonstrate suprabasilar exocytosis of lymphocytes with satellitosis to necrotic keratinocytes, slight or absent thickening of the basement membrane zone or follicular plugging, and no significant deep perivascular or periadnexal infiltrate. Atrophy is variable, but usually is present in lesions of SLE and SCLE. Lesions of DLE generally manifest a heavier superficial and deep perivascular and periappendageal lymphocytic infiltrate, basement membrane zone thickening, keratotic follicular plugging, and variable acanthosis and atrophy (Fig. 5-10).

Differential Diagnosis The differential diagnosis is that of lymphocytic interface dermatitis, and embraces dermatomyositis, Sjogren's syndrome, drug-related lupus erythematosus–like eruptions, polymorphous light eruption, Jessner's lymphocytic infiltrate, and certain delayed-type hypersensitivity reactions and viral exanthemata.[31,32,37] Lichen planus can be problematic pathologically if parakeratosis and atrophy are seen. Another potential pitfall is the distinction of lichenoid actinic keratoses from lesions of DLE in sun-damaged skin. Correlation with clinical, serologic, and immunofluorescence findings then becomes imperative. These conditions are discussed elsewhere.

Direct Immunofluorescence: The Lupus Band Test and Its Implications for Pathogenesis of Connective Tissue Diseases

The examination by fluorescence microscopy of frozen sections cut from lesional or nonlesional sun-exposed or non–sun-exposed skin received fresh, in saline or transport medium, and incubated with fluorescein-conjugated antibodies monospecific for IgG, IgA, IgM, and complement constitutes the lupus band test (LBT).[38] In order to be meaningful, a positive LBT should be strictly defined as an interrupted or continuous granular or homogeneous band of IgG of moderate intensity along the dermoepidermal junction (DEJ) or a continuous granular band of marked intensity for IgM with or without a similar pattern observed for IgA.[38] One should be reluctant to designate as positive an LBT showing only small quantities of IgM deposited along the DEJ, without either IgG or IgA, in biopsies obtained from sun-exposed skin. A continuous or interrupted homogeneous linear or granular band of IgG or IgM defines a positive LBT in non–sun-exposed skin. Although a skin lesion less than 2 months old may give negative direct immunofluorescence results, a positive LBT is seen in 90 percent of lesions of DLE and SLE. A negative LBT is almost invariably seen in nonlesional skin of DLE patients, whereas over 80 percent of nonlesional skin biopsies show a positive LBT in SLE patients.[39] The LBT is positive in over 90 percent of sun-exposed nonlesional skin biopsies from SLE patients with active disease versus only one-third of patients with inactive disease.[39] Patients with SCLE tend to manifest a positive LBT in 30 to 50 percent of cases.[30]

Indirect Immunofluorescence: The Membrane Attack Complex of Complement and Its Putative Pathogenetic Role

An indirect immunofluorescence methodology to detect the presence of the membrane attack complex of complement (C_{5b-9}) in frozen sections may be a helpful adjunct to the LBT.[30] Keratinocyte fluorescence for C_{5b-9} correlates with seropositivity for antibodies to extractable nuclear antigens Smith, Ro/SSA, La/SSB, or RNP (Fig. 5-11). Patients with antibodies to these antigens often manifest distinctive clinical features

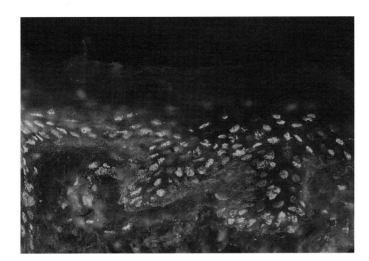

FIGURE 5-11 Mixed connective tissue disease. Positive staining of keratinocyte nuclei with C_{5b-9} correlates strongly with antibodies to extractable nuclear antigens Ro, La, Smith, or as in this case, RNP. A similar pattern may be seen in SCLE, Sjogren's syndrome, dermatomyositis, SLE, and very rare cases of DLE associated with antibodies to extractable nuclear antigens. (Mr. C. Chapman of Pathology Services, Inc, Cambridge MA, performed this study.)

and may be seronegative for antinuclear antibody.[30] Antibodies to La correlate with SICCA syndrome, and in the setting of SCLE, may be predictive of a higher incidence of pulmonary disease, whereas patients with SLE who have antibodies to Ro are at greater risk for photosensitive skin eruptions, interstitial pneumonitis, myositis, myocarditis, and complete heart block.[40] Patients with antibodies to RNP frequently have Raynaud's disease, sclerodactyly, and myopathy.[41] The Ro, La, Sm, and RNP antigens are small ribonucleoprotein macromolecules resident in nuclei, and, in the case of Ro, the cytoplasms of all eukaryotic cells.[41] Binding of the Ro autoantibody may be dependent on relocation of nuclear and cytoplasmic Ro antigens to the cell surface, an event that follows ultraviolet light exposure, viral infection, or estrogen therapy.[42–44] The presence of the membrane attack complex of complement in the basement membrane zone of skin lesions of patients with SLE and DLE and of renal tubules in patients with lupus nephritis, coupled with its absence in uninvolved skin, suggests a pathogenic role for C_{5b-9}.[30,45] The surface binding of anti-Ro antibodies may allow adherence of C_{5b-9}, the latter forming plasmalemmal pores that, in concert with antibody-dependent cellular cytotoxicity, may be an important mechanism of keratinocyte injury.[30,45,46]

Vascular deposition of C_{5b-9} is seen in dermatomyositis, in mixed connective tissue disease (MCTD), and in SLE patients who possess the lupus anticoagulant, antibodies to Ro, or biopsy proven lymphocytic vasculitis.[30,31,33,47,48] Vasculitis has been shown in skeletal muscle biopsy specimens of LE patients with anti-Ro and anti-La antibodies, perhaps reflecting localization of the Ro antigen to endothelia, as has been shown in vitro.[44,48,49] In addition to myositis, SLE patients with anti-Ro antibodies manifest cutaneous lesions virtually identical to those seen in dermatomyositis (see the following).[48]

Dermatomyositis

Clinical Features Dermatomyositis combines an inflammatory myopathy with characteristic skin lesions: the often subtle heliotrope rash, the Gottron's papule, a violaceous or hypopigmented papule over the joints of the fingers, erythema of the upper back (the "shawl sign"), extensive erythema of the extensor surfaces of the arms, and cuticular

TABLE 5-12

Criteria for Myopathic Dermatomyositis (after Bohan and Peter)[50]

Proximal symmetric muscle weakness
Elevated serum levels of muscle-derived enzymes
Abnormal electromyogram
Abnormal muscle biopsy
Cutaneous disease compatible with dermatomyositis

overgrowth with periungual telangiectasias.[31] Myopathic dermatomyositis is defined by the criteria listed in Table 5-12.[50] Although myositis usually eventuates, skin involvement may be unaccompanied initially by objective evidence of muscle disease; such cases are referred to as amyopathic dermatomyositis.[51] Coexistant malignancies are found in 6 to 60 percent of cases. Other manifestations include arthritis, myocarditis, and esophageal and pulmonary disease. Dermatomyositis appears to represent an aberrant immune response directed principally at endothelia in an immunogenetically predisposed individual following antigenic stimuli such as drugs, infections, or neoplasms.

Histopathological Features Although some observers doubt that dermatopathologic criteria exist to distinguish dermatomyositis from other connective tissue diseases, such as SLE, SCLE, and MCTD, a constellation of light-microscopic and immunofluorescent features, in concert with modern serology, is virtually pathognomonic for each of these entities.[30–33] Skin lesions of dermatomyositis manifest an atrophying cell-poor lymphocytic interface dermatitis accompanied by dermal mucinosis and vascular alterations that vary according to the age of the lesion biopsied and the presence or absence of myopathy: in patients with myopathic dermatomyositis, a characteristic injury pattern comprising a variably cell-poor thrombogenic lymphocytic vasculopathy principally affecting the dermal papillae capillaries is seen.

Immunofluorescence The immunofluorescent profile of dermatomyositis comprises a negative lupus band test in conjunction with membrane attack complex (C_{5b-9}) deposition along the dermoepidermal junction and within blood vessels.[31] Similar vascular deposition is seen in the setting of SLE with antibodies to Ro and MCTD in the setting of antibodies to RNP.[33,48] All three conditions manifest myopathy, interstitial lung disease, and vasculitis, perhaps reflecting the common localization of antibodies to endothelial RNA antigens, the expression of which is upregulated owing to endogenous or exogenous triggers.

Differential Diagnosis The differentiating points of dermatomyositis from most cases of lupus erythematosus include active vascular injury characterized by endothelial cell necrosis and intraluminal fibrin deposition along with the end sequelae of vasculopathy, namely, reduction of vascular density and vascular ectasia. Hypovascularity is more conspicuous in cases of myopathic versus amyopathic dermatomyositis, implying that cutaneous vascular changes mirror those in muscle, whereby a critical reduction in vascular density is necessary to generate objective evidence of myositis.[31,52,53] In MCTD, a lymphocytic interface injury pattern in concert with a lymphocytic vasculopathy can closely mimic dermatomyositis. However, sclerodermoid tissue alterations are fairly common in the former, but rare in the latter. Finally, eosinophils are observed in biopsies of dermatomyositis in approximately 10 to 20 percent of cases (personal observation), but are rare in idiopathic LE and MCTD, possibly reflecting a pathogenic role for aberrant delayed-type hypersensitivity in a minority of patients with dermatomyositis. The

TABLE 5-13

Diagnostic Criteria for Mixed Connective Tissue Disease (MCTD)

A diagnosis of MCTD is based on the presence of one criterion from category I, plus the criterion from category II, plus one or more criteria from category III.

I.   Common symptoms:
   Raynaud's phenomenon
   Swollen fingers or hands
II. Anti-nRNP antibody
III. Mixed findings:
   SLE-like findings:
      Polyarthritis
      Lymphadenopathy
      Facial erythema
      Pericarditis or pleuritis
      Leukocytopenia or thrombocytopenia
   PSS-like findings:
      Sclerodactyly
      Pulmonary fibrosis, restrictive changes of the lung, or
         reduced diffusion capacity
      Hypomotility or dilatation of the esophagus
   DM-like findings:
      Muscle weakness
      Increased serum level of myogenic enzymes (CPK)
      Myogenic pattern at electromyography

other causes of cell-poor vacuolopathic interface dermatitis, such as certain viral exanthems and hypersensitivity reactions, do not appear to produce the same vascular injury patterns.

Mixed Connective Tissue Disease

Clinical Features   Mixed connective tissue disease (MCTD) was first defined by Sharp as a distinct rheumatic disease syndrome associated with high titers of antibody to an extractable nuclear antigen (nRNP).[54] The typical features (see Table 5-13) include Raynaud's phenomenon, polyarthritis, polyserositis, myositis, sclerodactyly, restrictive lung disease, lymphadenopathy, and esophageal dysfunction. The cutaneous manifestations include SLE-like malar erythema, discoid plaques, an SCLE-like photodistributed eruption, swollen hands, sclerodactyly, and vasculitis.

Histopathological Features   Biopsies of the photodistributed eruptions show a cell-poor or lichenoid interface dermatitis with suprabasilar exocytosis around necrotic keratinocytes in the absence of deep periadnexal or perivascular extension or conspicuous follicular plugging.[33]

Immunofluorescence   Nuclear keratinocyte immunoreactivity with IgG and C_{5b-9} is demonstrated in all cases studied (Fig. 5-11), accompanied by a positive lupus band test in roughly one-half of cases. The in vivo speckled nuclear staining for IgG observed within keratinocytes of lesional and nonlesional skin correlates with antibodies to nRNP, the serologic hallmark of MCTD. Granular vascular deposition of immunoreactants including C_{5b-9} is also is seen.[33]

Differential Diagnosis   The histopathology of MCTD mimics SCLE by virtue of the lymphocytic interface dermatitis, but differs by showing vasculopathic alterations comprising ectasia, hypovascularity, and

luminal thrombosis confined to the superficial vascular plexus, and sometimes by a concomitant sclerodermoid tissue reaction.[33] As mentioned, distinction from dermatomyositis can be problematic. Perniosis can demonstrate a similar pattern of interface injury with associated lymphocytic vasculopathy, but the exocytosis of lymphocytes in perniosis tends to be directed to retia and acrosyringia.[20,21] The interface dermatitis of erythema multiforme often is accompanied by pronounced papillary dermal edema, tissue eosinophilia, and epidermal colloid body formation in the absence of atrophy or alterations of the stratum corneum.

REFERENCES

1. Greaves MW: Chronic urticaria. *N Engl J Med* 332:1767–1772, 1995.
2. Kobza Black A, Greaves MW, Champion RH, Pye RJ: The urticarias 1990. *Br J Dermatol* 124:100–108, 1991.
3. Doeglas HMG, Rijnten WJ, Schroder FP, Schirm J: Cold urticaria and virus infections: A clinical and serological study in 39 patients. *Br J Dermatol* 114:311–318, 1986.
4. Hide M, Francis DM, Grattan CEH, Hakimi J, Kochan JP, Greaves MW: Autoantibodies against the high affinity IgE receptor as a cause of histamine release in chronic urticaria. *N Engl J Med* 328:1599–1604, 1993.
5. Baty V, Hoen B, Hudziak H, Aghassian C, Jeandel C, Canton P: Schnitzler's syndrome: Two case reports and review of the literature. *Mayo Clin Proc* 70:570–572, 1995.
6. Mehregen DR, Hall MJ, Gibson LE: Urticarial vasculitis: A histopathologic and clinical review of 72 cases. *J Am Acad Dermatol* 26:441–448, 1992.
7. Alcalay J, Wolfe JE: Pruritic urticarial papules and plaques of pregnancy: The enigma and the confusion. *J Am Acad Dermatol* 19:1115–1116, 1988.
8. Zurn A, Celebi CR, Bernard P, Didierjean L, Saurat J-H: A prospective immunofluorescence study of 111 cases of pruritic dermatoses of pregnancy: IgM anti-basement membrane zone antibodies as a novel finding. *Br J Dermatol* 126:474–478, 1992.
9. Murray JC: Pregnancy and the skin. *Dermatol Clin* 8:327–334, 1990.
10. Champion RH. Annular erythemas, in Champion RH, Burton JL, Ebling FJG (eds): *Textbook of Dermatology*, 5th ed. Oxford: Blackwell Scientific, 1992, pp. 1839–1842.
11. Caputo R, Bencini PL, Vigo GP, Berti E, Veraldi S: Eruption resembling erythema gyratum repens in linear IgA dermatosis. *Dermatology* 190:235–237, 1995.
12. Lever WF, Schaumberg-Lever G: *Histopathology of the Skin*, 7th ed. Philadelphia: JB Lippincott, 1990, pp. 153–154.
13. Crowson AN, Magro CM: The clinical and histopathological spectrum of IgA-associated vasculitis (abstract). *Lab Invest* 76:43A, 1997.
14. Lever WF, Schaumberg-Lever G: *Histopathology of the Skin*, 7th ed. Philadelphia: JB Lippincott, 1990, pp. 177–178.
15. Lopez-Estebaranz JL, Vanaclocha F, Gil R, et al: Febrile ulceronecrotic Mucha-Habermann disease. *J Am Acad Dermatol* 29:903–906, 1993.
16. Benmaman O, Sanchez JL: Comparative clinicopathological study on pityriasis lichenoides chronica and small plaque parapsoriasis. *Am J Dermatopathol* 10:189–196, 1988.
17. Goette DK: Chilblains (Perniosis). *J Am Acad Dermatol* 23:257–262, 1990.
18. Champion RH: Reactions to cold, in Champion RH, Burton JL, Ebling FJG (eds): *Textbook of Dermatology*, 5th ed. Oxford, Blackwell Scientific, 1992, pp. 833–847.
19. Wall LM, Smith NP: Perniosis: A histopathological review. *Clin Exp Dermatol* 6:263–271, 1981.
20. Crowson AN, Magro CM: Perniosis: A forme fruste of connective tissue disease (abstract). *Lab Invest* 74:41A, 1996.
21. Crowson AN, Magro CM: Idiopathic perniosis and its mimics: A clinical and histological study of 38 cases. Perniosis and its mimics. *Hum Pathol* 28:478–484, 1997.
22. White KP, Roth MJ, Milanese A, Grant-Kels JM: Perniosis in association with anorexia nervosa. *Pediatr Dermatol* 11:1–5, 1994.
23. Crowson AN, Magro CM: Antidepressant therapy: A possible cause of atypical cutaneous lymphoid hyperplasia. *Arch Dermatol* 131:925–929, 1995.
24. Magro CM, Crowson AN: Behçet's disease. *Int J Dermatol* 34:159–165, 1995.
25. King R, Crowson AN, Murray E, Magro CM: Acral purpuric papulonodular lesions as a manifestation of Behcet's disease. *Int J Dermatol* 34:190–192, 1995.
26. Doutre MS, Beylot C, Beylot J, Pompougnac E, Royer P: Chilblain lupus erythematosus: Report of 15 cases. *Dermatology* 184:26–28, 1992.
27. Magro CM, Crowson AN, Mihm MC: Cutaneous manifestations of gastrointestinal disease and nutritional deficiency states, in Elder DE, Johnson BE, Jaworsky C, Elenitsas R (eds): *Lever's Histopathology of the Skin*, 8th ed. Philadelphia, JB Lippincott, 1997, pp. 353–368.
28. Ledo E: Photodermatoses. *Dermatol Clin* 12:797–803, 1994.
29. Hood AF: Superficial and deep infiltrates of the skin, in Farmer ER, Hood AF (ed): *Pathology of the Skin*. Norwalk, CT: Appleton and Lange, 1990, pp. 196–199.
30. Magro CM, Crowson AN, Harrist TJ: The use of antibody to C_{5b-9} in the subclassification of lupus erythematosus. *Br J Dermatol* 134:855–862, 1996.

31. Crowson AN, Magro CM: The role of microvascular injury in the pathogenesis of cutaneous lesion of dermatomyositis. *Hum Pathol* 1926:14–19, 1996.

32. Teramoto N, Katayama I, Arai H, et al: Annular erythema: A possible association with Sjogren's syndrome. *J Am Acad Dermatol* 20:596–601, 1989.

33. Magro CM, Crowson AN, Regauer S: The dermatopathology of mixed connective tissue disease. *Am J Dermatopathol* 19:205–212, 1997.

34. Tan EM, Cohen AS, Fries JF, et al:. The 1982 revised criteria for the classification of systemic lupus erythematosus. *Arthritis Rheum* 25:1271–1277, 1982.

35. David-Bajar KM:. Subacute cutaneous lupus erythematosus. *J Invest Dermatol* 100:2S–8S, 1993.

36. Jerdan MS, Hood AF, Moore GW, Callen JP: Histopathologic comparison of the subsets of lupus erythematosus. *Arch Dermatol* 126:52–55, 1990.

37. Crowson AN, Magro CM: Subacute cutaneous lupus erythematosus arising in the setting of calcium channel blocker therapy. *Hum Pathol* 28:67–73, 1997.

38. Harrist TJ, Mihm MC Jr: Cutaneous immunopathology: The diagnostic use of direct and indirect immunfluorescence techniques in diagnostic dermatopathology. *Hum Pathol* 10:625–653, 1979.

39. Lever WF, Schaumberg-Lever G: *Histopathology of the Skin*, 7th ed. Philadelphia, JB Lippincott, 1990, pp. 494–505.

40. Ben-Chetrit E: The molecular basis of the SSA/Ro antigens and the clinical significance of their autoantibodies. *Br J Rheumatol* 32:396–402, 1993.

41. McCauliffe DP, Sontheimer RD: Molecular characterization of the Ro/SS-A autoantigens. *J Invest Dermatol* 100:73S–79S, 1993.

42. Furukawa F, Kahihara-Sawami M, Lyons MB, Norris DA: Binding of antibodies to ENA SS-A/Ro and SS-B/La is induced on the surface of human keratinocytes by UVL: Implications for the pathogenesis of photosensitive cutaneous lupus. *J Invest Dermatol* 94:77–85, 1990.

43. Tesar JT, Armstrong J: Expression of Ro/SSA and La/SSB antigens on epithelial cell surface following in vitro adenovirus (AV) infection (abstr). *Arthritis Rheum* S74, C20, 1986.

44. Norris DA: Pathomechanisms of photosensitive lupus erythematosus. *J Invest Dermatol* 100:58S–68S, 1993.

45. Helm KF, Peters MS: Deposition of membrane attack complex in cutaneous lesions of lupus erythematosus. *J Am Acad Dermatol* 28:687–691, 1993.

46. Crowson AN, Magro CM: C_{5b-9} deposition at the dermoepidermal junction in lupus erythematosus. *J Am Acad Dermatol* 31:515–516, 1994.

47. Lim KL, Abdul-Wahab R, Lowe J, Powell RJ: Muscle biopsy abnormalities in systemic lupus erythematosus: Correlation with clinical and laboratory parameters. *Ann Rheum Dis* 53:178–182, 1994.

48. Magro CM, Crowson AN: A clinical and pathological study of 19 non-SCLE patients with anti-Ro antibodies (abstract). *Lab Invest* 76:45A, 1997.

49. Lanto B, Bohm F, Maffert W, Sonnichsen N: The cytotoxic effect of anti-Ro- (SS-A) antibodies and UVA light on human endothelial cells in vitro. *Dermatol Monatsschr* 176:305–311, 1990.

50. Bohan A, Peter JB: Polymyositis and dermatomyositis (first of two parts). *N Engl J Med* 292:344–347, 1975.

51. Euwer RL, Sontheimer RD: Amyopathic dermatomyositis: A review. *J Invest Dermatol* 100:124S–127S, 1993.

52. Kissel JT, Halterman RK, Rammohan KW, Mendell JR: The relationship of complement-mediated microvasculopathy to the histological features and clinical duration of disease in dermatomyositis. *Arch Neurol* 48:26–30, 1991.

53. Emslie-Smith AM, Engel AG: Microvascular changes in early and advanced dermatomyositis : A quantitative study. *Ann Neurol* 27:343–356, 1990.

54. Sharp GC, Irwin WS, Tan EM, Gould RG, Holman JR: Mixed connective tissue disease: An apparently distinct rheumatic disease syndrome associated with a specific antibody to an extractable nuclear antigen. *Am J Med* 52:148–159, 1972.

CHAPTER 6

NODULAR AND DIFFUSE CUTANEOUS INFILTRATES

Jeff D. Harvell / Wain L. White

Nodular and diffuse dermal infiltrates encompass a wide spectrum of infectious and noninfectious dermatitides, noninflammatory dermatoses, and neoplasms. Nodular infiltrates produce discrete cellular aggregations that are separated by relatively normal dermis. Diffuse infiltrates tend to involve the entire breadth of a biopsy. They may be relegated to either the upper, middle, or lower portion of a specimen or can be confluent. This chapter will focus on inflammatory diseases, dermatoses, and some entities in which the true nature of the infiltrate is not precisely defined (i.e., inflammatory vs. neoplastic). Although there are many neoplasms that display these patterns, they will be treated mainly as differential diagnoses that are discussed in depth in other sections of this text.

The conditions to be discussed are organized according to the predominant type of cutaneous inflammation seen histologically and include the following eight categories: granulomatous infiltrates, palisaded granulomatous infiltrates, suppurative granulomatous infiltrates, diffuse histiocytic infiltrates, neutrophilic infiltrates, lymphocytic-plasma cellular infiltrates, mast cell infiltrates, and eosinophilic infiltrates. Each category thus represents a fairly extensive differential diagnostic list, that is further subdivided into infectious and noninfectious conditions. Key histological/clinical features that differentiate one condition from another are provided.

A low threshold for use of special stains to demonstrate microorganisms cannot be overemphasized, especially in the case of granulomatous infiltrates (whether tuberculoid, sarcoidal, palisaded, or diffuse "histiocytic"). This same rule holds true for neutrophilic and sometimes lymphocytic-plasma cellular infiltrates seen in the setting of immunodeficiency, which often have unexpected histologic appearances. Since cutaneous infections are considered in detail elsewhere, they are presented only in tabular form here.

GRANULOMATOUS INFILTRATES

In general, all granulomatous infiltrates require the exclusion of infectious agents and foreign material through the judicious use of special stains for microorganisms and polarization microscopy. Rarely, more sophisticated techniques will be required, such as spectrophotometric or x-ray analysis. Table 6-1 lists infectious diseases whose histologic pattern is typically, but not exclusively, granulomatous. Granulomatous infiltrates in the skin can be broadly classified as conditions in which the tissue monocyte/macrophages, that is, histiocytes, are the predominating inflammatory cell. Because of their abundant cytoplasms, the infiltrate may have a pale appearance on scanning magnification, a clue to the granulomatous nature. In some granulomatous infiltrates, especially

in early disease, the aggregations of tissue macrophages are not well-defined, so it is difficult to identify a discrete granuloma. Traditionally, granulomas have been subdivided into aggregations of tissue macrophages having no or few surrounding lymphocytes ("naked" or sarcoidal granulomas), those rimmed by lymphocytes (tuberculoid granulomas), palisading granulomas in which the infiltrate forms around a central area of degeneration and/or necrosis, and foreign body type granulomas. These divisions have utility in defining a differential diagnosis, but there may be considerable overlap in any given case among these particular types.

Acne Rosacea (See also Chapter 10)

Synonyms: Rosacea; adult onset acne

The pathogenesis of acne rosacea is unknown. A disorder of dermal vessel regulation, possibly related to severe solar elastosis or, as recently suggested, to abnormal endothelial nitric oxide synthase, has been proposed.[1–3] Others consider it a sebaceous gland disorder or a folliculitis. The progression of rosacea from the telangiectatic patches to papules, pustules, and ultimately to rhinophyma remains an enigma.

Clinical Features   Patients present with erythematous papules, pustules, and/or telangiectases on the central face. Long-standing cases may eventuate into rhinophyma. An advanced granulomatous form (Lewandowsky's rosacea) presents as yellow-brown nodules. Patients may give a history of blushing or flushing with consumption of hot liquids, alcohol, or spicy foods.

Histopathological Features   The pathology of acne rosacea depends on the stage of the disease that is biopsied. Nonpustular lesions reveal a mixed perivascular and perifollicular inflammation with lymphocytes, plasma cells, macrophages (some multinucleated), and fewer scattered neutrophils and eosinophils.[2] There is usually spongiosis of the infundibular epithelium. Pronounced granulomatous inflammation often results from rupture of involved hair follicles (Fig. 6-1). In this instance, central necrosis may be present, producing caseation indistinguishable from that seen in mycobacterial infections.

The differential diagnosis of oral-facial granulomas includes perioral-periocular dermatitis, cheilitis granulomatosa, Crohn's disease, sarcoidosis, lupus vulgaris, and chronic granulomatous disease. The histologic features of acne rosacea and perioral dermatitis are identical. Lupus miliaris disseminatus faciei is probably a caricature of granulomatous acne rosacea with extensive caseation necrosis. Plasmacytic or granulomatous follicular-based inflammation should suggest acne

TABLE 6-1

Infectious Causes of Granulomatous Infiltrates

	Organism	Tissue morphology	Histopathological features
Primary cutaneous tuberculosis	M. tuberculosis	Ziehl-Neelsen-pos AFB	Caseation usually, but not always present
Lupus vulgaris	M. tuberculosis	Ziehl-Neelsen-pos AFB	Caseation usually, but not always present
Tuberculosis verrucosa cutis	M. tuberculosis	Ziehl-Neelsen-pos AFB	Pseudocarcinomatous hyperplasia
Tuberculids	Hypersensitivity reaction to M. tuberculosis	AFB not seen	Vasculitis; granuloma annulare–like
Tuberculoid leprosy	M. leprae	Acid-fast (Fite-pos)	Elongated, sausage-shaped granulomas; perineural
Chronic mucocutaneous candidiasis	C. albicans	Pseudohyphae and yeasts in stratum corneum and hair follicle (PAS-pos)	Presence of yeasts distinguishes from dermatophyte
Aspergillosis	A. flavus A. fumigatus A. niger	2–4μ septate hyphae; 45° angle branching; no yeasts	Present in blood vessel walls
Late cryptococcosis	Cryptococcus neoformans	5–15μ yeasts with thick capsule; no hyphae	Mucicarmine stains capsule red
Lobomycosis	Loboa loboi	10-μ yeast; form short linear chains, no hyphae	Mucicarmine-neg
Mucomycosis	Rhizopus Mucor Absidia	Large (30-μ) nonseptate hyphae; 90° angle branching; no yeasts	Easily seen in H&E
Secondary and tertiary syphilis	Treponema pallidum	Spirochete (Warthin-Starry-pos)	Plasma cells; lichenoid granulomatous
Brucellosis	Brucella sp.	Gram-negative, intracellular coccobacilli	Perivascular and periadnexal with plasma cells
Chronic leishmaniasis	Leishmania sp.	2–4μ round-oval protozoa with nucleus and kinetoplast (Giemsa-pos)	Oranisms within macrophages; nucleus and kinetoplast stain red with Giemsa
Tularemia	Francisella tularensis	Gram-negative coccobacillus	Not seen in H&E; may be visualized by immunomicros-copy
Prototheceosis	P. wickerhamii	5–10μ round spores; morulalike sporangia	

rosacea or perioral dermatitis. Although marked telangiectasia is a component of acne rosacea, histologically this feature often is difficult to assess objectively.

Perioral Dermatitis

Perioral dermatitis is most commonly seen among young women. The underlying etiology is not understood, but potent fluorinated topical steroids were implicated in the past. Some consider perioral dermatitis a distinct entity; others, a form of acne rosacea.[4,5]

Clinical Features   Patients present with relatively symmetric erythematous papules or pustules in a perioral distribution. Involvement of the nasolabial folds is fairly characteristic. Similar lesions may occur exclusively in a periocular distribution (periocular dermatitis).

Histopathological Features   Histology is identical to acne rosacea (see Acne Rosacea). Early lesions may show follicular spongiosis with infundibular hyperkeratosis. These changes are similar to topical steroid–induced rosacea and are indistinguishable from those of systemic steroid acne.[6]

Cheilitis Granulomatosa (Miescher-Melkersson-Rosenthal Syndrome)

Synonyms: Orofacial granulomatosis; granulomatous cheilitis

Cheilitis granulomatosa and Miescher-Melkersson-Rosenthal syndrome are overlapping clinical conditions with identical histology. The etiology is unclear.

Clinical Features   In Miescher-Melkersson-Rosenthal syndrome, patients present with a triad of lip swelling, unilateral facial paralysis, and furrowed tongue.[7] In some cases, there is more extensive facial swelling, involving the eyelids. Similar swelling may affect the penis and vulva. Mono- and oligo-symptomatic disease is the rule.[8] Patients with cheilitis granulomatosa have lip swelling alone.

Histopathological Features   There is prominent dermal edema and noncaseating poorly formed, "naked" granulomas adjacent to, and sometimes impinging on, dilated lymphatic channels (Fig. 6-2 A,B). A perivascular lymphocytic and plasma cell infiltrate also is present (Table 6-2).

The differential diagnosis of oral-facial granulomas includes acne rosacea, perioral dermatitis, Crohn's disease, sarcoidosis, lupus vul-

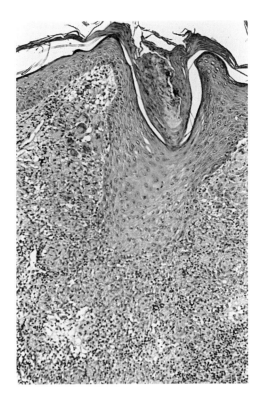

FIGURE 6-1 Acne rosacea. A perivascular and perifollicular granulomatous infiltrate focally disrupts a follicular infundibulum that contains a keratin plug with neutrophils.

garis, and chronic granulomatous disease. Poorly formed paralymphatic granulomas and dermal edema help to distinguish cheilitis granulomatosa and Miescher-Melkersson-Rosenthal syndrome.[7]

Cutaneous Crohn's Disease

Crohn's disease is a form of intrinsic inflammatory bowel disease. The pathogenesis is not understood, but it may be immunologically mediated. Unlike ulcerative colitis, all parts of the gastrointestinal tract are potentially affected, including oral and perianal areas.

Clinical Features   Oral involvement presents as cobblestoning, facial/lip swelling, or linear ulcers and may precede gastrointestinal involvement by many years. Perianal involvement presents as fistulas, sinus tracts, or ulcers.[9,10] Cutaneous involvement at sites distant from the anus or mouth has been termed "metastatic" Crohn's disease, a designation that should be avoided for it implies a malignancy. These disseminated lesions present as nodules or plaques in the flexural areas and tend to ulcerate. Lesions on the lower extremities (mimicking erythema nodosum) and the penis are common, and vulva disease also has been reported.[11] Finally, in patients with colostomies, peristomal lesions may be seen.[9,10] Rarely, patients may have quiescent bowel disease but active cutaneous lesions as the sole manifestation of persistent disease, even developing during sulfasalazine treatment. The cutaneous disease in these settings is very refractory to therapy.[11]

Histopathological Features   Regardless of site, histology reveals non-caseating granulomatous inflammation with lymphocytes and plasma cells (Fig. 6-3A), often extending deeply into the subcutaneous tissue, where it may produce an extensive septolobular panniculitis (Table 6-3). Palisaded granulomatous areas may be present as well as granulomatous vasculitis (Fig. 6-3B).[11] On genitalia, marked edema may accompany the granulomatous changes.

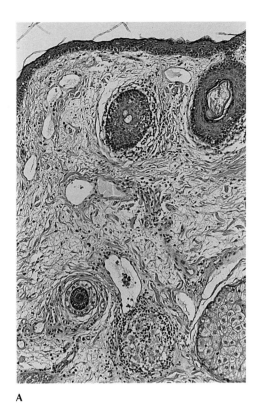

A

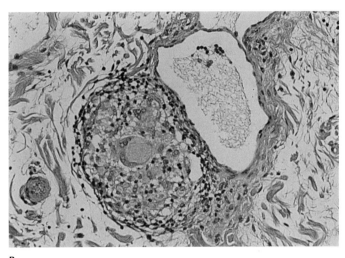

B

FIGURE 6-2 Cheilitis granulomatosa. (Miescher-Melkersson-Rosenthal syndrome.) (*A,B*) Marked edema of the dermis is accompanied by discrete granulomata that are positioned adjacent to dilated lymphatics.

The differential diagnosis of oral-facial granulomas includes acne rosacea, perioral dermatitis, cheilitis granulomatosa, sarcoidosis, lupus vulgaris, and chronic granulomatous disease. In cheilitis granulomatosa, the granulomas are paralymphatic. In the perianal or vulvar areas, hidradenitis suppurativa enters the differential diagnosis. The granulomas of hidradenitis suppurativa are folliculocentric and often are accompanied by suppuration. Granulomas in the deep dermis or subcutis, especially with granulomatous vasculitis, should suggest Crohn's disease.[10,11]

Sarcoidosis

Sarcoidosis is a systemic disease of unknown etiology that affects multiple organ systems, typically the lungs, lymph nodes, skin, and eyes.

TABLE 6-2

Cheilitis Granulomatosa
(Miescher-Melkersson-Rosenthal Syndrome)

Clinical Features

　Miescher-Melkersson-Rosenthal syndrome
　　Lip swelling
　　Unilateral facial paralysis
　　Furrowed tongue
　Cheilitis granulomatosa
　　Lip swelling, alone

Histopathological Features

　Noncaseating granulomas adjacent to and impinging on dilated
　　lymphatics
　Dermal edema
　Perivascular lymphocytes and plasma cells

Differential Diagnosis

　Oral-facial granulomas
　　Acne rosacea
　　Perioral dermatitis
　　Crohn's disease
　　Sarcoidosis
　　Lupus vulgaris and other infections
　　Chronic granulomatous disease

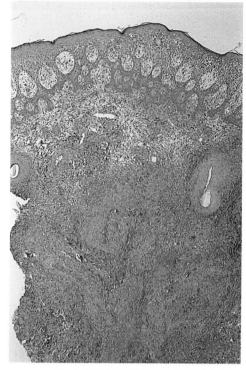

A

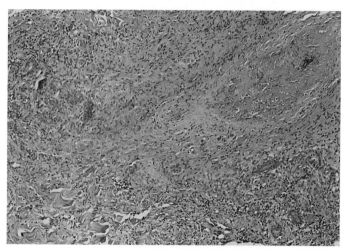

B

FIGURE 6-3 Crohn's disease. (*A,B*) A superficial and deep perivascular and interstitial mixed inflammatory cell infiltrate is associated with granulomata and vasculitis with necrosis and thrombosis. Marked edema of the papillary dermis and spongiosis are present.

Black females are the most commonly affected patient population. Approximately 25 percent of patients with systemic involvement have cutaneous involvement, and, rarely, the skin may be involved alone.[12]

Clinical Features　The clinical presentation of sarcoidosis may be extremely diverse. Smooth-surfaced violaceous nodules that develop on the nose, cheeks, or earlobes characterize lupus pernio. Other sites may show brown-purple indurated papules, nodules, or plaques with annular or serpiginous configurations. A diffuse maculopapular form also is recognized. Lesions may develop in scars or tattoos. Scalp involvement causes a scarring alopecia.[12]

Histopathological Features　Typically noncaseating epithelioid granulomas are scattered throughout the dermis without any relation to nerves, hair follicles, or blood vessels. The granulomas are usually "naked," having no or only a sparse surrounding lymphocytic infiltrate (Fig. 6-4 *A,B*). Although not frequently described, sarcoid granulomas may fill the papillary dermis and abut the epidermis, producing spongiosis, crusting, and irregular hyperplasia. The centers of some granulomas may demonstrate fibrinoid degeneration and even frank caseation necrosis when the panniculus is involved.[13]

　Asteroid bodies, Schaumann bodies, and Hamazaki-Wasserman bodies may be present but are nonspecific. One may see a number of cytoplasmic positively birefringent crystals on polarization, which probably are calcium oxalate and calcium carbonate degradation products of cell metabolism.[14] Although their appearance should make one consider a diagnosis of foreign body reaction, such crystals are a well-established phenomenon in both pulmonary and cutaneous sarcoidosis.[14–16] If the clinical picture is typical, the presence of a rare crystal by polarization microscopy should not negate a diagnosis of sarcoidosis (Table 6-4).[15,16]

Chalazion

Chalazia are eyelid lesions that are the result of a foreign body inflammatory reaction to lipid released from ruptured sebaceous glands (meibomian glands).

Clinical Features　Chalazia present as nodules of the eyelid, which are usually painless.

Histopathological Features　There is a nodular infiltrate consisting of lymphocytes, plasma cells, sometimes neutrophils, and noncaseating

TABLE 6-3

Cutaneous Crohn's Disease

Clinical Features

Facial or lip swelling
Oral mucosa cobblestoning/linear ulcers
Perianal ulcers, sinus tracts, fistulas
Ulcerating nodules/plaques in flexural areas, genitalia, or peri-
  colostomy sites
Erythema nodosum–like lesion

Histopathological Features

Noncaseating granulomas with deep dermal and subcutaneous
  extension
Granulomatous panniculitis, often

Differential Diagnosis

Oral-facial granulomas
  Acne rosacea
  Perioral dermatitis
  Cheilitis granulomatosa
  Sarcoidosis
  Lupus vulgaris and other infections
  Chronic granulomatous disease
Hidradenitis suppurativa

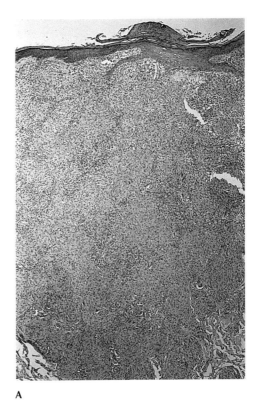

A

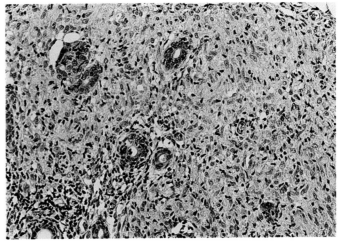

B

FIGURE 6-4   Sarcoidosis. (*A*) Confluent granulomata extend from the dermal-epidermal junction and are accompanied by only scattered lymphocytes. No caseation necrosis is identified. (*B*) The infiltrate disrupts the basement membrane zone superficially and encases the eccrine coil, deep.

granulomas centered around lipid vacuoles and/or meibomian glands (Fig. 6-5).

Granulomatous inflammation of the eyelid is most suggestive of chalazion. Acne rosacea may involve the lids, and some cases of Miescher-Melkersson-Rosenthal syndrome may primarily involve the eyelid. Recurrent chalazia should arouse suspicion for sebaceous carcinoma.[17] The presence of distinct vacuoles that represent lipid dissolved during processing in the center of the infiltrate distinguishes chalazion.

Lupus Miliaris Disseminatus Faciei

Synonyms: Acnitis; acne agminata

Lupus miliaris disseminatus faciei most likely represents a dramatic form of the granulomatous stage of acne rosacea.

Clinical Features   Like granulomatous acne rosacea, patients present with yellow-brown papules on the central face. Eyelid involvement is characteristic.

Histopathological Features   Histology is identical to granulomatous acne rosacea in which caseation necrosis may be prominent (see Acne Rosacea).

Foreign Body Granulomas

Granulomatous inflammation frequently forms around either endogenous or exogenous material that comes in direct contact with the dermis where it is perceived as foreign. This commonly occurs when cornified cells or hair, devoid of their epithelial cloaks, are extruded into the dermis. A foreign body type granulomatous infiltrate, frequently with suppuration, forms around these structures (see Ruptured Follicles and Follicular Cysts and Sinuses). Injected carbon, such as in carbon tattoos,

is inert, and if one sees granulomatous inflammation associated with a carbon tattoo, there are additional substances present (e.g., silica) that are responsible for the inflammatory response. Regardless of the origin, multinucleated giant cells, usually with nuclei conglomerated centrally or at one edge of the cell, form around the structure in an attempt to phagocytize and destroy the substance (Fig. 6-6). Table 6-5 lists both endogenous and exogenous foreign materials commonly encountered in skin specimens.

TABLE 6-4

Sarcoidosis

Clinical Features

Systemic disease with lung, eye, lymph node, and skin involvement
Lupus pernio
    violaceous nodules on nose, cheeks, earlobes
Brown-purple papules, nodules, plaques
Diffuse maculopapular form, rarely
Scarring alopecia
Development of lesions in scars, tattoos

Histopathological Features

"Naked" epithelioid granulomas, lacking well-developed lympho-
    cyte cuff
Asteroid bodies
Schaumann bodies
Hamazaki-Wasserman bodies

Differential Diagnosis

Oral-facial granulomas
    Acne rosacea
    Perioral dermatitis
    Cheilitis granulomatosa
    Crohn's disease
    Chronic granulomatous disease
Foreign body granulomas
    Tattoo pigments
    Silicates
    Zirconium
    Beryllium
Infectious agents
    Tuberculosis
    Tuberculoid leprosy
    Secondary and tertiary syphilis
    Leishmaniasis
Lymphoproliferative disorders

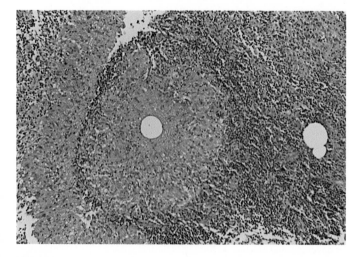

FIGURE 6-5 Chalazion. Granulomatous inflammation surrounds spherical aggregates of lipid.

Differential Diagnosis   In addition to distinguishing one type of granulomatous dermatitis from another, the other major differential diagnostic consideration is neoplastic disease that may have a granulomatous component or granulomatous appearance. Many are malignant lymphomas. Granulomatous mycosis fungoides is a histologic variant of mycosis fungoides, which features noncaseating granulomatous inflammation in addition to typical papillary dermal and epidermal changes of mycosis fungoides.[18] Granulomatous slack skin is a T-cell lymphoma and is probably a variant of granulomatous mycosis fungoides, which clinically presents as large pendulous folds of the skin in the axillae, groin, and elsewhere. Histology reveals noncaseating granulomatous inflammation with papillary dermal and epidermal changes suggesting mycosis fungoides. The multinucleated giant cells in the infiltrate are characteristic, containing large numbers of nuclei (up to 50) per cell. Elastic tissue stains reveal almost complete loss of connective tissue elastic fibers.[18]

Lethal midline granuloma and lymphomatoid granulomatosis are best considered as two variants of angiocentric T-cell lymphoma, which feature invasion of vascular walls by neoplastic and atypical T lymphocytes.[18,19] Of these two, lymphomatoid granulomatosis most frequently demonstrates cutaneous involvement. Angiocentric lymphoma should not be confused with angiotropic lymphoma, which also commonly involves the skin.[20] Angiotropic lymphoma (malignant angioendotheliomatosis; intravascular lymphomatosis) is a B-cell lymphoma, which features occlusion of vascular spaces by neoplastic B lymphocytes, and lacks the invasion of vascular walls seen in angiocentric lymphoma.[20]

Plexiform fibrohistiocytic tumor is a soft tissue neoplasm of intermediate malignancy, most commonly seen in children and young adults, and characterized by a plexiform arrangement of spindle cells in the deep dermis and subcutaneous tissue. There is a biphasic appearance with fascicles of spindle cells, merging with and surrounding small nodules composed of histiocytic cells and multinucleate osteoclastlike giant cells.[21] These nodules closely simulate granulomas but often contain erythrocytes, which is a helpful clue to the diagnosis.

Previously known as angiomatoid malignant fibrous histiocytoma, angiomatoid fibrous histiocytoma is now classified as a soft tissue neoplasm of intermediate malignancy.[22] The neoplasm most commonly occurs in children and is characterized by a well-circumscribed nodule of slightly pleomorphic spindled and epithelioid cells, irregular blood-filled spaces lined by flattened tumor cells, and lymphoid aggregates (sometimes with germinal center formation) situated at the periphery.[23] The epithelioid cells can simulate a granulomatous infiltrate.

The whorled configurations of meningocytes seen in cutaneous meningiomas and meningothelial hamartomas may bear a superficial resemblance to multinucleated giant cells. Both of these conditions occur on the scalp. Meningothelial hamartoma may be associated with alopecia. When present, psammoma bodies are a useful histologic clue.[24]

PALISADED GRANULOMATOUS INFILTRATES

Granuloma Annulare

The etiology and pathogenesis underlying granuloma annulare is unknown, but the following mechanisms have been suggested: cell-mediated immunity, immune-complex-mediated vasculitis, abnormalities of macrophage function, and primary collagen degeneration.[25] It is important to emphasize that an incomplete, early, or interstitial granuloma annulare–type histologic pattern—defined as a superficial and deep perivascular lymphocytic infiltrate with histiocytes splayed between collagen bundles—is a dermal reaction pattern that may be requisite for a specific diagnosis or simply an epiphenomenon to other events. (Also see Palisaded and Neutrophilic Granulomatous

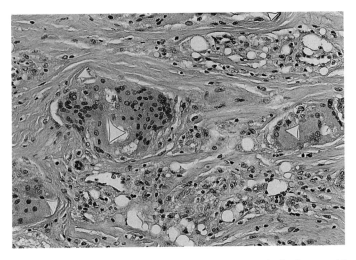

FIGURE 6-6 Foreign body granulomas. This reaction is to the foreign material from a breast implant capsule and silicone contents. Multinucleate giant cells contain fragments of the capsular wall, and foamy macrophages form small granulomas containing silicone.

Dermatitis.) For example, one can see this interstitial granuloma annulare–type reaction to resolving neutrophilic dermatitides and even insect bites with no clinical evidence of granuloma annulare. On the other hand, typical clinical lesions of granuloma annulare have been seen following herpes-virus infections and in the acquired immunodeficiency syndrome.[26,27]

Clinical Features Women are affected more often than men. Granuloma annulare presents as erythematous or flesh-colored discrete and coalescent papules in annular configurations, mainly on hands, feet, arms, and legs. Generalized, perforating, and subcutaneous forms have been described (see Deep Granuloma Annulare). Umbilicated clustered lesions simulate molluscum contagiosum.[28]

PALISADED GRANULOMATOUS FORM

Histopathological Features The fully developed lesion of granuloma annulare displays a palisaded granulomatous dermatitis surrounding an area of degenerated collagen (Fig. 6-7A). Connective tissue mucin deposition within the central degenerated collagen is a near constant

TABLE 6-5

Foreign Body Granulomas

Material	H&E features	Adjunctive techniques	Clinical/source
Suture material	Basophilic-yellow fibers	Polarizable	Prior surgery
Tattoo pigments	Black pigment granules		Chrome green; carbon; cobalt blue; cinnabar
Starch	10–20μ oval, particles	Polarizable; PAS-, GMS-pos; maltese cross birefringence	Surgical glove powder; IV drug abuse
Talc (magnesium silicate)	10–20μ particles	Polarizable, white particles; x-ray diffraction	
Oils (mineral oil, paraffin, cottenseed, sesame, camphor)	Round-ovoid clear spaces; "Swiss cheese" appearance	Sudan IV, oil red O stains reveal lipid on frozen tissue	Male genitalia (sclerosing lipogranuloma)
Silicone	Round-ovoid clear spaces; "Swiss cheese" appearance		Breast augmentation mammoplasty
Hair	Hair shaft		Interdigital web space; barbers; dog groomers
Silica (Silicon dioxide)	Sarcoidal granulomas; crystalline particles	Polarizable; spectrographic analysis	Contamination of wound from soil or glass
Zirconium	Sarcoidal granulomas	Nonpolarizable; spectrographic analysis, only	Deodorant sticks
Aluminum (adjuvant in vaccines)	Central basophilic granular material	X-ray microanalysis	Site of vaccinations
Beryllium	Sarcoidal with hyalinized central necrosis	Nonpolarizable; spectrographic analysis, only	Fluorescent light bulbs
Injectable steroid	Amphophilic granular/ amorphous material, sometimes with crystalline material	Weakly PAS-positive	Intralesional corticosteroids
Gout (sodium urate)	Amorphous amphophilic material; needle-shaped urate crystals seen in specimens fixed in alcohol	Alocohol fixation preserves crystals better than formalin; under polarized light, crystals are negatively birefringent	Big toe, helix of ear
Injectable collagen	May be sarcoidal or palisaded granulomatous	Electron microscopy	History of bovine collagen injection
Mercury	Spherical black globules with foreign body reaction, refractile brown-black granules in macrophages (up to 300μ)		Self-injection, thermometer accidents, topical mercurial preparations

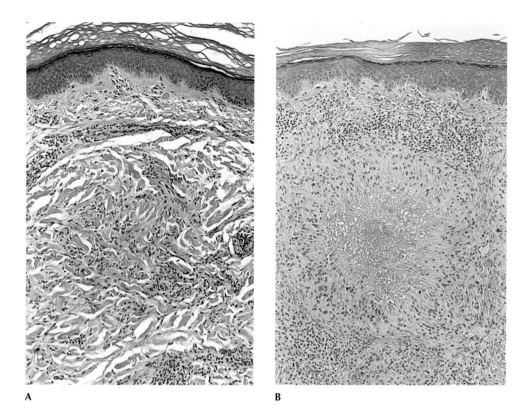

A   B

FIGURE 6-7   Granuloma annulare. (*A*) A fully developed lesion of granuloma annulare shows well-formed palisaded granulomas containing central mucin and degenerated collagen. (*B*) Early or so-called "interstitial" granuloma annulare consists of tissue macrophages (histiocytes) splayed between collagen bundles with a subtle increase in connective tissue mucin.

finding but may require special stains (i.e., alcian blue or colloidal iron) to demonstrate. In hematoxylin and eosin–stained sections, mucin appears as stringy and/or granular basophilic material. Away from the central palisade, there is a superficial and deep perivascular inflammatory cell infiltrate of lymphocytes and macrophages. Eosinophils occur in approximately 40 percent of cases.

INTERSTITIAL OR INCOMPLETE FORM

Histopathological Features   Some lesions of granuloma annulare lack typical palisading granulomatous dermatitis but, instead, show macrophages splayed between individual collagen bundles, increased connective tissue mucin deposition, and little to no collagen degeneration (Fig. 6-7*B*). This pattern has been labeled "interstitial" granuloma annulare but that term is not distinguishing, for all lesions are, in fact, interstitial. Early or incomplete lesions are a better designation.

The major differential diagnostic consideration is necrobiosis lipoidica (diabeticorum, NLD). The following features help distinguish granuloma annulare from NLD.

1. In granuloma annulare the dermis surrounding the primary focus of inflammation is normal. In NLD it is often altered.
2. NLD features a greater degree of central collagen degeneration. Sometimes the central collagen in granuloma annulare is not yet morphologically altered.
3. NLD lacks central mucin deposition as a rule. Central mucin in granuloma annulare usually is prominent, but may require special stains for demonstration.
4. The palisades in granuloma annulare are round to ovoid. In NLD, they are horizontally oriented tiers.
5. NLD features prominent plasma cells, whereas granuloma annulare does not.

6. NLD may demonstrate a granulomatous vasculitis not seen in granuloma annulare.[29]

The presence of central mucin and focal (as opposed to diffuse) dermal involvement of the dermis are distinguishing features. Eruptive xanthomas can mimic this pattern but are recognized by foamy macrophages, extracellular lipid, no mucin, and rarely uratelike crystals (see the following). Palisaded neutrophilic and granulomatous dermatitis features greater numbers of neutrophils and/or neutrophilic nuclear dust than is seen in granuloma annulare (Table 6-6).

Deep Granuloma Annulare

Synonyms: Pseudorheumatoid nodule; nodular granuloma annulare

Granuloma annulare may involve the subcutis, most often in children. Although first thought to represent a type of cutaneous involvement in rheumatoid arthritis, patients generally do not have rheumatoid arthritis. The pathogenesis is not fully understood, but local trauma may play a significant role.[30] Cell-mediated immunologic and vasculitic processes also have been implicated.

Clinical Features   Deep granuloma annulare affects children more often than adults. Subcutaneous nodules are found on the extensor aspects of hands, feet, lower legs, buttocks, scalp, and periorbitally.

Histopathological Features   Except for its subcutaneous locale, the histologic features of deep granuloma annulare are similar to the more superficial forms (Fig. 6-8). The deep reticular demis above the subcutaneous disease frequently shows focal involvement. The subcutaneous locale with central connective tissue mucin deposition is distinctive.

A subcutaneous palisaded granulomatous dermatitis with mucin deposition, especially in children, suggests deep granuloma annulare.

TABLE 6-6

Palisaded Granulomatous Dermatitis

	Granuloma Annulare (GA)	Necrobiosis Lipoidica	Rheumatoid Nodule	Rheumatic Fever Nodule	Palisaded Neutrophilic and Granulomatous Dermatitis	Necrobiotic Xanthogranuloma	Infection
Clinical Features	Annular papules Hands, feet, arms, legs	Plaques Shins	Adults with rheumatoid arthritis Subcutaneous nodules Elbows, knuckles, Achilles tendon	Children with rheumatic fever Subcutaneous nodules Elbows, knuckles	Many associated diseases Umbilicated papules Extremities	IgG paraproteinemia Papules, nodules, plaques Face, periorbital	Variable, according to specific infection Often immuno-compromised
Histopathological Features	Palisades Round/oval Discrete/focal Central mucin No plasma cells "Incomplete" form Macrophages splayed between collagen fibers Central mucin	Palisades Horizontally oriented Diffuse/full-thickness No central mucin Plasma cells Vasculitis, sometimes	Subcutaneous palisades Central eosinophilic fibrinoid necrosis No central mucin Vasculitis, sometimes Lipidized macrophages	Similar to rheumatoid nodule, sometimes with neutrophils/leukocytoclasis	Early GA-like, with prominent neutrophils/leukocyto-clasis Late Extravascular foci of degenerated stroma, mucin may be present	Central cholesterol clefts Foreign body and Touton-type giant cells Lymphocytes/plasma cells Lymphoid follicles, some-times	Central necrosis with numerous neutrophils

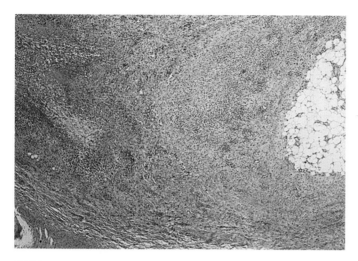

FIGURE 6-8 Subcutaneous/deep granuloma annulare. Palisaded granulomas are present in the subcutaneous septa and extend into the lobules. They contain central areas of connective tissue mucin.

Rheumatoid nodule and rheumatic fever nodule are also subcutaneous but lack mucin and instead feature central fibrinoid necrosis.[31]

Actinic Granuloma

Synonyms: Annular elastolytic granuloma; Miescher's granuloma; atypical necrobiosis lipoidica; granulomatosis disciformis of the face

Actinic granuloma is a controversial entity. Some consider it distinct.[32] Others believe it is simply granuloma annulare at sun-damaged sites, an opinion we support. Like granuloma annulare, its pathogenesis and inciting events are not understood. A cell-mediated immunologic reaction to altered elastotic fibers has been proposed.

Clinical Features   Adult patients present with expanding arciform papules and plaques, usually on the face, but also at other sun-exposed areas such as the chest, arms, and neck. Individual lesions tend to spontaneously resolve over time.

Histopathological Features   The peripheral, "active," part of the lesion demonstrates either an interstitial collection of macrophages between individual collagen bundles (similar to the incomplete pattern of granuloma annulare) (Fig. 6-9) or a prominent palisaded granulomatous dermatitis arranged around elastotic material in the superficial dermis. The giant cells contain blue-gray elastotic material, and asteroid bodies may be seen. Neither prominent mucin nor degenerated collagen typically is present. The central portion of the plaque demonstrates loss of both elastotic fibers and normal elastic fibers.[32]

The facial location and the presence of palisaded granulomas and phagocytized elastotic material (elastophagocytosis) are distinguishing features. One must be cautious, however, not to overinterpret the mere presence of elastophagocytosis, for it is a nonspecific mesenchymal reaction pattern in both sun-damaged and non-sun-damaged skin.[33,34]

Necrobiosis Lipoidica

Synonyms: necrobiosis lipoidica diabeticorum (NLD)

Approximately two-thirds of patients with necrobiosis lipoidica have diabetes mellitus. On the other hand, in patients with diabetes mellitus, necrobiosis lipoidica occurs in less than 1 percent. The etiology and

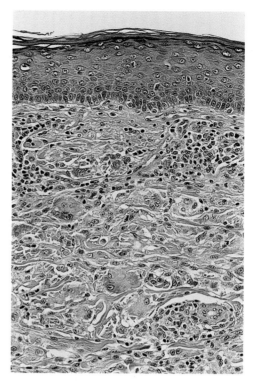

FIGURE 6-9 Actinic granuloma. This pattern is a granuloma annulare–type reaction on severely sun-damaged skin. There is extensive phagocytosis of elastic fibers (elastophagocytosis).

pathogenesis are not fully understood, but microangiopathic changes, immune complex–mediated vasculitis, and a thrombotic tendency have been implicated.[35,36]

Clinical Features   Females are affected more often than males (3:1). Adults present with waxy, indurated, yellow-brown patches or plaques with a surrounding erythematous, raised, and expanding margin. Lesions are characteristically found on the anterior shins but may also be seen on forearms, hands, and trunk.[35]

Histopathological Features   Biopsies of the erythematous margin show palisaded and granulomatous dermatitis, often involving full-thickness dermis and extending into subcutaneous fat (Fig. 6-10). In contrast to the circular palisades seen in granuloma annulare, the palisades in necrobiosis lipoidica assume a horizontal and parallel arrangement with respect to the overlying epidermis. The central portion of the palisade shows marked collagen degeneration without connective tissue mucin. The dermis to the periphery of the palisaded area is usually fibrotic (in contrast to a more normal dermis seen in granuloma annulare), sometimes with lipid deposition.[37] There is an accompanying superficial and deep perivascular inflammatory cell infiltrate featuring plasma cells. Vasculitis may be seen.[35] In some cases vessels at the junction of the dermis and subcutaneous fat show leukocytoclastic vasculitis in acute lesions and granulomatous vasculitis in chronic lesions. Involvement of the panniculus takes the form of a predominantly septal panniculitis. The atrophic centers of plaques demonstrate fibrosis.[35–37]

Horizontally oriented tiers of palisading granulomatous dermatitis with marked collagen degeneration, diffuse as opposed to focal dermal involvement, a lack of connective tissue mucin, and the presence of plasma cells are features that distinguish necrobiosis lipoidica from granuloma annulare and rheumatoid nodule. In addition, NLD usually involves the dermis and possibly the subcutis whereas the converse is true for rheumatoid nodule (Table 6-6).[37]

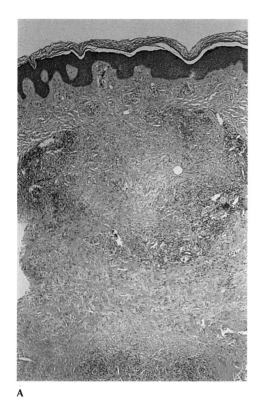

A

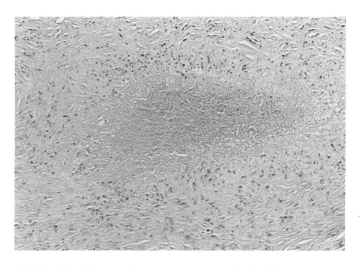

FIGURE 6-11   Rheumatoid nodule. Large areas of palisaded granulomatous inflammation surround degenerated collagen and sheets of fibrinoid material, which is in contrast to deep granuloma annulare that contains pools of connective tissue mucin.

Rheumatoid Nodule

Rheumatoid nodules are seen in approximately 20 percent of adults with rheumatoid arthritis. Nodules with similar histology may be seen in visceral sites, including lung, heart, and gastrointestinal tract. The pathogenesis is most likely an immune complex–mediated vasculitis, which results in ischemic damage to subcutaneous tissues and a palisaded granulomatous inflammatory reaction.[36,38]

Clinical Features   Rheumatoid nodules present in adults as subcutaneous nodules situated over joints, classically the elbows. Other common sites include the knuckles, Achilles tendon, and weight-bearing parts of the foot. Perforating variants are also known.

Histopathological Features   Within subcutaneous tissue and lower dermis there is palisaded granulomatous dermatitis surrounding a large area of homogeneous, eosinophilic fibrinoid necrosis (Fig. 6-11). The central area lacks pools of connective tissue mucin as a rule.[31,39] Vasculitic changes may or may not be apparent.[38]

The subcutaneous location and central fibrinoid necrosis (without pools of connective tissue mucin) are distinctive features of rheumatoid nodules.[31] As opposed to subcutaneous granuloma annulare, the general architecture of the subcutaneous fat is obliterated, the deep fat is involved, and there are no scattered interstitial histiocytes (Table 6-6).[39]

Rheumatic Fever Nodule

Rheumatic fever nodules are seen in patients with acute rheumatic fever and, early on, were more thoroughly studied than rheumatoid nodules.[38] The advent of effective antistreptococcal therapy resulted in a decrease in the disease, so few lesions are currently biopsied.[40] However, rheumatic heart disease is a major problem in developing countries, and recent reports have documented a rising increase of rheumatic fever in the United States and Europe.[41] Similar nodules are found in the heart and are known as Aschoff nodules. The cutaneous disease is a giant Aschoff nodule.[42] Like rheumatoid nodules, the pathogenesis is most likely an immune complex–mediated vasculitis, with subsequent ischemic damage, followed by a palisaded granulomatous repair reaction.

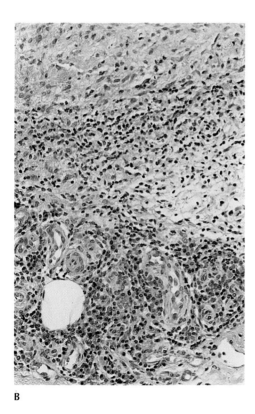

B

FIGURE 6-10   Necrobiosis lipoidica. (*A*) The perivascular granulomatous infiltrate alternates with degenerated collagen in a somewhat laminated display and extends in a confluent fashion from the upper reticular dermis to the base of the biopsy. (*B*) Numerous plasma cells are present around the deeper vessels.

Clinical Features   Rheumatic fever nodules typically develop in children with a history of acute rheumatic fever.[38] Sites of predilection include the bony prominences (humeral condyles, olecranon processes, knuckles) and occiput. Individual nodules spontaneously resolve.

Histopathological Features   In early lesions neutrophils may be admixed with histiocytes and lymphocytes. Otherwise, the histology is identical to rheumatoid nodule, although individual lesions may be smaller (see Rheumatoid Nodule).[36,38]

Necrobiotic Xanthogranuloma

Necrobiotic xanthogranuloma occurs in association with IgG paraproteinemia (usually kappa subtype) in approximately 80 percent of cases. Other laboratory findings include hypocomplementemia, cryoglobulinemia, anemia, and leukopenia. Although bone marrow examination may reveal plasmacytosis, true multiple myeloma is rare.[43]

Clinical Features   Indurated papules, nodules, or plaques (sometimes with ulceration/atrophy) most commonly occur periobitally but can involve the trunk and extremities. Systemic manifestations can include hepatosplenomegaly, arthritis/arthralgias, or neuropathy.

Histopathological Features   Necrobiotic xanthogranuloma demonstrates broad zones of collagen degeneration and cholesterol clefts surrounded by foamy macrophages with foreign body and Touton-type multinucleated giant cells (Fig. 6-12 *A,B*). Numerous lymphocytes and plasma cells (sometimes with lymphoid follicle formation) are conspicuous. These changes extend throughout the dermis, sometimes into the subcutaneous fat.[37,43]

Innumerable foam cells and cholesterol clefts distinguish necrobiotic xanthogranuloma.[37] Similar changes may be focally seen in plane xanthoma, suggesting a pathogenetic relationship between the two (Table 6-6).[44]

Palisaded Neutrophilic and Granulomatous Dermatitis

Synonyms: Churg-Strauss granuloma; cutaneous extravascular necrotizing granuloma; rheumatoid papules; superficial ulcerating rheumatoid necrobiosis; interstitial granulomatous dermatitis with arthritis

In 1983, Finan and Winkelmann reported a granulomatous condition seen in the setting of systemic disease, which they termed "Churg-Strauss granuloma" or "cutaneous extravascular necrotizing granuloma."[45] Recently, two reports have further delineated the clinicopathologic features.[46,47] An umbrella term of "palisaded neutrophilic and granulomatous dermatitis" has been suggested to encompass the conditions cited (see Synonyms), since all share granuloma annulare–like or necrobiosis lipoidica–like histology and most likely represent an inflammatory reaction to a primary vasculopathy/vasculitis.[46] Skin lesions in Wegener's granulomatosis may demonstrate identical granulomatous inflammation and, in fact, many noninfectious palisaded granulomas (from Aschoff nodules to some cases of granuloma annulare) probably reflect a similar pathogenesis.[48] Juxta-articular nodes of syphilis may also fall under this rubric.

Clinical Features   The associated systemic diseases include systemic lupus erythematosus, rheumatoid arthritis, Wegener's granulomatosis (and other ANCA-positive vasculitides), inflammatory bowel disease, lymphoproliferative disease, thyroid disease, diabetes mellitus, and infections (including bacterial endocarditis, EBV, HIV, *Mycoplasma pneumoniae*, parvovirus, Hepatitis C, and *Borrelia burgdorferi*).

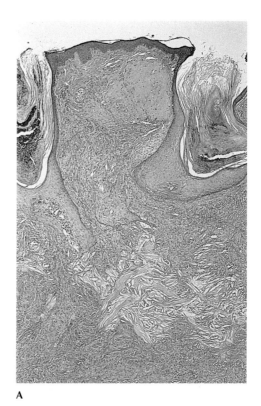

A

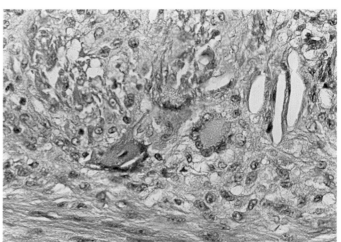

B

FIGURE 6-12   Necrobiotic xanthogranuloma. (*A,B*) Palisaded granulomatous inflammation composed of foamy macrophages surrounds large areas containing cholesterol clefts. The infiltrates focally disrupt follicular epithelium where there is an accompanying neutrophilic infiltrate.

Patients present with skin-colored to erythematous papules with overlying crust, ulceration, or umbilication. The papules are found predominantly on extremities and often are symmetrically distributed.[45–48]

Histopathological Features   The histology is variable and reflects the variable stages of repair to a primary vasculitis. Early lesions demonstrate collagen degeneration, pandermal infiltrates of neutrophils, nuclear debris, and focal leukocytoclastic vasculitis. The dermal vessels have characteristic broad collars of fibrin, surrounded by basophilic debris.[46] Fully developed lesions resemble granuloma annulare and demonstrate palisaded and granulomatous dermatitis surrounding zones of fibrin deposition and necrosis, collagen degeneration, neutrophils, and nuclear dust (Fig. 6-13). The central area contains connective tissue

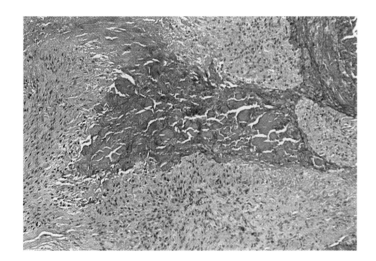

FIGURE 6-13   Palisaded neutrophilic and granulomatous dermatitis. A nodular granulomatous infiltrate is present around large stellate areas of degenerated collagen containing basophilic material and scattered neutrophils.

mucin. Late-stage lesions resemble necrobiosis lipoidica and demonstrate palisaded granulomas surrounding deeply eosinophilic fibrin with scattered neutrophils.[44–46]

Depending on stage of disease, the lesions of palisaded neutrophilic and granulomatous dermatitis may resemble granuloma annulare or necrobiosis lipoidica. At all stages, though, more neutrophils/leukocytoclasis are seen as compared to either granuloma annulare or necrobiosis lipoidica. Except for its dermal location and papular clinical appearance, palisaded neutrophilic and granulomatous dermatitis is virtually identical to rheumatoid or rheumatic fever nodules. All three conditions most likely represent a similar reaction to a primary immune complex–mediated vasculitis, which results in a fully developed granuloma annulare–like repair response (also see Introduction to Granuloma Annulare). Emphasis should be given to the fact that patients with lesions that are histologically identical to the palisaded neutrophilic and granulomatous dermatitis may only have skin disease, more typical of granuloma annulare.[49] It is incumbent on the physician to establish an associated systemic disease before more aggressive therapy is warranted, for patients with disease limited to the skin disease often respond to topical steroid therapy alone (Table 6-6).[50]

Infectious Palisaded Granulomatous Dermatitis

A palisaded granulomatous reaction pattern also occurs in response to infections caused by typical and atypical mycobacteria, phaeohyphomycosis, syphilis, sporotrichosis, cryptococcosis, coccidioidomycosis, cat-scratch disease, lymphogranuloma venereum, and schistosomiasis.[51,52] Infection-related palisaded granulomatous dermatitis is rare and in some series represented only 4.3 percent of all cases of palisading granuloma and less than 0.44 percent of all granulomas.[52]

Clinical Features   The clinical features are mostly those of the specific infection.

Histopathological Features   In the evaluation of palisaded and granulomatous dermatitis, central necrosis (not mucin or fibrin deposition) with numerous neutrophils should suggest an infectious etiology. A palisaded granulomatous reaction pattern in immunocompromised patients should prompt a search for infection.

Morphologic demonstration and/or microbiologic culture of the infectious agent is diagnostic (Table 6-6).

Differential Diagnosis   As discussed (see Granuloma Annulare), the histologic reaction pattern seen in the incomplete type of granuloma annulare may be a response to a plethora of insults, which are not necessarily associated with clinical lesions of granuloma annulare. Rare patients can develop lesions of granuloma annulare at sites of cutaneous involvement by herpes simplex or varicella zoster virus sometimes months to years after the primary infection. Typically, these lesions lack the cytopathic changes so characteristic of the earlier viral infection.[26] Eruptive xanthoma can also mimic this pattern, particularly those lesions with uratelike crystal formation (see Eruptive Xanthoma in the following).[53]

Some malignancies may also mimic palisaded granulomatous dermatitis. Epithelioid sarcoma is a malignant soft tissue neoplasm, which most frequently affects young adults and occurs on the extremities.[54] Histology reveals spindled and epithelioid cells surrounding central areas of necrosis in palisaded array. Lymphocytes and plasma cells may be seen. In contrast to tissue macrophages, the tumor cells of epithelioid sarcoma are cytologically atypical, with vesicular nuclei and prominent nucleoli, and are immunoreactive with antibodies to cytokeratin and epithelial membrane antigen.[54] Granulomatous mycosis fungoides is a histologic variant of mycosis fungoides that features deep granulomatous inflammation. The pattern of granulomatous inflammation is variable and may be diffuse or palisaded.[18]

SUPPURATIVE GRANULOMATOUS INFILTRATES

Aggregations of neutrophils commonly accompany granulomatous infiltrates. When infectious agents are found in this setting, it is often in the area of suppuration that the organisms are demonstrated. Table 6-7 lists infectious diseases whose histologic pattern is typically, but not exclusively, suppurative and granulomatous.

Blastomycosislike Pyoderma

Synonyms: Superficial granulomatous pyoderma; atypical plaquelike folliculitis in HIV; vegetative pyoderma gangrenosum

Blastomycosislike pyoderma represents an exaggerated inflammatory reaction to bacterial infection (particularly *Staphylococcus aureus*, but also *Pseudomonas aeruginosa*, and beta-hemolytic *Streptococcus*), usually seen in the setting of immunosuppression and/or lymphoproliferative disorders.[55,56] The condition is responsive to antibiotics, and in nearly all cases pathogenic bacteria are culturable, even though they may not be demonstrable in tissue sections. A similar exuberant inflammatory response to staphylococcal folliculitis is seen in the setting of HIV disease.[57]

Clinical Features   Patients with lymphoproliferative disorders or drug-induced/HIV-induced immunosuppression present with isolated or disseminated, well-marginated, verrucous plaques with multiple pustules. Plaques are distributed on head and neck, extremities, or intertriginous areas. The clinical differential diagnosis includes blastomycosis or other deep fungal infections, halogenodermas, pyoderma gangrenosum, and tuberculosis verrucosa cutis.

Histopathological Features   There is a diffuse mixed cellular infiltrate present in the superficial reticular dermis. Typically, a central nidus of numerous neutrophils with fewer numbers of eosinophils is surrounded by macrophages with multinucleated giant cells and a more peripheral rim of lymphocytes and plasma cells.[56] Pseudocarcinomatous hyperplasia is common. In some cases, the inflammation is folliculocentric and/or folliculo-destructive. Vasculitis is not seen.

TABLE 6-7

Infectious Causes of Suppurative Granulomatous Infiltrates

	Organism	*Tissue Morphology*	*Histopathological Features*
Atypical mycobacteria	*M. marinum* *M. kansasii* *M. fortuitum* *M. chelonei* *M. avium-intracellulare* *M. ulcerans* (Buruli ulcer)	Larger than *M. tuberculosis*	Variable inflammatory infiltrates
Blastomycosis	*Blastomyces dermatitidis*	8–15μ yeasts, broad-based budding; no hyphae	Pseudocarcinomatous hyperplasia
Chromomycosis	*Fonsecaea pedrosi* *Phialophora* sp. *Cladosporium* sp.	Brown, 6–12μ clustered yeast-like (copper pennies; medlar bodies); no hyphae	Pseudocarcinomatous hyperplasia
Phaeohyphomycosis	*Exophiala jeanselmei* *Wangiella dermatitidis*	Brown, septate hyphae and yeasts	May form a cystic cavity
Sporotrichosis	*Sporothrix schenckii*	4–8μ yeasts, some cigar-shaped; rare hyphae	Asteroid bodies suggestive, but nonspecific
Paracoccidioidomycosis	*Paracoccidioides brasiliensis*	10–60μ yeasts; multiple budding; no hyphae	Budding yeasts resemble "pilot's or mariner's wheel"
Coccidioidomycosis	*Coccidioides immitis*	Large 20–80μ sporangia containing 5–10μ endospores; no hyphae	Sporangia large and easily seen in H&E
Eumycetoma	*Allescheria boydii* *Madurella* sp.	Septate hyphae; Granules (Gram-neg, GMS-pos)	Filaments in granules are thick hyphae, not thin as in *Nocardia* and *Actinomyces*
Nocardiosis	*N. asteroides* *N. brasiliensis*	Thin, filamentous, Gram-positive bacteria; granules (Gram-pos, Ziehl-Neelsen-pos)	Filaments in granules are thin and partially acid-fast
Actinomycosis	*Actinomyces israelii*	Thin, filamentous gram-positive bacteria; granules (Gram-pos, Ziehl-Neelsen-neg)	Filaments in granules are same size as *Nocardia*, but are not acid-fast
Botryomycosis	*S. aureus* *P. aeruginosa*	Granules composed of numerous bacteria (Gram-pos)	No filaments
Tularemia	*Francisella tularensis*	Gram-negative coccobacillus	Immunomicroscopy required to visualize organism
Rhinosporidiosis	*Rhinosporidium seeberi*	Large (100–400μ) sporangia containing 7μ endospores; no hyphae	Sporangia easily seen in H&E
Cat-scratch disease	*Bartonella henselae*	Warthin-Starry-pos rods	Central PMNs surrounded by macrophages (stellate abscess)
Lymphogranuloma venereum	*Chlamydia trachomatis*	1–4μ Giemsa- or direct immunofluorescence-pos coccoid bodies	Intracellular
Alternariosis	*A. alternata* *A. dianthicola*	Brown, broad (5–7μ thick) septate hyphae; 3–10μ brown spores	Similar to phaeohyphomycosis
Scrofuloderma	*M. tuberculosis* and atypical mycobacteria	Ziehl-Neelsen-pos AFB	Caseation
Miliary tuberculosis	*M. tuberculosis*	Ziehl-Neelsen-pos AFB	Caseation may be absent in very small lesions

TABLE 6-8

Blastomycosislike Pyoderma

Clinical Features

Immunosuppressed patients
Lymphoproliferative diseases
Verrucous plaques with surface pustules
Head, neck, extremities, intertriginous sites
Normal serum halogen levels

Histopathological Features

Superficial infiltrates
Central neutrophils/eosinophils surrounded by
   multinucleated giant cells and lymphocytes
Pseudocarcinomatous hyperplasia
No vasculitis

Differential Diagnosis

Infection
Halogenodermas
Follicular occlusion triad
Ruptured follicles, follicular cysts, and sinuses

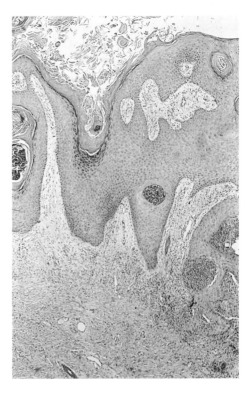

FIGURE 6-14   Halogenoderma. Suppurative granulomatous inflammation is accompanied by pseudocarcinomatous hyperplasia. Focal abscesses are seen in the epidermis.

In contrast to the pandermal inflammation seen in pyoderma gangrenosum, blastomycosislike pyoderma features mostly superficial infiltrates. The histology may be virtually identical to halogenodermas, but normal serum halogen levels exclude this possibility (Table 6-8).

Halogenodermas

Synonyms: Bromoderma; iododerma; fluoroderma

Halogenodermas are a group of dermatoses owing to chronic ingestion or application of iodine, bromide, or fluoride. The source of bromides and iodides often are expectorants and sedatives.[58]

Clinical Features   The large vegetative nodules or plaques of halogenodermas often are studded with pustules and clinically resemble deep fungal infections or blastomycosislike pyoderma.

Histopathological Features   The most striking and constant feature is pseudocarcinomatous hyperplasia, containing intraepidermal microabscesses, composed of neutrophils and fewer eosinophils (Fig. 6-14). In some cases, there are dermal abscesses composed of numerous neutrophils with fewer macrophages and multinucleated giants cells.[58]

Special stains for microorganisms are required to rule out infectious causes of suppurative granulomatous inflammation, especially deep fungal infections. The histologic appearances may resemble blastomycosislike pyoderma, and clinical history and/or serum halogen levels are necessary to distinguish the two (Table 6-9).

Follicular Occlusion Triad

Synonyms: Hidradenitis suppurativa; acne conglobata, dissecting cellulitis

Follicular occlusion triad is an umbrella term given to the mentioned three clinical conditions (see Synonyms), whose pathogenesis is related to a disorder of follicles resulting in subsequent occlusion, inflammation, and destruction. All three conditions may coexist in the same patient.[59]

Clinical Features   Dissecting cellulitis presents on the scalp as a boggy indurated plaque that may be associated with alopecia. Hidradenitis suppurativa typically presents in the axillae, groin, or perineum (areas rich in apocrine glands) as erythematous, tender, deep-seated nodules, sometimes with sinus tract formation. Acne conglobata presents on the chest, back, buttocks, or proximal extremities as erythematous, tender nodules or cysts, sometimes with sinus tract formation.

Histopathological Features   All three conditions demonstrate a common pathology and pathogenesis, as described by Brunsting in 1952.[59]

TABLE 6-9

Halogenodermas

Clinical Features

Ingestion/application of bromide, iodide, fluoride
Increased serum halogen levels
Verrucous plaques with surface pustules

Histopathological Features

Pseudocarcinomatous hyperplasia
Intraepidermal microabscesses
Dermal neutrophils amd multinucleated giant cells

Differential Diagnosis

Mycobacterial and fungal infections
Blastomycosislike pyoderma
Follicular occlusion triad
Ruptured follicles, follicular cysts, and sinuses

The features include perifollicular dermal abscesses composed of a mixed inflammatory cell infiltrate with a predominance of neutrophils, macrophages with multinucleated giant cells, and fewer lymphocytes, plasma cells, and eosinophils. The inflammation usually results in destruction of the follicle and sometimes the formation of epithelial-lined sinus tracts. Later stages of the disease demonstrate more lymphocytes, plasma cells, and fibrosis.

Clinical locale separates these three conditions from each other. The multiplicity of lesions distinguishes follicular occlusion triad from ruptured follicle/follicular cysts.

Ruptured Follicles and Follicular Cysts and Sinuses

The most common cause of a suppurative granulomatous infiltrate is a ruptured follicle or follicular cyst. Disruption of these structures releases hair and/or other cornified cells into the adjacent dermis, resulting in a foreign-body inflammatory response, admixed with neutrophils.

Clinical Features   Ruptured follicles or follicular cysts present as solitary erythematous, tender nodules. Alternatively, ruptured follicles may be the etiology underlying recent changes in melanocytic nevi, especially hair-bearing congenital nevi. Pilonidal sinus most commonly presents in the sacrococcygeal area of hirsute males, although other sites including the scalp and the finger webs of barbers' hands have been reported.[60]

Histopathological Features   There is a follicular-based, dense, nodular, mixed inflammatory cell infiltrate with a predominance of neutrophils, macrophages, and multinucleated giant cells. Keratin debris and/or hair is seen lying free within the infiltrate or within the cytoplasm of multinucleated giant cells (Fig. 6-15). In some cases the infiltrate may extend deep and affect the panniculus preferentially, giving rise to a lobular panniculitis. The latter is the rule in pilonidal sinus where hair shafts can usually be identified in the granulomatous inflammation.

Special stains for microorganisms to rule out infection are required if keratin debris is not visualized.

DIFFUSE HISTIOCYTIC INFILTRATES

The term "histiocyte" is admittedly controversial. Wood and Haber proposed that the term histiocyte "refers to all types of bone marrow–derived macrophages and immune-related dendritic cells. Similarly, the term histiocytosis refers to any proliferative disorder exhibiting the differentiation of these cells."[61] A similar definition is used to define the entities discussed, but in general, when the involvement remains as discrete cutaneous papules or nodules (single or multiple), the suffix oma is attached (i.e., histiocytoma, xanthoma). It is when lesions tend to coalesce, to progress relentlessly, and/or to involve extracutaneous sites, that the suffix osis is applied (i.e., histiocytosis, reticulohistiocytosis). As always, there are exceptions, and some entities demonstrate overlapping clinical pictures. Table 6-10 lists infectious diseases whose histologic pattern is typically, but not exclusively, a diffuse histiocytic infiltrate.

Xanthomas

Xanthoma (unmodified) is the generic term applied to a group of infiltrates of foamy macrophages (histiocytes). Those associated with hyperlipidemias have characteristic sites of predilection. These xanthomas include eruptive xanthoma, tuberous xanthoma, tendinous xanthoma, and xanthelasma (Table 6-11). The characteristic cell is the foam cell—a macrophage whose cytoplasm is stuffed with lipid and appears foamy

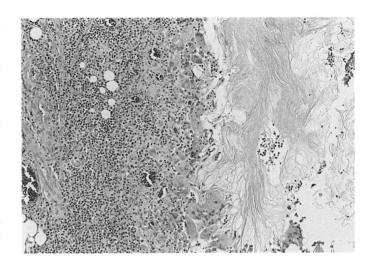

FIGURE 6-15 Ruptured follicular cyst. Suppurative granulomatous inflammation surrounds keratinous debris of a cyst content. The cyst wall has been destroyed by the inflammatory infiltrate.

in hematoxylin and eosin–stained sections. Aggregations of foam cells are the common denominator of other lesions called xanthomas—plane, verruciform, papular, plexiform—but that have distinctive clinical and/or pathological features. Xanthoma disseminatum is more closely related to xanthogranuloma. These latter five entities are discussed separately.

Clinical Features   Sites of predilection for the usual xanthoma types associated with hyperlipidemia are provided in Table 6-11. With the exception of the eruptive type, the histologic appearance for all types is virtually identical. The clinical locale is most helpful in distinguishing these (Table 6-11).

Histopathological Features   Tuberous xanthoma, tendinous xanthoma, and xanthelasma demonstrate virtually identical histology. There is an infiltrate almost exclusively of foam cells disposed between individual collagen bundles, in small clusters, or in large nodular aggregates (Fig. 6-16). Lymphocytes, neutrophils, and eosinophils are completely absent or present only in small numbers. Eruptive xanthomas are often smaller and more inflammatory, clinically. They demonstrate greater numbers of lymphocytes, neutrophils, and macrophages and fewer characteristic foam cells. One hallmark of eruptive xanthoma is

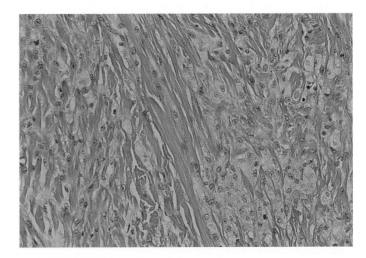

FIGURE 6-16 Xanthomas. Foamy macrophages form nests and sheets that are separated by coarse collagen bundles.

TABLE 6-10

TABLE 6-10

Infectious Causes of Diffuse Histiocytic Infiltrates

	Organism	Tissue morphology	Histopathological features
Lepromatous leprosy	M. leprae	Fite-pos AFB	Foamy lepra cells; grenz zone; globi
Histoid leprosy and atypical mycobacteria in HIV	M. leprae and atypical mycobacteria	Fite-pos AFB, Ziehl-Neelsen-pos AFB	Spindle cell pseudotumor confused with neoplasm
Histoplasmosis	H. capsulatum	2–4μ intracellular yeasts with clear halo; no hyphae	Organisms within macrophages
Leishmaniasis	L. tropica L. mexicana L. brasiliensis L. donovani	2–4μ round-oval protozoa with nucleus and kinetoplast (Giemsa-pos)	Organisms within macrophages; nucleus and kinetoplast stain red with Giemsa

the presence of both intracellular and extracellular lipid, producing a pattern similar to granuloma annulare (Fig. 6-17).[62] This palisaded granulomatous appearance is exaggerated in those eruptive xanthomas that also contain deposits of uratelike crystals.[53]

With the exception of eruptive xanthoma, the almost exclusive infiltrate of foam cells and lack of lymphocytes, neutrophils, and eosinophils are characteristic of these xanthomas and serve to differentiate them from the non-Langerhans cell histiocytoses (Table 6-11).

Diffuse Normolipemic Plane Xanthoma

Synonyms: Generalized plane xanthoma

Diffuse normolipemic plane xanthoma is commonly associated with multiple myeloma. Other less common associations are erythroderma, cryoglobulinemia, myelogenous leukemia, lymphomas (including mycosis fungoides) and, rarely, hyperlipoproteinemia types IIA, III, and IV. Some cases have no demonstrable associated disease.[44]

Clinical Features Well-demarcated yellow-orange plaques are distributed periorbitally and on the trunk and extremities in patients without elevated serum lipids.

Histopathological Features In addition to a perivascular lymphocytic infiltrate, there are clusters or sheets of foamy macrophages extending throughout the papillary and reticular dermis. Touton-type giant cells are variably present.

The presence of a perivascular lymphocytic infiltrate separates diffuse normolipemic plane xanthoma from other xanthomas. Some cases may demonstrate focal collagen degeneration and cholesterol clefts, suggesting a histologic (and with the dysproteinemia, a clinical) overlap with necrobiotic xanthogranuloma.[44]

Verruciform Xanthoma

Verruciform xanthoma is a solitary lesion encountered in the oral mucosa and rarely at extraoral sites. Similar histologic changes are encountered in a wide variety

of conditions including pemphigus vulgaris, lichen planus, epidermolysis bullosa, discoid lupus erythematosus, epidermal nevi, and inflammatory linear verrucous epidermal nevus (ILVEN).[63] The etiology is unknown, but there is no association with diabetes or hyperlipidemia. The theorized pathogenesis involves degeneration of keratinocytes followed by a macrophage inflammatory response.

Clinical Features Oral lesions may occur at any site, but the gingiva and hard palate are affected preferentially. They are described as soft, red, white, or yellow papules with a roughened surface. Cutaneous lesions have been described on the penis, the vulva, scrotum, groin, anus, and nostril.

Histopathological Features There is verrucous epithelial hyperplasia with tiers of parakeratosis and associated neutrophils in some cases (Fig. 6-18 *A,B*). Within an expanded submucosa (or papillary dermis),

TABLE 6-11

Xanthomas

Tuberous	Tendinous	Xanthelasma	Eruptive
Clinical Features			
Hypercholesterolemia (IIa) Dyslipoproteinemia (III) Hypertriglyceridemia (IV) Elbows Knees	Hypercholesterolemia (IIa) Extensor tendons of hands, feet Achilles tendon	Hypercholesterolemia (IIa) Dyslipoproteinemia (III) Idiopathic Eyelids	Lipoprotein lipase deficiency (I) Dyslipoproteinemia (III) Hypertriglyceridemia (IV/V) Diabetes mellitus Buttocks and other sites
Histopathological Features			
Foam cells arranged interstitially between collagen bundles, as small clusters, or in large nodular aggregates Few to no Lymphocytes, Neutrophils, Eosinophils	Same as tuberous	Same as tuberous	Fewer foam cells More Lymphocytes, Neutrophils, Eosinophils Intracellular and extracellular lipid

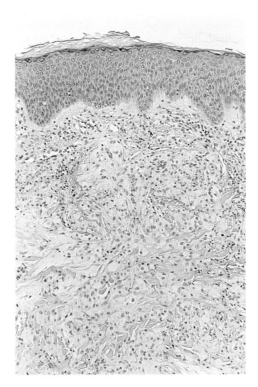

FIGURE 6-17 Eruptive xanthoma. This xanthoma shows a perivascular and interstitial pattern of foamy macrophages, some of which are disrupted. Their content is present as extracellular lipid which is focally accompanied by neutrophils.

there are collections of foam cells (lipid-rich macrophages) partially enclosed by hyperplastic rete pegs.[63] Collections of foam cells immediately below a verrucous mucosa are characteristic of verruciform xanthoma.

Papular Xanthoma

Papular xanthoma is a non-Langerhans cell histiocytosis that primarily affects infants and children. The etiology is unknown. Patients have normal serum lipid parameters.

Clinical Features Patients present usually in the first year of life with numerous yellow papules or nodules in a generalized distribution. The mucous membranes are occasionally involved. Viscera are spared, and there is no association with diabetes insipidus.[64]

Histopathological Features Individual lesions are composed almost entirely of lipidized, foamy histiocytes in a diffuse or nodular pattern. Foamy Touton-type giant cells are also seen, but unlike xanthogranuloma (and benign cephalic histiocytosis, generalized eruptive histiocytosis, xanthoma disseminatum), papular xanthoma lacks an accompanying inflammatory cell infiltrate of lymphocytes, plasma cells, or eosinophils. The histiocytes are S-100- and CD1a (OKT6)-negative.[64]

   Diffuse or nodular collections of S-100- and CD1a (OKT6)-negative foamy histiocytes and Touton-type giant cells and a conspicuous lack of lymphocytes, plasma cells, and eosinophils are suggestive of papular xanthoma. The generalized distribution and normal serum lipid parameters separate papular xanthoma from other xanthomas.

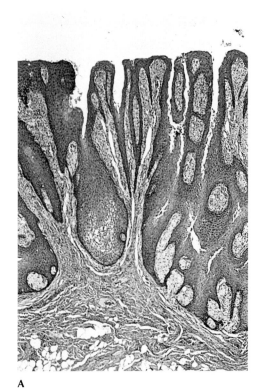

A

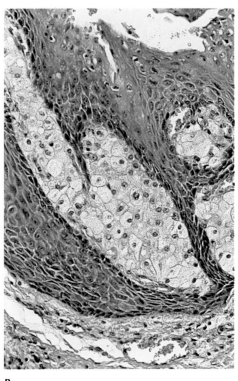

B

FIGURE 6-18 Verruciform xanthoma. (*A,B*) Digitated squamous hyperplasia overlies papillae containing foamy macrophages.

Plexiform Xanthoma

Plexiform xanthoma is a recently described dermal tumor of middle-aged adults composed of foam cells in a plexiform arrangement. Some consider it neoplastic, whereas others consider it inflammatory.[65] There may or may not be an association with hyperlipidemia (essential or secondary).

Clinical Features Reported cases have involved the chin, knee, and buttocks.

Histopathological Features There are nodular collections of foamy macrophages within the dermis, which gradually merge with spindle-shaped cells arranged in large sweeping fascicles. Variable features include foci of cholesterol clefts surrounded by dense collagen, nodules of spindle cells in a storiform arrangement, and a lymphocytic-plasma cellular infiltrate. Osteoclast-like giant cells (as seen in plexiform fibrohistiocytic tumor) are not seen in plexiform xanthoma. The cells are CD68 (KP1)-positive, muscle actin (HHF35)-negative, and S-100-negative.[62] This entity may represent a lipidized benign cutaneous histiocytoma.[66] The plexiform architecture and presence of foams cells are distinctive.

Langerhans Cell Histiocytosis

Synonyms: Histiocytosis X; Letterer-Siwe disease; Hand-Schüller-Christian disease; eosinophilic granuloma

Langerhans cell histiocytosis is a proliferative disorder of Langerhans cells with both cutaneous and extracutaneous involvement. The term Langerhans cell histiocytosis is preferred to histiocytosis X, since X was chosen to indicate a cell of unknown differentiation. The term histiocyte refers to a family of bone marrow–derived dendritic cells with phagocytic or immune-related activities, of which Langerhans cells are a member. Others in this family include indeterminate cells, interdigitating cells, and follicular-dendritic cells. Langerhans cells are S-100-positive, CD1a (OKT6)-positive, and contain Birbeck granules; indeterminate cells are S-100-positive, CD1a (OKT6)-positive, but lack Birbeck granules. Proliferative disorders of interdigitating and follicular-dendritic cells rarely affect the skin.[61,67]

The nosology of Langerhans cell histiocytosis remains unsettled. Some reports, based on molecular DNA techniques, support a monoclonal proliferation and a neoplastic disorder.[68,69] Others question this conclusion.[70] The definitive answer awaits further clarification. Owing to overlapping clinical features, the classic subtypes of Letterer-Siwe disease, Hand-Schüller-Christian disease, and eosinophilic granuloma are subsumed under the rubric of Langerhans cell histiocytosis.

Clinical Features Cutaneous lesions are variable and may include red-brown papules, nodules, plaques, vesicles, pustules, or ulcers. Lesions are distributed on the scalp, trunk, and intertriginous areas. Mucosal (especially gingival) involvement is characteristic. Extracutaneous involvement is frequently present in Langerhans cell histiocytosis and separates it from congenital self-healing reticulohistiocytosis. Commonly involved organs include bone, bone marrow, liver, spleen, hypothalamus-pituitary (diabetes insipidus), and lung.

Histopathological Features Hematoxylin and eosin–stained sections reveal perivascular or lichenoid infiltrates of Langerhans cells confined to the papillary and upper reticular dermis. Cytologic features are bland and characterized by cells with abundant eosinophilic or pale cytoplasms, and longitudinally grooved or reniform nuclei with small nucleoli (Fig. 6-19).[71] Epidermotropism is often seen. Eosinophils are sometimes prominent. Langerhans cells are S-100- and CD1a (OKT6)-positive and contain Birbeck granules by electron microscopy.[72]

A proliferation of Langerhans cells (cytologic features described earlier) with accompanying eosinophils and epidermotropism suggest Langerhans cell histiocytosis. Identical histology may be seen in congenital self-healing reticulohistiocytosis, and clinical workup to exclude extracutaneous involvement is required to separate the two. It must be underscored that one cannot predict the biology of Langerhans disease

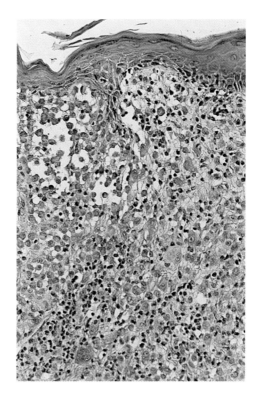

FIGURE 6-19 Langerhans cell histiocytosis. A diffuse infiltrate of mononuclear cells having abundant cytoplasm and reniform nuclei extend from the dermal-epidermal junction into the reticular dermis. A few multinucleate cells are also present in addition to scattered lymphocytes and numerous eosinophils. The cells are focally present within the epidermis.

from the histopathology, a tenet that has been well established in clinical oncology/hematology (Table 6-12).[72]

Congenital Self-Healing Langerhans Histiocytosis (Reticulohistiocytosis)

Synonyms: Hashimoto-Pritzker disease; pure cutaneous histiocytosis X; congenital spontaneously regressing histiocytosis

Congenital self-healing reticulohistiocytosis is a disease of infants/neonates, which represents the self-limited, benign end of the spectrum of Langerhans cell proliferative disorders. The disease is confined to the skin, and there is no (or only mild) systemic involvement. The skin lesions and histopathologic features can be virtually identical to other Langerhans cell histiocytoses; therefore, one must attempt to rule out systemic involvement through clinical evaluation of lymph nodes, liver, spleen, bone survey, CBC with differential, and liver function tests.[72,73] Although most cases spontaneously regress, these patients should be followed closely for the possible development of relapses or progression with skeletal involvement.[72,73] For those reasons the term congenital self-healing Langerhans histiocytosis is the most appropriate designation.

Clinical Features Neonates present with red-brown papules, nodules, or pustules in a generalized distribution. Mucous membrane involvement is more suggestive of the systemic variety of Langerhans cell histiocytosis. Multiple blue nodules resembling the "blueberry muffin baby" may also be encountered.

Histopathological Features The histologic features are identical to Langerhans cell histiocytosis, but some cases may have more of an

TABLE 6-12

Langerhans Cell Proliferative Disorders

Langerhans Cell Histiocytosis (Systemic)	Congenital Self-Healing Langerhans Histiocytosis (Reticulohistiocytosis)
Clinical Features	
Cutaneous and extracutaneous disease	Cutaneous involvement only
Red-brown papules, nodules, plaques	Cutaneous lesions similar to systemic
Vesicles, pustules, ulcers	Langerhans cell histiocytosis, but
Scalp, trunk, intertriginous	gingiva and other mucosal sites
Gingiva and other mucosal sites	less commonly affected
Histopathological Features	
Superficial perivascular or lichenoid	Identical to systemic Langerhans cell
infiltrates of Langerhans cells	histiocytosis
with grooved (reniform) nuclei	
Epidermotropism	
Eosinophils	
Langerhans cells S-100-, CD1a (OKT6)-	
positive	
EM: Birbeck granules	

admixture of foamy macrophages.[74] Langerhans cells (characterized as mononuclear cells with copious pale-eosinophilic cytoplasms and longitudinally grooved or reniform nuclei) occupy the papillary and upper reticular dermis and sometimes demonstrate epidermotropism. Eosinophils constitute a significant portion of the infiltrate. The cells are S-100- and CD1a (OKT6)-positive and contain Birbeck granules. Extensive areas of dermal necrosis (possibly indicative of involution) may be more common in congenital self-healing disease than in the systemic variety of Langerhans cell histiocytosis.[73] Clinical workup to rule out extracutaneous involvement is mandatory (Table 6-12).

Indeterminate Cell Histiocytosis

With the advent of immunohistochemical, electron microscopic, and molecular diagnostic techniques, new histiocytic subsets are being recognized. Histiocyte subsets include Langerhans cells, indeterminate cells, interdigitating cells, and follicular-dendritic cells. Proliferating disorders of interdigitating and follicular-dendritic cells usually affect lymph nodes and only rarely the skin.[61] Indeterminate cell histiocytoses are rare (approximately 10 cases reported to date) and represent proliferations of S-100- and CD1a (OKT6)-positive cells, which lack Birbeck granules.[61] The lesions may completely regress, partially regress, or (in two reported cases) involve lymph nodes and other extracutaneous sites. As some consider indeterminate cells to represent one stage of Langerhans cell differentiation, further study of these rare cases is needed to determine if indeterminate cell histiocytosis is indeed a distinct entity. At this juncture, this seems doubtful.

Rosai-Dorfman Disease

Synonyms: Sinus histiocytosis with massive lymphadenopathy; cutaneous sinus histiocytosis

The cause of Rosai-Dorfman disease is unknown. Patients develop massive cervical lymphadenopathy accompanied by fever, leukocytosis, hypergammaglobulinemia, and an elevated erythrocyte sedimentation rate.[75] Extranodal involvement is fairly common, and the skin is the most frequent site (approximately 30% of cases), with the respiratory tract, eyes, soft tissues, bones, and genitourinary tract and nervous system less commonly affected. There are also cases of skin-limited Rosai-Dorfman disease.[76] Black patients are more frequently affected than whites, and there is a slight male predominance. The disease spontaneously resolves.[75]

Clinical Features In both skin-limited disease and secondary cutaneous disease, the clinical lesions are similar with erythematous or yellow-red papules, nodules, or plaques, which may be solitary or multiple.

Histopathological Features There is a dense diffuse or nodular dermal infiltrate of histiocytes admixed with lymphocytes, plasma cells, and neutrophils. Eosinophils, if present at all, are seen in only small numbers. Although rare eosinophilic abscesses have been described, large numbers of eosinophils should suggest another histiocytic proliferation, especially Langerhans cell histiocytosis.[76] Emperipolesis of lymphocytes, plasma cells, and neutrophils by histiocytes is characteristic. (Fig. 6-20). At the periphery of histiocytic nodules, there are lymphoid aggregates with germinal centers and thick-walled vessels surrounded by plasma cells. In the centers of histiocytic nodules, dilated lymphatics containing intraluminal histiocytes are seen.[75,76] The histiocytes in Rosai-Dorfman disease are S-100-positive, CD1a (OKT6)-negative, and lack Birbeck granules. In some cases, the subcutis, rather than the dermis, is primarily affected.

Emperipolesis of inflammatory cells seen among an infiltrate of S-100-positive histiocytes, which have wispy cytoplasms, is characteristic of Rosai-Dorfman disease. Dilated lymphatic channels with intraluminal histiocytes and thick-walled vessels surrounded by plasma cells are distinctive in Rosai-Dorfman disease.[75,76]

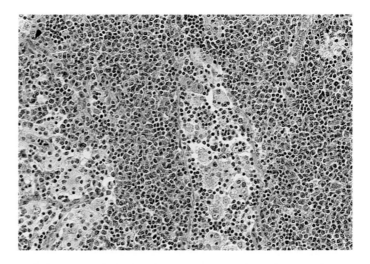

FIGURE 6-20 Rosai-Dorfman disease. A mixed infiltrate of lymphocytes and plasma cells surrounds sheets of large tissue macrophages that contain abundant eosinophilic cytoplasm. Many of these macrophages contain phagocytized lymphocytes, producing the so-called "beanbag" appearance.

Xanthogranuloma

Synonyms: Juvenile xanthogranuloma; adult xanthogranuloma

Juvenile xanthogranuloma is a non-Langerhans cell histiocytosis seen in infants or children usually before the age of 6 months. The etiology is not known. Although juvenile xanthogranuloma usually is limited to the skin, it may affect other organ systems.[77] The eye is the most frequently involved extracutaneous site, but others include liver, spleen, lymph nodes, lungs, heart, testes, ovary, colon, kidneys, and bones. Adults are sometimes affected by identical lesions (adult xanthogranuloma).[78] Deep subcutaneous or intramuscular forms also have been described.[79]

Clinical Features   Cutaneous lesions present as solitary or multiple yellow-red papules or nodules on the face, neck, or upper trunk. Individual lesions spontaneously regress over time.

Histopathological Features   The histologic picture is largely dependent on the stage of the lesion at the time of biopsy. Mature lesions demonstrate nodular, dense, sheet-like collections of histiocytes admixed with Touton-type giant cells (giant cells with a wreath of nuclei), lymphocytes, and eosinophils (Fig. 6-21).[77–79] In contrast to the monotonous infiltrate of macrophages with foamy cytoplasms (foam cells) seen in xanthomas, xanthogranulomas feature histiocytes with varied morphology. In addition to foam cells (which usually constitute the majority), there are histiocytes with vacuolated cytoplasms, histiocytes with eosinophilic granular cytoplasms, and spindle-shaped histiocytes.[78] Early lesions demonstrate few-to-no Touton-type giant cells and foam cells. Late lesions demonstrate areas of fibrosis. The histiocytes are positive for HAM56 (CD64), KP1 (CD68), vimentin, and fac-

tor XIIIa and negative for S-100.[77,78] Deep subcutaneous or intramuscular forms differ in only minor degree from the superficial forms. They are more circumscribed, contain fewer Touton-type giant cells, and contain more abundant eosinophils.[79]

The presence of Touton-type giant cells and an admixture of lymphocytes and eosinophils are distinctive. Touton-type giant cells may be absent in early lesions. Xanthogranulomas are HAM56 (CD64)-, KP1 (CD68)-, and factor XIIIa–positive and S-100-negative (Table 6-13).[77,78]

Benign Cephalic Histiocytosis

Benign cephalic histiocytosis is a non-Langerhans cell histiocytosis which affects infants and young children less than 3 years of age. The etiology is unknown, but overlapping clinical and histologic features suggest that benign cephalic histiocytosis, generalized eruptive histiocytosis, xanthoma disseminatum, and xanthogranuloma are closely related.[80]

Clinical Features   Infants or young children less than 3 years of age develop numerous brown-yellow papules distributed on the head, neck, and sometimes upper trunk. Mucous membranes and viscera are spared. Individual lesions spontaneously resolve over time.[80]

Histopathological Features   The histologic features of benign cephalic histiocytosis, generalized eruptive histiocytosis, xanthoma disseminatum, and xanthogranuloma are nearly identical (see Xanthogranuloma). The histiocytes are S-100- and CD1a (OKT6)-negative. Electron microscopy reveals coated vesicles and comma-shaped bodies, but this finding is of no diagnostic aid, since similar findings are present in xanthogranuloma, generalized eruptive histiocytosis, Langerhans cell histiocytosis, and congenital self-healing reticulohistiocytosis.[80]

The clinical locale and young age of the patient distinguish benign cephalic histiocytosis, but the histopathology is not distinctive, as generalized eruptive histiocytosis, xanthoma disseminatum, and xanthogranuloma are probably pathogenetically related conditions.

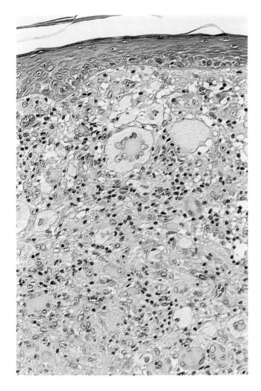

FIGURE 6-21   Xanthogranuloma. A diffuse infiltrate of macrophages, both single and multinucleate, are accompanied by a mixed inflammatory cell infiltrate of lymphocytes and scattered eosinophils. Foam cells containing a wreath of nuclei are present.

Generalized Eruptive Histiocytosis (Histiocytoma)

Generalized eruptive histiocytosis is a non-Langerhans cell histiocytosis, which affects adults. The etiology is unknown, but overlapping clinical and histologic features suggest that generalized eruptive histiocytosis, benign cephalic histiocytosis, xanthoma disseminatum, and xanthogranuloma are closely related.[80,81]

Clinical Features   Adult patients present with numerous, generalized, brown to dark blue papules or nodules symmetrically distributed on the trunk and extremities. Mucous membranes occasionally are involved, but there is no visceral involvement. Individual lesions spontaneously resolve over time.[81]

Histopathological Features   The histologic features of generalized eruptive histiocytosis, benign cephalic histiocytosis, xanthoma disseminatum, and xanthogranuloma are nearly identical (see Xanthogranuloma). The histiocytes are S-100- and CD1a (OKT6)-negative. As a rule, in generalized eruptive histiocytosis lipid stains are negative and giant cells are absent.[81]

The generalized distribution, older age of the patient, and lack of visceral involvement are helpful in distinguishing generalized eruptive histiocytosis from benign cephalic histiocytosis, xanthoma disseminatum, and xanthogranuloma; but all of these conditions are probably pathogenetically related. Recently, histiocytomas have been described with an eruptive, progressive presentation but with histopathology closest to xanthogranuloma, a fact that further supports the unifying concept.[82]

Xanthoma Disseminatum

Synonyms: Montgomery's syndrome

Xanthoma disseminatum is a non-Langerhans cell histiocytosis that may affect all ages. The etiology is unknown, but overlapping clinical and histologic features suggest that xanthoma disseminatum, benign cephalic histiocytosis, generalized eruptive histiocytosis, and xanthogranuloma are closely related.[80]

Clinical Features   Patients of any age present with numerous red-brown or yellow papules that frequently become confluent to form large plaques. Flexural areas of the neck, axillae, antecubital fossae, groin, and perianal region are preferentially affected. Mucous membrane involvement is fairly common, and lesions of the buccal mucosa or larynx may cause dysphagia or breathing difficulties. The conjunctiva and cornea are additional sites of potential involvement. Diabetes insipidus is seen in approximately 40 percent of cases. Individual lesions spontaneously resolve over time.

Histopathological Features   The histologic features of xanthoma disseminatum, benign cephalic histiocytosis, generalized eruptive histiocytosis, and xanthogranuloma are nearly identical (see Xanthogranuloma) (Fig. 6-22). The histiocytes of xanthoma disseminatum are S-100- and CD1a (OKT6)-negative.

The clinical features usually are distinctive. These include the confluence of individual lesions to form plaques, the flexural distribution, the association with diabetes insipidus, and the involvement of mucous membranes and other organs (i.e., eye).

Multicentric Reticulohistiocytosis

Synonyms: Lipoid dermatoarthritis

Multicentric reticulohistiocytosis defines a distinct clinical entity in which multiple cutaneous nodules are associated with a destructive

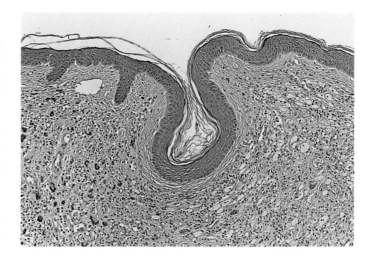

FIGURE 6-22   Xanthoma disseminatum. Tissue macrophages (histiocytes) form a diffuse infiltrate in a thickened papillary dermis accompanied by a lymphocytic infiltrate. Focally many foamy macrophages are present, and in other areas delicate fascicles of plump spindle cells are formed. This lesion, taken from the axilla of a patient with typical xanthoma disseminatum, shows the histologic overlap with xanthogranuloma.

polyarthritis. The arthritis most frequently involves the interphalangeal joints of the hands, but knees, ankles, wrists, elbows, and shoulders may also be affected. Adult females are affected more often than males, and the cutaneous nodules may precede, occur with, or postdate the onset of arthritis. In some cases multicentric reticulohistiocytosis is associated with malignancies (gastrointestinal or ovarian), thyroid disorders, tuberculosis, diabetes mellitus, dermatomyositis, celiac disease, and systemic lupus erythematosus.[83,84] The etiology is unknown.

Clinical Features   Yellow-brown cutaneous papules or nodules are distributed over the hands, forearms, and face. The oral mucosa may rarely be involved.

Histopathological Features   There is an interstitial, poorly circumscribed, infiltrate of histiocytes and large multinucleated giant cells with distinctive eosinophilic finely granular ("ground-glass") cytoplasms, scattered between collagen bundles of the dermis (Fig. 6-23). Lymphocytes are also present. The giant cells are relatively large (>50 μ) with randomly arranged nuclei.[83] The cytoplasms mono- and multinucleated cells are PAS-positive and diastase-resistant. Immunohistochemical studies have shown positive reactions with KP1 (CD68), HAM56, and vimentin; and negative reactions with S-100, factor XIIIa, and muscle actin (HHF35).[84]

The eosinophilic, finely granular, ground-glass cytoplasm is distinctive. Solitary reticulohistiocytoma shows nearly identical histologic features, with the following exceptions: the infiltrate in solitary reticulohistiocytoma is nodular, dense, and sheetlike (as opposed to interstitial), and the immunohistochemical profile is different (factor XIIIa- and muscle actin [HHF35]-positive).[83]

Reticulohistiocytoma

Reticulohistiocytomas are solitary cutaneous nodules with similar histology to that seen in multicentric reticulohistiocytosis (i.e., mono- and multinucleated histiocytes with characteristic ground-glass cytoplasm).[83,84] In fact, prior reports indicated that the two conditions were histologically identical. However, solitary reticulohistiocytomas are not associated with arthritis, and recent immunohistochemical investigations suggest that they may be variants of xanthogranulomas.[83,84]

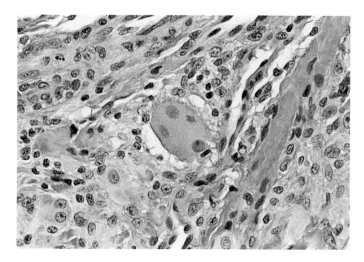

FIGURE 6-23 Multicentric reticulohistiocytoma. Mononuclear and multinucleated histiocytes form a diffuse infiltrate. The typical multinucleated cells contain three to ten nuclei and have ground-glass appearing cytoplasm.

Clinical Features Solitary reticulohistiocytomas are yellow-brown nodules without any site predilection. An acral location should suggest multicentric reticulohistiocytosis.

Histopathological Features There is a dense, nodular, sheetlike infiltrate of mono- and multinucleated histiocytes with eosinophilic, finely granular (ground-glass) cytoplasm, which is PAS-positive and diastase-resistant (Fig. 6-24 *A,B*). Scattered lymphocytes are also present. The multinucleated giant cells are large (50–100 μ) and often contain bizarre, randomly arranged nuclei. There are fewer numbers of Touton-type giant cells.[84] Based on the presence of Touton-type giant cells and a minority population of vacuolated, foamy, and spindle-shaped histiocytes (i.e., a heterogenous population of histiocytes, similar to that seen in xanthogranuloma), some consider solitary reticulohistiocytoma to be a variant of xanthogranuloma.[84]

A solitary cutaneous nodule composed of histiocytes with eosinophilic, ground-glass cytoplasm or large bizarre multinucleated giant cells with similar ground-glass cytoplasm is distinctive. A nonacral location and absence of associated arthritis are additional clinical features that allow distinction from multicentric reticulohistiocytosis. The immunohistochemical profile of solitary reticulohistiocytoma [KP1 (CD68)-, HAM56-, factor XIIIa–, muscle actin (HHF35)-positive; S-

100-negative] is identical to xanthogranuloma and different from multicentric reticulohistiocytosis [KP1 (CD68)-, HAM56-positive; S-100-, factor XIIIa–, muscle actin (HHF35)-negative].[84]

Fibrous Histiocytoma (Dermatofibroma) (See Chapter 30)

Progressive Nodular Histiocytoma

Progressive nodular histiocytoma is an extremely rare disorder with only two reported cases.[85,86] The etiology is unknown, but it shares some clinical and histologic features with eruptive dermatofibromas (histiocytomas).

Clinical Features The two reported cases occurred in a 9-year-old girl and a 29-year-old man who were otherwise healthy. Both presented with numerous, generalized lesions of two different morphologies: superficial yellow-brown papules and deep nodules with overlying telangiectases. These were distributed on the trunk, face, and extremities. Mucosal involvement was reported on the tongue, larynx, and conjunctiva.[85,86]

Histopathological Features The histology of lesions (whether superficial or deep) resembled the spectrum of histologic appearances encountered in dermatofibromas. Histology demonstrated either predominantly foamy, lipid-laden histiocytes or predominantly spindle cells in a vague storiform pattern. Like dermatofibroma, intracellular and extracellular hemosiderin were also present. Sudan black and oil red O stains of frozen tissue confirmed that the foamy material within histiocytes was lipid.[85,86]

Histology recapitulating the spectrum of dermatofibroma in the clinical setting of innumerable generalized papules and nodules is suggestive of progressive nodular histiocytoma. It may be related to generalized eruptive histiocytosis/histiocytoma (see the preceding).[81,82]

Hereditary Progressive Mucinous Histiocytosis

First described by Bork and Hoede in 1988, hereditary progressive mucinous histiocytosis is an extremely rare disorder with only nine affected patients reported.[87,88] It is most likely autosomal dominantly inherited. Unlike other non-Langerhans cell histiocytoses, there is no spontaneous involution. Histologically, individual lesions demonstrate copious connective tissue mucin.

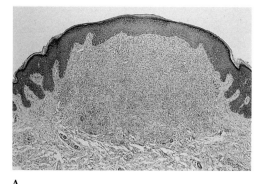

A

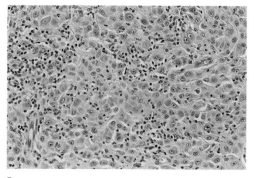

B

FIGURE 6-24 Reticulohistiocytoma. (*A,B*) A discrete infiltrate of histiocytes have glassy cytoplasms and single to multiple nuclei. They are accompanied by a mixed inflammatory cell infiltrate predominantly of lymphocytes.

Clinical Features The patients present in adolescence with numerous dark red, blue, or brown papules that increase in number over time. The lesions are distributed primarily on extremities, but the trunk, head, and face are also involved. Neither mucous membrane nor visceral involvement is seen.

Histopathological Features Histology reveals dilated vascular spaces and spindle-shaped and stellate histiocytes arranged either interstitially between collagen bundles or in vague, nodular aggregates. Preexisting collagen bundles are separated by abundant connective tissue mucin, which stains with alcian blue. Lymphocytes, plasma cells, and eosinophils are not seen.[87,88]

The presence of copious mucin surrounding aggregates of histiocytes and lack of accompanying lymphocytes, plasma cells, or eosinophils are distinctive.

Multinucleate Cell Angiohistiocytoma

Multinucleate cell angiohistiocytoma is a recently described condition that is thought to be inflammatory. Females are affected more often than males, and the average age in one series was 65 years.[89] The etiology is unknown, but trauma has been implicated.

Clinical Features The typical patient is an older female who presents with multiple unilateral or bilateral, smooth-surfaced, red-brown to violaceous papules of long duration. Papules are distributed on the extremities, backs of hands, and less commonly the face. A generalized form also has been described.[90]

Histopathological Features There are numerous dilated vessels with prominent, but not atypical endothelial cells. The most characteristic feature is that of numerous multinucleated giant cells with scalloped eosinophilic cytoplasms scattered interstitially between thickened collagen bundles of the reticular dermis.[89–91] The nuclei of the multinucleate giant cells are hyperchromatic and either clumped within the center of the cell or arranged to the periphery in a floret-type pattern. Perivascular lymphocytes, plasma cells, and neutrophils are also seen. Variable findings include overlying epidermal hyperplasia, basal cell hyperpigmentation, and compact hyperorthokeratosis.[89,90] The multinucleated giant cells are S-100- and CD1a (OKT6)-negative, but vimentin-positive. Staining with factor XIIIa reveals numerous interstitial factor XIIIa–positive dermal dendrocytes, but the multinucleated giant cells fail to react with factor XIIIa.[91]

The dilated vascular spaces and bizarre multinucleate giant cells are characteristic. The histologic appearances resemble dermatofibroma, fibrous papule, and the soft tissue neoplasm, giant cell fibroblastoma, but the clinical context usually is distinctive.

Malakoplakia

Malakoplakia is most commonly encountered in the setting of immunosuppression. Although the etiology is not entirely understood, it is hypothesized that it may represent a chronic bacterial infection, in which there is a defect in the ability of histiocytes to degrade ingested bacteria.[92] Coliform bacteria (especially *E. coli*) are most frequently isolated, but in skin lesions *Staphylococcus aureus* has been implicated. The urinary tract is most frequently affected, but the gastrointestinal tract, lymph nodes, genitalia, brain, bones, lungs, and adrenal glands are other potential sites of involvement. Skin lesions have been reported but are rare.[92]

Clinical Features Cutaneous lesions of malakoplakia are yellow-pink indurated or polypoid nodules that may ulcerate and are most commonly distributed in the groin or perianally.

Histopathological Features There are dense sheetlike collections of histiocytes with either foamy, granular, or vacuolated cytoplasms.[92] The most characteristic feature is Michaelis-Gutmann bodies. These are 5–15 µ, oval-to-spherical, concentrically laminated basophilic structures, found both extracellularly and intracellularly within histiocytes (von Hansemann histiocytes). Michaelis-Gutmann bodies are PAS-positive, diastase-resistant, and stain positively with von Kossa's calcium stain and with Perl's stain for iron. Michaelis Gutmann bodies are distinctive and diagnostic of malakoplakia.

Reaction to Granulocyte-Macrophage Colony-Stimulating Factor

Granulocyte-macrophage colony-stimulating factor (GMCSF) is a recombinant human hematopoietic growth factor used in the setting of bone marrow transplantation, systemic chemotherapy, and radiation therapy to amplify the numbers of circulating granulocytes and macrophages.[93]

Clinical Features Fairly common side effects from GMCSF include fever, myalgias, peripheral eosinophilia, and bone pain. Less commonly, patients develop a maculopapular eruption of the trunk and extremities, which begins within 3 days of initiation of therapy, and resolves within 10 days after discontinuation.[93–95] Some patients develop erythroderma after subcutaneous administration of GMCSF.

Histopathological Features There is a diffuse mixed inflammatory cell infiltrate of lymphocytes, eosinophils, and neutrophils present within the papillary and superficial reticular dermis.[93,94] Clustered and enlarged macrophages, sometimes with phagocytized elastin fragments, are characteristic. Variable findings include epidermal spongiosis and interface vacuolar changes. The erythrodermic cases demonstrate a spongiotic dermatitis with lymphocytes and eosinophils, but without macrophages.[95]

Clustered and enlarged macrophages are distinctive of the maculopapular reactions secondary to GMCSF. In many respects, this entity is similar to an incomplete granuloma annulare–like tissue reaction to mixed inflammatory cell dermatitis (see Granuloma Annulare) with elastophagocytosis.[33,34]

Clofazimine-Induced Hyperpigmentation

Leprosy patients and patients with mycobacterium avium-intracellulare treated with clofazimine sometimes develop a peculiar hyperpigmentation at sites of cutaneous disease, which begins as a pink macular discoloration and gradually darkens into brown over a 6- to 12-month period. The reaction is rarely biopsied by physicians familiar with the drug and its side effects.[96]

Clinical Features As discussed in the preceding section.

Histopathological Features There are large collections of dermal macrophages whose cytoplasm is foamy and contains brownish-pigment granules and needle-shaped crystals. The granules are PAS-positive, autofluorescent, and react with lipofuscin stains. Iron and melanin stains are negative. By electron microscopy, the brown granules represent lipofuscinlike material within lysosomes and are probably a breakdown product of clofazimine.[96] The clinical setting, history of clofazimine administration, and reaction with lipofuscin stains are distinctive.

Monsel's Solution Reaction

Monsel's solution (solution of ferric subsulfate) is a topical agent used for hemostasis after superficial biopsies. Monsel's solution reaction is encountered usually when examining sections of excised malignant skin lesions that have been previously biopsied and treated with Monsel's. At first glance, the reaction may be mistaken for malignant melanoma because of both the fine, dark, brown-black cytoplasmic granules and reactive atypia of macrophages.[97] Similar changes may occur from iron sesquioxide, an archaic therapy for skin ulcers.[98]

Clinical Features   Brown pigmentation in the area of application can occur.

Histopathological Features   Underlying an ulcer or scar of previous procedure, there is a diffuse, sometimes nodular infiltrate of macrophages containing dark brown or black, granular intracytoplasmic pigment (Fig. 6-25 A). The pigment is finer and less refractile than hemosiderin obtained from the breakdown of red blood cells and resembles intracytoplasmic melanin. Similar extracellular granules can be seen decorating dermal collagen bundles. The collagen bundles also may show amphophilic discoloration in sections stained with hematoxylin and eosin. Foreign-body type multinucleate giant cells are often seen. In some cases the macrophages exhibit atypia with large irregularly shaped hyperchromatic nuclei and prominent nucleoli. The intra- and extracellular pigment granules stain positively with special stains for iron (Perl's or Gomori's) (Fig. 6-25 B).[97,98]

The presence of scar or ulcer of previous procedure, intra- and extracellular pigment, and foreign body giant cells (sometimes seen) are helpful in differentiating Monsel's reaction. In cases of doubt, special stains for iron (Perl's or Gomori's) are very helpful. Monsel's solution reactions are, in effect, a foreign body reaction to a ferruginous tattoo.

Aluminum Chloride Solution Reaction

Synonyms: Aluminum tattoo

Aluminum chloride solution, like Monsel's solution, is a topical agent used for hemostasis following superficial shave biopsies. The aluminum particles induce a foreign-body macrophage response. The basophilic intracytoplasmic aluminum particles may bear a superficial resemblance to phagocytized Leishmania, *Calymmatobacterium granulomatis*, or histoplasmosis.[99]

Clinical Features   No clinical features are distinctive, purely a histologic finding.

Histopathological Features   Underlying an ulcer or scar of previous procedure, there is a diffuse infiltrate of macrophages containing intracytoplasmic basophilic particles. Multinucleate giant cells may or may not be present. In contrast to infectious organisms, the basophilic particles vary in size and shape, do not contain a nucleus or kinetoplast, and fail to stain with PAS, GMS, Giemsa, or Gram's stains.[99]

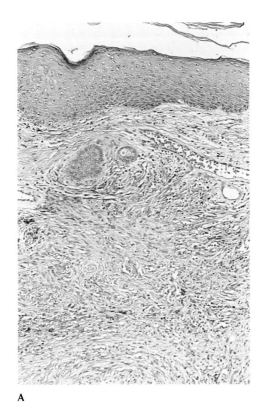
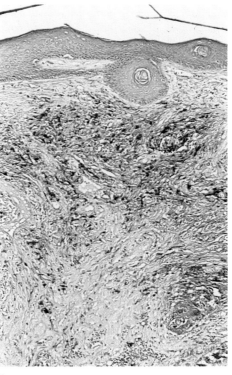

A   B

FIGURE 6-25   Monsel's solution reaction. (*A*) Diffuse nodular infiltrate of macrophages containing dark brown intracytoplasmic pigment. In addition there are extracellular granules associated with collagen bundles. (*B*) The pigment granules stain blue with special stains for iron (Perl's).

The variable size and shape of the intracytoplasmic particles, scar or ulcer of previous procedure, and history of prior biopsy are sufficient in distinguishing aluminum chloride solution reaction from infection.

Differential Diagnosis   High-grade large cell lymphomas of B- or T-cell type may bear a superficial resemblance to the diffuse histiocytic processes described earlier. This occurrence is particularly problematic when the lymphoma has a significant granulomatous inflammation component. The neoplastic lymphocytes of large cell lymphomas have vesicular nuclei with prominent nucleoli, numerous mitotic figures, and at times have associated areas of necrosis. The lymphoid cells usually are immunoreactive with LCA (CD 45) and B-(CD20) or T-(CD3) cell markers. Ki-1 (CD30)-positive anaplastic large cell lymphoma displays large epithelioid lymphocytes, some multinucleated with striking nuclear atypia.[100,101] Some forms of peripheral T-cell lymphoma, particularly subcutaneous T-cell lymphomas, are associated with benign histiocytes that engulf erythrocytes and inflammatory cells (cytophagocytosis).[102]

Phagocytosis of red blood cells, lymphocytes, plasma cells, neutrophils, and other inflammatory cell elements may be encountered in a variety of other conditions, including infection (most often viral, but also bacterial, fungal, and parasitic), multiple myeloma, hairy cell and other leukemias, Hodgkin's disease, some high-grade carcinomas, Rosai-Dorfman disease (see the preceding), reticulohistiocytoma (see the preceding), and a benign autosomal recessive familial condition.[103,104]

The differential diagnosis of diffuse "histiocytic" panniculitis also includes Rosai-Dorfman disease, rare cases of true histiocytic sarcoma, and cutaneous lesions of Whipple's disease.[104] Whipple's disease features PAS-positive bacteria (*Tropheryma whipelii*) within the cytoplasms of macrophages.[105]

Atypical fibroxanthoma (superficial malignant fibrous histiocytoma) is a soft tissue neoplasm that most commonly occurs on the head of elderly patients. Pleomorphic spindled and epithelioid cells with bizarre multinucleate giant cells and numerous mitotic figures, usually with foci of fascicle formation, help to distinguish this neoplasm from the inflammatory conditions described in the preceding.[91] Atypical fibroxanthoma lacks the cytokeratin immunoreactivity seen in spindle-cell squamous cell carcinomas, and the S-100 immunoreactivity seen in spindle-cell melanomas.

Benign or malignant neoplasms composed of granular cells may resemble diffuse histiocytic infiltrates. Examples include benign and malignant granular cell schwannoma, congenital gingival epulis, granular cell fibrous papule, granular cell leiomyoma and leiomyosarcoma,

granular cell basal cell carcinoma, granular cell angiosarcoma, granular cell dermatofibrosarcoma protuberans, and primitive polypoid granular cell tumor.[106,107]

Spitz's nevi, which lack a junctional component (intradermal Spitz's nevi, desmoplastic nevi), feature cells with abundant eosinophilic cytoplasm and large vesicular nuclei with prominent nucleoli, arranged in an interstitial pattern between thickened collagen bundles. The cells can particularly resemble the epithelioid histiocytes in reticulohistiocytoma. A nested arrangement of the cells offers a clue to this melanocytic nevus. These cells are S-100-positive, but HAM56-, and CD1a (OKT6)-negative. Invasive malignant melanoma, especially balloon cell melanoma, may demonstrate epithelioid cells with clear cytoplasms. Intranuclear cytoplasmic inclusions and pleomorphic nuclei with prominent nucleoli are suggestive of malignant melanoma. Cytoplasmic melanin may be abundant, scarce, or absent altogether. The cells are almost always S-100- and sometimes HMB45-positive. Melanocytic nevi also can have dominant balloon cell populations that simulate xanthomatous infiltrates.[108]

Metastatic poorly differentiated carcinomas assume either an interstitial or nodular pattern within the dermis. The most common metastases to the skin are from breast, lung, and colon cancers and from malignant melanoma. Stains for epithelial mucins and antibodies against low-molecular-weight cytokeratins are helpful in proving the epithelial nature of carcinomas.

Lysosomal storage diseases and other diseases associated with enzyme defects may demonstrate diffuse tissue macrophages in cutaneous lesions (Table 6-14).

NEUTROPHILIC INFILTRATES

Table 6-15 lists infectious diseases whose histologic pattern is typically, but not exclusively, diffuse neutrophilic.

Sweet's Syndrome (See also Chapter 9)

Synonyms: Acute febrile neutrophilic dermatosis

The etiology underlying Sweet's syndrome is unknown, but it is seen in association with myelogenous leukemia (10 to 15 percent of cases), lymphoma, multiple myeloma, polycythemia vera, adenocarcinomas, and upper respiratory tract infections. The pathogenesis is not known. A true vasculitis is not seen. A pathogenesis involving immune complexes and hyperchemotaxis of neutrophils has been proposed.[109]

Clinical Features   Adult females are most frequently affected. Patients present with tender erythematous-violaceous nodules or plaques on the face, neck, and arms. Patients also have a flulike illness with fever, malaise, arthralgias, and conjunctivitis. A peripheral leukocytosis usually is present.

Histopathological Features   Fully developed lesions demonstrate a diffuse neutrophilic infiltrate with marked papillary dermal edema. (Fig. 6-26 *A*) Fewer numbers of eosinophils, macrophages, and lymphocytes are present, and lymphocytes may increase in number in later stages. As a rule, plasma cells are not seen in Sweet's syndrome.[110] Vessels may demonstrate dilatation, prominent endothelial cells,

TABLE 6-14

Enzyme Deficiency Disorders

Disorder	Heredity	Clinical	Histology/EM
Disseminated lipogranulomatosis (Farber's disease)	Autosomal recessive; ceramidase deficiency	Subcutaneous nodules over wrist/ankles Hoarseness Pulmonary failure Mental retardation	Dense fibrosis and interstitial foamy histiocytes; EM: curvilinear bodies; zebra bodies; banana bodies
Niemann-Pick disease	Autosomal recessive; sphingomyelinase deficiency	Xanthomas CNS degeneration Hepatosplenomegaly	Foamy histiocytes, with lymphocytes, multinucleate giant cells
Mannosidosis	Mannosidase deficiency	Gargoyle facies Mental retardation Hyperplastic gingiva	Vacuolated histiocytes in gingival biopsies

TABLE 6-15

Infectious Causes of Diffuse Neutrophilic Infiltrates

	Organism	Tissue morphology	Histologic features
Bacillary angiomatosis	Bartonella henselae Bartonella quintana	Warthin-Starry-pos rods	Purple clumps of bacteria (H&E); pyogenic granuloma–like
Verruga peruana (Bartonellosis)	Bartonella bacilliformis	Warthin-Starry- or Giemsa-pos rods	Rocha-Lima bodies in endothelial cells; pyogenic granuloma–like
Toxic shock syndrome	S. aureus	Usually not seen	Clusters of necrotic keratinocytes and neutrophils
Amoeba	Entamoeba histolytica Acanthamoeba	12–20-μ round-ovoid cells sometimes with phagocytized RBCs (H&E)	May show leukocytoclastic vasculitis
Suppurative folliculitis	S. aureus	Gram-positive cocci in clusters	Folliculocentric and folliculodestructive
Erysipelas/cellulitis	Group A Strep. S. aureus H. influenzae	Gram-positive cocci in chains or clusters; Gram-negative rods	Dermal edema, sparse infiltrate
Atypical mycobacteria	M. fortuitum M. chelonei	Slightly larger than M. tuberculosis	Neutrophilic panniculitis
Anthrax	Bacillus anthracis	Large Gram-positive rod 6–10μ long	Numerous extravasated erythrocytes

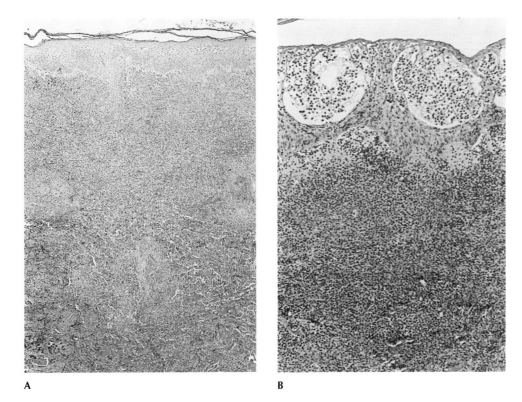

A   B

FIGURE 6-26 Sweet's syndrome. (A) A dense diffuse neutrophilic infiltrate fills the papillary dermis and extends deep into the reticular dermis. There is sparing of the epidermis. (B) Atypical Sweet's. This biopsy was taken from a patient with a myelodysplastic syndrome with evolving granulocytic leukemia. In addition to the dense infiltrate in the dermis, the epidermis is involved with intraepidermal pustules.

intramural and perivascular neutrophils, but fibrin deposition and intraluminal microthrombi are not seen. Thus, a true vasculitis (defined by the presence of intramural fibrin and/or intraluminal microthrombi) is not seen.[109] Leukocytoclasis may be prominent but should not be considered an indication of a primary vasculitis, for some leukocytoclasis may be encountered in any condition where neutrophils comprise a large bulk of the infiltrate. Papillary dermal edema may be so extensive that subepidermal vesiculation occurs. Intraepithelial spongiotic vesicles are sometimes seen.

Marked papillary dermal edema and an absence of vasculitis distinguish Sweet's syndrome. The presence of plasma cells should suggest a diagnosis other than Sweet's.[110]

Rheumatoid Neutrophilic Dermatitis

Rheumatoid neutrophilic dermatitis (dermatosis) is seen in the setting of severe rheumatoid arthritis. The pathogenesis is not understood, but in the few reports of this rare dermatosis, a true vasculitis has not been seen.[111,112]

Clinical Features Patients have severe, long-standing rheumatoid arthritis and present with symmetric, erythematous papules, plaques, and/or vesicles typically over the extensor surfaces of forearms and interphalangeal joints.[111,112]

Histopathological Features The histology is virtually identical to that seen in Sweet's syndrome, with the following exceptions: neutrophils tend to accumulate in and expand dermal papillae, causing histologic similarity to dermatitis herpetiformis; and plasma cells are present in the infiltrate. Like Sweet's syndrome, subepidermal bulla formation or intraepithelial spongiotic vesicles may be seen in some cases.[113]

The clinical setting of severe rheumatoid arthritis combined with Sweet's-like histology, plasma cells, and expansion of dermal papillae with large numbers of neutrophils should suggest rheumatoid neutrophilic dermatitis.

Pyoderma Gangrenosum (See also Chapter 9)

The pathogenesis of pyoderma gangrenosum is unknown, but immune complex–mediated neutrophilic vascular reactions and abnormalities in humoral and cell-mediated immunity have been suggested.[109] Disease associations include ulcerative colitis, Crohn's disease, paraproteinemia (most commonly IgA), seronegative arthritis, rheumatoid arthritis, myeloproliferative disorders (particularly chronic myelogenous leukemia and polycythemia vera), lymphoma, multiple myeloma, HIV infection, systemic lupus erythematosus, and chronic active hepatitis. Half of all cases, however, are unassociated with systemic disease.[114]

Clinical Features Lesions of pyoderma gangrenosum begin as erythematous papules/nodules which expand centrifugally into large ulcers with characteristic heaped up and undermined violaceous borders. The lower extremities are preferentially affected, but lesions may be seen at any site. In cases of pyoderma gangrenosum arising in the setting of leukemia, a bullous variant has been described (also known as atypical pyoderma gangrenosum, atypical Sweet's syndrome), which has overlapping clinical and histologic features with Sweet's syndrome (Fig. 6-26 *B*). Because of this overlap, Caughman et al. have suggested that neutrophilic dermatoses in the setting of myeloproliferative disorders be grouped under the term *neutrophilic dermatosis of malignancy*.[114]

Histopathological Features In well-developed lesions, there is a dense diffuse neutrophilic infiltrate, which characteristically begins as a folliculocentric and sometimes folliculodestructive process. Variable

numbers of lymphocytes, macrophages, and eosinophils also are present. True vasculitis as evidenced by intramural fibrin, intramural neutrophils, and intraluminal microthrombi may be seen, but when present, the vasculitic changes probably are secondary to the abscess rather than initiating events. As in any dermatitis with significant numbers of neutrophils, some leukocytoclasis invariably is present. As the infiltrate expands, the central epidermis ulcerates and the adjacent intact epidermis has an undermined appearance (Fig. 6-27). The more peripheral erythematous area displays a perivascular lymphocytic infiltrate.

A dense, deep, and diffuse folliculocentric neutrophilic infiltrate should suggest pyoderma gangrenosum. As already mentioned, in the setting of myeloproliferative disorders and leukemia, there is significant histologic overlap with Sweet's syndrome and a distinction between the two is not always possible. *Neutrophilic dermatosis of malignancy* has considerable utility for that clinical scenario.[114]

Bowel-Associated Dermatosis-Arthritis Syndrome (See also Chapter 9)

Synonyms: Bowel bypass syndrome, pustular pyoderma gangrenosum

The bowel-associated dermatosis-arthritis syndrome is seen among patients with inflammatory bowel disease, diverticular disease, or those who have undergone either jejunoileal bypass surgery for morbid obesity or Billroth II surgery, resulting in a blind loop of bowel.[115,116] A similar eruption can be seen among patients with liver disease such as chronic hepatitis (especially autoimmune hepatitis) and/or cholangitis (especially primary sclerosing cholangitis). Circulating immune complexes and hyperchemotaxis of neutrophils induced by enteropathic bacteria appear to be responsible for the clinical features.[116]

Clinical Features Patients with one of the mentioned clinical scenarios present with fever, gastrointestinal upset, and recurrent crops of pustules on purpuric bases that are distributed on the trunk and extremities.

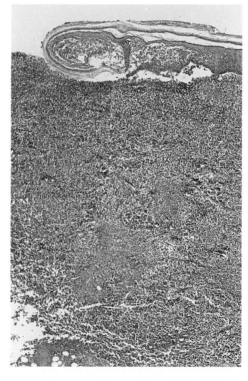

FIGURE 6-27 Pyoderma gangrenosum. A dense diffuse infiltrate extends from an ulcerated epidermis deep into the subcutaneous fat. Infiltrate undermines the adjacent epidermis, which is showing extensive spongiosis.

TABLE 6-16

Bowel-Associated Dermatosis-Arthritis Syndrome

Clinical Features

Patients with either
  Inflammatory bowel disease
  Diverticular disease
  Jejunoileal bypass surgery
  Billroth II surgery
  Chronic autoimmune hepatitis
  Primary sclerosing cholangitis
Fever
Gastrointestinal upset
Pustules on purpuric bases, or
Erythema nodosum–like lesions
Trunk/extremities
Nonerosive arthritis

Histopathological Features

Identical to Sweet's syndrome
  Diffuse neutrophils
  Papillary dermal edema
  Leukocytoclasis, but no true vasculitis

Differential Diagnosis

Sweet's syndrome
Rheumatoid neutrophilic dermatitis
Pyoderma gangrenosum
Behcet's disease
Infection

TABLE 6-17

Behcet's Disease

Clinical Features

Oral ulcers (aphthae)
Genital ulcers
Erythema nodosum–like lesions
Pseudofolliculitis
Pathergy-induced lesions
Papulopustular lesions
Acneiform nodules
Multiorgan involvement (including uveitis)
  is common

Histopathological Features

Early
  Superficial and deep perivascular and interstitial
    with many neutrophils
  Neutrophils and fewer lymphocytes
  Leukocytoclasis, but no true vasculitis
Late
  Superficial and deep perivascular with
    mostly lymphocytes

Differential Diagnosis

Sweet's syndrome
Rheumatoid neutrophilic dermatitis
Pyoderma gangrenosum
Bowel-associated dermatosis-arthritis syndrome
Infection

Erythema nodosum–like lesions also may be seen. Additional clinical manifestations may include a nonerosive arthritis or flulike symptoms of arthralgia, myalgias, and chills.

Histopathological Features   Histology is identical to that seen in Sweet's syndrome. However, like the situation encountered in atypical lesions of Sweet's and pyoderma gangrenosum in the setting of myeloproliferative disorders, there is some histologic overlap with pyoderma gangrenosum.[115,116] Thus, some lesions may demonstrate neutrophilic infiltrates that are distinctly folliculocentric.

The clinical scenario of pustular lesions with Sweet's-like histology in the setting of prior bowel surgery, inflammatory bowel disease, diverticular disease, liver disease, or cholangitis is distinctive (Table 6-16).

Behcet's Disease

Behcet's disease is a multisystem disease of unknown etiology. Hypersensitivity reactions to a previous streptococcal infection have been proposed. The pathogenesis may involve an immune complex–mediated vascular reaction with hyperchemotaxis of neutrophils.[109]

Clinical Features   The classic clinical triad consists of oral aphthae, genital aphthae, and uveitis. Behcet's disease can potentially affect many organ systems, including joints (arthritis), central nervous system (meningoencephalitis), kidney, heart, lung, and reproductive system. Although aphthae may involve any portion of the gastrointestinal tract, it should be emphasized that patients with inflammatory bowel disease (i.e., ulcerative colitis, Crohn's disease) do not have Behcet's disease.

Mucocutaneous manifestations consist of oral ulcers (aphthae), genital ulcers, erythema nodosum–like lesions, pseudofolliculitis, pathergy-induced lesions, and papulopustular lesions or acneiform nodules.[117]

Histopathological Features   The histology is controversial, but both pathergy-induced and spontaneous lesions demonstrate a spectrum of histologies, probably reflective of stage of disease at the time of biopsy. The infiltrate ranges from a perivascular mixed inflammatory cell infiltrate with neutrophils, to a perivascular infiltrate of lymphocytes only, to a diffuse neutrophilic infiltrate resembling Sweet's. The vascular changes range from intramural neutrophils without intramural fibrin or intraluminal microthrombi, to lymphocytic vasculitis, to true leukocytoclastic vasculitis; however, true leukocytoclastic vasculitis is rare.[118] On balance, a superficial and deep perivascular and interstitial mixed inflammatory cell infiltrate with numerous neutrophils and fewer lymphocytes probably best characterizes early lesions of Behcet's. Later, a predominantly perivascular lymphocytic infiltrate is seen. Early-induced pathergy lesions show a dense, but focal, aggregation of neutrophils at the immediate injury site.[119] As this histology is rather nonspecific, a diagnosis of Behcet's disease can only be made with clinicopathologic correlation (Table 6-17).

Granuloma Faciale (See Chapter 9)

Erythema Elevatum Diutinum (See Chapter 9)

Reactions to Granulocyte Colony–Stimulating Factor

Patients receiving granulocyte colony–stimulating factor (GCSF) may develop a neutrophilic dermatosis, which clinically and histologically resembles Sweet's syndrome with fever and tender erythematous plaques and nodules.[120] This neutrophilic dermatosis is a direct effect of GCSF, which increases absolute neutrophil counts after myelosuppressive therapy, and, unlike GMCSF (granulocyte-macrophage colony-stimulating factor), specifically targets the neutrophil cell line.

Clinical Features   See the preceding section.

Histopathological Features   Histology reveals dense dermal infiltrates of neutrophils with abundant nuclear dust and, in some cases, true leukocytoclastic vasculitis. Some cases histologically resemble bullous pyoderma gangrenosum (also known as atypical Sweet's syndrome, atypical pyoderma gangrenosum).[120] The clinical scenario and history of GCSF therapy is distinctive.

Differential Diagnosis   A photodistributed and photoexacerbated neutrophilic dermatosis clinically resembling Sweet's syndrome has been described in some HIV-infected patients. This neutrophilic dermatosis in HIV infection may be idiopathic or related to photosensitizing medications or GCSF therapy. The histology resembles bullous pyoderma gangrenosum (also known as atypical Sweet's syndrome).[121]

Venomous spider bites (i.e., brown recluse) feature prominent tissue necrosis, hemorrhage, and a mixed infiltrate with a predominance of neutrophils and fewer eosinophils. Vessels in the vicinity of the inflammation often demonstrate intraluminal thrombi.

Acute myelomonocytic (M4) and acute monocytic (M5) are the most common forms of granulocytic leukemia to involve the skin. Histology demonstrates a diffuse, often interstitial, infiltrate of immature granulocytes within the dermis and subcutaneous fat. Conversely, in patients with neutrophilic dermatitis who have the Pelger-Huët neutrophil anomaly, congenital or acquired (pseudo), the infiltrate can masquerade as leukemia cutis. The neutrophils are not segmented normally and can simulate leukemic blasts or other immature granulocytic precursors.[122] Granulocytic sarcomas (chloromas) are solitary cutaneous tumors composed of dense nodular aggregates of leukemic cells with admixed eosinophils.

Cutaneous extramedullary hematopoiesis is seen in neonates as part of the "blueberry muffin baby" syndrome or in adults as a consequence of myelofibrosis with myeloid metaplasia. Extramedullary hematopoiesis demonstrates a diffuse interstitial infiltrate of myeloid and erythroid elements in various stages of maturation, and fewer megakaryocytes, as would be seen in the bone marrow.

Leukocytoclastic vasculitis is a constituent of both erythema elevatum diutinum and granuloma faciale, but can be seen in a number of diverse clinical settings. The presence of leukocytoclasis, intraluminal thrombi, and vessels containing fibrin and inflammatory cells within their walls is diagnostic of leukocytoclastic vasculitis.

Neutrophilic eccrine hidradenitis is a side effect of chemotherapeutic agents (especially cytarabine) and is seen in the context of high-dose induction chemotherapy. It presents as tender erythematous papules and plaques with no particular distribution.[123] The neutrophilic infiltrate of neutrophilic eccrine hidradenitis is centered around the eccrine coils of the lower reticular dermis. Variable findings include vacuolar interface changes and dermal necrosis. Similar reactions may be seen with acetaminophen.[123] A condition not associated with chemotherapy or other drugs has been described as palmoplantar neutrophilic eccrine hidradenitis.[124,125] It is seen in otherwise healthy individuals, often children. It differs from the chemotherapy-related disease by the lack of both necrosis of the eccrine coil and syringosquamous metaplasia.[124,125] Actinomycin D–induced folliculitis also features numerous neutrophils. The folliculitis affects the face, trunk, and buttocks, typically occurs 1 week after induction chemotherapy with actinomycin D, and spontaneously resolves.[123]

The erysipelaslike skin lesions of familial Mediterranean fever demonstrate a mixed perivascular and interstitial inflammatory cell infiltrate with neutrophils, which resembles cellulitis. The differential diagnosis of panniculitis with neutrophils includes alpha-1 antitrypsin deficiency, infection, pancreatic fat necrosis, and gouty panniculitis.[105]

LYMPHOCYTIC-PLASMA CELLULAR INFILTRATES

Table 6-18 lists infectious diseases whose histologic pattern is typically, but not exclusively, diffuse lymphocytic-plasma cellular.

Plasmacytosis Mucosae

Synonyms: Zoon's balanitis; plasma cell vulvitis; plasmacytosis circumorificialis; orificial plasmacytosis; balanitis plasmacellularis; benign plasma cell erythroplasia; balanoposthitis chronica circumscripta plasmocellularis; plasma cell gingivitis

Plasmacytosis mucosae is an encompassing term for an inflammatory accumulation of plasma cells at mucosal sites. The term Zoon's balanitis is given to involvement of the prepuce or glans penis; plasma cell vulvitis to involvement of the vulva; and plasmacytosis circumorificialis, to involvement of the oral mucosa, lips, gums, or tongue in both sexes.[126] Most cases are idiopathic, but in oral mucosal lesions, immediate hypersensitivity reactions (often to chewing gum ingredients) have been implicated.

Clinical Features   The clinical presentation is similar at all three sites, consisting of well-marginated erythematous patches.

Histopathological Features   There is a dense, bandlike, mixed mononuclear inflammatory cell infiltrate with a predominance of plasma cells.[126] Dilated blood vessels, sometimes with red blood cell extravasation, also are seen. The epidermis may exhibit spongiosis with exocytosis of inflammatory cells.

The heterogeneous nature of the inflammatory cell infiltrate, with a predominance of plasma cells, in a typical locale should suggest plasmacytosis mucosae. Immunohistochemical study for light-chain restriction may be necessary to definitively rule out plasmacytoma.

Systemic and Cutaneous Plasmacytosis

Synonyms: Plasma cell type of giant lymph node hyperplasia; Castleman's disease; plasma cell type of angiofollicular hyperplasia; POEMS (polyneuropathy, organomegaly, endocrinopathy, M protein, skin lesions) syndrome

Systemic and cutaneous plasmacytosis is a disease spectrum typified by a polyclonal proliferation of plasma cells that lack atypia, arising in the absence of other chronic inflammatory or connective tissue diseases. By definition, the systemic variety affects more than two organ systems and typically produces lymphadenopathy.[127] Commonly affected organs include lymph nodes, lungs, and skin. A skin-limited form also exists (cutaneous plasmacytosis). Both the systemic and skin-limited forms are associated with polyclonal hypergammaglobulinemia. The etiology is unknown, but patients with both systemic and skin-limited forms have increased serum levels of IL-6, which may drive the plasma cell proliferation. Serum levels of IL-6 have proved useful in monitoring response to therapy.[127] There are several reports of Castleman's disease associated with POEMS syndrome, and in fact, POEMS may represent one aspect of this disease spectrum.

Clinical Features   Cutaneous lesions consist of multiple erythematous or red-brown nodules or plaques on the trunk and extremities.

TABLE 6-18

Infectious Causes of Diffuse Lymphocytic-Plasma Cellular Infiltrates

	Organism	Tissue morphology	Histopathological features
Syphilis	Treponema pallidum	Spirochete (Warthin-Starry-pos)	Psoriasiform hyperplasia; lichenoid and granulomatous
Yaws	Treponema pertenue	Spirochete (Warthin-Starry-pos)	Spirochetes in epidermis
Pinta	Treponema carateum	Spirochete (Warthin-Starry-pos)	Spirochetes in epidermis
Chancroid	Haemophilus ducreyi	Gram-negative bacillus (school of fish) (Warthin-Starry- or (Giemsa-pos)	Three-zone inflammation: PMN's and necrosis; granulation tissue; plasma cells
Granuloma inguinale	Calymmatobacterium granulomatosis	Intracellular gram-negative bacillus (Donovan bodies) (Giemsa- or Warthin-Starry-pos)	Organisms within macrophages
Lymphogranuloma venereum	Chlamydia trachomatis	1–4μ Giemsa- or direct immunofluorescence-pos coccoid bodies	Intracellular
Rhinoscleroma	Klebsiella rhinoscleromatis	Intracellular gram-negative rods (Frisch bacilli) (Warthin-Starry- or PAS-pos)	Organisms within macrophages (Mikulicz cells); Russell bodies
Lyme disease	Borrelia burgdorferi	Spirochete (larger than T. pallidum)	Superficial and deep perivascular or pseudolymphoma
Necrotizing fasciitis	Group A Strep, S. aureus	Gram-positive cocci in chains or clusters	Blood vessel thrombosis

Histopathological Features   There is a dense perivascular and periadnexal infiltrate of many plasma cells with fewer lymphocytes. The plasma cells lack atypia and are polyclonal, as evidenced by a lack of kappa or lambda light-chain restriction using immunoperoxidase techniques.

Dense perivascular and periadnexal infiltrates of benign plasma cells in the clinical setting of polyclonal hypergammaglobulinemia should suggest systemic or cutaneous plasmacytosis.

Differential Diagnosis   The major problem is differentiating these inflammatory conditions from neoplastic plasma cell infiltrates. Cutaneous plasmacytomas are monoclonal neoplastic proliferations of plasma cells. Cutaneous plasmacytomas may be primary (unassociated with multiple myeloma or extramedullary plasmacytoma) or secondary (arising in the setting of established multiple myeloma, extramedullary plasmacytoma, or plasma cell leukemia).[128] In general, the prognosis of primary cutaneous plasmacytomas is guarded, for primary cutaneous plasmacytomas may eventually progress to multiple myeloma (approximately 10 to 20 percent of cases) or develop metastases. The prognosis for secondary cutaneous plasmacytomas generally is very poor, indicating a large tumor cell burden.[128]

Cytologic features of plasmacytoma vary from mostly mature plasma cells, to mostly immature pleomorphic forms, to mixtures of the two. In cases composed of mostly well-differentiated plasma cells, clues to the neoplastic nature of the infiltrate include binucleated forms, many mitotic figures, and many Dutcher bodies (intranuclear PAS-positive inclusions). In poorly differentiated neoplasms, clues to the plasma cell nature of the infiltrate include eccentrically placed nuclei and peripherally placed dense chromatin (clock face chromatin). Immunohistochemical stains reveal light-chain restriction in all cases.[128]

In HIV-infected individuals, plasma cells may form a significant proportion of the inflammatory cell infiltrate in lesions of psoriasis, seborrheic dermatitis, and Kaposi's sarcoma (Table 6-18).[129]

Plasma cells may be prominent in some cases of nodular amyloidosis. The differential diagnosis of plasma cell panniculitis includes dermatomyositis, fasciitis with eosinophilia, morphea profunda, polymyositis, Sjögren's syndrome, and scleroderma.[130]

MAST CELL INFILTRATES

Cutaneous Mastocytosis

Synonyms: Solitary mastocytoma; urticaria pigmentosa; telangiectasia macularis eruptiva perstans (TMEP); systemic mastocytosis

Cutaneous mastocytosis is an umbrella term for four entities: solitary mastocytoma, urticaria pigmentosa, systemic mastocytosis, and TMEP.[131] In all four, there are excessive numbers of mast cells in the skin. Lesions of solitary mastocytoma and urticaria pigmentosa are limited to the skin and are more common in childhood. Urticaria pigmentosa may, over time, progress to systemic mastocytosis, in which excessive numbers of mast cells also are found in the viscera, such as the gastrointestinal tract (leading to diarrhea), bone marrow, liver, spleen, and lymph nodes. TMEP occurs in adults and rarely progresses to systemic mastocytosis. The release of vasoactive mediators (especially histamine) leads to the clinical manifestations of urticaria, wheal, and flare with pruritus.[131]

Clinical Features   The cutaneous lesions of solitary mastocytoma, urticaria pigmentosa, and systemic mastocytosis are reddish-brown macules, papules, or nodules that may be clinically confused with melanocytic lesions. Stroking of the lesion causes mast cell degranulation with the development of urticarial wheal and flare (Darier's sign). TMEP presents as pruritic lightly pigmented macules with surface telangiectases distributed on the trunk and proximal extremities.[131]

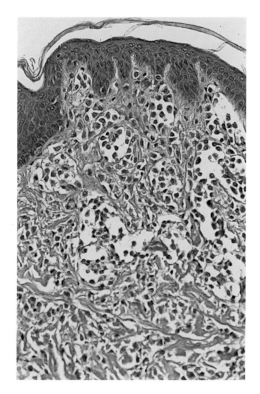

FIGURE 6-28   Cutaneous mastocytosis. Below an intact epidermis are sheets of uniform mononucleate cells with abundant amphophilic cytoplasms typical of mast cells.

Histopathological Features   In solitary mastocytoma, urticaria pigmentosa, and systemic mastocytosis, biopsy reveals either a perivascular or diffuse infiltrate of mast cells within the upper dermis (Fig. 6-28). Mast cells are round-oval cells with amphophilic-basophilic cytoplasm, centrally placed nuclei, and inconspicuous nucleoli (so-called fried-egg appearance). Mast cells stain with toluidine blue, chloracetate esterase, or Giemsa stains. Especially in childhood, excessive dermal edema may cause subepidermal bulla formation.[131] In TMEP, excessive numbers of

mast cells are distributed perivascularly around dilated superficial dermal vessels (similar to the distribution in normal skin) and are elongate-to-spindle-shaped (Table 6-19).[132,133]

Differential Diagnosis   The cells in papules and nodules are very uniform and on scanning magnification can resemble nevus cells, histiocytes or Langerhans cells, and leukemic infiltrates. The amphophilic cytoplasms and lack of nesting help to distinguish mast cell disease from melanocytic nevi. Histiocytic infiltrates may be characterized by cells with a monomorphous appearance; however, in contrast to mast cells, histiocytes usually have somewhat angulated or reniform nuclei. Special stains and immunohistochemistry may be needed to distinguish the latter conditions from mast cell disease.

In TMEP the low-power appearance resembles normal skin. As the histology of TMEP may be subtle, Giemsa or toluidine blue stains are helpful in highlighting the increased numbers of perivascular mast cells.[132,133] Normal skin may have up to ten mast cells per 40× field.[133] Dermatopathologists should always keep this diagnosis in mind when dealing with "normal skin" biopsies or patients with unexplained pruritus.

EOSINOPHILIC INFILTRATES

Table 6-20 lists parasitic diseases that produce large numbers of tissue eosinophils.

Well's Syndrome

Synonyms: Eosinophilic cellulitis

Well's syndrome (eosinophilic cellulitis) is an uncommon condition that is thought to be a hypersensitivity reaction. Most cases are completely idiopathic; others are associated with arthropod assaults, drug allergy, parasitic infestation, an atopic diathesis, internal malignancy, or dermatophyte infection.[134] Histology reveals eosinophilic infiltrates with flame figures and later granulomas (see the following). It should be emphasized that flame figures are not pathognomonic of Well's syndrome but constitute a dermal reaction pattern that may be seen in

TABLE 6-19

Cutaneous Mastocytosis

Solitary Mastocytoma	Urticaria Pigmentosa	Systemic Mastocytosis	TMEP
Clinical Features			
Infants, neonates	Infants, neonates	Adults, usually	Adults, usually
Single red-brown macule, papule, nodule	Multiple red-brown macules, papules, nodules	Multiple red-brown macules, papules, nodules	Lightly pigmented macules with telangiectases
Vesicle, bulla, sometimes	Vesicles, bullae, often	Extracutaneous involvement, as a rule	Rare progression to systemic mastocytosis
No extracutaneous involvement	No extracutaneous involvement		
	Rare progression to systemic mastocytosis		
Histopathological Features			
Perivascular or diffuse mast cells within upper dermis	Same as solitary mastocytoma	Same as solitary mastocytoma	Telangiectatic vessels with increased perivascular mast cells (>10 mast cells per 40× field)
Subepidermal bulla formation, sometimes			

TABLE 6-20

Parasitic Causes of Diffuse Eosinophilic Infiltrates

Disease	Organism
Schistosomiasis	S. haematobium
	S. japonicum
	S. mansoni
Cysticercosis	Taenia solium
Sparganosis	Spirometra sp.
Onchocerciasis	Onchocerca volvulus
Dirofilariasis	Dirofilaria immitis
Larva migrans	Ancylostoma braziliense
Strongyloidiasis	S. stercoralis
Gnathostomiasis	G. spinigerum
Trichinosis	Trichinella spiralis
Paragonimiasis	P. skrjabini
	P. westermani
Toxocariasis	T. canis
	T. cati
Dracunculosis	D. medinensis

any given lesion with numerous eosinophils, including allergic contact dermatitis, arthropod assault, bullous pemphigoid, and herpes gestationis.[135]

Clinical Features   Well's syndrome presents as arcuate erythematous, indurated plaques, typically on the upper back, extremities, or buttocks. As the lesions evolve they may become indurated and complete resolution usually occurs within 2 months.[134]

Histopathological Features   Histology reveals a diffuse and, early on, massive infiltrate of eosinophils with few lymphocytes (Fig. 6-29 A). In areas where eosinophils have degranulated, so-called "flame figures" are created (Fig. 6-29 B). These represent dermal collagen fibers that become coated with bright red, eosinophilic granules containing major basic protein surrounded by macrophages, sometimes with giant cells. Early lesions may result in subepidermal or intraepidermal vesicle/bulla formation. In later stages, macrophages with giant cells may predominate.[134,135] The panniculus may occasionally be involved, one cause of eosinophilic panniculitis.[105]

In the proper clinical setting, flame figures are very suggestive of Well's syndrome, but isolated lesions of common dermatoses with numerous eosinophils may feature flame figures.[135] A search to rule out associated conditions (especially internal malignancy, parasite infestation, and drug hypersensitivity) is warranted in patients with Well's syndrome (Table 6-21).

Hypereosinophilic Syndrome

The hypereosinophilic syndrome is a systemic disorder featuring peripheral eosinophilia and eosinophilic infiltration of numerous organs including heart, lungs, skin, kidneys, liver, gastrointestinal tract, and nervous system.[136] This syndrome encompasses Löeffler's endocarditis and eosinophilic leukemia but excludes other known causes for peripheral eosinophilia, such as parasite infestation or drug hypersensitivity. The skin is the second most common organ to be involved, preceded only by the heart.[136] The NIH inclusion criteria are as follows: (1) a persistent eosinophilia of 1500 eosinophils/mm^3 for greater than 6 months, or death before 6 months associated with the signs and symptoms of hypereosinophilic disease; (2) a lack of evidence for parasitic, allergic, or other known causes of eosinophilia; and (3) presumptive signs and symptoms of organ system involvement. Patients usually succumb to eosinophilic cardiomyopathy.

Clinical Features   The cutaneous lesions are either pruritic, erythematous, papules/nodules, or lesions of urticaria/angioedema, distributed on trunk, extremities, or face.[136]

Histopathological Features   Histology demonstrates a superficial and deep perivascular mixed inflammatory cell infiltrate of eosinophils and lymphocytes. In some cases neutrophils and plasma cells may be present. Flame figures typically are not seen, but cutaneous microthrombi may be present.[137] Cutaneous microthrombi most likely result from the large amounts of platelet activating factor released by eosinophils. Similar microthrombi are seen in other involved organs, and their presence portends a bad prognosis.[137]

Histologic diagnosis of this rare disorder requires clinicopathologic correlation, as similar histologic appearances may be seen in many of the entities discussed in the differential diagnosis that follows. Evidence of systemic involvement is suggestive of hypereosinophilic syndrome, but it is a diagnosis of exclusion (see NIH Inclusion Criteria). Cutaneous microthrombi may provide a valuable clue to the diagnosis.[137]

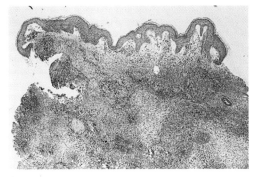

A

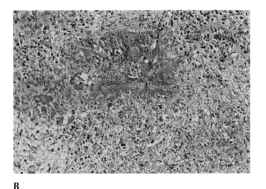

B

FIGURE 6-29   Well's syndrome. (*A*) A diffuse mixed inflammatory cell infiltrate containing numerous eosinophils extends into the subcutaneous fat. There is marked interstitial edema. (*B*) Numerous "flame figures" are formed by degenerated collagen produced by degranulation of eosinophils, which is rimmed by a wreath of macrophages.

Well's Syndrome

Clinical Features

Most cases idiopathic, but
Associations with:
    Drug hypersensitivity
    Parasites
    Internal malignancy
    Dermatophytes
Arcuate, erythematous, indurated plaques
Upper back, extremities, buttocks

Histopathological Features

Diffuse eosinophils
Flame figures
Eosinophilic panniculitis, sometimes
Granulomas, especially in late lesions

Differential Diagnosis

Hypereosinophilic syndrome
Arthropod assault
Allergic contact dermatitis
Bullous pemphigoid
Herpes gestationis
Pruritic urticarial papules and plaques of pregnancy (PUPPP)
Urticaria

Differential Diagnosis   Cutaneous arthropod assaults owing to insects (tungiasis, myiasis, pediculosis), scabies, ticks, and spiders demonstrate dense superficial and deep perivascular and interstitial mixed cell infiltrates with numerous eosinophils and are the most common demonstrable cause of clinical papular urticaria. Fortuitous sections may demonstrate embedded mouth or body parts, eggs, or excreta. Lesions of chronic urticaria or of physical urticaria demonstrate a perivascular lymphocytic infiltrate with scattered interstitial mixed cell infiltrates composed of lymphocytes, neutrophils, and eosinophils. Papular dermatitis (subacute prurigo) features a relatively sparse superficial and deep perivascular lymphocytic infiltrate with scattered interstitial eosinophils and, at times, overlying epidermal spongiosis.[138] Virtually identical appearances are seen in papular dermatitis of HIV.[129]

Changes to the side of eosinophilic folliculitis may resemble a primary perivascular dermatitis. Eosinophilic folliculitis may occur as an idiopathic condition in otherwise healthy individuals (Ofuji's disease) or in the setting of HIV. Often cutting deeper into the tissue blocks of tangential samples reveals a folliculocentric infiltrate of eosinophils and lymphocytes, which both surround and infiltrate the follicular epithelium, sometimes producing eosinophilic pustules.[139]

Urticarial lesions of bullous pemphigoid may feature slight psoriasiform hyperplasia, variable spongiosis with eosinophils in the epidermis (so-called eosinophilic spongiosis), and eosinophils in number in a slightly edematous papillary dermis. Both herpes gestationis and pruritic urticarial papules and plaques of pregnancy (PUPPP) (or the polymorphous eruption of pregnancy) are pregnancy-associated dermatoses that feature superficial perivascular lymphocytic infiltrates with interstitial eosinophils. Spongiosis with eosinophils, which is histologically indistinguishable from bullous pemphigoid, is common in herpes gestationis, but absent in PUPPP.[140] Additionally, the density of eosinophils is much greater in herpes gestationis and bullous pemphigoid, and in PUPPP they tend to involve the reticular dermis more than the papillary dermis.[140]

Type A lesions of lymphomatoid papulosis may feature eosinophils, but only rarely do they make up a significant part of the infiltrate. In addition to the superficial and deep perivascular mixed cell infiltrate, Ki-1 (CD30)-positive and LeuM1 (CD15)-negative large atypical cells are seen. A related condition called eosinophilic histiocytosis is thought by some to be a distinct Ki-1-negative entity that overlaps between lymphomatoid papulosis and Langerhans cell histiocytosis.[141]

Cutaneous lesions of Hodgkin's disease generally arise as a result of retrograde spread to the skin from involved lymph nodes, but primary cutaneous disease is well-documented.[142–144] The histology of cutaneous lesions mirrors that seen in lymph nodes with nodular or diffuse mixed cell infiltrates with eosinophils and either Hodgkin's cells or classic Reed-Sternberg cells.[142] The immunophenotype of Reed-Sternberg and Hodgkin's cells in cutaneous examples is similar to that observed in lymph nodes [Ki-1 (CD30)-positive, Leu-M1 (CD15)-positive, LCA (CD45)-negative]. Lymphocyte predominant forms of Hodgkin's disease are Leu-M1 (CD15)-negative.[142–144]

Angiolymphoid hyperplasia with eosinophilia is a vascular lesion that most commonly occurs on the head and neck. As its name implies, histology features a vascular proliferation with prominent endothelial cells, numerous eosinophils, and lymphoid aggregates, sometimes with germinal center formation. It is unclear as to whether this represents a reactive or neoplastic condition. Its relationship to Kimura's disease also is unsettled. The differential diagnosis of panniculitis with eosinophils includes erythema nodosum, vasculitis, Well's syndrome, drug reaction, atopic dermatitis, contact dermatitis, streptococcus infection, parasitic infection (*Gnathostoma* or *Toxocara canis*), atheromatous emboli, foreign-body, malignancy, or lupus erythematosus panniculitis.[145]

REFERENCES

1. Marks R: Concepts in the pathogenesis of rosacea. *Br J Dermatol* 80:170, 1968.
2. Marks R, Harcourt-Webster JN: Histopathology of rosacea. *Arch Dermatol* 100:683, 1969.
3. Qureshi AA, Lerner LH, Lerner EA: Nitric oxide and the cutis. *Arch Dermatol* 132:889, 1996.
4. Wilkinson DS, Kirton V, Wilkinson JD: Perioral dermatitis: A 12-year review. *Br J Dermatol* 101:245, 1979.
5. Cotterill JA: Perioral Dermatitis. *Br J Dermatol* 101:259, 1979.
6. Hurwitz RH: Steroid Acne. *J Am Acad Dermatol* 21:1179, 1989.
7. Greene RM, Rogers RS: Melkersson-Rosenthal syndrome: A review of 36 patients. *J Am Acad Dermatol* 21:1263, 1989.
8. Zimmer WM, Rogers RS, Reeve CM, Sheridan PJ: Orofacial manifestations of Melkersson-Rosenthal syndrome: A study of 42 patients and a review of 220 cases from the literature. *Oral Surg Oral Med Oral Pathol* 74:610, 1992.
9. Vettraino IM, Merritt DF: Crohn's disease of the vulva. *Am J Dermatopathol* 17:410, 1995.
10. Lattanoos RL, Appleton MAC, Hughes LE, et al: Granulomatous hidradenitis suppurativa and cutaneous Crohn's disease. *Histopathology* 23:111, 1993.
11. Hackzell-Bradley M, Hedbald M-A, Stephanssson EA: Metastatic Crohn's disease: Report of 3 cases with special reference to histopathologic findings. *Arch Dermatol* 132:928, 1996.
12. Hanno R, Callen JP: Sarcoidosis. A disorder with prominent cutaneous features and their interrelationship with systemic disease. *Med Clin North Am* 64(5):847, 1980.
13. Kuramoto Y, Shindo Y, Tagami H: Subcutaneous sarcoidosis with extensive caseation necrosis. *J Cutan Pathol* 15:188, 1988.
14. Katzenstein A-L A, Askin FB: *Surgical Pathology of Nonneoplastic Lung Disease. Major Problems in Pathology*, 2nd ed. Philadelphia: W.B. Saunders, 13:235, 1990.
15. Lowe L, Rapini RP: Polarizable foreign material in granulomas of sarcoidosis. *J Cutan Pathol (Abs)* 17:305, 1990.
16. Walsh NMG, Hanly JG, Tremaine R, Murray S: Cutaneous sarcoidosis and foreign bodies. *Am J Dermatopathol* 15:203, 1993.
17. Wolfe JT, Campbell RJ, Yeatts RP, et al: Sebaceous carcinoma of the eyelid: Errors in clinical and pathologic diagnosis. *Am J Surg Pathol* 8:597, 1984.
18. LeBoit PE: Variants of mycosis fungoides and related cutaneous T-cell lymphomas. *Semin Diag Pathol* 8:73, 1991.
19. Chan JKC, Ng CS, Ngan KC, et al: Angiocentric T-cell lymphoma of the skin. An aggressive lymphoma distinct from mycosis fungoides. *Am J Surg Pathol* 12:861, 1988.
20. Wick MR, Mills SE, Scheithauer BW, et al: Reassessment of malignant angioendothe-

liomatosis: Evidence in favor of its reclassification as intravascular lymphomatosis. *Am J Surg Pathol* 10:112, 1986.

21. Enzinger FM, Zhang R: Plexiform fibrohistiocytic tumor presenting in children and young adults: An analysis of 65 cases. *Am J Surg Pathol* 12:818, 1988.

22. Costa MJ, Weiss SE: Angiomatoid malignant fibrous histiocytoma: A follow-up study of 108 cases with evaluation of possible histologic predictors of outcome. *Am J Surg Pathol* 14:1126, 1990.

23. Enzinger FM, Weiss SW: *Soft Tissue Tumors*, 3rd ed. St. Louis: CV Mosby, 1995, p. 341.

24. David LR, White WL, Jain AK, Argenta LC: Meningothelial hamartoma of the scalp: Two case reports and literature review. *Eur J Plast Surg* 19:156, 1996.

25. Modlin RL, Vaccaro SA, Gottlieb B, et al: Granuloma annulare: Identification of cells in the cutaneous infiltrate by immunoperoxidase techniques. *Arch Pathol Lab Med* 108:379, 1984.

26. Zanolli MD, Powell BL, McCalmont T, White WL: Granuloma annulare and disseminated herpes zoster. *Int J Dermatol* 31:55, 1992.

27. Penneys NS, Hicks B: Unusual cutaneous lesions associated with acquired immunodeficiency syndrome. *J Am Acad Dermatol.* 13:845, 1985.

28. Lucky AW, Prose NS, Bove K, et al: Papular umbilicated granuloma annulare: A report of four pediatric cases. *Arch Dermatol* 128:1375, 1992.

29. Granuloma annulare vs. necrobiosis lipoidica, in Ackerman AB, Mendonça AMN, Guo Y (eds): *Differential Diagnosis in Dermatopathology I*, 2nd ed. Philadelphia: Lea & Febiger, 1992, p. 50.

30. Evans MJ, Blessing K, Gray ES: Pseudorheumatoid nodule (deep granuloma annulare) of childhood: Clinicopathologic features of twenty patients. *Ped Dermatol* 11:6, 1994.

31. Patterson JW: Rheumatoid nodule and subcutaneous granuloma annulare: A comparative histologic study. *Am J Dermatopathol* 10:1, 1988.

32. Steffen C: Actinic granuloma (O'Brien): *J Cutan Pathol* 15:66, 1988.

33. Barnhill RL, Goldenhersh MA: Elastophagocytosis: A nonspecific reaction pattern associated with inflammatory processes in sun-protected skin. *J Cutan Pathol* 16:199, 1989.

34. Kamino H: Elastophagocytosis with granulomatous inflammation is a nonspecific reactive pattern. (Abs) *J Cutan Pathol* 15:310, 1989.

35. Muller SA, Winkelmann RK: Necrobiosis lipoidica diabeticorum: Histopathologic study of 98 cases. *Arch Dermatol* 94:1, 1966.

36. Johnson WC: Necrobiotic granulomas. *J Cutan Pathol* 12:289, 1985.

37. Necrobiosis lipoidica vs. necrobiotic xanthogranuloma, in Ackerman AB, White WL, Guo Y, Umbert I (eds): *Differenial Diagnosis in Dermatopathology IV*. Philadelphia: Lea & Febiger, 1994, p. 38.

38. Bennett GA, Zeller JW, Bauer W: Subcutaneous nodules of rheumatoid arthritis and rheumatic fever: A pathologic study. *Arch Pathol* 30:70, 1940.

39. Subcutaneous granuloma annulare vs. rheumatoid nodule, in Ackerman AB, White WL, Guo Y, Umbert I (eds): *Differential Diagnosis in Dermatopathology IV*. Philadelphia: Lea & Febiger, 1994, p. 42.

40. Strutton G: The granulomatous reaction pattern, in Weedon D (ed): *The Skin. Systemic Pathology*, 3rd ed. Edinburgh: Churchill Livingstone: 1992, p. 195.

41. Fraser WJ, Haffejee Z, Cooper Z: Rheumatic Aschoff nodules revisited: An immunohistochemical reappraisal of the cellular component. *Histopathology* 27:457, 1995.

42. Cotran RS, Kumar V, Robbins SL (eds): *Pathologic Basis of Disease*, 5th ed. Philadelphia: WB Saunders: 1994, p. 547.

43. Mehregan DA, Winkelmann RK: Necrobiotic xanthogranuloma. *Arch Dermatol* 128:94, 1992.

44. Williford PM, White WL, Jorizzo JL, Greer K: The spectrum of normolipemic plane xanthoma. *Am J Dermatopathol* 15:572, 1993.

45. Finan MC, Winkelmann RK: The cutaneous extravascular necrotizing granuloma (Churg-Strauss granuloma) and systemic disease: A review of 27 cases. *Medicine* 62:142, 1983.

46. Chu P, Connolly K, LeBoit PE: The histopathologic spectrum of palisaded neutrophilic and granulomatous dermatitis in patients with collagen vascular disease. *Arch Dermatol* 130:1278, 1994.

47. Magro CM, Crowson AN, Regauer S: Granuloma annulare and necrobiosis lipoidica tissue reactions as a manifestation of systemic disease. *Hum Pathol* 27:50, 1996.

48. Barksdale SK, Hallahan CW, Kerr GS, et al: Cutaneous pathology in Wegener's granulomatosis: A clinicopathologic study of 75 biopsies in 46 patients. *Am J Surg Pathol* 19:161, 1995.

49. Winkelmann RK, Conolly SM, Quimby SR, Mertz LE: Cutaneous Churg-Strauss syndrome: Granuloma annulare-like histology in the spectrum of vasculitis. *Eur J Dermatol* 3:175, 1993.

50. Jorizzo JL: Personal communication, 1996.

51. Santa Cruz DJ, Strayer DS: The histologic spectrum of the cutaneous mycobacterioses. *Hum Pathol* 13:485, 1982.

52. Su WPD, Kuechle MK, Peters MS, Muller SA: Palisading granulomas caused by infectious diseases. *Am J Dermatopathol* 14:211, 1992.

53. Walsh NMG, Murray S, D'Intino Y: Eruptive xanthoma with urate-like crystals. *J Cutan Pathol* 21:350, 1994.

54. Zanolli MD, Wilmoth G, Shaw J, et al: Epitheliod sarcoma: Clinical and histologic characteristics. *J Am Acad Dermatol* 26:302, 1992.

55. Su WPD, Duncan SC, Perry HO: Blastomycosis-like pyoderma. *Arch Dermatol* 115: 170, 1979.

56. Winkelmann RK, Wilson-Jones E, Gibson LE, Quimby SR: Histopathologic features of superficial granulomatous pyoderma. *J Dermatol* 16:127, 1989.

57. Becker BA, Frieden IJ, Odom RB, Berger TG: Atypical plaque-like staphylococcal folliculitis in human immunodeficiency virus-infected persons. *J Am Acad Dermatol* 21:1024, 1989.

58. O'Brien TS: Iodic eruptions. *Aust J Dermatol* 28:119, 1987.

59. Brunsting HA: Hidradenitis and other variants of acne. *Arch Dermatol Syph* 65:303, 1952.

60. Moyer DG: Pilonidal cyst of the scalp. *Arch Dermatol* 105:578, 1972.

61. Wood GS, Haber RS: Novel histiocytoses considered in the context of histiocyte subset differentiation. *Arch Dermatol* 129:210–214, 1993.

62. Cooper PH: Eruptive xanthoma: A microscopic simulant of granuloma annulare. *J Cutan Pathol* 13: 207, 1986.

63. Smith KJ, Skelton HG, Angritt P: Changes of verruciform xanthoma in an HIV positive patient with diffuse psoriasiform skin disease. *Am J Dermatopathol* 17:185, 1995.

64. Sanchez RL, Raimer SS, Peltier F: Papular xanthoma: A clinical, histologic, and ultrastructural study. *Arch Dermatol* 121:626, 1985.

65. Michal M: Plexiform xanthomatous tumor: A report of three cases. *Am J Dermatopathol* 16:532, 1994.

66. Beham A, Fletcher CDM: Plexiform xanthoma: An unusual variant. *Histopathol* 19: 565, 1991.

67. Perez-Ordonez, Erlandson RA, Rosai J: Follicular dendritic cell tumor: Report of 13 additional cases of a distinctive entity. *Am J Surg Pathol* 20:944, 1996.

68. Willman CL, Busque L, Griffith BB, et al: Langerhans' cell histiocytosis (Histiocytosis X): A clonal proliferative disease. *N Eng J Med* 331:154, 1994.

69. Yu RC, Chu C, Buluwela L, Chu AC: Clonal proliferation of Langerhans' cells in Langerhans' cell histiocytosis. *Lancet* 343:767, 1994.

70. Yu RC, Chu AC: Lack of T-cell receptor gene arrangements in cells involved in Langerhans' cell histiocytosis. *Lancet* 343:767, 1994.

71. Favara BE, Jaffe R: Pathology of Langerhans' cell histiocytosis. *Hematol Oncol Clin N Am* 1(1):75, 1987.

72. Osband ME, Pochedly C: Histiocytosis-X: An overview. *Hematol Oncol Clin N Am* 1(1):1, 1987.

73. Longaker MA, Frieden IJ, LeBoit PE, Sherertz EF: Congenital "self-healing" Langerhans cell histiocytosis: The need for long-term follow-up. *J Am Acad Dermatol* 31:910, 1994.

74. Hashimoto K, Bale GF, Hawkins HK et al: Congenital self-healing reticulohistiocytosis (Hashimoto-Pritzker type). *Int J Dermatol* 25:516, 1986.

75. Foucar E, Rosai J, Dorfman R: Sinus histiocytosis with massive lymphadenopathy (Rosai-Dorfman disease): Review of the entity. *Semin Diagn Pathol* 7:19, 1993.

76. Chu P, LeBoit PE: Histologic features of cutaneous sinus histiocytosis (Rosai-Dorfman disease): Study of cases both with and without systemic involvement. *J Cutan Pathol* 19:201, 1992.

77. Sangueza OP, Salmon JK, White CR, Beckstead JH: Juvenile xanthogranuloma: A clinical, histopathlgic, and immunohistochemical study. *J Cutan Pathol* 22:327, 1995.

78. Zelger G, Cerio R, Orchard G, Wilson-Jones E: Juvenile and adult xanthogranuloma: A histological and immunohistochemical comparison. *Am J Surg Pathol* 18:126, 1994.

79. Janney CG, Hurt MA, Santa Cruz DJ: Deep juvenile xanthogranuloma: Subcutaneous and intramuscular forms. *Am J Surg Pathol* 15:150, 1991.

80. Gianotti R, Alessi E, Caputo R: Benign cephalic histiocytosis: A distinct entity or a part of a wide spectrum of histiocytic proliferative disorders of children? A histopathological study. *Am J Dermatopathol* 15:315, 1993.

81. Umbert IJ, Winkelmann RK: Eruptive histiocytoma. *J Am Acad Dermatol* 20:958, 1989.

82. Gibbs NF, O'Grady TC: Progressive eruptive histiocytoma. *J Am Acad Dermatol* 35:323, 1996.

83. Oliver GF, Umbert I, Winkelmann RK: Reticulohistiocytoma cutis: Review of 15 cases and an association with systemic vasculitis in two cases. *Clin Exp Derm* 15:1, 1990.

84. Zelger B, Cerio R, Soyer HP, et al: Reticulohistiocytoma and multicentric reticulohistiocytosis: Histopathologic and immunophenotypic distinct entities. *Am J Dermatopathol* 16:577, 1994.

85. Taunton OD, Yeshurun D, Jarratt M: Progressive nodular histiocytoma. *Arch Dermatol* 114:1505, 1978.

86. Burgdorf WHC, Kusch SL, Nix TE, Pitta J: Progressive nodular histiocytoma. *Arch Dermatol* 117:644, 1981.

87. Bork K, Hoede N: Hereditary progressive mucinous histiocytosis in women: Report of three members in a family. *Arch Dermatol* 124:1225, 1988.

88. Schroder K, Hettmannsperger U, Schmuth M, et al: Hereditary progressive mucinous histiocytosis. *J Am Acad Dermatol* 35:298, 1996.

89. Shapiro PE, Nova MP, Rosmarin LA, Halperin AJ: Multinucleate cell angiohistiocytoma: A distinct entity diagnosable by clinical and histologic features. *J Am Acad Dermatol* 30:417, 1994.

90. Chang SN, Kim HS, Kim S-C, Yang WI: Generalized multinucleate cell angiohistiocytoma. *J Am Acad Dermatol.* 35:320, 1996.

91. Annessi G, Girolomoni G, Giannetti A: Multinucleate cell angiohistiocytoma. *Am J Dermatopathol* 14:340, 1992.

92. Palazzo JP, Ellison DJ, Garcia IE, et al: Cutaneous malakoplakia simulating malignant lymphoma. *J Cutan Pathol* 17:171, 1990.

93. Horn TD, Burke PJ, Karp JE, Hood AF: Intravenous administration of recombinant human granulocyte-macrophage colony-stimulating factor causes a cutaneous eruption. *Arch Dermatol* 127:49, 1991.

94. Mehregan DR, Fransway AF, Edmonson JH, Leiferman KM: Cutaneous reaction to granulocyte-monocyte colony-stimulating factor. *Arch Dermatol* 128:1055, 1992.

95. Scott GA: Report of three cases of cutaneous reactions to granulocyte macrophage-colony-stimulating factor and a review of the literature. *Am J Dermatopathol* 17:107, 1995.

96. Fitzpatrick JE: New histopathologic findings in drug eruptions. *Dermatol Clin* 10:19, 1992.

97. Wood C, Severin GL: Unusual histiocytic reaction to Monsel's solution. *Am J Dermatopathol* 2:261, 1980.

98. Hanau D, Grosshans E: Monsel's solution and histological lesions. *Am J Dermatopathol* 3:418, 1981.

99. Elston DM, Bergfeld WF, McMahon JT: Aluminum tattoo: A phenomenon that can resemble parasitized histiocytes. *J Cutan Pathol* 20:326, 1993.

100. Motley RJ, Jasani B, Ford AM, et al: Regressing atypical histiocytosis, a regressing cutaneous phase of Ki-1 positive anaplastic large cell lymphoma. *Cancer* 70:476, 1992.

101. LeBoit PE: Lymphomatoid papulosis and cutaneous CD30+ lymphoma. *Am J Dermatopathol* 18:221, 1996.

102. Gonzalez CL, Medeiros LJ, Braziel RM, Jaffe ES: T-cell lymphoma involving subcutaneous tissue: A clinicopathologic entity commonly associated with hemophagocytic syndrome. *Am J Surg Path* 15:17, 1991.

103. White JW, Winkelmann RK: Cytophagic histiocytic panniculitis is not always fatal. *J Cutan Pathol* 16:137, 1989.

104. Suster S, Cartagena N, Cabello-Inchausti B, Robinson MJ: Histiocytic lymphophagocytic panniculitis: An unusual presentation of sinus histiocytosis with massive lymphadenopathy. (Rosai-Dorfman Disease). *Arch Dermatol* 124:1246, 1988.

105. Peters MS, Su WPD: Panniculitis. *Dermatol Clin* 10:37, 1992.

106. LeBoit PE, Barr RJ, Burall S, et al: Primitive polypoid granular cell tumor and other cutaneous granular cell neoplasms of apparent nonneural origin. *Am J Surg Pathol* 15:48, 1991.

107. Mentzel T, Wadden C, Fletcher CDM: Granular cell change in smooth muscle tumors of skin and soft tissue. *Histopathology* 24:223, 1994.

108. Balloon-cell nevus vs. balloon-cell melanoma, in Ackerman AB, White WL, Guo Y, Umbert I (eds): *Differential Diagnosis in Dermatopathology IV*. Philadelphia: Lea & Febiger, 1994, p. 98.

109. Jorizzo JL, Solomon AR, Zanolli MD, Leshin B: Neutrophilic vascular reactions. *J Am Acad Dermatol* 19:983, 1988.

110. Jordaan HF: Acute febrile neutrophilic dermatosis: A histopathological study of 37 patients and a review of the literature. *Am J Dermatopathol* 11:99, 1989.

111. Delaporte E, Graveau DJ, Piette FA, Bergoënd HA: Acute febrile neutrophilic dermatosis (Sweet's syndrome): Association with rheumatoid vasculitis. *Arch Dermatol* 125:1101, 1989.

112. Scherbenske JM, Benson PM, Lupton GP, Samlaska CP: Rheumatoid neutrophilic dermatitis. *Arch Dermatol* 125:1105, 1989.

113. Lowe L, Kornfeld B, Clayman J, Golitz LE: Rheumatoid neutrophilic dermatitis. *J Cutan Pathol* 19:48, 1992.

114. Caughman W, Stern R, Haynes H: Neutrophilic dermatosis of myeloproliferative disorders. *J Am Acad Dermatol* 9:751, 1983.

115. O'Loughlin S, Perry HO: A diffuse pustular eruption associated with ulcerative colitis. *Arch Dermatol* 114:1061, 1978.

116. Jorizzo JL, Apisarntharnarax P, Subrt P, et al: Bowel-bypass syndrome without bowel bypass: Bowel-associated dermatosis arthritis syndrome. *Arch Intern Med* 143:457, 1983.

117. International study group criteria in Behcet's disease: Criteria for diagnosis of Behcet's disease. *Lancet* 335:1078, 1990.

118. Jorizzo JL, Abernethy JL, White WL, et al: Mucocutaneous criteria for the diagnosis of Behcet's disease: An analysis of clinico-pathologic data from multiple international centers. *J Am Acad Dermatol* 32:968, 1995.

119. Harvell J, Ergun T, Gurbuz O, White W: The histopathology of pathergy: A chronological study of skin hyperreactivity in Behcet's disease. (Abs) *J Cutan Pathol* 23:77, 1996.

120. Peters MS, Argenyi Z, Cerio R, et al: Friday evening slide symposium. *J Cut Pathol* 20:465, 1993.

121. Berger TG, Dhar A, McCalmont TH: Neutrophilic dermatoses in HIV infection. *J Am Acad Dermatol* 31:1045, 1994.

122. Wade TR, Finan MC, Stahr BJ, et al: Self assessment: Neutrophilic dermatosis with pseudo-Pelger-Huët anomaly. *J Cutan Pathol* 20:513, 1993.

123. Fitzpatrick JE: The cutaneous histopathology of chemotherapeutic reactions. *J Cutan Pathol* 20:1, 1993.

124. Stahr BJ, Cooper PH, Caputo RV: Idiopathic plantar hidradenitis: A neutrophilic eccrine hidradenitis occurring primarily in children. *J Cutan Pathol* 21:289, 1994.

125. Rabinowitz LG, Cintra ML, Hood AF, Esterly NB: Recurrent palmoplantar hidradenitis in children. *Arch Dermatol* 131:817, 1995.

126. Nishimura M, Matsuda T, Muto M, Hori Y: Balanitis of Zoon. *Int J Dermatol* 29:421, 1990.

127. Kodama A, Tani M, Hori K, et al: Systemic and cutaneous plasmacytosis with multiple skin lesions and polyclonal hypergammaglobulinaemia: Significant serum interleukin-6 levels. *Br J Dermatol* 127:49, 1992.

128. Wong KF, Chan JKC, Li LPK, et al: Primary cutaneous plasmacytoma: Report of 2 cases and review of the literature. *Am J Dermatopathol* 16:392, 1994.

129. LeBoit PE: Dermatopathologic findings in patients infected with HIV. *Dermatol Clin* 10:59, 1992.

130. McGovern TW, Erickson AR, Fitzpatrick JE: Sjögren's syndrome plasma cell panniculitis and hidradenitis. *J Cutan Pathol* 23:170, 1996.

131. Roupe G: Urticaria pigmentosa and systemic mastocytosis. *Semin Dermatol* 6:334, 1987.

132. Kasper CS, Freeman RG, Tharp MD: Diagnosis of mastocytosis subsets using a morphometric point counting technique. *Arch Dermatol* 123:1017, 1987.

133. Sweet WL, Smoller BR: Perivascular mast cells in urticaria pigmentosa. *J Cutan Pathol* 23:247, 1996.

134. Aberer W, Konrad K, Wolff K: Wells' syndrome is a distinctive disease entity and not a histologic diagnosis. *J Am Acad Dermatol* 18:105, 1988.

135. Wood C, Miller AC, Jacobs A, et al: Eosinophilic infiltration with flame figures: A distinctive tissue reaction seen in Well's Syndrome and other diseases. *Am J Dermatopathol* 8:186, 1986.

136. Kazmierowski JA, Chusid MJ, Parrillo JE, et al: Dermatologic manifestations of the hypereosinophilic syndrome. *Arch Dermatol* 114:531, 1978.

137. Fitzpatrick JE, Johnson C, Simon P, Owenby J: Cutaneous microthrombi: A histologic clue to the diagnosis of hypereosinophilic syndrome. *Am J Dermatopathol* 9:419, 1987.

138. Sherertz EF, Jorizzo JL, White WL, et al: Papular dermatitis in adults: Subacute prurigo, American style? *J Am Acad Dermatol* 24:697, 1991.

139. McCalmont TH, Altemus D, Maurer T, Berger TG: Eosinophilic folliculitis: The histologic spectrum. *Am J Dermatopathol* 17:439, 1995.

140. Pruritic urticarial papules and plaques of pregnancy vs. herpes gestationis, urticarial stage, in Ackerman AB, White W, Guo Y, Umbert I (eds): *Differential Diagnosis in Dermatopathology IV*. Philadelphia: Lea & Febiger, 1994, p. 26.

141. Helton JL, Maize JC: Eosinophilic histiocytosis: Histopathology and immunohistochemistry. *Am J Dermatopathol* 18:111, 1996.

142. Kadin ME: Lymphomatoid papulosis, Ki-1[+] lymphoma, and primary cutaneous Hodgkin's disease. *Semin Dermatol* 10:164, 1991.

143. Cerroni L, Beham-Schmid C, Kerl H: Cutaneous Hodgkin's disease: An immunohistochemical analysis. *J Cutan Pathol* 22:229, 1995.

144. Sioutos N, Kerl H, Murphy SB, Kadin ME: Primary cutaneous Hodgkin's disease: Unique clinical, morphologic and immunophenotypic findings. *Am J Dermatopathol* 16:2, 1994.

145. Adame J, Cohen PR: Eosinophilic panniculitis: Diagnostic considerations and evaluation. *J Am Acad Dermatol* 34:229, 1996.

CHAPTER 7

INTRAEPIDERMAL VESICULOPUSTULAR DERMATITIS

Terence J. Harrist / Brian Schapiro / Lisa Lerner / Cynthia M. Magro

A wide variety of disorders may produce intraepidermal vesicles and pustules. Distinct diseases may have similar, or even identical, pathologic features. In addition, the histopathologic findings in each disease evolve over time. Thus, the algorithmic approach to diagnosis in this group is, of necessity, complex but facilitates the diagnosis in this complex group of disorders (Tables 7-1 to 7-4). Correlation of the clinical findings and historical data with the microscopic findings often is essential to derive a definitive diagnosis. The algorithm narrows the differential diagnosis to a few entities or a specific diagnosis through evaluation of the blister–cleft separation plane, the principal pathologic process and inflammatory cell complement—its presence, the type of cells, or its absence.

DEFINITIONS

A blister is a fluid-filled cavity within or beneath the epidermis containing tissue fluid, plasma, and a variable complement of inflammatory cells. Vesicles are blisters less than 0.5 cm in diameter, and bullae are blisters greater than 0.5 cm in diameter. A vesiculopustule is a vesicle in which there is a prominent component of neutrophils. Some diseases produce microscopic "slitlike" spaces within the epidermis that are known as clefts. Clefts characteristically occur in the group of diseases that have focal acantholytic dyskeratosis as their histologic reaction pattern and, as a rule, do not have clinically apparent blisters.

A pustule is a dense aggregate of neutrophils or eosinophils, viable and degenerated, with a small component of tissue fluid. A pustule is yellow-white clinically and resides intracorneally, within the stratum spinosum or at the dermoepidermal junction. A microabscess is a small aggregate of neutrophils or eosinophils observed histologically. Pustules or microabscesses composed virtually entirely of eosinophils are important diagnostically.

The Separation Plane

The separation plane is relatively constant in each vesiculobullous disease. Each process tends to reliably produce blisters in either the subcorneal-granular, spinous, or suprabasal zones in the epidermis. However, blisters occasionally may extend from one plane to another. Pustules tend to form in the subcorneal or intracorneal zone, but are not limited to those locations.

Spongiosis

Spongiosis is the accumulation of extracellular fluid within the epidermis that causes separation between adjacent keratinocytes. The keratinocytes often appear stellate with clear spaces separating them from their neighbors, producing a "spongy" appearance. As the degree of spongiosis increases, microscopic vesicles develop and may progress to macroscopic vesicles or bullae. In cases of severe spongiosis, ballooning degeneration (intracellular edema) with subsequent rupture of the cell membranes (a form of cytolysis) may lead to a "lacelike" appearance (reticular degeneration). Spongiosis develops primarily because of transudation of serum from damaged or inflamed vessels within the superficial plexus. Ballooning degeneration occurs when the keratinocytes lose osmotic control.

Acantholysis

Acantholysis is the result of loss of appropriate keratinocyte-keratinocyte adherence. This adherence is mediated by tight junctions, adherens junctions, gap junctions, and desmosomes. The role of desmosomes in keratinocytic adhesion is paramount and they are the last structures to split when acantholysis occurs. Those acantholytic disorders that have been well-characterized develop as sequelae of desmosomal dysfunction or disruption of the desmosomal connections with the intracellular keratin structural matrix. Keratinocyte-keratinocyte adhesion is by necessity a dynamic process, as the relationship of one keratinocyte to another must change during epidermal maturation. Thus, acantholysis may be viewed as the loss of the equilibrium between the formation and dissolution of junctions. This disequilibrium may occur primarily when the adhesion junctions are directly impaired, or secondarily when keratinocytic viability is affected. Acantholytic keratinocytes are rounded with condensed eosinophilic cytoplasm, large nuclei, peripherally marginated chromatin, and prominent nucleoli.

Cytolysis and Apoptosis

Cytolysis of keratinocytes, as well as apoptosis, may lead to blister formation. Cytolysis may occur in the normal epidermis when the structural matrix of the keratinocytes is overwhelmed by high levels of deleterious physical agents, such as mechanical forces or heat. Mechanical energy applied parallel to the epidermis (friction) may lead to shearing between keratinocytes and within keratinocytes themselves, that is, cytolysis. Minimal friction may lead to cytolysis when keratinocytes do not have a normal structural matrix, as in epidermolysis bullosa simplex. Immune-mediated cell necrosis in the context of antibody-dependent cell-mediated immunity or a delayed-type hypersensitivity reaction may lead to blister formation, which is most typically subepidermal in nature. The morphologic hallmark of this pattern of necrosis is karyolysis-producing colloid bodies. This is not to be confused with apoptosis, which is a unique form of cell death whereby individual scattered

TABLE 7-1

Intraepidermal Blistering and Pustular Diseases

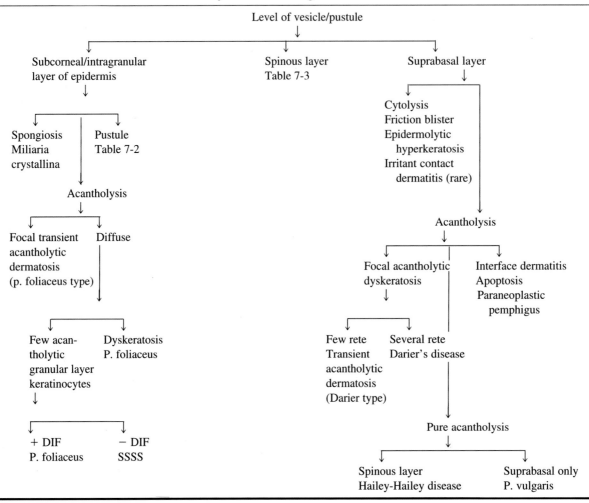

SPONGIOTIC DERMATITIS

Most forms of spongiotic dermatitis are characterized by an orderly progression of histologic changes that evolve over time. These changes are common to many of the spongiotic processes and do not establish a specific diagnosis. However, they do allow an assessment of the evolutionary stage of the spongiotic dermatitis: acute, subacute, or chronic (see Table 7-5; also see Chapter 2). Some histologic clues point to a specific diagnosis (Table 7-6). These clues and other important histologic features are outlined in Table 7-7.

Evolution

In the acute phase, a variable degree of spongiosis essentially is the only diagnostic feature (Fig. 7-1). If spongiosis is minimal, only clear spaces surrounding the stellate keratinocytes may be present. If spongiosis is severe, microvesicles and macroscopic vesicles form. Intracellular edema often parallels the degree of spongiosis such that in severe reactions reticular degeneration and cytolysis may develop. There is loss of

single cells die without release of cellular contents. Such a pattern of programmed cell death does not usually lead to epidermal disruption.

the granular layer with minimal parakeratosis. Crusts and scale-crusts may result from the rupture of the vesicles onto the surface or into the parakeratotic stratum corneum, respectively. The degree of papillary dermal and epidermal edema parallel one another. Almost invariably, there is a lymphohistiocytic infiltrate about the superficial vascular plexus and in the papillary dermal interstitium with exocytosis of lymphocytes into the spongiotic foci. Although the quantity of the infiltration is highly variable, it usually parallels the degree of spongiosis. Eosinophils may be present or absent. Erosions and ulcerations secondary to rubbing may develop in any phase.

In the subacute phase, the changes parallel the severity of the spongiotic dermatitis. If mild, there may be minimal spongiosis, variable parakeratosis, variable loss or thickening of the granular layer with slight psoriasiform acanthosis and a scant lymphohistiocytic infiltrate. If severe, there is prominent spongiosis with vesicles, confluent parakeratosis, loss of the granular layer, prominent psoriasiform acanthosis, and prominent lymphohistiocytic infiltration. Crust and scale-crusts usually are prominent in the severe reactions. Eosinophils may or may not be present. Overall, the changes reflect the specific causative agent (topical agent, drug, ingestant, etc.), its continued or repetitive exposure, and the immunologic and structural reaction to it. For example, topical caustic irritants or severe phototoxicity may produce confluent coagulative necrosis. In contrast, in some topical reactions, the psoriasiform hyperplasia may mimic psoriasis, whereas in others, such as in shoe dermati-

TABLE 7-2

Subcorneal/Intragranular Pustules

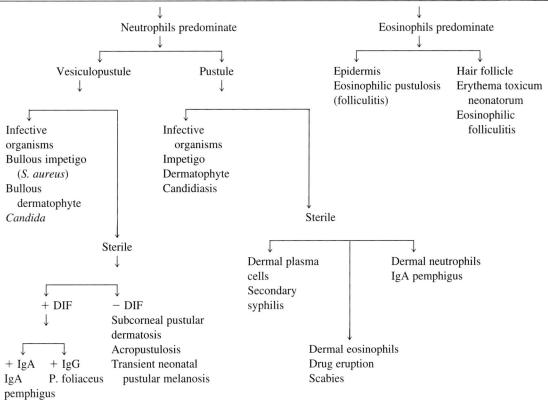

tis owing to rubber, there is only mild spongiosis and mild psoriasiform hyperplasia with minimal spongiosis and lymphocytic infiltrate.

In the chronic phase, there is hyperkeratosis with focal parakeratosis, hypergranulosis, and psoriasiform acanthosis. These changes may vary in severity. Spongiosis usually is minimal.

Contact Dermatitis, Allergic Type

Clinical Features   The prototype of allergic contact dermatitis is the reaction to poison ivy.[1] At the sensitization exposure, there is usually no visible reaction. On subsequent challenge of the oleoresin, onto the cutaneous surface to which it has come in contact, pruritic, edematous red papules, plaques, and vesicles develop in approximately 24 to 72 hours (Table 7-8). The shape and distribution of the lesions reflect the points of contact between the oleoresin and the skin. The vesicles, redness, and weeping evolve into scaly crusted papules and plaques that resolve in several weeks. In each allergic contact reaction the exact degree of reaction depends on the exact nature of the allergen and the individual's immunologic response to it. In contrast to poison ivy dermatitis, allergic contact reactions to such allergens as rubbers, nickel, fragrance, and preservatives tend to consist of only mild erythema and scaling.

Histopathological Features   The features are those described in the temporal evolution of acute to chronic spongiotic dermatitis (Table 7-8). The degree of the changes and their persistence are the function of properties of the allergen itself, its duration of application, and the immunologic response of the host. Thus, the changes may be minimal,

as in most cases of nickel allergy, or striking, in the case of Rhus oleoresin exposure. Intraepidermal vesicles in acute allergic contact dermatitis often are multiloculated and large, resulting from reticular degeneration of keratinocytes. That is to say, the keratinocytes are progressively stretched apart by intercellular edema with rupture of the cellular membranes and formation of tissue spaces. Usually one also observes exocytosis of eosinophils and intracellular and subepidermal edema.

Differential Diagnosis   Other forms of spongiotic dermatitis such as an irritant contact dermatitis (see the following), "id" reaction, dyshidrotic eczema, nummular eczema, photoallergic and other photodermatitides, infestation with an ectoparasite (e.g., scabies), cutaneous larva migrans, bullous pemphigoid, spongiotic drug reaction, and spongiotic bite reaction may be associated with intraepidermal vesicles. Distinction of allergic contact dermatitis from many of the latter entities may not be possible without clinical information. Allergic contact dermatitis often may show an acute spongiotic dermatitis with larger intraepidermal vesicles, more edema, and greater numbers of eosinophils than are observed in other forms of eczema. Irritant dermatitis may show greater intracellular edema of keratinocytes and infiltration by neutrophils than in allergic contact dermatitis.

Other diagnostic considerations include infective processes such as bacterial, fungal (e.g., candidal and dermatophyte infections), viral disorders, and erythema multiforme, which may exhibit prominent spongiosis and intraepidermal vesicles or vesiculopustules.

A particular problem may be the distinction of an intraepidermal from a subepidermal vesicular dermatitis. One must try to establish what is the predominant morphologic alteration, that is, intraepidermal

TABLE 7-3

Spinous Layer Blister/Pustule

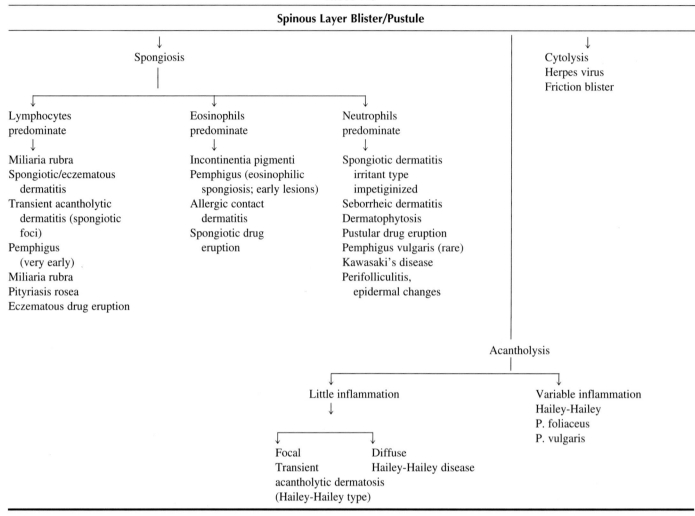

or subepidermal edema. In some cases this may not be possible since both of the changes may be prominent or the lesion may be old and show reepithelialization. Detailed clinical information may be necessary to resolve the differential diagnosis. In some instances such a distinction is moot because some inflammatory processes may present as either intraepidermal or subepidermal vesicles or with both, depending on where the accumulation of edema is greatest.

Contact Dermatitis, Irritant Type

Clinical Features   The clinical features essentially are identical to allergic contact dermatitis, spanning the full spectrum from mild erythema and slight scaling to erythematous papules and plaques with spongiotic vesicles and crusting (Table 7-9). No sensitization exposure is required. The overall response, however, is determined by the nature of the chemical itself, its concentration, type of exposure, the age of the patient, and the "irritability" of the skin itself.[2] Superficial necrosis and ulceration may develop after contact with highly concentrated alkalis and acids. However, most acute irritant reactions produce a monomorphic picture with scaling, redness, vesicles, pustules, or erosions and are caused by mild irritants such as detergents, water, or water with additives. Chronic irritant dermatitis is produced by repetitive exposure to mild irritants and usually is characterized by dryness and chapping, with no vesicles apparent clinically.

Histopathological Features   The histologic picture of irritant dermatitis and its evolution essentially is identical to allergic contact dermatitis in most instances (Table 7-9). Controlled studies comparing irritant and allergic contact reactions have supported this contention. However, necrosis, neutrophilic infiltration, and acantholysis are more frequent overall in irritant reactions (Fig. 7-2).[3] The degree of neutrophilic infiltration parallels the degree of necrosis. In mild reactions there is slight dermal edema, spongiosis, acanthosis, and parakeratosis with minimal lymphoid infiltrate. In severe reactions, spongiosis, keratinocyte ballooning degeneration, and cytolysis develop and are most prominent in the upper stratum spinosum and stratum granulosum. Coagulative necrosis may be present superficially and extend deeply in the epidermis, leading to ulcers in the case of highly concentrated alkalis and acids. The pathologic hallmarks of a delayed-type hypersensitivity reaction, namely eosinophils, Langerhans cell clusters, and extensive exocytosis of lymphocytes usually are not observed. Again, the variability of severity of the alterations must be stressed. In most instances, a definitive histologic determination of either an irritant or allergic dermatitis cannot be made.

Differential Diagnosis   The same considerations apply as discussed in the preceding for differential diagnosis of allergic contact dermatitis. Particularly for irritant dermatitis, the differential diagnosis includes other external insults, such as light, radiation, thermal injury, and viral infections.

TABLE 7-4

Intraepidermal Blistering and Pustular Diseases

Separation Plane	Pathologic Process	Inflammatory Cells	Disease
Subcorneal/intragranular	Spongiosis	Lymphocytes	Miliaria crystallina
	Acantholysis	—	Staphylococcal scalded skin syndrome
			Pemphigus foliaceus
			Transient acantholytic dermatosis (P. foliaceus–like foci)
	Pustules	Neutrophils	Impetigo
			Bullous impetigo
			Subcorneal pustular dermatosis
			IgA pemphigus
			Dermatophytosis
			Candidiasis
			Pustular secondary lues
			Pustular drug eruption
			Acropustulosis of infancy
			Transient neonatal pustular melanosis
			Pustular Id reaction
			Pemphigus vulgaris (rare)
			Pustular psoriasis
		Eosinophils	Scabies
			Erythema toxicum neonatorum
Spinous	Spongiosis	Lymphocytes	Miliaria rubra
			Spongiotic/eczematous dermatitis
			Transient acantholytic dermatitis (spongiotic foci)
			Pemphigus (very early)
			Miliaria rubra
			Pityriasis rosea
			Eczematous drug eruption
		Eosinophils	Incontinentia pigmenti
			Pemphigus (eosinophilic spongiosis; early lesions)
			Allergic contact dermatitis
			Spongiotic drug eruption
		Neutrophils	Spongiotic dermatitis
			irritant type
			impetiginized
			Seborrheic dermatitis
			Dermatophytosis
			Pustular drug eruption
			Pemphigus vulgaris (rare)
			Kawasaki's disease
			Perifolliculitis, epidermal changes
	Acantholysis	Little inflammation	Hailey-Hailey disease
			Transient acantholytic dermatosis (Hailey-Hailey-like foci)
		Variable inflammation	Hailey-Hailey disease
			Pemphigus foliaceus and variants (extension from subcorneal plane)
			Pemphigus vulgaris and variants (extension from suprabasal plane)
			Irritant contact dermatitis (rare)
	Cytolysis	Marked inflammation	Herpes virus infection
		Little inflammation	Friction blister
Suprabasal	Cytolysis		Friction blister
			Epidermolytic hyperkeratosis
			Irritant contact dermatitis (rare)
	Acantholysis		Pemphigus vulgaris and variants
			Darier's disease
			Transient acantholytic disease (Pemphigus vulgaris–like foci)

After Elder D, Elenitsas R, Jaworsky C, Johnson B: *Lever's Histopathology of the Skin: Algorithmic Classification of Skin Diseases for Differential Diagnosis*, 8th ed. Philadelphia: Lippincott-Raven, pp 61–116, 1997.

TABLE 7-5

Histologic Evolution of Spongiotic Dermatitis*

Phase	Acute		Subacute		Chronic	
Reaction Severity:	Mild	Severe	Mild	Severe	Mild	Severe
Features:						
Edema						
Spongiosis	+	+++	+	++	+/−	+
Vesiculation	+/−	+++	+/−	++	−	−
Dermal Edema	+	+++	+/−	++	+/−	0−+/−
Epithelial Alteration						
Hyperkeratosis	0−+	0−+	+	++	+	+++
Parakeratosis	0−+	0−+	0−+	+++	+/−	++
Crusts	0	+++	0	++	0	0
Hypergranulosis	+/−	0 +/−	0	0	+/−	+++
Hypogranulosis	+/−	+/−	+/−	++		
Acanthosis	0	0	+/−	++	+/−	+++
Langerhans Cell						
Clusters	+/−	0−++	+/−	++	+/−	0
Lymphocytic Infiltrate						
Epidermal	+	+++	+	++	0−+	0−++
Dermal	+	+++	+	++	+	0−+
Endothelial Activation	+	+++	+/− to +	++	−	−
Papillary Dermal Fibrosis	0	0	0	0	+	+++

Legend: 0 = no change; +/− = minimal change; may or may not be present; + = few; ++ = moderate; moderate numbers; +++ = severe; many.
*After Murphy, GF: *Dermatopathology: A Practical Guide to Common Disorders.* Philadelphia: W.B. Saunders, 1995, p. 53.

TABLE 7-6

Clues to Diagnosis in Spongiotic Dermatitis

Pattern of parakeratosis
The presence or absence of spongiotic vesicles
The size of spongiotic vesicles
Intraepidermal Langerhans cell clusters
Neutrophilic infiltration exocytosis
Eosinophilic spongiosis and pustulation
Keratinocyte necrosis and apoptosis
Dermal eosinophil infiltration
Depth and pattern of the dermal inflammatory infiltration
Erythrocyte extravasation
Follicular involvement

"Id" Reaction

Clinical Features   A secondary generalized or localized spongiotic dermatitis that develops in association with a defined local dermatitis or infection is known as "autoeczematization" (Table 7-10). Small, erythematous papules and vesicles often develop on the hands and forearms but may involve other sites. The most common types of underlying primary dermatitis include stasis dermatitis and dermatophytosis.[4]

Histopathological Features   The features are usually those of an acute spongiotic dermatitis (Table 7-10).[5] Eosinophils may be present.[6] Often the spongiotic dermatitis is relatively sharply circumscribed; however, no specific features allow a definitive diagnosis. Thus, clinical findings are critical in making a specific clinicopathologic diagnosis.

Differential Diagnosis   See the preceding discussion of allergic contact dermatitis.

Atopic Dermatitis

Clinical Features   Atopic dermatitis often begins in infancy and is characterized by pruritus, erythema, scaling, excoriation, lichenification, and superimposed lichen simplex chronicus. It is more common in females and there may be other associated allergic disorders, such as asthma and allergic rhinitis. In infancy and childhood, there is a characteristic involvement of the face and extensor surfaces of the extremities.[7] In older children and adults, the flexural surfaces, sides of the neck, and the popliteal and antecubital fossae are the most frequent sites. These patients have hypersensitive skin and often develop exaggerated responses to mild irritants.[7]

Histopathological Features   The histologic features of atopic dermatitis range from a subacute to chronic spongiotic dermatitis.[8] It may be extremely minimal to moderate in severity. Some observers believe there is no primary dermatitis and attribute all the changes to rubbing.[9] Eosinophils are uncommon.[10] Intense pruritus provokes rubbing, and lichen simplex chronicus ensues. The usual absence of eosinophils and lack of Langerhans cell clusters are important negative findings. Follicular eczematous changes may be observed and are prominent in some cases. Some patients have coexisting ichthyosis vulgaris or keratosis pilaris.

Differential Diagnosis   See the preceding discussion of allergic contact dermatitis.

TABLE 7-7

Differential Diagnostic Points in Spongiotic Dermatitis

Disease	ACD	ICD	Id	AtopicD	NumD	DysD	SebD	StasisD	Miliaria	Drug	PhotoAD	PhotoTD	K	TSS	PR	IP
Histologic feature:																
Eos der	0-+++	0	0/++	0	0/+	0	0	0	0	0/+	0/+	0	0	0	0/+	+/+++
Eos spon	0/+++	0	0/+	0/+	0	0	0	0	0	0/++	0/+	0	0	0	0	+/+++
LCC	++	0	0/+	0	0/+	0/+	0	0	0	+/-	++	0	0	0	+	0
SPI	+	+	+	+	+	+	+	+	+	+	+	+	+	+	+	+
DPI	0	0	0	0	0	0	0	0	0	0/+	+	0	0	0	0	0
Neut	0/+	0/+++	0	0	0	0	+/++	0	0/+	0/+	0	0/+	+	+	0	0
EN	0	0/+++	0	0	0	0	0	0	0	0	0	0/+	0	0	0	0
Vesicles	0/+++	+	+/+++	+	0/++	0/++	0	+	+	+/-	0/+++	0/+	0/+	0	0/++	++/+++
IH	0	+(some)	0	0	0	0	0	0	0	0	0	0	0	0	+	0
Apoptosis	0	0	0	0	0	0	0	0	0	0/++	0/+	0/++	0	+	+	0/+++
FI	0/++	+/-	0	0/++	0/+	0	+	0	0	0/+	0	0	0	0	0	0

Histologic features:
Eos der = Dermal eosinophil infiltrate   SPI = Superficial perivascular infiltrate   EN = Epidermal necrosis
Eos spon = Eosinophilic spongiosis   DPI = Deep perivascular infiltrate   IH = Intraepidermal hemorrhage
LCC = Langerhans cell clusters   Neut = Neutrophils   FI = Follicular involvement

Diseases:
ACD = Allergic contact dermatitis   DysD = Dyshidrotic dermatitis   K = Kawasaki's exanthem
ICD = Irritant contact dermatitis   SebD = Seborrheic dermatitis (non-AIDS) TSS = Toxic shock syndrome
Id = Id reaction   StasisD = Stasis dermatitis   PR = Pityriasis rosea
AtopicD = Atopic dermatitis   PhotoAD = Photoallergic dermatitis   IP = Incontinentia pigmenti
NumD = Nummular dermatitis   PhotoTD = Phototoxic dermatitis

Legend:
0 = absent/none   + = present, few; minimal change   ++ =moderate change; moderate numbers   +++ = marked change; many.

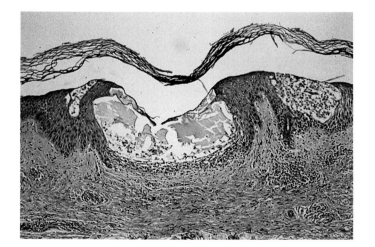

FIGURE 7-1 Spongiotic dermatitis, acute phase. Deep to a normal stratum corneum are intraepidermal vesicles filled with proteinaceous fluid. There is exocytosis of lymphocytes and papillary dermal edema with a superficial perivascular lymphohistiocytic infiltrate.

Nummular Dermatitis

Clinical Features   Nummular dermatitis is characterized by pruritic, oval, nummular (coin-shaped) erythematous or scaly crusted plaques on the extensor surface of the extremities, usually in older adults.[11] On occasion, clinical vesicles may supervene.

Histopathological Features   The histologic features are those of spongiotic dermatitis with no distinguishing features.[12,13] The early stages consist of an acute spongiotic dermatitis with microvesicles and macroscopic vesicles.

Differential Diagnosis   See the preceding discussion of allergic contact dermatitis.

Dyshidrotic Dermatitis

Clinical Features   Dyshidrotic eczema, representing about 5 percent of hand dermatitides, is recognized by its limitation to the palms and soles, with particular accentuation on the sides of the fingers and toes. In the early stages, large vesicles are clinically apparent beneath an intact stratum corneum. Later stages are characterized by the changes of subacute and chronic dermatitis, with superimposed lichen simplex chronicus and fissuring, leading to confusion with contact dermatitis.

TABLE 7-8

Contact Allergic Dermatitis with Vesicles, Bullae

Clinical Features

Reactions range from mild erythema and scaling to pruritic,
edematous red plaques and vesicles
Distribution reflects areas of contact with allergen
Evolution to scaly crusted papules and plaques

Histopathological Features

Spongiosis resulting in intraepidermal vesicles
Papillary dermal edema
Irregular psoriasiform epidermal hyperplasia in subacute and
chronic reactions
Often superficial perivascular exocytosis of lymphocytes
Exocytosis of eosinophils may be present
Scale-crust

Differential Diagnosis

Irritant contact dermatitis
Id reaction
Dyshidrotic eczema
Nummular eczema
Photoallergic eruption
Spongiotic drug eruption
Bite reaction
Infestation
Fungal and viral infections
Bullous pemphigoid

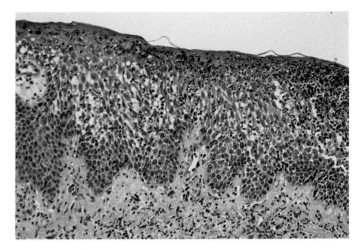

FIGURE 7-2 Contact dermatitis, irritant type. There is prominent spongiosis as well as exocytosis of neutrophils and a superficial perivascular mixed cell infiltrate.

Histopathological Features   Large intraepidermal vesicles reside beneath an intact stratum corneum. The lymphocytic infiltrate in dyshidrotic eczema is less than might be expected in other spongiotic dermatitides when large vesicles are present. The vesicle is composed principally of fluid with few Langerhans cells and possibly a rare acantholytic keratinocyte. Intraepidermal eosinophils and neutrophils are uncommon unless there is superinfection. Dermal eosinophils are absent to sparse. Superinfection may lead to vesiculopustules.

TABLE 7-9

Contact Dermatitis, Irritant Type, with Vesicles, Bullae

Clinical Features

Spectrum from mild erythema to papules and plaques with erosions
and vesicle formation
Ulceration may develop

Histopathological Features

Spongiosis resulting in intraepidermal vesicles
Variable cytolysis and coagulative necrosis
Papillary dermal edema
Irregular psoriasiform epidermal hyperplasia in subacute and
chronic reactions
Often superficial perivascular exocytosis of lymphocytes
Neutrophils may be prominent
Scale-crust

Differential Diagnosis

Allergic contact dermatitis
Id reaction
Dyshidrotic eczema
Nummular eczema
Photoallergic eruption
Spongiotic drug eruption
Bite reaction
Infestation
Fungal and viral infections
Bullous pemphigoid

TABLE 7-10

"Id" Reaction

Clinical Features

Erythematous papules and vesicles developing in association with
a defined dermatitis or infection

Histopathological Features

Spongiosis resulting in intraepidermal vesicles
Papillary dermal edema
Irregular psoriasiform epidermal hyperplasia in subacute and
chronic reactions
Often superficial perivascular exocytosis of lymphocytes
Eosinophils may be present
Scale-crust

Differential Diagnosis

Allergic and irritant contact dermatitis
Id reaction
Dyshidrotic eczema
Nummular eczema
Photoallergic eruption
Spongiotic drug eruption
Bite reaction
Infestation
Fungal and viral infections
Bullous pemphigoid

Differential Diagnosis See the preceding discussion of allergic contact dermatitis. Contact dermatitis usually has a greater complement of infiltrating lymphocytes when such degrees of spongiosis are present. Later-stage lesions are indistinguishable from other forms of subacute chronic spongiotic dermatitis.

Stasis Dermatitis

Clinical Features In older individuals with chronic venous insufficiency of the lower extremities, erythema, scaling, weeping, and occasional vesicles may develop on top of firm brownish plaques. Lichenification may result from rubbing.

Histopathological Features Superficially, the changes usually are those of subacute to chronic spongiotic dermatitis.[14] Eosinophils usually are absent. Later lesions may be dominated by the changes of lichen simplex chronicus with striking parakeratotic scale as well as spongiosis and spongiotic microvesicles and secondary impetigo.

Differential Diagnosis See the preceding discussion of allergic contact dermatitis and Chapter 2. The eosinophil infiltration and Langerhans cell clusters are important features, as they imply a contact allergy.

Miliaria

Clinical Features Miliaria has three subsets—miliaria crystallina, miliaria rubra, and miliaria profunda. Miliaria crystallina presents with asymptomatic, superficial, noninflammatory "dewdrop" vesicles, principally on the trunk after sunburn or profuse sweating. Miliaria rubra appears as inflammatory papules after excessive sweating in skin covered by clothing or occlusive wraps.[15,16] Pruritic papulovesicles and pustules surrounded by erythema may be present. Miliaria pustulosa is considered to be a variant of miliaria rubra exhibiting pustules that are localized to the acrosyringium. Miliaria profunda usually occurs in tropical climates after recurrent miliaria rubra has damaged the eccrine ducts, which leak in the dermis.

Occlusion of the sweat ducts at various levels and infection with Gram-positive cocci, usually staphylococci, are causal and lead to the three clinicopathologic subsets. In miliaria crystallina, the sweat duct is obstructed within the stratum corneum which is excessively hydrated.[17] In miliaria rubra, the sweat duct is obstructed within the lower stratum spinosum, and in miliaria profunda it is occluded at the level of the dermoepidermal junction. The exact cause of the blockage is unclear, but increased numbers of *Staphylococcus aureus* may be observed within the sweat ducts, particularly in those cases that develop after occlusive wrappings with an associated PAS-positive cast that may be a result of injury to the luminal cells and inflammation.[18] Also, it should be remembered that *Staphylococcus aureus* may also produce an epidermolysin that may play a role in separation of the cuticle away from the underlying eccrine poral cells.

Histopathological Features In miliaria crystallina, there are intracorneal/subcorneal vesicles in continuity with the adjacent sweat ducts.[19] Thus, the changes are those of acute spongiotic dermatitis limited to the areas around the ostium of the eccrine duct (Fig. 7-3). There is papillary dermal edema and sparse superficial lymphohistiocytic infiltrate. A few neutrophils may be present.

In miliaria rubra, the vesicles are present within the stratum spinosum and also are in continuity with the sweat duct.[20] Amorphous casts, which are PAS-positive and diastase-resistant, may be observed within

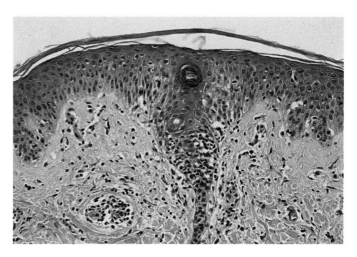

FIGURE 7-3 Miliaria crystallina. Areas of spongiosis surround the acrosyringium. There is superficial dermal edema and a sparse superficial perivascular mononuclear infiltrate.

the eccrine pore.[18] There is also perivascular and periductal lymphohistiocytic infiltrate and spongiosis, giving the picture of a localized acute to subacute spongiotic dermatitis.[20] Miliaria pustulosa is characterized by neutrophilic subcorneal pustules involving the acrosyringium. In miliaria profunda, the changes are similar to miliaria rubra, but with greater inflammation, spongiosis, and dermal edema. The inflammatory changes usually are more prominent and are accentuated in the lower epidermis and the superficial dermis. Eosinophils and Langerhans cell clusters are not present.

Spongiotic Drug Eruption

Clinical Features Drugs may produce a wide variety of patterns of dermatitis including vesicles and bullae (also see Chapters 8 and 12).[21] A spongiotic or eczematous drug reaction as a reactivation of a contact hypersensitivity already has been alluded to.

Topically applied medications characteristically produce an allergic contact dermatitis. Certain drugs contain substances to which the patient has launched a prior allergic sensitization response. Cell-mediated immune responses have been strongly suspected, but never have been documented to be associated with systemically administered drugs.

Histopathological Features The histologic features are essentially identical to that of an allergic contact dermatitis. There is a perivascular lymphohistiocytic infiltrate with a variable number of eosinophils that may produce eosinophilic spongiosis.[22] However, eosinophils are not always present. The infiltrate may reside only about the superficial plexus, but the deep plexus may be involved as well. There is edema, particularly prominent in the perivascular and papillary dermal zones. Mild spongiosis may be present, such that the lesions may be classified histologically as an acute mild spongiotic dermatitis. (Drug eruptions are biopsied early in their course.) Large spongiotic vesicles and Langerhans cell clusters are unusual. As the lesions age, the changes evolve to a subacute eczematous dermatitis. Many drug eruptions lack spongiosis and consist only of a perivascular dermatitis.

Differential Diagnosis See the preceding discussion of allergic contact dermatitis and Chapters 8 and 12.

Photoallergic Dermatitis

Clinical Features Photoallergic dermatitis refers to a rash that develops as a consequence of a presumed delayed-type hypersensitivity reaction.[23] Common causes are soaps and cleansers containing salicylanilides, perfumes including musk ambrette, benzones, benzocaine, and plants, particularly those containing coumarins (celery, parsnips, etc.). Common drug causes of photoallergic eruptions include thiazides, oral hypoglycemics, and phenothiazines. The clinical features mimic those of allergic contact dermatitis, but the eruption is confined to sun-exposed areas, such as the face, dorsal aspect of the arms, and "V" of the neck and upper chest.

Phototoxic reactions tend to be more indurated and exudative with scale-crust but often are indistinguishable from photoallergic dermatitis.

The topical agent or ingested drug is rendered immunogenic after exposure to light energy.[23] For example, photooxidation of sulfanilamide produces a derivative that functions as a hapten in photoallergic reactions in humans and experimental animals.

Histopathological Features The features are those of an acute to subacute spongiotic dermatitis, independent of whether the allergen is a topical agent or drug.[24] A dense angiocentric lymphocytic infiltrate, with concomitant endothelial swelling and mural edema, is common in photoallergic dermatitis, but it is not always present. Often, the intensity of the vascular reaction diminishes toward the base of the biopsy, the vasculopathic changes (i.e., endothelial swelling and mural edema) being most conspicuous superficially. As most photoallergens also may have phototoxic properties, if administered in sufficient doses, additional features characteristic of a phototoxic process may be present. Such features include keratinocyte necrosis, including so-called "sunburn cells," architectural disarray and dysmaturation, and, in later-stage lesions, irregular and increased melanization, transepidermal elimination of melanin pigment, and hypergranulosis.

Photodermatitis: Other Variants

Several acquired idiopathic photodermatoses have spongiotic components. This is in contrast to the porphyrias, disorders of DNA repair and tryptophan metabolism, and solar urticaria.

POLYMORPHOUS LIGHT ERUPTION

Polymorphous light eruption (PMLE) is an acquired abnormal cutaneous reaction to ultraviolet light. Nonscarring pruritic, erythematous papules, vesicles, or plaques develop on exposed skin hours to days after light exposure. Histologically, there is a superficial to middermal perivascular infiltrate of lymphocytes. The infiltrate is moderate to heavy and may extend to the deep plexus.[25] There are a few neutrophils apparent superficially and eosinophils may be observed, but they are few in number in the vast majority of cases. The vessels are prominent because of striking endothelial swelling and vacuolation. Mural edema leading to luminal attenuation and luminal fibrin deposition may be observed. Often there is striking upper dermal edema. Epidermal changes are frequently absent, although spongiosis, vesicles, and exocytosis of lymphocytes may develop.

ACTINIC PRURIGO

Actinic prurigo, probably a variant of PMLE, presents in children, more commonly in females, and usually resolves in adolescence.[26] The pruritic papules and nodules often are excoriated, lichenified, and crusted.

The histologic features are similar to those of PMLE, with superimposed lichen simplex chronicus.[27]

HYDROA VACCINIFORME

Hydroa vacciniforme is a rare, chronic photodermatosis of unknown pathogenesis. Recurrent crops of papules and vesicles, with subsequent varioliform scarring, begin in childhood. Unlike other photodermatides, large tense vesicles with ulceration and subsequent scarring occur, often on the face. Hydroa estivale is not well characterized and is considered a mild nonscarring form of hydroa vacciniforme by some, and by others a childhood variant of PMLE.

In hydroa vacciniforme-estivale, classic descriptions include a superficial to deep perivascular dermatitis, with striking dermal edema (Fig. 7-4). The epidermis develops microvesicles with reticular degeneration. Fibrin thrombi and erythrocyte extravasation may be present. Later stages reveal epidermal and superficial dermal necrosis, with resultant fibrosis. An interface dermatitis with follicular accentuation of lymphocytic satellitosis about apoptotic keratinocytes has been identified.

CHRONIC ACTINIC DERMATITIS (ACTINIC RETICULOID)

Chronic actinic dermatitis (actinic reticuloid) is a persistent, eczematous dermatitis with pruritic firm papules and plaques occurring on sun-exposed skin.[28] It appears to be an abnormal response to UVB irradiation that develops in middle-aged or elderly individuals, usually men. There are confluent eczematous changes on the exposed areas of the backs of the hands, face, and upper chest. The eruption may extend over into relatively non-sun-exposed skin. Histologically, there is a subacute to chronic spongiotic dermatitis.[29] In later-stage lesions, atypical lymphocytes may be present in perivascular, bandlike, and epidermotropic array. These are T lymphocytes with hyperconvoluted nuclei, mimicking mycosis fungoides.

Differential Diagnosis See the preceding discussion of allergic contact dermatitis and Chapters 2 and 13. Features peculiar to a photodermatitis may facilitate distinction from other intraepidermal vesicular dermatitides; these include keratinocyte necrosis with so-called sunburn cells, architectural disarray and dysmaturation, and, in later-stage le-

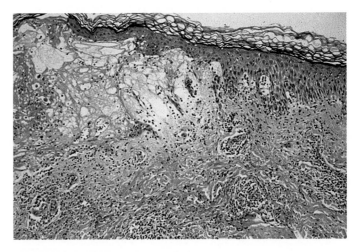

FIGURE 7-4 Hydroa vacciniforme. There is almost complete epidermal necrosis. There is marked dermal edema with a perivascular and interstitial lymphoid infiltrate with red blood cell extravasation.

sions, irregular and increased melanization, transepidermnal elimination of melanin pigment, and hypergranulosis.

Spongiotic Insect Bite Reaction

Clinical Features Three classes of arthropods bite or sting the skin (Chilopoda, Diplodica, and Insecta), producing inflammatory papules and nodules, with a central punctum, vesicles, and bullae. The lesions resolve over a period of weeks, but may persist for much longer periods of time, up to a year and possibly longer. The bites of arachnids and crustaceans produce a different histologic pattern and are not discussed here.

Histopathological Features A superficial to deep perivascular and interstitial dermatitis is apparent, broader superficially than deep, known as a wedge-shaped pattern.[30] In some reactions, one may observe only single eosinophils infiltrating between the reticular dermal collagen bundles. The lymphocytes, histiocytes, and eosinophils extend into the dermal interstitium.[30,31] Eosinophils usually are prominent. Encrustation of eosinophil granules on arthropod parts, or occasionally reticular dermal collagen bundles, the latter giving rise to flame figures, may be observed. The infiltration may be quite dense. Although the vast majority of lymphocytes appear normal, occasional large reactive lymphocytes may be present, producing a lymphomatoid hypersensitivity reaction. The bite or stinger parts may be present beneath the central punctum, which consists of a spongiotic focus or a small ulcer. Polarization may facilitate recognition of the stinger parts. Both intraepidermal and subepidermal vesiculation may occur secondary to the striking edema, and neutrophils may be prominent in this zone. As the biopsy specimen may not contain the punctum, the central changes of spongiosis, with exocytosis of lymphocytes, and of eosinophils (on occasion with eosinophilic spongiosis) may not be observed.

Some arthropod bites, particularly those caused by fleas, mosquitos, fire ants, and others, may produce primarily neutrophilic infiltration.

Differential Diagnosis See the preceding discussion of allergic contact dermatitis. It must be remembered that a standard reaction pattern of a bite reaction for any insect species cannot be given. The individual patient's immunologic response is an important confounding variable.

Pityriasis Rosea

Clinical Features The herald "patch" is a thin oval patch or minimally elevated plaque, usually located on the trunk. After a few days to 3 weeks, crops of 1- to 3-cm oval plaques develop on the trunk and proximal extremities in a "fir tree" pattern following the lines of tension.[32] They may be annular with a peripheral scale or may be nonscaly. Vesicles may be present on occasion.

Histopathological Features Pityriasis rosea usually is a mild subacute active spongiotic dermatitis.[33,34] Classically, small foci of "moundlike" parakeratosis in the stratum corneum develop above the papillae and alternate with orthokeratosis.[34,35] Often, one edge of the (lenticular) mound appears elevated. The spongiosis may be focal or generalized. Most commonly, the changes are limited to a papilla and surmounting epidermis with skipping of several papillae before another is involved. In some cases, clinically obvious spongiotic vesicles may be apparent. Spongiosis tends to be most intense above dermal papillae, into which there is exocytosis of lymphocytes and occasionally small numbers of red cells.[35] Papillary dermal hemorrhage is present in dermal papillae. Apoptotic cells and small intraepidermal clusters of Langerhans cells

may be apparent. The perivascular infiltrate consists of lymphocytes and histiocytes and usually is only superficial. Eosinophils are absent to few. Neutrophils are uncommon.

Differential Diagnosis Any subacute or pityriasiform variant of eczematous dermatitis, dermatophytosis, and superficial gyrate erythema (erythema annulare centrifugum) may have identical findings, as may pityriasiform drug eruptions such as those owing to captopril or gold. Plasma cells are absent, helping to exclude secondary lues, which often is a clinical diagnostic consideration.

Dermatophytosis

Clinical Features Dermatophytosis (tinea) is an infection of the stratum corneum by dermatophytes (see Chapter 21). The classic lesion for tinea corporis, an annular patch with scaling, may not develop when dermatophytes infect other body sites. The appearance of the lesions varies according to the type of organism present. Therefore, relatively noninflammatory lesions are produced by the anthropophilic fungi, whereas the zoophilic organisms produce a more inflammatory lesion with pustules and vesicles.

Histopathological Features Commonly, dermatophytosis leads to a subacute mild spongiotic eczematous dermatitis. There is slight psoriasiform epidermal hyperplasia, with focal mild spongiosis, exocytosis of lymphocytes, and few neutrophils.[36] Neutrophils enter the stratum corneum in which parakeratosis alternates with compact orthokeratosis scale.[37] There is a superficial perivascular lymphoid infiltrate, with few neutrophils and eosinophils, in association with dermal edema. The fungi vary in number, and may be visible as clear refractile small oval spaces on routine preparations. However, PAS stain always should be performed if dermatophytosis is a clinical possibility, as the hyphae sometimes may be of extremely low density (tinea occulta). Zoophilic fungal infection can give rise to a general spongiotic dermatitis with numerous neutrophils, spongiform pustulation, interface dermatitis, and a superficial and deep perivascular dermatitis. At times a florid intraepidermal response with marked neutrophilic and eosinophilic spongiosis and frank pustulation may develop in nonzoophilic fungal infections. Such cases are designated as representing inflammatory tinea.

Differential Diagnosis Any subacute or pityriasiform variant of eczematous dermatitis, bacterial and candidal infection, nutritional deficiency such as migratory necrolytic erythema, and superficial gyrate erythema (erythema annulare centrifugum) may have identical findings, as may pityriasiform drug eruptions such as those owing to captopril or gold.

Gianotti-Crosti Syndrome

Clinical Features Gianotti and Crosti described a childhood exanthem characterized by multiple nonpruritic flat-topped to vesicular erythematous papules, located principally on the face and extremities with sparing of the torso.[38,39] The rash lasts up to 2 to 4 weeks in contrast to other exanthems.

Originally, the rash was considered idiopathic. Subsequently, it has been associated with hepatitis B infection and now has been reported to occur in association with Epstein-Barr virus, enterovirus, cytomegalovirus, hepatitis A, and parainfluenza virus and may therefore be considered an eczematous "id" reaction.[40,41]

Histopathological Features   Early lesions are characterized by a mild acute spongiotic dermatitis, according to some.[39,42] Older lesions may be better developed and show subacute spongiotic changes. Essentially, there are no eosinophils. Some observers maintain that Gianotti-Crosti syndrome shows the characteristic morphology of a mixed spongiotic and vaculopathic interface dermatitis, in concert with a superficial to mild dermal perivascular lymphocytic infiltrate and red blood cell extravasation.[43]

Differential Diagnosis   One should consider subacute or pityriasiform types of spongiotic dermatitis such as pityriasis rosea and other viral exanthems in the differential diagnosis.

Toxic Shock Syndrome

Clinical Features   A diffuse, scarlatiniform exanthem, more prominent in the flexural areas, is present.[44] It may begin on the trunk, but usually spreads to the arms and legs. There is associated erythema and edema of the palms and soles. After 10 to 21 days, generalized desquamation usually develops. The rash is accompanied by high fever and severe constitutional symptoms.

Toxic shock syndrome is caused by localized infection (vaginitis, pharyngitis, wound infection, etc.) of toxin-producing strains of *Staphylococcus aureus*.[44,45] Toxic shock syndrome (TSS) toxin-1 is the most significant mediator, but other *Staphylococcus* enterotoxins may potentiate the disorder or produce it in the absence of TSS toxin-1.

Histopathological Features   There is a mild, acute spongiotic dermatitis associated with a superficial perivascular infiltrate of lymphocytes, neutrophils, and occasionally eosinophils.[46] There are small foci of spongiosis, which may be associated with clustered apoptotic keratinocytes and neutrophils. The neutrophils may be single or in small clusters. In later-stage lesions, a subacute spongiotic dermatitis is present without any distinguishing features.

Differential Diagnosis   Various subacute or pityriasiform variants of eczematous dermatitis, other bacterial and fungal infections, nutritional deficiency such as migratory necrolytic erythema, superficial gyrate erythema (erythema annulare centrifugum), and drug eruptions may have identical findings.

Kawasaki Disease

Clinical Features   Kawasaki syndrome is defined by a complex of cutaneous and mucosal lesions in association with cardiac abnormalities.[47] Diagnostic criteria include a fever of unexplained origin for at least 5 days, bilateral nonexudative conjunctival injection, oropharyngeal changes (injected or fissured lips, injected pharynx, or strawberry tongue) or extremity alteration (palmoplantar erythema, palmoplantar edema, periungual desquamation), polymorphous exanthem, and acute nonsuppurative cervical lymphadenopathy in order to make the diagnosis. The polymorphic exanthem is composed of macules, papules, a morbilliform eruption, or erythema multiforme–like lesions involving the trunk and the extremities. The cardiac findings include myocarditis and ischemia associated with coronary artery vasculitis.

Although the etiology is unknown, the clinical and pathologic features suggest an infectious etiology.

Histopathological Features   There is a superficial perivascular dermatitis of mixed-cell type with small foci of spongiosis, in which neutrophils may predominate. The vesicles usually are microscopic and are

not noted clinically. The superficial perivascular dermatitis usually is more prominent than the small zones of spongiosis. An erythema multiforme–like interface dermatitis may be present. Late-stage lesions may resemble psoriasis but without characteristic vascular changes.

Differential Diagnosis   See the preceding discussion of Gianotti-Crosti and toxic shock syndromes. Erythema multiforme also might be considered.

Incontinentia Pigmenti

Clinical Features   Incontinentia pigmenti is an X-linked genodermatosis that is believed to be lethal in males in utero.[48,49] The exact genetic defect, at this time, is not known. Characteristically there are three stages. Vesicles, principally on the extremities and often in linear array, are present at birth or begin within 2 weeks in 90 percent of cases. In 2 to 6 weeks, the vesicular lesions evolve to verrucous and papillomatous lesions, similar to those observed in ichthyosis histrix. In the last stage, there is whorled, brown to gray macular pigmentation that is most prominent on the trunk.

Histopathological Features   The first stage is characterized by an eosinophilic spongiosis (Table 7-11). Eosinophils usually are numerous, with intraepithelial eosinophilic abscesses (Fig. 7-5). As the lesions age, a subacute spongiotic dermatitis develops, with apoptotic, often clustered, keratinocytes. Within the dermis, there is a perivascular lymphohistiocytic infiltrate with interstitial extension. In the verrucous papules and plaques (second stage), there is hyperkeratosis, papillomatosis, and acanthosis, with whorled grouped and single apoptotic keratinocytes. A vaculopathic basal vaculopathy also may be apparent as well as epidermal dysmaturation. There is at most minimal spongiosis. The dermal edema observed in the first stage is almost absent. Dermal melanophages are present and may be numerous. In the pigmentary stage (third stage), dermal melanophages often are numerous. There is no inflammatory infiltrate. There is variable epidermal atrophy and single apoptotic keratinocytes.

Differential Diagnosis   Although the clinical findings usually are distinctive, the differential diagnosis includes causes of intraepidermal vesicles with eosinophilic spongiosis, such as allergic contact dermatitis, spongiotic drug eruptions, bite reactions, infestations, and primary blistering conditions, such as bullous pemphigoid. The presence of clustered apoptotic keratinocytes and other concomitant features, such as verrucous changes and pigment incontinence, also may aid in discriminating incontinentia pigmenti from the described entities.

TABLE 7-11

Eosinophilic Spongiosis: Differential Diagnosis

Drug eruption
Insect bite reaction
Scabetic infestation
Incontinentia pigmenti (+ pustules)
Pemphigoid
Pemphigus
Allergic contact dermatitis
Transient acantholytic dermatosis

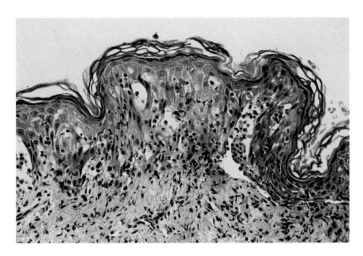

FIGURE 7-5   Incontinentia pigmenti, vesicular stage. Eosinophilic spongiosis and early intraepithelial eosinophilic pustules are present.

ACANTHOLYTIC DERMATITIS (SEE TABLES 7-1 TO 7-4 AND 7-12)

Pemphigus Vulgaris and Variants

Clinical Features   Large and flaccid bullae develop on the oral mucosa, face, scalp, central chest, and intertriginous zones in older individuals (Table 7-13). Oral lesions are the first manifestation in 10 to 15 percent of cases and almost invariably develop during the course of the disease.[50]

In 1 to 2 percent of cases of pemphigus vulgaris, vegetative plaques containing pustules may develop principally in the intertriginous areas.[51] Referred to as pemphigus vegetans, it is thought by many to be a "reactive state" in pemphigus.[51,52]

Polyclonal IgG develops against the pemphigus vulgaris antigen, desmoglein 3, a desmosomal cadherin that mediates cell binding.[53,54] Desmoglein 3 appears to be in greater concentration in the lower epidermis, the location of the suprabasal acantholytic blister of pemphigus vulgaris. The antigen-antibody union results in desmosomal dysfunction and potentiates dyshesion by causing production of a cytoplasmic proteinase, plasminogen activator, which is released into the squamous intercellular substance. Complement fixation may potentiate the acantholysis.

About 80 to 90 percent of patients have circulating IgG antibodies detectable by indirect immunofluorescence that show a general (but imperfect) correlation with disease activity.

Histopathological Features   The earliest stage most often is a paucicellular spongiotic dermatitis with edema most prominent in the lower epidermis (Table 7-13). Less commonly the early phase is eosinophilic spongiosis. Later, acantholysis supravenes, leading first to the formation of clefts and then to clinically apparent blisters that arise in suprabasal location (Fig. 7-6). They frequently extend into follicular external root sheaths. The basal keratinocytes separate from one another, but remain attached to the basal lumina, reminiscent of a "row of tombstones."[55] The acantholytic blister may be limited to the suprabasal plane or may extend higher within the epidermis. The acantholysis extends into appendages. The acantholytic keratinocytes are of relatively large size, with prominent eosinophilic glassy cytoplasm, prominent nuclei with large nucleoli, and perinuclear clearing. There is a superficial perivascular lymphohistiocytic infiltrate with dermal edema. As the lesions

TABLE 7-12

Important Differential Diagnostic Features of Acantholytic Dermatoses

	P. Foliaceus	SSSS	Hailey-Hailey D.	P. Vulgaris	P. Vegetans	Darier's D.	Grover's D.
Subcorneal cleavage	+++	+++	−	−	−	−	−
Intraspinous cleavage	0/+	−	+++	0/+	−	−	−
Suprabasal cleavage	−	−	0/+	+++	+++	+++	+(small)
Cleft	−	−	−	−	−	++	++
Blister	+	+	+	+	+	−	−
Dyskeratosis	+ (some)	−	−	−	−	++	+(some lesions)
Villi	−	−	+	+/+++	+++	+/+++	+
Tombstone basal keratinocyte	−	−	−	+++	+	−	−
Follicular involvement	+	−	−	++	+	+	−
Epidermal hyperplasia	−	−	+/++	0/+	+++	+	−
Spongiotic early change	+	−	−	+	+	−	+
Eosinophilic spongiosis	0/+	−	−	0/+ (some)	+++ (abscesses)	−	−

Legend:
0 = none; + = present; ++ = moderate change; +++ = marked change.

TABLE 7-13

Pemphigus Vulgaris and Variants

Clinical Features

Flaccid bullae on skin; face, scalp, chest and intertriginous areas (especially pemphigus vegetans)
Oral mucosa involved in 100%
Older individuals

Histopathological Features

Suprabasal acantholysis with blister formation
Involvement of hair follicles by acantholysis
Spongiosis early
Superficial perivascular mononuclear cell infiltrate
Direct immunofluorescence: squamous epithelial intercellular deposition of IgG and possibly C3

Differential Diagnosis

Other forms of pemphigus
Benign familial pemphigus (Hailey-Hailey disease)
Transient acantholytic dermatosis (Grover's disease)
Focal acantholytic dyskeratosis
Acantholytic variants of actinic keratosis
Herpesvirus infection

erode and ulcerate, a mixed infiltrate composed principally of neutrophils may develop. Older blisters may exhibit necrosis of the blister roof, with several keratinocytic layers lining the blister cavity on its lowermost aspect, owing to keratinocyte migration and proliferation. As well, epidermal reti may elongate, giving rise to the so-called villi. A neutrophilic spongiotic dermatitis may be present in some cases of pemphigus vulgaris. In these, spongiosis is a much more prominent feature than acantholysis.

All patients with active pemphigus have IgG autoantibodies against the cell surface of keratinocytes detectable by direct and often indirect immunofluorescence (also see Appendix). The pattern of intercellular space deposition of IgG may be identical in pemphigus vulgaris (PV), pemphigus foliaceus (PF) (and their closely related variants pemphigus

vegetans and erythematosus, respectively), and the majority of patients with drug-induced pemphigus. Rarely, the site of predominant immunoreactivity may correspond to the location of intraepidermal cleavage, that is, the suprabasal epidermis in PV and the superficial spinous layer in PF. The latter patterns of immunofluorescence provide evidence of PV versus PF, but final diagnosis should be based on the level of cleavage observed by light microscopy and the clinical context. In addition to IgG, C3 and other complement components often (up to 50% of cases) are found on direct immunofluorescence and exhibit a similar intercellular pattern of immunoreactivity as with IgG. Pemphigus should not be diagnosed if only C3 is present.

In pemphigus vegetans, the initial lesions are identical to those of pemphigus vulgaris. As the lesions age, verrucous epidermal hyperplasia develops (Fig 7-7), with prominent eosinophilic spongiosis and eosinophilic pustules. Rarely, neutrophil-rich intraepidermal pustules may be present. Acantholysis often is focal and may be difficult to identify.

Differential Diagnosis Although the clinical and histopathologic features of pemphigus vulgaris often are distinctive, other acantholytic disorders, such as pemphigus foliaceus and variants, drug-induced pemphigus, IgA pemphigus, paraneoplastic pemphigus, familial benign pemphigus, focal acantholytic dyskeratosis, herpesvirus infection, and acantholytic variants of actinic keratosis, may enter into the differential diagnosis. Pemphigus vulgaris is distinguished from pemphigus foliaceus and variants only by the suprabasal location of cleavage in PV versus the superficial cleavage in PF, that is, a subcorneal-granular blister, with or without dyskeratosis. Rarely, pemphigus erythematosus also may show basal layer vacuolopathy of the epidermis and deposition of IgG and possibly C3 in the basement membrane zone (BMZ) (as in lupus erythematosus), whereas PV usually does not. A clear association with a drug may be necessary to separate drug-induced pemphigus from PV; however, a minority of cases with drug-induced pemphigus do not have detectable antibodies by immunofluorescence. IgA pemphigus differs from PV by demonstrating subcorneal or intraepidermal neutrophilic pustules with minimal or no acantholysis and positive immunoreactivity for IgA in an intercellular pattern in the epidermis. Paraneoplastic pemphigus is distinctive because of a close relationship with cancer, the usual widespread nature of the eruption and striking mucocutaneous involvement, histologically the presence of interface

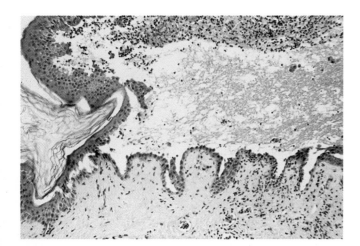

FIGURE 7-6 Pemphigus vulgaris. In this well-developed lesion there is a suprabasal cleft with acantholytic cells present in the blister cavity. Also seen are elongated epidermal reti below a single row of basal keratinocytes.

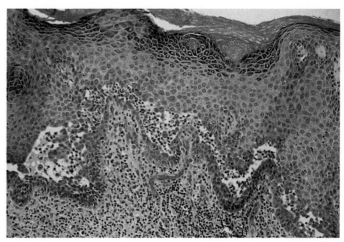

FIGURE 7-7 Pemphigus vegetans. In this early lesion, there is irregular epidermal hyperplasia with hyperkeratosis and hypergranulosis. In the suprabasal zone and lower stratum spinosum, there is acantholysis and accumulation of eosinophils, which may progress to eosinophilic pustules.

alterations and dyskeratosis resembling erythema multiforme, and both intercellular and BMZ patterns of immunofluorescence, in addition to acantholysis. Familial benign pemphigus (Hailey-Hailey disease) is discriminated from pemphigus by the usual presence of acanthosis, acantholysis involving at least half of the epidermis in a diffuse pattern, possibly some dyskeratosis, the lack of appendageal involvement, and finally negative immunofluorescence results. Pemphigus differs from focal acantholytic dyskeratosis (i.e., Darier and Grover diseases) by exhibiting greater breadth of involvement of the epidermis and involvement of appendages by the acantholysis versus only focal epidermal involvement in FAD, and the usual absence of dyskeratosis. On occasion, pemphigus may mimic herpesvirus infection by showing, in addition to acantholysis, alterations suggesting viral cytopathic changes of herpes; "ground-glass" nuclear changes, multinucleolation, and perinucleolar chromatin clearing, mimicking Type A Cowdry inclusions. Acantholytic variants of actinic keratosis usually are distinguished from pemphigus by the presence of parakeratosis, crowding, atypia of the basilar keratinocytes, and clinical presentation.

The presentation of pemphigus as eosinophilic spongiosis without vesicles raises a rather extensive differential diagnosis the principal entities of which are mentioned in Table 7-3 (also refer to Chapter 2). Clinical information and immunofluorescence studies are needed for definitive diagnosis in most instances.

Pemphigus Foliaceus and Variants

Clinical Features   Flaccid fragile bullae rupture to leave shallow crusted erosions and crusted patches and plaques on the trunk, intertriginous areas, proximal extremities, head, and neck of middle-aged and older individuals (Table 7-14). Most patients experience a chronic generalized course, although some patients present with an exfoliative dermatitis.

TABLE 7-14

Pemphigus Foliaceus and Variants

Clinical Features

  Crusted erosions and patches
  Very fragile flaccid bullae
  Middle-aged and elderly
  Trunk, head and neck, intertriginous areas, and proximal extremities
  "Butterfly rash" mimicking lupus erythematosus seen in pemphigus
    erythematosus

Histopathological Features

  Subcorneal/granular blister with acantholytic keratinocytes or
    dyskeratotic granular cells
  Variable eosinophilic spongiosis
  Direct immunofluorescence: squamous epithelial intercellular
    deposition of IgG and possibly C3
    Possible accentuation in superficial epidermis
    Pemphigus erythematosus usually shows linear or granular IgG
      and possibly C3 at the epidermal basement membrane zone

Differential Diagnosis

  Other forms of pemphigus
  Impetigo
  Staphylococcal scalded skin syndrome
  Subcorneal pustular dermatosis

FOLGO SELVAGEM

Fogo selvagem is similar clinically to pemphigus foliaceus, but develops in people who live adjacent to rivers and streams in Brazil.[56,57] An arthropod (*Simulium* sp.) vector may mediate this disorder.

PEMPHIGUS ERYTHEMATOSUS

Pemphigus erythematosus is characterized by erythematous plaques and papules in a butterfly distribution on the face, mimicking lupus erythematosus.

Polyclonal IgG within the serum is directed against desmoglein 1, a desmosomal cadherin.[54,58] Desmoglein 1 may be of a greater concentration in the upper epidermis. This distribution likely explains the subcorneal–granular layer cleavage plane of the blisters.

Histopathological Features   Three characteristic histologic patterns occur: eosinophilic spongiosis and abscesses, subcorneal–granular blisters with few acantholytic keratinocytes, and subcorneal–granular blisters with dyskeratotic granular cells (Table 7-14).[59,60] The latter pattern is diagnostic of this disorder (Fig. 7-8). As in pemphigus vulgaris, the cleavage plane is not exact and may extend to the suprabasal zone, on occasion rendering histologic distinction of the two principal pemphigus variants difficult.[61] There is an associated superficial perivascular dermatitis with edema. As the lesions erode and age, a mixed infiltrate may appear. Bacterial suprainfection may lead to a picture identical to that of impetigo. The histologic features of pemphigus erythematosus are identical to those of pemphigus foliaceus; however, in rare cases an interface dermatitis similar to that of lupus erythematosus has been present.

As discussed previously for PV, all patients with active PF have positive direct immunofluorescence for IgG and to a lesser degree C3 in a typical intercellular pattern that is indistinguishable from other forms of pemphigus or concentrated in the superficial epidermis. In the vast majority of cases, indirect immunofluorescence also is positive. As mentioned previously, pemphigus erythematosus usually exhibits BMZ deposition of IgG and occasionally C3 in addition to the intercellular immunoreactivity.

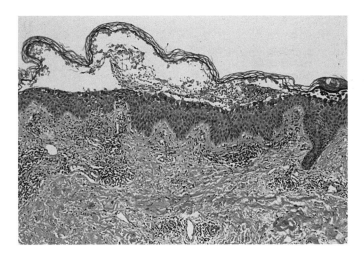

FIGURE 7-8   Pemphigus foliaceus. There is a subcorneal split with few viable acantholytic keratinocytes present (left). In the superficial dermis a perivascular mononuclear infiltrate with a few eosinophils is seen. Accumulation of neutrophils in the acantholytic blister may lead to confusion with bullous impetigo.

Differential Diagnosis   See the preceding discussion on differential diagnosis for pemphigus vulgaris. Other considerations not already mentioned include bacterial and fungal infections, especially impetigo and bullous impetigo, pustular drug eruption, IgA pemphigus, and subcorneal pustular dermatosis. Impetigo is distinguished from PF by a Gram-positive stain (may not be present in bullous impetigo) and cultures and negative immunofluorescence findings. PF is separated from the other disorders by IgA or lack of any positivity on immunofluorescence studies. Both pemphigus erythematosus and paraneoplastic pemphigus usually demonstrate deposition of immunoreactants, that is, IgG, in intercellular and BMZ patterns and must be discriminated by other findings (clinical, histopathologic, and laboratory).

Drug-Induced Pemphigus

Clinical Features   Drug-induced pemphigus usually begins as a non-specific eruption of morbilliform, annular, or urticarial plaques, without blisters (Table 7-15). Patients with penicillamine-induced pemphigus have a characteristic generalized toxic erythema that has been labeled "a toxic pre-pemphigus rash."[62,63] After a variable period of time, blisters develop on scaly crusted patches, similar to those of pemphigus foliaceus in most cases. The most common causative drugs include penicillamine and captopril.[64]

Drug-induced pemphigus can be separated into two subsets. In the first group, representing 10 percent of cases, pemphigus antibodies are produced and cause acantholysis identical to that of idiopathic pemphigus.[55] Direct binding of the drugs to the pemphigus antigens may render the antigens immunogenic in such cases. In the second group, the drugs or metabolites, rich in sulfhydryl groups, accumulate within the epidermis. They may cleave the disulfide bonds of keratin, incorporate into the keratin molecule itself because of their similarity to cystine, leading to dyshesion. Another possible mechanism is the direct binding of the drugs to the pemphigus vulgaris and foliaceus antigen, disrupting their interchain disulfide bonds.

TABLE 7-15

Drug-Induced Pemphigus

Clinical Features

Morbilliform, annular, or urticarial plaques progress to blisters
Scaly crusted plaques
Penicillamine and captopril are common causative agents

Histopathological Features

Plane of blister separation may occur in either subcorneal or
   suprabasal plane
Subacute eczematous dermatitis seen in early lesions
Direct immunofluorescence study: intercellular deposition of IgG
and possibly C3 in epidermis in almost all active cases

Differential Diagnosis

Other forms of pemphigus
Benign familial pemphigus (Hailey-Hailey disease)
Transient acantholytic dermatosis (Grover's disease)
Focal acantholytic dyskeratosis
Acantholytic variants of actinic keratosis
Herpesvirus infection
Impetigo
Staphylococcal scalded skin syndrome
Subcorneal pustular dermatosis

Histopathological Features   In the early eruption, there is an acute to subacute eczematous dermatitis (Table 7-15). Eosinophils may be present, on occasion giving rise to eosinophilic spongiosis. The blister separation plane may be either in the subcorneal or suprabasal zones, such that in well-developed lesions the histologic features are identical to pemphigus foliaceus or vulgaris. The immunofluorescence findings also may be indistinguishable from other forms of pemphigus.

Differential Diagnosis   See the preceding discussions on pemphigus vulgaris and foliaceus.

IgA Pemphigus

Synonyms: IgA pemphigus foliaceus; IgA herpetiform pemphigus; intercellular IgA vesiculopustular dermatosis; intercellular IgA dermatosis; intraepidermal IgA pustulosis

Clinical Features   IgA pemphigus is a pruritic, vesiculopustular eruption that develops in middle-aged to older individuals, often involving the axilla, trunk, and extremities (Table 7-16). Many cases of subcorneal pustular dermatosis, in which immunologic investigation was not undertaken, may represent IgA pemphigus. Flaccid vesicles, pustules, or bullae arise on erythematous bases similar to the lesions of pemphigus foliaceus. Patients have been segregated into two groups, one with a subcorneal pustular dermatosis and the other with an intraepidermal pustular eruption.

Circulating IgA is directed against adhesion molecules within the epidermis. The antigens against which the antibodies are directed are neither the pemphigus foliaceus nor vulgaris antigen, but rather desmocollins.[65] The differing clinical presentation of the patients likely relates to the fact that the antibodies are directed against two separate desmocollins, which have differing distributions within the epidermis.

Histopathological Features   Two variants, a subcorneal pustular dermatosis and an intraepidermal pustular eruption, are observed (Table 7-16).[65–67] In the former, there are subcorneal vesiculopustules with minimal acantholysis. In the latter, there are intraepidermal pustules containing small to moderate numbers of neutrophils throughout the breadth of the epidermis (Fig. 7-9). Suprabasal separation is not apparent. Minimal acantholysis is apparent such that the histologic reaction pattern is best considered an intraepidermal pustular dermatosis. In one case, no neutrophil infiltration was present.[68] IgA pemphigus is defined by the presence of IgA intercellular deposition on direct immunofluorescence examination.

TABLE 7-16

IgA Pemphigus

Clinical Features

Flaccid vesicles, pustules, and bullae arise on an erythematous base
Middle-aged to elderly patients

Histopathological Features

Subcorneal or intraepidermal pustules
Direct immunofluorescence: intercellular IgA in epidermis

Differential Diagnosis

Other forms of pemphigus
Impetigo
Staphylococcal scalded skin syndrome
Subcorneal pustular dermatosis

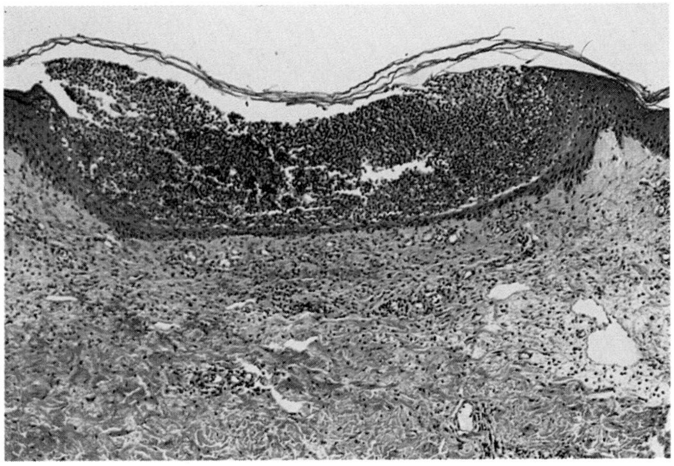

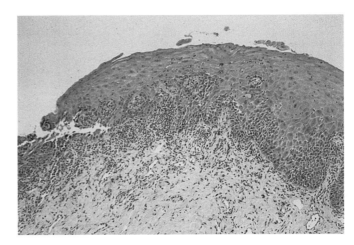

FIGURE 7-9 IgA pemphigus, subcorneal pustular variant. There is a large sub-corneal pustule with spongiform pustulation. This picture is similar to Sneddon-Wilkinson disease, pustular psoriasis, and a pustular drug eruption.

Differential Diagnosis The major entities to be considered include pemphigus foliaceus, subcorneal pustular dermatosis, bacterial and fungal infection (particularly impetigo), pustular psoriasis, pustular drug eruption, nutritional deficiency such as migratory necrolytic erythema, and on occasion Hailey-Hailey disease. Systematic evaluation with clinical history for evidence of psoriasis, drug ingestion, special stains and cultures for infective organisms, and immunofluorescence studies should facilitate making a specific diagnosis.

Paraneoplastic Pemphigus

Clinical Features Paraneoplastic pemphigus recently has been described by Anhalt et al.[69] It is characterized by a generalized polymorphous eruption of blisters and lichenoid papules (Table 7-17).[69,70] Painful oral ulcerations are a prominent feature and have been present in all cases. The ulcerations often are extensive over the lower lips, mimicking those of Stevens-Johnson syndrome. With one possible exception, all patients have had known or occult malignancies, including Hodgkin's disease, thymoma, chronic lymphocytic leukemia, other hematopoietic malignancies, as well as bronchogenic carcinoma and retroperitoneal sarcoma.[71,72] The disorder is aggressive and generally refractory to treatment. Successful treatment of the underlying malignancy may induce a remission of the pemphigus.

A panoply of autoantibodies is directed against a number of epidermal antigens and bind to simple, columnar, and transitional epithelia in addition to epidermis. The target antigens include desmoplakin-1, desmoplakin-2, the bullous pemphigoid antigen (BPAg1), and an antigen of 190 kDa that remains uncharacterized.[69]

Histopathological Features The hallmarks include suprabasal acantholysis, with principally basal layer keratinocyte apoptosis and an interface dermatitis that resembles erythema multiforme or lichen planus (Table 7-17; Fig. 7-10).[73] Some cases may appear identical to pemphigus vulgaris without interface dermatitis and apoptosis. It is important to note that acantholysis may be focal or not present at all in a single lesion. Thus the lesions may appear as either a purely erythema multiforme–like interface dermatitis or cell-rich lichenoid interface dermatitis.[74] Thus, biopsies of more than one lesion or level sections of a biopsy specimen may be necessary in order to make the diagnosis.

Direct immunofluorescence studies usually reveal both intercellular IgG (and possibly C3) and BMZ IgG, C3, and occasionally IgM (in both

---

TABLE 7-17

Paraneoplastic Pemphigus

Clinical Features

Polymorphous eruption of blisters and lichenoid papules
Painful oral ulcerations
Remission may be seen following successful treatment of underlying malignancy

Histopathological Features

Suprabasal acantholysis
Interface dermatitis; either vacuolar or lichenoid type
Direct immunofluorescence: squamous epithelial intercellular deposition of IgG, or IgM, and possibly C3 usually shows linear or granular IgG, or IgM, and possibly C3 in epidermal basement membrane zone

Differential Diagnosis

Other forms of pemphigus
Benign familial pemphigus (Hailey-Hailey disease)
Transient acantholytic dermatosis (Grover's disease)
Focal acantholytic dyskeratosis
Acantholytic variants of actinic keratosis
Lichen planus
Erythema multiforme

FIGURE 7-10 Paraneoplastic pemphigus. There is an interface dermatitis (right) in association with a suprabasal acantholytic blister (left). (Courtesy of Thomas D. Horn MD and Grant J. Anhalt MD.)

granular and linear patterns). Indirect immunofluorescence demonstrates intercellular IgG in all cases studied.

Differential Diagnosis See the preceding discussion of pemphigus vulgaris.

Generalized Staphylococcal Scalded Skin Syndrome (Ritter's Disease)

Clinical Features Affected infants develop a painful tender, orange-tinged erythematous rash associated with a purulent conjunctivitis, otitis media, or occult nasopharyngeal infection.[75] Within 2 days, large flaccid bullae develop in the axillae, groin, and around body orifices and become generalized. Healing usually is complete within 5 to 7 days.

The associated infection is usually caused by staphylococci of group II phage type 71. They produce two epidermolysins that enter the circulation and deposit in the skin, producing a subcorneal–granular layer separation plane.[76] In adults these epidermolysins usually are rapidly cleared owing to the presence of neutralizing antibodies. Neonates do not have these neutralizing antibodies and have a decreased renal clearance of the epidermolysin.

Histopathological Features   There is a subcorneal separation without dyskeratosis and only a few acantholytic keratinocytes. Few inflammatory cells are present initially, but later, neutrophilic infiltration may be striking, producing a histologic picture identical to that of impetigo.

Differential Diagnosis   The histologic appearance of P. foliaceous may be identical.

Darier's Disease

Synonym: Keratosis follicularis

Clinical Features   Darier's disease is an autosomal dominant genodermatosis presenting in the first two decades of life (Table 7-18).[77] Skincolored papules covered by a tenacious scale coalesce into large plaques that involve the chest, back, head, and groin. Cobblestone papules are present on the oral mucosa. Warty papules are present acrally. Several variants have been described, including a hyperkeratotic form involving the intertriginous zones, a vesiculobullous form in which true clinical blisters may develop, and a linear pattern that likely represents an epidermal nevus with the histologic features of focal acantholytic dyskeratosis.

The Darier disease gene has been localized to chromosome 12q23-q24.1.[78] The function of the abnormal gene has not been clarified. Cultured keratinocytes from Darier disease patients become acantholytic.

Histopathological Features   Darier's disease is the prototype of focal acantholytic dyskeratosis (Table 7-18; Figs. 7-11 A,B).[79] Over a broad zone within the epidermis there is an acantholytic suprabasal cleft, beneath which the basal cell layer is intact. The rete may be elongated, giving rise to so-called villi. Within the cleft (lacuna) are occasional acantholytic keratinocytes. Above the acantholytic cleft the compact,

---

TABLE 7-18

Darier's Disease

Clinical Features

   Scaly papules and plaques of the head, back, chest, and groin
   Autosomal dominant

Histopathological Features

   Acantholytic dyskeratosis with suprabasal split
   Corps ronds and corps grains
   Acanthosis and parakeratosis
   Direct immunofluorescence: nonspecific pattern of granular C3 at
     the epidermal basement membrane zone

Differential Diagnosis

   Hailey-Hailey disease
   Transient acantholytic dermatosis (Grover's disease)
   Pemphigus vulgaris

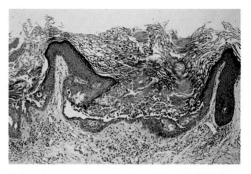

A

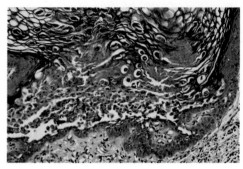

B

FIGURE 7-11   (*A, B*) Darier's disease. There is an epidermal invagination filled with ortho- and parakeratotic debris. A suprabasal lacuna with dyskeratotic acantholytic cells is present. At higher power the typical large keratinocytes with perinuclear halos and clumped keratohyalin granules in eosinophilic cytoplasm (corps ronds), and the small seed-shaped cells with pyknotic nuclei and dense eosinophilic cytoplasm (corps grains) are noted.

enlarged keratinocytes of the stratum granulosum are surmounted by parakeratotic keratinocytes within the hyperkeratotic stratum corneum. Dyskeratosis may be apparent in the acantholytic cells, above or lateral to the acantholytic cleft. Large keratinocytes contain clumped keratohyalin granules in an eosinophilic cytoplasm, have large nuclei with perinuclear chromatin clumping, and halos about prominent nucleoli. At the other end of the spectrum are small, seed-shaped cells with pyknotic elongated nuclei and dense eosinophilic, oftentimes elongated, cytoplasm. The dyskeratotic acantholytic granular cells are referred to as "corps ronds" and the dyskeratotic parakeratotic cells are referred to as "corps grains." Intermediate forms may be observed. The focal acantholytic dyskeratosis occurs in the background of a papillary epidermal hyperplasia, with the dells between the papillae filled by keratotic debris. In other zones of papillary epidermal hyperplasia, there may be small foci of ill-defined focal acantholytic dyskeratosis.

In Darier's disease, there may be epidermal basement membrane zone deposition of C3 in granular array and spotty granular C3 within the epidermis, a nonspecific finding.

Differential Diagnosis   The principal conditions to be considered include transient acantholytic dermatosis (TAD) (Grover's disease), Hailey-Hailey disease, and on occasion other acantholytic processes such as herpesvirus infection and pemphigus. TAD may be indistinguishable from Darier's disease but usually shows additional histologic patterns resembling pemphigus, Hailey-Hailey disease, and spongiotic dermatitis (see the following). Hailey-Hailey disease differs from Darier's disease by demonstrating more diffuse or full-thickness acantholysis and less dyskeratosis (usually minimal). Pemphigus shows more diffuse suprabasilar acantholysis with involvement of appendages, usually no dyskeratosis (except for p. foliaceus), and uniform squamous intercellular substance deposition of IgG and C3, in contrast to the non-specific pattern in Darier's disease. Herpesvirus is discriminated by clear-cut viral cytopathic changes, that is, multinucleate keratinocyte giant cells with molding of nuclei and ground-glass chromatin.

Hailey-Hailey Disease

Synonym: Familial benign pemphigus

Clinical Features   This autosomal dominant genodermatosis presents in adolescence or adulthood with localized, recurrent vesicles arising on erythematous bases (Table 7-19). The vesicles often become eroded and develop scale-crust. The plaques expand serpiginously with healing or ensuing vegetation. Lesions usually are limited to the intertriginous areas, sides of the neck, and less commonly, the antecubital, perianal, and inframammary zones.[80] Lesions may extend elsewhere and in rare cases become widespread. Maceration and fissuring may be prominent, particularly in intertriginous areas.

The Hailey-Hailey disease gene has been mapped to chromosome 3q.[81] It is unclear how the gene products result in keratinocyte dyshesion. Culture of Hailey-Hailey epidermis reveals suprabasal blisters. Friction and superinfection may augment the acantholysis.

Histopathological Features   Full-thickness acantholysis of the stratum spinosum develops in a hyperplastic epidermis, resulting in an appearance resembling a "dilapidated brick wall," without a discrete supra-basal cleft (Table 7-19; Fig. 7-12).[82] The acantholysis does not extend down follicles. Basal layer budding and villi are usually less prominent than those observed in Darier's disease.

Dyskeratosis usually is minimal. The roof of the blister consists of intact upper stratum spinosum or stratum granulosum. In the later lesions, the upper portion of the epidermis degenerates into a parakeratotic crust above the residual acantholytic epidermis. In some cases a subacute to chronic eczematous dermatitis may be present.

Immunofluorescence studies also are nonspecific as in Darier's disease.

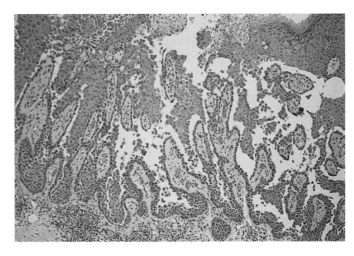

FIGURE 7-12   Hailey-Hailey disease. There is extensive acantholysis of the stratum spinosum in a floridly hyperplastic epidermis. The extent of the acantholysis of the stratum spinosum excludes pemphigus vulgaris.

Differential Diagnosis   One must primarily consider pemphigus and Darier's disease (see the preceding discussions for the differential diagnosis for each respective condition).

Transient Acantholytic Dermatosis

Synonym: Grover's disease

Clinical Features   Also known as Grover's disease, transient acantholytic dermatosis (TAD) is characterized by pruritic discrete papulovesicles on the chest, back, and thighs, usually in middle-aged or elderly men (Table 7-20) often following sun exposure.[83] The appellation "transient" is appropriate in some cases; however, in others, the process may persist for several years.[84]

The pathogenesis is unknown. Some recent work suggests an association with miliaria.[85]

TABLE 7-19

Hailey-Hailey Disease

Clinical Features

Fragile flaccid blisters give rise to scale-crust
Intertriginous areas, neck, perianal, inframammary, and antecubital
   regions
Autosomal dominant

Histopathological Features

Acantholysis giving rise to dilapidated brick wall appearance in at
   least half of epidermis
Acanthosis
Often slight dyskeratosis
Direct immunofluorescence: nonspecific pattern

Differential Diagnosis

Darier's disease
Transient acantholytic dermatosis (Grover's disease)
Pemphigus vulgaris

TABLE 7-20

Transient Acantholytic Dermatosis (Grover's Disease)

Clinical Features

Pruritic papulovesicles on chest, back, and thighs
Middle-aged or elderly men

Histopathological Features

Acantholytic dyskeratosis in small foci
Four histological patterns:
   Focal acantholytic dyskeratosis as in Darier's disease
   Hailey-Hailey disease pattern
   Pemphigus vulgaris or foliaceus pattern
   Spongiotic dermatitis pattern
Any or all four patterns may be present in a single biopsy
Direct immunofluorescence: nonspecific pattern

Differential Diagnosis

Darier's disease
Hailey-Hailey disease
Pemphigus vulgaris or foliaceus
Spongiotic dermatitis

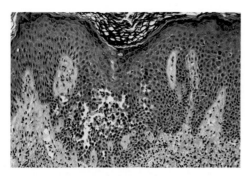

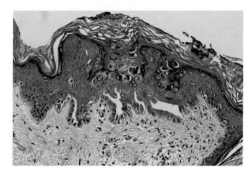

FIGURE 7-13   (*A*) Grover's disease, pemphigus pattern. There is lower epidermal acantholysis with an underlying superficial perivascular mononuclear infiltrate. (*B*) Grover's disease, Darier's pattern. A suprabasal split is present with acantholysis and dyskeratosis of the sloughed keratinocytes. There is an overlying zone of hyperkeratosis. A similar picture may be seen as an incidental finding or in some forms of epidermal nevi.

Histopathological Features   Any of four histologic patterns may be observed in small foci, often only several rete wide (Table 7-20; Fig. 7-13): focal acantholytic dyskeratosis resembling Darier's disease, full-thickness acantholysis mimicking Hailey-Hailey disease, small suprabasal clefts as observed in pemphigus vulgaris, and a spongiotic dermatitis. Any or all of these histologic patterns may be present in an individual biopsy from an individual patient.[84]

Differential Diagnosis   Because the four histologic patterns described may occur in TAD, the differential diagnosis includes Darier's disease, Hailey-Hailey disease, pemphigus, and a spongiotic dermatitis. TAD is distinguished from the latter entities based on the presence of two or more histologic patterns and their limitation to small foci, often only several rete wide. On occasion, these foci may be larger, rendering it difficult to make a specific diagnosis without clinical information.

CYTOLYTIC DERMATITIS

Epidermolytic Hyperkeratosis

Clinical Features   Epidermolytic hyperkeratosis is an autosomal dominantly inherited genodermatosis that presents at birth with widespread blistering followed by a generalized ichthyosis (also see Chapter 14). Other milder phenotypes also occur, including localized annular hyperkeratotic plaques and palmoplantar keratoderma.

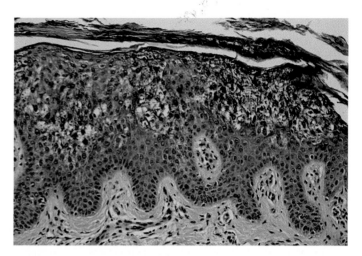

FIGURE 7-14   Epidermolytic hyperkeratosis. Beneath diffuse hyperorthokeratosis there is vacuolization of the suprabasal keratinocytes. The vacuolated keratinocytes have a characteristic appearance with large keratohyalin granules. Trichohyalin granules often are present as well.

Recent studies have shown mutations on chromosome 12 and chromosome 17, the respective sites of the keratin 1 gene and keratin 10 gene complexes.[86] It is thought that the abnormal keratins cannot form a normal cytoskeleton and result in the aggregated tonofilaments that have been observed on electron microscopic evaluation.

Histopathological Features   Beneath compact hyperorthokeratosis, there is striking keratinocytic cytoplasmic vacuolization, extending from the granular layer to the suprabasal zone (Fig. 7-14). At the periphery of the vacuoles, there is condensation of cytoplasmic elements, including markedly enlarged keratohyalin granules, and dense eosinophilic granules that resemble trichohyalin. The irregularly shaped shrunken nuclei are preserved. The blisters occur in irregular fashion throughout the stratum malpighii owing to coalescence of the vacuoles. The background epidermis exhibits irregular psoriasiform hyperplasia, but this feature may not be present in early lesions. It should be remembered that these exact histologic events can occur as a part of congenital ichthyosiform bullous erythroderma, as the principal histologic findings of epidermal nevi, and as incidental small foci within the epidermis, analogous to focal acantholytic dyskeratosis.

Differential Diagnosis   Although the clinical and histologic features are distinctive, one might consider verruca, a viral vesicle, or a spongiotic dermatitis as other diagnostic possibilities.

Friction Blisters

Clinical Features   These blisters develop mainly on the soles and palms as a result of repetitive actions producing energy applied parallel to the cutaneous surface in normal individuals (Table 7-21). In the mechanobullous diseases, only minimal friction will produce blisters owing to a lack of appropriate structural integrity of the epidermis and dermis.

Friction blisters are caused by shearing forces within the epidermis. They tend to occur where the epidermis is thick and firmly attached to the underlying tissues.[87]

Histopathological Features   The intraepidermal cleavage, a result of cytolysis of keratinocytes, may be present in the superficial or lower

TABLE 7-21

Friction Blister

Clinical Features

  Palms and soles most common sites affected
  History of mechanical injury at site affected

Histopathological Features

  Blister with intraepidermal cleavage
  Individual necrotic keratinocytes
  Hemorrhage is common

Differential Diagnosis

  Epidermolysis bullosa simplex superficialis

stratum spinosum (Table 7-21).[88] There are individual necrotic keratinocytes, with cytoplasmic strands of disrupted keratinocytes. Pale degenerated keratinocytes, which have been sheared, are located on the superior and inferior aspect of the blister.[87-89] The blister fluid is usually clear owing to transudation. When the shearing force extends into the dermis, hemorrhage into the blister cavity is common.

Differential Diagnosis   The differential diagnosis includes epidermolysis bullosa simplex superficialis (see Chapter 14).

Thermal Burns

First-degree burns are those in which the lower epidermis is intact and only the upper epidermis is necrotic. The nuclei appear pyknotic and the cytoplasm pale giving the upper epidermis a mummified ghostlike appearance. Extensive dermal edema leads to transudation of fluid above the intact lower epidermis into intraepidermal spinous blisters. The dermis is edematous, with neutrophils exiting the superficial vessels and forming a purulent layer beneath the necrotic epidermis.[90] Second- and third-degree burns are not discussed because they do not give rise to intraepidermal blisters or pustules.

VESICULOPUSTULAR DISEASES

Impetigo and Bullous Impetigo

Clinical Features   In impetigo, red papules that transform into vesicles and pustules develop at sites where abrasions, insect bites, or excoriations disrupt the cutaneous barrier. Honey-colored crusts develop rapidly. Secondary impetigo may develop in all varieties of eczematous dermatitis, particularly atopic eczema. Ordinary impetigo is caused by infection by group A streptococci.[91] Bullous impetigo is almost entirely owing to infections by *Staphylococcus aureus*, primarily phage group 2, type 71, which produces an epidermolysin that causes staphylococcal scalded skin syndrome.

In bullous impetigo, vesicles, bullae and vesiculopustules form on erythematous macules and plaques.

Histopathological Features   In ordinary nonbullous impetigo, neutrophils migrate throughout the epidermis to form subcorneal pustules. The exocytosis of neutrophils as single cells and clusters into the hyperplastic and spongiotic epidermis resembles psoriasis. There usually is prominent edema in the upper dermis and diapedesis of neutrophils from the superficial vessels.

In contrast, bullous impetigo begins as a fluid-filled acantholytic blister in subcorneal location. Few acantholytic keratinocytes are present, and neutrophils may be sparse. As the vesiculopustule ages, it usually becomes filled with neutrophils. Otherwise, the features are similar to those of nonbullous impetigo, although the inflammatory infiltrate and reactive epidermal changes usually are less intense.

Bacterial cocci, often few in number, may be noted within the stratum corneum, pustules, or vesiculopustules and are best demonstrated by a tissue Gram stain.

Differential Diagnosis   The major entities to be considered include other infective processes, such as dermatophytosis, candida, syphilis; pemphigus foliaceus; IgA pemphigus; subcorneal pustular dermatosis; pustular psoriasis; pustular drug eruption; pustular bite reaction; pustular vasculitis; a neutrophilic dermatosis, such as pyoderma gangrenosum; and a nutritional deficiency as to zinc or an amino acid resulting in an eruption such as migratory necrolytic erythema. Systematic evaluation with clinical history for evidence of psoriasis, drug ingestion, and so forth; special stains and cultures for infective organisms; and immunofluorescence studies should facilitate making a specific diagnosis.

Candidiasis

Clinical Features   Red papules and plaques develop, most frequently in the intertriginous areas. Pustules may develop at the surface, often at the edges. Satellite pustules also may develop around the spreading plaque.

Candida albicans is the most frequent infectious agent. It is a dimorphic fungus that produces both yeasts (2 to 5 μm) and pseudohyphae. Local disruption of the integrity of the upper epidermis, such as maceration and abrasion, facilitates infection. Although other mechanisms are at play, mannin in the fungal cell walls fixes complement, which then leads to neutrophilic infiltration.

Histopathological Features   There is neutrophilic permeation of the parakeratotic stratum corneum.[92] Beneath the stratum corneum, micropustules coalesce into larger pustules. Neutrophils, as single cells and small clusters, permeate the underlying stratum spinosum, which is spongiotic. The underlying dermis is edematous, with a perivascular and interstitial infiltrate composed principally of neutrophils. Although the yeasts and branching pseudohyphae, that are 2 to 5 μm in diameter, may be demonstrable on routine hematoxylin and eosin stains, PAS stain is more reliable in revealing the organisms. It may be difficult to specifically identify the agent as *Candida albicans*, leading to the necessity of culture in selected cases.

Differential Diagnosis   See the preceding discussion of impetigo.

Pustular Secondary Lues

Clinical Features   Approximately 3 to 6 weeks after the chancre, secondary lesions may develop. Macules and papules (mimicking pityriasis rosea) develop on the trunk, extremities, and the palms and soles. Mucous patches are common. Pustules usually are a later development.

Dissemination of *Treponema pallidum* to distant sites is the etiology. They are spiral bacteria that range from 7 to 15 μm in length and 0.25 μm in width. Intact spirochetes are demonstrated in histologic sections in up to 30 percent of secondary lesions using Warthin-Starry or Dieterle stains.

TABLE 7-22

Subcorneal Pustular Dermatosis (Sneddon-Wilkinson)

Clinical Features

Pustules develop in erythematous skin
Predilection for flexural skin, axillary and inguinal folds

Histopathological Features

Subcorneal neutrophil-rich pustules
Superficial and deep perivascular mononuclear cell infiltrates
Direct immunofluorescence: negative

Differential Diagnosis

Impetigo
Candida
Dermatophytosis
Staphylococcal scalded skin syndrome
Psoriasis
Keratoderma blenorrhagicum (Reiter disease)
IgA pemphigus
Pemphigus foliaceus
Pustular drug eruption

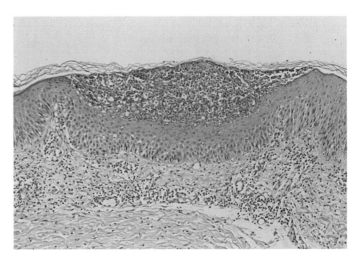

FIGURE 7-15 Subcorneal pustular dermatosis (Sneddon-Wilkinson disease). There is a florid subcorneal pustule containing neutrophils. This tense pustule is distinct from the flaccid pustule of bullous impetigo.

Histopathological Features   Subcorneal pustules surmount a variably platelike acanthotic or psoriasiform epidermis. Numerous neutrophils transverse the stratum spinosum. In the dermis, there is a variable perivascular and lichenoid lymphohistiocytic infiltrate often rich in plasma cells. In fact, plasma cells are observed in up to 75 percent of these late-stage lesions. This is in contrast to early lesions of secondary syphilis, in which only a perivascular lymphohistiocytic infiltrate may be observed. The infiltration extends into the interstitium in some lesions with numerous macrophages.

Differential Diagnosis   See the preceding discussion of impetigo.

Subcorneal Pustular Dermatosis/ Sneddon-Wilkinson Disease

Clinical Features   Pustules and vesiculopustules develop on erythematous skin (Table 7-22). The lesions may be annular or serpiginous and have a predilection for flexural surfaces as well as axillary and inguinal folds. Subcorneal pustular dermatosis may occur in association with IgA gammopathy, multiple myeloma, or in association with other neutrophilic dermatoses. It has been described also in association with rheumatoid arthritis and inflammatory bowel disease.[93–95]

Although unknown, at this time it is presumed that the neutrophils are responding to chemotactic factors present in the subcorneal zone. Those cases of subcorneal pustular dermatosis with squamous intercellular deposits of IgA are best classified as IgA pemphigus.

Histopathological Features   Subcorneal neutrophil-rich pustules and scale-crust are present (Table 7-22; Fig. 7-15). The pustules tend to be tense rather than flaccid. In most cases the underlying edematous spongiotic stratum malpighii contains only few neutrophils, and eosinophils are absent or rare. Occasional acantholytic keratinocytes may be present at the lower edge of the pustule, primarily in older lesions. These

changes surmount a psoriasiform epidermis with little change, or, in older lesions, a psoriasiform eruption with exocytosis of lymphocytes as well. There is a superficial and deep perivascular infiltrate of lymphocytes and histiocytes that may on occasion give rise to a bandlike pattern.

Differential Diagnosis   See the preceding discussion of IgA pemphigus and impetigo.

Pustular Drug Reaction

Clinical Features   Drug-induced pustular eruptions have been infrequently reported. Drugs implicated include antibiotics (including streptomycin, cotrimoxazole, and oxytetracycline) and other drugs, including chloramphenicol, pyrimethamine, diltiazem, furosemide, and carbamazepine. Patients usually present 3 to 10 days after initiation of therapy with diffuse macular erythema and multiple non-follicular-based pustules. In addition, malaise, chills, and low-grade fever may be present. The dermatitis rapidly resolves after withdrawal of the offending drug.

Histopathological Features   Foci of neutrophilic spongiosis with or without subcorneal or intraepidermal pustules are seen. The process may be based around the acrosyringium or follicle.[96,97] There is underlying papillary dermal edema and a perivascular infiltrate usually containing eosinophils.

Differential Diagnosis   See the preceding discussions of IgA pemphigus and impetigo. The differential diagnosis includes pustular psoriasis, Reiter disease, subcorneal pustular dermatosis, impetigo, pemphigus foliaceus, and a pustular id reaction.[98] The presence of eosinophils excludes pustular psoriasis, Reiter disease, subcorneal pustular dermatosis, and impetigo. In Reiter disease, vasculitis is usually present. In pustular psoriasis a background of conventional psoriasis may or may not be present. Pemphigus foliaceus shows acantholysis. In difficult cases, immunofluorescence study will help distinguish neutrophil-rich pemphigus foliaceus from a pustular drug reaction.

Infantile Acropustulosis

Clinical Features   Recurrent crops of intensely pruritic vesicles or pustules develop most commonly in African-American infants at birth or during the first year of life.[99,100] The lesions involve predominantly the distal extremities, particularly the palms and soles, dorsum of the hands and feet, and the sides of the fingers and toes. Individual lesions heal with hyperpigmentation, and the process resolves within 2 years in most cases. Some patients have a history of atopic dermatitis, and in several patients there has been associated scabetic infestation.

The etiology is unknown.

Histopathological Features   Early lesions reveal spongiosis and small foci of epidermal necrosis, apoptosis, and exocytosis of neutrophils and eosinophils. Later lesions reveal subcorneal and intraepidermal vesiculopustules containing numerous neutrophils and admixed eosinophils.[101,102] A few cases have shown a predominance of eosinophils. There is minimal papillary dermal edema and a sparse mixed-cell perivascular infiltration. As in all intraepidermal pustular disorders, PAS stain and tissue Gram stain should be performed in order to exclude infection.

Differential Diagnosis   See the preceding discussions of IgA pemphigus and impetigo.

Transient Neonatal Pustular Melanosis

Clinical Features   Flaccid vesiculopustules on the trunk and diaper area are present at birth.[103] The vesiculopustules rupture after 1 to 2 days, leaving hyperpigmented macules with collarettes of scale.

The pathogenesis is unknown.

Histopathological Features   Vesiculopustules in the intracorneal or subcorneal zones contain neutrophils with an admixture of eosinophils. There is slight spongiosis. The papillary dermis is edematous with an infiltrate of neutrophils and eosinophils around superficial vessels. Later lesions consist only of basal hypermelaninosis.

Differential Diagnosis   See the preceding discussion of impetigo. Some have suggested that erythema toxicum neonatorum and neonatal pustular melanosis are related disorders.[104]

Erythema Toxicum Neonatorum

Clinical Features   Erythema toxicum neonatorum is characterized by pustules that develop on macules, papules, or wheals distributed on the face, torso, and proximal extremities (Table 7-23). The pustules arise within the first 2 days of life and occasionally are present at birth. On occasion, vesicles precede the development of the pustules.

The pathogenesis is unknown.

Histopathological Features   In macular lesions, a sparse perivascular infiltrate is associated with mild papillary dermal edema. The papules reveal numerous eosinophils and some neutrophils in the outer root sheath of hair follicles, giving rise to eosinophilic pustules overlying follicular orifice (Table 7-23). Intraepidermal subcorneal pustules consisting predominantly of eosinophils also are present.[105]

Differential Diagnosis   See the preceding discussion of neonatal pustular melanosis. One might also consider eosinophilic pustular folliculitis/pustulosis in the differential diagnosis.

TABLE 7-23

Erythema Toxicum Neonatorum

Clinical Features

Pustules and macules arise in the first few days of life
Face, torso, and extremities

Histopathological Features

Intraepidermal and subcorneal eosinophilic pustules in hair follicles

Differential Diagnosis

Scabies
Incontinentia pigmenti
Eosinophilic folliculitis

REFERENCES

1. Dvorak HF, Mihm MC Jr, Dvorak AM: Morphology of delayed-type hypersensitivity reactions in man. *J Invest Dermatol* 67:391–401, 1976.
2. Kligman AM: Cutaneous toxicology: An overview from the underside. *Cur Prob Dermatol* 7:1–25, 1978.
3. Lachapelle JM: Comparative histopathology of allergic and irritant patch test reactions in man. *Arch Belg Dermatol* 28:83–92, 1973.
4. Kasteler JS, Petersen MJ, Vance JE, Zone JJ: Circulating activated T lymphocytes in autoeczematization. *Arch Dermatol* 128:795–798, 1992.
5. Abell E: Spongiotic dermatitis, in Farmer ER, Hood AF (eds): *Pathology of the Skin.* Norwalk, CT: Appleton & Lange, 1990, pp. 74–75.
6. Ackerman AB: *Histologic Diagnosis of Inflammatory Diseases.* Philadelphia: Lea & Febiger, 1976, p. 499.
7. Diepgen TL, Fartasch M: Recent epidemiological and genetic studies in atopic dermatitis. *Acta Derm Venereol* (Stockh) 176 (suppl):13–18, 1992.
8. Hurwitz RM, DeTrana C: The cutaneous pathology of atopic dermatitis. *Am J Dermatopathol,* 12:544–551, 1990.
9. Caputo R, Ackerman AB, Sison-Torre EQ: *Pediatric Dermatology and Dermatopathology: A Text and Atlas.* Philadelphia: Lea & Febiger, 1990, p. 172.
10. Leiferman KM, Ackerman SJ, Sampson HA, et al: Dermal deposition of eosinophil-granule major basic protein in atopic dermatitis. Comparison with onchocerciasis. *N Engl J Med,* 313:282–285, 1985.
11. Sirot G: Nummular eczema. *Semin Dermatol* 2:68–74, 1983.
12. Braun-Falco O, Petry G: On the fine structure of the epidermis in chronic nummular eczema. II. Stratum spinosum. *Arch Klin Exp Dermatol* 224:63–80, 1966.
13. Ackerman AB: *Histologic Diagnosis of Inflammatory Skin Diseases: A Method by Pattern Analysis.* Philadelphia: Lea & Febiger, 1978, pp. 227, 260, 275.
14. Ackerman AB: *Histologic Diagnosis of Inflammatory Skin Diseases: A Method by Pattern Analysis.* Philadelphia: Lea & Febiger, 1978, p. 246.
15. Pandolf KB, Griffin TB, Munro EH, Goldman RF: Heat intolerance as a function of percent of body surface involved with miliaria rubra. *Am J Physiol* 239:233–240, 1980.
16. Sulzberger MB, Harris DR: Miliaria and anhidrosis III. Multiple small patches and the effects of different periods of occlusion. *Arch Dermatol* 105:845–850, 1972.
17. Lillywhite LP: Investigation into the environmental factors associated with the incidence of skin disease following an outbreak of miliaria rubra at a coal mine. *Occup Med* 42:183–187, 1992.
18. Lyons RE, Levine R, Auld D: Miliaria rubra: A manifestation of staphylococcal disease. *Arch Dermatol* 86:282–286, 1962.
19. Straka BF, Cooper PH, Greer KE: Congenital miliaria crystallina. *Cutis* 47:103–106, 1991.
20. Loewenthal LJA: The pathogenesis of miliaria. *Arch Dermatol* 84:2–17, 1961.
21. Bigby M, Jick S, Jick H, Arndt K: Drug-induced cutaneous reactions. A report from the Boston collaborative drug surveillance program on 15,438 consecutive inpatients, 1975 to 1982. *JAMA* 256:3358–3363, 1986.
22. Fellner MJ, Prutkin L: Morbilliform eruptions caused by penicillin. A study by electron microscopy and immunologic tests. *J Invest Dermatol* 55:390–395, 1970.
23. Harber LC, Baer RL: Pathogenic mechanisms of drug-induced photosensitivity. [Review] *J Invest Dermatol* 58:327–342, 1972.
24. Ackerman AB: *Histologic Diagnosis of Inflammatory Skin Diseases: A Method by Pattern Analysis.* Philadelphia: Lea & Febiger, 1978, pp. 226–227.

25. Ackerman AB: *Histologic Diagnosis of Inflammatory Skin Diseases: A Method by Pattern Analysis.* Philadelphia: Lea & Febiger, 1978, pp. 611–612.

26. Frain-Bell W: The idiopathic photodermatoses, in *Cutaneous Photobiology.* New York: Oxford University Press, 1985, p. 24.

27. Addo HA, Frain-Bell W: Actinic prurigo: A specific photodermatosis? *Photodermatology* 1:119–128, 1984.

28. Norris PG, Hawk JL: Chronic actinic dermatitis. A unifying concept. *Arch Dermatol* 126:376–378, 1990.

29. Hawk JLM, Norris PG: Abnormal responses to ultraviolet radiation: Idiopathic, in Fitzpatrick TB, Eisen AZ, Wolff K, et al (eds): *Dermatology in General Medicine,* 4th ed. New York: McGraw-Hill, 1993, p. 1661.

30. Ackerman AB: *Histologic Diagnosis of Inflammatory Skin Diseases: A Method by Pattern Analysis.* Philadelphia: Lea & Febiger, 1978, p. 294–296.

31. Shaffer B, Jacobson C, Beerman H: Histopathologic correlation of lesions of papular urticaria and positive skin test reactions to insect antigens. *Arch Dermatol* 70:437, 1956.

32. Björnberg A, Hellgren L: Pityriasis rosea: A statistical, clinical and laboratory investigation of 826 patients and matched healthy controls. *Acta Derm Venereol* 42(suppl. 50):1–68, 1962.

33. Bunch LW, Tilley JC: Pityriasis rosea: A histologic and serologic study. *Arch Dermatol* 84:129–136, 1961.

34. Ackerman AB: *Histologic Diagnosis of Inflammatory Skin Diseases: A Method by Pattern Analysis.* Philadelphia: Lea & Febiger, 1978, pp. 233–235.

35. Verbov J: Purpuric pityriasis rosea. *Dermatologica* 160:142–144, 1980.

36. Ackerman AB: *Histologic Diagnosis of Inflammatory Skin Diseases: A Method by Pattern Analysis.* Philadelphia: Lea & Febiger, 1978, pp. 266–267, 574.

37. Gottlieb GJ, Ackerman AB: The "sandwich sign" of dermatophytosis. *Am J Dermatopathol* 8:347–350, 1986.

38. Gianotti F: Papular acrodermatitis of childhood and other papulo-vesicular acrolocated syndromes. *Br J Dermatol* 100:49–59, 1979.

39. Caputo R, Gelmetti C, Ermacora E, et al: Gianotti-Crosti syndrome: A retrospective analysis of 308 cases. *J Am Acad Dermatol* 26:207–210, 1992.

40. Gianotti F: Papular acrodermatitis of childhood. An Australia antigen disease. *Arch Dis Child* 48:794–799, 1973.

41. Draelos ZK, Hansen RC, James WD: Gianotti-Crosti syndrome associated with infections other than hepatitis B. *JAMA* 256:2386–2388, 1986.

42. Ackerman AB: *Histologic Diagnosis of Inflammatory Skin Diseases: A Method by Pattern Analysis.* Philadelphia: Lea & Febiger, 1978, p. 238.

43. Magro CM, Crowson AN, Mihm MC: Cutaneous manifestations of gastrointestinal disease, in Elder DE, Johnson BE, Jaworsky C, Elenitsas R (eds): *Lever's Histopathology of the Skin,* 8th ed. Philadelphia: J.B. Lippincott, 1997, pp. 353–368.

44. Resnick SD: Staphylococcal toxin-mediated syndromes in childhood. *Semin Dermatol* 11:11–18, 1992.

45. Parsonnet J: Mediators in the pathogenesis of toxic shock syndrome: Overview. *Rev Infect Dis* 11(suppl)1:S263–S269, 1989.

46. Hurwitz RM, Ackerman AB: Cutaneous pathology of the toxic shock syndrome. *Am J Dermatopathol* 7:563–578, 1985.

47. Leung DYM, Lucky AW: Kawasaki disease, in Fitzpatrick TB, Eisen AZ, Wolff K, et al (eds): *Dermatology in General Medicine,* 4th ed. New York: McGraw-Hill, 1993, pp. 2689–2697.

48. Wiklund DA, Weston WL: Incontinentia pigmenti. A four-generation study. *Arch Dermatol* 116:701–703, 1980.

49. Carney RG Jr: Incontinentia pigmenti: A world statistical study. *Arch Dermatol* 112:535, 1976.

50. Younus J, Ahmed AR: The relationship of pemphigus to neoplasm. *J Am Acad Dermatol* 23:482–502, 1990.

51. Korman NJ: Pemphigus. *J Am Acad Dermatol* 18:1219–1238, 1988.

52. Korman NJ: Pemphigus. *Immunodermatology* 8:689–700, 1990.

53. Thivolet J: Pemphigus: Past, present, and future. *Dermatology* 189(suppl.):26–29, 1994.

54. Stanley JR, Koulu L, Thivolet C: Pemphigus vulgaris and pemphigus foliaceus autoantibodies bind different molecules (abstr). *J Invest Dermatol* 82:439, 1984.

55. Korman NJ, Eyre RW, Zone J, et al: Drug-induced pemphigus: Autoantibodies directed against the pemphigus antigen complexes are present in penicillamine and captopril-induced pemphigus. *J Invest Dermatol* 96:273–276, 1991.

56. Beutner EH, Prigenzi LS, Hale LS, et al: Immunofluorescent studies of autoantibodies to intracellular areas of epithelia in Brazilian pemphigus foliaceus. *Proc Soc Exp Biol Med* 127:81–86, 1968.

57. Crosby DL, Diaz LA: Endemic pemphigus foliaceus in bullous diseases, in Crosby DL, Diaz LA (eds): *Dermatologic Clinics.* Philadelphia: W.B. Saunders, 1993, pp. 453–462.

58. Koulu L, Kusumi A, Steinberg MS, et al: Human antibodies against a desmosomal core protein in pemphigus foliaceus. *J Exp Med* 160:1509–1518, 1984.

59. Emerson RW, Wilson Jones E: Eosinophilic spongiosis in pemphigus. *Arch Dermatol* 97:252–257, 1968.

60. Jablonska S, Chorzelski TP, Beutner EH, et al: Herpetiform pemphigus: A variable pattern of pemphigus. *Int J Dermatol* 14:353–359, 1975.

61. Perry HO: Pemphigus foliaceus. *Arch Dermatol* 83:57–72, 1961.

62. Pisani M, Ruocco V: Drug induced pemphigus. *Clin Dermatol* 4:118–132, 1986.

63. Ruocco V, De Luca M, Pisani M, et al: Pemphigus provoked by D-penicillamine: An experimental approach using in vitro tissue cultures. *Dermatologica* 164:236–248, 1982.

64. Ruocco V, Sacerdoti G: Pemphigus and bullous pemphigoid due to drugs. *Int J Dermatol* 30:307–312, 1991.

65. Ebihara T, Hashimoto T, Iwatsuki K, et al: Autoantigens for IgA anti-intercellular antibodies of intercellular IgA vesiculopustular dermatosis. *J Invest Dermatol* 97:742–745, 1991.

66. Hodak E, David M, Ingber A, et al: The clinical and histopathological spectrum of IgA-pemphigus: A report of two cases. *Clin Exp Dermatol* 15:433–437, 1990.

67. Teraki Y, Amagai Z, Hashimoto T, et al: Intercellular IgA dermatosis of childhood. *Arch Dermatol* 127:221–224, 1991.

68. Neumann E, Dmochowski M, Bowszyc M, et al: The occurrence of IgA pemphigus foliaceus without neutrophilic infiltration. *Clin Exp Dermatol* 19:56–58, 1994.

69. Anhalt GJ, Kim SC, Stanley JR, et al: Paraneoplastic pemphigus. An autoimmune mucocutaneous disease associated with neoplasia. *N Engl J Med* 323:1729–1735, 1990.

70. Mutasim DF, Pelc NJ, Anhalt GJ: Paraneoplastic pemphigus. *Dermatol Clin* 11:473–481, 1993.

71. Ostezan LB, Fabre VC, Caughman W, et al: Paraneoplastic pemphigus in the absence of a known neoplasm. *J Am Acad Dermatol* 33:312–315, 1995.

72. Camisa C, Helm TN, Valenzuela R, et al: Paraneoplastic pemphigus: Three new cases [abstr]. *J Invest Dermatol* 98:590, 1992.

73. Horn TD, Anhalt GJ: Histologic features of paraneoplastic pemphigus. *Arch Dermatol* 128:1091–1095, 1992.

74. Stevens SR, Griffiths EM, Anhalt GJ, Cooper KD: Paraneoplastic pemphigus presenting as a lichen planus pemphigoides-like eruption. *Arch Dermatol* 129:866–869, 1993.

75. Resnick SD: Staphylococcal toxin-mediated syndromes in childhood. [Rev] *Semin Dermatol* 11:11–18, 1992.

76. Florman AL, Holzman RS: Nosocomial scalded skin syndrome. Ritter's disease caused by phage group 3 *Staphylococcus aureus. Am J Dis Child* 134:1043–1045, 1980.

77. Burge SM, Wilkinson JD: Darier-White disease: A review of the clinical features in 163 patients. [Rev] *J Am Acad Dermatol* 27:40–50, 1992.

78. Parfitt E, Burge S, Craddock N, et al: The gene for Darier's disease maps between D12S78 and D12S79. *Hum Mol Genet* 3:35–38, 1994.

79. Ackerman AB: *Histologic Diagnosis of Inflammatory Skin Diseases: A Method by Pattern Analysis.* Philadelphia: Lea & Febiger, 1978, p. 534–537.

80. Wilkin JK: Chronic benign familial pemphigus. Minimal involvement mimicking chronic perianal candidiasis. *Arch Dermatol* 114:136, 1978.

81. Ikeda S, Welsh EA, Peluso AM, et al: Localization of the gene whose mutations underlie Hailey-Hailey disease to chromosome 3q. *Hum Mol Genet* 3:1147–1150, 1994.

82. Ackerman AB: *Histologic Diagnosis of Inflammatory Skin Diseases: A Method by Pattern Analysis.* Philadelphia: Lea & Febiger, 1978, pp. 532–534.

83. Grover RW: Transient acantholytic dermatosis. *Arch Dermatol* 101:426–434, 1970.

84. Chalet M, Grover R, Ackerman AB: Transient acantholytic dermatosis. *Arch Dermatol* 113:431–435, 1977.

85. Hu C-H, Michel B, Farber EM: Transient acantholytic dermatosis (Grover's disease). A skin disorder related to heat and sweating. *Arch Dermatol* 121:1439–1441, 1985.

86. Syder AJ, Yu QC, Paller AS, et al: Genetic mutations in the K1 and K10 genes of patients with epidermolytic hyperkeratosis. Correlation between location and disease severity. *J Clin Invest* 93(4):1533–1542, 1994.

87. Sulzberger MB, Cortese TA Jr, Fishman L, et al: Studies on blisters produced by friction. *J Invest Dermatol* 47:456–465, 1966.

88. Naylor PFD: Experimental friction blisters. *Br J Dermatol* 67:327–342, 1955.

89. Brehmer-Anderson E, Göransson K: Friction blisters as a manifestation of pathomimia. *Acta Derm Venereol* (Stockh) 55:65–71, 1975.

90. Sevitt S: Histological changes in burned skin, in *Burns: Pathology and Therapeutic Application.* London: Butterworth & Co, 1957, pp. 18–27.

91. Dajani AS, Ferrieri P, Wannamaker LW: Natural history of impetigo. II. Etiologic agents and bacterial interactions. *J Clin Invest* 51:2863–2871, 1972.

92. Lever W, Schaumburg-Lever G: *Histopathology of the Skin,* 7th ed. Philadelphia: J.B. Lippincott, 1990, p. 368.

93. Dal Tio R, Di Vito F, Salvi F: Subcorneal pustular dermatosis and IgA myeloma. *Dermatologica* 170:240–243, 1985.

94. Wilkinson MDS (Londres): Subcorneal pustular dermatosis. *Bull de la Societe Francaise de Dermatologie et de Syphiligraphie* 69:674–679, 1962.

95. Burns RE, Fine G: Subcorneal pustular dermatosis. *Arch Dermatol* 80:72, 1959.

96. Burrows NP, Russell Jones R: Pustular drug eruptions: A histopathological spectrum. *Histopathology* 22:569–573, 1993.

97. Fitzpatrick JE: New histopathologic findings in drug eruptions. *Dermatol Clin* 10:19–36, 1992.

98. Spencer JM, Silvers DN, Grossman ME: Pustular eruption after drug exposure: Is it pustular psoriasis or a pustular drug eruption? *Br J Dermatol* 130:514–519, 1994.

99. Jarratt M, Ramsdell W: Infantile acropustulosis. *Arch Dermatol* 115:834–836, 1979.

100. Newton JA, Salisbury J, Marsden A, McGibbon DH: Acropustulosis of infancy. *Br J Dermatol* 115:735–739, 1986.

101. Bundino S, Zina AM, Ubertalli S: Infantile acropustulosis. *Dermatologica* 165:615–619, 1982.

102. Palungwachira P: Infantile acropustulosis. *Aust J Dermatol* 30:97–100, 1989.

103. Ramamurthy RS, Reveri M, Esterly NB, et al: Transient neonatal pustular melanosis. *J Pediatr* 88:831–835, 1976.

104. Ferrandiz C, Coroleu W, Ribera M, et al: Sterile transient neonatal pustulosis is a precocious form of erythema toxicum neonatorum. *Dermatology* 185:18–22, 1992.

105. Freeman RG, Spiller R, Knox JM: Histopathology of erythema toxicum neonatorum. *Arch Dermatol* 82:586–589, 1960.

SUBEPIDERMAL VESICULAR DERMATITIS

B r u c e   R .   S m o l l e r   /   S a b i n e   K o h l e r

The histologic diagnosis of a blistering disorder begins with several determinations that are made most easily at scanning magnification. The parameters which should be examined initially include the level of the blister, the nature of the inflammatory infiltrate, if any, and the process responsible for the blister formation, if this can be determined. Determination of these simple criteria will allow an algorithmic approach to blistering disorders which greatly simplifies the microscopic differential diagnosis (Tables 8-1 and 8-2). As this chapter is limited to subepidermal vesicular disorders, we will not discuss blisters occurring at sites other than beneath the basal keratinocytes and will ignore those branches of the algorithm. These entities will be found in other chapters.

After determining that the blister is occurring in a subepidermal location, it is important to identify the cellular infiltrate involved in the process. As can be seen in Table 8-1, the inflammatory cellular component of these processes varies between entities. Thus, the differential diagnosis of a subepidermal blister with abundant eosinophils is quite different from the differential diagnosis of a subepidermal blister with abundant neutrophils. There is some overlap in this list of entities, but these diseases often can be separated based on more specific characteristics which will be addressed later in the chapter. Many diseases which are characterized by subepidermal blisters do not have any apppreciable inflammatory component. These entities can also be found in Table 8-1 and are distinguishable by more specific histologic features.

Following the determination of the site of the blister and the nature of the inflammatory infiltrate, it is often helpful to assess the process by which the blister has formed. The best place to examine for this process is at the newest portion of the blister, adjacent to intact skin. Here secondary inflammation and necrosis are less likely to confound the observations than they are in the oldest, most centrally located portions of the separation. In some cases, necrosis of keratinocytes (i.e., erythema multiforme) has led to separation of the epidermis from the dermis. In other diseases, marked dermal edema has eventuated in the formation of a subepidermal blister (i.e., Sweet's syndrome). In other cases, marked inflammation seems to be the main histologic features associated with the blister formation (i.e., linear IgA dermatosis). Simple observation for these types of histologic features will further narrow the histologic differential diagnosis as seen in Table 8-1. Nevertheless, the histologic differential diagnosis of subepidermal blisters is based on relatively subtle differences, and individual entities often show significant overlap of histologic features. Careful clinical-pathologic correlation and further studies (direct immunofluorensense, electron microscopy, determination of serum porphyrins) are often required for a definitive diagnosis.

Biopsy Technique

Proper selection of the biopsy site and appropriate handling of the biopsy specimen are of critical importance in the diagnosis of blistering disorders. Independent of the underlying disease, biopsy of an early blister will provide the best chance at obtaining important diagnostic clues. In older lesions the histologic picture is often confounded by secondary changes such as impetiginization, excoriation, and reepithelialization. In addition, infected blisters may contain neutrophils and may then mimic a primary neutrophilic dermatosis. Similarly, reepithelialization of a subepidermal blister may result in a seemingly intraepidermal location of the split. After an early lesion is identified, the biopsy ideally should be obtained from the edge of the blister. This usually requires a 4-mm punch biopsy. Perilesional skin and blister should be represented in the biopsy diameter in approximately equal parts. This approach maximizes the chances to include the newest portion of the blister adjacent to intact skin. If the differential diagnostic considerations for an individual patient include an autoimmune blistering disorder, tissue for direct immunofluorescence studies should be obtained at the time of initial biopsy. The biopsy for direct immunofluorescence should include mostly or entirely perilesional skin. The area of blistering should represent less than one-third of the biopsy diameter. Dividing the tissue after biopsy with a scalpel into a portion for histologic examination and a portion for direct immunofluorescence is not optimal, because cutting fresh tissue often introduces crush artifact and may lead to shearing of the epidermis. Two separate 4-mm punch biopsies are the preferred method. Tissue for direct immunofluorescence should be placed immediately into transport medium. If transport medium is not available, tissue should be placed on gauze soaked in physiologic saline, kept cool (on ice or in a refrigerator), and immediately delivered to the immunofluorescence laboratory.

The Epidermal Basement Membrane Zone

To understand the pathogenesis of many of the inherited diseases and autoimmune processes involved in subepidermal blistering disorders, it is necessary to understand the anatomic structure of the basement membrane zone (BMZ). A schematic representation of the basement membrane zone is depicted in Fig. 8-1. This region is demarcated superficially by the lowermost pole of the basal keratinocyte. The deepest margin is in the superficial papillary dermis, in the region of the anchoring plaques. Many proteins have now been isolated which comprise the basement membrane zone, contribute to the functional status of the region, and are the target antigens when disease states arise. The following is a description of the BMZ components moving from the outside (basal keratinocyte) toward the dermis.

Electron microscopy demonstrates four distinct basement membrane regions: the plasma membrane and hemidesmosomes of the basal keratinocyte, the lamina lucida, the lamina densa, and the sublamina densa fibrillar zone.[1] Functionally, all constituents of the BMZ are interdependent, and separation into distinct layers is arbitrary. Basal keratinocyte intermediate filaments (keratins 5 and 14) insert into

TABLE 8-1

Subepidermal Blistering Diseases Algorithm

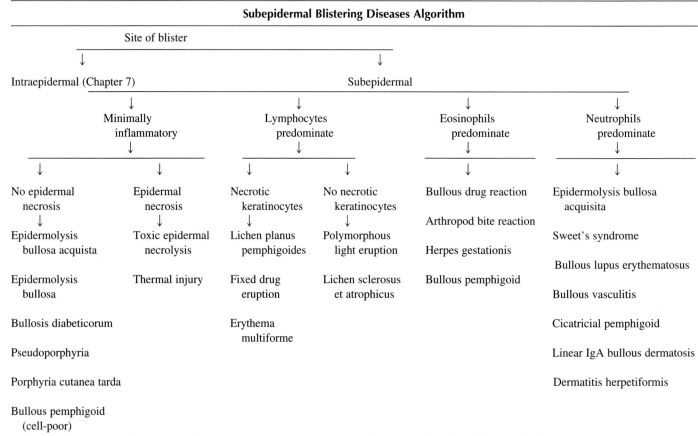

hemidesmosomes. On electron microscopy hemidesmosomes appear as electron-dense plaques located on the inner surface of the plasma membrane of basal keratinocytes. Recently, a number of intracellular hemidesmosomal proteins have been identified and are currently the target of further characterization. BP230 (bullous pemphigoid antigen 1, BPAg1) is a constitutive component of basal keratinocytes. It is a glycoprotein of 230 to 240 kD and shows significant homology to desmoplakin I, a desmosomal component.[2] BPAg1 is one of the target antigens in bullous pemphigoid. HD1 and a 200-kD protein are other intracellular hemidesmosome components but are less well characterized. All three proteins are candidate proteins for interaction points of intermediate filaments (keratins 5 and 14) with hemidesmosomes. In addition to the intracellular proteins, hemidesmosomes also contain transmembrane proteins that extend into the lamina lucida. The best characterized transmembrane proteins to date are BP180 (bullous pemphigoid antigen 2, BPAg2), a second target antigen in bullous pemphigoid, and the integrin α6β4. The lamina lucida contains laminin 1 as its major component. Laminin 1 binds to the collagen (type IV collagen) and to the heparan sulfate proteoglycan in the lamina densa. In addition to playing an active role in cell trafficking, laminin 1 seems to stabilize the BMZ. The lamina lucida is traversed by anchoring filaments which appear to connect the hemidesmosomes to the lamina densa. Anchoring filaments are more conspicuous underneath hemidesmosomes. A number of anchoring filament molecules have been described, including epiligrin,[3] BM600/nicein,[4] and kalinin.[5,6] These proteins are the target of the GB3 antibody, and recent research has shown them to be identical or at least very similar.[7] They are now collectively termed laminin 5. Epiligrin is

the target for autoantibodies in a subset of patients with cicatricial bullous pemphigoid. Laminin 5 has been shown to be absent or significantly reduced in individuals with the Herlitz (gravis) form of junctional EB (JEB). Several recent reports have identified mutations of the laminin 5 gene in patients with JEB.[8] UNCein is recognized by the antibody 19-DEJ-1 and is another protein associated with anchoring filaments. UNCein appears distinct from laminin 5 and is located closer to the keratinocyte plasma membrane. UNCein is absent in the gravis and the milder forms (mitis) of JEB. The antigen recognized by the monoclonal antibody 123 is named LAD-1 and has been a component of anchoring filaments and is located in the upper lamina lucida, more superficial than laminin 5. It recently has been identified as the autoantigen in the majority of patients with linear IgA disease.[55] The lamina densa contains type IV collagen, heparan sulfate proteoglycan, chondroitin-6-sulfate proteoglycan, and various other components. Anchoring fibrils are hooklike filamentous structures of approximately 800 nm. They attach in the lamina densa, extend into the papillary dermis, and either loop back into the lamina densa or attach to electron-dense structures in the papillary dermis, termed anchoring plaques. Anchoring fibrils entrap extracellular matrix molecules and insert in anchoring plaques. They are thought to anchor the BMZ to the papillary dermis. Anchoring fibrils contain collagen VII,[9,10] a basement-membrane-specific collagen. Collagen VII is the target for autoantibodies in patients with epidermolysis bullosa acquisita. Individuals with dystrophic epidermolysis bullosa have a genetic defect leading to fewer or no anchoring fibrils. The above discussion is summarized in Fig. 8-1 and Table 8-3.

TABLE 8-2

Subepidermal Blistering Diseases: An Overview

Disease	Clinical Features	Histopathological Features	Immunologic Features	Other Features
Porphyria cutanea tarda	Tense, noninflammatory acral blisters	Noninflammatory, vascular wall thickening	Linear IgG, IgM, C3 around vessels and dermal-epidermal junction	Elevated urine porphyrins
Toxic epidermal necrolysis	Extensive desquamation	Full-thickness epidermal necrosis, minimally inflammatory	Negative	
Erythema multiforme	Targetoid lesions, commonly acral	Necrotic keratinocytes, lymphocytic infiltrate	Negative	
Bullous pemphigoid	Tense blisters on erythematous base, often extremities	Abundant eosinophils, no keratinocyte necrosis	Linear IgG and C3 in lamina lucida	Circulating immune complexes common
Herpes gestationis	Tense blisters, late pregnancy	Abundant eosinophils, rare necrotic keratinocytes	Linear IgG and C3 in lamina lucida	Circulating immune complexes
Dermatitis herpetiformis	Intensely pruritic vesicles, extensors of extremities	Neutrophilic abscesses in papillary dermal tips	Granular IgA and C3 in papillary dermal tips	Gastrointestinal findings
Linear IgA bullous dermatosis	Vesicles at periphery of annular erythematous lesions	Neutrophils diffusely along dermal-epidermal junction	Linear IgA and C3 in lamina lucida	
Cicatricial pemphigoid	Tense blisters, heal with scarring, often mucosal	Neutrophils in blister cavity, dermal scarring	Linear IgG and C3 in lamina lucida	Rare circulating immune complexes
Bullous lupus erythematosus	Vesicular lesions on sun-exposed skin	Neutrophils in blister cavity and papillary dermis	Granular IgG, IgM, and C3 along dermal-epidermal junction	Other signs and symptoms of lupus

The remainder of the chapter will follow the algorithmic approach described above, discussing each of the clinical and histologic features of each of the entities that give rise to subepidermal bullae.

SUBEPIDERMAL BLISTERS WITH LITTLE INFLAMMATION

Epidermolysis Bullosa

Epidermolysis bullosa is a heterogeneous family of inherited blistering disorders caused by structural defects in the basement membrane zone.

Classification of the disease is based on the mode of inheritance, the precise location of the blister within the skin, and the clinical phenotype. As is seen in Table 8-4, some types of epidermolysis bullosa are inherited in an autosomal dominant manner, whereas others are autosomal recessive.[11] Three general classes of epidermolysis bullosa are based on the level of separation within the skin: simplex type, junction type, and dystrophic type. Epidermolysis bullosa simplex is caused by separation of the epidermis from the dermis at the level of the lower portion of the basal keratinocyte. This has recently been shown to be due to abnormal keratins 5 and 14 in these patients.[12] This type of EB is usually transmitted in an autosomal dominant manner and is a relatively mild disorder in most patients. The junctional form of EB has been shown to be

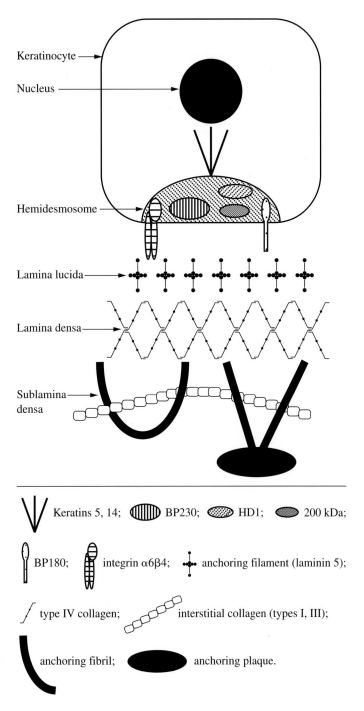

Keratinocyte

Nucleus

Hemidesmosome

Lamina lucida

Lamina densa

Sublamina densa

Keratins 5, 14;   BP230;   HD1;   200 kDa;

BP180;   integrin α6β4;   anchoring filament (laminin 5);

type IV collagen;   interstitial collagen (types I, III);

anchoring fibril;   anchoring plaque.

FIGURE 8-1   Schematic representation of the basement membrane zone.

due to defects in the structure of hemidesmosomal and anchoring filament proteins, resulting in blister formation at the level of the lamina lucida. Depending upon the severity of the defect, this can cause mild or lethal disease in patients. The final group of EB variants is the dystrophic form which is caused by structurally abnormal anchoring fibrils or decreased numbers of anchoring fibrils (type VII collagen) in the superficial papillary dermis. The recessive form of dystrophic EB is often associated with severe blistering throughout life, whereas the dominant form is often less intense.

Clinical Features   The clinical features vary greatly depending on the site of the blister. In epidermolysis bullosa simplex, the blister is located within the lower half of the basal keratinocytes. The disease is usually inherited in an autosomal dominant manner with complete penetrance.

There is no disruption of the basement membrane zone, and no scarring occurs. These patients tend to have mild blister formation in response to minor trauma, often limited to acral locations. Within the group, variants are distinguished by their clinical characteristics.[11] For reasons that are not entirely understood, the disease tends to improve with age.

Junctional epidermolysis bullosa is a group of diseases that show blistering at the level of the lamina lucida and are inherited in an autosomal recessive manner. Variants are distinguished by their clinical characteristics and range from a very severe, rapidly lethal form to milder forms. The most severe subtype, Herlitz or gravis form of junctional epidermolysis bullosa, presents at birth as extensive blisters and erosions. The mucosal membranes of the gastrointestinal and urogenital tract are commonly affected. Laryngeal and bronchial lesions may cause respiratory distress. Perioral skin involvement and pitted enamel hypoplasia are characteristic. Blisters heal without scarring or milia formation unless complicated by secondary factors. Some patients form vegetative lesions as a result of exuberant granulation tissue formation. Growth retardation secondary to malnutrition is common, and few individuals survive beyond 3 years. Patients with the mitis form of generalized junctional epidermolysis bullosa (generalized atrophic benign epidermolysis bullosa) initially present with symptoms similar to patients with the gravis form but show less involvement of mucosal surfaces. The patients improve with age and have an overall favorable prognosis. Much progress has been made in understanding the molecular basis of junctional epidermolysis bullosa. The heterogeneous clinical presentation of the disease is reflected on the molecular level. Recently mutations and deletions in several genes coding for proteins associated with hemidesmosomes and the lamina lucida have been reported (e.g., laminin 5 in some patients with the gravis form, BP180 in some patients with the mitis form).

Dystrophic epidermolysis bullosa is characterized by repeated blistering at all sites of mechanical trauma with subsequent extensive scarring and milia formation. The separation occurs beneath the lamina densa in the superficial papillary dermis. Scarring deformities often lead to the complete loss of functional use of the extremities and ectropion and esophageal abnormalities. The disorders comprising this heterogeneous group are classified based on morphology, distribution, and mode of inheritance. The two forms of autosomal dominant epidermolysis bullosa dystrophica are the hyperplastic Cockayne-Touraine variant and the albopapuloid Pasini variant. Common features of both entities are onset during infancy, blisters mainly localized to the extremities, healing with milia and scars, and dystrophic nails. The albopapuloid variant shows more extensive blistering, involves the oral mucosa, and is characterized by albopapuloid lesions on the trunk. Albopapuloid lesions are hypopigmented scarlike papules. Recessive dystrophic epidermolysis bullosa includes a wide range of clinical presentations ranging from localized forms to severe varieties. Generalized severe (gravis) recessive dystrophic epidermolysis bullosa is the most clinically distinct form. The first blisters appear during infancy and diffusely affect the skin surface and mucous membranes. Repeated cycles of blistering and healing with scar formation result in digital fusions, flexural contractures, esophageal strictures, phimosis, and conjunctival and corneal scarring. All forms of dystrophic epidermolysis bullosa, the generalized forms in particular, predispose to the development of squamous cell carcinomas with locally aggressive and metastatic potential. On ultrastructural examination, skin from patients with dystrophic epidermolysis bullosa shows the anchoring fibrils to be absent, markedly decreased, or morphologically abnormal. Type VII collagen is the major anchoring fibril component. Recently over 50 types of mutations in the gene coding for collagen VII have been discovered.

Histopathological Features   Epidermolysis bullosa of all types is characterized by a noninflammatory subepidermal blister (Fig. 8-2). Although the simplex variants are not truly subepidermal, but rather intraepidermal, in many cases the scant keratinocyte cytoplasm located on the floor of the blister is not apparent on routine histologic sections and can be identified only with ultrastructural examination. In older lesions of dystrophic EB, dermal scarring may be apparent (Fig. 8-3). Precise histologic subtyping of EB requires ultrastructural analysis with electron microscopy and/or extensive immunomapping using a panel of newly described antibodies directed against basement membrane zone proteins.[11] Understanding of the molecular events underlying different forms of epidermolysis bullosa has provided DNA-based techniques as a new adjunct to the diagnosis of epidermolysis bullosa. These techniques can also be applied to prenatal diagnosis through chorionic villi sampling or amniocentesis.[13]

Differential Diagnosis   The histologic differential diagnosis of epidermolysis bullosa includes entities which demonstrate a minimally inflammatory subepidermal blister. Porphyria cutanea tarda and pseudoporphyria most commonly exhibit prominent solar elastosis and vascular wall thickening not observed in epidermolysis bullosa. The clinical history is very helpful in distinguishing epidermolysis bullosa acquisita, traumatic blisters, and penicillamine dermopathy from hereditary epidermolysis bullosa. A few eosinophils along the dermal-epidermal junction support a diagnosis of cell-poor bullous pemphigoid. Toxic epidermal necrolysis also enters the histologic differential diagnosis, but the presence of diffuse epidermal necrosis helps to distinguish it from epidermolysis bullosa.

Porphyria

The porphyrias are a heterogeneous group of disorders, each arising from a genetically determined partial enzyme defect in heme biosynthesis.[14–17] The heme biosynthetic pathway is shown in Fig. 8-4. The characteristic clinical features result from excessive accumulation of precursors of porphyrins, porphyrin by-products, or both. The site of deposition and the type of accumulating substance determine the clinical symptoms. Traditionally, the porphyrias have been classified into hepatic and erythropoietic forms, depending on whether the excess production of porphyrin precursors and/or porphyrins is located in the liver or bone marrow. The acute porphyrias are all hepatic porphyrias and are characterized by neurovisceral symptoms and elevated plasma and urine concentrations of δ-aminolevulinic acid (ALA) and porphobilinogen

TABLE 8-3

Overview of Genetic and Autoimmune Blistering Diseases

Ultrastructural Target	Molecular Target	Genetic Disease	Autoimmune Disease
Hemidesmosome	BPAg1 BPAg2	? JEB mitis	Bullous pemphigoid Herpes gestationis
Anchoring filament	UNCein	JEB gravis et mitis	Cicatricial pemphigoid (subset)
Anchoring filament	LAD-1	?	Linear IgA disease (subset)
Anchoring filament	Laminin 5	JEB gravis	Cicatricial pemphigoid (subset)
Anchoring fibril	Type VII collagen	Dystrophic EB	Epidermolysis bullosa acquisita

BPAg = bullous pemphigoid antigen; JEB = junctional epidermolysis bullosa; EB = epidermolysis bullosa.

TABLE 8-4

Epidermolysis Bullosa—Subtypes

Subtype	Inheritance	Clinical	Defect
Simplex			
Dowling-Meara (herpetiformis)	Autosomal dominant	Herpetiform distribution; milia common; nail dystrophy	Keratins 5 and 14
Weber-Cockayne (localized)	Autosomal dominant	Limited to hands and feet	Keratins 5 and 14
Koebner (generalized)	Autosomal dominant	Extremities > elsewhere	Keratins 5 and 14
Junctional			
Generalized benign atrophic (mitis)	Autosomal recessive	Generalized blisters, scarring and atrophy; dystrophic nails, baldness	Reduced hemidesmosomes and anchoring filaments (variable)
Herlitz (gravis)	Autosomal recessive	Generalized blisters, limited scarring, granulation tissue, enamel defects	Reduced hemidesmosomes and anchoring filaments
Dystrophic			
Dominant	Autosomal dominant	Generalized blisters with scarring; dystrophic nails; albopapuloid lesions	Type VII collagen
Recessive	Autosomal recessive	Generalized blisters with extensive scarring and milia; dystrophic nails; severe oral cavity involvement	Type VII collagen

(PBG). Erythropoietic porphyrias result in elevated bone marrow and red blood cell porphyrins. This classification system generally holds true in patients who are heterozygous for the defective gene. Patients who are homozygous for autosomal dominant hepatic porphyrias, however, may also have erythropoietic features. Hepatoerythropoietic por-

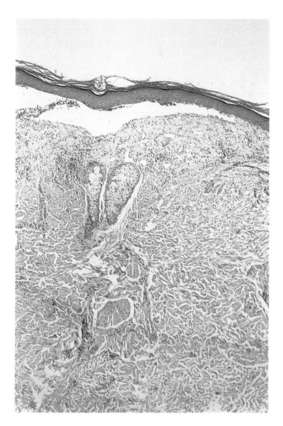

FIGURE 8-2 Epidermolysis bullosa, dystrophic type. Routine histologic sections in the dystrophic type of epidermolysis bullosa show a noninflammatory subepidermal split.

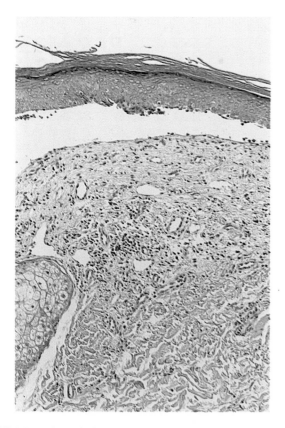

FIGURE 8-3 Epidermolysis bullosa, dystrophic type. Scarring can be seen in the superficial papillary dermis.

phyria, the homozygous form of porphyria cutanea tarda, for example, resembles congenital erythropoietic porphyria, clinically. A more accurate classification is based on the specific enzyme deficiency. Seven types of porphyrias are currently recognized (Table 8-5). For therapy, medical management, and genetic counseling, determining which type of porphyria is present in a given patient is important. Intermediates of the heme biosynthetic pathway that accumulate in porphyrias may be excreted unchanged or following chemical modification. Urinary and fecal porphyrins can be separated and quantitated, allowing a precise diagnosis in conjunction with demonstration of the specific enzyme defect.

In addition to neurovisceral symptoms, most porphyrias have cutaneous manifestations. Plasma porphyrin levels are increased, leading to deposition in the skin and cutaneous photosensitivity. Porphyrins are highly photoactive and strongly absorb light in the visible range with maximum absorption between 400 and 410 nm. Acute intermittent porphyria and ALA-dehydratase deficiency are the only forms of porphyria that do not produce skin lesions.

Clinical Features   Porphyria cutanea tarda (PCT) is the most common form of porphyria (Table 8-6) and results from decreased activity of URO-decarboxylase. It occurs as sporadic (type I) and familial forms (types II and III). PCT is the only porphyria that can be induced by exposure to chemicals (e.g., halogenated aromatic hydrocarbons). Cutaneous photosensitivity is the major feature of PCT. Cutaneous blisters occur at sites of sun exposure such as dorsa of hands, face, and forearms. These blisters frequently heal with scarring and milia formation. Although the exact pathogenesis of the blister formation has not yet been determined, it has been hypothesized that increased levels of photosensitizing porphyrins are located in the skin. When the skin is exposed to sunlight, the activated porphyrins lead to the release of cytokines which subsequently damage vascular walls. Immunoglobulins deposit in the vascular walls. The subepidermal blisters which form are thought to be secondary events. Minor trauma may precede blister formation. Thickening of the skin and scarring are often striking and can resemble scleroderma. Other cutaneous manifestations include facial hypertrichosis and hyperpigmentation, alopecia, and photo-onycholysis. PCT is commonly associated with chronic liver disease, such as chronic hepatitis (viral or alcoholic). PCT has also been reported in association with estrogenic hormone therapies and lupus erythematosus. Patients with PCT are at increased risk for the development of hepatocellular carcinoma, possibly related to longstanding liver damage (4 to 47 percent incidence). Hepatoerythrocytic porphyria is the homozygous form of familial PCT, shows an earlier onset, and clinically resembles congenital erythropoietic porphyria.

Acute intermittent porphyria (AIP) is characterized by recurrent bouts of severe abdominal pain and peripheral neuropathy. Mental symptoms ranging from anxiety to hallucinations may be observed. This form of porphyria lacks skin manifestations.

The skin lesions in variegate porphyria and hereditary coproporphyria may be indistinguishable from PCT. The neurovisceral manifestations of both forms closely resembly AIP.

ALA-dehydratase-deficient porphyria is the most recently described form of porphyria. It is rare (four cases in the literature), and the clinical presentations have been remarkably different in individual patients.

Marked photosensitivity starting in early infancy characterizes congenital erythropoietic porphyria (Günther's disease). The skin in sun-exposed areas is friable, and repeated blister formation leads to extensive scarring and photomutilation. The teeth of these patients are brown-red. Hemolytic anemia is common.

Erythropoietic protoporphyria is the most common cutaneous porphyria after PCT. Photosensitivity in sun-exposed areas usually begins in childhood. Within minutes following sun exposure, burning, itching, and edema develop. Vesicles or bullae are uncommon. After repeated attacks the skin may become thickened and show pigmentary changes and scarring. Photoonycholysis may occur. The skin changes of this disease are distinct from other forms of porphyria. Progressive life-threatening hepatic failure may develop in rare patients.

Histopathological Features   The histologic features are similar in all forms of cutaneous porphyrias and vary only in degree. Scanning magnification reveals a minimally inflammatory subepidermal blister (Fig. 8-5). Scattered lymphocytes may be seen surrounding vessels of the superficial vascular plexus. The blood vessels in the papillary dermis have markedly thickened, hyalinized walls in which periodic acid–Schiff (PAS) positive, diastase-resistant material can be seen (Fig. 8-6). These homogenous eosinophilic deposits are particularly prominent in erythropoietic protoporphyria, can become almost confluent in the papillary dermis, and may also affect deeper vessels and eccrine glands. On electron microscopic examination, this hyalinized material corresponds to replicated redundant basal lamina around dermal blood vessels. Increased dermal elastosis is common. Due to the increased rigidity of the hyalinized vessel walls, the papillary dermal tips often retain their configuration and festoon into the blister cavity. Caterpillar bodies are segmented eosinophilic structures which are comprised of basement membrane material. They are seen within the blister roof in many cases.[18] No basal vacuolization or spongiosis is seen in most cases.

Direct immunofluorescence studies can be helpful in the diagnosis of cutaneous porphyrias. They reveal linear staining around vessels within the superficial vascular plexus with antibodies directed against C3 and immunoglobulins. IgG is the most frequently seen immunoglobulin, but IgM and IgA have been reported in a similar distribution. There is also linear staining along the dermal-epidermal junction with the same immunoreactants. Immunomapping studies have revealed that the split occurs in the lamina lucida.

Differential Diagnosis   The histologic differential diagnosis is that of the minimally inflammatory subepidermal blistering disorders and includes hereditary and acquired epidermolysis bullosa, pseudoporphyria, penicillamine dermopathy, cell-poor bullous pemphigoid, traumatic blisters, bullosis diabeticorum, and blisters overlying recent scars.

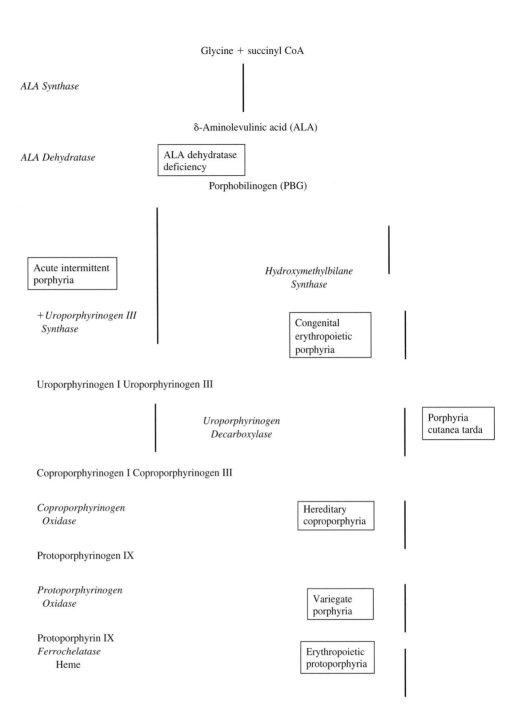

FIGURE 8-4   The heme biosynthetic pathway.

The markedly thickened papillary dermal vessel walls and the prominent dermal elastosis are helpful in making a diagnosis of porphyria. Direct immunofluorescence demonstrating linear deposits of IgG and C3 around the papillary dermal vessels and less frequently along the dermal epidermal junction is also helpful in confirming the diagnosis and ruling out epidermolysis bullosa acquisita and cell-poor bullous pemphigoid. The histologic and immunologic findings in pseudoporphyria are identical to those of porphyria. The distinction between the two entities hinges on porphyrin studies, which are negative in pseudoporphyria.

TABLE 8-5

The Porphyrias

Type	Enzyme	Heredity	Onset	Skin	Other Symptoms	Urine	Feces	Red Blood Cells
Hepatic								
ALA-dehydratase deficiency	ALA-dehydratase	AR	Variable	None	Variable COPRO III	ALA,	—	PROTO IX
Acute intermittent porphyria (AIP)	HMB-synthase	AD	Young adulthood	None	Abdominal pain neuropathy, psychoses	ALA, PBG	—	—
Porphyria cutanea tarda (PCT)	URO-decarboxylase	AD	Middle age	Bullae, scarring, thickening, hypertrichosis	↓ liver function, siderosis	URO I, 7-carboxylate	ISO-COPRO	—
Hereditary coproporphyria	COPRO-oxidase	AD	Young adulthood	Same as PCT	Same as AIP	ALA, PBG COPRO III	COPRO III	—
Variegate porphyria	PROTO-oxidase	AD	Young adulthood	Same as PCT	Same as AIP	ALA, PBG, COPRO III	COPRO III, PROTO IX	—
Erythropoietic								
Congenital erythropoietic porphyria	URO-synthase	AR	Infancy	Blisters, marked scarring	Red teeth, hemolytic anemia	URO I	COPRO I	URO I
Erythropoietic protoporphyria	Ferrochelatase	AD	Childhood	Bullae rare, edema, burning, thickening	Rarely fatal liver disease	—	PROTO IX	PROTO IX

AR = autosomal recessive; AD = autosomal dominant; ALA = δ-aminolevulinic acid; PBG = porphobilinogen; COPRO I = coproporphyrin I; COPRO III = coproporphyrin III; ISOCO-PRO = isocoproporphyrin; URO I = uroporphyrin I; URO III = uroporphyrin III; PROTO IX = protoporphyrin IX.

TABLE 8-6

Porphyria Cutanea Tarda

Clinical Features

Sporadic or familial
Blisters at sites of sun exposure
Scarring and milia
Facial hypertrichosis
Hyperpigmentation
Often associated with liver disease

Histopathological Features

Subepidermal blister
Minimal inflammation
Thickening of vessel walls in papillary dermis
Marked solar elastosis
Caterpillar bodies

Laboratory Evaluation

Direct immunofluorescence positive
Serum, urine, fecal porphyrins

Differential Diagnosis

Cell-poor bullous pemphigoid
Epidermolysis bullosa (hereditary and acquired)
Thermal injury
Toxic epidermal necrolysis
Bullosis diabeticorum
Pseudoporphyria
Traumatic blisters

Pseudoporphyria

Pseudoporphyria is synonymous with bullous disease of dialysis and describes a rare self-limited skin eruption that is virtually identical to that of porphyria cutanea tarda.[19] Pseudoporphyria affects patients receiving hemodialysis for chornic renal failure. Porphyrin studies in these patients are negative. A similar, if not identical, disorder has been described in patients receiving furosemide, nalidixic acid, tetracycline, and naproxen.

Clinical Features   Tense bullae develop spontaneously or in response to minor trauma on the sun-exposed skin of the dorsal hands, dorsal feet, face, and ears. Lesions range from 0.5 to 5.0 cm and are filled with serous or serosanguinous fluid. Bullae usually heal without scarring or milia formation. Eruptions are more common in summer than in winter. The cutaneous presentation is indistinguishable from porphyria cutanea tarda. Analysis of serum, feces, urine, and red blood cells, however, is negative for porphyrins. In drug-induced cases of pseudoporphyria, withdrawal of the drug is curative.

Histopathological Features   The histologic picture and findings on immunofluorescence are indistinguishable from cases of porphyria (see above). A noninflammatory blister forms in a subepidermal location. The vessels of the superficial dermal plexus are markedly thickened by concentric hyalinized PAS-positive and diastase-resistant material.

Differential Diagnosis   The differential diagnosis is identical to that of porphyria and is discussed above.

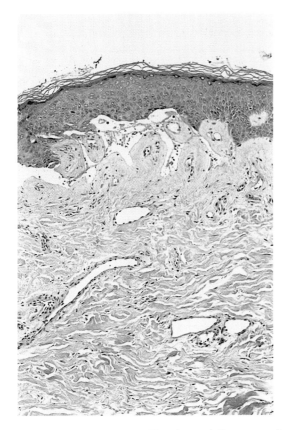

FIGURE 8-5   Porphyria cutanea tarda. There is a noninflammatory subepidermal split.

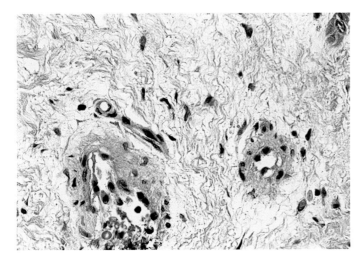

FIGURE 8-6   Porphyria cutanea tarda. Blood vessels with markedly thickened walls are present in the papillary dermis.

Cell-Poor Bullous Pemphigoid

On rare occasions, lesions of bullous pemphigoid may lack a significant inflammatory infiltrate (Fig. 8-7). In those cases, other minimally inflammatory subepidermal blisters may enter the histologic differential diagnosis. However, in all other aspects, cell-poor bullous pemphigoid resembles classic bullous pemphigoid, probably representing an extreme at one end of a continuous spectrum rather than a distinct entity.

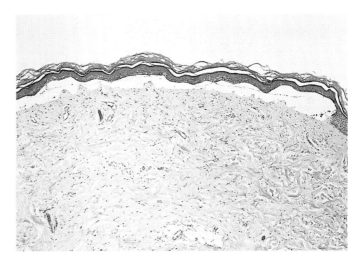

FIGURE 8-7   Cell-poor bullous pemphigoid. A subepidermal blister is present with minimal inflammation.

An in-depth discussion of bullous pemphigoid can be found in the section of this chapter on subepidermal blisters with eosinophils.

Burns

Thermal injury manifests itself with damage to the skin, and the damage depends on the magnitude of the injury.[20] A three-degree grading system exists which is helpful in standardizing severity of injury and assessing likelihood of reepithelialization. First-degree burns involve only the epidermis and are associated with full, and usually rapid, reepithelialization. Second-degree burns extend into the papillary dermis and occasionally into the superficial reticular dermis. However, the deepest portions of the follicular and eccrine epithelia are spared. Reepithelialization occurs as keratinocytes from the follicular bulbs and the deeper components of the eccrine duct grow upward and repopulate the overlying epidermis. There is concomitant scar formation due to the damage to the surrounding dermal collagen. Third-degree burns involve the epidermis, underlying papillary and reticular dermis, and all appendageal epithelium. Thus, extensive scar formation occurs, and there is no chance of reepithelialization as all keratinocytes in the region have been destroyed. This degree of thermal injury necessitates skin grafting.

Histopathological Features   The earliest manifestations of thermal injury include spongiosis within the epidermis. Keratinocyte nuclei become elongated, and hyperchromatic and basal cells appear vacuolated. In more extensive injury, a blister forms at the dermal-epidermal junction. Edema is present within the papillary dermis, and there is a minimal inflammatory infiltrate. As thermal damage becomes more extensive, homogenization of the papillary and reticular dermal collagen becomes apparent. The collagen becomes amphophilic and loses its fibrillar appearance. In the most extensive thermal injury, dermal blood vessels demonstrate coagulative necrosis, and the appendageal epithelium shows changes identical to that seen in the overlying epidermis, with elongation of nuclei, vacuolization of cells, and separation of the epithelium from the surrounding basement membrane.

Differential Diagnosis   The main histologic differential diagnosis in the diagnosis of a burn injury is injury due to freezing and/or electrocautery. This is most commonly seen in the setting of a biopsy performed following recent local therapy. In this setting, similar changes of basal keratinocyte vacuolization with nuclear pyknosis and underlying dermal homogenization can be seen. The clinical history usually provides the information necessary to arrive at a correct diagnosis.

Toxic Epidermal Necrolysis

Toxic epidermal necrolysis (Lyell's disease) is a controversial, yet life-threatening disorder (Table 8-7).[21,22] This rare blistering disorder is thought by some to be a severe variant of erythema multiforme and by others to be a discrete entity.[23] The pathogenesis of the extensive blister formation which occurs in toxic epidermal necrolysis remains elusive, although many workers believe the disease to be immunologically mediated.[24,25] Direct immunofluorescence studies are almost always negative for immunoreactants.

Clinical Features   Patients with toxic epidermal necrolysis present with rapidly progressive blister formation which eventuates in extensive desquamation. Over the course of 24 to 48 h, patients can progress from fever and malaise, with a single small blister, to loss of the majority of their epidermis. In these situations, patients may develop infection and problems with fluid maintenance and thermal regulation that constitute a medical emergency, frequently requiring hospitalization. In most patients, a relationship to proximal drug ingestion can be determined. Some of the most frequent drugs implicated include phenytoin, barbiturates, sulfonamides, ampicillin, butazones, and nonsteroidal anti-inflammatory drugs.[26] In a smaller group of patients, a history of antecedent infection is ascertained. In some cases, toxic epidermal necrolysis has been reported to occur in association with administration of vaccines and graft-versus-host disease.[27] However, in many patients with toxic epidermal necrolysis, no specific precipitating factors can be isolated. The mortality rate has been assessed at approximately 30 percent and remains high even with extensive medical intervention.

Histopathological Features   Toxic epidermal necrolysis is characterized by full-thickness epidermal necrosis, usually without or with only

---

TABLE 8-7

Toxic Epidermal Necrolysis

Clinical Features

Rapid onset
Fever, malaise
Frequent drug history
30% mortality

Histopathological Features

Full-thickness epidermal necrosis
Minimal inflammation
Extensive basal vacuolization

Laboratory Evaluation

Negative direct immunofluorescence

Differential Diagnosis

Thermal injury
Erythema multiforme
Graft-vs-host disease
Staphylococcal scalded-skin syndrome

---

minimal underlying inflammatory infiltrate. A blister is present beneath the basal keratinocytes. Extensive basal vacuolization is present. A variable but usually small number of lymphocytes and eosinophils may be seen. In the earliest lesions, a scant mononuclear cell infiltrate with sparse exocytosis is present in the dermis. Scattered necrotic keratinocytes may be seen.

Differential Diagnosis   The histologic differential diagnosis of toxic epidermal necrolysis includes severe thermal injury, in which full-thickness epidermal necrosis is seen. However, in the thermally damaged skin, there is an elongation of keratinocyte nuclei not seen in toxic epidermal necrolysis, and the dermal homogenization characteristic of thermal injury is not present. Severe erythema multiforme also enters the histologic differential diagnosis for those who believe that to be a separate entity. There is generally slightly more of a lymphocytic infiltrate within the papillary dermis accompanied by exocytosis in erythema multiforme than is seen in toxic epidermal necrolysis. In the earliest lesions of toxic epidermal necrolysis, distinction from erythema multiforme may be impossible. Graft-versus-host disease, grade III, also has a subepidermal blister with abundant necrotic keratinocytes but in most cases has a more prominent inflammatory infiltrate. The presence of necrotic keratinocytes within eccrine structures is also more commonly seen in graft-versus-host disease than in toxic epidermal necrolysis.

Another entity which enters into the clinical differential diagnosis and must be distinguished from toxic epidermal necrolysis is staphylococcal scalded skin syndrome. Clinically, toxic epidermal necrolysis and staphylococcal scalded skin syndrome may present in a very similar manner with extensive blistering and denudation. Both entities constitute potentially life-threatening diseases but require different lines of therapy. Frozen-section diagnosis is therefore often required for rapid therapeutic intervention. Full-thickness epidermal necrosis is characteristic for toxic epidermal necrolysis and differentiates this disorder from staphylococcal scalded skin syndrome which shows an intraepidermal blister with a cleavage plane in the uppermost epidermis.

Bullosis Diabeticorum

Bullosis diabeticorum is used synonymously with *bullous eruption of diabetes mellitus* and *bullous disease of diabetes*.[28] It occurs most frequently in patients with poorly controlled insulin-dependent diabetes mellitus and evidence of renal insufficiency or other diabetic complications. Ultrastructurally, destruction of anchoring fibrils has been seen in lesions in some patients with bullosis diabeticorum, whereas other lesional skin has shown the cleavage plane to be within the lamina lucida. Direct immunofluorescence studies are negative in most cases or nonspecific, showing immunoglobulin and complement in dermal vessel walls.

Clinical Features   Bullosis diabeticorum is characterized by non-inflammatory tense bullae which are most often limited to the hands and feet. Blisters occur spontaneously and may be recurrent. Some lesions heal with atrophy and scarring and others resolve without sequelae. Patients who develop these blisters often display signs of diabetic neuropathy but have good circulation in the affected extremity. The clinical differential diagnosis primarily includes porphyria cutanea tarda, bullous pemphigoid, and epidermolysis bullosa acquisita.

Histopathological Features   Bullosis diabeticorum is characterized by a minimally inflammatory subepidermal blister. The underlying vessels within the papillary dermis have markedly thickened walls, similar to those seen in porphyria cutanea tarda. A sparse perivascular lymphocytic infiltrate may be present. Intraepidermal bullae at various levels ranging from suprabasilar to subcorneal have been described. It is unclear whether these cases represent a true intraepidermal split or are the result of regeneration of epidermis at the floor of the blister.

Differential Diagnosis   The histologic differential diagnosis of bullosis diabeticorum includes epidermolysis bullosa acquisita, which would not demonstrate thickened papillary dermal blood vessel walls, and porphyria cutanea tarda. Porphyria cutanea tarda demonstrates a minimally inflammatory subepidermal blister with thickening of the papillary dermal vessel walls but would also frequently have extensive solar elastosis that is not as prominent in bullosis diabeticorum.

Blisters Overlying Scars

Several other conditions, not ordinarily considered to be primary blistering disorders, can appear as subepidermal blistering processes on histologic sections. A minimally inflammatory subepidermal blister can occur overlying a scar. Although the blister is not ordinarily apparent clinically, the incompletely formed basement membrane zone remains a region of relative weakness for an extended period following scar formation and is vulnerable to separation during routine histologic processing. This same region is also susceptible to shear forces clinically. The explanation for the relative weakness of this zone is incomplete regrowth of type VII collagen anchoring fibrils into the region for an extended period following injury.[29]

Bullous Amyloidosis

Skin involvement is frequent in primary (idiopathic) amyloidosis and in amyloidosis associated with multiple myeloma. The most common lesions consist of papules and purpura, often in the periorbital area. Rare patients develop bullae. Histologic examination shows amyloid as dense, homogeneous deposits in the papillary and reticular dermis. If the disease results in blisters, the separation typically occurs within the deposits of amyloid, i.e., in the papillary dermis. The split can be very superficial and create the impression of a noninflammatory subepidermal blister. The presence of dermal amyloid deposits should enable a correct diagnosis and distinguish this entity from other noninflammatory subepidermal blisters. Amyloidosis will be discussed more extensively elsewhere.

SUBEPIDERMAL BLISTERS WITH LYMPHOCYTES

Erythema Multiforme

Erythema multiforme (Table 8-8) is discussed in more detail in Chapter 3.[30] Depending on the extent of mucosal involvement, erythema multiforme is divided into minor and major subsets. Patients with the common minor variety of erythema multiforme most often have self-limited, short-lived disease which requires minimal therapy.

The more severe variant of erythema multiforme (major) involves mucous membranes and is designated *Stevens-Johnson syndrome*. This form of the disease is usually accompanied by fever and affects children more commonly. Patients with this variant have much more extensive disease which can result in scarring of mucosal surfaces. These patients often require hospitalization and extensive therapy. Toxic epidermal necrolysis is considered another variant of erythema multiforme by some authors and is discussed above.

Clinical Features   Patients with erythema multiforme of the less severe or minor variant typically present with targetoid lesions which are primarily acral in distribution. More extensive cases will have sim-

---

TABLE 8-8

Erythema Multiforme

Clinical Features

Most common in young adults
Strong association with herpes virus infection
Drug association also common
Severe forms involve mucous membranes
Target lesions
Acral sites and symmetric involvement common

Histopathological Features

Individual necrotic keratinocytes
Mild lymphohistiocytic inflammatory infiltrate
No parakeratosis

Laboratory Evaluation

Direct immunofluorescence usually negative

Differential Diagnosis

Fixed drug eruption
Toxic epidermal necrolysis
Pityriasis lichenoides et varioliformis acuta

---

ilar appearing lesions widely distributed on the trunk as well as the extremities, including palms and soles. The extremities often show symmetric involvement. In virtually all cases, a history of a nonspecific prodrome can be elicited from patients. Lesions start as erythematous, slightly edematous patches. As they develop, each lesion forms a central necrotic or white area which is surrounded by a rim of erythema. Well-developed lesions are fairly characteristic in appearance. Lesions last for a matter of days, and in most cases the eruption resolves within 7 to 10 days. Mucosal involvement is uncommon in the minor variant of erythema multiforme.

Patients with Stevens-Johnson syndrome present with a more extensive and febrile eruption which, in addition, involves several mucosal surfaces. In particular, oral mucosa and conjunctiva are frequently affected. This form of the disease is a systemic illness and resolves over a much longer period than does the minor variant.

Histopathological Features   The histologic findings of erythema multiforme vary with the clinical severity of the disease and the age of the individual lesion. In its earliest diagnostic stage, the epidermis contains rare necrotic keratinocytes within and above the basal layer. There is frequently a mild lymphohistiocytic inflammatory response centered around the superficial vascular plexus, with some lymphocytes present within the epidermis. These lymphocytes are often in proximity to the dying keratinocytes. Mild spongiosis is seen in conjunction with slight papillary dermal edema. In most cases, there is no overlying parakeratotic scale, and the inflammatory infiltrate does not extend into the deep reticular dermis. Occasional eosinophils may be present, especially in drug-related cases of erythema multiforme.[31]

In more severe cases, the number of necrotic keratinocytes increases to the point where a subepidermal blister is often present, and there is full-thickness epidermal necrosis. The inflammatory infiltrate may be slightly more intense than in the less severe cases. In older lesions, small foci of parakeratosis can be seen.

Differential Diagnosis   Pityriasis lichenoides et varioliformis acuta (PLEVA) has some histologic similarities to erythema multiforme. In PLEVA, confluent parakeratosis is seen in virtually all cases. The inflammatory infiltrate extends deeper into the reticular dermis than that usually seen in erythema multiforme, and eosinophils are not characteristically seen. Hemorrhage is not seen in most cases of erythema multiforme and is a common feature of PLEVA.

A fixed drug eruption also bears a strong histologic resemblance to erythema multiforme, and some investigators regard these entities as closely related. In fixed drug eruptions, the papillary dermis contains a dense collection of melanophages, reflecting the repeated nature of the basal keratinocyte necrosis. In addition, neutrophils can be seen in fixed drug eruptions and are not a common finding in erythema multiforme.

Toxic epidermal necrolysis is also in the histologic differential diagnosis for those who believe it to be an entity separate from severe erythema multiforme. In general, there is more epidermal necrosis and less inflammation in toxic epidermal necrolysis than is ordinarily seen in erythema multiforme, but there is marked overlap, and this distinction can be histologically impossible.

Fixed Drug Eruption

Fixed drug eruption is an uncommon cutaneous reaction to ingestion of various medications or other antigenic materials. The most commonly implicated medications include phenolphthalein, sulfa derivatives (particularly trimethoprim-sulfamethoxazole), tetracycline, barbiturates, and aspirin.

Clinical Features   Patients present with edematous and erythematous patches or plaques which recur on various parts of the body following repeated exposures to the offending drug. The most common sites include lips, sacral region, and genitalia. The lesions become dusky and ultimately necrotic over a several-day period and heal with postinflammatory pigmentation changes. In more florid lesions, vesicles and bullae may be apparent.

Histopathological Features   Histologic sections demonstrate an interface dermatitis. The basal layer shows extensive vacuolization and necrosis of keratinocytes that, in severe cases, results in a subepidermal blister. Exocytosis of lymphocytes into the epidermis is usually present. Epidermal lymphocytes are often associated with single necrotic keratinocytes. The inflammatory infiltrate is primarily composed of lymphocytes and is localized around vessels in the papillary and at least mid-dermis. In many cases, a mixed cellular inflammatory infiltrate can be seen. Melanin pigment incontinence with abundant melanophages in the papillary dermis is usually a prominent feature and is histologic evidence of repeated injury to the basal layer.

Differential Diagnosis   The histologic differential diagnosis of fixed drug eruption includes erythema multiforme. The presence of melanophages is more commonly seen in fixed drug eruptions; however, they may also be seen in recurrent lesions of erythema multiforme.

Lupus erythematosus may bear some histologic resemblance to a fixed drug eruption, but biopsies of lupus also demonstrate a deep perivascular and periappendageal inflammatory infiltrate not characteristically seen in fixed drug eruptions.

Lichen Sclerosus

Lichen sclerosus is an inflammatory dermatosis of unknown pathogenesis.[32] This entity is discussed in more detail elsewhere in this book. In most cases, clinical bullae are not observed; however, on histologic sectioning a subepidermal blister may be apparent.

Clinical Features   Lichen sclerosus occurs in people of any age. Up to 15 percent of cases occur in children. Genital lesions are more common than extragenital lesions. The reported female preponderance is likely related to the special interest in vulvar lesions in the literature, and the actual female-to-male ratio may approach 1 to 1. Pruritus is the most common symptom for genital lesions, whereas extragenital lesions are usually asymptomatic. The neck and shoulders are the most frequent extragenital site of involvement. Lesions appear as white, hyperkeratotic polygonal papules that eventually form plaques. Central dells may be seen. In rare bullous lesions, hemorrhage may be present.

Histopathological Features   Lichen sclerosus demonstrates an atrophic epidermis underlying dense hyperkeratosis. Follicular plugging is often seen. There is extensive basilar vacuolar degeneration which may lead to blister formation. The papillary dermis is edematous and homogenized, and a variably intense lymphocytic infiltrate is present. The inflammatory component is most marked in early lesions. In more fully developed lesions, the infiltrate becomes less lichenoid, and a sparse perivascular lymphocytic infiltrate may underlie the thickened and homogenized papillary dermis. Plasma cells may be seen, but abundant eosinophils are uncommon.

Differential Diagnosis   The histologic differential diagnosis of lichen sclerosus depends largely on the stage of the lesion biopsied. In its earliest stages, lichen sclerosus is very lichenoid and resembles lichen planus to a large degree. At this stage, lupus erythematosus also could resemble lichen sclerosus. A dense perieccrine infiltrate would favor a diagnosis of lupus, as would positive staining on direct immunofluorescence examination. As lichen sclerosus becomes more atrophic and sclerotic and less lichenoid, morphea and chronic radiation dermatitis enter the histologic differential diagnosis. Involvement of the deep reticular dermis favors a diagnosis of morphea. The presence of radiation fibroblasts, swollen endothelial cells, or deep dermal elastosis favors a diagnosis of radiation dermatitis over that of lichen sclerosus. A clinical history would also be helpful in distinguishing these entities.

Lichen Planus Pemphigoides

Lichen planus pemphigoides is an ill-defined and somewhat controversial entity which has clinical, histologic, and immunologic features of both lichen planus and bullous pemphigoid. Many suggest that distinguishing this entity from bullous lichen planus requires that lesions of lichen planus coexist with bullous lesions occurring on normal-appearing skin. Direct immunofluorescence of skin adjacent to blisters in patients with lichen planus pemphigoides demonstrates linear IgG and C3 along the dermal-epidermal junction, identical to the pattern seen in bullous pemphigoid. Salt-split skin has shown the antibodies to localize to the lamina lucida; however, immunoelectron microscopy has localized the antibodies to the floor of the blister, unlike the situation in bullous pemphigoid. Circulating autoantibodies have been found in about half of these patients. It has been proposed that lesions resembling lichen planus are the earliest manifestations of this disease and that, as a result of damage to the basement membrane zone in these lichenoid lesions, autoantibodies against basement membrane zone proteins are formed and result in blister formation. In some cases, the antigen has been shown to be identical by Western blotting to the 180-kD bullous pemphigoid antigen seen in bullous pemphigoid, but this has not been seen in every case.[33] In addition, Western blotting demonstrates a unique 200-kD protein.[34]

Clinical Features   This uncommon autoimmune blistering disorder is primarily a disease of adults, but rare cases have been reported in childhood.[35] Patients with lichen planus pemphigoides present with lesions indistinguishable from lichen planus occurring in conjunction with tense bullae which are arising from skin clinically normal in appearance or from a preexisting lesion of lichen planus.

Histopathological Features   Biopsies taken from lesions clinically resembling lichen planus show histologic features indistinguishable from ordinary lichen planus, namely hyperkeratosis, hypergranulosis, sawtoothed acanthosis, colloid bodies, and a dense lichenoid, lymphohistiocytic inflammatory infiltrate with marked exocytosis.

Bullous lesions reveal a subepidermal split with an inflammatory infiltrate that is less lichenoid, more perivascular, and may contain eosinophils. A subepidermal blister is seen overlying an edematous papillary dermis. Other findings of lichen planus are not observed.

Differential Diagnosis   The histologic differential diagnosis of lichen planus pemphigoides depends on the type of lesion biopsied. A biopsy from a lichenoid lesion will be difficult to distinguish from lichen planus, and one from a blister will be indistinguishable from bullous pemphigoid. Clinical history in conjunction with direct immunofluorescence studies should enable accurate distinction.

Polymorphous Light Eruption

Polymorphous light reaction (Table 8-9) is the most common photodermatosis. It is separated from other photodermatoses known as *chronic actinic dermatoses* on the basis of its acute, intermittent, and recurrent presentation. Polymorphous light eruption is generally believed to have an immunologically mediated mechanism and can be induced by a combination of UVA and UVB or by either type of light alone.

TABLE 8-9

Polymorphous Light Eruption

Clinical Features

Acute, intermittent, recurrent eruption
Induced by UVA and/or UVB
Slight female preponderance
More common in younger adults
Usual onset in spring
Papules, vesicles, bullae, plaques

Histopathological Features

Dense perivascular superficial and deep lymphocytic infiltrate
Minimal epidermal changes
Papillary dermal edema
Eosinophils uncommon

Laboratory Evaluation

Direct immunofluorescence negative

Differential Diagnosis

Lupus erythematosus
Jessner's lymphocytic infiltrate

Clinical Features   The majority of cases of polymorphous light eruption arise within the first three decades. There is a slight female preponderance, and there appears to be some familial predisposition. Most cases are seen in the spring and early summer, shortly following the first extensive sun exposure each year. Lesions present within hours to several days after exposure to ultraviolet light. They take multiple different clinical appearances, thus giving rise to the name. The most common type of lesion is a pruritic erythematous papule which occurs at sites of sun exposure. Less common types of lesions include vesicles, bullae, and plaques. Lesions heal without scarring. The severity of the disease varies greatly from patient to patient, but each patient tends to have a similar appearing eruption each time it recurs.

Histopathological Features   The histologic features of polymorphous light eruption vary with the clinical appearances of the lesions. A dense perivascular lymphocytic infiltrate surrounding vessels of the superficial vascular plexus is the unifying pathologic change. In more plaque-like lesions, lymphocytes are also seen extending deep into the dermis. There is little exocytosis, and basal vacuolization is not seen. Vesicular and bullous lesions demonstrate marked papillary dermal edema, in some cases resulting in subepidermal blister formation. It is unusual to find eosinophils or neutrophils in this condition.

Differential Diagnosis   The main histologic differential diagnosis of polymorphous light eruption is lupus erythematosus. Lupus is characterized by more of an interface dermatitis, with vacuolization of basal keratinocytes, a feature that is not seen in polymorphous light eruption. Further, a dense periappendageal infiltrate, basement membrane thickening, and epidermal atrophy are features of lupus and are not associated with polymorphous light eruption. Mucin may be present within the reticular dermis in lupus and is absent or at most minimal in polymorphous light eruption. Direct immunofluorescence may further help in the differential diagnosis. In contrast to lupus erythematosus, direct immunofluorescence studies in polymorphous light eruption are negative.

Jessner's lymphocytic infiltrate also enters the histologic differential diagnosis. Marked papillary dermal edema is not an expected finding in this entity. Clinical correlation is also important in distinguishing these entities.

Bullous Mycosis Fungoides

Bullous mycosis fungoides is a rare presentation of mycosis fungoides and is caused by a massive population of epidermotropic lymphocytes entering the epidermis and destroying the basement membrane zone. Other features of mycosis fungoides are readily apparent on the biopsy specimen.

Bullous Fungal Infections

Occasional fungus infections in the skin can have marked papillary dermal edema and a dense inflammatory infiltrate as part of the histologic appearance. The dermal inflammatory infiltrate is generally lymphocyte predominant but has an admixture of eosinophils, plasma cells, and occasional neutrophils. In most cases, parakeratosis and spongiosis in the overlying epidermis are present. A fungal stain readily establishes the diagnosis, if the organisms cannot be visualized on routine stained sections.

SUBEPIDERMAL BLISTERS WITH EOSINOPHILS

Bullous Pemphigoid

Bullous pemphigoid (Table 8-10) is mainly a disease of the elderly; however, cases have been reported in patients of all ages. The disease is believed to be an autoimmune blistering disease.[36,37] On direct immunofluorescence examination, nearly 100 percent of perilesional biopsies will display linear deposits of C3 along the dermal-epidermal junction. Linear immunoglobulin deposition along the dermal-epidermal junction is also present in most cases. IgG is the most common immunoglobulin, occurring in 60 to 90 percent of cases. Occasional biopsies will demonstrate IgM, IgA, IgD, or IgE deposits. In cases with IgG autoantibodies, IgG4 is the predominant subclass. The incidence of positive staining is slightly lower for biopsies taken from the lower extremity[38] and markedly lower when examining lesional skin as opposed to perilesional skin. Immunoblotting and immunoprecipitation with patient sera recognize one or two antigens in human skin extracts, with molecular mass of 230 kD (bullous pemphigoid antigen 1, BPAg1) or 180 kD (bullous pemphigoid antigen 2, BPAg2), respectively. Immunoelectron microscopic studies have localized BPAg1 to the hemidesmosome, whereas BPAg2 localizes both to the hemidesmosome and the upper lamina lucida. Both molecules have been cloned, and sequence analysis suggests that BPAg1 is an intracellular protein and BPAg2 is a transmembrane protein (Fig. 8-1). Autoantibodies from patients with the generalized form of bullous pemphigoid recognize the same 230-kD protein (BPAg1) as do autoantibodies from patients with clinical variants of bullous pemphigoid (i.e., childhood bullous pemphigoid, vesicular and localized forms). The BPAg2 band is usually weaker, and not all patients with bullous pemphigoid have autoantibodies against this antigen. Nevertheless, there seems to be no correlation between the autoantibodies present in individual patients and their clinical presentation. In diagnostic dermatopathology, the hemidesmosomal location of the bullous pemphigoid antigens is corroborated with direct immunofluorescence studies performed on salt-split skin. Incubation of human skin in 1 M NaCl leads to separation of the epidermis from the dermis at the level of the lamina lucida with hemidesmosomes localizing to the roof of the split. Indirect immunofluorescence on salt-split skin reproducibly demonstrates immunoreactant deposits in the roof of the blister. Immunofluorescence studies on salt-split skin also help differentiate bullous pemphigoid from epidermolysis bullosa acquisita and cicatricial pemphigoid, its closest clinical and histologic mimics. Animal models of bullous pemphigoid have proved difficult to establish, and the full pathogenesis of the disease is still under investigation. The current model postulates attachment of IgG autoantibodies (IgG4 subclass) to the basement membrane, followed by activation of the complement cascade. Inflammatory mediators attract mast cells, which in turn release chemotactic factors that recruit neutrophils and eosinophils. Lysosomal proteolytic enzymes released by neutrophils and eosinophils then contribute to the formation of a subepidermal blister.

Clinical Features   Bullous pemphigoid is characterized by the presence of tense bullae arising on normal skin or on an erythematous base. The blisters have a predilection for the extremities but often spread to the trunk and become generalized. The blisters frequently remain intact and are not enlarged with subtle pressure. The lesions may be mildly or intensely pruritic or asymptomatic. The mucosal membranes of the oral cavity, pharynx, urethra, and conjunctiva may be involved but are less frequently affected than in pemphigus vulgaris. In some patients, the lesions appear urticarial and do not form discrete bullae. Several clinical variants of the disease exist: Dyshidrosiform pemphigoid affects predominantly the palms and soles and resembles dyshidrotic eczema; this variant may remain limited to the palms and soles or eventually disseminate to resemble generalized bullous pemphigoid. Vesicular pemphigoid is characterized by small vesicles rather than bullae. Nodular pemphigoid is distinguished by nodular and hyperkeratotic lesions resembling prurigo nodularis. Childhood localized vulvar pemphigoid has been reported in rare cases. Pretibial localized pemphigoid affects mainly older women and remains limited to the lower legs. Pemphigoid vegetans clinically resembles pemphigus vegetans but has the histologic and immunofluorescence characteristics of bullous pemphigoid. The association of bullous pemphigoid with malignancy has been controversial. Recent case-controlled studies, however, have failed to show a statistically increased incidence of malignancy in patients with bullous pemphigoid.[39]

Histopathological Features   The histologic features of bullous pemphigoid include the presence of a subepidermal blister with a moderately dense accumulation of eosinophils and other inflammatory cells within and beneath the blister cavity (Fig. 8-8). There is no necrosis of the overlying epidermis, except at the middle portion of the blister roof, where the blister is oldest. In some cases, eosinophils can be seen in a linear array in close approximation to the basement membrane zone (Fig. 8-9). Lymphocytes are also frequently seen in bullous pemphigoid. In rare cases, neutrophils may predominate, and, in exceptional cases, the inflammatory infiltrate can be almost nonexistent (so-called cell-poor bullous pemphigoid). The inflammatory infiltrate is usually confined to the papillary dermis and the superficial portion of the reticular dermis. Papillary dermal edema may be present. Urticarial pemphigoid is characterized by a papillary dermal infiltrate composed predominantly of eosinophils with extension of the eosinophils into the epidermis. This epidermotropism is accompanied by spongiosis (eosinophilic spongiosis) but does not result in a subepidermal blister. Immunofluorescence studies show linear C3 and IgG along the dermal-epidermal junction like in regular bullous pemphigoid and aid in the differential diagnosis.

Differential Diagnosis   Epidermolysis bullosa acquisita may be indistinguishable from bullous pemphigoid on clinical and histologic

---

TABLE 8-10

Bullous Pemphigoid

Clinical Features

Usually elderly patients
Tense blisters on erythematous base
Blisters intact
Predilection for extremities
Mucosal surfaces sometimes involved

Histopathological Features

Subepidermal blister
Dense inflammatory infiltrate in papillary dermis
Abundant eosinophils in most cases
No necrosis of overlying epidermis

Laboratory Evaluation

Linear IgG and C3 at dermal-epidermal junction in most cases
Indirect immunofluorescence positive in most patients
Immune complexes localize to roof with salt-split skin

Differential Diagnosis

Epidermolysis bullosa acquisita
Herpes gestationis
Bullous arthropod bite
Bullous drug eruption

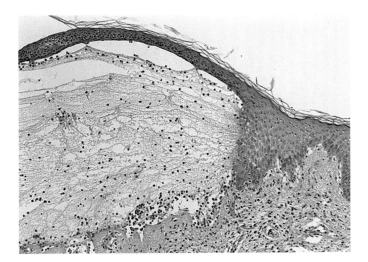

FIGURE 8-8 Bullous pemphigoid displays a subepidermal blister with abundant eosinophils in the blister cavity. Necrotic keratinocytes are not seen.

grounds and on routine direct immunofluorescence. In the routine laboratory setting, the differential diagnosis hinges on direct immunofluorescence studies performed on salt-split skin. IgG is deposited on the floor of the blister in epidermolysis bullosa acquisita and localizes almost exclusively to the roof of the blister in bullous pemphigoid. The more specialized techniques that differentiate between the two entities, such as immunoblotting, immunoprecipitation, and immunoelectron microscopy, are limited to few facilities. The histopathologic alterations and direct immunofluorescence findings in cicatricial pemphigoid are the same as those seen in bullous pemphigoid. Clinical features usually differentiate the two diseases. The usual variant of cicatricial pemphigoid affects almost exclusively the mucous membranes as opposed to bullous pemphigoid that mainly involves the skin. Direct immunofluorescence performed on salt-split skin is of little help, because cicatricial pemphigoid is a heterogeneous disease on the molecular level, and the majority of antigens targeted by the autoantibody localize to the roof of the blister as in bullous pemphigoid.

The histologic differential diagnosis also includes herpes gestationis. This entity is best distinguished by the clinical presentation. Direct immunofluorescence may be of some help: C3 is deposited in a linear fashion along the dermal-epidermal junction in nearly 100 percent of

cases of herpes gestationis and bullous pemphigoid. IgG, in contrast, can be seen in 60 to 80 percent of cases of bullous pemphigoid but only in 30 to 50 percent of patients with herpes gestationis. On histology the presence of necrotic basal keratinocytes may also favor a diagnosis of herpes gestationis over bullous pemphigoid. Occasional cases of dermatitis herpetiformis and linear IgA dermatosis may have increased numbers of eosinophils. Conversely, occasional cases of bullous pemphigoid may display increased numbers of neutrophils. In these situations, direct immunofluorescence is probably the easiest way to distinguish these entities. Other conditions which may give rise to a subepidermal blister with abundant eosinophils include bullous arthropod bite reaction and bullous drug eruption. Bullous arthropod bite reactions tend to have an inflammatory infiltrate which is more intense, extends deeper into the reticular dermis and subcutaneous fat, and may have eosinophils individually dispersed between collagen bundles. Bullous drug eruptions may also have a deeper infiltrate, but can be histologically indistinguishable from bullous pemphigoid. Bullous arthropod bite reactions and bullous drug eruptions will be negative or demonstrate only nonspecific features of vascular leakage on direct immunofluorescence examination. Lesions of cell-poor bullous pemphigoid must be distinguished from each of the entities described as subepidermal blisters with minimal inflammation. These distinctions are best made on the basis of clinical and immunologic methods.

Herpes Gestationis

Herpes gestationis (Table 8-11) is a subepidermal blistering disorder of pregnancy. Similar to bullous pemphigoid, it is an autoimmune disorder in which patients develop autoantibodies to a component of the basement membrane zone. As with bullous pemphigoid, immune complexes can be detected along the basement membrane in a linear distribution. In contrast to bullous pemphigoid, however, linear deposition of IgG is of lesser intensity and is less commonly seen in conjunction with C3.

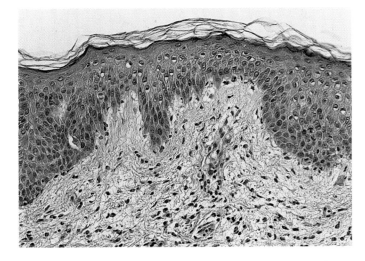

FIGURE 8-9 Bullous pemphigoid. The urticarial phase without blister formation. Eosinophils are characteristically present near the basement membrane zone.

TABLE 8-11

Herpes Gestationis

Clinical Features

Uncommon
Usually in second or third trimesters of pregnancy
Recurs with subsequent pregnancies
Most lesions on trunk and extremities
Newborn may have blisters
Mucosal lesions uncommon

Histopathological Features

Subepidermal blister
Abundant eosinophils
Papillary dermal edema
Rare necrotic keratinocytes

Laboratory Evaluation

Linear C3 at dermal-epidermal junction in most cases
Linear IgG present at dermal-epidermal junction in a minority of cases

Differential Diagnosis

Bullous pemphigoid
Bullous arthropod bite
Bullous drug eruption
Pruritic urticarial papules and plaques of pregnancy

IgG, which is of the IgG1 subtype, fixes complement but is only seen in 30 to 50 percent of cases with routine direct immunofluorescence testing. The target antigen appears to be the same 180-kD protein (bullous pemphigoid antigen 2, BPAg2) that is also recognized by the autoantibodies of some bullous pemphigoid patients. BPAg2 is a transmembrane protein located within the hemidesmosome and extending into the lamina lucida.[40]

In approximately 10 percent of cases, the newborn infant is affected with mild, self-limited blisters caused by the transplacental passage of autoantibodies. There seems to be a slight increase in small-for-gestational-age births in patients with herpes gestationis, but most studies now suggest that there is no increase in fetal mortality in this patient population.[41]

The occurrence of herpes gestationis has been associated with the presence of other autoimmune diseases, most commonly Graves disease. There is an association with HLA types -DR3 and -DR4.[42]

Clinical Features　Herpes gestationis is an uncommon disease of pregnancy. It may begin at any time during pregnancy or in the postpartum period. The majority of cases occur during the second and third trimester. Lesions appear rapidly over the trunk and extremities. The abdomen is the usual site of the earliest lesions. Lesions may be urticarial or frankly bullous and often arise on an inflammatory base. The face is usually spared. Mucosal involvement is extremely uncommon. There may be a clinical exacerbation immediately postpartum. Typically, lesions resolve over a few weeks and recur with subsequent pregnancies in the majority of cases.[43]

Histopathological Features　The histologic features of herpes gestationis include a subepidermal blister with marked papillary dermal edema (Fig. 8-10) and abundant eosinophils within the papillary dermis and blister cavity (Fig. 8-11). Spongiosis is present. Individually necrotic keratinocytes may be seen within the basal layer of the epidermis. Within the dermis, a mixed perivascular infiltrate of eosinophils, histiocytes, and lymphocytes is present. In some cases, eosinophils line up along the dermal-epidermal junction (Fig. 8-12).

Differential Diagnosis　The histologic differential diagnosis includes bullous pemphigoid, bullous arthropod bite, bullous drug eruption, and pruritic urticarial papules and plaques of pregnancy. On histologic sections, the presence of individually necrotic keratinocytes would favor

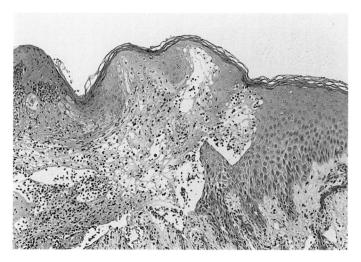

FIGURE 8-11　Herpes gestationis. There are numerous eosinophils in the blister space.

herpes gestationis over bullous pemphigoid, but in most cases these two entities can most easily be distinguished by the clinical setting as well as differences in immunologic findings (see above). Bullous arthropod bite reactions usually have a more dense infiltrate which extends deeper into the dermis. Direct immunofluorescence examinations are invariably negative for immune complexes in arthropod bite reactions and bullous drug eruptions.

Subepidermal blisters are not seen in pruritic urticarial papules and plaques of pregnancy, but, in some cases of herpes gestationis, eosinophilic spongiosis without fully formed blisters may be present. In these cases the histologic features of these two entities may be identical. The

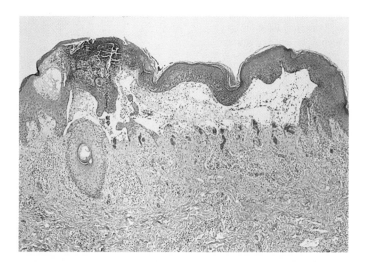

FIGURE 8-10　Herpes gestationis demonstrates a subepidermal blister. In some cases, rare necrotic keratinocytes may be seen near the blister edge.

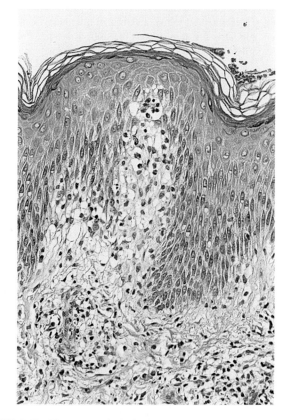

FIGURE 8-12　Herpes gestationis. Urticarial lesion with eosinophils near the dermal-epidermal junction.

clinical features are most often different, and pruritic urticarial papules and plaques of pregnancy are always negative on direct immunofluorescence examination.

Arthropod Bite Reactions

Arthropod bite reactions are dermal hypersensitivity reactions to a wide range of arthropods. They represent a host response to antigens in the saliva of the insect and as such are no different from other reactions of delayed type hypersensitivity.

Clinical Features   Bullous arthropod bite reactions usually appear as grouped papules with surrounding erythema. In some cases, puncta are readily apparent. In florid cases, the papules may become vesicular. The lower extremities are the most common sites for arthropod bite reactions, but they may occur in any location.

Histopathological Features   A bullous arthropod bite reaction is characterized by focal parakeratosis overlying a spongiotic epidermis. In the region of the punctum, epidermal disruption and focal keratinocyte necrosis can be seen. Within the dermis, there is a superficial and deep perivascular inflammatory infiltrate which is most commonly comprised of lymphocytes, histiocytes, and abundant eosinophils. In some lesions, however, eosinophils may be sparse. The inflammatory infiltrate can extend into the subcutaneous fat. Some authors regard the presence of eosinophils in the interstitium between collagen bundles and away from vessels helpful in making the diagnosis of an arthropod bite reaction. In bullous lesions, there is abundant papillary dermal edema which leads to a subepidermal blister. In older lesions, the lymphocytic infiltrate can be quite dense, with germinal center formation.

Differential Diagnosis   The differential diagnosis of a bullous arthropod bite reaction includes other subepidermal blisters containing abundant eosinophils. The most commonly encountered situations are bullous pemphigoid, herpes gestationis, and bullous drug eruptions. The first two conditions usually do not display a deep component to the dermal infiltrate and may have eosinophils linearly arrayed along the dermal-epidermal junction. Further, direct immunofluorescence studies are positive in nearly all perilesional biopsies in patients with these disorders and are negative in bullous arthropod bites. A bullous drug eruption can be very difficult to distinguish from a bullous arthropod bite reaction. In general, drug eruptions are not as prone to extend into the subcutaneous fat, and eosinophils are not as frequently seen within the interstitium. However, in individual cases, either observation may be present, and the history may be the only discriminating feature. If present, histologic evidence of a punctum favors an arthropod bite reaction.

Bullous Drug Eruptions

Drug eruptions can occur in response to virtually all medications and present with a myriad of clinical appearances. Fixed drug eruptions and erythema multiforme and their relationships to drug ingestion have already been discussed in this chapter. In some circumstances, the clinical presentation of a drug eruption is that of a blistering disorder indistinguishable from a primary blistering process. These types of reactions occur most frequently in conjunction with severe morbilliform eruptions. Furosemide is commonly associated with this type of reaction. Similar eruptions can be seen with penicillamine and clonidine.[44] Other types of drug reactions will be discussed in other chapters in this book.

Clinical Features   Patients with a bullous drug eruption usually present within days of ingestion of a drug. The clinical presentation largely

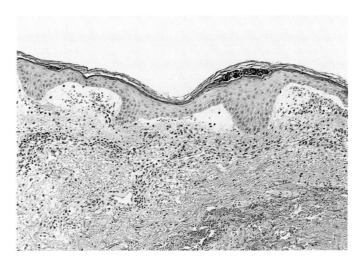

FIGURE 8-13   Bullous drug eruption. Subepidermal blister with inflammatory cell infiltrate and hemorrhage.

depends on the drug. Bromides and iodides are the most common causes of drug-induced vesiculobullous eruptions. Furosemide, sulfones, ibuprofen, penicillin, and 5-fluorouracil have caused clinical eruptions indistinguishable from bullous pemphigoid. Naproxen, tetracycline, furosemide, and nalidixic acid have been shown to cause a porphyria cutanea tarda–like eruption (see above, pseudoporphyria).[45]

Histopathological Features   The histologic features of a bullous drug eruption are nonspecific and depend upon the type of reaction present. In many cases, there is a subepidermal blister with abundant papillary dermal edema and a moderately intense superficial and deep mixed inflammatory infiltrate (Figs. 8-13 and 8-14). Eosinophils are frequently seen but are not required for the diagnosis. Keratinocyte necrosis may be seen in some cases but is often absent. In other situations, the inflammatory infiltrate may be sparse or absent.

Differential Diagnosis   The histologic differential diagnosis is based on the histologic features of any particular drug eruption. In many cases, the closest histologic mimic is bullous pemphigoid. Bullous pemphigoid most often does not involve a deep infiltrate, a feature commonly seen in bullous drug eruptions. Further, direct immunofluorescence is almost always positive in bullous pemphigoid and variable in

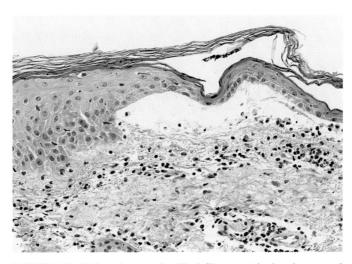

FIGURE 8-14   Bullous drug eruption. The infiltrate contains lymphocytes and eosinophils.

drug eruptions. The immunofluorescence patterns vary from case to case in bullous drug eruptions. Some cases are entirely negative, others show linear IgG and C3 along the dermal-epidermal junction, and still others show an intercellular staining pattern, resembling pemphigus vulgaris. Furosemide has been reported to cause an autoimmune bullous process with immunoglobulin deposition in a pattern identical to bullous pemphigoid.[46] Keep in mind that bullous drug eruptions may mimic primary blistering diseases on all levels.

In less inflammatory lesions, the main histologic differential diagnosis is porphyria cutanea tarda. This entity is characterized by hyaline thickening of blood vessel walls and increased solar elastosis not usually seen in drug eruptions and often by a different clinical presentation. Drug-induced pseudoporphyria, however, has histologic and immunologic findings identical to porphyria cutanea tarda. Clinical history and negative porphyrin studies help in the differential diagnosis.

SUBEPIDERMAL BLISTERS WITH NEUTROPHILS

Dermatitis Herpetiformis

Dermatitis herpetiformis (Table 8-12) is an intensely pruritic papulovesicular dermatitis which usually manifests during the second and third decades of life.[47] Virtually, 100 percent of these patients will have IgA deposits along the dermal-epidermal junction in biopsies taken from perilesional skin. These deposits are granular in nature and tend to cluster within papillary tips, sparing the areas around the base of rete ridges. C3 deposition is also seen in most cases. The incidence of immunoglobulin deposits in normal skin is only slightly lower; however, biopsies taken from lesional skin will frequently fail to demonstrate IgA deposits, possibly due to the increased degradation caused by the dense neutrophilic infiltrates in lesional skin. At one time, investigators believed that a small percentage of patients with dermatitis her-

petiformis displayed a linear deposition of IgA along the dermal-epidermal junction. It is now most widely believed, however, that this subset of patients is best classified as having linear IgA bullous dermatosis and not dermatitis herpetiformis because these patients do not have the associated gluten-sensitive enteropathy seen to some degree in virtually all patients with dermatitis herpetiformis. The gluten-sensitive enteropathy is histologically indistinguishable from celiac sprue. However, patients are rarely symptomatic from their small intestinal disease, and symptoms are invariably mild for patients who experience them. Further, the HLA haplotypes of -A1, -B8, -DR3 that are so frequently seen in patients with dermatitis herpetiformis are not seen to any significant degree in patients with linear IgA dermatosis. The pathogenesis for the cutaneous lesions in dermatitis herpetiformis remains largely unknown.

Patients with dermatitis herpetiformis have a higher rate of autoimmune thyroid disease and gastric atrophy and/or gastric hypochlorhydria. There is also an increase in the rate of gastrointestinal lymphoma.[48]

Clinical Features Dermatitis herpetiformis presents as a symmetrically distributed eruption usually concentrated on the extensor surfaces of the extremities. In more severe cases, lesions may be widespread. The individual vesicular lesions are quite small and are often entirely excoriated on the basis of the intense pruritus that they engender. Pruritus frequently precedes the onset of a new lesion by 12 to 24 h. Mucous membrane involvement is uncommon.

Histopathological Features Dermatitis herpetiformis is characterized by small subepidermal blisters. The epidermis is mildly spongiotic and is often excoriated. Within the papillary dermal tips, small aggregates of neutrophils and cellular debris can be seen, frequently underlying the areas of blister formation (Fig. 8-15). In most cases, there is a discontinuous distribution of neutrophils (Fig. 8-16), in contrast to the linear distribution seen in linear IgA bullous dermatosis. Frequently a lymphocytic inflammatory infiltrate surrounds vessels of the superficial vascular plexus. Occasional eosinophils can be seen within the inflammatory infiltrate but are not the predominant cell type.

Differential Diagnosis The histologic differential diagnosis of dermatitis herpetiformis includes linear IgA bullous dermatosis, epidermolysis bullosa acquisita, bullous lupus erythematosus, cicatricial pemphigoid, pustular drug eruptions, and occasional cases of bullous pemphigoid. Dermatitis herpetiformis is the only one of these entities in which the neutrophils tend to aggregate within papillary dermal tips. The blister spaces tend to be smaller in dermatitis herpetiformis than in the other entities. Epidermolysis bullosa acquisita is less inflammatory in many cases, and bullous pemphigoid demonstrates a predominantly eosinophilic infiltrate in most cases. Pustular drug eruptions may exhibit papillary dermal collections of neutrophils similar to dermatitis herpetiformis but, in contrast to dermatitis herpetiformis, also show evidence of leukocytoclastic vasculitis with fibrinoid necrosis of vessel walls.[49] The direct immunofluorescence staining patterns will be different for each of the disorders in this differential diagnosis and probably represent the most reliable method of distinguishing between them.

Linear IgA Bullous Dermatosis

Linear IgA disease (Table 8-13) is now generally thought to be a spectrum of heterogeneous IgA1-mediated autoimmune blistering disorders that also includes chronic bullous disease of childhood.[50–53] Linear IgA disease and chronic bullous dermatosis of childhood are both characterized by the presence of IgA deposits within the basement membrane zone. In a minority of cases IgG may be present. Immunoelectron

---

TABLE 8-12

Dermatitis Herpetiformis

Clinical Features

Intensely pruritic
Usual onset in early adulthood
Symmetric vesicles on extensor surfaces of extremities
Mucous membrane involvement uncommon
Gluten-sensitive enteropathy
   associated with HLA-A1, -B8, -DR3

Histopathological Features

Subepidermal blister
Neutrophilic microabscesses in papillary dermal tips
Lymphocytic infiltrate around superficial vascular plexus

Laboratory Evaluation

Granular IgA and C3 in papillary dermal tips on direct immunofluorescence

Differential Diagnosis

Linear IgA bullous dermatosis
Epidermolysis bullosa acquisita
Bullous lupus erythematosus
Cicatricial pemphigoid
Bullous pemphigoid
Pustular drug eruption

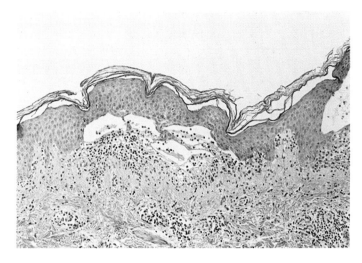

FIGURE 8-15 Dermatitis herpetiformis. Neutrophilic abscesses in papillary dermal tips and subepidermal blister formation are seen in dermatitis herpetiformis.

microscopy reveals two subtypes of linear IgA disease. In most cases, the IgA deposits are found in the lamina lucida and localize to the epidermal side of the blister in salt-split skin. In a minority of cases, the immunoglobulin deposits are in the sub–lamina densa area and localize to the floor of the blister cavity. The autoantigen in the lamina lucida form of IgA disease has been determined to be the LAD-1 antigen.[54,55] This is a component of the anchoring filaments of the lamina lucida. The protein has a mass of 120 kD when synthesized by keratinocytes in culture and runs as a 97-kD band after being processed in the skin. The antigen in the sub–lamina densa form of linear IgA disease has not been identified, yet. Circulating IgA anti–basement membrane zone antibodies can be demonstrated in 60 to 70 percent of patients with either subtype of the disease. Unlike dermatitis herpetiformis, no association with specific HLA subtypes has been found in patients with both linear IgA disease and chronic bullous disease of childhood. Linear IgA disease has been associated with vancomycin and captopril ingestion in several cases, and other drugs in more sporadic reports. Linear IgA disease has also been reported with malignancy in rare cases. The association of linear IgA disease and gluten-sensitive enteropathy is controversial, although some authors believe there to be a weak link.

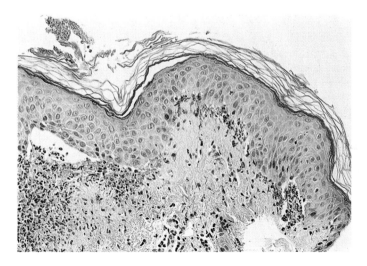

FIGURE 8-16 Dermatitis herpetiformis. There are discrete papillary dermal microabscesses as well as confluence of abscesses.

TABLE 8-13

Linear IgA Bullous Dermatosis

Clinical Features

Childhood disease has onset within 5–6 years of birth
Adult onset in sixth to eighth decades
Often antecedent infection
Annular erythematous patches with tense blisters at edges
Trunk and extremities most commonly affected sites

Histopathological Features

Subepidermal blister
Neutrophils linearly aligned along dermal-epidermal junction
Papillary dermal edema
Occasional eosinophils present

Laboratory Evaluation

Linear IgA and C3 along dermal-epidermal junction
Immune deposits localize to roof of blister in most cases

Differential Diagnosis

Dermatitis herpetiformis
Bullous arthropod bite reaction
Sweet's syndrome
Bullous lupus erythematosus
Epidermolysis bullosa acquisita

Clinical Features Chronic bullous disease of childhood generally presents in children within the first 5 to 6 years of life. Linear IgA disease presents in adults in the sixth to eighth decades, in most cases. In many patients, an antecedent infection such as a viral respiratory illness, tetanus, or streptococcal pharyngitis has been reported. Rather than clinical parameters, linear deposition of IgA along the dermal-epidermal junction on direct immunofluorescence is definitional for this disease. The clinical findings are variable and may resemble those of dermatitis herpetiformis or bullous pemphigoid in adults. In children the clinical presentation is more characteristic. Patients with both disorders present with annular erythematous patches with tense bullae scattered at the edges of the lesions. The distribution of lesions is variable. In patients with a bullous pemphigoid–like distribution, the trunk and extremities are most commonly affected. Patients with a dermatitis herpetiformis–like eruption present with lesions mainly on the extensor surfaces. Oral involvement may be present in up to 70 percent of patients. Lesions continue to occur for many years. Symptoms can be controlled with appropriate therapy, and spontaneous remissions occur in 30 to 60 percent of adult patients and in almost all pediatric patients.

Histopathological Features Linear IgA dermatosis and chronic bullous disease of childhood have identical histologic patterns. In early lesions, neutrophils are aligned along the dermal-epidermal junction accompanied by basal vacuolization (Fig. 8-17). Eventually a subepidermal blister forms, with an intact overlying epidermis. Within the blister cavity and along the dermal-epidermal junction, abundant neutrophils are present, frequently admixed with smaller numbers of eosinophils and lymphocytes. As the lesion ages, eosinophils become more prominent. There is papillary dermal edema. Vasculitis is not seen.

Differential Diagnosis The major histologic differential diagnosis is dermatitis herpetiformis. In the classic situation, dermatitis herpetiformis has a less diffuse and more abscesslike distribution of neu-

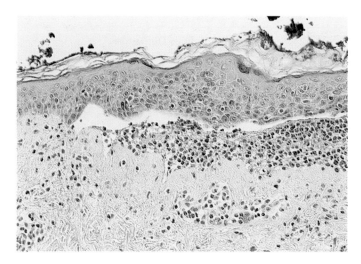

FIGURE 8-17 Linear IgA dermatosis. A linear distribution of neutrophils along the dermal-epidermal junction and a subepidermal blister are seen in linear IgA dermatosis.

trophils, confined to papillary dermal tips, whereas linear IgA dermatosis and chronic bullous disease of childhood display neutrophils in a more evenly distributed pattern along the dermal-epidermal junction. However, there is great overlap in these cases, and direct immunofluorescence demonstrating a linear or granular staining pattern with IgA is frequently the only way to distinguish these entities. Clinical parameters such as HLA-B8/DR3 haplotype and small-bowel abnormalities in dermatitis herpetiformis may further aid in the differential diagnosis.

Occasional arthropod bite reactions can display neutrophil predominant infiltrates, and these cases resemble linear IgA dermatosis. The presence of a punctum, or a deep component to the inflammatory infiltrate, as well as a negative or nonspecific direct immunofluorescence study would favor a bite reaction.

The neutrophilic infiltrate in Sweet's syndrome is usually far more florid and diffuse than that seen in linear IgA dermatosis or chronic bullous disease of childhood. In addition, Sweet's syndrome is characterized by much more papillary dermal edema.

Bullous lupus erythematosus can present with a histologic picture similar to linear IgA disease. Patients with bullous lupus erythematosus have serologic findings of systemic lupus. On direct immunofluorescence the staining pattern of lupus is granular and bandlike and is usually observed with several immunoglobulins and not just IgA.

Epidermolysis bullosa acquisita, cicatricial pemphigoid, and bullous pemphigoid may have histologic features similar to linear IgA disease but can be discerned by direct immunofluorescence. Cases with neutrophilic blisters and with linear deposition of IgA and IgG along the dermal-epidermal junction are more problematic. One approach is to classify the disease according to the stronger staining immunoglobulin, i.e., as linear IgA disease if IgA is the predominant immunoglobulin or as bullous pemphigoid when IgG predominates. Some authors accept as linear IgA disease only cases with exclusive staining with IgA and classify all others as bullous pemphigoid or epidermolysis bullosa acquisita.

Cicatricial Pemphigoid and Localized Cicatricial Pemphigoid

Cicatricial pemphigoid (Table 8-14) is a rare autoimmune blistering disorder with a predilection for mucosal surfaces.[56,57] More than 80 percent of biopsies from perilesional skin will demonstrate linear IgG and C3 along the dermal-epidermal junction. IgA and IgM may also be present, albeit less commonly. On immunoelectron microscopy cicatricial

TABLE 8-14
Cicatricial Pemphigoid

Clinical Features

Elderly patients
More common in women
Vesiculobullous eruption primarily involves mucous membranes
Extensive scarring
Skin involvement in only 25% of cases

Histopathological Features

Subepidermal blister
Moderately intense mixed inflammatory infiltrate
Dense dermal fibrosis in older lesions

Laboratory Evaluation

Linear IgG and C3 along dermal-epidermal junction in most patients
Immune complexes may localize to roof or floor of blister
Only 25% of patients demonstrate circulating autoantibodies

Differential Diagnosis

Sweet's syndrome
Linear IgA bullous dermatosis
Dermatitis herpetiformis
Bullous lupus erythematosus
Epidermolysis bullosa acquisita

pemphigoid autoantibodies localize to the lamina densa. Immunologic studies, however, reveal a more heterogeneous picture and several different autoantigens have been identified in small subsets of patients. For the majority of patients the autoantigen is unclear. The heterogeneous nature of this entity is further supported by immunofluorescence studies on salt-split skin that reveal the autoantibody on the roof of the blister in the majority of cases. In approximately 20 percent of patients, the autoantibody localizes either to the roof and the floor or exclusively to the floor of the blister.

Only about 25 percent of patients have circulating antibodies against basement membrane proteins, and following antibody titers has not proven useful in monitoring disease activity.

Clinical Features   Cicatricial pemphigoid is most commonly seen in elderly patients and is twice as frequent in women. Rare cases have been reported in children. The disease is characterized by a vesiculobullous eruption that affects mucosal membranes primarily. Individual lesions are slow to heal and result in extensive scarring. Skin involvement occurs in only 25 percent of cases and is usually limited. The disease follows a chronic course and may result in extensive scarring if not treated. In 85 percent of cases, the oral cavity is involved. The eye is another common site of involvement (65 percent) and, if left untreated, can progress to blindness. It is most unusual to have cutaneous lesions in the absence of mucosal involvement. This variant, known as *localized cicatricial pemphigoid* or *Brunsting-Perry cicatricial pemphigoid*, is more common in men. It mainly affects the head and neck region and may lead to scarring alopecia. Penicillamine has been implicated in producing a disease with clinical, histologic, and immunologic features to cicatricial pemphigoid.

Histopathological Features   Cicatricial pemphigoid is characterized by a subepidermal blister with a moderately intense, mixed inflammatory infiltrate present within the blister cavity (Fig. 8-18) and in a perivascular distribution within the underlying dermis. The proportion

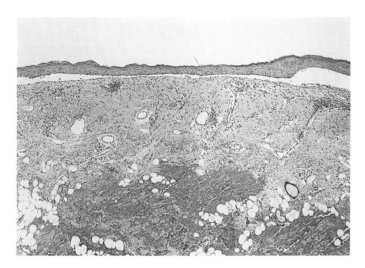

FIGURE 8-18   Cicatricial pemphigoid is characterized by a subepidermal split.

of eosinophils is variable, and, in many cases, there is a neutrophilic predominance within the infiltrate. In mucosal lesions, mononuclear cells may predominate. Acantholysis is not seen. In well-developed lesions, granulation tissue or dense dermal fibrosis indicates chronicity and scarring. The histologic features closely resemble bullous pemphigoid.

Differential Diagnosis   The histologic differential diagnosis depends upon the degree of dermal inflammatory infiltrate. In lesions which are intensely inflammatory, the differential diagnosis would include Sweet's syndrome and linear IgA bullous dermatosis, neither of which is associated with dermal scarring. Dermatitis herpetiformis could also be in the differential diagnosis but usually has neutrophils which are more localized to dermal papillae than is seen in cicatricial pemphigoid. Bullous lupus could appear quite similar to cicatricial pemphigoid on routine histology. The differences in direct immunofluorescence staining patterns is helpful in discriminating between these diseases. Epidermolysis bullosa acquisita would also be in the differential diagnosis and can produce dermal scarring. Direct immunofluorescence on salt-split skin probably offers the most reliable method for distinguishing between these two entities.

Bullous Acute Vasculitis

Leukocytoclastic vasculitis is an immune complex–mediated process (type III hypersensitivity reaction) which is described more completely in another chapter. Evidence for the immunologic basis for this disorder is the presence of IgG or IgM and C3 in the vessel walls in virtually all lesions less than 24 h old.

Clinical Features   Leukocytoclastic vasculitis can present with clinical and histologic features resembling a primary blistering process. In addition to the typical purpuric and ulcerated lesions, tense blisters can be seen. These most commonly occur on an erythematous base. The lower extremities are the most common site for blisters to appear in a patient with leukocytoclastic vasculitis.

Histopathological Features   The histologic features of bullous leukocytoclastic vasculitis are similar to other cases of leukocytoclastic vasculitis. There is a perivascular neutrophilic infiltrate with transmural involvement of the vessel walls. Fibrin deposits are seen within the vas-

cular walls of affected vessels, and there is evidence of endothelial cell swelling and destruction. Extravasated red blood cells are frequently present. In bullous lesions, there is marked papillary dermal edema, resulting in a subepidermal blister. In cases with ischemic changes secondary to vascular occlusion, there may be necrosis of the overlying keratinocytes; however, bullous lesions may occur in the absence of keratinocyte necrosis in cases with marked dermal edema.

Differential Diagnosis   The main histologic differential diagnosis is Sweet's syndrome, which is also characterized by a dense neutrophilic infiltrate and marked papillary dermal edema. In Sweet's syndrome, vascular destruction is not seen, and the neutrophils are more diffusely scattered throughout the papillary dermis. Direct immunofluorescence demonstrating perivascular immune complexes is also helpful in making a diagnosis of leukocytoclastic vasculitis.

Bullous Lupus Erythematosus

Bullous lupus erythematosus is a rare variant of lupus. It is believed to be an autoimmune disease in which patients display autoantibodies to basement membrane proteins. In some cases, these antibodies appear to be directed against type VII collagen, similar to the situation in epidermolysis bullosa acquisita.[58,59] Granular or linear deposition of IgG, IgA, IgM, and C3 along the dermal-epidermal junction in lesional as well as clinically normal skin provides immunologic confirmation of this hypothesis. These deposits have been localized to the lamina densa and sublamina densa region of the papillary dermis. In addition to the characteristic cutaneous findings, a firm diagnosis requires other clinical and laboratory findings of systemic lupus erythematosus.

Clinical Features   Patients with the bullous form of lupus erythematosus present with widespread vesicles and bullae which occur most frequently on sun-exposed skin but may occur at any site. The trunk and flexural surfaces are most commonly involved. The blisters may be preceded by plaques and tend to occur on erythematous bases. The disease is encountered most often in young black women. The eruption may resemble either dermatitis herpetiformis or bullous pemphigoid. It is unusual to see classic discoid lesions in patients with this variant of lupus erythematosus.[60]

Histopathological Features   Bullous lesions of lupus erythematosus do not resemble discoid lesions of lupus histologically. The salient pathologic changes are a subepidermal blister with abundant neutrophils present within the papillary dermis (Figs. 8-19 and 8-20). The neutrophils may be confined to the papillae or may form a bandlike pattern within the entire papillary dermis and into the blister cavity. There is marked dermal edema. A moderate perivascular inflammatory infiltrate surrounds the vessels of the superficial and middle dermis, which consists predominantly of lymphocytes; however, neutrophils and occasional eosinophils can be seen. In some cases, leukocytoclastic vasculitis and hemorrhage are present. Basal vacuolization, epidermal atrophy, and a thickened basement membrane so typical of discoid lupus lesions are only occasionally seen.[61]

Differential Diagnosis   The histologic differential diagnosis of bullous lupus erythematosus includes dermatitis herpetiformis, linear IgA bullous dermatosis, Sweet's syndrome, epidermolysis bullosa acquisita, and cicatricial pemphigoid. The presence of leukocytoclastic changes favors the diagnosis of lupus over the other entities listed. The most compelling diagnostic information is found on direct immunofluorescence examination which separates out each of these entities.

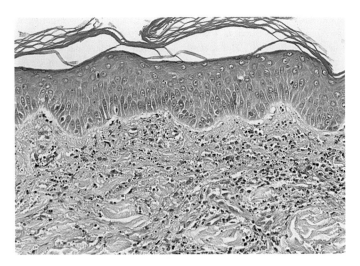

FIGURE 8-19   Bullous systemic lupus erythematosus. Although there is no blister, there are neutrophils in the papillary dermis.

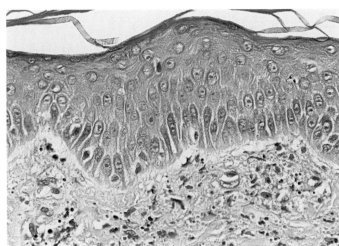

FIGURE 8-20   Bullous systemic lupus erythematosus. Vacuolization at dermal-epidermal junction with neutrophils and erythrocytes in papillary dermis.

Sweet's Syndrome

Acute febrile neutrophilic dermatosis (Sweet's syndrome) is an acute, self-limited disorder of unknown etiology.[62] Sweet's syndrome is described more completely in another chapter.

Clinical Features   Sweet's syndrome occurs about twice as often in women as men and has a peak incidence in the fourth to seventh decades. Patients typically present with fever and malaise. Lesions present as multiple, painful plaques. The most common locations include the face, neck, upper chest, and upper extremities. Pseudovesiculation is commonly seen, and, in severe cases, blistering may occur. Arthralgias are reported in about half of patients. Most patients have elevated erythrocyte sedimentation rates and peripheral leukocytosis.

Histopathological Features   Sweet's syndrome histologically demonstrates a dense dermal inflammatory infiltrate consisting of lymphocytes and abundant neutrophils in a bandlike distribution. There is vasodilatation, but no vascular destruction is seen. Leukocytoclasis is prominent. Marked papillary edema leads to a subepidermal blister in severe cases. In the earliest lesions, lymphocytes may be the predominant cell type, whereas in late-resolving lesions, histiocytes may be the predominant cell type. Intraepidermal clusters of neutrophils forming pustules are seen in a minority of cases.

Differential Diagnosis   The histologic differential diagnosis is that of a subepidermal blister with abundant neutrophils. The closest histologic mimic, in most cases, is leukocytoclastic vasculitis, which is differentiated from Sweet's syndrome on the basis of vascular destruction. Other entities such as linear IgA bullous dermatosis can be distinguished by the presence of neutrophils more closely adherent to the basement membrane zone and less papillary dermal edema. Direct immunofluorescence studies are negative in Sweet's syndrome, further helping in this distinction. The neutrophils are distributed in a more bandlike fashion in Sweet's syndrome than is usually seen in dermatitis herpetiformis.

Epidermolysis Bullosa Acquisita

Epidermolysis bullosa acquisita (Table 8-15) is a putative autoimmune disease in which afflicted individuals develop antibodies directed against type VII collagen.[63] Destruction of the anchoring fibrils comprised of type VII collagen within the superficial papillary dermis gives rise to subepidermal blisters. Evidence for the autoimmune nature of the process is found on direct immunofluorescence studies which demonstrate linear staining with IgG and C3 in perilesional skin in virtually all patients with the disease. Immunofluorescence studies performed on 1M NaCl split skin further localize the autoantibodies to the floor of the blister, a finding which is confirmed with immunoelectron miscroscopy showing immune deposits on anchoring fibrils deep to the lamina densa. Indirect immunofluorescence studies demonstrate circulating immune complexes in approximately half of the patients with epidermolysis bullosa acquisita. Epidermolysis bullosa acquisita occurs in association with systemic lupus erythematosus and inflammatory bowel disease in some cases.

TABLE 8-15

Epidermolysis Bullosa Acquisita

Clinical Features

Usually affects middle-aged to elderly adults
Blisters on noninflammatory skin
Scarring and milia
Predilection for trauma-prone sites
Nail dystrophy may be present

Histopathological Features

Subepidermal blister
Most cases with minimal inflammation
Occasional cases with mixed inflammatory infiltrate
No keratinocyte necrosis
Dermal scarring may be present

Laboratory Evaluation

Linear C3 and IgG along dermal-epidermal junction in most cases
Immune complexes localize to floor of blister in salt-split skin
About 50% of patients demonstrate circulating autoantibodies

Differential Diagnosis

Porphyria cutanea tarda
Cell-poor bullous pemphigoid
Bullous lupus erythematosus

Clinical Features   Patients with epidermolysis bullosa acquisita are usually in their fifth through seventh decades. The disease is quite rare in children but has been reported. Three clinical variants of epidermolysis bullosa acquisita exist. In the most common noninflammatory mechanobullous form, blisters arise on a nonerythematous base and heal with scarring and milia formation. The lesions have a predilection for trauma-prone areas such as elbows, knees, hands, and feet but may be quite widely distributed. Nail dystrophy is also present in many cases. This variant of the disease clinically resembles porphyria cutanea tarda or recessive dystrophic epidermolysis. A second presentation consists of widespread vesicles and bullae arising on erythematous skin. This inflammatory vesiculobullous eruption shows marked similarities with bullous pemphigoid. The lesions may be very pruritic. Scarring and milia formation is less prominent than in the mechanobullous form of the disease. A third variant clinically resembles cicatricial pemphigoid and is characterized by prominent mucosal involvement.[64]

Histopathological Features   The histologic picture parallels the clinical presentation. A clean subepidermal blister with minimal inflammatory reaction is seen in many cases of the mechanobullous variant of epidermolysis bullosa acquisita. The inflammatory vesiculobullous variant demonstrates a moderately intense inflammatory infiltrate, comprised of predominantly neutrophils with admixed lymphocytes and eosinophils. The infiltrate is largely confined to the papillary dermis and superficial vascular plexus. Keratinocyte necrosis is not seen. Dermal scar formation may be present.

Differential Diagnosis   The histologic differential diagnosis depends on the histologic subtype of epidermolysis bullosa acquisita. In relatively noninflammatory lesions, the differential diagnosis includes porphyria cutanea tarda and cell-poor bullous pemphigoid. These two conditions can be distinguished from epidermolysis bullosa acquisita on the basis of immunofluorescence staining patterns (requiring salt-split skin to differentiate bullous pemphigoid and epidermolysis bullosa acquisita). Porphyria cutanea tarda can be further distinguished with urine, fecal, and blood porphyrin studies.

   In more inflammatory cases of epidermolysis bullosa acquisita with abundant dermal neutrophils, bullous lupus erythematosus is the major differential diagnostic possibility. Bullous lupus erythematosus may display other histologic features of lupus such as a superficial and deep perivascular and periappendageal lymphocytic infiltrate, but these features are often absent. In fact the histologic features of epidermolysis bullosa acquisita and bullous lupus erythematosus may be indistinguishable. Patients with the latter disease meet the criteria of the American Rheumatologic Association for systemic lupus erythematosus. Further, the granular nature of the immunoglobulin deposits seen in lupus erythematosus on direct immunofluorescence often differentiates this entity from the linear deposits seen in epidermolysis bullosa acquisita.

Erysipelas

Erysipelas may yield a histologic picture of a subepidermal blister with a predominantly neutrophilic inflammatory infiltrate. In comparison with the primary blistering processes, the inflammatory infiltrate is more widely dispersed between collagen bundles and extends deep into the reticular dermis and the subcutaneous fat. Blisters arise as a result of massive dermal edema. Epidermal changes are uncommon.

Bullous Urticaria

Bullous urticaria may also reveal the histologic picture of a subepidermal blister with a predominantly neutrophilic inflammatory infiltrate.

The infiltrate in bullous urticaria may be scant but is generally mixed and includes eosinophils, lymphocytes, and mast cells, as well as the neutrophils. The infiltrate tends to be confined to the dermis immediately surrounding vessels of the superficial vascular plexus. Marked papillary dermal edema leads to a subepidermal blister, and epidermal changes are not seen.

SUBEPIDERMAL BLISTERS WITH MAST CELLS

Bullous Mastocytosis

Bullous mastocytosis (Table 8-16) is a form of urticaria pigmentosa which occurs almost exclusively in children.[65] The exact pathogenesis of this group of mast cell proliferations is unknown. The prognosis is excellent when the disease presents within the first 2 years of life, with the vast majority of children experiencing complete resolution of their disease by puberty.[66] Systemic involvement is quite rare in this population. Urticaria pigmentosa is discussed more extensively in other chapters.

Clinical Features   Bullous lesions present usually by the age of 6 months. Lesions are most common on the extremities but not in acral locations.[67] In most cases of bullous mastocytosis, the number of lesions is smaller than in other forms of urticaria pigmentosa, but each individual lesion is larger, ranging up to several centimeters. Stroking of the lesions will result in marked urticaria (Darier's sign), but caution should be exercised to avoid provoking massive mast cell degranulation and anaphylaxis.

Histopathological Features   Bullous mastocytosis is characterized by an intense and diffuse mast cell infiltrate. There is marked papillary dermal edema, resulting in a subepidermal blister. Exocytosis of mast cells into the overlying epidermis and keratinocyte necrosis are generally not seen. Mast cells display a "fried egg" appearance in most bullous lesions and contain abundant granules which stain metachromatically with Giemsa and toluidine blue stains.

Differential Diagnosis   The histologic differential diagnosis of bullous mastocytosis is quite limited. Once the infiltrating cells have been identified as mast cells, no other conditions have this histologic appearance.

TABLE 8-16

Bullous Mastocytosis

Clinical Features

Almost exclusively in children
Excellent prognosis when child is less than 2 years of age
Only rare systemic involvement
Most common on extremities
Positive Darier's sign

Histopathological Features

Intense mast cell infiltrate
Marked papillary dermal edema

Laboratory Evaluation

None

Differential Diagnosis

Histiocytic infiltrate

MISCELLANEOUS SUBEPIDERMAL BLISTERING PROCESSES

Ischemia and Drug-Overdose-Related Bullae

Subepidermal blisters can also be seen in a myriad of situations in which the skin is secondarily involved. Blisters may form as a result of ischemia. Bullous vasculitis (see above) is one of the forms of ischemic blister formation. Less commonly, occlusion of a larger vessel that may not even be represented in the biopsy specimen can lead to a subepidermal split, often accompanied by epidermal necrosis. Hypoxia in conjunction with pressure cause bullae formation in pressure necrosis secondary to drug- or alcohol-induced coma. In this setting, compression of skin leads to necrosis of the eccrine glands and preservation of the ducts. There is marked papillary dermal edema, and a slight lymphocytic response may be present. The overlying epidermis may show a variable degree of necrosis or may be entirely intact.

PUVA-Induced Bullae

Treatment with PUVA (oral psoralens with ultraviolet A light therapy) may result in a subepidermal blister identical to that seen in acute sunburns or other thermal injury. There is a subepidermal blister with pyknosis and elongation of the basal keratinocytes. A minimal lymphocytic infiltrate may be present. Keratinocyte necrosis is present and dose-dependent.

Etretinate-Induced Bullae

Recently, subepidermal hemorrhagic subepidermal blisters have been reported in a patient with Darier's disease being treated with etretinate. With the current widespread use of this medication, it is important to document its implication in causing a blistering process.[68]

REFERENCES

1. Briggaman RA, Wheeler CE: The epidermal-dermal junction. *J Invest Dermatol* 65:71–84, 1975.
2. Stanley JR, Tanaka T, Mueller S, et al: Isolation of complimentary DNA for bullous pemphigoid antigen by use of patients' autoantibodies. *J Clin Invest* 82:1864–1870, 1988.
3. Carter WG, Ryan MC, Gahr PJ: Epiligrin, a new cell adhesion ligand for integrin α3β1 in epithelial basement membranes. *Cell* 65:599–610, 1991.
4. Verrando P, Bae-Li H, Chang-Jing Y, et al: Monoclonal antibody GB3, a new probe for the study of human basement membranes and hemidesmosomes. *Exp Cell Res* 170:116–128, 1987.
5. Rouselle P, Lunstrum GP, Keene DR, Burgeson RE: Kalinin: An epithelium-specific basement membrane adhesion molecule that is a component of anchoring filaments. *J Cell Biol* 114:567–576, 1991.
6. Marinkovich MP, Lunstrum GP, Burgeson RE: The anchoring filament protein kalinin is synthesized and secreted as a high molecular weight precursor. *J Biol Chem* 267:17900–17906, 1992.
7. Marinkovich MP, Verrando P, Keene DR, et al: Basement membrane proteins kalinin and nicein are structurally and immunologically identical. *Lab Invest* 69:295–299, 1993.
8. McGrath JA, Pulkkinen L, Christiano AM, et al: Altered laminin 5 expression due to mutations in the gene encoding the beta 3 chain (LAMB3) in generalized atrophic benign epidermolysis bullosa. *J Invest Dermatol* 104:467–474, 1995.
9. Keene DR, Sakai LY, Lunstrum GP, et al: Type VII collagen forms an extended network of anchoring fibrils. *J Biol Chem* 104:611–621, 1987.
10. Parente MG, Chung LC, Ryynänen J, et al: Human type VII collagen: cDNA cloning and chromosomal mapping of the gene. *Proc Natl Acad Sci* 88:6931–6935, 1991.
11. Fine JD, Bauer EA, Briggaman RA, et al: Revised clinical and laboratory criteria for subtypes of inherited epidermolysis bullosa. *J Am Acad Dermatol* 24:119–135, 1991.
12. Bonifas JM, Rothman AL, Epstein EH: Epidermolysis bullosa simplex: Evidence in two families for keratin gene abnormalities. *Science* 254:1202–1205, 1991.
13. Uitto J, Christiano AM: Molecular genetics of the cutaneous basement membrane zone: Perspectives on epidermolysis bullosa and other blistering skin diseases. *J Clin Invest* 90:687–692, 1992.
14. Poh-Fitzpatrick MB: The porphyrias. *Dermatol Clin* 5:55–61, 1987.
15. Elder GH: The cutaneous porphyrias. *Semin Dermatol* 9:63–69, 1990.
16. Maynard B, Peters MS: Histologic and immunofluorescence study of cutaneous porphyrias. *J Cutan Pathol* 19:40–47, 1992.
17. Dabski C, Beutner EH: Studies of laminin and type IV collagen in blisters of porphyria cutanea tarda and drug-induced pseudoporphyria. *J Am Acad Dermatol* 25:28–32, 1991.
18. Egbert BM, LeBoit PE, McCalmont T, et al: Caterpillar bodies: Distinctive, basement-membrane containing structures in blisters of porphyria. *Am J Dermatopathol* 15:199–202, 1993.
19. Kekzces K, Farr M: Bullous dermatosis of chronic renal failure. *Br J Dermatol* 95:541–546, 1976.
20. Pearson R: Response of human epidermis to graded thermal stress. *Arch Environ Health* 11:498–507, 1965.
21. Avakian R, Flowers FP, Araujo OE. Ramos-Caro FA: Toxic epidermal necrolysis: A review. *J Am Acad Dermatol* 25:69–79, 1991.
22. Roujeau J-C, Chosidow O, Saiag P, Guillaume J-C: Toxic epidermal necrolysis (Lyell syndrome). *J Am Acad Dermatol* 23:1039–1058, 1990.
23. Assier H, Bastuji-Garin S, Revuz J, Roujeau JC: Erythema multiforme with mucous membrane involvement and Stevens-Johnson syndrome are clinically different disorders with distinct causes. *Arch Dermatol* 131:539–543, 1995.
24. Correia O, Delgado L, Ramos JP, et al: Cutaneous T-cell recruitment in toxic epidermal necrolysis: Further evidence of CD8+ lymphocyte involvement. *Arch Dermatol* 129:466–468, 1993.
25. Villada G, Roujeau J-C, Clerici T, et al: Immunopathology of toxic epidermal necrolysis. Keratinocytes, HLA-DR expression, Langerhans cells and mononuclear cells: An immunologic study of five cases. *Arch Dermatol* 128:50–53, 1992.
26. Guillaume JC, Roujeau JC, Revuz J, et al: The culprit drugs in 87 cases of toxic epidermal necrolysis (Lyell's syndrome). *Arch Dermatol* 123:1166–1170, 1987.
27. Peck GL, Herzig GP, Elias PM: Toxic epidermal necrolysis in a patient with graft-vs-host reaction. *Arch Dermatol* 105:561–569, 1972.
28. Perez MI, Kohn SR: Cutaneous manifestations of diabetes mellitus. *J Am Acad Dermatol* 30:519–531, 1994.
29. Compton CC, Gill JM, Bradford DA, et al: Skin regenerated from cultured epithelial autografts on full-thickness burn wounds from 6 days to 5 years after grafting: A light, electron microscopic and immunohistochemical study. *Lab Invest* 60:600–612, 1989.
30. Fabbri P, Panconesi E: Erythema multiforme ("minus" and "maius") and drug intake. *Clin Dermatol* 11:479–489, 1993.
31. Patterson JW, Parsons JM, Blaylock K, Mills AS: Eosinophils in skin lesions of erythema multiforme. *Arch Pathol Lab Med* 113:36–39, 1989.
32. Meffert JJ, Davis BM, Grimwood RE: Lichen sclerosus. *J Am Acad Dermatol* 32:393–416, 1995.
33. Archer CB, Cronin E, Smith NP: Diagnosis of lichen planus pemphigoides in the absence of bullae on normal-appearing skin. *Clin Exp Dermatol* 17:433–436, 1992.
34. Davis AL, Bhogal BS, Whitehead P, et al: Lichen planus pemphigoides: Its relationship to bullous pemphigoid. *Br J Dermatol* 125:263–271, 1991.
35. Paige DG, Bhogal BS, Black MM, Harper JI: Lichen planus pemphigoides in a child—immunopathological findings. *Clin Exp Dermatol* 18:552–554, 1993.
36. Stanley JR: Cell adhesion molecules as targets of autoantibodies in pemphigus and pemphigoid, bullous diseases due to defective epidermal cell adhesion. *Adv Immunol* 53:291–325, 1992.
37. Helm KF, Peters MS: Immunodermatology update: The immunologically mediated vesiculobullous diseases. *Mayo Clin Proc* 66:187–202, 1991.
38. Weigand DA: Effect of anatomic region on immunofluorescence diagnosis of bullous pemphigoid. *J Am Acad Dermatol* 12:274–278, 1985.
39. Venning VA, Wojnarowska F: The association of bullous pemphigoid and malignant disease: A case control study. *Br J Dermatol* 123:439–445, 1990.
40. Eady RA: The hemidesmosome: A target in auto-immune bullous disease. *Dermatology* 189 Suppl 1:38–41, 1994.
41. Shornick JK, Black MM: Fetal risks in herpes gestationis. *J Am Acad Dermatol* 26:63–68, 1992.
42. Black MM: New observations on pemphigoid "herpes" gestationis. *Dermatology* 189 Suppl 1:50–51, 1994.
43. Shornick JK: Herpes gestationis. *J Am Acad Dermatol* 17:539–556, 1987.
44. Wintroub BU, Stern R: Cutaneous drug reactions: Pathogenesis and clinical classification. *J Am Acad Dermatol* 13:167–179, 1985.
45. Shelley ED, Shelley WB, Burmeister V: Naproxen-induced pseudoporphyria presenting a diagnostic dilemma. *Cutis* 40:314–316, 1987.
46. Fellner MJ, Katz JM: Occurrence of bullous pemphigoid after furosemide therapy. *Arch Dermatol* 112:75–77, 1976.
47. Hall RP: Dermatitis herpetiformis. *J Invest Dermatol* 99:873–881, 1992.
48. Bose SK, Lacour JP, Bodokh I, Ortonne JP: Malignant lymphoma and dermatitis herpetiformis. *Dermatology* 188:177–181, 1994.

49. Burrows NP, Russell Jones R: Pustular drug eruptions: A histopathological spectrum. *Histopathology* 22:569–573, 1993.

50. Wojnarowska F, Bhogal BS, Black MM: Chronic bullous disease of childhood and linear IgA disease of adults are IgA1-mediated diseases. *Br J Dermatol* 131:210–214, 1994.

51. Wojnarowska F, Allen J, Collier P: Linear IgA disease: A heterogeneous disease. *Dermatology* 189 Suppl 1:52–56, 1994.

52. Collier PM, Wojnarowska F, Millard PR: Variation in the deposition of the antibodies at different anatomical sites in linear IgA disease of adults and chronic bullous disease of childhood. *Br J Dermatol* 127:482–484, 1992.

53. Kuechle MK, Stegemeir E, Maynard B, et al: Drug-induced linear IgA bullous dermatosis: Report of six cases and review of the literature. *J Am Acad Dermatol* 30:187–192, 1994.

54. Zone JJ, Taylor TB, Kadunce DP, Meyer LJ: Identification of the cutaneous basement membrane zone antigen and isolation of antibody in linear immunoglobulin A bullous dermatosis. *J Clin Invest* 85:812–820, 1990.

55. Marinkovich MP, Taylor TB, Keene DR, et al: LAD-1, the linear IgA bullous dermatosis autoantigen, is a novel 120-kDa anchoring filament protein synthesized by epidermal cells. *J Invest Dermatol* 106:734–738, 1996.

56. Ahmed AR, Kurgis BS, Rogers RS III: Cicatricial pemphigoid. *J Am Acad Dermatol* 24:987–1001, 1991.

57. Sarrett Y, Hall R, Cobo M, et al: Salt-split skin substrate for the immunofluorescent screening of serum from patients with cicatricial pemphigoid and a new method of immunoprecipitation with IgA antibodies. *J Am Acad Dermatol* 24:952–958, 1991.

58. Gammon WR, Briggaman RA: Bullous SLE: A phenotypically distinctive but immunologically heterogeneous bullous disorder. *J Invest Dermatol* 100:28S–34S, 1993.

59. Yell JA, Allen J, Wojnarowska F, et al: Bullous systemic lupus erythematosus: Revised criteria for diagnosis. *Br J Dermatol* 132:921–928, 1995.

60. Fleming MG, Bergfeld WF, Tomecki KJ, et al: Bullous systemic lupus erythematosus. *Int J Dermatol* 28:321–326, 1989.

61. Burrows NP, Bhogal BS, Black MM, et al: Bullous eruption of systemic lupus erythematosus: A clinicopathological study of four cases. *Br J Dermatol* 128:332–338, 1993.

62. Von den Driesch P: Sweet's syndrome (acute febrile neutrophilic dermatosis). *J Am Acad Dermatol* 31:535–556, 1994.

63. Woodley DT, Briggaman RA, Gammon WR: Acquired epidermolysis bullosa: A bullous disease associated with autoimmunity to type VII (anchoring fibril) collagen. *Dermatol Clin* 8:717–726, 1990.

64. Stewart MI, Woodley DT, Briggaman RA: Epidermolysis bullosa acquisita and associated symptomatic esophageal webs. *Arch Dermatol* 127:373–377, 1991.

65. Longley J, Duffy TP, Kohn S: The mast cell and mast cell disease. *J Am Acad Dermatol* 32:545–561, 1995.

66. Stein DH: Mastocytosis: A review. *Pediatr Dermatol* 3:365–375, 1986.

67. Soter NA: The skin in mastocytosis. *J Invest Dermatol* 96:32S–39S, 1991.

68. Gebauer K, Holgate C, Navaratnam A: Retinoid-induced haemorrhagic bullae in Darier's disease. *Austral J Dermatol* 31:99–103, 1990.

CHAPTER 9

VASCULITIS AND RELATED DISORDERS

Klaus J. Busam / Sarah K. Barksdale / Raymond L. Barnhill

This chapter addresses cutaneous diseases with vascular damage, which includes a heterogeneous group of inflammatory and noninflammatory clinical conditions whose common denominator is damage to cutaneous vessels. It cannot be emphasized enough at the beginning of this chapter that vascular injury is dynamic and its spectrum of clinical and histologic reaction patterns is limited.

Vascular injury can occur in a great number of clinical settings. It may be limited to the skin; however, in many instances it is the hallmark of systemic disease with variable involvement of other organs. Vascular damage may be the principal event of a disease process, such as in polyarteritis nodosa; a significant component of a complex disease, such as connective tissue disease; or it may simply be a secondary effect to a localized clinical phenomenon, such as an arthropod bite or traumatic ulcer.

The clinical manifestations of vascular damage include edema, livedo reticularis, and various forms of hemorrhage (purpura). Hemorrhagic lesions less than 3 mm in diameter are called petechiae. If they are larger, they are called ecchymoses. Palpable purpura generally indicates the presence of an inflammatory cell infiltrate. If vascular damage is severe, vascular occlusion may lead to ischemic injury resulting in necrosis and/or ulceration.

DEFINITIONS

In principle, vascular injury may occur with or without inflammation, and the extent of vascular damage is variable as is the composition and cellularity of the inflammatory cell infiltrate (Table 9-1).

Those processes that generally show inflammation and clear-cut vascular damage are defined as vasculitis. As would be expected, the criteria for recognizing microvascular injury are somewhat arbitrary, and the minimal criteria for vasculitis remain controversial. Simplistically, vasculitis must have two components: an inflammatory cell infiltrate and evidence of vascular injury (Table 9-1, Fig. 9-1). Vasculitis thus is defined as an inflammatory process. The absence of inflammation would preclude the diagnosis, even though vascular alterations may be present. To some extent the type of infiltrating cell (neutrophils, lymphocytes, or macrophages) may correlate with the chronology of the process, but not always. In the late, healing stage, the inflammatory cell infiltration may be minimal.

The histologic features that are thought to be indicative of vascular injury may vary from observer to observer (Table 9-2). Certain changes, including edema, extravasation of erythrocytes, infiltration of vessel walls by inflammatory cells, leukocytoclasis, and thrombosis, may occur without actual damage to the structural integrity of the vessel. Vessels become leaky from time to time for physiologic reasons, leading to edema or even extravasation of erythrocytes. Leukocytoclasis

TABLE 9-1
Definitions of Vascular Injury

Primary Vascular Injury
  Vasculitis
    Inflammatory cell infiltrate
    Clear-cut vascular damage (e.g., fibrinoid necrosis of vessel wall)
  Inflammatory vascular reaction
    Inflammatory cell infiltrate
    Limited vascular damage (insufficient for vasculitis)
  Vasculopathy
    Lack of inflammation
    Vascular damage of any degree
Secondary Vascular Injury
  May present as vasculitis, inflammatory vascular reaction, or vasculopathy
  Secondary to another insult such as external trauma, ulceration
  Variable vascular alterations with sparing of some vessels
  Peripheral perivascular fibrinoid deposition

may result from the breakdown of a perivascular neutrophilic infiltrate during the resolution of an inflammatory process unrelated to vasculitis. Similarly, fibrin thrombi may be present in essentially uninjured vessels in the setting of a hypercoagulable state. Unequivocal injury to the vascular wall is manifested by deposition of fibrinoid material and/or necrosis. In other words, a diagnosis of vasculitis is established histologically if vascular inflammation is accompanied by fibrinoid alterations of the vessel wall. Is the presence of fibrinoid necrosis an absolute prerequisite for the pathologist to render a diagnosis of vasculitis? For didactic purposes, it is tempting to answer the question with an unambiguous "yes." Yet, there may be individual situations in which other features of vascular damage, such as leukocytoclasis or intraluminal thrombi, are developed to such a degree that the constellation of findings favors vasculitis in spite of the lack of clear-cut fibrinoid necrosis. As a general rule, however, we advise the application of strict criteria for the diagnosis of vasculitis and caution in diagnosing vasculitis in the absence of fibrinoid necrosis.

The term vasculopathy is used to describe evidence of vascular damage in the absence of inflammation. The degree of vascular damage is variable. The spectrum of clinical settings in which noninflammatory vascular injury commonly occurs includes mainly coagulopathies and other vascular occlusive conditions. Intraluminal fibrin (thrombi) is a common histologic finding in these disorders (Fig. 9-2).

There is a third group of reactions in which inflammation is present, but the extent of vascular injury usually is limited and appears insuffi-

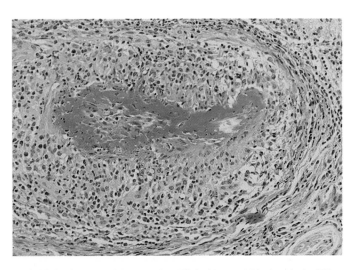

FIGURE 9-1 Fibrinoid degeneration. Fibrinoid material is deposited within a vessel. There is also a polymorphonuclear infiltrate.

cient for vasculitis. This is the least defined group of disorders and encompasses a great number of heterogeneous inflammatory conditions, which may regularly or occasionally manifest vascular injury. Accordingly, it may be rather arbitrary to decide which conditions should be included in this section of the chapter. We have included those diseases whose histologic or clinical presentation warrants a differential diagnosis from "true" vasculitis. Since the only common denominator for these disorders is the presence of an inflammatory infiltrate and some limited vascular damage, we designate them inflammatory vascular reactions (Fig. 9-3). This term is an adaptation and generalization of the more established term neutrophilic vascular reactions, which was coined to define a group of inflammatory disorders that showed histologic overlap with neutrophilic small-vessel vasculitis.[1]

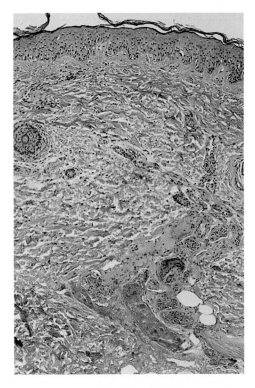

FIGURE 9-2 Vasculopathic reaction. Fibrin thrombi in small dermal vessels and ischemic damage of the skin are seen. An inflammatory cell infiltrate is lacking.

TABLE 9-2

Histological Manifestations of Vascular Damage

Necrosis of vessel wall with deposition of fibrinoid material*
    Leukocytoclasis
    Extravasation of erythrocytes
    Endothelial cell swelling
    Luminal thrombosis
    Edema

*Generally required for a diagnosis of vasculitis.

In discussing definitions of vascular injury, it is important to realize that vascular damage may be a primary or secondary process. Primary vascular injury implies that the vascular insult is the predominant disease process. Secondary vascular injury indicates that another disease process outside the vessels is the primary pathologic process. An example of the latter would be vessels engulfed by the necrotizing inflammation around an ulceration initiated by external insult or infection. In many instances a clear distinction between a primary versus a secondary vascular insult may not be possible. However, secondary vascular injury often is variable with sparing of some vessels in the zone of tissue injury. Other indications of secondary vascular injury include deposition of fibrinoid material at the periphery of the vessel wall or focal thrombosis without significant infiltration by inflammatory cells.

Vasculitis

The classification of vasculitis is difficult for a number of reasons.[2–5] Clinically different entities lack histologic specificity and the same disease process may show a spectrum of histologic changes depending on the stage of the disease, its level of activity, and the type of treatment that might have modified its course. Moreover, advances in research have led to redefinitions or expanded definitions of certain disease processes with subsequent loss of histologic criteria previously thought to be specific.

In an attempt to standardize nomenclature for the vasculitides, an international conference has proposed a system primarily based on the size of vessels (Table 9-3).[4] Classification based on vessel size is helpful because there is some correlation with the clinical presentation. Purpura typically reflects small-vessel injury, whereas cutaneous nodules suggest the involvement of medium-sized arteries. However, classification based on vessel size alone is of limited value in dermatopathology, since most cutaneous vasculitides affect primarily small dermal vessels. In addition, medium-sized vessel vasculitis frequently will show some degree of small-vessel involvement and vice versa. Classification by etiology or pathogenetic mechanism is difficult since much remains to be learned about the causes of vasculitis. The discovery of anti-neutrophil cytoplasmic antibodies (ANCAs) has recently led to a category of ANCA-associated vasculitis.

A practical approach (Table 9-4) to evaluating vascular inflammatory reactions is first to decide whether or not clear-cut vascular damage is present and sufficient for a designation as vasculitis, then to assess the composition of the inflammatory infiltrate (neutrophilic/leukocytoclastic vs. lymphocytic vs. granulomatous), its distribution (superficial, superficial and deep, or deep only), and to look for associated findings, such as microorganisms, that might narrow the differential diagnosis. It is important to consider the context of the histologic findings; that is, vasculitic changes may merely be secondary events in the setting of an ulcer resulting from nonvasculitic causes, such as viral infection or

TABLE 9-3

Names and Definitions of Vasculitis Adopted by the Chapel Hill (NC) Consensus Conference on the Nomenclature of Systemic Vasculitis*

Condition	Definition
	Large-Vessel Vasculitis[†] (>10 mm in diameter)
Giant cell (temporal) arteritis	Granulomatous arteritis of the aorta and its major branches, with a predilection for the extracranial branches of the carotid artery; often involved the temporal artery; usually occurs in patients older than 50 years and often is associated with polymyalgia rheumatica.
Takayasu arteritis	Granulomatous inflammation of the aorta and its major branches; usually occurs in patients younger than 50 years
	Medium-Sized Vessel Vasculitis[†] (about 0.3–10mm)
Polyarteritis nodosa (classic polyarteritis nodosa)	Necrotizing inflammation of medium-sized or small arteries without glomerulonephritis or vasculitis in arterioles, capillaries, or venules
Kawasaki disease	Arteritis involving large, medium-sized, and small arteries, and associated with mucocutaneous lymph node syndrome; coronary arteries are often involved; aorta and veins may be involved; usually occurs in children
	Small-Vessel Vasculitis[†] (10–300 μm)
Wegener's granulomatosis[‡]	Granulomatous inflammation involving the respiratory tract, and necrotizing vasculitis affecting small- to medium-sized vessels, for example, capillaries, venules, arterioles, and arteries; necrotizing glomerulonephritis is common
Churg-Strauss syndrome[‡]	Eosinophil-rich and granulomatous inflammation involving the respiratory tract and necrotizing vasculitis affecting small- to medium-sized vessels, and associated with asthma and blood eosinophilia
Microscopic polyangiitis (microscopic polyarteritis)[‡]	Necrotizing vasculitis with few or no immune deposits affecting small vessels, that is, capillaries, venules, or arterioles; necrotizing arteritis involving small- and medium-sized arteries may be present; necrotizing glomerulonephritis is very common; pulmonary capillaritis often occurs
Henoch-Schoenlein purpura	Vasculitis with IgA-dominant immune deposits affecting small vessels, that is, capillaries, venules, or arterioles; typically involves skin, gut, and glomeruli, and is associated with arthralgias or arthritis
Essential cryoglobulinemic vasculitis	Vasculitis with cryoglobulin immune deposits affecting small vessels, that is, capillaries, venules, or arterioles, and associated with cryoglobulins in serum, skin, and glomeruli often are involved

*Modified from Jennette et al.[4]
[†]Larger artery refers to the aorta and the largest branches directed toward major body regions (e.g., to the extremities and the head and neck); medium-sized artery refers to the main visceral arteries (e.g., renal, hepatic, coronary, and mesenteric arteries); and small artery refers to the distal arterial radicals that connect with arterioles (e.g., renal arcuate and interlobular arteries). Note that some small- and large-vessel vasculitides may involve medium-sized arteries; but large- and medium-sized vessel vasculitides do not involve vessels smaller than arteries.
[‡]Strongly associated with antineutrophil cytoplasmic autoantibodies. May be accompanied by glomerulonephritis and can manifest as nephritis or pulmonary-renal vasculitis syndrome.

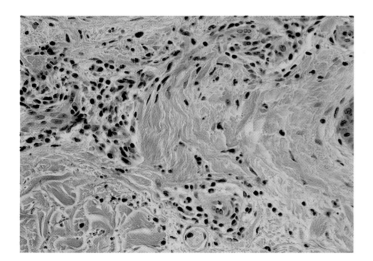

FIGURE 9-3   Inflammatory vascular reaction. Occasional perivascular karyor-rhectic debris and endothelial cell swelling are noted. However, no fibrinoid necrosis is present.

trauma. One should also realize that lesions have a life span and, for example, a lesion that shows a leukocytoclastic vasculitis at one point may show a predominantly lymphocytic or even granulomatous infiltrate at another point in time.

The following sections discuss the histologic features and differential diagnoses of vasculitides affecting the skin (focusing on small-vessel vasculitides). As suggested, classification of these disease entities into discrete categories is somewhat arbitrary, as significant overlap of features exists. It is also important to remember that some of the histologic entities discussed are not actual diseases per se but are reaction patterns to a wide variety of etiologic stimuli. As an organizing principle for discussing small-vessel vasculitides, we follow mainly morphologic criteria, that is, the composition of the inflammatory cell infiltrate (neutrophilic vs. lymphocytic vs. granulomatous). After reviewing small-vessel vasculitides and other inflammatory vascular reactions that need to be distinguished from vasculitis, we discuss ANCA-associated vasculitides and vasculitides of medium- and large-sized vessels separately.

TABLE 9-4

Approach to Vasculitis

Determine if vasculitis or vasculopathy is present or absent
Determine if primary or secondary vascular injury, if possible
Size of vessel and type
    Large
    Medium
    Small
Composition of infiltrate
    Neutrophilic/leukocytoclastic
    Lymphocytic
    Histiocytic/granulomatous
Evaluation for infection (special stains for microorganisms and
    cultures)
Additional histologic clues:
    Intravascular PAS-positive bright red material (suspicious for
        cryoprecipitates)
    Viral cytopathic changes (e.g., HSV*-associated vascular damage)
    Plasma cells (spirochetes)
    Presence of eosinophils (r/o drug, hypersensitivity reaction)
    Changes suggestive of connective tissue disease (e.g., interface
        dermatitis, dermal mucin)
    Edema (urticarial reaction)
Serologic and immunopathologic evaluation
    ANCA, ANA, rheumatoid factor, cryoglobulins, immunofluores-
        cence, and other studies for the detection of immune complexes,
        for example, IgA fibronectin aggregates
Clinical context
    Cutaneous involvement only
    Extent of systemic involvement

*HSV, herpes simplex virus

TABLE 9-5

Differential Diagnosis of Cutaneous Neutrophilic Small-Vessel Vasculitis

Infection-associated
    Bacterial
        (Gram-positive/-negative organisms, mycobacteria, spirochetes)
    Rickettsial
        Rocky Mountain spotted fever
        Scrub typhus
    Fungal
    Viral
Immunologic injury associated
    Immune-complex-mediated
        Henoch-Schoenlein purpura
        Urticarial vasculitis
        Cryoglobulinemia
        Serum sickness
        Connective tissue diseases
        Autoimmune diseases
            Infection-induced immunologic injury (e.g., hepatitis B or C,
                streptococcal)
            Drug-induced
            Paraneoplastic processes
            Behçet's disease
            Erythema elevatum diutinum
Antineutrophil antibody–associated
    Wegener's granulomatosis
    Microscopic polyangiitis
    Churg-Strauss syndrome
    Some drug-induced vasculitis
No known association
    Polyarteritis nodosa

SMALL-VESSEL NEUTROPHILIC/ LEUKOCYTOCLASTIC VASCULITIS

A large number of different disease processes can be accompanied by small-vessel vasculitis with predominantly neutrophilic infiltrates. The main diseases to be considered are listed in Table 9-5.[5]

Clinical Features The clinical manifestations are related to the depth of vascular involvement and degree of vascular injury. Vasculitis confined to the superficial dermis may exhibit lesions ranging from urticarial lesions to erythematous and purpuric macules, papules, and pustules. Involvement of the deep reticular dermal vascular plexus and subcutaneous fat by small-vessel vasculitis may result in hemorrhagic bullae, livedo reticularis, erythematous nodules, and cutaneous infarcts and necrosis. The single most common manifestation of this form of vasculitis is "palpable purpura," that is, small papules associated with purpura. The distal lower extremities are the most common location, although any site may be involved.

Histopathological Features Neutrophilic small-vessel vasculitis is a reaction pattern of small dermal vessels, almost exclusively postcapillary venules, characterized by a combination of vascular damage and an infiltrate composed largely of neutrophils (Fig. 9-4). Since there is often fragmentation of nuclei (karyorrhexis or leukocytoclasis) the term leukocytoclastic vasculitis (LCV) is used frequently. Depending on its severity, this process can be subtle and limited to the superficial dermis or pandermal and florid and associated with necrosis and ulceration. If edema is prominent, a subepidermal blister may form. In a typical case of LCV, the dermal vessels show swelling of the endothelial cells and

deposits of strongly eosinophilic strands of fibrin within and around their walls. The deposits of fibrin and the marked edema together, give the walls of the vessels a "smudgy" appearance referred to as fibrinoid degeneration (Fig. 9-1). Actual necrosis of the perivascular collagen, however, is seen primarily in conjunction with lesions of vasculitis showing ulceration. Luminal occlusion of vessels by an expanded, inflamed, edematous vessel wall or by microthrombi might be observed. The cellular infiltrate is present predominantly around or within dermal blood vessels, blurring the vascular outlines. Neutrophils and varying numbers of eosinophils and mononuclear cells are found in the infiltrate. Karyorrhectic nuclear debris, or "nuclear dust," gives these infiltrates a dirty appearance. If neutrophils are numerous and densely packed, micropustules are formed. If large pustules are found, the process can be termed pustular vasculitis (Fig. 9-5). Inflammatory cells may also be scattered throughout the upper dermis in association with fibrin deposits between and within collagen bundles. Extravasation of erythrocytes is almost invariably present.

As with any inflammatory process, the appearance of the reaction pattern depends on the stage at which the biopsy is taken. In older lesions, the number of neutrophils may be decreased and the number of mononuclear cells increased so that mononuclear cells may predominate and a designation of a lymphocytic or even granulomatous vasculitis or vascular reaction might be made.

Many infectious and immunologically mediated processes are associated with vasculitis (Table 9-5). In many cases, the pathogenesis is unknown. The final common pathway typically involves neutrophils and monocyte activation with adherence to endothelial cells, infiltration of the vessel wall, and release of lytic enzymes and toxic radicals. The

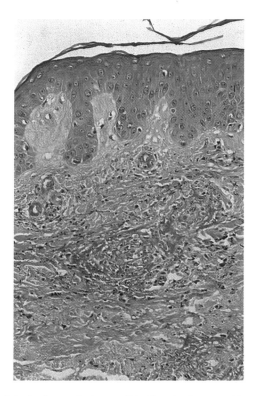

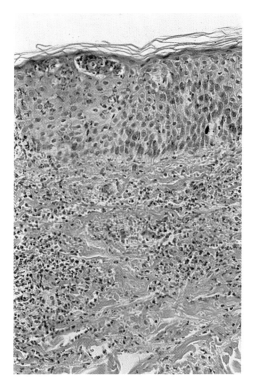

FIGURE 9-4   Leukocytoclastic vasculitis. Vascular damage with perivascular neutrophilic infiltrate and nuclear debris are seen.

FIGURE 9-5   Pustular vasculitis. Subepidermal blister formation with many polymorphonuclear cells and vascular damage are present.

cascade leading to vascular injury may be initiated by (1) the deposition of immune complexes, (2) direct binding of antibodies to antigens in vessel walls, and (3) activation of leukocytes by antibodies with specificity for leukocyte antigens (ANCAs). T cell–mediated inflammation has been implicated as an important pathogenic factor in large-vessel vasculitides, while antibody-mediated inflammation seems to play a prominent role in small-vessel vasculitis. It must be stressed that an immune-complex etiology has been invoked much too often to explain all forms of vasculitis but in particular small-vessel vasculitis. In many instances immune complexes are not the primary event in vascular injury but simply epiphenomena.

Diagnostic Approach to Neutrophilic Small-Vessel Vasculitis
The cutaneous and histologic manifestations are largely nonspecific for the small-vessel vasculitides. For example, palpable purpura may be the clinical appearance of dermal leukocytoclastic small-vessel vasculitis secondary to infection (e.g., gonococcal sepsis), immune-complex-mediated vasculitis (e.g., cryoglobulinemia or Henoch-Schoenlein purpura), ANCA-associated vasculitis (e.g., Wegener's granulomatosis), allergic vasculitis (e.g., reaction to a drug), vasculitis associated with connective tissue, or a paraneoplastic phenomenon. It is important, therefore, to search for additional histologic clues (Table 9-4) and to interpret the histologic findings only in the context of clinical information to reach an appropriate diagnosis. Often, additional laboratory data, such as from microbiologic cultures, special stains for organisms, or immunofluorescence or serologic studies, are needed. Because the treatment for infectious vasculitides is so radically different from immune-mediated diseases, the most important diagnostic step in the evaluation of a vasculitis is to rule out an infectious process. If noninfectious vasculitis is suspected, evidence for systemic vasculitis must be sought. Clinical findings, such as hematuria, arthritis, myalgia, enzymatic assays for muscle or liver enzymes, and serologic analysis for ANCAs, antinuclear antibodies, cryoglobulins, hepatitis B and C antibodies, IgA-fibronectin aggregates, and complement levels, are important to further delineate the disease process. Exposure to a potential allergen, such as

a drug, that might have elicited a hypersensitivity reaction should be sought. Evidence of an allergic pathogenesis is reassuring because it suggests that the vasculitic process may be self-limited and not associated with systemic vasculitis. As mentioned previously, it is also important to address the possibility that the histologic findings of vasculitis may be a secondary phenomenon, for example, to ulceration from localized trauma.

The following paragraphs discuss the main clinical settings in which LCV occurs.

Infectious Vasculitis
An infectious process needs to be ruled out early in the evaluation of a LCV.[2,4] Clinically, the spectrum of findings ranges from small macules to papules, pustules, and purpura. Histologically, infection-related vasculitis probably shows a greater frequency of the following changes: subcorneal, intraepidermal, and subepidermal neutrophilic pustules and abscesses, that is, pustular vasculitis; dermal infiltrates with more neutrophils relative to other cell types, such as eosinophils and lymphocytes; intravascular fibrin thrombi, some of which will contain microorganisms on occasion. Infection-related vasculitis may show a lesser degree of vascular damage compared to noninfectious vasculitides. Microorganisms may invade vessels directly or damage them by an immune-mediated mechanism. *Neisseria meningitidis* is a common cause of infectious cutaneous leukocytoclastic vasculitis. Meningococci may be found within endothelial cells and neutrophils at sites of vascular inflammation. However, other Gram-positive or -negative bacteria and fungi also may cause cutaneous small-vessel vasculitis. Staphylococcal sepsis can lead to neutrophilic vasculitis with purpura or nodular lesions that may contain microabscesses (Fig. 9-6). Rickettsial infections, such as Rocky Mountain spotted fever (RMSF), are characterized by invasion of endothelial cells by organisms causing vascular damage. Inflammation, however, often is minimal in RMSF. The Brown-Hopp stain and direct immunofluorescence microscopy may demonstrate the organism.

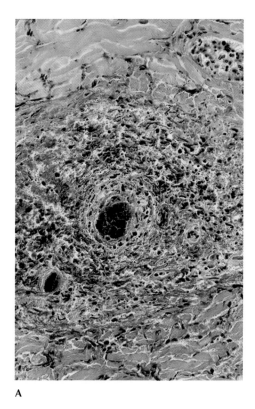

A

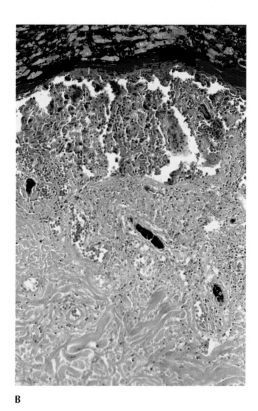

B

FIGURE 9-6 Septic vasculitis. (*A*) Small dermal vessel filled with coccal forms and surrounded by a neutrophilic infiltrate. (*B*) Gram-positive cocci are present within small dermal vessels.

ANCA-Associated Vasculitides

Microscopic polyarteritis nodosa, Wegener's granulomatosis (WG), and Churg-Strauss syndrome may be associated with LCV and are discussed at length in the following under ANCA-associated vasculitides.

Henoch-Schoenlein Purpura

Henoch-Schoenlein purpura is clinically characterized by palpable purpura of the buttocks and lower extremities, abdominal pain, and hematuria. It typically affects children (but may be seen at any age) after a streptococcal upper respiratory tract infection and usually is self-limited with a resolution expected 6 to 16 weeks after the onset of symptomatology. Complications generally arise from renal involvement.

Henoch-Schoenlein purpura (HSP) cannot be distinguished histologically from other forms of LCV, although the vascular damage in HSP often is more subtle. The limited extent of vascular damage is similar to that observed in infectious vasculitis or urticarial vasculitis (see the following), and clinical information may be needed to distinguish these entities. In HSP, immunofluorescence studies typically demonstrate deposition of IgA in capillaries. Interestingly, Jennette and colleagues have recently reported that serologic detection of IgA-fibronectin aggregates may be associated with greater likelihood of renal or systemic disease in patients with cutaneous LCV.[6]

Urticarial Vasculitis

Urticarial vasculitis is not a specific disease but is a pattern of often minimal vasculitis associated with increased vascular permeability. Persistent wheals (lasting more than 24 h by convention) with faint purpura is a typical clinical finding. Often there is residual purpura after resolution of the urticarial lesions.[7] The histology of urticarial vasculitis ranges from mild vascular damage with swollen endothelial cells and a sparse infiltrate composed of neutrophils, eosinophils, and lymphocytes to fully developed LCV (Fig. 9-7). Approximately one-third of

patients with vasculitic urticaria have decreased complement levels (hypocomplementemic vasculitis). They may have systemic findings, such as arthralgias and adenopathy. The clinical course generally is benign and episodic, lasting several months. Urticarial vasculitis occurs with some frequency in lupus erythematosus and may be the initial clinical manifestation of the disease.

Cryoglobulinemias and Other Small-Vessel Vasculitides Associated with Paraproteins

Small-vessel vasculitis may be associated with paraproteins, that is, abnormal serum proteins, including cryoglobulins, cryofibrinogens, macroglobulins, and gamma heavy chains.[2,8] Type I cryoglobulinemia most commonly leads to an occlusive vasculopathy as discussed later in this chapter, but can also be associated with LCV. Types II and III or mixed cryoglobulinemia frequently are associated with connective tissue disorders or infection, in particular, hepatitis C infection. The latter patients and patients with essential cryoglobulinemia commonly develop a cutaneous LCV but may occasionally have PAS-positive intramural and intravascular cryoprecipitate (Fig. 9-8).

Serum Sickness

This is a self-limited syndrome typified by a morbilliform urticarial eruption, fever, arthralgias-myalgias, and lymphadenopathy, occurring 7 to 10 days after a primary antigen exposure or 2 to 4 days after a repeat exposure. The offending antigen may be a drug, an arthropod sting, an antecedent infection, or therapeutic serum globulins.[9] The LCV of serum sickness is not distinctive. Drugs and sera commonly associated with serum sickness are listed in Table 9-6.

Connective Tissue Disease

Rheumatoid arthritis, lupus erythematosus, dermatomyositis, and other diseases in the spectrum of connective tissue disease may develop LCV.

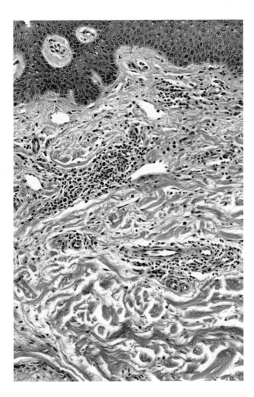

FIGURE 9-7   Urticarial vasculitis. There is dermal edema and a sparse predominantly polymorphonuclear vascular reaction.

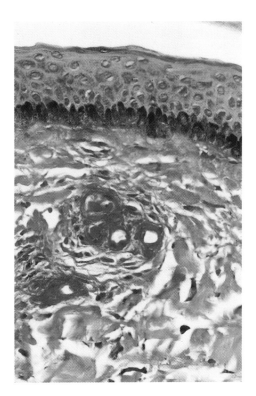

FIGURE 9-8   Cryoglobulinemia. PAS-positive bright red cryoprecipitates are seen in small superficial dermal vessels.

Clinical and serologic information is critical to arrive at the correct interpretation of the cutaneous findings in these clinical settings.

Autoimmune Diseases
Primary Sjogren's syndrome, not associated with connective tissue disease, may present with purpura in addition to ocular and glandular involvement.[2] Skin biopsy commonly shows a LCV in these cases.

Drug-Induced Vasculitis
A hypersensitivity reaction to a drug may result in a LCV or even a pustular vasculitis.[2,5] Penicillin, thiazides, and sulfonamides are the most common drugs to induce LCV (Table 9-7).

Recently, immunotherapeutic agents (IL-2, G-CSF), retinoids, and quinolones have been implicated.[10] A comprehensive list of drugs alleged to cause cutaneous vasculitis was reported by Jain.[11]

Paraneoplastic Vasculitis
A wide spectrum of vasculitic processes has been associated with neoplastic disorders.[12] The most common associations include polyarteritis nodosa with hairy cell leukemia and cutaneous small-vessel vasculitis with lymphoproliferative disorders and some carcinomas.

Behçet's Disease

Clinical Features   Behçet's disease is a multisystem disease characterized by oral aphthous lesions and at least two of the following criteria: genital aphthae, synovitis, posterior uveitis, superficial thrombophlebitis, cutaneous pustular vasculitis, and meningoencephalitis (Table 9-8).[11] It is common in the Middle East and Japan, but rare in northern Europe and the United States. An association with HLA-B51

has been reported. The clinical presentation is extremely variable and so is the vascular involvement. Vascular lesions include not only active inflammatory lesions but also aneurysms, arterial or venous occlusions, and varices. The etiology of Behçet's disease remains unknown. The vascular injury presumably is immune-mediated, since immune-

TABLE 9-6

Drugs and Sera Associated with Serum Sickness Reactions

Cefaclor
Minocycline
Penicillins
Propanolol
Streptokinase
Horse serum diphtheria antitoxin
Horse serum antithymocyte globulins
Human diploid cell rabies vaccine

*Adapted from Wollenstein and Revuf, 1995.[10]

TABLE 9-7

Common Examples of Drugs Associated with Vasculitis*

Allopurinol
Penicillin and aminopenicillins
Sulphonamides
Thiazide diuretics
Pyrazolones
Hydantoins
Propylthiouracil

*Adapted from Wollenstein and Revuf, 1995.[10]

TABLE 9-8

Behçet's Syndrome

Clinical Features

Oral and genital aphthae
Synovitis
Posterior uveitis
Meningoencephalitis
Vascular lesions: cutaneous pustular vasculitis, aneurysms, arterial
  or venous occlusions, varices
Middle East and Japan, rare in northern Europe and the United States
HLA-B51 associated

Histopathological Features

Early: Neutrophilic, fully developed necrotizing leukocytoclastic
  vasculitis or pustular vasculitis
Late: Lymphocytic and granulomatous vascular reactions

Differential Diagnosis

Infection and infectious vasculitis
Vasculitis in connective tissue disease
Paraneoplastic vasculitis
Neutrophilic vascular reactions
  Sweet's syndrome
  Pyoderma gangrenosum
Inflammatory bowel disease
Other pustular vasculitides
Bowel-bypass-associated process

TABLE 9-9

Erythema Elevatum Diutinum

Clinical Features

Red to violaceous, soft papules
Nodules and plaques evolving into brown to yellow fibrous nodules
  primarily on the extensor surfaces of the extremities

Histopathological Features

Early: LCV
Mature: Granulation tissue
  Fibrosis with vertical vessels
  A diffuse mixed-cell infiltrate with neutrophils
  Capillaries with fibrinoid necrosis or fibrous thickening
Late: Fibrosis
  Lipid material may also be present as cholesterol clefts
  Active vasculitis may still be observed

Differential Diagnosis

Early: Sweet's syndrome
  Other causes of LCV
  Rheumatoid neutrophilic dermatitis
  Bowel-bypass-associated dermatosis
  Neutrophilic drug reaction
  Behçet's syndrome
Mature: Granuloma faciale
Late: Kaposi's sarcoma
  Dermatofibroma
  Granuloma annulare

complex deposition has been demonstrated in vessel walls. A functional disorder of neutrophils also has been hypothesized.

Histopathological Features   The histopathologic spectrum of mucocutaneous inflammatory vascular lesions, depending on the stage and activity of the lesion, includes neutrophilic, lymphocytic, and granulomatous vascular reactions. Biopsy specimens of early lesions typically show a neutrophilic vascular reaction. However, fully developed necrotizing leukocytoclastic vasculitis, pustular vasculitis, or lymphocytic vasculitis may develop (Fig. 9-5).

Erythema Elevatum Diutinum (EED)

Clinical Features   This rare condition is characterized by persistent, initially red to violaceous and later brown to yellow papules, nodules, and plaques.[13] The lesions, typically located on the extensor surfaces of the extremities, initially are soft and then evolve into fibrous nodules (Table 9-9). EED probably is not a distinct disease entity, but rather a clinicopathologic reaction pattern that can be seen in a number of different disease processes, such as inflammatory bowel disease, rheumatoid arthritis, and systemic lupus erythematosus. HIV-infected patients also develop EED, which can clinically mimic Kaposi's sarcoma.[14] EED is most often associated with either a monoclonal or polyclonal gammopathy, in particular IgA hyperglobulinemia.

Histopathological Features   In its early stage, a LCV is observed. In later stages, there is formation of granulation tissue and fibrosis with a diffuse mixed-cell infiltrate with predominance of neutrophils (Fig. 9-9). The capillaries may still show deposits of fibrinoid material or merely fibrous thickening. Vertically oriented vessels, as noted in scars,

suggest EED. In the late fibrotic stage, lipid material also may be present as cholesterol clefts. Serial sections may be required to demonstrate vascular damage in late lesions.

Differential Diagnosis   Early lesions of EED show nonspecific LCV. Fully developed lesions of EED may be indistinguishable from Sweet's syndrome, rheumatoid neutrophilic dermatitis, bowel bypass–associated dermatosis, neutrophilic drug reaction, and Behçet's syndrome. Granuloma faciale may also resemble EED but is distinguished by clinical localization to the face, sparing of the superficial papillary dermis (a "grenz zone"), and prominence of eosinophils and plasma cells in addition to neutrophils. Older lesions of EED must be differentiated from Kaposi's sarcoma, dermatofibroma, or granuloma annulare. In old, fibrotic lesions of EED there is an orderly array of spindle cells and collagen bundles often parallel to the skin surface with vertically arranged capillaries similar to a scar (Fig. 9-9). Many of the spindle cells have the immunohistochemical and electron microscopic features of macrophages. Neutrophils, nuclear dust, and fibrin owing to persistent vascular damage may be present, helping to distinguish these lesions from dermatofibromas or scars. The irregularly arranged, jagged vascular spaces of Kaposi's sarcoma are absent. Focal areas of basophilic collagen caused by nuclear dust in EED can resemble the mucin seen in granuloma annulare, but do not stain with alcian blue.

Lucio's Phenomenon and Erythema Nodosum Leprosum

Lucio's phenomenon (erythema necroticans) and erythema nodosum leprosum (ENL) are syndromes that may arise during the course of lepromatous leprosy. These entities are discussed in Chapter 19. In both

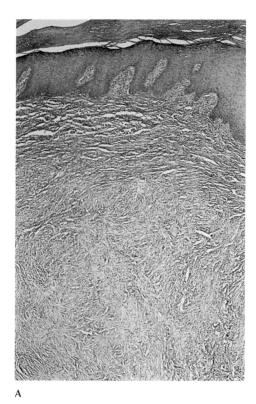

A

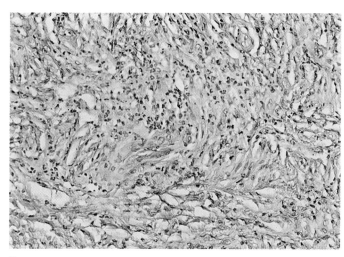

B

FIGURE 9-9 Erythema elevatum diutinum. (*A*) Fibroplasia and vertically arranged capillaries are noted. (*B*) Higher magnification shows neutrophilic infiltrates and fibroplasia.

cases, biopsies show vascular damage, including LCV. Immunoglobulins and/or complement may be demonstrated by immunofluorescence in dermal and subcutaneous blood vessels in both of these syndromes. Serologic studies detect immune complexes in these patients as well.[15] Despite these similarities, the two syndromes are distinctive.

Patients with Lucio's phenomenon are most often from Mexico or Central America. Cutaneous findings include painful bluish-red macules that form ulcers or occasionally bullae within days of onset. Nodules typically are absent.

On the other hand, in ENL, nodules are common and may be painful. They rarely ulcerate but often are accompanied by severe systemic symptoms.

Histologically, Lucio's phenomenon shows necrotizing small-vessel vasculitis, and Fite-Faraco staining reveals large aggregates of acid-fast bacilli within the vascular walls and endothelium and throughout the dermis. Some researchers have suggested that the massive endothelial mycobacterial burden in Lucio's phenomenon may directly lead to vascular damage.[16] In ENL, only occasional fragments of bacilli are identified. In Lucio's phenomenon there is ischemia and necrosis of the epidermis, dermis, and adnexal structures often with ulceration. ENL rarely ulcerates, and tissue necrosis thus is rarely observed.

Granuloma Faciale

Clinical Features   Clinically granuloma faciale (GF) presents as one or several asymptomatic, soft, brown-red, slowly enlarging papules or plaques, almost always on the face of older individuals (Table 9-10).

Histopathological Features   A dense polymorphous infiltrate is present (Table 9-10) mainly in the upper half of the dermis, but may extend into the lower dermis and occasionally even into the subcutaneous tissue. Quite characteristically, the infiltrate does not invade the epidermis or the pilosebaceous appendages but is separated from them by a nar-

row "grenz" zone of normal collagen (Fig. 9-10*A*). The pilosebaceous structures tend to remain intact. The polymorphous infiltrate consists in larger part of neutrophils and eosinophils, but mononuclear cells, plasma cells, and mast cells also are present. Vascular damage in GF is seen but often is limited, and thus perhaps GF is best termed a

TABLE 9-10

Granuloma Faciale

Clinical Features

Asymptomatic, soft, brown-red, slowly enlarging papules or plaques
   usually on the face

Histopathological Features

Dense polymorphous dermal infiltrate primarily of neutrophils but
   also eosinophils, plasma cells
Grenz zone beneath epidermis and around pilosebaceous appendages
Intact pilosebaceous structures
Subtle evidence of vascular damage
Nuclear dust
Fibrinoid material within and around vessels
Foam cells and fibrosis in older lesions

Differential Diagnosis

Infections
Erythema elevatum diutinum
Acne vulgaris or rosacea
Acute folliculitis
Other neutrophilic dermatoses
Sweet's syndrome

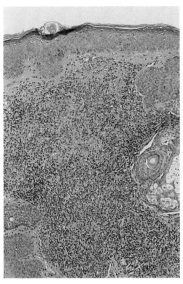

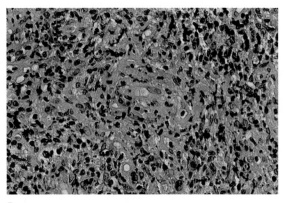

B

A

FIGURE 9-10 Granuloma faciale. (*A*) There is a small grenz zone between epidermis and dermal mixed inflammatory cell infiltrate, (*B*) composed of neutrophils, eosinophils, lymphocytes, and histiocytes.

neutrophilic vascular reaction (Fig. 9-10*B*).[17] However, vascular damage may be important to the pathogenesis of this lesion as direct immunofluorescence data suggest an immune complex–mediated event with deposition of mainly IgG in and around vessels. Frequently, the nuclei of some of the neutrophils are fragmented, especially in the vicinity of the capillaries, thus forming nuclear dust. Often, there is some evidence of vasculitis with deposition of fibrinoid material within and around vessel walls. Occasionally, some hemorrhage is noted. Foam cells and fibrosis frequently are observed in older lesions.

Differential Diagnosis Granuloma faciale can appear similar to erythema elevatinum diutinum, although a grenz zone and prevalence of eosinophils and plasma cells favors granuloma faciale. Other neutrophilic dermatoses can be distinguished from granuloma faciale by the lack of a grenz zone and clinical features. Frank leukocytoclastic vasculitis should not be seen in granuloma faciale. In acneiform lesions and folliculitides, pilosebaceous units are invaded by inflammatory cells and may be destroyed or disrupted.

Neutrophilic Vascular Reactions

In many clinical conditions, there are reactions characterized by a neutrophilic infiltrate with variable leukocytoclasis and some vascular damage (Fig. 9-11).[1] However, the extent of vascular damage is insufficient for necrotizing vasculitis, that is, fibrinoid necrosis is lacking. This histologic pattern needs to be distinguished from necrotizing vasculitis. Occasionally a neutrophilic vascular reaction may be a precursor to or associated with full-blown necrotizing vasculitis. Conditions with a neutrophilic vascular reaction that rarely develop necrotizing vasculitis generally are categorized as neutrophilic dermatoses.

The term "neutrophilic dermatosis" includes a number of conditions characterized: (1) histologically by a neutrophilic infiltrate, (2) by the lack of microorganisms on special stains and cultures, and (3) clinical improvement on systemic steroid treatment. The differential diagnosis of these lesions is outlined in Table 9-11. Vascular damage has been observed in these conditions, but it remains unclear whether the vascular injury plays an etiologic role or is merely an epiphenomenon.

ACUTE FEBRILE NEUTROPHILIC DERMATOSIS (CLASSIC SWEET'S SYNDROME)

Clinical Features Sweet described in 1964 a disease process that he termed "acute febrile neutrophilic dermatosis," that was characterized by acute onset of fever, leukocytosis, and erythematous plaques infiltrated by neutrophils.[18–20] This condition classically occurs in middle-aged women after a non-specific infection of the respiratory or gastrointestinal tract (Table 9-12). Abrupt onset of painful or tender erythematous plaques, nodules, vesicles, and pustules on the face, extremities, and rarely the trunk is characteristic. Involvement of noncutaneous sites, such as the eyes, joints, oral mucosa, as well as visceral sites (lung, liver, kidney) has been reported. A variety of disorders have been associated with neutrophilic dermatoses similar to those seen in Sweet's syndrome: myeloproliferative disorders, malignancy in general, Sjogren's syndrome, pustular psoriasis, rheumatoid arthritis, subacute lupus erythematosus, subacute thyroiditis, and pregnancy. Sweet's syndrome may be a hypersensitivity reaction, but its etiology is unknown. Current hypotheses include altered T-cell activation and altered function of neutrophils. The vascular alterations seen in Sweet's may be secondary to the massive extravasation of activated neutrophils, and a primary immune complex vasculitis is likely. Direct immunofluorescence studies are generally negative in Sweet's syndrome.[19]

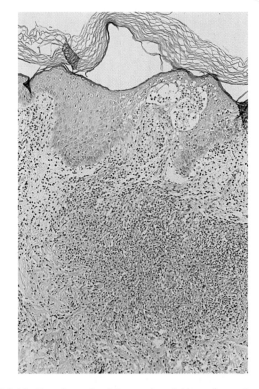

FIGURE 9-11 Bowel-associated dermatosis arthritis syndrome. In addition to a dense superficial dermal infiltrate composed of neutrophils and mild vascular damage, there is an intraepidermal pustule.

TABLE 9-12

Sweet's Syndrome

Clinical Features

Women > men
Adults, but patients of any age
Fever
Leukocytosis
Elevated erythrocyte sedimentation rate
Erythematous plaques
Vesicles and pustules of the face or extremities, rarely trunk
Response to systemic steroids or potassium iodide
Involvement of noncutaneous sites: eye, joints, oral mucosa, visceral
    sites
Associations: Gastrointestinal or upper respiratory tract infection,
    (Classic Sweet's) malignancy, especially myeloproliferative
    disorders
    Sjogren's syndrome
    Pustular psoriasis
    Rheumatoid arthritis
    Subacute lupus erythematosus
    Subacute thyroiditis
    Pregnancy

Histopathological Features

Superficial dermal neutrophilic infiltrate with some leukocytoclasis
Vascular alterations, including vasodilation and swelling of
    endothelium
Erythrocyte extravasation
Prominent edema with subepidermal blister formation

Differential Diagnosis

Infection
Vasculitis
Other neutrophilic dermatoses
Dermatitis herpetiformis or linear IgA disease
Neutrophilic drug reaction
Leukemia cutis
Suppurative panniculitides
Neutrophilic arthropod bite
Secondary syphilis

Histopathological Features   A dense bandlike and perivascular infiltrate composed largely of neutrophils occupies the superficial dermis. Some of the neutrophils may show leukocytoclasis. Lymphocytes, histiocytes, and occasionally eosinophils may be included in the infiltrate. The density of the infiltrate varies and may be limited in a small proportion of cases. Although extensive vascular damage is not a feature of Sweet's syndrome, common vascular alterations include vasodilation, swelling of endothelium, erythrocyte extravasation, and occasional karyorrhectic debris. Frank fibrinoid necrosis may occur but is rare.[20] Prominent edema of the upper dermis may result in subepidermal blister formation. As expected, the histologic appearance varies depending on the stage of the process. In later stages, lymphocytes and histiocytes may predominate.

Differential Diagnosis   Since neutrophils are prominent in Sweet's lesions, infection (bacterial or fungal especially) must be excluded by special stains and tissue cultures. Vasculitis should be considered but necrotizing vasculitis, that is, fibrinoid necrosis, should not be observed in the Sweet's or Sweet's-like lesions. The findings overlap with other neutrophilic dermatoses such as early or bullous pyoderma gangrenosum, EED, and bowel-associated dermatosis arthritis. Clinical features should distinguish these entities. A neutrophilic vesicular disease such as dermatitis herpetiformis or linear IgA disease may be suspected in cases of Sweet's syndrome with vesicle formation. Clinical features and immunofluorescence should differentiate between these possibilities. Some cases of lupus erythematosus or polymorphous light eruption with an unusual neutrophilic component may resemble Sweet's syndrome. Clinicopathologic and immunofluorescence studies should distinguish these entities. Secondary syphilis may also mimic Sweet's syndrome. Other considerations include a neutrophilic drug reaction. Leukemia cutis must be excluded in the appropriate clinical setting.

BOWEL-ASSOCIATED DERMATOSIS–ARTHRITIS SYNDROME

Clinical Features   Initially described in patients after jejunoileal bypass surgery, the syndrome has been expanded to include neutrophilic cutaneous lesions associated with many bowel diseases.[1] Patients may have inflammatory bowel disease or a blind loop after peptic ulcer surgery (Table 9-13). The cutaneous lesions are characterized by initial small macules that develop through a papular phase into pustules on a purpuric base. This evolution usually occurs within a 2-day period. The lesions commonly reach a size of 0.5 to 1.5 cm. They are typically distributed on the upper part of the body, especially arms, rather than the dependent sites of the legs and often occur in episodic, recurrent crops. Fever, myalgias, and arthralgias may accompany the disease process. An immune complex–mediated reaction triggered by intestinal bacterial-derived antigens may lead to the initiating vascular insult.

Histopathological Features   The histopathologic changes are usually those of a neutrophilic vascular reaction with minimal or no vascular damage, as seen in Sweet's syndrome and the other neutrophilic dermatoses (Fig. 9-11). However, frank necrotizing small-vessel vasculitis occasionally may be noted. In fully developed lesions, the neutrophilic infiltrate and papillary dermal edema may be florid, and subepidermal pustules form. If vascular damage is observed in such a context, the term pustular vasculitis is applied.

PYODERMA GANGRENOSUM

Pyoderma gangrenosum (PG) is included in this chapter as well, because in these and other authors' opinions, it falls within the spectrum

TABLE 9-13

Bowel-Associated Dermatosis–Arthritis Syndrome

Clinical Features

Status-postjejunoileal bypass
Inflammatory bowel disease
Blind loop syndrome
Associated fever, myalgias, and arthralgias
Episodic, recurrent crops of cutaneous lesions on upper body, especially arms
Initial small macules developing into papules, then pustules on a purpuric base

Histopathological Features

Neutrophilic dermal infiltrate with minimal or no vascular injury
Occasional frank necrotizing small-vessel vasculitis
Papillary dermal edema with subepidermal pustule formation

Differential Diagnosis

As for Sweet's-like neutrophilic dermatoses

TABLE 9-14

Pyoderma Gangrenosum

Clinical Features

Tender papulopustules or folliculitis
Ulcerated lesions with bluish borders
Vegetating lesions
Associated diseases: Inflammatory bowel disease
    Malignancy (especially leukemia)
    Connective tissue disease
    Immunologic abnormalities
    Monoclonal gammopathy (hypogammaglobulinemia, hyperimmunoglobulin E, iatrogenic immunosuppression)

Histopathological Features

Possible lymphocytic infiltrates early
Extensive neutrophilic infiltrates often involving follicular structures
Neutrophilic vascular reaction with variable vascular damage
Pustular vasculitis
Ulceration
Necrosis
Occasional granulomatous inflammation

Differential Diagnosis

Deep fungal infection
Mycobacterial lesions
Traumatic deep ulceration (factitial diseases)
Sweet's and Sweet's-like dermatosis
Subcorneal pustular dermatosis
Erythema elevatum diutinum
Bowel-associated dermatosis
Spider bite
Pustular drug reactions
Blastomycosislike pyoderma (from vegetative PG)

---

of neutrophilic dermatoses.[1] As with other neutrophilic dermatoses, it is critical to rule out an infection to arrive at the correct diagnosis.

Clinical Features   Several clinical types have been described: ulcerative PG, with an undermined border; pustular PG with discrete, painful pustules; painful bullae with progression to a superficial ulceration; vegetative PG with a painless ulcer, a nonundermined exophytic border.[21]

Classically, lesions begin as tender papulopustules or folliculitis that eventually may ulcerate. Again, as with other neutrophilic dermatoses, pyoderma gangrenosum, especially the vegetative form, may occur as an isolated cutaneous phenomenon or may be a cutaneous manifestation associated with a number of systemic disease processes, such as inflammatory bowel disease, connective tissue disease, or a lymphoproliferative disorder (Table 9-14). Bullous PG, when associated with leukemia, is an indicator of poor prognosis.[21]

Histopathological Features   The histologic findings are nonspecific and depend on the type of lesion and timing of the biopsy. The diagnosis primarily is clinical. Most authors studying early lesions have reported a primarily neutrophilic infiltrate, which frequently involves follicular structures. Other authors, however, have stated that the lesions begin with a lymphocytic reaction. Degrees of vessel involvement range from none to fibrinoid necrosis. In the majority of biopsied lesions, a neutrophilic vascular reaction is present with limited vascular damage. The infiltrate tends to be deeper and more extensive than in classic Sweet's syndrome. The pattern of pustular vasculitis may be present. Fully developed lesions show ulceration, necrosis, and a mixed inflammatory cell infiltrate. Involvement of the deep reticular dermis and subcutis may exhibit primarily mononuclear cell and granulomatous inflammatory reactions.

Lymphocytic Vasculitides and Vascular Reactions

A histologic diagnosis of a lymphocytic vasculitis may be made, if there is sufficient evidence of vascular damage and the inflammatory infiltrate is predominantly lymphocytic (Fig. 9-12). Often, the vascular damage is subtle, and in many cases there may be disagreement among dermatopathologists on whether the term vasculitis is warranted or not.[22] Clear-cut evidence of vasculitis again is indisputable, if an inflammatory infiltrate is present together with fibrinoid necrosis of the vascular wall. A diagnosis of lymphocytic vasculitis may still be rendered in the absence of fibrinoid necrosis, if the constellation of findings suggest clear-cut vascular damage. Features indicative of vascular damage include lamination of the adventitia of venules by concentrically arranged pericytes and basement membrane material, lymphocytic nuclear fragmentation, and subendothelial or intramural infiltration of arterioles by lymphocytes. Lymphocytic vasculitis, if rigidly defined as here, is rare. However, in the majority of conditions to manifest lymphocytic vasculitis, "true vasculitis" is the exception rather than the rule. In instances one might use the term lymphocytic vascular reaction to indicate that a lymphocytic infiltrate is accompanied by some, albeit limited, vascular injury.

The disease processes in which lymphocytic vasculitis is commonly seen include pernio (chilblains), arthropod bites, hypersensitivity reactions to drugs, urticarial vasculitis, pigmented purpuric dermatitis, autoimmune diseases (e.g., Sjogren's syndrome), connective tissue diseases, polymorphous light eruption, livedoid vasculitis (atrophie blanche), viral and some Rickettsial (Mediterranean spotted or boutonneuses fever) processes, and papulonecrotic tuberculid and cutaneous T-cell infiltrates, such as pityriasis lichenoides et varioliformis acuta (PLEVA), pityriasis lichenoides chronica (PLC), and lymphomatoid papulosis (LYP) (see Table 9-15). Lymphocytic vasculitis/lymphocytic vascular reactions also may be seen as a stage of leukocytoclastic vasculitis, (e.g., drug reaction), neutrophilic vascular reaction (e.g., pyoderma gangrenosum), or in a process that at other times may even be

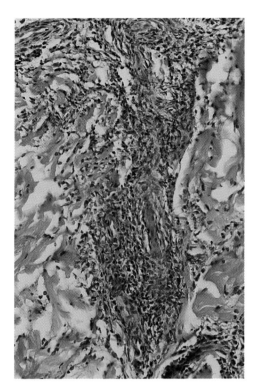

FIGURE 9-12 Lymphocytic vasculitis. A dermal vessel is affected by fibroid degeneration and infiltrated by lymphocytes.

noninflammatory and manifest perhaps as a vasculopathy (e.g., atrophie blanche). Most of these entities are discussed at greater length elsewhere in this text.

PERNIOSIS

Pernio (chilblains) is perhaps the most commonly biopsied condition in which lymphocytic vasculitis is observed. It is clinically characterized by erythematous to purpuric lesions that are prone to develop in cold damp air. Most patients are young or middle-aged women, and the most common sites involved are acral surfaces. Histologically, a biopsy typically shows a superficial and possibly deep dermal perivascular lymphocytic infiltrate accompanied by variable degrees of vascular damage,

TABLE 9-15

Differential Diagnosis of Lymphocytic Vasculitis and Lymphocytic Vascular Reactions

Pernio (chilblains)
Arthropod bites
Drug-induced or other hypersensitivity reactions
Infection-associated reactions (e.g., viral)
Connective tissue diseases
Behçet's disease
Pigmented purpuric dermatitides
Pityriasis lichenoides (acute and chronic)
Lymphomatoid papulosis
Cutaneous lymphoma
Autoimmune diseases
Polymorphous light eruption
Atrophie blanche
Infestations (e.g., scabies)

most commonly in the form of fibrin in the walls of venules. There may be associated papillary dermal edema or an interface dermatitis.

PIGMENTED PURPURIC DERMATITIS

Synonyms Purpura pigmentosa chronica, pigmented purpura, capillaritis, purpura annularis telangiectoides of Majocchi, progressive pigmentary dermatosis of Schamberg, pigmented purpuric dermatitis of Gougerot and Blum, and eczematidlike purpura of Doucas and Kapetanakis.

Table 9-16 lists the various clinical presentations that have been described. However, it is important to realize that they are closely related and often cannot be reliably distinguished on clinical and histologic grounds.[23] Their precise classification as distinct entities may not be necessary dermatopathologic practice, but some knowledge of the spectrum of their various appearances is helpful. Lichen aureus is a closely related variant, since the clinical lesion has a purpuric component and the histologic findings are similar to the other four variants of pigmented purpuric dermatitis (PPD). The general terms pigmented purpuric dermatitis, chronic purpuric dermatitis, or purpura pigmentosa chronica appear suitable for this disease spectrum. The etiology of PPD is essentially unknown, and there are probably a number of different factors involved. Some degree of venous insufficiency or stasis is present in most or many patients with PPD. In some instances PPD also may be related to drug or contact hypersensitivity. Eruptions with the clinical and histologic appearance of a pigmented purpuric dermatitis also have been associated with subsequent development of a T-cell lymphoproliferative disorder. Thus, it is possible that some PPD may be the initial manifestation of T-cell lymphoproliferative disease.[24]

Clinical Features Clinically, the primary lesion consists of discrete puncta. Telangiectatic puncta may appear as a result of capillary dilatation, and pigmentation as a result of hemosiderin deposits. In some cases, telangiectasia predominates (Majocchi's disease), and in others, pigmentation (Schamberg's disease). In Majocchi's disease, the lesions usually are irregular in shape and occur predominantly on the lower legs. In some cases, the findings may mimic those of stasis. Frequently, clinical signs of inflammation are present, such as erythema, papules, and scaling (Gougerot-Blum disease) or papules, scaling, and lichenification (eczematidlike purpura). The disorder often is limited to the lower extremities, but it may be extensive. Mild pruritus may be present but usually there are no systemic symptoms.

Lichen aureus, a localized persistent variant of PPD, most commonly involves the lower extremities but may occur anywhere.[25] One or a few patches are composed of closely set, flat papules of rust, copper, or orange color. In some cases, petechiae are present within the patches. Lichen aureus shows a male predilection and its peak incidence is in the fourth decade.

Histopathological Features The principal histological finding is a lymphocytic perivascular infiltrate limited to the papillary dermis (Fig. 9-13). The pattern of the infiltrate often is not strictly confined to the perivascular area and may infiltrate the adjacent papillary dermis between vessels. In some instances, the infiltrate may assume a bandlike or lichenoid pattern (Fig. 9-14), particularly in the lichenoid variant of Gougerot-Blum, and may involve the reticular dermis in a perivascular distribution. Epidermal alterations are variable and include parakeratosis, slight acanthosis, spongiosis, exocytosis, and basal layer vacuolopathy. Evidence of vascular damage may be present, and the reaction pattern then may be termed lymphocytic vasculopathy or vasculitis. However, the extent of vascular injury usually is mild and often insufficient to justify the term vasculitis. Vascular damage commonly

TABLE 9-16

Pigmented Purpuric Dermatoses

Clinical Features

Orange/brown pigmentation
Interspersed pinpoint (cayenne pepper–like) purpura

Histopathological Features

Superficial dermal perivascular lymphocytic infiltrate
Vascular damage (usually limited, e.g., endothelial cell swelling,
   focal karyorrhectic debris)
Extravasation of red blood cells
Hemosiderin
Occasional epidermal changes
   Spongiosis
   Basal layer vacuolopathy

Clinicopathological Patterns

Schamberg's Disease

Clinical: Male predominance
   Ill-defined lesions, pinhead-sized reddish purpura
   Predilection for lower leg
Histopathological Features: Usually moderately dense perivascular
   lymphocytic infiltrate and hemorrhage

Majocchi's Disease

Clinical: Discrete annular lesions
   Associated telangiectasia
   Often symmetric involvement beginning on lower
      extremities
Histopathological Features: Telangiectasia may be prominent

Lichenoid Dermatitis of Gougerot and Blum

Clinical: Male predominance
   Purpuric lesions with lichenoid papules, erythema
   Predilection for legs
Histopathological Features: Lichenoid, more densely cellular infiltrate

Eczematidlike Purpura of Doucas and Kapetanakis

Clinical: Papules, scale, lichenification
Histopathological Features: Spongiosis, parakeratosis more prominent

Lichen Aureus

Clinical: Male predominance
   Younger individuals
   Discrete confluent macules and papules (golden-yellow,
      dark brown, or bruiselike)
   Variable purpura
   Persistent clinical course
   Predilection for lower legs
   Usually unilateralHistopathological Features: Bandlike
lymphocytic infiltrate
   Increase in vascularity
   Prominent hemosiderin-laden macrophages
   Usually no or minimal vascular damage

Differential Diagnosis

Stasis dermatitis
Eczematous dermatitis
Drug eruptions
Abnormal T-cell process

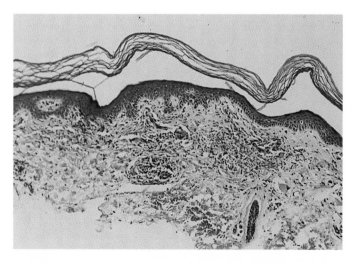

FIGURE 9-13 Pigmented purpuric dermatitis. There is a papillary dermal lymphocytic perivascular infiltrate and extravasation of red blood cells.

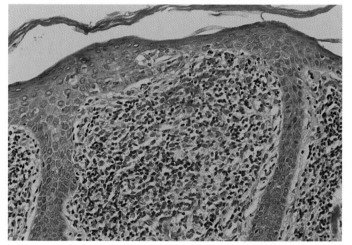

FIGURE 9-14 Pigmented purpuric dermatitis. A lichenoid infiltrate of lymphocytes and hemorrhage is seen.

consists only of endothelial cell swelling and dermal hemorrhage. Extravasated red blood cells usually are found in the vicinity of the capillaries. However, less commonly one may observe deposition of fibrinoid material in vessel walls. This may be observed particularly in pigmented purpuric lichenoid dermatitis of Gougerot and Blum and eczematidlike purpura of Doucas and Kapetanakis.

In older lesions, the capillaries often show dilatation of their lumen and proliferation of their endothelium. Extravasated red blood cells may no longer be present, but one frequently finds hemosiderin deposition. The inflammatory infiltrate is less pronounced than in the early stage.

Lichen aureus is characterized by a dense mononuclear cell in the papillary dermis, typically distributed in a bandlike fashion. Scattered within the infiltrate are hemosiderin-laden macrophages. The epidermal changes are variable, as are the other forms of PPD.

Differential Diagnosis   PPD may resemble stasis dermatitis since inflammation, dilatation of capillaries, extravasation of erythrocytes, and deposits of hemosiderin occur in both. However, stasis dermatitis usually extends much deeper into the dermis and exhibits more pronounced epidermal changes and fibrosis of the dermis than PPD. In addition, intravascular sludging of erythrocytes and fibrin are indicative of stasis. PPD also may resemble an abnormal T-cell process. Careful evaluation of the lesion for epidermotropism and lymphoid atypia, and clinicopathologic correlation are needed to arrive at the correct diagnosis. However, patients with suspicious or equivocal lesions require monitoring and possibly further evaluation to exclude a cutaneous T-cell lymphoproliferative disorder. The scarcity of Civatte bodies or basal layer vacuolopathy facilitates the differential diagnosis of lichen aureus from lichenoid dermatitides, such as lichen planus.

LYMPHOMATOID VASCULITIS AND VASCULAR REACTIONS

The terms lymphomatoid vasculitis or lymphomatoid vascular reaction may be used if there is a lymphocytic vasculitis or lymphocytic vascular reaction with significant cytologic atypia of the lymphoid cells. Although lymphoid nuclear irregularities of some degree may be present in many lymphocytic vascular reactions, probably as a reflection of an activated state of the lymphocytes, lymphoid atypia tends to be particularly well-developed in lymphomatoid papulosis (LYP) and some viral processes (Table 9-17). The differential diagnosis includes, then,

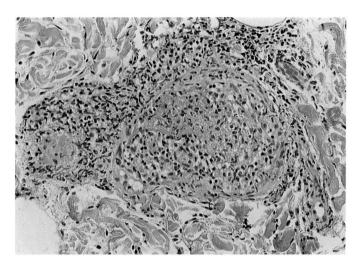

FIGURE 9-15   Granulomatous vasculitis. There is a perivascular histiocytic/granulomatous infiltrate and focal vascular damage.

vascular damage in the context of cutaneous lymphoma, such as angiocentric T-cell lymphoma and other T-cell lymphomas.[26]

Vasculitis with Granulomatosis

In the life span of many inflammatory reactions involving blood vessels, histiocytes may predominate at a certain stage and form granulomas (Fig. 9-15).[27] This may occur with little or no vascular wall damage, or it may be associated with fibrinoid degeneration of the vessel wall. In the latter situation, a granulomatous vasculitis is present. In several diseases (e.g., Takayasu's arteritis, Wegener's granulomatosis, Churg-Strauss syndrome), a granulomatous vasculitis can be found in large visceral vessels, whereas cutaneous biopsies show extravascular granulomas, leukocytoclastic vasculitis, or ulcerative lesions. Granulomatous vasculitis is only rarely seen in a cutaneous biopsy. Adequate clinical information is essential to an accurate assessment of the skin biopsy in such situations. The main disease processes that need to be considered in the differential diagnosis of a granulomatous vascular reaction are listed in Table 9-18.

TABLE 9-17

Differential Diagnosis of Lymphomatoid Vasculitis and Vascular Reaction

T-cell lymphoproliferative disorders
Peripheral T-cell lymphoma
Angiocentric T-cell lymphoma
Lymphomatoid papulosis
Lymphomatoid granulomatosis
Angioimmunoblastic lymphadenopathy
Pigmented purpuric dermatitis–like eruptions
Lymphomatoid drug eruptions
Lymphomatoid contact dermatitis
Connective tissue disease
Viral processes
Florid hypersensitivity reactions
   Arthropod bite
   Scabies infestation

TABLE 9-18

Differential Diagnosis of Vasculitides Associated with Granulomatous Inflammation

Temporal arteritis
Infection
Wegener's granulomatosis
Churg-Strauss syndrome
Polyarteritis nodosa
Cutaneous Crohn's disease
Drug reaction
Connective tissue disease
Granuloma annulare
Necrobiosis lipoidica
Paraneoplastic phenomena
Angiocentric T-cell lymphoma (lymphomatoid
   granulomatosis)
Erythema nodosum and erythema nodosumlike reactions

ANCA-Associated Systemic Vasculitides

A major recent advance in our understanding and classification of vasculitides has been the recognition that antineutrophil cytoplasmic antibodies (ANCAs) are associated with certain vasculitides.[27–29] Indirect immunofluorescence assays reveal two staining patterns: cytoplasmic (c-ANCA) and perinuclear (p-ANCA). The majority of c-ANCAs react with proteinase 3, and most p-ANCAs are specific for myeloperoxidase (MPO). Although a number of different vasculitic processes can be associated with ANCA, these antibodies are especially helpful in the differential diagnosis of Wegener's syndrome (WG), Churg-Strauss syndrome (CSS), and microscopic polyarteritis (MPA). WG is usually associated with c-ANCA, MPA with either p- or c-ANCA, and CSS with p-ANCA (Table 9-19). ANCAs may play a role in inducing vasculitis by activating circulating neutrophils and monocytes, causing them to adhere to vessels, degranulate, and release toxic metabolites, thereby causing vascular injury. On the other hand, ANCA may be an epiphenomenon unrelated to the pathogenesis of these diseases. CSS and WG most often are classified as granulomatous vasculitides in textbooks. However, the most common cutaneous histologic finding in both diseases is leukocytoclastic vasculitis. The granulomatous inflammation seen in the skin usually is not angiodestructive. Although MPA does not have a significant granulomatous component, it is discussed here, since there is significant overlap, histologically and clinically, with WG and CSS patients who show an extensive vasculitic diathesis.

CHURG-STRAUSS SYNDROME

Synonyms   Allergic granulomatosis.

The classic clinicopathologic syndrome of Churg-Strauss is characterized by asthma, fever, hypereosinophilia, eosinophilic tissue infiltrates, necrotizing vasculitis, and extravascular granuloma formation (Table 9-20). Short of an autopsy, the classic pathologic triad of necrotizing vasculitis, eosinophilic tissue infiltration, and extravascular granulomas is extremely difficult to demonstrate because of the focality of the process.[30] A broader definition of CSS requiring asthma, hypereosinophilia $>1.5 \times 10^9$/L, and systemic vasculitis involving two or more extrapulmonary organs has been suggested. There is considerable overlap of this disease process with other systemic vasculitides, such as polyarteritis nodosa (PAN) and WG, and with other inflammatory disorders associated with eosinophils, such as eosinophilic pneumonitis. Hence, there is some confusion surrounding the definition of this syndrome and even its very legitimacy.

Clinical Features   Despite multiple reports on the CSS, it appears to be rare. Between 1950 and 1974, only 30 cases were identified at the Mayo clinic.[31] The incidence of CSS is similar in males and females. It typically presents in the third and fourth decade of life. Patients tend to move through several phases of disease development, from nonspecific

TABLE 9-20

Churg-Strauss Syndrome

Clinical Features

Men and women equally affected 20 to 40 years of age
Asthma
Allergic rhinitis
Eosinophilia
Petechiae, extensive ecchymoses
Necrotic ulcers
Cutaneous-subcutaneous nodules

Histopathological Features

Leukocytoclastic vasculitis
Tissue eosinophilia
Churg-Strauss granulomata (extravascular granulomas with
     numerous eosinophils)

Differential Diagnosis

Infection
Connective tissue disease
Wegener's granulomatosis
Microscopic polyarteritis nodosa

signs and symptoms such as asthma and allergic rhinitis (prodromal phase), to a phase of hypereosinophilia with eosinophilic pneumonitis or gastroenteritis (second phase), and finally, systemic vasculitis (third phase). The three disease phases are not always sequential, and may on occasion occur simultaneously.

Two types of cutaneous lesions occur in about two-thirds of patients: (1) hemorrhagic lesions varying from petechiae to extensive ecchymoses, sometimes accompanied by necrotic ulcers and often associated with areas of erythema (similar to Henoch-Schoenlein purpura); and (2) cutaneous-subcutaneous nodules. The most common sites of skin lesions are the extremities, followed by the trunk. In some instances, the petechiae and ecchymoses are generalized. A limited form of allergic granulomatosis is characterized by preexisting asthma and lesions confined to the conjunctiva, skin, and subcutaneous tissue.

The internal organs most commonly involved are the lungs, the gastrointestinal tract, and less commonly, the peripheral nerves and heart. In contrast to PAN, renal failure is rare.

Diagnostically helpful laboratory findings include an elevated peripheral eosinophil count. Patients with active CSS have anti-MPO (p-ANCA) in the majority of cases (approx 70%). The levels of anti-MPO have been found to correlate with disease activity. Anti-MPO are less often found in patients with limited forms of the disease. Antiserine proteinase antibodies (c-ANCA) are uncommon in patients with CSS (approx 7%).

Histopathological Features   The areas of cutaneous hemorrhage typically show small-vessel LCV often with numerous eosinophils. In some instances, the dermis shows a distinctive granuloma typified by radially arranged histiocytes and multinucleated giant cells centered around degenerated collagen fibers (Fig. 9-16). The central portion of these granulomas contain not only degenerated collagen fibers but also disintegrated cells, particularly eosinophils, in great numbers. These granulomas initially were thought to be characteristic and were referred to as Churg-Strauss granulomas. However, they are not always present and are not a prerequisite for the diagnosis. Moreover, recent studies have shown that similar findings also can be observed in other disease processes, such as connective tissue disease (rheumatoid arthritis and

TABLE 9-19

ANCA-Positive Vasculitides

Disease process	Antimyeloperoxidase (p-ANCA)	Antiserine proteinase (c-ANCA)
Wegener's granulomatosis	Rare (5%)	Common (80%)
Microscopic polyarteritis	Common (50–60%)	Common (45%)
Churg-Strauss syndrome	Common (70%)	Rare (7%)

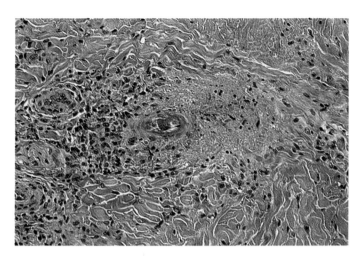

FIGURE 9-16 Palisading necrotizing granuloma. An area of fibrinoid dermal necrosis is surrounded by epithelioid histiocytes.

lupus erythematosus), Wegener's granulomatosis, PAN, lymphoproliferative disorders, subacute bacterial endocarditis, chronic active hepatitis, and inflammatory bowel disease (Crohn's disease and ulcerative colitis).[32]

The extravascular granulomas may involve subcutaneous fat where they may attain considerable size through expansion and confluence, thus giving rise to the clinically apparent cutaneous-subcutaneous nodules. The palisading granulomas are embedded in a diffuse inflammatory exudate rich in eosinophils.

Differential Diagnosis CSS is a clinicopathologic entity whose diagnosis depends on the presence of respiratory disease, in particular, a history of asthma, p-ANCA-positivity, and particular histologic features such as extravascular granulomas described earlier, necrotizing vasculitis, and eosinophilia. The differential diagnosis includes all varieties of small-vessel LCV but in particular, PAN, MPA, and WG, and the conditions mentioned earlier that may show extravascular necrotizing granulomas. Although Churg and Strauss initially characterized allergic granulomatosis as a "strikingly uniform clinical picture," there is less clarity today about its distinction from other vasculitic processes, particularly WG and PAN.[33] It is well known that particular patients may shift from one disease category to another over time.

WEGENER'S GRANULOMATOSIS

Wegener's granulomatosis was first recognized as a distinct clinicopathologic disease process in 1936, when Wegener reported three patients with a "peculiar rhinogenic granulomatosis."[34] Goodman and Churg summarized postmortem studies in 1954, from which the classic triad of this clinicopathologic complex evolved, which is characterized by (1) necrotizing and granulomatous inflammation of the upper and lower respiratory tracts, (2) glomerulonephritis, and (3) systemic vasculitis.[35] Limited variants of the disease involving the respiratory tract only have been described. In the protracted, superficial variant, ulcerated, necrotizing lesions remain localized to the mucosa and skin for many years, with pulmonary and renal involvement eventually developing in some of these patients.

With the recognition of an association between ANCAs and WG, the concept of WG has been modified and the necessity of demonstrating granulomatous inflammation as a prerequisite for the diagnosis of WG has been challenged. A less restrictive definition has been proposed (The Third International Workshop on ANCA) as Wegener's vasculitis.[4] Subsumed under this less restrictive category are ANCA-positive

---

TABLE 9-21

Wegener's Granulomatosis

Clinical Features

Sinusitis
Recurrent pneumonitis
Glomerulonephritis
Myalgia, arthralgia, fever
Palpable purpura, nodules, and ulcers

Histopathological Features of Skin Lesions

Leukocytoelastic vasculitis (LCV)
Granulomatous inflammation with suppuration and necrosis
Cutaneous extravascular necrotizing granuloma
Erythema elevatum diutinum, granuloma annulare, or erythema nodosum
Nonspecific acute or chronic inflammatory lesions and ulcerations

Differential Diagnosis

Vasculitic component
   Microscopic polyarteritis (MPA), Churg-Strauss syndrome (CSS), other causes of LCV
   Metastatic Crohn's disease
Granulomatous component
   Granulomatous infections
   CSS
   Sarcoidosis
   Granulomatous rosacea
   Foreign body reactions
   Ruptured cysts

patients with clinical presentations of WG, such as sinusitis, pulmonary infiltrates, and nephritis, and documented necrotizing vasculitis, but without biopsy-proven granulomatous inflammation. Both classic WG and Wegener's vasculitis are considered different manifestations of Wegener's syndrome, a more generic term proposed by the Working Classification of ANCA-Associated Vasculitides.

Clinical Features Two-thirds of patients with WG are male, and the mean age of diagnosis is 35 to 54 years.[35] The vast majority of patients are Caucasians. The clinical presentation is extremely variable, ranging from an insidious course with a prolonged period of nonspecific constitutional symptoms and upper respiratory tract findings to abrupt onset of severe pulmonary and renal disease (Table 9-21). The most commonly involved anatomic sites include the upper respiratory tract, lower respiratory tract, and kidney. Other organs systems that are commonly affected include joints and skin. Migratory, polyarticular arthralgia of large and small joints are found in up to 85 percent of patients with WG. Cutaneous involvement is extremely variable in different series, ranging from less than 20 percent to over 50 percent of patients. Cutaneous manifestations include macular erythematous eruptions, palpable purpura, papulonecrotic lesions, and nodules with and without ulceration. Cutaneous lesions may be the first indication of WG.

Histopathological Features The majority of skin biopsies in patients with WG are nonspecific, as for example, perivascular lymphocytic infiltrates.[37] However, in about 25 to 50 percent of patients, the histopathologic findings are fairly characteristic. The most frequent reaction patterns that are distinctive include necrotizing/leukocytoclastic small-vessel vasculitis and granulomatous inflammation. The small-vessel vasculitis is characterized by neutrophilic infiltrates and is indistinguishable from LCV secondary to many other processes (Fig. 9-17).

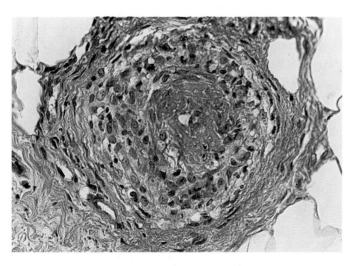

FIGURE 9-17 Wegener's granulomatosis. A subcutaneous small artery shows fibrinoid necrosis and a florid inflammatory cell infiltrate.

Eosinophils can be as numerous in LCV lesions from patients with WG as in those with CSS. The granulomatous reactions contain histiocytes, lymphocytes, and giant cells and show suppurative necrosis. Minute foci of tissue necrosis are surrounded by histiocytes and are similar to lesions described in open lung biopsies from WG patients. True granulomatous vasculitis (Fig. 9-15), erythema elevatum diutinum, and erythema-nodosum-like reaction patterns have been described and may be coincidental. The palisading granulomas of WG resemble those of Churg-Strauss syndrome, except that the center of the WG granuloma contains necrobiotic collagen and basophilic fibrillar necrotic debris admixed with neutrophils. Tissue eosinophilia and eosinophilic debris are observed less frequently in WG. These lesions, also referred to as cutaneous extravascular necrotizing granuloma or, confusingly, Churg-Strauss granuloma, may be associated with systemic vasculitis, connective tissue disease, or lymphoproliferative disease.[32] In a recent clinicopathologic study of 46 patients with WG, the authors suggested that the cutaneous findings characteristic of WG might correlate to some degree with disease activity, distribution, and course of the disease. The patients with leukocytoclastic vasculitis of the skin tended to have a more aggressive course than patients with cutaneous granulomatous inflammation. LCV commonly presented as palpable purpura or papulonecrotic lesions on the lower extremities. Its presence was often associated with active multiorgan disease. However, patients with cutaneous LCV and limited disease forms also have been reported.

Patients with granulomatous inflammation tended to be younger, had visceral manifestations of WG less frequently, and their disease progressed at a slower rate than patients with leukocytoclastic vasculitis. However, the presence of granulomatous inflammation does not assure a benign course, since such findings also have been reported in patients with severe multiorgan WG. Both granulomatous inflammation and necrotizing vasculitis have been reported to coexist frequently in the context of cutaneous ulcers, which may show secondary vascular damage.

Differential Diagnosis   The histologic differential diagnosis includes numerous entities causing LCV and palisading granulomas. Infective processes causing granulomatous inflammation and possibly vasculitis should be excluded; the list of such agents is large and includes mycobacteria, deep fungi, viruses, and syphilis, among others. Other conditions causing LCV and granulomatous reactions include CSS,

metastatic Crohn's disease, and sarcoidosis. Tightly packed, nonnecrotizing granulomas characteristic of sarcoid are not typical of WG.

The distinction between WG and these other diseases relies primarily on the clinical findings. In contrast to WG, CSS is associated with asthma, lacks lesions in the upper respiratory tract, rarely shows severe renal involvement, and typically is accompanied by eosinophilia or eosinophilic infiltrates and p-ANCA-positivity.

MICROSCOPIC POLYARTERITIS NODOSUM

Synonyms   Microscopic polyangiitis, ANCA-positive leukocytoclastic angiitis, MPA.

Microscopic polyarteritis nodosa, also termed MPA, is a systemic small-vessel vasculitis that is typically associated with focal necrotizing glomerulonephritis with crescents. In contrast, ischemic glomerular lesions are common, but glomerulonephritis is rare in classic polyarteritis nodosa.

Clinical Features   The majority of patients with MPA are male and over 50 years of age (Table 9-22). Prodromal symptoms include fever, myalgias, arthralgias, and sore throat. The most common clinical feature is renal disease, manifesting as microhematuria, proteinuria, or acute oliguric renal failure. Although cutaneous involvement is rare in classic PAN, 30 to 40 percent of patients with MPA have skin changes. These include palpable purpura, splinter hemorrhages, and ulcerations. Tender erythematous nodules and livedo reticularis typical of classic PAN are exceedingly rare in MPA. Pulmonary involvement without granulomatous tissue reaction occurs in approximately one-third of patients. Other organ systems (e.g., gastrointestinal tract, central nervous system, serosal and articular surfaces) also may be affected, but this is less common. Serious clinical complications usually arise from renal and pulmonary disease.

Histopathological Features   A leukocytoclastic vasculitis primarily affecting arterioles, venules, and capillaries is observed (Fig. 9-17). Necrotizing vasculitis of medium-sized arteries typical of classic PAN is present on occasion (Fig. 9-1). Cutaneous granulomatous inflammation is not a feature of MPA.

TABLE 9-22

Microscopic Polyarteritis Nodosa (MPA)

Clinical Features

Males over 50 years of age
Virallike prodrome
Renal disease:
   Microhematuria, proteinuria, or acute oliguric renal failure
Cutaneous symptoms:
   Palpable purpura, splinter hemorrhages, and ulcerations
   Pulmonary involvement without granulomas

Histopathological Features

Leukocytoelastic vasculitis (LCV)

Differential Diagnosis

Wegener's granulomatosis
Churg-Strauss syndrome
PAN
Other causes of LCV

Differential Diagnosis At present pathologists continue to distinguish classic and microscopic polyarteritis, although the rationale for this separation has been challenged by an increasing number of cases with overlapping features. This has led to the introduction of the term "overlapping syndrome of vasculitis" to encompass vasculitis affecting both small and medium-sized arteries.[38] For patients presenting with cutaneous small-vessel vasculitis only (no arteriolar or arterial involvement) and elevated ANCA titers, Jennette has proposed the term ANCA-positive leukocytoclastic angiitis.[4] However, the differential diagnosis of ANCA-positive, pauci-immune leukocytoclastic angiitis still includes MPA, since the failure to detect arteriolar involvement could be related to sampling error. The differential diagnosis also includes Wegener's vasculitis and other small-vessel vasculitides that are occasionally ANCA-positive, such as certain drug reactions. Some are of the opinion that the distinction of MPA from WG is largely artificial.[39]

VASCULITIS OF MEDIUM- AND LARGE-SIZED VESSELS

This section on vasculitides concludes with a brief review of conditions that preferentially affect medium- and large-sized vessels. Wegener's granulomatosis and Churg-Strauss syndrome can affect medium-sized arteries, but they have been discussed previously as ANCA-associated vasculitis. The remaining topic for discussion include polyarteritis nodosa and processes that characteristically affect visceral vessels or large veins with rather nonspecific cutaneous findings.

Polyarteritis Nodosa

Synonyms Periarteritis nodosa, PAN.

The first report of PAN in 1885 describes a 27-year-old man with fever, abdominal pain, muscle weakness, peripheral neuropathy, and renal disease.[40] The fatal illness was termed periarteritis nodosa (PAN), referring to nodular protuberances along the course of medium-sized muscular arteries. Ferrari in 1903 emphasized the characteristic presence of inflammatory cells within all levels of the affected vessels (panarteritis) and suggested the term polyarteritis instead of periarteritis.[41]

The pathogenesis of PAN is poorly understood. Direct immunofluorescence testing of skin lesions of PAN shows some immune deposits in dermal vessels. However, they may reflect a secondary event after vascular injury from another cause. PAN may be related to the ANCA-associated vasculitides previously discussed. However, the relationship between ANCA and PAN is still not clearly delineated. Patients with exclusively medium-sized (classic PAN) may be ANCA-negative, whereas those with both medium-sized vessel arteritis and small-vessel arteritis (as seen in microscopic polyarteritis nodosa) sometimes are ANCA-positive.[4]

Clinical Features PAN is more common in men than women, usually occurring between the ages of 20 and 60 years. Clinical manifestations are protean and may reflect the systemic nature of the illness or infarction of specific organs (Table 9-23). Fever, malaise, weight loss, weakness, myalgias, arthralgias, and anorexia are common systemic symptoms. Renal involvement, present in about 75 percent of patients, is the most common cause of death. Hematuria, proteinuria, hypertension, and azotemia may result from both infarction owing to disease of renal arteries or focal, segmental necrotizing glomerular lesions suggesting involvement of small vessels. Acute abdominal crises, strokes, myocardial infarction, and mononeuritis multiplex result from involvement of

---

TABLE 9-23

Polyarteritis Nodosa

Clinical Features

Fever, malaise, weight loss, weakness, myalgias, arthralgias, and anorexia
Hematuria, proteinuria, hypertension, and azotemia
Acute abdominal crises, strokes, myocardial infarction, and mononeuritis multiplex
Subcutaneous nodules that may pulsate or ulcerate
Ecchymoses and gangrene of fingers and toes
Livedo reticularis, bullae, papules, scarlatiniform lesions, and urticaria

Histopathological Features

Early: Leukocytoclastic vasculitis of small- to medium-sized arteries
Late: Intimal proliferation and thrombosis, chronic inflammatory infiltrate, fibrosis

Differential Diagnosis

Infection (bacterial, e.g., *Pseudomonas*; viral, e.g., hepatitis B or HIV)
Connective tissue disease (lupus erythematosus, rheumatoid arthritis)
Vasculitides with granulomatosis
Wegener's granulomatosis
Churg-Strauss syndrome

---

the relevant arteries. Arteriography of visceral arteries often shows multiple aneurysms that are highly suggestive of PAN. Symptoms such as asthma, Löffler's syndrome, and rashes may be related to the hypereosinophilia sometimes seen in these patients. Cutaneous manifestations include subcutaneous nodules that may pulsate or ulcerate, ecchymoses, and gangrene of fingers and toes. Livedo reticularis, bullae, papules, scarlatiniform lesions, and urticaria occur in some patients. It is still an unresolved issue whether a form of PAN exists that is limited to the skin.[42]

Histopathological Features Although affected skin often shows only a small-vessel necrotizing vasculitis, the characteristic lesion of classic PAN is a panarteritis involving medium-sized and small arteries in visceral sites (Fig. 9-17). A panarteritis of the larger arteries in deeper dermis or panniculus most commonly is observed in patients presenting with cutaneous nodules. Lesions typically are in different stages of development. Early lesions show degeneration of the arterial wall with deposition of fibrinoid material. There is partial to complete destruction of the external and internal elastic laminae. An infiltrate present within and around the arterial wall is composed largely of neutrophils showing evidence of leukocytoclasis, although eosinophils often are admixed. At a later stage, intimal proliferation and thrombosis lead to complete occlusion of the lumen with subsequent ischemia and possibly ulceration. The subacute infiltrate often contains lymphocytes, histiocytes, and some plasma cells. The healing stage is distinguished by a fibroblastic proliferation extending into the perivascular area. The small vessels of the middle and upper dermis often show a nonspecific lymphocytic perivascular infiltrate.

Differential Diagnosis Vasculitis indistinguishable from PAN may be observed in infection (bacterial, e.g., *Pseudomonas*; viral, e.g., hepatitis B or HIV), connective tissue disease (lupus erythematosus, rheumatoid arthritis), Wegener's granulomatosis, Churg-Strauss syndrome, and in other settings without explanation, for example, acute myelogenous leukemia. As with all vasculitides, one must systematically evaluate the disease process by ruling out infection (special stains, cultures, other studies), specific systemic diseases such as lupus erythematosus, and then document the extent of systemic involvement and presence of other findings (serologic and other laboratory as well as clinical findings).

Buerger's Disease

Synonym   Thromboangiitis obliterans.

Clinical and Histopathological Features   This is a distinctive but rare condition observed most frequently in men ranging in age from 20 to 40 years who are tobacco smokers (Table 9-24). This disorder is characterized by a painful segmental, thrombosing inflammatory process of intermediate and small arteries and sometimes veins. The vessels of the upper and lower extremities primarily are affected. The cutaneous findings are manifestations of ischemic injury, and include claudication, cyanosis, painful ulcers, and gangrene. The ischemic injury often is so extreme that amputation is needed to control the process.

Active lesions show luminal thrombotic occlusion, a mixed inflammatory cell infiltrate of the vessel wall, and luminal microabscesses that are thought to be characteristic. A granulomatous reaction may be present as well.

Differential Diagnosis   The histologic findings in Buerger's disease have been thought to be unique; however, they are likely to be nonspecific and probably occur in other processes, including nonspecific thrombosis and inflammation of intermediate-sized arteries and veins. Peripheral vascular disease from arteriosclerosis must be excluded.

Superficial Thrombophlebitides

Synonyms   Mondor's disease, nonsclerosing lymphangitis of the penis.

Clinical Features   Superficial thrombophlebitis of small- to medium-sized veins may be seen at many anatomic sites, but especially the lower extremities. The clinical presentation usually includes tenderness and erythema of the overlying skin. Some thrombophlebitides occurring at particular anatomic sites have been given specific names. Mondor's disease is a thrombophlebitis of the subcutaneous veins of the chest region and often is manifested clinically by a cordlike induration.[42] It usually is not accompanied by general symptoms and tends to resolve within weeks. In the majority of cases, the etiology remains unknown. However, Mondor's disease has been associated with trauma, connec-

---

TABLE 9-24

Buerger's Disease, Thromboangiitis Obliterans

Clinical Features

Men > women, 20 to 40 years of age
Smokers
Lower extremities > upper extremities
Painful ulcers, gangrene

Histopathological Features

Mixed inflammatory cell infiltrates of intermediate and small-vessel
   walls with microabscesses ± a granulomatous reaction
Luminal thrombi

Differential Diagnosis

Infection

---

tive tissue disease, rarely with breast carcinoma, and a variety of other conditions. Nonvenereal sclerosing lymphangitis of the penis arises acutely and has features similar to Mondor's disease. Despite the name, the involved vessel is most likely a vein, and some refer to this condition as Mondor's phlebitis of the penis.[44] Clinically, a firm, tender, wormlike cord lying just behind the corona of the glans penis in the coronary sulcus suddenly appears. Resolution usually occurs in 4 to 6 weeks regardless of therapy. Proposed etiologic factors include trauma during coitus and infectious agents such as viruses or chlamydiae.

Histopathological Features   In early lesions, a polymorphonuclear infiltrate may be present. However, the majority of biopsied lesions show subcutaneous veins with organizing thrombi and fibrous thickened walls, giving them a cordlike appearance at scanning magnification.

Kawasaki Disease

Synonym   Mucocutaneous lymph node syndrome.

Clinical Features   Kawasaki disease is a necrotizing arteritis that usually affects young children with a peak age incidence at 1 year.[45] Mucocutaneous findings are common and include a polymorphous exanthematous macular rash, conjunctival congestion, dry reddened lips, "strawberry tongue," oropharyngeal reddening, and swelling of the hands and feet, especially the palms and soles. There is typically an associated nonpurulent cervical lymphadenopathy. Desquamation of the skin of the fingers typically occurs after 1 to 2 weeks, often followed by thrombocytosis. The most serious clinical complications are related to arteritis and thrombosis of coronary arteries.

Histopathological Features   Cutaneous vasculitis is rare. The macular rash usually is accompanied by nonspecific histologic changes, such as a perivascular infiltrate of lymphocytes and histiocytes. Characteristic arteritis typically is seen in visceral sites, such as the coronary arteries.

Takayasu's Arteritis

Synonyms   Pulseless disease.

Clinical Findings   Takayasu's arteritis primarily affects the aorta and its main branches in young Asian women (Table 9-25). Chronic granulomatous vascular inflammation with fibrosis and thickening of the vessel walls is the predominant pathologic feature. The resulting vascular stenosis leads to symptoms such as upper extremity claudication, visual symptoms, and Raynaud's phenomenon. Arterial bruits and diminished arterial pulses are found. Cutaneous findings include erythema nodosum–like nodules and ulcers with features of pyoderma gangrenosum.

Histopathological Features   Nodular cutaneous lesions potentially related to Takayasu's disease have shown necrotizing vasculitis of both small and large vessels, granulomatous vasculitis, acute panniculitis, and sarcoidal noncaseating tuberculoid granulomas.[46] A distinctive granuloma similar to the Churg-Strauss granuloma has been also described in a skin nodule in Takayasu's arteritis (see the preceding). The latter lesion was characterized by radially arranged histiocytes and multinucleated giant cells centered around degenerated collagen fibers and has been referred to as "cutaneous extravascular granuloma."

TABLE 9-25

Takayasu's Arteritis

Clinical Features

Young Asian women
Upper extremity claudication
Visual symptoms and Raynaud's phenomenon
Arterial bruits and diminished arterial pulses
Cutaneous findings:
    Erythema nodosum–like nodules
    Ulcers with features of pyoderma gangrenosum and papular lesions

Histopathological Features

Necrotizing vasculitis of both small and large vessels
Granulomatous vasculitis
Sarcoidal noncaseating tuberculoid granulomas
Acute panniculitis
Cutaneous extravascular granulomas

Differential Diagnosis

Infection similar to that described under Wegener's granulomatosis

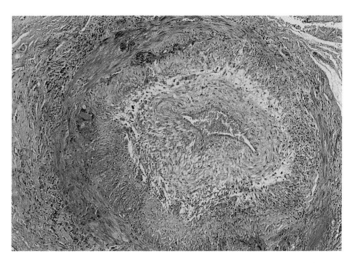

FIGURE 9-18   Giant cell arteritis. A biopsy of the temporal artery shows a panmural predominantly mononuclear infiltrate with giant cells and fragmentation of elastic fibers (elastic stain).

Differential Diagnosis   None of the pathologic findings in the skin are specific for Takayasu's arteritis. A host of vasculitic or granulomatous diseases are included in the differential diagnosis of the lesions described earlier. Infection must be excluded. The appropriate clinical context is required before the possibility of Takayasu's arteritis can be entertained.

Temporal Arteritis

Synonyms   Giant cell arteritis, giant cell arteritis of the elderly, cranial arteritis, Horton's disease.

Clinical Features   Temporal arteritis affects primarily large or medium-sized arteries in the temporal region of elderly people. Other arteries of the head and neck, particularly retinal arteries, may be involved and cases with generalized arterial involvement have been described. The clinical presentation may include pain and tenderness of the forehead or scalp and possible sudden visual impairment. There may be systemic symptoms, such as fever and malaise. Erythema and edema of the skin overlying the involved arteries may be noted, and, occasionally, ulcerations of the scalp occur.[47] The involved artery may be palpable. Clinical laboratory findings include a significantly elevated erythrocyte sedimentation rate (ESR) and sometimes a normochromic, microcytic, or normocytic anemia. Although the clinical presentation strongly suggests the diagnosis, a biopsy often is performed for confirmation prior to the initiation of systemic steroid therapy. Long segments of the artery, preferably nodular or tender areas, should be biopsied since skip lesions are common.

Histopathological Features   Involved arteries show partial destruction by an inflammatory infiltrate composed mainly of lymphocytes and macrophages (Fig. 9-18). In some instances neutrophils may be present, but this finding should not dissuade one from the diagnosis. The inflammatory infiltrate may extend throughout the entire arterial wall but is unevenly distributed and step sections often are needed for identification. Some of the macrophages are multinucleated and intimately associated with the internal elastic lamina. Fragmentation of the elastic lam-

ina and elastophagocytosis by the multinucleated giant cells may even be observed. An elastica–van Gieson stain greatly facilitates the evaluation of elastic fibers. Depending on the stage of the disease process, giant cells may not be present. In late stages, there only may be thickening of the intima by deposits of fibrinlike material and myofibroblastic proliferation with subsequent luminal narrowing or obliteration.

Differential Diagnosis   Not all cases of arteritis involving the temporal artery represent examples of temporal arteritis. Biopsy of the temporal artery may show necrotizing vasculitis, such as polyarteritis nodosa, hypersensitivity angiitis, or vasculitis associated with infection or connective tissue disease. Serologic studies, the exclusion of infection, and the appropriate clinical findings along with the histopathologic requisite features lead to the correct diagnosis.

VASCULOPATHIC REACTIONS

A vasculopathic reaction as defined in Table 9-1 refers to vascular damage without inflammation. Conditions leading to vascular occlusion, alterations of the vessel wall, or to structural deficiencies of the perivascular connective tissue can be classified as vasculopathies and are discussed in the following.

Vascular Occlusive Conditions

In these conditions, thrombi are present in blood vessels of dermis and subcutis. There may be little or no associated inflammation. In general, extensive infarctions and necrosis may be more characteristic of some coagulopathies, cryoglobulinemias, early livedoid vasculitis (atrophie blanche), cholesterol emboli, and calciphylaxis. Livedo reticularis and late atrophie blanche present a more fibrotic chronic picture. Usually, the various conditions can be distinguished by other distinctive pathologic findings, such as calcification in calciphylaxis, needle-shaped crystals in cholesterol emboli, or the wedge-shaped dermal alteration of Degos' syndrome. Characteristic clinical findings or serologic tests (cryoglobulinemia, cryofibrinogenemia, coagulopathy) further narrow the differential diagnosis. A differential diagnosis is provided in Table 9-26.

TABLE 9-26

Differential Diagnosis of Cutaneous Vascular Occlusive Conditions

TABLE 9-26

Differential Diagnosis of Cutaneous Vascular Occlusive Conditions

Coagulopathy
Cryoglobulinemia
Cholesterol embolism
Livedo reticularis
Atrophie blanche
Degos' syndrome
Calciphylaxis
Oxalosis
Secondary vasculopathy

Coagulopathies

Any coagulopathy may be accompanied by vasculopathic changes, although the extent of vascular damage is variable. Vascular damage may occur in the setting of altered platelet counts, such as in idiopathic thrombocytopenic purpura, in coagulation factor deficiencies (e.g., inherited or acquired protein C and S deficiencies), coagulopathies associated with connective tissue disease (e.g., lupus anticoagulant, antiphospholipid antibody syndrome), and platelet thrombosis in heparin necrosis. Extensive vascular damage with luminal occlusion by thrombotic material may develop in coumarin necrosis, thrombotic

TABLE 9-27A

Type I Cryoglobulinemia

Clinical Features

Cutaneous: Palpable purpura, urticarialike lesions, livedo reticularis,
    acrocyanosis, digital gangrene, leg ulcers, Raynaud's phenomenon
Systemic: Arthralgia, hepatosplenomegaly, lymphadenopathy,
    glomerulonephritis

Histopathological Features

Amorphous, PAS-positive thrombi, cracking of thrombi
Extensive extravasation of erythrocytes

Differential Diagnosis

Coagulopathies

thrombocytopenic purpura, and in disseminated intravascular coagulation, in particular, in the setting of purpura fulminans.[48]

Clinical Features   In mild forms, the clinical manifestations may be subtle and limited to petechiae. Severe forms of coagulopathy may show palpable purpura or large areas of ecchymoses, often on the extremities. Large hemorrhagic bullae may overlie the ecchymoses, and in some instances, necrosis may supervene.

Histopathological Features   The histologic findings are nonspecific. In mild forms of coagulopathy, dermal hemorrhage with extravasation of red blood cells into perivascular connective tissue may be the only histologic manifestation. With increasing severity of the coagulopathic process, intravascular fibrin thrombi may be found (Fig. 9-2). In the severe coagulopathies (e.g., thrombotic thrombocytopenic purpura, coumarin necrosis, or purpura fulminans), thrombotic vascular occlusion may lead to hemorrhagic infarcts, epidermal and dermal necroses, or subepidermal bullae formation. Systemic intravascular coagulation, with widespread thrombosis of the small vessels of internal organs leading to hemorrhagic necrosis, also may develop.

Cryoglobulinemia

Cryoglobulins are serum immunoglobulins that precipitate when the serum is cooled and redissolve with rewarming. There are three major types of cryoglobulinemia (Tables 27A and 27B). In type I cryoglobulinemia, monoclonal IgG or IgM cryoglobulins are found. This type of cryoglobulinemia may be idiopathic but often is associated with lymphoma, leukemia, Waldenstroem's macroglobulinemia, or multiple myeloma. In type II cryoglobulinemia, the cryoprecipitate consists of both monoclonal and polyclonal cryoglobulins, with one cryoglobulin acting as an antibody against the other. These cryoglobulins are circulating immune complexes. The most common combination is IgG-IgM. In type III cryoglobulinemia, the immunoglobulins are polyclonal. Types II and III or mixed cryoglobulinemias are frequently associated with connective tissue disorders, such as lupus erythematosus, rheumatoid arthritis, Sjogren syndrome, or may be related to infection, in particular, hepatitis C infection. Idiopathic forms of types II and III cryoglobulinemias also are termed essential mixed cryoglobulinemia.

Clinical Features   Cutaneous lesions in patients with cryoglobulinemia may manifest as chronic palpable purpura, urticarialike lesions, livedo reticularis, Raynaud's phenomenon, acrocyanosis, digital gangrene, and leg ulcers (Table 9-27A). Systemic manifestations may include arthralgia, hepatosplenomegaly, lymphadenopathy, and glomerulonephritis.

TABLE 9-27B

Clinicopathological Associations of Cryoglobulinemias (after Cohen et al[8])

	Immunoglobulin	*Associations*	*Site*	*Clinical Findings*	*Histopathological Features*
Type I	Monoclonal IgG or IgM	Lymphoma, leukemia, Waldenstroem's macroglobulinemia, or multiple myeloma	Head, neck, oral or nasal mucosa	Hemorrhagic crusts, skin ulcerations	Noninflammatory hyaline thrombosis, cutaneous infarction
Types II and III	Monoclonal and polyclonal immune complexes	Connective tissue disorders idiopathic (essential) infection autoimmune diseases	Legs	Erythematous to purpuric macules or papules	Leukocytoclastic vasculitis

Histopathological Features   In type I cryoglobulinemia, amorphous material (precipitated cryoglobulins) is deposited subjacent to endothelium, throughout the vessel wall and within the vessel lumen, resulting in a thrombuslike appearance. These precipitates stain pink with hematoxylin and eosin and bright red with PAS stain, as opposed to less intense staining of fibrinoid material (Fig. 9-8). Cracking of the precipitate may be a prominent feature. Some capillaries are filled with red blood cells, and extensive extravasation of erythrocytes may be present. An inflammatory infiltrate is usually lacking in contrast to the vascular injury seen in mixed cryoglobulinemias, which typically show a vasculitis, as previously discussed. PAS-positive intramural and intravascular cryoprecipitate may be found also in mixed cryoglobulinemia (Fig. 9-8), however, less frequently than in type I cryoglobulinemia.[8]

Cutaneous Cholesterol Embolism

Synonym   Atheroembolism.

Cholesterol crystal embolization is usually a disease of the elderly with significant atherosclerosis (Table 9-28).[49] Atheromatous plaque material may detach spontaneously or, more commonly, may follow an invasive procedure, such as arterial catheterization. Microemboli, composed of cholesterol crystals and/or other components of atheromatous plaque, often result in ischemic changes, most commonly involving the lower extremities. The cutaneous manifestations include livedo reticularis, purple discoloration, gangrene of toes, small, painful ulcerations, and on occasion, nodules or indurated plaques. The latter findings often closely mimic vasculitis, cryoglobulinemia, and chilblains. A helpful feature is the presence of intact arterial pulses on examination of the affected extremity, indicating that the ischemia is secondary to small-vessel involvement rather than major arteries.

Histopathological Features   Cholesterol emboli may be found as needle-shaped clefts within the lumina of small vessels (Fig. 9-19). The intravascular clefts that are in effect dissolved crystals may be single or multiple and are commonly associated with amorphous eosinophilic material, macrophages, or a foreign body–giant cell reaction. Vascular walls exhibit intimal fibrosis and often obliteration of lumina in older lesions. In many instances only fibrin thrombi are observed. Often a deep biopsy is needed to reveal such emboli, which are distributed focally and therefore difficult to find.

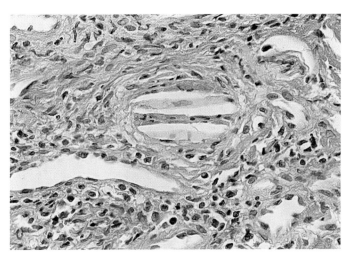

FIGURE 9-19   Cholesterol emboli. Needle-shaped clefts are present within the lumin of a small vessel.

Livedo Reticularis

Clinical Features   Livedo reticularis is persistent red-blue mottling of the skin in a netlike pattern (Table 9-29). It is a nonspecific sign of sluggish blood flow from any cause. It differs from cutis marmorata by not subsiding with warming of the skin. It may occur in association with a vasculitis or a vasculopathy in the context of a number of different systemic or localized disease processes, such as infection, atrophie blanche, cholesterol emboli, calciphylaxis, oxalosis, or connective tissue disease. However, frequently the condition is idiopathic and limited to the lower extremities. A generalized form of livedo reticularis has also been described as part of a potentially severe arterio-occlusive syndrome (Sneddon's syndrome) that often is complicated by cerebrovascular disease.[50]

Histopathological Features   Biopsy specimens taken from erythematous areas may be normal, whereas a biopsy specimen from a white area may show a vessel with a thickened wall and lumen occluded by a thrombus. In other cases, deeply situated dermal arterioles have shown obliterative changes. Other changes observed in livedo reticularis are intravascular aggregates of red blood cells, suggesting a low flow state.

TABLE 9-28

Cutaneous Cholesterol Embolism

Clinical Features

Elderly patient with significant atherosclerosis
Often status postarterial catheterization
Often lower extremities affected
Extremity with adequate pulsation
Livedo reticularis, purple discoloration, gangrene of toes, and small, painful ulcerations on the legs, nodules or indurated plaques

Histopathological Features

Emboli with needle-shaped clefts in the lumina of small vessels associated with amorphous eosinophilic material
Macrophages
Foreign body–giant cell reaction
Intimal fibrosis
Obliteration of lumina
Fibrin thrombi

TABLE 9-29

Livedo Reticularis

Clinical Features

Persistent red-blue mottling of the skin in a netlike pattern

Histopathological Features

Erythematous areas: no distinct findings
White areas: Thick vessel walls, thrombi, arteriole obliteration, red blood cell sludging

Associations

Vasculitis or vasculopathies owing to infection
Atrophie blanche
Cholesterol emboli
Connective tissue disease
Calciphylaxis and oxalosis
Idiopathic
Sneddon's syndrome

Atrophie Blanche

Synonyms   Livedoid vasculitis, segmental hyalinizing vasculitis.

Clinical Features   Atrophie blanche is a common condition that may be seasonal, with greatest disease activity in the summer and winter months. Usually middle-aged or elderly females are affected.[51] Initially, purpuric macules and papules develop into small, painful ulcers with a tendency to recur. Healing of the ulcers results in the white atrophic areas that have given the disease its name. Typically lesions are located on the lower portions of the legs, particularly on the ankles and the dorsa of the feet. In the fully developed state, there are irregularly outlined, whitish atrophic areas with peripheral hyperpigmentation and telangiectasia. Many of the patients have associated livedo reticularis. The etiology of atrophie blanche is unknown. Immune-complex deposits that have been observed in late lesions are likely secondary changes. A primary disturbance of fibrinolysis in the endothelium of affected microvessels has been postulated.

Histopathological Features   The histologic findings are nonspecific and vary with the stage of the lesion (Table 9-30). However, in all stages, vascular changes are present. In early lesions, fibrinoid material may be noted in vessel walls or vessel lumina (Fig. 9-20). Infarction with hemorrhage and an inflammatory infiltrate may be present as well. In late atrophic lesions, the epithelium is thinned, and the dermis is sclerotic with little, if any, cellular infiltrate. The walls of the dermal vessels may show thickening and intimal hyalinization. Occlusion of vessel lumina by intimal proliferation and/or fibrinoid material and sometimes recanalized thrombotic vessels may be seen. In some cases, the vessels in the superficial dermis are predominantly affected; in others, the vessels in the middle and even deep dermis are mostly affected.

Degos' Syndrome

Synonyms   Malignant atrophic papulosis (MAP), Degos' disease.

Degos initially described a cutaneointestinal syndrome, in which distinct skin findings ("drops of porcelain") were associated with recurrent attacks of abdominal pain that often ended in death from intestinal perforations.[52] He chose the name malignant atrophic papulosis (MAP) to emphasize the serious clinical course of the disease. Originally, the cutaneous lesions were thought to be specific and pathognomonic for a unique disease entity (Degos' disease). Currently, MAP is considered to be a clinicopathologic reaction pattern that can be associated with a number of conditions other than the cutaneointestinal syndrome

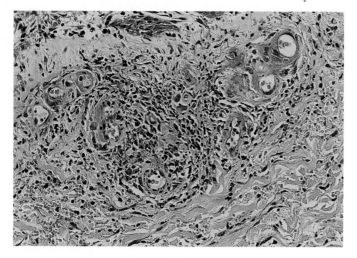

FIGURE 9-20   Atrophie blanche. The microvessels show deposition of fibrinoid material in their walls and an associated lymphoid infiltrate.

described by Degos and others.[53] Lesions similar, if not identical, to MAP have been noted, in particular, in connective tissue diseases, such as lupus erythematosus, dermatomyositis, and progressive systemic sclerosis; in atrophie blanche; and in Creutzfeldt-Jakob disease. The etiology of Degos' syndrome is unclear. The findings have been ascribed to a coagulopathy, vasculitis, or mucinosis. However, convincing evidence to support any single causal factor is lacking.

Clinical Features   The cutaneous manifestations of Degos' syndrome include crops of asymptomatic, slightly raised, yellowish-red or pale-rose papules (Table 9-31). Gradually, the papules become umbilicated and develop an atrophic porcelain-white center with a livid red, telangiectatic margin. These papules tend to affect the trunk and proximal extremities. Symptoms of an acute abdomen or less commonly of a cerebral infarction may supervene.

Histopathological Features   A typical lesion shows a wedge-shaped area of altered dermis covered by atrophic epidermis with slight hyperkeratosis. Dermal alterations may include frank necrosis. However, more commonly edema, extensive mucin deposition, and slight sclerosis are seen (Fig. 9-21A). Typically, vascular damage is noted in the vessels at the base of the "cone of necrobiosis." Vascular alterations may be subtle and manifest as endothelial swelling only. However, more characteristically, intravascular fibrin thrombi may be noted (Fig. 9-21B). Their presence suggests that the dermal and epidermal changes result from ischemia. Altered vessels usually lack an inflammatory infiltrate.

Calciphylaxis

Clinical Features   Widespread calcification with vascular thrombosis or calciphylaxis is an uncommon complication of renal failure (Table 9-32). Usually secondary or tertiary hyperparathyroidism is found in these patients. Painful violaceous lesions that may be indurated often develop

TABLE 9-31

Degos' Syndrome

Clinical Features

Crops of asymptomatic, slightly raised, yellowish-red or pale-rose
   papules that umbilicate and develop an atrophic porcelain-white
   center with a livid red, telangiectatic surrounding
Trunk and proximal extremities commonly affected
Acute abdominal crisis
Cerebral infarction

Histopathological Features

Atrophic epidermis with hyperkeratosis
Wedge-shaped area of altered dermis
Necrosis or edema
Mucin deposition and slight sclerosis
Vascular damage at the base of the wedge, fibrin thrombi common

Differential Diagnosis

Coagulopathies
Cryoglobulinemia
Atrophie blanche
Pityriasis lichenoides

TABLE 9-32

Calciphylaxis

Clinical Features

Renal failure with secondary hyperparathyroidism
Primary hyperparathyroidism
Hypercalcemia of malignancy
Livedo reticularis
Firm, indurated, painful, violaceous lesions
Progression to bullae, ulcers, eschars, and gangrene
Trunk and extremities involved

Histopathological Features

Calcium deposition in soft tissue and small blood vessels
Intimal proliferation and luminal occlusion
Thrombi in uncalcified, noninflamed small vessels of the subcutis
Full-thickness ischemic necrosis of skin

Differential Diagnosis

Coagulopathies
Calcinosis cutis
Panniculitis with calcification

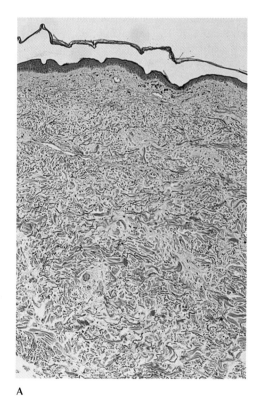

A

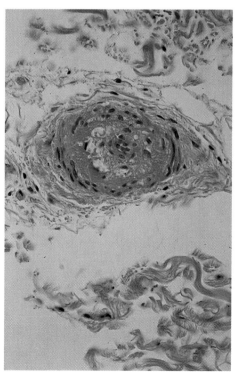

B

FIGURE 9-21   Degos lesion. (*A*) Atrophic epidermis overlies a wedge-shaped area of dermis with mucin deposition and (*B*) a thrombosed vessel at the base. This Degos lesion was seen in a patient with dermatomyositis.

in areas of livedo reticularis on the trunk and extremities and can rapidly progress to form bullae, ulcers, eschars, and gangrene. The prognosis is extremely poor even with aggressive treatment by parathyroidectomy.[54] The relationships between the calcification, thrombosis, and ischemic necrosis in calciphylaxis are unclear. Although vascular calcification is common in uremic patients, calciphylaxis is rare. Elevation of the calcium and phosphorous product along with a poorly defined precipitating or challenging event or agent are hypothesized to be necessary for calcium deposition in cutaneous tissues. However, the list of putative sensitizing agents is long and the calcium and phosphorus product may be within normal limits. The development of a hypercoagulable state may be an additional important element in the pathogenesis of this entity but is not present in all cases.[55]

Histopathological Features   The principal histological findings include: (1) calcification of soft tissue and small vessels (Fig. 9-22), (2) nonspecific intimal proliferation of small vessels, often resulting in luminal narrowing, (3) variable fibrin thrombi, and (4) frequent ischemic necrosis of skin and subcutis (see Chap. 11). The small vessels involved by this process cannot be identified as either arterial or venous. Often one observes foreign body–giant cell reaction to calcium and mixed inflammatory cell infiltrates that are neutrophil-rich.

Differential Diagnosis   Cutaneous calcium deposits may be seen in a number of other conditions, especially cutaneous calcinosis and metastatic calcifications. In contrast to calciphylaxis (see Chap. 16) the calcinosis usually lacks prominent vascular involvement. Other crystal-induced inflammatory diseases such as gout, pseudogout, or oxalosis that are associated with a giant cell reaction to crystal deposits and surrounding fibrosis may resemble calciphylaxis.[54] Histopathologically, pancreatic panniculitis may suggest calciphylaxis. However, the polymorphous infiltrate and ghost-like cells are absent in calciphylaxis, in contrast to pancreatic panniculitis.[56] If the sampling lacks significant calcium deposits, the biopsy may mimic ischemic damage or a coagulopathy.

Oxalosis

Clinical Findings   Oxalosis is characterized by the deposition of calcium oxalate crystals in multiple organs, most frequently the kidneys and myocardium. The disease may be primary, owing to inborn errors of metabolism, or secondary. The most common cause of secondary oxalosis is hyperabsorption of dietary oxalate secondary to intestinal disease or ileal resection, or excessive intake of oxalates or oxalate precursors, such as ethylene glycol. Deposition of calcium oxalate in small vessels of the dermis and subcutis may result in livedo reticularis, whereas involvement of larger peripheral blood vessels may lead to peripheral gangrene.[57,58]

Histopathological Features   Calcium oxalate is a light yellow-brown birefringent crystal exhibiting a number of shapes, including rosettes, ellipses, prisms, and radial patterns. The latter crystals may be deposited in the wall or occlude the lumina of small vessels with or without fibrin thrombi or localize to the media of larger vessels. There may be infiltration of vessel walls by neutrophils. Varying degrees of ischemic necrosis of skin often are the end result.

Differential Diagnosis   The histopathologic findings may resemble calciphylaxis. However, the calcium oxalate crystal morphology and birefringence allow discrimination from calcium phosphate. Although both oxalosis and calciphylaxis patients exhibit renal failure, the cutaneous clinical findings are distinct. Other crystal deposition syndromes, such as gout, may resemble oxalosis. However, urate crystals are dissolved during routine processing, unlike oxalate crystals, and are not deposited in vascular walls with associated thrombi. Oxalate thrombi may be confused with a cholesterol embolus; however, cholesterol is removed by routine processing and is not birefringent. Calcium oxalate can be identified histochemically by the method of Johnson and Pani.[59]

Conditions Leading to Alteration of the Vessel Wall

Metabolic disorders may lead to the deposition of endogenously produced material within the walls of the small vessels supplying the skin. Ischemic damage may result. Examples of such disorders include diabetes mellitus, amyloidosis, or porphyria, which are discussed in more detail in Chapters 8 and 16. The salient histologic vascular alteration in the above mentioned disorders is the deposition of amorphous material in the walls of dermal capillaries. Atherosclerosis is by far the most common type of metabolic vasculopathy. However, it is not discussed in detail because it is primarily a disease of large vessels supplying visceral organs. Cutaneous changes usually are rare and secondary manifestations of peripheral ischemia. Luminal occlusion may result from intimal thickening and lipid deposition, superimposed thrombosis, or less frequently, cholesterol emboli (discussed earlier).

Vasculopathies Owing to Deficiencies of Connective Tissue

Last, structural deficiencies of the perivascular connective tissue may contribute to vascular fragility and the attendant extravasation of erythrocytes. Such alterations underlie the hemorrhage in senile purpura and scurvy. This group of conditions can be described as noninflammatory purpura.

Histopathological Features   In senile purpura, extravasation of red blood cells occurs in atrophic skin with solar elastosis and normal-appearing capillaries. Scurvy is characterized by dermal hemorrhage predominantly in the vicinity of hair follicles without evidence of vascular damage, hemosiderin-laden macrophages, follicular keratotic plugs, and coiled hair.[60]

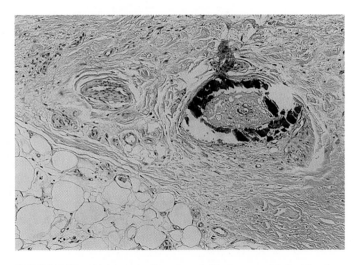

FIGURE 9-22 Calciphylaxis. Vascular calcification associated with microvessel in dermis.

REFERENCES

1. Jorizzo JL, Solomon AR, Zanolli MD, et al: Neutrophilic vascular reactions. *Arch Dermatol* 19:983–1005, 1988.
2. Callen JP: Cutaneous vasculitis: Relationship to systemic disease and therapy. *Curr Probl Dermatol* 5:45–80, 1993.
3. Fauci AS: The spectrum of vasculitis. *Ann Intern Med* 89:660–676, 1978.
4. Jennette JC, Falk RJ, Andrassy K, et al: Nomenclature of systemic vasculitides: Proposal of an international consensus conference. *Arthritis Rheum* 37:187–192, 1994.
5. Jennette JC: Vasculitis affecting the skin. *Arch Dermatol* 130:899–906, 1994.
6. Jennette JC, Tuttle R, Falk RJ: The clinical serologic and immunopathologic heterogeneity of cutaneous leukocytoclastic angiitis. *Immunol Clin Asp* 323–326, 1993.
7. Mehregan DR, Hall MJ, Gibson LE: Urticarial vasculitis: A histopathologic and clinical review of 72 cases. *J Am Acad Dermatol* 26:441–448, 1992.
8. Cohen SJ, Pittelkow MR, Su WPD: Cutaneous manifestations of cryoglobulinemia: Clinical and histopathologic study of 72 patients. *J Am Acad Dermatol* 26:38–44, 1992.
9. Patel A, Prussick R, Buchanan WW, Sauder DN: Serum sickness–like illness and leukocytoclastic vasculitis after intravenous streptolinase. *J Am Acad Dermatol* 24:652–653, 1991.
10. Wollenstein P, Revuf J: Drug-induced severe skin reactions. *Pharmacoepidemiology* 13:56–68, 1995.
11. Jain KK: Drug-induced cutaneous vasculitis. *Adverse Drug React Toxicol Rev* 12:263–276, 1993.
12. Sanchez-Guerro J, Gutierrez-Urena S, Vidaller A, et al: Vasculitis as a paraneoplastic syndrome: Report of 11 cases and review of the literature. *J Rheumatol* 17:1458–1462, 1990.
13. LeBoit PE, Yen TSB, Wintroub B: The evolution of lesions in erythema elevatum diutinum. *Am J Dermopathol* 8:392–402, 1986.
14. Requena L, Yus ES, Martin L, et al: Erythema elevatum diutinum in a patient with acquired immunodeficiency syndrome. *Arch Dermatol* 127:1819–1822, 1991.
15. Quismorio FP, Rea T, Chandor S, et al: Lucio's phenomenon: An immune complex deposition syndrorme in lepromatous leprosy. *Clin Immunol Immunopathol* 9:184–193, 1978.
16. Pursley TV, Jacobson RR, Apisarnthanarax P: Lucio's phenomenon. *Arch Dermatol* 116:201–204, 1980.
17. Pinkus H: Granuloma faciale. *Dermatologica* 105:85–99, 1952.
18. Sweet RD: Acute febrile neutrophilic dermatosis. *Br J Dermatol* 74:349–356, 1964.
19. von den Driesch P: Sweet's syndrome (acute febrile neutrophilic dermatosis). *J Am Acad Dermatol* 31:535–556, 1994.
20. Jordan HF: Acute febrile neutrophilic dermatosis: A histopathologic study of 37 patients and a review of the literature. *Am J Dermatopathol* 11:99–111, 1989.
21. Powell FC, Su WPD, Perry HO: Pyoderma gangrenosum: Classification and management. *J Am Acad Dermatol* 34(3):395–409, 1996.
22. Massa MC, Su WPD: Lymphocytic vasculitis: Is it a specific clinicopathologic entity? *J Cut Pathol* 11:132–139, 1984.
23. Randall SJ, Kierland RR, Montgomery H: Pigmented purpuric eruptions. *Arch Dermatol Syph* 64:177–191, 1951.
24. Barnhill RL, Bravermann IM: Progression of pigmented purpura-like eruptions to mycosis fungoides: Report of 3 cases. *J Am Acad Dermatol* 19:25–31, 1988.
25. Waisman M: Lichen aureus. *Arch Dermatol* 112:696–697, 1976.
26. Thomas R, Vuitch F, Lakhanpl S: Angiocentric T-cell lymphoma masquerading as cutaneous vasculitis. *J Rheumatol* 21:760–762, 1994.
27. Jennette JC, Falk RJ: Anti-neutrophil cytoplasmic antibodies and associated diseases: A review. *AM J Kidney Dis* 15:517–529, 1990.
28. Jennette JC, Falk RJ: Diagnostic classification of antineutrophil cytoplasmic autoantibody-associated vasculitides. *Am J Kidney Dis* 16:184–187, 1991.
29. Goeken J: Antineutrophil cytoplasmic and anti-endothelial cell antibodies: New mechanisms for vasculitis. *Curr Opin Dermatol* 75–82, 1995.
30. Lanham JG, Elhon KB, Pusey CD, Hughes GR: Systemic vasculitis with asthma and eosinophilia: A clinical approach to Churg-Strauss syndrome. *Medicine* 63:65–81, 1984.
31. Chumbley LC, Harrison EG Jr, Dereme RA: Allergic granulomatosis and angiitis (Churg-Strauss syndrome): Report and analysis of 30 cases. *Mayo Clin Proc* 52:477–484, 1977.
32. Finan MC, Winkelman RK: The cutaneous extravascular necrotizing granuloma (Churg-Strauss granuloma) and systemic disease: A review of 27 cases. *Medicine* (Baltimore) 62:142–158, 1983.
33. Churg J, Strauss L: Allergic granulomatosis, allergic angiitis, and periarteritis nodosa. *Am J Pathol* 27:277–301, 1951.
34. Wegener F: Ueber generalisierte, septische Gefaesserkrankungen. *Verh Dtsch Ges Pathol* 29:202, 1936.
35. Goodman GC, Churg J: Wegener's granulomatosis: Pathology and review of the literature. *Arch Pathol* 58:533, 1954.
36. Fauci AS, Wolff SM: Wegener's granulomatosis: Studies in 18 patients and a review of the literature. *Medicine* (Baltimore) 52:535–561, 1973.
37. Barksdale SK, Hallahan CW, Kerr GS, et al: Cutaneous pathology in Wegener's granulomatosis. *Am J Surg Pathol* 19:161–172, 1995.
38. deShazo RD, Levinson AI, Lawless OJ, Weisbaum G: Systemic vasculitis with co-existent large and small-vessel involvement: A classification dilemma. *JAMA* 238:1940–1942, 1977.
39. Modesto A, Keriven O, Dupre-Goudable C, et al: There is no real difference beween Wegener's granulomatosis and micropolyarteritis. *Contrib Nephrol* 94:191–194, 1991.
40. Kussmaul A, Maier K: Ueber eine bisher nicht beschriebene eigentuemliche Arterien veraenderung (periarteritis nodosa), die mit Morbus Briggti und rapide fortschreitender all gemeiner Muskellaehmung einhergeht. *Dtsch Akad Klin Med* 1:484–517, 1885.
41. Ferrari E: Veber Polylarteritis acuta nodosa (sogerannte Periarteritis nodosa) undihre Beziehurgen zur polylmyositis und polyneuritis acuta. *Beitr Pathol Anat* 34:350–386, 1903.
42. Diaz-Perez JL, Winkelman RK: Cutaneous periarteritis nodosa. *Arch Dermatol* 110:407–414, 1974.
43. Johnson WC, Wallrich R, Helwig EB: Superficial thrombophlebitis of the chest wall. *JAMA* 180:103–108, 1962.
44. Findlay GH, Whiting DA: Mondor's phlebitis of the penis: A condition miscalled "non-venereal sclerosing lymphangitis." *Clin Exp Dermatol* 2:65–67, 1977.
45. Landing BH, Larson EJ: Pathologic features of Kawasaki disease (mucocutaneous lymph node syndrome). *Am J Cardiovasc Pathol* 4:75–84, 1987.
46. Perniciaro CV, Winkelmann RK, Hunder GG: Cutaneous manifestations of Takayasu's arteritis. *J Am Acad Dermatol* 17:998–1005, 1987.
47. Baum EW, Sams WM Jr, Payne RR: Giant cell arteritis: A systemic disease with rare cutaneous manifestations. *J Am Acad Dermatol* 6:1081–1088, 1982.
48. Robboy SJ, Mihm MC, Colman RC, et al: The skin in disseminated intravascular coagulation. *Br J Dermatol* 88:221–229, 1973.
49. Falanga V, Fine MJ, Kapoor WN: The cutaneous manifestations of cholesterol crystal embolization. *Arch Dermatol* 122:1194–1198, 1986.
50. Sneddon IB: Cerebro-vascular lesions and livedos reticularis. *Br J Dermatol* 77:180–185, 1975.
51. Stiefler RE, Bergfeld WF: Atrophie blanche (review). *Int J Dermatol* 21:1–7, 1982.
52. Degos R, Delort J, Tricot R: Dermatite papulo-squameuse atrophiante. *Bull Soc Fr Dermatol Syph* 49:148–150, 281, 1942.
53. Doutre MS, Beylot C, Bioulac P, et al: Skin lesion resembling malignant atrophic papulosis in lupus erythematosus. *Dermatologica* 175:45–46, 1987.
54. Fischer AH, Morris DJ: Pathogenesis of calciphylaxis: Study of 3 cases with literature review. *Hum Pathol* 26:1055–1064, 1995.
55. Mehta RL, Scott G, Sloand JA, Francis CW: Skin necrosis associated with acquired protein C deficiency in patients with renal failure and calciphylaxis. *Am J Med* 88:252–257, 1990.
56. Lugo-Somolinos A, Sanchez JL, Menedez-Coll J, Joglar F: Calcifying panniculitis associated with polycystic kidney disease and chronic renal failure. *J Am Acad Dermatol* 22:743–747, 1990.
57. Greer KE, Cooper PH, Campbell R, Westervelt FB: Primary oxalosis with livedo reticularis. *Arch Dermatol* 116:213–214, 1980.
58. Arbus GS, Sniderman S: Oxalosis with peripheral gangrene. *Arch Pathol* 97:107–110, 1974.
59. Johnson FB, Pani K: Histochemical identification of calcium oxalate. *Arch Pathol Lab Med* 74:347–351, 1962.
60. Walker A: Chronic scurvy. *Br J Dermatol* 80:625–630, 1968.

CHAPTER 10

DISORDERS OF CUTANEOUS APPENDAGES

David A. Whiting / Stephen F. Templeton / Alvin R. Solomon

The interpretation of scalp biopsies from patients with hair loss can be difficult (Table 10-1). The pathologist depends on accurate clinical information when assessing scalp biopsies. The commonest causes of hair loss or shedding are nonscarring and include androgenetic alopecia, diffuse alopecia, alopecia areata, trichotillomania, and other types of traumatic alopecia (Table 10-2).[1]

A basic understanding of the hair follicle and the hair cycle is needed to interpret scalp biopsies.[1] The human hair follicle consists of a permanent upper segment, comprised of infundibulum and isthmus, and an impermanent lower segment, comprised of lower follicle and hair root. The infundibulum is lined with keratinized skin surface epithelium and ends at the entry of the sebaceous duct into the follicle. The isthmus extends down from the sebaceous duct and ends at the bulge where the arrector pili muscle inserts into the follicle. It is lined by trichilemma (external root sheath) and trichilemmal keratin. The lower segment surrounds a growing hair with internal and external root sheaths, hyaline membrane, and fibrous sheath. The bulb consists of the dermal papilla surrounded by hair matrix cells. It generates the growing hair.

Human scalp hair follicles cycle continuously through periods of growth and rest. Asynchronous follicular growth produces an ever-changing mosaic pattern of growing follicles on the scalp. The growth or anagen phase lasts 2 to 7 years, 1000 days on average, and the resting or telogen phase lasts 2 to 4 months, an average of 100 days. The end of telogen is signalled by the appearance of a new anagen hair and the shedding of the telogen hair. Assuming an average 100,000 hairs on the human scalp, with 5 to 10 percent in telogen at any one time, then up to 10,000 hairs are shed every 100 days, an average loss of 100 hairs per day.

Large hairs with a diameter exceeding 0.03 mm, growing more than 1 cm in length, often pigmented and medullated, are classified as *terminal* hairs. Small hairs with a diameter less than 0.03 mm, growing less than 1 cm in length, and with no pigment or medullary cavity, are classified as *vellus* (*downy*) hairs. Depigmented hairs less than 0.03 mm in diameter which have been miniaturized by androgenetic alopecia, alopecia areata, or any other cause, can be classified as *velluslike* hairs. The designation *vellus hairs* used in this chapter includes true vellus hairs and velluslike hairs. Terminal hairs are rooted in the subcutaneous tissue, but vellus hairs are rooted in the dermis. Terminal-to-vellus ratios therefore denote the proportions of large hairs to small hairs, and a normal scalp averages 7 terminal hairs per vellus hair. Less than 4 terminal hairs to 1 vellus hair denotes a relative increase in vellus hairs, perhaps indicating a miniaturization process.

The termination of anagen is signalled by the onset of catagen. Catagen is the short, 10- to 14-day, intermediate phase between anagen and telogen which really indicates the onset of telogen, since it irrevocably commits the growing follicle to a resting phase. In catagen, the hair shaft retracts upward, the hyaline basement membrane thickens and corrugates, and individual cell necrosis or apoptosis occurs in the outer root sheath or trichilemma. The hair displacement and volumetric reduction of root sheath leads to the progressive disappearance of the lower or impermanent part of the hair follicle, so that in telogen the resting hair root is seen near the insertion of the arrector pili muscle, where the permanent follicle begins. A telogen bulb lacks pigment and internal and external root sheaths and is surrounded by trichilemmal keratin. An angiofibrotic strand extending down from the permanent follicle, known variously as a *fibrous tract*, *streamer*, or *stela*, indicates the former position of the retracted follicle.

Histopathologic examination is helpful for diagnostic purposes and for evaluating the capacity for future hair regrowth. If possible the biopsy should be taken from an area of active alopecia. For predictive purposes an area of maximum hair loss can be sampled. Punch biopsies of the scalp are adequate substitutes for excisional biopsies. A sharp trephine of at least 4 mm diameter is used. The biopsy is angled in the direction of any emerging hairs and taken deep enough to include subcutaneous tissue and therefore hair bulbs. For additional information, two 4-mm punch biopsies are taken from comparable sites. One biopsy is bisected vertically parallel to the direction of any hairs, and both halves are placed in a cassette for formalin fixation and standard staining with hematoxylin and eosin (H&E). If necessary, one-half of the vertical biopsy can be reserved for immunofluorescence or any other purpose which requires different processing. The other 4-mm punch is carefully bisected horizontally (transversely) parallel to the epidermis and 1 to 1.5 mm below it.[2] Both segments are embedded in paraffin side by side with the cut surfaces face down in the block.[3] Sectioning will progress down toward the subcutaneous tissue in the one half and up toward the epidermis in the other. The pathologist who uses this technique and is familiar with the transverse anatomy of the hair follicle can then count the hair bulbs, terminal anagen, catagen and telogen hairs, telogen germinal units, and stelae (fibrous tracts or streamers) in sections through reticular dermis (Table 10-3).[4,5] Terminal hairs, vellus hairs (which include true vellus hairs and miniaturized or velluslike hairs), and follicular units can be counted in sections of the papillary dermis (Table 10-3). From these data, total follicular counts are derived with anagen:telogen ratios, terminal:vellus hair ratios, and follicular concentration per square millimeter. Comparative data for controls versus androgenetic alopecia, chronic telogen effluvium, alopecia areata, and trichotillomania are shown in Table 10-4.[6] For pathologists who rely only on vertical sections, multiple sections may be required to estimate the total follicular counts and the terminal:vellus and anagen:telogen ratios which are helpful in the diagnosis of nonscarring alopecia. The presence or absence of inflammatory changes and fibrosis are also important in establishing the diagnosis. Some of the histopathologic dif-

TABLE 10-1

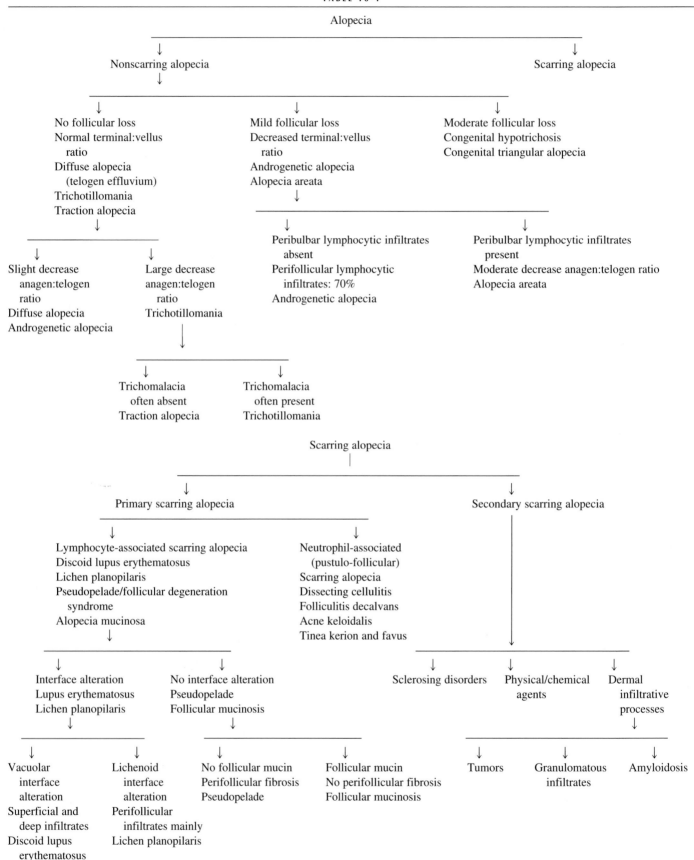

TABLE 10-2

Common Causes of Alopecia*

Androgenetic alopecia	618	68.8%
Diffuse alopecia	101	11.3
Alopecia areata	89	9.9
Cicatricial alopecia	44	4.9
Trichotillomania	12	1.3
Trauma, traction	10	1.1
Other	24	2.7
	898	100.00

*An analysis of the 898 cases of alopecia out of the first 1000 patients seen in 1987 to 1988 at Baylor Hair Research and Treatment Center, Dallas, Texas.
SOURCE: Whiting DA: *The Diagnosis of Alopecia, Current Concepts.* Kalamazoo, MI, Upjohn, 1990, p 14.

ferences in the common forms of nonscarring alopecia are set out in Table 10-5.

NONSCARRING VERSUS SCARRING ALOPECIA

Determining whether a patient clinically has a scarring or nonscarring alopecia can be challenging, and in these cases scalp biopsy is a very useful tool for specific diagnosis and prognosis for possible regrowth. The terms *scarring* and *nonscarring* are firmly entrenched in the dermatologic lexicon and are helpful for classification and prognosis in many cases of alopecia. However, many traditionally designated nonscarring alopecias may eventuate in permanent follicular drop-out and hair loss. Androgenetic alopecia, alopecia areata, traction alopecia, and trichotillomania are examples of nonscarring alopecias that may progress to complete permanent hair loss that is typically considered "scarring." Thus the terms *scarring* and *nonscarring* as they have been used historically do not always correlate with prognosis for hair regrowth.

NONSCARRING ALOPECIA

Androgenetic Alopecia

Androgenetic alopecia, or common baldness, affects at least 50 percent of the population by age 50 years in males[7] and a decade later in females. The familiar pattern of frontoparietal hair loss is due to a genetically determined end-organ sensitivity of the hairs on the crown to androgens. The affected terminal hairs are replaced by progressively finer and shorter hairs.[8]

Clinical Features   Androgenetic alopecia predominantly affects the top of the scalp in both sexes, with relative sparing of the back and sides (Table 10-6). It is of dominant inheritance with variable penetrance.[9]

Hair thinning occurs in males at any time after puberty. It often begins with bitemporal hair recession followed by a circular patch of hair loss over the vertex and then thinning of the frontal hairline.[7]

In females hair thinning can also begin after puberty, but an onset between 25 and 35 years is more common. Female pattern alopecia causes diffuse thinning over the top of the scalp, with an intact frontal hair margin,[10,11] without total baldness. In females severe bitemporal recession, vertex baldness, acne, hirsutism, and abnormal menses reflect significant hyperandrogenism, which needs investigation.[12,13]

Histopathological Features   The histopathologic changes in androgenetic alopecia are similar in males and females and reflect the pathogenesis of the condition (Table 10-6).[14] With progressively shorter hair cycles, terminal hairs become velluslike. The hair roots retreat upward toward the epidermis so that many of the miniaturized hair bulbs are found in mid- or papillary dermis. Residual follicular stelae (fibrous tracts or streamers) extending from the subcutaneous tissue up the old follicular tract to the miniaturized hair mark the former position of the original terminal follicle (Fig. 10-1). Thus, the expected findings in androgenetic alopecia are decreased terminal hairs, increased follicular stelae, and increased vellus hairs (Fig. 10-2).[14–17] A varying number of intermediate hairs, with a shaft diameter less than the average 0.06-mm terminal-hair diameter but more than the 0.03-mm vellus hair diameter, may be present[18]; for simplicity, these intermediate hairs are classified as terminal hairs in follicular counts quoted in this chapter. The progressive reduction in duration of anagen, but not telogen, causes a relative increase in telogen hairs. The average follicular counts in horizontal sections of a 4-mm punch biopsy of androgenetic alopecia are 23 terminal hairs + 12 vellus hairs = 35 total hairs, with a terminal:vellus ratio of 1.9:1, and a ratio of 83 percent anagen to 17 percent telogen (Table 10-4).[14] These counts contrast with those in normal controls which are 35 terminal hairs + 5 vellus hairs = 40 total hairs, with a terminal:vellus ratio of 7:1 and a ratio of 93.5 percent anagen to 6.5 percent telogen (Table 10-4).[14] A terminal:vellus ratio of less than 4:1 indi-

TABLE 10-3

Description of Follicular Structures

Terminal (big) hair	Shaft diameter exceeds 0.03 mm and is thicker than its inner root sheath. A medullary cavity and/or pigment may be present. This definition includes "intermediate" hair shafts of diameter 0.03 to 0.06 mm, commonly seen in androgenetic alopecia.
Vellus (small)	Shaft diameter equals 0.03 mm or less and is thinner hair than its inner root sheath. Shaft lacks pigment and medullary cavity, and arrector pili muscle is usually not found. All hairs of this size are counted as *vellus* hairs, whether true vellus hairs or velluslike hairs secondary to miniaturization from any cause.
Hair bulb	The hair bulb comprises root sheath, hair matrix, and dermal papilla.
Anagen hairs	Hair bulbs or hair shafts surrounded by inner and outer root sheaths. Only identifiable in lower follicle below bulge area.
Telogen hairs	Catagen hairs with trichilemmal apoptosis and thickened, corrugated, vitreous membrane, telogen hairs containing trichilemmal keratin, and telogen germinal units (resting telogen follicles containing basaloid cells). Only identifiable in lower follicle below bulge area.
Follicular stelae	Residual fibrous tracts or streamers representing the impermanent lower third of the hair follicle below the bulge area. Not counted as extra hair-forming structures because they are either downward prolongations of follicular structures which are counted in horizontal sections of the papillar dermis anyway or are permanently fibrosed follicles.
Follicular units	Hexagonal areas seen in horizontal sections at sebaceous duct level, surrounded by collagen and containing terminal and vellus hairs, sebaceous glands and ducts, and arrector pili muscles. Not counted as follicular structures, but if fibrosed represent severe cicatricial alopecia.

SOURCE: Whiting DA: Chronic telogen effluvium: Increased scalp shedding in middle-aged women *J Am Acad Dermatol* 35:899–906, 1996.

TABLE 10-4

Horizontal Sections of 4-mm Scalp Biopsies: Mean Follicular Counts in Differential Diagnosis of Alopecia.

Diagnosis Anagen:Telogen	No. of Pts.	Age	Sex (M:F)	Terminal(T) + Hairs	Vellus(V) = Hairs*	Total Hairs	T:V Ratio	Ratio %
Normal controls	22	43	1.4:1	35 +	5 =	40	7:1	93.5:6.5
Androgenetic alopecia	412	40	1:1.1	23 +	12 =	35	1.9:1	83:17
Chronic telogen effluvium	355	44	1:38	35 +	4 =	39	9:1	89:11
Alopecia areata	290	32	1:1.7	14 +	13 =	27	1.1:1	73:27
Trichotillomania	34	22	1:5	32 +	7 =	39	5:1	58:42

SOURCE: Adapted from Whiting DA: Horizontal sections of scalp biopsies, in Burgdorf WHC, Katz SI (eds), *Dermatology: Progress and Perspectives. The Proceedings of the 18th World Congress of Dermatology*, New York, June 12–18, 1992. New York, Parthenon, 1993, pp 215–216, with permission.
*Vellus = vellus hairs and velluslike hairs miniaturized from any cause.

TABLE 10-5

Histopathological Features of Nonscarring Alopecias

	Follicular loss	Terminal: vellus ratio	Anagen:telogen ratio	Perifollicular lymphoid infiltrates	Peribulbar lymphoid infiltrates	Trichomalacia
Congenital hypotrichosis	Moderate	NA	Large decrease	Usually absent	Absent	Absent
Congenital triangular alopecia	Moderate	Decreased	Large decrease	Usually absent	Absent	Absent
Androgenetic alopecia	Mild	Decreased	Slight decrease	70%*	Absent	Absent
Alopecia areata	Mild	Decreased	Moderate decrease	Usually absent	Present	Absent
Diffuse alopecia (telogen effluvium)	None	Normal	Slight decrease	40%*	Absent	Absent
Trichotillomania	None	Normal	Large decrease	Usually absent	Absent	Often present
Traction alopecia	None	Normal	Large decrease	Usually absent	Absent	Often absent

NA = Not applicable
*Percentage of patients with mild to moderate infiltrates; 40% of normal controls have mild to moderate infiltrates.

cates increased follicular miniaturization. A significant reduction in the total follicular count is seen in 10 percent of cases of androgenetic alopecia, indicating a decreased capacity for follicular regrowth in these cases.[14] A mild, perifollicular, lymphohistiocytic infiltrate, usually around upper follicles, is present in one-third of cases of androgenetic alopecia, as it is in one-third of normal controls. A moderate, perifollicular, lymphohistiocytic infiltrate, perhaps with concentric layers of collagen deposition, is present in 40 percent of cases of androgenetic alopecia but only in 10 percent of normal controls.[14] Occasional mast cells and even eosinophils are seen. Despite the inflammatory changes, sebaceous glands remain intact in androgenetic alopecia. Routine stains are adequate to evaluate androgenetic alopecia, but periodic acid–Schiff (PAS) stains apoptotic cells and vitreous layer to highlight catagen, and elastic stains show up Arao-Perkins bodies in follicular stelae.

Differential Diagnosis Androgenetic alopecia must be distinguished from diffuse alopecia, alopecia areata, and trichotillomania. Hair miniaturization does not occur in diffuse alopecia or in trichotillomania but is present in alopecia areata, often with a peribulbar lymphocytic infiltrate. Increased catagen hairs are present in trichotillomania and alope-

cia areata. Trichomalacia is characteristic of traction alopecia, notably trichotillomania, but can occur in alopecia areata.

Diffuse Alopecia

Diffuse alopecia implies generalized hair loss or shedding involving the back, sides, and top of the scalp. Common causes are listed in Table 10-7.[19] The underlying mechanism is often a telogen effluvium.[20]

Headington has described five functional types of telogen effluvium based on changes occurring in different phases of the hair cycle.[21] These comprise immediate anagen release (postfebrile), delayed anagen release (postpartum), short anagen cycle (inability to grow long hair), immediate telogen release (minoxidil), and delayed telogen release (molting).

Basically, an abnormal number of hairs go into the telogen phase and only fall out 1 to 3 months later when new anagen hairs grow in.[22] Classic acute telogen effluvium, often occurs after childbirth, severe illness, operation, stress, crash diet, or various drugs (Table 10-8).[22] In chronic telogen effluvium, the trigger factor may be obscure and any one of Headington's functional types can be implicated.

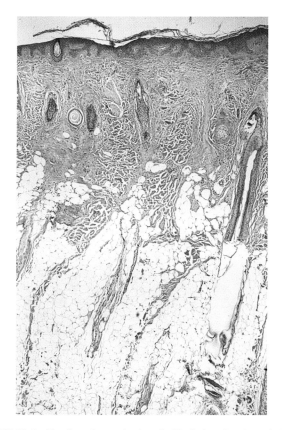

FIGURE 10-1 Female androgenetic alopecia. Vertical section: 2 terminal hairs and 5 follicular stelae (streamers or fibrous tracts) project down into the subcutaneous tissue; 4 vellus (velluslike or miniaturized) hairs are seen in the upper dermis, 2 of which are connected to follicular stelae extending down to subcutaneous tissue. There is no inflammation and no fibrosis.

Anagen effluvium is a severe condition, often resulting from antimitotic drugs, in which large amounts of hair fall out within a few weeks of impaired DNA synthesis.[23,24]

Clinical Features   In an acute phase of diffuse alopecia, hair pull tests are positive from all over the scalp (Table 10-9). In telogen effluvium,

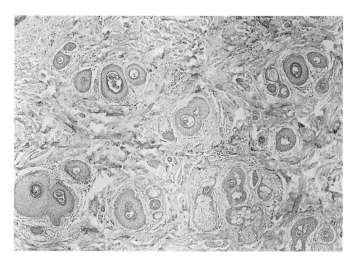

FIGURE 10-2 Male androgenetic alopecia. Horizontal section, papillary dermis: relatively few terminal hairs and many vellus hairs are visible. A mild lymphohistiocytic infiltrate is present around a few follicular infundibula, and no fibrosis is seen.

TABLE 10-6

Androgenetic Alopecia

Clinical Features

Progressive miniaturization of hairs on crown, with relative sparing of hair on back and sides of scalp.
   Male: Onset from puberty to 50 years; marked bitemporal recession with balding of vertex
   Female: Onset often one decade later than males; intact frontal hairline with diffuse thinning over crown

Histopathological Features

Increased miniaturized, vellus hairs
Increased follicular stelae
Decreased terminal hairs
Increased telogen hairs
Mild to moderate perifollicular lymphohistiocytic inflammation in 70% of cases
Intact sebaceus glands

Differential Diagnosis

Diffuse alopecia, especially telogen effluvium
Diffuse alopecia areata
Diffuse trichotillomania

the extracted hairs show depigmented club roots and no root sheaths.[22] In anagen effluvium, extracted hairs show a proximal taper with a fracture[24]; when the antimitotic influence is removed, hairs grow back promptly with a distal taper due to reversal of the pencil-pointing process.

Classic acute telogen effluvium affecting any age group has an abrupt onset and a short course of 3 to 6 months.[22] Chronic telogen effluvium can last from 6 months to 6 years or more, with an abrupt or gradual onset and a cyclical course.[25] It is often idiopathic, usually affects middle-age women, and does not cause severe baldness.

Histopathological Features   The histopathology of telogen effluvium is often similar to that seen in a normal scalp, except for the definite increase in telogen hairs seen during an active phase of hair loss (Table 10-9).[26] In vertical sections many terminal hairs are present, few vellus hairs are seen, and follicular stelae are uncommon (Fig. 10-3). Follicular counts in horizontal sections of a 4-mm punch biopsy of the crown in

TABLE 10-7

Causes of Diffuse Alopecia

Classic acute telogen effluvium	Nutritional causes
Chronic telogen effluvium	Malabsorption
Anagen effluvium	Renal failure
Drugs	Hepatic failure
Other chemicals	Systemic disease
Thyroid disorders	Miscellaneous causes
Iron deficiency	Idiopathic

SOURCE: After Simpson NB: Diffuse alopecia: Endocrine, metabolic and chemical influences on the follicular cycle, in Rook A, Dawber R (eds), *Diseases of the Hair and Scalp*, 2d ed. Oxford, Blackwell Scientific, 1991, chap 5, pp 136–166.

TABLE 10-8

TABLE 10-8

Drugs Causing Diffuse Alopecia

Allopurinol	Alpha receptor blockers	Amiodarone
Amoxapine	Amphetamine[TE]	Androgens
ACE inhibitors*[TE]	Anticancer drugs[AE]	Anticoagulants[TE]
Anticonvulsants[TE]	Antithyroid drugs[TE]	Arsenicals[TE]
Aspirin[TE]	Azathioprine	Azulfidine
Beta blockers[TE]	Birth control drugs[TE]	Bismuth[AE]
Boric acid[AE]	Bromocriptine[TE]	Calcium channel blockers[TE]
Carbamazepine	Cholesterol reducers[TE]	Cimetidine[TE]
Clomiphene	Clonidine	Colchicine[AE]
Danazol[TE]	Estrogen	Ethambutol
Ethionamide	Fluoxetine	Gentamycin
Gold[AE]	Haloperidol	Histamine 2 blockers
Levodopa[TE]	Lithium[TE]	Mercury
Methyldopa	Methysergide[TE]	Methyrapone[TE]
Nitrofurantoin[TE]	NSAIDS**[TE]	Omerprazole
Para amino salicylic acid	Penicillamine	Prazosin
Probenecid	Pyridostigimine bromide[TE]	Retinoids[TE]
Retinol[TE]	Salicylates[TE]	Sulfasalazine
Terfenadine	Thallium salts[AE]	Tricyclic antidepressants

*Angiotensin-converting enzyme inhibitors
**Nonsteroidal anti-inflammatory drugs
[AE]Cause of anagen effluvium
[TE]Cause of telogen effluvium

chronic telogen effluvium average 35 terminal hairs + 4 vellus hairs = 39 total hairs, with a terminal:vellus ratio of 9:1 and a ratio of 89 percent anagen to 11 percent telogen (Table 10-4).[25] These findings are the same as in normal controls except that the 11 percent telogen hairs exceeds the 6.5 percent telogen hairs found in normals (Figs. 10-4, 10-5). The telogen count can increase to 20 to 30 percent or higher in active phases of telogen effluvium. Inflammatory changes are similar to controls in that mild perifollicular lymphohistiocytic infiltration occurs in one-third and moderate infiltration in 10 percent of cases of telogen effluvium. Normal numbers of follicular stelae are found.[25]

The diffuse alopecia caused by hypothyroidism, other systemic diseases, and many drugs and chemicals results from a telogen effluvium and shows a similar histology.

Anagen effluvium involves the 90 percent of scalp hairs in anagen.[27] The diagnosis is usually simple, since there is a clear history of the drug or influence which interferes with DNA synthesis. Examination of plucked hairs is diagnostic, so biopsies are not indicated. The proximal tapering of a plucked hair in anagen effluvium is shown in Fig. 10-6.

Differential Diagnosis   Diffuse alopecia can usually be diagnosed on clinical grounds but is sometimes confused with female androgenetic alopecia, diffuse alopecia areata, or congenital hypotrichosis, and biopsies may be necessary. There is no reduction in terminal hair numbers in diffuse alopecia, but there is a definite reduction in terminal hairs, with increased vellus hairs, in androgenetic alopecia, diffuse alopecia areata, and congenital hypotrichosis. Peribulbar lymphocytes are often present in alopecia areata.

Alopecia Areata

Alopecia areata presents with patchy hair loss.[28,29] It is not uncommon and may affect 1 in 100 Americans by age 50.

The etiology of alopecia areata is unknown, and many believe it to be an autoimmune disease. Helper T cells are consistently found in the predominately lymphocytic infiltrate around affected hair bulbs. A family history is present in 20 percent of cases. Recent studies have shown the importance of the HLA class II antigens DQ3, DR4, and DR11 genes[30,31] in susceptibility to alopecia areata, and of DRW52A in resistance to the condition.[30] Long-standing alopecia totalis or universalis patients have unique associations with HLA antigens DR4, DR11, and DQ7.[31] Trigger factors include seasonal variation, emotional stress, and infections.

Clinical Features   The initial patch of alopecia areata on the scalp is often barely noticeable,[32] but it may enlarge and further patches may appear (Table 10-10). Disease activity is indicated by "exclamation point" hairs at the spreading margin of lesions. Specific forms of alopecia areata include ophiasis, a persistent bandlike loss of hair; diffuse alopecia areata; and reticular alopecia areata with multiple patches of hair loss.[28] In some cases the alopecia primarily involves beard, eyebrow, eyelash, or, rarely, body hair. In the most severe cases all scalp (alopecia totalis) and body (alopecia universalis) hair is lost. Alopecia areata is more common in females, except in children. Its course is unpredictable.

Histopathological Features   In the active stage of alopecia areata there is a characteristic cluster of mononuclear cells around follicular bulbs which has been likened to a swarm of bees[28] (Table 10-10) (Figs. 10-7, 10-8). Alopecia areata consists primarily of CD4 lymphocytes and Langerhans' cells, but some eosinophils and plasma cells may be

TABLE 10-9

Diffuse Alopecia

Clinical Features

Diffuse shedding, all over scalp, often abrupt
Classic acute telogen effluvium: moderate hair thinning, within months of childbirth, severe illness, accident or operation, crash diets, drugs, etc.
Chronic telogen effluvium: mild-to-moderate hair thinning, often idiopathic
Anagen effluvium: severe hair thinning within weeks of cytostatic drugs, etc.

Histopathological Features

Normal numbers of terminal hairs
Normal numbers of vellus hairs
Normal numbers of follicular stelae
Increased numbers of telogen hairs in active phases of telogen effluvium

Differential Diagnosis

Female pattern androgenetic alopecia
Diffuse alopecia areata
Congenital hypotrichosis

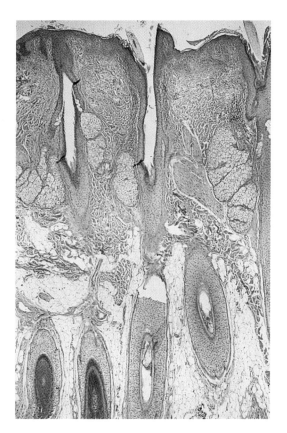

FIGURE 10-3   Diffuse alopecia, chronic telogen effluvium, vertical section: 5 terminal hairs and no follicular stelae are seen projecting into the subcutaneous tissue. A mild lymphohistiocytic infiltrate is present around a few upper follicles. The epidermis is normal.

seen.[33] This lymphocytic infiltrate can invade the hair bulb and cause pigment incontinence.[34] The infiltrate can also surround the adjacent suprabulbar portion of the hair shaft. Inflammatory cells invading bulbar epithelium can cause inter- and intracellular edema; nuclear pyknosis; apoptosis of matrix and outer sheath keratinocytes, melanocytes,

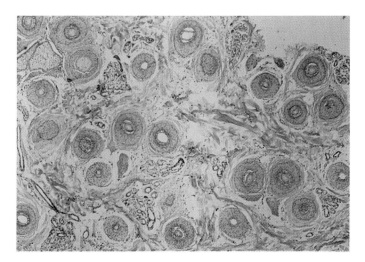

FIGURE 10-4   Diffuse alopecia, chronic telogen effluvium, horizontal section, reticular dermis: Many terminal hairs are seen with relatively few vellus hairs; 1 telogen hair and 4 telogen germinal units are present. There is no inflammation of note.

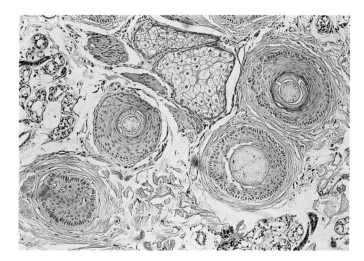

FIGURE 10-5   Diffuse alopecia, chronic telogen effluvium, horizontal section, reticular dermis: 2 terminal hairs, 1 telogen germinal unit (left lower margin), and 1 telogen hair (right lower margin) are visible.

Langerhans' cells, and dermal dendrocytes; and necrosis and microvesicle formation in the upper bulb above the dermal papilla.[35] In the initial stages the disease usually involves terminal hairs, but later on vellus hairs can be involved as well. As the disease progresses follicular stelae infiltrated with lymphocytes (Fig. 10-7) and containing melanin pigment are common. The inflammatory process involves anagen hairs which either become tapered and dystrophic, sometimes progressing to trichomalacia,[18] or, more commonly, are projected through catagen into premature telogen (Fig. 10-9). The increased number of catagen hairs which results (Figs. 10-10, 10-11) is exceeded only by the number of catagen hairs found in trichotillomania. Persistent disease results in miniaturization of hairs with decreased terminal hairs, and increased vellus hairs and follicular stelae. The average follicular count found in horizontal sections of a 4-mm punch biopsy comprises 14 terminal hairs + 13 vellus hairs = 27 total hairs, with a terminal:vellus ratio of 1.1:1

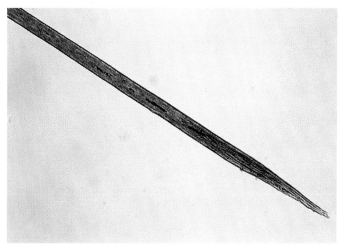

FIGURE 10-6   Anagen effluvium. The broken-off hair shaft shows proximal tapering adjacent to the fracture.

Alopecia Areata

Clinical Features

Periodic attacks of circumscribed patches of hair loss
Unpredictable course: patches may regrow or progress to confluent
patches, alopecia totalis or alopecia universalis

Histopathological Features

Peribulbar and intrabulbar mononuclear cell infiltrate
Degenerative changes in hair matrix
Decreased numbers of terminal anagen hairs
Increased numbers of terminal catagen and telogen hairs
Increased numbers of follicular stelae
Increased numbers of miniaturized vellus hairs
Pigment incontinence of hair bulbs and follicular stelae

Differential Diagnosis

Other causes of patchy alopecia include tinea capitis, trichotillomania,
traction and pressure alopecia, loose anagen syndrome, secondary
syphilis, congenital triangular alopecia, familial focal alopecia, aplasia cutis, pseudopelade, tick bite alopecia, etc.

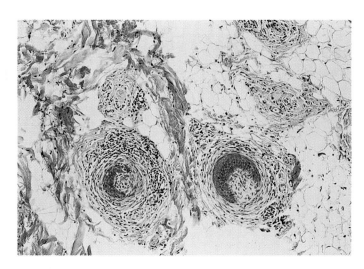

FIGURE 10-8 Alopecia areata, horizontal section, reticular dermis: 2 hair bulbs surrounded by lymphocytes and 3 follicular stelae infiltrated by lymphocytes are visible.

and an anagen:telogen ratio of 73 percent to 27 percent (Table 10-4).[36] The reduction in total hairs and the increase in vellus and telogen hairs contrast with normal controls. Contrary to general belief, there is a definite follicular dropout with fibrosis in about 10 percent of cases with a long history of attacks of alopecia areata.[6] Peribulbar lymphocytic infiltration may not be prominent between acute attacks. In such cases the reduced anagen:telogen and terminal:vellus ratios, and the possible presence of catagen hairs, may be useful indicators of alopecia areata.[6] Melanin incontinence, trichomalacia, and foreign-body tissue reaction may be further diagnostic pointers.[28] It is surprising, however, that in some chronic and apparently inactive cases of alopecia areata, perifollicular mononuclear cell infiltrates are still found.[18]

Differential Diagnosis Causes of patchy alopecia, which may be confused with alopecia areata, include tinea capitis, trichotillomania, trac-

tion alopecia, pressure alopecia, congenital triangular alopecia, loose anagen syndrome, familial focal alopecia,[37] secondary syphilis,[18] tick bite alopecia, and scarring alopecia such as aplasia cutis and pseudopelade. These can usually be distinguished by the history and clinical appearance, but biopsies may be necessary. Tinea capitis shows chronic folliculitis, often granulomatous, with intrafollicular neutrophils; fungal spores and hyphae may still be present. Inflammation and miniaturized hairs are lacking in trichotillomania and other forms of traumatic alopecia, but catagen hairs occur. Inflammation is absent in congenital triangular alopecia and loose anagen syndrome and in familial focal alopecia in which a marked increase of telogen germinal units with no scarring indicates telogen arrest; terminal hairs are reduced in congenital triangular alopecia but not in loose anagen syndrome. Plasma cells may be sparse or plentiful in the diffuse inflammation of secondary syphilis. Cicatricial alopecia is characterized by permanent destruction of hair follicles with replacement by fibrosis. Follicles are undamaged in tick bite alopecia, which is a localized telogen effluvium caused by an anticoagulant in tick saliva.

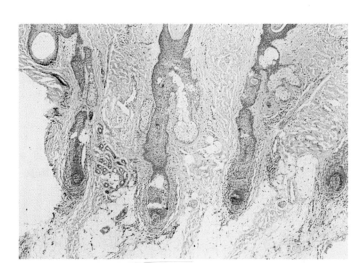

FIGURE 10-7 Alopecia areata, vertical section: 4 hair bulbs are seen surrounded by lymphocytes, with follicular stelae beneath them, also infiltrated by lymphocytes. A lymphocytic infiltration is also present around lower hair follicles.

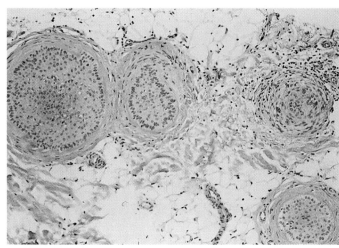

FIGURE 10-9 Alopecia areata, horizontal section, reticular dermis: 1 catagen hair (left lateral margin), 1 follicular stela infiltrated by lymphocytes (right lateral margin), and 2 telogen germinal units are visible.

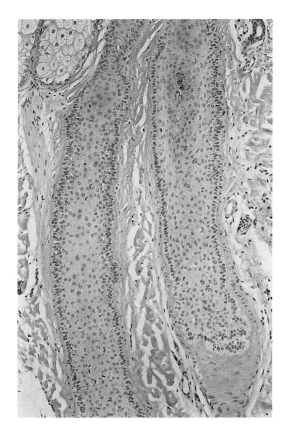

FIGURE 10-10   Alopecia areata, vertical section: 2 catagen hairs are present showing a thickened vitreous membrane and central apoptotic cells.

Trichotillomania

Trichotillomania is an abnormal compulsion to pull out hair. It affects more children than adults and after age 6 years is commoner in females. Two polar forms of trichotillomania occur: The juvenile type peaks between 2 and 6 years, and the adult between 11 and 17 years of age.[38] In children the habit may develop subconsciously and replace thumb sucking or represent an effort to gain attention. Mental retardation or severe psychologic disturbances are more common in adults.

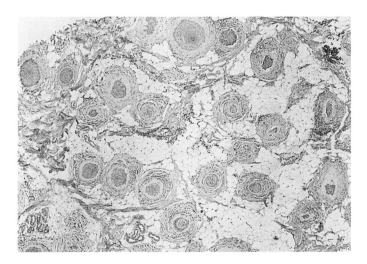

FIGURE 10-11   Alopecia areata, horizontal section, reticular dermis: Several hair bulbs surrounded by lymphocytes, a large number of catagen hairs surrounded by thickened vitreous membrane and lymphocytes, several telogen germinal units, and some follicular stelae infiltrated by lymphocytes are visible.

TABLE 10-11
Trichotillomania

Clinical Features

Recurrent attacks of patchy hair loss—chronic course
Affected hairs broken off at different lengths
Underlying scalp usually normal

Histopathological Features

Normal follicular counts with normal terminal:vellus ratio
Marked increase in catagen and telogen hairs
Follicular damage may be present
Follicles may contain pigmented casts
Trichomalacia can occur
Inflammatory changes usually absent

Differential Diagnosis

Other causes of patchy alopecia include alopecia areata, tinea capitis, loose anagen syndrome, traction and pressure alopecia, secondary syphilis, tick bite alopecia, aplasia cutis, congenital triangular alopecia, familial focal alopecia, pseudopelade, etc.

Clinical Features   Trichotillomania presents with one or more patches of hair thinning (Table 10-11).[39] The patches are characterized by an irregular stubble due to hair breakage at different times.[40] In severe patches, only newly growing anagen hairs remain.[41] The underlying scalp is usually normal. Trichotillomania can involve eyebrows and lashes. The onset is often sudden, and the course is fluctuating and prolonged.

Histopathological Features   Normal numbers of hair follicles are present (Fig. 10-12), although some may be distorted by hair shaft avulsion and show perifollicular shearing and hemorrhages (Table 10-11). Follicular plugging and pigment casts are common, but true trichomalacia, or softened, twisted hair, is less frequent. Hair plucking induces telogen via catagen, accounting for the high catagen and telogen counts seen in trichotillomania (Figs. 10-13, 10-14). Miniaturized hairs are not seen.[42] Inflammatory changes are not a feature of trichotillomania, unless excoriations are complicated by secondary bacterial infection with infiltration of neutrophils, lymphocytes, and histiocytes.[18] The average follicular count in horizontal sections of a 4-mm punch biopsy of trichotillomania comprises 32 terminal hairs + 7 vellus hairs = 39 total hairs, with a terminal:vellus ratio of 5:1, similar to normal controls; however, a ratio of 58 percent anagen to 42 percent telogen and an average of 5 catagen hairs are strikingly abnormal (Table 10-4).[6] Catagen hairs are rare in normal controls.

Differential Diagnosis   Other causes of patchy alopecia must be excluded. Trichotillomania is often misdiagnosed as tinea capitis, alopecia areata, or even loose anagen syndrome. Other conditions to be excluded include other forms of traction alopecia, pressure alopecia, secondary syphilis, congenital triangular alopecia, tick bite alopecia, and subtle forms of scarring alopecia such as pseudopelade and congenital aplasia cutis. The history and appearance are often diagnostic, but in some cases scalp biopsies are necessary. The lack of inflammation, fungal elements, and scarring and the presence of terminal hairs, catagen hairs, and trichomalacia exclude most other conditions (see discussion of differential diagnosis of alopecia areata). Differentiation from other forms of traction alopecia may depend on clinical history.

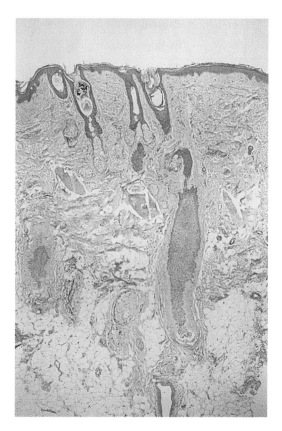

FIGURE 10-12 Trichotillomania, vertical section: 1 terminal hair, 1 telogen hair, and 2 follicular stelae are seen projecting into the subcutaneous tissue. Another telogen hair is seen in the middle dermis; 1 follicular infundibulum shows trichomalacia.

Traction and Pressure Alopecia

There are many other causes of traction alopecia besides trichotillomania. Acute traction alopecia results from sudden, painful avulsion in accidental or intentional hair pulling or domestic or industrial accidents. Chronic traction alopecia is more common and insidious and results from hair weaves, other hair additions glued or clipped in place, excessive brushing, backcombing, braiding, or tight ponytails.

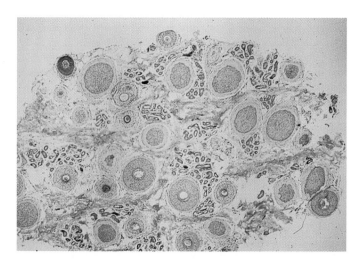

FIGURE 10-13 Trichotillomania, horizontal section, reticular dermis: 1 hair bulb, some terminal hairs, many catagen hairs, a telogen hair, and a telogen terminal unit are visible.

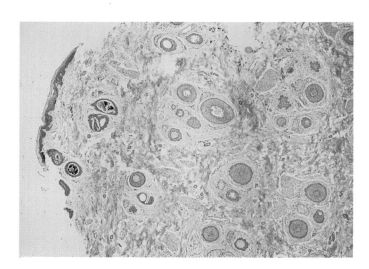

FIGURE 10-14 Trichotillomania, horizontal section, papillary dermis: Terminal hairs, telogen hairs, telogen germinal units and vellus hairs are visible. Several follicular infundibula show pigment casts or trichomalacia. There is no inflammation.

Prolonged pressure on the scalp from prolonged immobility can cause alopecia.

Clinical Features   Bandlike traction alopecia involving frontal, temporal, and occipital scalp hair margins is usually due to ponytails with the maximum pull on peripheral hairs (Table 10-12).

Traction alopecia from hair weaves, and other hair additions, occurs at the point of attachment.[43] Traction alopecia can occur between tight braids and in areas where hair is wound too tightly on rollers.[44] Sustained traction usually induces telogen in affected hairs, which eventually fall out.

Pressure alopecia can occur in the newborn and in patients of any age who are severely injured, very ill, or anesthetized or who have sustained blunt trauma to the scalp. It usually results from prolonged immobilization of the patient on a hard operating table, bed, or floor. The soft-tissue compression over underlying skull causes ischemia.[45] A patch of alopecia develops over the compressed scalp within 2 to 4 weeks but regrows within a few months, unless permanent scarring has resulted from necrosis and ulceration.[44]

Histopathological Features   The histopathology of traction alopecia is similar to trichotillomania. Due to the sustained traction many catagen and telogen hairs are seen which reduce the anagen:telogen ratio (Table 10-12) (Figs. 10-15, 10-16). There is usually a lack of inflammation. Total follicular counts on horizontal section are identical to normal controls. Pigment casts and trichomalacia are rare (Fig. 10-17).[18] In chronic traction alopecia affecting hair margins, dense fibrosis may be present around upper and lower follicles.

In the early stages of pressure alopecia, vascular thrombosis, and tissue necrosis, with a mild lymphohistiocytic infiltrate, may be present. Most of the terminal hairs are then projected into a catagen or telogen phase. Fat necrosis with foamy macrophages, and varied degrees of dermal fibrosis, may eventuate.[18]

Differential Diagnosis   The diagnosis of an acute traction or avulsion alopecia is usually easy from the history and physical appearance. Marginal alopecia must be distinguished from ophiasis and tinea capitis. Other forms of patchy hair loss such as loose anagen syndrome, secondary syphilis, alopecia from chemical trauma, congenital triangular alopecia, tick bite alopecia, and subtle forms of scarring such as pseudopelade and congenital aplasia cutis may also have to be excluded.

TABLE 10-12

Traction and Pressure Alopecia

Clinical Features

Acute traction alopecia from avulsion: easily diagnosable from history and clinical findings

Obvious linear alopecia at scalp hair margins, caused by chronic traction from ponytails

Chronic traction alopecia under points of attachment of hair weaves or other hair additions more subtle

Pressure alopecia: localized to the area of pressure and usually transient

Histopathological Features

Normal follicular counts with normal terminal:vellus ratio

Marked increase in catagen and telogen hairs

Occasional pigmented casts; trichomalacia uncommon

Inflammatory changes usually absent

In late cases of marginal alopecia, terminal hairs decreased due to follicular fibrosis

Catagen and telogen hairs increased from pressure alopecia

Differential Diagnosis

Common causes of patchy alopecia to be differentiated from traumatic alopecia include trichotillomania, alopecia areata—especially ophiasis, tinea capitis, loose anagen syndrome, and other causes of localized alopecia.

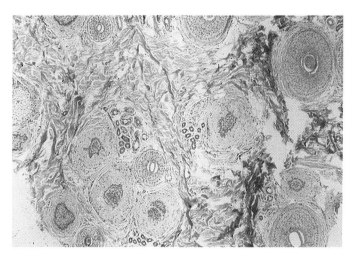

FIGURE 10-16 Traction alopecia, horizontal section, reticular dermis: 3 terminal hairs, 3 vellus hairs, and 7 telogen germinal units are visible. There is no inflammation.

This can usually be done on clinical grounds, but in some cases scalp biopsies are helpful. The frequent presence of scarring with increased catagen and telogen hairs in chronic cases, and the lack of inflammation and fungal elements, should exclude alopecia areata and tinea capitis. For discussion of other causes of patchy hair loss see discussion of differential diagnosis of alopecia areata.

Miscellaneous Causes of Nonscarring Alopecia

Rarer causes of nonscarring alopecia include alopecia due to infections and infestations, alopecia due to hair shaft abnormalities, alopecia due to hereditary and congenital conditions such as ectodermal dysplasias, and alopecia due to various dermatoses involving the scalp which are sometimes accompanied by hair loss. Some of these conditions are discussed elsewhere and others are beyond the scope of this chapter.

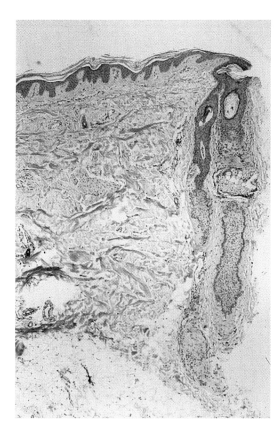

FIGURE 10-15 Traction alopecia, vertical section: 1 terminal catagen hair and 1 terminal telogen hair are seen. A mild lymphohistiocytic infiltrate is present around 1 follicular infundibulum.

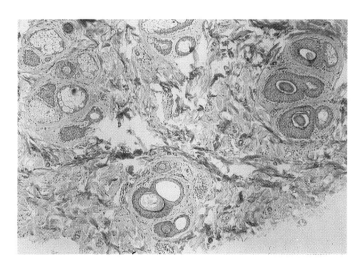

FIGURE 10-17 Traction alopecia, horizontal section, papillary dermis: Terminal and vellus hairs are seen. Several follicular infundibula are empty. No trichomalacia is present. There is a mild lymphohistiocytic infiltrate around a few follicular infundibula.

Clinical Features   A common cause of patchy alopecia in small children is tinea capitis.[46] This produces circumscribed areas of hair loss with inflammation, scaling, crusting, and broken-off hairs. Black dots from hairs broken off flush with the skin indicate endothrix ringworm, due to *Trichophyton tonsurans* in the United States. Whitish-gray hairs broken off a few millimeters away from the scalp and fluorescent to Wood's light are caused by an ectothrix infection such as *Microsporum canis* or *M. audouini*. Most cases of tinea capitis occur in children, peaking at 5 to 6 years of age, but endothrix ringworm caused by *T. tonsurans* and favus caused by *T. schoenleinii* can occur in adults. The diagnosis can usually be confirmed by a potassium hydroxide preparation or by culture, and a biopsy is rarely necessary.

Bacterial infections such as syphilis and viral infections such as herpes zoster, which are capable of causing alopecia, will not be discussed here.[46]

Broken-off hairs can result from hair shaft abnormalities. Only the histopathology of loose anagen syndrome will be discussed in this chapter. The reader is referred to other source material for a discussion of hair shaft anomalies.[47–50]

There are many different forms of congenital or inherited hair loss.[51,52] These include congenital hypotrichosis with or without associated defects, congenital triangular alopecia, and a large variety of ectodermal dysplasias affecting the hair, teeth, nails, and sweat glands. There are also major congenital hypotrichoses which occur in hereditary syndromes such as the hereditary hypotrichosis of Marie Unna, Hallerman-Streiff syndrome, and atrichia with papular lesions. Major congenital hypotrichosis also occurs in premature aging syndromes and with skeletal abnormalities. Minor hypotrichosis can occur in other hereditary syndromes and in chromosomal abnormalities. In general, the diseases causing congenital or inherited hypotrichosis are associated with hair loss due to a reduction in hair follicles which may be patchy or patterned or generalized.

Various dermatoses which do not directly cause alopecia may lead to pruritus, erythema, scaling, crusting, and excoriations. A secondary alopecia may result which is usually reversed by treating the underlying cause. Such dermatoses include seborrheic dermatitis, psoriasis, tinea amiantacea, and prurigo and lichen simplex.[18,46]

Histopathological Features   If the alopecia is produced by an infection, the histopathology should reflect the pathology of that particular infection. Sometimes unsuspected fungal infections are seen on histopathologic examination and confirmed with a PAS stain. Secondary syphilis can be difficult to diagnose.[18]

Hair shaft abnormalities are usually diagnosed by microscopic examination of the hair shaft. In loose anagen syndrome the hair shafts may show absent inner and outer root sheaths, a ruffled cuticle, and longitudinal grooving[53]; in biopsies, loss of adhesion between follicular sheaths may only be seen with transmission electron microscopy. However, splits between follicular sheaths are sometimes seen with light microscopy and may represent real changes due to loose anagen syndrome rather than to fixation and sectioning artifacts (Fig. 10-18); inflammation is absent, but premature keratinization of the inner root sheath may be seen.[54]

Congenital triangular alopecia is distinguished by a normal follicular count, with a reduction in the total number of terminal anagen hairs, although many vellus hairs are seen.[18] However, a frequent feature of these cases is the presence of many telogen hairs. This arrested state of hair cycling also appears to be common in various types of congenital hypotrichosis (Figs. 10-19, 10-20) and ectodermal dysplasia (Fig. 10-21).

Associated dermatoses such as seborrheic dermatitis, psoriasis, or lichen simplex may be diagnosed by their specific pathologic appearance.

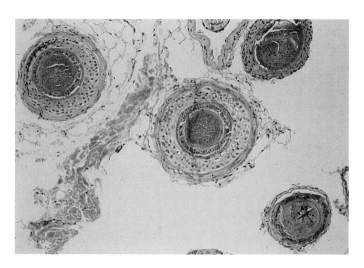

FIGURE 10-18   Loose anagen syndrome, horizontal section, reticular dermis: In many follicles clefts are present between the hair shaft and the internal root sheath, within the layers of the internal root sheath, between the internal root sheath and the external root sheath, or between the external root sheath and the surrounding connective tissue layer. One hair bulb shows a cleft between the matrix of the bulb and the surrounding connective tissue sheath.

Differential Diagnosis   The differential diagnosis of infections, congenital and inherited causes of alopecia, hair shaft abnormalities, and miscellaneous dermatoses includes most of the conditions discussed in this chapter. The diagnosis can usually be made on clinical grounds or by examination of hair shafts, but scalp biopsies may be necessary to clarify diagnoses.

SCARRING ALOPECIA

Clinically, scarring alopecias are characterized by loss of follicular orifices. Distinguishing characteristics that aid in diagnosis include the pattern of alopecia, pigmentary alteration, follicular prominence, keratinous plugs, follicular pustules, and any other associated nonscalp cutaneous findings. Histologic evaluation of progressive, "active" alopecia is very helpful for diagnosis of specific scarring alopecias.

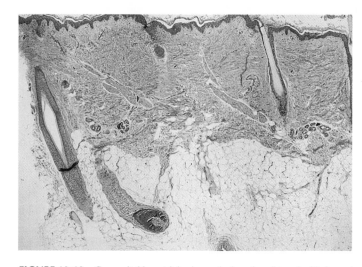

FIGURE 10-19   Congenital hypotrichosis, vertical section: 2 terminal hairs and 4 follicular stelae are seen in the subcutaneous tissue; 1 telogen hair is seen in the dermis. There is no inflammation.

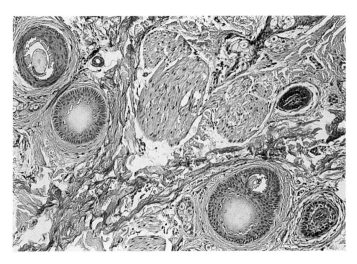

FIGURE 10-20   Congenital hypotrichosis, horizontal section, middle dermis: 1 terminal hair, 2 telogen hairs, 2 telogen germinal units and 1 vellus are visible.

However, biopsies from patients with inactive, "burned out" scarring alopecia infrequently yield a specific diagnosis, but microscopic evaluation for the extent of follicular destruction is helpful in evaluating the chance of regrowth.

Biopsy Site and Technique

Appropriate biopsy site selection is essential for histologic diagnosis of alopecia.[3,4–6,18,55] If present, primary lesions such as pustules, vesicles,

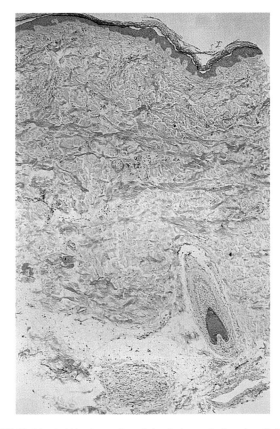

FIGURE 10-21   Anhidrotic ectodermal dysplasia, vertical section: Only 1 terminal hair is present, and no mature eccrine glands are seen. Primordial eccrine glands are present at the inferior margin of the specimen.

TABLE 10-13
Advantages and Disadvantages of Transverse Sections

Advantages
  More follicles per section
  Rapid, accurate assessment of follicle density, the number of terminal follicles and the preservation or loss of normal follicular unit morphology
  Easy assessment of follicle and shaft diameters
  Most accurate anagen:telogen ratios
Disadvantages
  Must be familiar with scalp microanatomy in a different plane of sectioning
  Gross tissue-specimen processing requires a different protocol
  The epidermis and dermal-epidermal interface is more easily evaluated in vertical sections
Limitations of both methods
  The 4 to 6 mm of scalp biopsy is a small sample compared to the total scalp area
  Biopsy site selection is critical
  The specificity of the histopathologic diagnosis decreases with the duration and extent of follicular destruction

SOURCE: Adapted from Templeton SF, Solomon AR: Alopecia: histologic diagnosis by transverse section. *Sem Diagn Pathol* 13:2–18, 1996, with permission.

or follicular papules should be sampled. In patterned alopecia, the biopsy should be taken at the boundary between alopecia and normal scalp with special care to include areas of erythema, empty follicular orifices, and small or abnormal shafts. Biopsy of an area completely devoid of hair is usually not advisable but can be helpful in some instances to evaluate the extent of follicular destruction and potential for regrowth for treatment purposes.[56]

A round punch biopsy tool (at least 4 mm, preferably 6 mm) should be used and positioned parallel to the direction of hair shaft growth. The biopsy specimen should include abundant subcutaneous fat, as the bulb and lower portion of the follicle are present in the subcutis. Occasionally two specimens may be helpful, as one can be processed using transverse sections and the other using traditional vertical sections.[57]

Transverse versus Vertical Section Techniques

Much has been written about the utility of transverse sections in evaluating alopecia, and the advantages of this technique are many (Table 10-13).[5,56] Familiarity with follicular microanatomy is essential when evaluating transverse sections (Table 10-14), and several recent reviews describe this in detail.[4,5,9,56] The follicular units are encompassed by fine adventitial dermis and separated by coarse reticular dermis.

TABLE 10-14
Normal Transverse Section Microanatomy—4-mm Punch Biopsy

Follicular unit composition	2–4 terminal follicles
	2–4 vellus follicles
	Sebaceous lobules
	Arrector pili
Follicular unit density	10–12 follicular units
Hair follicle density	20–40 terminal follicles
Anagen follicles	90%
Telogen follicles	10%

Transverse sections allow for rapid detection of pathologic alteration of this normal follicular microanatomy, especially follicular density.

Transverse sectioning provides for semiquantitative evaluation of numerous follicles and follicular units in one section, thus allowing for a rapid, accurate assessment of whether the specimen represents a scarring or nonscarring alopecia. By definition, scarring alopecias show diminished follicular density (complete follicular dropout) and disruption of follicular unit morphology. Evaluation of follicular density is more difficult using traditional vertical sections, since multiple serial sections must be examined. Furthermore, follicular unit morphology cannot be accurately assessed with vertical sections. The dermal epidermal junction is more easily evaluated in vertical sections but can also be viewed in transverse sections, although in tangential orientation.

Primary or Secondary Scarring Alopecia

Scarring alopecia is either primary or secondary depending on the pattern of follicular destruction.[5,55] *Primary scarring alopecia* occurs as the result of preferential destruction of follicular epithelium and/or its associated adventitial dermis with relative sparing of the intervening reticular dermis. In primary scarring alopecia, the hair follicle is the primary target of destruction. The interfollicular epidermis may be affected as in lupus erythematosus and lichen planopilaris, but the epidermal changes in and of themselves do not result in follicular destruction. Primary scarring alopecias are a diverse group of diseases with differing or uncertain etiologies. The unifying feature of these varied disorders is destruction of sufficient follicles to yield permanent alopecia.

Many classification systems of scarring alopecia have been proposed according to clinical, histologic, and pathogenic factors. Microscopically, primary scarring alopecia is easily categorized into two groups according to the predominant inflammatory cell type: (1) *lymphocyte-associated scarring alopecia* and (2) *neutrophil-associated (pustulofollicular) scarring alopecia.*

Secondary scarring alopecia occurs as the result of nonfollicular events that impinge upon and eventually destroy the follicle.[5,55] Follicular destruction and subsequent permanent scarring alopecia is not the primary pathologic process but occurs secondarily due to the close anatomic location of follicles to the primary pathologic event, i.e., dermal sclerosis in coup de sabre linear morphea.

Lymphocyte-Associated Primary Scarring Alopecia

Discoid lupus erythematosus (DLE), *lichen planopilaris* (LPP), *pseudopelade of Brocq* (PPOB), *follicular degeneration syndrome* (FDS), and *alopecia mucinosa* (AM) are lymphocyte-associated scarring alopecias that may be distinguished by the presence and type of interface alteration, pattern and density of lymphocytic infiltrates, and intrafollicular mucin deposits (Table 10-15).

DISCOID LUPUS ERYTHEMATOSUS

Clinical Features   Scalp involvement in DLE is common, and 30 to 50 percent of patients develop scarring alopecia.[58,59] DLE typically occurs in young to middle-aged females (2:1 female predominance), and lesions occur on sun-exposed sites, especially the face, scalp, and conchal bowel of the ear. Early lesions are scaly erythematous papules, and late lesions are sclerotic plaques with follicular plugging, telangiectasia, and pigmentary alteration. Patients with DLE uncommonly progress to systemic lupus erythematosus.[60] Diffuse, nonscarring alopecia may occur in patients with systemic lupus erythematosus but is best categorized as *inflammatory telogen effluvium.*[21]

Histopathological Features   *Vacuolar interface alteration* at the level of the epidermis and hair follicle is the primary feature of DLE (Table 10-15). Epidermal and follicular dyskeratosis is also present, but less than in LPP. The epidermis is often atrophic with overlying orthokeratotic hyperkeratosis, but the hypertrophic variant of DLE is characterized by marked acanthosis and hyperkeratosis. Focal parakeratosis may be seen in some lesions. Laminated keratin fills dilated follicular ostia corresponding to the clinical follicular plugs. The basement membrane zone of the epidermis and/or follicle may be thickened with a corrugated appearance. This finding is best seen with the PAS stain and ultrastructurally represents a multilayered basal lamina.

Superficial and deep, perivascular and periadnexal lymphocytic infiltrates of variable density are present (Figs. 10-22 and 10-23). Occasional admixed plasma cells can be found. Lymphocyte exocytosis into the epidermis and follicular epithelium may be present but is usually not prominent. Pigment incontinence with melanophagocytosis is commonly seen in the papillary dermis. Increased dermal mucin (hyaluronic acid) is present both superficially and deep and is best detected in colloidal iron- or alcian blue-stained sections. Dermal sclerosis and complete follicular dropout occurs in advanced lesions and is similar to end-stage microscopic findings of other primary scarring alopecias.

Biopsies of well-established clinical lesions for immunofluorescence usually show granular immunoglobulin and complement at the dermal-epidermal junction. IgM deposits are more common but less specific for DLE than IgG deposits.[61] The incidence of lesional immunoglobulin deposition in DLE is about 75 percent with older, sun-exposed lesions more likely to be positive.[61–63]

Differential Diagnosis   LPP and pseudopelade are the primary differential diagnostic considerations as described below (Table 10-15). Both are also lymphocyte-associated scarring alopecias, and end-stage biopsies from all these entities can be identical. However, in "active" clinical lesions, interface alteration in DLE is primarily vacuolar rather than lichenoid as in LPP. The superficial and deep infiltrate is both perivascular and periadnexal in DLE as opposed to tightly perifollicular in LPP. PPOB and FDS lack interface alteration around follicles.

LICHEN PLANOPILARIS

Clinical Features   LPP is an uncommon scarring alopecia. First described in 1895 by Pringle, LPP presents as acuminate, spinous, and hyperkeratotic follicular papules with perifollicular erythema (Table 10-15).[64] LPP is more common in women, and onset ranges from young adulthood to elderly age. As follicles are destroyed, smooth, atrophic, polygonal-shaped patches of complete alopecia result. Typical lichen planus papules and plaques are present elsewhere on the body in 50 to 70 percent of patients. The clinical triad of typical lichen planus, spinous or accuminate lesions, and alopecia of the scalp or other nonglabrous skin is known as the *Graham-Little syndrome.* Noninflammatory end-stage lesions closely resemble PPOB. Drug-induced LPP, especially gold, rarely occurs.[65]

Histopathological Features   *Lichenoid interface alteration* of follicular epithelium is the primary microscopic feature of LPP (Table 10-15) (Figs. 10-24 and 10-25). Although not always completely distinct from vacuolar interface alteration, lichenoid interface alteration of the follicle is characterized by disruption of the epithelial-adventitial dermal junction with angular glassy basal keratinocytes and a tight perifollicular lymphocytic infiltrate that is largely confined to the follicular adventitial dermis. (Figs. 10-24, 10-25) Exocytosis into the follicular epithelium and dyskeratosis are more prominent in LPP than DLE. Artifactual

TABLE 10-15

Lymphocyte-Associated Primary Scarring Alopecia

	Discoid lupus erythematosus	Lichen planopilaris	Pseudopelade of Brocq	Follicular mucinosis
Clinical Features	Young to middle-aged Women > men Erythematous papules to sclerotic plaques Follicular plugging, telangiectasia, dyspigmentation	Adults Women > men Acuminate, spinous hyperkeratotic follicular papules Perifollicular erythema Smooth atrophic polygonal-shaped patches of alopecia	Young to middle-aged Women >> men Slowly progressive, irregularly shaped alopecic patches ("footprints in the snow") Confluence of patches Noninflammatory	All ages Head and neck > trunk, extremities Erythematous infiltrate Sometimes boggy plaques with scaling, expression of mucin Adults have lymphoproliferative disorder in about 30% of cases
Histopathological Features				
Interface alteration at DEJ	Primarily vacuolar	Primarily lichenoid if present	Absent	Absent
at follicle	Primarily vacuolar	Primarily lichenoid	Absent	Absent
Dyskeratosis	Minimal to moderate	Moderate to prominent	Absent	Absent
Inflammation type	Lymphocytic	Lymphocytic	Lymphocytic	Lymphocytic
Perivascular pattern	Superficial and deep	Minimal superficial perivascular, primarily perifollicular	Mostly superficial	May be superficial and deep in lymphoma
Perifollicular infiltrates	Present, prominent	Present, prominent	Present, sparse	Present, variable
Perieccrine infiltrates	Present	Absent	Absent	Absent
Epidermal mucin	Minimal	Absent	Absent	Prominent
Dermal mucin	Moderate to prominent	Absent	Absent	Minimal
Concentric lamellar fibrosis	End-stage finding	Yes in advanced lesions	Prominent	No
Pigment incontinence	Yes	Yes	Minimal	No

SOURCE: Adapted from Templeton SF, Solomon AR. Scarring alopecia: A classification based on microscopic criteria. *J Cutan Pathol* 21:97–109, 1994, with permission.

clefting similar to that seen at the dermal epidermal junction in lichen planus (Max Joseph space) can also occur around hair follicles in LPP. In a minority of cases, lichenoid interface alteration typical of lichen planus may affect the intervening epidermis. Superficial and deep perivascular lymphocytic infiltrates and dermal mucin typical of DLE is lacking in LPP.

Complete follicular dropout with scattered naked hair shafts surrounded by sparse histiocytic and granulomatous infiltrates occurs in late lesions. These end-stage features are not specific for LPP but may occur in all scarring alopecias.

Lesional biopsy for direct immunofluorescence reveals globular IgM deposits on cytoid bodies and fibrin at the dermal-epidermal junction and infundibular-adventitial dermal junction.[62,63,66] However these immunofluorescent findings are not specific for LPP and may be seen in other dermatoses with interface dermatitis.

Differential Diagnosis   DLE, PPOB, and FDS are considered in the differential diagnosis (Table 10-15). See discussion of these entities for details.

PSEUDOPELADE OF BROCQ/FOLLICULAR DEGENERATION SYNDROME

Much controversy surrounds pseudopelade. Brocq first described this form of alopecia in 1885 as a clinically noninflammatory, progressive,

idiopathic scarring alopecia.[67] Since then, conflicting opinions have arisen as to whether pseudopelade is a disease *sui generis* or just end-stage scarring alopecia due to other diseases such as DLE, LPP, and folliculitis decalvans.[1,5,64,68–72] There is evidence that PPOB is a unique primary scarring alopecia given the relatively distinct clinical and histologic features of well-established lesions. However, it is clear that end-stage LPP, DLE, and folliculitis decalvans can clinically result in a pseudopeladelike state which microscopically consists of nonspecific, permanent follicular ablation.[72]

The *follicular degeneration syndrome* (FDS) as described by Sperling and colleagues[72,74] is considered by many to be a variant of PPOB. Considerable clinical overlap exists between classic PPOB and FDS, and the microscopic findings are virtually identical.

Clinical Features   Classically described PPOB is a patterned alopecia that begins as small, round to irregularly shaped alopecic patches that progress to large, irregular, smooth-surfaced zones with rare scattered hairs (Table 10-15). The appearance of early lesions has been described as "foot prints in the snow." Perifollicular erythema is common in active disease but absent in the burned-out quiescent state. The clinical course involves slow but unrelenting progression that eventually ceases after several years, leaving large areas of permanent alopecia. PPOB is most common in young to middle-aged women and uncommon in men.

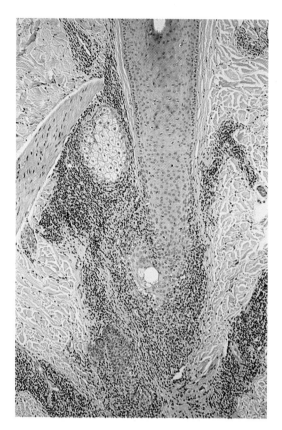

FIGURE 10-22 Discoid lupus erythematosus, vertical sections: Superficial and deep perifollicular and perivascular lymphocytic infiltrates with vacuolar interface alteration of follicular epithelium.

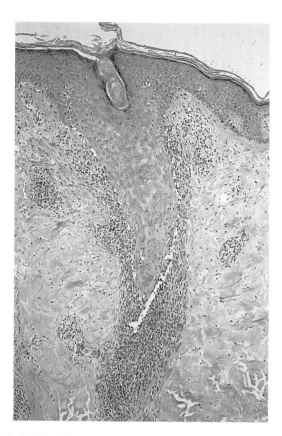

FIGURE 10-24 Lichen planopilaris, vertical sections: Infundibular keratinocytes are glassy with lichenoid interface alteration and perifollicular lymphocytic infiltrate. The epidermis is largely spared.

The FDS variant of PPOB is almost exclusively seen in black patients and more commonly affects women.[73] The alopecia begins on the crown and in severe cases expands centrifugally to involve the entire vertex. As in classic PPOB, no epidermal changes are present, leaving a smooth skin surface, and variable perifollicular erythema is seen. Scattered hairs, some exhibiting polytrichea, are present in the alopecic regions.

Histopathological Features The earliest findings are perifollicular lymphocytic infiltrates and perifollicular fibroplasia *without* interface

alteration (Table 10-15) (Fig. 10-26). The infiltrate is more dense in these early lesions and present from the level of the follicular infundibulum to the middle segment of the follicle. Sparse adjacent perivascular lymphocytic infiltrates may also be present. Follicular density is diminished, and the follicular unit morphology is disrupted. Scattered residual fibrous tracts indicating the site of destroyed follicles are present.

In more advanced areas, the predominant finding is *concentric lamellar fibroplasia* and follicular epithelial atrophy (Fig. 10-27). Frequently the follicular canal is eccentrically located, and premature disintegration of the inner root sheath is emphasized in FDS.[73] Finally,

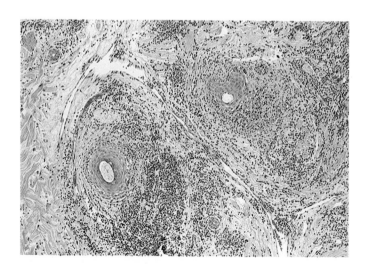

FIGURE 10-23 Discoid lupus erythematosus, horizontal sections.

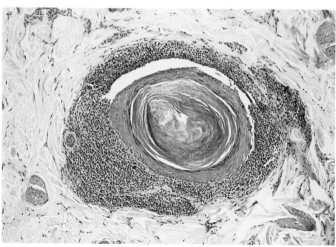

FIGURE 10-25 Lichen planopilaris, horizontal sections: Dense perifollicular lichenoid infiltrates with artifactual clefting.

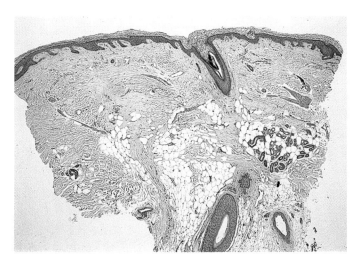

FIGURE 10-26 Pseudopelade of Brocq/Follicular degeneration syndrome, vertical sections: Diminished follicular density with vertically oriented residual fibrous tracts and sparse lymphocytic infiltrates.

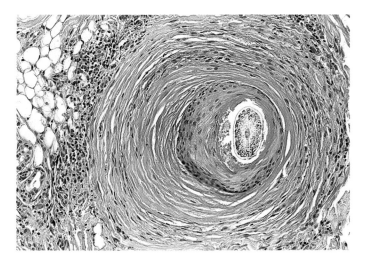

FIGURE 10-27 Pseudopelade of Brocq/Follicular degeneration syndrome, horizontal sections: Concentric lamellar fibroplasia surrounds a follicle with eccentric thinning of follicular epithelium. Only sparse lymphocytes are seen.

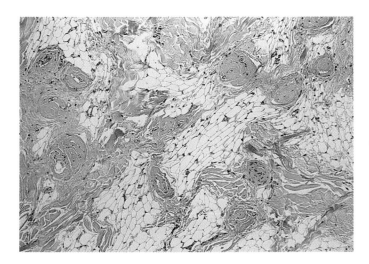

FIGURE 10-28 End-stage scarring alopecia, horizontal sections: Complete follicular dropout with numerous residual fibrous tracts. These end-stage features occur in many primary scarring alopecias and are not diagnostic of a specific entity.

the follicular epithelium becomes so atrophic as to rupture, and a foreign-body giant cell reaction ensues. In end-stage PPOB, only rare viable, though somewhat miniaturized, follicles are present, and numerous residual fibrous tracts are present. These end-stage changes are similar to those seen in other primary scarring alopecias, including DLE and LPP (Fig. 10-28).

Direct immunofluorescence is usually negative, but occasional, minimal nonspecific IgM deposits may be seen around the follicular infundibulum.[62,69]

Differential Diagnosis   DLE, LPP, and end-stage folliculitis decalvans may be considered (Table 10-15). The lack of interface dermatitis in PPOB is the primary distinguishing microscopic feature from DLE and LPP. The neutrophil is the predominant inflammatory cell in active folliculitis decalvans, but end-stage folliculitis decalvans and PPOB are similar.

ALOPECIA MUCINOSA (AM)

Clinical Features   AM most commonly involves the head and neck, but involvement of the trunk and extremities may occur (Table 10-15). Lesions are erythematous, scaling, infiltrated plaques devoid of hair. When AM affects children and young adults, it is usually self-limited without permanent alopecia; however, follicular destruction by extensive mucin deposits can occasionally lead to permanent alopecia in some patients.[75] An associated lymphoproliferative disorder, most commonly mycosis fungoides, occurs in approximately 30 percent of cases, especially older patients with numerous lesions.[76,77]

Histopathological Features   Mucin (hyaluronic acid) deposition in hair follicle epithelium is the cardinal microscopic feature of AM and is termed *follicular mucinosis* (Table 10-15). Follicular keratinocytes are stellate-shaped and splayed apart by extracellular mucin. The mucin is initially deposited in the infundibulum but involves the entire follicle in advanced lesions with intrafollicular mucin-filled cystic spaces (Fig. 10-29). The mucin can be identified in hematoxylin and eosin stained sections but is best appreciated with colloidal iron or alcian blue stains. Variably dense perifollicular lymphocytic infiltrates with admixed eosinophils are present. Folliculo-tropism of lymphocytes can be seen in both lymphoma-associated and non-lymphoma-associated AM. Although it is difficult to distinguish the banal form from the lymphoma-associated form, pronounced epidermotropism, cellular atypia and confluent papillary dermal infiltrates are usual markers of coexisting cutaneous T-cell lymphoma.

Differential Diagnosis   *Follicular mucinosis* is considered by some to be a synonym of AM, but this term is best used as a microscopic description of intrafollicular mucin deposits and not the clinical pathologic entity, AM.[78] Focal, limited follicular mucinosis outside of the setting of AM occurs and likely represents a reactive follicular process. Follicular spongiosis in follicular eczema and seborrheic dermatitis may mimic early AM, and mucin stains help differentiate follicular mucin from follicular spongiosis.

Pustulofollicular, Neutrophil-Associated Primary Scarring Alopecia

The pustulofollicular, neutrophil-associated primary scarring alopecias are *dissecting cellulitis of the scalp* (DCS), *folliculitis decalvans* (FD), *acne keloidalis* (AK), *erosive pustular dermatosis of the scalp* (EPDS), and *tinea capitis* (TC) (Table 10-16). Common features include early comedonal dilatation and predominately neutrophilic infiltrates. Early lesions have overlapping clinical and microscopic features, but well-developed cases are distinct.

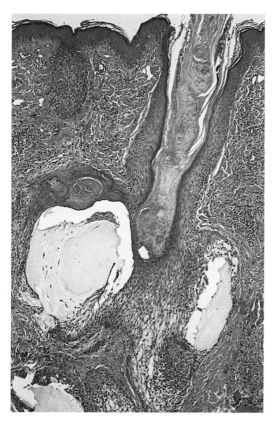

FIGURE 10-29 Alopecia mucinosa, vertical sections: Extensive mucin deposits are present including mucin-filled cystic spaces.

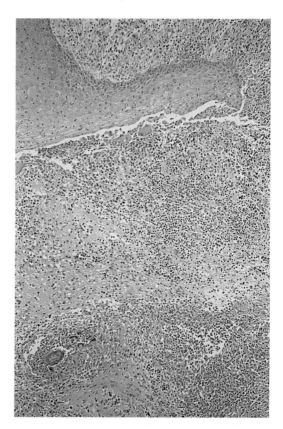

FIGURE 10-30 Dissecting cellulitis of the scalp, vertical sections: Partially squamous lined abscess with naked hair shaft. Follicles are destroyed by fibroinflammatory process.

DISSECTING CELLULITIS OF THE SCALP (PERIFOLLICULITIS CAPITIS ABSCEDENS ET SUFFODIENS)

Clinical Features   In 1908 Hoffman and colleagues described perifolliculitis capitis abscedens et suffodiens (Table 10-16).[79] It was later renamed *dissecting cellulitis of the scalp*,[80] and synonyms include *dissecting perifolliculitis* and *dissecting folliculitis* of the scalp. It is most common in young black men and begins as fluctuant scalp nodules that progressively coalesce to form complex, interconnected, crusted abscesses and sinus tracts that drain spontaneously or with slight pressure. Well developed lesions are painful and result in extensive scarring of the scalp.[81] Some patients with DCS also have acne conglobata and hidradenitis suppurativa and are said to have the follicular occlusion triad.

Histopathological Features   As in other pustulofollicular alopecias, the earliest finding is acneiform dilatation with neutrophilic infiltrates (Table 10-16). Biopsies from fluctuant nodules and sinuses reveal large dermal and subcutaneous abscesses. Well developed lesions are abscesses and sinus tracts partially lined with squamous epithelium derived from the overlying epidermis or follicular epithelium (Fig. 10-30). Bacteria may be seen superficially in follicular infundibula but not in abscesses, and the pathogenic significance is unclear. Dense dermal and subcutaneous fibrosis eventually surrounds the sinus tracts, and the follicles are destroyed by the fibro-inflammatory process. The infiltrate in older, more scarred lesions is primarily lymphoplasmacytic and histiocytic with few neutrophils.

Differential Diagnosis   Other pustulofollicular scarring alopecias are to be considered (Table 10-16). The microscopic features of DCS are very similar to those in hidradenitis suppurativa. PAS and gram stains should be done to rule out fungal and bacterial infection.

FOLLICULITIS DECALVANS

Clinical Features   FD is a rare pustulofollicular alopecia that presents as round to irregular-shaped patches of alopecia with follicular pustules at the peripheral, advancing edge (Table 10-16). FD occurs in both sexes and primarily affects the scalp, but involvement of the beard, axillae, pubic area, arms, and legs may also occur.[5,55,56,81] End-stage FD without pustules may resemble PPOB.

Histopathological Features   The earliest finding is comedonal dilatation with intra- and perifollicular neutrophilic infiltrates (Table 10-16) (Fig. 10-31). Follicular rupture ensues with resulting perifollicular fibrosis and eventual permanent follicular destruction. Localized perifollicular dermal abscesses are often present but are not as extensive or deep as seen in DCS. Sinus tracts are not seen in FD. In later stages, the infiltrate is mixed with lymphocytes, plasma cells, and neutrophils. Naked hair shafts surrounded by foreign-body giant cells are present after the follicular epithelium has been destroyed, and, as in all primary scarring alopecias, numerous residual fibrous tracts mark sites of destroyed follicles.

TABLE 10-16

Pustulofollicular, Neutrophil-Associated Primary Scarring Alopecia

	Dissecting Cellulitis	Folliculitis Decalvans	Acne Keloidalis	Tinea Kerion & Favus
Clinical Features				
	Young black men Fluctuant scalp nodules Progression to extensive interconnected abscesses, sinus tracts Spontaneous drainage Painful, prominent scarring Associated follicular occlusion triad	Adults Round or irregularly shaped patches of alopecia with follicular pustules Other sites may be affected	Young black men Occipital scalp, neck Follicular papules, pustules progress to large, exophytic, keloidal alopecic plaques	Children, adolescents Boggy, erythematous, crusted, scaling nodules and plaques with variable alopecia. Zoophilic and geophilic forms of dermatophyte. Yellow, cup-shaped crusts (scutula) with favus
Histopathological Features				
Acneiform follicular dilatation	Early finding, persists	Early finding, persists	Early finding, persists	Early finding, persists
Follicular rupture	Present	Present	Present	Present
Abscess formation	Extensive dermal and subcutaneous	Present in dermis	Less prominent in dermis	Variable, may be prominent
Sinus tract formation	Yes, partially squamous lined	Absent	Largely absent	Absent
Location of fibrosis	Dense fibrotic scar around sinus tracts in dermis and subcutis	Less dense perifollicular fibrosis in dermis	Dense dermal hypertrophic scar and/or keloid	Perifollicular dermal scar, may be extensive in favus
Infectious agents	Occasional staph within follicular infundibulum	Occasional staph within follicular infundibulum	Occasional propionibacteria acnes	Endothrix and ectothrix
Inflammation type	Neutrophilic initially, later mixed granulomatous with plasma cells	Neutrophilic initially, later mixed	Neutrophilic initially, later mixed with lymphocytes and prominent plasma cells	Neutrophilic initially, later mixed granulomatous
Location	Initially peri-infundibular, progresses to involve entire follicle and subcutis	Primarily peri-infundibular, may extend to involve entire follicle	Primarily peri-infundibular, may extend to involve entire follicle	Primarily peri-infundibular, may extend to involve entire follicle

SOURCE: Adapted from Templeton SF, Solomon AR: Scarring alopecia: A classification based on microscopic criteria. *J Cutan Pathol* 21:97–109, 1994, with permission.

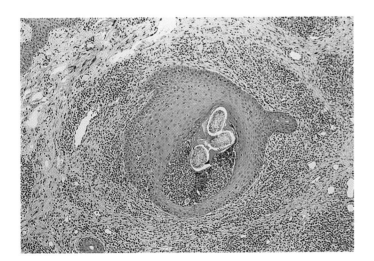

FIGURE 10-31   Folliculitis decalvans, horizontal sections: Pustular folliculitis with incipient rupture and adjacent mixed dermal infiltrates.

Differential Diagnosis   See Table 10-16. PAS and gram stains are suggested to rule out dermatophyte and bacterial folliculitis.

ACNE KELOIDALIS

Clinical Features   AK is a destructive pustulofollicular process that primarily affects the occipital scalp and neck of young black men (Table 10-16). Lesions begin as discrete follicular papules or pustules and may progress to large exophytic keloidal plaques devoid of hair.[81,82] Similar lesions may occur in the beard region in patients with pseudofolliculitis barbae.

Histopathological Features   Early lesions display comedonal dilatation and pustular folliculitis as in other pustulofollicular alopecias (Table 10-16). Follicular rupture with subsequent mixed neutrophilic infiltrates occurs. Well developed lesions are characterized by dense dermal scar with many entrapped naked hair shafts surrounded by lymphohistiocytic infiltrates with admixed neutrophils and abundant plasma cells (Fig. 10-32). Variable numbers of broad eosinophilic hyalinized

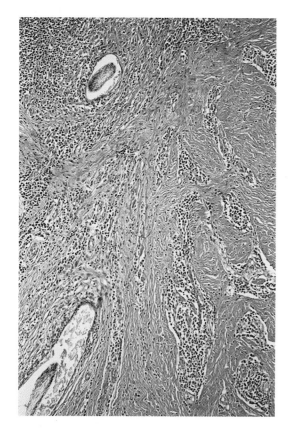

FIGURE 10-32   Acne keloidalis, vertical sections: Chronic lesion with dense dermal scar, recent follicular rupture, naked hair shafts, and mixed infiltrates including neutrophils and numerous plasma cells.

keloidal collagen bundles may be present but are not essential for diagnosis.[56,83]

Differential Diagnosis   See Table 10-16 for differential diagnosis. Special stains are suggested to rule out bacterial and dermatophyte infections. The extensive dermal fibrosis typical of hypertrophic or keloidal scar is the most distinctive microscopic feature of AK.

EROSIVE PUSTULAR DERMATOSIS OF THE SCALP

Clinical Features   EPDS is an uncommon erosive and pustular process that may lead to permanent alopecia. It generally begins on the crown as a localized area of crusted erosion with occasional pustules and occurs most commonly in elderly white women.[84,85]

Histopathological Features   The histology is not specific and consists of ulcer with subjacent mixed inflammatory infiltrates and abscess.

TINEA CAPITIS/KERION/FAVUS

Clinical Features   Kerion and favus subtypes of tinea capitis can result in permanent alopecia and are most commonly seen in children. Kerion is inflammatory tinea capitis caused by a zoophilic or geophilic follicular dermatophyte infection and presents as boggy, erythematous, scaling, crusted partially alopecic plaques with regional adenopathy. Favus is an uncommon follicular dermatophyte infection of the scalp seen in rural regions and associated poor nutrition and poor hygiene. Yellow, cup-shaped crusts termed *scutula* are present on the scalp and often result in permanent alopecia. The causative organism is *Trichophyton schoenleinii*.[86] In adults noninflammatory endothrix dermatophyte infections, usually *Trichophyton tonsurans*, can occasionally cause a

more diffuse alopecia mimicking female pattern androgenetic alopecia or follicular degeneration syndrome.

Histopathological Features   The follicular infundibula are generally dilated and often hyperkeratotic. Pustular folliculitis with incipient or complete rupture is commonly seen in kerion. Dense mixed inflammatory infiltrates including many neutrophils surround the affected follicles. Endothrix (hyphae within hair shafts) and ectothrix (hyphae around hair shafts) patterns of follicular dermatophytosis may be seen and are best appreciated in PAS-stained or silver-impregnated sections (Fig. 10-33). Hyphae are not usually seen in the overlying epidermis. Some endothrix infections do not illicit a brisk inflammatory response but result in a relatively noninflammatory diffuse alopecia with broken shafts and perifollicular fibroplasia.

Thick parakeratotic and orthokeratotic hyperkeratosis overlying an atrophic dermis with lymphoplasmacytic and granulomatous dermal infiltrates and follicular dermatophytosis is seen in favus.

Differential Diagnosis   Other infectious and noninfectious folliculitides have similar findings. Gram and PAS stains as well as culture of plucked hairs are for diagnosis.

Secondary Scarring Alopecia

Hair loss in secondary scarring alopecias is the result of non-folliculocentric skin disease. The pilosebaceous apparatus is not the focus of disease but is only secondarily involved. The clinical and microscopic features of secondary scarring alopecia are characteristic for the specific disease involved. Some examples include hair loss produced by neoplasms, nonfollicular sarcoidal granulomas, dermal sclerosis from morphea, and external trauma (Table 10-17).

FOLLICULAR HYPERKERATOSIS

Follicular hyperkeratosis includes keratosis pilaris, lichen spinulosus, phrynoderma, and scarring follicular keratosis.

Clinical Features   Keratosis pilaris (KP) is a very common follicular dermatosis often associated with ichthyosis and atopic dermatitis. Onset occurs in the first and second decades of life with persistence into adult-

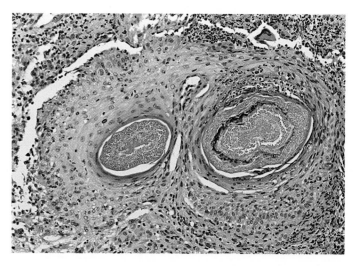

FIGURE 10-33   Tinea capitis, horizontal sections: Dermatophyte hyphae extensively permeate (endothri.) and surround (ectothri.) hair shafts in this patient treated with topical steroids. Numerous neutrophils are seen.

Sclerosing disorders
    Morphea
    Sclerodermoid Porphyria Cutanea Tarda
    Lichen Sclerosis et Atrophicus
    Parry-Romberg Syndrome
Physical/chemical agents
    Mechanical trauma, laceration
    Thermal burns
    Chemical burns
    Radiation dermatitis
Dermal infiltrative processes
    Tumors
        Basel cell carcinoma
        Squamous cell carcinoma
        Metastatic Carcinoma
        Lymphoma
        Adnexal Tumors
        Dermatofibrosarcoma Protuberans
        Others
    Granulomatous
        Sarcoidosis
        Necrobiosis Lipoidica
        Miecher's Granuloma
        Actinic Granuloma
        Infections
            Syphilis (tertiary)
            Tuberculosis
            Viral
            Protozoal
            Other
    Amyloidosis

SOURCE: Adapted from Templeton SF, Solomon AR: Scarring alopecia: A classification based on microscopic criteria. *J Cutan Pathol* 21:97–109, 1994, with permission.

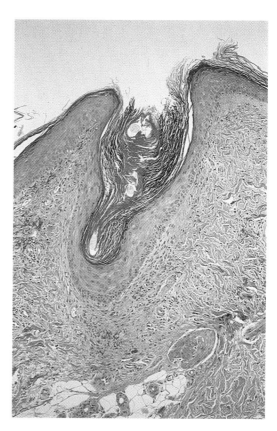

FIGURE 10-34 Keratosis pilaris: Follicular hyper keratosis with slight perifollicular fibroplasia and sparse lymphocytic infiltrates are seen.

hood.[87] Lesions consist of patches of follicular hyperkeratosis with variable perifollicular erythema commonly affecting the upper outer arm, thighs, and buttocks. Lichen spinulosus is a closely related follicular hyperkeratotic condition presenting in children as patches of minute horny follicular spines. Patients with vitamin A deficiency develop numerous follicular hyperkeratotic lesions termed *phrynoderma* that begin on thighs and posterolateral arms with subsequent involvement of extensor surfaces. Night blindness, xerophthalmia, keratomalacia, diarrhea, weakness, and generalized wasting may occur in hypovitaminosis A.

Several genetically determined syndromes characterized by keratosis pilaris, follicular destruction, and typical clinical findings have been described.[88,89] This group of disorders is often termed *scarring follicular keratosis*. Three major variants include keratosis pilaris spinulosa decalvans (KPSD), keratosis pilaris atrophicans (KPA, also known as *ulerythema oophryogenes*) and atrophoderma vermiculata (AV, also known as *acne vermiculata, folliculitis ulerythematosa reticulata*). Scarring alopecia with keratosis pilaris-like lesions occurs in KPSD with onset during the teenage years. Loss of eyebrow hair with atrophy and follicular hyperkeratosis is characteristic of KPA. AV is characterized by reticulate, ice-pick scarring of the cheeks with follicular hyperkeratosis. Overlapping clinical findings may be seen in these three clinical subtypes of scarring follicular keratosis.

Histopathological Features Follicular dilatation with compact follicular hyperkeratosis, at times tightly adherent to the hair shaft, is seen in KP and lichen spinulosus (Fig. 10-34). Follicular infundibular atrophy with slight perifollicular lymphocytic infiltrates is also present. Follicular rupture with subsequent inflammatory folliculitis may occur.

Similar findings are seen in the scarring follicular keratosis.[88] Early lesions display typical KP features but may have more prominent infundibular hypergranulosis. Inflammatory and pustular lesions show follicular rupture and folliculitis. Late lesions are no different from other end-stage scarring alopecias with complete follicular dropout, numerous residual fibrous tracts, and scattered naked hair shafts.

FOLLICULITIS

Inflammation within and around the hair follicle is characteristic of folliculitis. There are many nonalopecic diseases characterized by folliculitis, and these can be grouped as *infectious*, *acneiform*, and *eosinophilic folliculitis* (Table 10-18).

Infectious Folliculitis

Bacterial, fungal, parasitic, and viral follicular infections comprise the infectious folliculitides (Table 10-18).

BACTERIAL FOLLICULITIS

Clinical Features Bacterial folliculitis may be superficial or deep and begins as a pustule on an erythematous base. Superficial bacterial folliculitis, also known as *Bockhart's impetigo*, is usually caused by

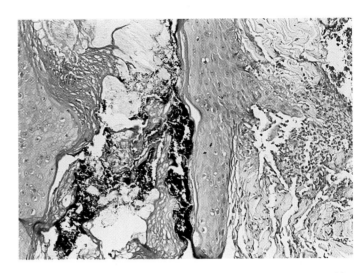

FIGURE 10-35   Bacterial folliculitis: Numerous intrafollicular gram positive bacteria are seen as well as early follicular rupture.

Staphylococcus aureus. Furuncles, or deep folliculitis, are larger tender, warm, erythematous plaques and nodules with central pustules generally caused by *Staphylococcus aureus.* Furuncles may occur on any nonglabrous skin but are more common on legs, buttocks, posterior neck, and axillae. Carbuncles are more common in diabetics and are composed of two or more coalescing furuncles.

"Hot tub" folliculitis is a less common gram-negative folliculitis, usually caused by *Pseudomonas aeruginosa*[90] and acquired through exposure to inadequately chlorinated water in swimming pools and hot tubs. Lesions are generally distributed over areas covered by the bathing suit. "Mud-wrestling" folliculitis caused by soil bacteria, *Enterobacteriaceae*, also occurs on covered skin in individuals participating in this activity.[91]

FUNGAL FOLLICULITIS

Fungal folliculitis is caused by *Malassezia furfur*, formerly termed *Pityrosporum ovale* (pityrosporum folliculitis) or *dermatophytes* (Majocchi's granuloma and tinea capitis). Pityrosporum folliculitis occurs on the trunk as pruritic acneiform papules and pustules most commonly in young adults.[92] Majocchi's granuloma is a form of follicular dermatophytosis that occurs on nonglabrous skin, most commonly on extremities.[93] The lesions present as grouped, somewhat annular inflammatory papulopustules or as deep furunclelike nodules. Topical corticosteroid usage prior to correct diagnosis is common in Majocchi's granuloma and may allow for more extensive infection of hair shafts.

Histopathological Features   Bacterial and fungal folliculitis have similar microscopic features of intra- and perifollicular infiltrates rich in neutrophils. Follicular rupture with dense mixed infiltrates, abscess, and granulation tissue is common. Bacterial organisms may be seen in infundibula in bacteria folliculitis and at a deeper follicular level in furuncles and carbuncles (Fig. 10-35). Acneiform dilatation with budding yeast and follicular hyperkeratosis is seen in pityrosporum folliculitis (Fig. 10-36). The histology of Majocchi's granuloma is similar to tinea capitis/kerion with follicular rupture, abscess, and dermatophyte-infected hair shafts (Fig. 10-37).

DEMODEX FOLLICULITIS

Clinical Features   The ectoparasites *Demodex folliculorum* and *Demodex brevis* are hair follicle mites frequently found in normal adult skin. The pathogenicity of the mites in folliculitis, especially acne

rosacea, is controversial.[94] However, in some cases facial rosacealike papules and pustules respond to topical acaricidal therapy, suggesting *Demodex* mites may play a role in some instances.

Histopathological Features   *Demodex* mites are elongate eosinophilic ectoparasites and are more numerous on the head and neck.[95] One or more mites may be found in normal follicular infundibula. Mites may also be seen within the sebaceous duct. Follicular spongiosis with perifollicular lymphohistiocytic infiltrates can occur in rosacealike lesions, especially on the face (Fig. 10-38).

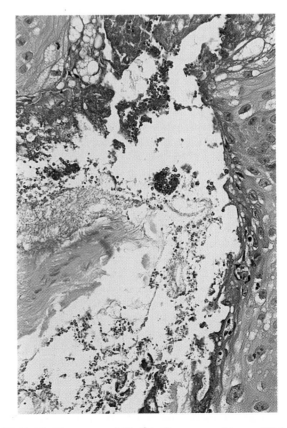

FIGURE 10-36   Pityrosporum folliculitis: Numerous oval to round Malassezia furfur organisms are present within an inflamed follicle.

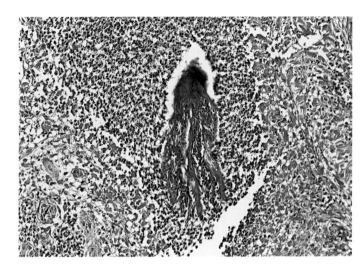

FIGURE 10-37   Majocchi's granuloma: A disintegrating hair shaft with numerous endothrix dermatophyte hyphae is present in a dermal abscess.

HERPES FOLLICULITIS

Clinical Features   Although not typically a follicular process herpesvirus, infections (herpes simplex and herpes zoster) can involve hair follicles especially in early lesions. In addition, chronic cutaneous herpesvirus infections can involve follicles and present as persistent hyperkeratotic papules in immunocompromised patients, especially patients infected with the human immunodeficiency virus.[96]

Histopathological Features   Viral cytopathic changes of herpesvirus infection may initially be seen in follicular infundibulum. These

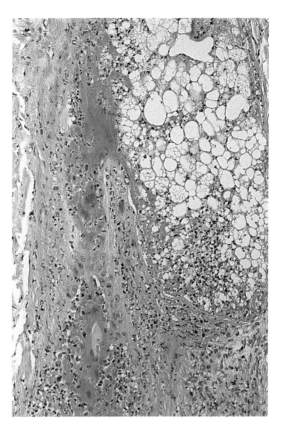

FIGURE 10-39   Herpes folliculitis: Multinucleate herpetic keratinocytes are present in a necrotic follicular infundibulum. The adjacent sebaceous lobule is also necrotic.

changes include pale keratinocytes with dysmaturation, acantholysis, dyskeratosis, and multinucleate keratinocytes. In papular chronic herpesvirus infections, typical viral cytopathic changes are seen in the epidermis and hair follicles with prominent overlying hyperkeratosis.[96] Extensive necrosis occurs in some cases (Fig. 10-39). The dermal infiltrate is typical of cutaneous herpes with dense perivascular and occasionally perineural lymphocytic infiltrates. In addition, dense, atypical but reactive lymphocytic infiltrates simulating lymphoma can occur in herpesvirus folliculitis.[97]

Acneiform Folliculitis

Acne vulgaris, other acne subtypes, pseudofolliculitis barbae, hidradenitis suppurativa, and pustulofollicular scarring alopecias are all acneiform folliculitides. Some forms of rosacea are included in this group of diseases (Table 10-19).

ACNE VARIANTS

Clinical Features   Acne can be comedonal, papular, pustular, nodular, or cystic. The face, chest, and back are involved, and this disorder primarily affects adolescents and young adults (Table 10-19).[98,99] Comedonal, papular, and pustular acne are the most common variants termed *acne vulgaris*. Comedones are either open (blackheads) or closed (whiteheads). *Acne conglobata* is a severe form of nodulocystic acne that usually involves back, chest, and posterior neck and consists of numerous coalescing large comedones, acne cysts, and nodules. Extensive irregular-shaped scars and epidermoid cysts occur in the latter stage, and association with the *follicular occlusion triad* is common.

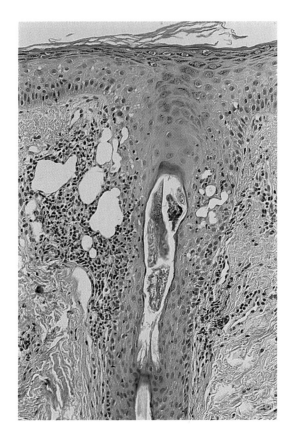

FIGURE 10-38   Demodex folliculitis: Elongate demodex folliculorum mites are present in the follicular infundibulum with perifollicular infiltrates.

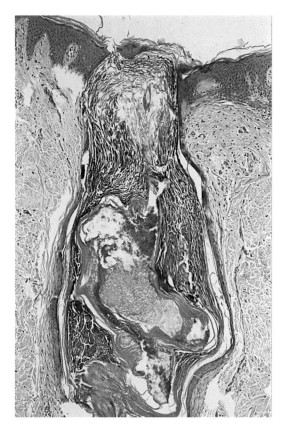

FIGURE 10-40 Comedone: A large comedone is pictured and consists of a keratin-filled dilated follicle with atrophy of infundibular epithelium. Inflammation is variable.

Chloracne is a rare acne variant occurring after exposure to halogenated aromatic compounds, especially dioxin.[100] Patients using systemic and topical corticosteroids may develop a monomorphic acneiform follicular eruption termed *steroid acne*.[101] Acne cosmetica (pomade acne) is more common in woman and occurs on the face as the result of persistent follicular occlusion by cosmetics and applied hair oils.[98] Noninflammatory comedones and cysts associated with nodular solar elastosis is termed the *Favre-Racouchot syndrome* and generally occurs on the upper to lateral cheeks and temples near the eyes.[102]

Histopathological Features   The follicular infundibulum is thinned, dilated, and filled with compact hyperkeratosis in comedones (Table 10-19) (Fig. 10-40). Inflammatory comedones, papules, and pustules show mixed infiltrates of increasing density within and around dilated follicles. Follicular rupture with dermal abscess is seen in nodulocystic acne lesions, and subsequent scarring is common. Extensive abscesses and partially squamous lined sinuses with prominent scarring is seen in acne conglobata. Focal dystrophic calcification may occur in old, scarred acne lesions. Extensive solar elastosis, open comedones, and small epidermoid cysts are seen in the Favre-Racouchot syndrome.

PSEUDOFOLLICULITIS BARBAE

Clinical Features   Pseudofolliculitis barbae is an acneiform eruption of the bearded area most common in men with thick tightly curled hair, especially blacks. Concomitant acne keloidalis often occurs in these patients.

Histopathological Features   Pseudofolliculitis barbae results from close shaving in individuals with thick, tightly curled hair. Closely shaven hair shafts either penetrate their own follicular infundibulum or curl back and penetrate the adjacent epidermis after exiting the acrotrichium. A follicular and perifollicular mixed foreign-body inflammatory response ensues.

HIDRADENITIS SUPPURATIVA

Clinical Features   Hidradenitis suppurativa is a painful deep-scarring folliculitis of the axillae and groin often associated with nodulocystic acne and dissecting cellulitis of the scalp (Table 10-20).

Histopathological Features   The histology of hidradenitis is very similar to DCS and consists of extensive scarring of the dermis and subcutis with deep abscesses and sinuses partially lined with squamous epithelium (Table 10-20) (Fig. 10-41).[103] Follicular occlusion occurs initially with subsequent superficial and deep folliculitis with abscess. A persistent fibro-inflammatory response occurs as the result of continuous keratin production by ruptured squamous-lined sinuses. Abundant granulation tissue is seen in some cases. Suppurative inflammation of apocrine glands occurs secondarily and only in a minority of cases.[104]

ROSACEA

Clinical Features   Rosacea is an acneiform disorder that most commonly affects the middle-aged and elderly (Table 10-21). Telangiectatic, papulopustular, granulomatous, and rhinophyma variants occur.[105] The nose, cheeks, and chin are typically affected, but extrafacial involvement can occur rarely. Transient and persistent flushing of the face is common and may be aggravated by external and psychologic factors. Inflammatory papular and granulomatous lesions can clinically mimic basal cell carcinoma and therefore are often biopsied. Though once considered a tuberculid, lupus miliaris disseminata facei is now

---

TABLE 10-19

Acne Vulgaris

Clinical Features

Adolescence, early adulthood
Men ≥ women
Face >> back, chest, shoulder
Comedones
Erythematous papules, pustules, nodules, cysts
Occasional scarring
Association with hidradenitis suppurativa and dissecting cellulitis

Histopathological Features

Comedone: dilated follicular infundibulum with keratinous plug, open to surface or closed
Follicular pustule with or without rupture into surrounding dermis
Neutrophilic and foreign-body granulomatous reaction to keratin and follicular contents in dermis
Epithelial cyst and sinus tract formation
Dermal scarring

Differential Diagnosis

Keratosis, pilaris and related conditions
Other forms of folliculitis, e.g., bacterial, fungal, viral

TABLE 10-20
Hidradenitis Suppurativa

Clinical Features

Onset after puberty
Axillae, inguinal, and perineal areas, other sites
Erythematous nodules followed by draining abscesses, sinus tracts,
    prominent scarring
Association with severe acne, dissecting cellulitis of scalp

Histopathological Features

Early lesions
    Follicular plugging, folliculitis
Chronic lesions
    Features of chronic folliculitis
    Abscesses within apocrine glands and in the dermis and subcutis
    Prominent foreign body granulomatous reaction
    Dermal scarring often extensive
Sinus tract and cyst formation

Differential Diagnosis

Other chronic active deep folliculitides, infectious and noninfectious
Pyoderma gangrenosum
Crohn's disease

---

considered a variant of granulomatous rosacea and consists of discrete red-brown papules distributed over the face and eyelids.[106,107] Rhinophyma is an end-stage variant of rosacea that results in enlargement of the nose, especially the nasal tip, due to sebaceous gland hypertrophy.[108] On occasion other areas of the face or ears may be involved by a phyma.

The pathogenesis is poorly understood, but the vascular flushing reaction is one of the earliest stages in the development of rosacea. Aggravating factors include hot, spicy foods and liquids, alcohol, certain vasodilatory drugs, and sunlight.[109] Ocular rosacea is relatively common.[106]

Perioral dermatitis is a relatively common facial eruption consisting of acneiform papules and pustules distributed around the mouth of young women.[110] Use of topical fluorinated corticosteroids on the face is often the inciting cause, but idiopathic cases occur. Clinically, perioral dermatitis has features of acne, rosacea, and seborrheic dermatitis. Granulomatous variants of perioral dermatitis occur, especially in children, and in these cases involvement of the eyelids and neck is common.

Histopathological Features   Microscopic features vary according to clinical subtype (Table 10-21).[111,112] In telangiectatic rosacea, increased numbers of ectatic venules with sparse perivascular lymphocytic infiltrates are seen. Solar elastosis is common. Papular rosacea lesions have perivascular and perifollicular lymphohistiocytic infiltrates involving the superficial to middle dermis (Fig. 10-42). Admixed multinucleate histiocytes and loose granulomas are seen in papular and granulomatous rosacea (Fig. 10-43). Nonfollicular epithelioid granulomas that occasionally exhibit caseation necrosis occur less frequently. The inflammatory infiltrate in papular rosacea is often not centered around hair follicles but commonly has a perivascular to nodular pattern. Suppurative folliculitis with admixed lymphohistiocytic infiltrates including foreign-body giant cells is characteristic of pustular rosacea. Extensive hypertrophy of mature sebaceous glands, follicular dilatation, and hyperkeratosis with variable inflammation is characteristic of rhinophyma. In contrast to discrete lesions of sebaceous hyperplasia in which

TABLE 10-21
Rosacea and Rhinophyma

Clinical Features

Age 20–50 years common
Women > men
Fair-skinned individuals
Central face: nose, cheek, chin, glabella, forehead; rarely neck,
    upper trunk
Blushing, flushing
Erythema, telangiectasia, edema
Papules, pustules
Rhinophyma, other phymas involving forehead, chin

Histopathological Features

Variable degrees of the following:
    Vascular ectasia
    Perivascular and perifollicular lymphoid infiltrates
    Folliculitis
    Solar elastosis
    Edema
    Granulomatous inflammation
    Epithelioid granulomas, especially perifollicular
    Sebaceous hyperplasia
Rhinophyma and other phymas show variable degrees of the
    following:
    Florid sebaceous gland hyperplasia
    Diffuse fibroplasia
    Ectatic venular vessels
Nodular solar elastosis

Differential Diagnosis

Lupus erythematosus
Perioral dermatitis
Acne vulgaris
Sarcoidosis
Other granulomatous dermatitides

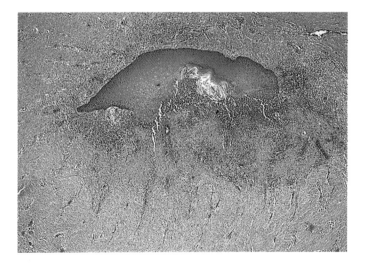

FIGURE 10-41   Hidradenitis suppurativa: Extensive dermal scarring is present with a partially squamous lined sinus tract and associated suppurative infiltrates.

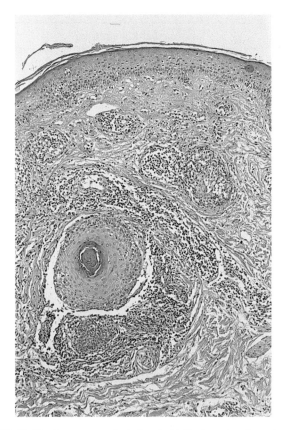

FIGURE 10-42   Rosacea, papular lesion: Perifollicular and perivascular lymphohistiocytic infiltrates are characteristic of papular rosacea.

sebaceous lobules radiate around a central dilated sebaceous duct, rhinophyma is characterized by more extensive and diffuse sebaceous gland hypertrophy, diffuse fibroplasia, fibrovascular hypertrophy (fibroplasia and prominent vascular ectasia), nodular accumulation of solar elastotic material, or any combination of the latter alterations.

The role of *Demodex* mites in the pathogenesis of rosacea is unclear. Increased numbers of mites have been repeatedly observed in rosacea and rosacealike conditions,[113] and occasional patients have reported success with topical acaricides.

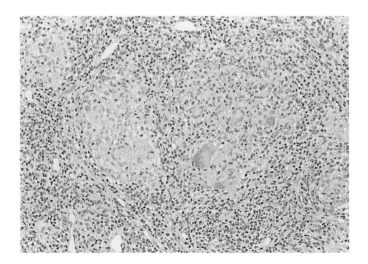

FIGURE 10-43   Granulomatous rosacea: Loose to well-formed granulomas comprised of histiocytes and multinucleate giant cells are seen. Granulomas may or may not be perifollicular.

The histology of *perioral dermatitis* is very similar to papular, pustular, and granulomatous variants of rosacea.[110]

PERFORATING FOLLICULITIS

Clinical Features   Perforating folliculitis was defined as a clinicopathologic entity in 1968 by Mehregan and Coskey.[114] The primary lesion was described as a follicular-centered erythematous papule perforated by a central hair shaft. The papules were typically located on the thighs and buttocks of young adults, anatomic sites where chronic friction, presumably secondary to close-fitting clothing on hair-bearing surfaces, could induce the lesion. The perforating hair shaft may be encompassed by a keratotic plug. Other than the postulated role of chronic rubbing and friction, no pathogenesis is known.

In addition to the above described clinicopathologic entity, the microscopic finding of infundibular perforation is common to several types of folliculitis.[115–117] The microscopic findings of perforating folliculitis may be seen in bacterial and fungal folliculitis, acneiform folliculitis such as acne vulgaris, keratosis pilaris and pustulo-follicular forms of alopecia including folliculitis decalvans and acne keloidalis. Perforating folliculitis may also occur in patients with chronic renal failure and hemodialysis,[118] and in this clinical setting, the disease can be considered part of the spectrum of acquired perforating dermatosis, previously termed *Kyrle's disease*.[119] Given the diversity of these types of folliculitis, infundibular perforation appears to be a nonspecific event occurring in the course of inflammatory follicular destruction. Consequently, the microscopic finding of perforating folliculitis should not be considered indicative of the clinicopathologic entity of the same name without appropriate cutaneous lesions present.

Histopathological Features   The diagnostic microscopic changes of perforating folliculitis, the clinical entity, consist of an eccentric infundibular perforation. A plug of hyperkeratotic stratum corneum is usually present within the acrotrichium. The infundibular epithelium is variably hyperplastic, but attenuation of the epithelium is usually evident adjacent to the site of rupture. The dilated infundibulum is filled with necrotic basophilic debris, sebaceous material, keratin, and inflammatory cells. Intact and karyorrhectic neutrophils predominate. A hair shaft may be present within the follicular canal at or near the site of perforation, but it is not invariably present. A mixed inflammatory cell infiltrate composed of neutrophils, lymphocytes, and plasma cells is present in the dermis adjacent to the ruptured infundibular epithelium. Granulomatous inflammation may be present in older lesions. The reticular dermal collagen near the site of perforation is frequently basophilic and granular.

Infundibular perforation is seen in addition to the other diagnostic findings of specific forms of folliculitis. For example, hyphae are present in the follicular canal in fungal folliculitis, and bacteria are found in this location in bacterial folliculitis. Comedonal distortion of the infundibulum is present in acne vulgaris. A dense hyperkeratotic plug is found in the acrotrichium and infundibulum in keratosis pilaris. Perifollicular abscess is evident in folliculitis decalvans, and perifollicular scarring is invariably present in acne keloidalis. In contrast to elastosis perforans serpiginosa, no alteration of perifollicular elastic fibers is seen in perforating folliculitis. The epidermis is the location of the perforation site in reactive perforating collagenosis, not the follicular infundibulum.

Eosinophilic Folliculitis

Clinical Features   Eosinophilic folliculitis (EF) occurs in three clinical settings: (1) young to middle-aged adult men, mainly Japanese, (2) neonates and young children and (3) HIV-infected patients (Table

TABLE 10-22

Eosinophilic Folliculitis

Clinical Features

Adult young to middle-aged men, mainly Japanese
Neonates and young children
HIV-infected patients
Face, trunk, upper extremities
Erythematous follicular pustules
Polycyclic plaques often with centripetal extension, central clearing
Urticarial follicular papules often in HIV patients
Low CD4 counts (usually < 200 cells/mm^3)

Histopathological Features

Peri and intrafollicular eosinophilic infiltration
Occasional subcorneal eosinophilic pustules
Follicular spongiosis often
Perivascular and interstitial lymphocytic infiltrates
Flame figures rare

Differential Diagnosis

Other folliculitides, especially infectious
Arthropod bite reaction
Papular urticaria
Papular eruption of HIV

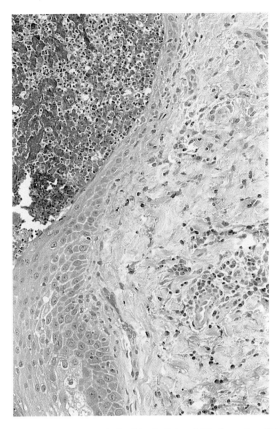

FIGURE 10-44   Eosinophilic folliculitis: Both intrafollicular and perifollicular eosinophils are seen in this case of eosinophilic folliculitis.

20-22). Ofuji first described EF in adults[120–125] as erythematous follicular pustules and polycyclic plaques with centripetal extension and central clearing with postinflammatory hyperpigmentation. The lesions may be pruritic and most commonly affect the face, trunk, and upper extremities. Patients often have a mild leukocytosis and peripheral eosinophilia.

The neonatal and young childhood variant occurs predominately on the scalp as pruritic indurated erythematous plaques with pustules.[121,122] Lesions typically crust over and resolve after days to weeks, but recurrence is common. Ninety percent of patients are male, and most are Caucasian. Blood eosinophilia is often present.

HIV-associated EF occurs primarily on the trunk, head, and neck as numerous discrete urticarial follicular papules that are often excoriated.[123,124] Frank pustules are less commonly seen. Pruritus is often severe. CD4 counts are almost always low (less than 200 cells/mm^3), and the presence of EF in a patient typically suggests more advanced HIV disease. Serum IgE levels are frequently elevated.

Histopathological Features   Peri- and intrafollicular infiltrates rich in eosinophils are characteristic of EF (Table 10-22) (Fig. 10-44).[125] Follicular spongiosis of the infundibula and sebaceous lobules is commonly present. Subcorneal eosinophilic pustules may also be seen. In many cases, the infiltrate is not limited to the follicle, but variably dense perivascular and interstitial lymphocytic superficial and deep dermal infiltrates are seen. Flame figures may rarely occur.

Differential Diagnosis   Gram and PAS stains are helpful in differentiating the above folliculitides. Perforating folliculitis and perforating dermatosis should be considered in some instances. Papular urticaria, arthropod bite reaction, papular eruption of HIV, and scabies infestation should be considered in cases of eosinophilic folliculitis.

Sarcoidosis may be considered in cases of granulomatous rosacea, but in general, the granulomas of granulomatous rosacea are more inflammatory with numerous lymphocytes, plasma cells, and neu-

trophils and are less organized with fewer true tuberculoid granulomas. Infectious granulomas due to mycobacteria, deep fungi, and follicular dermatophytosis (Majocchi's granuloma) can be ruled out with special stains and tissue culture.

MISCELLANEOUS DISORDERS

Fox-Fordyce Disease (Apocrine Miliaria)

Clinical Features   First described in 1902,[126] Fox-Fordyce disease is an uncommon persistent, pruritic papular eruption that affects adolescent and young women and is localized to skin containing apocrine glands.[127] It most commonly affects the axilla but can be seen in the pubic area, labia, perineum, areola, presternal area, umbilicus, and medial aspect of the upper thigh. Severe paroxysmal pruritus initiated by emotional stimuli, sexual activity, excitement, and exercise is common.[128]

Histopathological Features   The histology is usually not specific. The most reproducible findings are follicular hyperkeratosis and spongiosis.[127] Overlying epidermal acanthosis and spongiosis as seen in subacute to chronic eczematous dermatitis are common. Hyperkeratotic plugging of the distal apocrine duct that enters the follicular infundibulum can occasionally be seen if multiple serial sections are examined. Spongiosis and apocrine sweat retention vesicle are also occasionally observed in the distal apocrine duct. A sparse perivascular, perifollicular, and periductal lymphocytic infiltrate with exocytosis is present.

The pathogenesis is unknown. Genetic and hormonal factors may play a role. Experimental plugging of apocrine glands produces microscopic apocrine ductal dilatation but not clinical disease.[128]

Differential Diagnosis　Keratosis pilaris and lichen spinulosus also have prominent follicular hyperkeratosis and should be considered in the differential diagnosis. Disseminate and recurrent infundibulo-folliculitis of Hitch and Lund can be considered but generally has less prominent follicular hyperkeratosis. Eczematous dermatitis with prominent follicular spongiosis that may be seen in atopic dermatitis should also be considered.

Apocrine Chromhidrosis

Clinical Features　Apocrine chromhidrosis, the localized secretion of colored sweat, is a rare disorder that is restricted to skin containing apocrine glands.[129] The face and axilla are the most common sites, but involvement of the areola has also been reported.[130] Emotional stimuli and mechanical stimulation prompt secretion of colored sweat which is usually black or brown. Less common, blue, green, yellow, or red sweat may be secreted.

Histopathological Features　Apocrine secretory cells are more basophilic than usual and contain variably sized yellow-brown intracytoplasmic granules consistent with lipofuscin. These lipofuscin granules show a positive Schmorl reaction and are autofluorescent with fluorescent microscopy. The differing clinical color of the sweat has been suggested to be due to varying amounts of lipofuscin in differing states of oxidation.

Neutrophilic Eccrine Hidradenitis

Clinical Features　First described by Harrist and colleagues in 1982,[131] neutrophilic eccrine hidradenitis (NEH) is a polymorphous cutaneous eruption consisting of tender erythematous macules, papules, plaques, or purpuric nodules in patients receiving systemic chemotherapy for a variety of neoplasms (Table 10-23). Cytarabine and bleomycin are the most common chemotherapy agents, and the pathogenesis is thought to be due to direct drug effect on eccrine units.[132,133] NEH also occurs in association with other non-cytotoxic drugs and myeloid

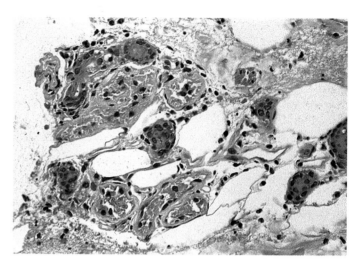

FIGURE 10-45　Neutrophilic eccrine hidradenitis. Note infiltration of sweat glands by neutrophils.

leukemia prior to chemotherapy.[134] An idiopathic variant of NEH occurs on the palms and soles of children.[135]

Squamous metaplasia and necrosis of eccrine glands and ducts occurs in association with systemic chemotherapy and has been termed *eccrine squamous syringometaplasia*.[134] Squamous metaplasia without necrosis and eccrine duct hyperplasia can be seen in association with skin neoplasms,[136] especially keratoacanthoma and skin trauma. When occurring in the setting of systemic chemotherapy, it is considered a cutaneous sweat gland reaction in the histologic spectrum of neutrophilic eccrine hidradenitis.[134]

Histopathological Features　The predominant microscopic finding in classic NEH is sparse-to-dense neutrophilic infiltrates surrounding eccrine units (Table 10-23) (Fig. 10-45). Secretory coils in the superficial subcutis are generally more extensively involved by the infiltrate, and epithelial cell necrosis and vacuolization are present. Focal degenerative mucinous changes are often seen in the surrounding subcutis. The coiled and straight dermal ducts are variably involved by the neutrophilic infiltrate, and dyskeratotic vacuolization in these ducts is also variable. Spongiosis without prominent infiltrates is often seen in the straight dermal duct.

Similar microscopic features are seen in idiopathic NEH of the palms and soles. More extensive neutrophilic abscesses at the dermal subcutaneous junction may be present and efface and replace eccrine coils.

Squamous metaplasia with variable dyskeratosis of eccrine epithelial cells may affect all or select portions of the eccrine unit in chemotherapy-associated eccrine squamous syringometaplasia. Often minimal inflammatory infiltrates are identified, but sparse neutrophilic and lymphocytic infiltrates may be present.

Differential Diagnosis　The microscopic differential diagnosis includes infectious hidradenitis, neutrophilic dermatosis, small-vessel leukocytoclastic vasculitis, and coma- or pressure-induced eccrine necrosis. Infectious hidradenitis has very similar microscopic features, but special stains and/or tissue culture are positive. Some have considered NEH to be in the spectrum of neutrophilic dermatosis, given its association with myeloid leukemia. In contrast to classic Sweet's syndrome, the neutrophilic infiltrate is confined to the eccrine unit. At scanning power, the linear pattern of the infiltrate with some necrosis can mimic vasculitis, but closer inspection shows that eccrine ducts and not vessels are affected.

T A B L E 1 0 - 2 3

Neutrophilic Eccrine Hidradenitis

Clinical Features

Onset a few days after administration of chemotherapeutic agents such as cytarabine,
　　bleomycin
Neck, trunk, extremities
Tenderness
Erythematous macules, papules, plaques
Spontaneous resolution

Histopathological Features

Neutrophilic infiltrates associated with eccrine sweat coil
Eccrine epithelial cells show vacuolar degeneration and necrosis
Mucin deposition in peri-eccrine adipose tissue
Dermal edema
Sparse dermal infiltrates composed of lymphocytes and neutrophils

Differential Diagnosis

Infectious hidradenitis and pyoderma
Other neutrophilic dermatitides

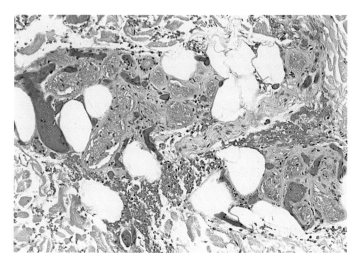

FIGURE 10-46   Sweat gland necrosis: Extensive noninflammatory necrosis of eccrine units is seen in coma-associated sweat gland necrosis.

Sweat Gland Necrosis

Clinical Features   Patients in a comatose state due to carbon monoxide poisoning,[137] drug overdose,[138] especially barbiturates,[139] severe illness, or trauma may develop bullae with sweat gland necrosis at pressure sites. The cause of these blisters is thought to be related to pressure-induced ischemia and possible toxic effect of offending drugs.

Histopathological Features   Intra- and subepidermal vesicle with variable dyskeratosis and necrosis is present in the epidermis. Eosinophilic coagulative necrosis of the eccrine secretory coils with minimal inflammatory infiltrates is the most characteristic finding in this entity (Fig. 10-46). Similar necrotic changes can be observed in adjacent hair follicles and sebaceous lobules. The dermis may be acellular or contain degenerating fibroblasts. Generally, the inflammatory infiltrate is minimal, but sparse neutrophils can be seen around necrotic adnexal structures.

Differential Diagnosis   Other causes of cutaneous necrosis such as coumarin necrosis, purpura fulminans, and vascular insufficiency-induced necrosis should be considered, but occlusion of vessels by fibrin, thrombi, or embolic material is identified in these cases. Chemotherapy-associated squamous metaplasia and necrosis can also be considered but lack the homogenized eosinophilic necrosis seen in coma-associated sweat gland necrosis.

REFERENCES

1. Whiting DA: *The Diagnosis of Alopecia, Current Concepts.* Kalamazoo, MI, Upjohn, 1990.
2. Headington JT: Transverse microscopic anatomy of the human scalp. *Arch Dermatol* 120: 449–56, 1984.
3. Whiting DA: The value of horizontal sections of scalp biopsies. *J Cutan Aging Cosmet Dermatol* 1:165, 1990.
4. Sperling LC: Hair anatomy for the clinician. *J Am Acad Dermatol* 25:1, 1991.
5. Solomon AR: The transversely sectioned scalp biopsy specimen: The technique and an algorithm for its use in the diagnosis of alopecia. *Adv Dermatol,* 9:127, 1994.
6. Whiting DA: Horizontal sections of scalp biopsies. In Burgdorf WHC, Katz SI (eds), *Dermatology: Progress and Perspectives. The Proceedings of the 18th World Congress of Dermatology.* New York, June 12–18, 1992. New York, Parthenon, 1993.
7. Hamilton JB: Patterned loss of hair in man: Types and incidence. *Ann NY Acad Sci* 53:708, 1951.
8. Olsen EA: Androgenetic alopecia, in Olsen EA (ed), *Disorders of Hair Growth: Diagnosis and Treatment.* New York, McGraw-Hill, 1995, chap 11.
9. Smith MA, Wells RS: Male-type alopecia, alopecia areata, and normal hair in women: Family histories. *Arch Dermatol* 89:95, 1964.
10. Ludwig E: Classification of the types of androgenetic alopecia (common baldness) occurring in the female sex. *Br J Dermatol* 97:247, 1977.
11. DeVillez RL, Jacobs JP, Szpunar CA, Warner ML: Androgenetic alopecia in the female. Treatment with 2% minoxidil solution. *Arch Dermatol* 130:303, 1994.
12. Sperling LC, Heimer WL: Androgen biology as a basis for the diagnosis and treatment of androgenic disorders in women. *J Am Acad Dermatol* 28:669, 1993.
13. Sperling LC, Heimer WL: Androgen biology as a basis for the diagnosis and treatment of androgenic disorders in women. *J Am Acad Dermatol* 28:901, 1993.
14. Whiting DA: Diagnostic and predictive value of horizontal sections of scalp biopsy specimens in male pattern androgenetic alopecia. *J Am Acad Dermatol* 28:755–763, 1993.
15. Sperling LC, Winton GB: The transverse anatomy of androgenetic alopecia. *J Dermatol Surg Oncol* 16:1127, 1990.
16. Whiting DA: Diagnostic and predictive value of horizontal sections of scalp biopsies in female androgenetic alopecia (Abstr). *Br J Dermatol* 125:94, 1991.
17. Fiedler VC, Storrs PA, Abell E: Histologic evaluation of the evolution and response to treatment of female pattern androgenetic alopecia (Abstr). *J Invest Derm* 102:566, 1995.
18. Sperling LC, Lupton GP: Histopathology of non-scarring alopecia. *J Cutan Pathol* 22:97, 1995.
19. Simpson NB: Diffuse alopecia: Endocrine, metabolic and chemical influences on the follicular cycle in Rook A, Dawber R (eds), *Diseases of the Hair and Scalp,* 2d ed. Oxford, Blackwell Scientific, 1991, chap 5.
20. Fiedler VC, Hafeez A: Diffuse alopecia: Telogen hair loss, in Olsen EA (ed), *Disorders of Hair Growth: Diagnosis and Treatment.* New York, McGraw-Hill, 1994, chap 10.
21. Headington JT: Telogen effluvium: New concepts and review. *Arch Dermatol* 129:356, 1993.
22. Kligman AM: Pathologic dynamics of human hair loss. I: Telogen effluvium. *Arch Dermatol* 83:175, 1961.
23. Van Scott EJ, Ekel TM, Auerbach R: Determinants of rate and kinetics of cell division in scalp hair. *J Invest Dermatol* 41:269, 1963.
24. Grossman KL, Kvedar JC: Anagen hair loss, in Olsen EA (ed), *Disorders of Hair Growth: Diagnosis and Treatment.* New York, McGraw-Hill, 1994, chap 9.
25. Whiting DA: Chronic telogen effluvium: Increased scalp hair shedding in middle-aged women. *J Am Acad Derm* 35:899–906, 1996.
26. Sperling LC: Transverse anatomy of telogen effluvium. *J Assoc Mil Dermatol* 16:3, 1990.
27. Crounse RG, Van Scott EJ: Changes in scalp hair roots as a measure of toxicity from cancer chemotherapeutic drugs. *J Invest Dermatol* 35:83, 1960.
28. Duvik M, Hordinsky MK, Fiedler VC, et al: HLA-D locus associations in alopecia areata. *Arch Dermatol* 127:64, 1991.
29. Colombe BW, Price VH, Khoury EL, et al: HLA class II antigen associations help to define two types of alopecia areata. *J Am Acad Dermatol* 33:757, 1995.
30. Hordinsky MK: Alopecia areata, in Olsen EA (ed), *Disorders of Hair Growth: Diagnosis and Treatment.* New York, McGraw-Hill, 1994, chap 8.
31. Muller SA, Winkelmann RK: Alopecia areata: An evaluation of 736 patients. *Arch Dermatol* 88:290, 1963.
32. Mitchell AJ, Krull EA: Alopecia areata: Pathogenesis and treatment. *J Am Acad Dermatol* 11:763, 1984.
33. McDonald-Hull SP, Hull SM, Nutbrown M, Pepall L, Thornton MJ, Randal VA, Cunliffe WJ, et al: Immunohistologic and ultrastructural comparison of the dermal papilla and hair follicle bulb from "active" and normal areas of alopecia areata. *J Invest Dermatol* 96:673, 1991.
34. Tobin DJ, Fenton DA, Kendall MD: Ultrastructural observations on the hair bulb melanocytes and melanosomes in acute alopecia areata. *J Invest Dermatol* 94: 803, 1990.
35. Tobin DJ, Fenton DA, Kendall MD: Cell degeneration in alopecia areata. *Am J Dermatopathol* 13:248, 1991.
36. Whiting DA: Diagnostic and predictive value of transverse sections of scalp biopsies in alopecia areata (Abstr). *J Cutan Pathol* 15:350, 1988.
37. Headington JT, Astle N: Familial focal alopecia. A new disorder of hair growth clinically resembling pseudopelade. *Arch Dermatol* 123–234, 1987.
38. Dawber R: Self-induced hair loss. *Semin Dermatol* 4:53, 1985.
39. Sanderson KV, Hall-Smith P: Tonsure trichotillomania. *Br J Dermatol* 82:343, 1970.
40. Muller SA: Trichotillomania. *Dermatol Clin* 5:595, 1987.
41. Steck WD: The clinical evaluation of pathologic hair loss with a diagnostic sign in trichotillomania. *Cutis* 24:293, 1979.
42. Muller SA: Trichotillomania: A histopathologic study of sixty-six patients. *J Am Acad Dermatol* 23:56, 1990.
43. Perlstein HH: Traction alopecia due to hair weaving. *Cutis* 5:440, 1969.
44. Lopresti P, Papa CM, Kligman AM: Hot comb alopecia. *Arch Dermatol* 98:234, 1968.

45. Wiles JC, Hansen RC: Postoperative (pressure) alopecia. *J Am Acad Dermatol* 12:195, 1985.

46. DeVillez RL: Infections, physical and inflammatory causes of hair and scalp abnormalities, in Olsen EA (ed), *Disorders of Hair Growth: Diagnosis and Treatment*. New York, McGraw-Hill, 1994, chap 5.

47. Whiting DA: Structural abnormalities of the hair shaft. *J Am Acad Dermatol* 16:1–25, 1987.

48. Whiting DA: Hair shaft defects, in Olsen EA (ed), *Disorders of Hair Growth: Diagnosis and Treatment*. New York, McGraw-Hill, 1994, chap 6.

49. Rook AJ, Dawber RPR: Defects of the hair shaft, in Rook A, Dawber R (eds), *Diseases of the Hair and Scalp*, 2d ed. Oxford, Blackwell Scientific, 1991, chap 7.

50. Price VH: Structural anomalies of the hair shaft, in Orfanos CE, Happle R (eds), *Hair and Hair Diseases*. Berlin, Springer-Verlag, 1990.

51. Rook AJ, Dawber RPR: Hereditary and congenital alopecia and hypotrichosis, in Rook A, Dawber R (eds) *Diseases of the Hair and Scalp*, 2d ed. Oxford, Blackwell Scientific, 1991, chap 6.

52. Olsen EA: Hair loss in childhood, in Olsen EA (ed), *Disorders of Hair Growth: Diagnosis and Treatment*. New York, McGraw-Hill, 1994, chap 7.

53. Price VH, Gummer CL: Loose anagen syndrome. *J Am Acad Dermatol* 20:249, 1989.

54. O'Donnell B, Sperling LC: The loose anagen syndrome. *Int J Dermatol* 31:107, 1992.

55. Templeton SF, Solomon AR. Scarring alopecia: A classification based on microscopic criteria. *J Cutan Pathol* 21:97–109, 1993.

56. Templeton SF, Santa Cruz DJ, Solomon AR: Alopecia: Histologic diagnosis by transverse sections. *Sem Diag Pathol* 3:2–18, 1996.

57. Elston DM, McCollough ML, Angeloni VL: Vertical and transverse sections of alopecia biopsy specimens: Combining the two to maximize diagnostic yield. *J Am Acad Dermatol* 32:454–457, 1995.

58. Callen JP: Chronic cutaneous lupus erythematosus. *Arch Dermatol* 118:412–416, 1982.

59. Wilson CL, Burge SM, Dean D, Dawber RPR: Scarring alopecia in discoid lupus erythematosus. *Br J Dermatol* 126:307–314, 1992.

60. Callen JP. Systemic lupus erythematosus in patients with chronic cutaneous (discoid) lupus erythematosus. *J Am Acad Dermatol* 12:278–288, 1985.

61. Dahl MV, Gilliam JN: Direct immunofluorescence in lupus erythematosus, in Beutner EH, Chorzelski TP, Kumar V (eds): *Immunopathology of the Skin*, 3d ed. New York, John Wiley, 1987.

62. Abell E: Immunofluorescent staining technics in the diagnosis of alopecia. *Southern Med J* 10:1407–1410, 1977.

63. Jordan RE: Subtle clues to diagnosis by immunopathology. *Am J Dermatopathol* 2:157–159, 1980.

64. Mehregan DA, Van Hale HM, Muller SA: Lichen planopilaris: Clinical and pathologic study of forty-five patients. *J Am Acad Dermatol* 27:935–942, 1992.

65. Burrows NP, Grant JW, Crisp AJ, Roberts SO: Scarring alopecia following gold therapy [letter]. *Acta Derm Venereol* 74:486, 1994.

66. Bergfeld WF, Valenzuela R, Beutner EH: Lichen planus, in Beutner EH, Chorzelski TP, Kumar V (eds), *Immunopathology of the Skin*, 3d ed. New York, John Wiley, 1987.

67. Brocq L: Alopecia. *J Cutan Vener Dis* 3:49–50, 1885.

68. Ronchese F: Pseudopelade. *Arch Dermatol* 82:336–341,1960.

69. Braun-Falco O, Imai S, Schmoeckel C, et al: Pseudopelade of Brocq. *Dermatologica* 172:18–23, 1986.

70. Pierard-Franchimont C, Pierard GE: Massive lymphocyte mediated apoptosis during the early stage of pseudopelade. *Dermatologica* 172:254–257, 1986.

71. Prieto JG: Pseudopelade of Brocq: Its relationship to some forms of cicatricial alopecias and to lichen planus. *J Invest Dermatol* 24:323–335,1955.

72. Anderson RL, Cullen SI: Pseudopelade of Brocq secondary to lichen planus. *Cutis* 17:916–918, 1976.

73. Sperling LC, Sau P: The follicular degeneration syndrome in black patients: Hot comb alopecia revisited and revised. *Arch Dermatol* 128:68–74, 1992.

74. Sperling LC, Skelton III MC, Smith KJ, et al: Follicular degeneration syndrome in men. *Arch Dermatol* 130:763–769, 1994.

75. Gibson LE, Muller SA, Peters MS: Follicular mucinosis of childhood and adolescence. *Pediatr Dermatol* 5:231–235, 1988.

76. Gibson LE, Muller SA, Leiferman KM, Peters MS. Follicular mucinosis: Clinical and histopathologic study. *J Am Acad Dermatol* 20:441–446, 1989.

77. Mehregan DA, Gibson LE, Muller SA: Follicular mucinosis: Histopathologic review of 33 cases. *Mayo Clin Proc* 66:387–390, 1991.

78. Hempstead RW, Ackerman AB: Follicular mucinosis: A reaction pattern in follicular epithelium. *Am J Dermatopathol* 7:245–257, 1985.

79. Hoffman E: Perifolliculitis capitis abscedens et suffodiens: Case presentation. *Derm Ztschr* 15:122–123, 1908.

80. Wise F, Parkhurst HJ: A rare form of suppurating cicatrizing disease of the scalp (perifolliculitis capitis abscedens et suffodiens). *Arch Dermatol* 4:750–758, 1921.

81. Newton RC, Hebert AA, Freese TW, Solomon AR: Scarring alopecia. *Dermatol Clin* 603–618, 1987.

82. Dinehart SM, Herzberg AJ, Kerns BJ, Pollack SV: Acne keloidalis: A review. *J Dermatol Surg Oncol* 15:642–647, 1989.

83. Herzberg AJ, Dinehart SM, Kerns BJ, Pollack SV: Acne keloidalis. Transverse microscopy, immunohistochemistry, and electron microscopy. *Am J Dermatopathol* 12:109–121, 1990.

84. Pye RJ, Peachey RDG, Burton JL: Erosive pustular dermatosis of the scalp. *Br J Dermatol* 100:559–566, 1979.

85. Caputo R, Veraldi S: Erosive pustular dermatosis of the scalp. *J Am Acad Dermatol* 28:96–98, 1993.

86. Dvoretzky I, Fisher BK, Movshovitz M, Schewach-Millet M: Favus. *Int J Dermatol* 19:89–92, 1980.

87. Poskitt L, Wilkinson JD: Natural history of keratosis pilaris. *Br J Dermatol* 130:711–713, 1994.

88. Baden HP, Byers R: Clinical findings, cutaneous pathology, and response to therapy in 21 patients wih keratosis pilaris atrophicans. *Arch Dermatol* 130:469–475, 1994.

89. Oranje AP, van Osch LDM, Oosterwijk JC: Keratosis pilaris atrophicans. One heterogeneous disease or a symptom in different clinical entities? *Arch Dermatol* 130:500–502, 1994.

90. Zacherle BJ, Silver DS: Hot tub folliculitis. *West J Med* 137:191–194, 1982.

91. Adler AI, Altman J: An outbreak of mud-wrestling-induced pustular dermatitis in college students. *JAMA* 269:502–504, 1993.

92. Bäck O, Faergemann J, Hörnqvist R: Pityrosporum folliculitis: A common disease of the young and middle-aged. *J Am Acad Dermatol* 12:56–61, 1985.

93. Smith KJ, Neafie RC, Skelton III HG, et al: Majocchi's granuloma. *J Cutan Pathol* 18:28–35, 1990.

94. Bonnar E, Eustace FC, Powell FC: The Demodex mite population in rosacea. *J Am Acad Dermatol* 28:443–448, 1993.

95. Aylesworth R, Vance C: Demodex folliculorum and Demodex brevis in cutaneous biopsies. *J Am Acad Dermatol* 7:583–589, 1982.

96. Smith KJ, Skelton HG, Frissman DM, Angritt P: Verrucous lesions secondary to DNA viruses in patients infected with the human immunodeficiency virus in association with increased factor XIIIa-positive dermal dendritic cells. *J Am Acad Dermatol* 27:943–950, 1992.

97. Sexton M: Occult herpesvirus folliculitis clinically simulating pseudolymphoma. *Am J Dermatopathol* 13:234–240, 1991.

98. Kaminer MS, Gilchrest BA: The many faces of acne. *J Am Acad Dermatol* 32:S6–14, 1995.

99. Leyden JJ: New understandings of the pathogenesis of acne. *J Am Acad Dermatol* 32:S15–25, 1995.

100. Tindall JP: Chloracne and chloracnegens. *J Am Acad Dermatol* 13:539–558, 1985.

101. Kligman AM, Frosch PJ: Steroid addiction. *Int J Dermatol* 18:23–31, 1979.

102. Goeteyn M, Mestdagh M, Aelbrecht M: Elastoidosis with cysts and comedones. *Dermatologica* 180:194, 1990.

103. Jemec GB, Hansen U: Histology of hidradenitis suppurativa. *J Am Acad Dermatol* 34:994–999, 1996.

104. Attanoos RL, Appleton MAC, Douglas-Jones AG: The pathogenesis of hidradenitis suppurativa: a closer look at apocrine and apoeccrine glands. *Br J Dermatol* 133:254–258, 1995.

105. Jansen T, Plewig G: Rosacea: classification and treatment. *J R Soc Med* 90:144–150, 1997.

106. Kligman AM: Ocular rosacea. Current concepts and therapy. *Arch Dermatol* 133:89–90, 1997.

107. Snapp RH: Lewandowsky's rosacea-like eruption: A clinical study. *J Invest Dermatol* 13:175–189, 1949.

108. Tope WD, Sanguexa OP: Rhinophyma's fibrous variant. Histopathology and immunochemistry. *Am J Dermatopathol* 16:307–310, 1994.

109. Medandsky RS, Bronson DM, Jacobson C, et al: Management of rosacea. *J Geriatr Dermatol* 4(A):1–8, 1996.

110. Hogan DJ: Perioral dermatitis. *Curr Probl Dermatol* 22:98–104, 1995.

111. Marks R, Harcourt-Webster JN: Histopathology of rosacea. *Arch Dermatol* 100:683–691, 1969.

112. Helm KF, Menz J, Gibson LE, Dicken CH: A clinical and histopathologic study of granulomatous rosacea. *J Am Acad Dermatol* 25:1038–1043, 1991.

113. Sahn EE, Sheridan DM: Demodicidosis in a child with leukemia. *J Am Acad Dermatol* 27:799–801, 1992.

114. Meheragan AH, Coskey RJ: Perforating folliculitis. *Arch Dermatol* 97:394–399, 1968.

115. Sehgel WN, Jain S, Thappa DM, Bhattacharya SN, Logani K: Perforating dermatoses: A review and report of four cases. *J Dermatol* 20:329–340, 1993.

116. Golitz L: Follicular and perforating disorders. *J Cutan Pathol* 12:282–288, 1985.

117. Patterson JW: The perforating disorders. *J Am Acad Dermatol* 10:561–581, 1984.

118. Hurwitz RM: The evolution of perforating folliculitis in patients with chronic renal failure. *Am J Dermatopathol* 7:231–239, 1985.

119. Moss HV: Kyrle's disease. *Cutis* 33:463–466, 1979.

120. Ofuji S, Ogino A, Horio T, et al: Eosinophilic pustular folliculitis. *Acta Derm Venereol (Stockh)* 50:195–203, 1970.

121. Lucky AW, Esterly NB, Heskel N, et al: Eosinophilic pustular folliculitis in infancy. *Pediatr Dermatol* 1:202–206, 1984.

122. Taïeb A, Bassan-Andrieu L, Maleville J: Eosinophilic pustulosis of the scalp in childhood. *J Am Acad Dermatol* 27:55–60, 1992.

123. Rosenthal D, LeBoit PE, Klumpp L, Berger TG: Human immunodeficiency virus-associated eosinophilic folliculitis. *Arch Dermatol* 127:206–209, 1991.

124. Blauvelt A, Plott RT, Spooner K, et al: Eosinophilic folliculitis associated with the acquired immunodeficiency syndrome responds well to permithrin. *Arch Dermatol* 131:360–361, 1995.

125. McCalmont TH, Altemus D, Maurer T, Berger TG: Eosinophilic folliculitis. The histologic spectrum. *Am J Dermatopathol* 17:439–446, 1995.

126. Fox GH, Fordyce JA: Two cases of a rare papular disease affecting the axillary region. *J Cutan Genito-Urinary Dis* 20:1, 1902.

127. Shelley WB, Levy EJ: Apocrine sweat retention in man. *Arch Dermatol* 73:38–49, 1956.

128. Miller ML, Harford RR, Yeager JK: Fox-Fordyce disease treated with topical clindamycin solution. *Arch Dermatol* 131:1112–1113, 1995.

129. Shelley WB, Hurley HJ: Localized chromhidrosis: a survey. *Arch Dermatol & Syphilol* 69:449–471, 1954.

130. Saff DM, Owens R, Kahn TA: Apocrine chromhidrosis involving the areolae in a 15-year-old amateur figure skater. *Pediatr Dermatol* 12:48–50, 1995.

131. Harrist TJ, Fine JD, Berman RS, et al: Neutrophilic eccrine hidradenitis. A distinctive type of neutrophilic dermatosis associated with myelogenous leukemia and chemotherapy. *Arch Dermatol* 118:263–266, 1982.

132. Fitzpatrick JE, Bennion SD, Reed OM, et al: Neutrophilic eccrine hidradenitis associated with induction chemotherapy. *J Cutan Pathol* 14:272–278, 1987.

133. Templeton SF, Solomon AR, Swerlick RA: Intradermal bleomycin injections into normal human skin, a histologic and immunohistologic study. *Arch Dermatol* 130: 577–583, 1994.

134. Hurt MA, Halvorson RD, Petr C, et al: Eccrine squamous syringometaplasia. A cutaneous sweat gland reaction in the histologic spectrum of chemotherapy-associated eccrine hidradenitis and neutrophilic eccrine hidradenitis. *Arch Dermatol* 126:73–77, 1990.

135. Stahr BJ, Cooper PH, Caputo RV: Idiopathic plantar hidradenitis: A neutrophilic eccrine hidradenitis occurring primarily in children. *J Cutan Pathol* 21:289–296, 1994.

136. Mehregan AH: Proliferation of sweat ducts in certain diseases of the skin. *Am J Dermatopathol* 3:27–31, 1981.

137. Leavell UW, Farley CH, McIntire JS: Cutaneous changes in a patient with carbon monoxide poisoning. *Arch Dermatol* 99:429–433, 1969.

138. Mandy S, Ackerman AB: Characteristic traumatic skin lesions in drug-induced coma. *JAMA* 213:253–256, 1970.

139. Leavell UW: Sweat gland necrosis in barbituate poisoning. *Arch Dermatol* 100: 218–221, 1969.

CHAPTER 11

PANNICULITIS AND FASCIITIS

Raymond L. Barnhill

Inflammatory processes involving the subcutaneous fat constitute one of the most difficult and confusing areas in all of dermatopathology.[1–6] Why does panniculitis pose such a problem for the dermatopathologist? On the whole, many of these conditions have not been sufficiently studied, and thus adequate information is not available concerning their pathogenesis. Some of the reasons for the lack of data include the following: (1) in general, panniculitis is relatively uncommon, (2) dermatologists and other physicians are often reluctant to biopsy subcutaneous nodules, since poor wound healing is common, (3) biopsies are often too small and do not adequately sample the condition (Table 11-1), (4) the clinical findings for many panniculitides are fairly similar, (5) the response of adipose tissue to injury is limited, and (6) the histopathological findings depend on when the biopsy is obtained in the time course of the disease process. Because of the lack of data, skin pathologists have often ascribed too much specificity to morphologic observations made on limited samplings taken from limited numbers of patients, often without considering when the specimen was obtained in the natural history of the panniculitis.

In order to gain a better understanding of the nature of pathological processes in subcutaneous tissue, it is necessary to review briefly (1) the microanatomy of adipose tissue and (2) the reactions of subcutaneous fat to injury.

THE MICROANATOMY OF SUBCUTANEOUS FAT

In general, the subcutaneous tissue consists of depot fat sandwiched between the reticular dermis above and superficial fascia below.[1,2] Adipose tissue is organized into two compartments: (1) discrete round or ovoid lobules composed of confluent aggregates of the clear-appearing fat cells and (2) fibrous trabeculae (or *septa*) that form a meshwork separating the individual fat lobules. The fibrous septa are continuous with collagen of the reticular dermis and the superficial fascia and contain all the blood vessels, lymphatics, and nerves of the subcutaneous fat. In one sense, the fibrous septa simply serve as scaffolding for vascular and nerve plexi traversing the subcutis from deeper tissue to supply the skin. Thus, inflammatory conditions affecting the fat often involve the reticular dermis and fascia, and vice versa. Arterial vessels in the fat are small to medium in size and are categorized as muscular arteries. Thus, it is not possible to develop large-vessel arteritis in the subcutaneous fat but rather an arteritis affecting vessels of the caliber noted in polyarteritis nodosa.

Each fat lobule is vascularized by a single arteriole, and, in effect, is an end-organ with no collateral blood supply.[1,2] There are no lymphatics within the lobules. Any interruption to this arterial supply will eventuate in ischemia or infarction of the fat lobule, depending upon the speed with which vascular compromise develops. The individual fat cells are supplied by arterial capillaries with drainage to venous capil-

laries and venules at the peripheries of the fat lobules. Based on these vascular patterns, in very general terms pathologic processes affecting arterial vessels may result in a *lobular* pattern of panniculitis versus a *septal* pattern associated with venular or venous inflammatory disorders.

THE REACTIONS OF SUBCUTANEOUS FAT TO INJURY

Many of the morphologic changes observed in "panniculitis" are simply nonspecific reparative reactions of the fat to injury, often irrespective of the particular etiologic agent (Table 11-2).[1–5] For some time it has been recognized that injury to the fat cell results in the release of lipid which becomes a foreign body or irritant. The ensuing host response is thus involved in removing this "foreign" substance and restoring the tissue to normal. The initial reaction is local proliferation of the blood vessels and an influx of neutrophils (acute inflammation). The next phase of the tissue reaction is characterized by the arrival of mononuclear cells, i.e., lymphocytes and monocyte-macrophages. The latter cells are primarily concerned with the phagocytosis of lipid and other debris, often resulting in the formation of lipidized macrophages (foamy histiocytes) and multinucleate giant cells. The final stage in this reparative response is fibroplasia and the reconstitution of tissue integrity. The ultimate outcome in many instances is a scarring process. These three stages of the host reaction—acute inflammation, chronic inflammation, and fibrosis—are fairly constant but will obviously vary depending upon the intensity and nature of the insult to the fat.

APPROACH TO THE INTERPRETATION OF PANNICULITIS

Major problems with the traditional classification of panniculitis include (1) the tendency to place too much emphasis on categorizing a process as either a septal or lobular panniculitis and (2) the application of often arcane terminology, such as *Weber-Christian disease* or *erythema induratum*, to the condition rather than looking for a specific cause. In fact, many panniculitides may be either septal or lobular, and probably most are *both* septal *and* lobular. Thus, this pattern approach often adds little additional information to the diagnostic evaluation when looking for a cause of the panniculitis is more important (Tables 11-3 to 11-5). The objectives of this chapter are to emphasize the systematic evaluation of panniculitis for a specific etiology and to discourage the use of outdated terminology that if anything obfuscates the rational investigation of disorders of adipose tissue.

The objectives of the histopathologist confronted with a disease process in subcutaneous fat are (1) to identify the predominant pattern

233

TABLE 11-1

Evaluation of Panniculitis

1. Excisional wedge biopsy is necessary for adequate sampling.
2. Punch biopsies are to be discouraged and may be misleading.
3. Biopsy an active rather than a late-stage lesion.
4. Special stains for infectious organisms include Gram's, acid-fast, fungal, Warthin-Starry, Fite-Faraco.
5. Examine specimen under polarized light for foreign material.
6. Laboratory investigation includes cultures and other techniques, such as immunostaining and polymerase chain reaction, for infection; serologic testing for syphilis, borreliosis, connective tissue disease, vasculitis, alpha-1-antitrypsin deficiency, calcium, phosphorus, oxalate, coagulopathy, lipase, amylase.
7. Directed clinical history for isolated lesion (e.g., ruptured cyst), trauma, factitial causes, psychiatric illness, drug abuse, cold exposure, recent medications, systemic disease, e.g., vasculitis, connective tissue disease, sarcoidosis, infections, malignancy.

TABLE 11-2

Manifestations of Fat Necrosis

Lipophages—macrophages containing phagocytosed lipid following necrosis of adipocytes
Microcysts—coalesced tissue spaces in fat following fat necrosis
Liquefactive alterations—granular cellular debris
Hyalinizing (sclerosing) alterations—intact mummified lipocytes with a grainy and later glassy amorphous appearance
Membranous (lipomembranous) microcyst formation—microcysts lined by feathery, almost ciliated membranes
Ischemic alterations—pallor of adipocytes with loss of nuclei and microvessels, hemorrhage, hemosiderin deposits, karyorrhexis

as septal or lobular, or both septal and lobular, without placing too much emphasis on this exercise (Table 11-6); (2) to identify whether there is any alteration of the epidermis, dermis, or fascia; and (3) to look for particular histologic findings that would indicate or suggest a specific diagnosis (Table 11-5). The histopathologic findings must then be correlated with clinical history and laboratory studies. The evaluation of panniculitis should use the major categories of septal panniculitis and lobular panniculitis, realizing that this categorization is often of limited value, since many processes may be septal or lobular or show varying degrees of both septal and lobular involvement.

SEPTAL PANNICULITIS

As discussed above, the goals for the histopathologist are to systematically evaluate a mainly septal process (Fig. 11-1), looking for histopathologic findings or clues leading to a specific diagnosis if at all possible (Tables 11-5 and 11-7).[1–10] Such entities include vasculitis; prominent sclerosis of septa as in morphea, scleroderma, and eosinophilic fasciitis; lymphoid infiltrates or nodules, as in connective tissue disease; lymphoid infiltrates and hyalinization, as in lupus panniculitis; infectious agents; foreign bodies; and palisading granulomas.

If the latter are not observed, one is often left with a nonspecific panniculitis. Based on the cellular composition and degree of fibrosis, the septal panniculitis may be categorized as (1) an acute process, e.g., neutrophils, eosinophils, edema, little or no septal thickening, (2) a subacute panniculitis (predominantly mononuclear cells), e.g., presence of lymphocytes, monocyte-macrophages, some septal thickening, and fibrosis, or (3) a chronic or late-stage septal panniculitis.

TABLE 11-3

Algorithmic Approach to Diagnosis of Panniculitis

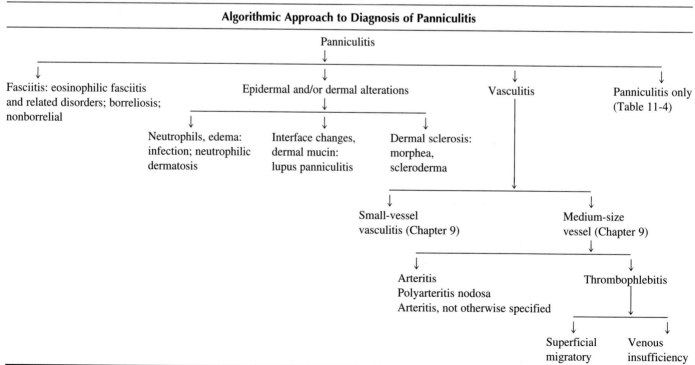

TABLE 11-4

Algorithmic Approach to Diagnosis of Panniculitis

Panniculitis only

- **Septal**
  - Erythema nodosum reactions
    - Short duration reactions
    - Chronic reactions
  - Other, early
- **Septal, Lobular**
  - Lymphoplasma cellular infiltrates: connective tissue disease
    - Septal sclerosis: morphea; scleroderma
  - Ghost cells saponification: pancreatic panniculitis
    - Cytophagocytosis: cytophagic histiocytic panniculitis; immunosuppression: infection; malignancy
  - Crystals
    - Inflammation; crystals in macrophages; lipocytes: subcutaneous fat; necrosis; poststeroid panniculitis
    - Little or no inflammation; crystals in lipocytes: sclerema neonatorum
- **Lobular**
  - Granulomatous inflammation: infection; physical panniculitis; metastatic Crohn's disease; pyoderma gangrenosum
  - Neutrophilic infiltrates: EN reactions; infection; neutrophilic dermatosis; pyoderma gangrenosum; physical panniculitis

---

Many processes may produce a nonspecific predominantly septal panniculitis, particularly in the early stages (Table 11-6). In many cases, thorough evaluation of the patient and of the clinical history and follow-up will make it possible to identify a cause or presumed cause.

Erythema Nodosum

Thought by many clinicians to be a distinctive clinicopathologic entity,[2–4,6–12] erythema nodosum (EN) is a relatively nonspecific hypersensitivity reaction and a diagnosis of exclusion associated with a variety of causes (Table 11-7), eventuating in fairly short-lived tender red nodules.[7–15] EN may be thought of as a nonspecific clinical finding, perhaps analogous to urticaria or a maculopapular erythematous eruption. A major problem is that the clinical lesions are thought to be distinctive, almost regardless of the histopathologic findings. Histologic examination of the red nodules most commonly discloses a (predominantly) septal panniculitis, but in some instances, lobular infiltrates are observed. Thus, the histologic spectrum associated with EN has expanded and now includes neutrophilic,[8] eosinophilic,[16] and granulomatous lobular infiltrates.[9] Furthermore, the clinical spectrum of EN has been extended to encompass long-standing or chronic forms of panniculitis, termed *chronic EN*, *EN migrans*, or *subacute nodular migratory panniculitis of Villanova*.[17–21] However, some authors believe that chronic EN and EN migrans are related but have clinical and histopathologic differences.[21]

The term *EN* should probably be reserved for panniculitides that have been thoroughly investigated and monitored for a specific etiology and show the appropriate clinical and pathologic features.

Clinical Features   Typical EN is strictly defined as symmetric crops of tender, reddish nodules lasting approximately 3 to 6 weeks and often resolving with a bruiselike appearance, but without ulceration or scarring (Table 11-8).[3,4,7–12] The lesions may occur anywhere but characteristically involve the anterior shins. Women with EN outnumber men about 3 to 1, and patients are typically 20 to 50 years of age. Often, the lesions are accompanied by fever, malaise, and arthralgias.[10]

Chronic EN and EN migrans appear to represent hypersensitivity reactions of longer duration, often 1 to 4 years or more.[17–21] Some authors maintain that chronic EN is characterized by fairly discrete persistent nodules that are symmetric and not migratory, whereas EN migrans tends to show nodules that coalesce into spreading plaques that are commonly unilateral.[21]

Histopathological Features   Although erythema nodosum may be thought of as a nonspecific reaction resulting from a wide variety of agents, the histopathologic findings may be categorized as principally early, intermediate and/or established, or late-stage (Figs. 11-1 to 11-5) (Table 11-6).[7–12] Early or acute lesions commonly show changes primarily confined to the fibrous trabeculae: edema, hemorrhage, and variable inflammatory cell infiltrates composed primarily of neutrophils,

TABLE 11-5

Histopathologic Findings Suggesting a Particular Category or Type of Panniculitis

Vasculitis
 Small-vessel vasculitis
 Thrombophlebitis
 Polyarteritis and other arteritides
Calcification of vessels
 Calciphylaxis
Thrombotic occlusion of vessels
 Coagulopathy
 Cryoprecipitate
Septal sclerosis
 Morphea profunda
 Scleroderma
 Eosinophilic fasciitis
Lymphoplasma cellular infiltrates
 Connective tissue disease
  Lupus panniculitis
  Dermatomyositis
  Connective tissue panniculitis
 Lipoatrophy
 Necrobiosis lipoidica
Hyalinization and lymphoplasmacellular infiltrates
 Lupus panniculitis
Infectious organisms
Palisading granulomas
 Granuloma annulare
 Rheumatoid nodule
 Necrobiosis lipoidica
Panniculitis with crystal formation
 Subcutaneous fat necrosis
 Sclerema neonatorum
 Poststeroid panniculitis
 Oxalosis
 Gout
Ghost cells, saponification
 Pancreatic (enzymic) panniculitis
Cytophagocytosis
 Cytophagic histiocytic panniculitis
  Infection
  Lymphoma
Sclerosing lipogranuloma
 Injected or implanted lipids
Foreign bodies
 Chemical and factitial panniculitis
Atypical cellular infiltrates
 Lymphoma
 Leukemia

TABLE 11-6

Predominant Patterns of the Panniculitides

Condition	Pattern of Panniculitis
Hypersensitivity reactions	
Short duration (erythema nodosum reactions)	Septal → lobular
Longer duration (chronic EN)	Septal → lobular
Vasculitis	
Small-vessel vasculitis	Septal → lobular
Medium- to large-vessel vasculitis	Septal and lobular
Lipodermatosclerosis	Septal and lobular Septal early
Calciphylaxis	Septal and lobular
Oxalosis	Septal and lobular
Morphea profunda, scleroderma, eosinophilic fasciitis	Septal → lobular Septal early
Palisading granulomas	Septal → lobular
Alpha-1-antitrypsin deficiency	Septal and lobular
Cytophagic histiocytic panniculitis	Lobular → septal
Pancreatic panniculitis	Lobular → septal
Subcutaneous fat necrosis	Lobular → septal
Sclerema neonatorum	Lobular → septal
Poststeroid panniculitis	Lobular → septal
Infection-related panniculitis	Septal and lobular
Physical panniculitis	
Cold panniculitis	Septal and lobular
Trauma-related	Lobular → septal
Chemical and factitial	Lobular → septal
Connective tissue disease	
Lupus panniculitis	Septal and lobular
Dermatomyositis	Septal and lobular
Connective tissue panniculitis	Septal and lobular
Eosinophilic panniculitis	Septal and lobular
Noninfectious granulomatous panniculitis	
Sarcoidosis	Septal and lobular
Metastatic Crohn's disease	Septal and lobular
Lymphoma and leukemia	Lobular → septal

possibly with some admixture of lymphocytes and eosinophils (Fig. 11-2). This infiltrate often extends into the peripheries of the fat lobules. Otherwise, the fat lobules are largely unaffected. Older lesions often exhibit some thickening of the septa and a predominance of mononuclear cells, lymphocytes in particular (Fig. 11-3). There may be greater encroachment into the fat lobules by the inflammatory cell infiltrates. Often at this stage, one begins to encounter mononuclear cells arranged in a radial array and somewhat later multinucleated histiocytic giant cells in the thickened fibrotic septa, the so-called Miescher's granulomas (Figs. 11-3 and 11-4).[22] The latter feature is considered by some authors to be diagnostic of EN. However, this granulomatous reaction involving the fibrous trabeculae is likely to be a nonspecific reparative response associated with phagocytosis of collagen and other materials.

With evolution of lesions, there is greater thickening and fibrosis of the septa. The infiltrate becomes more granulomatous, and there is a general tendency to greater involvement of the lobules.[4,7,9] With time, there is gradual obliteration of fat lobules by the septal fibrosis. Although some fat necrosis is occasionally observed, this is not a prominent feature in EN. To the extent that fat necrosis does occur, lipophages and granulomatous inflammation are present.

Two additional reaction patterns observed in this setting of EN include: (1) acute (neutrophilic) panniculitis (Fig. 11-5)[8] and (2) eosino-

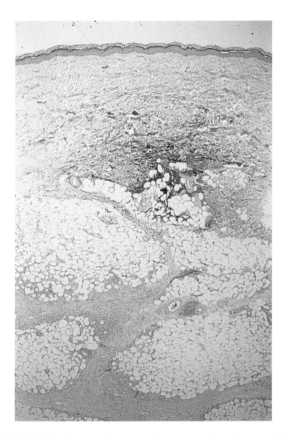

FIGURE 11-1 Erythema nodosum reaction pattern. Scanning magnification shows thickening of the fibrous trabeculae and predominantly lymphocytic infiltrates at the peripheries of the fat lobules.

philic panniculitis[16] (see below). Both present as predominantly lobular infiltrates of neutrophils and eosinophils, respectively. The inclusion of panniculitides with the above histologic features speaks to the nonspecific nature of EN.

By definition, vasculitis is not a major feature of EN. However, low-grade vascular injury and thrombophlebitis have been emphasized as findings commonly encountered in the EN reaction pattern.[7] One must determine whether septal panniculitis or thrombophlebitis is the predominant finding and consider the clinical features in order to arrive at a final interpretation of their significance.

Chronic EN and EN migrans have been reported to have histopathologic as well as clinical differences.[21] Chronic EN has been described as showing discrete perivascular lymphocytic infiltrates and lacking fibrosis and thickening of fibrous trabeculae. However, EN migrans may have septal thickening and fibrosis, epithelioid granulomas, and vascular proliferation resembling granulation tissue.

Differential Diagnosis   As already discussed, this reaction pattern is nonspecific, since a number of processes may begin or present as a septal panniculitis. Thus, one must consider connective tissue disease, infection, neutrophilic dermatoses (Sweet's syndrome and pyoderma gangrenosum),[15,23] physical insults, fibrosing panniculitides, and palisading granulomas in this differential diagnosis. Careful scrutiny of the specimen for histologic findings leading to one of the latter diagnoses, special stains for organisms, evaluation with polarized light, serologic evaluation, and clinical history are needed to exclude specific causes of the panniculitis.

TABLE 11-7

Causes of Septal Panniculitis (Erythema Nodosum Reactions)

Sarcoidosis
Streptococcal infection
Mycobacteria
   Tuberculosis
   Leprosy
Gastrointestinal infections and infestations
   Yersiniosis
   Salmonellosis
   Campylobacter colitis
   Shigellosis
Deep fungal infections
   Coccidioidomycosis
   Histoplasmosis
   Blastomycosis (North American)
   Deep trichophytosis
Other infections
   Ornithosis
   Cat-scratch disease
   Syphilis
   Gonorrhea
   Lymphogranuloma inguinale
   Other chlamydial infections
   Infectious mononucleosis
Inflammatory bowel disease
   Crohn's disease
   Ulcerative colitis
Hormonal causes
   Pregnancy
   Contraceptive pills
Malignancies
   Leukemias
   Carcinomas
   Sarcomas
   Hodgkin's disease
Drugs
   Iodine
   Bromine
   Sulphathiazole
   Penicillin
   Phenacetin
   Pyritinol
Other causes
   Periarteritis nodosa
   Sweet's syndrome
   Behçet's disease

Vasculitis, Vasculopathy, and Ischemic Necrosis of Subcutaneous Fat

As previously discussed, vascular injury is a common component and cause of panniculitis. Vessels ranging from capillaries to medium-size arteries or veins may be involved.[1–4,7] Thus the subcutis should be examined for leukocytoclastic venulitis; arteritis, as in polyarteritis nodosa; or thrombophlebitis. Vasculitis is discussed in detail in Chapter 9 and is beyond the scope of this chapter. In general, vasculitis should

TABLE 11-8

Erythema Nodosum

Clinical Features

Women > men
Age 20–50 years
Tender reddish nodules
3 to 6 weeks' duration
No ulceration or scarring—anterior shins most often
Fever
Malaise
Arthralgias
Bilateral hilar lymphadenopathy (Löfgren's syndrome)

Histopathological Features

Septal panniculitis
  Neutrophils, occasional eosinophils, followed by lymphocytes,
    mononuclear cells
  Edema, hemorrhage
  Thickening of septa
  Peripheral involvement of fat lobules
  Usually no fat necrosis
  Thrombophlebitis on occasion
Lobular panniculitis
  Acute neutrophilic panniculitis
  Granulomatous panniculitis
  Usually minimal fat necrosis

Differential Diagnosis

Septal panniculitis
  Sclerosing panniculitis
  Connective tissue disease
  Many conditions early
Lobular panniculitis
  Infection
  Neutrophilic dermatosis
    Sweet's syndrome
    Pyoderma gangrenosum
  Vasculitis
  Calciphylaxis
  Physical and factitial panniculitis
  Alpha-1-antitrypsin deficiency
  Subcutaneous fat necrosis of newborn

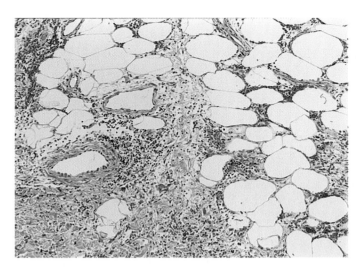

FIGURE 11-2 Erythema nodosum reaction pattern. Inflammatory cell infiltrates and extravasation of erythrocytes are present at the periphery of a fat lobule.

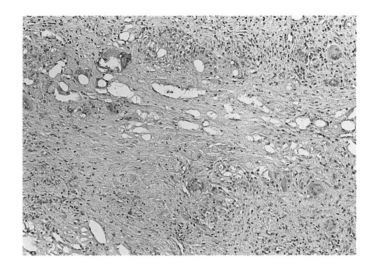

FIGURE 11-3 Erythema nodosum reaction pattern. A thickened fibrous septum contains Miescher's granulomas.

be assessed with respect to the caliber of the vessel involved; the type of vessel, e.g., venule, arteriole, vein, medium-size artery; the composition of the infiltrate, e.g., the presence of neutrophils, eosinophils, lymphocytes, granulomatous elements. The vasculitis must be correlated with the extent of systemic involvement, i.e., other organs involved. The patient must be evaluated for infection, connective tissue disease, inflammatory bowel disease, or other systemic disease. Use of terms such as *nodular vasculitis* should be discouraged, since they may impede thorough investigation of the patient for a specific etiology. A vasculitis or arteritis without obvious cause is best designated as such and the patient followed with the goal of eventually identifying a cause of the process.

Ischemic fat necrosis is the result of interruption of the vascular supply to fat lobules from any cause. Potentially any type of vasculitis or intravascular occlusive process can result in ischemic necrosis of fat.

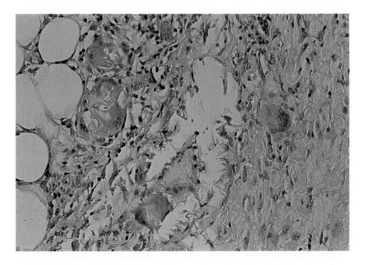

FIGURE 11-4 Erythema nodosum reaction pattern. High magnification showing multinucleated giant cells that form Miescher's granulomas. There is also focal lipomembranous alteration.

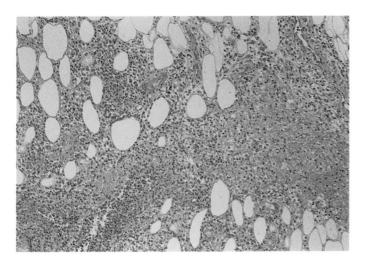

FIGURE 11-5 Acute neutrophilic lobular panniculitis associated with a clinical presentation of erythema nodosum.

The latter entities, which include hypercoagulable states and other occlusive vasculopathies, are discussed in Chapter 9. However, three distinctive forms of ischemic fat necrosis will be discussed in this chapter: lipodermatosclerosis (sclerosing panniculitis), calciphylaxis, and oxalosis.

LIPODERMATOSCLEROSIS

Lipodermatosclerosis is a distinctive clinicopathologic entity associated with striking induration of the distal third of the lower extremity and ischemic fat necrosis.[24–26] This entity has been clinically recognized for many years under a variety of terms, including *hypodermitis sclerodermiformis*, *lipomembranous change in chronic panniculitis*,[26–28] and recently, *(stasis-related) sclerosing panniculitis*.[26]

Clinical Features   The condition is most commonly observed in adult women with a history of venous insufficiency and stasis of the lower extremities, often resulting from superficial or deep thromboses or varicosities (Table 11-9).[24–26] Characteristically, the distal third of the lower extremities is affected by circumferential erythematous edematous plaques that give place to hyperpigmented indurated depressed lesions that have a characteristic "inverted bottle" appearance.

Histopathological Features   The epidermis and dermis commonly show stasis dermatitis with variable acanthosis, spongiosis, lobular vascular proliferation, fibroplasia, dermal atrophy, and hemosiderin deposition.[24–26] The panniculitis is septal and lobular, and the histopathologic findings are related to the age of the lesion (Table 11-9). Early lesions show perivascular lymphocytic infiltrates involving the fibrous trabeculae and the peripheries of fat lobules. At this stage, ischemic fat necrosis is typified by pallor of and loss of nuclei in adipocytes in the central part of the fat lobule; loss of lobular vessels; and variable karyorrhexis, extravasation and degeneration of erythrocytes, and hemosiderin deposits.[26] With time, there is progressive fibrosis and sclerosis of septa and gradual obliteration of fat lobules (Figs. 11-6 and 11-7). The inflammatory infiltrates show an admixture of lymphocytes; macrophages, some lipidized; and plasma cells. Necrosis of fat with microcysts are also observed with evolution of the process. A finding commonly observed in this context but not specific for this entity is membranous (lipomembranous or membranocystic) fat necrosis (Fig.

11-7).[26–29] The latter change refers to cystic spaces in areas of fat necrosis that are lined by eosinophilic feathery crenulated membranous structures suggesting the cuticle of a parasite. These membranes stain with periodic acid–Schiff (PAS) diastase stain and the lipid stains Sudan black and Luxol fast blue. Ultrastructurally, the membranes are composed of tubular structures containing neutral fat, corresponding to the breakdown and collapse of lipocytes.

Although membranous fat necrosis is perhaps most commonly observed in ischemia, it also has been reported in a variety of other settings, including traumatic injury and connective tissue disease.[28,29]

Differential Diagnosis   Early lesions may be histologically confused with almost any septal panniculitis; however, the clinical features with evidence of venous insufficiency and stasis should provide evidence in favor of lipodermatosclerosis and the exclusion of other conditions. More developed lesions may be difficult to distinguish from lupus profundus and other fibrosing panniculitides. Lipodermatosclerosis shows ischemic fat necrosis, whereas lupus profundus is notable for prominent lymphoplasmacytic infiltrates and hyalinizing fat necrosis. Morphea and related conditions should not show stasis changes, dermal atrophy, and ischemic necrosis to the degree of that observed in lipodermatosclerosis. The clinical manifestations should easily allow distinction of even late-stage sclerosing panniculitis from collagen vascular disease.

CALCIPHYLAXIS

Calciphylaxis (also known as *vascular calcification–cutaneous necrosis syndrome*)—a rare syndrome of vascular calcification and ischemic necrosis—has been recognized for almost a hundred years, yet its pathophysiology remains poorly understood.[30–39] Patients presenting with

---

TABLE 11-9

Lipodermatosclerosis

Clinical Features

Adult women > men
Venous insufficiency
Stasis
Thromboses
Erythematous, edematous indurated plaques with "inverted bottle" appearance, distal lower extremities above ankles

Histopathological Features

Stasis dermatitis
Septal and lobular involvement
    Perivascular lymphocytic infiltrates
    Ischemic fat necrosis
        Pallor of adipocytes, loss of nuclei
        Karyorrhexis, hemorrhage, hemosiderin deposition
        Progressive fibrosis, obliteration of fat lobules and vessels
        Lipomembranous fat necrosis
        Fat microcysts

Differential Diagnosis

Septal panniculitides (erythema nodosum)
Other fibrosing panniculitides
    Lupus panniculitis
    Morphea profunda, fasciitis
Physical panniculitis

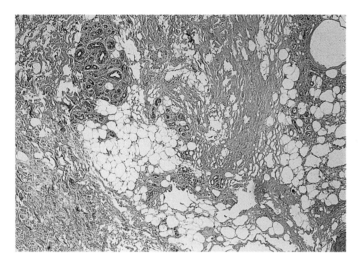

FIGURE 11-6 Lipodermatosclerosis. There is obliteration of fat lobules by hyalinized fibrous tissue. There is relatively little inflammation at this late stage.

this dramatic condition often have a systemic disease commonly associated with perturbation of calcium and/or phosphorus metabolism, such as chronic renal failure, primary or secondary hyperparathyroidism, idiopathic hypercalcemia, or hypervitaminosis D.[31–35,38,39] However, rare patients without any of the latter conditions or abnormal calcium or phosphorus levels have been reported.[38] Patients with both acquired immunodeficiency syndrome[37] and protein C deficiency[36] have developed calciphylaxis. Although Selye described many features of the syndrome in an animal model,[30] the mechanisms responsible for triggering ischemia necrosis have yet to be fully elucidated.[38] Possible etiologic factors include (1) endovascular fibrosis and calcification of small vessels, (2) a hypercoagulable state, and (3) luminal narrowing by calcification.

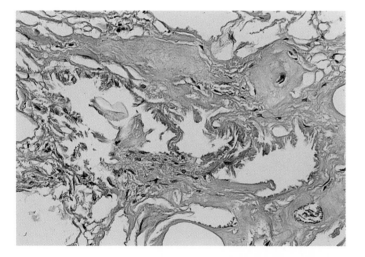

FIGURE 11-7 Lipodermatosclerosis. There is prominent lipomembranous alteration resulting in a feathery membrane in this fat lobule. The latter changes are nonspecific.

TABLE 11-10

Calciphylaxis

Clinical Features

Abnormalities of calcium and/or phosphorus metabolism
Chronic renal failure
Primary or secondary hyperparathyroidism
Protein C deficiency
Livedo reticularis
Painful inflammatory nodules that ulcerate
Vascular calcification

Histopathological Features

Small vessels (30 to 600 μm) show:
   Mural calcification
   Intimal proliferation
Soft-tissue calcification
Fibrin thrombi, variable
Ischemic fat necrosis
Mixed inflammatory cell infiltrates involving panniculus with
   neutrophils and mononuclear cells

Differential Diagnosis

Other calcifying panniculitides (dystrophic and metastatic
   calcification)
Connective tissue disease
Peripheral vascular disease, sclerosing panniculitis
Cholesterol emboli
Marantic and septic emboli
Oxalosis
Intravascular thrombotic and occlusive vasculopathies
Vasculitis
Infection
Pyoderma gangrenosum

Clinical Features   The clinical manifestations in calciphylaxis are distinctive.[31–39] Patients usually develop painful erythematous to dusky lesions that undergo necrosis in a background of livedo reticularis (Table 11-10). The lesions are often bilateral and may involve the trunk and extremities. Radiographic examination commonly reveals vascular calcification of large vessels, the so-called pipe-stem pattern of calcific medial stenosis, which is nonspecific. Small-vessel (less than 0.5 mm) calcification is more specific.[38,39] The mortality rate is approximately 60 percent.

Histopathological Features   In general, early lesions have not been biopsied, and thus the initial findings have not been clearly delineated.[38] In established lesions, mural calcification of small vessels ranging in size from 30 to 600 (average about 100) μm is observed (Table 11-10).[38,39] The sizes of these vessels correspond to arterioles and smaller vessels. The vessels also exhibit a distinctive yet nonspecific intimal proliferation but, in general, are too damaged to be clearly identified as either arterial or venous. A regular finding is the presence of fibrin thrombi in vessels. The adipose tissue generally shows foci of ischemic fat necrosis with calcification and variable mixed inflammatory cell infiltrates containing neutrophils and mononuclear cells.

Differential Diagnosis   The differential diagnosis includes peripheral vascular disease; atheroemboli; Monckeberg's medial calcific sclerosis;

marantic and septic emboli; oxalosis; intravascular thrombotic and occlusive vasculopathies (protein C deficiency, coumadin necrosis, circulating lupus anticoagulant, cryoprecipitates, disseminated intravascular coagulation); vasculitis including livedoid vasculitis, pyoderma gangrenosum, lipodermatosclerosis, and infection-related panniculitis; and other variants of dystrophic and metastatic calcifying panniculitis. The clinical presentation, presence of small-vessel calcification with endovascular proliferation, and fat necrosis should allow distinction from the latter entities.

OXALOSIS

An extremely rare form of panniculitis associated with deposition of the crystalline material calcium oxalate in vessels may closely resemble calciphylaxis.[40–42] Oxalosis may occur as a primary inherited defect or as a secondary metabolic condition resulting from the excessive ingestion of oxalate and other substances. The clinical manifestations include hyperoxaluria, nephrolithiasis, nephrocalcinosis, renal failure in many cases, and widespread tissue deposition of calcium oxalate.

Clinical and Histopathological Features   Patients often have late-stage renal failure, manifest livedo reticularis, and ulcerated lesions.[40–42] Histologically the findings are similar to calciphylaxis; there is ischemic fat necrosis with birefringent oxalate crystals in the walls of small blood vessels situated in the deep dermis and subcutaneous fat. The crystals are yellow-tan, have a diamond-shaped or radial appearance, and are often associated with thrombosis. The microscopic appearance of the crystals is characteristic; however, the nature of the crystals must be confirmed by a histochemical method (oxalate is incinerated to carbonate and the resulting calcium carbonate stained with alizarin red S),[40,41] infrared spectroscopy, x-ray diffraction, or scanning electron microscopy.

Differential Diagnosis   In general, one should consider the disorders mentioned under the differential diagnosis for calciphylaxis.

Thrombophlebitis

Two principal forms of thrombophlebitis are associated with panniculitis: (1) superficial migratory thrombophlebitis and (2) thrombophlebitis secondary to venous insufficiency.[43,44] The first condition occurs more often in men than in women and is characterized by multiple discrete tender nodules most commonly involving the lower extremities but occurring anywhere. These lesions tend to develop in crops and last 1 to 3 weeks. The nodules tend to be smaller than those in conventional panniculitis, e.g., erythema nodosum, and to have a linear pattern. In general, patients have few complaints, and ulceration does not occur. This form of thrombophlebitis often develops in association with malignancy (commonly gastric or pancreatic carcinoma), hypercoagulable states, Behçet's syndrome, and Winiwarter-Buerger disease. Histologically, small to medium-size veins show thrombosis, prominent infiltration of the vessel wall by mixed inflammatory cell infiltrates, and with time, varying degrees of fibrosis of the wall. The veins affected are usually larger than those involved by other forms of panniculitis. This form of thrombophlebitis is notable for little or no inflammatory reaction (panniculitis) in the surrounding fat.

Thrombophlebitis associated with venous insufficiency is more common in women and usually characterized by much more extensive panniculitis involving fat lobules.[4,44]

Morphea Profunda, Scleroderma, Eosinophilic Fasciitis

Morphea, scleroderma, and eosinophilic fasciitis may show prominent involvement of subcutaneous fat as well as the dermis and fascia.[2,4,45–55] Although morphea, scleroderma, and eosinophilic fasciitis share clinical and histopathologic features, there are also substantial differences among these diseases.[46–49] There is still no consensus as to whether eosinophilic fasciitis is simply a deep variant of morphea-scleroderma or a distinct entity. Recently the term *fasciitis-panniculitis* syndrome has been proposed to describe this sclerosing reaction pattern which occurs in a number of conditions, including morphea profunda, eosinophilic fasciitis, toxic oil syndrome, tryptophan-related fasciitis, sclerodermoid graft-versus-host reaction, and cancer-associated fasciitis panniculitis.[55–57] The authors proposing the latter reaction pattern have suggested this syndrome is distinct from scleroderma.[55] Although this hypothesis has merit, further study is needed to validate the extent of this reaction pattern. *Tryptophan-related fasciitis* (the eosinophilia-myalgia syndrome) refers to a disorder with features of morphea, scleroderma, and eosinophilic fasciitis occurring after ingestion of L-tryptophan.[56] Cancer-associated fasciitis panniculitis appears to be a rare paraneoplastic phenomenon occurring in adult patients with a predominance of hematopoietic malignancies.[57] In addition, morphea and eosinophilic fasciitis in some patients may be related to borrelial infection.[58,59]

Clinical Features   These conditions usually present with pitting edema followed by cutaneous indurations and a typical "bound-down" quality (Table 11-11). In the case of morphea, the lesions are generally well circumscribed guttate (droplike) or oval plaques or occasionally linear processes (coup de sabre). The plaques are often described as having an ivory appearance with an erythematous or purple border. Scleroderma is characterized by diffuse cutaneous induration, principally involving the

---

TABLE 11-11

Morphea Profunda, Scleroderma, Eosinophilic Fasciitis

Clinical Features

Pitting edema early
Cutaneous induration
   Plaques, linear lesions
   Sleevelike circumferential pattern
   Diffuse

Histopathological Features

Lymphoplasma cellular infiltrates, occasionally dense, involving
   fibrous trabeculae
Sclerosis, thickening of fibrous trabeculae
Progressive obliteration of fat lobules
Variable sclerosis of dermis, fasciitis
Occasional eosinophils, mucinosis
Lymphocytic vasculopathy, vasculitis

Differential Diagnosis

Lupus panniculitis
Borrelial infection
Other fibrosing panniculitides, sclerosing panniculitis
Necrobiosis lipoidica

trunk. Eosinophilic fasciitis is distinctive and usually typified by a sudden onset following stress or intense exercise. The extremities are most frequently involved and demonstrate an extensive sleevelike circumferential induration with dimpling on the skin. A peripheral eosinophilia is often present.[46-48]

Histopathological Features   The involvement of the panniculus by these disorders is characterized by two principal features (Figs. 11-8 to 11-10)[46-59]: (1) inflammatory infiltrates localized to the fibrous trabeculae, composed principally of lymphocytes and plasma cells with a variable admixture of eosinophils, neutrophils, and mucinous edema and (2) a progressive sclerosis of the fibrous trabeculae (Fig. 11-8) resulting in the obliteration of the fat lobules in the final stages (Table 11-11). The septal sclerosis is often continuous with sclerosis involving the reticular dermis, fascia, and perimysium. The septa and fascia show progressive hypertrophy and hyalinization of the collagen fibers as in the dermis. Edema and inflammatory infiltrates are generally most prominent in the initial stages and have a perivascular and septal localization with involvement of the peripheries of the fat lobules. The lymphoplasma cellular infiltrates also vary in density from sparse infiltrates to large nodules with germinal centers. Although the "center of gravity" for the disease activity of morphea and scleroderma is frequently the interface of the reticular dermis and subcutis, the focus of eosinophilic fasciitis and related processes is the fascia (Figs. 11-9 and 11-10) and immediately contiguous deep adipose tissue. Morphea and scleroderma often show progressive involvement of the entire panniculus and occasionally the fascia (termed *morphea profunda*). Conversely, eosinophilic fasciitis commonly progresses to involve the upper subcutaneous fat and reticular dermis.

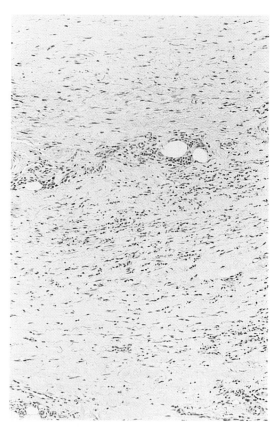

FIGURE 11-9   Eosinophilic fasciitis. The fascia is thickened and shows infiltration by inflammatory cells.

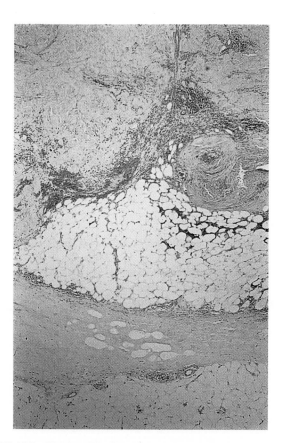

FIGURE 11-8   Morphea. The fibrous septa are markedly thickened and sclerotic with inflammation at the periphery of the fat lobules.

Tissue eosinophilic infiltrates range from none to marked. There also is frequent edema, hemorrhage, and variable mucin deposition. Vascular damage is commonly observed as fibrinoid deposition, thrombosis, lymphocytic vasculitis, or uncommonly as a necrotizing vasculitis.

On occasion, spirochetes consistent with borrelial organisms can be demonstrated with silver stains, such as the Warthin-Starry reaction.[58-59]

Differential Diagnosis   Long-standing septal panniculitis of any cause may result in septal thickening and fibrosis that may suggest morphea or scleroderma. However, other septal panniculitides generally do not show the degree of septal thickening or sclerosis, associated involvement of the dermis or fascia, or the frequency of lymphoplasma cellular infiltrates observed in morphea and related processes. Lupus panniculitis may show considerable similarity on occasion because of dermal and septal sclerosis, lymphoplasma cellular infiltrates, mucin deposition, and a vasculopathy.[60] However, lupus panniculitis differs from morphea-scleroderma because of prominent hyalinization of connective tissue, adipocytes, and vessels and a lesser degree of septal sclerosis (see below). Epidermal and dermal involvement by lupus and clinical information are also helpful in distinguishing lupus panniculitis from morphea.

Panniculitis Associated with Palisading Granulomas

Granuloma annulare, necrobiosis lipoidica, rheumatoid nodules, and rheumatic nodules may localize to the panniculus with the fibrous trabeculae the initial site of involvement.[4] The disease process often

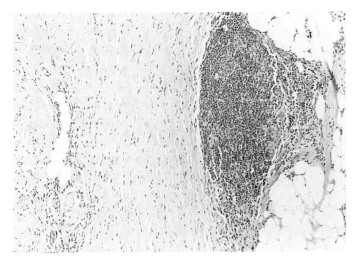

FIGURE 11-10 Eosinophilic fasciitis. There is marked sclerosis of the fascia and an adjacent nodular inflammatory cell infiltrate at the periphery of a fat lobule.

extends into the periphery of fat lobules and can obliterate the lobules. See Chapter 6 for a more detailed discussion.

Differential Diagnosis Necrobiosis lipoidica in some instances may prove difficult to distinguish from morphea profunda–fasciitis and lupus panniculitis because of septal fibrosis and degenerative changes, lymphoplasma cellular infiltrates, and vascular injury. Pandermal involvement by zonal necrosis ("necrobiosis") with palisading infiltrates and the typical clinical features of necrobiosis lipoidica should facilitate this discrimination.

LOBULAR PANNICULITIS

Many disease processes may eventuate in a predominantly lobular panniculitis.[1–5,8,9,61–63] However, as already mentioned, many of these panniculitides also may be septal initially, may remain septal, or may display both septal and lobular patterns. In a large proportion of cases, the lobular panniculitis is entirely nonspecific. However, the particular features observed in any given biopsy, although nonspecific, may be influenced by when the biopsy is taken in the natural history of the panniculitis and the severity of the insult to the fat. Early lesions tend to show predominantly neutrophilic infiltrates; older lesions, mononuclear cell infiltrates with lymphocytes, lipid-laden macrophages, granulomatous elements, and finally, fibrosis.

Weber-Christian Disease

The histopathologist must look for certain histopathologic features that are clues to diagnosis (Table 11-5). The section will outline the recognizable causes of predominantly lobular panniculitis. Historically, *Weber-Christian disease*, or idiopathic lobular panniculitis, refers to recurrent crops of erythematous nodules accompanied by fever, malaise, arthralgias, and fatigue.[2,4,62–65] These nodules occasionally discharge oily material and, hence, have been termed *liquefying panniculitis*.[63] Women aged 30 to 60 years have been most commonly affected. Histopathologically, Weber-Christian disease has been reported to show a predominantly lobular panniculitis, and the presence of numerous lipophages has been considered diagnostic.

It is likely that Weber-Christian disease is entirely a nonspecific reaction pattern whose histologic picture varies according to the age of the lesion biopsied, i.e., neutrophils followed by mononuclear cells/lipophages, granulomas, and fibrosis (Figs. 11-5 and 11-11 to 11-14). As will be outlined in the following sections, over the years specific causes of Weber-Christian disease have been recognized and probably will continue to be identified. Beyond acknowledging Weber-Christian disease as a historical entity, this author recommends that the term be abandoned. If no cause of a particular panniculitis can be established, the process should be designated "lobular panniculitis of unknown etiology," and the patient should continue to be evaluated and monitored.

Alpha-1-Antitrypsin Deficiency

This section details specific causes of predominantly lobular panniculitis (or mixed septal and lobular panniculitis). As mentioned below, many of these conditions may show septal panniculitis as the predominant finding. Severe homozygous deficiency of the protease inhibitor alpha-1-antitrypsin may result in a recurrent ulcerating lobular panniculitis thought in the past to be Weber-Christian disease.[66–68] Alpha-1-antitrypsin, which is synthesized in the liver, is the major inhibitor of serine proteases circulating in the blood. The deficiency of alpha-1-antitrypsin is thought to result in unopposed proteolytic activity and the promotion of inflammatory reactions.

Clinical Features There is often a history of tender, recurrent, erythematous nodules associated with ulceration that involves the trunk, buttocks, and proximal extremities (Table 11-12).[66–68] The nodules commonly follow trauma and exhibit drainage of clear or serosanguinous material. In some instances, the clinical picture suggests cellulitis. Patients may have other manifestations of the protease inhibitor deficiency such as emphysema, hepatitis, and acquired angioedema. Laboratory evaluation usually discloses a reduction in level of the serum alpha-1-antitrypsin activity.

Histopathological Features Two patterns of panniculitis have been described: (1) a lobular panniculitis with fat necrosis and (2) a septal panniculitis with proteolysis of collagen and necrosis of the fibrous trabeculae (Table 11-12).[67] The first pattern is commonly characterized by

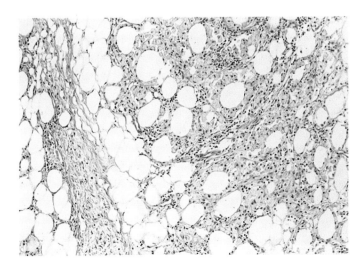

FIGURE 11-11 Lobular panniculitis. The fat lobule shows prominent infiltration by mononuclear cells. These changes are nonspecific and may be associated with a wide variety of etiologies.

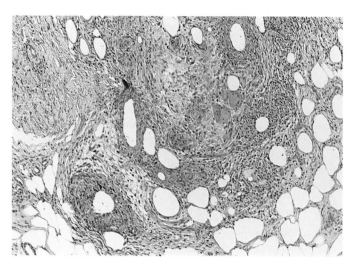

FIGURE 11-12 Lobular panniculitis. This fat lobule shows granulomatous inflammation as well as infiltration by mononuclear cells. These changes are nonspecific.

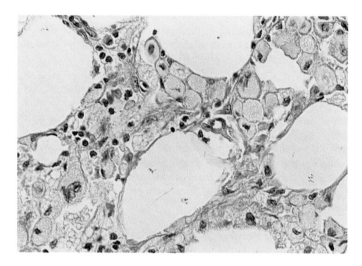

FIGURE 11-13 Lobular panniculitis. There is nonspecific infiltration of a fat lobule by lipidized macrophages.

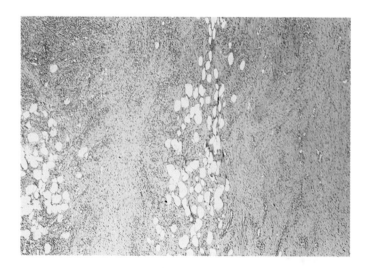

FIGURE 11-14 Late-stage septal and lobular panniculitis. There is obliteration of fat lobules by inflammation and fibrosis. The changes are nonspecific.

TABLE 11-12
Alpha-1-Antitrypsin Deficiency

Clinical Features

Tender recurrent erythematous nodules
  Ulceration
  Drainage
Cellulitislike presentation
Trunk, buttocks, proximal extremities
Emphysema
Hepatitis
Acquired angioedema

Histopathological Features

Lobular panniculitis
  Fat necrosis
  Neutrophilic infiltrates
Septal panniculitis
  Liquefactive necrosis of septa, dermis
  Neutrophilic and macrophage infiltrates

Laboratory Evaluation

Reduced serum alpha-1-antitrypsin activity

Differential Diagnosis

Infection
Physical and factitial panniculitis

neutrophilic infiltration of fat lobules that may be focal but is often indistinguishable from other forms of lobular panniculitis. The entire fat lobule may be destroyed. The septal pattern of panniculitis also shows neutrophilic infiltration of fibrous septa but is usually accompanied by prominent numbers of macrophages. Concomitant lobular involvement with fat necrosis may or may not be present. An important feature is the presence of liquefactive necrosis of the dermis, which, along with a similar pattern in the fibrous septa, is thought to be characteristic of alpha-1-antitrypsin deficiency panniculitis.

Differential Diagnosis The lobular form of alpha-1-antitrypsin deficiency may be indistinguishable from other lobular panniculitides, particularly those associated with infection and physical or factitial agents. Cultures, special stains, polaroscopy, clinical history, and laboratory evaluation of serum alpha-1-antitrypsin activity are needed to sort out these possibilities.

Cytophagic Histiocytic Panniculitis

This extremely rare form of panniculitis usually presents in patients as a systemic disorder, characterized by recurrent subcutaneous nodules, fever, generalized lymphadenopathy, hepatosplenomegaly, pancytopenia, liver dysfunction, a hemorrhagic diathesis, and purpura.[69–77] The panniculitis is usually part of a hemophagocytic syndrome with proliferation and infiltration of subcutaneous fat and other organs by benign histiocytes that show phagocytosis of erythrocytes, lymphocytes, and other cells.[78–79] Patients often die of fatal hemorrhages, hepatic failure, pancytopenia, or possibly an associated malignancy.[80–82] The etiology of this disorder is poorly understood but in many cases is related to immunosuppression or immune dysregulation.[79] Many of the manifestations may be explained by a proliferation of T lymphocytes, either

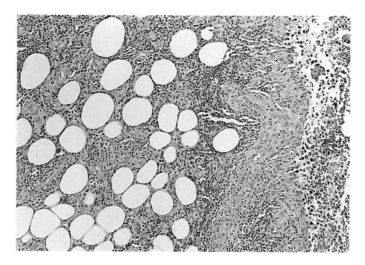

FIGURE 11-15   Cytophagic histiocytic panniculitis. This field shows a lobular panniculitis with infiltration of fat by an inflammatory cell infiltrate and some necrosis of adipocytes.

neoplastic or secondary to viral infection, and reactive phagocytic macrophages. A cytokine phagocytosis-inducing factor (PIF) secreted by CD4-positive T lymphocytes may be responsible for the prominent phagocytic properties of monocytes-macrophages in this syndrome.[79] This process has been associated with (1) viral infections, particularly cytomegalovirus, Epstein-Barr virus, and HIV, (2) other infections, including bacterial, fungal, and protozoal agents, (3) a number of lymphoproliferative disorders: T-cell lymphomas, including subcutaneous T-cell lymphoma and angiocentric lymphoproliferative lesions, B-cell lymphoma, and true histiocytic lymphoma, (4) allogeneic bone marrow transplantation, and (5) connective tissue disease, including lupus erythematosus and Sjogren's syndrome.[79]

Clinical Features   Patients usually present with recurrent, large erythematous nodules involving the extremities but also occasionally the face and trunk (Table 11-13). The nodules may ulcerate and show ecchymoses.

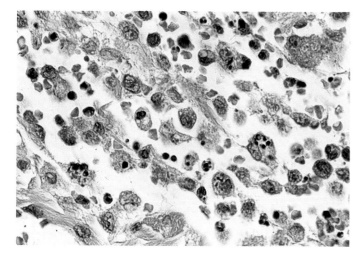

FIGURE 11-16   Cytophagic histiocytic panniculitis. High magnification shows phagocytosis of erythrocytes and leukocytes by macrophages in a fat lobule.

Histopathological Features   The epidermis and dermis are usually uninvolved. In most cases, the principal finding is a lobular infiltration of the subcutaneous fat by benign monocyte-macrophages (histiocytes) (Fig. 11-15) that show phagocytosis of other cellular elements: erythrocytes, platelets, lymphocytes, and neutrophils (Fig. 11-16) (Table 11-13).[69–79] The latter cells have been termed *beanbag* cells. In general, this cellular population is cytologically banal, although occasional cells may show some nuclear atypia or activation. These changes are usually accompanied by prominent extravasation of erythrocytes in the fat lobules; karyorrhectic debris; variable infiltration by other cells, such as lymphocytes, lipophages, plasma cells, and granulocytes; and possibly some fat necrosis. On occasion, the panniculitis shows a mainly septal pattern. Prominent cytologic atypia may be observed in some cases and should prompt full evaluation for a lymphoproliferative disorder. However, hemophagocytosis occurring in association with malignancies such as true histiocytic lymphoma, T-cell lymphomas, acute leukemia, and some carcinomas is usually minimal.[78–82]

Differential Diagnosis   Although the histologic findings of cytophagocytosis are distinctive, the patient and such lesions should be carefully assessed for infection, connective tissue disease, lymphoproliferative disease, and other systemic disorders.

TABLE 11-13

Cytophagic Histiocytic Panniculitis

Clinical Features

Hemophagocytic syndrome often
Immunosuppression, immune dysregulation
Recurrent subcutaneous nodules—extremities commonly involved
Fever
Lymphadenopathy
Hepatosplenomegaly
Pancytopenia
Liver dysfunction
Hemorrhagic diathesis
Often fatal
Associated diseases:
    Infections, particularly viral
    Lymphoproliferative disorders, usually T-cell
    Connective tissue disease

Histopathological Features

Lobular panniculitis
    Monocyte-macrophage infiltration
    Phagocytosis of erythrocytes, platelets, lymphocytes by
        macrophages ("beanbag" cells)
    Extravasation of erythrocytes
    Infiltration by other cell types
Septal panniculitis
Atypical infiltrates in lymphoproliferative disorders

Differential Diagnosis

Infection
Connective tissue diseases
Lymphoproliferative disorder

Pancreatic Panniculitis

A syndrome including pancreatic disease, subcutaneous fat necrosis, arthritis, lytic bone lesions, eosinophilia, and polyserositis has been recognized for over a century.[83–89] This syndrome is most commonly associated with alcohol-related acute pancreatitis but has also been associated with chronic pancreatitis, cholelithiasis, traumatic panniculitis, pancreatic cysts and pseudocysts, calculi of the pancreatic duct, acinar cell carcinoma, pancreatic adenocarcinoma, pancreatic divisum, and unusual pancreatic infections, including a syphilitic gumma and tuberculosis. The clinical lesions occurring in various organs are secondary to widespread or metastatic fat necrosis. The pathogenesis of these lesions, including those in the panniculus, is poorly understood but thought to be secondary to lipolytic enzymes released into the systemic circulation from the diseased pancreas.[85] In particular, elevations of serum lipase and, to a lesser extent, amylase and other enzymes have been reported. The resemblance of the syndrome to connective tissue disease has prompted studies to identify an immune mechanism for tissue injury.[86] The deposition of immunoglobulin and complement in the pleura and a reduced complement level in one patient provided some evidence for possible immune injury.

Clinical Features   In contrast to other forms of panniculitis, pancreatic panniculitis is more common in men than women (a ratio of 3 to 1) and generally presents as tender erythematous nodules on the lower extremities, resembling or indistinguishable from EN (Table 11-14).[4,83–88] The nodules often measure about 1 to 2 cm and commonly involve the anterior shins. The distribution of lesions, however, is often more widespread than typical EN. These lesions also may break down and drain a creamy oily substance. The ages of patients most commonly afflicted

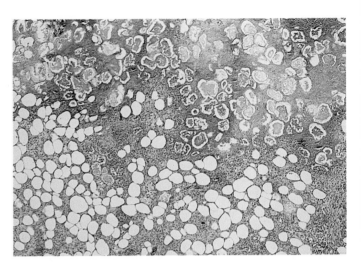

FIGURE 11-17   Pancreatic panniculitis. A lobular panniculitis shows basophilic necrosis of fat and saponification.

are in the range of 30 to 50 years. Patients commonly exhibit systemic involvement with fever, arthralgias, arthritis, and occasionally widespread necrosis of fat including the bone marrow.

Histopathological Features   In their fully developed state, the histologic findings in pancreatic panniculitis are diagnostic (Table 11-14).[4,83–88] The fat lobules show a characteristic form of necrosis with formation of *ghost cells* (Figs. 11-17 and 11-18). The latter finding refers to necrotic adipocytes with intact but thickened eosinophilic cell walls and absence of nuclei. At the peripheries of necrotic foci with ghost cells, there is variable calcification, resulting in a basophilic lamellation which constitutes saponification, i.e., formation of calcium soaps from the reaction of free fatty acids with ionizable calcium. Neutrophilic infiltration of fat lobules accompanies the fat necrosis and later gives place to mononuclear cells and granulomatous inflammation.

The earliest lesions have been reported to show perivascular lymphocytic infiltrates without evidence of fat necrosis in a pattern resembling erythema nodosum.[84]

TABLE 11-14

Pancreatic Panniculitis

Clinical Features

Men > women
Age 30–50 years
Alcohol-related pancreatitis
Pancreatic carcinoma
Traumatic pancreatitis
Fluctuant tender erythematous nodules
   Extremities, especially pretibial
   Buttocks
Arthritis
Polyserositis

Histopathological Features

Early septal panniculitis with perivascular lymphocytic infiltrates
Fat necrosis with ghost cells
Basophilic alteration (saponification)
Calcification
Neutrophilic infiltration of fat lobules
Mononuclear cells later

Laboratory Evaluation

Elevated lipase, amylase levels

Differential Diagnosis

Early septal panniculitides
Infection

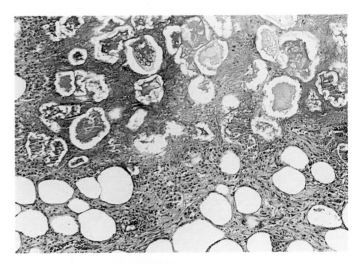

FIGURE 11-18   Pancreatic panniculitis. The outlines of necrotic adipocytes are still maintained as so-called ghost cells.

Differential Diagnosis As mentioned above, early lesions may show nonspecific change suggesting a broad differential diagnosis. Typical lesions showing fat necrosis with ghost cells and saponification are characteristic and should not be confused with other forms of panniculitis.

Crystal-Related Panniculitis (Panniculitis in Neonates and Children Associated with Crystal Formation)

Subcutaneous fat necrosis of the newborn (SFN),[90–98] sclerema neonatorum (SN),[83,93,95,99,100] and poststeroid panniculitis (PSP)[101,102] are three forms of panniculitis occurring either in neonates or in children and showing crystallization of subcutaneous fat. The pathogenesis of this crystal formation remains poorly understood, but certain factors may contribute to its development. At least with respect to SFN and SN, the composition of the subcutaneous fat in infants differs from that in older individuals. In infants, there is a higher ratio of saturated to unsaturated fatty acids. Since saturated fatty acids have a higher melting point than unsaturated fatty acids, solidification (or crystallization) of fat may occur at lower temperatures. Additional factors that have some bearing on this phenomenon include prematurity, trauma, infection, fetal asphyxia, hypothermia, and other stresses. However, none of the latter factors has been consistently implicated in precipitating these diseases.

SUBCUTANEOUS FAT NECROSIS OF THE NEWBORN

Clinical Features Full-term or postmature infants develop variable-size red to violaceous indurated nodules that are reasonably well circumscribed and not bound down to deep tissue (Table 11-15). The lesions are primarily localized to the cheeks, shoulders, back, buttocks, and thighs. The lesions usually develop in the first few days or weeks of life and generally resolve over 3 to 5 months with an excellent outcome in most newborns. Occasional infants develop an associated hypercalcemia which can potentially result in extensive calcification.

Histopathological Features The epidermis and dermis are generally uninvolved. The most characteristic findings are patchy fat necrosis with crystallization of fat (Fig. 11-19) (Table 11-15). Typically macrophages and, to a lesser extent, lipocytes contain radially oriented needle-shaped clefts that correspond to triglyceride crystals dissolved during processing (Fig. 11-20). In addition to macrophages and foreign-body giant cells, other inflammatory cells, including neutrophils, lymphocytes, and plasma cells, may be observed. Early lesions may exhibit prominent neutrophilic infiltrates. The panniculitis is often septal and lobular, and it is important to emphasize that one may not detect the needle-shaped clefts in all cases of SFN. Furthermore, prominent calcification of the fibrous trabeculae may occur in some specimens. Frozen specimens or those not yet subjected to paraffin-embedding show positive staining with lipid stains such as oil red O, and birefringent crystals may be observed when examined with polarized light.

Differential Diagnosis Poststeroid panniculitis is histologically indistinguishable from SFN, and thus one depends on clinical history to distinguish the two conditions. SN characteristically shows crystal formation in lipocytes and lacks inflammation (see below). If crystals are not detected in SFN, one must exclude other forms of panniculitis, particularly infection or cold panniculitis. However, the clinical features of SFN should enable one to make the diagnosis without too much difficulty.

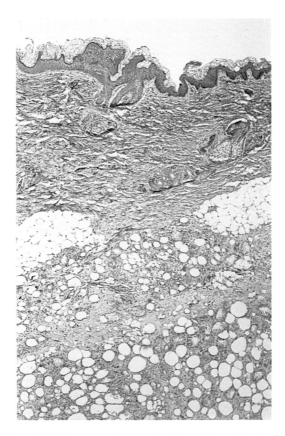

FIGURE 11-19 Subcutaneous fat necrosis of the newborn. There is a prominent lobular panniculitis.

SCLEREMA NEONATORUM

Clinical Features Neonates developing SN are often premature and develop the process within 1 week of birth (Table 11-15). These newborns are usually seriously ill at the onset of SN, and many are dehydrated or undernourished. In general, a widespread boardlike induration involves the entire cutaneous surface except the palms, soles, and scrotum. The process commonly begins on the lower extremities and progresses upward. There is a high mortality rate, often resulting from sepsis.

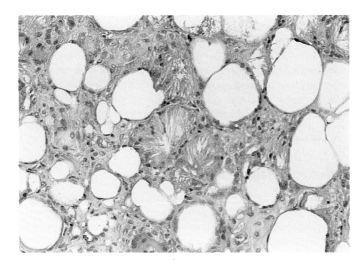

FIGURE 11-20 Subcutaneous fat necrosis of the newborn. The characteristic stellate clefting from triglyceride crystals is evident in the center of the field.

TABLE 11-15

Crystal-Related Panniculitis

Subcutaneous fat necrosis (SFN) of the newborn	Sclerema neonatorum	Poststeroid panniculitis
Clinical Features		
Full- or postterm	Often premature	Young children
Healthy	Seriously ill	Healthy
Onset first few days or weeks	Onset within 1 week of birth	Onset days after stopping high-dose steroids
Reddish indurated nodules	Widespread boardlike induration	
Cheeks, shoulder, back, buttocks	Often fatal	
Good prognosis		
Histopathological Features		
Inflammation	Little or no inflammation	Similar to SFN
Needle-shaped clefts in macrophages and lipocytes	Crystals mainly in adipocytes	
Variable fat necrosis		

Histopathological Features   The findings in SN are fairly distinctive, although there may be considerable histologic overlap with SFN. On gross examination, the subcutaneous fat is greatly thickened and has a firm lard-like consistency. The expanded fat lobules are separated by thickened fibrous trabeculae. Histologically, the expanded fat lobules show lipocytes containing the characteristic needle-shaped clefts with a radial or starburst pattern, as described above for SFN. In general, there is little or no associated inflammation. However, occasional neutrophils, lymphocytes, eosinophils, macrophages, and multinucleated giant cells, some containing the needle-shaped clefts, are observed. Older lesions may show thickening of fibrous trabeculae and rarely calcification.

Differential Diagnosis   As discussed above, SFN differs from SN by showing radial clefts predominantly in macrophages, greater inflammation, and fat necrosis in contrast to SN, which shows crystals primarily in lipocytes and little or no inflammation or fat necrosis.

POSTSTEROID PANNICULITIS

An extremely rare form of panniculitis, poststeroid panniculitis has thus far only been observed in young children 1 to 13 days after the rapid discontinuation of high doses of oral corticosteroids (Table 11-15).[101,102] Subcutaneous nodules develop particularly in areas of fat accumulation, especially the cheeks, secondary to steroid therapy. The lesions are generally asymptomatic and resolve without scarring over a period of weeks to months. The histologic findings are similar to SFN with needle-shaped clefts occurring within both macrophages and adipocytes.

Infection-Related Panniculitis

As already emphasized, infection is a relatively frequent cause of panniculitis.[103–105] Bacterial organisms are probably the most common agents, especially conventional and atypical mycobacteria, followed by fungi, *Nocardia*, and recently, acanthamoeba. A particularly important predisposing factor to infection-related panniculitis is immunosuppression (Table 11–16). Many predisposed patients have undergone organ transplantation and have received immunosuppressive agents such as

TABLE 11-16

Infection-Related Panniculitis

Clinical Features

Immunosuppression
   Organ transplantation
   Corticosteroid and cytotoxic therapy
   Cancer
   Connective tissue disease
Diabetes mellitus
Inflammatory nodules—lower extremities most common

Histopathological Features

Epidermal and dermal changes common
   Neutrophil-rich infiltrate
   Edema
Septal and lobular panniculitis often
   Septal changes frequent with bacterial infection
   Neutrophilic infiltrates
   Abscess formation
   Basophilic necrosis
   Hemorrhage
   Granulomatous inflammation in nonbacterial panniculitis
   Vascular damage and vasculitis

Differential Diagnosis

Acute neutrophilic panniculitis (erythema nodosum syndromes)
Neutrophilic dermatoses
   Sweet's syndrome
   Pyoderma gangrenosum
Inflammatory bowel disease—metastatic Crohn's disease
Physical and factitial panniculitis

systemic corticosteroids and other cytotoxic drugs. Other conditions associated with this form of panniculitis include diabetes mellitus, acquired immunodeficiency syndrome, cancer, and connective tissue disease.

Clinical Features   Most patients are adults, but individuals of any age may be affected. Patients most commonly present with inflammatory subcutaneous nodules involving the lower extremities, but any site may be affected.

Histopathological Features   Epidermal and dermal changes are more frequent in infection-related panniculitis than in the other panniculitides (Table 11–16). Often there is parakeratosis, acanthosis, and spongiosis. In addition, dermal edema and a neutrophil-rich inflammatory infiltrate are commonly encountered in the dermis. In general, the panniculitis is both septal and lobular. A predominantly septal panniculitis with infiltration of fibrous trabeculae and the peripheries of fat lobules may be noted with bacterial infection. Other notable features include a prominent neutrophilic infiltrate with occasional abscess formation, hemorrhage, basophilic necrosis (Fig. 11-21), and associated necrosis of sweat glands. Bacterial panniculitis as a general rule does not exhibit granulomatous inflammation. However, granulomatous inflammation is a common finding in other forms of infection-related panniculitis, particularly those with mycobacterial infection (Fig. 11-22). Both small- and medium-size vessel vasculitis may be observed.

Differential Diagnosis   The differential diagnosis includes causes of acute neutrophilic panniculitis as might be associated with short-lived hypersensitivity reactions (the erythema nodosum reaction pattern); vasculitis; a primary neutrophilic dermatosis, as in Sweet's syndrome and pyoderma gangrenosum; inflammatory bowel disease; and physical and factitial forms of panniculitis. Infection can be confirmed by special stains, cultures, and possibly special techniques, including immunostaining and the polymerase chain reaction (PCR).

Erythema Induratum and Nodular Vasculitis (Bazin's Disease)

Since the description of this entity by Bazin in 1861,[106] there has been continued controversy as to its relationship to tuberculosis as a "tuberculide," the relationship to and the nature of the vasculitis described in many cases ("nodular" vasculitis), and its very legitimacy. Nonetheless, many clinicians maintain that erythema induratum/nodular vasculitis is a distinctive clinical entity, characterized by dusky, bluish nodules, principally localized to the posterior calves of obese adult women.

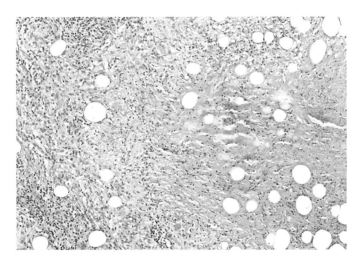

FIGURE 11-22   Septal and lobular panniculitis with caseation necrosis. These changes are nonspecific but may be associated with infectious agents such as mycobacteria.

These nodules seem to have some relationship to cold exposure and are often associated with ulceration and scarring. Variants which are clearly related to cold exposure have been termed *erythema induratum of Whitfield* and are likely to be a form of perniosis (Whiting DA, personal communication, 1996). A pattern of livedo reticularis has been described in many cases.

The relationship of erythema induratum–nodular vasculitis to mycobacterium tuberculosis (MBT) has remained controversial over the past century.[107–110] Some authors have provided convincing evidence for a relationship to MBT based on documentation of tuberculosis at other sites, positive Mantoux (tuberculin-purified protein derivative) tests, and response to antituberculous therapy. Others have disavowed any relationship, and Montgomery and his colleagues[43] emphasized the presence of vasculitis in these lesions and proposed the term *nodular vasculitis* to describe nodules not having any clear association with MBT. A relationship to perniosis was suggested for some lesions. Nonetheless, recent studies utilizing molecular diagnostic techniques (polymerase chain reaction) have isolated MBT DNA from lesions considered to be erythema induratum. Furthermore, patients with these lesions have responded to treatment for MBT.

Histopathological Features   The histopathologic features described in these lesions are entirely nonspecific and often are related to the age of the lesion biopsied. Vasculitis of small- and medium-size arterial and venous vessels has been observed. Montgomery and colleagues[43] reported features similar to polyarteritis nodosum in some lesions. Often there is prominent ischemic fat necrosis, extensive inflammatory infiltrates with granulomatous inflammation, and caseation necrosis affecting fat lobules (Fig. 11-22). Vasculitis is not always identified.

Increasing evidence indicates that many cases of erythema induratum are likely to be a form of infection-related panniculitis in which a florid hypersensitivity reaction has probably resulted in the death of MBT organisms, since they cannot be cultured from such lesions. Nonetheless, the structure of some organisms remains intact, since they can be detected by PCR amplification. Further studies are needed to confirm the infectious etiology of erythema induratum.

Although there will be resistance to this recommendation, the author proposes that the terms *erythema induratum* and *nodular vasculitis* be abandoned in favor of more objective morphologic descriptions. For example, such panniculitides are best designated as *granulomatous pan-*

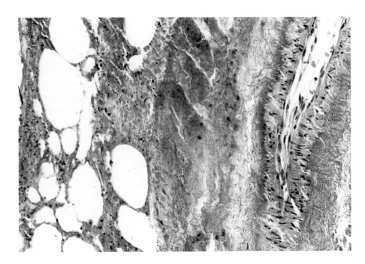

FIGURE 11-21   Bacterial panniculitis. There is granular basophilic necrosis of fat.

niculitis associated with MBT detection; *granulomatous panniculitis without specific cause* (failure to detect an infective agent); or *panniculitis associated with small or medium-size vessel vasculitis*. Patients should have thorough evaluation for a local or systemic cause of their panniculitis.

Erythema Nodosum Leprosum

Erythema nodosum leprosum (ENL) is characterized by tender erythematous papules or nodules developing in patients with lepromatous or borderline lepromatous leprosy after initiating treatment for leprosy or from other factors such as pregnancy or bacterial or viral infections.[111] A necrotizing small-vessel vasculitis with associated neutrophilic infiltrates usually involves the dermis and/or subcutis. The panniculitis is often septal and lobular with variable fat necrosis. Although macrophages generally contain lepra bacilli, the vasculitis appears to be immune-complex-related.

Physical and Factitial Panniculitis

This category of panniculitis refers to injury to fat secondary to various physical insults, such as cold, pressure, external trauma, chemical agents, and self-induced injury.

COLD PANNICULITIS

Cold-related panniculitis was first described in 1902 by Hochsinger in children 4 to 10 years of age, primarily involving the face.[112–118] The propensity to develop cold panniculitis is inversely correlated with age. Thus, as with crystal-associated panniculitis, cold panniculitis has been attributed to a higher ratio of saturated to unsaturated fatty acids and generally presents in infants and young children.

Clinical Features   The exposed skin, especially the cheeks and submental area of the chin, of neonates and young children are most commonly affected (Table 11-17). Typically patients develop tender, often indurated, erythematous plaques and nodules about 2 to 3 days after cold exposure from cold air, ice cubes, cold fluids, or ice pops.

Histopathological Features   In general, the epidermis and dermis are unaffected. The most prominent findings often are perivascular lymphocytic infiltrates at the dermal-subcutaneous interface with features observed in chilblains, i.e., the "fluffy" edema involving the walls of blood vessels (Table 11-17). However, as with many other insults to the fat, the panniculitis is nonspecific with variable fat necrosis and inflammatory cell infiltrates, including neutrophils, lymphocytes, macrophages, and other inflammatory cells involving fat lobules and, to a lesser extent, fibrous trabeculae.

TRAUMA-RELATED PANNICULITIS

Physical trauma, whether self-inflicted (factitial) or otherwise, is a major cause of injury to fat.[1–5,119,120] Common locations include the breasts of women and accessible sites, such as the extremities, and purpura and scarring may be important clinical features. Secrétan's syndrome and *l'oedeme bleu* are forms of factitial panniculitis resulting from blunt trauma to the dorsal hand and forearm and upper arm, respectively, or any site. Clinically one observes traumatic edema and hemorrhage, often resulting in brawny, discolored, indurated plaques or

---

TABLE 11-17

Cold Panniculitis

Clinical Features

Infants and young children
Young women
Exposed skin, cheeks
Tender, indurated plaques, nodules
Onset 2 to 3 days after cold exposure

Histopathological Features

Perivascular lymphoid infiltrates
   Histologic features of chilblains
   Dermal-subcutis interface
   "Fluffy" edema of vessels
Lobular and septal panniculitis
   Fat necrosis
   Mixed infiltrates

Differential Diagnosis

Other physical panniculitides

---

nodules. Histologically, there is prominent hemorrhage, organizing hematoma, granulation tissue, focal fat necrosis, and, often in the late stage, fibrosis.

CHEMICAL AND FACTITIAL PANNICULITIS

Injection of various foreign or organic substances and medications are also common causes of panniculitis.[119–125] *Sclerosing lipogranuloma* describes the reaction of adipose tissue to various mineral, animal, and vegetable oils; silicone; and other hydrocarbons injected into the subcutaneous fat for cosmetic and other reasons. Almost every conceivable substance, including milk, feces, and blood, has been injected into the subcutis. Many medications, including meperidine, pentazocine, povidone iodine, morphine, and tetanus toxoid have been associated with panniculitis.

Clinical Features   The injection or implantation of various oils, paraffin, and other hydrocarbons may involve any site (Table 11-18). However, particularly common locations include the male genitalia, face and scalp, female breasts, and hands ("greasegun" granuloma). Such lesions are often indurated, may break down, and drain oily material. The clinical manifestations associated with injections of other substances, e.g., feces or medications, relate to the properties of the particular substance. Many such patients have health-profession backgrounds, psychiatric histories, and exhibit unusual or bizarre manifestations. There may be systemic signs, such as fever and, in some instances, a liquefying panniculitis.

Histopathological Features   Sclerosing lipogranuloma shows a rather characteristic constellation of findings involving fat lobules: the so-called Swiss cheese pattern with variable-size vacuoles corresponding to lipid removed with tissue processing, variable foreign-body giant cell reaction associated with vacuolated spaces, dense hyalinized fibrous tissue, and variable inflammatory cell infiltrates (Table 11-18). The histologic features associated with injection or implantation of other substances are in general nonspecific but vary with the particular agent

TABLE 11-18

Chemical and Factitial Panniculitis

Clinical Features

Injection of foreign or organic substances, oils, paraffin, silicone, medications
Psychiatric history
Health care professionals
Unusual or bizarre manifestations
Indurated lesions—drainage

Histopathological Features

Sclerosing lipogranuloma
    Variable-size vacuoles ("Swiss cheese" pattern).
    Foreign body reaction
    Dense hyalinized fibrous tissue
    Variable inflammation
Fat necrosis
Microcyst formation
Mixed and granulomatous inflammation
Fibrosis
Calcification
Birefringent material, often

Differential Diagnosis

Infection
Alpha-1-antitrypsin deficiency
Pancreatic panniculitis

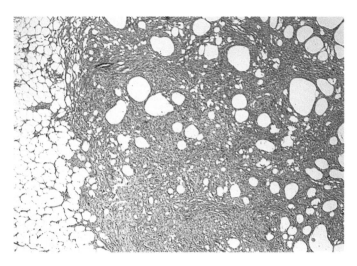

FIGURE 11-23 Traumatic fat necrosis. These changes are nonspecific and may follow a number of insults.

(Fig. 11-23). Commonly there is patchy, sometimes focal fat necrosis accompanied by microcyst formation and inflammatory infiltrates composed of neutrophils, mononuclear cells, and granulomatous elements. Birefringent material may be demonstrated with polarized light. Some agents such as meperidine may result in exuberant fibrotic reactions.

Differential Diagnosis   In many instances, the cause of physical panniculitis is obvious. However, factitial panniculitis may present considerable difficulties in diagnosis. Unusual forms of panniculitis, particularly persistent or recurrent, should raise suspicion for factitial etiologies. The differential diagnosis includes infection, alpha-1-antitrypsin deficiency, pancreatic panniculitis, and superficial thrombophlebitis. Evaluation for birefringent material and calcification may provide evidence for self-administered local injections.

Lupus Panniculitis (Lupus Profundus)

The first recorded observation of subcutaneous nodules in lupus erythematosus (LE) was by Kaposi in 1883.[126–133] Reports over the past half-century have confirmed the rarity of lupus profundus (incidence about 2 to 5 percent of patients with LE). Lupus panniculitis occurs commonly without evidence of systemic lupus erythematosus (approximately 50 to 60 percent of patients). Patients with systemic involvement seem to have a milder course, often exhibiting only arthralgias, polyserositis, and Raynaud's phenomenon.

Clinical Features   In general, lupus panniculitis is a disease of adults aged 20 to 60 years but children as young as 3 years may be affected (Table 11-19). Women are afflicted twice as often as men. Patients com-

TABLE 11-19

Lupus Panniculitis

Clinical Features

Women > men
Age 20–60 years
Multiple indurated subcutaneous nodules or plaques—proximal extremities, buttocks, trunk, or face
Ulceration
Overlying discoid lupus erythematosus, poikiloderma
Lipoatrophy, depressed scars late

Histopathological Features

Epidermis and dermis may or may not show features of lupus erythematosus
Septal and lobular panniculitis
    Hyaline necrosis of fat lobules
    Hyalinization of adipocytes, connective tissue, blood vessels ("onion-skin" pattern)
    Karyorrhectic material
    Lymphocytic infiltrates and nodules at peripheries of fat lobules
    Plasma cells often
    Lymphocytic vasculopathy and vasculitis
    Occasional fibrin thrombi
    Mucin deposition
    Variable fibrous thickening of septa

Differential Diagnosis

Septal panniculitis
Panniculitis in connective tissue disease
    Morphea/scleroderma
    Eosinophilic fasciitis
    Dermatomyositis
Lipoatrophy, not otherwise specified
Borreliosis
Necrobiosis lipoidica

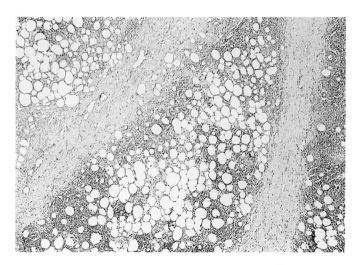

FIGURE 11-24 Lupus panniculitis. A septal and lobular panniculitis is present. There is some hyalinization of the fibrous septa and fat lobules. Fat lobules also exhibit infiltration by rather dense mononuclear cell infiltrates.

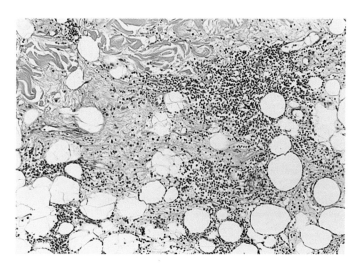

FIGURE 11-25 Lupus panniculitis. Higher magnification shows hyalinizing necrosis of fat with mononuclear cell infiltrates.

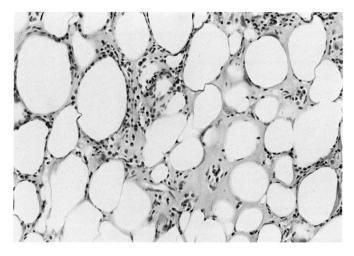

FIGURE 11-26 Lupus panniculitis. There is hyalinization of the fat lobule accompanied by lymphocytic infiltrates.

monly present with multiple indurated, subcutaneous nodules or plaques involving the proximal extremities, buttocks, trunk, breasts (lupus mastitis), or face. Ulceration may occur, and the lesions often heal with lipoatrophy and depressed scars. Cutaneous manifestations overlying the panniculitis may include discoid LE, poikiloderma, atrophy, telangiectasia, and dyspigmentation.

Histopathological Features The epidermis and dermis may or may not show features typical of LE, such as hyperkeratosis, follicular plugging, epidermal atrophy, basal layer vacuolization, basement membrane thickening, perivascular and periadnexal lymphoid infiltrates, and dermal mucin.

In general, lupus panniculitis shows distinctive changes involving septal and lobular areas (Figs. 11-24 to 11-26) (Table 11-19). The principal findings include (1) hyaline necrosis (Fig. 11-25) involving primarily fat lobules but extending to the fibrous trabeculae in many instances and (2) lymphocytic infiltrates often forming nodules and occasionally containing germinal centers (Figs. 11-24 and 11-25). The *hyaline necrosis* refers to the degeneration of fat lobules and connective tissue with development of a progressive glassy eosinophilic appearance. This alteration is often accompanied by karyorrhectic debris and mucin deposition. The fat lobules are commonly characterized by the formation of hyalinized microcysts (Fig. 11-26), and involved blood vessels exhibit a characteristic onion-skin-like concentric layering of eosinophilic fibrils. The lymphocytic infiltrates are variable and primarily localized to the peripheries of fat lobules or septal-lobular interface but rarely involve the entire lobule. The lymphocytic infiltrates are often present between vessels as well as having a perivascular disposition. Almost without exception, plasma cells are an integral part of the infiltrate.

Variable degrees of vascular injury are commonly observed, with lymphocytic vasculitis the most frequent finding. Fibrinoid necrosis and fibrin thrombi are noted on occasion. Other more variable features include fibrous thickening of septa, deposition of elastic fibers in the septa, calcification (which may be extensive), mucin deposition, granulomas involving septa, and occasional eosinophils in the infiltrate. On occasion, the histopathologic findings are nonspecific.

Differential Diagnosis Early lesions of lupus panniculitis may be confused with septal patterns of panniculitis (the erythema nodosum reaction pattern). However, the major entities to be considered include connective tissue disease–related panniculitis, i.e., morphea, eosinophilic fasciitis, and allied conditions; dermatomyositis; necrobiosis lipoidica; lipoatrophy; and borreliosis. The greatest difficulty may be distinguishing lupus panniculitis from morphea profunda–eosinophilic fasciitis. Both may present as clinically indurated plaques or nodules, and both exhibit prominent lymphoplasmacellular infiltrates, thickening of fibrous septa, lymphocytic vasculitis, mucinosis, and occasional eosinophilic infiltrates. As discussed above (see Morphea), lupus panniculitis is distinguished from morphea by the frequent presence of the epidermal changes of hyperkeratosis, atrophy, basal layer vacuolopathy, basement membrane thickening, prominent dermal mucin, hyalinizing necrosis of adipose tissue, and less prominent sclerosis of the subcutis and dermis compared to morphea profunda (and eosinophilic fasciitis).

Panniculitis in Dermatomyositis and Polymyositis

Panniculitis is rarely observed in both children and adults with dermatomyositis.[131–136] Patients may present with painful indurated nodules or plaques, or the panniculitis may be asymptomatic and diagnosed coincidentally with skin or muscle biopsy. Histologically, one often observes features noted in the other connective tissue diseases, particularly lymphoplasmacytic infiltrates of variable density affecting fat lobules. Other features noted less commonly include hyalin necrosis of fat, mucinosis, calcification, and lymphocytic vasculitis. Overlying features of dermatomyositis may affect the epidermis and dermis.

Connective Tissue Panniculitis

Winkelmann and Padilha-Goncalves reported an unusual form of panniculitis which they considered to be closely related to lupus panniculitis and morphea.[137] However, "connective tissue panniculitis" was distinguished from the latter conditions by florid lymphocytic infiltration and extensive caseation necrosis of fat lobules. There was no hyaline necrosis or vasculitis according to these authors, and the lesions resolved with lipoatrophy.

Lipoatrophy and Lipodystrophy

This category includes a highly heterogenous and confusing group of conditions, perhaps only related by the clinical finding of loss of subcutaneous fat.[2,131,138–145] This atrophy or disappearance of fat may be localized, partial, or generalized (total) (Table 11-20). Much more work is needed to characterize the pathogenesis of these various disorders.

The localized lipoatrophies probably encompass the most heterogeneous grouping of conditions. One well-recognized outcome of panniculitis occurring in connective tissue disease, e.g., lupus panniculitis and morphea profunda, is localized lipoatrophy which has been designated *atrophic connective tissue panniculitis.* However, other autoimmune diseases such as diabetes mellitus, Hashimoto's thyroiditis, and juvenile rheumatoid arthritis may result in localized lipoatrophic panniculitis. Localized lipoatrophy may be secondary to a variety of local insults to fat, such as injections of depot corticosteroids and insulin, and factitial disease. Other unusual and poorly understood variants include centrifugal lipodystrophy and the annular and semicircular lipoatrophies. Centrifugal lipodystrophy is characterized by round, depressed lesions having a raised erythematous border, often involving the trunk and groin areas of children. The annular and semicircular variants show circumscribed bands of lipoatrophy involving the upper extremities and thighs, respectively, of adult patients. Annular lipoatrophy of the ankles is typified by a broad (about 10 cm) annulus of lipoatrophy involving the distal leg above the ankle.

The partial lipodystrophies most commonly show progressive loss of facial fat that may gradually extend to the upper trunk and arms (cephalothoracic lipodystrophy) of female children. Many patients have reduced serum complement (C3) levels, a circulating immunoglobulin that activates C3 (the C3 nephritic factor), membranoproliferative glomerulonephritis, hypertriglyceridemia, insulin resistance, and diabetes.

The generalized or total lipodystrophies may present at birth or develop later in life. They are more common in females and show a number of cutaneous signs, including acanthosis nigricans, hypertrichosis, and hyperpigmentation. Endocrine abnormalities including diabetes and hypothalamic dysfunction are often present.

Histopathological Features All forms of lipoatrophy are characterized by loss of subcutaneous fat in their established or fully developed stages, i.e., fat lobules are greatly diminished in size and associated with prominent microvessels and myxoid alteration. Early lesions, particularly those associated with inflammation, autoimmune or connective tissue disease in localized lipoatrophy, have been reported to show infiltration of fat lobules by lymphocytes, plasma cells, and macrophages.

An involutional phase of localized lipoatrophy has been described and may have a relationship to antecedent inflammation. This stage is characterized by diminished sizes of fat lobules, variation in the sizes of adipocytes, prominent vascularity, and a hyaline or myxoid stromal alteration. The latter findings greatly resemble fetal adipose tissue.

Eosinophilic Panniculitis

Eosinophilic panniculitis is a distinctive but nonspecific histopathologic reaction pattern associated with a wide variety of processes that may be localized or systemic.[16,146–148] Review of 18 patients with eosinophilic panniculitis included the following associations: drug dependency, atopy, cancer (particularly lymphoma), vasculitis, local injections, and Wells' syndrome (eosinophilic cellulitis, a closely related nonspecific reaction).

TABLE 11-20

Lipoatrophies and Lipodystrophies

Condition	Clinical Features
Localized lipoatrophies	
Atrophic connective tissue panniculitis; lipotrophic panniculitis	Children or adults with connective tissue and autoimmune diseases
Secondary localized lipoatrophies	Localized lipoatrophy secondary to local processes such as injections, factitial disease
Centrifugal lipodystrophy (lipodystrophia centrifugalis, abdominalis infantilis)	Annular erythematous lesions involving abdomen and other sites of children, possibly related to Kawasaki disease
Annular lipoatrophy, semicircular lipoatrophy, annular lipoatrophy of the ankle	Circumferential band of lipoatrophy affecting circumscribed areas of the extremities
Localized lipoatrophy	Localized lipoatrophy without evidence of inflammation
Partial lipoatrophies, dystrophies; cephalothoracic lipodystrophy	Progressive loss of fat from the face and upper trunk; relationship to hypocomplementemia, C3 nephritic factor, glomerulonephritis, and diabetes; often inherited
Generalized lipodystrophies	Congenital or acquired; generalized loss of fat; diabetes and other endocrine abnormalities; often inherited

Clinical and Histopathological Features In general, adults are affected and present with inflammatory nodules, occasionally associated with other cutaneous findings, including vesicles, pustules, and urticaria (Table 11-21). The panniculitis is characterized by prominent infiltration of fat lobules by eosinophils, possibly with an admixture of other inflammatory cells, including lymphocytes, neutrophils, plasma cells, and macrophages. Vasculitis, "flame figures" (deposition of eosinophilic granules on connective tissue), and palisading granulomas may be seen in some instances. Associated eosinophilic cellulitis and fasciitis also may be present. If relevant, silver stains (e.g., Warthin-Starry) and serologic evaluation may be considered to rule out borrelial infection.

Neutrophilic Dermatitides and Vascular Reactions

The neutrophilic dermatitides, including Sweet's syndrome and pyoderma gangrenosum, may involve the panniculus.[15,23] These conditions often show varying degrees of septal and/or lobular infiltration by neutrophils and possibly microvascular injury. There may be some admixture of other inflammatory cells. Infections must be excluded by special stains and culture. These disorders are discussed in more detail in Chapter 9.

Noninfectious Granulomatous Panniculitis

A number of (presumed) noninfectious processes may involve the subcutaneous fat eventuating in varying degrees of septal and/or lobular panniculitis, in addition to the palisading-necrobiotic granulomatous disorders.[2,4] These conditions include sarcoidosis, metastatic Crohn's disease, and granulomatous reactions secondary to arthropod bites, rupture of pilosebaceous units, and epithelial cysts.

Lymphoma and Leukemia

Cutaneous lymphoid infiltrates, lymphoma, and leukemia may involve the subcutaneous fat. These entities are discussed in more detail in Chapter 35. Nonetheless, because of its importance in differential diagnosis, subcutaneous T-cell lymphoma will be mentioned briefly.

Patients with leukemia on occasion may develop erythematous subcutaneous nodules (resembling EN) that histologically suggest an inflammatory septal panniculitis.[13] The number of leukemic cells in such infiltrates varies from none to many.

This rare form of peripheral T-cell lymphoma presents as subcutaneous nodules mimicking conventional panniculitis in both children and adults.[149–153] Patients often develop the hemophagocytosis syndrome. Histologically, the lymphoid cells most commonly infiltrate the fat lobules in a lacelike pattern or in sheets. There is usually an admixture of small and large atypical lymphocytes with karyorrhexis, necrosis of fat and fibrous trabeculae, and erythrophagocytosis. In general, there is little or no involvement of the epidermis and dermis. The course of the lymphoma may be protracted with multiple recurrences or may be rapidly progressive.

REFERENCES

1. Elliot RIK: Pathological reactions in subcutaneous tissue: function and structure of the subcutaneous tissue, in Rook A, and Champion RH (eds): *Progress in the Biological Sciences in Relation to Dermatology*, Cambridge, Cambridge University Press, 1964.

TABLE 11-21

Eosinophilic Panniculitis

Clinical Features

Many etiologies
  Atopy
  Local injections
  Cancer (especially lymphoma)
  Vasculitis
  Borrelial infection
Inflammatory subcutaneous nodules
Vesicles, pustules, urticarias

Histopathological Features

Infiltration of fat lobules by eosinophils
Other inflammatory cells to variable extent
Occasional "flame figures"
Occasional eosinophilic cellulitis and fasciitis

Laboratory Evaluation

Special stains and serologic evaluation for Borrelial infection

Differential Diagnosis

Lymphoma

---

2. Reed RJ, Clark WH, Mihm MC: Disorders of the panniculus adiposus. *Hum Pathol* 4(2):219–229, 1973.
3. Niemi KM, Förström L, Hannuksela M, et al: Nodules on the legs: A clinical, histological and immunohistological study of 82 patients representing different types of nodular panniculitis. *Acta Dermatovener* 57:145–154, 1977.
4. Black MM: Panniculitis. *J Cutan Pathol* 12:366–380, 1985.
5. Panush RS, Yonker RA, Dlesk A, et al: Weber-Christian disease: Analysis of 15 cases and review of the literature. *Medicine* 64:181–191, 1985.
6. Patterson JW: Panniculitis. *Arch Dermatol* 123:1615–1618, 1987.
7. Winkelmann RK, Förström L: New observations in the histopathology of erythema nodosum. *J Invest Dermatol* 65:441–446, 1975.
8. Förström L, Winkelmann RK: Acute panniculitis: A clinical and histopathologic study of 34 cases. *Arch Dermatol* 113:909–917, 1977.
9. Förström L, Winkelmann RK: Granulomatous panniculitis in erythema nodosum. *Arch Dermatol* 111:335–340, 1975.
10. Hannuksela M: Erythema nodosum. *Clin Dermatol* 4:88–95, 1986.
11. Vesey CMR, Wilkinson DS: Erythema nodosum. *Br J Dermatol* 71:139–155, 1959.
12. Gordon H: Erythema nodosum: A review of 115 cases. *Br J Dermatol* 73:394–409, 1961.
13. Sumaya C, Babu S, Reed RJ: Erythema nodosum-like lesions of leukemia. *Arch Dermatol* 110:415–418, 1974.
14. Kaneko F, Takahashi Y, Muramatsu Y, Miura Y: Immunological studies on aphthous ulcer and erythema nodosum-like eruption in Behçet's disease. *Br J Dermatol* 113:303–312, 1985.
15. Cohen PR, Holder WR, Rapini RP: Concurrent Sweet's syndrome and erythema nodosum: A report, world literature review and mechanism of pathogenesis. *J Rheumatol* 19:814–820, 1992.
16. Winkelmann RK, Frigas E: Eosinophilic panniculitis: A clinicopathologic study. *J Cutan Pathol* 13:1–12, 1986.
17. Vilanova X, Aguade J: Subacute nodular migratory panniculitis. *Br J Dermatol* 71:45–50, 1959.
18. Bafverstedt B: Erythema nodosum migrans. *Acta Derm Venereol* 48:381–384, 1968.
19. Fine RM, Meltzer HD: Chronic erythema nodosum. *Arch Derm* 100:33–38, 1969.
20. Hannuksela M: Erythema nodosum migrans. *Acta Derm Venereol* 53:313–317, 1973.
21. De Almeida Prestes C, Winkelmann RK, Su Daniel WP: Septal granulomatous panniculitis: Comparison of the pathology of erythema nodosum migrans (migratory panniculitis) and chronic erythema nodosum. *J Am Acad Dermatol* 22:477–483, 1990.
22. Yus ES, Vico MDS, de Diego V: Miescher's radial granuloma: A characteristic marker of erythema nodosum. *Am J Dermatopathol* 11:434–442, 1989.

23. Cooper PH, Frierson HF, Greer KE: Subcutaneous neutrophilic infiltrates in acute febrile neutrophilic dermatosis. *Arch Dermatol* 119:610–611, 1983.

24. Kirsner RS, Pardes JB, Eaglstein WH, Falanga V: The clinical spectrum of lipodermatosclerosis. *J Am Acad Dermatol* 28:623–627, 1993.

25. Cantwell AR Jr, Kelso DW, Rowe L: Hypodermitis sclerodermiformis and unusual acid-fast bacteria. *Arch Dermatol* 115:449–452, 1979.

26. Jorizzo JL, White WL, Zanolli, MD, et al: Sclerosing panniculitis: A clinicopathologic assessment. *Arch Dermatol* 127:554–558, 1991.

27. Nasu T, Tsukahara Y, Terayama K: A lipid metabolic disease "membranous lipodystrophy." *Acta Path Jap* 23:539–558, 1973.

28. Poppiti RJ, Margulies M, Cabella B, Rywlin AM: Membranous fat necrosis: Case report. *Am J Surg Pathol* 10:62–69, 1986.

29. Alegre VA, Winkelmann RK, Aliaga A: Lipomembranous changes in chronic panniculitis. *J Am Acad Dermatol* 19:39–46, 1988.

30. Selye H: *Calciphylaxis*. Chicago, University of Chicago Press, 1962.

31. Adrogué HJ, Frazier MR, Zeluff B, Suki W: Systemic calciphylaxis revisited. *Am J Nephrol* 1:177–183, 1981.

32. Richens G, Piepkorn MW, Krueger GG: Calcifying panniculitis associated with renal failure. *J Am Acad Dermatol* 6:537–539, 1982.

33. Rubinger D, Friedlaender MM, Silver J, et al: Progressive vascular calcification with necrosis of extremities in hemodialysis patients: A possible role of iron overload. *Am J Kidney Dis* 2:125–129, 1986.

34. Lugo-Somolinos A, Sánchez JL, Mendez-Coll J, Joglar F: Calcifying panniculitis associated with polycystic kidney disease and chronic renal failure. *J Am Acad Dermatol* 22:743–747, 1990.

35. Khafif RA, DeLima C, Silverberg A, et al: Calciphylaxis and systemic calcinosis. *Arch Intern Med* 150:956–959, 1990.

36. Mehta RL, Scott G, Sloand JA, et al: Skin necrosis associated with acquired protein C deficiency in patients with renal failure and calciphylaxis. *Am J Med* 88:252–257, 1990.

37. Cockerell CJ, Dolan ET: Widespread cutaneous and systemic calcification (calciphylaxis) in patients with the acquired immunodeficiency syndrome and renal disease. *J Am Acad Dermatol* 26:559–562, 1992.

38. Fischer AH, Morris DJ: Pathogenesis of calciphylaxis: Study of three cases with literature review. *Human Pathol* 26:1055–1064, 1995.

39. Dahl PR, Winkelmann RK, Connolly SM: The vascular calcification-cutaneous necrosis syndrome. *J Am Acad Dermatol* 33:53–58, 1995.

40. Arbus GS, Sniderman S: Oxalosis with peripheral gangrene. *Arch Pathol* 97:107–110, 1974.

41. Olusegun-Fayemi A, Ali M, Braun EV: Oxalosis in hemodialysis patients: A pathologic study of 80 cases. *Arch Pathol Lab Med* 103:58–62, 1979.

42. Greer KE, Cooper PH, Campbell F, Westervelt FB Jr: Primary oxalosis with livedo reticularis. *Arch Dermatol* 116:213–214, 1980.

43. Montgomery H, O'Leary PA, Barker NW: Nodular vascular disease of the legs. *JAMA* 128:335–341, 1945.

44. Ackerman AB: *Histologic Diagnostic of Inflammatory Skin Diseases*, Philadelphia, Lea and Febiger, 1979.

45. Moore CP, Willkens RF: The subcutaneous nodule: Its significance in the diagnosis of rheumatic disease. *Semin Arthritis Rheum* 7:63–79, 1977.

46. Torres VM, George WM: Diffuse eosinophilic fasciitis: A new syndrome or variant of scleroderma? *Arch Dermatol* 113:1591–1593, 1977.

47. Krauser RE, Tuthill RJ: Eosinophilic fasciitis. *Arch Dermatol* 113:1092–1093, 1977.

48. Fleischmajer R, Jacotot AB, Shore S, Binick SA: Scleroderma, eosinophilia, and diffuse fasciitis. *Arch Dermatol* 114:1320–1325, 1978.

49. Barnes L, Rodnan GP, Medsger TA, Short D: Eosinophilic fasciitis. *Am J Pathol* 96:493–518, 1979.

50. Lupton GP, Goette DK: Localized eosinophilic fasciitis. *Arch Dermatol* 115:85–87, 1979.

51. Su WPD, Person JR: Morphea profunda: A new concept and a histopathologic study of 23 cases. *Am J Dermatopathol* 3:251–260, 1981.

52. Benedek TG, Rodnan GP: The early history and nomenclature of scleroderma and of its differentiation from sclerema neonatorum and scleredema. *Semin Arthritis Rheum* 12:52–67, 1982.

53. Vincent F, Prokopetz R, Miller RA: Plasma cell panniculitis: A unique clinical and pathologic presentation of linear scleroderma. *J Am Acad Dermatol* 21:357–360, 1989.

54. Peters MS, Su WPD: Eosinophils in lupus panniculitis and morphea profunda. *J Cutan Pathol* 18:189–192, 1991.

55. Naschitz JE, Yeshurun D, Zuckerman E, et al: The fasciitis-panniculitis syndrome: Clinical spectrum and response to cimetidine. *Semin Arthritis Rheum* 21:211–220, 1992.

56. Connolly SM, Quimby SR, Griffing WL, Winkelmann RK: Scleroderma and L-tryptophan: A possible explanation of the eosinophilia-myalgia syndrome. *J Am Acad Dermatol* 23:451–457, 1990.

57. Naschitz JE, Yeshurun D, Zuckerman E, et al: Cancer-associated fasciitis panniculitis. *Cancer* 73:231–235, 1994.

58. Granter SR, Barnhill RL, Hewins ME, Duray PH: Identification of *Borrelial burgdorferi* in diffuse fasciitis with peripheral eosinophilia: Borrelial fasciitis. *JAMA* 272: 1283–1285, 1994.

59. Granter SG, Barnhill RL, Duray PH: Borrelial fasciitis: Diffuse fasciitis and peripheral eosinophilia associated with Borrelia infection. *Am J Dermathol* 18:465–473, 1996.

60. Stork J, Vosmik F: Lupus erythematosus panniculitis with morphea-like lesions. *Clin Exp Dermatol* 19:79–82, 1994.

61. LeBoit PE, Schneider S: Gout presenting as lobular panniculitis. *Am J Dermatopathol* 9:334–338, 1987.

62. Christian HA: Relapsing febrile nodular nonsuppurative panniculitis. *Arch Intern Med* 41:338, 1928.

63. Hoyos N, Shaffer B, Beerman H: Liquefying nodular panniculitis. *Arch Derm* 94:436–439, 1966.

64. MacDonald A, Feiwel M: A review of the concept of Weber-Christian panniculitis with a report of five cases. *Br J Dermatol* 80:355–361, 1968.

65. Ciclitira PJ, Wight DGD, Dick AP: Systemic Weber-Christian disease: A case report with lipoprotein profile and immunological evaluation. *Br J Dermatol* 103:685–692, 1980.

66. Smith KC, Pittelkow MR, Su WPD: Panniculitis associated with severe alpha 1-antitrypsin deficiency. *Arch Dermatol* 123:1655–1661, 1987.

67. Su WPD, Smith KC, Pittelkow MR, Winkelmann RK: Alpha 1-Antitrypsin deficiency panniculitis: A histopathologic and immunopathologic study of four cases. *Am J Dermatopath* 9(6):483–490, 1987.

68. Smith KC, Su WP, Pittelkow MR, Winkelmann RK: Clinical and pathologic correlations in 96 patients with panniculitis. *J Am Acad Dermatol* 21:1192–1196, 1989.

69. Crotty CP, Winkelmann RK: Cytophagic histiocytic panniculitis with fever, cytopenia, liver failure, and terminal hemorrhagic diathesis. *J Am Acad Dermatol* 4:181–194, 1981.

70. Barron DR, Davis BR, Pomeranz JR, et al: Cytophagic histiocytic panniculitis. *Cancer* 55:2538–2542, 1985.

71. Peters MS, Winkelmann RK: Cytophagic panniculitis and B cell lymphoma. *J Am Acad Dermatol* 13:882–885, 1985.

72. Willis SM, Opal SM, Fitzpatrick JE: Cytophagic histiocytic panniculitis: Systemic histiocytosis presenting as chronic, nonhealing, ulcerative skin lesions. *Arch Dermatol* 121:910–913, 1985.

73. Alegre VA, Winkelmann RK: Histiocytic cytophagic panniculitis. *J Am Acad Dermatol* 20:177–185, 1989.

74. Matsue K, Itoh M, Tsukuda K, et al: Successful treatment of cytophagic histiocytic panniculitis with modified CHOP-E. *Am J Clin Oncol* 17:470–474, 1994.

75. Galende J, Vasquez ML, Almeida J, et al: Case report: Histiocytic cytophagic panniculitis: A rare late complication of allogeneic bone marrow transplantation. *Bone Marrow Transp* 14:637–639, 1994.

76. Tsukahara T, Horiuchi Y, Iidaka K: Cytophagic histiocytic panniculitis in systemic lupus erythematosus. *Hiroshima J Med Sci* 44:13–16, 1995.

77. Takeshita M, Akamatsu M, Ohshima K, et al: Angiocentric immunoproliferative lesions of the skin show lobular panniculitis and are mainly disorders of large granular lymphocytes. *Human Pathol* 26:1321–1328, 1995.

78. Risdall RJ, McKenna RW, Nesbit ME, et al: Virus-associated hemophagocytic syndrome: A benign histiocytic proliferation distinct from malignant histiocytosis. *Cancer* 44:993–1002, 1979.

79. Smith KJ, Skelton HG, Yeager J, et al: Cutaneous histopathologic, immunohistochemical, and clinical manifestations in patients with hemophagocytic syndrome. *Arch Dermatol* 128:193–200, 1992.

80. Risdall RJ, Sibley RK, McKenna RW, et al: Malignant histiocytosis: A light- and electron-microscopic and histochemical study. *Am J Surg Pathol* 4:439–450, 1980.

81. Jurco S, Starling K, Hawkins E: Malignant histiocytosis in childhood: Morphologic considerations. *Human Pathol* 14:1059–1065, 1983.

82. Pileri S, Mazza P, Rivano MT, et al: Malignant histiocytosis (true histiocytic lymphoma) clinicopathological study of 25 cases. *Histopathology* 9:905–920, 1985.

83. Schrier RW, Melmon KL, Fenster LF: Subcutaneous nodular fat necrosis in pancreatitis. *Arch Intern Med* 116:832–836, 1965.

84. Mullin GT, Caperton EM, Crespin SR, Williams RC Jr: Arthritis and skin lesions resembling erythema nodosum in pancreatic disease. *Ann Int Med* 68:75–87, 1968.

85. Förström L, Winkelmann RK: Acute, generalized panniculitis with amylase and lipase in skin. *Arch Dermatol* 111:497–502, 1975.

86. Potts DE, Mass MF, Iseman MD: Syndrome of pancreatic disease, subcutaneous fat necrosis and polyserositis. *Am J Med* 58:417–423, 1975.

87. Bennett RG, Petrozzi JW: Subcutaneous fat necrosis. *Arch Dermatol* 111:896–898, 1975.

88. Good AE, Schnitzer B, Kawanishi H, et al: Acinar pancreatic tumors with metastatic fat necrosis. *Dig Dis* 21:978–987, 1976.

89. Fine RM: The fine page: Subcutaneous fat necrosis, pancreatitis and atrophy. *Int J Dermatol* 22:575–576, 1983.

90. Noojin, RO, Pace BF, Davis HG: Subcutaneous fat necrosis of the newborn: Certain etiologic considerations. *J Invest Dermatol* 331–334, 1949.

91. Oswalt GC Jr, Montes LF, Cassady G: Subcutaneous fat necrosis of the newborn. *J Cutan Pathol* 5:193–199, 1978.

92. Chen TH, Shewmake SW, Hansen DD, Lacey HL: Subcutaneous fat necrosis of the newborn. *Arch Dermatol* 117:36–37, 1981.

93. Silverman AK: Panniculitis in infants. *Arch Dermatol* 121:834, 1985.

94. Silverman AK, Michels EH, Rasmussen JE: Subcutaneous fat necrosis in an infant, occurring after hypothermic cardiac surgery. *J Am Acad Dermatol* 15:331–336, 1986.

95. Fretzin DF, Arias AM: Sclerma neonatorum and subcutaneous fat necrosis of the newborn. *Pediatr Dermatol* 4(2):112–122, 1987.

96. Friedman SJ, Winkelmann RK: Subcutaneous fat necrosis of the newborn: Light, ultrastructural and histochemical microscopic studies. *J Cutan Pathol* 16:99–105, 1989.

97. Chuang SD, Chiu HC, Chang CC: Subcutaneous fat necrosis of the newborn complicating hypothermic cardiac surgery. *Br J Dermatol* 132:805–810, 1995.

98. Sharata H, Postellon DC, Hashimoto K: Subcutaneous fat necrosis, hypercalcemia and prostaglandin E. *Pediatr Dermatol* 12:43–47, 1995.

99. Horsfield GI, Yardley HJ: Sclerema neonatorum. *J Invest Dermatol* 44:326–332, 1965.

100. Kellum RE, Ray TL, Brown GR: Sclerema neonatorum. *Arch Dermatol* 97:372–380, 1968.

101. Roenigk HH Jr, Haserick JR, Arundell FD: Poststeroid panniculitis. *Arch Dermatol* 90:387–391, 1964.

102. Silverman RA, Newman AJ, LeVine MJ, Kaplan B: Poststeroid panniculitis: A case report. *Pediatr Dermatol* 5:92–93, 1988.

103. Sanderson TL, Moskowitz L, Hensley GT, et al: Disseminated mycobacterium avium-intracellulare infection appearing as a panniculitis. *Arch Pathol Lab Med* 106:112–114, 1982.

104. Santa Cruz DJ, Strayer DS: The histopathologic spectrum of the cutaneous mycobacterioses. *Human Pathol* 13:485, 1982.

105. Patterson JW, Brown PC, Broecker AH: Infection-induced panniculitis. *J Cutan Pathol* 16:183–193, 1989.

106. Rademaker M, Low DG, Munro DD: Erythema induratum (Bazin's disease). *J Am Acad Dermatol* 21:740–745, 1989.

107. Schneider JW, Geiger DH, Rossouw DJ, et al: Mycobacterium tuberculosis DNA in erythema induratum of bazin. *Lancet* 342:747–748, 1993.

108. Degitz K, Steidl M, Thomas P, et al: Aetiology of tuberculids. *Lancet* 341:239–240, 1993.

109. Roblin D, Kelly R, Wansbrough-Jones M, Harwood C: Case report: Papulonecrotic tuberculide and erythema induratum as presenting manifestations of tuberculosis. *J Infect* 28:193–197, 1994.

110. Degitz K: Detection of mycobacterial DNA in the skin: etiologic insights and diagnostic perspectives. *Arch Dermatol* 132:71–75, 1996.

111. Murphy G, Sanchez NP, Flynn TC, et al: Erythema nodosum leprosum: Nature and extent of the cutaneous microvascular alterations. *J Am Acad Dermatol* 14:59–69, 1986.

112. Haxthausen H: Adiponecrosis e frigore. *Br J Dermatol* 53:83–89, 1941.

113. Solomon LM, Beerman H: Cold panniculitis. *Arch Dermatol* 88:265–268, 1963.

114. Rotman H: Cold panniculitis in children [case reports]. *Arch Dermatol* 94:720–721, 1966.

115. Duncan WC, Freeman RG, Heaton CL: Cold panniculitis. *Arch Dermatol* 494:722–724, 1966.

116. Lowe LB Jr: Cold panniculitis in children. *Am J Dis Child* 115:709–113, 1968.

117. Epstein EH, Oren ME: Popsicle panniculitis. *N Engl J Med* 282:966–967, 1970.

118. Beacham BE, Cooper PH, Buchanan CS, Weary PE: Equestrian cold panniculitis in women. *Arch Dermatol* 116:1025–1027, 1980.

119. Förström L, Winkelmann RK: Factitial panniculitis. *Arch Dermatol* 110:747–750, 1974.

120. Winkelmann RK, Barker SM: Factitial traumatic panniculitis. *J Am Acad Dermatol* 13:988–994, 1985.

121. Ackerman BA, Mosher DT, Schwamm HA: Factitial Weber-Christian Syndrome. *JAMA* 198(7):731–736, 1966.

122. Kossard S, Ecker RI, Dicken CH: Povidone panniculitis. *Arch Dermatol* 116:704–706, 1980.

123. Castillo-Oertel Y, Johnson FB: Sclerosing lipogranuloma of male genitalia. *Arch Pathol Lab Med* 101:321–326, 1977.

124. Hirst AE, Heustis DG, Rogers-Neufeld B, Johnson FB: Sclerosing lipogranuloma of the scalp. *Am J Clin Pathol* 82:228–231, 1984.

125. Henrichs WD, Helwig EB: Grease gun granulomas. *Mil Med* 151:78–82, 1986.

126. Tuffanelli DL: Lupus erythematosus panniculitis (profundus): Clinical and immunological studies. *Arch Derm* 103:231–242, 1971.

127. Sanchez NP: The histology of lupus erythematosus panniculitis. *J Am Acad Dermatol* 5:673–680, 1981.

128. Koransky JS, Esterly NB: Lupus panniculitis (profundus). *J Pediatr* 98:241–244, 1981.

129. Winkelmann RK, Peters MS: *Lupus Panniculitis. Dermatology Update: Reviews for Physicians.* New York, Elsevier, 1982.

130. Izumi AK, Takiguchi P: Lupus erythematosus panniculitis. *Arch Dermatol* 119:61–64, 1983.

131. Winkelmann RK: Panniculitis in connective tissue disease. *Arch Dermatol* 119:336–344, 1983.

132. Fox JN, Klapman MH, Rowe L: Lupus profundus in children: Treatment with hydroxychloroquine. *J Am Acad Dermatol* 16:839–844, 1987.

133. Peters MS, Su WP: Lupus erythematous panniculitis. *Med Clin North Am* 73:1113–1126, 1989.

134. Raimer SS, Solomon AR, Daniels JC: Polymyositis presenting with panniculitis. *J Am Acad Dermatol* 13:366–369, 1985.

135. Neidenbach PJ, Sahn EE, Helton J: Panniculitis in juvenile dermatomyositis. *J Am Acad Dermatol* 33:305–307, 1995.

136. Ishikawa O, Tamura A, Ryuzaki K, et al: Membranocystic changes in the panniculitis of dermatomyositis. *Br J Dermatol* 134:773–776, 1996.

137. Winkelmann RK, Padilha-Goncalves A: Connective tissue panniculitis. *Arch Dermatol* 116:291–294, 1980.

138. Jablonska S, Szczepanski A, Gorkiewicz A: Lipo-atrophy of the ankles and its relation to other lipo-atrophies. *Acta Dermatovener* 55:135–140, 1975.

139. Peters MS, Winkelmann RK: Localized lipoatrophy (atrophic connective tissue disease panniculitis). *Arch Dermatol* 116:1362–1368, 1980.

140. Peters MS, Winkelmann RK: The histopathology of localized lipoatrophy. *Br J Dermatol* 114:27–36, 1986.

141. Billings, JK, Milgraum SS, Gupta AK, et al: Lipoatrophic panniculitis: A possible autoimmmune inflammatory disease of fat. *Arch Dermatol* 123:1662–1666, 1987.

142. Tsuji T, Kosaka K, Terao J: Localized lipodystrophy with panniculitis: Light and electron microscopic studies. *J Cutan Pathol* 16:359–364, 1989.

143. Zachary CB, Wells RS: Centrifugal lipodystrophy. *Br J Dermatol* 110:107–110, 1984.

144. Nelson HM: Atrophic annular panniculitis of the ankles. *Clin Exp Dermatol* 13:111–113, 1988.

145. Rongioletti F, Rebora A: Annular and semicircular lipoatrophies: Report of three cases and review of literature. *J Am Acad Dermatol* 20:433–436, 1989.

146. Burket JM, Burket BJ: Eosinophilic panniculitis. *J Am Acad Dermatol* 12:161–164, 1985.

147. Samlaska CP, de Lorimier AJ, Heldman LS: Eosinophilic panniculitis. *Pediatr Dermatol* 12(1):35–38, 1995.

148. Adame J, Cohen PR: Eosinophilic panniculitis: Diagnostic considerations and evaluation. *J Am Acad Dermatol* 34:229–234, 1996.

149. Aronson IK, West DP, Variakojis D, et al: Panniculitis associated with cutaneous T-cell lymphoma and cytophagocytic histiocytosis. *Br J Dermatol* 112:87–96, 1985.

150. Gonzalez CL, Medeiros LJ, Braziel RM, Jaffe ES: T-cell lymphoma involving subcutaneous tissue. *Am J Surg Path* 15:17–27, 1991.

151. Prescott RJ, Banerjee SS, Cross PA: Subcutaneous T-cell lymphoma with florid granulomatous panniculitis. *Histopathol* 20:535–537, 1992.

152. Perniciaro C, Zalla MJ, White JW Jr, Menke DM: Subcutaneous T-cell lymphoma: Report of two additional cases and further observations. *Arch Dermatol* 129:1171–1176, 1993.

153. Chan YF, Lee KC, Llewellyn H: Subcutaneous T-cell lymphoma presenting as panniculitis in children: Report of two cases. *Pediat Pathol* 14:595–608, 1994.

CHAPTER 12

CUTANEOUS DRUG ERUPTIONS

Neil Crowson / Cynthia M. Magro

Adverse clinical manifestations resulting from administration of medicinal agents account for 2 percent of hospital admissions,[1] affect 1 to 2 percent of the population, and are said to generate roughly $3 billion of annual expense in the United States.[2] Although many organ systems may be involved, cutaneous manifestations are frequent and offer an ideal window for diagnosis. Drug reactions may be immunologic or nonimmunologic in nature, the latter comprising overdosage, intolerance, teratogenicity, facultative effects which result from disruption of bacterial flora in mucous membranes and skin, and toxicity, the latter either delayed (i.e., carcinogenic) or cumulative (i.e., pigmentary disturbances due to deposition of gold or silver). Other nonimmunologic mechanisms of drug toxicity include anaphylactic reactions due to agents which degranulate mast cells (i.e., opiates) or impair arachidonic acid metabolism (i.e., cyclooxygenase inhibitors such as acetylsalicylic acid or other nonsteroidal anti-inflammatory agents). Recent advances in our understanding of perturbational effects of drugs upon the immune system indicate that classes of drugs which alter immune function may dramatically modify the cutaneous response to exogenous antigens, including drugs of alternate classes. Synergistic and cumulative effects of different agents may exacerbate the cutaneous manifestations of a drug reaction, often making it difficult to implicate one agent in isolation. The diagnosis of drug reaction is thus challenging and requires a thorough history, often aided by clinical algorithms. It is essential to know whether the drug in question has an established adverse effect, whether an alternative explanation for an eruption is possible, whether the timing of the eruption can plausibly be attributed to drug ingestion, whether the eruption resolves after drug therapy is stopped, and whether the rash recurs following rechallenge.[1,2,3,4] This chapter focuses on those drug eruptions in which the dermatopathologist, by implicating a specific agent, can offer most help to the clinician.

IMMUNOLOGIC DRUG REACTIONS

Allergic reactions to drugs encompass immediate hypersensitivity (type I) reactions, type II reactions in which antibodies are directed against cell surface antigens, immune-complex-mediated (type III) reactions, and delayed-type hypersensitivity (type IV) reactions. As the histomorphology of each pattern is distinctive, the pathogenetic basis of the reaction can often be inferred. The first step in the evolution of the cutaneous drug reaction is primary sensitization, often via topical exposure to contactants which cross-react with an offending oral agent. Following primary sensitization a reaction may occur within seconds to hours after subsequent antigenic rechallenge. Factors which influence the development of hypersensitivity include the nature of the allergen (i.e., lipid versus water solubility), the antigenic load (i.e., drug dose), individual genetic variations in absorption or metabolism of the drug, immunomodulatory effects of concurrently administered drugs or systemic diseases, environmental factors such as sun exposure, and route of administration.

IMMEDIATE HYPERSENSITIVITY (TYPE I) REACTIONS

Most dramatic are the drug reactions of immediate hypersensitivity type (type I), mediated by the in vivo cross-linkage by polyvalent drug-protein complexes of IgE molecules on the surface of sensitized mast cells or basophils, provoking the release of histamine, leukotrienes, and other proinflammatory molecules which result in vasodilation, increased vascular permeability, angioedema, pruritus, urticaria, bronchospasm, laryngeal edema, and, in some cases, death. The prototype is that due to penicillin.[5]

ANTIBODY-MEDIATED (TYPE II) REACTIONS

Antibody binding to cells leads to damage through complement-mediated lysis. One example is hemolytic anemia associated with methyldopa, mediated by the induction of autoantibodies directed against red cell antigens; another is autoimmune thrombocytopenic purpura, mediated through antibodies against platelets, provoked by pyrazolone derivatives (i.e., phenylbutazone and allopurinol), sulphonamides, penicillin, salicylates, thiazides, diuretics, and chloramphenicol.

IMMUNE COMPLEX (TYPE III) REACTIONS

Immune-complex-mediated reactions encompass urticaria; the Arthus reaction, a localized form of immune-complex-mediated leukocytoclastic vasculitis; urticarial vasculitis, Henoch-Schonlein purpura, and serum sickness.

DELAYED-TYPE HYPERSENSITIVITY (TYPE IV) REACTIONS

The initial event in the delayed-type hypersensitivity (DTH), or cell-mediated immune response, endocytosis by Langerhans' cells of an exogenous antigen (hapten), of drug, viral, or other derivation, is followed by complexing with tissue proteins. The latter leads to the recruitment of a subset of skin-seeking T lymphocytes which attach to high endothelial venules via interaction between lymphocyte function antigens and their respective endothelial receptors.[6,7] These T cells in turn migrate into the perivascular dermis, where they may encounter antigen-presenting Langerhans' cells. The sensitized lymphocytes then

257

TABLE 12-1
Clinical Forms of Drug Reactions

Exanthematous (maculopapular)
Lichenoid
Fixed
Photosensitivity
Pustular
Eczematous
Bullous
   Porphyria and pseudoporphyria
   Drug-induced pemphigoid
   Drug-induced pemphigus
Erythema multiforme and Stevens-Johnson syndrome
Toxic epidermal necrolysis
Psoriasiform
Pityriasiform
Lymphomatoid
Drug-induced lupus erythematosus
Collagen and elastic tissue alterations
   Elastosis perforans serpiginosa
   Sclerodermoid
Alopecia
Ichthyosiform
Purpuric
Annular erythema
Erythrodermic/exfoliative
Urticarial or anaphylactic
Pigmentary abnormalities
Vasculitis
   Serum sickness
Halogenoderma
Eosinophilia-myalgia syndrome
Erythema nodosum
Erythromelalgia
Drug-induced hypertrichosis
Drug-induced nail abnormalities
Drug-induced oral abnormalities
Acanthosis nigricans
Hidradenitis
Panniculitis
Dermatomyositis

migrate to the peripheral lymph nodes, where proliferation of memory and effector cells occurs. The circulating effector lymphocytes return to sites of cutaneous sensitization via homing receptors for tissue-specific endothelial ligands. The expression of these ligands is up-regulated, as is that of corresponding endothelial adhesion markers, in sites of DTH reactions[8]; memory or previously activated lymphocytes return to the tissue or lymphatic bed in which they were first activated. Drug reactions where this mechanism is operative include erythema multiforme and morbilliform, fixed, eczematous, pustular, lichenoid, lymphomatoid, and pigmentary purpuralike drug reactions.

CLINICAL FORMS OF DRUG REACTIONS AND THEIR HISTOPATHOLOGIC EXPRESSION

The types of clinical drug reactions are listed in Table 12-1.[1,9,10]

TABLE 12-2
Exanthematous Drug Reactions

Clinical Features

Salmon-colored macular or papular eruption
Often polycyclic, gyrate, or reticular patterns
Trunk → acral areas in symmetric distribution
Dependent areas may manifest purpura
Clear following drug withdrawal
May progress to exfoliative erythroderma if drug continued

Histopathological Features

Cell-poor lymphocytic interface dermatitis with basilar vacuolopathy
Basket-weave orthokeratosis overlying epidermis of normal thickness
Mixed lymphohistiocytic, eosinophilic, and/or plasmacellular dermal infiltrate
Papillary dermal edema

Differential Diagnosis

Viral exanthemata
Erythema multiforme

Exanthematous (Morbilliform) Drug Eruptions

Clinical Features   The most frequent of all cutaneous drug eruptions, the exanthematous or morbilliform eruptions are characterized by red to salmon-colored macular or papular eruptions which may form polycyclic, gyrate, or reticular patterns resembling a viral exanthem (Table 12-2). Lesions often appear first on the trunk and spread peripherally in a symmetric fashion. Dependant areas, such as the lower extremities, may manifest purpura. Lesions clear with withdrawal of the causative agent but may progress to a generalized exfoliative dermatitis if the drug is continued. Pruritus and fever may be present. Lesions may fade following drug cessation or resolve with a residuum of postinflammatory hyperpigmentation. The commonly implicated agents are listed in Table 12-3. One unusual cause is the lymphocyte recovery state in patients receiving chemotherapeutic drugs for leukemia and lymphoma following the nadir of their peripheral lymphocyte counts.[11]

TABLE 12-3
Drugs Causing Exanthematous (Morbilliform) Eruptions

Penicillin and synthetic derivatives
Phenylbutazone
Sulfonamide
Phenytoin and carbamazepine
Gold
Amphotericin B
Oral hypoglycemic agents
Thiazides
Barbiturates
Benzodiazepines
Phenothiazines
Allopurinol
Quinidine
Captopril
Nonsteroidal anti-inflammatory agents
Gentamicin
Lithium

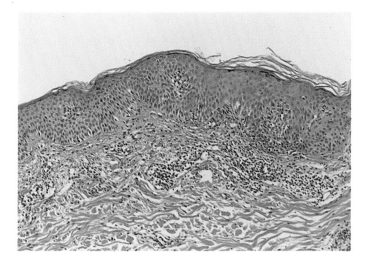

FIGURE 12-1 Morbilliform drug eruption: A basket-weave pattern of ortho-keratinization surmounts a slightly acanthotic epidermis showing a cell-poor lymphocytic interface dermatitis.

Histopathological Features   The major findings (Fig. 12-1) include a cell-poor lymphocytic interface dermatitis with basilar and suprabasilar vacuolopathy in an epidermis of normal thickness surmounted by a bas-ket-weave pattern of orthokeratinization. Scattered cytoid bodies may be seen along the lower layers of the epithelium with patchy paraker-atosis and slight acanthosis in lesions of several days' duration. Scattered eosinophils, histiocytes, and plasma cells are seen around the superficial vascular plexus (Fig. 12-2), often accompanied by papillary dermal edema. Some examples, particularly the scarlatiniform erup-tions, may show no epithelial alterations.

Differential Diagnosis   Viral exanthemata and erythema multiforme closely mimic exanthematous drug eruptions. Tissue eosinophilia is unusual in the former, and keratinocyte necrosis is pronounced in the latter.

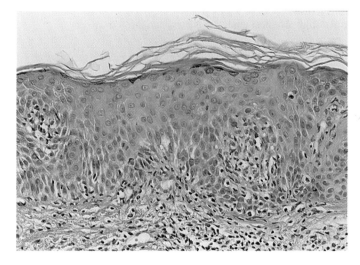

FIGURE 12-2 Morbilliform drug eruption due to fluvoxamine, an antidepres-sant: A vacuolar lymphocytic interface dermatitis is associated with a superficial perivascular lymphohistiocytic and eosinophilic infiltrate.

TABLE 12-4

Lichenoid Drug Reactions

Clinical Features

Extensive violaceous papular eruption, sometimes with psoriasiform
  appearance
Individual lesions resemble lichen planus
Postinflammatory hyperpigmentation more pronounced than lichen
  planus
Clear following drug withdrawal

Histopathological Features

Bandlike lymphocytic infiltrate hugs dermoepidermal junction
Basilar vacuolopathy of keratinocytes and colloid body formation
Patchy parakeratosis often seen
Mixed lymphohistiocytic, eosinophilic, and/or plasmacellular dermal
  infiltrate
Middermal perivascular extension

Differential Diagnosis

Lichen planus
Connective tissue diseases with lichenoid infiltrates
    Subacute cutaneous lupus erythematosus
    Discoid lupus erythematosus
    Systemic lupus erythematosus in the setting of anti-Ro antibodies
    Mixed connective tissue disease
Postherpetic eruptions
Other lichenoid hypersensitivity reactions, including:
    Some insect bite reactions
    Lichenoid contact reactions (i.e., color photodeveloper fluids)
Erythema multiforme

Lichenoid Drug Eruptions

Clinical Features   Lichenoid drug eruptions (Table 12-4) resemble lichen planus. Eruptions may develop in weeks or months and tend to be extensive, presenting as violaceous papular eruptions which develop a psoriasiform appearance. Oral involvement is uncommon. Resolution following cessation of therapy is slow, and postinflammatory pigmenta-tion is more pronounced than in idiopathic lichen planus. Implicated drugs are listed in Table 12-5.

Histopathological Features   A bandlike lymphocytic infiltrate along the dermoepidermal junction associated with vacuolopathic basal layer keratinocyte degeneration and colloid body formation is cognate to lichen planus (Fig. 12-3). Eosinophils and plasma cells are frequently present (Fig. 12-4). Perivascular lymphoid infiltrates in addition to the papillary dermal bandlike infiltrate are commonly observed.

Differential Diagnosis   Compared to lichen planus, acanthosis is often less striking in the lichenoid drug eruption, and the wedge-shaped hypergranulosis of lichen planus, although present in some cases (Fig. 12-3), is uncommon. Eosinophils and parakeratosis, common in lichenoid drug eruptions (Fig. 12-4), are rare in lichen planus. Lichenoid patterns of inflammation may be seen in certain connective tissue dis-eases, namely, mixed connective tissue disease, some cases of discoid and subacute cutaneous lupus erythematosus, and cases of systemic lupus erythematosus in the setting of anti-Ro antibodies (personal observation). However, such cases often manifest at least focal epider-mal atrophy and virtually never exhibit tissue eosinophilia.

TABLE 12-5

Causes of Lichenoid Drug Eruptions

Beta blockers
Captopril
Methyldopa
Thiazides
Lasix
Gold
Antimalarials
Quinidine
Oral hypoglycemic agents
Phenytoin and carbamazepine
Antituberculous agents
Phenylbutazone
Antipsychotics (including phenothiazines)
Bismuth
p-aminosalicylic acid
Lithium

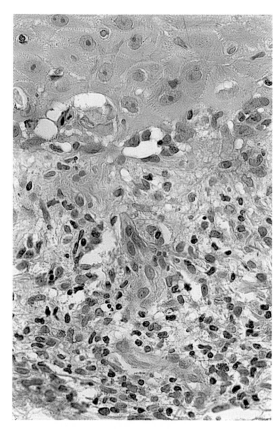

FIGURE 12-4 Lichenoid drug eruption due to a beta blocker (same patient as illustrated in Fig. 12-3): vacuolar interface injury pattern with cytoid bodies, and a dermal perivascular lymphocytic and eosinophilic infiltrate.

Fixed Drug Eruption

Clinical Features Fixed drug eruptions (Table 12-6) are associated with the drugs listed in Table 12-7. The eruptions characteristically recur in the same locations following antigenic rechallenge, with areas of involvement often increasing in size and distribution with each recurrence. The mechanism appears to reflect up-regulated keratinocyte expression of ICAM-1 and endothelial expression of E-selectin and vascular adhesion molecule-1.[12] Lesions occur more often on acral and anogenital sites than on the trunk. The acute lesion, a sharply circumscribed round or oval patch of violaceous or dusky erythema, generally arises within 30 min to several hours following drug administration. Vesiculation or blistering may ensue. Multifocal and extensive eruptions may resemble erythema multiforme and toxic epidermal necrolysis, respectively. Lesions may progress to scaling and resolve with striking postinflammatory pigmentary alteration.

TABLE 12-6

Fixed Drug Eruption

Clinical Features

Oval or round, sharply demarcated violaceous or dusky macule
Arises 30 min to several hours after drug ingestion
Anogenital areas, especially glans penis, and acral sites most common
Vesiculation and blistering may ensue
Areas of involvement tend to expand and multiply with drug rechallenge
Postinflammatory hyperpigmentation
Clear following drug withdrawal

Histopathological Features

Variably bandlike lymphocytic interface infiltrate
Basilar vacuolopathy of keratinocytes and colloid body formation, often accentuated at tips of retia
Acanthosis more pronounced than erythema multiforme
Patchy parakeratosis often seen
Mixed lymphohistiocytic, eosinophilic, plasmacellular, and neutrophilic dermal infiltrate

Differential Diagnosis

Erythema multiforme
Viral exanthema
Connective tissue disease
Graft-versus-host disease

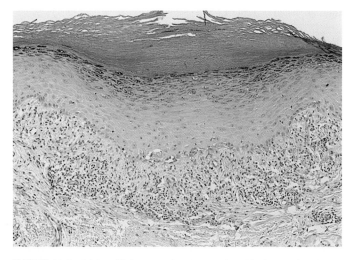

FIGURE 12-3 Lichenoid drug eruption due to a beta blocker: wedge-shaped hypergranulosis overlying an acanthotic epidermis with a lichenoid lymphocytic infiltrate.

TABLE 12-7

Drugs Associated with Fixed Drug Eruptions

Antibiotic agents
    Sulfonamides
    Tetracycline
    Penicillin and synthetic penicillins
    Trimethoprim
    Antifungal agents
    Dapsone
    Arsenicals
    p-aminosalicylic acid
    Antimalarials
    Flagyl
Sedatives
    Barbiturates
    Opiates
    Benzodiazepines
    Anticonvulsants
    Dextromethorphan
Nonsteroidal anti-inflammatory agents
    Acetylsalicylic acid
    Phenylbutazone
    Ibuprofen
Miscellaneous agents

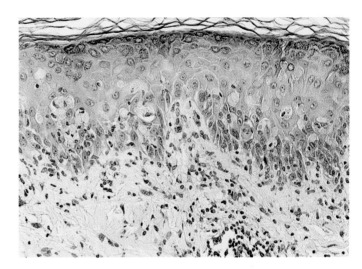

FIGURE 12-5 Fixed drug eruption: A lymphocytic interface dermatitis is present, showing focal accentuation at tips of retia, associated with striking colloid body formation and a dermal perivascular and bandlike lymphocytic and eosinophilic infiltrate.

Histopathological Features   The fixed drug eruption manifests a lymphocytic interface dermatitis with rete accentuation associated with marked colloid body formation, often with a dermal lymphocytic and eosinophilic infiltrate (Fig. 12-5). There may be an admixture of neutrophils or plasma cells or both. Later in lesional evolution, more pronounced epithelial necrosis and pigment incontinence may be seen (Fig. 12-6).

Differential Diagnosis   Fixed drug eruptions can be distinguished from erythema multiforme by virtue of relatively greater epithelial hyperplasia, pigment incontinence, and more frequent tissue eosinophilia and neutrophilia, inclusive of intraepithelial eosinophilic microabscesses. Graft-versus-host disease and viral exanthemata are usually pauci-inflammatory.

Photosensitivity Drug Eruptions

Clinical Features   Drugs that induce photosensitivity absorb electromagnetic radia in the ultraviolet (UV) and visible ranges, the former mainly comprising UVA (320 to 400 nm) and UVB (290 to 320 nm) (Table 12-8). In phototoxic reactions, the drug absorbs radiation and enters an excited state, producing species which react with other cellular constituents including reactive oxygen species. In photoallergic reactions the drug is converted into an immunologically active compound. Interactions between drugs and UV light produce eruptions in a photodistribution sparing the submental and retroauricular areas and upper eyelids. Phototoxic eruptions characteristically occur within 5 to 20 h of first exposure to a drug and resemble an exaggerated sunburn reaction, being characterized by erythema with blistering, vesiculation, desquamation, and hyperpigmentation of sun-exposed skin. Photoallergic eruptions require a latent period for sensitization and characteristically appear within 24 h of repeat antigenic challenge with both drug and ultraviolet light. Unlike purely phototoxic reactions, photoallergic erup-

tions may also be seen on non-sun-exposed sites. Most drugs associated with photoallergy, if given in sufficient quantities, can induce a phototoxic reaction. Combined photallergic-phototoxic eruptions are common. Implicated drugs are represented in Table 12-9.

Histopathological Features   The phototoxic eruption manifests keratinocyte injury at all levels of the epidermis with architectural disarray and dysmaturation (Fig. 12-7). Parakeratosis may surmount areas of epithelial injury, the patterns of which include apoptosis and reticular degeneration. Neutrophils may infiltrate the epidermis at sites of injury. There is a variable perivascular mononuclear cell–predominant infiltrate which is accentuated around the superficial vascular plexus and manifests exocytosis. Blood vessels are usually dilated and show endothelial swelling or necrosis which diminishes in the depths of the biopsy and is accompanied by hemorrhage. The photoadaptive reaction

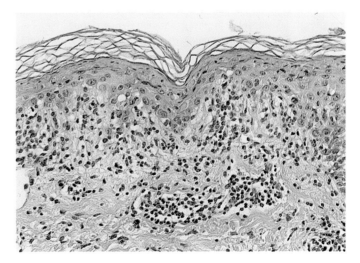

FIGURE 12-6 Fixed drug eruption in a patient on Premarin: More pronounced epidermal necrosis and colloid body formation is seen, and a bandlike dermal lymphocytic and eosinophilic infiltrate is associated with pigment incontinence.

TABLE 12-8

Photosensitivity Drug Reactions

Clinical Features

Erythematous macular, papular, or vesicular eruptions in a
   photodistribution, sparing submental and retroauricular areas
Phototoxic: occur 5–20 h after exposure to drug and light
Photoallergic: occur within 24 h of repeat antigenic challenge with
   drug and sunlight and may occur on non-sun-exposed skin
Combined phototoxic/photoallergic eruptions common

Histopathological Features

Phototoxic
   Keratinocyte injury (apoptosis or reticular degeneration) at all levels
      with architectural disarray and dysmaturation
   Neutrophilic epidermotropism at sites of injury
   Perivascular lymphocytic infiltrate in dermis
   Superficial vasculature ectatic with endothelial swelling
Photoadaptive: Hypergranulosis, hyperkeratosis, and melanocytic
   hyperplasia
Photoallergic
   Spongiosis and vesiculation with adherent scale-crust
   Mixed lymphohistiocytic and eosinophilic dermal infiltrate
   Papillary dermal edema

Differential Diagnosis

Phototoxic
   Viral exanthemata
      Erythema multiforme
         Graft-versus-host disease
Photoallergic: Delayed-type hypersensitivity reactions of diverse cause

TABLE 12-9

Drugs Associated with Photosensitivity Eruptions

Common
   Amiodarone (PA)
   Phenothiazines (PA, PT, pigmentation)
   Psoralens (PT)
   Sulfonamides
   Tetracyclines (PT)
   Thiazide diuretics (lichenoid, LE-like)
   Nonsteroidal anti-inflammatory agents (PA, PT, PCT-like)
   Nalidixic acid (PA, PT, PCT-like)
   Coal tar
   Quinidine (lichenoid, eczematous)
Uncommon
   Antihistamines (PA)
   Synthetic penicillins
   Antidepressants (PA, PT)
   Antifungal agents (PA)
   Beta blockers
   Anticonvulsants (PA)
   Benzodiazepines (PA)
   Methyldopa
   Oral contraceptives (PA)
   Antimalarials (PA, PT)
   Retinoids (PA, PT)
   Sun screens (PA)
   Oral hypoglycemics (PA)

PA = predominately photoallergic
PT = predominately phototoxic
PCT = porphyria cutanea tarda
LE = lupus erythematosus

(Fig. 12-8) shows hypergranulosis, hyperkeratosis, melanocytic hyperplasia, suprabasilar melanization, and transepidermal elimination of melanin. The photoallergic eruption is characterized by epidermal spongiosis and vesiculation, which frequently eventuates in an adherent plasma-rich scale crust. Eosinophils are a frequent component of the infiltrate. In eruptions of combined phototoxic-photoallergic type, variable expressions of these two prototypic morphologies are seen. Some patients develop persistent photosensitivity at exposed and nonexposed skin sites. If accompanied by skin infiltration by transformed lymphocytes, the designation *chronic photosensitivity dermatitis* may be appropriate. Histologically, the presence of intraepithelial cerebriform lymphocytes arranged into groups surrounded by a clear halo reminiscent of Pautrier's microabscesses results in a histologic pattern mimicking mycosis fungoides.

Differential Diagnosis   Subacute and chronic dermatitides of diverse causes mimic photoallergic eruptions but generally lack the scattered epidermal cytoid bodies and vascular alterations of phototoxic states and the photoadaptive changes in melanocytes. The nodular perivascular distribution of the infiltrates, psoriasiform hyperplasia, multinucleated stromal giant cells, and perivascular elastolysis, in concert with the clinical history, enable distinction of the chronic photosensitivity dermatitides from mycosis fungoides.

Pustular Eruptions

Clinical Features   Acute generalized exanthematous pustulosis (AGEP) is a distinctive generalized toxic pustular erythema associated

with reactions to drugs, including calcium channel blockers, nonsteroidal anti-inflammatory agents, anticonvulsants, and beta-lactam and macrolide antimicrobials.[13] Less common associations are with antiarrhythmic agents including quinidine and contact with mercury. Typically, patients present with a generalized scarlatiniform eruption of sudden onset which is studded with sterile pustules, is associated with fever, and follows a self-limited course of 4 to 17 days.[14]

Histopathological Features   Biopsies show spongiform pustulation of the epidermis typically with follicular and acrosyringeal accentuation (Fig. 12-9). There may be an accompanying leukocytoclastic vasculitis.

Differential Diagnosis   The main considerations include variants of pustular psoriasis. A leukocytoclastic vasculitis is not seen in lesions of psoriasis, however, except in the setting of concomitant hypersensitivity reactions, such as to drugs. When a psoriasiform diathesis is seen in concert with a leukocytoclastic vasculitis, Reiter's disease merits strong consideration.[15] It has been suggested that some patients with AGEP have latent psoriasis[16] or underlying immune dysregulation, such as that due to human immunodeficiency virus infection.[14,17] The other pustular eruptions, such as Sneddon-Wilkinson syndrome, impetigo, and pustular vasculitis, are nonspongiform in nature.

Eczematous Drug Reactions

Clinical Features   Oral ingestion, inhalation, or transcutaneous application of a drug to which a person has been previously sensitized via contact exposure may elicit an eczematous drug reaction (Table 12-

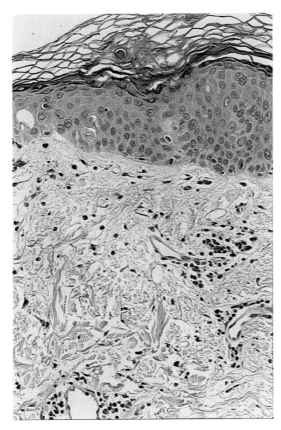

FIGURE 12-7 Phototoxic drug eruption: Cytoid bodies are present along the basal layer, in suprabasilar epidermis, and in the cornified layer. Ectasia of superficial blood vessels, associated with endothelial swelling, is characteristic.

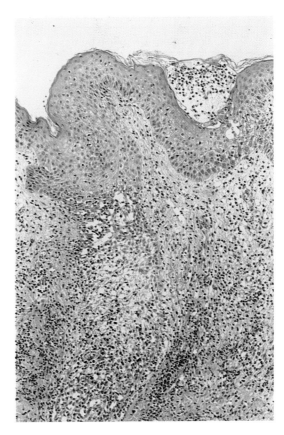

FIGURE 12-9 Pustular drug eruption: spongiform pustulation involving a hair follicle is accompanied by a subcorneal pustule in the adjacent interfollicular epidermis and a perivascular and diffuse dermal infiltrate of lymphocytes and eosinophils.

10).[18] Affected sites frequently correspond to those involved in a prior contact dermatitis, the onset of symptoms being within 2 to 24 h after an oral dose. The term *baboon syndrome* has been used to describe bright red, well-demarcated anogenital lesions associated with a symmetric eczematous eruption involving elbow flexures, axillae, eyelids,

and the sides of the neck. Among the classic drugs associated with eczematous reactions are antibiotics and ethylenediamine-containing antihistaminic and aminophylline preparations. Oral administration of sulfonyl urea hypoglycemic drugs in patients sensitized to para-amino compounds such as sulfanilamide results in flare-ups of dermatitis.

Histopathological Features Biopsies show spongiosis with intraepidermal vesiculation (Fig. 12-10) and a moderately dense lymphoeosinophilic infiltrate with variable exocytosis of lymphocytes and eosinophils.[18]

Differential Diagnosis Hypersensitivity reactions to a variety of antigenic triggers will look similar.

Blistering Drug Eruptions

The blistering drug eruptions include pseudoporphyria cutanea tarda, bullous erythema multiforme, bullous fixed drug eruption, and drug-induced pemphigus, pemphigoid, and linear IgA dermatosis.[19–21]

Drug-Induced Pseudoporphyria Cutanea Tarda

Pseudoporphyria cutanea tarda is a blistering disorder reminiscent of porphyria cutanea tarda by virtue of clinical, histologic, and immunofluorescent findings[22] but in which porphyrin metabolism is normal. Patients often have an underlying connective tissue disease.[21] This process is discussed in Chapter 7.

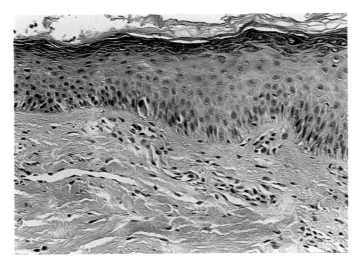

FIGURE 12-8 Photoallergic drug eruption in a patient on amiodarone: Hypergranulosis, hyperkeratosis, and acanthosis are seen, and a plump, photoactivated melanocyte is present in the basal layer.

TABLE 12-10

Eczematous Drug Reactions

Clinical Features

Erythematous, papular, or vesicular eruption in patients exposed to an agent to which they were previously sensitized
Sites often correspond to those previously affected

Histopathological Features

Spongiosis and intraepidermal vesiculation
Moderately dense dermal lymphocytic and eosinophilic infiltrate with variable exocytosis

Differential Diagnosis

Other delayed-type hypersensitivity reactions of diverse cause

TABLE 12-11

Drug Classes Associated with Drug-Induced Lupus Erythematosus

Antihypertensive
Antipsychotic
Anticonvulsant
Anti-inflammatory
Antimicrobial
Immunosuppressive
Antihormonal
Recombinant cytokines

Drug-Induced Pemphigus, Pemphigoid, and Linear IgA Dermatosis

A variety of drugs can produce a picture closely mimicking these idiopathic blistering conditions, the clinical and histologic features and differential diagnosis of which are discussed in Chapter 8.

Drug-Associated Lupus Erythematosus–like Eruptions

Clinical Features   Drug-induced lupus erythematosus (DIL) occurs with a variety of medication classes (see Table 12-11) and should be suspected in patients who, in the absence of underlying lupus erythematosus (LE), develop antinuclear antibodies and at least one clinical manifestation of LE while ingesting a drug, and in whom symptoms abate after its discontinuance. Although the clinical stigmata of DIL vary somewhat with drugs from different classes, skin disease in general is less frequent and pulmonary manifestations more common. A systemic LE-like syndrome is characteristic, although some cases resemble discoid LE clinically. Recently described is drug-induced subacute cutaneous lupus erythematosus (SCLE) associated with calcium channel blockers.[23] The prototypic drugs associated with DIL generate two distinctive serologic profiles; chlorpromazine and hydralazine are

associated with antihistone antibodies, and procainamide and quinidine generate anti-H2a-H2b-DNA antibodies, the latter directed at a histone-DNA complex. Predisposition to development of DIL tends to be in part genetically determined; patients are often slow acetylators and thus metabolize hydralazine and procainamide slowly. Although the mechanisms by which these agents provoke DIL are not fully elucidated, we know that procainamide and hydralazine inhibit T-cell DNA methylation, provoking autoreactivity in cloned T-helper (Th) lymphocytes, and perhaps share the capacity to induce autologous B-cell differentiation. Passive transfer of Th cells treated with procainamide or other DNA methyltransferase inhibitors causes a lupuslike illness in syngeneic mice. Agents most closely associated with DIL, including methyldopa, procainamide, chlorpromazine, and hydralazine, are known to disturb a variety of lymphocyte functions, as do calcium channel blockers. This may create an immunologic milieu permissive of the development of autoantibodies against ribonucleoproteins.[24]

With respect to the calcium channel blockers, most patients are women with photoinduced annular papulosquamous eruptions held clinically to represent SCLE, in whom serologic studies demonstrate a positive ANA with or without anti-Ro, anti-La, and anti-centromere antibodies.[24]

Histopathological Features   Light microscopic and direct immunofluorescent studies tend to show features typical for lupus erythematosus,[25] namely, systemic lupus erythematosus in the case of methyldopa, procainamide, chlorpromazine, and hydralazine, and SCLE in patients receiving calcium channel blockers[24,25] (Fig. 12-11). The histologic features of lupus erythematosus are discussed elsewhere (Chapters 3 and 5).

Differential Diagnosis   Concomitant features typically associated with delayed-type hypersensitivity reactions, namely, tissue eosinophilia and epithelioid histiocytic granulomata, may be seen, and are distinguishing features from idiopathic lupus erythematosus.

Lymphomatoid Drug Eruptions

Clinical Features   Lymphomatoid drug reactions are a type of lymphomatoid hypersensitivity reaction,[26] a spectrum which also encompasses aberrant and excessive immune reactions to other antigenic stimuli inclusive of insect bites,[27] viruses, bacteria, contactants, and light.[28] The most frequently encountered drugs are listed in Table 12-12.[26,29–33] Patients often receive two or more such drugs, suggesting a synergistic or cumulative effect on lymphoid function. Although the iatrogenic causes of immune dysregulation usually reflect the ingestion of one or more drugs with immune-dysregulating properties,[33] patients often have underlying systemic immune dysregulatory states such as those seen in

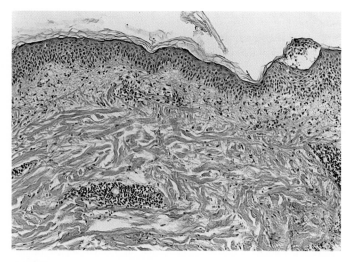

FIGURE 12-10 Eczematous drug eruption: A Langerhans' cell–containing vesicle is associated with epidermal spongiosis.

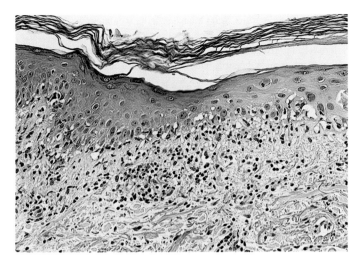

FIGURE 12-11 Drug-induced subacute lupus erythematosus in a patient on diltiazem: A lymphocytic interface dermatitis is associated with epidermal atrophy, vacuolar basal layer degeneration, cytoid body formation, and suprabasilar lymphocytic satellitosis around degenerating keratinocytes.

TABLE 12-12
Drugs Implicated in Pseudolymphomata

ACE inhibitors
Alpha antagonists
Anticonvulsants
Antidepressants
Benzodiazepines
Beta blockers
Calcium channel blockers
H1 Antagonists
H2 Antagonists
Lithium
Lipid-lowering agents
Nonsteroidal anti-inflammatory agents
Phenothiazines
Sex steroids

ACE—Angiotensin converting enzyme
H1—Histamine receptor, type 1
H2—Histamine receptor, type 2

the setting of malignant lymphoma, human immunodeficiency virus infection, or connective tissue disease.[26] Lesions present as one or more plaques resembling mycosis fungoides (MF), as multiple papules, or as a solitary nodule. Long-term clinical follow-up is necessary, as distinction from lymphoma can be difficult and as progression from pseudolymphoma to malignant lymphoma can occur.[26] As immune dysregulation may persist for weeks after a drug is discontinued, failure of an eruption to resolve within several weeks should not be considered indicative of malignant lymphoma; lesional persistence several months after appropriate drug modulation should prompt consideration of malignant lymphoma.[26]

Histopathological Features   Distinctive patterns seen in the context of the lymphomatoid drug reaction (Table 12-13) include the MF-like pattern (Fig. 12-12), the lymphomatoid vascular reaction (Fig. 12-13), follicular mucinosis, and lymphocytoma cutis. The MF-like pattern combines features of epidermotropic cutaneous T cell lymphoma (CTCL) with histologic hallmarks of delayed type hypersensitivity,[26,29,30] including basilar vacuolopathy, spongiosis, vesiculation, keratinocyte necrosis, and papillary dermal edema. Epithelial infiltration is frequently only mild and is of maximal intensity in suprapapillary plates and adnexae, sites of preferential antigenic processing.[26] The lymphomatoid vascular reaction manifests an angiocentric infiltrate of atypical lymphocytes that obscures the vessel architecture, usually without fibrinoid necrosis (Fig. 12-13).

Differential Diagnosis   The mycosis fungoides–like lymphomatoid hypersensitivity pattern is distinguished from MF by virtue of the architecture of the lymphoid infiltrate, the lack of epidermal Sézary cells, infrequent individual cell necrosis (apoptosis) of lymphocytes, low mitotic rates, tingible body macrophages, polyphenotypy, and polygenotypy. The lymphomatoid vascular reaction pattern may be seen in a variety of neoplastic and nonneoplastic lesions

inclusive of angioimmunoproliferative lesions (AIL) ranging from low-grade lymphomatoid granulomatosis to angiocentric T-cell lymphoma, adult T-cell leukemia/ lymphoma, lymphomatoid papulosis, angioimmunoblastic lymphadenopathy, delayed-type hypersensitivity reactions, and lymphomatoid connective tissue disease.[34,35]

Drug-Associated Alopecia

Drugs induce alopecia primarily through two mechanisms: induction of telogen effluvium or mitotic arrest of anagen hair (anagen effluvium) (see Chapter 10). Causes of the former include anticoagulants, lithium, and boric acid, whereas chemotherapeutic agents cause the latter. Although virtually any drug may induce alopecia, only a few are routinely associated with hair loss. Exacerbation of hair loss with re-exposure and hair recovery following withdrawal is the best evidence to incriminate a specific drug. Other drugs associated with diffuse hair loss through unclear mechanism include naproxen, colchicine,

TABLE 12-13	
Histologic Features of the Lymphomatoid Hypersensitivity Reaction	
Mycosis Fungoides–like pattern of Lymphomatoid hypersensitivity	*Features common to Mycosis Fungoides and lymphomatoid hypersensitivity*
Infiltration of the epidermis by mildly atypical lymphocytes or by cells with a comparable cytomorphology to the small- and intermediate-size atypical dermal lymphocytes	Dermal Sézary cells
Sézary cells	Atrophy
Directed pattern of epidermal infiltration with maximal involvement of suprapapillary plates/adnexae*	Vascular ectasia
	Dermal fibrosis, either vertical or laminated
Vesiculation*	
Papillary dermal edema*	
No Pautrier's microabscesses	
Vascular fibrin deposition*	

*histologic features characteristic of delayed-type hypersensitivity reactions

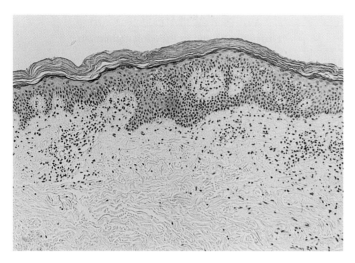

FIGURE 12-12 Lymphomatoid hypersensitivity reaction (mycosis fungoides–like) in a patient on amitriptyline: A bandlike dermal lymphocytic infiltrate is present and shows haphazard epidermotropism with minimal spongiosis; in other areas not shown, the epidermis was spared, unlike mycosis fungoides, where epidermal involvement is continuous in shave biopsy specimens.

thiamphenicol, amiodarone, levodopa, anticonvulsants, and estrogen therapy following withdrawal.[36,37]

Histopathological Features Drugs associated with a lichenoid reaction, the prototype being quinidine, can produce a scarring alopecia (see Chapter 10).

Differential Diagnosis Distinction of drug-induced from idiopathic anagen and telogen effluvium may be impossible. The lichenoid infiltrate provoked by quinidine mimics lichen planopilaris but lacks hypergranulosis of the interfollicular epidermis and may manifest tissue eosinophilia.

Sclerodermoid Tissue Reactions

Drugs implicated in the pathogenesis of fibrosing disorders include serotonin, methysergide and other ergot alkaloids, practolol, and

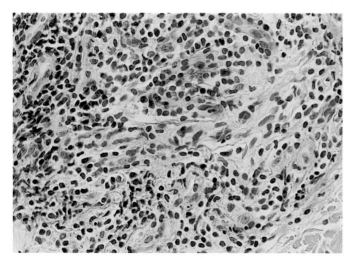

FIGURE 12-13 Lymphomatoid vascular reaction in a patient on diazepam: A perivascular and transmural infiltrate of mature and transformed lymphocytes is present and is unaccompanied by vascular fibrin deposition.

hydralazine. Among the drugs that can induce cutaneous sclerosis are bromocriptine, lithium, valproic acid, hydantoins, and L-tryptophan. Sclerodermoid tissue reactions localized to injection sites are associated with corticosteroids, heparin, vitamin K1, pentazocine, and prior radiotherapy. With respect to pathobiology, the ergot derivatives provoke peripheral vasoconstriction which damages capillary endothelium. A reduction in cyclic AMP levels promotes collagen synthesis and is the proposed mechanism of fibrosis in patients receiving beta blockers. Trytophan-associated eosinophilic fasciitis is addressed elsewhere.

Histopathological Features Sclerodermoid tissue reactions demonstrate widened collagen fibers with diminished fibrillar striations and interstitial infiltrates of lymphocytes and plasma cells.

Differential Diagnosis The morphology is indistinguishable from idiopathic morphea and from sclerodermoid alterations associated with connective tissue disease and Borrelia infection.

Alterations of Collagen and Elastic Fibers (Other than Sclerodermoid Alterations) Associated with Drug Therapy

Cutis laxa, anetoderma, elastosis perforans serpiginosa, and pseudoxanthoma elasticum, the clinical and histopathologic features and differential diagnosis of which are considered elsewhere, can be provoked by drugs (see Table 12-14).

Side Effects of Chemotherapeutic Agents

Clinical Features Chemotherapy-induced reactions include *acral erythema*,[38] characterized by erythema and swelling of the hands after administration of fluorouracil, doxorubicin, and arabinoside; *neutrophilic hidradenitis*[39]; and *radiation recall dermatitis* provoked by doxorubicin and methotrexate, in which an eruption occurs in a previously quiescent radiation field.[40]

Histopathological Features Acral erythema manifests as basilar vacuolopathy accompanied by focal dyskeratosis.[38] In radiation recall dermatitis, an atrophying interface dermatitis characterized by basilar vacuolopathy and superficial vascular ectasia is observed (personal observation). *Neutrophilic eccrine hidradenitis* manifests neutrophilic infiltrates surrounding and permeating the eccrine apparatus with epithelial cell degeneration and necrosis.[38,39] Eccrine ducts may exhibit *squamous syringometaplasia*, manifesting comma-shaped structures showing mature squamous epithelium[41] in response to a variety of chemotherapeutic agents.

Differential Diagnosis Connective tissue diseases, erythema multiforme, and viral exanthemata mimic acral erythema lesions; the incipient lesion is often indistinguishable from acute graft-versus-host disease. Neutrophilic eccrine hidradenitis may be a manifestation of the administration of other drugs, such as lithium,[38] or of id reactions to microbial pathogens.

Drug-Associated Vasculitis Including Serum Sickness

Clinical Features Drug-associated vasculitis in the skin is expressed as palpable purpura or a maculopapular rash. Some implicated drugs and their associated vascular injury patterns are listed in Table 12-15.

TABLE 12-14

Alterations of Collagen and Elastic Fibers by Drugs

Elastosis perforans serpiginosa
  Tiopronine
  D-Penicillamine
Cutis laxa/pseudoxanthoma elasticum–like
  Penicillin
  Isoniazid
  L-Tryptophan
  D-Penicillamine
Anetoderma
  Penicillamine

TABLE 12-15

Drug-Associated Vasculitis

Leukocytoclastic vasculitis, not otherwise specified
  Phenylbutazone
  Indomethacin
  Allopurinol
  Penicillins
  Erythromycin
  Sulfonamides
  Thiazide diuretics
  Hydantoins
Henoch-Schonlein purpura
  Acetylsalicylic acid
  Penicillins
  Quinine
  Thiouracil
  Gold
Pustular vasculitis
  Naproxen
  Penicillins
  Ampicillin
  Amoxicillin
  Furosemide
  Diltiazem
  Carbamazepine
  Mercury
Pigmentary purpuras
  Bromhexine
  Carbromal
  Bromisoval
Polyarteritis nodosa–like
  Acetylsalicylic acid
  Sulfasalazine
  Allopurinol
  Sulfamethoxazole
  Sulfonamides
  Quinidine
  Phenytoin
  Meprobamate
  Thiouracil
  Potassium

Histopathological Features Characteristic is a leukocytoclastic vasculitis confined to the superficial vascular plexus, the histopathology and differential diagnosis of which are discussed elsewhere.

Psoriasiform Drug Reactions

A variety of drugs can be associated with a psoriasiform eruption and/or with the induction or exacerbation of psoriasis (see Table 12-16).[43]

Histopathological Features Psoriasiform epidermal hyperplasia, granular cell layer diminution, and foci of neutrophil-imbued parakeratosis are seen, variably accompanied by an interface dermatitis, spongiotic epithelial changes, eosinophilia, and focal dyskeratosis (Fig. 12-14). Some cases also manifest a lichenoid infiltrate, particularly those associated with beta blockers.

Differential Diagnosis The hallmark of a true psoriasiform diathesis, namely, tortuous dermal papillae capillaries in apposition to thinned suprapapillary plates, is not seen. Reactions associated with induction or aggravation of underlying psoriasis manifest a histomorphology indistinguishable from psoriasis, which is discussed elsewhere.

Pityriasiform Eruptions

Clinical Features Drugs associated with eruptions resembling pityriasis rosea are listed in Table 12-17.

Histopathological Features These reactions are morphologically indistinguishable from pityriasis rosea, the hallmarks of which are a subacute dermatitis with focal parakeratosis, superficial erythrocyte extravasation, dyskeratosis, and tissue eosinophilia.

Differential Diagnosis The histopathology of pityriasis lichenoides chronica can look similar to the pityriasiform drug eruption but is

TABLE 12-16

Drugs which Induce or Aggravate Psoriasiform Eruptions

ACE inhibitors
Acetylsalicylic acid
Morphine
Ibuprofen
Codeine
Ampicillin
Chloroquin
Quinidine
Beta blockers
  Propanolol
  Pindolol
  Practolol
Lithium
Cyclosporine
Gold
Arsenic
Iodine
Penicillamine
Interleukins
Interferon
Etretinate
Methoxsalen

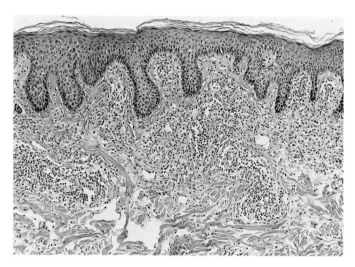

FIGURE 12-14 Psoriasiform drug eruption in a patient of African extraction: psoriasiform hyperplasia of epidermis with a nodular perivascular dermal lymphocyte-predominant infiltrate; unlike true psoriasis, tortuous dermal papillae capillaries in apposition to thinned suprapapillary plates are not seen.

usually separable by the presence of eosinophils in the latter. The epithelial injury of pityriasis lichenoides et varioliformis acuta is usually greater, and the dermal infiltrate, like in pityriasis lichenoides chronica, is usually purely lymphocytic.

Drug-Associated Ichthyosiform Dermatoses

Clinical Features   Certain classes of drugs may provoke ichthyosiform reactions (see Table 12-18).

Histopathological Features   The histopathology resembles ichthyosis vulgaris by virtue of laminated orthohyperkeratosis, a diminished or absent granular cell layer, and, in some cases, attenuation of the epidermis.

Differential Diagnosis   Distinction from ichthyosis vulgaris under the microscope can be impossible, although the presence of eosinophils tends to point toward a drug-based etiology. The remainder of the heritable ichthyosis states manifest a normal or increased granular cell layer, as discussed elsewhere.

Erythema Multiforme, Including Stevens-Johnson Syndrome and Toxic Epidermal Necrolysis

Drugs implicated in erythema multiforme and toxic epidermal necrolysis are listed in Tables 12-19 and 12-20. The clinical and histologic features are discussed in Chapter 3.

Halogenodermas

Clinical Features   Iodides, bromides, and fluorine can induce vegetative, fungating, papulopustular, and ulcerating lesions[44] (Table 12-21). Iododermas tend to manifest as a pustular facial eruption, often with ulceration. Bromodermas present as nodules or plaques with a verrucous or granulating surface, most commonly on the lower extremities; some cases manifest panniculitis.[45] The pathophysiology of the halogenodermas is not well understood, although underlying systemic diseases may predispose to their development.[46]

TABLE 12-17

Drugs Associated with Pityriasiform Reactions

Acetylsalicylic acid
Griseofulvin
Metronidazole
Captopril
Clonidine
Gold
Arsenic

TABLE 12-18

Drugs Inducing Ichthyosiform Dermatoses

Allopurinol
Clofazimine
Hydrochlorothiazide
Nicotinic acid (Niacin)
Dyrazine
Ergocalciferol
Lipid-lowering agents

TABLE 12-19

Erythema Multiforme and Stevens-Johnson Syndrome

Pyrazolone derivatives including phenylbutazone and oxyphenbutazone
Penicillins
Slowly excreted sulfonamides
Ampicillin
Salicylates
Salazopyrin
Barbiturates
Phenobarbital
Hydantoins
Carbamazepine
Phenothiazine derivatives
D-Penicillamine

TABLE 12-20

Toxic Epidermal Necrolysis

Sulfonamides
Trimethoprim and sulfadoxine
Trimethoprim and sulfamethoxazole
Pyrazalones including phenybutazone and allopurinol
Barbiturates
Anti-inflammatory drugs
Tetracycline
Nitrofurantoin
Antituberculous drugs
Hydantoins
Carbamazepine

TABLE 12-21
Halogenodermas
Iodides
Amiodarone
Potassium iodide
Iodized radiographic contrast media
Iodized salt
Iodine in seaweed and other food
Bromides
Fluorides

TABLE 12-22
Drugs Associated with Erythroderma
Acetylsalicylic acid
Sulfasalazine
Fenbufen
Oxytetracycline
Gentamicin
Nystatin
Ketoconazole
Sulfonamides
Co-trimoxazole
Clofazimine
Quinidine
Captopril
Timolol
Minoxidil
Phenobarbital
Methotrexate
Granulocyte macrophage colony–stimulating factor
Etretinate

Histopathological Features   The epidermis shows pseudoepitheliomatous hyperplasia with neutrophilic intraepidermal and dermal microabscesses (Fig. 12-15) and superficial dermal edema.[46] In lesions of iododerma, epithelial proliferation is less prominent, but vascular alterations may be more conspicuous and likely account for the ulceration that may be observed.

Differential Diagnosis   Other causes of pseudoepitheliomatous hyperplasia associated with tissue neutrophilia and intraepidermal pustulation include infections with atypical mycobacteria or fungi, which may be distinguished from halogenodermas by special stains and culture; pyostomatitis vegetans of Crohn's disease, separable by clinical history and by proximity to a mucosal orifice[47]; and blastomycosislike pyoderma of the immunocompromised, a bacterial infection.[48]

Erythroderma

Clinical Features   Erythroderma due to drugs must be distinguished from other causes such as pityriasis rubra pilaris, psoriasis, seborrheic dermatitis, and cutaneous T-cell lymphoma. The common drugs associated with erythroderma are listed in Table 12-22.

Histopathological Features   Characteristic is psoriasiform hyperplasia with granular cell layer diminution, variable spongiosis, and a diffuse parakeratotic scale which may contain neutrophils. Additional features include a vacuolopathic interface dermatitis, focal dyskeratosis, and a mixed inflammatory cell infiltrate often containing lymphocytes, eosinophils, and neutrophils.

Differential Diagnosis   The constellation of findings diagnostic of a true psoriasiform diathesis, namely, the direct apposition of ectatic capillaries to thinned suprapapillary plates, is not seen. Tissue eosinophilia may be observed in pityriasis rubra pilaris, erythrodermic psoriasis, and cutaneous T-cell lymphoma and is not in isolation a discriminating feature. Mycosis fungoides can usually be distinguished by virtue of continuous epidermotropism of atypical lymphoid forms in concert with epidermal atrophy.

Dilantin Hypersensitivity Syndrome

Clinical Features   In addition to its perturbative effects upon lymphocyte function, namely, enhancement of blast transformation and abrogation of T-suppressor function, phenytoin and its analogues also may function as antigens in some patients. In concert, these two processes promote a variety of clinical consequences, including the *dilantin hypersensitivity syndrome* which is seen in 2 to 20 percent of patients who consume the drug.[49] The manifestations of dilantin hypersensitivity syndrome include fever, lymphadenopathy, hepatosplenomegaly, mucositis, a rash which characteristically manifests as patchy erythema which may progress to generalized erythroderma, a folliculocentric pustular eruption, erythema multiforme, and toxic epidermal necrosis. Dilantin also perturbs collagen synthesis, resulting in gingival hyperplasia in roughly 50 percent of patients receiving the drug. The types of phenytoin-induced exanthems are listed in Table 12-23.

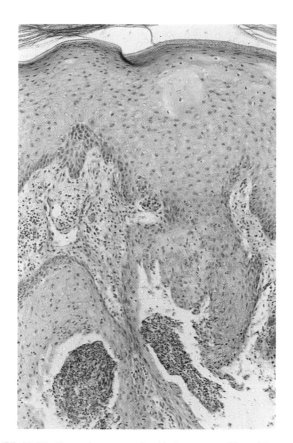

FIGURE 12-15 Bromoderma: pseudoepitheliomatous epidermal hyperplasia with intraepidermal neutrophilic abscesses.

TABLE 12-23

Phenytoin-Induced Exanthems

Acneiform eruptions
Exfoliative dermatitis
Hyper- and hypopigmentation
Maculopapular eruptions
Erythema multiforme
Toxic epidermal necrolysis
Vasculitis
Pseudolymphoma

Histopathological Features Histologic features reflect the type of eruption biopsied. The pustular lesions exhibit intraepidermal vesiculo-pustules, often accentuated in hair follicles, whereas the erythema multiforme–like eruptions manifest lymphocytic interface inflammation with keratinocyte necrosis and the maculopapular eruptions demonstrate a mild perivascular lymphocytic infiltrate with variable interface injury.

Differential Diagnosis Depending upon the type of lesion biopsied, dilantin-induced eruptions may mimic mycosis fungoides and other mycosis fungoides–like pseudolymphomata, other pustular drug eruptions and pustular bacterid, and other causes of erythema multiforme and vasculitis.

REFERENCES

1. Weedon D: Cutaneous drug reactions, in Weedon D (ed): *The Skin*. Edinburgh, Churchill Livingston, 1992, pp. 559–569.
2. Rieder MJ: Mechanisms of unpredictable adverse drug reactions. *Drug Safety* 11:196–212, 1994.
3. Shear NH: Diagnosing cutaneous adverse reactions to drugs. *Arch Dermatol* 126:94–97, 1990.
4. Alanko K, Stubb S, Kauppinen K: Cutaneous drug reactions: Clinical types and causative agents. *Acta Derm Venereol (Stockh)* 69:223–226, 1989.
5. Wintroub BU, Stern R: Cutaneous drug reactions: Pathogenesis and clinical classification. *J Am Acad Dermatol* 13:167–179, 1985.
6. Wawryk SO, Novotny JR, Wicks IP, et al: The role of LFA-1/ICAM-1 interaction in human leukocyte homing and adhesion. *Immunol Rev* 108:135–161, 1989.
7. Picker LJ, Butcher EC: Physiological and molecular mechanisms of lymphocyte homing. *Ann Rev Immunol* 10:561–591, 1992.
8. Colditz IG, Watson DL: The effect of cytokines and chemotactic agonists on the migration of T lymphocytes into the skin. *Immunology* 76:272–278, 1992.
9. Breathnach SM, Hintner H: *Adverse Drug Reactions and the Skin*. Oxford, Blackwell Scientific, 1992.
10. Zurcher K, Krebs A: *Cutaneous Drug Reactions*. Basel, Karger, 1992.
11. Horn TD, Redd JV, Karp JE, et al: Cutaneous eruptions of lymphocyte recovery. *Arch Dermatol* 125:1512–1517, 1989.
12. Teraki Y, Moriya N, Shiohara T: Drug-induced expression of intracellular adhesion molecule-1 on lesional keratinocytes in fixed drug eruption. *Am J Pathol* 145:550–560, 1994.
13. Moreau A, Dompmartin A, Castel B, et al: Drug-induced generalized exanthematous pustulosis with positive patch tests. *Int J Dermatol* 34:263–266, 1995.
14. Sawhney RA, Dubin DB, Otley CC, et al: Generalized exanthematous pustulosis induced by medications. *Int J Dermatol* 35:826–827, 1996.
15. Magro CM, Crowson AN, Regauer S: Vasculitis as the basis of cutaneous lesions of Reiter's disease. *Hum Pathol* 26:633–638, 1995.
16. Roujeau JC, Bioulac-Sage P, Bourseau C, et al: Acute generalized exanthematous pustulosis. *Arch Dermatol* 127:1333–1338, 1991.
17. Coopman S, Johnson RA, Platt R, Stern RS: Cutaneous disease and drug reactions in HIV infection. *N Engl J Med* 328:1670–1674, 1993.
18. Menne T, Veien NK, Maibach HI: Systemic contact-type dermatitis due to drugs. *Semin Dermatol* 8:144–148, 1989.
19. Breathnach SM, Hintner H: *Adverse Drug Reactions and the Skin*. Oxford, Blackwell Scientific, 1:99–109, 1992.
20. Geissmann C, Beylot-Barry M, Doutre M-S, Beylot C: Drug-induced linear IgA bullous dermatosis. *J Am Acad Dermatol* 32:296, 1995.
21. Magro CM, Crowson AN, Regauer S: The dermatopathology of mixed connective disease. *Am J Dermatopathol* 19:205–212, 1997.
22. Gately LE, Nesbitt LT: Update on immunofluorescent testing in bullous diseases and lupus erythematosus. *Dermatol Clin* 12:133–142, 1994.
23. Crowson AN, Magro CM: Diltiazem and subacute cutaneous lupus erythematosuslike lesions. *N Engl J Med* 333:1429, 1995.
24. Crowson AN, Magro CM: Subacute cutaneous lupus erythematosus–like eruptions associated with calcium channel blocker therapy. *Hum Pathol* 28:67–73, 1997.
25. Magro CM, Crowson AN, Harrist TJ: The use of antibody to C5b-9 in the subclassification of lupus erythematosus. *Br J Dermatol* 134:855–862, 1996.
26. Magro CM, Crowson AN: Drug-induced immune dysregulation as a cause of atypical cutaneous lymphoid hyperplasia: A hypothesis. *Hum Pathol* 27:50–58, 1996.
27. Crowson AN, Magro CM: Woringer-Kolopp disease: A lymphomatoid hypersensitivity reaction. *Am J Dermatopathol* 16:542–548, 1994.
28. Crowson AN, Magro CM: Cutaneous pseudolymphoma: A review. *Fitzpatrick's J Clin Dermatol* 3:43–55, 1995.
29. Crowson AN, Magro CM: Antidepressant therapy: A possible cause of atypical cutaneous lymphoid hyperplasia. *Arch Dermatol* 131:925–929, 1995.
30. Magro CM, Crowson AN: Drugs with antihistaminic properties as a cause of atypical cutaneous lymphoid infiltrates. *J Am Acad Dermatol* 32:419–28, 1995.
31. Rijlaarsdam U, Scheffer E, Meijer CJLM, et al: Mycosis fungoides-like lesions associated with phenytoin and carbamazepine therapy. *J Am Acad Dermatol* 24:216–222, 1991.
32. Rijlaarsdam JU, Scheffer E, Meijer CJLM, Willemze R: Cutaneous pseudo-T-cell lymphomas: A clinicopathologic study of 20 patients. *Cancer* 69:717–724, 1992.
33. Rao VR: Binary combination effects of some pharmacologically active chemicals as promotors of tumorigenesis. *J Pharm Sci* 81:403–407, 1992.
34. Magro CM, Tawfik N, Crowson AN: Lymphomatoid granulomatosis. *Int J Dermatol* 33:157–160, 1994.
35. Magro CM, Crowson AN, Harrist TJ: Lymphomatoid reactions in lesions of connective tissue disease. *Am J Dermatopathol* (in press).
36. Zurcher K, Krebs A: *Cutaneous Drug Reactions*. Basel, Karger, 1:318–324, 1992.
37. Stroud JD: Drug induced alopecia. *Semin Dermatol* 4:29–34, 1985.
38. Kerker BJ, Hood AF: Chemotherapy-induced cutaneous reactions. *Semin Dermatol* 8:173–181, 1989.
39. Harrist TJ, Fine JD, Berman RS, et al: Neutrophilic eccrine hidradenitis: A distinctive type of neutrophilic dermatosis associated with cytarabine therapy and acute leukemia. *Arch Dermatol* 118:263–266, 1982.
40. Shenkier T, Gelman K: Paclitaxel and radiation-recall dermatitis. *J Clin Oncol* 12:439, 1994.
41. Bhawan J, Malhotra R: Syringosquamous metaplasia: A distinctive eruption in patients receiving chemotherapy. *Am J Dermatopathol* 12:1–6, 1990.
42. Gupta AK, Knowles SR, Gupta MA, et al: Lithium therapy associated with hidradenitis suppurativa: Case report and review of the dermatological side effects of lithium. *J Am Acad Dermatol* 32:382–386, 1995.
43. Zurcher K, Krebs A: *Cutaneous Drug Reactions*. Basel, Karger, 331–333, 1992.
44. Noonan MP, Williams CM, Elgart ML: Fungating pustular plaques in a patient with Graves' disease: Iododerma. *Arch Dermatol* 130:786–787, 789–790, 1994.
45. Diener W, Kruse R, Berg P: [Halogen-induced panniculitis caused by potassium bromide]. *Monatsschr Kinderheilkd* 141:705–707, 1993.
46. Soria C, Allegue F, Espana A, et al: Vegetating iododerma with underlying systemic diseases: Report of three cases. *J Am Acad Dermatol* 22:418–422, 1990.
47. Magro CM, Crowson AN, Mihm MC: Cutaneous manifestations of gastrointestinal disease, in Elder DE, Johnson BE, Jaworsky C, Elenitsas R (eds): *Lever's Histopathology of the Skin*, 8th ed. Philadelphia, Lippincott, 353–368, 1997.
48. Rongioletti F, Semino M, Drago F, et al: Blastomycosislike pyoderma (pyoderma vegetans) responding to antibiotics and topical disodium chromoglycate. *Int J Dermatol* 35:828–830, 1996.
49. Silverman AK, Fairley J, Wong RC: Cutaneous and immunologic reactions to phenytoin. *J Am Acad Dermatol* 18:721–741, 1988.

CHAPTER 13

CUTANEOUS REACTIONS TO EXOGENOUS AGENTS

Neal S. Penneys / Julia LaGuette

REACTIONS TO TRAUMA AND IRRITATION

Clinical Features   The skin is the interface that protects the internal milieu from an endless potential array of external irritants. The continuum of external stimuli ranges from minimal to severe, and the objective result follows the same continuum. Minimal stimuli may result in redness, mild scale, and symptoms such as pruritus. More severe irritations can lead to blisters, eczematous changes, and ulceration, along with more provocative symptoms. Clinical patterns associated with external trauma and irritation include artifactual dermatitis, ulceration, friction blisters, and calcaneal petechia, to name but a few.

Histopathological Features   The histologic panoply associated with trauma and irritation follow the continuum observed clinically. Minimal trauma may result in superficial parakeratosis, crust, mild spongiosis, superficial vasodilatation, and mild papillary dermal inflammation. More severe changes include prominent intracellular edema, spongiosis with overlying parakeratosis and crust and possible vesicle formation, superficial ulceration, and polymorphous dermal inflammation with hemorrhage. Severe traumas may have all the preceding in addition to ulceration, necrosis, and dermal hemorrhage. The histopathology of ulceration is not specific and contains a dense polymorphous inflammatory infiltrate, varying degrees of vascular damage, hemorrhage, dermal necrosis, and overlying crust (Fig. 13-1). If foreign material is part of the process, it may be detected within the necrotic mass or in the dermis. Foreign material may be detected directly, through the use of special stains, and by polarization microscopy. Location may be helpful in arriving at a clinicopathologic correlation; for example, transepidermal elimination of hemorrhage with intracorneal collections in a biopsy specimen from a plantar site would be compatible with the shear injury that produces calcaneal petechiae.

Differential Diagnosis   Most of the pathologic pictures associated with the continuum of external trauma and irritation require clinicopathologic correlation. Most of the histologic patterns associated with irritation and trauma are not diagnostic alone. Certain gross clinical and histologic features, e.g., a very deep decubitus ulceration located on the sacrum of an elderly person, may favor a more precise diagnosis.

REACTIONS TO RADIATION

Ionizing radiation in its many forms can affect the skin. For the purposes of this text, radiation dermatitis is divided into three clinical groups: acute radiation dermatitis, subacute radiation dermatitis, and chronic radiation dermatitis (Table 13-1).

Clinical Features   Acute radiation dermatitis follows exposure to a threshold dose of ionizing radiation. The multiphasic response is dose-dependent and is characterized initially by transient redness, hair loss, and possibly vesiculation. In the second phase, redness develops 7 to 9 days following radiation exposure. Finally, redness and pigmentary changes may recur weeks after radiation exposure. Intense exposure may produce ulceration, generally after several weeks. Healing of the acute phase occurs with scaling and pigmentary changes. Subacute radiation dermatitis develops several months following exposure, producing scaling and postinflammatory changes.[1] Chronic radiation dermatitis develops months to years following exposure and is associated with atrophy, telangiectasia, and pigmentary changes. Late radiation necrosis can occur over bony or cartilaginous prominences, generally beginning 1 or more years following exposure and precipitated by trauma.

Histopathological Features   The location of the pathologic change in radiation-induced cutaneous injury will depend on the radiation penetration. In acute radiation dermatitis, keratinocytes have intracellular edema as well as variation in nuclear size and tinctorial qualities. Spongiosis, vacuolar change, and individual cell necrosis are also features. Dermal injury is variable and includes degenerative effects in the adnexae, dermal edema, ectasia of vessels, and scattered thrombus formation. Inflammatory infiltrates are variable and can be composed of all cell types.

In subacute radiation dermatitis, epidermal changes include vacuolar alteration, necrosis of keratinocytes, focal atypia of keratinocytes, hypergranulosis, and compact hyperkeratosis. Dermal changes may contain a variably dense infiltrate of lymphocytes and histiocytes in the papillary dermis, telangiectatic vessels, and reparative changes.[1]

In chronic radiation dermatitis, epidermal changes vary and may include alterations in the stratum corneum, epidermal thinning and/or thickening, edema of the epidermis with possible vacuolar alteration of the basal cell layer and ulceration (Fig. 13-2). There may be cytologic atypia of keratinocytes, dyskeratosis, and loss of the rete ridge pattern. The dermis may be hyalinized and sclerotic. Dermal fibroblasts may exhibit variation in the size and tinctorial qualities of their nuclei (Fig. 13-3). Ectasia, proliferative changes, hyalinization of media, and occasional thrombosis of dermal vessels also may be present. Adnexal structures may be diminished or absent. With penetrating radiation, similar changes can be seen in the subcutis. Inflammatory infiltrates are variable and may be associated with dermal pigmentary alteration.

Differential Diagnosis   Histologically, radiation dermatitis will evoke a number of differential diagnostic paths depending on the specific findings in a specimen. Epidermal changes may suggest an interface

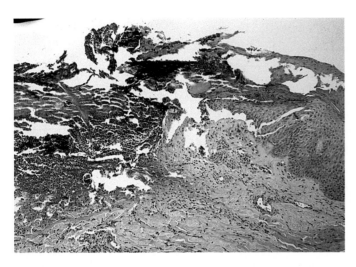

FIGURE 13-1 Decubitus ulcer. Ulcerated epidermis with impetiginized neutrophilic scale crust, underlying acute and chronic inflammation, and granulation tissue formation.

process, raising the possibility of cytotoxic effects from chemotherapy, burn injury, lupus erythematosus, lichen sclerosus, erythema multiforme, fixed drug eruption, acute graft-versus-host eruption, and dermatomyositis. Dermal changes raise the possibility of cicatrix, sclero-

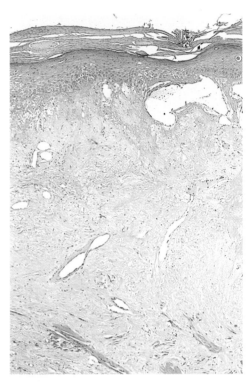

FIGURE 13-2 Chronic radiation dermatitis. Hyperkeratotic and parakeratotic epidermal hyperplasia with vacuolar interface change. Full-thickness dermal sclerosis with lymphatic dilation and loss of adnexa is characteristic.

derma, morphea, lichen sclerosus, and nonspecific sclerosis and fibrosis. The dermal changes in the late stages of burns may be indistinguishable from those in chronic radiation dermatitis, with the exception of "radiation fibroblasts." Markedly atypical dermal fibroblasts may raise the possibility of a neoplasia. In general, the array of histologic findings associated with biopsies of radiation change are sufficient to suggest the proper diagnosis.

TABLE 13-1

Radiation Dermatitis

Clinical Features

Acute
  Erythema
  Hair loss
  Vesicle formation
Chronic
  Atrophy
  Telangiectasia
  Pigmentary changes

Histopathological Features

Acute
  Spongiosis
  Epidermal necrosis
  Dermal edema
  Vascular ectasia and thrombosis
Chronic
  Epidermal hypoplasia and/or hyperplasia
  Squamous epithelial atypia
  Dermal sclerosis/hyalinization
  Deeply located elastotic material in dermis
  Loss of adnexae
  Bizarre "radiation fibroblasts"
  Hyalinization of vessel walls and thrombosis

Differential Diagnosis

Scar
Thermal burn
Lichen sclerosus
Morphea/scleroderma
Chronic graft-versus-host reaction

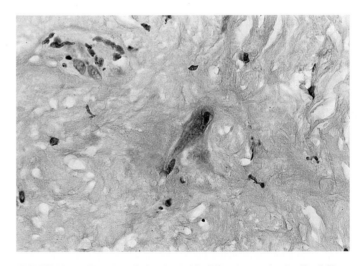

FIGURE 13-3 Chronic radiation dermatitis. Bizarre-appearing "stellate" fibroblast with features of radiation effect: pleomorphic hypochromatic nuclei, abundant cytoplasm, and intranuclear and intracytoplasmic vacuoles.

REACTIONS TO HEAT AND COLD

As an interface between the internal milieu and the environment, skin may be subjected to extreme conditions. Both thermal stress and electrical injury produce tissue damage. These external stresses have been studied in animal systems and the histologic changes associated with degree of damage identified.

Clinical Features   Thermal burns range in clinical appearance from faint erythema to vesiculation and necrosis (Table 13-2). Electrical injury produces three zones: a central zone of carbonization, a pale ischemic intermediate zone, and an erythematous peripheral zone. Cold injury presents in a similar fashion to thermal injury, the clinical lesion ranging from mild redness to vesiculation and necrosis. Chilblains (perniosis) are pruritic, burning, recurrent red vesicular or ulcerative patches or plaques that occur symmetrically in acral locations following exposure to cold or a drop in temperature. Lesions result from a spasm of dermal arterioles. The diagnosis is suggested by the temporal relationship between cool weather and symptom onset in patients without occlusive peripheral arterial disease. Spontaneous healing is common when spring arrives. Females are more commonly affected than males.

Histopathological Features   Mild thermal and cold injuries produce epidermal and dermal edema, vacuolated keratinocytes, and vascular dilatation with engorgement.[2] More severe injury leads to necrosis of keratinocytes, vesicle formation, dermal thrombosis, and hemorrhage. Traditionally, the extent (depth) of cutaneous injury following a burn has been categorized as first degree—predominantly epidermal damage only; second degree—both epidermal and partial dermal injury; or third degree—full-thickness necrosis of the epidermis and dermis. The histopathologic features of burns are highly dependent on the severity of the thermal insult. The changes vary from focal epidermal cell necrosis, vascular ectasia, and dermal edema to full-thickness necrosis of the dermis (Figs. 13-4 to 13-6). Second-degree burns are characterized by subepidermal vesicle and bullae formation. In third-degree burns, extensive necrosis of the dermis is present. Some lesions show carbonized debris. Severe burns may be associated with a "mummified" appearance of the dermis; the dermal collagen is subtly swollen and eosinophilic, and nuclei are lost. Diagnosis in such cases may not be possible by inspection of the dermis alone; however, necrosis of the overlying epidermis provides evidence of thermal injury. In lesions with significant inflammation, superinfection should be considered, and special stains for organisms should be obtained to evaluate this possibility.

Electrical injury produces vascular thrombosis in the intermediate and peripheral zones and necrosis in the central area. These changes vary in degree and depth depending on the severity of the electrical burn. Chilblains shows perivascular lymphoid infiltrates with edema and thickening of blood vessel walls.[3,4] However, published histologic descriptions of chilblains also include a lymphocytic vasculitis,[5] endothelial proliferation with necrosis,[6] and leukocytoclastic vasculitis.[7]

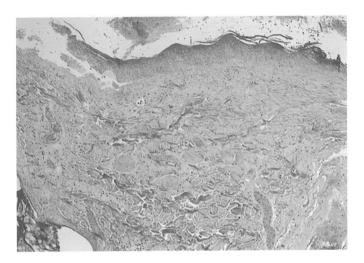

FIGURE 13-4   Partial-thickness thermal burn. Coagulative necrosis of epidermis and superficial dermis with focal involvement of superficial adnexa.

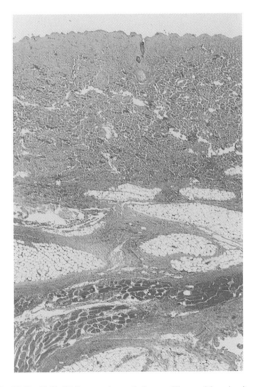

FIGURE 13-5   Full-thickness thermal burn. The epidermis is detached. Coagulative necrosis involves the entire dermis with extension into the subcutaneous adipose tissue and focally into underlying skeletal muscle.

TABLE 13-2

Thermal Burns

Clinical Features

Erythema
Vesiculation
Necrosis

Histopathological Features

Degree and thickness of injury are highly variable
Epidermal necrosis
Necrosis and "mummification" of dermis
Reepithelialization of epidermis in less severe burns

Differential Diagnosis

Cicatrix resulting from trauma or iatrogenic injury
Lichen sclerosus
Morphea/scleroderma
Radiation dermatitis

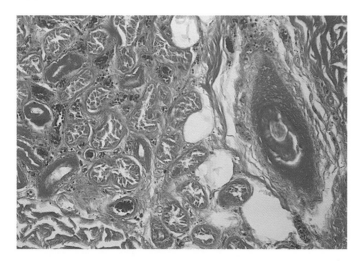

FIGURE 13-6   Necrotic hair follicle and eccrine glands in thermal burn.

Differential Diagnosis   The histologic features of thermal, electrical, and cold injury are similar and characterized by evidence of external trauma leading, if sufficiently severe, to vesiculation and necrosis. External trauma may be suggested in limited injuries by necrosis of keratinocytes limited to the outermost portions of the epidermis. The histologic picture of chilblains is not specific and is considered in the differential diagnosis of perivascular lymphoid infiltrates, although other patterns of inflammation also have been described.

REACTIONS TO LIGHT

Light-related eruptions offer a spectrum of clinical morphologies, etiologies, and histologic patterns. All require absorption of light energy. Recognized syndromes related to light exposure include phototoxic reactions (i.e., a photoactive chemical agent plus light), photoallergic reactions (i.e., an allergen that requires alteration by light to generate the antigen), and entities where the etiologic agent is unknown; however, light exposure is required for development (hydroa vacciniforme, polymorphous light eruption, actinic prurigo, chronic photodermatoses, persistent light reactions, photosensitive eczema, and actinic reticuloid).

Clinical Features   Clinical features of these light-related eruptions are listed in Table 13-3. Photoaccentuation of the exposed areas of the face, neck, chest, arms, and hands is most common. Phototoxic eruptions follow exposure to phototoxic chemicals that increase the skin's reactivity to light. If the concentration of the chemical is sufficient and the wavelength of the light appropriate, a sunburnlike reaction will ensue. Photoallergic reactions occur in sensitized persons, simulate contact dermatitis, and are characterized by redness, edema, and on occasion, vesiculation. Polymorphous light eruption is an acquired process in which skin lesions develop in exposed areas after ultraviolet light exposure. The eruption is frequently recurrent and usually resolves spontaneously. Hydroa vacciniforme primarily affects children, can be induced by ultraviolet A (UVA),[8-10] and heals with scarring. Actinic prurigo is an idiopathic familial photodermatosis in Native Americans.[11] The face is affected most commonly, and cheilitis occurs. Chronic photodermatoses or chronic actinic dermatitis is a poorly defined group in which there is a persistent eczematous eruption in the sun-exposed areas. Lim and coworkers[12] included as part of their defi-

nition the following: (1) present for greater than 3 months, (2) decreased minimal erythema dose to either UVA and/or ultraviolet B (UVB), and (3) histologic changes, including an infiltrate of lymphocytes and macrophages, with or without epidermal spongiosis and atypical mononuclear cells in the dermis and epidermis. Actinic reticuloid can be regarded as the most severe variant of chronic actinic dermatitis.[13] There may be multiple etiologies, including chronic contact dermatitis, photoallergic contact dermatitis, and phototoxic, immunologic, and other factors. A clinical diagnosis of actinic reticuloid should be made when the following criteria are present: (1) infiltrated papules and plaques extending to covered areas, sometimes erythroderma,[14] (2) a broad spectrum of photosensitivity, and (3) a dermal infiltrate containing atypical lymphoid cells.

Histopathological Features   There is an overlapping spectrum of histopathologic findings in light-related eruptions that precludes specific identification in many cases (see Table 13-3; see also Chap. 5). Photoallergic and phototoxic reactions may have similar histologies as may a variety of spongiotic processes not related to light exposure. In these cases, the most common pattern includes a component of epidermal change, usually including spongiosis. In severe phototoxic reactions, epidermal necrosis may be present. The dermal components of phototoxic and photoallergic dermatitis may be similar and are composed of perivascular lymphocytoid infiltrates with varying numbers of macrophages and other cell types. Photoallergic reactions, from topical or systemic agents, have histologic pictures similar to other spongiotic dermatitides. Hydroa vacciniforme is characterized by keratinocytic edema, spongiosis, and necrosis that may progress to panepidermal necrosis. There is a variable infiltrate of lymphocytes and mononuclear phagocytes that is occasionally associated with hemorrhage and vascular thrombosis. The histology of actinic prurigo includes spongiotic epidermal changes and a lymphocytoid perivascular infiltrate in the superficial dermis; the acute form is said to be indistinguishable from polymorphous light eruption. The chronic forms of actinic prurigo exhibit hyperkeratosis, acanthosis, and signs of tissue repair.[15] Chronic actinic dermatitis has a nonspecific pattern including a dermal perivascular and sometimes bandlike infiltrate of lymphocytes and macrophages, with or without epidermal spongiosis and atypical mononuclear cells in the dermis and epidermis.[12] Actinic reticuloid may have a pattern similar to chronic actinic dermatitis and, by definition, must have atypical lymphoid cells within the infiltrate. There is usually a prominent component of lichen simplex chronicus. Multinucleated giant cells often are noted in the papillary dermis but are in fact related to the lichen simplex chronicus and are nonspecific. Immunophenotyping of the infiltrate may show dominance of CD8+ cells.[13]

Differential Diagnosis   The differential diagnosis for this group lies primarily in the spectrum of either spongiotic or superficial dermal inflammatory processes. The spongiotic forms of light-related eruption are not histologically distinguishable from other forms of spongiotic dermatitis. Photo-related eruptions characterized by few epidermal changes and a well-defined cuffed lymphocytoid infiltrate need to be differentiated from superficial forms of gyrate erythema, dermal contact allergy, chilblains, and collagen vascular disease.

REACTIONS TO MARINE AGENTS

There is an endless array of potential interactions between the marine environment and skin. Possible reactions include granulomatous reactions to foreign materials such as sea urchin spines, envenomations, toxic exposures following discharge of nematocysts (Portuguese man-

TABLE 13-3

Reactions to Light

Disorder	Clinical Findings	Histopathological Features
Polymorphous light eruption	Acquired; recurrent; worse in spring and early summer; in sun-exposed areas hours to days after exposure; burning or pruritus; lesions vary from papules to plaques and vesicles	Spectrum of changes; epidermal changes ranging from minimal to spongiotic; dermal changes range from superficial and deep perivascular cuffed lymphocytoid patterns to polymorphous infiltrates with neutrophils and other cell types; prominent papillary dermal edema may be present
Photoallergic dermatitis	Acute or chronic papular and/or vesicular eruption following exposure to photosensitive agent and light; pruritic	Variable epidermal changes including edema and spongiosis; a superficial polymorphous infiltrate including lymphocytes, eosinophils, neutrophils, and edema
Hydroa vacciniforme	A chronic eruption with redness, vesicles, necrosis, and varicelliform scars generally in children; absence of laboratory abnormalities; eye involvement has been reported; resolves in adolescence	Intraepidermal reticular degeneration and cellular necrosis; spongiosis and epidermal necrosis with dense lymphohistiocytic infiltrates with hemorrhage and thrombosis of small vessels
Phototoxic eruption	Nonimmunologic; can be elicited in majority of persons exposed; redness, burning, edema in affected areas, possibly with vesiculation	Variable epidermal changes including edema and spongiosis; there is minimal inflammatory infiltrate; neutrophils may be present
Actinic prurigo	Familial in Native Americans; acute and chronic phases; eczematous; cheilitis and pruritus are common	Epidermal spongiosis with a superficial and deep lymphocytic perivascular infiltrate and dermal edema; chronic forms show hyperkeratosis, acanthosis, and signs of tissue repair
Chronic photodermatoses	Present for 3 months or longer; decreased MED to UVA, UVB, or both	A dermal infiltrate of lymphocytes and macrophages, with or without epidermal spongiosis and atypical mononuclear cells in the dermis and epidermis
Persistent light reaction	May be a form of photoallergic contact dermatitis; musk ambrette and oxybenzone are frequently implicated; the MED is shortened	The histology is that of a spongiotic dermatitis and similar to that seen in photoallergic and allergic contact dermatitis
Photosensitive eczema Actinic reticuloid	Severe variant of chronic actinic dermatitis; persistent infiltrated papules and plaques, often extending to covered areas; broad-banded photosensitivity; usually, a prominent component of lichen simplex chronicus is present	Usually, a prominent component of lichen simplex chronicus; dermal lymphoid infiltrate with atypical cells; CD8+ lymphoid cells dominate in the infiltrate; reversed CD4+ to CD8+ ratio in peripheral blood

of-war reactions), contact allergic dermatitis to many agents such as coral exposure, and infections. The clinical and histologic pictures will vary depending on the inciting agent.

Clinical Features   The clinical features of the most common marine reactions are presented in Table 13-4. Seabather's eruption is a highly pruritic eruption under swimwear that occurs after bathing in the ocean.[16] The average duration of the eruption and pruritus is 12.5 days. Cnidarian larvae of the thimble jellyfish, *Linuche unguiculata*, appear to be the cause. The problem occurs in sporadic epidemics. Reaction to the coelenterate, *Physalia physalis*, is a common medical problem.[17] Contact with humans results in extrusion of nematocysts from tentacles that adhere to the skin and inject toxin. Acute lesions are painful, red, and edematous. The linear array of lesions marks the path of the tentacle. The lesions may resolve with hyperpigmentation. Swimmer's itch affects exposed parts and is produced by cutaneous penetration by shistosomal cercariae.[18] The lesions are transient urticarial lesions that evolve into pruritic papules. A wide array of additional potential reactions can follow exposure to venomous marine agents; however, histologies of these reactions have been poorly documented. Contact aller-

gic dermatitis may follow exposure to a coral and many other marine substances.

Histopathological Features   Histopathologic changes of seabather's eruption include a dermal infiltrate around superficial and deep vessels composed of lymphocytes, neutrophils, and eosinophils. The histopathology of sea urchin spine penetration is that of a polymorphous inflammatory infiltrate coupled with a foreign-body granulomatous tissue reaction. The mixed infiltrate may contain neutrophils, occasional eosinophils and plasma cells, lymphocytoid cells, and mononuclear phagocytes. Prominent edema and hemorrhage may be present. Foreign-body-type giant cells and foreign material also may be present. Portuguese man-of-war stings exhibit vascular dilatation, hemorrhage, and a lymphocytoid infiltrate. Nematocysts are found rarely in the stratum corneum. The pathologic changes of swimmer's itch include dermal edema and a polymorphous infiltrate containing eosinophils.[18]

Differential Diagnosis   Seabather's eruption, swimmer's itch, and envenomation can produce nonspecific histologic features characterized by polymorphous inflammation. The presence of exogenous material,

TABLE 13-4

Reactions to Marine Agents

Disorder	Etiology	Clinical Features	Histopathological Features
Seabather's eruption	Cnidarian larvae of the thimble jellyfish, *Linuche unguiculata*	Confined to bathing suit areas; chills and fever may be present; erythema, macules, and papules may be present	There is a superficial and deep perivascular infiltrate of lymphocytes, neutrophils, and eosinophils
Sea urchin spines	Penetration by the spines of the sea urchin (Echinoidea).	There is immediate burning pain and bleeding, variable swelling, and tender red swollen papules and nodules at site of penetration; delayed reactions can follow 2–4 months after injury	Polymorphous inflammation with foreign-body granuloma; foreign material may be identified; a wide spectrum of pathologies, including sarcoidal granulomas
Portuguese man-of-war	*Physalia physalis*	At points of contact, there is burning, pain, redness, and whealing; systemic signs also may be present	Nematocysts may be present in the stratum corneum; superficial vascular dilatation, focal hemorrhage, and lymphocytoid infiltrate
Swimmer's itch	Cercariae of avian and mammalian forms of *Trichobilharzia*	Itching as water evaporates; urticarial reaction progresses to itchy papules	Dermal edema with a polymorphous infiltrate containing eosinophils

e.g., a portion of nematocyst or sea urchin spine, coupled with the appropriate history, leads to the correct association. In these cases, the history is the most important factor to narrow the histologic differential diagnosis. The histopathologic features of contact allergic dermatitis as from coral exposure (Fig. 13-7) are nonspecific and include spongiotic dermatitis with dermal perivascular lymphocytic infiltrates usually containing eosinophils (see Chap. 2).

REACTIONS TO ARACHNIDS

There are three orders of arachnids that can produce cutaneous reactions; they are spiders, scorpions, and ticks and mites. These organisms are distinct from insects in that they do not have wings or antennae and the body is not divided into distinct segments.

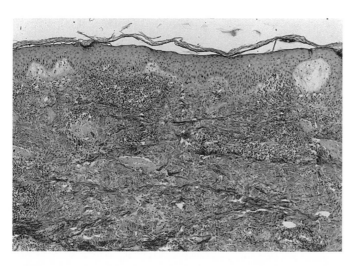

FIGURE 13-7   Coral dermatitis. There is a spongiotic dermatitis with papillary dermal edema, subepidermal blister formation, and a cuffed perivascular lymphocytic infiltrate. Some cases exhibit numerous eosinophils.

Clinical Features   The constellation of signs and symptoms that follows spider bite is called *arachnidism*. In the United States, arachnidism most often follows the bite of either the black widow spider (*Latrodectus mactans*) or the loxoscelese (brown recluse) spider (*Loxosceles reclusa*). In general, redness develops rapidly around the bite site, and there is pain. Tissue injury is usually trivial; however, it can progress to induration and necrosis.[19,20] Systemic signs such as nausea, fever, and vomiting may be present. Scorpions carry a venom apparatus in their tails. There is rapid onset of local burning pain and induration. Local tissue necrosis may follow. Systemic signs and symptoms include diaphoresis, vomiting, and nausea. Tick bite reactions follow implantation of an ectoparasite of the Ixodoidea superfamily.[21,22] There are two family groups: soft-bodied ticks and hard-bodied ticks. The species of tick will vary based on geographic and exposure characteristics. The tissue reaction to implantation represents response to salivary materials secreted by the tick after implantation. Included in the salivary material is an adhesive that cements the mouthpart to the tissue. Attachment sites are edematous and erythematous. Persistent inflammatory reactions can remain at attachment sites. Mites, from a variety of families, are capable of producing dermatitis by biting and sensitizing their targets. Baker's itch, grocer's itch, copra itch, and other colorful names have been applied to the clinical syndrome that follows the bite of a mite.[23] Diagnosis is made by recognition of the proper occupational exposure that explains the distribution. *Cheyletiella* dermatitis is an infrequently reported eruption caused by an ectoparasite, *Cheyletiella*, whose normal hosts are household pets.[24,25] Because the mites do not remain on human skin, support for the diagnosis is obtained by identification of mites detected on the patient's pet. Trombiculid mites, known as chiggers, feed on humans only in their larval stage. The larvae, which are very small, attach to a host and seek a soft area, constricted by clothing in humans. The lesion is a macule that evolves into a pruritic red papule, and some lesions may vesiculate.

Histopathological Features   The histopathologic changes that follow spider bite are those of an infarct with thrombosis, vascular injury, hemorrhage, necrosis, and inflammation. Often there is a superficial and deep perivascular and interstitial infiltrate containing lymphocytes and

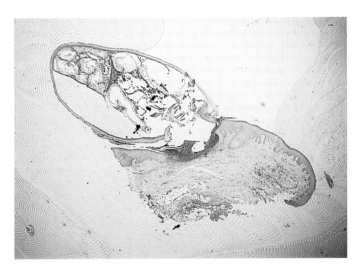

FIGURE 13-8   Tick body still attached to epidermis.

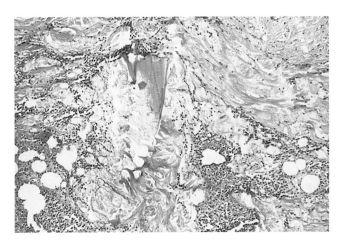

FIGURE 13-10   Tick mouthpart. Refractile mouthparts are embedded in the superficial dermis. There is an associated marked lymphoeosinophilic infiltrate and reactive fibrosis.

neutrophils with variable numbers of eosinophils. Reparative changes are seen during resolution of the injury. The histopathology of a tick attachment site may include sections through the attached ectoparasite (Figs. 13-8 to 13-10). There are varying degrees of spongiosis, dermal edema, and a superficial and deep intense infiltrate containing a polymorphous infiltrate including eosinophils and hemorrhage. Mast cells may be increased.[21] Epidermal hyperplasia and chronic dense lymphocytoid infiltrates may persist at the attachment site.[22]

Differential Diagnosis   Spider bites need to be separated from the large spectrum of causes associated with focal necrosis, including infections, pyoderma gangrenosum, vasculitides, trauma, and thrombotic or embolic causes.

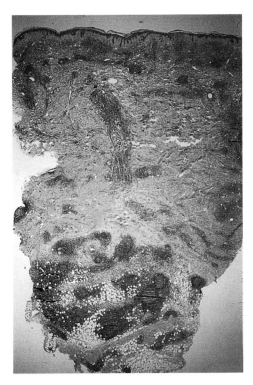

FIGURE 13-9   Tick bite reaction. Dense, superficial and deep, perivascular and periadnexal, lymphohistiocytic infiltrate with scattered eosinophils. This process extends deeply into the lobular panniculus and shows prominent germinal center formation.

REACTIONS TO INSECTS

The outcome of an insect bite is usually trivial; however, occasionally bites result in clinically significant reactions. The mosquito bite is the most common clinical lesion. It follows contact with a female mosquito whose mouth parts have penetrated into the dermis, where a complex array of foreign material in saliva is deposited. A variety of biochemical reactions ensues, including local anticoagulation, protease release, and cellular infiltration. The type and degree of tissue reaction depend on the immunologic state of the individual. Pediculosis is produced by infestation with either of two species, *Phthirus pubis* or *Pediculus humanus*. *P. humanus* exists as either the body louse or the head louse. Bed bugs are members of the family Cimicidae and are blood-sucking insects about 3 to 4 mm in size. The bed bug emerges from crevices in floors, walls, and furniture to feed in darkness. They are attracted to the body temperature of the host, feed for several minutes, and then depart. A variety of species of Cimicidae will attack humans. Myiasis is the infestation by larvae of Diptera. There are numerous genera capable of producing myiasis in humans, including *Dermatobia*, *Callitroga*, *Chrysomyia*, *Cordylobia*, and *Wohlfahrtia*. Tungiasis is caused by infestation of the skin by a fertilized female sand flea, *Tunga penetrans*.

Clinical Features   Infestation with either the head or body louse produces pruritus. Secondary changes from excoriation are common. There may be matting of hair and secondary infection. Diagnosis of head lice is made by identifying the oval egg capsules attached to hair shafts. Mobile head lice are seen frequently. The bite site of the body louse is macular and red. Persistent wheals and papules may develop. Eggs are laid in clothing, and infestation is transmitted by clothing and bedding. Diagnosis is made by identifying lice and their eggs in the seams of clothing. Pubic lice produce a blue-gray macular lesion on the lower abdomen and upper thighs. Secondary infection may be present. Cutaneous myiasis occurs on exposed skin. The skin lesions are either furuncular or form a tortuous red line of papules and vesicles if the lesions are clinically creeping eruption. Flea bites in a sensitized person produce a pruritic papule. Lesions may be clustered and rarely bullous. The sand flea, *T. penetrans*, generally penetrates the skin on the toes or between the toes. The flea appears initially as a black dot; eventually, inflammation and pustules develop.

Insect bite reactions span a wide spectrum—depending on the immune status of the host and the type and contents of the bite. The insect inserts its proboscis and releases salivary material into the dermis. In this mixture are proteases, ATPases, anticoagulants, and other materials—all of which may serve as antigenic and/or locally destructive agents. The range of clinical reactions extends from little or no response to the first exposure to intense inflammation with associated clinical signs and symptoms. For the most part, pruritus is the chief symptom. Lesions generally are papular but also can be vesicular. Because of trauma, the lesions may be excoriated and covered by crust.

Histopathological Features   The histopathology of all these clinical lesions almost always contains superficial and middermal to deep inflammation with varying degrees of edema. The infiltrate often has a predominately perivascular and wedge-shaped pattern with extension into the deep dermis. The components of the infiltrate may vary; however, the presence of eosinophils, particularly in an interstitial pattern, is a strongly suggestive feature. Neutrophils, lymphocytes, and other forms also may be present. If the biopsy sections are taken in the vicinity of mouthpart penetration, there will be a vertical area of amphophilic tissue necrosis extending through the epidermis for a variable distance into the dermis. Necrotic inflammatory cells and hemorrhage also may be present in this area. Epidermal changes are variable and range from intraepidermal vesicle formation to minimal acanthosis. Most reactions have some degree of epidermal spongiosis, occasionally with exocytosis of eosinophils (eosinophilic spongiosis). Rarely, there will be both intraepidermal and subepidermal vesicle formation simultaneously in the same section; this is a strongly supportive finding for an insect bite reaction. The histology of tungiasis may contain portions of the ectoparasite surrounded by a dense polymorphous host response and with epidermal spongiosis and acanthosis.

Differential Diagnosis   Because these reactions represent response to a potpourri of toxic and immunologic stimuli, the possible histologic diagnoses are legion. Generally, the depth of the pattern, coupled with the presence of eosinophils, is suggestive of insect bite reaction, but do not exclude other forms of hypersensitivity reactions.

REFERENCES

1. LeBoit PE: Subacute radiation dermatitis: A histologic imitator of acute cutaneous graft-versus-host disease. *J Am Acad Dermatol* 20:236–241, 1989.
2. Schoning P: Frozen cadaver: Antemortem versus postmortem. *Am J Forensic Med Pathol* 13:18–20, 1992.
3. Vayssairat M: Chilblains. *J Mal Vasc* 17:229–231, 1992.
4. Wall LM, Smith NP: Perniosis: A histopathologic review. *Clin Exp Dermatol* 6:263–271, 1981.
5. Herman EW, Kezis JS, Silvers DN: A distinctive variant of pernio. *Arch Dermatol* 117:26–28, 1981.
6. McGovern T, Wright IS, Kruger E: Pernio: A vascular disease. *Am Heart J* 22:583–606, 1941.
7. Klapman MH, Johnston WH: Localized recurrent postoperative pernio associated with leukocytoclastic vasculitis. *J Am Acad Dermatol* 24:811–813, 1991.
8. Halasz CLG, Leach EE, Walther RR, et al: Hydroa vacciniforme: Induction of lesions with ultraviolet A. *J Am Acad Dermatol* 8:171–176, 1983.
9. Leenutaphong V: Hydroa vacciniforme: An unusual clinical manifestation. *J Am Acad Dermatol* 25:892–895, 1991.
10. Goldgeier MH, Nordlund JJ, Lucky AW, et al: Hydroa vacciniforme: Diagnosis and Therapy. *Arch Dermatol* 118:588–591, 1982.
11. Lane PR, Hogan DJ, Martel MJ, et al: Actinic prurigo: Clinical features and prognosis. *J Am Acad Dermatol* 26:683–692, 1992.
12. Lim HW, Morison WL, Kamide R, et al: Chronic actinic dermatitis: An analysis of 51 patients evaluated in the United States and Japan. *Arch Dermatol* 130:1284–1289, 1994.
13. Toonstra J: Actinic reticuloid. *Semin Diagn Pathol* 8:109–116, 1991.
14. Healy E, Rogers S: Photosensitivity dermatitis/actinic reticuloid syndrome in an Irish population: A review and some unusual features. *Acta Derm Venereol (Stockh)* 75: 72–74, 1995.
15. Lane PR, Murphy F, Hogan DJ, et al: Histopathology of actinic prurigo. *Am J Dermatopathol* 15:326–331, 1993.
16. Wong DE, Meinking TL, Rosen LB, et al: Seabather's eruption: Clinical, histologic and immunologic features. *J Am Acad Dermatol* 30:399–406, 1994.
17. Ioannides G, Davis JH: Portuguese man-of-war stings. *Arch Dermatol* 91:488–451, 1965.
18. Brackett S: Pathology of schistosome dermatitis. *Arch Dermatol Syphilol* 42:410–418, 1940.
19. Norment BR, Foil LD: Histopathology and physiological action of venom from the brown recluse spider, *Loxosceles reclusa. Toxicon* 17(suppl 1):131, 1979.
20. Pucevich MV, McChesney T: Histopathologic analysis of human bites by the brown recluse spider. *Arch Dermatol* 119:851, 1983.
21. Winer LH, Strakosch EA: Tick bites: *Dermacentor variabilis* (Say). *J Invest Dermatol* 4:249, 1941.
22. Goldman L: Tick bite granuloma: Failure of prevention of lesion by excision of tick bite area. *Am J Trop Med Hyg* 12:246, 1963.
23. Krinsky W: Dermatoses associated with the bites of mites and ticks (Arthroposi: *Acari*). *Int J Dermatol* 22:75–91, 1983.
24. Rivers JK, Martin J, Pukay B: Walking dandruff and *Cheyletiella* dermatitis. *J Am Acad Dermatol* 1130–1133, 1986.
25. Lee BW: *Cheyletiella* dermatitis. *Arch Dermatol* 117:677–678, 1981.

PART TWO

PREDOMINANTLY NON-INFLAMMATORY CONDITIONS

CHAPTER 14

ALTERATIONS OF THE STRATUM CORNEUM AND EPIDERMIS

Michael W. Piepkorn / Philip Fleckman

An exceptionally diverse group of disorders that are both heterogeneous in their genetic basis and pleiotropic in their phenotypic expression can be assembled under the general category of alterations of the stratum corneum and epidermis. These disorders reflect a wide range of acquired and hereditary pathologic processes. Two distinct themes, however, unite many of the entities described here. One common pathophysiologic feature reflects defects in the keratinization process that manifest clinicopathologically as ichthyoses; the other feature involves molecular defects in keratin genes and other genes yet to be determined that confer defective epidermal integrity and that present clinically as the mechanobullous disorders.

Many of the disorders discussed here, particularly the ichthyoses, have similar microscopic features, which complicates the histopathologic differential diagnosis and highlights the importance of clinical correlation. Accurate diagnosis may also involve special procedures, including immunocytochemistry. Indeed, for the hereditary cytolytic (mechanobullous) disorders, immunolabeling of basement membrane components and/or electron microscopy to delineate the level of the separation within the tissue is necessary for adequate diagnosis. The histopathologic algorithms offered here, therefore, can only serve in many situations to resolve the differential diagnosis to a limited level, beyond which one must resort to supplemental strategies.

The organization of this chapter follows the two major schemata of defects in the process of keratinization and defective epidermal integrity often due to mutations in keratin genes. Pathways for differential diagnosis of the nonbullous ichthyoses are discussed first, followed by disorders with epidermolytic change.

HYPERKERATOSIS WITHOUT EPIDERMOLYTIC CHANGE: THE NONBULLOUS ICHTHYOSES AND RELATED DISORDERS

The designation *ichthyosis* is fundamentally a descriptive term covering a variety of keratinization disorders that are usually genetic in nature. All share the common feature of scaling skin, which is usually generalized, but, as in the instances of the palmoplantar keratodermas and the erythrokeratodermas, can be localized. This section covers those disorders with significant hyperkeratosis due to defective keratinization but with no cytolytic (epidermolytic) alterations. The organization of these hyperkeratotic disorders, which has been adapted from the work of Traupe,[1] follows the diagnostic algorithm presented in Fig. 14-1. This scheme focuses initial attention on whether the predominant mode of keratinization is ortho- or parakeratotic and then on the morphologic

status of the stratum granulosum. The features that assist with the differential diagnosis of the entities are summarized in Table 14-1.

Disorders with Hyperorthokeratosis and Reduced-to-Absent Stratum Granulosum

The following entities share the common features of hyperorthokeratosis and a general thinning or absence of the stratum granulosum.

ICHTHYOSIS VULGARIS

Ichthyosis vulgaris was first delineated from X-linked recessive ichthyosis, the other common form of ichthyosis, in the 1960s by Wells and coworkers on the basis of inheritance and clinical appearance.[2,3] The disorder is the most common ichthyosis, with an estimated prevalence of between 1 in 250 and 1 in 5300.[2] Ichthyosis vulgaris is inherited as an autosomal dominant trait. Granular layer abnormalities by microscopic examination have led to investigations of the role of profilaggrin, the predominant keratohyalin protein in human epidermis, in ichthyosis vulgaris. Profilaggrin expression in affected epidermis is decreased or absent, depending on disease severity.[4] A subset of individuals with the clinical findings of ichthyosis vulgaris and with no granular layer has been identified (Fleckman, Brumbaugh, submitted); keratinocytes cultured from such individuals have very little detectable profilaggrin protein, and profilaggrin mRNA level is reduced by approximately one-half in these cells. A posttranscriptional defect in which profilaggrin mRNA half-life is reduced appears responsible for the changes.[5]

Clinical Features The disorder manifests early in life, usually within the first year, but is rarely present at birth (Table 14-2). Fine, white scales are found on the trunk and extensor surfaces of the extremities, in association with superficial fissuring in severe cases. The central face and cheeks may be involved, but the sides of the neck are almost always spared. The condition is associated with the atopic diathesis and with keratosis pilaris. Hyperlinearity and chafing of the palms and soles are often present, although whether this is linked to the atopy or the ichthyosis is disputed. Because of the overlap in clinical phenotype, ichthyosis vulgaris and X-linked recessive ichthyosis are often confused clinically; the usual mistake in diagnosis is labeling X-linked recessive ichthyosis as ichthyosis vulgaris.[6] Assay for reduced levels of steroid sulfatase activity, however, can currently be used to confirm the diagnosis of X-linked recessive ichthyosis.

FIGURE 14-1

Hyperkeratosis without Epidermolytic Change: The Nonbullous Ichthyoses and Related Disorders: Diagnostic Algorithm

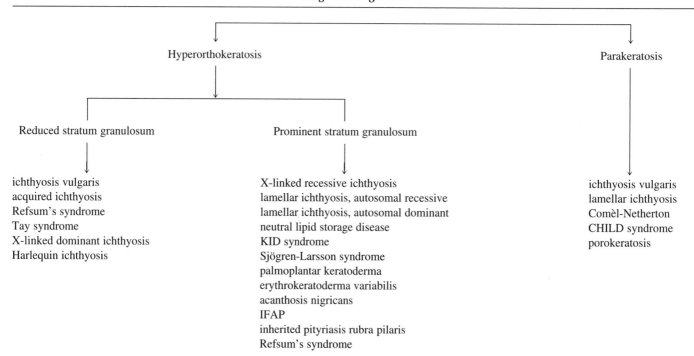

FIGURE 14-1   Hyperkeratosis without epidermolytic change: Diagnostic algorithm for the nonbullous ichthyoses and related disorders. The pathway for differential diagnosis is dichotomized on the preponderant mode of hyperkeratosis, whether ortho- or parakeratotic, and, if the former, whether the stratum granulosum is reduced or retained

Histopathological Features   Microscopic examination of the stratum corneum in ichthyosis vulgaris reveals compact hyperorthokeratosis.[1,7] The degree of hyperkeratosis varies from mild to moderate. This alteration is associated with a uniformly reduced granular layer that is absent in at least some foci (Figure 14-2). Parakeratosis is generally not observed. Follicular dilatation and hyperkeratosis are regularly present. The epidermis is usually found to be of normal thickness,[7] but on occasion there can be acanthosis or even atrophy. The rete ridge pattern is not accentuated. Sebaceous glands are atrophic. No or slight perivascular inflammation is found in the papillary dermis.

Differential Diagnosis   The differential diagnosis may include lamellar ichthyosis and X-linked recessive ichthyosis in cases where the granular layer is not especially thinned. However, the usual case will manifest an absent, or at least clearly thinned, granular layer. Keratohyalin granules appear crumbly or degenerated when viewed by electron microscopy, allowing distinction from the other ichthyoses in which the granular layer is thinned. In the differential diagnosis of nonbullous ichthyosis with reduced granular layer, many of the remaining disorders, such as Refsum's disease and X-linked dominant ichthyosis,[1] are syndromes in which the ichthyotic change is one component associated with other signs and symptoms in a recognizable pattern that collectively allows assignment of the diagnosis (see below). The diagnostic consideration of an acquired ichthyosis is discussed below.

ACQUIRED ICHTHYOSIS

Acquired ichthyosis has been described in association with a number of systemic disorders (including thyroid disease, sarcoidosis, systemic lupus erythematosus, and malnutrition), drugs, and malignancies.[8]

Although solid tumors have rarely been found,[9] lymphoproliferative disorders, particularly Hodgkin's disease, prevail. Speculation regarding the possible role of vitamin A deficiency caused by liver involvement or malabsorption has not been substantiated. Thus, the causes of acquired ichthyosis are unknown.

Clinical Features   The clinical findings are reported to resemble those of ichthyosis vulgaris, although large, platelike or hyperpigmented scales are sometimes observed. Hyperlinearity of the palms and soles is not a feature, but palmoplantar keratoderma has been described.[8]

Histopathological Features   The histologic pattern also resembles that of ichthyosis vulgaris, with hyperorthokeratosis, compaction of the stratum corneum, and thinning of the granular layer in some cases. No cases of a totally absent granular layer have been reported, and staining with antiprofilaggrin-filaggrin antibody in two cases has demonstrated the presence of profilaggrin-filaggrin (Dale BA and Fleckman P, unpublished).

Differential Diagnosis   Clinicopathologic overlap exists among ichthyosis vulgaris, acquired ichthyosis, and dry skin (xerosis). Distinction between ichthyosis vulgaris and acquired ichthyosis is essentially founded on the clinical history and physical findings. Xerosis is poorly understood and loosely defined; other than an association with winter weather and aging, few distinguishing features are present. The distinction of the dry skin seen in atopic eczema from ichthyosis vulgaris has been made on the basis of other clinical findings associated with the two disorders and appears distinct histologically.[10]

TABLE 14-1

Differential Diagnosis for Nonbullous Ichthyoses and Related Disorders

	Histologic Feature					
	Hyper-keratosis	Acanthosis	Follicular keratosis	Spongiosis	Peri-vascular infiltrates	Other
Disorders with hyperorthokeratosis and reduced granular layer						
Ichthyosis vulgaris	+−++	0	+	0	0−+	
Refsum's syndrome	+	0−+	0	0	0	Vacuolized keratinocytes
Tay syndrome	+−++	+	0	0	+	
X-linked dominant ichthyosis	+−++	+−++	+−++	+	+−++	Follicular atrophoderma (late)
Harlequin ichthyosis	+++	+	+	0	+	Parakeratosis (some cases)
Disorders with hyperorthokeratosis and normal to thickened granular layer						
X-linked recessive ichthyosis	+−++	+	0−+	0	+−++	
Lamellar ichthyosis	+	+	+	0	+	
Dorfman's syndrome	+	+	+	+	+	Foamy kera-tinocytes
KID syndrome	+−++	Variable	+−++	0	Variable	
Sjögren-Larsson syndrome	+−++	0−+	+	+	+	
Palmoplantar keratoderma	++	+	−	0	+	Keratolysis, in some cases
Erythrokeratoderma variabilis	+	++	−	Variable	+−++	
IFAP syndrome	++	0	++	−	+	Follicular atrophy
Pityriasis ruba pilaris	++− +++	++	++	0	+	Alternating parakeratosis
Disorders with hyperparakeratosis						
CHILD syndrome	+−++	+	0	0	0−+	
Comèl-Netherton syndrome	++− +++	+−++	0	+	++	PAS-positive debris & neutrophils in corneum

REFSUM'S SYNDROME (HEREDOPATHIA ATACTICA POLYNEURITIFORMIS)

Refsum's syndrome is an uncommon disorder affecting eye, nervous system, and skin.[11] The condition is inherited as an autosomal recessive trait. Accumulation of phytanic acid from chlorophyll results in altered epidermal metabolism, with an increased thymidine-labeling index, increased incorporation of precursors into DNA and protein, and altered lipid metabolism.[12] How accumulation of the long-chain, branched fatty acid effects such changes is unclear. The underlying defect lies in the alpha-oxidation of phytanic acid.[13]

Clinical Features   Refsum's syndrome initially presents with night blindness caused by retinal degeneration. Sequential involvement with relapsing peripheral neuropathy, cerebellar ataxia, cataracts, and nerve deafness is seen.[14] Skin changes occur after the eye and neurologic

TABLE 14-2

Ichthyosis Vulgaris

Clinical Features
Onset within first year
Fine, white scales, trunk and extensor extremities, sparing sides of neck and flexural areas
Hyperlinearity and chafing of the palms and soles
Association with atopy and keratosis pilaris

Histopathological Features
Compact hyperorthokeratosis, mild to moderate in extent
Diminished to absent stratum granulosum
Follicular dilatation and hyperkeratosis
Epidermis usually of normal thickness

Differential Diagnosis
Acquired ichthyosis
Xerosis
Syndromes with associated ichthyosis: Refsum's, ichthyosis and trichothiodystrophy, X-linked dominant ichthyosis with chondrodysplasia punctata

---

changes and vary from mild scaling of the palms and soles to widespread, severe scaling resembling lamellar ichthyosis.[1]

Histopathological Features The stratum corneum exhibits slight hyperorthokeratosis, which is associated with a thinned to normal granular layer. There may be slight acanthosis. Vacuolization of basal and suprabasal keratinocytes, due to lipid accumulation with phytanic acid, may not be evident by routine histologic examination but will be shown with histochemical lipid stains such as Sudan red.

Differential Diagnosis The routine histopathologic findings will resemble those of ichthyosis vulgaris and related disorders. The accumulation of phytanic acid within keratinocytes and other cutaneous cells such as melanocytes, however, is the hallmark of the disorder and can be demonstrated by lipid staining. The presence of elevated phytanic acid levels will serve to discriminate Refsum's disease from most other ichthyoses with similar histologic features, although neutral lipid storage disease will show similar lipid accumulations.

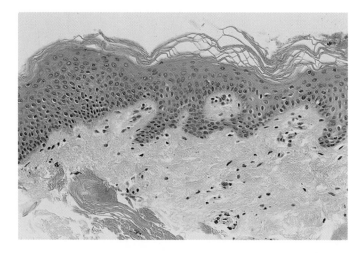

FIGURE 14-2 Ichthyosis vulgaris. A moderately hyperorthokeratotic stratum corneum overlies a mildly acanthotic spinous layer, without an intervening stratum granulosum.

SYNDROMES OF ICHTHYOSIS AND TRICHOTHIODYSTROPHY— TAY SYNDROME, BIDS, IBIDS, PIBI(D)S

The syndromes of ichthyosis and trichothiodystrophy, including BIDS (brittle hair, impaired intelligence, decreased fertility, short stature), IBIDS (ichthyosis, brittle hair, impaired intelligence, decreased fertility, short stature), and PIBI(D)S (photosensitivity, ichthyosis, brittle sulfur-deficient hair, impaired intelligence, decreased fertility, short stature), are a heterogeneous group with no firm criteria allowing for absolute categorization.[1] All are thought to be inherited as autosomal recessive traits. The defect is unknown, although cystine content of hair is decreased, and one subset, those with photosensitivity [PIBI(D)S], is linked to xeroderma pigmentosum complementation group D.

Clinical Features The syndromes have in common the features of ichthyosis, brittle hair, and short stature. The ichthyosis varies from mild to severe congenital erythroderma with collodion membrane, which evolves to more platelike scaling with little erythema, similar to lamellar ichthyosis. The hair is often fractured, with varied microscopic findings and characteristic banding when viewed with polarized light; cystine and proline content are reduced. Additional findings include psychomotor and mental retardation and unusual sociability. Photosensitivity with abnormal DNA excision repair and retarded sexual development with decreased fertility are variable findings.

Histopathological Features Microscopic sections of skin show moderate hyperorthokeratosis and thinning of the granular layer.[1] The spinous layer is moderately acanthotic and mildly papillomatous. There is slight perivascular lymphocytic inflammation within the papillary dermis.

Differential Diagnosis The histopathologic findings are nonspecific and similar to those of autosomal dominant ichthyosis vulgaris and related conditions. Although the differential diagnosis may not be resolvable by the cutaneous histopathology, microscopic examination of hair will show trichoschisis (transverse breaks), and polarized light reveals alternating (tigertail) light and dark bands.

X-LINKED DOMINANT ICHTHYOSIS WITH CHONDRODYSPLASIA PUNCTATA (CONRADI-HÜNERMANN SYNDROME)

This uncommon disorder is inherited as an X-linked dominant trait. An autosomal recessive form with more severe involvement has also been described, but the skin findings have not been reported. An autosomal dominant form without skin changes is postulated. A defect in peroxisomes or other cellular organelles may underlie the X-linked dominant form.[15]

Clinical Features Generalized ichthyosiform erythroderma with linear areas of thickened hyperkeratosis are seen in the X-linked dominant form.[1] The erythema resolves within weeks to months, leaving atrophic follicular involvement, ichthyosis, and hyperpigmentation following the lines of Blaschko. Patchy areas of cicatricial alopecia with nonspecific microscopic hair shaft abnormalities, sparse eyebrows and eyelashes, and nail dystrophy are also seen. Cataracts and skeletal defects are additional components of the Conradi-Hünermann syndrome.

Histopathological Features In this disorder, moderate hyperorthokeratosis is associated with a thinned granular layer and slight acanthosis.[16] A mild perivascular lymphocytic infiltrate may be present in the papillary dermis. Prominent follicular hyperkeratosis is found in young patients, with late follicular atrophoderma in adults. Some reports have suggested the presence of a variable neutrophilic reaction in the epidermis.

Differential Diagnosis   The findings are those of disorders sharing the histologic phenotype of autosomal dominant ichthyosis vulgaris. The differential diagnosis in suspected cases can be resolved by identification of the other components of the syndrome, particularly chondrodysplasia punctata, supplemented by special histologic studies. Mainly, the latter rests with the demonstration of calcium within the epidermis by von Kossa's stain. Reduced density of epidermal Langerhans' cells can also be shown by immunostaining with specific markers. A vacuolated granular layer may also be observed, along with spicules, by electron microscopic examination. All these findings, however, are seen early in the course of the disease and may resolve over time, leaving the residual, linear areas of pigmentary change, follicular atrophoderma, and cicatricial alopecia with no characteristic histologic features.

HARLEQUIN ICHTHYOSIS

Harlequin ichthyosis is a rare keratinizing disorder thought to be variously inherited as an autosomal recessive trait or a new dominant mutation.[17] The disorder is phenotypically heterogeneous.[18] The defects underlying the different histologic and biochemical phenotypes are unknown, but abnormal lamellar granules and absent filaggrin protein have been observed in all forms, and etiologic defects in epidermal protein phosphatases have been postulated.[17]

Clinical Features   The condition is the most severe of the congenital ichthyoses. Newborns are incarcerated in a massively thick, platelike scale affecting the entire integument, which produces ectropion and eclabium, restricts respiration and feeding, and alters development of the ears, nose, eyes, and mouth. The cuirass cracks soon after birth, resulting in deep fissures in geometric patterns. Death often ensues. If the affected infant survives beyond the newborn period, the phenotype evolves into that of a severe nonbullous congenital erythroderma.

Histopathological Features   The histologic pattern in Harlequin ichthyosis varies between reports, which probably reflects genetic heterogeneity.[17,18] Across all categories, however, there is massive compact hyperorthokeratosis, creating a stratum corneum that is much thicker than the spinous layer (Fig. 14-3). Changes in the granular layer are variable. This zone is usually thinned, with keratohyalin granules either reduced in density or totally absent, but it may be normal.[17,18] The follicles are dilated and hyperkeratotic. Inconstant and less striking changes include mild acanthosis and papillomatosis. Pronounced parakeratosis can be observed in patients who completely lack keratohyalin granules. A superficial perivascular lymphocytic infiltrate is an inconstant feature.

Differential Diagnosis   The massive hyperorthokeratosis is distinctive and not simulated as a rule by any of the other ichthyoses. Clinical correlation will, of course, resolve histologic ambiguities, if any, because of the distinctive clinical phenotype.

Disorders with Hyperorthokeratosis and Prominent Stratum Granulosum

A separate pathway of differential diagnosis is suggested when histologic examination indicates a normal to expanded stratum granulosum (Fig. 14-1). The prototypes for these disorders are X-linked recessive ichthyosis and the lamellar ichthyoses. These and most of the other entities included here look alike histologically. In addition, a number of multisystem syndromes enter the differential diagnosis, wherein the specific diagnosis is made by the corresponding clinical context.

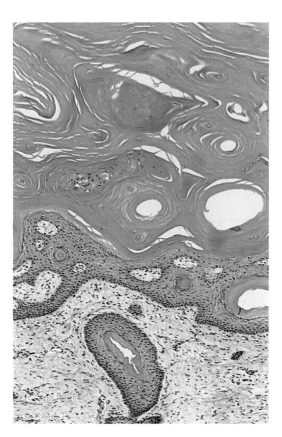

FIGURE 14-3   Harlequin ichthyosis. There is massive orthokeratotic thickening of the stratum corneum, in association with a thinned stratum granulosum and a spinous layer that is mildly acanthotic and papillomatous. The follicular ostia are dilated and plugged with keratin.

X-LINKED RECESSIVE ICHTHYOSIS

X-linked recessive ichthyosis is the second "common" ichthyosis (ichthyosis vulgaris being the other). Distinction between the two was clarified by Wells, Kerr, and coworkers on the basis of inheritance,[2] clinical findings,[19] and histology.[3] However, definitive diagnosis depends on steroid sulfatase determination, as the two disorders may be confused clinically in 10 to 15 percent of cases.[6] The disorder occurs in between 1 out of 4152 and 1 out of 9500 individuals.[2,20] Mutations (most commonly complete gene deletions) in the steroid sulfatase gene, a locus that maps to the telomeric short arm of the X chromosome,[21] are responsible for the defect. The resulting accumulation of cholesterol sulfate in keratinocytes is thought to result in retention hyperkeratosis and scaling. Due to presumptive contiguous gene defects, some cases are associated with Kallmann's syndrome, mental retardation, chondrodysplasia punctata, and short stature.[21]

Clinical Features   Affected individuals present at birth or soon thereafter (Table 14-3). Collodion membrane is seen infrequently, and affected infants more commonly manifest fine, relatively mild scaling at birth. The scaling worsens in the first 2 to 6 months as larger, pigmented scales appear on the trunk, extremities, axillae, sides of the neck, and the popliteal and antecubital fossae. Associated findings may include cryptorchidism and asymptomatic corneal opacities. Obstetric complications, such as late-for-dates pregnancy, weak labor, and prolonged delivery, occur in as many as 30 percent of affected pregnancies because of blocked placental estrogen synthesis.

TABLE 14-3

X-Linked Recessive Ichthyosis

Clinical Features
    Present at birth, or shortly thereafter
    Generalized fine scaling, especially at flexural sites
    Progresses over first 6 months to large pigmented scales
Histopathological Features
    Marked hyperorthokeratosis, with occasional parakeratotic foci
    Granular layer usually thickened
    Variable acanthosis and papillomatosis
Differential Diagnosis
    Lamellar ichthyosis

Histopathological Features There is marked hyperorthokeratosis, with occasional foci of parakeratosis.[7] The granular layer is usually thickened (Fig. 14-4), although this can vary, and in some sections it may be thinned. The spinous layer is variably acanthotic and papillomatous. Perivascular lymphoid infiltrates within the papillary dermis range from mild to marked. Follicular dilatation and plugging are usually absent but can occasionally be observed.

Differential Diagnosis Although, in contrast to autosomal dominant ichthyosis vulgaris, the granular layer is thickened, this feature is variable, and in those cases with a reduced stratum granulosum, distinction from ichthyosis vulgaris may not be possible from histologic criteria. Cases with thickening of the granular layer will resemble lamellar ichthyosis. Biochemical analysis for steroid sulfatase activity may be necessary to resolve the differential diagnosis.

LAMELLAR ICHTHYOSIS

Clinical Features Lamellar ichthyosis is clinically and genetically a heterogeneous disease. Most cases are transmitted as an autosomal recessive trait, but cases of dominant transmission occur.[1] The recessively inherited form is a severe and often generalized dermatosis, usually presenting at birth and accounting for the majority of cases of collodion baby (Table 14-4). The spectrum of clinical involvement

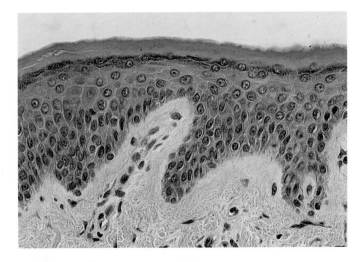

FIGURE 14-4 X-linked recessive ichthyosis. A continuous granular layer of normal-to-slightly-increased thickness separates the densely compact, orthokeratotic corneum from the histologically unremarkable stratum spinosum.

TABLE 14-4

Lamellar Ichthyosis

Clinical Features
    Presents at birth with generalized involvement, often with collodion membrane
    Erythrodermic or nonerythrodermic
    Large platelike scale to fine white scale
    Ectropion
Histopathological Features
    Mild to moderate hyperorthokeratosis
    Normal to widened stratum granulosum
    Acanthosis and papillomatosis, often
Differential Diagnosis
    X-linked recessive ichthyosis

varies from large, platelike scale to fine white scale in the presence or absence of erythroderma. Milder phenotypes may have involvement of only flexural sites and the palms and soles. Mutations in keratinocyte (type I) transglutaminase, which cross-links cornified envelopes of terminally differentiating keratinocytes, are associated with some cases of lamellar ichthyosis.[22]

Histopathological Features The histologic patterns are indistinguishable across all clinical variants of lamellar ichthyosis of autosomal recessive type, as well as those cases with autosomal dominant transmission. One observes mild to marked compact hyperorthokeratosis and a normal to increased stratum granulosum (Fig. 14-5).[1,7] Often acanthosis and occasionally papillomatosis are seen. Parakeratotic foci associated with a focally thinned granular layer are less commonly observed, and parakeratosis with a thickened granular layer is seen in the autosomal dominant variant. The papillary dermis may contain a perivascular lymphocytic infiltrate of variable intensity.

Differential Diagnosis The histopathology is nonspecific, mimicking that of X-linked recessive ichthyosis, but will serve to exclude clinical look-alikes, especially those disorders with epidermolytic hyperkeratosis (bullous ichthyosiform erythrodermas). Distinction from the Comèl-Netherton syndrome, which clinically resembles erythrodermic autosomal recessive lamellar ichthyosis, is resolved by the presence of marked inflammation, with spongiosis, lymphocytic exocytosis, parakeratosis, and thinned-to-absent granular cell layer in the former syndrome.

NEUTRAL LIPID STORAGE DISEASE WITH ICHTHYOTIC (ICHTHYOSIFORM) ERYTHRODERMA (DORFMAN'S SYNDROME)

Clinical Features Neutral lipid storage disease has been reported in fewer than 20 cases, primarily in individuals of Arabic background. The disorder is inherited as an autosomal recessive trait. It presents in the skin as diffuse nonbullous ichthyosiform erythroderma,[23] which is not distinguishable from other ichthyoses of that phenotype. Hepatomegaly with abnormal liver function tests, myopathy, cataracts, and lipid vacuolization of leukocytes and keratinocytes are other components of the syndrome.

Histopathological Features The routine histologic findings are nonspecific, with acanthosis and hyperorthokeratosis. There are variable parakeratotic foci. The stratum granulosum may be thickened or thinned. A slight perivascular infiltrate can be observed in the papillary dermis. The most distinctive feature is the presence of foamy cytoplasm within keratinocytes of the basal and granular layers; by histochemical staining this is shown to be lipid accumulation.

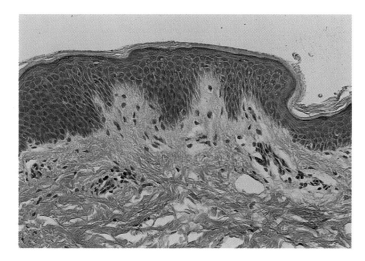

FIGURE 14-5   Lamellar ichthyosis. The compact and mildly thickened, orthokeratotic corneum is separated from the slightly acanthotic stratum spinosum by a continuous granular layer of normal thickness.

Differential Diagnosis   The microscopic features are not distinguishable from other nonbullous congenital ichthyoses, but the observation of lipid droplets in the keratinocytes by careful microscopic examination of hematoxylin and eosin (H&E)–stained sections, with confirmation by histochemical lipid staining, may allow discrimination from lamellar ichthyosis.

ICHTHYOSIS AND DEAFNESS SYNDROMES: HYSTRIXLIKE ICHTHYOSIS WITH DEAFNESS (HID); KERATITIS, ICHTHYOSISLIKE HYPERKERATOSIS, AND DEAFNESS (KID)

Although similar in name, the two are distinct clinically and histologically. All HID cases have been sporadic; although X-linked recessive inheritance has been excluded, autosomal dominant or recessive transmission are possible. Most KID cases have also been sporadic, but some evidence supports autosomal dominant inheritance. The underlying defects are unknown.

Clinical Features   HID presents with patches of erythema soon after birth that progress to generalized, dark gray, scaly skin resembling ichthyosis hystrix. Palms and soles can be mildly affected, and alopecia and nail dystrophy can be seen. In KID, erythroderma at birth disappears within a few days; erythematous, sharply marginated, keratotic plaques develop at about 1 year and increase until puberty. The face, elbows and knees, palms and soles are involved, but the trunk is spared. In both syndromes sensorineural hearing loss, frequent bacterial and fungal infections, and scarring alopecia are seen.[24] Severe palmoplantar involvement and vascularizing keratopathy are observed in KID, but in HID palmoplantar involvement is mild, and only punctate keratitis is seen.

Histopathological Features   Microscopic examination shows nonspecific findings of hyperorthokeratosis and acanthosis, although the hyperkeratosis can be marked. The granular layer is generally thickened. There can be prominent follicular plugging.[7]

Differential Diagnosis   The diagnosis is made by the clinical recognition of the other components of the syndrome. Vacuolated keratinocytes with the nucleus surrounded by an empty halo and ringed by keratohyalin granules have been reported in some cases of HID syndrome, which along with the characteristic differences in clinical presentation of KID and HID, are helpful in distinguishing the two disorders.

SJÖGREN-LARSSON SYNDROME

Clinical Features   Sjögren-Larsson syndrome is a severe, autosomal recessive, neurocutaneous disease consisting of mental retardation, spasticity, and ichthyosis. Affected individuals exhibit an enzymatic deficiency in fatty aldehyde dehydrogenase, and recent studies have confirmed deletional and point mutations in the gene.[25] The generalized, yellow-brown, lichenified ichthyosis associated with Sjögren-Larsson syndrome appears early[26] and is not specifically distinguishable from other widespread ichthyoses of lamellar type. Erythema is mild and fades with age.

Histopathological Features   Histologic sections exhibit acanthosis and some papillomatosis. Moderate compact hyperorthokeratosis characterizes the stratum corneum, although there may be scattered foci of parakeratosis. The granular layer is retained and may be thickened. Follicular hyperkeratosis is variably observed.[1,7]

Differential Diagnosis   Sjögren-Larsson syndrome cannot be discriminated histologically from autosomal recessive lamellar ichthyosis. The diagnosis is made by identification of the other components of the syndrome.

PALMOPLANTAR KERATODERMA

As the isolated phenotype or an associated component of a syndrome, the palmoplantar keratodermas comprise a heterogeneous group of inherited diseases sharing the common feature of aberrant volar keratinization.[27,28] The common forms are dominantly inherited; some less prevalent cases represent recessive transmission. Autosomal dominant palmoplantar keratoderma of Unna-Thost is considered the most common form of this group, but the nomenclature has been clouded by the discovery that the family originally described by Thost in the last century exhibits epidermolytic hyperkeratosis on microscopic examination, indicating overlap with the phenotype of palmoplantar keratoderma type Voerner.[29] Palmoplantar keratodermas of the Meleda type and of the Papillon-Lefevre syndrome are recessive traits. Some affected kindreds with nonepidermolytic palmoplantar keratoderma link genetically to the type I or II keratin gene clusters on chromosomes 17q and 12q.[30] The epidermolytic form of palmoplantar keratoderma cosegregates with keratin 9 mutations in several families, while the nonepidermolytic form has been associated with a K1 mutation in one family.

A large kindred with the Vohwinkel syndrome (palmoplantar hyperkeratosis in a honeycomb pattern, strictures on the hands, and constricting bands encircling the fifth digits leading to autoamputation) links to chromosome 1q21 and is associated with mutations in the loricrin gene.

Clinical Features   Cases exhibit localized or diffuse, and often marked, hyperkeratosis of the palms and soles.[31] Onset may occur from birth to the fourth decade. The callouslike lesions are often well demarcated. The borders of the hyperkeratotic plaques may be erythematous. Spread onto the extensor surfaces can occur, especially in the Meleda type, and there may be hyperhidrosis, constricting bands with autoamputation, thickening of the nails, and psoriaticlike lesions on other parts of the body. Keratoderma in the Papillon-Lefevre syndrome is associated with periodontosis resulting in shedding of the permanent dentition.

Histopathological Features   In all clinical varieties of palmoplantar keratodermas, there is marked hyperorthokeratosis of the corneum, in association with thickening of the stratum granulosum. Acanthosis and some papillomatous change are also seen. Mild perivascular chronic inflammation is found in the papillary dermis. Variably, some cases will display epidermolytic hyperkeratosis of the upper spinous and granular cell layers and scattered dyskeratotic cells. A compact column of para-keratosis within the stratum corneum is observed in the subtype of keratosis palmoplantaris punctata.

Differential Diagnosis   The histologic pattern of nonepidermolytic cases is similar to that of the nonbullous lamellar ichthyoses, whereas those with epidermolytic hyperkeratosis can be distinguished from the bullous ichthyosiform erythrodermas by correlation with the clinical features (see below). Distinction from pityriasis rubra pilaris is on the basis of associated clinical findings.

ERYTHROKERATODERMA VARIABILIS AND PROGRESSIVE SYMMETRIC ERYTHROKERATODERMA

Erythrokeratoderma variabilis and progressive symmetric erythrokeratoderma are rare, usually autosomal dominant diseases that present from birth to early adulthood. Preliminary study supports linkage of erythrokeratoderma variabilis to the Rh system on chromosome 1p36-34.

Clinical Features   Transient, polycyclic, bright patches of erythema are seen that change in size, shape, and distribution over hours to days. The areas are bounded by a trailing scale and may be ringed by a thin, white line. They are commonly found on the extremities and buttocks, but trunk and abdomen may be involved. Affected areas are exacerbated by temperature extremes and stress. More stable, fixed, erythematous, hyperkeratotic plaques develop on the extensor surface of the extremities. Mild palmoplantar keratoderma may be seen in up to 50 percent of cases, and CNS abnormalities have been reported in some families. The lesions of progressive symmetric erythrokeratoderma resemble those of erythrokeratoderma variabilis, but their distribution is strikingly symmetric and limited to the extremities and buttocks, and they remain fixed once they appear. Although the two disorders are usually distinct, occurrence of both, one each in sisters, suggested that they may represent variants of the same process.[32]

Histopathological Features   A normal granular cell layer underlies a hyperorthokeratotic stratum corneum. The epidermis is acanthotic and shows papillomatosis. The suprapapillary zones of the stratum spinosum may be thinned. The papillary dermis contains a perivascular lymphocytic dermatitis of variable intensity.

Differential Diagnosis   The histologic pattern of erythrokeratoderma variabilis is nonspecific, resembling many of the nonbullous ichthyoses. The diagnosis rests with the clinicopathologic correlation. Progressive symmetric erythrokeratoderma histologically shows hyperkeratosis with focal parakeratosis. The granular cell layer is normal to increased. There may be perinuclear granular cell vacuolization. The spinous layer is acanthotic.

ACANTHOSIS NIGRICANS

A relatively prevalent mucocutaneous disorder, acanthosis nigricans occurs in several clinically defined types, but most often it is found in association with obesity and insulin resistance and less commonly in an exuberant, paraneoplastic form.[33] The eruption is probably caused in most instances by circulating insulin and insulinlike growth factors acting on keratinocytes and other cutaneous cells that express the cognate growth factor receptor(s).

Clinical Features   Whereas acanthosis nigricans can occur anywhere on the skin, the characteristic velvety hyperpigmented plaques of this disorder exhibit a predilection for flexural sites of the axillae, the nape, groin, and popliteal and antecubital fossae. Associated palmoplantar keratoderma (tylosis) may rarely occur in those cases induced by inter-

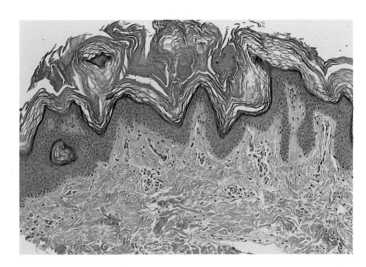

FIGURE 14-6   Acanthosis nigricans. Pronounced hyperorthokeratosis in a basket-weave pattern overlies the papillomatous epidermis, but there is little acanthosis.

nal malignancy. Papillomatous epithelial hyperplasia on occasion can affect the conjunctiva and the stratified squamous mucosae of the oropharynx and anal canal.

Histopathological Features   Despite the impression created by this disorder's name, there is usually little acanthosis; the epidermis is more often somewhat thinned and rather moderately to markedly papillomatous (Fig. 14-6). The papillomatosis has a blunted, hill-and-dale silhouette. The hyperkeratotic stratum corneum often retains the normal basket-weave architecture. There is little, if any, perivascular lymphocytic infiltration of the papillary dermis.

Differential Diagnosis   Distinction from seborrheic keratosis and hamartomatous epidermal nevi may occasionally be necessary when the papillomatosis is pronounced; the usual absence of significant acanthosis helps to rule out these considerations. Confluent and reticulate papillomatosis of Gougerot and Carteaud is generally not distinguishable histologically, but the flexural distribution of lesions of acanthosis nigricans compared with the more generalized distribution of confluent and reticulate papillomatosis will permit the clinical distinction of the two.

ICHTHYOSIS FOLLICULARIS WITH ATRICHIA AND PHOTOPHOBIA (IFAP) SYNDROME

Clinical Features   The essential phenotypic components of the syndrome are follicular ichthyosis, generalized congenital nonscarring alopecia, and photophobia. Other common findings include mild generalized scaling with erythema, psychomotor and growth retardation, susceptibility to pyodermas, dentition abnormalities, and nail dystrophy.[34] The strong gender predilection for males suggests X-linked recessive inheritance.

Histopathological Features   Microscopic examination discloses moderate hyperorthokeratosis, with follicular dilatation and plugging. The granular layer is preserved and may be thickened. Specimens of scalp skin will reveal atrophy of the folliculosebaceous units and thinning of the dermis.

Differential Diagnosis   The retention of the granular layer allows distinction from autosomal dominant ichthyosis vulgaris and related disorders. The absence of epidermolytic hyperkeratosis will exclude bullous ichthyosiform erythrodermas. Clinical features allow distinction from the keratosis pilaris syndromes.

INHERITED PITYRIASIS RUBRA PILARIS

Clinical Features   Whereas most instances of the uncommon disease, pityriasis rubra pilaris, are sporadic, an inherited form exists and is observed most often in juvenile cases.[35] Inheritance is autosomal dominant. The underlying defect is unknown. The clinical lesions of pityriasis rubra pilaris are thick, erythematous, salmon-colored plaques that are localized to sites of predilection, such as scalp, volar surfaces, and elbows and knees, or more generalized, eventuating into an exfoliative erythroderma.[36]

Histopathological Features   The epidermis is acanthotic and papillomatous, with elongation of the rete ridges that may create a psoriasiform pattern of hyperplasia.[35] There may be widening of the intercellular spaces within the spinous layer. The stratum corneum is remarkable for marked hyperkeratosis, which in some foci will exhibit horizontally alternating zones of ortho- and parakeratosis. The stratum granulosum is usually hypergranular. Dilatation and keratotic plugging of the follicular infundibulae are often reliably prominent features of pityriasis rubra pilaris and should be searched for in additional recuts if the diagnosis is unclear from the original sections. The stratum corneum adjacent to the follicular ostia may show parakeratosis. A slight perivascular lymphocytic infiltrate is observed in the papillary dermis.

Differential Diagnosis   The psoriasiform hyperplasia of pityriasis rubra pilaris can make distinction from psoriasis difficult, especially considering that alternating parakeratotic foci and variably thickened or absent stratum granulosum can be observed in the latter. However, the presence of neutrophilic foci within the corneum (Munro abscesses) and dermal papillae with lymphocytic infiltrates and dilated capillaries will favor the interpretation of psoriasis, and there should be few if any dilated and keratotic follicular infundibulae in the latter. Follicular plugging, although not an invariable feature, is helpful in resolving the differential diagnosis of other papulosquamous diseases when present. Discrimination from cases of nonbullous ichthyosiform erythrodermas may not be possible on histologic grounds alone.

Disorders with Hyperparakeratosis

In few entities is prominent parakeratosis a clue to the diagnosis. More often, parakeratosis is found as a transient or inconstant feature in a disorder with hyperkeratosis developing in an orthokeratotic fashion, including some cases of autosomal dominant ichthyosis vulgaris, lamellar ichthyoses, and Harlequin ichthyosis. Those entities are discussed under the sections reflecting their more constant histopathologic patterns.

CHILD (CONGENITAL HEMIDYSPLASIA, ICHTHYOSIFORM ERYTHRODERMA, LIMB DEFECTS) SYNDROME

Clinical Features   This rare, congenital dermatosis is defined by unilateral nevoid skin lesions with features of ichthyosiform erythroderma and ipsilateral limb underdevelopment. The nevoid lesions, which can occur in the absence of the other components of the syndrome,[37] may develop later in childhood and manifest as linear or diffuse erythematous plaques with waxy yellow-brown scale. The lesions can expand or resolve spontaneously. Because nearly all cases are female, inheritance is hypothesized to be X-linked dominant and lethal in hemizygous males.[37] A peroxisomal abnormality in affected fibroblasts has been postulated.

Histopathological Features   Histologic sections show epidermal acanthosis, associated with papillomatous hyperplasia. Prominent foci of parakeratosis are found within a compact, hyperkeratotic stratum corneum.[38] The granular layer is normal to thinned. Foamy histiocytes may be found in the dermal papillae, simulating verruciform xanthoma.

Differential Diagnosis   The histopathologic features are nonspecific. Pityriasis rubra pilaris, epidermal nevi, and erythrodermic psoriasis may need to be considered diagnostically. The presence of alternating zones of para- and orthokeratosis within the stratum corneum and follicular plugging and minimal inflammatory infiltrates will permit the diagnosis of pityriasis rubra pilaris, whereas Munro abscesses within the corneum and inflammatory infiltrates and capillary ectasia within the dermal papillae will suggest the diagnosis of psoriasis.

COMÈL-NETHERTON SYNDROME, WITH ICHTHYOSIS LINEARIS CIRCUMFLEXA OR CONGENITAL ICHTHYOSIFORM ERYTHRODERMA

Clinical Features   A rare, autosomal recessive disorder of unknown etiology, Comèl-Netherton syndrome presents clinically with a distinctive hair abnormality designated *trichorrhexis invaginata* ("bamboo hair") and cutaneous signs of exfoliative ichthyosiform erythroderma and/or ichthyosis linearis circumflexa, which consists of migratory or evanescent, erythematous patches fringed by a double-edged scale. The other clinical manifestations are variable but often include an associated atopic diathesis, recurrent infections, failure to thrive in infancy, enteropathy, and mild palmoplantar keratoderma.[39,40]

Histopathological Features   The microscopic findings in skin specimens are similar across the variable clinical phenotype of either ichthyosis linearis circumflexa (most often) or ichthyotic (ichthyosiform) erythroderma.[1] Accumulation of eosinophilic periodic acid–Schiff (PAS)-positive material within the stratum corneum is the most characteristic criterion.[1] Parakeratotic hyperkeratosis is marked, and the corneal layer often contains masses of pyknotic neutrophils. Although disputed in some reports, the granular layer is usually thinned and may be focally absent. A subcorneal cleft created by separation of much of the stratum corneum is frequently observed. The spinous layer is acanthotic, and papillomatosis is well-developed (Fig. 14-7).[7] The papillary dermis contains a marked perivascular lymphocytic infiltrate, which

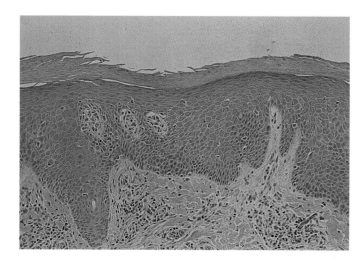

FIGURE 14-7   Comèl-Netherton syndrome. A moderately thickened stratum corneum with parakeratotic foci is associated with a hyperplastic epidermis and a brisk superficial perivascular lymphocytic infiltrate.

may be associated with spongiosis of the overlying epidermis and lymphocytic exocytosis. Electron microscopy reveals cytoplasmic inclusion bodies, probably lysosomes, in spinous and granular cells that are not seen in other ichthyoses.

Differential Diagnosis The psoriasiform epidermal hyperplasia of ichthyosis linearis circumflexa may resemble psoriasis. The PAS-positive stratum granulosum, irregular elongation of the rete ridges, and subcorneal clefting, when present, will serve to distinguish the two disorders. Nodose swelling of hair shafts, due to trichorrhexis invaginata, taken in context with the combined clinicopathologic phenotype of ichthyosis linearis circumflexa or ichthyotic erythroderma, should permit reliable diagnosis in questionable cases.

POROKERATOSIS

Clinical Features Whereas the clinical spectrum of porokeratosis is diverse, the characteristic feature of all types, except for punctate porokeratosis, is the distinctive, fine threadlike ring at the perimeter of the lesions that corresponds to the histologic cornoid lamella. The clinical varieties consist of the isolated, plaque-type lesions in porokeratosis of Mibelli; the common disseminated superficial porokeratosis; linear porokeratosis; porokeratosis plantaris, palmaris, et disseminata; and a punctate form restricted to the palms and soles. It has been suggested that the cornoid lamella is formed by atypical keratinocytes that are hyperproliferative and defective in keratinization, resulting in aberrant desquamation.[41]

Histopathological Features The histologic hallmark of all clinical varieties of porokeratosis is the cornoid lamella. It consists of a layered column within the corneum created by parakeratotic corneocytes. This tier of cells is often obliquely oriented to the epidermal surface and appears to arise from a dell in the upper viable layers of the epidermis, in association with a focal absence of the stratum granulosum (Fig. 14-8). Dyskeratotic cells are frequently observed in the subjacent upper spinous layer.

Differential Diagnosis The cornoid lamella is a distinctive structure not usually confused with other processes, although its presence in tissue sections may be subtle and easily overlooked. Although the cornoid lamella is the characteristic finding in porokeratosis, it is not completely specific to the diagnosis. A cornoid lamella can occasionally be found in a variety of other conditions, such as wart, solar keratosis, seborrheic keratosis, squamous cell carcinoma, and basal cell carcinoma. Clinicopathologic correlations and/or observation of other pathologic processes in the tissues are necessary to resolve the differential diagnosis in those instances associated with incidental cornoid lamellae.

EPIDERMOLYTIC DISORDERS

The unifying feature in the disorders included under this section is epidermal separation, due either to shearing through various levels of the basement membrane zone or to vesiculation resulting from cytolysis or acantholysis of epidermal keratinocytes. The basal and/or suprabasal spinous cells are most often affected in the cytolytic and acantholytic diseases. These usually genetic disorders range from bullous variants of certain ichthyoses to the mechanobullous diseases associated with mutations in genes for keratins and other structural proteins. The diagnostic algorithm (Fig. 14-9) principally exploits the level of the separation within the epidermal layers and, secondarily, associated histologic changes of defective keratinization, if any. Table 14-5 summarizes the salient histologic features that can be used to facilitate the differential diagnosis of the epidermolytic diseases.

Disorders with Basal Layer or Basement Membrane Zone Lysis

The entities described here are limited to the clinicopathologic varieties of epidermolysis bullosa, which are mechanobullous diseases that have in common heritable lesions in genes coding for structural proteins of basal keratinocytes or for components of the basement membrane zone.

EPIDERMOLYSIS BULLOSA SIMPLEX

The genetically heterogeneous diseases grouped under *epidermolysis bullosa simplex* share autosomal dominant inheritance, pathophysiologic changes of minor trauma-induced cytolysis within the basal or suprabasal keratinocytes, and the tendency for lesions to heal without scarring. Tonofilament clumps within basal and suprabasal keratinocytes are observed by electron microscopy in the Dowling-Meara variant; these structures contain the keratin pair 5 and 14 by immunolabeling.[42] Point mutations have been demonstrated in either gene (K5 or K14) in all clinical variants of epidermolysis bullosa simplex.[43] The clinical severity is evidently determined in each affected kindred by the extent to which the specific mutation disrupts the functional properties of the gene product.[44]

Clinical Features The phenotypes include the generalized Koebner, the Dowling-Meara, which is characterized by herpetiform clustering of blisters, and the localized (usually acral) Weber-Cockayne variants. The first two types usually present early in infancy with blisters and erosions induced by minor trauma, whereas onset of the latter is often delayed. Mucosal lesions, minor scarring, nail shedding, and widespread erosions with risk of secondary pyogenic infection occur in severely affected patients.[45] Spontaneous improvement is sometimes seen in later childhood and adult years.

Histopathological Features In all variants of epidermolysis bullosa simplex, vesicles form by cytolysis within the basal or lower spinous cell layers (Fig. 14-10).[46] Histologic sections thus show focal dissolution of the basal or spinous keratinocytes, resulting in epidermal separation through that layer. Dyskeratotic changes may manifest histologically within the cells, especially in the Dowling-Meara variant.[47] On

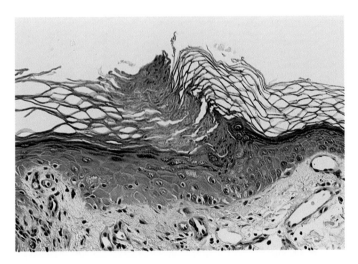

FIGURE 14-8 Porokeratosis. The obliquely oriented cornoid lamella, containing parakeratotic corneocytes, has arisen from a superficial dell, the base of which contains several dyskeratotic cells.

FIGURE 14-9

Epidermolytic Disorders:
Diagnostic Algorithm

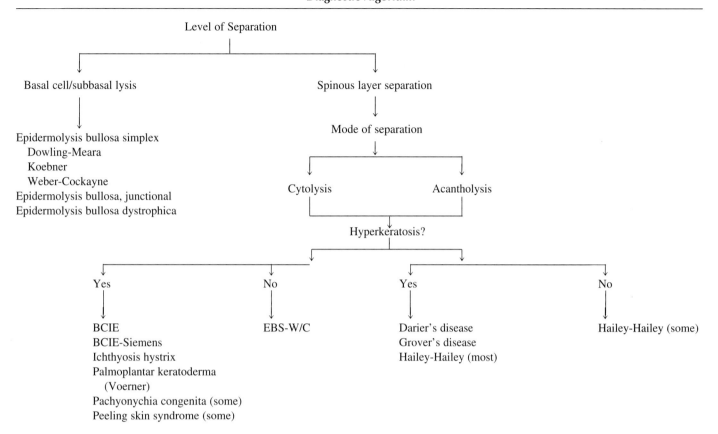

FIGURE 14-9 Diagnostic algorithm for the epidermolytic disorders. The hierarchy for differential diagnosis follows primarily from the level of separation within the epidermis or basement membrane zone and secondarily from the mode of separation, whether cytolysis or acantholysis.

occasion, epidermolysis bullosa simplex Dowling-Meara and Koebner have been associated with palmoplantar keratoderma,[48] where the histologic sections will exhibit compact hyperorthokeratosis and a variably thickened granular layer in addition to the cytolytic changes within the keratinocytes.

Differential Diagnosis In the Dowling-Meara subtype, the separation can occur deep in the basal layer such that when seen by light microscopy the entire epidermis appears to have formed the roof of the blister; this may simulate the findings in junctional epidermolysis bullosa and may require electron microscopy or immunomapping of basement membrane components for resolution of the level of the separation. Epidermolysis bullosa simplex of Dowling-Meara is distinguished from the other two varieties by herpetiform clustering of the clinical lesions and by keratin filament clumping on electron microscopy of lesional skin samples.

EPIDERMOLYSIS BULLOSA, JUNCTIONAL (LETALIS)

Junctional epidermolysis bullosa includes several genetically heterogeneous diseases that, although phenotypically variable, share autosomal recessive transmission and subepidermal separation through the lamina lucida of the basement membrane zone due to reduced numbers of hemidesmosomes.[49] Mutations in the peptide subunits of laminin 5 (epiligrin) and the 180 kDa bullous pemphigoid antigen, which are lamina lucida components, appear to be etiologic in some cases.[50]

Clinical Features The most severe clinical presentation occurs in the Herlitz syndrome (epidermolysis bullosa letalis), which exhibits widespread cutaneous and mucosal blisters and erosions soon after birth, usually proving fatal within the first 1 to 2 years of life. Less severe forms of junctional epidermolysis bullosa exhibit qualitatively similar changes but differ in the extent of the cutaneous and mucosal blisters and erosions, allowing survival into adulthood. Many of the latter display abnormal dental enamel development, which imparts a cobblestone appearance to the teeth.

Histopathological Features Separation occurs beneath the basal cell layer, but above the lamina densa (Fig. 14-11), due to dissolution of the lamina lucida, as shown by electron microscopy. Histologic sections reveal a plane of separation formed between the epidermis and the basement membrane zone. By PAS staining or immunomapping the basement membrane remains on the dermal side of the split.

Differential Diagnosis By light microscopy, junctional epidermolysis bullosa may be simulated by dystrophic variants of that disease spectrum or by subepidermal autoimmune vesiculobullous disorders such as bullous pemphigoid. The clinical context will direct the histopathologic interpretations along the appropriate pathways. Resolution of the differential diagnosis for the mechanobullous disorders is usually obtained by immunolabeling for markers of basement membrane components, such as type IV collagen and laminin, to localize the plane of separation or by electron microscopy. The autoimmune disorders are confirmed diag-

TABLE 14-5

Differential Diagnosis for Epidermolytic Disorders

	Histologic Feature					
	Level of separation	*Mechanism of separation*	*Hyper-keratosis*	*Status of granular layer*	*Acanthosis*	*Other*
Epidermolysis bullosa simplex	Basal and/or spinous layer	Cytolysis	+ (occasional)	Normal − +	0	Focal dyskeratotic cells
Epidermolysis bullosa junctional	Basement membrane zone	Shearing through lamina lucida	0	Normal	0	
Epidermolysis bullosa dystrophica	Beneath basement membrane	Shearing through anchoring fibril zone	0	Normal	0	
Bullous ichthyosiform erythroderma	Spinous and granular layers	Epidermolytic hyperkeratosis	+ + − + + +	+ − + +	+ − + +	Perivascular lymphocytic infiltrates
Palmoplantar keratoderma (Voerner)	Spinous and granular layers	Epidermolytic hyperkeratosis	+ +	+	+	Perivascular lymphocytic infiltrates
Pachyonychia congenita	Upper spinous layer	Cytolysis	+ + − + + +	+ +	+ − + +	Follicular plugging, in some cases
Darier's disease	Suprabasal layer	Acantholysis	+ − + +	+ − + +	+	Corp ronds and grains
Hailey-Hailey	Spinous layers	Acantholysis	0 − +	Normal − +	+ − +	Dilapidated brick wall
Grover's disease	Suprabasal layer	Acantholysis	+	+	0 − +	
Peeling skin syndrome	Subcorneal	Inter-, intracellular cleavage	+	Normal or thinned	+ − + +	Perivascular lymphocytic infiltrates

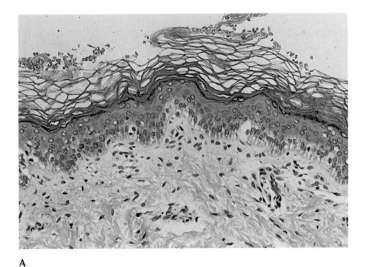

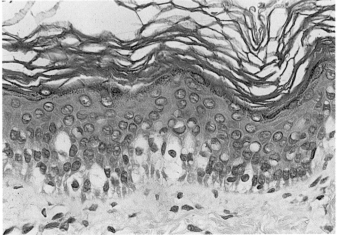

A   B

FIGURE 14-10 Epidermolysis bullosa of Dowling-Meara. (*A*) Basal and suprabasal keratinocytes display prominent cytolytic degeneration. (*B*) The more superficial epidermal layers appear normal.

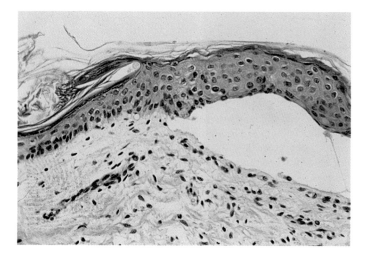

FIGURE 14-11   Epidermolysis bullosa, junctional. Separation has occurred beneath the basal keratinocyte layer, but superficial to the eosinophilic basement membrane.

nostically from the characteristic patterns of autoantibody deposition as shown by direct immunofluorescence methods.

EPIDERMOLYSIS BULLOSA DYSTROPHICA

Epidermolysis bullosa dystrophica is genetically heterogeneous, with either autosomal dominant or recessive inheritance. Cases of dystrophic epidermolysis bullosa have long been known to demonstrate morphologic abnormalities of the anchoring fibrils, which are structures distributed below the basal lamina.[51] Type VII collagen was an early candidate for the etiologic molecular defect because it is a major collagenous component of the anchoring fibrils. Immunolabeling for type VII collagen demonstrates either reduced content or disarrayed organization of this component.[52] Genetic studies confirmed linkage between markers for the collagen VII locus on chromosome 3 and both the dominantly and recessively inherited clinical phenotype[53,54]; mutational analyses subsequently confirmed mutations in the gene.[55]

Clinical Features   As a reflection of genetic heterogeneity, the clinical severity of epidermolysis bullosa dystrophica varies widely. On one hand, the recessive form presents in infancy with extensive blistering and scarring of the entire cutaneous and squamous mucosal surfaces of the oropharynx, anus, and esophagus, eventuating in mutilating deformities, shedding of nails, joint contractures, pseudosyndactyly, and enteric strictures. On the other hand, the phenotype of the dominant form, while also exhibiting mechanically induced blisters and secondary scarring, is much less severe.

Histopathological Features   Due to molecular defects in the subepidermal anchoring fibrils, histologic sections show separation of the entire epidermis from the dermis, with the PAS-positive basement membrane and type IV collagen or laminin segregating to the epidermal roof of the blister cavity.

Differential Diagnosis   Ambiguities in the differential diagnosis will be resolved by immunostaining for type IV collagen and/or electron microscopy to localize the plane of separation, which confirms that the basal lamina remains attached to the epidermis. The blister thus forms beneath the lamina densa. Immunostaining will also demonstrate reduced labeling for collagen type VII in the anchoring fibril zone.

Disorders with Spinous Layer Vesiculation due to Cytolysis or Acantholysis

The entities grouped under this category range from hereditary ichthyoses featuring the distinctive histologic change of epidermolytic hyperkeratosis to vesiculobullous disorders displaying the common feature of spinous layer acantholysis.

BULLOUS CONGENITAL ICHTHYOSIFORM ERYTHRODERMA (BCIE; EPIDERMOLYTIC HYPERKERATOSIS, EHK)

This dominantly inherited, uncommon dermatosis presents with generalized erythroderma, severe scaling, and blistering. Corn-row-like scaling accumulates in the antecubital fossae, axillae, and over the knees and dorsal ankles. Early ultrastructural studies of ichthyosiform erythroderma indicated clumping and aggregation of suprabasal keratin filaments,[56] suggesting molecular defects in keratin genes. Genetic linkage studies demonstrated cosegregation of the trait and markers for the type I and II keratin loci on chromosomes 17q and 12q.[57] Mutational analyses showed that point mutations in the critical rod domains of both keratins 1 and 10 associate with the phenotype.[58] The etiologic role of the keratin mutations has been established experimentally by expression of mutant keratin alleles in transgenic mice, which reproduces the phenotype.[59] In some families, somatic mutations with associated epidermal nevi exhibiting the histologic changes of epidermolytic hyperkeratosis have resulted in generalized BCIE in subsequent generations as a result of gonadal mosaicism.

Clinical Features   Epidermolytic hyperkeratosis is clinically heterogeneous, although within an affected kindred the phenotype is relatively uniform[60] (Table 14-6). In most cases, widespread erythema, blistering, and hyperkeratotic verrucous plaques are noted at birth or during childhood.[61] Clinical blistering often abates after the first few years of life. The presence or absence of palmoplantar keratoderma distinguishes some pedigrees.[60]

Histopathological Features   Microscopically, all cases exhibit massive hyperorthokeratosis, in either a compact or, more often, a basket-weave pattern.[1,7] The granular layer is thickened and contains coarse keratohyalin granules. The acanthotic epidermis is distinctive for cytoplasmic edema and perinuclear vacuolization affecting the keratinocytes of the granular and spinous cell layers. The basal and, occasionally, the suprabasal keratinocytes appear normal. The hydropic changes create indistinct boundaries between the epidermolytic cells and a reticular pattern of degeneration, referred to as *epidermolytic hyperkeratosis* or

TABLE 14-6

Bullous Congenital Ichthyosiform Erythroderma

Clinical Features
   Onset at birth or early childhood
   Erythema, blistering, and verrucous plaques, usually widespread
   Abatement of blistering with age
Histopathological Features
   Massive hyperorthokeratosis
   Thickened granular layer with coarse keratohyaline granules
   Acanthotic spinous layer with epidermolytic changes
Differential Diagnosis
   Ichthyosis bullosa of Siemens
   Palmoplantar keratoderma, type Voerner
   Incidental finding in hyperproliferative epidermal disorders

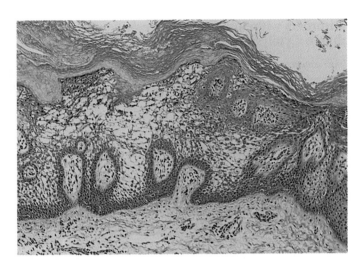

FIGURE 14-12   Bullous ichthyosiform erythroderma. The markedly acanthotic and hyperkeratotic epidermis exhibits prominent epidermolysis at the levels of the middle to upper spinous and granular cell layers. The widened stratum granulosum contains coarsely clumped keratohyalin granules.

acanthokeratolysis (Fig. 14-12). When fully evolved, vesiculation occurs through the upper spinous to granular layers, the roof of which is formed by thickened stratum corneum and the floor by edematous keratinocytes. A slight-to-moderate perivascular lymphoid infiltrate is found in the superficial dermis.

Differential Diagnosis   Bullous congenital ichthyosiform erythroderma is distinguished from ichthyosis bullosa of Siemens by clinical differences and by involvement of the entire suprabasal epidermal compartment, whereas the cytolytic changes in the latter disorder are restricted to the upper spinous and granular layers. Epidermolytic hyperkeratosis is not specific to these bullous ichthyoses because it is not uncommonly observed as an incidental finding contiguous to melanocytic nevi and hyperproliferative disorders of the epidermis,[62] including linear epidermal nevus, verrucae, actinic keratosis, squamous cell carcinoma, seborrheic keratosis, solitary epidermolytic acanthoma, sundry inflammatory conditions, and some palmoplantar keratodermas. Diagnosis in those situations is contingent on recognition of the associated findings distinctive for each disorder. The epidermolytic palmoplantar keratodermas are diagnosed from the appropriate clinical presentation.

ICHTHYOSIS BULLOSA OF SIEMENS

This mechanobullous condition is an autosomal dominant disease characterized by a mild, nonerythrodermic clinical phenotype with microscopic changes of epidermolytic hyperkeratosis limited to the granular layer and upper stratum corneum in lesional skin.[63] Clinical and histologic overlap with bullous congenital ichthyosiform erythroderma suggests that they may be variants of the same disease process.[64] Ichthyosis bullosa links genetically to the type II keratin gene cluster on chromosome 12q,[63] and most cases appear to be caused by point mutations in the differentiation-specific keratin, K2e.[65]

Clinical Features   Dark gray, hyperkeratotic lesions are restricted to certain sites of predilection, which include shins, para-articular, and periumbilical areas. Characteristic, superficial blistering with subsequent shedding of the affected skin ("molting") and erosions can occur after mild trauma and with sweating.[66]

Histopathological Features   The principal histologic change is that of epidermolytic hyperkeratosis, which is limited to the upper strata of the epidermis and is generally less well developed and less extensive than in bullous congenital ichthyosiform erythroderma.[66] Acanthosis of mild extent may be observed.

Differential Diagnosis   The histologic differential diagnosis is essentially that for bullous congenital ichthyosiform erythroderma (above). Ichthyosis bullosa of Siemens is discriminated clinically from the former by the absence of erythroderma, by the more limited distribution of the keratotic lesions, and by the characteristic formation of superficial blisters.

ICHTHYOSIS HYSTRIX OF CURTH AND MACKLIN

This rare ichthyotic disease is inherited as an autosomal dominant trait. Ultrastructurally, the hyperkeratotic lesions show disruption of the keratin filament network of the suprabasal keratinocytes. Immunolabeling studies for keratin expression have shown that both normal appearing and lesional skin persistently express fetal keratins.[67] The condition, however, does not link genetically to keratin gene loci.[68]

Clinical Features   The clinical onset of ichthyosis hystrix is usually in childhood. The hyperkeratotic and papillomatous, coalescent papules can be localized or distributed extensively and bilaterally in whorled or arborizing arrays of thickened, darkened (hystrixlike) scale anywhere on the skin surface. Palmoplantar involvement is variable.

Histopathological Features   The distinctive pattern of epidermolytic hyperkeratosis is found against the backdrop of mild orthohyperkeratosis, acanthosis, papillomatosis, and elongation of the rete ridges. The former is comprised of perinuclear vacuolization of granular and upper spinous layer keratinocytes and irregularity of cell borders leading to reticular degeneration. There is hypertrophy of the granular layer, which contains coarse keratohyalin granules. A slight-to-moderate perivascular lymphoid infiltrate is present in the superficial dermis.

Differential Diagnosis   Ichthyosis hystrix (Curth-Macklin) is distinguished by a discrete, dark shell around the nuclei of spinous cells and by the presence of binucleate cells.[1] By electron microscopy, there is a continuous shell of intermediate filaments separating the perinuclear compartment, which often will contain vacuoles, from an outer, cytoplasmic compartment. Otherwise, the differential diagnosis is that discussed under *bullous ichthyosiform erythroderma*.

PALMOPLANTAR KERATOSIS OF VOERNER
(EPIDERMOLYTIC PALMOPLANTAR KERATODERMA)

Some kindreds with the autosomal dominant form of diffuse palmoplantar keratoderma will show epidermolytic hyperkeratosis on biopsy of affected skin, to which the designation *Voerner* is eponymously assigned. The condition has been linked to mutations in the keratin 9 gene, the expression of which is restricted to the suprabasal zone of the palms and soles.[56,69]

Clinical Features   The clinical presentation of diffuse palmoplantar keratoderma does not allow distinction of the epidermolytic variant of Voerner from the ostensibly nonepidermolytic variety described by Unna and Thost. The volar lesions typically are sharply demarcated with erythematous borders. The lesions can be associated with knuckle-pad-like changes and nail clubbing.[70]

Histopathological Features   Changes of epidermolytic hyperkeratosis in the upper spinous and granular cell layers are associated with mild orthohyperkeratosis, acanthosis, and papillomatosis.[71] A slight-to-moderate perivascular lymphoid infiltrate is present in the superficial dermis. Clumping of suprabasal keratins is seen with electron microscopy.

Differential Diagnosis   The differential diagnosis is that discussed under *bullous congenital ichthyosiform erythroderma*. The clinical presentation, however, will appropriately focus the diagnostic considerations to the palmoplantar keratodermas.

PACHYONYCHIA CONGENITA

Heterogeneous dyskeratotic and dysplastic alterations of ectodermal tissues are found in pachyonychia congenita, a rare, genetically heterogeneous trait that is transmitted in an autosomal dominant manner with variable expressivity.[72] Genetic linkage analyses have established that the loci for the more common Jadassohn-Lewandowsky variant and the rarer Jackson-Lawler subtype map to chromosome 17q, in close proximity to the type I keratin gene cluster[73]; mutations in keratins 6 and 16 account for some cases of the former variant,[74] and defective alleles for keratin 17 are etiologic for the latter subtype.[75] The seemingly pleiotropic phenotype reflects the tissue-specific distributions of the variously defective keratin gene products.

Clinical Features   Onset of pachyonychia congenita is usually in early infancy, but delayed presentation into the teenage years occurs in tardive cases.[76] Symmetrically thickened nails are present in all patients, but the other components of the clinical syndrome are variable.[77] The nail involvement, termed *pachyonychia*, consists of subungual hyperkeratosis in which keratinous material sequentially lifts the nail plate from the bed in a proximal-to-distal gradient, resembling a ski jump. The more common Jadassohn-Lewandowsky variant exhibits pachyonychia, palmoplantar keratoderma with tender blisters and erosions, follicular hyperkeratosis, and leukokeratotic changes of the oral mucosa, resembling white sponge nevus. The rarer Jackson-Lawler subtype is characterized by multiple epidermoid inclusion cysts, natal teeth, and hair abnormalities, including alopecia.

Histopathological Features   The principal histologic changes of involved skin are marked hyperorthokeratosis, papillomatosis, acanthosis, and moderate hypergranulosis; there can be focal parakeratosis and follicular plugging.[77] Sections may display an upper spinous layer vesicle created by intracellular edema. The papillary dermis contains a sparse perivascular lymphocytic infiltrate.

Differential Diagnosis   In cases without intraspinous vesiculation, the histologic pattern may not be distinguishable from lamellar and X-linked recessive ichthyoses. However, the clinical presentation, especially the pachyonychia, is distinctive.

DARIER'S DISEASE (DARIER-WHITE DISEASE; KERATOSIS FOLLICULARIS)

An uncommon, dominantly inherited dermatosis, Darier's disease manifests as focal keratinocyte defects in intercellular adhesions that are restricted to the sites of the clinical lesions.[78] Fine structure studies have suggested that the initial event in the lesions is separation of the paired desmosomal plaques, followed by retraction of the tonofilaments from their attachment sites in the plaques and redistribution to a perinuclear pattern; dyskeratosis follows the initiating acantholytic event. The

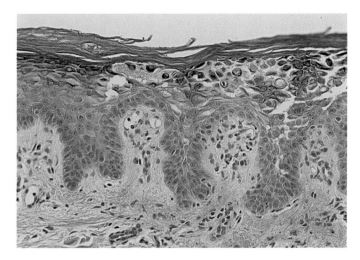

FIGURE 14-13   Darier's disease. Prominent suprabasal acantholysis is present in association with dyskeratotic cells (the corp ronds and grains), hypergranulosis, and hyperkeratosis.

mutant genetic locus responsible for Darier's disease is highly penetrant[79] and has been mapped to chromosome 12q,[80] but genes for keratins and other known epidermal proteins have been excluded as candidate loci. New spontaneous mutations are prone to occur.

Clinical Features   Clinical onset of Darier's disease ranges from childhood to the early adult years. The lesions are hyperkeratotic, crusted, erythematous papules, often with a follicular localization, that are predisposed to seborrheic areas, especially the presternal skin; however, flexural and oral mucosal lesions occur occasionally.[81] Clinical variants include hypertrophic, vesicular, and linear lesions. Distinctive nail changes are present in most patients and are often associated with palmar pits and keratoses.[79] Neuropsychiatric disorders cosegregate in some families. The condition typically pursues an unremitting course.

Histopathological Features   The characteristic pattern of acantholytic dyskeratosis in Darier's disease occurs in association with epidermal papillomatosis, acanthosis, and hyperkeratosis. Acantholytic changes giving rise to microscopic lacunae and dyskeratosis develop in the immediate suprabasal zone (Fig. 14-13). Villus structures lined by solitary layers of basal cells are created by the apparent upward proliferation of the dermal papillae into these lacunae. Lying free within the lacunae are dyskeratotic spinous keratinocytes, which have lost their intercellular bridges and may have prematurely keratinized. In the upper epidermis the acantholytic cells take the morphologic forms of corp ronds and grains. Corp ronds reside in the upper spinous and granular layers and consist of acantholytic cells with homogeneously pyknotic nuclei and a clear pericellular halo. Grains are smaller counterparts within the stratum granulosum or higher, displaying pericellular halos and resembling, but more plump than, parakeratotic corneocytes. The folliculosebaceous elements may show infundibular dilatation and plugging. A perivascular mixed lymphocytic infiltrate occurs in the superficial dermis. Variants of Darier's disease include vesiculobullous lesions, created by large lacunae, and hypertrophic lesions, with accentuation of downward proliferation by the rete.

Differential Diagnosis   The pattern of acantholytic dyskeratosis is not specific to Darier's disease, as it is often found in warty dyskeratoma, Grover's disease, and focal acantholytic dyskeratoma and may reside as an incidental finding in diverse lesions, such as verrucae, basal cell carcinoma, keratoacanthoma, psoriasis, and angiomata.[82] Although also evident on occasion in Hailey-Hailey disease, the latter disorder usually exhibits few corp ronds or grains and more widespread acantholysis; this differential diagnosis is further discussed under *Hailey-Hailey disease*.

HAILEY-HAILEY DISEASE

Hailey-Hailey disease represents a widespread, subclinical abnormality of cell adhesion mediated by dissolution of desmosomal plaques.[83,84] Its clinical manifestations, however, are usually restricted to intertriginous anatomic regions that are subject to friction and maceration.[85] Although the etiology is unknown, the disorder is genetic, segregating as an autosomal dominant trait, and the responsible locus has been mapped to chromosome 3q.[86] As with Darier's disease, genes coding for known epidermal proteins have been excluded as candidate loci.

Clinical Features   The disease often presents in the second to fourth decades with vesicles, bullae, and chronic erosive lesions in flexural sites, especially the axillae and groin, that are subject to exacerbation by friction or heat[87] (Table 14-7). Uncommon morphologic variants include dermatitic, verrucoid, and papular lesions. Although the condition is chronic, remissions occur. With rare exceptions, the mucous membranes are unaffected. The erosions are often secondarily infected. Longitudinal white bands may be found in the nail beds.

Histopathological Features   The most typical finding in Hailey-Hailey disease is widespread acantholysis of the spinous layer, which characteristically involves at least one-half of the thickness of the epidermis. Acanthosis is usually present. Whereas numerous completely acantholytic cells can be found free within the resulting intraspinous vesicles, other regions of contiguously affected cells are not completely separated but rather remain partially tethered to one another (Fig. 14-14). When fully developed, this suprabasal change gives an appearance that has been aptly likened to a "dilapidated brick wall." As in Darier's disease, villus projections lined by a single row of basal cells often project into the lacunae and bullae. The acantholytic cells generally retain an otherwise normal appearance without morphologically apparent dyskeratosis, but focally the latter can develop and may resemble the corp ronds and grains of Darier's disease.

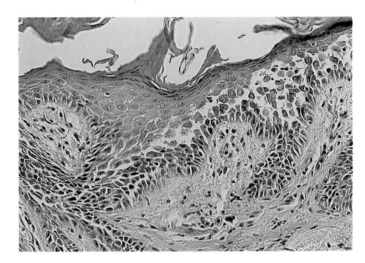

FIGURE 14-14   Hailey-Hailey disease. Acantholysis affects the suprabasal to middle spinous layers in an incomplete fashion that has resulted in keratinocytes remaining partially tethered to one another, giving the impression of a "dilapidated brick wall."

Differential Diagnosis   Both Hailey-Hailey and Darier's diseases share common features of suprabasal acantholysis and formation of villus structures that protrude into separations created by acantholytic keratinocytes. In Darier's disease, however, the separations take the form of small lacunae, in contrast to the larger vesicles and bullae resulting from more widespread acantholysis in Hailey-Hailey disease. Moreover, dyskeratosis is typically a feature of Darier's disease and is associated with the development of corp ronds and grains. The discrimination of Hailey-Hailey disease from pemphigus vulgaris can be difficult because the initial pathologic process in each disorder is suprabasal acantholysis. In pemphigus, however, there is less acantholysis overall, and the separations are often strikingly restricted to the cell layer immediately superficial to the basal keratinocytes, lacking the "dilapidated brick wall" effect of Hailey-Hailey disease. When present, the finding of intralesional eosinophils supports the diagnosis of pemphigus vulgaris. Resolution of the differential diagnosis requires direct immunofluorescence assay for display of the characteristic intercellular autoantibody deposition in pemphigus but not in Hailey-Hailey disease.

GROVER'S DISEASE (TRANSIENT ACANTHOLYTIC DERMATOSIS)

An apparently acquired abnormality, Grover's disease is a non-immune-mediated acantholytic disorder of the epidermis that afflicts middle-aged or elderly men most often.[88] The onset is often acute, and the duration may be transient or persistent. Structural alterations and dysfunction of keratinocyte adhesion molecules are found in the lesions. Fine structure studies have described dissolution of the components of the desmosomal attachment plaque.[83]

Clinical Features   Intensely pruritic papules, and occasionally papulovesicles, occur predominantly on the trunk and less often on the buttocks and thighs. A history of sun exposure, excessive perspiration, or occlusion of the affected skin, such as from enforced bed rest, can occasionally be elicited.

Histopathological Features   The principal microscopic finding consists of small foci of spinous layer acantholysis (Fig. 14-15). The spectrum of acantholysis in Grover's disease includes both superficial and deep variants, which respectively mimic pemphigus foliaceus and vul-

---

TABLE 14-7

Hailey-Hailey Disease

Clinical Features
   Onset second to fourth decades
   Bullae, erosions at flexural sites, exacerbated by friction and heat
   Dermatitic, verrucoid, and papular variants
Histopathological Features
   Widespread acantholysis affecting more than half of spinous layer
   Dilapidated brick wall
   Villus projections into lacunae
   Acanthosis
Differential Diagnosis
   Grover's disease
   Darier's disease
   Pemphigus vulgaris

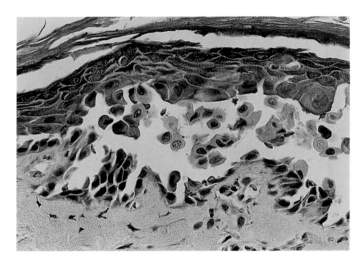

FIGURE 14-15 Grover's disease. This microscopic lacuna, which has been created by acantholysis restricted to the suprabasal keratinocytes, contains dyskeratotic cells and is lined at the base by cells anchored to the basement membrane.

garis. Most often, however, the acantholytic change takes the form of that found in either pemphigus vulgaris or Darier's disease (see above), with acantholytic dyskeratosis. On occasion, the histologic image of Hailey-Hailey disease is simulated, or, uncommonly, the predominant feature can be spongiosis, but with little acantholysis.

Differential Diagnosis   The histopathologic pattern found in Grover's disease generally differs from that of each disease it simulates by the multifocal presentation of small microscopic foci of acantholysis. In dubious instances, the differential diagnosis can be resolved by reference to the clinical presentation, which generally is distinctive for each of the entities simulated histologically by Grover's disease.

PEELING SKIN SYNDROME

Several rare syndromes have been described that share the cardinal feature of peeling of the skin.[1,89,90] Two distinct phenotypes, A and B, have been described. In type A, there are no associated abnormalities, but in type B, variable findings include decreased plasma tryptophan levels, elevated serum copper and iron, aminoaciduria, and elevated serum IgE levels. The presentation is frequently congenital, and inheritance patterns have suggested autosomal recessive transmission, often with a history of parental consanguinity. The disorders are not mediated by autoreactive antibodies.

Clinical Features   Peeling skin syndrome of type A displays generalized, asymptomatic, noninflammatory skin peeling. In contrast, type B presents clinically with generalized patches of peeling skin, in association with inflammation and pruritus. The palms and soles may exhibit keratoderma, and dystrophic nail changes and easily plucked hair are commonly observed.

Histopathological Features   Hyperorthokeratosis is noted microscopically. There characteristically is separation of the upper epidermis, with the histologic split forming between stratum corneum and stratum granulosum or in the lower stratum corneum. One report documents splitting within keratinocytes in a type A subject, whereas the split appears to be intercellular in type B cases. In the type B cases, psoriasiform epidermal hyperplasia, with both hyperkeratosis and parakeratosis, has been

observed. The granular layer may be either retained or lacking, and there can be considerable acanthosis with elongated rete ridges and an underlying chronic perivascular lymphocytic dermatitis in the papillary dermis.

Differential Diagnosis   In histologic sections not displaying the subcorneal separation, the differential diagnosis for disorders histologically resembling autosomal dominant ichthyosis vulgaris will need consideration. Epidermal separation at or near that found in peeling skin syndrome may be observed in staphylococcal scalded skin syndrome and pemphigus foliaceus, but acantholytic cells can be found focally in the latter disorders.

THE PERFORATING DERMATOSES

Four primary perforating dermatoses have traditionally been included among the conditions displaying transepidermal elimination of stromal elements: Kyrle's disease, perforating folliculitis, reactive perforating collagenosis, and elastosis perforans serpiginosa.[91,92] There are, in addition, numerous reports of secondary transepidermal elimination in association with a clearly identifiable primary cutaneous process.[91] The prototype for the primary perforating diseases is Kyrle's disease, as described early in this century.[93] With further studies, however, it has become evident that there are more clinicopathologic similarities than there are differences between Kyrle's disease and the other entities, which has obscured the criteria that were originally advanced for their recognition. Kyrle's disease itself may not be a distinct entity but rather the extreme phenotype of a more common pathophysiologic process.[91,94] Perforating folliculitis and reactive perforating collagenosis, according to the current trend for unification, may be phenotypic variants of a disease spectrum or merely different stages in lesional development. Because of these considerations and in view of their common clinical association with renal disease and diabetes mellitus, Kyrle's disease, reactive perforating collagenosis, and perforating folliculitis have been incorporated for the present purposes under the general designation *acquired perforating dermatosis*, as suggested by others.[94,95] Elastosis perforans serpiginosa is segregated on the basis of its association with disorders of connective tissues and its rather distinctive clinical presentation.

ACQUIRED PERFORATING DERMATOSIS

Acquired perforating dermatosis (including Kyrle's disease, perforating folliculitis, and reactive perforating collagenosis) is commonly associated with chronic renal failure, hemodialysis, and diabetes mellitus.[94–96] Its pathogenesis is poorly understood and has been the subject of wide-ranging conjecture, which has included theories of alterations in vitamin A metabolism, accumulation of nondialyzable metabolic products recognized as foreign by the skin, disordered keratinocyte maturation (e.g., keratinization occurring at the expense of proliferation), and an unusual effect of humoral and cell-mediated immunity. The pathophysiologic mechanism may not be the same for all cases of acquired perforating dermatosis, but rather the mechanism may represent a common response pathway to a variety of epidermal and dermal alterations, acting alone or in combination. The common association with uremia during the early phases of hemodialysis[97] tends to support the theory of dermal deposition of a toxic metabolite that is not dialyzable. Autosomal recessive inheritance has been suggested in some kindreds diagnosed with reactive perforating collagenosis, raising the possibility of a genetic diathesis in those instances.

TABLE 14-8

Acquired Perforating Dermatosis

Clinical Features
  Onset at any age, with few to many lesions, with predilection for
    extensor surfaces
  Common association with chronic renal failure or diabetes mellitus
  Pruritic, follicular or extrafollicular papules, nonconfluent
  Central, conical keratinaceous plug

Histopathological Features
  Keratotic plug within epidermal invagination, over focus of per-
    foration
  Bordered by acanthotic, hyperkeratotic epidermis
  Inflammatory debris in channel, with basophilic collagen and/or
    eosinophilic elastin
  Granulomatous reaction at base

Differential Diagnosis
  Elastosis perforans serpiginosa
  Acneiform eruptions
  Keratosis pilaris

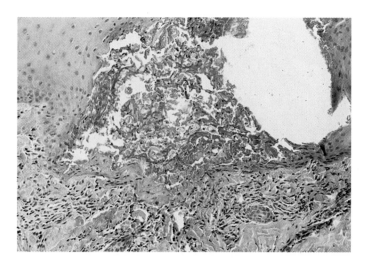

FIGURE 14-16   Acquired perforating dermatosis. The perforation in this follicular lesion has occurred through the infundibulum. Brightly eosinophilic
elastin fibers are present within the basophilic debris filling the transepithelial
channel. The adjacent stroma contains a sparse, mixed mononuclear infiltrate.

Clinical Features   The florid (Kyrle's-disease-like) presentation is
rare, but the milder phenotype is rather common in the setting of chronic
renal failure,[96–99] diabetes,[100,101] or, less commonly, liver disease
(Table 14-8). At clinical presentation, which can occur at any age, there
may be few to many lesions, which are often localized to the legs, or the
onset may be more generalized to all extremities and the torso, with a
predilection for extensor surfaces. Mucous membranes and volar surfaces are spared. The lesions are characteristically pruritic but not
invariably so. The early lesions are pinhead-sized follicular and extrafollicular papules that resemble keratosis pilaris.[93] With progression,
the lesions evolve into larger, red-brown or purplish papules and nodules, or occasionally plaques, tending to remain nonconfluent. Mature
lesions display a central cuplike depression containing a conical, keratinaceous plug. An isomorphic (Koebner) response is frequent. It is
uncommon for the condition to remit spontaneously, but improvement
has been reported following renal transplantation.

Histopathological Features   Early lesions are associated with variable
acanthosis, follicular and perifollicular hyperkeratosis, neutrophils in
the subjacent dermis, and, variably, tinctorial changes in the connective
tissue fibers. Some foci are clearly follicular (Fig. 14-16), others perifollicular.[97] The central cuplike keratotic plug within the epidermal
invagination overlies the locus of epithelial perforation, with its apex
oriented downward.[99,100,102] Some reports describe vacuolar changes in
the keratinocytes at the base of the plug and breaks in the basement
membrane, prior to channelization. The basophilic material undergoing
transepidermal elimination is composed of a mixture of inflammatory
cells and leukocytic debris, a parakeratotic column of keratinaceous
material, and fragments of basophilic collagen and/or eosinophilic
elastin.[94,102,103] At the base can be found a foreign-body granulomatous
reaction, with or without a suppurative component, after the epithelium
has been breached.[100,104] The walls of the channels are bordered by flattened, anucleate, and variably glycogenated keratinocytes, which has
suggested premature keratinization; these altered keratinocytes follow
the outflow of material through the epidermis.[95,102] Extracellular lysosomal enzymes derived from the neutrophils may play an initiating role
by altering elastin and collagen (with its basophilic degeneration) and
possibly opening up the channel[104]; under this model, however, what
initiates chemoattraction of the neutrophils is unclear.

Differential Diagnosis   No absolute criteria discriminate the classic
perforating dermatoses of Kyrle's disease, perforating folliculitis, and
reactive perforating collagenosis because transepidermal elimination of
altered collagen and/or elastin via a central, cuplike invagination can
occur in each. The locus of the elimination may be both follicular and
extrafollicular. Moreover, each can be associated with chronic renal
failure or diabetes mellitus. Observation of an infundibular locus with
hair material for transepidermal elimination, as defined for perforating
folliculitis,[98] may depend on the stage of disease or the extent of the histologic sampling of the biopsy specimen.[94] For these reasons, it seems
arbitrary to separate them. Elastosis perforans serpiginosa also exhibits
histologic similarities, but this condition is distinctive clinically, and it
exhibits microscopically a definite increase in the number and thickness
of the papillary dermal elastic fibers on elastin stains.[105] A cuplike
invagination plugged with keratinaceous material is observed in keratosis pilaris, but there should be no epithelial breach nor elimination of
degenerated collagen or elastin in the latter condition.

ELASTOSIS PERFORANS SERPIGINOSA

An uncommon but clinically distinctive disorder recognized since the
early 1950s, elastosis perforans serpiginosa is characterized by the
transepidermal elimination of altered elastic fibers. Its pathogenesis
remains unclear, but some cases are familial, with an autosomal dominant pattern of inheritance, indicating a genetic basis.[106] The frequent
association in approximately 25 percent of cases with either Down syndrome or an inborn disorder of connective tissue metabolism, such as
Ehlers-Danlos syndrome, osteogenesis imperfecta, pseudoxanthoma
elasticum, or Marfan's syndrome,[105] suggests that the pathophysiology
is based on a defect in the connective tissues. Some cases have been
coincident with penicillamine therapy. From these associations, hyperplastic connective tissue fibers may act as local irritants, provoking epidermal hyperplasia that envelops the altered material, which is then
carried upward by the process of keratinocyte differentiation for
transepidermal elimination.[105]

Clinical Features   The lesions of elastosis perforans serpiginosa,
which are often asymptomatic, occur in arcuate-to-annular arrays that
are characteristically localized to one region of the body, most often the

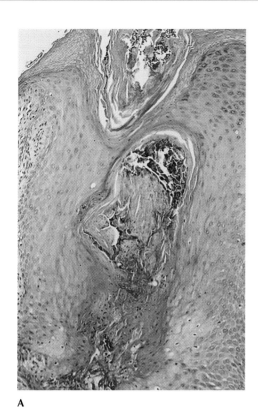

A

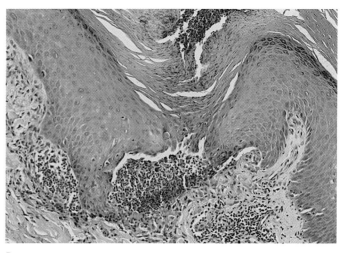

B

FIGURE 14-17   Elastosis perforans serpiginosa. (*A*) A channel breaches the acanthotic, hyperkeratotic epidermis and is covered by a wedge-shaped, parakeratotic plug containing aggregates of leukocytic debris. (*B*) The stroma subjacent to the perforation contains a neutrophil-rich inflammatory infiltrate, within which are several eosinophilic elastic fibers.

nape but on occasion the face or upper extremities (Table 14-9). The lesions are coalescent flesh-colored or erythematous, keratotic papules with central invaginations. There can be clinical resemblance to granuloma annulare or porokeratosis of Mibelli. Spontaneous remissions occur.

Histopathological Features   The lesions, which may be either follicular or extrafollicular, are associated with hyperplasia and hyperkeratosis of the contiguous epidermis. Transepidermal elimination of altered elastin occurs through a central, narrow channel with a funnellike or corkscrew configuration, which is delimited by a collarette formed from the acanthotic epidermis. Within the channel there is basophilic necrotic material, comprised of parakeratotic keratin, degenerated keratinocytes, inflammatory cells, and, most distinctively, brightly eosinophilic elastic fibers[105] (Fig. 14-17*A* and *B*). At the base of the perforation, there is a

chronic inflammatory infiltrate containing multinucleate macrophages. With specific elastin stains of early and fully evolved lesions, increased numbers and sizes of elastic fibers can be shown in the subjacent dermis, from which a stream of fibers enters the perforating channel, losing their normal staining quality as they do so.

Differential Diagnosis   The differential diagnosis of the primary perforating dermatoses is most reliably resolved by the differences in their clinical presentations and disease associations, as the elimination of altered, eosinophilic elastic fibers via a central keratotic channel can be observed in any of the four classic perforating diseases. The finding of increased numbers and sizes of elastic fibers in the subjacent papillary dermis in elastosis perforans serpiginosa by special staining, however, may offer a criterion for its histologic discrimination.[105] The clinical differential diagnosis of elastosis perforans serpiginosa from granuloma annulare and porokeratosis of Mibelli is discriminated histologically by necrobiotic dermal changes and the cornoid lamella, respectively, in the latter two diseases, as well as by the usual absence of transepidermal elimination.

REFERENCES

1. Traupe H: *The Ichthyosis. A Guide to Clinical Diagnosis, Genetic Counseling, and Therapy.* Berlin, Heidelberg, Springer-Verlag, 1989.
2. Wells RS, Kerr CB: Clinical features of autosomal dominant and sex-linked ichthyosis in an English population. *Br Med J* 1:947–950, 1966.
3. Wells RS, Kerr CB: The histology of ichthyosis. *J Invest Dermatol* 46:530–535, 1966.
4. Sybert VP, Dale BA, Holbrook KA: Ichthyosis vulgaris: Identification of a defect in synthesis of filaggrin correlated with an absence of keratohyaline granules. *J Invest Dermatol* 84:191–194, 1985.
5. Nirunsuksiri W, Presland RB, Lewis SP, et al: Decreased profilaggrin expression in ichthyosis vulgaris is a result of selectively impaired post-transcriptional control. *J Biol Chem* 270:871–876, 1995.
6. Mevorah B, Krayenbuhl A, Bovey EH, Van Melle GD: Autosomal dominant ichthyosis and X-linked ichthyosis. *Acta Derm Venereol Stockh* 71:431–434, 1991.
7. Scheimberg I, Harper JI, Malone M, Lake BD: The inherited ichthyoses: A review of the histology of the skin. *Pediatr Pathol Lab Med*, 16:359–378, 1996.

TABLE 14-9

Elastosis Perforans Serpiginosa

Clinical Features
  Typically solitary or few lesions, with predilection for nape
  Common association with Down syndrome or disorders of connective tissue
  Arcuate lesions, formed by coalescence of keratotic papules with central plugs
Histopathological Features
  Increased number and sizes of elastin fibers at base
  Narrow transepithelial channel, delimited by acanthotic, hyperkeratotic epidermis
  Brightly eosinophilic elastin amongst basophilic debris in channel
  Granulomatous reaction at base
Differential Diagnosis
  Acquired perforating dermatosis

8. Kaplan MH, Sadick NS, McNutt NS, et al: Acquired ichthyosis in concomitant HIV-1 and HTLV-II infection: A new association with intravenous drug abuse. *J Am Acad Dermatol* 29:701–708, 1993.

9. Polisky RB, Bronson DM: Acquired ichthyosis in a patient with adenocarcinoma of the breast. *Cutis* 38:359–360, 1986.

10. Uehara M, Miyauchi H: The morphologic characteristics of dry skin in atopic dermatitis. *Arch Dermatol* 120:1186–1190, 1984.

11. Refsum S: Heredopathia atactica polyneuritiformis: Familial syndrome not hitherto described: Contribution to clinical study of hereditary diseases of nervous system. *Acta Psychiatr Scand Suppl* I, 1–303, 1946.

12. Dykes PJ, Marks R, Davies MG, Reynolds DJ: Epidermal metabolism in heredopathia atactica polyneuritiformis (Refsum's disease). *J Invest Dermatol* 70:126–129, 1978.

13. Herndon JH, Steinberg D, Uhlendorf BW, Fales HM: Refsum's disease: Characterization of the enzyme defect in cell culture. *J Clin Invest* 48:1017–1032, 1969.

14. Steinberg D, Vroom FQ, Engel WK, et al: Refsum's disease—a recently characterized lipidosis involving the nervous system. *Ann Intern Med* 66:365–395, 1967.

15. Emami S, Hanley KP, Esterly NB, et al: X-linked dominant ichthyosis with peroxisomal deficiency: An ultrastructural and ultracytochemical study of the Conradi-Hunermann syndrome and its murine homologue, the bare patches mouse. *Arch Dermatol* 130:325–336, 1994.

16. Hamaguchi T, Bondar G, Siegfried E, Penneys NS: Cutaneous histopathology of Conradi-Hunermann syndrome. *J Cutan Pathol* 22:38–41, 1995.

17. Dale BA, Kam E: Harlequin ichthyosis: Variability in expression and hypothesis for disease mechanism. *Arch Dermatol* 129:1471–1477, 1993.

18. Dale BA, Holbrook KA, Fleckman P, et al: Heterogeneity in Harlequin ichthyosis, an inborn error of epidermal keratinization: Variable morphology and structural protein expression and a defect in lamellar granules. *J Invest Dermatol* 94:6–18, 1990.

19. Merrett JD, Wells RS, Kerr CB, Barr A: Discriminant function analysis of phenotype variates in ichthyosis. *Am J Hum Genet* 19:575–585, 1967.

20. Ziprkowski L, Feinstein A: A survey of ichthyosis vulgaris in Israel. *Br J Dermatol* 86:1–8, 1972.

21. Paige DG, Emilion GG, Bouloux PM, Harper JI: A clinical and genetic study of X-linked recessive ichthyosis and contiguous gene defects. *Br J Dermatol* 131:622–629, 1994.

22. Huber M, Rettler I, Bernasconi K, et al: Mutations of keratinocyte transglutaminase in lamellar ichthyosis. *Science* 267:525–528, 1995.

23. Judge MR, Atherton DJ, Salvayre R, et al: Neutral lipid storage disease: Case report and lipid studies. *Br J Dermatol* 130:507–510, 1994.

24. Langer K, Konrad K, Wolff K: Keratitis, ichthyosis and deafness (KID)-syndrome: Report of three cases and a review of the literature. *Br J Dermatol* 122:689–697, 1990.

25. DeLaurenzi V, Rogers GR, Hamrock DJ, et al: Sjögren-Larsson syndrome is caused by mutations in the fatty aldehyde dehydrogenase gene. *Nat Genet* 12:52–57, 1996.

26. Rizzo WB: Sjögren-Larsson syndrome. *Semin Dermatol* 12:210–218, 1993.

27. Kimonis V, DiGiovanna JJ, Yang J-M, et al: A mutation in the V1 end domain of keratin 1 in non-epidermolytic palmar-plantar keratoderma. *J Invest Dermatol* 103:764–769, 1994.

28. Lucker GPH, Kerkhof Van de MPC, Steijlen PM: The hereditary palmoplantar keratoses: An updated review and classification. *Br J Dermatol* 131:1–14, 1994.

29. Kuster W, Becker A: Indication for the identity of palmoplantar keratoderma type Unna-Thost with type Vorner: Thost's family revisited 110 years later. *Acta Derm Venereol* 72:120–122, 1992.

30. Kelsell DP, Stevens HP, Ratnavel R, et al: Genetic linkage studies in non-epidermolytic palmoplantar keratoderma: Evidence for heterogeneity. *Hum Mol Genet* 4:1021–1025, 1995.

31. Itin PH, Lautenschlager S: Palmoplantar keratoderma and associated syndromes. *Semin Dermatol* 14:152–161, 1995.

32. Macfarlane AW, Chapman SJ, Verbov JL: Is erythrokeratoderma one disorder? A clinical and ultrastructural study of two siblings. *Br J Dermatol* 124:487–491, 1991.

33. Schwartz RA: Acanthosis nigricans. *J Am Acad Dermatol* 31:1–19, 1994.

34. Hamm H, Meinecke P, Traupe H: Further delineation of the ichthyosis follicularis, atrichia, and photophobia syndrome. *Eur J Pediatr* 150:627–629, 1991.

35. Vanderhooft SL, Francis JS, Holbrook KA, et al: Familial pityriasis rubra pilaris. *Arch Dermatol* 131:448–453, 1995.

36. Piamphongsant T, Akaraphant R: Pityriasis rubra pilaris: A new proposed classification. *Clin Exp Dermatol* 19:134–138, 1994.

37. Happle R, Mittag H, Kuster W: The CHILD nevus: A distinct skin disorder. *Dermatology* 191:210–216, 1995.

38. Hashimoto K, Topper S, Sharata H, Edwards M: CHILD syndrome: Analysis of abnormal keratinization and ultrastructure. *Pediatr Dermatol* 12:116–129, 1995.

39. Greene SL, Muller SA: Netherton's syndrome: Report of a case and review of the literature. *J Am Acad Dermatol* 13:329–337, 1985.

40. Judge MR, Morgan G, Harper JI: A clinical and immunological study of Netherton's syndrome. *Br J Dermatol* 131:615–621, 1994.

41. Ito M, Fujiwara H, Maruyama T, et al: Morphogenesis of the cornoid lamella: Histochemical, immunohistochemical, and ultrastructural study of porokeratosis. *J Cutan Pathol* 18:247–256, 1991.

42. Ishida-Yamamoto A, McGrath JA, Chapman SJ, et al: Epidermolysis bullosa simplex (Dowling-Meara type) is a genetic disease characterized by an abnormal keratin-filament network involving keratins K5 and K14. *J Invest Dermatol* 97:959–968, 1991.

43. Fuchs E, Coulombe P, Cheng J, Chan Y: Genetic bases of epidermolysis bullosa simplex and epidermolytic hyperkeratosis. *J Invest Dermatol* 103:25S–30S, 1994.

44. Chan YM, Yu QC, Fine JD, Fuchs E: The genetic basis of Weber-Cockayne epidermolysis bullosa simplex. *Proc Natl Acad Sci USA* 90:7414–7418, 1993.

45. McGrath JA, Ishida-Yamamoto A, Tidman MJ, et al: Epidermolysis bullosa simplex (Dowling-Meara): A clinicopathological review. *Br J Dermatol* 126:421–430, 1992.

46. Smith LT: Ultrastructural findings in epidermolysis bullosa. *Arch Dermatol* 129:1578–1584, 1993.

47. Pearson RW: Clinicopathologic types of epidermolysis bullosa and their nondermatological complications. *Arch Dermatol* 124:718–725, 1988.

48. Haber RM, Ramsay CA, Boxall LBH: Epidermolysis bullosa simplex with keratoderma of the palms and soles. *J Am Acad Dermatol* 12:1040–1044, 1985.

49. Gil SG, Brown TA, Ryan MC, Carter WG: Junctional epidermolysis bullosis: Defects in expression of epiligrin/nicein/kalinin and integrin β4 that inhibit hemidesmosome formation. *J Invest Dermatol* 103:31S–38S, 1994.

50. Vidal F, Baudoin C, Miquel C, et al: Cloning of the laminin alpha 3 chain gene (LAMA3) and identification of a homozygous deletion in a patient with Herlitz junctional epidermolysis bullosa. *Genomics* 30:273–280, 1995.

51. Uitto J, Pulkkinen L, Christiano AM: Molecular basis of the dystrophic and junctional forms of epidermolysis bullosa: Mutations in the type VII collagen and kalinin (laminin 5) genes. *J Invest Dermatol* 103:39S–46S, 1994.

52. McGrath JA, Ishida-Yamamoto A, O'Grady A, et al: Structural variations in anchoring fibrils in dystrophic epidermolysis bullosa: Correlation with type VII collagen expression. *J Invest Dermatol* 100:366–372, 1993.

53. Ryynanen M, Knowlton RG, Parente MG, et al: Human type VII collagen: Genetic linkage of the gene (COL7A1) on chromosome 3 to dominant dystrophic epidermolysis bullosa. *Am J Hum Genet* 49:797–803, 1991.

54. Dunnill MG, Richards AJ, Milana G, et al: Genetic linkage to the type VII collagen gene (COL7A1) in 26 families with generalised recessive dystrophic epidermolysis bullosa and anchoring fibril abnormalities. *J Med Genet* 31:745–748, 1994.

55. Christiano AM, Suga Y, Greenspan DS, et al: Premature termination codons on both alleles of the type VII collagen gene (COL7A1) in three brothers with recessive dystrophic epidermolysis bullosa. *J Clin Invest* 95:1328–1334, 1995.

56. Anton-Lamprecht I: Ultrastructural identification of basic abnormalities as clues to genetic disorders of the epidermis. *J Invest Dermatol* 103:6S–12S, 1994.

57. Bonifas JM, Bare JW, Chen MA, et al: Linkage of the epidermolytic hyperkeratosis phenotype and the region of the type II keratin gene cluster on chromosome 12. *J Invest Dermatol* 99:524–527, 1992.

58. Rothnagel JA, Dominey AM, Dempsey LD, et al: Mutations in the rod domains of keratins 1 and 10 in epidermolytic hyperkeratosis. *Science* 257:1128–1130, 1992.

59. Fuchs E, Esteves RA, Coulombe PA: Transgenic mice expressing a mutant keratin 10 gene reveal the likely genetic basis for epidermolytic hyperkeratosis. *Proc Natl Acad Sci USA* 89:6906–6910, 1992.

60. DiGiovanna JJ, Bale SJ: Clinical heterogeneity in epidermolytic hyperkeratosis. *Arch Dermatol* 130:1026–1035, 1994.

61. Bale SJ, Compton JG, DiGiovanna JJ: Epidermolytic hyperkeratosis. *Semin Dermatol* 12:202–209, 1993.

62. Mahaisavariya P, Cohen PR, Rapini RP: Incidental epidermolytic hyperkeratosis. *Am J Dermatopathol* 17:23–28, 1995.

63. Steijlen PM, Kremer H, Vakilzadeh F, et al: Genetic linkage of the keratin type II gene cluster with ichthyosis bullosa of Siemens and with autosomal dominant ichthyosis exfoliativa. *J Invest Dermatol* 103:282–285, 1994.

64. Murdoch ME, Leigh IM: Ichthyosis bullosa of Siemens and bullous ichthyosiform erythroderma—variants of the same disease? *Clin Exp Dermatol* 15:53–56, 1990.

65. Rothnagel JA, Traupe H, Wojcik S, et al: Mutations in the rod domain of keratin 2e in patients with ichthyosis bullosa of Siemens. *Nat Genet* 7:485–490, 1994.

66. Steijlen PM, Perret CM, Schuurmans-Stekhoven JH, et al: Ichthyosis bullosa of Siemens: Further delineation of the phenotype. *Arch Dermatol Res* 282:1–5, 1990.

67. Niemi KM, Virtanen I, Kanerva L, Muttilainen M: Altered keratin expression in ichthyosis hystrix Curth-Macklin: A light and electron microscopic study. *Arch Dermatol Res* 282:227–233, 1990.

68. Bonifas JM, Bare JW, Chen MA, et al: Evidence against keratin gene mutations in a family with ichthyosis hystrix Curth-Macklin. *J Invest Dermatol* 101:890–891, 1993.

69. Navsaria HA, Swensson O, Ratnavel RC, et al: Ultrastructural changes resulting from keratin-9 gene mutations in two families with epidermolytic palmoplantar keratoderma. *J Invest Dermatol* 104:425–429, 1995.

70. Kuster W, Zehender D, Mensing H, et al: Vorner keratosis palmoplantaris diffusa: Clinical, formal genetic and molecular biology studies of 22 families. *Hautarzt* 46:705–710, 1995.

71. Requena L, Schoendorff C, Sanchez-Yus E: Hereditary epidermolytic palmo-plantar keratoderma (Vorner type)—report of a family and review of the literature. *Clin Exp Dermatol* 16:383–388, 1991.

72. Dahl PR, Daoud MS, Su WP: Jadassohn-Lewandowski syndrome (pachyonychia congenita). *Semin Dermatol* 14:129–134, 1995.

73. Munro CS, Carter S, Bryce S, et al: A gene for pachyonychia congenita is closely linked to the keratin gene cluster on 17q12-q21. *J Med Genet* 31:675–678, 1994.

74. Bowden PE, Haley JL, Kansky A, et al: Mutation of a type II keratin gene (K6a) in pachyonychia congenita. *Nat Genet* 10:363–365, 1995.

75. McLean WH, Rugg EL, Lunny DP, et al: Keratin 16 and keratin 17 mutations cause pachyonychia congenita. *Nat Genet* 9:273–278, 1995.

76. Paller AS, Moore JA, Scher R: Pachyonychia congenita. *Arch Dermatol* 127:701–703, 1991.

77. Su WPD, Chun SI, Hammond DE, Gordon H: Pachyonychia congenita: A clinical study of 12 cases and review of the literature. *Pediatr Dermatol* 7:33–38, 1990.

78. Burge SM, Millard PR, Wojnarowska F, Ryan TJ: Darier's disease: A focal abnormality of cell adhesion. *J Cutan Pathol* 17:160–164, 1990.

79. Munro CS: The phenotype of Darier's disease: Penetrance and expressivity in adults and children. *Br J Dermatol* 127:126–130, 1992.

80. Richard G, Wright AR, Harris S, et al: Fine mapping of the Darier's disease locus on chromosome 12q. *J Invest Dermatol* 103:665–668, 1994.

81. Burge SM, Wilkinson JD: Darier-White disease: A review of the clinical features in 163 patients. *J Am Acad Dermatol* 27:40–50, 1992.

82. Sanchez YE, Requena L, Simon P, deHijas CM: Incidental acantholysis. *J Cutan Pathol* 20:418–423, 1993.

83. Hashimoto K, Fujiwara K, Harada M, et al: Junctional proteins of keratinocytes in Grover's disease, Hailey-Hailey's disease and Darier's disease. *J Dermatol* 22:159–170, 1995.

84. Burge SM, Cederholm-Williams SA, Garrod DR, Ryan TJ: Cell adhesion in Hailey-Hailey disease and Darier's disease: Immunocytological and explant-tissue-culture studies. *Br J Dermatol* 125:426–435, 1991.

85. Hailey H, Hailey H: Familial benign chronic pemphigus. *Arch Dermatol* 39:679–685, 1939.

86. Ikeda S, Welsh EA, Peluso AM, et al: Localization of the gene whose mutations underlie Hailey-Hailey disease to chromosome 3q. *Hum Mol Genet* 3:1147–1150, 1994.

87. Burge SM: Hailey-Hailey disease: The clinical features, response to treatment and prognosis. *Br J Dermatol* 126:275–282, 1992.

88. Grover RW: Transient acantholytic dermatosis. *Arch Dermatol* 101:426–434, 1970.

89. Levy SB, Goldsmith LA: The peeling skin syndrome. *J Am Acad Dermatol* 7:606–613, 1982.

90. Aras N, Sutman K, Tastan HB, et al: Peeling skin syndrome. *J Am Acad Dermatol* 30:135–136, 1994.

91. Mehregan AH: Perforating dermatoses: A clinicopathologic review. *Int J Dermatol* 16:19–27, 1977.

92. Sehgal VN, Jain S, Thappa DM, et al: Perforating dermatoses: A review and report of four cases. *J Dermatol* 20:329–340, 1993.

93. Kyrle J: Hyperkeratosis follicularis et parafollicularis in cutem penetrans. *Arch Dermatol Syphilol* (Berlin) 123:466–493, 1916.

94. Rapini RP, Hebert AA, Drucker CR: Acquired perforating dermatosis: Evidence for combined transepidermal elimination of both collagen and elastic fibers. *Arch Dermatol* 125:1074–1078, 1989.

95. Patterson JW, Brown PC: Ultrastructural changes in acquired perforating dermatosis. *Int J Dermatol* 31:201–205, 1992.

96. Hood AF, Hardegen GL, Zarate AR, et al: Kyrle's disease in patients with chronic renal failure. *Arch Dermatol* 118:85–88, 1982.

97. Garcia-Bravo B, Rodriguez-Pichardo A, Camacho F: Uraemic follicular hyperkeratosis. *Clin Exp Dermatol* 10:448–454, 1985.

98. Mehregan AH, Coskey RJ: Perforating folliculitis. *Arch Dermatol* 97:394–399, 1968.

99. Stone RA: Kyrle-like lesions in two patients with renal failure undergoing dialysis. *J Am Acad Dermatol* 5:707–709, 1981.

100. Abele DC, Dobson RL: Hyperkeratosis penetrans (Kyrle's disease). *Arch Dermatol* 83:277–283, 1961.

101. Carter VH, Constantine VS: Kyrle's disease: I. Clinical findings in five cases and review of literature. *Arch Dermatol* 97:624–632, 1968.

102. Constantine VS, Carter VH: Kyrle's disease: II. Histopathologic findings in five cases and review of the literature. *Arch Dermatol* 97:633–639, 1968.

103. Mehregan AH, Schwartz OD, Livingood CS: Reactive perforating collagenosis. *Arch Dermatol* 96:277–282, 1967.

104. Zelger B, Hintner H, Aubock J, Fritsch PO: Acquired perforating dermatosis: Transepidermal elimination of DNA material and possible role of leukocytes in pathogenesis. *Arch Dermatol* 127:695–700, 1991.

105. Mehregan AH: Elastosis perforans serpiginosa: A review of the literature and report of 11 cases. *Arch Dermatol* 97:381–393, 1968.

106. Langeveld-Wildschut EG, Toonstra J, van Vloten WA, Beemer FA: Familial elastosis perforans serpiginosa. *Arch Dermatol* 129:205–207, 1993.

CHAPTER 15

DISORDERS OF PIGMENTATION

Ken Hashimoto / Raymond L. Barnhill

The source of pigment which causes hyperpigmentation of the skin ranges from endogenous products such as melanin and hemosiderin to exogenous agents such as dyes for tattoos, ingested metals, and drugs. In some instances these agents are combined to produce hyperpigmentation; for example, in argyria- and chlorpromazine-related hyperpigmentation, silver particles plus melanin and drug metabolites and melanin contribute to the dyschromasia. Ultraviolet rays often enhance these pigmentations, and, therefore, sun-exposed skin shows more intense discoloration. When the basal layer of the epidermis is heavily melanized, incontinence of melanin results in upper dermal melanization as well. Disorders of hypopigmentation and depigmentation are mainly caused by damage to and dysfunction of epidermal melanocytes (Tables 15-1 and 15-2). In some congenital diseases melanocytes are absent (piebaldism). The circulation of blood through the superficial capillary plexus may influence the skin color as evidenced by nevus anemicus. Both hyper- and hypopigmentations may be congenital and/or hereditary, may occur after inflammation, or may be induced by chemicals and foreign materials.

Melanocytes from all sites (skin, hair bulb, eye, etc.) produce melanosomes which in the normal process mature into electron-dense stage IV melanosomes in dark-skinned races. The maturation is arrested at stage I or II in fair-skinned Caucasians (Fig. 15-1). In leukodermic conditions, various dysfunctions of tyrosinase or damage to melanocytes produce less-pigmented melanosomes or a decreased number of them (Figs. 15-2, 15-3). These changes are more visible in dark-skinned races. Conversely, hyperactivity of melanocytes results in various hyperpigmented conditions, and in such disorders the lesions of dark-skinned individuals are again more striking than those of Caucasians. In some conditions the transfer of melanosomes from normal melanocytes to the surrounding basal keratinocytes is disturbed (Fig. 15-4). This causes an uneven light color of the lesion (e.g., nevus depigmentosus) or in some instances hyperpigmentation (e.g., Peutz-Jegher syndrome). In many hyperpigmented conditions (e.g., lentigo simplex and senilis) the rete ridges are elongated, and a heavy aggregation of melanocytes and heavy pigmentation occur along the basal layer and particularly at the tips (Fig. 15-5).

The DOPA stain has long been the standard method to demonstrate melanin-synthesizing melanocytes (Table 15-3) (Fig. 15-3). Silver stains such as the Fontana-Masson stain have been used to demonstrate melanin granules (aggregated melanosomes) (Figs. 15-2, 15-6). More recently pathology laboratories routinely perform immunoperoxidase stains, and this method is universally available. Today, it is much more convenient to use melanocyte-specific monoclonal antibodies such as MEL-5 (Fig. 15-7), which is applicable to formalin-fixed, paraffin-embedded tissues, than to use conventional DOPA stain.

HYPOPIGMENTATION DISORDERS

In these disorders the histopathology is mostly nonspecific (Tables 15-1 and 15-4). Epidermal melanocytes are either absent or inactive; accordingly the epidermis is hypomelanized or totally depigmented.

Piebaldism (Patterned Leukoderma)

Clinical Features   There are congenital patches of depigmentation (leukoderma), a white forelock, or poliosis (white hairs) in 85 percent of patients, and the occasional association of Hirschprung disease (aganglionic megacolon).[1–3] Hyperpigmented macules may occur in the depigmented lesions or in normal skin. The disease is dominantly inherited. Unlike vitiligo, the leukoderma is mostly permanent, because melanocytes are largely absent in the lesion. Occasionally repigmentation may occur at the periphery of a lesion or, rarely, within the depigmented macule. In a similar disorder of mice, i.e., dominant white spotting, a mutation or deletion of the C-KIT gene has been detected. The C-KIT proto-oncogene was originally found in HZ4-feline sarcoma virus (hence *kit*). It is an important gene for the production of cell-surface receptors for embryonic growth factors (stem cell factor, mast cell growth factor, and so on) and seems to promote development, migration, and survival of melanocytes. The human piebaldism gene locus has been mapped to chromosome 4q12, a site near the human KIT gene locus.

In the Klein-Waardenburg syndrome,[4] also dominantly inherited, the white forelock (in 50 percent of patients) and congenital patches of leukoderma are associated with hypertelorism and heterochromia of irides.

Histopathological Features   The DOPA reaction and antimelanocyte antibody (MEL-5) stain are negative in the leukoderma and white hair of the forelock. Electron microscopy does not reveal melanocytes with melanosomes. The hyperpigmented macules contain normal numbers of melanocytes.

Differential Diagnosis   The depigmented macules in piebaldism cannot be histologically distinguished from established lesions of vitiligo and leukodermas resulting from chemicals, trauma, or burns that show loss of all epidermal melanocytes (see discussion for vitiligo) without clinical details. Most other leukodermas are distinguished from piebaldism by the presence of melanocytes.

303

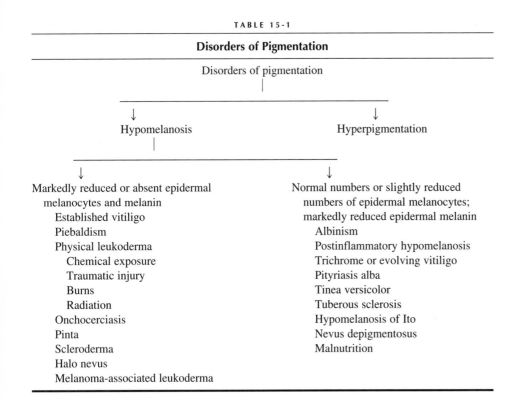

TABLE 15-1

Disorders of Pigmentation

Disorders of pigmentation	
Hypomelanosis	Hyperpigmentation
Markedly reduced or absent epidermal melanocytes and melanin	Normal numbers or slightly reduced numbers of epidermal melanocytes; markedly reduced epidermal melanin
Established vitiligo	Albinism
Piebaldism	Postinflammatory hypomelanosis
Physical leukoderma	Trichrome or evolving vitiligo
Chemical exposure	Pityriasis alba
Traumatic injury	Tinea versicolor
Burns	Tuberous sclerosis
Radiation	Hypomelanosis of Ito
Onchocerciasis	Nevus depigmentosus
Pinta	Malnutrition
Scleroderma	
Halo nevus	
Melanoma-associated leukoderma	

Vitiligo and Vogt-Koyanagi-Harada Syndrome

Vitiligo is an acquired patchy pigment loss of the skin and, rarely, of the hairs that may develop at any age; it is rarely congenital (Table 15-5).[5] Up to 30 percent of cases have a familial basis. Vitiligo may present with focal lesions, i.e., one or more isolated macules, segmental lesions which are unilateral and often show a dermatomal pattern, generalized symmetric lesions commonly periorificial, and with universal involvement. Individual macules of established vitiligo often measure several centimeters, are completely depigmented with a milk-white color, and have well-defined often scalloped borders. *Trichrome vitiligo* refers to three types of lesions: white (established vitiligo), light tan (transitional areas that will become depigmented), and normal brown areas.

When serum IgG from the vitiligo patient is injected into nude mice to which normal human skin has been grafted, melanocytes of the grafted skin are damaged, and DOPA stain–positive melanocytes are significantly decreased, suggesting an autoimmune mechanism in the etiology. Electron microscopy shows cytolysis of melanocytes. Vitiligo is probably an autoimmune disease in which autoantibodies are formed against the melanocyte or melanosome and destroy them via antibody-mediated cytotoxicity and complement-mediated cytolysis. The titers of autoantibody seem to correlate with the disease activity. In the Vogt-Koyanagi-Harada syndrome, not only the skin (vitiligo) but other melanocyte-bearing tissues such as leptomeninges (meningitis), uveal tract (uveitis), and stria vascularis of the ear (dysacousia) are attacked by autoantibodies.

Histopathological Features   In well-established lesions neither melanocytes nor melanin can be detected in the epidermis with the hematoxylin and eosin (H&E) stain as well as with various other staining methods including the DOPA stain, silver impregnation, and MEL-5. Likewise, melanosome-containing melanocytes are not detected with electron microscopy. At the periphery of the lesion large melanocytes with long dendritic processes and many melanosomes are present

TABLE 15-2

Disorders of Hyperpigmentation

Disorders of hyperpigmentation			
Predominantly increased epidermal melanin (some pigment incontinence)	Predominantly increased dermal melanin (pigment incontinence)	Both epidermal and dermal melanin increased	Increased melanin, epidermal and/or dermal, and other pigments
	Postinflammatory hypermelanosis	Postinflammatory hypermelanosis	Tattoo
Diffuse hypermelanosis Patterned or circumscribed hypermelanosis	Melasma (dermal)	Melasma	Hemochromatosis
Addison's disease Freckle	Incontinentia pigmenti		Argyria
Myxedema CALM	Prurigo pigmentosa		Chrysiasis
Grave's disease Melanotic macule			Mercury
Malnutrition of Albright			Arsenic
Hemochromatosis, Lentigo			Lead
early Melasma (epidermal)			Bismuth
Chemotherapeutic Becker's melanosis			Minocycline
agents			Antimalarials
			Amiodarone
			Clofazimine
			Phenothiazine

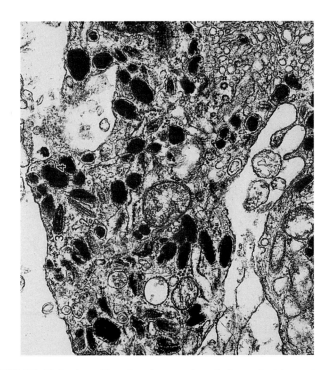

FIGURE 15-1 An epidermal melanocyte is actively synthesizing melanosomes. Stage I melanosome contains amorphous material and is not dark (electron-lucent). In stage II, cristae are formed, and melanin begins to deposit on them. In stage III, melanin polymers become denser and in stage IV the increased density masks underlying structure of cristae.

(Figs. 15-2, 15-3), as if they were trying to cover the depigmented areas. Lymphocytic infiltration and basal cell vacuolization may be seen at the advancing border of vitiligo. The light tan areas of trichrome vitiligo show both basilar melanocytes and melanin.

Differential Diagnosis The differential diagnosis of vitiligo is related to the distribution and extent of the hypopigmentation encountered as well as other clinical factors. Other conditions to be considered include leukoderma from chemicals, trauma, burns, halo nevi, melanoma,

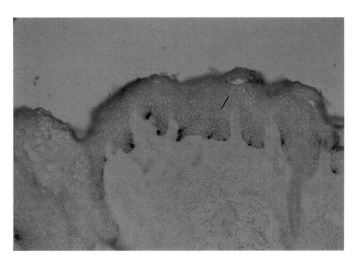

FIGURE 15-3 DOPA stain of the edge of vitiligo lesion. DOPA-positive melanocytes are regularly distributed in the basal layer in the normal skin on the right, and those with negative DOPA reaction are in the lesion on the left.

piebaldism, and Waardenburg's syndrome, all of which may show absence of epidermal melanocytes and melanin and thus be histologically indistinguishable from established vitiligo without clinical information. In addition, the following entities may be clinically confused with vitiligo: lupus erythematosus, postinflammatory hypopigmentation, tuberous sclerosis, pityriasis alba, tinea versicolor, leprosy, idiopathic guttate hypomelanosis, and nevus depigmentosus. In general, the latter processes will show basilar melanocytes, diminished epidermal melanin, and distinctive features in some of the diseases, e.g., lupus erythematosus, leprosy, and tinea versicolor.

It must be emphasized that the presence of some basilar melanocytes and epidermal melanin does not necessarily rule out vitiligo, since skin adjacent to vitiligo, trichrome vitiligo, and repigmenting vitiligo may show the latter changes.

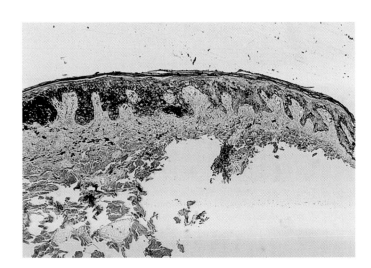

FIGURE 15-2 Silver stain (cf. Fig. 15-6) of the edge of vitiligo. Heavily melanized normal skin on the left makes a striking contrast to less melanized vitiliginous skin. With this stain all melanin granules, either within melanocytes or outside of them, are stained.

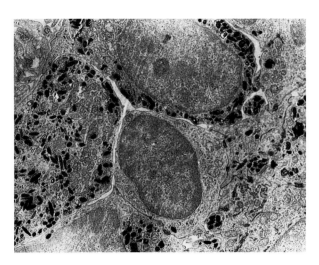

FIGURE 15-4 Blockade of melanosome transfer from two heavily melanized melanocytes to a basal keratinocyte in center is seen. This keratinocyte contains only a few transferred melanosomes.

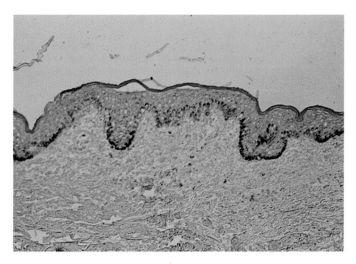

FIGURE 15-5 Lentigo simplex. A heavy melanization of rete ridges, particularly around the tip, is seen. H&E stain.

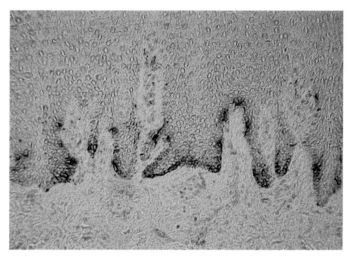

FIGURE 15-7 MEL-5 stain. Formalin-fixed, paraffin-embedded tissue section is stained to demonstrate melanocytes. This monoclonal antibody labels melanosome membrane. The stained pattern of basal melanocytes are comparable to that shown in Fig. 15-3.

Oculocutaneous Albinism

Clinical Features Total loss of pigment from the skin and hair occurs with associated blue irides and red fundi of the eyes (Table 15-6).[6] This condition is also called simply *albinism*. It is congenital and recessively inherited. There are two subtypes, i.e., tyrosinase-positive and tyrosinase-negative. In the former, a plucked hair bulb becomes dark after incubation in DOPA solution. These patients may develop freckles and pigmented nevi. In the latter the hair bulb does not become dark after incubation in DOPA solution and will never become pigmented. However, the degree of skin pigmentation such as the ability to tan is variable among both types, depending upon the mutant alleles. Optical findings such as foveal hypoplasia, misrouting of optic nerve to the brain, and reduced visual acuity are universal for all types of albinism.

The tyrosinase-negative type is now further subclassified into OCA-1A, in which there is no tyrosinase activity; OCA-1B (yellow OCA) and OCA-1MP (minimal pigment OCA), in which some tyrosinase activity is present; and OCA-2TS (temperature sensitive). Various mutations of tyrosinase gene on chromosome 11q14-21 are responsible for these different clinical phenotypes.

Histopathological Features In all types basal clear cells (melanocytes) are observed, but epidermal melanin content is greatly diminished or absent. Electron microscopy proves the presence of normal melanocytes. In the tyrosinase-positive type some melanosomes mature to stages III and IV, whereas in the tyrosinase-negative type, the melanosomes are not pigmented even after the incubation with DOPA.

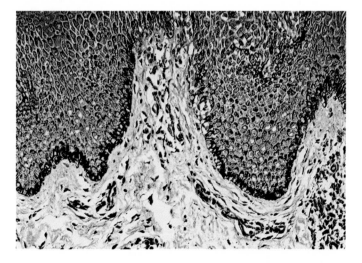

FIGURE 15-6 Silver stain of a lesion of postinflammatory hyperpigmentation. A linear hypermelanization of the basal layer and a moderate melanization of prickle cell layer are noticed. Melanin particles are scattered in the papillary dermis.

TABLE 15-3

Evaluation of Disorders of Pigmentation

1. Hematoxylin and eosin–stained sections of lesional and uninvolved skin for basilar melanocytes, melanin, other changes such as inflammation, granulomas
2. Silver stains, such as Fontana-Masson for melanin, dendritic melanocytes
3. Other stains, such as PAS, acid-fast bacillus, Fite-Faraco for infectious organisms; Prussian blue for iron, hemosiderin
4. DOPA reaction to demonstrate melanocytes (specific for tyrosinase) not practical—special fixation and development required
5. MEL-5 antibody to demonstrate melanocytes by immunohistochemistry
6. Examination by electron microscope to demonstrate quantitative and qualitative aspects of melanosomes
7. Clinical information, such as congenital or acquired onset, diffuse or circumscribed nature of process, distribution of disorder, history of trauma, chemical exposure, other dermatoses, infectious disease

TABLE 15-4

Disorders of Hypopigmentation: Principal Histopathological Features

Disorder	Basilar melanocytes	Melanin in basal layer	Other findings
Established vitiligo	Absent	Absent	
Vitiligo margin	Present, enlarged	Present, reduced in number	Basal layer vacuolization, lymphocytic infiltrates
Trichrome vitiligo (light tan skin)	Present	Present	
Piebaldism, Waardenburg's syndrome, Woolf's syndrome	Absent	Absent	
Albinism	Normal number, morphology	Greatly reduced or absent	
Chédiak-Higashi syndrome	Present	Greatly reduced or absent	Large pigment granules (giant melanosomes)
Tuberous sclerosis (ash-leaf macules)	Present	Reduced	Reduced number, size, and melanization of melanosomes
Hypomelanosis of Ito	Normal or decreased in number	Decreased	Underdeveloped dendrites
Nevus depigmentosus	Normal numbers	Decreased	Poorly developed dendrites, decreased melanosomes
Postinflammatory hypomelanosis	Normal or slightly reduced numbers	Decreased	Block in transfer of melanosomes to keratinocytes
Pityriasis alba	Reduced	Decreased	Fewer and smaller melanosomes
Tinea versicolor	Normal	Decreased	Defective melanosome maturation and transfer block
Idiopathic guttate hypomelanosis	Slightly decreased	Decreased	Atrophic epidermis immature melanosomes, stages I and II
Physical, chemical depigmentation	Absent	Absent	Possible scarring

Chédiak-Higashi Syndrome

This autosomal recessive disorder resembles oculocutaneous albinism because of the fair color of skin, hair, and irides; nystagmus; and photophobia.[7,8] Patients rarely survive beyond childhood because of an increased susceptibility to bacterial infections. The skin is creamy white, but the degree of depigmentation is not very striking. The hair is light blond to brown and has a silver-green sheen.

Histopathological Features   As with OCA mentioned above, basilar melanocytes are present, but epidermal melanin is diminished. With a silver stain one can detect large melanin granules throughout the epidermis and in the melanophages in the upper dermis. Electron microscopy reveals that these granules are localized to membrane-bound giant melanosomes. Hair contains the same giant melanosomes. Giemsa stain of a blood smear shows numerous large granules in leukocytes. These granules are formed by the fusion of abnormal phagosomes which are not capable of killing bacteria in normal fashion.

Ash Leaf Spots of Tuberous Sclerosis

In this autosomal dominant disease one may find ash-leaf-shaped hypopigmented spots in 50 to 98 percent of the patients.[9] These spots are scattered over the trunk and extremities from birth or early childhood. They are therefore a significant early sign of the disease, like axillary freckling of neurofibromatosis. The combination of these congenital hypopigmented lesions with seizures and mental retardation is highly suggestive of tuberous sclerosis. Additional depigmentations are poliosis and depigmentation spots of the iris and retina.

The gene for tuberous sclerosis has been mapped to chromosomes 9q33-34 (tuberous sclerosis 1) and 16p13.3 (tuberous sclerosis 2), and the gene product tuberin is believed to be abnormal in the latter.

Histopathological Features   A normal to reduced density of melanocytes is present, but the DOPA reaction is weak compared to the surrounding normal skin. By electron microscopy, the size of melanosomes and degree of melanization are less than the normal counterparts. In addition, the dendrites of melanocytes are less well developed.

Differential Diagnosis   The principal entities to be considered include: piebaldism, vitiligo, nevus depigmentosus, hypomelanosis of Ito, and postinflammatory hypopigmentation. The ash-leaf macules are discriminated from piebaldism and vitiligo by the presence of melanocytes in the former and differing clinical features. Nevus depigmentosus may be difficult to distinguish from ash-leaf macules, since both lesions are usually congenital and show basilar melanocytes in hypopigmented

TABLE 15-5

Vitiligo

Clinical Features

Onset any age, especially adolescents, young adults
Patterns:
    Generalized-periorificial, bony prominences, extensor surfaces
    Segmental-dermatomal
    Localized
Milk-white macular lesions
    Well-defined, scalloped borders
Trichrome lesions
    Light tan
Associations:
    Thyroid disease, diabetes mellitus, Addison's disease, pernicious
        anemia

Histopathological Features

Established (depigmented) lesions
    Absence of epidermal melanocytes and melanin
Marginal (normal) skin
    Epidermal melanocytes and melanin present
    Basal layer vacuolization often
    Sparse lymphocytic infiltrates
Trichrome vitiligo
    Epidermal melanocytes and melanin present but usually reduced

Differential Diagnosis

Piebaldism
Chemical, physical depigmentation
Postinflammatory hypopigmentation
Lupus erythematosus
Pityriasis alba
Tinea versicolor
Tuberous sclerosis
Leprosy
Melanoma-associated leukoderma
Idiopathic guttate hypomelanosis
Nevus depigmentosus

TABLE 15-6

Albinism

Clinical Features

Abnormalities of optic system
    Nystagmus, photophobia, decreased visual acuity
    Blue and translucent iris (blue eyes)
Hair white to yellow
White skin
Often greatly increased risk for skin cancer
Autosomal recessive
    Numerous variants

Histopathological Features

Melanocytes normal in number and structure
Greatly reduced or absent epidermal melanin

Differential Diagnosis

Rare genetic disorders with hypopigmentation
Universal vitiligo

---

skin. However, the clinical findings of seizures and mental retardation are indicative of tuberous sclerosis. Postinflammatory hypopigmentation is an acquired and more clinically variable condition as compared to ash-leaf macules.

Idiopathic Guttate Hypomelanosis (IGH)

This condition is relatively common among older (>50 years) African-American men and women (Table 15-7).[10] It may be equally frequent among Caucasians but is not as noticeable as in blacks. Numerous well-demarcated depigmented and hypopigmented ("porcelain white") macules 2 to 10 mm in diameter are seen on the shins and less frequently on the extensor aspects of the arms.

Histopathological Features   The epidermis is atrophic with flattened rete ridges and shows decreased melanin content. Basilar melanocytes are observed but are reduced in number with the DOPA reaction. Examination with an electron microscope reveals that most melanosomes are immature at stages I and II and the dendrites of melanocytes

are less well-developed than normal. Normal melanocytes may be intermingled with these less active ones.

Differential Diagnosis   Vitiligo, chemical and traumatic depigmentation, postinflammatory hypopigmentation, tuberous sclerosis, and tinea versicolor enter into the differential diagnosis. IGH differs from vitiligo and chemical and traumatic depigmentation by the presence of melanocytes in IGH. IGH is primarily discriminated from other leukodermas by its distinctive clinical features and distribution.

Hypomelanosis of Ito or Incontinentia Pigmenti Achromians

Hypopigmented bands or streaks are found on the trunk at birth or during first year of life.[11] The pattern of hypopigmented bands follow, as in incontinentia pigmenti, the lines of Blaschko. Repigmentation may occur in some cases. Mental retardation or seizure disorders may be present. Karyotyping of blood lymphocytes, skin fibroblasts, and/or keratinocytes of 115 patients has revealed abnormalities in 60, but these abnormalities are neither uniform nor specific. Chromosomal alterations reported with some frequency include mosaicism for tetrasomy 12p and for trisomy 18. Somatic cell line mosaicism obviously is responsible for the hypopigmentation. Diploidy/triploidy 45, X/46, X, r(X) or 45, X/46, X + mar and chimerism of 46, XX/46, XY are also relatively frequent. Single-gene inheritance has not been proved in this disease.

Histopathological Features   The hypopigmented area has fewer and smaller melanocytes than the normal skin, as detected by DOPA stain. Examination by electron microscopy demonstrates significantly decreased numbers of melanosomes in the melanocytes and basal keratinocytes. Some melanocytes show degenerative changes and contain no melanosomes.

Differential Diagnosis   The major conditions to be considered are nevus depigmentosus and postinflammatory hypopigmentation. The clinical findings of symmetric swirled lesions in patients with seizures,

TABLE 15-7

Idiopathic Guttate Hypomelanosis

Clinical Features

Older individual (especially older than 50 years)
Sun-exposed surfaces of extremities
Discrete, usually round, white macules about 5 mm in diameter; multiple, often numerous

Histopathological Features

Hyperkeratosis
Effacement of epidermis
Reduction in number of melanocytes
    Poorly developed dendrites
Significant reduction in epidermal melanin
Electron microscopy
    Stage I and stage II melanosomes

Differential Diagnosis

Vitiligo
Physical leukoderma
Postinflammatory hypopigmentation
Tinea versicolor

---

mental retardation, and other developmental abnormalities should facilitate this discrimination, since the histologic findings in these disorders may be similar and not definitive.

Nevus Depigmentosus

A solitary congenital patch of hypopigmentation occurs on the trunk and neck and in other locations.[12] Such a lesion may be systematized in a quasidermatomal distribution. In contrast to vitiligo or piebaldism, depigmentation is not complete, and the contour is usually not smooth as in vitiligo but is rather ragged.

Histopathological Features   The number of basilar melanocytes is normal, and the amount of epidermal melanin is decreased with a silver stain. The DOPA stain shows a normal population of melanocytes but the reaction is reduced in intensity. Examination by electron microscopy reveals poorly developed, less dendritic melanocytes. However, they contain normal melanosomes with normal to decreased melanosome count. The abnormality seems to be their abnormal aggregation within the melanocytes and failure to be transferred to the basal keratinocytes, since melanosomes in these keratinocytes are reduced in number.

Differential Diagnosis   Conditions to be excluded include piebaldism, segmental vitiligo, tuberous sclerosis, postinflammatory hypopigmentation, and hypomelanosis of Ito. Nevus depigmentosus is congenital, differs from the first two disorders histologically because of normal numbers of epidermal melanocytes and from the latter three entities based primarily on clinical features, since the histologic features may be quite similar.

Pityriasis Alba

This condition causes hypopigmented patchy macules around the nose, cheeks, and eyebrow areas of children, particularly in blacks, and is often misdiagnosed as tinea faciae because fine scales may cover the

lesion.[13] The condition may be equally common among white children but may be less noticeable. This condition is probably a variant of seborrheic dermatitis or atopic dermatitis, and pityrosporum infection may be a contributing factor.

Histopathological Features   The principal findings include hyperkeratosis, patchy parakeratosis, slight acanthosis, possibly slight spongiosis, and a superficial perivascular lymphocytic infiltrate. The lack of pigmentation is due to decreased basal layer melanin; the number of basilar melanocytes is normal or decreased, and these cells produce fewer and smaller melanosomes. Transfer of melanosomes to the keratinocytes is normal. Many authors have attributed the loss of pigment to a screening of light by a thick epidermis and postinflammatory phenomenon. However, many inflammatory dermatoses with hyperkeratosis lack hypomelanosis. Pityrosporum species may be involved in the etiology, and the tyrosinase inhibitor azelaic acid as in tinea versicolor is produced by these lipophilic yeasts.

Differential Diagnosis   The major conditions to be considered are postinflammatory hypopigmentation, tinea versicolor, vitiligo, and leprosy. In general, the clinical features and identification of microorganisms should allow discrimination of pityriasis alba from other leukodermas. In reality, pityriasis alba may be a form of postinflammatory pigment loss.

Postinflammatory Leukoderma or Hypomelanosis

Hypomelanotic macular lesions may follow a number of inflammatory dermatitides such as eczematous dermatitis, seborrheic dermatitis, psoriasis, drug eruptions, pityriasis lichenoides chronica, lupus erythematosus, lichen planus, alopecia mucinosa, sarcoidosis, and mycosis fungoides (not an inflammatory process per se) (Table 15-8). In general, the latter type of leukoderma is fairly similar irrespective of the antecedent

TABLE 15-8

Postinflammatory Hypopigmentation

Clinical Features

Widespread or localized
Usually follows dermatitis, such as eczematous dermatitis, psoriasis, pityriasis lichenoides, lichen planus, lupus erythematosus, seborrheic dermatitis, mycosis fungoides
Off-white (not fully depigmented)
    Macular lesions with ill-defined margins
Repigmentation occurs

Histopathological Features

Basilar melanocytes present
Reduced melanin in epidermis (blocked transfer to keratinocytes, often)
Evidence of antecedent inflammatory process may be present in early lesions

Differential Diagnosis

Vitiligo
Chemical, physical depigmentation
Tinea versicolor
Pityriasis alba
Leprosy

TABLE 15-9

Physical Leukoderma (Depigmentation)

Clinical Features

Physical injury
Thermal injury
Radiation
Chemical exposure
    Phenols
    Catechols
    Sulfhydryl compound
Depigmented macular lesions of sites of exposure, injury

Histopathological Features

Absence of melanocytes and melanin
Reparative changes (depending on agent)

Differential Diagnosis

Vitiligo
Scleroderma
Onchocerciasis
Pinta
Melanoma-associated leukoderma

inflammatory condition. The clinical lesions are usually off-white (not fully depigmented), often have indistinct margins, and show gradual repigmentation.

Melanocytes also may be severely damaged by various physical, chemical, thermal, and other pathologic injuries (Table 15-9). Hypopigmentation may be temporary or permanent. Repigmentation may occur rapidly on sun-exposed sites and in less severely damaged areas. The repigmentation is irregular and often shows a mottled pattern. Total destruction of melanocytes in burns, exposure to certain chemicals (Table 15-8), infectious diseases such as pinta or onchocerciasis, discoid lupus erythematosus, scleroderma, halo nevi may leave a permanent leukoderma.

Histopathological Features   In general, reversible forms of leukoderma show basilar melanocytes—often in normal numbers but in some instances reduced in number or damaged—and reduced epidermal melanin. Some pigment incontinence may be present as well as features of the antecedent dermatitis such as lupus erythematosus.

The melanocytes may or may not be detected with the DOPA stain and other methods depending upon the degree of melanocyte damage. Permanent forms of leukoderma are characterized by an absence of epidermal melanocytes and a corresponding absence of epidermal melanin. In old scars, the melanocytes may have recovered, but fibrosis and relative paucity of blood vessels contribute to the white color. Poor blood supply to the superficial dermis in such scars may contribute to the whitish color of the skin. Some examples include atrophie blanche, lichen sclerosus et atrophicus, and nevus anemicus (see below).

Differential Diagnosis   The differential diagnosis includes conditions with detectable (normal or slightly reduced numbers of) basilar melanocytes and those with absence of epidermal melanocytes. Entities to be considered in the first group include early or trichrome vitiligo, tuberous sclerosis, hypomelanosis of Ito, nevus depigmentosus, leukoderma secondary to infectious processes (tinea versicolor, leprosy, syphilis, and the like), and pityriasis alba. The differential diagnosis for the second group (not mutually exclusive) is that of established vitiligo, piebaldism, and any form of depigmentation not otherwise specified.

Diagnosis is predicated upon confirming a relationship to an antecedent dermatosis, chemical exposure, or trauma; exclusion of an infectious agent; and clinical features.

Nevus Anemicus

Nevus anemicus is characterized by a congenital white patch with an irregular border and is found most commonly on the trunk, particularly the chest.[14,15] Familial cases have been reported. Rubbing the border makes the normal skin erythematous while the lesion remains white. The abnormality seems to be a focal hypersensitivity of blood vessels to catecholamines resulting in vasoconstriction, since the intralesional injection of adrenergic blocker may induce erythema.

Histopathological Features   Epidermal melanocytes and dermal blood vessels are normal in number and size. Other dermal components are likewise normal.

HYPERPIGMENTATION DISORDERS

In this group of diseases the epidermal melanocytes are hyperactive or increased in number or both; accordingly the epidermis is hypermelanized, and excess pigment drops into upper dermis and either remains free or is phagocytosed by macrophages (melanophages) (Figs. 15-8, 15-9). Vacuolar degeneration of basal cells releases melanin granules into upper dermis to cause hyperpigmentation, particularly in dark-skinned patients (Fig. 15-10). Disorders of hyperpigmentation may thus be classified histologically according to the predominant pattern as (1) epidermal, (2) dermal (pigment incontinence), or (3) mixed epidermal and dermal. The predominant location of the excess melanin correlates with the color of the hyperpigmentation: (1) brown (epidermal), (2) blue-gray (dermal), and (3) brown-gray (mixed epidermal and dermal). In reality, attempting to classify such disorders may not be very helpful in many cases, since many of these conditions show varying degrees of both epidermal and dermal hyperpigmentation. These disorders are also classified by their clinical distribution as (1) generalized or diffuse and (2) patterned or circumscribed.

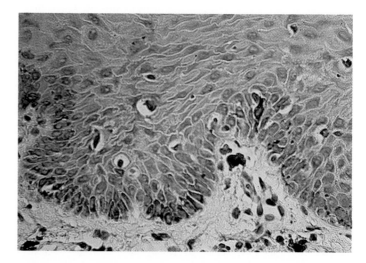

FIGURE 15-8   Solitary labial lentigo. There are a heavy melanization of the basal layer, scattered clear cells (melanocytes), and incontinence of melanin in the papillary dermis. A combination of these causes clinical hyperpigmentation.

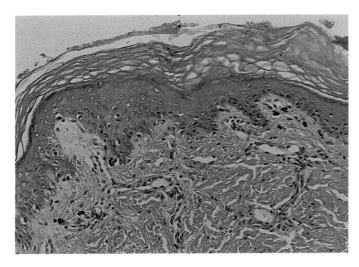

FIGURE 15-9 ANOTHER syndrome. A biopsy from reticular pigmentation of foot shows an increased basal clear cells and a mild basal hyperpigmentation.

Generalized or Diffuse Hyperpigmentations

Although the patient is diffusely hyperpigmented in the following conditions, disease-specific, preferential areas of hyperpigmentation may be seen (Table 15-2). Sun-exposed areas are more frequently affected in many of these conditions.

Addison's Disease

This is a primary disease of adrenocortical insufficiency. Hyperpigmentation is most pronounced in the sun-exposed areas; areas exhibiting dark skin normally, such as the axillae, nipples, genitalia, and other skin folds (joints); and oral mucous membranes, including tongue.[16,17] Fatigue, nausea, loss of appetite and weight, low blood sugar and sodium, low blood pressure, decreased plasma cortisol and ACTH, urinary 17-OHCS and 17-KS, and little or no response of

plasma cortisol levels to the ACTH stimulation test are of diagnostic importance.

With a decreasing incidence of tuberculosis, idiopathic cases are increasing. Antiadrenal autoantibodies causing adrenocortical atrophy are currently the most common cause of Addison's disease. Metastatic tumors, bilateral hemorrhage due to anticoagulant therapy, histoplasmosis, and sarcoidosis destroying adrenal cortex may be etiologic factors. The mechanism of hyperpigmentation is thought to be related to the elevated ACTH secretion which is accompanied by the by-products α- and β-MSH which stimulate melanocytes.

Histopathological Features The number of melanocytes is normal but their activity is increased, resulting in heavily melanized basal cells and malpighian cells. Pigment dropping to upper dermis and melanophages are observed.

Differential Diagnosis This pattern of increased epidermal melanin with some degree of pigment incontinence is entirely nonspecific and may be associated with a wide variety of etiologies. Some examples include Grave's disease, malnutrition, hemochromatosis (especially early), argyria, arsenic ingestion, many drugs (particularly photosensitizing drugs) such as minocycline, psychotropic and chemotherapeutic agents.

Nelson's Syndrome

Clinical Features An ACTH-producing pituitary adenoma is seen in 10 to 47 percent of adrenalectomized patients with Cushing's syndrome.[18,19] By the same feedback inhibition mechanism as discussed in Addison's disease, β-MSH and ACTH are increased concomitant with pituitary hyperplasia or development of adenoma. Hyperpigmentation is similar to Addison's disease and consists of generalized darkening of skin and hair. In addition, multiple lentigines and pigmented bands involving nails may be seen.

Histopathological Features Increased melanin production in the normal population of basal melanocytes is observed.

POEMS or Crow-Fukase Syndrome

Clinical Features In this syndrome an M protein–producing plasmacytoma or multiple myeloma occurs.[20] It has been argued that the M protein itself is responsible for all symptoms in this condition. Otherwise, the plasma cell may produce other substances contributing to the disease manifestations. The acronym *POEMS* derives from *p*olyneuropathy, *o*rganomegaly, *e*ndocrinopathies, *M* protein, and *s*kin lesions. The skin pigmentation is diffuse or more prominent on the extensor surfaces of the arms, neck, and back. Hirsutism and cherry hemangiomas may be present. Treatment of plasmacytoma may decrease the hyperpigmentation.

OTHER CONDITIONS

Generalized or diffuse hypermelanosis can occur in the disorders listed below and in other conditions. In the following disorders, hypermelanosis of the epidermis with or without incontinence of melanin to the upper dermis is responsible for the pigmentation: porphyria cutanea tarda, dermatomyositis, progressive systemic sclerosis, Whipple's intestinal lipodystrophy, primary biliary cirrhosis, vitamin B_{12} deficiency, and folate deficiency.

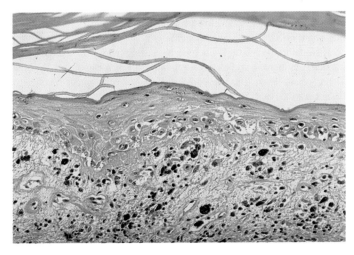

FIGURE 15-10 Lupus erythematosus. Vacuolization of the basal cells and incontinence of the released melanin into upper dermis are seen. These melanin granules are tattooed in the dermis semipermanently. Hyaline degeneration (cytoid body formation) of the epidermis causes atrophy. Thin epidermis makes these pigment granules more readily visible.

Acromelanosis

Several names for dyschromic conditions similar or identical to acromelanosis have been used. Because these conditions are rare and variable in their presentations, a consensus on their identity has not been reached. A hyper- or hypopigmented epidermis shows increased or decreased melanocyte activity and variable basal layer melanization. Incontinence of melanin in the upper dermis is seen in the former.

DYSCHROMATOSIS SYMMETRICA (DOHI-KOYAMA), ACROPIGMENTATIO SYMMETRICA (DOHI), LEUCOPATHIA PUNCTATA ET RETICULARIS SYMMETRICA (MATSUMOTO)

The dorsal hands, feet, and extensor surface of the forearms and lower legs are involved with punctate to reticulated hyper- and hypopigmentation.[21] Distal lesions are more prominent than proximal ones. The face shows ephelides (freckles). Because patients have photosensitivity, some authors believe that these are from frustes of xeroderma pigmentosum. Inheritance is autosomal dominant.

DYSCHROMATOSIS UNIVERSALIS HEREDITARIA (TOYAMA-ICHIKAWA-HIRAGA)

In this variant, the lesions are generalized.[21-23] Sharply demarcated brown macules occur on hypopigmented skin.

ACROPIGMENTATIO RETICULARIS OR RETICULATE ACROPIGMENTATION (KITAMURA)

The dorsal hands, feet, and, rarely, neck and shoulder show irregular, polygonal brown eruptions which are depressed or atrophic.[24] The skin may become rough. The onset is from childhood to adolescence, and familial incidence has been recorded in an autosomal dominant pattern.

DIFFUSE ACROMELANOSIS

Diffuse and not reticular pigmentation of fingers is seen in children of dark-skinned races.[21-23] Pigmentation may extend proximally as the patient becomes older.

ANOTHER SYNDROME

Reticulated hyperpigmentation appears during infancy, often on the hands and feet, including palms and soles.[25,26] The trunk is probably more involved with reticular pigmentation. The patient exhibits ectodermal dysplasialike skin symptoms, hypothyroidism, growth retardation, and frequent respiratory infection. The acronym *ANOTHER* stands for *a*lopecia, *n*ail dystrophy, *o*phthalmic complications, *t*hyroid dysfunction, *h*ypohidrosis, *e*phelides and enteropathy, and *r*espiratory tract infection. Mild basal cell hyperpigmentation and incontinence of melanin in the upper dermis are seen (Fig. 15-9).

Circumscribed or Patterned Hypermelanosis

In this group of hyperpigmentation disorders, patterned or special regional increase of skin pigmentation occurs (Table 15-10). The pigmentations are often reticulated, punctate, or spotty.

ZOSTERIFORM HYPERPIGMENTATION

Lentiginous, cribriform, or macular hyperpigmentations are present at birth or in the second to fourth decade.[27-29] The pattern of pigmentation is dermatomal or zosteriform on various parts of the body. Histopathologic features range from nevus cells at the tip of rete ridges to increased basal layer pigmentation only. Dermal melanophages may be present.

INHERITED PATTERNED LENTIGINOSIS IN BLACKS

Multiple small pigmented spots are scattered mainly on sun-exposed areas such as the face and the outer arm but also on the buttocks and sometimes palmoplantar surfaces of blacks.[30] The onset is in infancy or early childhood, and the condition is transmitted in an autosomal dominant pattern. Light-colored blacks or lighter-colored siblings tend to develop this disease. The abnormality is limited to the skin. Histopathology involves prominent hyperpigmentation of the lower epidermis, particularly the basal layer, and effaced rete ridges.

LEOPARD, MOYNAHAN'S, OR MULTIPLE LENTIGINES SYNDROME

This is an autosomal dominant disease typified by multiple lentigines affecting any part of the body from the scalp to the feet.[31,32] In addition to *l*entigines, there are *E*CG abnormalities, *o*cular hypertelorism, *p*ulmonic stenosis, *a*bnormal genitalia, growth *r*etardation, and *d*eafness (hence the *LEOPARD* syndrome). The inheritance is autosomal dominant.

Histopathologic features include elongation of rete ridges with increased melanocytes and an increased melanization of the epidermis. Examination by electron microscope reveals giant melanosomes and complex melanosomes with a granular matrix probably representing lysosomes.

PEUTZ-JEGHERS SYNDROME

In this autosomal dominant disorder, the pattern of pigmentation is characterized by small irregular-shape macules localized to the oral mucosa, lips, perioral skin, and dorsal skin of the fingers.[33-35] In the majority of cases multiple polyps develop in the small intestines which become malignant in 2 to 3 percent of patients.

Histopathologic features include basal cells which are heavily pigmented, but there is no increase in the number of melanocytes with the DOPA stain. There may be some disturbance of pigment transfer to basal keratinocytes.

DOWLING-DEGOS DISEASE OR RETICULATE PIGMENTED DERMATOSIS OF THE FLEXURES

This is a dominantly inherited pigmentation involving flexural or frictional surfaces such as the axillae, neck, groin, and, in women, inframammary folds with slowly spreading reticular hyperpigmentation.[36,37] Perioral, comedolike follicular keratosis and pitted scars may be present. The distribution of hyperpigmentation is similar to acanthosis nigricans, but there is no velvety texture present. The age of onset is usually late (30 to 40 years of age). In Haber's syndrome, rosacealike facial erythema and telangiectasia are associated with black keratotic papules of the axillae, neck, and occasionally trunk. This disease may be the same as Dowling-Degos disease.

TABLE 15-10

Circumscribed Hypermelanosis

Disorder	Clinical Features	Epidermal Configuration	Basilar Melanocytes	Other Features
Freckle	Sunlight responsive, 1- to 3-mm macules Light to medium brown	Normal	Reduced, normal, increased	Melanocytes larger with increased development of dendrites
Lentigo	Persistent 1- to 5-mm macule Light to dark brown	Elongated, club-shaped, epidermal rete ridges	Increased	
Solar lentigo	Sun-exposed skin 5- to 15-mm macules Medium to brown	Elongated, club-shaped rete ridges, often anastomosing	Normal or increased	
Café-au-lait macule	2- to 5-cm oval macule, uniform tan to dark brown	Normal	Normal or slightly increased	Association with neurofibromatosis, melanin macroglobules
Melasma	Patterned macular pigmentation on face	Normal	Normal or slightly increased	Pigment incontinence may be prominent
Becker's melanosis	Macular or raised lesion, a few to several cm Tan to dark brown, often hairy	Elongated rete ridges to papillomatous	Normal or slightly increased	Smooth muscle hamartoma in dermis often

Histopathologic features include characteristic elongated, tapered, and heavily melanized epidermal cords (Fig. 15-11). There may be small horn cysts or follicular plugs (Fig. 15-11). The overall appearance may, therefore, be similar to adenoid seborrheic keratosis. Haber's syndrome shows similar histologic findings.

FRANCESCHETTI-JADASSOHN-NAEGELI SYNDROME

In this rare autosomal dominant disease of childhood onset, punctate pigmentation occurs involving the axillae, neck, and trunk.[21] Hypohidrosis, palmoplantar hyperkeratosis, and abnormalities of teeth and nails may be present. Histopathology involves increased epidermal melanization and melanophages in the upper dermis.

DERMATOPATHIA PIGMENTOSA RETICULARIS

This is a heterogeneous autosomal dominant disease.[38] A constant finding is reticulated pigmentation over the trunk and extremities. Loss of the fingernails and toenails, hypohidrosis, and atrophy of the skin of elbows, knees, and extremities may occur.

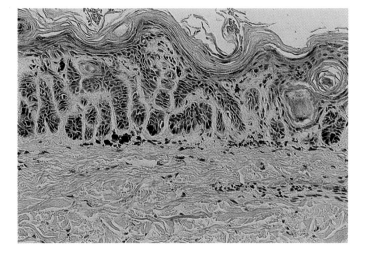

FIGURE 15-11   Dowling-Degos disease. Irregularly elongated, slender rete ridges are heavily pigmented. There are a few keratin cysts and keratin plugs.

involve the face, forearms, and feet. Hyperkeratosis of palms and soles may be associated.

CANTU'S SYNDROME

This is an autosomal disorder with the onset in adolescence.[39] Small punctate hyperpigmented macules that often have a reticular pattern

CENTROFACIAL NEURODYSRAPHIC LENTIGINOSIS

This is also an autosomal dominant disease.[40] It is characterized by centrofacial lentigines without mucous membrane involvement. There are no lentigines present in areas other than the face. Associated abnormalities include seizures, mental retardation and psychiatric disorders, endocrine disorders, and bone abnormalities. In addition, lentigines regress over time, and there are no reports of lesions in patients older than 54 years.

CARNEY'S SYNDROME

Carney's syndrome is also called *lentiginosis with cardiocutaneous myxomas* or *NAME syndrome* (*n*evi, *a*trial myxoma, *m*yxoid neuroma, and *e*phelides).[41,42] This is another autosomal dominant syndrome with lentiginosis. There may be mucous membrane involvement and associated cardiac abnormalities (classically with cardiac myxomas) and endocrine abnormalities.

GENERALIZED LENTIGINOSIS

This term is used to describe patients with many lentigines that appear at birth, in a generalized dense distribution, yet sparing mucous membranes and without associated abnormalities.[43]

Incontinentia Pigmenti (Bloch-Sulzberger Syndrome)

This is mainly an X-linked dominant disorder that is usually lethal in hemizygous males.[44–47] The disease is 37 times more common in females. The gene loci have been mapped either to Xp11.21 or Xq28 regions. Variable expressions and severity of disease are explained by X-inactivation (Lyon hypothesis) in females. For example, if the affected allele is inactivated, amelioration of the disease may occur. There are three major stages, each of which may overlap or be skipped. The first stage is vesicular, erythematous lesions occurring in groups, often distributed along Blaschko's lines on the trunk and extremities. These resolve in a few weeks, and the second stage of verrucous lesions follow the previous vesicular lesions, particularly heavy on extremities. As these subside in a few weeks to months, whorled hyperpigmentation develops corresponding to previous verrucous lesions, i.e., in Blaschko's pattern. The late stage of this disease may exhibit atrophic lesions with hypo- or depigmentation on the extremities. Alopecia, nail dystrophy, dental defects, eye findings (cataracts, blindness, and so on), and central nervous system abnormalities (seizures, mental retardation, and the like) are common disease manifestations.

Histopathological Features   In vesicular lesions, one observes intraepidermal spongiosis and, commonly, vesicle formation with numerous eosinophils. In the verrucous stage hyperkeratosis and acanthosis with many cytoid bodies are present. In the lesions of whorled or linear hyperpigmentation, the most prominent alteration is pigment incontinence. The basal cells of the epidermis are vacuolated, and melanosomes are released into papillary dermis subsequently phagocytosed by macrophages. When prominent vesicular lesions occur, the epidermis is atrophic and depigmented by the loss of melanocytes. The appendages may also be absent.

Differential Diagnosis   The lesions exhibiting hyperpigmentation show nonspecific pigment incontinence indistinguishable from other forms of predominantly dermal postinflammatory hyperpigmentation without clinical information. However, on occasion one may observe the concomitant features of eosinophilic spongiosis and/or a whorled pattern of dyskeratosis that will suggest IP.

Dyskeratosis Congenita

This rare disease is mostly transmitted as an X-linked recessive trait affecting males with the gene mapped to Xq28.[48,49] Occasionally an autosomal dominant mode of inheritance, affecting also females, has been observed. The triad is (1) pterygiumlike nail dystrophy, (2) leukoplakia of oral and occasionally anal mucosa, and (3) extensive reticulated hyperpigmentation. Leukoplakia may degenerate into squamous cell carcinoma. The hair is thin and lusterless in approximately half the cases. Fanconi's anemia, an autosomal recessive disease, and dyskeratosis congenita share several features, e.g., reticulated hyperpigmentation, progressive anemia, mental retardation, hypoplastic genitalia, and increased risk of malignancy. However, each condition is a distinct disease.

Histopathological Features   The nonspecific findings include increased basal layer melanization with slightly increased melanocytes. The most constant finding is the presence of melanophages in the upper dermis. Oral leukoplakia may show squamous cell carcinoma in situ or invasive.

Melasma or Chloasma

This disorder is most commonly observed on the faces of women of dark-skinned races living in tropical or subtropical locations where ultraviolet irradiation is intense.[50] Increased estrogen and progesterone levels seem to be causative in susceptible women; pregnancy, contraceptives, estrogen replacement therapy, and ovarian tumors are often linked to the onset. This condition involves the face symmetrically in one of three patterns: a centrofacial pattern involving the forehead, nose, cheeks, upper lip, and chin; a malar pattern; and a mandibular pattern. The hyperpigmentation may be predominantly epidermal, and consequently brown, dermal, and bluish, or both epidermal and dermal (brown and blue).

Histopathological Features   Epidermal melanocytes are usually slightly increased in number and activity. Corresponding to the clinical patterns, increased melanin may be localized primarily to the epidermis, upper dermis, or both.

Differential Diagnosis   The major entities to be considered include postinflammatory hyperpigmentation, café-au-lait macule, and lentigo. Melasma may be histologically indistinguishable from postinflammatory hyperpigmentation and café-au-lait macule; the clinical presentation of melasma should readily allow its discrimination from the latter two entities in most instances.

Ephelides or Freckles

Small brown or tan macules are distributed on sun-exposed locations, typically on the face, upper back, and shoulders.[51,52] Fair-skinned races are more affected; in northern Sweden the prevalence among children of ages 12 to 16 years is 18.4 percent. An autosomal dominant trait is suggested.

Histopathological Features   The epidermis has a normal appearance, and the number of melanocytes are not increased but may be normal or decreased. Melanization of the basal layer occurs because of larger and more active melanocytes which produce stage IV melanosomes even in fair-skinned individuals.

Differential Diagnosis   The freckle must be distinguished from the simple lentigo and solar lentigo. The simple lentigo demonstrates elongated epidermal rete ridges with increased numbers of basilar melanocytes and basal layer melanin, both of which are most accentuated at the tips of the elongated rete, in contrast to the lack of these features in the freckle. In general, the solar lentigo differs from the freckle by also showing elongated and hypermelanotic club-shaped rete; however, the number of melanocytes may or may not be increased. The freckle may be histologically indistinguishable from the café-au-lait macule and melasma without clinical information.

Café-au-Lait Spots and Axillary Freckling

Café-au-lait macules (CALM) are one of the hallmarks of neurofibromatosis 1 (NF1) or von Recklinghousen's multiple neurofibromatosis.[53,54] "Coffee with milk" color is only applicable for white skin; in pigmented races, the color is much darker. The border is smooth ("coast of California") in contrast to the "coast of Maine" border of the macule of McCune-Albright syndrome. These macules are not influenced by ultraviolet rays; the most common locations are the covered areas of the body. CALM are found in 90 percent of NF1 patients. If one has six café-au-lait macules of 1.5 cm or larger, the development or the presence of NF1 is 100 percent. Axillary freckles are not darkened by sun exposure and are different from facial freckles both clinically and histologically. The inguinal and inframammary folds may show similar freckles. Axillary or inguinal freckles are observed in 81 percent of affected children under 6 years of age and often precede the appearance of neurofibromas.

Histopathological Features   The epidermis is of normal thickness and exhibits basal layer hyperpigmentation. Although the number of basilar melanocytes appears normal, an increased number and activity of melanocytes can be demonstrated with silver and DOPA stains. Examination by electron microscope reveals giant or macromelanosomes measuring up to 5 μm in these active melanocytes (Fig. 15-12). Giant melanosomes are absent in the lesions of children. These large melanosomes are also found in melanotic macules of McCune-Albright syndrome, lentigo simplex, melanocytic nevi, multiple lentiginosis, and other conditions and therefore are not diagnostic for NF1.

Differential Diagnosis   CALM cannot be histologically discriminated from the melanotic macule of Albright's syndrome, the freckle, melasma, or perhaps rarely postinflammatory hyperpigmentation without the reliance on clinical characteristics and history. The CALM does not exhibit the elongated epidermal rete ridges and clearly increased numbers of melanocytes observed in simple lentigo.

Macules of McCune-Albright Syndrome

Large pigmented macules with an irregular border (coast of Maine type) and unilateral distribution, unilateral (often on the same side as the macules) polyostotic fibrous dysplasia, and precocious puberty in females are the usual triad in this syndrome.[55,56] The pigmented macules are darker than the café-au-lait macules in neurofibromatosis 1. These pigmented macules are located on the head, neck, shoulder, lower back, and buttocks. Although two possible familial cases have been reported, all others are sporadic. It is more common in females. Postzygotic somatic mutation causing functional mosaicism and mutations of Gs α subunit of G protein which stimulate adenosine 3',5'-cyclic phosphate (cAMP) formation in affected endocrine organs such as gonadal glands have been proposed. Gs mutation has also been found in the pigmented

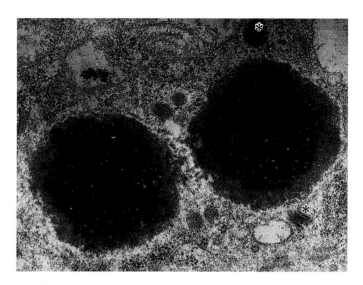

FIGURE 15-12   Giant or macromelanosomes of café-au-lait spot. Ill-defined dense melanosomes are formed in a melanocyte. These are extraordinarily large compared with the normal ones. Within the macromelanosomes there are many electron-light granules or vacuoles.

macules. In support of the mosaicism hypothesis, some macules are formed according to the lines of Blaschko.

Histopathological Features   The basal layer of the epidermis is hyperpigmented. The melanocytes are not increased in number but contain giant or macromelanosomes.

Differential Diagnosis.   See differential diagnosis for CALM.

Becker's Pigmented Hairy Nevus or Melanosis

Clinical Features   A large unilateral patch of pigmentation with varying degrees of hypertrichosis develops most commonly during adolescence on the shoulder or chest of males.[57,58] Among 280 reported cases, about 50 have occurred in women. Occasionally, the onset is earlier in life, in different locations, or in multiple numbers. Hairs become coarse as patient grows older. When a smooth-muscle hamartoma is present, follicular papules, slight induration, and occasional pain are observed.

Histopathological Features   The epidermal changes vary from almost normal to showing acanthosis, papillomatosis, elongation of rete ridges, and hyperpigmentation of the basal layer. Melanocytes may be slightly increased in number in the epidermis. Becker's pigmented hairy "nevus" therefore refers to the hamartomatous combination of hair, increased melanocytes, and smooth muscle. Dermal melanophages are often present. Hair follicles are usually normal but on occasion may be increased in number and enlarged. Increased smooth muscle is almost always found to varying degree in the reticular dermis (Fig. 15-13). Sebaceous gland hyperplasia and thickening of dermal connective tissue may occur.

Differential Diagnosis   Becker's nevus must be distinguished from an epidermal nevus, a large variety of lentigo, and other papillomatous lesions, such as confluent and reticulated papillomatosis (of Gougerot-Carteaud) on occasion. The clinical features of a unilateral hyperpigmented and often hairy patch or plaque and frequent smooth-muscle

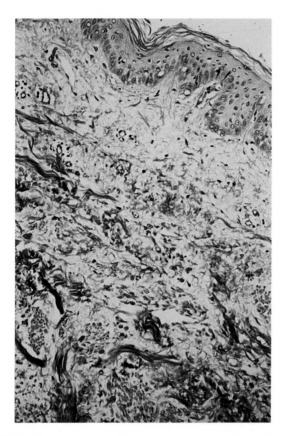

FIGURE 15-13 Becker's nevus. Masson's trichrome stain. Hypermelanosis of the basal layer and an increased number of dermal smooth-muscle bundles (red) are seen.

hamartoma histologically are distinctive and should facilitate discrimination from the other entities.

Prurigo Pigmentosa

The majority of cases of prurigo pigmentosa reported thus far have been young Japanese women in their second and third decades.[59,60] The eruption begins acutely with erythematous papules which become confluent to form linear or anastomosing elevated lesions which are intensely pruritic. Vesicular or exudative papular lesions have also been described in the initial acute stage. The upper back, shoulders, neck, and chest are common sites of involvement. A familial basis has been reported. Potential etiologic factors include diabetes mellitus, friction with underwear, and contact with cosmetic and antiseptic agents.

Histopathological Features In the inflammatory stage one observes features of an interface dermatitis with vacuolization of basal cells and cytoid bodies, as well as spongiosis and exocytosis. In chronic pigmented lesions incontinence of melanin is the predominant feature.

Differential Diagnosis The histologic findings are nonspecific and indistinguishable from other forms of (predominantly dermal) postinflammatory hyperpigmentation following an interface dermatitis.

Postinflammatory Melanosis or Hyperpigmentation

Any damage to the basal keratinocytes may result in the incontinence of pigment in the upper dermis and a tattoolike effect. Such damage could be a stimulus for melanocytes to overproduce melanin and overcom-

pensate for the loss; thus more melanin is produced and epidermal hypermelanization occurs (Table 15-11) (Fig. 15-6). Another mechanism may be an active melanosome transfer from stimulated epidermal melanocytes through their dendrites into dermal melanophages. Melanin polymers may act as antioxidants, and, therefore, epidermal melanocytes may actively transfer melanosomes to the dermal foci of inflammation.

Pigmented races are more prone to these changes in a florid form because the epidermal melanocytes are easily stimulated to produce more melanin granules. In blacks the discoloration may be permanent. The primary conditions vary from lichenoid eruptions to chronic exogenous irritations and friction. Examples are lichen planus, lichenoid drug eruption, discoid lupus erythematosus (Fig. 15-10), dermatomyositis, Riehl's melanosis, and mycosis fungoides. In fixed drug eruption and erythema dyschromicum perstans, the repeated episodes of acute interface dermatitis eventually produce gray-blue dyspigmentation as the amount of incontinent melanin accumulates in large amount and in somewhat deeper location in the dermis ("ashy" dermatosis for the latter).

Histopathological Features Varying degrees of epidermal inflammatory change such as interface dermatitis are still visible in early lesions together with melanin deposition in the upper dermis, either free or in melanophages. Increased epidermal melanin content also may be present. Long-standing lesions usually show pigment incontinence without any active inflammation.

Differential Diagnosis Unless active inflammation is present, the pigmentary alteration alone is entirely nonspecific. Diagnosis of a specific etiology depends on identification of the antecedent inciting agent. Other considerations might include regression of a pigmented lesion and amyloidosis.

Friction Melanosis (Nylon Towel Melanosis)

Ill-defined light brown to "dirty brown" hyperpigmentation may occur over the bony prominences such as the clavicle, shoulder blades, frontal neck, and shins.[61] Over the nonbony areas pigmentation occurs in a rippled pattern similar to that of macular amyloidosis. Most of the early cases have been reported from Japan. These patients used more durable

TABLE 15-11

Postinflammatory Hypermelanosis

Clinical Features

Usually follows inflammatory process
Localized or widespread
Common dermatoses include: lichen planus, lupus erythematosus, eczematous dermatitis, psoriasis, phytophoto dermatitis, drug eruptions
Gradual loss of pigmentation, may be permanent

Histopathological Features

Variable degrees of epidermal hypermelanosis, pigment incontinence

Differential Diagnosis

Melasma
Endocrine dysfunction
    Addison's disease
Malnutrition

nylon towels or brushes for a long time which replaced traditional cotton towels or plant fiber brushes in postwar Japan. No evidence of contact hypersensitivity has been found, and it has been concluded that chronic frictional trauma of thin skin over the hard bony structures causes epidermal damage and subsequent pigment incontinence. The mechanism seems to be similar to that involved in friction amyloidosis in which tonofilaments of damaged keratinocytes are transformed into amyloid filaments.

Histopathological Features   Epidermal atrophy, basal cell vacuolization leading to dermal-epidermal cleavage in severe cases, and pigment incontinence in the upper dermis are observed. No amyloid deposition has been documented.

Generalized Melanosis in Metastatic Melanoma

Generalized melanosis in metastatic melanoma is associated with a widespread metastasis of malignant melanoma.[62] In such cases the urine is black (melanuria). Slate-blue diffuse discoloration of the skin, including mucous membranes and conjunctiva, may occur. Neutrophils and monocytes in the circulation also contain melanin. The intima of arteries and many visceral organs are black.

Histopathological Features   Macrophages of the entire dermis, particularly in perivascular spaces, contain a large number of melanin granules which are often DOPA-positive, indicating that melanin synthesis is still active in the phagocytosed melanosomes which most likely are derived from melanoma cells and carried to the skin by blood. The dermal blood vessels may be occluded with DOPA-positive dark materials. In some cases only melanophages are present, but in other cases both melanoma cells and melanophages are admixed in the dermis.

Pigment Deposits Other Than Melanin

Miscellaneous pigmented substances may deposit in the skin and produce various discolorations (Tables 15-12 and 15-13).

OCHRONOSIS

Endogenous ochronosis is an autosomal recessive disease of homogentisic acid oxidase deficiency.[63,64] A slow accumulation of homogentisic acid, which is an intermediate product of metabolism of phenylalanine to tyrosine, causes pigmentation of cartilages and eventually the skin. An affected child's urine is pink to brown (alkaptonuria), and the staining of diaper is the first sign of the disease. This is a rare disease in the United States (1:250,000) but is more frequent in the Dominican Republic and in the Czech Republics (1:25,000). Since the cartilage of ear is covered with thin skin, a bluish-gray to dark brown color is readily noticed. A butterfly pattern of pigmentation of the face including nose may suggest a photosensitivity of the patient. Axillary sweat may be variously colored from greenish-blue to greenish-yellow-brown. The sclera and teeth may also be pigmented.

EXOGENOUS OCHRONOSIS OR PSEUDO-OCHRONOSIS

This disorder is caused by the chronic topical use of high-concentration (6 to 8%) hydroquinone, resorcinol, phenol, quinine injection, systemic antimalarial therapy, or exposure to benzene.[65,66] In hydroquinone-induced ochronosis, blue-black pigmentation is seen most prominently on prominent parts of the face, i.e., cheeks, forehead, nose, and in some cases on the chin, suggesting the photo-induced nature of the disease. The discoloration is usually permanent despite discontinuation of hydroquinone. Annular lesions similar to actinic granuloma may occur.

Histopathological Features   The pigment in the dermis is a yellow-brown or "ochre" color with the H&E stain, hence *ochronosis*. Blue-gray-brown color is produced by scattering of light from deep-seated ochre-colored pigment (Tindall effect). The pigment is also observed in the endothelial cells of blood vessels and basement membranes, the secretory cells of eccrine glands, and dermal macrophages. However, the most diagnostic form of deposition is the banana-shaped dermal collagen fibers which become swollen, rigid, and fragmented with jagged ends. The same pigment is deposited on elastic fibers, which also degenerate. The epidermis is normally pigmented. In annular lesions sarcoidal granulomas occur. Transepidermal elimination of degenerated collagen may occur.

TATTOO

A professional tattoo is deeper and more difficult to remove than an amateur tattoo.[67] Tattoos may occur secondary to accidental introduction of pigments into the skin such as the graphite of lead pencils. Blue-black tattoos of miners are commonly due to the traumatic inoculation of carbon (coal). Common dyes used in professional tattoos are cinnabar or mercuric sulfide (red), chromic oxide (green), cobaltous albuminate (light blue), cadmium sulfide (yellow), and iron oxide or ochre (brown).

Histopathological Features   After an acute inflammatory reaction, these inert pigments elicit little or no tissue reaction in the majority of cases. Pigments are found scattered in the upper dermis, particularly around blood vessels. Late-stage reactions include dermal contact der-

TABLE 15-12

Metal Deposition and Dyspigmentation

Condition	Epidermal Hypermelanosis	Dermal Alteration	Other Findings
Hemochromatosis	Present	Hemosiderin	
Argyria (silver deposition)	Present, sun-exposed skin	Silver particles, basement membranes of sweat glands, elastic fibers	Refractile granules on dark-field examination
Chrysiasis (gold deposition)	May be present	Gold particles in macrophages and endothelium	Refractile granules on dark-field microscopy
Mercury	May be present	Brown-black mercury granules either free or in macrophages	
Arsenic	Present	Arsenic particles	
Lead		Lead particles	
Bismuth		Bismuth granules in papillary and reticular dermis	

TABLE 15-13

Drug-Related Dyspigmentation

Drug	Epidermal Hypermelanosis	Dermal Alteration	Other Findings
Minocycline			
Facial, blue-black pigmentation	Usually not present	Drug metabolite–protein complex in macrophages that stains for iron but not melanin	
Extremities, blue-gray pigmentation	Usually not present	Drug metabolite–protein complex that stains for iron and is positive by the Fontana reaction but fails to bleach (and thus is not melanin)	
Sun-exposed skin, brown pigmentation	Present	Melanin, negative iron stain	
Antimalarials			
Chloroquine		Ochronosislike material	
Quinacrine		Drug-melanin complex, hemosiderin	
Amiodarone		Drug metabolite in endothelium, macrophages	Drug metabolite–pigment granules in phagolysosomes
Clofazimine	Present	Melanin, ceroidlike material	
Psychotropic drugs	Present	Drug metabolite–melanin in macrophages, endothelial cells	
Chemotherapeutic drugs	Present	Melanin	

matitis, lichenoid dermatitis, foreign-body reaction with giant cells, and sarcoidal granulomatous reactions (Fig. 15-14). Several patients have developed hilar lymphadenopathy together with sarcoidal reactions at tattoo sites. It is not clear if these patients had a sarcoidosis.

Differential Diagnosis   The major conditions to be considered include blue nevi and dermal melanocytoses and iron and other metal depositions. Most tattoos are clinically evident. The usual histologic appearance for the common carbon tattoo is that of a jet-black material rather than the granular brown character of melanin in dermal melanocytic lesions.

IDIOPATHIC HEMOCHROMATOSIS

Skin pigmentation, liver cirrhosis, cardiac failure, and diabetes mellitus are the tetrad of this rare autosomal recessive disease.[68,69] In white skin, discoloration varies from bronze (bronze diabetes) to blue-gray, whereas in pigmented skin it is brown to black. Pigmentation is most pronounced in the sun-exposed areas, skin creases and folds and nipples, similar to that of Addison's disease. Pigmentation precedes other

symptoms and is an important sign, because early treatment with phlebotomy and chelating agents improves the prognosis significantly. Systemic symptoms appear only after sufficient iron storage (20 to 60 g), usually between 35 to 60 years of age. Repeated blood transfusions may cause this disease. However, gene mapping suggests the abnormal gene is present on chromosome 6p, and frequent HLA types are HLA-A3,11 and B-5, 7, 11. Normal regulation of intestinal absorption of iron seems to be disrupted.

Histopathological Features   In early cases without systemic symptoms, only atrophy of epidermis and hypermelanosis of the lower layers of the epidermis but no deposition of hemosiderin are observed. It is therefore believed that the main cause of discoloration is hypermelanosis, which may be modified by the dermal hemosiderosis. Hemosiderin deposition is seen in the cytoplasm of eccrine secretory cells as well as periglandular connective tissue. Perivascular macrophages also contain hemosiderin.

Differential Diagnosis   (See discussion for differential diagnosis for Addison's disease). The golden refractile appearance of hemosiderin

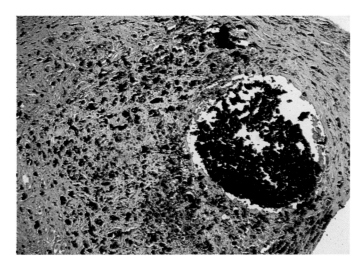

FIGURE 15-14   Tattoo with graphite (pencil). Black pigment particles are scattered from the main body of accidentally inoculated graphite. Granulomatous reaction is seen.

and a Prussian blue stain usually allows separation from melanin and other pigments.

HEMOSIDERIN FROM OTHER SOURCES

Any hemorrhage leaves erythrocytes in the tissue, and their degradation causes temporary or long-term hemosiderosis. Yellowish-brown discoloration follows chronic, repeated bleeding such as in stasis dermatitis, Henoch-Schönlein's purpura, and pigmented purpuric dermatosis (Schamberg's disease, Majocchi's disease, lichen aureus, and others).

Histopathology is related to the individual conditions. Hemosiderin is most often seen in perivascular spaces and is demonstrable with iron stains such as Berlin blue or Prussian blue stains.

"BRONZE BABY" SYNDROME

Since blue light effectively oxidizes bilirubin, infants with hyperbilirubinemia (>15 mg/dl) due to various causes including extrahepatic biliary atresia are treated with blue light.[70] Within 3 to 4 days after the phototherapy, the patient's serum, urine, and skin become gray-brown-black, which disappears in about 6 weeks after the discontinuation of the treatment. It is assumed that photodegradation products of bilirubin are not metabolized properly due to hepatic dysfunction and are retained in the skin.

Histopathological Features   The nature of the pigment causing skin discoloration has not been elucidated. It may be a photoisomer of bilirubin or photoproducts of copper-bound porphyrins which have been elevated in the serum of some patients.

SILVER DEPOSITION (ARGYRIA)

Slate-gray pigmentation, particularly on sun-exposed sites, and the azure lunula of nails develop after a prolonged ingestion or application to mucous membranes of silver salts.[71–73] Absorption from mucous membranes may cause local as well as systemic argyria. Visceral organs accumulate silver and show blue discoloration. Localized argyria can

occur by wearing earrings with silver backs, by application of silver sulfadiazine cream for the treatment of burns, after acupuncture, with the use of silver wire for suture, and after traumatic implantation of silver ring.

Histopathological Features   Silver particles which have a dark brown to black granular appearance are scattered extracellularly in the dermis and concentrated in the basement membrane of eccrine sweat glands (Figs. 15-15, 15-16). Perifollicular sheath, nerves, capillary walls, and elastic fibers are also impregnated with silver particles in a high concentration. Silver particles are best demonstrated with dark-field microscopy as white refractile particles standing out against dark background (Fig. 15-15). Silver particles are absent in the epidermis but hypermelanosis of the epidermis particularly in exposed areas is evident. Actinic elastosis of sun-exposed skin also attracts silver particles.

GOLD DEPOSITION (CHRYSIASIS) OR CHRYSODERMA

A prolonged treatment with injection of gold salts induces slate-gray-blue discoloration of the exposed skin.[74] In such patients laser treatment of skin conditions may elicit chrysiasis in the normal colored skin.

Histopathological Features   In contrast to silver, gold particles are found in the cells of vascular endothelium and dermal phagocytes. Dark-field microscopy demonstrates large refractile particles in those locations. Light seems to intensify the color by making gold particles larger.

MERCURY

Mercury-containing cream (ammoniated mercury) was once used extensively by dermatologists for the treatment of microbial and fungus infections and to bleach hyperpigmentation of face and neck areas.[75] The chronic use of such cream caused slate-gray pigmentation. Filling teeth with silver-mercury amalgam also causes tattooing of mercury in the gingiva. The pigmentation is most pronounced in skin folds of the eyelids, neck, and nasolabial folds. Amalgam pigmentation may occur locally near the filled tooth or at some distance from it. (See tattoo section for red cinnabar inoculation.)

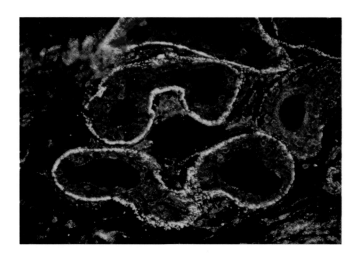

FIGURE 15-15   Argyria. Dark-field examination of eccrine gland reveals refractile silver grains in the basement membrane.

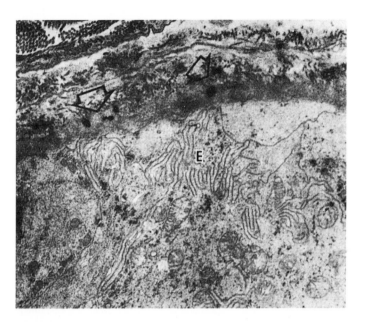

FIGURE 15-16   Argyria. Examination by electron microscopy of the basal lamina of eccrine gland reveals electron-dense particles (arrow). *E*: clear cell of eccrine gland.

Histopathological Features   The upper dermis contains brown-black small mercury granules either free or in macrophages. Dark-field microscopy shows these granules best as refractile particles. The epidermal pigmentation is either normal or slightly increased.

ARSENIC

Diffuse, bronze discoloration of the skin, prominent on the trunk, may be one of the sequelae of chronic ingestion of inorganic arsenics.[75] In less pigmented areas, these pigment spots are described as "raindrops on a dusty road." Dermal deposition of arsenic stimulates epidermal melanocytes, and the clinical hyperpigmentation is mainly due to hypermelanosis.

LEAD

A lead line at the gingival margin and nail pigmentation are associated with lead poisoning.[76] The lead line is caused by submucosal deposition of lead.

BISMUTH

Generalized blue-gray discoloration resembling argyria has been reported following the prolonged use of oral bismuth.[77] A gingival pigment line, oral, conjunctival, and vaginal pigmentations have been reported. Small granules are found in the papillary and reticular dermis.

TITANIUM

A topical cream containing 13.5% titanium dioxide has been applied to erosive herpes simplex lesion of glans, sulcus, and prepuce, resulting in the development of yellowish lesions at the sites of cream application.[78] Titanium dioxide is currently used as a light-scattering agent in some facial moisturizing and sunscreening creams and sold over the counter. Pigmentation from these has not been reported.

Histopathological Features   Many brown granules are found in the dermis which are brightly refractile by dark-field microscopy. Examination by electron microscope shows granular electron-dense bodies both in dermal macrophages and free in the connective tissue. Energy dispersive analysis with x-rays of these dense granules has demonstrated a peak corresponding to titanium spectrum.

Drug Deposits and Pigmentation

There are many systemic and topical medications which deposit in the skin and cause discoloration by themselves or by their metabolites and photoproducts.[79] Many of these simultaneously stimulate melanocytes, and the discolorations observed are a combined effect of both drug and hypermelanosis. Many of these drugs are photosensitizers or photostimulators, and the hyperpigmentation is a nonspecific postinflammatory phenomenon. In the following section, only selected drugs will be discussed. Readers are referred to Chapter 12 and to general reviews for a more comprehensive listing.

MINOCYCLINE

The most common discoloration is blue-black pigmentation of old acne scars or inflammation, because this antibiotic is routinely used for acne.[80,81] This complication is usually seen in patients who have taken this medication for 1 to 3 years in high dosages of 100 to 200 mg per day. Bluish macules also develop on previously normal skin of the anterior lower legs, around eyes, or anywhere else and are accentuated by sun exposure. Generalized gray-brown discoloration, i.e., "muddy skin syndrome," may occur particularly in exposed areas, the gingiva, hard palate, teeth, and nails. These varieties of color changes may occur individually or in combination.

Histopathological Features   Lesions associated with acne scars contain pigmented macrophages which are iron-stain-positive and negative for melanin by the Fontana-Masson stain. Macular lesions of leg contain pigmented macrophages which are positive for iron and positive for the Fontana reaction but fail to bleach with potassium permanganate, indicating that melanin is not present. The generalized muddy skin shows an increased basal melanization of the epidermis and melanophores in the upper dermis but is negative on staining for iron.

ANTIMALARIALS

Quinacrine produces a diffuse lemon-yellow color if taken for a long period, particularly in fair-skinned patients.[82–84] The yellow color is probably the direct stain of quinacrine itself. Chloroquine may cause irregular grayish macules of the shins and diffuse pigmentation of the face. Hard palate and nail discoloration may occur after chronic ingestion. The pigment is found in the dermis as a drug-melanin complex. Hemosiderin is deposited around capillaries.

CAROTENOIDS

Oranges, apricots, carrots, and green vegetables contain carotenoids.[85] Excessive intake of these causes yellowish discoloration of the palms, soles, and the postauricular skin. Synthetic carotene is commonly used for photoprotection, as cancer preventative drug, and a "tanning" agent (this tan is not sun-protective). The synthetic carotene does not produce the same degree of discoloration as natural carotenoids. The pigment is deposited in subcutaneous fat, skin, and retina.

AMIODARONE

This is an antiarrhythmia drug.[86] One of the many complications of chronic use of this drug is a sun-sensitive blue-gray discoloration which occurs almost always over the exposed skin areas such as face and hands. At least 20 months of continuous medication totaling about 250 g seem to be necessary.

Histopathological Features   Perivascular and endothelial cells and dermal macrophages accumulate pigments. Examination by electron microscope reveals these pigment granules in phagolysosomes in the form of lipid membranous structures. They are probably drug metabolites which were undigested and stored as residual bodies.

CLOFAZIMINE

This drug is currently used for leprosy.[87] Reddish discoloration which represents the color of the drug occurs in conjunctiva and skin within 4 weeks of beginning the medication in 49 to 65 percent of patients. After 2 to 3 months of therapy the lepromatous lesions and occasionally even normal skin turn brown-violaceous. This color may be due to a combination of epidermal and dermal melanin and a ceroidlike substance in the dermis.

PSYCHOTROPIC DRUGS

Prolonged use of phenothiazine and the tricyclic antidepressant imipramine can cause blue-gray to slate-gray discoloration mainly in sun-exposed locations.[88,89]

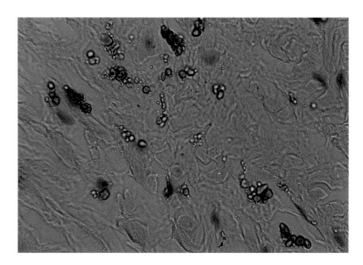

FIGURE 15-18 Imipramine pigmentation. Under semipolarized light, imipramine granules are seen as refractile yellow granules.

Histopathological Features   The dark granules associated with chlorpromazine discoloration and scattered golden pigments in imipramine pigmentation are noted in the upper dermis and perivascular spaces (Figs. 15-17, 15-18). Both melanosomes and electron-dense substances representing drug metabolites are found in dermal macrophages (Fig. 15-19), fibroblasts, vascular endothelial cells, and dermal dendrocytes. The epidermis is hyperpigmented.

CHEMOTHERAPEUTIC DRUGS

The ingestion of agents such as bleomycin, busulphan, cyclophosphamide, doxorubicin, and 5-fluorouracil or topical application of nitro-

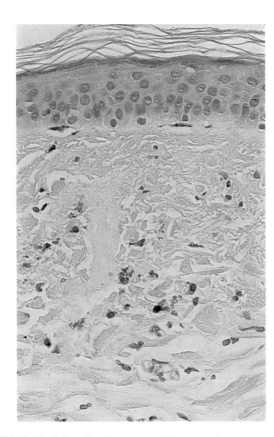

FIGURE 15-17   Imipramine pigmentation. Yellow granules are scattered in the upper and middle dermis.

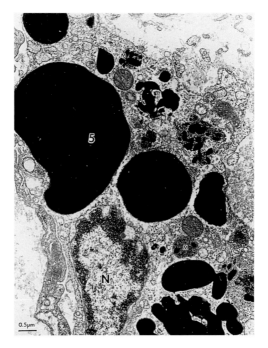

FIGURE 15-19 Imipramine pigmentation. In a dermal phagocyte a large imipramine granule (5) is seen alongside of normal, aggregated melanosomes (m). *N*: nucleus of the phagocyte.

gen mustard (mechlorethamine) and carmustine (BCNU) may result in diffuse hypermelanosis or, in the case of bleomycin, so-called flagellate streaks after long-term ingestion.[90]

Histopathological Features   The epidermis shows increased melanin usually with some pigment incontinence (Table 15-13).

REFERENCES

1. Spritz RA: Molecular basis of human piebaldism. *J Invest Dermatol* 103:137S, 1994.
2. Spritz RA, Ho L, Strunk KM: Inhibition of proliferation of human melanocytes by KIT antisense oligodeoxynucleotide: Implications for human piebaldism and mouse dominant white spotting (W). *J Invest Dermatol* 103:148, 1994.
3. Chang T, McGrae JD Jr, Hashimoto K: Ultrastructural study of two patients with piebaldism and neurofibromatosis 1. *Pediatr Dermatol* 10:224, 1993.
4. Chang T, Hashimoto K, Bawle EV: Spontaneous contraction of leukodermic patches in Waardenburg syndrome. *J Dermatol* 20:707, 1993.
5. Gilhar A, Zelickson B, Ulman Y, Etzioni A: In vivo destruction of melanocytes by the IgG fraction of serum from patients with vitiligo. *J Invest Dermatol* 105:683, 1995.
6. Oetting WS, King RA: Molecular basis of oculocutaneous albinism. *J Invest Dermatol* 103:131S, 1994.
7. Blume RS, Wolff SM: The Chédiak-Higashi syndrome: Studies in four patients and a review of the literature. *Medicine* 51:247, 1972.
8. Holcombe RF, Strauss W, Owens FL, et al: Relationship of the genes for Chédiak-Higashi syndrome (beige) and the T-cell receptor g chain in mouse and man. *Genomics* 1:187, 1987.
9. Harris R, Moynahan EJ: Tuberous sclerosis with vitiligo. *Br J Dermatol* 78:149, 1966.
10. Falabella R, Escobar C, Giraldo N, et al: On the pathogenesis of idiopathic guttate hypomelanosis. *J Am Acad Dermatol* 16:35, 1987.
11. Sybert VP: Hypomelanosis of Ito: A description, not a diagnosis. *J Invest Dermatol* 103:141S, 1994.
12. Pinto FJ, Bolognia JL: Disorders of hypopigmentation in children. *Pediatr Clin North Am* 38:991, 1991.
13. Zaynoun ST, Aftimos BG, Tenekjian KK, et al: Extensive pityriasis alba: A histological, histochemical and ultrastructural study. *Br J Dermatol* 108:83, 1983.
14. Greaves MW, Birkett D, Johnson C: Nevus anemicus: A unique catecholamine-dependent nevus. *Arch Dermatol* 102:172, 1970.
15. Cardosa H, Vignale R, de Sastre A: Familial naevus anemicus (abstract). *Am J Hum Genet* 27:24A, 1975.
16. Dunlop D: Eighty-six cases of Addison's disease. *Br J Med* 12:8987, 1963.
17. Blizzard RM, Chandler RW, Kyle MA, Hung W: Adrenal antibodies in Addison's disease. *Lancet* 2:901, 1962.
18. Feingold KR, Elias DM: Endocrine-skin interactions. *J Am Acad Dermatol* 19:1, 1988.
19. Bilton RN, Cobbs R, Schneider BS: Development of Nelson's syndrome in a patient with recurrent Cushing's disease. *Am J Med* 84:319, 1988.
20. Kanitakis J, Roger H, Soubrier M, et al: Cutaneous angiomas in POEMS syndrome. *Arch Dermatol* 124:695, 1988.
21. Fulk CS: Primary disorders of hyperpigmentation. *J Am Acad Dermatol* 10:1, 1984.
22. Findlay GH, Whiting DA: Universal dyschromatosis. *Br J Dermatol* 85:66, 1971.
23. Witkop CJ Jr: Inherited disorders of pigmentation. *Clin Dermatol* 3:90, 1985.
24. Mizoguchi M, Kukita A: Behavior of melanocytes in reticulate acropigmentation of Kitamura. *Arch Dermatol* 121:659, 1985.
25. Pinheiro M, Penna JF, Freire-Maia N: Two other cases of ANOTHER syndrome? Family report and update. *Clin Genet* 35:237, 1989.
26. Pike MG, Baraitser M, Dinwiddie R, Atherton DJ: A distinctive type of hypohidrotic ectodermal dysplasia featuring hypothyroidism. *J Pediatr* 108:109, 1986.
27. Matsudo H, Reed WB, Homme D, et al: Zosteriform lentiginous nevus. *Arch Dermatol* 107:903, 1973.
28. Rawer JM, Carr RD, Lowney ED: Progressive cribriform and zosteriform hyperpigmentation. *Arch Dermatol* 114:98, 1978.
29. Simoes GA, Piwa N: Progressive zosteriform macular pigmented lesions (letter). *Arch Dermatol* 116:20, 1980.
30. O'Neill JF, James WD: Inherited patterned lentiginosis in blacks. *Arch Dermatol* 125:1231, 1989.
31. Voron DA, Hatfield HH, Kalkhoff RK: Multiple lentigines syndrome: Case report and review of the literature. *Am J Med* 60:447, 1976.
32. Bhawan J, Purtilo DT, Riordan JE, et al: Giant and "granular melanosomes" in leopard syndrome: An ultrastructural study. *J Cutan Pathol* 3:207, 1976.
33. Utsunomiaya J, Gocho H, Miyanaga T, et al: Peutz-Jeghers syndrome: Its natural course and management. *Johns Hopkins Med J* 136:71, 1975.
34. Gregory B, Ho VC: Cutaneous manifestations of gastro-intestinal disorders. *J Am Acad Dermatol* 26:153, 1992.
35. Yamada K, Matsukawa A, Hori Y: Ultrastructural studies on pigmented macules of the Peutz-Jeghers syndrome. *J Dermatol* 8:367, 1981.
36. Wilson-Jones E, Grice K: Reticulate pigmented anomaly of the flexures (Dowling-Degos): A new genodermatosis. *Br J Dermatol* 91:36, 1974.
37. Rebova A, Crovato F: The spectrum of Dowling-Degos disease. *Br J Dermatol* 110:627, 1984.
38. Gablen W: Dermatopathia pigmentosa reticulosa hypohidrotica et atrophica. *Dermatol Wochenschr* 34:193, 1964.
39. Cantu JM, Sanchez-Corona J, Fragoso R: A new autosomal-dominant genodermatosis characterized by hyperpigmented spots and palmoplantar hyperkeratosis. *Clin Genet* 14:165, 1978.
40. Touraine A: Une nouvelle neuroectodermose congeniale: La lentiginose centrofaciale et les dysplasie associée. *Ann Dermatol Syphiligre* (Paris) 8:453, 1941.
41. Rees JR, Ross FGM, Keen G: Lentiginosis and left atrial myxoma. *Br Heart J* 35:874, 1973.
42. Atherton DJ, Pitcher DW, Wells RS, MacDonald DM: A syndrome of various cutaneous pigmented lesions, myxoid neurofibromata and atrial myxoma: The NAME syndrome. *Br J Dermatol* 103:421, 1980.
43. Uhle P, Norvell SS: Generalized lentiginosis. *J Am Acad Dermatol* 18:444, 1988.
44. Sefani A, M'rad R, Simard L, et al: Linkage relationship between incontinentia pigmenti (IP2) and nine terminal X long arm markers. *Hum Genet* 86:297, 1991.
45. Hodgson SV, Neville B, Jones RWA, et al: Two cases of X/autosome translocation in females with incontinentia pigmenti. *Hum Genet* 71:231, 1985.
46. Midgeon BR, Axelman J, Jan deBeur S, et al: Selection against lethal alleles in females heterozygous for incontinentia pigmenti. *Am J Hum Genet* 44:100, 1989.
47. Carney RG: Incontinentia pigmenti: A world statistical analysis. *Arch Dermatol* 112:535, 1976.
48. Cheesbrough MJ: Dyskeratosis congenita. *Br J Dermatol* 99:29, 1978.
49. Connor JM, Gatherer D, Gray FC, et al: Assignment of the gene for dyskeratosis congenita to Xq28. *Hum Genet* 72:348, 1986.
50. Smith AG, Shuster S, Thoday AJ, Peberdy M: Chloasma, oral contraceptives, and plasma immunoreactive-melanocyte-stimulating hormone. *J Invest Dermatol* 68:169, 1977.
51. Larsson P, Lidén S: Prevalence of skin diseases among adolescents 12 to 16 years of age. *Acta Derm Venereol* 60:415, 1980.
52. Nicholls EM: Genetic susceptibility and somatic mutation in the production of freckles, birthmarks, and moles. *Lancet* 1:71, 1968.
53. Riccardi VM: Neurofibromatosis: Past, present, and future. *N Engl J Med* 324:1283, 1991.
54. Obringer AC, Meadows AT, Zackai EH: The diagnosis of neurofibromatosis I in the child under the age of 6 years. *Am J Dis Child* 143:717, 1989.
55. Weinstein LS, Shenker A, Gejman PV, et al: Activating mutations of the stimulatory G protein in the McCune-Albright syndrome. *N Engl J Med* 325:1688, 1991.
56. Riccardi VM: Neurofibromatosis and AlBright's syndrome. *Dermatol Clin* 5:193, 1987.
57. Glinick SE, Alper JC, Bogaars H, Brown JA: Becker's melanosis: Associated abnormalities. *J Am Acad Dermatol* 9:509, 1983.
58. Tate PR, Hodge SJ, Owen LG: A quantitative study of melanocytes in Becker's nevus. *J Cutan Pathol* 7:404, 1980.
59. Nagashima J: Prurigo pigmentosa: Clinical observations of our 14 cases. *J Dermatol* 5:61, 1978.
60. Shimizu H, Yamasaki Y, Harada T, Nishkawa T: Prurigo pigmentosa. *J Am Acad Dermatol* 12:165, 1985.
61. Tanigaki T, Hata S, Kitano Y, et al: Unusual pigmentation on the skin over trunk bones and extremities. *Dermatologica* 170:235, 1985.
62. Konrad K, Woolf K: Pathogenesis of diffuse melanosis secondary to malignant melanoma. *Br J Dermatol* 91:635, 1974.
63. O'Brien WM, LaDu BN, Bunim JJ: Biochemical, pathologic and clinical aspects of alkaptonuria, ochronosis and ochronotic arthropathy. *Am J Med* 34:813, 1963.
64. Wyre HW: Alkaptonuria with extensive ochronosis. *Arch Dermatol* 115:461, 1979.
65. Laurence N, Bigard CA, Reed R, Perret WJ: Exogenous ochronosis in the United States. *J Am Acad Dermatol* 18:1207, 1988.
66. Jacyk WK: Annular granulomatous lesions in exogenous ochronosis are manifestations of sarcoidosis. *Am J Dermatopathol* 17:18, 1995.
67. Goldstein N: Tattoos. *J Dermatol Surg & Oncol* 5:11, 1979.
68. Igarashi H, Ogai M, Kumaoka H: Idiopathic hemochromatosis in brothers. *Hifubyo Shinryo* 16:409, 1984.
69. Fairbanks VF, Baldus WP: Hemochromatosis: The neglected diagnosis. *Mayo Clinic Proc* 61:296, 1986.
70. Ashley JR, Littler CM, Burgdorf WHC, Brann BS: Bronze baby syndrome. *J Am Acad Dermatol* 12:325, 1985.
71. Kaplan BS: Azure lunulae due to argyria. *Arch Dermatol* 94:333, 1966.
72. Prose PH: An electron microscopic study of human generalized argyria. *Am J Path* 42:293, 1963.
73. Espinel MC, Ferrando L: Asymptomatic blue nevus-like macule. *Arch Dermatol* 132:459, 1996.
74. Trotter MJ, Tron VA, Hollingdale J, Rivers JK: Localized chrysiasis induced by laser therapy. *Arch Dermatol* 131:1411, 1995.
75. Granstein RD, Sober AJ: Drug- and heavy metal-induced hyperpigmentation. *J Am Acad Dermatol* 5:1, 1981.

76. Zhu WY, Xia MY, Huang SD, Du D: Hyperpigmentation of the nail from lead deposition (letter). *Int J Dermatol* 28:273, 1989.

77. Leuth HC, Sutton DC, McMullen CJ, Meuhlberger CW: Generalized discoloration of skin resembling argyria following prolonged oral use of bismuth: A case of "bismuthia." *Arch Intern Med* 57:1115, 1936.

78. Dupre A, Touron P, Daste J, et al: Titanium pigmentation: An electron probe microanalysis study. *Arch Dermatol* 121:656, 1985.

79. Kang S, Lerner EA, Sober, AJ, Levine N: Pigmentary disorders from exogenous causes, in Levine N (ed): *Pigmentation and Pigmentary Disorders.* Boca Raton, FL, CRC Press, pp 417–438, 1993.

80. Gordon B, Sparano BM, Iatropoulos MJ: Hyperpigmentation of the skin associated with minocycline therapy. *Arch Dermatol* 121:618, 1985.

81. Argenyi ZB, Finelli L, Bergfeld WF, et al: Minocycline-related cutaneous hyperpigmentation as demonstrated by light microscopy, electron microscopy, and X-ray energy spectroscopy. *J Cutan Pathol* 14:176–180, 1987.

82. Lutterloh CC, Shallenberger PL: Unusual pigmentation developing after prolonged suppressive therapy with quinacrine hydrochloride. *Arch Dermatol Venereol* 53:349, 1946.

83. Tuffanelli D, Abraham RK, Dubois EI: Pigmentation from antimalarial therapy: Its possible relation to the ocular lesions. *Arch Dermatol* 88:419, 1963.

84. Levantine A, Almeyda J: Drug induced changes in pigmentation. *Br J Dermatol* 89:105, 1973.

85. Gupta AK, Haberman JF, Pawlowski D, et al: Canthaxanthine. *Int J Dermatol* 24:528, 1985.

86. Waitzer S, Britany J, From L, et al: Cutaneous ultrastructural changes and photosensitivity associated with amiodarone therapy. *J Am Acad Dermatol* 16:779, 1987.

87. Levy L: Pharmacologic studies of clofazimine. *Am J Trop Med Hyg* 23:1097, 1974.

88. Hashimoto K, Wiener W, Albert J: An electron microscopic study of chlorpromazine pigmentation. *J Invest Dermatol* 47:296, 1966.

89. Hashimoto K, Joselow SA, Tye MJ: Imipramine hyperpigmentation: A slate-gray discoloration caused by long-term imipramine administration. *J Am Acad Dermatol* 25:357, 1991.

90. Fitzpatrick JE: The cutaneous histopathology of chemotherapeutic reactions. *J Cutan Pathol* 20:1–14, 1993.

CHAPTER 16

DEPOSITION DISORDERS

CHAPTER 16

DEPOSITION DISORDERS

Ken Hashimoto / Raymond L. Barnhill

Various substances may form deposits in the skin, and this chapter will discuss abnormal endogenous substances. Exogenous materials such as tattoo and heavy metals and the special category of endogenous deposition such as melanin depositions are discussed in Chapter 15.

Abnormal deposition of endogenous substances exhibits particular colors. However, different substances may have a similar color with the hematoxylin and eosin (H&E) stain (Table 16-1). These substances are often grouped together and were once considered the same chemical substances. Examples are mucin, hyalin, and colloid. A dermatopathologist examining H&E-stained tissue sections will notice the color characteristics and common texture of a substance in one of these three groups and will place focus analysis within the group of diseases which produces these characteristics. The dermatopathologist's analysis will be fine-tuned to more specific entities based upon the clinical data. Special stains, immunostains, and electron microscopy will aid further differentiation. In many instances, clinical knowledge is essential in the final synthesis of all data to reach a reasonable conclusion. This process is always at work in the experienced pathologist's mind. A model of algorithmic sequence of differential elimination is presented in Table 16-1. Tables 16-2 through 16-8 will assist in this analytical process.

DERMAL MUCINOSIS

In most instances, mucin depositions occur in dermal connective tissue as bluish-gray material with the H&E stain (Table 16-2). Epithelial mucin deposition occurs in hair follicles (follicular mucinosis). Mucin or protein–hyaluronic acid complex is a normal component of the dermal connective tissue produced by fibroblasts and mast cells. In disease conditions, the amount of mucin is increased, and, since hyaluronic acid holds water (hygroscopic), the dermal connective tissue is swollen (myxedema). If this condition persists, the dermis and sometimes the subcutaneous connective tissues react with production of excessive collagen, leading to sclerodermalike fibrosis (scleromyxedema). Mucin is usually present in early lesions and may diminish or even disappear in late stages. Also, during tissue processing mucin may largely be washed out. If one suspects mucin deposition because of light blue staining between widely separated collagen bundles or empty spaces, special stains should be utilized such as alcian blue at pH 2.5 (negative at 0.5), toluidine blue at pH 4.0 and 7.0 (negative below 2), and colloidal iron. The periodic acid–Schiff (PAS) stain is negative.

Generalized Myxedema

This condition is associated with a severe form of chronic hypothyroidism.[1,2] The face, particularly the eyelids and lips, are prominently swollen but not pitted with pressure.

Histopathological Features Histopathologic features include hyperkeratosis, occasional keratinous cysts, only slight edema (mucinosis) of the dermis in most cases, usually requiring mucin stains. The mucin is often deposited around blood vessels and hair follicles of the upper and middle dermis only. In some instances, there is massive accumulation of mucin resulting in the disruption of collagen bundles and accompanied by perivascular mononuclear cell infiltrates. In the late stages, fibrosis in the deep dermis and subcutis may simulate scleroderma.

Differential Diagnosis Myxedema may be difficult to discriminate from other mucinoses with slight deposition of mucin (Table 16-2). Lesions with prominent mucin deposits may suggest pretibial myxedema, reticular erythematous mucinosis, and tumid forms of lupus erythematosus.

Pretibial Myxedema

This is most commonly observed in patients with established hyperthyroidism who have been treated.[1–3] These patients are usually euthyroid by the time they develop this condition, although they may still exhibit exophthalmos. With regard to pathophysiology, thyroid-stimulating hormone (TSH) appears to have lost its normal target organ and now stimulates fibroblasts of the lower extremities.

Clinical Features The anterior shins and occasionally dorsal feet are involved by elevated, knobby plaques or dome-shaped nodules. The cutaneous surface is shiny or waxy, and peau d'orange–type follicular openings with follicular plugging are noted in new lesions. In severe cases one may observe marked edema and verrucoid surface changes, possibly resembling elephantiasis nostras verrucosa. After biopsy transparent viscous fluid continues to ooze.

Histopathological Features The lower two-thirds of the dermis are expanded by mucin which may be seen as bluish threads and granules in the spaces between collagen bundles (Fig. 16-1). Spindle-shaped and large stellate fibroblasts appear to float in edematous areas. In chronic lesions, increased collagen production occurs in the deep dermis and subcutaneous fat, resulting in the replacement of fat lobules by fibrosis. Alcian blue stain is strongly positive and differentiates mucin from conventional lymphedema (Fig. 16-2).

Differential Diagnosis See Table 16-2.

Papular Mucinosis and Scleromyxedema

This disorder is also known as *lichen myxedematosus* because in severe cases lichenified plaques develop in thickened, edematous skin. In some

TABLE 16-1

Abnormal Dermal and Epidermal Depositions

Abnormal Dermal and Epidermal Depositions (H&E stain)

Pink-gray, amorphous PAS+				Pale blue-grayish blue, edematous	Pale blue-gray
Hyalin	Amyloid	Colloid		Colloidal iron +	Multicolor
EM: amorphous	EM: filaments	EM: amorphous	EM: filaments	Alcian blue +, pH 2.5;	birefringence
PAS ++	Congo	Amyloid P+	Antikeratin ++	−, pH 0.5	
↓	red +++	↓		Toluidine blue	↓
Hyalinosis cutis	Greenish	Adult colloid	Congo red +	metachromasia +, >pH 2.0	Gouty tophi
et mucosae	birefrin-	milium	↓	PAS −	
	gence of		Juvenile colloid milium	Aldehyde fuchsin −	
	Congo red		or cytoid body		
	stain+		(cytoid body: IgM++)	Mucin	
	↓				
	Various			See Table 16-2	
	amyloidoses				

Ig λ or κ chain	Potassium	Antikeratin
	permanganate	antibody +
AL amyloid	treatment	↓
	PAS −	Amyloid K
Primary systemic,	↓	
nodular, or	AA amyloid	
Waldenstrom's macroglobulinemia		
	Secondary systemic	
	amyloidosis	

Lichenoid macular	Epithelial tumor	Juvenile colloid
or concha amyloidosis	amyloidoses	milium
	(basal cell carcinoma, actinic	
	keratosis, seborrheic keratosis,	
	Bowen's disease, etc.)	

lesions, particularly on the upper back, differentiation from scleredema is difficult. In a typical case of papular mucinosis, closely set papules and sometimes nodules involve the arms and face. In scleromyxedema, coalesced papulonodules form large, thick, often erythematous plaques on the face, upper back, and peripheral extremities.[4] In this group of cutaneous mucinosis, paraproteinosis of the IgG λ light chain is frequently present.

Papulonodular dermal mucinosis may be associated with systemic lupus erythematosus and the albopapuloid variant (Pasini) of dominant dystrophic epidermolysis bullosa. Such forms of mucinosis are commonly found on the upper back.

Histopathological Features The amount of mucin deposition and reactive fibrosis are quite variable depending upon the type of lesion present (papules, nodules, or plaques) and the age of the lesion. In general, the upper reticular dermis shows fraying and rarefaction of dermal collagen and the bluish-gray deposition of mucin. Stellate and spindled fibroblasts are present in the milieu of mucinous substances. Normal fibroblasts are increased in number in the fibrotic periphery.

Differential Diagnosis This condition can only be distinguished from other mucinoses by clinical features and the dermal fibrosis, which is not observed in the other mucinoses until the late stages. Scleredema shows distinctive features as discussed below.

Reticular Erythematous Mucinosis (REM)

Clinical Features Predominantly adult females are affected by reticulated erythematous macules and plaques in the central chest and upper back.[5] The arms and face may be involved. More infiltrated papular lesions are called *plaquelike cutaneous mucinosis*.

Histopathological Features Perivascular and perifollicular lymphohistiocytic infiltrates with plasma cells, variable amounts of bluish-gray mucin deposition, and stellate fibroblasts between collagen bundles are observed.

Differential Diagnosis Other entities with both mucin deposition and inflammatory infiltrates include: connective tissue disease, especially

TABLE 16-2

Mucin Depositions in the Dermis

Disorders	Distribution Characterization	Associated Disorders	Special Stains	Histopathological Features
Generalized myxedema	Nonpitting, waxy facial edema	Hypothyroidism	Colloidal iron, alcian blue	Scant mucin, upper dermis around blood vessels, hair follicles
Pretibial myxedema	Shin, dorsal feet	Thyrotoxicosis, treated	Alcian blue, toluidine blue, Giemsa	Prominent mucin, lower two-thirds of dermis
Papular mucinosis, lichen myxedematosus, scleromyxedema	Face, upper back, distal extremities	IgG paraproteinosis	Alcian blue	Diffuse mucin, upper dermis, proliferation of fibroblasts
Reticulated erythematous mucinosis (REM)	Female chest, upper back		Alcian blue, Giemsa	Dermal mucin, lymphoplasma cellular infiltrates
Scleredema	Upper back, nape	Diabetes, acute infection	Toluidine blue	Dermis two to three times normal thickness, fenestrated collagen, mucin may be absent on H&E stain
Focal mucinosis	Solitary or multiple papulonodules	Systemic mucinosis (LAMB)	Alcian blue	Focal accumulation of mucin
Digital mucous cyst	Distal interphalangeal joint, posterior nailfold		Alcian blue	Focal accumulation of mucin
Mucocele of the lip, oral mucous cyst	Mucosal side of lower lip		Alcian blue, PAS	Sialomucin with inflammatory reaction
Cutaneous myxoma	Widespread, small lesions, more often in eyelid, ears, nipples	LAMB or NAME syndrome	Alcian blue	Somewhat poorly defined margins, fine collagen fibers in mucin
Follicular mucinosis	Face, head/neck	Mycosis fungoides	Colloidal iron, alcian blue, Giemsa	Mucin within pilosebaceous unit, inflammatory cell infiltrates
Acral persistent papular mucinosis	Multiple discrete papules (2–5 mm)—dorsal aspects of hands and extensor surfaces		Alcian blue	Abundant mucin, upper dermis, no fibroblast proliferation
Papular and nodular mucinosis associated with lupus erythematosus	Lumpy papules; nodules—neck, trunk, upper extremities		Alcian blue, colloidal iron	Mucin deposition, papillary and upper reticular dermis
Self-healing juvenile cutaneous mucinosis	Children—linear infiltrated plaques, head and neck, trunk, thighs; deep nodules, face, elbows, knees, fingers		Alcian blue	Mucin, upper reticular dermis, increased fibroblasts, mast cells
Cutaneous mucinosis of infancy	Firm papules—elbows, dorsa of hands, upper arms		Alcian blue	Mucin, papillary dermis
Hurler/Hunter's Disease	Thickened skin of face, upper back; pebbled papules; gargoylism	Dwarfism, ankylosing joints, hepatosplenomegaly, mental retardation	Giemsa, toluidine blue, colloidal iron, alcian blue	EM: lamellar inclusion bodies in dermal fibroblasts

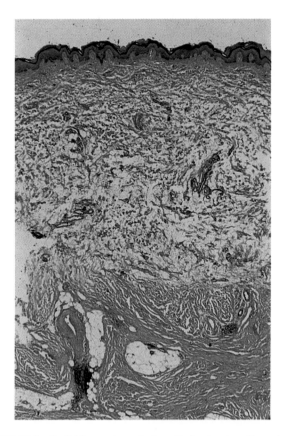

FIGURE 16-1 Pretibial myxedema. In the reticular dermis, collagen bundles are widely separated by edema. Subcutaneous fat tissue is largely replaced with sclerotic collagen.

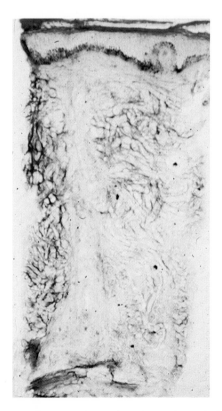

FIGURE 16-2 Pretibial myxedema. Alcian blue stain at pH 2.5 reveals an abundant mucin throughout the dermis.

"tumid" forms of lupus erythematosus (probably including so-called Jessner's lymphocytic infiltrate); pretibial or localized myxedema and the gyrate erythemas on occasion; and in a variety of other inflammatory dermatoses uncommonly as a reactive phenomenon. In general, REM does not show other distinguishing features of connective tissue disease such as epidermal atrophy, interface dermatitis, basement membrane thickening, or infiltration of appendages and nerves by lymphoid infiltrates.

Scleredema Adultorum

Clinical Features   The most common cause of this disorder is chronic, adult-onset diabetes.[6] Other causes such as acute respiratory infection are rare in the United States. The onset of scleredema related to diabetes is insidious and often begins on the upper back with subsequent extension to the neck and occipital scalp. In advanced cases, nonpitting indurated edema elevates the skin of the shoulder blade area with associated deep vertebral folds. Such patients are usually obese, and the mobility of the neck and head may be severely restricted. The skin is shiny and often uneven. In chronic lesions the skin becomes verrucoid, and acanthosis nigricans may develop around the neck. Groups of small papules resembling papular mucinosis may develop in the lesion. The course is often chronic. Similar lesions may be observed occasionally in nondiabetics, and the course is chronic. On occasion, scleredema may follow acute respiratory infection. This type of scleredema is often acute and resolves rapidly. Very rarely the tongue, skeletal muscle, pleura, or pericardium are involved.

Histopathological Features   The dermis is significantly thickened, sometimes up to two to three times normal, by increased collagen, which sometimes replaces subcutaneous fat (Fig. 16-3). In general, one observes thick hyalinized collagen bundles reminiscent of hypertrophic scar or even keloid except that the collagen bundles are widely separated (resulting in so-called fenestrations) (Fig. 16-4). After the early stage of disease, mucin stains may become negative. However, frozen sections may be stained with alcian blue at pH 2.5 or toluidine blue at pH 7.0. Mucin, if present, is found in the spaces (fenestrations) between collagen bundles.

Differential Diagnosis   Scleredema differs from other forms of mucinosis by showing marked thickening of the dermis, hypertrophied collagen bundles, the fenestrations between collagen bundles, and the frequent absence of mucin in H&E-stained sections. Scleredema is distinguished from lichen myxedematosus by the above features and by the lack of fibroblastic proliferation that often typifies the latter condition. Morphea and scleroderma in contrast to scleredema tend to exhibit tightly packed hypertrophied collagen bundles without fenestrations or mucin deposition.

Focal Dermal Mucinosis

Clinical Features   This condition is typified by solitary or grouped papules or nodules without the underlying induration, encountered in lichen myxedematosus or scleromyxedema.[7] Spontaneous resolution may occur. In rare instances there may be systemic myxomatosis involving the heart.

Histopathological Features   Mucin deposition replaces the dermal collagen focally. Stellate fibroblasts are noted in such mucinous materials. Essentially the histologic features are similar to lichen myxedematosus, and only clinical correlation establishes the diagnosis.

Differential Diagnosis   The focal nature of the mucin deposition is usually distinctive compared to other forms of mucinosis which are

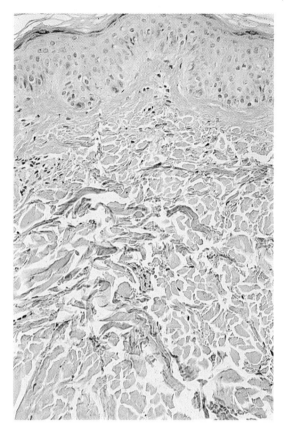

FIGURE 16-3 Scleredema. Thick, sclerotic collagen bundles are separated in reticular dermis.

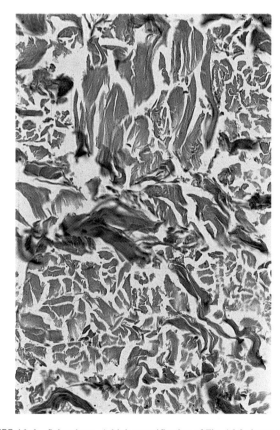

FIGURE 16-4 Scleredema. A high magnification of Fig. 16-3 shows sclerotic collagen bundles which are separated by edema.

TABLE 16-3

Focal Cutaneous Mucinosis and Cutaneous Myxoma

Focal cutaneous mucinosis	Cutaneous myxoma
Clinical Features	
Common	Rare
Discrete whitish papule	Ill-defined papule, nodule associated with Carney syndrome, cardiac myxoma
Histopathological Features	
Well-circumscribed	Less well-defined; gradual transition to surrounding tissue
No inflammatory cells, mast cells	No inflammatory cells, mast cells
No fine collagenous fibers in general	Fine collagenous fibers present
Uniform mucin deposition	Uniform mucin deposition

commonly diffuse. The major entity to be discriminated is cutaneous myxoma (Table 16-3). Myxoma is perhaps less well-defined with a gradual transition to the surrounding tissue.

Digital Mucous (Myxoid) Cyst

Clinical Features A dome-shaped elevation with or without visible semitransparent contents forms on the dorsal skin on or near the distal interphalangeal joint of the finger.[8] The cyst may erupt near the nail. Puncture or biopsy results in the drainage of viscous, stringy mucin from the cyst. Some cysts may represent a herniation of synovial cavity and thus a ganglion.

Histopathological Features The accumulation of mucin in the dermis results in collagen fibers that are widely spaced and thin (Fig. 16-5). Thus the reticular network of collagen is embedded in pale blue mucin with the H&E stain (Fig. 16-6). Alcian blue at pH 2.5 stains the mucin intensely. Stellate fibroblasts are abundant. As the production of mucin continues, the reticular meshwork of thin collagen fibers is obliterated, and a cyst is formed.

Differential Diagnosis See Table 16-2.

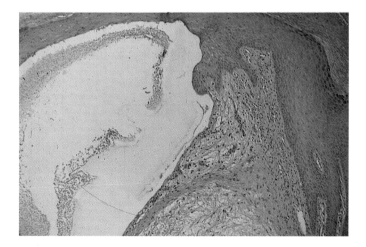

FIGURE 16-5 Digital mucous cyst. Subepidermal cyst and a severe mucinous edema are stained bluish gray, a typical color of mucin in H&E stain.

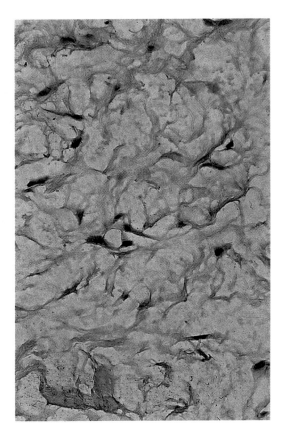

FIGURE 16-6 Digital mucous cyst. An enlargement of edematous area of Fig. 16-5. Stringy remnant of collagen fibers and stellate fibroblasts with long, tapering processes (mucoblasts) are embedded in pale blue mucin.

Mucocele of the Lip

This is an oral mucous cyst.[9] (See Chapter 37.)

Histopathological Features   Multiple edematous pockets of extravasated sialomucin are present in the submucosa. An inflammatory cell reaction surrounds these foci. In an old lesion one large cavity filled with faintly eosinophilic material is observed. Sialomucin is an epithelial mucin (secreted by salivary glands) which is PAS-positive and diastase-resistant. Alcian blue stain is also positive, but hyaluronidase does not abolish this staining.

Cutaneous Myxoma

Clinical Features   Cutaneous myxoma and myxoid neurofibromas may be a part of LAMB syndrome, i.e., pigmented skin lesions (*l*entigines), cardiac *a*trial myxoma, cutaneous papular *m*yxoma, *b*lue nevus, and sometimes endocrine tumors.[10] Subcutaneous large nodular myxomas may coexist. Cardiac myxoma is fatal, and cutaneous myxoma may be an important first indication of this serious condition. Focal mucinosis (see above) may be part of the LAMB syndrome.

Histopathological Features   Dermal or subcutaneous mucinous degeneration is more localized rather than diffuse and contains stellate and elongated fibroblasts (Fig. 16-7).

Differential Diagnosis   The major process to be distinguished is focal cutaneous mucinosis (Table 16-3). Both lesions are reasonably well defined, but myxoma perhaps shows more ill-defined margins and contains fine collagenous elements as compared to focal mucinosis.

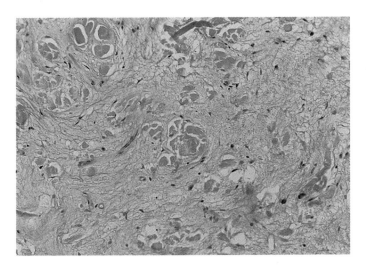

FIGURE 16-7   Myxoma. Dermal collagen bundles are disrupted by an accumulation of pale blue mucin. H&E stain.

Follicular Mucinosis

Clinical Features   This condition affects predominantly face and head-neck region of middle-aged individuals.[11] If terminal hairs of the beard or head are affected, a localized hair loss is noticed, hence alopecia mucinosa. Vellous hairs may be lost but are not noticeable. It may occur as a group of individual follicular papules with prominent follicular openings or as a large indurated plaque in which coalesced follicular and nonfollicular papules are present. Follicular mucinosis of either variety may heal spontaneously after a few months to a few years, may have a chronic but benign course, or may be associated with mycosis fungoides from the beginning or follow it. The chronic benign type may eventuate in mycosis fungoides.

Histopathological Features   Early changes consist of intra- and intercellular edema of follicular epithelium due to accumulation of mucin. The intercellular edema produces a reticular network pattern from the cell walls of the outer root sheath keratinocytes. The increased mucin eventually destroys cell walls and makes a pool of mucin within the hair follicle and sebaceous gland. The mucin in this disease can be stained with colloidal iron, alcian blue, and Giemsa but is mostly negative with the PAS stain. Hyaluronidase digestion abolishes all staining. In severe cases the accumulated mucin extravasates to form perifollicular mucinosis. The inflammatory reaction is variable, and in florid reactions it resembles mycosis fungoides. The presence of numerous eosinophils in the infiltrate speaks in favor of benign course of the disease. Atypia and hyperchromasia of lymphocyte nuclei, Pautrier's microabscesses in the epidermis, and convoluted nuclear contours of CD4-positive lymphocytes revealed by electron microscopy are features supporting a diagnosis of mycosis fungoides.

Differential Diagnosis   Follicular eczema and staphylococcal folliculitis may resemble follicular mucinosis but do not show staining with alcian blue and other stains for hyaluronic acid.

HYALINE DEPOSITIONS

Hyaline is not a single substance. Traditionally, this term included a variety of skin deposits which appeared eosinophilic and somewhat glassy by the refraction of light. Therefore, the recognition of hyaline is

TABLE 16-4

Amyloid-Hyaline-Colloid Deposition

Disorders	Distribution and Characterization	Associated Disorder	Special Stains
Amyloidoses Systemic AL amyloidosis	Periorbital papules and ecchymosis, macroglossia pinch hemorrhage	Kidney, liver, heart, muscle deposition	Congo red (green birefringence), crystal violet, thioflavine-T fluorescence
Systemic AA amyloidosis (secondary systemic amyloidosis)	Subcutaneous fat, rectal submucosa	Kidney, liver, spleen	Same
Familial amyloidotic neuropathy	Leg ulcers, atrophic scars, pinch hemorrhage	Peripheral nerve, kidney, pancreas, testes	Same
β_2-microglobulin amyloid	Lichenoid papules on arms and trunk	Long-term hemodialysis	Same
Colloid milium	Face, hands, neck	None	Adult type: amyloid P component Juvenile type: antikeratin Ab
Hyalinosis cutis et mucosae	Oral mucous membrane, edges of eyelids and nostrils (string of beads), over joints	Epilepsy	PAS (diastase-resistant)
Porphyria	Sun-exposed areas (face, dorsum of hands, arms)	Hepatitis C in PCT, hepatic fibrosis and gallstones in EPP, neuropathy in variegated and hereditary coproporphyria	PAS (diastase-resistant)
Gout (tophi)	Auricle, finger, elbow	Arthritis (big toe), kidney stones, neuropathy	Birefringence in alcohol-fixed tissue
Waldenstrom's macroglobulinemia (storage papule)	Semitranslucent papules	IgM gammopathy	Anti-IgM stain

the beginning point to consider a group of limited but still diverse conditions (Tables 16-4 and 16-5). All hyalines described below are PAS-positive, Congo red–positive, and thioflavine T–positive.

Systemic Amyloidoses

Amyloid was once considered to be the same substance regardless of the differences in clinical presentations.[12–14] We now know that the origin and chemical nature of amyloid is quite diverse (Table 16-4). Why then do we still use the term *amyloid*? So-called amyloid defined by Virchow as a starchlike, iodine-stainable substance shares several common characteristics: an eosinophilic amorphous appearance with the H&E stain (Table 16-5), Congo red staining resulting in doubly refractile green color under polariscopy, thioflavine-T fluorescence, and straight, non-branching filaments (6 to 10 nm in diameter) revealed by electron microscope (Figs. 16-8 to 16-11). Keratin, immunoglobulin, insulin, thyrocalcitonin, and other chemical substances can produce beta-pleated antiparallel polypeptide sheets and therefore are amyloidogenic. The current classification of amyloidoses is based on the chemical nature of the amyloids with significant consideration of the conventional clinical subclassification (Table 16-4).

Systemic Amyloid Light Chain (AL) Amyloidosis

Clinical Features If multiple myeloma can be identified as the source of immunoglobulin light chain, the amyloidosis should properly be classified as myeloma-associated AL amyloidosis. If no gammopathy is

found, it should be designated as primary (idiopathic) systemic amyloidosis. This form of amyloidosis is mainly a systemic deposition disease (kidney, liver, heart), but cutaneous lesions are observed in 30 to 40 percent of the patients. Pinch hemorrhages, periorbital waxy papules and plaques with hemorrhage, enlargement of the tongue (macroglossia), and hardening of oral mucous membranes are the most common signs.

Histopathological Features Amyloid deposition begins in the perivascular areas and surrounding sweat glands, hair follicles, and fat cells (amyloid rings). It eventually fills the papillary dermis and diffusely involves the entire dermis (Figs. 16-8 to 16-10). Pinch hemorrhages occur because blood vessels are involved without visible skin lesions. In extensive infiltrates, diffuse or nodular eosinophilic deposits are often fissured and cracked into smaller aggregates. Fibroblasts are often attached to the fissured edges. Although these depositions of immunoglobulins with associated polysaccharides are, in fact, foreign to the skin, inflammatory reaction to such deposits is usually absent.

Differential Diagnosis See Tables 16-4 to 16-6.

Systemic AA Amyloidosis

Clinical Features Systemic AA amyloidosis, or *secondary systemic amyloidosis*, occurs in association with a variety of chronic inflammatory diseases such as rheumatoid arthritis, familial Mediterranean fever, or chronic infectious diseases such as osteomyelitis, bronchiectasis, and lepromatous leprosy. Visible skin lesions are rare except in Muckle-

TABLE 16-5

Summary of Special Stains for Pink Amorphous Deposits

	Amyloid	Colloid	Lipoid proteinosis	Porphyria	Waldenstrom's macroglobulinemia
Congo red	+	+	+	−	−
Apple green birefringence	+	−	Weak	−	−
Thioflavine T	+	+	+	−	−
Yellow-green birefringence			Weak		
Crystal violet metachromasia	+	+	+	−	−
Methyl violet (red)	+	−	Weak	−	−
Pagoda red 9 (Dylon)	+	−	−	−	−
Scarlet red 5 (RIT)	−	−	+	−	−
PAS+ diastase	+	+	+	+	+
Amyloid P component antibody	+	+	−	−	−
Keratin antibody	Cutaneous +	Juvenile +	−	−	−
IgM antibody	−	−	−	−	+
Colloidal iron pH 2.5	−	−	+	−	−
Alcian blue	−	−	+	−	−
Sudan black (frozen sections)	−	−	+	−	−
Oil red O	−	−	+	−	−

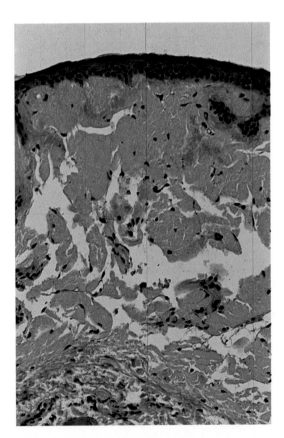

FIGURE 16-8 Systemic AL amyloidosis. A hyaline substance, i.e., amyloid, occupies the entire dermis. There are many fissures and cracks caused by processing artefact due to the lack of elasticity in amyloid.

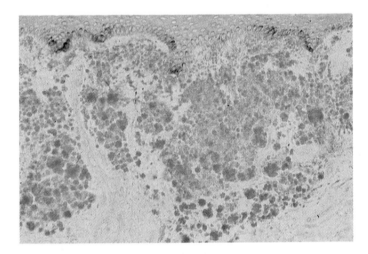

FIGURE 16-9 Systemic AL amyloidosis. Congo red stain is strongly positive in dermal amyloid.

Wells syndrome, in which geographic skin lesions are seen (probably not containing amyloid). The major sites of AA amyloid deposition are not the skin but rather parenchymatous organs such as kidney, liver (speckle or wax liver), and spleen (sago spleen). The AA amyloid is not immunoglobulin but instead is derived from globulin called *serum amyloid A* (SAA) which is split into AA amyloid in chronic febrile conditions.

Histopathological Features   Deep-needle biopsy of the lower abdomen shows amyloid deposition around the subcutaneous fat cells (amyloid rings) and eccrine glands. As the amount of amyloid increases, the dermis may be diffusely infiltrated. Rectal biopsy shows amyloid deposition in the submucosa. After treatment with potassium permanganate, AA amyloid become nonreactive for alkaline Congo red stain.

Differential Diagnosis   See Tables 16-4 to 16-6.

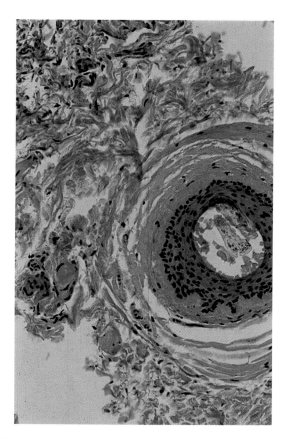

FIGURE 16-10 Systemic AL amyloidosis. A thick perifollicular coat of amyloid deposition is seen.

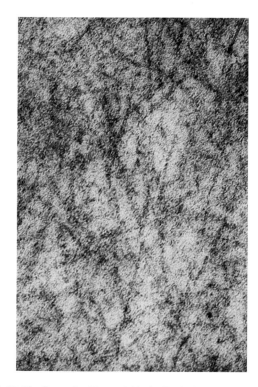

FIGURE 16-11 Systemic AL amyloidosis. Typical amyloid filaments are straight, nonbranching, nonanastomosing, and 6 to 10 nm in diameter ($\times$ 15,000).

Familial Amyloidotic Polyneuropathy

Clinical Features Skin changes consist of trophic leg ulcers and atrophic scars due to the accumulation of prealbumin type (AFP) amyloid in peripheral nerves. This autosomal dominant variety has long been confused with leprosy because of its nerve involvement and deformity of joints. There are Portuguese, Japanese, and Swedish subtypes.

Histopathological Features Amyloid infiltrates blood vessels, arrector pili muscles, and elastic fibers in the skin, in addition to cutaneous nerves. The kidney, pancreas, and testes may be affected, but the liver and spleen are usually spared.

β_2-Microglobulin Amyloid

Clinical Features Small shiny lichenoid papules develop on the arms and trunk of the patients who have had long-term hemodialysis. Dermal deposition of amyloid is similar to AL amyloid.

Skin-Limited Amyloidoses

All skin-limited amyloid depositions are of keratin type except nodular amyloidosis, which is derived from the light chain of immunoglobulins[12–15] (Table 16-6). The source of keratins is either epidermal or tumors of epidermal or hair follicle origin. Dark-colored races such as African-Americans, Asians, Latin Americans, and those of Middle Eastern extraction are more frequently affected than Caucasians.

MACULAR AMYLOIDOSIS

Clinical Features The upper back and scapular areas of middle-aged, dark-skinned women are most commonly affected. Pigmentation is not uniform but "rippled," often corresponding to the stream lines of hairs. Clinical symptoms are commonly absent but may include mild pruritus.

LICHEN AMYLOIDOSUS

Clinical Features Typical lesions are hyperkeratotic papules and plaques involving the shins and, in severe cases, the extensor surface of the arms including shoulders. Severe pruritus is often a feature.

BIPHASIC AMYLOIDOSIS

Clinical Features Both lichenoid and macular amyloidoses are present in the same area or separate locations in the same patient. The lichenoid lesions are commonly pruritic.

FRICTION AMYLOIDOSIS

Clinical Features The constant use of a nylon brush or towel may produce the macular-type amyloidosis commonly on the back. Friction melanosis clinically resembles this condition.

Histopathological Features The histologic findings in macular amyloidosis are usually subtle, and it may be difficult to demonstrate amyloid in many cases. Although cytoid bodies or other evidence of keratinocyte degeneration are not routinely observed in the epidermis, a careful search may identify such cells. They are the source of amyloid in these varieties of amyloidoses. These cells in the epidermis are Congo red–positive and exhibit greenish birefringence under polarized light. These epidermal cytoid bodies drop into the dermis, breaking through the basement membrane. Small numbers of eosinophilic globular bodies accumulate initially in the papillary dermis in macular

TABLE 16-6

Skin-Limited Amyloidoses

Disorder	Clinical features	Histopathological features	Differential diagnosis
Keratin-derived amyloidoses			
Macular amyloidosis	Rippled pigmentation, upper back, scapular areas, often middle-aged women of color, pruritus mild	Scant eosinophilic globules in papillary dermis, pigment incontinence, occasional dyskeratotic cells	Postinflammatory hypermelanosis
Lichen amyloidosus	Hyperkeratotic papules, plaques; shins, extensor surfaces; pruritus often severe	Hyperkeratosis, papillomatous epidermal hyperplasia, aggregates of eosinophilic globules in papillary dermis	Colloid milium, lipoid proteinosis
Biphasic amyloidosis (macular and lichen amyloidoses in the same patient)			
Friction amyloidosis (see macular amyloidosis)			
Epithelioma-associated keratin amyloidosis	Various cutaneous neoplasms: basal cell carcinoma, Bowen's disease, actinic keratosis, seborrheic keratosis	Deposition of eosinophilic globules in both the parenchyma and stroma	
Actinic amyloidosis: Juvenile colloid milium Disseminated superficial actinic porokeratosis	Waxy or pearly papules, nodules, sun-exposed skin; annular hyperkeratosis	Large aggregates of pink eosinophilic material, pink globular deposits	
Insulin-derived amyloidosis			
Insulin amyloidosis	Sites of repeated insulin injection	Eosinophilic globules, reparative changes	
Immunoglobulin-derived amyloidosis			
Nodular amyloidosis	Single or multiple nodules on face, scalp, legs of middle-aged women	Massive accumulation of pink amorphous material in dermis and occasional subcutis	Primary amyloidosis, Waldenstrom's macroglobulinemia

amyloidosis and expand dermal papilla, pressing the rete ridges into thin septae in lichen amyloidosus. In later stages, diffuse homogeneous eosinophilic amyloid fills the papillary dermis and infiltrates the upper reticular dermis (Figs. 16-12, 16-13). Usually some degree of pigment incontinence is present in both forms of cutaneous amyloidosis. Keratin amyloids (amyloid K) are strongly stained (Fig. 16-14) with polyclonal antikeratin antibodies which contain a combination of antibodies against basal cell keratins (K5, 14) and upper epidermal keratins (K1, 10). Amyloid P component is always positive. Maturation of degenerated keratin proteins into amyloid may require a digestion process in the lysosomes of dermal macrophages.

Routine Congo red (Fig. 16-9), Dylon, thioflavine T (Fig. 16-13), toluidine blue, or crystal violet stains are not reliable in formalin- or alcohol-fixed tissue sections. These stains are more reliable in fresh frozen sections. Electron microscopic demonstration of 6- to 10-nm straight filaments is the most specific and reliable diagnostic method (Figs. 16-15 to 16-17).

Differential Diagnosis The major conditions confused with macular amyloidosis include friction (nylon towel) melanosis (see Chapter 15), postinflammatory hypermelanosis, and melasma. Macular amyloidosis

and friction (nylon towel) melanosis are essentially the same process except that amyloid cannot be demonstrated in the latter. Postinflammatory hypermelanosis and melasma also do not exhibit amyloid and are usually characterized by different clinical features compared to macular amyloidosis.

The differential diagnosis of lichen amyloidosus includes nodular amyloidosis, colloid milium and colloid degeneration, lipoid proteinosis, and Waldenstrom's macroglobulinemia (Tables 16-4 to 16-7). Nodular amyloidosis usually shows much more extensive amyloid accumulation in the dermis (and possibly the subcutis) and waxy or translucent nodules of the head and neck versus lichen amyloidosus. In addition, immunoglobulin light chains can be demonstrated in nodular amyloidosis. Juvenile colloid milium may be histologically indistinguishable from lichen amyloidosus except by distribution and clinical features. Adult colloid milium differs from lichen amyloidosus by the features outlined in Table 16-7. Lipoid proteinosis (and erythropoietic porphyria) shows a perivascular pattern of accumulation of amorphous pink material that is PAS+D– and Congo red–positive. The storage papules of Waldenstrom's macroglobulinemia may closely resemble adult colloid milium and lichen amyloidosus because of the presence of clefts and fissures. The material is PAS+D–positive and Congo red–negative and reacts with antibodies against IgM.

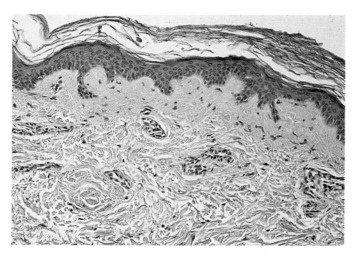

FIGURE 16-12 Lichen amyloidosus. Under the hyperkeratotic epidermis, pale-pink hyaline substance, i.e., amyloid, is deposited mainly in the papillary dermis.

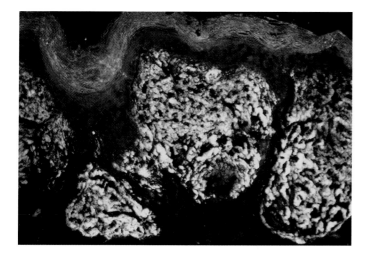

FIGURE 16-13 Lichen amyloidosus. Thioflavine-T fluorescence is seen in amyloid deposition in papillary dermis.

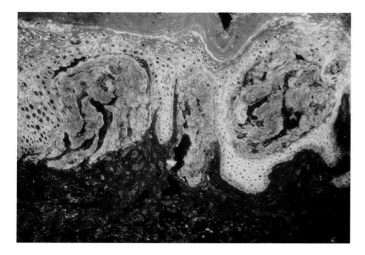

FIGURE 16-14 Lichen amyloidosus. Polyclonal antikeratin antibody stains the epidermal keratinocytes strongly and amyloid deposition in the papillary dermis moderately.

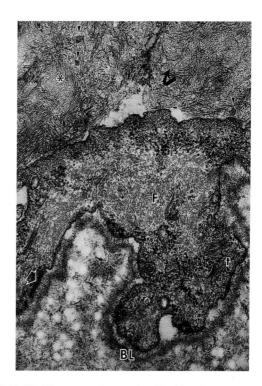

FIGURE 16-15 Filamentous degeneration (F) of keratinocytes is observed in the lower epidermis. Normal tonofilaments (t) lose their electron density (*) and become wavy (curved arrow). Some cellular organelles such as hemidesmosome (arrowheads) are intact (× 2000). (BL: basal lamina.)

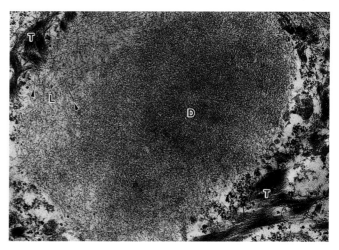

FIGURE 16-16 Filamentous degeneration of tonofilaments (T) produces amyloid filaments (arrowheads) which are more visible in the light area (L) of the cytoplasm than in the dense (D) portion (× 2000).

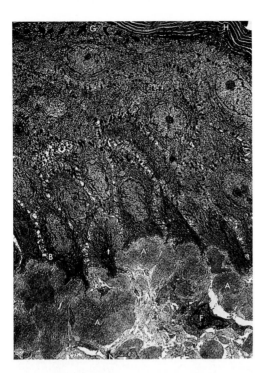

FIGURE 16-17 Lichen amyloidosus. The initial deposition of amyloid in the papillary dermis is globular (cytoid) in shape. These amyloid islands are of similar sizes to epidermal keratinocytes. *A*: represents cytoid bodies or amyloid bodies dropped off from the epidermis. *B*: basal cell. *F*: fibroblast. *G*: granular cell. *H*: horny cell. *N*: nuclear remnant in one of the amyloid islands (× 1500).

EPITHELIOMA-ASSOCIATED KERATIN AMYLOIDOSIS

Skin tumors derived from the epidermis or hair follicle produce keratin amyloid. Clinically there is no special way to differentiate amyloid-containing tumors from others. The same keratin species which are found in lichenoid and macular amyloidoses (keratin 5, 10, 14, and 15) are found in these tumors, in both the parenchyma and stroma. Common tumors which produce amyloid are basal cell carcinoma, Bowen's dis-

ease, actinic keratosis, seborrheic keratosis (Fig. 16-18), and premalignant epithelial tumor of Pinkus. The growth control of the tumor cell population by apoptosis induces filamentous degeneration of keratin intermediate filaments to form cytoid bodies which become amyloidogenic. It is probably necessary for such cytoid bodies to persist without perturbation such as from an inflammatory reaction; similar keratin cytoid bodies occurring in the lichenoid dermatoses, such as lupus erythematosus (LE), do not transform into amyloid. When apoptotic cells are eliminated from the epidermis or tumor parenchyma to the dermis or stroma, the components of basement membrane become entangled in the amyloidogenic filament mass and can be demonstrated within the mature amyloid; thus, PAS-positive substances, laminin, and types IV and VII collagens can be stained in mature keratin amyloid.

ACTINIC AMYLOIDOSIS

Clinical Features   Ultraviolet rays have a severely injurious effect on keratinocytes as evidenced in sunburn cells. Chronic sun exposure of the skin leads to the amyloidal degeneration of the epidermal keratinocytes.[16,17] For example, actinic keratosis is often associated with the deposition of keratin amyloid (Fig. 16-19). The "colloid" substance (Fig. 16-19) in juvenile colloid milium is actually keratin amyloid (Figs. 16-20, 16-21), whereas adult-type colloid milium contains severely degenerated elastic fibers. Concha amyloidosis of the inner auricle or helix of the ear is clinically an aggregation of cobblestonelike waxy or pearly papulonodules. Severe keratinocyte degeneration into cytoid bodies is present in the epidermis.

Histopathological Features   Epidermal cytoid bodies and dermal amyloid can be stained with polyclonal antikeratin antibodies in addition to standard amyloid stains. The filaments derived from these cytoid bodies meet the ultrastructural criteria for amyloid filaments (Fig. 16-21).

INSULIN AMYLOIDOSIS

Insulin can be converted into amyloid in insulinoma or pancreatic islet of diabetics. Such amyloid is designated islet amyloid polypeptide (IAPP). In the skin insulin amyloid is formed at the site of repeated insulin injection.

NODULAR AMYLOIDOSIS

Clinical Features   Single and sometimes multiple nodules may occur anywhere on the cutaneous surface, but the face, scalp, and leg of middle-aged women are the most common sites.[12–18] Individual nodules either are firm, waxy, and tumorlike or appear semitransparent, amber-colored, or hemorrhagic. Nodular amyloidosis may be associated with Sjögren's syndrome and subacute cutaneous lupus erythematosus (SCLE). In such cases serum autoantibodies SSA/SSB are positive.

Histopathological Features   A massive deposition of weakly eosinophilic amorphous amyloid substance is noted throughout the entire dermis, often extending into the subcutis. A Congo red stain (Fig. 16-22) elicits greenish birefringence under polarized light (Fig. 16-23). Collagen

TABLE 16-7

Lichen Amyloidosus and Colloid Milium of the Adult

Lichen Amyloidosus	*Colloid Milium of the Adult*
Small deposits within broadened dermal papillae	Large deposits within the upper half of the dermis
Amyloid in small globules	Colloid in large, nodular accumulations
Amyloid is amphophilic or eosinophilic in sections stained with hematoxylin and eosin	Colloid is amphophilic or basophilic in sections stained with hematoxylin and eosin
Stellate fibroblasts and melanophages are intimately associated with globules of amyloid	A few thin fibroblasts are associated with colloid, but no macrophages
There are no clefts within the globules of amyloid	There are clefts within the nodules of colloid
Vascular proliferation associated with amyloid	No vascular proliferation associated with colloid
Papillary epidermal hyperplasia usually with hyperkeratosis overlies amyloid	Thin epidermis with loss of the rete pattern and grenz zone overlies colloid
Solar elastosis is not usually seen	Solar elastosis always present

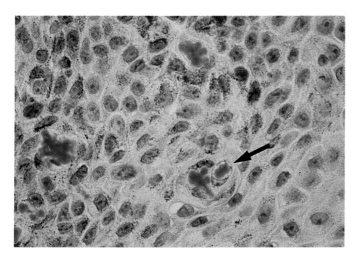

FIGURE 16-18   Cytoid bodies in seborrheic keratosis. Congo red stain is already positive in the cytoid bodies in the parenchyma, indicating amyloidal transformation of keratin (tonofilaments).

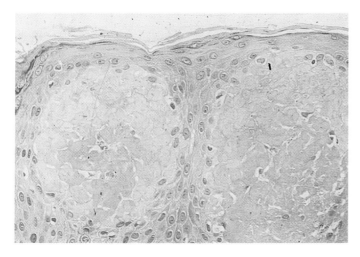

FIGURE 16-19   Juvenile colloid milium. Pink-stained hyaline substance, i.e., amyloid, occupies widened dermal papillae. Round, cytoid body–like amyloid globules can be recognized at the periphery.

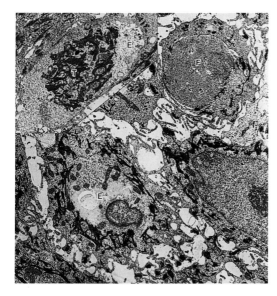

FIGURE 16-20   Juvenile colloid milium. Epidermal keratinocytes in the lesion show clumping of tonofilaments (*T*), edema (*E*), and filamentous degeneration (*F*), the first step of amyloid degeneration (× 2500).

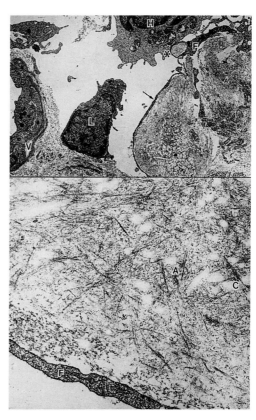

FIGURE 16-21   Juvenile colloid milium. In upper picture, round amyloid islands (*A*) are surrounded and phagocytosed (*) by fibroblast (*F*). Histiocyte (*H*), lymphocyte (*L*), and blood vessel (*V*) are present in the vicinity. Collagen (*C*) and fibrin (*F*) are admixed in these amyloid islands in lower micrograph (× 2500). The area indicated by an arrow in the upper picture is enlarged in the lower picture. Straight amyloid filaments (*A*), ghosts of collagen fibers (*C*), and an extended cytoplasmic process of fibroblast are seen (× 10,000).

bundles are often intimately admixed with amyloid. Immunoglobulin κ or λ light chains are demonstrable in the lesion. In all types of amyloid, immunoglobulins are present, probably passively trapped in the meshwork of amyloid filaments. These immunoglobulins can be eluted in acidic buffer without disrupting the filamentous nature of amyloid or altering the standard amyloid stains. In nodular amyloidosis the same elution procedure abolishes amyloid staining, suggesting that this amyloid is immunoglobulin itself. However, the origin of immunoglobulin is not always elucidated. Systemic AL amyloidosis of multiple myeloma may develop in these patients. Local production of κ or λ chains is possible in those lesions in which many plasma cells are present.

Differential Diagnosis   See Tables 16-5 and 16-6.

THE CYTOID BODY

The cytoid body, hyaline body, or Civatte body is a degenerated keratinocyte in which IgM and other immunoglobulins are deposited.[19] With electron microscopy it consists of a ball of wavy tonofilaments (10 nm) which are different from the thinner (6 to 10 mm) and straight amyloid filaments. These wavy bundles of tonofilaments are the first step of degeneration of tonofilaments (or keratin filaments). The antikeratin and anti-IgM antibody stains are always positive. Depending upon the

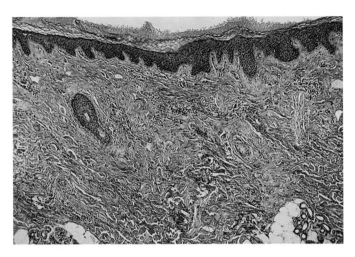

FIGURE 16-22 Nodular amyloidosis. Congo red stain. The area of amyloid infiltration is positively stained.

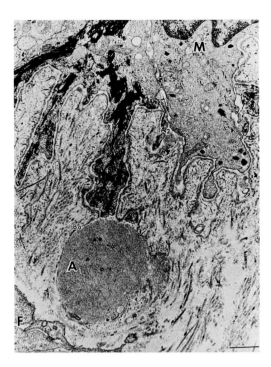

FIGURE 16-24 Cytoid body in epidermal-dermal junction in PUVA-treated skin. A ball of amyloid (A_1) is descending from the basal layer, still wrapped around with basal lamina (Ba). A_2: another small mass of amyloid. F: fibroblast. M: melanocyte ($\times$ 2000).

stages of degeneration, some cytoid bodies have intact nuclei, desmosomes, and cell membranes, and others do not. Cytoid bodies are found in various conditions in which keratinocytes are damaged, such as lichen planus, discoid LE (Fig. 16-20), erythema multiforme, graft-versus-host reaction, toxic epidermal necrolysis, the verrucous stage of incontinentia pigmenti (see Chapter 16), sunburn ("sunburn cell"), PUVA-treated skin (Fig. 16-24), and juvenile colloid milium. Cytoid bodies formed in epitheliomas, e.g., basal cell carcinoma, are often amyloidogenic, whereas those associated with inflammation as mentioned above are not. Why the former become amyloid is not known; however, it is postulated that a lymphocytic reaction is usually absent or minimal and cytoid bodies are allowed to mature into amyloid. In contrast, in lichen planus and discoid LE an intense tissue reaction destroys preamyloid cytoid bodies, and macrophages remove the keratin debris from the scene.

Hyalinosis Cutis Et Mucosae or Lipoid Proteinosis

Clinical Features This is a rare autosomal recessive or sporadic (new mutation) disease. In the hereditary form the initial symptom is hoarseness due to hyaline infiltration of vocal cords.[20-22] A diffuse infiltration of the pharynx, larynx, and oral mucosa including tongue produces extensive induration of the mouth. Early lesions consist of bullae and varicelliform scars on the face and arms which are similar to those of erythropoietic protoporphyria. The free edges of the eyelids and nostrils show small waxy, semitransparent papulonodules resembling a string of beads. Large plaque-type infiltration can occur on the face and over the joints. The nonfamilial type occurs in an older age group and is typified by similar lesions except bullae and scars on face.

Histopathological Features Hyaline deposition begins around dermal blood vessels and eccrine glands where PAS-positive diastase-resistant hyaline is demonstrated in concentric rings. Hyaline gradually fills the entire dermis (Figs. 16-25, 16-26). Small lipid droplets may be demonstrated with the scarlet red stain, particularly around the blood vessels. Electron microscopy demonstrates multiplication of lamina densa (basal lamina) in perivascular (Fig. 16-27) and periglandular spaces. The hyaline substance is mainly homogeneous, but some filament components are also admixed. Calcified foci are often observed (Fig. 16-28). Significant degeneration of collagen fibers is seen as longitudinal splitting or fragmentation of fibers.

Differential Diagnosis See differential diagnosis for lichen amyloidosus; also, lipoid proteinosis shows findings very similar to those in erythropoietic protoporphyria except that the deposits are often beyond the perivascular area in lipoid proteinosis.

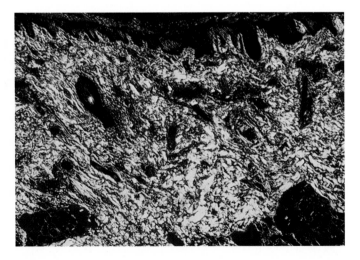

FIGURE 16-23 Nodular amyloidosis. Congo red stain observed under polarized light. Greenish birefringence of Congo red–stained amyloid makes contrast to white birefringence of collagen fibers. The same section as shown in Fig. 6-22.

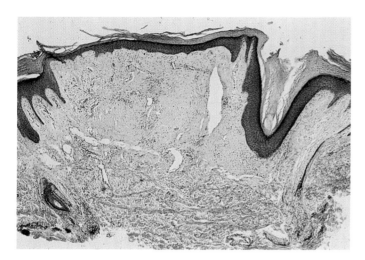

FIGURE 16-25 Hyalinosis cutis et mucosae. A widened dermal papilla is entirely occupied by hyaline material. Several dilated blood vessels are seen. The tissue reaction against this massive deposition is very minimal.

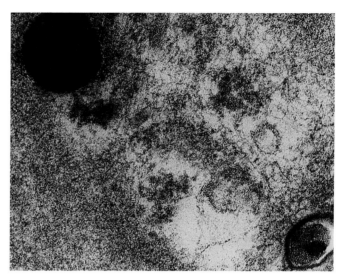

FIGURE 16-28 Hyalinosis cutis et mucosae. Hyaline in this disorder is mostly amorphous with a small number of very fine, wavy filaments. There are two calcified foci at upper-left and lower-right corners ($\times$ 15,000).

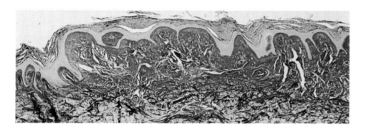

FIGURE 16-26 Hyalinosis cutis et mucosae. PAS stain is strongly positive in the hyaline deposition in the upper dermis.

Colloid Milium of the Adult

Clinical Features Yellowish semitransparent papules and plaques occur on the face and dorsum of the hands. Interestingly, the left side of the face and left hand are more frequently and severely affected because of more sun exposure on that side while driving.[23] Colloid milium usually occurs in older males with fair skin, particularly farmers or outdoor workers, sportsmen, and truck drivers. The lesions are soft, and a small incision and pressure allows the expression of the gelatinous substance. Hemorrhage is common in large lesions.

Histopathological Features Colloid in colloid milium of the adult type is the final degeneration product of elastic fibers. H&E-stained sections show a hyaline substance in large sheets occupying the papillary and upper reticular dermis (Figs. 16-29, 16-30). There are many cracks and fissures within the colloid material. A narrow grenz zone of normal collagen separates the atrophic epidermis from the colloid substance. An elastic fiber stain is largely negative in the main body of colloid and positive in the grenz zone and at the periphery of the colloid deposition. Amyloid P component, which is present in normal elastic fibers, is strongly stained in the lesion by the immunoperoxidase method.

By electron microscopy the colloid substance is resolved into a medium electron-dense amorphous substance with some granules and fine filaments (Figs. 16-31, 16-32). This is in contrast to colloid of juvenile colloid milium (Fig. 16-21) in spite of the clinical and histologic similarity of the juvenile and adult types. As discussed above, juvenile colloid milium contains typical amyloid filaments.

Differential Diagnosis See Table 16-7.

Nodular Colloid Degeneration

Clinical Features Single or multiple, large nodules occur on the face and/or head-neck region. Sun-protected skin of the trunk may be involved.[24]

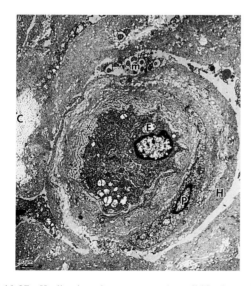

FIGURE 16-27 Hyalinosis cutis et mucosae. A small blood vessel is thickly surrounded with multiplied basal lamina and hyaline (*H*). Endothelial cells (*E*) are swollen and the lumen is occluded. *C*: collagen. *m*: mast cell. *p*: pericyte ($\times$ 1500).

Histopathological Features Colloid material occupies the entire dermis. Scattered fibroblasts, dilated blood vessels, clefts, and fissures are present. These features are similar to amyloid deposition of the dermis.

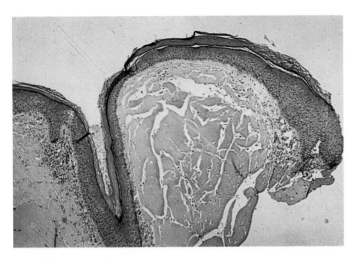

FIGURE 16-29 Adult colloid milium. Hyaline substance, i.e., colloid, occupies dilated dermal papillae. There are many fissures in these masses.

However, on electron microscopy, predominantly amorphous substance is admixed with fine filaments of 3 to 4 nm in diameters which are smaller than amyloid filaments (6 to 10 nm).

Waldenstrom's Macroglobulinemia

Clinical Features   In this condition extramedullary lymphatic tissues are invaded by a B-cell lymphoma which produces monoclonal IgM.[25] The lymph nodes, liver, and spleen are enlarged, and skin may show purpura. Large plaques and nodules develop in the skin. In some patients semitransparent small "storage papules" are seen.

Histopathological Features   The storage papules in this condition are similar to the amyloid deposition in lichen amyloidosus or the colloid in adult colloid milium, since the substance contained in these papules is eosinophilic and amorphous with the H&E stain and occupies the papillary and upper reticular dermis. Furthermore, large deposits show clefts and fissures. The material is PAS-positive and strongly reactive with anti–human IgM antibody. The large plaques or nodules show involvement by lymphoma.

Differential Diagnosis   See Tables 16-4 to 16-6.

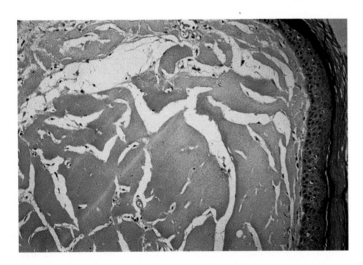

FIGURE 16-30 Adult colloid milium. A higher magnification of Fig. 16-29.

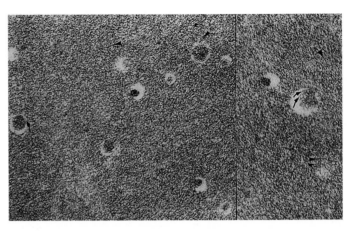

FIGURE 16-31 Adult colloid milium. Colloid in this disorder is largely amorphous with a small number of very fine filaments admixed. These filaments are found free in amorphous material (arrowheads) or frazzling out of degenerating collagen fibers (arrows) ($\times$ 20,000).

Porphyria

These diseases are caused by defective enzymes involved in heme synthesis.[26] Seven out of eight subtypes, except the acute intermittent type, exhibit a variety of photosensitivity and related skin changes. The most common subtype is porphyria cutanea tarda (PCT) in which serum uroporphyrin is elevated due to the deficiency of uroporphyrinogen decarboxylase. Vesicles and blisters occur on the face and dorsum of the hands. Hypertrichosis of the face may be pronounced and may account for the appearance suggesting a "wolfman." Hepatitis C may be a major factor in the etiology of PCT. Erythropoietic protoporphyria shows blisters and thickening of facial skin and the dorsum of the hands and may

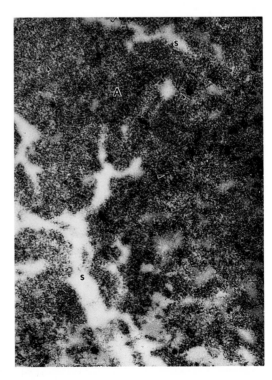

FIGURE 16-32 Adult colloid milium. Mainly amorphous colloid (*A*) embeds skeleton fibrils (*s*) of degenerated elastic fibers. Arrowheads: filament components ($\times$ 25,000).

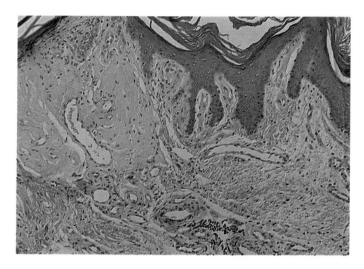

FIGURE 16-33   Erythropoietic protoporphyria. Upper dermis is filled with amorphous pinkish-gray hyaline. Capillaries are dilated.

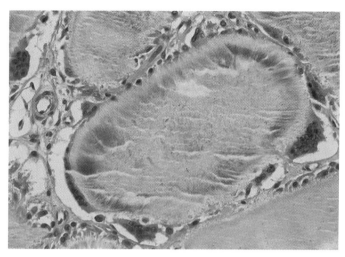

FIGURE 16-34   Gouty tophus. The deposition of urate is surrounded with foreign-body giant cells. (*Courtesy of Min W. Lee, M.D.*)

be caused mainly by an autosomal dominant mutation of heme synthase gene located on chromosome 18q21.3.

Histopathological Features   The histopathologic features are similar among all photosensitive subtypes. The primary change in all types of porphyrias is a perivascular deposit of hyaline material stainable with PAS; this staining is resistant to diastase digestion (neutral polysaccharides). In mild cases the hyaline deposition is limited to the capillaries of the upper dermis, and in severe cases the deposition fills the papillary dermis and extends into the lower dermis. Subepidermal blisters develop (Fig. 16-33). The dermal papillae are hardened by this deposition, and when subepidermal blister occurs, the stiff dermal papillae remain in place instead of collapsing; this has been termed *festooning* of dermal papillae. Sclerodermalike diffuse thickening of the dermal collagen may occur in chronic lesion.

Differential Diagnosis   See Tables 16-4 and 16-5.

Gout

Clinical Features   This dominantly inherited abnormality of purine metabolism produces a high level of serum uric acid, which deposits in small joints, typically those of the great toe.[27] Increased serum purine levels may be secondary to decreased renal function, diuretic therapy, or an increased purine synthesis in lymphomas. Skin deposition of uric acid, called *gouty tophi*, occurs most frequently on the auricle. Elbow and finger joints are also commonly affected.

Histopathological Features   Grayish amorphous material in the dermis is surrounded with palisading granulomas (Fig. 16-34). If fixed in alcohol, uric acid crystals are preserved and yield characteristic multicolor birefringence under the polarized light (Fig. 16-35). In formalin-fixed tissues the crystals are less obvious, and no birefringence is present.

Corticosteroid Injection Sites

The injection sites of corticosteroids often show multiple pools of eosinophilic hyaline material between collagen bundles (Fig. 16-36). Without any clinical history, such deposition is puzzling. Old injection sites show loosely bound thin collagen bundles with edema.

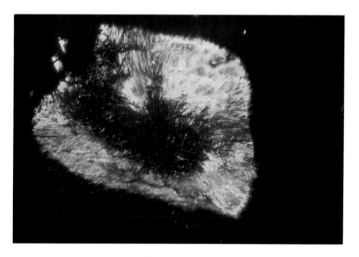

FIGURE 16-35   Gouty tophus. Under the polarized light, urate crystals give rise to multicolored birefringence. (*Courtesy of Min W. Lee, M.D.*)

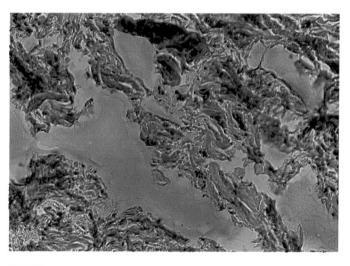

FIGURE 16-36   Corticosteroid injection site. Pale pink-blue homogenous, somewhat refractile material is pooled between collagen fibers which appear swollen and disrupted.

CALCIUM, BONE, AND CARTILAGE

Calcinosis Cutis

Calcium deposition in the skin may result from hypercalcemia due to hyperparathyroidism including an adenoma, hypervitaminosis D, milk alkali syndrome, or hyperphosphatemia caused by renal failure or renal dialysis in which excretion of phosphorus is inadequate (Table 16-8).[28-30] Because the production of calcium and phosphorus should be constant, this causes a drop in the serum calcium ion, which stimulates parathyroid secretion to mobilize calcium from bone.

Direct destruction of bone and the release of calcium may occur in sarcoidosis, osteomyelitis, bone metastases in cancer, and multiple myeloma. The released calcium "metastasizes" to the skin.

METASTATIC CALCINOSIS CUTIS

Clinical Features   Calcinosis resulting from the latter mechanism is called *metastatic calcinosis cutis*. The clinical appearance of metastatic calcification in the skin ranges from hard papules and nodules to subcutaneous diffuse hardening. When these lesions are ulcerated, chalky white material may be discharged. When blood vessels are calcified, hard, linear cords can be palpated.

Histopathological Features   Calcium is stained deep blue to violet in H&E-stained tissue sections (Fig. 16-37). Another stain commonly used is the von Kossa stain, which actually stains phosphates rather than calcium (which, nonetheless, is almost always present). Calcium deposition in the skin can be massive in the deep dermis to subcutaneous tissue and in small foci in upper dermis. Vascular involvement is present in the calcinosis cutis caused by hyperparathyroidism secondary to renal failure (calciphylaxis). It usually occurs in subcutaneous arteries and arterioles. Internal organs may also be involved.

DYSTROPHIC CALCINOSIS CUTIS

Clinical Features   In this type of calcinosis cutis, serum calcium and phosphorus are normal, and the internal organs are spared, i.e., this is strictly a cutaneous phenomenon secondary to local-tissue degeneration or "dystrophy." Widespread cutaneous calcification (calcinosis universalis) may occur in collagen vascular diseases such as childhood dermatomyositis, progressive systemic sclerosis, particularly the CREST syndrome, and systemic lupus erythematosus. Localized forms (calcinosis circumscripta) may also occur in the diseases mentioned above, particularly in the digits of patients with acrosclerosis. Pseudoxanthoma elasticum is always calcified, whereas subcutaneous nodules of calcifi-

TABLE 16-8

Calcium and Bone Deposits

Disorders	Distribution and Characterization	Associated Disorder	Special Stains
Calcinosis cutis	Any location	Hypercalcemia due to	H&E (blue-purple)
Metastatic	Deep dermis to subcutaneous tissue	hyperparathyroidism, hyperphosphatemia, hypervitaminosis D, milk-alkali syndrome	Von Kossa
Dystrophic	Any location	Normal serum calcium,	Von Kossa
	Deep dermis to subcutaneous tissue, preceding tissue damage, skin tumors, and cysts	collagen vascular disease	
Idiopathic	Any location	None	Von Kossa
	Deep dermis to subcutaneous tissue		
Calciphylaxis	Thick adipose tissues; abdomen, buttocks, thighs	Sensitizer: hyperparathyroidism	Von Kossa
		Challenger: albumin, metallic salts, Vit. D, parathyroid hormone	
Ossification of the skin			
Primary	Scalp, extremities in plaque type and in multiple miliary type in face; other types anywhere	None; in younger variety of multiple miliary osteoma may be related to acne	Von Kossa
Secondary	Any location depending on preceding condition	Skin appendage tumors, collagen vascular disease	Von Kossa
Albright's hereditary osteodystrophy	Short stature, round faces, absence of some knuckles (dimple sign)	Mental retardation Hypercalcemia (pseudohypoparathyroidism) or normocalcemia (pseudopseudohypoparathyroidism)	Von Kossa
Subungual exostosis	Distal toe and finger	None	Von Kossa
Cartilaginous lesions			
Enchondroma	Distal toe and finger		
Cutaneous cartilaginous tumor	Hand and foot		
Chondroid syringoma	Head and neck		Alcian blue, Giemsa

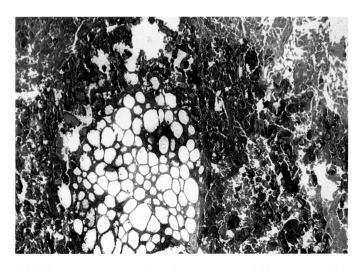

FIGURE 16-37   Metastatic calcinosis cutis due to renal failure. An extensive calcium deposition is present in the subcutaneous fat tissue.

cation rarely occur in the atrophic scars noted in the joints from patients with the Ehlers-Danlos syndrome, gravis-type. Subcutaneous fat necrosis of the newborn, frostbite or trauma of auricle, old lesions of nodular amyloidosis, and repeated venipuncture of the heels of infants for blood tests are followed by localized calcification. Many appendage tumors of the skin, notably calcifying epithelioma or pilomatricoma, trichilemmal (pilar) cysts, basal cell epithelioma, and trichoepithelioma (Fig. 16-38), often show calcium deposition. These tumors are mainly of hair follicle origin; epidermal cyst, for example, is much less frequently calcified than trichilemmal cyst. Calcified nodules may occur in the scrotum in varying numbers; they may be preceded by trichilemmal cysts or have an idiopathic origin.

Histopathological Features   Calcium deposition is usually mild in the upper dermis with localized granular deposits. The deposition in deep dermis and subcutaneous tissue is usually large or massive. Individual preceding conditions usually determine the pattern of calcification. For example, necrotized fat cells are primarily calcified in subcutaneous fat necrosis of the newborn, and tumor parenchyma is initially calcified in pilar tumors. Leakage of calcium into connective tissue elicits various degrees of foreign-body reactions.

IDIOPATHIC CALCINOSIS CUTIS

Clinical Features   Calcification of skin may occur without apparent causes or preceding tissue degeneration. *Tumoral calcinosis* is usually a familial condition in which numerous subcutaneous calcified nodules can be palpated. Hyperphosphatemia may be associated. Papular and nodular skin lesions may be present. This condition resembles clinically dystrophic calcinosis universalis of dermatomyositis and tends to affect bony prominences. It is more common in Africa and Papua-New Guinea than North America and Europe.

Localized, solitary nodular calcification (subepidermal calcified nodule or cutaneous calculus) is found in infants as a congenital tumor. It is covered with hyperkeratotic epidermis. The face or limbs are common sites. In rare instances multiple lesions occur. Such nodules may occur in adults.

Histopathological Features   As dystrophic type, the massive calcification is present in the subcutaneous tissue in tumoral calcinosis. In subepidermal calcified nodules (Fig. 16-39), multiple granules and islands of calcification are seen just beneath the epidermis. Transepidermal elimination through hair canals and eccrine sweat ducts may be observed.

CALCIPHYLAXIS

In calciphylaxis, a rare condition defined by Hans Selye in 1962, specific tissues of the body are sensitized by certain calcifying events, such as hyperparathyroidism secondary to renal failure. (See Chaps. 9 and 11.)[31-36] There is a latency period between the sensitizer and the discrete challenging conditions. Successful challengers in Selye's experiments were subcutaneous, intramuscular, and/or intravenous administration of metallic salts, albumin, egg yolk, parathyroid hormone, and vitamin D. Local trauma was also an important precipitating factor in calciphylactic reactions after appropriate sensitization.

Cutaneous Ossification

Ossification of the skin can occur in a variety of unrelated disorders.[37,38] It may be a primary event or be secondary to local (e.g., skin tumors) or systemic (Albright's hereditary osteodystrophy) conditions. The osteoblast, a modified fibroblast, produces type I collagen in a similar fashion to dermal fibroblasts. However, posttranslational alterations of

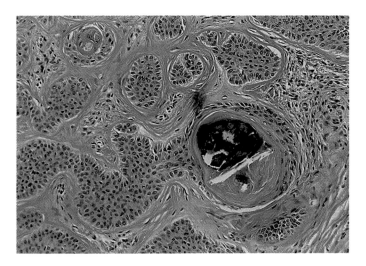

FIGURE 16-38   Dystrophic calcinosis cutis in trichoepithelioma. A large keratin cyst is calcified.

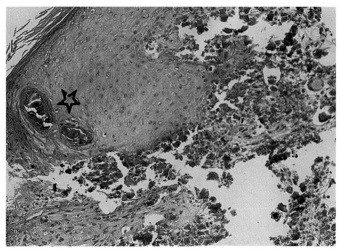

FIGURE 16-39   Subepidermal calcified nodule. Subepidermal calcification occurs in numerous small globular bodies which are stained deep purple. Amorphous calcium is being expelled through the eccrine duct (*). H&E stain.

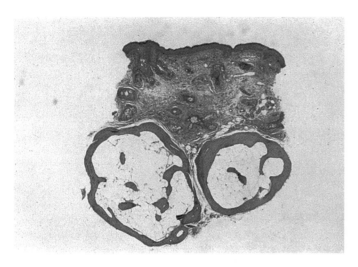

FIGURE 16-40   Multiple miliary osteoma of the face. Two small bones with trabecular projections.

osteoblast-derived type I collagen probably make it more suitable for phosphorylation to initiate ossification. Activators of bone formation such as osteonectin and transforming growth factor are produced by osteoblasts.

PRIMARY CUTANEOUS OSSIFICATION (OSTEOMA CUTIS)

Clinical Features   This condition may occur in early life or since birth as widespread multiple lesions or as a single, large plaque of ossification. The late onset varieties occur as a single, small nodule anywhere in the skin or as multiple miliary osteoma of the face. The latter lesions are most commonly encountered in older women, but recently the condition has been observed in elderly men. The face, particularly the forehead, is involved by multiple, hard, tiny papules of normal to blue color. One can extract small pebbly bone chips from these papules.

Histopathological Features   Fragments of bone that vary in size and shape are present in the deep dermis or subcutaneous tissue (Fig. 16-40). This type of bone is called *lamellar bone* and exhibits a laminated fibrous structure (cement lines) indicating underlying collagen bundles (Fig. 16-41). Osteoblasts are embedded within the bone and are noted

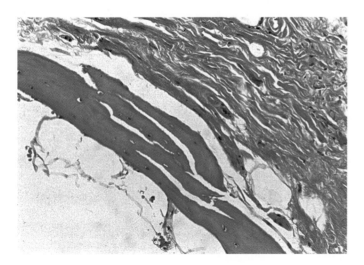

FIGURE 16-41   Multiple miliary osteoma of the face. Condensed, hyalinized collagen layers (osteoid) surround the outer surface of the cortex.

along the periphery where nonmineralized, condensed collagen islands (osteoid) are still present.

Connective tissue accompanied by blood vessels is enclosed in the bone and forms haversian canals. However, osteoclasts, multinucleated giant cells resembling foreign-body giant cells, are only rarely observed.

SECONDARY (METAPLASTIC) CUTANEOUS OSSIFICATION

Many conditions in which calcium deposition occurs (i.e., calcinosis cutis) are prone to ossification. Some examples are skin appendage tumors, notably calcifying epithelioma (pilomatricoma) and chondroid syringoma; collagen vascular diseases, particularly the CREST syndrome; and childhood dermatomyositis. The chronic stage of fibrosis, i.e., scars and scleroderma, seems to induce ossification.

Histopathological Features   The laminated layers of eosinophilic bone are the result of mineralization of type I and, to a lesser extent, types III and V collagens. Osteoblasts are found within and along the periphery of the bone. In larger lesions haversian canals with collagen and blood vessels are present. In chondroid syringoma, ossification occurs by the replacement of preformed cartilage, i.e., enchondral bone formation.

SUBUNGUAL EXOSTOSIS

This is a solitary tender nodule under the distal end of the nail, most commonly at the free edge of great toe. It may be multiple, and it may be asymptomatic.

ALBRIGHT'S HEREDITARY OSTEODYSTROPHY

Clinical Features   This dominantly inherited disorder of bone is also called *pseudohypoparathyroidism* or *pseudopseudohypoparathyroidism*, depending upon whether abnormal or normal calcium metabolism is present.[39] The former is characterized by hypocalcemia that does not respond to parathyroid hormone, whereas in the latter the response is unaltered. These patients show characteristic round faces, diminished stature, and shortened metacarpal bones. Ossifications of any size may occur anywhere in the skin and subcutaneous tissue. Bone may be extruded through cutaneous ulcerations.

Histopathological Features   The bone formation is of lamellar type, i.e., through the ossification of compacted collagen (osteoid) in which lamellar sheets are still visible.

Cartilaginous Lesions of the Skin

Clinical Features   The *enchondroma* is often associated with subungual exostosis (see above). *Cutaneous cartilaginous tumors* or *soft-tissue chondromas* arise independently of the normal cartilage of the hands and feet of older men, where they are found asymptomatic as small, freely movable nodules.[40] *Chondroid syringomas* or *mixed tumors* of the skin occur in head and neck region as a firm subcutaneous nodule.[41]

Histopathological Features   The enchondroma shows typical pale blue cartilage that contains large chondrocytes with halos. The cutaneous cartilaginous tumor exhibits an irregular mass of hyaline cartilage also containing chondrocytes (Fig. 16-42). Degenerative changes and calcification are often observed along with foreign body reaction. Large chondrocytes may demonstrate nuclear hyperchromasia, atypia, and mitoses. However, if the tumor is not connected to the underlying bone, the prognosis is good, although the tumor may recur after excision. The chondroid syringoma has less mature cartilage or a mucinous stroma that contains tubular or glandular epithelial components showing eccrine, apocrine, or follicular differentiation. Chondrocytes with typi-

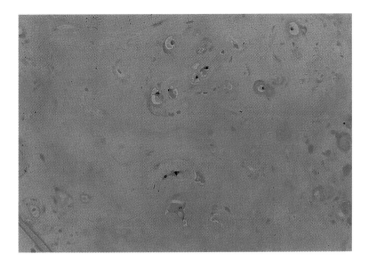

FIGURE 16-42 Cutaneous cartilaginous tumor. Large polygonal chondrocytes have hyperchromatic nucleus and are surrounded with empty halo.

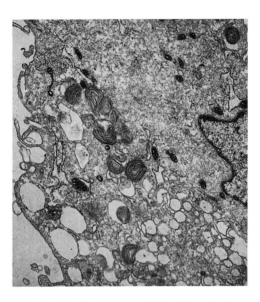

FIGURE 16-43 Hurler's disease. A large histiocyte has numerous empty vacuoles and several dense inclusion bodies ($\times$ 3000).

cal halos may or may not be present. In most cases, large stellate cells can be detected. However, in rare cases, even bone formation is observed.

MUCOPOLYSACCHARIDOSES (MPS)

Clinical Features Among the many types of MPS, the Hurler and Hunter types show significant skin changes.[42–44] The other varieties exhibit—in common with Hurler and Hunter disease—dwarfism, skeletal deformities, corneal opacity, hepatosplenomegaly, hirsutism, and coarse facial features (gargoylism). In severe cases the nervous system is affected, resulting in mental retardation. The basic defect in these diseases is a genetic mutation of lysosomal enzymes involved in the degradation of mucopolysaccharides (glycosaminoglycans). Unmetabolized large molecules of MPS accumulate in many organs, and the unavailability of essential metabolites disturbs the normal growth of bones and cartilages. There seem to be slightly different variations in these mutations, and, therefore, the clinical severity of the same disease may vary from case to case. For example, Hurler's and Hunter's diseases share similar enzyme deficiencies (α_1-iduronidase and α_1-iduronate sulfatase, respectively) resulting in an accumulation of dermatan and heparan sulfate; however, only Hunter's disease shows "pebbling" of the skin, i.e., closely set or coalescent ivory-white (in white patients) papules and nodules in the scapular region. In Hurler's disease only thickened plaques with hyperpigmentation are observed. In both diseases dermatan sulfate and heparan sulfate are detected in the urine, and this test is used for the diagnosis. Hurler's disease is inherited as an autosomal recessive, whereas Hunter's disease is transmitted in an X-linked recessive mode; there are mild and severe forms.

Histopathological Features In the thickened skin or pebbled areas, large, plump fibroblasts contain metachromatic granules demonstrated by the Giemsa or toluidine blue stain. Alcian blue or colloidal iron stains are also positive. Sometimes these fibroblasts therefore resemble mast cells. Metachromatic granules may be noted in the epidermis and eccrine gland and duct. Electron microscopy is probably most helpful, because it identifies unmetabolized MPS in the lysosomes of dermal fibroblasts and perivascular macrophages as electron-dense laminated membrane structures (Figs. 16-43 and 16-44). These cells also contain many vacuoles and electron-dense granular substances. The dermal Schwann cells also contain laminated dense bodies which resemble "zebra bodies" as described in the brain of these patients.

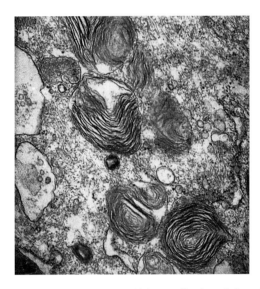

FIGURE 16-44 Hurler's disease. A high magnification of dense inclusion bodies reveals lamellar nature of these bodies ($\times$ 10,000).

REFERENCES

1. Heymann WR: Cutaneous manifestation of thyroid disease. *J Am Acad Dermatol* 26:885, 1992.
2. Truhan AP, Roenigk HH Jr: The cutaneous mucinoses. *J Am Acad Dermatol* 14:1, 1986.
3. Rosen I, Kleman GA: Thyroid and the skin, in Callen JP, Jorizzo JL, Greer KE, et al (eds): *Dermatological Signs of Internal Disease*, 2d ed. Philadelphia, Saunders, 1995.
4. Dinneen A, et al: Scleromyxedema. *J Am Acad Dermatol* 33:37, 1995.
5. Cohen PR, Rabinowitz AD, Ruszkowski AM, et al: Reticular erythematous mucinosis syndrome: Review of the world literature and report of the syndrome in a prepubertal child. *Pediatr Dermatol* 7:11, 1990.
6. McNaughton F, Keczkes K: Scleredema adultorum and diabetes mellitus (scleredema diutinum). *Clin Exp Dermatol* 8:41, 1983.
7. Wiek M, Schmoeckel C: Cutaneous focal mucinosis: A histopathological and immunohistochemical analysis of 11 cases. *J Cutan Pathol* 21:446, 1994.
8. Salasche SJ: Myxoid cysts of the proximal nail fold. *J Dermatol Surg Oncol* 10:35, 1984.
9. Lattand A, Johnson WC, Graham JH: Mucous cyst (mucocele). *Arch Dermatol* 101:673, 1970.
10. Carney JA, et al: The complex of myxoma, spotty pigmentation and endocrine overactivity. *Medicine* 64:270, 1985.

11. Gibson LE, Muller SA, Leiferman, KN, et al: Follicular mucinosis: Clinical and histopathologic study. *J Am Acad Dermatol* 20:441, 1989.

12. Hashimoto K: Cutaneous amyloidoses, in *Demis Clinical Dermatology*, vol 2, unit 12-21. Philadelphia, Lippincott, 1992.

13. Hashimoto K: Amyloidosis, in Arndt KA, LeBoit PE, Robinson JK (eds): *Clinical Medicine and Surgery*, vol 2. Philadelphia, Saunders, 1996.

14. Breathnach SM: Amyloid and amyloidosis. *J Am Acad Dermatol* 18:1, 1988.

15. Ito I, Hashimoto K: Reactivity of immunoglobulins on amyloid in lichenoid and macular amyloidoses with epidermal keratin, in Isobe T, Araki S, Uchino F (eds): *Amyloid and Amyloidosis*. New York, London, Plenum Press, 1988.

16. Hashimoto K, Nakayama H, Chimenti S, et al: Juvenile colloid milium: Immunohistochemical and ultrastructural studies. *J Cutan Pathol* 16:164, 1989.

17. Hicks BC, Weber PJ, Hashimoto K, et al: Primary cutaneous amyloidosis of the auricular concha. *J Am Acad Dermatol* 18:19, 1988.

18. Ito K, Hashimoto K, Kambe N, Van S: Roles of immunoglobulins in amyloidogenesis in cutaneous nodular amyloidosis. *J Invest Dermatol* 89:415, 1987.

19. Hashimoto K: Apoptosis in lichen planus and several other dermatoses *Acta Derm Venereol (Stockh)* 56:182, 1976.

20. Hashimoto K, Klingmuller G, Rodermund OE: Hyalinosis cutis et mucosae: An electron microscopic study. *Acta Derm Venereol (Stockh)* 52:179, 1972.

21. Konstantinov K, Kabakciev P, Karchev T, et al: Lipoid proteinosis. *J Am Acad Dermatol* 27:293, 1992.

22. Moy LS, Moy RI, Matsuoka LY, et al: Lipoid proteinosis: Ultrastructural and biochemical studies. *J Am Acad Dermatol* 16:1193, 1987.

23. Hashimoto K, Katzman RL, Kang AH, Kanzaki T: Electron microscopic and biochemical analysis of colloid milium. *Arch Dermatol* 111:49, 1975.

24. Kawashima Y, Matsubara T, Kinbara T: Colloid degeneration of the skin. *J Dermatol (Tokyo)* 4:115, 1977.

25. Kyle RA, Gleich GJ, Bayrd ED, et al: Benign hypergammaglobulinemic purpura of Waldenstrom. *Medicine* 50:113, 1971.

26. Cormane RH, Szabò E, Hoo TT: Histopathology of the skin in acquired and hereditary porphyria cutanea tarda. *Br J Dermatol* 85:531, 1972.

27. King DF, King LA: The appropriate processing of tophi for microscopy. *Am J Dermatopathol* 4:239, 1982.

28. Mehregan AH: Calcinosis cutis: A review of the clinical forms and report of 75 cases. *Semin Dermatol* 3:53, 1984.

29. Tezuka T: Cutaneous calculus: Its pathogenesis. *Dermatologica* 161:191, 1980.

30. Fisher AH, Morris D: Pathogenesis of calciphylaxis: Study of three cases with literature review. *Hum Pathol* 1055, 1995.

31. Ivker RA, Woosley J, Briggamon RH, et al: Calciphylaxis in three patients with end-stage renal disease. *Arch Dermatol* 131:63, 1995.

32. Walsh JS, Fairley JA: Calcifying disorders of the skin. *J Am Acad Dermatol* 33:693, 1995.

33. Hafner J, Keusch G, Wahl C, et al: Uremic small-artery disease with medial calcification and intimal hyperplasia (so-called calciphylaxis): A complication of chronic renal failure and benefit from parathyroidectomy. *J Am Acad Dermatol* 33:954, 1995.

34. Selye H: *Calciphylaxis*. Chicago, University of Chicago Press, 1962.

35. Gipstein RM, Coburn JW, Adams DA, et al: Calciphylaxis in man. *Arch Intern Med* 136:1273, 1976.

36. Lowry LR, Tschen JA, Wolf JE, Yen A: Calcifying panniculitis and systemic calciphylaxis in an end-stage renal patient. *Cutis* 51:245, 1993.

37. Roth SI, Stowell RE, Helwig EB: Cutaneous ossification. *Arch Pathol* 76:44, 1963.

38. Kotliar SN, Roth SI: Cutaneous mineralization and ossification, in Fitzpatrick et al (eds): *Cutaneous Lesions in Nutritional, Metabolic and Heritable Disorders, Dermatology in General Medicine*. New York, McGraw-Hill, 1993.

39. Eyre WG, Reed WB: Albright's hereditary osteodystrophy with cutaneous bone formation. *Arch Dermatol* 104:636, 1971.

40. Weinrauch L, Katz M, Pizov G: Primary benign chondro-blastoma cutis: Extraskeletal manifestation without bone involvement. *Arch Dermatol* 123:24, 1987.

41. Paslin DA: Cartilaginous papule of the ear. *J Cutan Pathol* 18:60, 1991.

42. Hers H: Inborn lysosomal disease. *Gastroenterology* 48:625, 1965.

43. LeGuern E, Couillin P, Oberle I, et al: More precise localization of the gene for Hunter syndrome. *Genomics* 7:358, 1990.

44. Clarke J, Greer WL, Strasberg PM, et al: Hunter disease (MPS type II) associated with unbalanced inactivation of the X-chromosomes in a karyotypically normal girl. *Am J Hum Genet* 49:289, 1991.

CHAPTER 17

ALTERATIONS OF COLLAGEN AND ELASTIN

Clifton R. White, Jr.

The major function of skin is to serve as a barrier to various exogenous substances, chemicals, and microbes. Collagen, ground substance, and elastic fibers are the three major components of the dermis and are crucial to maintaining the integrity and elasticity of the skin. Collagen is the most abundant of the three components of the dermis (80 percent by dry weight), consisting primarily of type I collagen, one of more than 19 distinct collagens now recognized (types I to XIX).[1,2]

ALTERATIONS OF COLLAGEN

Dermal collagen consists of fibers of 2 to 15 μm in diameter. In the papillary and periadnexal (adventitial) dermis, collagen consists of delicate interwoven fibers, whereas collagen of the reticular dermis consists of thick bundles. Type I collagen, distributed throughout the dermis, provides tensile strength to skin, whereas type III collagen (15 percent of the dermis by dry weight) is primarily a constituent of the adventitial dermis, where it participates in anchoring the epidermis and adnexae to the dermis.[3] Collagen is composed of three polypeptides, or alpha chains, that assume a stabilizing triple-helical conformation dependent on glycine residues located at every third position of the polypeptides. Hydroxyproline (synthesized from proline) is necessary for triple-helix stability at physiologic temperatures.[4] Conditions resulting in decreased levels of reducing agents such as ascorbic acid and oxygen, which are required for hydroxylation of prolyl residues, lead to deficient collagen production, resulting in scurvy (poor wound healing, skin fragility, easy bruising, and bleeding) and, perhaps, stasis ulcers.[4,5]

Alterations of collagen, which often exist in concert with deficient elastin and ground substance, are present in a diverse group of diseases, manifesting in some as sclerosis, including scleroderma and a number of diseases that produce changes histologically indistinguishable from scleroderma (sclerodermoid disorders). In other conditions, such as those preceding scar and keloid formation, collagen is produced in greater quantities than normal, and in still others, such as aplasia cutis congenita and focal dermal hypoplasia, collagen is deficient, resulting in atrophy. Rarely, cutaneous diseases may result from the loss of connective-tissue fibers to the skin surface (e.g., "perforating" diseases), whereas others are characterized by collagen defects on a molecular level (e.g., Ehlers-Danlos syndrome, osteogenesis imperfecta).

Scleroderma

Scleroderma ("hard skin") is the result of a deposition of excess collagen in the dermis and may be classified as primary, including morphea and its variants, such as atrophoderma of Pasini and Pierini and eosinophilic fasciitis (Shulman's syndrome), and systemic scleroderma (progressive systemic sclerosis), or secondary scleroderma (i.e., sclerodermoid disorders), as in sclerodermoid porphyria cutanea tarda, sclerodermoid graft-versus-host reaction, and acro-osteolysis, among others.

MORPHEA (LOCALIZED SCLERODERMA)

Morphea ("localized" or "circumscribed scleroderma") is the most common form of scleroderma and has diverse clinical presentations, including localized (guttate or plaque), generalized, linear, segmental, and subcutaneous. In some cases, systemic involvement, such as of the musculoskeletal system, may occur. Rarely, patients with morphea may develop systemic scleroderma.[6] As with systemic scleroderma, morphea affects women with greater frequency than men and white patients more than black patients, most cases beginning between the second and fifth decades. The cause of morphea, while unknown, is considered (like scleroderma) by some to be immunologic in nature; e.g., morphea coexists with other autoimmune diseases, and antinuclear antibodies are found in patients with morphea, particularly those with linear morphea. Other controversial evidence suggests a causative relationship between *Borrelia burgdorferi* and morphea, including the presence of spirochetes in histologic sections of morphea as well as their recovery from cultured lesional tissue,[7] findings not confirmed by other investigators.[8]

Clinical Features Morphea presents as indurated, smooth-surfaced, whitish to dusky-appearing plaques, often with a peripheral violaceous rim ("lilac ring") suggesting inflammation. Plaques vary from small (guttate) to large, confluent or generalized lesions and may be hyper- or hypopigmented. Unusual presentations of morphea include nodular (keloid),[9] bullous,[10] linear (en coup de sabre),[11] and facial hemiatrophy,[12] as well as aggressive mutilating (pansclerotic) morphea[13] and morphea profunda.[14] Most likely, atrophoderma of Pasini and Pierini and eosinophilic fasciitis also represent variants of morphea.

Histopathological Features The epidermis may be uninvolved, atrophic, or hyperplastic. Characteristically, there is thickening and sclerosis of the reticular dermis with increased width of collagen bundles, narrowing or obliteration of interbundle spaces, and a superficial and deep perivascular lymphocytic infiltrate containing plasma cells and occasionally eosinophils (Figs. 17-1 through 17-3). As sclerosis increases, collagen replaces small fat lobules encircling eccrine glands, which become "entrapped," pilosebaceous units may be atrophic, and the cellular infiltrate often diminishes. Subcutaneous septa and fasciae are sclerotic, and there often are nodular lymphoplasmacytic aggregates at the dermal-subcutaneous and septal-lobular junctions (Table 17-1). Small blood vessels may develop thickened walls and narrowed lumina. In some instances, subcutaneous (morphea profunda) or fascial (eosinophilic fasciitis) involvement may predominate.

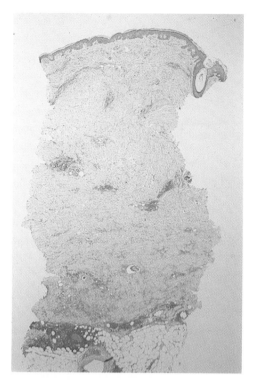

FIGURE 17-1 Morphea. At scanning magnification, there is dermal sclerosis throughout the reticular dermis and fat septa as well as a dense, superficial, and deep perivascular and interstitial lymphocytic infiltrate containing plasma cells with nodular accumulations at the dermal-subcutaneous junction.

Differential Diagnosis   Morphea and cutaneous scleroderma are indistinguishable histologically. However, early lesions of morphea, termed *inflammatory morphea*, exhibit greater edema and more prominent inflammatory cell infiltrates. These inflammatory infiltrates usually involve the reticular dermis in perivascular and interstitial patterns.

On occasion, the histologic features of morphea may be quite similar to that of lichen sclerosus et atrophicus (diseases reported to co-exist in some patients[15]), including prominent papillary dermal edema and

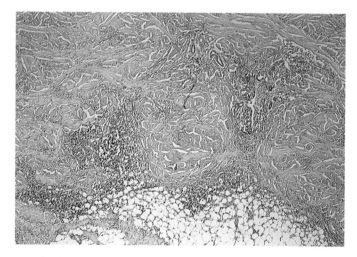

FIGURE 17-2 Morphea. Closer view of the lower reticular dermis demonstrates thickened, sclerotic collagen bundles with eccrine glands (*right*) completely entrapped. Note the nodular collections of lymphocytes and plasma cells at the dermal-subcutaneous junction and a sclerotic, thickened septum in the subcutis.

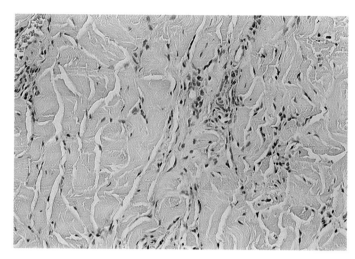

FIGURE 17-3 Morphea. High power of collagen sclerosis with perivascular lymphocytes and plasma cells.

sclerosis; in these cases, reticular dermal sclerosis present in morphea distinguishes it from the uninvolved reticular dermis of lichen sclerosus et atrophicus, in which changes are limited to papillary dermal sclerosis. Nonetheless, it must be emphasized that morphea and lichen sclerosus et atrophicus may be closely related such that the latter constitutes a superficial expression of the same disease process that results in morphea and eosinophilic fasciitis.

SYSTEMIC SCLERODERMA (PROGRESSIVE SYSTEMIC SCLEROSIS)

Systemic scleroderma (progressive systemic sclerosis, PSS) involving the skin develops in limited[16] as well as diffuse cutaneous patterns,[17] each resulting from excess deposition of collagen. While the cause of scleroderma is unknown, collagen synthesis, deposition, and degradation are elevated, as is collagen urinary excretion.[18] Collagen fibrils in scleroderma have smaller diameters than normal (30 to 40 nm versus 70

TABLE 17-1

Morphea (Localized Scleroderma)

Clinical Features

Adult women > men
Sclerotic plaques with "lilac ring"
Localized, generalized, linear (en coup de sabre),
   segmental, subcutaneous, nodular (keloid), bullous, facial hemiatrophy, pansclerotic, morphea profunda

Histopathological Features

Epidermis uninvolved or atrophic (rarely, hyperplastic)
Sclerosis of reticular dermis and fat septa
Superficial and deep lymphoplasmacytic infiltrate with occasional eosinophils
Nodular lymphocytic collections at dermal-subcutaneous junction

Differential Diagnosis

Scleroderma
Eosinophilic fasciitis
Atrophoderma of Pasini and Pierini
Sclerodermoid disorders

to 140 nm),[19] and scleroderma fibroblast cultures show a higher than normal rate of DNA synthesis.[20] Other potential etiologic factors are autoimmune causes (speckled or nucleolar pattern antinuclear antibodies are present in 80 to 95 percent of patients with PSS).[21] Finally, dermal vessels show alterations by electron microscopy, including formation of gaps between and destruction of endothelial cells with basal lamina reduplication and perivascular lymphocytes, often preceding fibrosis.[22]

Clinical Features   Systemic scleroderma involving skin is an uncommon disease frequently presenting initially as nonpitting edema of the extremities, especially the fingers ("sausage fingers"), or face and trunk, areas that become indurated, then atrophic, and sclerotic with a "bound down" palpable quality. Involvement may be limited to acral locations (acrosclerosis), or less commonly, rapid, progressive, diffuse cutaneous sclerosis may develop, often associated with significant involvement of internal organs (Table 17-2). The indurated cutaneous plaques of systemic scleroderma are not as sharply demarcated as those in morphea and may be hypo- or hyperpigmented. The skin becomes taut, immobile, and difficult to grasp. Involvement of overlying joints often leads to ulcerations, flexion contractures, and bone resorption. Raynaud's phenomenon and internal organ involvement often occur.[17] Digital soft-tissue calcification may accompany Raynaud's phenomenon, esophageal dysmotility, sclerodactyly, and telangiectasia (CREST syndrome).[23]

Histopathological Features   Systemic scleroderma and morphea are characterized by similar histologic changes, including a superficial and deep primarily perivascular, predominantly lymphocytic infiltrate usually containing plasma cells and eosinophils, which extends into the subcutaneous fat. As lesions evolve, the inflammatory infiltrate decreases, and collagen bundles thicken throughout the dermis, often more prominently in the middle to deep reticular dermis, with characteristic involvement of subcutaneous fat septa by sclerosis. Increasing sclerosis occurs coincident with loss of adnexal epithelial structures. Presumably, the involvement of the subcutaneous fat and fasciae result in the "bound down" clinical character of skin in scleroderma. Dermal calcification

TABLE 17-2

Scleroderma

Clinical Features

Adult women > men
Nonpitting edema of extremities and digits
Acrosclerosis versus diffuse sclerosis of face and trunk
Internal organ involvement
CREST syndrome

Histopathological Features

Epidermis uninvolved, hypo- or hyperpigmented
Dermal sclerosis often accentuated in lower half of
   reticular dermis and fat septa
Superficial and deep lymphoplasmacytic infiltrate with
   eosinophils
Atrophic to absent adnexal structures

Differential Diagnosis

Morphea
Mixed connective tissue disease
Eosinophilic fasciitis
Sclerodermoid disorders

develops rarely. Vascular changes may include intimal and adventitial fibrosis and thrombosis of small arteries and arterioles.[24] The epidermis often shows either a diminished number or absence of melanocytes or increased basal layer melanin.

Differential Diagnosis   Distinction histologically between systemic scleroderma and morphea is not possible on a consistent basis (see preceding discussion under "Differential Diagnosis" of morphea), whereas virtually identical histologic changes may occur in other sclerodermoid conditions such as sclerodermoid porphyria cutanea tarda or sclerodermoid graft-versus-host disease. Conventional scleroderma/morphea differs from sclerodermoid graft-versus-host disease by the usual development of sclerosis in the deep reticular dermis near the interface with the subcutis, whereas the sclerosis in graft-versus-host disease develops initially in the superficial dermis (the papillary and superficial reticular dermis).

Other entities to be considered in the differential diagnosis include radiation dermatitis and sclerosis secondary to other physical injury such as thermal burns. Chronic radiation dermatitis is distinguished from scleroderma by the presence of hyperkeratosis, usually concomitant epidermal hyperplasia and/or atrophy, enlarged "radiation" fibroblasts, and perivascular foamy histiocytes on occasion. Scarring from other injuries such as thermal burns is nonspecific and must be discriminated by clinical history.

Mixed Connective Tissue Disease

Clinical Features   As the name implies, mixed connective tissue disease (MCTD) presents with combined clinical features of systemic lupus erythematosus, scleroderma, and dermatomyositis. Circulating antibodies to ribonucleoprotein (extractable nuclear antigen, ENA) are typically present,[25] whereas those directed against Sm antigen and double-stranded DNA are not.[26] Patients characteristically develop acrosclerosis, Raynaud's phenomenon, and arthritis. Mixed connective tissue disease usually responds to systemic corticosteroids.

Histopathological Features   Reticular dermal sclerosis indistinguishable from PSS characterizes well-developed acrosclerotic lesions with some vessel wall thickening.

Eosinophilic Fasciitis (Shulman's Syndrome)

Clinical Features   Eosinophilic fasciitis (Shulman's syndrome) is characterized by rapid development, often following vigorous exercise, of sclerodermalike cutaneous, subcutaneous, and fascial changes, usually involving extremities, but lacking Raynaud's phenomenon and visceral involvement, with a typical clinical course of spontaneous remissions, relapses, and recurrences. Patients frequently have peripheral eosinophilia, elevated sedimentation rate, and hypergammaglobulinemia.[27] Systemic corticosteroid therapy, at times, provides improvement (Table 17-3). In the opinion of some observers, eosinophilic fasciitis represents a "deep" variant of morphea or morphea profunda, just as atrophoderma of Pasini and Pierini is considered to be an "atrophic" form of morphea.

Histopathological Features   Histologic characteristics of eosinophilic fasciitis include thickened, sclerotic fascia, often accompanied by a mixed inflammatory cell infiltrate of lymphocytes, plasma cells, and eosinophils (which may be few in number or absent), with sclerosis of the overlying dermis and subcutaneous fat septa indistinguishable from that seen in morphea and systemic scleroderma.[28]

Eosinophilic Fasciitis (Shulman's Syndrome)

Clinical Features

Rapid onset
Exercise related often
Sclerodermalike changes on extremities
Absent Raynaud's phenomenon and visceral involvement
Steroid responsive

Histopathological Features

Indistinguishable from morphea/scleroderma
Sclerosis of dermis, fat septa, and fascia
Peripheral and tissue eosinophilia

Differential Diagnosis

Morphea
Scleroderma (PSS)
Sclerodermoid disorders

Sclerodermoid Disorders

Sclerodermoid changes may be seen in a group of exceedingly heterogeneous conditions (Table 17-4) including Winchester's syndrome, a rare inherited disorder of connective tissue in which patients develop thick leathery skin,[29] and pachydermoperiostosis (primary hypertrophic osteoarthropathy), which affects both skin and bones of the extremities, face, and scalp, where thickened, deeply furrowed skin (cutis verticis gyrata) develops. Both diseases are characterized by a thickened dermis with hyalinized collagen and prominent subcutaneous fibrous septa. Recent studies have revealed accumulation of acid mucopolysaccharides and dermal fibrillary material apparently representing disorganized elastic tissue microfibrils with collagen synthesis and degradation markers not altered.[30] Porphyria cutanea tarda, on occasion, may result in sclerodermoid changes of sun-exposed skin that histologically are indistinguishable from scleroderma except for the usual presence of solar elastosis in porphyria.[31] Extensive sclerodermoid changes may occur in the skin and subcutaneous tissue after pentazocine,[32] bleo-

Sclerodermoid Disorders

Clinical Features

Variable induration of skin

Histopathological Features

Indistinguishable from morphea/scleroderma

Differential Diagnosis

Winchester's syndrome
Pachydermoperiostosis (cutis verticis gyrata)
Sclerodermoid porphyria cutanea tarda
Sclerodermoid graft-versus-host reaction
Sclerodermoid reaction to injections [pentazocine, bleomycin, phytonadione (vitamin K), silicone]
Acro-osteolysis, inherited and acquired
Sclerodermoid reaction to ingestion of olive oil substitute (denatured rapeseed oil) and L-tryptophan
Sequela of phenylketonuria

mycin,[33] or phytonadione (vitamin K) injections[34,35]; following injection or leakage of silicone for augmentation mammaplasty[36]; in acro-osteolysis, both inherited and acquired, including spontaneous[37] and occupationally induced[38]; in some graft-versus-host reactions[39,40]; and following ingestion of an olive oil substitute (rapeseed oil), denatured with aniline[41,42] or L-tryptophan.[43–45] Finally, sclerodermalike changes may be one sequela of phenylketonuria.[46] In each, the pathologic changes precisely mimic those of idiopathic scleroderma.

Lichen Sclerosus et Atrophicus

Lichen sclerosus et atrophicus primarily affects the anogenital region, extra-genital lesions occasionally occurring in females and rarely in males. Lichen sclerosus et atrophicus of the vulvar region is also termed *kraurosis vulvae* and of the glans penis as *balanitis xerotica obliterans*. According to some observers, lichen sclerosus et atrophicus represents a "superficial" form of morphea.[47,48] Squamous cell carcinoma develops within preexisting lichen sclerosus et atrophicus rarely. The cause of lichen sclerosus et atrophicus is unknown, although recent studies suggest an autoimmune pathogenesis. There is a slightly increased incidence of autoimmune-related diseases in patients with lichen sclerosus et atrophicus, including thyroid disease and pernicious anemia in women and vitiligo and alopecia in men.[49,50]

Clinical Features   Lichen sclerosus et atrophicus is characterized by white to pink, polygonal, hyperkeratotic macules and papules that coalesce to form atrophic plaques. Follicular plugging is prominent within the dry, atrophic, "cigarette paper–wrinkled" lesions (Table 17-5).

Histopathological Features   Lichen sclerosus et atrophicus involves changes primarily of the epidermis and papillary dermis while sparing the reticular dermis. Early features include a bandlike infiltrate of lymphocytes and histiocytes beneath the epidermis obscuring the dermal-epidermal junction. Over time, edema and subsequently "homogeneous" sclerosis develop over a broad zone and thicken the papillary dermis, "displacing" the lichenoid infiltrate toward the reticular dermis.[51] The epidermis frequently is atrophic, with hyperkeratotic plug-

Lichen Sclerosus et Atrophicus

Clinical Features

White to pink, flat-topped polygonal papules with follicular plugging
"Cigarette paper" atrophy
Anogenital region (kraurosis vulvae, balanitis xerotica obliterans)
Association with squamous cell carcinoma (rare)

Histopathological Features

Hyperkeratosis
Follicular plugging
Epidermal atrophy with vacuolar alteration
Papillary dermal edema and sclerosis
Telangiectasias
Lichenoid infiltrate beneath thickened papillary dermis

Differential Diagnosis

Morphea (certain examples with papillary edema)
Chronic radiodermatitis

ging of adnexal ostia and vacuolar alteration of the basal layer. Occasionally the vacuolar alteration may lead to subepidermal separation and blister formation. Numerous telangiectatic vessels in the upper dermis may lead to extravasation of red cells and hemorrhagic bullae. Elastic tissue stains of the sclerotic papillary dermis in lichen sclerosus et atrophicus show a marked diminution of elastic fibers unlike the normal elastic tissue findings in the reticular dermis of scleroderma.

Differential Diagnosis   In some instances, morphea may be characterized by papillary edema and sclerosis strikingly similar to lichen sclerosus et atrophicus but which can be distinguished from it by sclerosis of the reticular dermis and fat septa.[48] Similarly, chronic radiodermatitis may demonstrate epidermal hyperkeratosis, atrophy, papillary dermal edema, and sclerosis quite similar to lichen sclerosus et atrophicus. Radiodermatitis may be distinguished by sclerosis of the reticular dermis, absence of a lichenoid infiltrate, and, at times, the presence of pleomorphic endothelial or fibroblast nuclei.

Other Hypertrophic Collagenoses

CONNECTIVE TISSUE NEVI

Connective tissue nevi are rare hamartomas that involve alterations of collagen, elastic tissue, glycosaminoglycans (ground substance), or all three substances.[52] Collagen may be increased in amount ("collagenoma"), whereas elastic tissue may be increased ("elastoma"), normal, or decreased. Connective tissue nevi usually are present at birth or appear in childhood but uncommonly in adult life. They may be inherited or acquired.[53] Familial connective tissue nevi may occur as solitary lesions or associated with osteopoikilosis (radiographic bone densities or "stippling") in the Buschke-Ollendorff syndrome, an autosomal dominant condition.[54] Patients with tuberous sclerosis often have a type of connective tissue nevus called *collagenous plaques* (*shagreen patches*) over the lower back as well as other fibrous skin lesions including angiofibromas (adenoma sebaceum) of the central face and periungual or subungual locations (Koenen's tumor).

Clinical Features   Connective tissue nevi typically involve the chest, back, buttocks, or arms, presenting as small papules or plaques, at times multiple, distributed in a zosteriform or systematized fashion. Plaques are composed of coalescent papules with an ivory or light tannish color, sometimes having an orange peel (peau d'orange) or cobblestone appearance, at times with perifollicular orientation (Table 17-6).

Histopathological Features   Microscopically, connective tissue nevi often show extremely subtle changes, with the increased amount of collagen difficult to ascertain with routinely stained specimens. In most instances, the epidermis is normal in appearance, but the changes of epidermal nevus have been reported. The dermis may be increased in thickness, and there may be involvement of the subcutaneous fat by the hamartomatous process. Some lesions are characterized by thickened and homogenized collagen bundles; in some instances, the collagen bundles appear disordered and haphazardly arranged.[55] There may be concomitant alterations in the elastic tissue, including a dilutional effect; i.e., the elastic fibers are more widely spaced, they may be increased in quantity as in elastoma (see below), and finally, they may be fragmented and attenuated. Connective tissue nevi in the Buschke-Ollendorff syndrome, which are of the elastic tissue type (dermatofibrosis lenticularis disseminata), show a characteristic increase in elastic fibers that are broad and interlacing, often apparent with hematoxylin and eosin–stained specimens (Fig. 17-4). In some cases, the elastic fibers take on a clumped morphology.

TABLE 17-6
Connective Tissue Nevi

Clinical Features

Papules or plaques
Solitary or multiple
Zosteriform or systematized
Ivory to tan color
Orange peel (peau d'orange) or cobblestone surface

Histopathological Features

Thickened homogenized collagen bundles ("collagenoma")
Increased elastic tissue ("elastoma")—need elastic tissue stains
Comparison to uninvolved skin helpful

Differential Diagnosis

Normal skin
Dermatofibroma
Pseudoxanthoma elasticum
Scar
Fibrous hamartoma of infancy

Differential Diagnosis   The most common difficulty is distinguishing connective tissue nevi from normal skin, and a biopsy of uninvolved skin for comparison as well as special stains for collagen (trichrome) and elastic fibers are often very helpful. Elastic tissue type connective tissue nevi are distinguished from pseudoxanthoma elasticum because the elastic fibers are usually not fragmented and distorted and show no calcium deposition.

Other entities to be considered include reparative changes or scars, scleroderma/morphea, systemic scleredema, and fibrous hamartoma of infancy. Scars usually differ from connective tissue nevi by being well-defined and showing a horizontal disposition of collagen. Scleroderma/morphea usually exhibits diffuse homogenization of collagen, obliteration of appendageal structures, and possibly inflammatory infiltrates. Systemic scleredema displays much greater dermal thickening

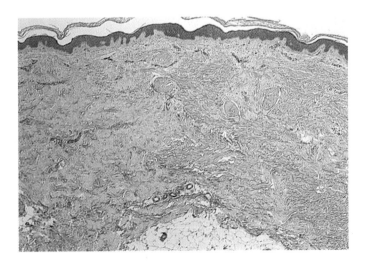

FIGURE 17-4   Connective tissue nevus (Buschke-Ollendorff syndrome). At scanning power, there are thickened, distorted elastic tissue fibers arranged in haphazard fashion throughout the reticular dermis (dermatofibrosis lenticularis disseminata).

(often two to three times normal), separation of collagen bundles ("fenestration"), and frequent but not invariable mucin deposition. Fibrous hamartoma shows three components to variable extent: distinct bands of collagen, whorled foci of mesenchymal cells, and an intimate admixture of adipose tissue.

FIBROSIS, HYPERTROPHIC SCARS, AND KELOIDS

Fibrosis characteristically represents the late stage of an intense inflammatory process, perhaps resulting in collagen destruction due to the inflammation. Fibrosis may be merely microscopic or, when more prominent, can result in a clinically visible scar. Typically, elastic fibers are reduced in quantity and in appearance in fibrosing conditions. Hypertrophic scars and keloids are manifestations of abnormal wound-healing responses that share some clinical similarities.[56] Both are raised, flesh-colored to red, firm nodules. Hypertrophic scars are usually symptomless and confined to the site of injury. Keloids are often symptomatic (including pruritus and tenderness) and frequently extend beyond the area of healing trauma. The cause of keloids is unknown, various hypotheses suggesting associations with race, age, skin tension lines, trauma, and hormonal factors.

Histopathological Features Hypertrophic scars, like their more common atrophic relatives, are characterized by fibrillary collagen arranged parallel to the skin surface, with associated numbers of increased fibroblasts having the same alignment (Fig. 17-5). Blood vessels are typically prominent with a vertical arrangement perpendicular to the skin surface and the predominant collagen bundle pattern. Usually, the epidermis overlying hypertrophic or atrophic scars is thinned, lacking rete ridges. Newly developed scars have increased mucin content, imparting a bluish to amphophilic color with routine stains.

A keloid differs from a hypertrophic scar by the presence of distinctive, characteristically thickened, eosinophilic, homogeneous collagen

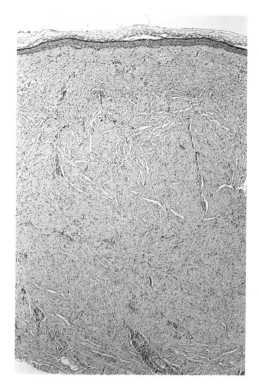

FIGURE 17-6 Keloid. Within the background of fibrosis (scar), there are broad collagen bundles arranged haphazardly throughout the middermis.

bundles associated with fibroblasts having plumper nuclei than those seen in scars. Mucin may be present between the thickened collagen bundles in a keloid that frequently displays evidence of a preexisting scar, often at the periphery of the lesion (Figs. 17-6 and 17-7). Rarely, calcification may develop in keloids. Elastic tissue is diminished to absent in both scars and keloids.[57]

Differential Diagnosis The differential diagnosis of hypertrophic scars and keloids includes dermatofibroma, morphea and cutaneous scleroderma, connective tissue nevus, fibromatosis, and other desmoplastic tumors, especially desmoplastic melanoma. In general, scars are distinctive because of the constellation of features present: effacement of the epidermis, horizontally displaced fibrillary collagen, vertically oriented microvessels, and the sharply delimited character of the process. Older scars may be more difficult to distinguish from some of the preceding entities. Dermatofibroma is typically a dermal nodular lesion with overlying epidermal hyperplasia and a characteristic storiform pattern in the dermis with entrapment of collagen bundles by spindle cells. Connective tissue nevi usually exhibit a normal epidermis, are poorly defined, and may show abnormal collagen, elastic fibers, or both. A fibromatosis differs from a scar by demonstrating fairly distinct linear bands of mature collagen. Desmoplastic melanoma enters into the differential diagnosis of some scarring processes and is an important entity to exclude. The presence of an intraepidermal melanocytic proliferative component, the presence of melanin, and immunostaining with S-100 protein and other markers for melanocytes may aid in this discrimination (see also Chap. 27).

STRIAE DISTENSAE

Striae distensae ("stretch marks") are the result of a variety of factors, including mechanical stretching of the skin such as from heavy lifting and pregnancy, as well as the effects of corticosteroids, both topically and systemically administered.

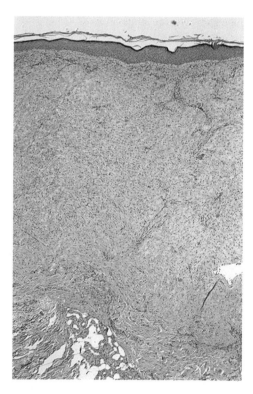

FIGURE 17-5 Scar. A scar at low power shows numerous spindled fibroblasts associated with collagen bundles arranged primarily parallel to the skin surface with vertically oriented blood vessels. The scar has replaced virtually the entire reticular dermis.

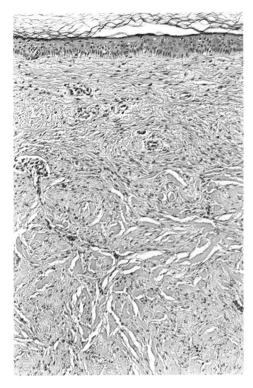

FIGURE 17-7   Keloid. Higher power shows the contrast between the broad, pale-staining keloidal collagen bundles surrounded by fibrotic collagen of the preexisting scar.

Clinical Features   Newly developed striae are linearly arranged, reddish to purplish, fibrosing lesions that, with age, become atrophic and whitish. There is a predilection for development on the buttocks, thighs, back, abdomen, and breasts.

Histopathological Features   Striae distensae in their early stages are characterized by fragmented collagen bundles separated by edema and altered elastic fibers that have a short and fragmented appearance. There is a sparse, predominately lymphocytic infiltrate around dilated blood vessels, the latter imparting the characteristic livid color. In chronic striae, collagen bundles are arranged parallel to the skin surface as in other scarring processes, while elastic tissue stains show increased numbers of elastic fibers, apparently newly formed, and dilated vessels, particularly in the upper dermis.[58]

Differential Diagnosis   In contrast to hypertrophic and atrophic scars, increased amounts of elastic tissue, best visualized with elastic tissue stains, are present in later-stage striae distensae as opposed to little to no elastic tissue in scars.[59] Blood vessels may be horizontally rather than vertically oriented in striae as well.

Fibroblastic Rheumatism

Fibroblastic rheumatism (FR) is a rare, relatively recently described idiopathic dermatosis-arthritis syndrome. In one patient, studies demonstrated an increase in fibronectin and tenascin deposition in both involved and uninvolved skin.[60] Some of the dermal cells in FR have ultrastructural features suggesting mild fibroblastic differentiation. Biochemical studies of cultured fibroblasts revealed a reduction in collagen and noncollagen protein synthesis distinguishing FR from other fibrotic skin conditions such as scleroderma.

Clinical Features   Fibroblastic rheumatism, a rare disease involving a combination of rheumatologic and cutaneous manifestations, presents with symmetric polyarthralgia leading to joint stiffness, as well as cutaneous nodules and sclerodactyly.

Histopathological Features   Biopsies of nodular lesions demonstrate increased numbers of fibroblasts associated with collagen fibers arranged in a whorled fashion extending into the subcutaneous fat.[61] A zone of uninvolved papillary dermis separates the epidermis from the deeper fibrosis. Dermal appendages are reportedly present, while elastic tissue stains show a marked decrease in elastic tissue in some areas and irregularly clumped elastic fibers in others.

Differential Diagnosis   The differential diagnosis of FR includes scleroderma, which shares some clinical similarities. Fibroblastic rheumatism shows characteristic whorled fibrosis rather than sclerosis as in scleroderma. Skin nodules also have been reported in localized and generalized morphea and Shulman's syndrome. Finally, some pediatric fibromatoses have similarities to FR, including juvenile hyaline fibromatosis, Winchester syndrome, and François's syndrome.

Collagenosis Nuchae

Clinical Features   Collagenosis nuchae was first described in 1988 as diffuse induration and swelling of the posterior neck areas of two adult men with some suggestion of accompanying inflammation.[62]

Histopathological Features   In the two reported cases, there were dense masses of disordered and thickened collagen bundles with few fibroblasts or inflammatory cells. There was no evidence of increased acid mucopolysaccharide with special stains. The histologic appearance resembled "hyalinized scar tissue."

Radiation Dermatitis

Ionizing radiation may produce radiodermatitis. Previously, most skin reactions occurred as a result of ionizing radiation at orthovoltage levels (90 to 100 kV), whereas radiation dermatitis now is seen less frequently owing to the use of deeper-penetrating megavoltage (2 to 4 MV).

Clinical Features   Radiodermatitis typically is divided into acute (early) and chronic (late) stages. Acute radiodermatitis is characterized by the sequential appearance of erythema, vesicle formation, and hyperpigmentation with frequent ulceration. In chronic radiodermatitis, there are shiny, atrophic patches with numerous telangiectases imparting a poikilodermatous appearance. Within areas of chronic radiodermatitis, cutaneous carcinomas may develop, including basal and squamous cell carcinomas, adnexal carcinomas, melanoma, and sarcomas.

Histopathological Features   Chronic radiodermatitis is characterized by sclerosing changes throughout the dermis, often with prominent edema in the papillary dermis. The quality of sclerosis and edema in chronic radiodermatitis has marked similarity to lichen sclerosus et atrophicus. Prominent fibroblasts, some with large, hyperchromatic, and in some cases bizarre nuclei, are scattered throughout the dermis beneath an epidermis thinned in some areas and hyperplastic in others. Fibrin deposition may be present subepidermally and within and around dermal vessel walls as well.

Differential Diagnosis   As mentioned, lichen sclerosus et atrophicus shares many histologic similarities with chronic radiodermatitis in the epidermis and superficial dermis, the latter distinguished by reticular dermal sclerosis as well as scattered stellate and atypical fibroblasts and endothelial cells.

Atrophic Collagenoses

APLASIA CUTIS CONGENITA

Aplasia cutis congenita (congenital localized absence of skin) is a focal absence of skin noted at the time of delivery, most commonly manifested as a solitary or a few ulcers of the scalp that heal following birth. Occasionally, intrauterine healing occurs, and the involved area presents as a scar. Aplasia cutis congenita represents a heterogeneous group of diseases including genetic disorders and those related to chromosomal abnormalities, teratogens, and intrauterine insults (infections, vascular accident), while the majority are due to unknown causes.[63]

Clinical Features   The scalp lesions vary in size from a few millimeters to many centimeters in diameter and may extend as deeply as the dura or meninges. Most lesions are solitary, whereas approximately one-fifth are multiple and have an eroded to ulcerated, frequently crusted membranous covering over the defect. Healed areas (scars) typically have permanent alopecia. Rarely, aplasia cutis congenita may present with other abnormalities, including cleft lip and palate, tracheoesophageal fistula, double cervix and uterus, vascular abnormalities, limb defects, mental retardation, and epidermolysis bullosa.[63]

Histopathological Features   Ulcers are characterized by a loss of epidermis and dermis extending to and through the subcutaneous fat, which may be absent as well. Healed areas show reepithelialized epidermis overlying a dermal scar with diminished elastic tissue and an absence of rudimentary adnexal structures[64] (Fig. 17-8).

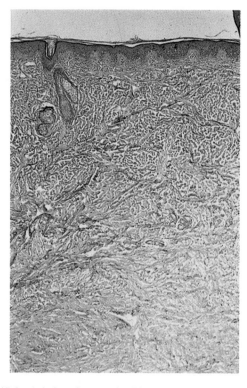

FIGURE 17-8   Aplasia cutis congenita. Biopsy from a healed site of previous aplasia cutis shows fibrosis throughout the dermis with almost complete loss of follicles, sebaceous glands, and eccrine glands.

FOCAL DERMAL HYPOPLASIA

Focal dermal hypoplasia (Goltz syndrome, Goltz-Gorlin syndrome), which is likely due to an X-linked dominant gene lethal in hemizygous males, is seen mainly in females. Male patients may be the result of a new rather than inherited mutation.[65]

Clinical Features   Focal dermal hypoplasia is characterized by linear areas of dermal thinning giving reticular or cribriform patterns, often with hyper- or hypopigmentation. In addition, soft, yellow nodules, which also may be in linear arrangement, and ulcers, due to congenital absence of skin, may be present and heal with atrophic scars (Table 17-7). There is frequently an absence of a digit, at times associated with syndactyly, which results in the characteristic "lobster-claw deformity," and loss of or abnormal hair, nails, and teeth. Osteopathia striata, representing radiographic longitudinal striations in long bone metaphyses, is a diagnostic marker of Goltz syndrome.[66,67]

Histopathological Features   Beneath a normal epidermis, there is marked thinning of the dermis with loose collagen bundles. The soft, yellow nodules histologically represent adipocytes extending upward from subcutaneous lobules that replace most of the dermis, resulting in fat located close to the undersurface of the epidermis, imparting the characteristic color.[67]

Differential Diagnosis   Nevus lipomatosus of Hoffmann and Zurhele also is characterized by subcutaneous fat extending into the upper dermis, whereas it lacks the marked attenuation of collagen bundles seen in focal dermal hypoplasia.

FOCAL FACIAL DERMAL DYSPLASIA

Clinical Features   Focal facial dermal dysplasia is a rare genodermatosis presenting as symmetric scarred areas involving the temple, typically present at birth, at times associated with other facial abnormalities. Most likely, focal facial dermal dysplasia represents a variant of aplasia cutis congenita with similar histopathology.[68]

PSEUDOAINHUM CONSTRICTING BANDS

Pseudoainhum constricting bands are fibrous constrictions of the digits (or rarely limbs) that occasionally develop in patients with severe, usu-

---

TABLE 17-7

Focal Dermal Hypoplasia (Goltz Syndrome, Goltz-Gorlin Syndrome)

Clinical Features

Cribriform or retiform linear dermal thinning
Soft yellow nodules
Ulcers
"Lobster-claw" deformity with syndactyly
Abnormal (or absence of) hair, nails, teeth
Osteopathia striata

Histopathological Features

Markedly thinned dermis
Loose collagen bundles
Superficial extension of adipocytes (yellow nodules)

Differential Diagnosis

Nevus lipomatosus superficialis (Hoffmann and Zurhele)

ally inherited, keratoderma and frequently result in autoamputation.[69] Pseudoainhum also refers to the development of constricting bands around the toes in nonhereditary conditions such as leprosy, syphilis, and scleroderma. Mutilating keratoderma of Vohwinkel, an autosomal dominant trait characterized by onset in infancy of keratoderma having a diffuse, honeycomb pattern, may lead to these digital fibrous constrictions.[70] Ainhum refers to similar bandlike constrictions, usually leading to spontaneous amputation of the fifth toe, affecting West African natives.

Histopathological Features   The constricting bands are characterized by a depression at the site of the constriction beneath which is fibrosis composed of increased numbers of fibroblasts and collagen bundles within a thinned dermis.

KERATOSIS PILARIS ATROPHICANS

Keratosis pilaris atrophicans more than likely represents a group of disorders (Table 17-8) characterized by follicular hyperkeratotic papules and perifollicular atrophy, including keratosis pilaris atrophicans facie (ulerythema ophryogenes), which is characterized by lesions located adjacent to and within lateral eyebrow regions where there is perifollicular erythema, follicular hyperkeratosis, and perifollicular fibrosis, with similar changes extending onto the cheeks. Keratosis follicularis spinulosa decalvans also begins at an early age as marked follicular plugging on cheeks and nose with resulting perifollicular atrophy as well as a scarring scalp alopecia, generalized keratosis pilaris, hyperkeratosis of the palms and soles, photophobia, and corneal abnormalities. Finally, atrophoderma vermiculatum (folliculitis ulerythematosa reticulata) develops in later childhood, again on the cheeks and preauricular skin with tiny, follicular plugging leading to atrophy that develops in a reticular pattern. Atrophoderma vermiculatum may represent an end stage of the preceding two diseases.[71]

Histopathological Features   Histologically, the group of diseases known as keratosis pilaris atrophicans shows typical changes of keratosis pilaris, including patulous follicular orifices often in the shape of an inverted cone, filled with basket weave to laminated cornified cells that characteristically protrudes above the surrounding cornified surface, and perifollicular fibrosis with atrophy of follicular and sebaceous epithelium. Comedones and milia may develop.

Differential Diagnosis   When keratosis pilaris atrophicans is associated with scarring alopecia, lichen planopilaris, discoid lupus erythematosus, and pseudopelade of Brocq are in the histologic differential diagnosis (see also Chap. 10).

CORTICOSTEROID ATROPHY

Clinical Features   Corticosteroid atrophy characteristically develops at injection sites of corticosteroids as well as from long-term topical application.[72,73] The atrophy may be related to diminished production as well as increased degradation of collagen.

Histopathological Features   A thinned epidermis with effacement of rete ridges overlies dilated superficial vessels with atrophy of the reticular dermis in severe cases. Individual collagen bundles may be attenuated or homogenized in appearance.

ATROPHODERMA OF PASINI AND PIERINI

Atrophoderma of Pasini and Pierini, in most observers' opinion, represents a variant of morphea.[74,75] However, some observers do not believe that such an entity exists.

Clinical Features   Atrophoderma lesions are typically on the trunk and present as areas of slight depression having a slate-gray color but no other epidermal changes. Usually up to 10 cm in diameter, the lesions are sharply demarcated, imparting (by palpation) a "cliff drop" edge with central induration similar to morphea.

Histopathological Features   In well-developed plaques of atrophoderma, there may be epidermal depression with a slightly thinned dermis (compared with nonlesional skin) showing sclerosis, diminished interbundle spaces, and eosinophilia of collagen bundles.

Differential Diagnosis   Since atrophoderma of Pasini and Pierini represents morphea, the diseases are virtually indistinguishable histologically.

ACRODERMATITIS CHRONICA ATROPHICANS

Acrodermatitis chronica atrophicans is a manifestation of late-stage borreliosis typically seen in Europe. Consequently, a history of preceding erythema chronicum migrans may be available in some patients. High titers of IgG antibodies against *Borrelia* usually are found in the serum of patients with acrodermatitis chronica atrophicans. Occasionally, spirochetes may be identified by dark-field examination or tissue culture.

Clinical Features   Acrodermatitis chronica atrophicans almost always involves the extensor surfaces of the lower extremities. Initially, the skin becomes red and slightly edematous and then subsequently atrophic with a bluish-red to brown, atrophic, wrinkled appearance. As a result of dermal and adipocyte atrophy, subcutaneous veins are clinically apparent. Occasionally, fibrosis develops in linear or plaquelike distribution as indurated bands over the legs or dorsum of the feet or as nodules near joints.

TABLE 17-8

Keratosis Pilaris Atrophicans

Clinical Features

Follicular hyperkeratotic papules with perifollicular
  atrophy involving:
    Early childhood, lateral eyebrows and cheeks
      (keratosis pilaris atrophicans facie, ulerythema ophryogenes)
    Early childhood, cheeks and nose with scalp alopecia,
      generalized keratosis pilaris, palmoplantar hyperkeratosis, photo-
      phobia, and corneal abnormalities
      (keratosis folliculosis spinulosa decalvans)
    Later childhood, cheeks and preauricular skin
      (atrophoderma vermiculatum, folliculitis ulerythematosa reticulata)

Histopathological Features

Horn-filled patulous follicular orifices
Perifollicular fibrosis
Atrophy of follicular and sebaceous epithelium

Differential Diagnosis

Lichen planopilaris
Discoid lupus erythematosus
Pseudopelade of Brocq

Histopathological Features Following an initial inflammatory stage characterized by a perivascular lymphocytic infiltrate mixed with plasma cells, the more classic findings include a thinned epidermis overlying an uninvolved papillary dermis, while collagen bundles in the midreticular dermis appear degenerated and split into smaller fibers. Destruction of elastic fibers may be demonstrated by elastic tissue stains. Adnexal structures including follicles and sebaceous glands become atrophic, as do, eventually, eccrine glands. Subcutaneous fat likewise becomes atrophic. The indurated bands and plaques are characterized histologically by fibrosis. There is a dense superficial and middermal infiltrate of lymphocytes, histiocytes, and many plasma cells. Warthin-Starry silver stains may reveal perivascular spirochetes.

Perforating Collagenoses

REACTIVE PERFORATING COLLAGENOSIS

Reactive perforating collagenosis, a controversial entity, has been described as showing autosomal recessive inheritance occurring in siblings.[76] An acquired, spontaneously developing variant in adult life also has been described, whereas a second variant termed *collagenoma perforans verruciforme* (perforating verruciforme collagenoma) has similar clinical and histologic features to reactive perforating collagenoses, although only a single occurrence, without genetic influence and due to more severe trauma, is characteristic.[77]

Clinical Features The lesions appear first in early childhood, apparently in response to superficial trauma, and consist of dome-shaped papules with a central umbilication filled with an adherent, firm, cornified plug. The lesions heal spontaneously within a few months, while new lesions may continue to appear in haphazard distribution.

Histopathological Features Well developed dome-shaped lesions show a central crusted ulceration adjacent to which there is irregular epidermal hyperplasia. At the base of the ulceration, collagen bundles have a basophilic appearance and may be present within the "epidermal perforation" or the ulcer bed, often oriented perpendicular to the surface. Elastic tissue stains show no increase in elastic fibers in the adjacent dermis and no evidence of elastic fibers in the keratotic plug or areas of epidermal perforation.

Differential Diagnosis More than likely, reactive perforating collagenosis represents ulceration secondary to trauma with a pronounced epidermal hyperplasia response simulating prurigo nodule–like changes.

CHONDRODERMATITIS NODULARIS CHRONICA HELICIS

Clinical Features Chondrodermatitis nodularis chronica helicis presents as one or two and rarely several, at times bilateral, small 2- to 3-mm dome-shaped papules, usually at the apex of the helix or antihelix.[78] The nodules are remarkably tender for their bland clinical appearance, and attempts to examine them frequently are met with a prominent withdrawal response by the patient. A central, small crusted or plugged umbilication is usually present.

Histopathological Features Within the center of a lesion of chondrodermatitis usually is a dilated, horn-filled follicular infundibulum, often with perforation of the infundibular epithelium at its base.[79] Scale crust also may overlie an epidermal ulceration adjacent to which are features simulating prurigo nodularis or lichen simplex chronicus, including hyperkeratosis, hypergranulosis, irregular epidermal hyperplasia, and dense fibrosis of the papillary dermis. At the base of the ulceration or

perforation is prominent fibrin deposition. The dermis, at times, has a chondroid appearance with fibroblasts simulating chondrocytes, and there is adjacent fibrosing granulation tissue. Ear cartilage at the base of the lesion often is uninvolved.

Differential Diagnosis The histologic appearance of chondrodermatitis is distinctive, and because of the absence of definitive changes within the cartilage, the disorder may be diagnosed with a superficial shave biopsy.

Variable Collagen Changes

EHLERS-DANLOS SYNDROME (CUTIS HYPERELASTICA)

Ehlers-Danlos syndrome is a heterogeneous group of inherited connective tissue disorders affecting primarily the skin, gastrointestinal tract, and musculoskeletal system. The syndrome is now divided into 11 subtypes based on clinical, genetic, and biochemical information (Table 17-9). Molecular or enzyme abnormalities of collagen synthesis have now been identified in more than half the subtypes, although precise classification of individual patients remains challenging.

Clinical Features Common to many patients with Ehlers-Danlos syndrome are skin fragility, hyperextensibility, velvety texture and a tendency to bruise easily, delayed wound healing leading to "cigarette paper" scars, and hypermobile joints.[80] While most forms of the disorder usually are compatible with normal life span, the so-called ecchymotic form of Ehlers-Danlos syndrome often leads to premature death from arterial or intestinal rupture. Occasionally, raisinlike (molluscoid) pseudotumors, raised, soft, and with a wrinkled surface, develop at the sites of trauma. Finally, in some patients, firm, spheroid subcutaneous nodules form at sites of traumatic fat necrosis.

Histopathological Features Other than areas of skin altered by trauma, patients with Ehlers-Danlos types I through III show no abnormalities histologically, either in skin thickness or in appearance of collagen or elastic fibers. Occasionally, patients show thin collagen fibers not united in bundles, with a reduction in thickness and a relative increase in numbers of elastic fibers. These changes tend to be more prominent in type I (gravis) than in types II and III. Ehlers-Danlos type IV is characterized by the most pronounced dermal thinning, usually resulting in a one-half to three-quarters normal thickness dermis with an abundance of elastic fibers that appear shortened and fragmented. The latter change may be secondary to changes in collagen fiber morphology. Electron microscopy reveals nonspecific changes in collagen fiber morphology and distribution, including "collagen flowers" loosely associated fibrils. Raisinlike pseudotumors that develop at hematoma sites demonstrate fibrosis and numerous capillaries as well as occasionally multinucleated histiocytes. Spheroid subcutaneous nodules are composed of fat lobules with a thick surrounding collagen layer that may contain aggregates of calcium (nodulocystic fat necrosis).

OSTEOGENESIS IMPERFECTA

Clinical Features Osteogenesis imperfecta is characterized by bone fragility as well as short stature, loose joints, blue sclerae, and occasionally, thin skin. Osteogenesis imperfecta represents a group of genetically inherited disorders with defects of various types of type I collagen.[81]

Histopathological Features There is a markedly thinned dermis seen in severely affected patients with clinically atrophic skin.

TABLE 17-9

Ehlers-Danlos Syndrome (Cutis Hyperelastica)

Clinical Features

Type I (gravis type)
  Autosomal dominant
  Hyperextensibility, skin fragility
  Atrophic scars, molluscoid pseudotumors
  Biochemical defect unknown
Type II (mitis type)
  Autosomal dominant
  Hyperextensibility
  Aortic dilatation
  Biochemical defect unknown
Type III (benign hypermobile type)
  Autosomal dominant
  Minimal skin changes
  Marked joint hypermobility
  Biochemical defect unknown
Type IV (arterial, ecchymotic type)
  Autosomal recessive (four subtypes)
  Aortic rupture, GI hemorrhage and rupture
  Ecchymoses, skin fragility, and mild
    hyperextensibility
  Absent or reduced type III collagen due to
    genetic mutation
Type V
  X-linked
  Clinical features similar to type I
  Easy bruisability
  Lysyl oxidase deficiency (reduced collagen cross-
    linking)
Type VI (ocular type)
  Autosomal recessive
  Ocular rupture
  Kyphoscoliosis and joint laxity
  Lysyl hydroxylase deficiency

Type VII (arthrochalasis type; corresponds to
    dermatosparaxis in cows, sheep)
  Autosomal recessive or dominant
  Marked joint and ligament laxity and
    dislocations
  Hyperextensible and velvety skin
  Deficient conversion of procollagen to collagen
  Procollagen N peptidase deficiency
Type VIII (periodontal type)
  Autosomal dominant
  Severe periodontosis
  Skin fragility and scarring
  Biochemical defect unknown
Type IX (X-linked cutis laxa)
  X-linked
  Joint laxity and hyperextensibility
  Diverticulosis
  Defective copper metabolism leads to lysyl oxidase
    deficiency and defective collagen cross-linking
Type X (fibronectin type)
  Autosomal recessive
  Skin extensibility and striae
  Platelet aggregation defect
  Plasma fibronectin deficiency and dysfunction
Type XI
  Unknown inheritance pattern
  Familial joint instability syndrome
  Biochemical defect unknown

Histopathological Features

Normal skin by light microscopy
Variably sized and distorted collagen fibrils, "collagen
  flowers" by electron microscopy

Differential Diagnosis

Normal skin
Anetoderma

MARFAN SYNDROME

Clinical Features   Patients with Marfan syndrome rarely have prominent cutaneous findings, although they are characteristically tall with skeletal malformations, arachnodactyly, lens dislocations, and aortic aneurysms and mitral valve prolapse. The findings are explained by abnormalities in the primary structure of fibrillin-1, a component of elastic tissue normally present in large quantities in muscular vessels, periosteum, skin, and lens ligaments.[82]

Histopathological Features   Occasionally, patients with Marfan syndrome may have dermal atrophy characterized by a diminished amount of collagen with morphologically thinner collagen bundles.

RELAPSING POLYCHONDRITIS

Relapsing polychondritis is typically a progressive, episodic inflammatory process involving most commonly auricular cartilage in up to 90 percent of patients who also have polyarthritis, nasal chondritis, ocular inflammation, and respiratory tract chondritis. Mortality may be up to 25 percent, usually the result of respiratory tract involvement or from cardiac valvular chondritis.

Clinical Features   Painful erythema and edema involving both the ears and nose develop intermittently, ultimately leading to soft and flabby ears and saddle-nose deformity due to cartilage degeneration. Cutaneous lesions occur rarely and are described as purpuric or erythema nodosum–like.

Histopathological Features   There is characteristically a mixed inflammatory infiltrate of lymphocytes, neutrophils, and plasma cells in the dermis surrounding deeper cartilage structures (Figs. 17-9 and 17-10). Cartilage changes include vacuolization and pyknosis of chondrocytes with eventual loss of cartilage basophilia. Elastic stains reveal destruction of elastic fibers within cartilage. With each succeeding attack, more chondrocytes are destroyed and replaced by fibrous tissue. Cutaneous lesions have shown vasculitis with fibrin deposition involving vessels that are surrounded by lymphocytes and eosinophils.

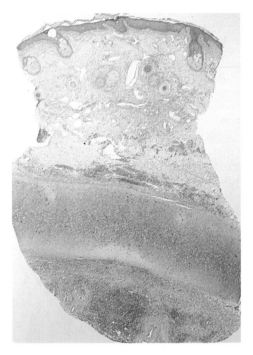

FIGURE 17-9 Relapsing polychondritis. At low power, there is a mixed inflammatory infiltrate in the perichondrial connective tissue.

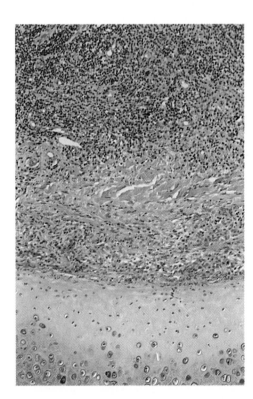

FIGURE 17-10 Relapsing polychondritis. At higher power, adjacent to the auricular cartilage there is a mixed inflammatory infiltrate of neutrophils, lymphocytes, plasma cells, and eosinophils with some loss of normal staining (devitalization) of the cartilage.

Syndromes of Premature Aging (Table 17-10)

WERNER SYNDROME (ADULT PROGERIA)

Werner syndrome is an autosomal recessive trait that first appears in patients in their teens or twenties, whereas death typically occurs in the fifth decade due to atherosclerosis.[83]

Clinical Features Patients with Werner syndrome are of short stature and develop atrophy of subcutaneous fat and extremity musculature, presenting with birdlike facies and thin arms and legs. Extremity skin gradually becomes taut, and leg ulcers may develop. Premature senility, graying of the hair and pattern alopecia, cataracts, and atherosclerosis develop in early adult life, whereas late-onset-type diabetes and hypogonadism due to interstitial fibrosis of the testes are common. The cause of Werner syndrome is unknown, some reports suggesting altered control of collagen synthesis.[84]

Histopathological Features In patients with well-developed changes, there is atrophic epidermis lacking rete ridges, whereas the dermis shows fibrosis and, at times, hyalinization of the collagen in sclerodermoid areas as well as loss of pilosebaceous units. The subcutaneous fat is replaced by collagen.

TABLE 17-10

Premature Aging Syndromes

Clinical Features

Werner's syndrome (adult progeria)
  Autosomal recessive
  Onset second–third decade
  Premature death due to atherosclerosis
  Birdlike facies
  Thin arms and legs
  Premature senility, pattern alopecia
  Hypogonadism
Progeria (Hutchinson-Gilford syndrome)
  Autosomal recessive
  Onset 6–12 months
  Growth retardation
  Alopecia
  Atrophy of muscle, fat
  Birdlike facies
  Normal intelligence
  No sexual maturation
Acrogeria (Gottran's syndrome)
  Onset early childhood
  Thin, dry, wrinkled skin
  Elastosis perforans serpiginosa
  ?Subgroup of Ehlers-Danlos type IV

Histopathological Features

Epidermal atrophy
Fibrosis and collagen hyalinization
Atrophy of subcutaneous fat

Differential Diagnosis

Scleroderma

Differential Diagnosis   Distinguishing skin of patients with Werner syndrome from scleroderma is exceedingly difficult, and clinical-pathologic correlation may be necessary.

PROGERIA (HUTCHINSON-GILFORD SYNDROME)

Progeria is a rare disease transmitted as an autosomal recessive trait, first described by Hutchinson in 1886. There is no sexual predilection, and rarely only a single family member is affected. Conflicting results have occurred following attempts to culture skin fibroblasts, some cultured cells showing a normal life span and others surviving only briefly.[85]

Clinical Features   Patients with progeria appear prematurely aged, and all show a striking resemblance to one another. Onset typically begins between 6 and 12 months of age and is characterized by growth retardation; scalp, eyebrow, and lash alopecia; prominent scalp veins; and generalized atrophy of muscle and subcutaneous tissues. The face is small, the chin is shortened, and the nose reveals prominent nasal cartilage resulting in a birdlike appearance. Frequently there is nasolabial and circumoral cyanosis. Nails may be atrophic and the skin thin except for areas with sclerodermalike plaques. Skeletal changes include prominent joints, thin bones, small clavicles, and defective ossification of the skull.[86] Although intelligence is normal and thyroid, parathyroid, pituitary, and adrenal gland function is normal, there is absence of sexual maturation.

Histopathological Features   In areas of sclerodermalike plaques, the dermis shows thickened homogenized collagen bundles extending into subcutaneous tissue with atrophic or absent follicles. Eventually, subcutaneous tissue atrophy occurs with only a few small fat lobules surrounded by connective tissue.

ACROGERIA (GOTTRAN SYNDROME)

A rare disease appearing first in early childhood, acrogeria is characterized by thin, dry, and wrinkled skin most prominently affected on the face and extremities.[87] Some bony abnormalities as well as elastosis perforans serpiginosa and perforating elastomas have been described. Acrogeria may represent a subgroup of Ehlers-Danlos syndrome type IV.[88]

Histopathological Features   Dermal atrophy with collagen abnormalities is characteristic, including thickened and homogeneous bundles extending into subcutaneous fat.

ALTERATIONS OF ELASTIN

Elastic tissue is one of the three major components of the dermis, with collagen and ground substance, and is crucial to maintaining the integrity and elasticity of the skin. Elastic fibers constitute approximately 3 percent of the dermis by dry weight, measuring 1 to 3 μm in diameter.[89,90] Elastic fibers are wavy and appear fragmented when examined by light microscopy, where visualization requires special stains such as silver, orcein, or resorcin-fuchsin. Abnormalities of elastic tissue often result in dramatic clinical changes.

Three types of elastic fibers can be identified: oxytalan, elaunin, and elastic fibers. Elastic tissue of the papillary dermis is composed of a plexus of elaunin fibers that are oriented primarily parallel to the dermal-epidermal junction, to which they are connected by oxytalan fibers, which are thin and oriented perpendicular to the junction. The thickest

fibers, elastic fibers, are the predominant elastic tissue component in the reticular dermis, where they appear fragmented and are arranged parallel to the surface.[89,90]

Increased Elastic Tissue

ELASTOMA

Elastoma (juvenile elastoma, nevus elasticus) is a variant of connective tissue nevus discussed above.

ELASTOFIBROMA

Elastofibroma is a peculiar, unilateral, asymptomatic proliferation of collagen and abnormal elastic tissue with an anatomic predilection for the subcutaneous tissue inferior to the scapulae (elastofibroma dorsi) usually found in older patients.[91,92] Elastofibromas present as flesh-colored nodules that may reach significant size (5 to 10 cm in diameter).

Histopathological Features   Elastofibromas are characterized by prominent, thickened collagen bundles within which are many, more darkly eosinophilic, irregularly shaped, and fragmented elastic fibers. There are often adipocytes scattered throughout the nodule. The elastic fibers stain characteristically with elastic tissue reagents.

ELASTOSIS PERFORANS SERPIGINOSA

Elastosis perforans serpiginosa is an uncommon, noninherited disorder characteristically affecting younger individuals. Commonly, elastosis perforans serpiginosa may be associated with other connective tissue disorders, including pseudoxanthoma elasticum, Ehlers-Danlos syndrome, osteogenesis imperfecta, Marfan syndrome, and Down syndrome[93] (Table 17-11). Clinically similar lesions may develop in patients receiving penicillamine, although the histologic characteristics are distinctive and allow differentiation from idiopathic elastosis perforans serpiginosa.

TABLE 17-11

Elastosis Perforans Serpiginosa

Clinical Features

Rare, noninherited
Associated with pseudoxanthoma elasticum, Ehlers-Danlos syndrome, osteogenesis imperfecta, Marfan syndrome, Down syndrome
Dome-shaped hyperkeratotic papules
Annular or circinate configuration on neck, face, arms

Histopathological Features

Increased elastic fibers in papillary dermis
Epidermal or follicular hyperplasia forming transepidermal channels
Perforation from channels into papillary dermis
Altered elastic fibers within perforations and channels

Differential Diagnosis

Kyrle's disease/perforating folliculitis
Reactive perforating collagenosis

Clinical Features   Numerous small 4- to 6-mm keratotic papules, many with peripheral erythema, develop in unusual annular or circinate configurations, most commonly around the nape of the neck, on the face and arms, and rarely, widely disseminated.

Histopathological Features   Numerous elastic fibers, increased in number, are present in the papillary dermis, frequently in aggregations ("papillary elastoma"). The elastic fibers are thickened, fragmented, and eosinophilic. The clinical papules are reflected histologically by transepidermal channels, most likely representing portions of follicular infundibulae, which are hyperplastic and often characterized by focal perforation into the papillary dermis with abnormal elastic fibers present not only in the surrounding dermis but also within the epithelial perforation and transepidermal channel.[94]

Differential Diagnosis   Kyrle's disease/perforating folliculitis has striking clinical and histopathologic similarities to elastosis perforans serpiginosa, including dome-shaped papules with central keratotic plugs that histologically reveal infundibular hyperplasia and perforations. However, the clinical distribution of Kyrle's disease/perforating folliculitis is more generalized, frequently on the extremities, with individual lesions scattered discretely. Histologically, Kyrle's disease/perforating folliculitis shows no evidence of increased or abnormal elastic tissue, particularly in dermal papillae or within the epidermal perforations.[94]

PSEUDOXANTHOMA ELASTICUM

Pseudoxanthoma elasticum may be inherited as an autosomal recessive or dominant trait, with the inheritance pattern and disease severity varying widely from patient to patient. Apparently two recessive and two dominant forms of pseudoxanthoma elasticum exist.[95] In pseudoxanthoma elasticum, genetically abnormal elastic fibers develop prominent calcium deposition and are present in skin, retina, and arterial walls, including those supplying gastric mucosa and myocardium, as well as larger peripheral arteries. Rupture of Bruch's membrane results in angioid streaks of the ocular fundus, while calcification and degeneration of elastic tissue fibers in internal organs lead to gastrointestinal bleeding, renal hypertension, angina pectoris, and intermittent claudication of the extremities.[96]

Clinical Features   Patients with pseudoxanthoma elasticum develop yellowish plaques with pebbly surfaces ("chicken skin") primarily involving flexures, such as the anticubital fossae, groin, axillae, and especially the lateral neck. In white skin, the cutaneous lesions may be mistaken for actinic elastosis or xanthomas.

Histopathological Features   With hematoxylin and eosin stain, the middle third of the reticular dermis is filled with numerous short, wavy, fragmented, irregularly shaped, and granular elastic fibers that frequently are deeply basophilic due to prominent calcium deposition (Figs. 17-11 and 17-12). Consequently, the fibers stain deeply black with both elastic (orcein or Verhoef) or calcium (von Kossa) stain. Some cases with marked elastic fiber calcification result in a granulomatous infiltrate.

Electron microscopy shows abnormalities of small elastic fibers, even those spared calcification, while most of the larger fibers show dense calcium deposition.

Differential Diagnosis   Solar elastosis also demonstrates abnormal elastic tissue located in the upper third of the dermis, usually beneath a small zone of spared papillary dermis, rather than the midreticular der-

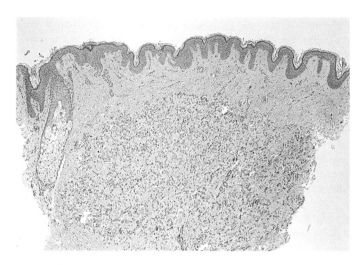

FIGURE 17-11   Pseudoxanthoma elasticum. Within the middle third of the dermis there are numerous small fragmented, distorted elastic fibers.

mal location characteristic of the abnormal elastic fibers of pseudoxanthoma elasticum. Calcium deposition does not occur in solar elastosis.

ELASTIC GLOBES

Elastic globes are small amphophilic collections present within the upper dermis of clinically normal skin that stain positively for elastic fibers. Elastic globes in large numbers have been reported in an epidermolysis bullosa patient with wrinkled skin and in one patient with cartilage-hair hypoplasia syndrome with hyperextensible skin.[97,98] Most likely, elastic globes represent a variation of solar elastosis.

Solar Elastotic Syndromes

SOLAR ELASTOSIS (ACTINIC ELASTOSIS)

Actinic elastosis, as the name implies, develops on sun-exposed skin, most prominately the lateral forehead, malar cheeks, neck, and extensor surfaces of the forearm and dorsal hands. Genetic pigmentation provides some protection from development of actinic elastosis.

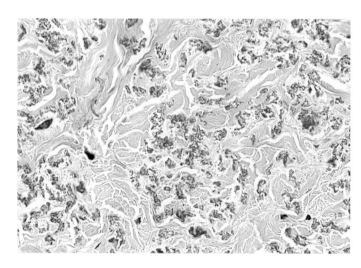

FIGURE 17-12   Pseudoxanthoma elasticum. Higher magnification shows the characteristic fragmented elastic fibers with calcium deposition.

Clinical Features   Actinic elastosis presents as papular to plaquelike areas with a distinctly yellowish hue, often separated by exaggerated skin folds and furrows. Patulous follicular orifices around the lateral forehead and cheeks as well as open and closed comedones (nodular elastosis with cysts and comedones, Favre-Racouchot syndrome) are frequently present, while geometric shapes may result from prominent and deeply fissured skin folds on the posterior and lateral neck (cutis rhomboidalis nuchae).[99]

Histopathological Features   Elastic fibers in solar elastosis have an eosinophilic to amphophilic to gray-blue appearance with hematoxylin and eosin stain. Solar elastosis stains prominently with elastic tissue stains, which reveal thick, tangled elastic fibers within amorphous ground substance beneath a thin subepidermal zone of apparently uninvolved dermis. Electron microscopy shows irregularly aggregated electron-dense material rather than characteristic arrangement in septa with ultimately complete degeneration of elastic material and transformation into an amorphous substance identical to colloid, as seen in colloid milium.[100,101]

ELASTOTIC NODULES OF THE EARS

Elastotic ear nodules are another manifestation of solar elastosis that are small, skin-colored papules predominantly found on the antihelix, frequently bilaterally. Occasionally, elastotic nodules may be painful, simulating chondrodermatitis nodularis.[102,103]

Histopathological Features   Elastotic nodules are characterized by prominent solar elastosis, including coarse elastotic fibers intermixed with larger accumulations.

COLLAGENOUS AND ELASTOTIC PLAQUES OF THE HANDS

Collagenous and elastotic plaques of the hands (keratoelastoidosis marginalis, degenerative collagenous plaques of the hands) are irregular, linear plaques that occur at the junction of the palmar and dorsal skin of the hands, particularly along the medial thumb and lateral index finger, where they resemble acrokeratoelastoidosis.[104] Most likely, collagenous and elastotic plaques of the hands represent another manifestation of marked solar elastosis.

Histopathological Features   With routine stains, there are increased numbers of thick collagen bundles arranged haphazardly throughout the dermis, some perpendicular to the epidermis, intermixed with solar elastotic fibers, which may be confirmed by elastic tissue stains.

ERYTHEMA AB IGNE

Erythema ab igne is a pattern of persistent reticulated pigmentation and telangiectasia over anatomic sites that have been exposed repeatedly to a heat source insufficient to cause burning. Use of and close approximation to space (gas or electric) heaters, electric heating pads, or hot water bottles is commonly implicated.[105] Rarely, squamous cell carcinoma may evolve within preexisting erythema ab igne.[106]

Histopathological Features   Histopathologic changes in erythema ab igne may be subtle, including epidermal atrophy with occasional atypical keratinocytes, focal vacuolar changes, telangiectasias, and often prominent elastotic fibers in the middermis. A sparse mixed cell infiltrate containing melanophages and hemosiderin is often present in the upper dermis.

Decreased Elastic Tissue

NAEVUS ANELASTICUS

Naevus anelasticus most likely represents localized anetoderma, discussed below.[107]

PERIFOLLICULAR ELASTOLYSIS

Perifollicular elastolysis is characterized by tiny, pinpoint lesions with finely wrinkled perifollicular atrophy that may bulge outward with lateral pressure. Most likely, perifollicular elastolysis results from preceding follicular inflammation, explaining its common occurrence in patients with follicular diseases such as acne vulgaris and its anatomic distribution involving the face and upper back.[108]

Histopathological Features   As the name implies, elastic stains demonstrate a markedly diminished number to absence of elastic fibers within the dermis immediately surrounding hair follicles associated with little inflammation.

MACULAR ATROPHY (ANETODERMA)

Macular atrophy may be classified as primary, where either it may be preceded by inflammation (Jadassohn-Pellizzari type) in which the atrophic cutaneous lesions appear initially red and, on histologic examination, demonstrate an inflammatory infiltrate, or the lesions may lack clinical and histologic evidence of inflammation (Schweninger-Buzzi type).[109] Secondary anetoderma has been reported following numerous cutaneous conditions. No hereditary forms of macular atrophy have been established. The cause of anetodermas is controversial, although elastolysis is a likely candidate.[110]

Clinical Features   In all forms of macular atrophy, round to oval atrophic patches primarily involving the upper trunk develop and are characterized by thin skin that bulges with movement. Palpation of macular atrophy transmits the sensation of a soft depression suggesting an orifice (Table 17-12).

Histopathological Features   In inflammatory macular atrophy, early lesions show a moderately dense perivascular, predominately lymphocytic infiltrate; occasionally, plasma cells and eosinophils predominate, and rarely neutrophils and epithelioid histiocytes may be present. In

---

TABLE 17-12

Macular Atrophy (Anetoderma)

Clinical Features

May develop following inflammatory rash (Jadassohn-Pellizzari) or spontaneously (Schweninger-Buzzi)
Round to oval atrophic patches on trunk
Skin bulges with movement
Palpation suggests orifice

Histopathological Features

Absence of elastic tissue (elastic stains)
Early lesions may have plasma cells, eosinophils, neutrophils, or epithelioid histiocytes

Differential Diagnosis

Atrophoderma

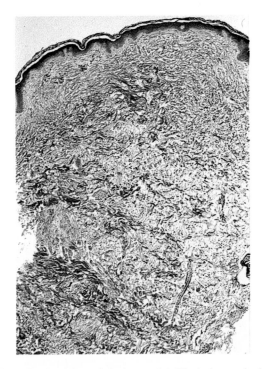

FIGURE 17-13   Anetoderma (macular atrophy). Elastic tissue stain shows loss of normal elastic tissue throughout the papillary and upper reticular dermis that allows the skin to bulge (elastic stain).

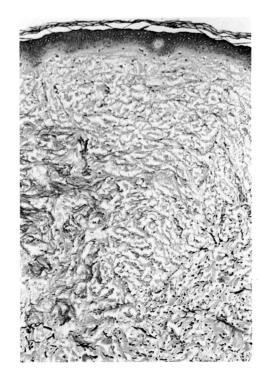

FIGURE 17-14   Anetoderma (macular atrophy). Higher power shows markedly reduced elastic tissue (elastic stain).

chronic noninflammatory lesions, elastic tissue stains show a virtually complete loss of elastic tissue either in the upper reticular and papillary dermis or confined to the upper reticular dermis (Figs. 17-13 and 17-14). Inflammatory cells may surround degenerated elastic fibers.

CUTIS LAXA (GENERALIZED ELASTOLYSIS)

Cutis laxa (dermatochalasis, generalized elastolysis, dermatomegaly) may be congenital or acquired, affecting both sexes, with autosomal dominant, recessive, and linked forms described. Cutis laxa is characterized by degenerative changes in elastic fibers; some cases show normal microfibrils and a deficiency of elastin, whereas in others elastin is preserved and microfibrils are absent. Cutis laxa may be preceded by an inflammatory rash or may develop spontaneously[111–113] (Table 17-13).

Clinical Features   Cutis laxa is characterized by loose, pendulous skin imparting a prematurely aged appearance. In both congenital and acquired types, systemic involvement is seen frequently, involving lungs (pulmonary emphysema), bladder, and gastrointestinal tract (diverticula and rectal prolapse) with inguinal, umbilical, and hiatal hernias. In some congenital cases, growth retardation and multiple joint dislocations involving hip joints also may be present.

Histopathological Features   The elastic fiber abnormalities vary depending on the stage and severity of the disease, either with elastic fibers diminished throughout the dermis or the decrease in elastic tissue confined to the upper or the lower dermis (Figs. 17-15 and 17-16). The remaining elastic fibers may be shortened, fragmented, and strikingly variable in diameter. Elastic tissue stains may be used to demonstrate the abnormalities. In severe examples, no elastic fibers may be present but only fine, dustlike or dotlike particles scattered through the dermis.[114,115] In cases preceded by an inflammatory eruption such as

urticaria, erythematous plaques, or vesicles, the inflammatory infiltrate may be mononuclear (lymphocytes and histiocytes) or mixed, containing neutrophils. When vesicles are present, they are subepidermal, with papillary collections of neutrophils and eosinophils mimicking dermatitis herpetiformis. Involved internal organs show granular changes in elastic fibers similar to those seen in the skin.

Collagen abnormalities also have been described but are ultrastructurally nonspecific.

TABLE 17-13

Cutis Laxa (Generalized Elastolysis)

Clinical Features

Congenital or acquired
Autosomal dominant, recessive, or X-linked
Loose, pendulous skin giving prematurely aged appearance
May be preceded by inflammatory eruption
Systemic involvement (lungs, bladder, GI tract, hernias)

Histopathological Features

Elastic fibers diminished throughout dermis or loss confined
   to upper or lower dermis (elastic stains)
Remaining elastic fibers short and fragmented
Lymphocytes, histiocytes, or neutrophils may be present

Differential Diagnosis

Granulomatous slack skin
Anetoderma

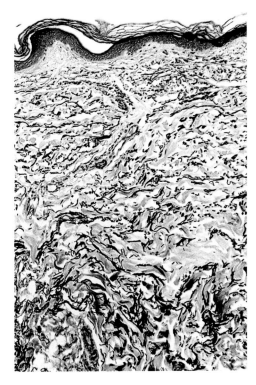

FIGURE 17-15   Cutis laxa. Elastic tissue stain of normal skin from patient with cutis laxa showing expected pattern of elastic tissue (elastic stain).

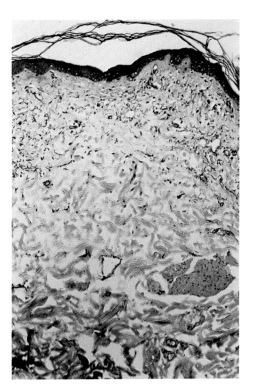

FIGURE 17-16   Cutis laxa. Elastic tissue stain from involved skin of patient with cutis laxa in contrast shows virtually no elastic tissue remaining with little evidence of an inflammatory infiltrate (elastic stain).

MENKES' SYNDROME

Menkes' kinky hair syndrome is a rare X-linked deficiency of copper metabolism resulting either in increased or decreased intracellular copper metabolism in various tissues, the latter leading to decreased activity of certain copper-dependent enzymes (tyrosinases, dopamine hydroxylase, cytochrome oxidase, lysil oxidase). Diminished enzyme activity results in the clinical features of Menkes' syndrome, such as twisted (kinky, steely) and hypopigmented hair.[116,117] Other changes include mental retardation, degeneration of elastic tissue within the walls of large blood vessels, and hypopigmentation involving Blaschko's lines in female carriers.

Histopathological Features   Diminished activity of lysil oxidase, necessary for elastin cross-linking, may result in fragmentation of internal elastic lamina of vessels, although dermal elastic tissue is not affected. There are a number of hair shaft abnormalities such as pili torti, monilethrix, and trichorrhexis nodosa.

FRAGILE X SYNDROME

Fragile X syndrome is another X-linked disorder resulting in mental retardation, characteristic facies, and connective tissue abnormalities similar to those seen in cutis laxa and Ehlers-Danlos syndromes.[118]

Histopathological Features   Fragile X syndrome results in diminished dermal elastic tissue with fragmented and curled elastic fibers as well as diminished ground substance (mucopolysaccharides).

GRANULOMATOUS DISEASES

Anetoderma in rare instances may result from preceding granulomatous inflammation such as sarcoidosis, leprosy, or tuberculosis. In addition, diminished elastic fibers may result from other granulomatous disorders, at times lacking clinical evidence of the underlying elastolysis, such as in actinic granuloma (elastolytic giant cell granuloma) and Meischer's granulomatous disciformis of the face (atypical necrobiosis lipoidica of the face and scalp). Elastotic fibers frequently are present within the cytoplasm of mononuclear and multinucleated epithelioid histiocytes in these conditions, presumably resulting in the focal elastolysis.

GRANULOMATOUS SLACK SKIN

It is now appreciated that granulomatous slack skin, initially termed *progressive, atrophying, chronic granulomatous dermohypodermatitis*,[119] represents a peculiar, rare presentation of cutaneous T-cell lymphoma in most patients, who develop striking, pendulous flexural skin folds indistinguishable from cutis laxa.[120] Diminshed elastic tissue is present similar to idiopathic cutis laxa.

MYXEDEMA

Dermal elastic tissue is prominently diminished in both hypothyroid and hyperthyroid (pretibial) myxedema. Ultrastructurally, elastic fibers show a marked variability in diameter as well as a decrease in microfibrils.[121]

ACROKERATOELASTOIDOSIS

Acrokeratoelastoidosis is an autosomal dominant condition characterized by small, hyperkeratotic papules of the hands and feet. Small shiny papules develop over the dorsal surfaces, usually in groups overlying the knuckles as well as the margins of the palms and soles.

Histopathological Features   There is slight hyperkeratosis overlying an epidermal dell with diminished, fragmented elastic fibers within the reticular dermis.

Variable or Minor Elastic Tissue Changes

LEPRECHAUNISM

Leprechaunism is a rare syndrome characterized by unusual facies, phallic enlargement, and diminished subcutaneous fat as well as wrinkled skin resulting in prominent periorificial folds. There also may be acanthosis nigricans and hypertrichosis.[122]

Histopathological Features   Both diminished collagen and elastic fibers have been reported in leprechaunism, although thickened elastic fibers involving the dermis and subcutaneous fat septa also have been reported.

SYNDROMES OF PREMATURE AGING

Elastic tissue may be increased in Werner syndrome, where ultrastructural changes have been described as granular and filamentous alterations of elastic tissue. Acrogeria may be characterized by diminished elastic fibers as well as elastosis perforans.

MARFAN SYNDROME

Marfan syndrome is a rare autosomal dominant disease characterized by abnormalities in tissues containing elastic fibers, such as the skin and aorta, as well as ocular and skeletal abnormalities. Cutaneous manifestations include elastosis perforans serpiginosa and striae distensae, which are of little clinical significance in contrast to the systemic findings. The underlying cause of the protean manifestations of Marfan syndrome has been determined to be abnormalities in the primary structure of fibrillin-1, a large protein forming part of the elastic fiber–microfibrillar complex as well as capable of independent microfibrillar bundle formation within the dermis.[82] Fibrillin-1 is present in periosteum, lens ligaments, and elastic tissue within cardiovascular structures and skin, explaining the clinical manifestations.

Histopathological Features   Elastosis perforans serpiginosa and striae distensae occurring in Marfan syndrome patients have characteristic features described previously. Clinically uninvolved skin in patients with Marfan syndrome shows no apparent abnormalities.

REFERENCES

1. Kielty CM, Hopkinson I, Grant ME: The collagen family: Structure, assembly, and organization in extracellular matrix, in Royce PM, Steinmann B (eds): *Connective Tissue and Its Heritable Disorders*. New York, Wiley-Liss, 1993:103–147.
2. Kivirikko KI: Collagens and their abnormalities in a wide spectrum of diseases. *Ann Med* 25:113–126, 1993.
3. Mauch C, Kreig T: Collagens: Their structure and metabolism, in Lapiere CM, Kreig T (eds): *Connective Tissue Diseases in the Skin* (Clinical Dermatology Series No. 9). New York, Marcel Dekker, 1993:1.
4. Prockop DJ, Berg RA, Kivirikko KI, et al: Intracellular steps in the biosynthesis of collagen, in Ramachandran GN, Reddi AJ (eds): *Biochemistry of Collagen*. New York, Plenum Press, 1976:163–273.
5. Uitto J, Prockop DJ: Synthesis and secretion of underhydroxylated procollagen at various temperatures by cells subject to temporary anoxia. *Biochem Biophys Res Commun* 60:414–423, 1974.
6. Jablonska S, Rodnan GP: Localized forms of scleroderma. *Clin Rheum Dis* 5:215–241, 1979.
7. Aberer E, Klade H, Stanek G, et al: *Borrelia burgdorferi* and different types of morphea. *Dermatologica* 182:145–154, 1991.
8. Halkier-Sorensen L, Kragballe K, Hansen K: Antibodies to the *Borrelia burgdorferi* flagellum in patients with scleroderma, granuloma annulare and porphyria cutanea tarda. *Acta Derm Venereol (Stockh)* 69:116–119, 1989.
9. Jablonska S, Rodnan GP: Localized forms of scleroderma. *Clin Rheum Dis* 5:215–241, 1979.
10. Su WPD, Greene SL: Bullous morphea profunda. *Am J Dermatopathol* 8:144–147, 1986.
11. Hulsmans RFHJ, Asghar SS, Siddiqui AH, Cormane RH: Hereditary deficiency of C2 in association with linear scleroderma "en coup de sabre." *Arch Dermatol* 122:76–79, 1986.
12. Lakhani PJ, David TJ: Progressive hemifacial atrophy with scleroderma and ipsilateral limb wasting (Parry-Romberg syndrome). *J R Soc Med* 77:138–139, 1984.
13. Cantwell AR Jr, Jones JE, Kelso DW: Pleomorphic, variably acid-fast bacteria in an adult patient with disabling pansclerotic morphea. *Arch Dermatol* 120:656–661, 1983.
14. Su WPD, Person JR: Morphea profunda: A new concept and a histopathologic study of 23 cases. *Am J Dermatopathol* 3:251–260, 1981.
15. Uitto J, Santz Cruz DJ, Bauer EA, Eisen AZ: Morphea and lichen sclerosus et atrophicus. *J Am Acad Dermatol* 3:271–279, 1980.
16. LeRoy EC, Black C, Fleischmajer R, et al: Scleroderma (systemic sclerosis): Classification, subsets and pathogenesis. *J Rheumatol* 15:202–205, 1988.
17. Krieg T, Meurer M: Systemic scleroderma: Clinical and pathophysiologic aspects. *J Am Acad Dermatol* 18:457–481, 1988.
18. Haustein UF, Herrmann K, Bohme HJ: Pathogenesis of progressive systemic sclerosis. *Int J Dermatol* 25:286–293, 1986.
19. Perlish JS, Lemlich G, Fleischmajer R: Identification of collagen fibrils in scleroderma skin. *J Invest Dermatol* 90:48–54, 1988.
20. Kahari V-M, Sandberg M, Kalimo H, et al: Identification of fibroblasts responsible for increased collagen production in localized scleroderma by in situ hybridization. *J Invest Dermatol* 90:664–670, 1988.
21. Kleinsmith DM, Heinzerling RH, Burnham TK: Antinuclear antibodies as immunologic markers for a benign subset and different clinical characteristics of scleroderma. *Arch Dermatol* 118:882–885, 1982.
22. Silverstein JL, Steen VD, Medsger TA Jr, Falanga V: Cutaneous hypoxia in patients with systemic sclerosis (scleroderma). *Arch Dermatol* 128:1379–1382, 1988.
23. Velayos EE, Masi AT, Stevens MB, Shulman LE: The "CREST" syndrome: Comparison with systemic sclerosis (scleroderma). *Arch Intern Med* 139:1240–1244, 1979.
24. Rodnan GP, Myerowitz RL, Justh GO: Morphologic changes in the digital arteries of patients with progressive systemic sclerosis (scleroderma) and Raynaud phenomenon. *Medicine* 59:393–408, 1980.
25. Sharp GC, Irvin WS, Tan EM, et al: Mixed connective tissue disease: An apparently distinct rheumatic disease syndrome associated with a specific antibody to an extractable nuclear antigen (ENA). *Am J Med* 52:148–159, 1972.
26. Sharp GC, Anderson PC: Current concepts in the classification of connective tissue diseases: Overlap syndromes and mixed connective tissue disease. *J Am Acad Dermatol* 2:269–279, 1980.
27. Chanda JJ, Callen JP, Taylor WB: Diffuse fasciitis with eosinophilia. *Arch Dermatol* 114:1522–1524, 1978.
28. Falanga V, Medsger TA Jr: Frequency, levels, and significance of blood eosinophilia in systemic sclerosis, localized scleroderma, and eosinophilic fasciitis. *J Am Acad Dermatol* 17:648–656, 1987.
29. Dunger DB, Dicks-Mireaux C, O'Driscoll P, et al: Two cases of Winchester syndrome: With increased urinary oligosaccharide excretion. *Eur J Pediatr* 146:615–619, 1987.
30. Oikarinen A, Palatsi R, Kylmaniemi M, et al: Pachydermoperiostosis: Analysis of the connective tissue abnormality in one family. *J Am Acad Dermatol* 31:947–953, 1994.
31. Friedman SJ, Doyle JA: Sclerodermoid changes of porphyria cutanea tarda: Possible relationship to urinary uroporphyrin levels. *J Am Acad Dermatol* 13:70–74, 1985.
32. Parks DL, Perry HO, Muller SA: Cutaneous complications of pentazocine injections. *Arch Dermatol* 104:231–235, 1971.
33. Mountz JD, Downs Minor MB, Turner R, et al: Bleomycin-induced cutaneous toxicity in the rat: Analysis of histopathology and ultrastructure compare with progressive systemic sclerosis (scleroderma). *Br J Dermatol* 108:679–686, 1983.
34. Janin-Mercier A, Mosser C, Souteyrand P, Bourges M: Subcutaneous sclerosis with fasciitis and eosinophilia after phytonadione injections. *Arch Dermatol* 121:1421–1423, 1985.
35. Sanders MN, Winkelmann RK: Cutaneous reactions to vitamin K. *J Am Acad Dermatol* 19:699–704, 1988.
36. Spiera H: Scleroderma after silicone augmentation mammoplasty. *JAMA* 260:236–238, 1988.
37. Meyerson LB, Meier GC: Cutaneous lesions in acroosteolysis. *Arch Dermatol* 106:224–227, 1972.
38. Markowitz SS, McDonald CJ, Fethiere W, Kerzner MS: Occupational acroosteolysis. *Arch Dermatol* 106:219–223, 1972.
39. Hood AF, Soter NA, Rappeport J, Gigli I: Graft-versus-host reaction. *Arch Dermatol* 113:1087–1091, 1977.
40. Chosidow O, Bagot M, Vernant JP, et al: Sclerodermatous chronic graft-versus-host disease. *J Am Acad Dermatol* 26:49–55, 1992.

41. Iglesias JL, De Moragas JM: The cutaneous lesions of the Spanish toxic oil syndrome. *J Am Acad Dermatol* 9:159–160, 1983.

42. Martinez-Tello FJ, Navas-Palacios JJ, Ricoy JR, et al: Pathology of a new toxic syndrome caused by ingestion of adulterated oil in Spain. *Virchows Arch [A]* 397: 261–285, 1982.

43. Silver RM: The eosinophilia-myalgia syndrome. *Clin Dermatol* 12:457–465, 1994.

44. Oursler JR, Farmer ER, Roubenoff R, et al: Cutaneous manifestations of the eosinophilia-myalgia syndrome. *Br J Dermatol* 127:138–146, 1992.

45. Guerin SB, Schmidt JJ, Kulik JE, Golitz LE: L-Tryptophan syndrome: Histologic features of scleroderma-like skin changes. *J Cutan Pathol* 19:207–211, 1992.

46. Nova MP, Kaufman M, Halperin A: Scleroderma-like skin indurations in a child with phenylketonuria: A clinicopathologic correlation and review of the literature. *J Am Acad Dermatol* 26:329–333, 1992.

47. Perry HO: Diseases that present as cutaneous sclerosis. *Aust J Dermatol* 23:45–52, 1982.

48. Patterson JAK, Ackerman AB: Lichen sclerosus et atrophicus is not related to morphea. *Am J Dermatopathol* 6:323–335, 1984.

49. Meyrick Thomas RH, Ridley CM, Black MM: The association of lichen sclerosus et atrophicus and autoimmune-related disease in males. *Br J Dermatol* 109:661–664, 1983.

50. Meyrick Thomas RH, Ridley CM, McGibbon DH, Black MM: Lichen sclerosus et atrophicus and autoimmunity: A study of 350 women. *Br J Dermatol* 118:41–46, 1988.

51. Mihara V, Mihara M, Hagari Y, Shimao S: Lichen sclerosus et atrophicus: A histological, immunohistochemical and electron microscopic study. *Arch Dermatol Res* 286: 434–442, 1994.

52. Uitto J, Santa Cruz DJ, Eisen AZ: Connective tissue nevi of the skin. *J Am Acad Dermatol* 3:441–461, 1980.

53. Uitto J, Santa Cruz DJ, Eisen AZ: Familial cutaneous collagenoma: Genetic studies on a family. *Br J Dermatol* 101:185–195, 1979.

54. Atherton DJ, Wells RS: Juvenile elastoma and osteopoikilosis (the Buschke-Ollendorf syndrome). *Clin Exp Dermatol* 7:109–113, 1982.

55. Pierard GE, Lapiere CM: Nevi of connective tissue: A reappraisal of their classification. *Am J Dermatopathol* 7:325–333, 1985.

56. Ketchum LD: Hypertrophic scars and keloids. *Clin Plast Surg* 4:301–310, 1977.

57. Ackerman AB, Ragaz A: The lives of lesions, in *Chronology in Dermatopathology*. New York, Masson, 1984:58–61.

58. Zheng P, Lavker RM, Kligman AM: Anatomy of striae. *Br J Dermatol* 112:185–193. 1985.

59. Tsuji T, Sawabe M: Elastic fibers in striae distensae. *J Cutan Pathol* 15:215–222, 1988.

60. Lacour JPH, Maquart FX, Bellon G, et al: Fibroblastic rheumatism: Clinical, histological, immunohistological, ultrastructural and biochemical study of a case. *Br J Dermatol* 128:194–202, 1993.

61. Vignon-Pennamen M-D, Naveau B, Foldes C, et al: Fibroblastic rheumatism. *J Am Acad Dermatol* 14:1086–1088, 1986.

62. Lister DM, Graham-Brown RAC, Burns DA, et al: Collagenosis nuchae: A new entity? *Clin Exp Dermatol* 13:263–264, 1988.

63. Frieden IJ: Aplasia cutis congenita: A clinical review and proposal for classification. *J Am Acad Dermatol* 14:646–660, 1986.

64. Harari Z, Pasmanik A, Dvoretzky I, et al: Aplasia cutis congenita with dystrophic nail changes. *Dermatologica* 153:363–368, 1976.

65. Staughton RCD: Focal dermal hypoplasia (Goltz's syndrome) in a male. *Proc R Soc Med* 69:232–233, 1976.

66. Goltz RW, Henderson RR, Hitch JM, Ort JE: Focal dermal hypoplasia syndrome: A review of the literature and report of two cases. *Arch Dermatol* 101:1–11, 1970.

67. Howell JB, Freeman RG: Cutaneous defects of focal dermal hypoplasia: An ectomesodermal dysplasia syndrome. *J Cutan Pathol* 16:237–258, 1989.

68. Magid ML, Prendiville JS, Esterly NB: Focal facial dermal dysplasia: Bitemporal lesions resembling aplasia cutis congenita. *J Am Acad Dermatol* 18:1203–1207, 1988.

69. Raque CJ, Stein KM, Lane JM, Reese EC Jr: Pseudoainhum constricting bands of the extremities. *Arch Dermatol* 105:434–438, 1972.

70. Rivers JK, Duke EE, Justus DW: Etretinate: Management of keratoma hereditaria mutilans in four family members. *J Am Acad Dermatol* 13:43–49, 1985.

71. Rand R, Baden HP: Keratosis follicularis spinulosa decalvans: Report of two cases and literature review. *Arch Dermatol* 119:22–26, 1983.

72. Stevanovic DV: Corticosteroid-induced atrophy of the skin with telangiectasia. *Br J Dermatol* 87:548–556, 1972.

73. Fritsch WC: Deep atrophy of the skin of the deltoid area *Arch Dermatol* 101:585–587, 1970.

74. Berman A, Berman GD, Winkelmann RK: Atrophoderma (Pasini-Pierini): Findings on direct immunofluorescent, monoclonal antibody, and ultrastructural studies. *Int J Dermatol* 27:487–490, 1988.

75. Miller RF: Idiopathic atrophoderma: Report of a case and nosologic study. *Arch Dermatol* 92:653–660, 1965.

76. Mehregan AH, Schwartz OD, Livingood CS: Reactive perforating collagenosis. *Arch Dermatol* 96:277–282, 1967.

77. Detlefs RL, Goette DK: Collagenome perforant verruciforme. *Arch Dermatol* 122:1044–1046, 1986.

78. Burns DA, Calnan CD: Chondrodermatitis nodularis antihelicis. *Clin Exp Dermatol* 3:207–208, 1978.

79. Hurwitz RM: Painful papule of the ear: A follicular disorder. *J Dermatol Surg Oncol* 13:270–274, 1987.

80. Sidhu-Malik NK, Wenstrup RJ: The Ehlers-Danlos syndrome and Marfan syndrome: Inherited diseases of connective tissue with overlapping clinical features. *Semin Dermatol* 14:40–46, 1995.

81. Pope FM, Nicholls AC, McPheat J, et al: Collagen genes and proteins in osteogenesis imperfecta. *J Med Genet* 22:466–478, 1985.

82. Dietz HC, McIntosh I, Sakai LY, et al: Four novel FBN1 mutations: Significance for mutant transcript level and EGF-like domain calcium binding in the pathogenesis of Marfan syndrome. *Genomics* 17:468–475, 1993.

83. Beauregard S, Gilchrest BA: Syndromes of premature aging. *Dermatol Clin* 5:109–121, 1987.

84. Arakawa M, Hatamochi A, Takeda K, Ueki H: Increased collagen synthesis accompanying elevated m-RNA levels in cultured Werner's syndrome fibroblasts. *J Invest Dermatol* 94:187–190, 1990.

85. Sephal GC, Sturrock A, Giro MG, Davidson JM: Increased elastin production by progeria skin fibroblasts is controlled by the steady-state levels of elastin mRNA. *J Invest Dermatol* 90:643–647, 1988.

86. Jimbow K, Kobayashi H, Ishii M, et al: Scar and keloidlike lesions in progeria. *Arch Dermatol* 124:1261—1266, 1988.

87. De Groot WP, Tafelkruyer J, Woerdeman MJ: Familial acrogeria (Gottron). *Br J Dermatol* 103:213–223, 1980.

88. Pope FM, Nicholls AC, Narcici P, et al: Type III collagen mutations in Ehlers-Danlos syndrome type IV and other related disorders. *Clin Exp Dermatol* 13:285–302, 1988.

89. Uitto J, Olsen DR, Fazio MJ: Extracellular matrix of the skin: 50 years of progress. *J Invest Dermatol* 92:61S–77S, 1989.

90. Uitto J, Fazio M, Kahari V-M: Elastic fibers, in Lapiere CM, Kreig T (eds): *Connective Tissue Diseases in the Skin* (Clinical Dermatology Series No 9). New York, Marcel Dekker, 1993:31.

91. Madri JA, Dise CA, LiVolsi VA, et al: Elastofibroma dorsi: An immunochemical study of collagen content. *Hum Pathol* 12:186–190, 1981.

92. Schwarz T, Oppolzer G, Duschet P, et al: Ulcerating elastofibroma dorsi. *J Am Acad Dermatol* 21:1142–1144, 1989.

93. Mehregan AH: Elastosis perforans serpiginosa: A review of the literature and report of 11 cases. *Arch Dermatol* 97:381–393, 1968.

94. White CR Jr: The dermatopathology of perforating disorders. *Semin Dermatol* 5: 359–366, 1986.

95. Pope FM: Historical evidence for the genetic heterogeneity of pseudoxanthoma elasticum. *Br J Dermatol* 92:493–509, 1975.

96. Mendelsohn G, Bulkley BH, Hutchins GM: Cardiovascular manifestations of pseudoxanthoma elasticum. *Arch Pathol Lab Med* 102:298–302, 1978.

97. Nakayama H, Hashimoto K, Kambe N, Eng A: Elastic globes: Electron microscopic and immunohistochemical observations. *J Cutan Pathol* 15:98–103, 1988.

98. Brennan TE, Pearson RW: Abnormal elastic tissue in cartilage-hair hypoplasia. *Arch Dermatol* 124:1411–1414, 1988.

99. Taylor CR, Stern RS, Leyden JJ, Gilchrest BA: Photoaging/photodamage and photoprotection. *J Am Acad Dermatol* 22:1–15, 1990.

100. Danielson L, Kobayasi T: Degeneration of dermal elastic fibres in relation to age and light-exposure: Preliminary report on electron microscopic studies. *Acta Derm Venereol (Stockh)* 52:1–10, 1972.

101. Ledoux-Corbusier M, Achten G: Elastosis in chronic radiodermatitis: An ultrastructural study. *Br J Dermatol* 91:287–295, 1974.

102. Carter VH, Constantine VS, Poole WL: Elastotic nodules of the antihelix. *Arch Dermatol* 100:282–285, 1969.

103. Weedon D: Elastotic nodules of the ear. *J Cutan Pathol* 8:429–433, 1981.

104. Rahbari H: Acrokeratoelastoidosis and keratoelastoidosis marginalis: Any relation? *J Am Acad Dermatol* 5:348–3350. 1981.

105. Shahrad P, Marks R: The wages of warmth: changes in erythema ab igne. *Br J Dermatol* 97:179–186, 1977.

106. Arrington JH III, Lockman DS: Thermal keratoses and squamous cell carcinoma in situ associated with erythema ab igne. *Arch Dermatol* 115:1226–1228, 1979.

107. Bordas X, Ferrandiz C, Ribera M, Galofre E: Papular elastorrhexis: A variety of nevus anelasticus? *Arch Dermatol* 123:433–434, 1987.

108. Varadi DP, Saqueton AC: Perifollicular elastolysis. *Br J Dermatol* 83:143–150, 1970.

109. Venenci PY, Winkelmann RK, Moore BA: Anetoderma: Clinical findings, associations, and long-term follow-up evaluations. *Arch Dermatol* 120:1032–1039, 1984.

110. Oikarinen AI, Palatsi R, Adomian GE, et al: Anetoderma: Biochemical and ultrastructural demonstration of an elastin defect in the skin of three patients. *J Am Acad Dermatol* 11:64–72, 1984.

111. Schreiber MM, Tilley JC: Cutis laxa. *Arch Dermatol* 84:266–272, 1961.

112. Ledoux-Corbusier M: Cutis laxa, congenital form with pulmonary emphysema: An ultrastructural study. *J Cutan Pathol* 10:340–349, 1983.

113. Mehregan AH, Lee SC, Nabai H: Cutis laxa (generalized elastolysis): A report of four cases with autopsy findings. *J Cutan Pathol* 5:116–126, 1978.

114. Sephel GC, Byers PH, Holbrook KA, Davidson JM: Heterogeneity of elastin expression cutis laxa fibroblast strains. *J Invest Dermatol* 93:147–153, 1989.

115. Kitano Y, Nishida K, Okada N, et al: Cutis laxa with ultrastructural abnormalities of elastic fiber. *J Am Acad Dermatol* 21:378–380, 1989.

116. Menkes JH, Alter M, Steigleder GK, et al: A sex-linked recessive disorder with retardation of growth, peculiar hair, and focal cerebral and cerebellar degeneration. *Pediatrics* 29:764–779, 1962.

117. Hart DB: Menke's syndrome: An updated review. *J Am Acad Dermatol* 9:145–152, 1983.

118. Waldstein G, Mierau G, Ahmad R, et al: Fragile X syndrome: skin elastin abnormalities. *Birth Defects* 23:103–114, 1987.

119. Convit J, Kerdel F, Goihman M, et al: Progressive, atrophying, chronic granulomatous dermohypodermitis. *Arch Dermatol* 107:271–274, 1973.

120. LeBoit PE, Beckstead JH, Bond B, et al: Granulomatous slack skin: Clonal rearrangement of the T-cell receptor B gene is evidence for the lymphoproliferative nature of a cutaneous elastolytic disorder. *J Invest Dermatol* 89:183–186, 1987.

121. Matsuoka LY, Wortsman J, Uitto J, et al: Altered skin elastic fibers in hypothyroid myxedema and pretibial myxedema. *Arch Intern Med* 145:117–121, 1985.

122. Roth SI, Schedewie HK, Herzberg VK, et al: Cutaneous manifestations of leprechaunism. *Arch Dermatol* 117:531–535, 1981.

CHAPTER 18

ECTOPIC TISSUE

Jacqueline Junkins-Hopkins / Raymond L. Barnhill

A specimen submitted to the dermatopathologist or pathologist with the clinical diagnosis of tag or nodule may, on occasion, have histologic features which may be normal or characteristic, but not *for a particular location*. Such a lesion could be considered *ectopic* (from the Greek *ektopos*, meaning "out of place") and may be benign and of no systemic consequence, or it may herald an ongoing or potentially more serious condition. Various types of ectopic tissue and characteristic locations are listed in Table 18-1.

ACCESSORY TRAGUS

Synonyms for *accessory tragus* include *preauricular tag*, *polyotia*, *accessory auricle anomaly*, *rudimentary ear*, *supernumery pinna*, and *wattle*. The tragus is the portion of the external ear derived from the first pharyngeal arch, and accessory tragi are congenital lesions which result from defects in development of this arch.[1] Some synonyms for this anomaly, such as *accessory auricle*, are less appropriate, since the external ear is derived from the second branchial arch.[2]

Clinical Features   Accessory tragi are most commonly located in the preauricular region, slightly above or below the level of the tragus. Rarely, they may present more anteriorly on the cheek along the line of the mandible or on the neck between the sternocleidomastoid muscle and the suprasternoclavicular region.[3] The latter lesions are referred to by some as *wattles*.[4] Accessory tragi typically present as pedunculated soft to cartilagenous papules, may be solitary or multiple, unilateral or bilateral, and are often diagnosed clinically as skin tags. Vellus hairs may cover the surface. The lesions are asymptomatic, unless they become infected or ulcerated. Associated developmental abnormalities of the pharyngeal arch may be seen in at least 5 percent of patients with accessory tragi.[3] Accessory tragi are a consistent feature in Goldenhar's syndrome, which also includes epibulbar dermoids and auricular pits.[1]

Histopathological Features   Histologically, the features are similar to those of the fetal external ear. At scanning magnification, accessory tragi are easily recognized by their polypoid appearance and central core of elastic cartilage present in most specimens (Fig. 18-1). The surface may be smooth or slightly rugated with a thin compact or basket-weave stratum corneum. The papillary dermis consists of collagen intermingled with adipose tissue and dilated vessels. Vellus hair follicles are scattered throughout the papillary dermis (Fig. 18-1). The associated sebaceous glands are hormonally responsive and vary in prominence depending on the age of the patient. Eccrine glands and ducts are often present, although apocrine glands are rarely seen.[3] In rare cases, an associated nevus may be seen.[1]

Differential Diagnosis   An accessory tragus may be confused with a fibroepithelial polyp or a soft fibroma, if cartilage is not present, and a

chondroma if cartilage is included. These lesions would not be present from birth, and the multiple vellus hairs and other associated adenexal structures support the diagnosis of an accessory tragus.

ACCESSORY NIPPLE

Accessory nipples, also known as *polythelia* or *supernumerary nipples*, may occur as an isolated finding or in association with supernumerary breasts or ectopic breast tissue.[5] Embryologically, the breasts develop from mammary ridges (milk lines) which are thickened areas of ectoderm extending ventrally from the base of the forelimb to the base of the hindlimb. Normally, the breast develops in the pectoral region of the ridge, while the remainder regresses. A variety of anomalies may result from failure of this regression, including supernumerary breasts—complete (polymastia) or incomplete, supernumerary nipples (polythelia), nipple and areola with the gland replaced by fat (pseudomamma), areola alone (polythelia areola), and a patch of hair (polythelia pilosis).[5]

Clinical Features   Supernumerary nipples may be solitary or multiple. The most common site is the left thoracic region inferior to the normal nipple.[5] However, they may be found anywhere along the milk line, i.e., the anterior axillary fold to the inner inguinal fold. Unusual sites include the scapula, posterior aspect of the thigh, face, neck, and labia majora.[6] In infancy, the nipples may be pigmented to pearl-colored macules which may be wrinkled or concave. In adulthood, if not associated with ectopic breast tissue, they may remain macular. However, they may become pigmented or raised, simulating nevi or skin tags.

Accessory nipples, themselves, usually do not pose a problem, unlike polymastia or ectopic breast tissue, which are subject to the same benign and malignant processes that afflict normal breast tissue.[5] The main concern related to supernumerary nipples is the possible association with urologic and possibly other developmental anomalies,[7,8] especially in familial polythelia.[7]

Histopathological Features   Histologically, accessory nipples closely resemble normal breast tissue. These lesions have a characteristic low-power silhouette that is dome-shaped and, if sectioned centrally, umbilicated (Fig. 18-2). The epidermis shows slight papillomatosis and acanthosis and variable hyperpigmentation. These features often involve the nonelevated epidermis and correspond to the areolar portion. Atrichial sebaceous glands and/or mammary ducts may open into the epidermis. The dermis immediately beneath the central portion of the nipple consists of fine bundles of collagen and a decrease in elastic fibers. However, the adjacent aureolar portion exhibits collagen that is similar to normal dermis.[9] Scattered smooth-muscle bundles are characteristic, and these are admixed with multiple vessels and nerves. In most cases, scattered mammary ducts are present in the lower dermis.

TABLE 18-1

Typical Anatomic Sites of Ectopic Tissue

Site	Lesion
Preauricular cheek	Accessory tragus
Lateral chest	Supernumerary nipple
First or fifth digit	Supernumerary/rudimentary digit
Umbilicus	Endometriosis
	Omphalomesenteric/urachal duct remnants
	Metastatic tumors (Sister Joseph's nodule)

Differential Diagnosis   When all the features are present, the diagnosis is straightforward, with the only possible exception being a normal nipple. If only a portion of the specimen is available for study, the differential diagnosis includes a benign keratosis, lentigo, fibroepithelial polyp, or soft fibroma. In the absence of mammary tissue, the presence of multiple smooth-muscle bundles helps to confirm the diagnosis. Atrichial sebaceous glands are also helpful supportive microscopic features. Clinical information would differentiate an accessory nipple from a Becker's nevus or smooth-muscle hamartoma, both of which are characterized by epidermal hyperpigmentation and elongation of epidermal rete ridges overlying smooth-muscle proliferation.

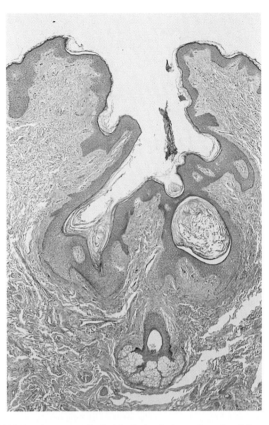

FIGURE 18-2   Accessory nipple. The lesion is dome-shaped and shows central invagination. The central invagination exhibits some papillomatosis and slight epithelial hyperplasia, with atrichial sebaceous glands.

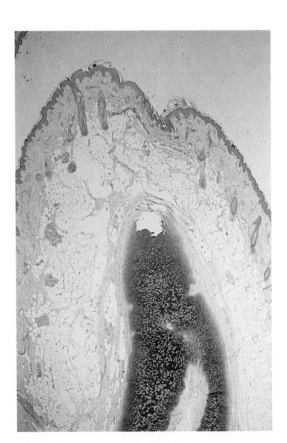

FIGURE 18-1   Accessory tragus. The structure is polypoid with a central core of elastic cartilage. Vellus hairs and adipose tissue are present between the epidermis and cartilage.

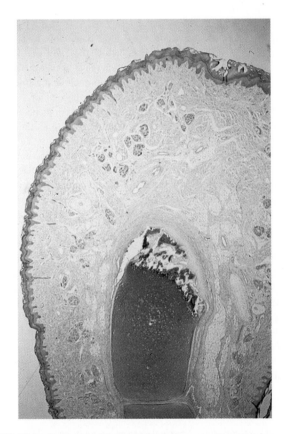

FIGURE 18-3   Supernumerary digit. This bulbous structure contains a central core of cartilage with the presence of a joint and osteoid formation.

SUPERNUMERARY DIGIT

Also known as *polydactyly*, *rudimentary digit*, *rudimentary polydactyly*, *accessory digit*, a supernumerary digit is a relatively common congenital deformity which probably results from the duplication of a single embryologic bud.[10] This deformity has been classified according to the extent of normal components of the digit present.[10] Type I polydactyly describes an extra soft-tissue mass unattached to the underlying skeletal structure, which may variably contain nail, bone, cartilage, or tendons. In type II, some portion of the digit is duplicated with its normal components. Type III consists of a complete digit, including the metacarpal and associated soft tissues. This discussion will be limited to type I polydactyly, which is the type most frequently encountered by dermatopathologists. Rudimentary polydactyly refers to a probable amputation stump of a supernumerary digit, resulting from intrauterine trauma.[11] These lesions may also result from purposeful strangulation during the neonatal period.

Clinical Features Supernumerary digits may occur in a medial (preaxial) or lateral (postaxial) location and may involve the hands or feet. Postaxial polydactyly, which may be autosomal dominantly inherited, is seen frequently in blacks, with an incidence of approximately 1 in 300, versus 1 in 3000 in Caucasians.[10] Often, polydactyly is associated with other anomalies or syndromes.[10,12] The most common site of duplication is the fifth digit, and bilaterality is common.[10] The gross morphology varies depending upon the structural composition of the lesion. Lesions submitted to the dermatopathologist may have a clinical differential which includes a skin tag, wart, fibroma, digital fibrokeratoma, or other similar flesh-colored papules.

Histopathological Features The histologic features correspond to the digital components present. There is compact keratin similar to that of normal acral skin. The epidermis shows elongation of rete ridges and numerous acrosyringeal structures (Fig. 18-3). The usual components of dermis are present along with numerous eccrine apparati. Nerve bundles may be present at the base. A central core of cartilage with or without joint or osteoid formation (Fig. 18-3) and abrupt keratinization, consistent with nail formation, may be present (Fig. 18-4). In what has been referred to as *rudimentary digit*, there is compact hyperkeratosis and rete elongation, similar to polydactyly (Fig. 18-5A and B). Only a few eccrine glands may be present, and the dermis contains numerous nerve bundles associated with mucin and surrounded by perineural sheaths.

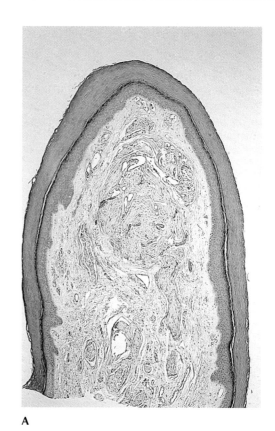

A

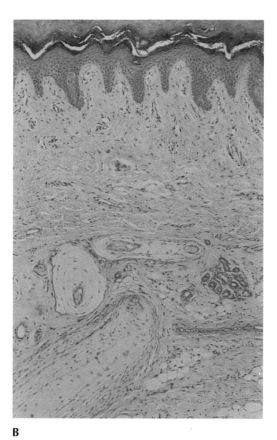

B

FIGURE 18-5 Rudimentary digit. *A*) Scanning magnification. *B*) The epidermis shows elongated rete ridges with compact hyperkeratosis. An eccrine coil and Meissner corpuscle can be observed in the dermis.

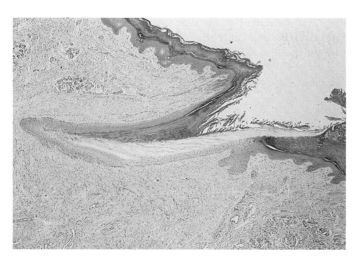

FIGURE 18-4 Supernumerary digit. There is focal nail formation.

Scattered Meissner corpuscles may be seen. Cartilage is not typically present.

Differential Diagnosis If cartilage or bone is present, the diagnosis of a supernumerary digit is not difficult. A skin tag or wart does not contain the adnexal structures or nerve bundles characteristic of a supernumerary digit. An acquired digital fibrokeratoma contains thick vertically oriented collagen bundles devoid of adnexal structures and elastic tissue. The rudimentary digit may be difficult to differentiate from a traumatic neuroma without appropriate clinical history.

ENDOMETRIOSIS

Endometriosis, also known as *endometrioma, menstruating tumor*, is defined as the presence of endometrial tissue outside the uterine cavity and affects up to 10 percent of women of childbearing age.[13] Men on estrogen therapy and postmenopausal women may rarely be affected.[14] Extrapelvic endometriosis may occur in the intestines, skin and subcutaneous tissue, and lung, among other less common sites.[13] Possible mechanisms for endometriosis include: (1) transportation, via tubal regurgitation, surgical manipulation, or hematogenous or lymphatic dissemination, and (2) local dedifferentiation or metaplasia of embryonic celomic mesothelium into endometrial tissue.[15]

Clinical Features Common locations for cutaneous endometriosis include gynecologically induced abdominal or pelvic scars, including episiotomy and laparoscopy scars,[13,14] and the umbilicus, which is involved in up to 1 percent of cases.[15] Nonsurgical related sites of endometriosis include the vulva, perineum, groin, and extremities.[13] Clinical presentations vary. A painful swelling is one of the most common presentations of scar endometriosis.[15] Endometriomas, distinct masses of endometrial tissue, occur in scars and in other sites. They appear as firm nodules ranging from a few millimeters to several centimeters in size and may be flesh-colored or various shades of red, blue, or purple depending on the amount of blood present, the depth of the lesion, and the duration. Waxing and waning pain are characteristic local symptoms. A *menstruating tumor* refers to the rare occurrence of bleeding or secretion from an endometrioma during menses.[12]

Cutaneous endometriosis is often an isolated event; however, occasionally dysmenorrhea, infertility, and other conditions associated with pelvic endometriosis may be seen. Endometrioid carcinoma associated with endometriosis has been reported.[14,15]

Histopathological Features Ectopic endometrial tissue variably responds to the same hormonal fluctuations as eutopic endometrial tissue, and the microscopic features vary accordingly, demonstrating proliferative, secretory, and menstrual changes. Different glandular morphology may be seen within the same specimen.[17] Within the dermis, subcutaneous tissue or muscle are irregular glandular lumina embedded within a cellular and vascular stroma (Fig. 18-6).

The glands are typically lined by columnar, cuboidal, or flat cells, and cystic dilation may be seen. Decapitation secretion characterizes the secretory phase, whereas interluminal erythrocytes and degenerative epithelial cells suggest menstrual changes. Numerous epithelial mitoses may be found in the proliferative phase.[18] The stroma consists of spindled cells admixed with vessels, lymphocytes, histiocytes, and a variable admixture of neutrophils, plasma cells, and mast cells. In the secretory phase, two stromal cell types may be present: a large cell and a small clear cell.[18] Erythrocyte extravasation and scattered hemosiderin deposits, highlighted with Perls' stain, are important diagnostic features. Pseudoxanthoma cells, histiocytic cells containing fine brown-gray pigment representing blood degradation products, are also characteristic.

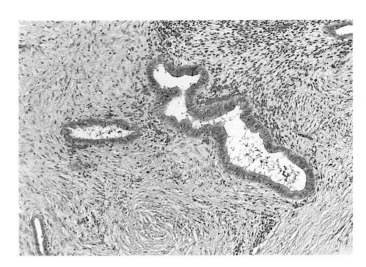

FIGURE 18-6 Endometriosis. There are glandular lumina embedded in a cellular and vascular stroma.

These demonstrate periodic acid–Schiff (PAS) and oil red O positivity characteristic of ceroid (lipofuscin).[17]

Differential Diagnosis The histologic differential diagnosis of cutaneous endometriosis includes ectopic cutaneous endosalpingiosis, a rare condition which may present with periumbilical papules which histologically demonstrate fallopian tube–like epithelium. The latter epithelium is composed of three cell types: ciliated columnar cells; nonciliated columnar, secretory, and mucinous cells; and intercalary dark cells intercalated between the two. Papillary projections into the lumen may be observed. Endosalpingiosis lacks the cellular stroma, hemorrhage, and hemosiderin noted in endometriosis. In addition, endometriosis has fewer ciliated cells.[19] Omphalomesenteric duct remnants, which also have an umbilical location, contain glands lined by gastrointestinal epithelium. Endometrial carcinoma can usually be differentiated from endometriosis by its higher degree of nuclear atypia. Metaplastic changes, such as tubal (ciliary), squamous, hobnail, and mucinous metaplasia, may occur in cutaneous endometriosis, possibly suggesting other metastatic neoplasms. Catamenial symptoms and characteristic stromal changes are helpful in supporting a diagnosis of endometriosis.

Rarely, massively decidualized tissue may be present. The presence of groups of polygonal cells with abundant and often vacuolated cytoplasm floating in pools of mucin and a lack of glandular components may make differentiation from carcinoma difficult. The presence of PAS-negative signet ring–type cells and vimentin-positive and keratin-negative decidual cells and the absence of significant nuclear atypia and mitoses support the diagnosis of myxoid change in decidualized endometriosis over carcinoma.[20]

OMPHALOMESENTERIC DUCT REMNANTS

The omphalomesenteric duct is an embryonic structure which joins the midgut to the yolk sac. Around the fifth week of gestation, this duct becomes incorporated into the umbilical cord, and by the ninth week of gestation, the duct detaches from the midgut and is obliterated.[21,22] Disturbances of this process may result in a variety of anomalies, determined by the portion of the duct which remains (Table 18-2). A combination of these anomalies, individually known as *vitello-intestinal anomaly, umbilical granuloma, umbilical polyp, enteroteratoma*, or *raspberry tumor*, may coexist.

TABLE 18-2

Omphalomesenteric Duct Anomalies

Anomaly	Remnant	Clinical Features
Patent OM* duct	Entire portion, patent	Umbilical-intestinal fistula with feculant, serous, mucous, purulent, or bilious drainage Small bowel umbilical herniation with or without intussusception
OM band	May be entire portion, nonpatent	Volvulus Intussusception (if with Meckel's diverticulum) Asymptomatic
Meckel's diverticulum	Proximal portion: diverticulum in small bowel with or without attachment to abdominal wall	Intussusception Ulceration (especially if ectopic gastric mucosa present) Volvulus
OM polyp	Distal, umbilical portion	Bright red, sticky, umbilicated nodule/polyp May be associated with OM sinus
OM sinus	Distal portion	Sinus of varying depth with or without drainage Often associated with OM polyp
OM cyst	Middle portion, any site	Subcutaneous cyst/nodule Intraabdominal cyst with or without attachment to abdominal wall and intestine GI complications as in Meckel's and OM band

*OM = omphalomesenteric

Clinical Features   Omphalomesenteric duct anomalies occur in approximately 2 percent of the population. The age of presentation ranges from infancy to adulthood. Male predominance has been noted.[22,23] This is particularly true with patent omphalomesenteric duct anomalies, which may also be associated with prematurity and other congenital anomalies. The clinical features of the various anomalies are outlined in Table 18-3. The umbilical lesions tend to be polypoid and range from a few millimeters to a few centimeters in size. Local symptoms include irritation of the overlying or adjacent skin, drainage if a sinus or fistula is present, and, on rare occasions, pain.

The clinical differential diagnosis for umbilical lesions includes pyogenic granuloma, foreign body granuloma, granulation tissue, fibroepithelial polyp, and epithelial inclusion cysts. Except for patent ducts, umbilical omphalomesenteric remnants are generally of minimal consequence. The main concern is to rule out a coexisting intestinal or intraabdominal remnant, which may be associated with fatal consequences.

Histopathological Features   The capacity of the omphalomesenteric remnants to differentiate into all types of enteric epithelium is reflected in the histologic features. The demonstration of ectopic epithelium from any portion of the gastrointestinal tract within an umbilical polyp or lining a cyst, sinus tract, or fistula from this site is sufficient for the diagnosis (Fig. 18-7). Gastric mucosa is recognized by columnar epithelium and the presence of chief, zymogenic, and parietal cells. Brunner's glands and changes of intestinal metaplasia may occasionally be seen. Small intestinal mucosa may be admixed with gastric mucosa and contains goblet cells and submucosal lymphoid follicles. Colonic mucosa contains glandular crypts lined by goblet cells interspersed with colum-

TABLE 18-3

Benign Neoplasms of the Umbilicus*

Melanocytic nevi
Seborrheic keratosis
Epidermal nevus
Endometriosis
Pyogenic granuloma
Epithelial inclusion cyst
Hemangioma
Dermatofibroma
Neurofibroma
Condyloma accuminatum
Granular cell tumor
Teratoma
Keloid
Desmoid tumor
Lipoma

*Adapted from ref. 27.

nar cells. Muscularis layers are present in all mucosal types. Rarely, pancreatic tissue may be observed.[22] The surrounding skin may show various inflammatory and reparative changes due to irritation.

Differential Diagnosis   These lesions need to be differentiated from gastrointestinal carcinoma metastatic to the umbilicus. Endometriosis, which may also occur in the umbilicus, also contains glandular struc-

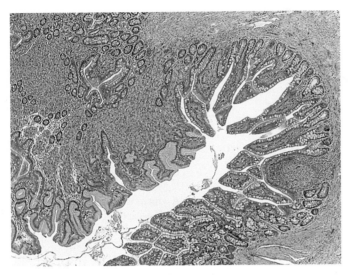

A

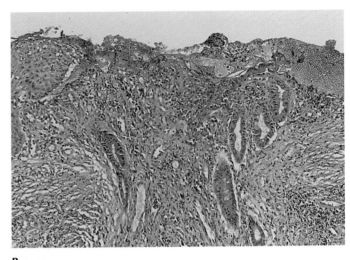

B

FIGURE 18-7 Omphalomesenteric duct remnant. *A*) Note lumen lined by glandular epithelium. *B*) This remnant shows ulceration and gastrointestinal mucosa beneath the area of ulceration.

tures. However, ciliated columnar cells do not predominate, and goblet cells and gastric enzymatic cells are not present.

UMBILICAL LESIONS

The anatomy of the umbilicus makes it vulnerable to numerous inflammatory, anomalous, and malignant conditions. Its crevasse-like nature predisposes it to intertrigo, psoriasis, seborrheic dermatitis, foreign-body granulomas, pilonidal sinus, omphaliths, and infections such as candidiasis and, in neonates, beta-hemolytic streptococcus and staphylococcal aureus. Other dermatoses which have a predilection for the umbilicus include Fabry's disease and herpes gestationis. Numerous benign and malignant neoplasms can also be found in this location (Tables 18-3, 18-4).[24] In infants, pyogenic granulomas are common. In adulthood, melanocytic nevi are frequently seen. The histologic features of these conditions are described elsewhere in this text.

The base of the umbilicus is comprised of the stump of the umbilical cord, which may include remnants of embryologic structures that may give rise to various anomalies. The umbilicus is also richly vascularized with an extensive venous drainage system,[25] and lymphatic channels from the axillary, external, and deep inguinal, and paraaortic lymph nodes pass through the umbilical region,[25–27] allowing exposure to metastatic disease.

Urachal Remnants

The urachus is a tube which extends from the umbilicus to the urinary bladder in the developing fetus. By the fourth or fifth gestational month, the tube atrophies to a fibromuscular cord called the *medial umbilical ligament*.[28] This cord is contained in a preperitoneal fascial space.[29] Persistence of any portion of the urachal duct may result in a variety of anomalies (Table 18-5).

Clinical Features   In the newborn, the most common urachal anomaly is the patent urachal duct, which classically presents with umbilical micturition. Enlargement of the umbilicus or erythema of the umbilical region may also occur.[30] In adulthood, urachal cysts predominate.

TABLE 18-4

Primary Malignant Tumors of the Umbilicus

Basal cell carcinoma
Squamous cell carcinoma
Malignant melanoma
Adenocarcinoma of urachal remnants
Adenocarcinoma of omphalomesenteric duct remnants
Primary papillary psammomatous adenocarcinoma[24]

These frequently become infected and present as an infraumbilical midline mass associated with fever, abdominal pain, and, occasionally, urinary symptoms.[30] A reopening of the canal may then result in purulent umbilical or bladder drainage (alternating sinus).[31] Other less common cutaneous presentations of urachal remnants include umbilical retraction during micturition[30] and a suprapubic sinus.[32,33]

The clinical relevance of urachal remnants pertains to the potential urologic and infectious complications with which they are associated.[28] In addition, malignant degeneration of these remnants may occur.[28,34–37]

TABLE 18-5

Urachal Duct Remnants

Remnant	Anomaly
Entire tubular duct	Patent urachal duct connecting urinary bladder and umbilicus
Superior portion	Urachal sinus with drainage to inferior umbilicus
Inferior portion	Vesicourachal diverticulum
Middle portion	Urachal cyst: usually lower third
Middle portion	Alternating sinus: usually with urachal cyst with intermittent umbilical or bladder drainage

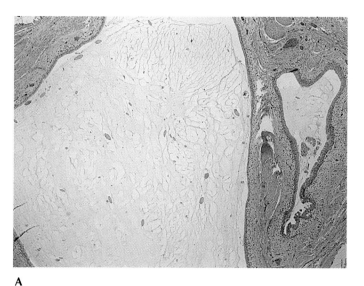
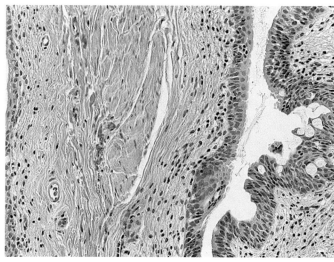

A   B

FIGURE 18-8   Urachal duct remnant. *A*) Large cystic structure with adjacent smaller lumen lined by glandular epithelium. *B*) The luminal structure exhibits both transitional and cuboidal epithelium.

Histopathological Features   Urachal remnants are most readily diagnosed radiologically and rarely present to the dermatopathologist. Occasionally, portions of a remnant may be present at the base of other lesions involving the umbilicus.[38,39] Histologically, the urachus is characterized by three layers: luminal cuboidal or transitional epithelium, submucosal connective tissue, and an outer smooth-muscle layer (Fig. 18-8A and B).[40] In the majority of cases, uroepithelium (cuboidal or transitional cells) is present, but columnar epithelium may occur adjacent to the uroepithelium or alone, at times with papillary projections.[34]

Rarely, malignant degeneration occurs, with the most common neoplasm being adenocarcinoma, but signet ring, transitional, neuroendocrine, and sarcomatous tumors have been reported.[28,34–37]

Differential Diagnosis   With the appropriate clinical information, the diagnosis is straightforward. An omphalomesenteric duct remnant, which frequently has a similar clinical presentation, can be differentiated from urachal processes by the presence of gastrointestinal epithelium rather than uroepithelium. The glands of endometriosis, although they occasionally contain cuboidal epithelium, are distinguished by the associated cellular stroma with scattered areas of hemorrhage and hemosiderin deposition.

Omphalith

An omphalith is an accumulation of compacted keratin and sebaceous material within the umbilicus.

Clinical Features   The umbilical anatomy and poor hygiene are predisposing factors for the development of omphaliths. They typically present as long-standing asymptomatic, black, firm nodules attached to the base of the umbilicus. Discomfort may arise from secondary inflammation or infection of the surrounding skin.[38] Because many clinicians may be unfamiliar with this condition, this lesion may be biopsied to rule out a seborrheic keratosis, epithelial or melanocytic nevus, malignant melanoma, or metastatic carcinoma (Sister Joseph's nodule).

Histopathological Features   Dense laminated keratin is intermingled with sebum, interspersed hair fragments, and clusters of gram-positive

cocci and pleomorphic gram-positive rods. Although the pigment observed clinically is thought to be due, in part, to oxidation of lipids, Fontana Masson positivity suggests the presence of melanin.[38]

Metastatic Disease

As described above, the venous and lymphatic systems of the umbilicus make it subject to metastatic disease. Endometriosis and metastatic disease each account for approximately one-third of umbilical tumors.[41] Metastasis to the umbilicus is an infrequent but unique and ominous condition. Commonly referred to as *Sister (Mary) Joseph's nodule*, after the surgical assistant to Dr. William Mayo who first noted this sign of internal malignancy,[42] these tumors are most frequently associated with stomach and other gastrointestinal carcinomas, including pancreatic and gall bladder, and ovarian carcinoma. Less common neoplasms include other gynecologic malignancies; penile, breast, and renal carcinomas; myeloma[42]; leiomyosarcoma[43]; transitional bladder carcinoma[44]; mesothelioma[45]; vaginal squamous cell carcinoma[46]; liver carcinoma[41]; small cell carcinoma of the lung[47]; and Paget's disease associated with prostate carcinoma.[48]

Clinical Features   Tumors metastatic to the umbilicus typically present as a firm vascular plaque or nodule which may be be ulcerated or fissured and exhibit a mucous or purulent discharge.[43] In some instances, the process may resemble cellulitis.[25] Such tumors may be the first sign of malignancy and usually portend a poor prognosis.

Histopathological Features   The histology varies with the malignancy. In up to 20 percent of cases, the histologic features may be nonspecific.[43]

PILONIDAL SINUS AND FOREIGN BODY GRANULOMA

The pathophysiology of the pilonidal (nest of hair) sinus remains controversial.[49] In most cases, it is an acquired condition in men and characterized by a hair shaft that becomes embedded within the skin and elicits an inflammatory reaction. Factors contributing to this situation include hirsutism and obesity.[50] Hairs are often found perpendicular to the skin surface with the distal end pointing outward and the cuticle scales oriented in a direction that resists outward movement. Negative subcutaneous pressure and a pit or a deep umbilical cleft may promote penetration of the hair.[49–51]

Clinical Features   The umbilicus is a rare site of involvement by a pilonidal sinus, which classically occurs in the sacrococcygeal region. Symptoms may include intermittent pain and purulent drainage. Rarely, malignant degeneration to squamous cell carcinoma may occur.[52]

Histopathological Features   Microscopically, within the dermis, there is a sinus lined by slightly acanthotic keratinizing epithelium, surrounded by dense acute and chronic inflammatory cells, occasional multinucleated giant cells, and a stroma with fibrosis and granulation tissue-type vascular proliferation. The sinus cavity contains hair shafts, keratin, and other debris.

Differential Diagnosis   The differential diagnosis includes a ruptured epidermoid cyst or pilosebaceous unit. In contrast to the latter entities, pilonidal sinuses contain longer hairs unassociated with hair follicles and longer, noncystic sinus tracts.

Other foreign-body reactions should be differentiated from the pilonidal sinus, especially the talc granuloma, a condition now rarely observed in infants following the now obsolete application of talc-containing hexachlorophene powders to the umbilical stump. These present clinically as a nodule or polyp with a denuded granulating surface, indistinguishable from a pyogenic granuloma. Histologically, there is dense fibrous tissue with numerous foreign-body giant cells, many of which contain the doubly refractile crystals of talc. Vascular proliferation, similar to that of a pyogenic granuloma may be seen in association with the foreign-body reaction.[53]

REFERENCES

1. Resnick KI, Soltani K, Bernstein JE, Fathizadeh A: Accessory tragi and associated syndromes involving the first branchial arch. *J Dermatol Surg Oncol* 7:39–41, 1981.
2. Sebben JE: The accessory tragus—No ordinary skin tag. *J Dermatol Surg Oncol* 15:304–307, 1989.
3. Brownstein MH, Wanger N, Helwig EB: Accessory tragi. *Arch Dermatol* 104:625–631, 1971.
4. Christensen P, Barr RJ: Wattle: An unusual congenital anomaly. *Arch Dermatol* 121:22–23, 1985.
5. Velanovich V: Ectopic breast tissue, supernumerary breasts, and supernumerary nipples. *South Med J* 88:903–906, 1995.
6. Cellini A, Offidani A: Familial supernumerary nipples and breasts. *Dermatology* 185:56–58, 1992.
7. Leung AK, Robson WL: Renal anomalies in familial polythelia (letter; comment): *Am J Dis Child* 144:619–620, 1990.
8. Leung AK, Robson WL: Accessory nipples and urinary tract malformation (to the editor). *Pediatr Dermatol* 10(3):300–301, 1993.
9. Mehregan AH: Supernumerary nipple: A histologic study. *J Cutan Pathol* 8:96–104, 1981.
10. Dobyns JH, Wood VE, Bayne LG, Frykman GK: Congenital hand deformities, in Green DP (ed): *Operative Hand Surgery.* New York, Churchill Livingstone, 1982, pp. 213–450.
11. Chung J, Nam IW, Ahn SK, et al: Rudimentary polydactyly. *J Dermatol* 21:54–55, 1994.
12. Coppolelli BG, Ready JE, Awbrey BJ, Smith LS: Polydactyly of the foot in adults: Literature review and unusual case presentation with diagnostic and treatment recommendations. *J Foot Surg* 30(1):12–18, 1991.
13. Albrecht LE, Tron V, Rivers JK: Cutaneous endometriosis. *Int J Dermatol* 34(4):261–262, 1995.
14. Firilas A, Soi A, Max M: Abdominal incision endometriomas. *Am Surg* 60:259–261, 1994.
15. Igawa HH, Ohura T, Sugihara T, et al: Umbilical endometriosis. *Ann Plast Surg* 29:266–268, 1992.
16. Purvis RS, Tyring SK: Cutaneous and subcutaneous endometriosis. *J Dermatol Surg Oncol* 20:693–695, 1994.
17. Clement PB: Pathology of endometriosis. *Pathol Ann* 25:245–295, 1990.
18. Tidman MJ, MacDonald DM: Cutaneous endometriosis: A histopathologic study. *J Am Acad Dermatol* 18:373–377, 1988.
19. Dore N, Landry M, Cadotte MS, Church W: Cutaneous endosalpingiosis: *Arch Dermatol* 116:909–912, 1980.
20. Nogales FF, Martin F, Linares J, et al: Myxoid change in decidualized scar endometriosis mimicking malignancy. *J Cutan Pathol* 20:87–91, 1993.
21. Kamii Y, Zaki AM, Honna T, Tsuchida Y: Spontaneous regression of patient omphalomesenteric duct: From a fistula to Meckel's diverticulum. *J Pediatr Surg* 27:115–116, 1992.
22. Steck WD, Helwig EB: Cutaneous remnants of the omphalomesenteric duct. *Arch Dermatol* 90:463–470, 1964.
23. Benson JM, Sparnon AL: Double intussusception of ileum through a patent vitellointestinal duct: Report of a case and literature review. (Review) *Aust NZ J Surg* 62(5):411–413, 1992.
24. Hernandez N, Medina V, Alvarez-Arguelles H, et al: Primary papillary psammomatous adenocarcinoma of the umbilicus. *Histol Histopathol* 8:593–598, 1993.
25. Raymond PL: The ubiquitous umbilicus: What it can reveal about intra-abdominal disease. *Postgrad Med* 87:175–181, 1990.
26. Majmudar B, Wiskind AK, Croft BN, Dudley AG: The Sister (Mary) Joseph nodule: Its significance in gynecology. *Gynecol Oncol* 40:152–159, 1991.
27. Powell FC, Su WPD: Dermatoses of the umbilicus. *Int J Dermatol* 27(3):150–156, 1988.
28. Binkovitz LA: Case of the month: Urachal carcinoma. *Mayo Clin Proc* 68:393–394, 1993.
29. Ward TT, Saltzman E, Chiang S: Infected urachal remnants in the adult: Case report and review. *Clin Infect Dis* 16:26–29, 1993.
30. Rowe PC, Gearhart JP: Retraction of the umbilicus during voiding as an initial sign of a urachal anomaly. *Pediatrics* 91:153–154, 1993.
31. MacNeily AE, Koleilat N, Kiruluta HG, Homsy YL: Urachal abscesses. Protean manifestations, their recognition, and management. *Urology* 40:530–535, 1992.
32. Groff DB: Suprapubic dermoid sinus. *J Pediatr Surg* 28:242–243, 1993.
33. Lawson A, Corkery JJ: Prepubic sinus: An unusual urachal remnant. *Br J Surg* 79:573, 1992.
34. Munichor M, Szvalb S, Cohen H, Bitterman W: Mixed adenocarcinoma and neuroendocrine carcinoma arising in the urachus: A case report and review of the literature. *Eur Urol* 28:345–347, 1995.
35. Chen KT, Workman RD, Rainwater G: Urachal signet-ring cell carcinoma. *Urology* 36:339–340, 1990.
36. Lyth DR, Booth CM: Transitional cell carcinoma of the urachus. *Br J Urol* 65:544–545, 1990.
37. Ravi R: Signet-ring cell carcinoma of urachus: A case report and review of literature. *Arch Esp Urol* 43:927–929, 1990.
38. Swanson SL, Woosley JT, Fleischer AB Jr, Crosby DL: Umbilical mass: Omphalith. *Arch Dermatol* 128:1267–1270, 1992.
39. Thompson NP, Stoker DL, Springall RG: Urachal abscess as a complication of tinea corporis. *Br J Urol* 73:319, 1994.
40. Risher WH, Sardi A, Bolton J: Urachal abnormalitites in adults: The Ochsner experience. *South Med J* 83:1036–1039, 1990.
41. Patel KS, Watkins RM: Recurrent endometrial adenocarcinoma presenting as an umbilical metastasis (Sister Mary Joseph's nodule). *Br J Clin Pract* 46:69–70, 1992.
42. Shetty MR: Metastatic tumors of the umbilicus: A review 1830–1989. *J Surg Oncol* 45:212–215, 1990.
43. Powell FC, Cooper AJ, Massa MC, et al: Sister Mary Joseph's nodule: A clinical and histologic study. *J Am Acad Dermatol* 10:610–615, 1984.
44. Edoute Y, Ben-Haim SA, Malberger E: Umbilical metastasis from urinary bladder carcinoma. *J Am Acad Dermatol* 26(4):656–657, 1992.
45. Chen KT: Malignant mesothelioma presenting as Sister Joseph's nodule: *Am J Dermatopathol* 13:300–303, 1991.
46. Bakri YN, Subhi J, Hashim E, Senoussi M: Umbilical metastasis (Sister Joseph's nodule) from carcinoma of the vagina. *Acta Obstet Gynecol Scand* 70:509–510, 1991.
47. Saito H, Shimokata K, Yamada Y, et al: Umbilical metastasis from small cell carcinoma of the lung. *Chest* 101(1):288–289, 1992.
48. Remond B, Aractingi S, Blanc F, et al: Umbilical Paget's disease and prostatic carcinoma. *Br J Dermatol* 128(4):448–450, 1993.
49. Sondenaa K, Pollard ML: Histology of chronic pilonidal sinus. *APMIS* 103(4):267–272, 1995.
50. Eby CS, Jetton RL: Umbilical pilonidal sinus. *Arch Dermatol* 106:893, 1972.
51. Ohtsuka H, Arashiro K, Watanabe T: Pilonidal sinus of the axilla: Report of five patients and review of the literature. *Ann Plast Surg* 33(3):322–325, 1994.
52. Davis KA, Mock CN, Versaci A, Lentrichia P: Malignant degeneration of pilonidal cysts. (Review) *Am Surg* 60(3):200–204, 1994.
53. McCallum DI, Hall GF: Umbilical granulomata—with particular reference to talc granuloma. *Br J Derm* 83:151–156, 1970.

PART THREE

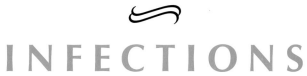

INFECTIONS

CHAPTER 19

BACTERIAL INFECTIONS

Ronald P. Rapini

Definitive diagnosis of most bacterial diseases depends on specific identification of the offending organisms. This must often be accomplished by appropriate cultures because special bacterial stains often fail to demonstrate sparse bacteria at all. Studies of infectious cellulitis show that even cultures yield organisms in less than 10 percent of cases. Culture of actual biopsies has a higher yield than culturing injected saline aspirates. Swab cultures from pustules, ulcers, or crusted lesions are suitable for only the most superficial infections, such as impetigo. An ideal method for deeper infections is to send half of a biopsy for culture, and send the other half for hematoxylin and eosin (H&E) and special stains. Prior to biopsy, excess antiseptic, such as chlorhexidine or povidone-iodine, which might inhibit the culture, should be wiped off the skin. Cultures are best performed on tissue that is rushed to the laboratory before it desiccates. It should be minced and immediately added to the culture media. If there is a chance a biopsy might dry out during transport, it may be placed on sterile gauze soaked in normal saline (without preservatives such as benzyl alcohol).

Even if the organisms are stained, it may be impossible to distinguish between similar pathogens or normal flora. The location of the bacteria is important to note. Gram-positive cocci and coccobacilli, such as staphylococci and *Corynebacteria*, are normal flora within the follicles or secondarily on the surface of crusted, eroded, or ulcerated conditions. By contrast, Gram-positive cocci in the dermis or deeper tissue are indicative of a significant infectious process such as infectious cellulitis (dermis), panniculitis (fat), or fasciitis (fascia). If the follicles are disrupted and infiltrated by neutrophils, then bacteria in the follicles may be pathogenic. They also can be secondary invaders in cases of fungal folliculitis and noninfectious folliculitis; therefore, in such cases it is important for pathologists finding bacteria to consider looking for other etiologic agents and to remember that the primary condition might not even be owing to infection. In immunosuppressed patients, particularly those with acquired immunodeficiency syndrome (AIDS), it is well known that a single biopsy specimen may contain more than one pathogen, so the pathologist should not stop after identifying one organism.[1,2]

Smears or touch preparations from tissue may improve the chances of staining the organisms. This is particularly true of acid-fast bacillus infections, chancroid, and granuloma inguinale, where stains of tissue sections have a lower yield. The Fite modification of the acid-fast bacillus (AFB) stain may be better than the more routine Ziehl-Neelson method, because the Fite has enhanced ability to stain *Mycobacterium leprae* and some of the atypical mycobacteria. The Fite stain also will stain the organisms stained by the other AFB methods. The auramine fluorescent method may also enhance the ability to find AFB.[3] Modifications of the tissue Gram stain, such as Brown-Brenn and Brown-Hopps, are modestly satisfactory for staining Gram-positive organisms in tissue sections, but are poor for demonstrating Gram-negatives. Immunoperoxidase staining methods are available for staining some pathogens, such as certain Rickettsia.[4]

Molecular genetic techniques, such as the polymerase chain reaction (PCR) method, and in situ hybridization are beginning to become commercially available for some organisms, but many of them are available only in research laboratories or at special facilities, such as the Centers for Disease Control and Prevention in Atlanta, Georgia.[5] These methods will be very important in the future because of their exquisite sensitivity, but occasionally there can be false-positive results if careful techniques are not followed in the laboratory.

There are a limited number of histologic patterns seen with bacterial infections in the skin (Table 19-1), and none of them are specific for bacterial infections or for any particular pathogens.[6] Most bacterial infections exhibit neutrophils or plasma cells as valuable etiologic clues. Even though neutrophils or plasma cells may not be numerous, either one or both usually are present in a majority of bacterial infections. Only exceptional examples of infections caused by bacteria, such as Lyme disease, exhibit a predominance of lymphocytes. Even in most cases of Lyme disease, a few scattered plasma cells often are found amongst the lymphocytes. Plasma cells are famous for their presence in secondary syphilis. It is less often appreciated that scattered plasma cells are a clue toward diagnosing the subtle foamy infiltrates of some cases of lepromatous leprosy.

Some bacterial diseases are granulomatous. This is defined as an infiltrate with predominant macrophages, also known as true histiocytes, with or without multinucleated giant cells. Even those bacterial diseases that are well known to be granulomatous (Table 19-1) may be somewhat suppurative (neutrophils prominent) in their early stages. It is important to realize that bacterial diseases evolve with time, just like most other skin conditions, so that the stereotypical histologic presentations emphasized in textbooks such as this one vary according to the age of the lesions.[7]

IMPETIGO

This common superficial bacterial infection occurs most often in children, especially around the mouth, nose, and groin (Table 19-2). It may follow trauma to the skin, such as abrasions or insect bites. The etiologic agents are *Staphylococcus aureus* and *Streptococcus pyogenes*, either alone or together.[8] In rare instances, glomerulonephritis or cellulitis may complicate impetigo.[9] Impetigo is often diagnosed on clinical grounds, with or without culture, so that biopsies are not often performed.

Clinical Features   Lesions characteristically are "honey-color crusts" of acute onset.[10] Certain forms of staphylococci may produce toxins that induce bullous lesions.[11] Mild infections may be self-limited. The usual treatment involves topical mupirocin or oral antibiotics such as cephalexin, erythromycin, or dicloxacillin.

TABLE 19-1

Histological Patterns Seen with Bacterial Infections and Their Differential Diagnosis

Subcorneal pustules	Lyme disease
Impetigo	Lupus erythematosus
Tinea and *Candida*	Rhinoscleroma
Scabies	Leprosy
Psoriasis and subcorneal pustular dermatosis	Necrobiosis lipoidica
Drug eruptions	Folliculitis of many types
Neonatal pustular melanosis	Human immunodeficiency virus infection
Acropustulosis of infancy	Inflammatory conditions of mucous membranes and genitals
Pemphigus (various types)	Many other infections as minor component
Gonococcemia	Granulomatous dermatitis
Mucha-Habermann disease	Noninfectious granulomas (see Chapter 6)
Late stages of intraepidermal blistering diseases	Acid-fast bacillus infections (atypical, tuberculosis, leprosy)
Pseudoepitheliomatous diseases listed herein	Deep fungal infections
Dermal neutrophils	Syphilis and yaws
Infectious cellulitis (bacterial or fungal)	Granuloma inguinale and lymphogranuloma venereum
Infectious vasculitis (especially Rickettsia, gonococcemia, meningococcemia)	Tularemia and brucellosis
Noninfectious vasculitis	Leishmaniasis
Dermatitis herpetiformis	Granulomatous dermatitis with pseudoepitheliomatous hyperplasia and intraepithelial microabscesses
Bullous lupus erythematosus	Botryomycosis
Pemphigoid (sometimes)	Acid-fast bacillus infections
Areas of necrosis attract neutrophils	Deep fungal infections
Inflamed cysts or follicles	Halogenodermas (bromoderma, iododerma)
Granuloma faciale	Pyoderma vegetans
Urticaria	Pemphigus vegetans
Neutrophilic eccrine hidradenitis	Foamy infiltrates
"Neutrophilic dermatoses" (must exclude infection)	Leprosy
Sweet's syndrome	Leishmaniasis
Behçet's syndrome	Atypical mycobacteria
Pyoderma gangrenosum	Xanthomas of many types
Erythema elevatum diutinum	Histiocytosis X
Rheumatoid neutrophilic dermatitis	Panniculitis
Bowel bypass syndrome	Granular cell tumor (more granular than foamy)
Plasma cells in inflammatory conditions	Some neoplasms (such as atypical fibroxanthoma, hibernoma, liposarcoma, balloon cell nevus and melanoma, sebaceous cell tumors)
Syphilis, yaws, pinta	
Granuloma inguinale	

Histopathological Features Subcorneal pustules are present in the subcorneal zone (Figs. 19-1 and 19-2) (Table 19-2).[12] As with any subcorneal pustules, occasional acantholytic keratinocytes may be found. Sometimes Gram-positive cocci may be identified. The epidermis may be spongiotic. The dermal infiltrate usually is perivascular lymphocytes and neutrophils.

Differential Diagnosis Other conditions that may produce subcorneal pustules are listed in Table 19-1. Most can be eliminated mainly on clinical grounds, but in some cases cultures or fungal stains may be needed. If acantholytic cells are prominent, pemphigus foliaceus or erythematosus may cause confusion, and can be identified with direct immunofluorescence. Occasional cases of impetigo have been reported with a confusing positive immunofluorescence pattern similar to pemphigus. Positive identification of organisms by histology or culture does not exclude the possibility of secondary impetiginization of another dermatologic condition.

ECTHYMA

Clinical Features In this variant of impetigo, patients present with punched-out crusted excavations of the skin (Table 19-2), usually caused by *Streptococcus pyogenes*.

Histopathological Features A crust is present within the ulceration. Gram-positive cocci may be present.

Differential Diagnosis Ecthyma can be confused with any secondarily impetiginized ulceration.

ECTHYMA GANGRENOSUM

The adjective "gangrenosum" on the end of the word "ecthyma" generally refers to severe disseminated ulcerative lesions in very ill patients

TABLE 19-2

Impetigo and Ecthyma

Clinical Features

"Honey-colored" crusted lesions, usually acute onset
Bullae in "bullous impetigo"
Ulceration in "ecthyma"
Children more commonly affected
Paranasal, axilla, groin are common sites

Histopathological Features

Subcorneal pustule filled with neutrophils and sometimes occasional
  acantholytic cells
Subcorneal bullae in bullous form, with few inflammatory cells
Ulceration in ecthyma
Sometimes Gram-positive cocci found in the pustule or on the
  surface of crusts or ulcers
Variable dermal infiltrate (usually sparse)

Differential Diagnosis

Other diseases with subcorneal pustules (see Table 19-1)
Pemphigus foliaceus and erythematosus

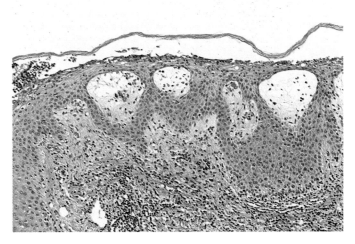

FIGURE 19-2   Bullous impetigo. Subcorneal blister containing few neutrophils and acantholytic keratinocytes. Prominent papillary dermal edema.

owing to sepsis with *Pseudomonas aeruginosa.*[13,14] This type of sepsis often occurs in those who are immunosuppressed from a wide variety of causes, and the condition often is fatal.

Clinical Features   The ulcers may start out as red macules, bullae, or pustules, but eventually they become covered with black eschars.

Histopathological Features   In most cases, the most striking change is extensive necrosis or ulceration of the epidermis, with infarction of the dermis (Fig. 19-3). The inflammatory infiltrate usually is sparse lymphocytes or neutrophils, sometimes with vessel wall changes compatible with vasculitis. The Gram-negative bacilli sometimes may be seen swarming in the dermis in huge numbers as subtle light blue rods with routine H&E staining.

Differential Diagnosis   Cultures or special stains allow a definitive diagnosis. Extensive necrosis of the epidermis may occur in toxic epidermal necrolysis and in herpes simplex. Extensive dermal infarction is common with pyoderma gangrenosum and certain deep fungal infections, such as *Mucor, Rhizopus, Aspergillus,* and *Fusarium,* but hyphae are demonstrated with special stains.

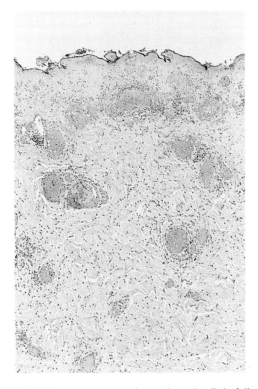

FIGURE 19-3   Ecthyma gangrenosum in a patient who died of disseminated intravascular coagulation. Epidermis and dermis are pale because of necrosis and infarction. There are numerous thrombi and only sparse inflammation.

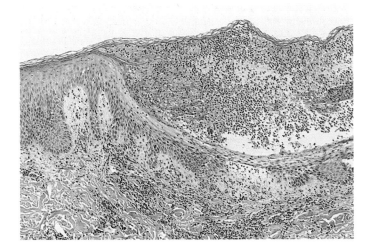

FIGURE 19-1   Impetigo. Subcorneal pustule containing neutrophils and occasional acantholytic keratinocytes.

STAPHYLOCOCCAL SCALDED SKIN SYNDROME

Staphylococcal "scalded skin" syndrome (SSSS), also known as Ritter's disease, is a generalized systemic illness, caused by strains of *Staphylococcus aureus* (phage group II) that produce an exfoliative exotoxin.[15]

Clinical Features   The disease most commonly affects children under the age of 5 years (Table 19-3). It is rare in adults, and most adults with the disease are immunosuppressed or have renal insufficiency, probably lacking an ability to excrete the toxin.[16,17] Patients develop mild constitutional symptoms while the facial skin becomes red, as in scarlet fever, eventually becoming superficially blistered.[18] The trunk and extremities usually are involved later. Conjunctivitis is common. Flaccid bullae with fragile roofs develop, leaving denuded skin after friction causes expansion of the blisters (Nikolsky's sign). The eruption is self-limited, resolving in a few weeks without scarring. A variant known as staphylococcal scarlet fever differs in that the bright red erythroderma becomes desquamative instead of producing the blistering seen with SSSS.

Histopathological Features   The blistering is at the subcorneal zone through the granular layer (Fig. 19-4). There is often very little inflammation, and epidermal necrosis generally is not seen. Acantholytic keratinocytes may be present. Dermal edema may be present.

Differential Diagnosis   Toxic epidermal necrolysis (TEN, Lyell's disease) usually is drug induced, is more common in adults, and involves full-thickness epidermal necrosis instead of the more superficial subcorneal peeling seen with SSSS. TEN is more likely to involve mucous membranes, and is more serious. The distinction usually is apparent clinically, but sometimes this can be an indication for a quick frozen section. An invasive biopsy is not necessary, as a frozen section easily can be prepared by rolling up some of the sloughed skin to determine the depth of separation. Bullous impetigo differs in that the site of the proliferation of the bacteria is in the skin, whereas in SSSS it is generally at remote sites such as the nose, conjunctiva, groin, or even in the blood of very sick patients. Kawaski's disease and toxic shock syndrome mainly differ by their clinical presentation.

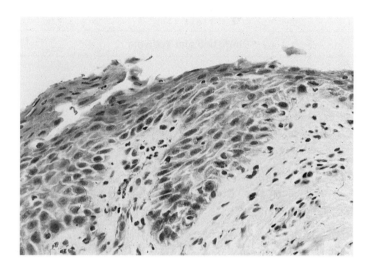

FIGURE 19-4   Staphylococcal scalded skin syndrome. Sloughing of the stratum corneum, with acantholytic keratinocytes. Sparse lymphocytic dermal infiltrate.

TOXIC SHOCK SYNDROME

This rare syndrome was first described in the late 1970's as an acute illness owing to *Staphylococcus aureus* (phage group I) toxin. Most cases at that time were caused by intravaginal growth of the bacteria in tampons.[19,20] At present, about 45 percent of cases are nonmenstrual, and the sites of growth of bacteria in those cases include abscesses, empyema, osteomyelitis, or surgical wound infections.[21] Certain strains of *Streptococcus pyogenes* also cause a toxic shock syndrome and the closely related scarlet fever.[8,22–25] Many of the toxic effects are thought to be owing to bacterial toxins and various cytokines, such as interleukin-1 and tumor necrosis factor.[18]

Clinical Features   Patients become acutely ill with high fever, a generalized sunburnlike rash that eventually desquamates (especially on the palms and soles), hypotension, and involvement of at least three or more organ systems (Table 19-4).

Histopathological Features   Histology is not crucial in making the diagnosis, since the syndrome is mainly defined by clinical features and the culture of the bacteria. Biopsies of skin may show nonspecific changes observed with any "toxic erythema" such as spongiosis, exocytosis of lymphocytes and neutrophils, necrotic keratinocytes, intraepithelial microabscesses, perivascular dermal inflammation with lymphocytes, neutrophils, and extravasated erythrocytes.

Differential Diagnosis   Toxic shock syndrome may resemble streptococcal scarlet fever, Rocky Mountain spotted fever, meningococcemia, toxic epidermal necrolysis, Kawasaki's syndrome, staphylococcal scalded skin syndrome, and drug eruptions.

ERYSIPELAS

Clinical Features   Erysipelas is a special type of infectious cellulitis that occurs most commonly on the face, with a more demarcated rapidly advancing red elevated margin.[26,27] There may be enough edema as to produce vesicles or bullae. It is owing to *Streptococcus pyogenes* and rarely other streptococci or *Staphylococcus aureus*. As with other forms of cellulitis, the organisms may be difficult to demonstrate or culture.

TABLE 19-3

Staphylococcal "Scalded Skin" Syndrome

Clinical Features

   Superficial peeling of bright red skin
   Head and neck most common
   Children usually
   Constitutional symptoms, usually acute onset
   Occult source of staphylococci in nonlesional sites (conjunctiva, nares, groin, blood, etc.)

Histopathological Features

   Pauci-inflammatory subcorneal blister that may contain few acantholytic keratinocytes
   Minimal perivascular inflammatory infiltrate
   Bacteria not present in lesional skin

Differential Diagnosis

   Pemphigus erythematosus or foliaceus
   Toxic epidermal necrolysis (clinical)
   Kawasaki's disease

TABLE 19-4

Toxic Shock Syndrome

Clinical Features

Acute onset systemic illness
Toxin-producing staphylococci or streptococci at remote sites (tampons, surgical wound, etc.)
Fever, hypotension, involvement of other organs
Bright red diffuse patches that later desquamate

Histopathological Features

Spongiosis, necrotic keratinocytes
Perivascular inflammation

Differential Diagnosis

Cellulitis
Exfoliative erythroderma
Erythema multiforme and toxic epidermal necrolysis
Drug eruption
Streptococcal scarlet fever and toxic shock–like syndrome
Kawasaki's disease
Meningococcemia
Rocky Mountain spotted fever
Staphylococcal scalded skin syndrome

Constitutional symptoms, such as fever, malaise, headache, and vomiting, may occur. Erysipelas is prone to recurrence.

Histopathological Features   The histology is similar to any other examples of cellulitis, discussed later, but dermal edema and lymphatic dilation often is exceptionally prominent, even to the point of subepidermal blister formation. Fibrosis may occur in recurrent cases.

Differential Diagnosis   Erysipelas may clinically resemble many other inflammatory conditions, such as lupus erythematosus, seborrheic dermatitis, rosacea, photodrug reactions, and contact dermatitis. Most of these do not cause fever or diffuse infiltration of the dermis by neutrophils. Other causes of infectious cellulitis may be similar histologically, but the difference depends on the demonstration of the offending agent by various methods described in the introduction to this chapter. Other diseases with diffuse infiltration of the dermis by neutrophils are listed in Table 19-1.

ERYSIPELOID

This is a relatively rare cellulitis owing to the Gram-positive bacillus *Erysipelothrix rhusiopathiae* (*E. insidiosa*). Although it grows in routine culture medias, definitive identification is dependent on the clinician's alerting the laboratory to the possibility of the isolation of this organism, which otherwise may resemble streptococci and diphtheroids. The culture is best made from a skin biopsy taken from the advancing edge of the cellulitis.

Clinical Features   Erysipeloid is mainly seen arising on the hands and fingers of those who are injured after handling fish or other animal products. A purplish macule may develop at the site of injury. The lesions are otherwise erythematous macules or slightly elevated plaques as with other forms of cellulitis, but there tends to be a central pallor or clearing and a slowly advancing edge. Constitutional symptoms are less common than with cellulitis owing to streptococci and staphylococci.

Lymphangitis and lymphadenitis are rare. In rare cases, endocarditis may develop.[28] If untreated, erysipeloid tends to spontaneously resolve within 3 weeks, although relapse may occur.

Histopathological Features   Biopsies of erysipeloid are similar to other examples of infectious cellulitis, as described later.

Differential Diagnosis   Staphylococcal and streptococcal infections are more common and are similar to erysipeloid histologically. Cultures may allow a distinction, but the treatment often is the same. Other hand infections may be worth considering. Brucellosis typically occurs as erythema, papules, or pustules on the hands of veterinarians who handle infected placentas, or other animal workers. Hand infections with tularemia usually are ulcerated, and occur after contact with infected rabbits, ticks, or occasionally other animals. Since cultures are hazardous, the diagnosis of brucello-sis and tularemia often are made serologically. Both brucellosis and tularemia eventually become more granulomatous than erysipeloid. Anthrax is also more likely to ulcerate; the histology may resemble erysipeloid but the exceptionally large Gram-positive rods usually are numerous and easily demonstrated. Early lesions of orf, milker's nodule, and erythema multiforme may cause some confusion with erysipeloid, but later the clinical manifestations are quite different, and the histology also is much different. Herpetic whitlow also may present initially as erythema, but vesicles form later. The biopsy would show herpetic cytopathic changes, and viral cultures or Tzanck smears may be positive.

BLISTERING DISTAL DACTYLITIS

This is a superficial infection of the anterior fat pad on the volar surface usually of one distal finger by *Streptococcus pyogenes* or *Staphylococcus aureus*.

Clinical Features   Patients present with acute swelling, redness, crusting, and blistering of the finger.[29,30] It is most common in children and adolescents, some of whom have an upper respiratory infection as well.

Histopathological Features   The patients often are not biopsied, since the diagnosis is made from the clinical presentation or by cultures and Gram stains of smears. The histology shows overlapping features of impetigo and cellulitis, depending on the stage of the lesion biopsied. A diffuse dermal neutrophilic infiltrate may extend into adipose tissue. Edema may be prominent enough to produce blistering or pustule formation. Epidermal necrosis may be present.

CELLULITIS

Although cellulitis is loosely defined as inflammation of cellular tissue, the term usually refers to infectious cellulitis, indicating a diffusely spreading infection of the dermis or underlying soft tissues, usually by bacteria. Infections by other agents such as fungi occasionally have been designated cellulitis when they present with the clinical features described in the following. As stated in the introduction to this chapter, the causative organisms may be difficult to identify in many cases despite special stains and cultures of biopsies.[31] Group A streptococci and *Staphylococcus aureus* rank among the more common offenders. *Haemophilus influenzae* causes an uncommon but distinct form of cellulitis in children between 6 months and 3 years of age. Marine vibrios can cause a fulminant form of cellulitis or necrotizing fasciitis after a wound or laceration while swimming.

TABLE 19-5

Infectious Cellulitis

Clinical Features

Bright red erythematous patches or plaques without epidermal
change
Low yield of positive cultures after biopsy
Sharply demarcated raised edge on the facial "erysipelas" variant

Histopathological Features

Diffuse dermal interstitial neutrophils
Dermal edema
Gram stain uncommonly demonstrates bacteria in dermis
Possible epidermal necrosis in later stages if severe

Differential Diagnosis

Other diseases with dermal neutrophils (see Table 19-1)

Clinical Features   The most common presentation is a warm and tender bright red macule or indurated plaque (Table 19-5). Epidermal
changes such as scaling, pustules, and ulcers are not present in most
cases, but may occur in later stages. Fever, chills, and regional lymphadenopathy may occur.

Histopathological Features   Biopsies usually show diffuse infiltration
of the dermis or underlying soft tissue by neutrophils (Figs. 19-5 and
19-6). Edema and extravasation of erythrocytes may be present. The
epidermis is unremarkable except in the later stages, where intraepidermal pustules or necrotic foci may be present.

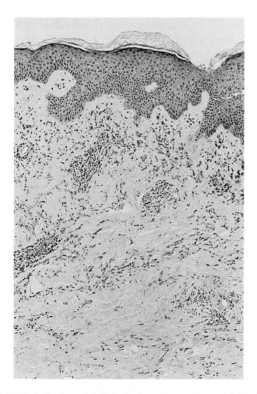

FIGURE 19-5   Infectious cellulitis. Perivascular and interstitial infiltrate of
neutrophils and lymphocytes.

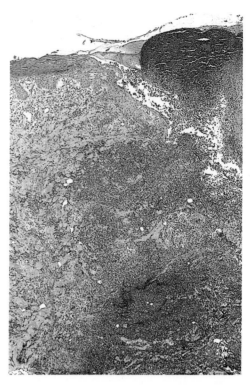

FIGURE 19-6   Staphylococcal furuncle. As in cellulitis, neutrophils are predominant in the dermis, but here they are dense and form a dermal abscess. Most
are centered on follicles, which has been largely destroyed here.

Differential Diagnosis   Erysipelas, described earlier, is considered to
be a variant of cellulitis with a more sharply demarcated elevated
advancing edge. Erysipeloid, also described in the preceding, is another
special type of cellulitis. Other diseases with diffuse dermal infiltration
by neutrophils are described in Table 19-1. The neutrophilic dermatoses
primarily are distinguished by the clinical presentation and negative cultures and special stain.

NECROTIZING FASCIITIS

This is an acute, rapidly progressive deep infection of the fascia and soft
tissue. Initially, it tends to relatively spare the skin and underlying muscle. It usually occurs as a result of an injury, diabetes, alcoholism,
peripheral vascular disease, malignancy, drug abuse, or immunosuppression.[32] The origin of some cases is idiopathic, as it can appear suddenly in young healthy individuals. A variety of different organisms
have been implicated, often growing synergistically. Streptococci,
enterococci, *Staphylococcus aureus*, *Proteus*, and anaerobes such as
Peptostreptococcus, *Bacteroides*, and *Clostridium* are common.[33]
When a mixed infection is present, the term type I necrotizing fasciitis
has been used.[31,34] Meleney's synergistic gangrene is a term used for a
similar type of mixed infection when it occurs in surgical wounds.
Fournier's gangrene is also a related condition involving the scrotum
idiopathically, or following trauma, surgery, urinary infection, appendicitis, or pancreatitis.

Type II necrotizing fasciitis infections are caused by group A streptococci or sometimes *Staphylococcus aureus*.[22,31,34] Some authors have
more strictly defined necrotizing fasciitis as this type only. The lay press
has recently coined the term "flesh-eating bacteria" (usually referring to
Streptococcus) for some of these rapidly progressive infections.[35]

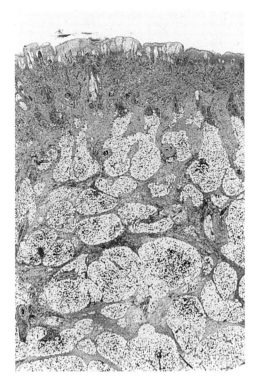

FIGURE 19-7   Necrotizing fasciitis. Epidermal necrosis and perivascular dermal infiltrate. The most striking changes are the fibrosis and diffuse inflammation in the adipose septa and in the fascia.

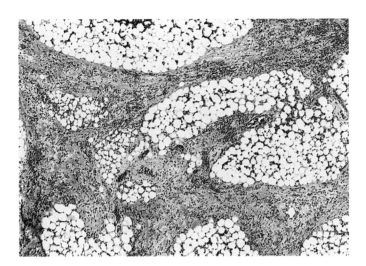

FIGURE 19-8   Necrotizing fasciitis. Higher power of Fig. 19-7 showing diffuse hemorrhage and mixed inflammatory infiltrate in the fibrosing adipose septa and fascia.

A third type of necrotizing fasciitis is the fulminant form caused by marine organisms, such as *Vibrio vulnificans*, *V. parahemolyticus*, and *V. alginolyticus*, either spontaneously or after a puncture wound.[31]

Early antibiotic therapy, aggressive surgical debridement of necrotic tissue, and fasciotomy are important for successful treatment of necrotizing fasciitis.[36] Magnetic resonance imaging and computed tomography scanning may help to determine the depth of tissue necrosis for surgical management.[37,38] The mortality rate is as high as 50 percent.

Clinical Features   Necrotizing fasciitis presents as a rapidly advancing painful indurated erythema, progressing to necrosis, blistering, and ulceration. The abdominal wall, perineum, and extremities are most commonly involved. Anaerobic infections may be foul smelling.

Histopathological Features   There is diffuse infiltration of the soft tissue and fascia with neutrophils and lymphocytes, with areas of necrosis, hemorrhage, and thrombosis (Figs. 19-7 and 19-8). Special stains may reveal organisms.

Differential Diagnosis   Necrotizing fasciitis may initially be confused with any type of panniculitis or deep inflammatory condition, but the rapidly aggressive course makes the diagnosis more obvious. Lupus panniculitis and eosinophilic fasciitis seldom are mistaken for very long. Special stains and cultures are key to the latter distinction.

PYODERMA VEGETANS ("BLASTOMYCOSISLIKE" PYODERMA)

The terminology used for this condition has been confusing. Hallopeau used the term pyoderma vegetans to refer to what is now called pemphigus vegetans, but this is a different disease. Pyoderma vegetans is now used to refer to a vegetating pustular skin reaction to a bacterial infection or as a variant of pyoderma gangrenosum.[39] The most common organism isolated is *Staphylococcus aureus*, and it is often difficult to determine whether it is the primary agent causing the vegetating epithelial proliferation or whether it is a secondary colonizer.[40]

Clinical Features   Verrucous or vegetating plaques with pustules are present. This process may occur anywhere, but the intertriginous areas, face, and legs are most commonly involved.

Histopathological Features   There are pseudoepitheliomatous hyperplasia and intraepithelial and dermal microabscesses (Fig. 19-9). As in pemphigus vegetans, eosinophils may be prominent in the abscesses.

Differential Diagnosis   Other diseases with pseudoepitheliomatous hyperplasia and intraepithelial microabscesses are listed in Table 19-1. Pemphigus vegetans ordinarily will show positive direct immunofluorescent staining, unlike pyoderma vegetans.

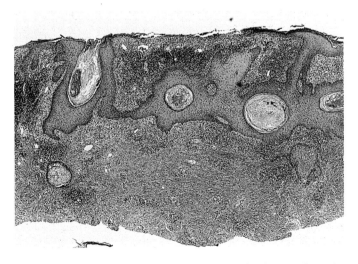

FIGURE 19-9   Blastomycosislike pyoderma. Pseudoepitheliomatous hyperplasia, intraepithelial microabscesses, and diffuse mixed dermal infiltrate.

DIPHTHERIA

Diphtheria is a localized infection of the skin or mucous membrane by the Gram-positive rod *Corynebacterium diphtheriae*.[41] Because of widespread immunization in the United States, the disease is rare, except for imported cases and those in older Americans who have lost their immunity. Since one-fourth to one-half of older adults are susceptible, local outbreaks in the United States have resulted in several hundred to 1000 cases in recent years.[42] The diagnosis is made by alerting the laboratory to use special media to insure isolation of the organism.

Clinical Features   Infection of the tonsils and pharynx results in a characteristic thick gray pseudomembrane. Systemic effects are mostly owing to toxin elaborated by the bacteria. Skin infection is more common in the tropics, but has increasingly been seen in the United States. It is usually a result of secondary infection complicating other skin diseases such as scabies or impetiginized eczema. It can occur almost anywhere on the skin. Punched-out ulcers are a common presentation, often covered with necrotic membranes.

Histopathological Features   Ulcerations contain a prominent amount of fibrin, necrotic material, and neutrophils on the surface. There may be evidence of an underlying skin disease such as scabies or eczema. Special stains may reveal the Gram-positive bacilli.

Differential Diagnosis   Since diphtheria can resemble many cutaneous infections and other dermatoses, a high index of suspicion is necessary so that the appropriate cultures can be obtained.

ERYTHRASMA

This is a superficial infection caused by the Gram-positive coccobacillus *Corynebacterium minutissimum* and possibly other corynebacteria.[43,44]

Clinical Features   Erythematous or brownish-red patches are found in moist intertriginous areas, such as the groin, axillae, inframammary areas, and interdigital spaces between toes (Table 19-6). A slight amount of scale may be present. Most lesions are asymptomatic. A coral-red fluorescence is seen with Wood's light examination (ultraviolet A).

Histopathological Features   Pathologic changes are primarily restricted to the stratum corneum, in which the organisms proliferate without significant host inflammatory response. The coccobacilli and thin bacterial filaments may be barely visible with H&E stain, but are more easily seen with the Gram or Giemsa stains or with electron microscopy.[45]

Differential Diagnosis   Erythrasma may resemble contact dermatitis, nonspecific intertrigo, tinea, *Candida*, and other superficial fungal infections. None of these conditions are characterized by the thin bacterial filaments in the stratum corneum. The organisms of tinea and *Candida* are larger.

TRICHOMYCOSIS

This condition is most commonly thought to be owing to *Corynebacterium tenuis*, but other members of this genus may be involved as well. The identification of specific species of this genus is not well worked out, and is not done routinely, so the diagnosis generally is made clinically without culture or biopsy.[44]

TABLE 19-6

Erythrasma

Clinical Features

   Red or brownish-red patches in moist intertriginous areas
   Characteristic coral-red fluorescence with Wood's lamp

Histopathological Features

   Filamentous Gram-positive rods in stratum corneum seen with
      H&E, PAS, or Giemsa stains
   Minimal inflammation

Differential Diagnosis

   Nonspecific intertrigo
   Tinea, *Candida*
   Contact dermatitis

Clinical Features   Asymptomatic nodular concretions form on the axillary or pubic hair shafts. These are most commonly yellow, but may be black or reddish.[46]

Histopathological Features   Corynebacteria (coccobacilli and filaments) are seen within the concretion stuck to the hair. They stain weakly with H&E, and are better seen with Giemsa or electron microscopy.

Differential Diagnosis   Concretions on the hairs are also seen with white piedra (*Trichosporon cutaneum*) on the scalp, mustache, or groin hairs. In black piedra (*Piedraia hortae*), concretions form on the scalp. Both of these fungi are larger than *Corynebacteria*, and can be distinguished microscopically or by culture. Both white and black piedra mainly occur in South America. Tinea also most commonly involves scalp hair rather than axillary or groin hair; the endothrix hyphae or spores tend to invade the hair shaft and are not present on the outside in concretions in the more common species.

PITTED KERATOLYSIS

This is a superficial skin infection caused by various *Corynebacterium* species, *Micrococcus sedentarius*, *Dermatophilus congolensis*, or *Actinomyces*.[47,48] It is owing to excessive moisture and prolonged occlusion of the feet. The organisms apparently elaborate a proteinase that produces hundreds of tiny pits in the skin.

Clinical Features   Numerous 1- to 2-mm or larger asymptomatic pits occur in the macerated stratum corneum of the soles. The feet may have a strong odor.

Histopathological Features   Coccobacilli and filaments are seen within the stratum corneum in the pits (Fig. 19-10). They may be seen with H&E stain, but are more clearly seen as Gram-positive and Giemsa stain–positive. There is no significant inflammatory reaction.

Differential Diagnosis   The diagnosis usually is clinically straightforward, and should not easily be confused with other causes of pits on the palms and soles, such as Darier's disease and basal cell nevus syndrome. The hyphae of tinea pedis are larger. Cultures could be done if necessary.

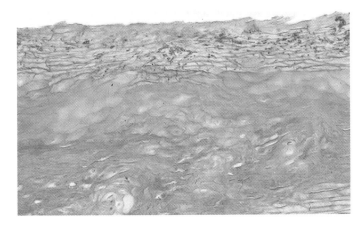

FIGURE 19-10 Pitted keratolysis. Coccobacilli and bacterial filaments infiltrating the superficial stratum corneum.

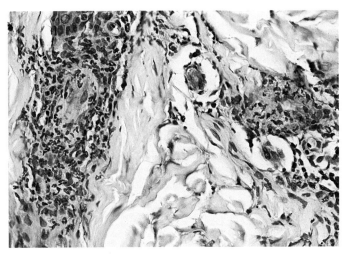

FIGURE 19-11 Meningococcemia. Vasculitis (necrosis of small blood vessel walls with infiltration by neutrophils and lymphocytes) in the dermis.

MENINGOCOCCAL INFECTIONS

Neisseria meningitidis occurs naturally in the throats of a minority of the population who serve as asymptomatic carriers. Sporadic epidemics of bacteremia and meningitis occur. Meningitis is more common in children.

Clinical Features Patients with meningococcemia, with or without meningitis, are febrile and acutely ill, developing petechiae or ecchymoses (Table 19-7).[49] The Waterhouse-Friderichsen syndrome is a fulminant form of the disease with adrenocortical insufficiency, vasomotor collapse, and shock. Cultures are positive from the blood and cerebrospinal fluid (if there is meningitis) in a majority of cases, from the skin in 50 percent of cases, and from the pharynx in a minority of cases. In the rare form of chronic meningococcemia, fever and arthritis appear along with a recurring maculopapular or petechial eruption.[50,51]

Histopathological Features The petechiae and ecchymoses exhibit microthrombi in the dermal blood vessels, with dermal hemorrhage (Fig. 19-11). In cases of disseminated intravascular coagulation, there may be very little inflammation. Sometimes frank vasculitis is found, with necrosis of vessel walls, neutrophils in and around vessels, with nuclear dust. Meningococcal infection as with many other bacterial infections may present as pustular vasculitis. The Gram-negative diplococci can sometimes be found in and around vessels. Intraepidermal and subepidermal pustules and epidermal necrosis sometimes occur.

In chronic meningococcemia, a nonspecific perivascular infiltrate of lymphocytes and a few neutrophils is more commonly found, and organisms are less frequently discovered. Petechial lesions may show neutrophilic (leukocytoclastic) vasculitis.

Differential Diagnosis Meningococcemia may resemble viral exanthems, gonococcemia, Rocky Mountain spotted fever, other forms of septicemia, and other purpuric eruptions. The histologic differential diagnosis includes other infection-related small vessel vasculitides associated with fibrin thrombi and neutrophil-rich infiltrates, pustular vasculitis, septic or sterile thrombi, or leukocytoclastic vasculitis from any cause. The chronic form of meningococcemia without vasculitis exhibits nonspecific features, suggesting infection in general, connective tissue disease, Still's disease, or a neutrophilic dermatosis.

GONOCOCCAL INFECTIONS

Gonorrhea is a common venereal disease caused by *Neisseria gonorrhoeae*.[52] Males usually develop acute purulent urethritis and less commonly proctitis or oropharyngitis. Females most often develop endocervicitis.

Clinical Features Gonococcemia has sometimes been called the dermatitis-arthritis syndrome, although meningococcemia and other bacteremias can produce a similar picture (Table 19-8). Patients develop fever, oligoarthritis, and skin lesions. The skin lesions most commonly are sparse acral necrotic hemorrhagic pustules, but red macules, papules, furuncles, ulcers, cellulitis, and bullae also have been described.

Histopathological Features Biopsies of skin lesions show neutrophilic (leukocytoclastic) vasculitis (Fig. 19-12). There often are hemorrhage, thrombosis, focal epidermal necrosis, intraepidermal or subepidermal pustules, and pustular vasculitis. The Gram-negative diplococci are seldom found.

Differential Diagnosis Reiter's syndrome, meningococcemia, and other bacteremias may resemble gonococcemia. Other causes of pustules are listed in Table 19-1.

TABLE 19-7

Meningococcemia

Clinical Features

    Febrile multisystem illness
    Acute onset of petechiae or ecchymoses

Histopathological Features

    Septic neutrophilic vasculitis
    Gram-negative diplococci sometimes demonstrated

Differential Diagnosis

    Neutrophilic (leukocytoclastic) vasculitis
    Viral exanthems
    Gonococcemia
    Rocky Mountain spotted fever
    Other septicemias

TABLE 19-8

Gonococcemia

Clinical Features

Acute onset of necrotic pustules, usually sparse in number, especially acral

Acute septic arthritis

Histopathological Features

Neutrophilic (leukocytoclastic) vasculitis

Gram-negative diplococci rarely demonstrated

Pustules vary in site of formation (subcorneal, intraepidermal, subepidermal)

Differential Diagnosis

Meningococcemia and other causes of septic and nonseptic vasculitis

Rickettsial infections

Other pustular conditions (see Table 19-1)

Pustular vasculitis

TUBERCULOSIS

Mycobacterium tuberculosis primarily affects the lungs, but many other organs including the skin can be involved. Tuberculosis (TB) had been decreasing in incidence in North America and Europe until the advent of AIDS. It has been estimated that half of the earth's population is infected with this bacterium, and it is responsible for 6 percent of all deaths worldwide. Bacterial resistance to antibiotics is a growing concern. In the United States, 95 percent of individuals who are infected recover completely from their primary TB in the lung, with no further evidence of disease. With any worsening in health status or immunosuppression, the quiescent bacteria persisting within macrophages may proliferate and cause clinical disease. In some parts of the world, immunity results from vaccination with bacille Calmette-Guerin (BCG). Skin testing with tuberculin-purified protein derivative (PPD) is commonly used in patients who have not been vaccinated with BCG as a reliable means of confirming previous mycobacterial infection. Cultures and

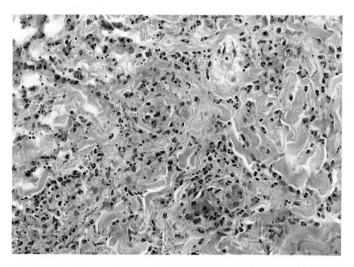

FIGURE 19-12 Gonococcemia. Vasculitic picture with necrosis, fibrin, and neutrophils in the vessel walls, nuclear dust, extravasated erythrocytes, and microthrombi.

acid-fast stains of biopsies, sputum, or other fluids are required to make a diagnosis of active disease. When these are negative, polymerase chain reaction (PCR) testing may be helpful.[53,54]

Clinical Features TB of the skin almost always means long-standing active disease elsewhere, with the rare exception of primary inoculation TB.[55–58] There are many different types, as outlined in Table 19-9.[59,60]

Histopathological Features TB classically causes caseating granulomas, but in some forms the granulomas do not caseate, and suppuration or purulence may be prominent, depending on the patient's immune status (Figs. 19-13 to 19-15).[61] Different patterns are described in Table 19-9.

Differential Diagnosis Other granulomatous conditions listed in Table 19-1 should be considered. Cultures and acid-fast stains are definitive.

ATYPICAL MYCOBACTERIA

There are many different *Mycobacterium* species that may infect humans besides *M. tuberculosis* and *M. leprae* (Table 19-10).[62–64] The Runyon classification into four groups of atypical mycobacteria is not as useful as it once was. Common organisms include *M. marinum* (common "swimming pool granuloma"), *M. ulcerans* (Buruli ulcer in Central Africa), *M. avium-intracellulare* (MAI, especially with AIDS), *M. fortuitum* and *M. chelonei* (rapid growers).

Clinical Features Clinical lesions include solitary or multiple erythematous nodules, abscesses, ulcers, verrucous plaques, or sinus tracts (Table 19-10).

Histopathological Features Typical biopsies show suppurative granulomatous inflammation, with or without caseation (Fig. 19-16). The epidermis may be hyperplastic or ulcerated. Fibrosis and granulation tissue may be prominent. Various modifications of the Ziehl-Neelson acid-fast stain or Fite stain may reveal the acid-fast bacilli (AFB).[3] The AFB most frequently are found in microabscesses or within vacuoles in the sections, rather than within multinucleated giant cells. Fluorescent antibodies or PCR may be used for detection of the organism.[65]

Differential Diagnosis Other diseases associated with granulomas or neutrophilic infiltrates in the dermis are listed in Table 19-1.

LEPROSY (HANSEN'S DISEASE)

Hansen's disease, caused by *Mycobacterium leprae*, affects millions of people worldwide. In the United States, it occurs mainly in immigrants from endemic areas, but some cases originate in Texas and Louisiana, perhaps from armadillo exposure. Leprosy affects multiple organs of the body, but clinical disease is most apparent in the skin, eyes, and peripheral nerves. Neuropathies may result in deformities of the distal extremities.

Clinical Features Leprosy is divided into several types, based on the immune status of the patient (Table 19-11). The tuberculoid form occurs in those with intact immunity, and patients tend to develop one or few lesions with prominent hypoesthesia and palpable peripheral nerves. The lesions may be annular or scaly or macular and hypopigmented.

Patients with lepromatous leprosy are anergic, and they tend to develop widespread cutaneous lesions. Although they are less likely to have hypoesthesia in the lesions, peripheral nerves may still be enlarged with consequent neuropathies. Lepromatous lesions include hypopig-

Tuberculosis

Clinical Features

Miliary: Rare papulopustular eruption as a result of widespread hematogenous dissemination owing to poor immunity (PPD-negative) or steroid treatment

Primary inoculation: Rare crusted ulcer with regional adenopathy following infection of the skin by laboratory accidents, performance of autopsies, or tatooing

TB cutis orificialis: Mucosal ulcers in patients with poor immunity

Scrofuloderma (TB colliquativa cutis): Nodular swelling or ulceration resulting from direct extension of underlying bone or lymph node TB

TB verrucosa cutis: Solitary purulent verrucous plaque seen in patients with high immunity

Lupus vulgaris: Reddish-brown apple jelly patches or plaques, usually on the head or neck, resulting from reactivation in a patient with good immunity

Tuberculids: (hypersensitivity reactions to active TB elsewhere; lesions improve after treatment of the TB)

    Papulonecrotic tuberculid:

        Multiple crusted papules

    Lichen scrofulosorum:

        Lichenoid papules, sometimes follicular or annular, mostly on the trunk

    Erythema induratum (Bazin's disease):

        Indurated nodules on the calves. Questionable whether this is related to TB (see Chapter 11)

Histopathological Features

Miliary TB, primary inoculation TB, TB cutis orificialis, scrofuloderma

    Variable epidermal ulceration

    Diffuse mixed infiltrate with many neutrophils

    Variable granulomatous component

    Acid-fast bacilli often present

Tuberculosis verrucosa cutis

    Hyperkeratosis, papillomatosis, acanthosis

    Sometimes neutrophilic microabscesses in the epidermis

    Diffuse mixed infiltrate in the dermis, neutrophils prominent

    Tuberculoid granulomas, sometimes with caseation

    Acid-fast bacilli sometimes present

Lupus vulgaris

    Epidermal atrophy, hyperplasia, or ulceration

    Tuberculoid granulomas in the superficial dermis

    Minimal or no caseation

    Predominance of Langhans-type giant cells

    Acid-fast bacilli usually cannot be demonstrated

Papulonecrotic tuberculid

    Lymphocytic or neutrophilic vasculitis

    Microthrombi frequent

    Wedge of dermal necrosis

Lichen scrofulosorum

    Granulomatous inflammation with or without caseation

    Often around follicles

Differential Diagnosis

Leprosy

Atypical mycobacterial infection

Lymphoma

Tertiary syphilis

Other granulomatous diseases (see Table 19-1)

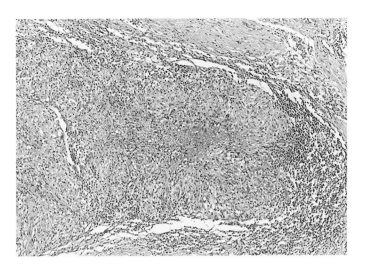

FIGURE 19-13   Primary inoculation tuberculosis. Caseating granuloma in the dermis.

mented or erythematous macules, infiltrated erythematous nodules or plaques, leonine (lionlike) facies with loss of eyebrows and eyelashes, and diffuse macular involvement of the skin resulting in a smooth surface.

In borderline leprosy, combined features of tuberculoid and lepromatous disease are seen.

Indeterminant leprosy represents early disease in patients living in populations where leprosy is prevalent; it is difficult to establish a definite diagnosis in some of these patients. They tend to have only a single or few hypopigmented or erythematous macules, with or without hypoesthesia. The disease may spontaneously heal or may evolve into one of the other forms.

Histoid leprosy refers to dermatofibromalike nodules of leprosy.

There are three types of reactional leprosy, which occur with or without treatment, usually as a result of a change in the patient's immune status. The type I reaction (Lepra reaction) is called a reversal reaction when the patient is under treatment and has shifted toward the tuberculoid spectrum with greater immunity.[66] It is called a downgrading reaction when untreated patients shift toward the lepromatous pole. Type I reactions involve swelling of previously existing cutaneous and neural lesions, with associated constitutional symptoms.

Type II reactions (erythema nodosum leprosum) occur in lepromatous and borderline lepromatous leprosy patients. Tender new red

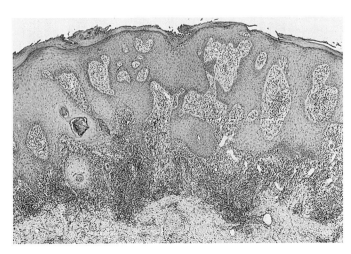

FIGURE 19-14   Tuberculosis verrucosa cutis. Pseudoepitheliomatous hyperplasia with granulomatous inflammation.

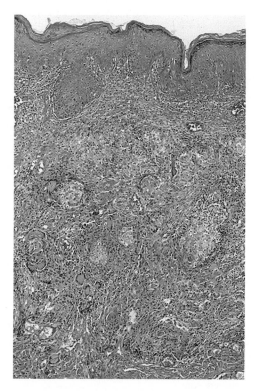

FIGURE 19-15   Lupus vulgaris. Noncaseating granulomas in the dermis with prominent Langhans giant cells.

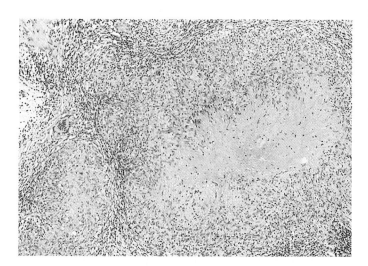

FIGURE 19-16   Atypical mycobacterial infection. Caseating granuloma in the dermis.

plaques and nodules develop on normal skin, accompanied by constitutional symptoms. This type of reaction involves immune complexes.

Type III reactions (Lucio's phenomenon) occur only in patients with the diffuse form of lepromatous leprosy. Hemorrhagic plaques occur on the legs, arms, or buttocks. These may eventually ulcerate. There are usually no constitutional symptoms.

Histopathological Features   The histologic findings are summarized in Table 19-11 (Figs. 19-17 to 19-22).[67,68] The Fite stain or modifications of it are recommended, because the Ziehl-Neelson method used for other AFB does not work as well.[3]

Differential Diagnosis   Other diseases with granulomatous infiltrates or foamy infiltrates are listed in Table 19-1.

ANTHRAX

Anthrax is an acute infection caused by *Bacillus anthracis*.[69]

Clinical Features   About 95 percent of human infections occur after primary inoculation of the skin by contact with infected animals, such as goats, sheep, or other herbivores. About 5 percent of cases are inhalation anthrax (woolsorter's disease). In cutaneous anthrax exposed skin typically is involved. Adults tend to have more involvement of the hands, whereas children under 5 years of age often acquire head and neck infections after being bitten by flies that carry the organism. The initial lesion is a red macule, evolving through papular and pustular stages and eventually ulcerating, often with a black eschar. The latter clinical appearance has been called the "malignant pustule." Patients usually are afebrile, with mild or no constitutional symptoms. The lesions heal spontaneously in 80 to 90 percent of cases.

Histopathological Features   Biopsies generally show edema, necrosis, hemorrhage, and scattered diffuse dermal neutrophils (Fig. 19-23). The histology may resemble other forms of cellulitis, but the exceptionally large Gram-positive rods (up to 10 μm long) usually are numerous and easily demonstrated.

Differential Diagnosis   Clinical lesions of anthrax may resemble staphylococcal infections, sporotrichosis, orf, or tularemia. Other hand infections, discussed under the topic of erysipeloid, might also be considered.

BRUCELLOSIS

There are four species of *Brucella* that may cause infection in humans.[70,71] The organism is a Gram-negative coccobacillus. Human infection occurs after contact with infected milk or animal products. The diagnosis of brucellosis is usually made serologically, because the laboratory cultures are hazardous. The antibodies may cross-react with those to *Vibrio cholerae*, *Francisella tularensis*, and *Yersinia enterocolitica*.

Clinical Features   Brucellosis usually is an acute multisystemic febrile condition, occurring after the ingestion of food or inhalation of the organisms. About 10 percent of the patients develop nonspecific erythematous macular, morbilliform, or eczematous eruptions or erythema

---

TABLE 19-10

Atypical Mycobacteria

Clinical Features

Ulcers, cysts, sinus tracts, or purulent nodules
Multiple or solitary, systemic or cutaneous only
May be sporotrichoid

Histopathological Features

Epidermis hyperplastic or ulcerated
Suppurative granulomatous inflammation with or without necrosis
Acid-fast bacilli may be present
Sometimes prominent fibrosis or granulation tissue

Differential Diagnosis

Other granulomatous conditions (or others with dermal neutrophils), see Table 19-1

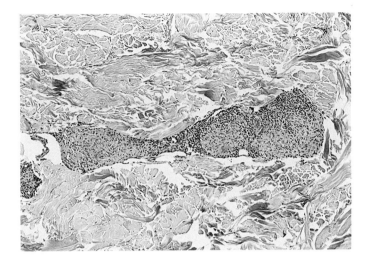

FIGURE 19-17   Tuberculoid leprosy. Linear granuloma following the course of a nerve.

multiforme, ulcers, bullae, or petechiae along with such a systemic infection. Primary inoculation of brucellosis into the skin may present as erythema, papules, or pustules on the hands or arms of veterinarians and other animal workers who handle infected placentas or other infected animal products. The latter exposure often results in a contact hypersensitivity reaction to *Brucella* antigens.

Histopathological Features   The histology of skin lesions has seldom been described in the literature. Superficial and deep perivascular dermatitis and lobular panniculitis have been reported. Necrotic foci are common, and there may be suppurative granulomatous inflammation with plasma cells.

Differential Diagnosis   The differential diagnosis of similar infections acquired from animals is discussed in the preceding for erysipeloid.

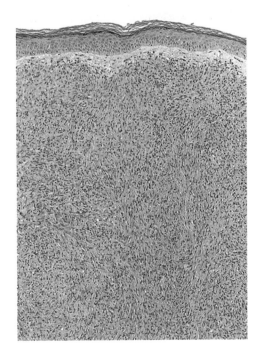

FIGURE 19-18   Lepromatous leprosy. Diffuse infiltration of the dermis by foamy macrophages, separated from the dermis by a grenz zone.

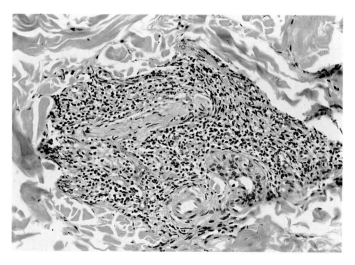

FIGURE 19-19 Lepromatous leprosy. Nodular dermal aggregate of foamy macrophages and lymphocytes surrounding a nerve.

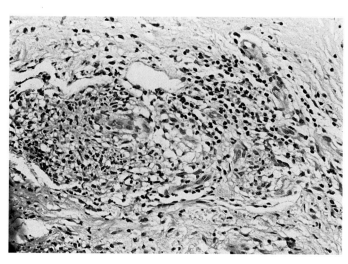

FIGURE 19-22 Erythema nodosum leprosum. Leukocytoclastic vasculitis combined with foamy infiltrates of macrophages in the dermis.

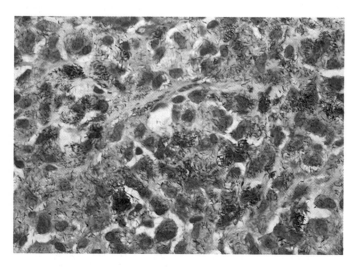

FIGURE 19-20 Lepromatous leprosy. Fite stain of numerous acid-fast bacilli, often clumped into globi.

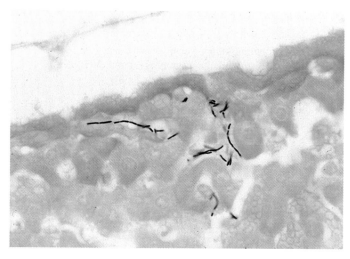

FIGURE 19-23 Anthrax. Exceptionally large Gram-positive bacilli.

YERSINIOSIS

There are three species in the Gram-negative genus *Yersinia*, all of which are zoonotic, and are acquired in humans from various rodents, farm animals, and birds. The term yersiniosis usually is used for infections by *Y. enterocolitica* and *Y. pseudotuberculosis*, whereas *Y. pestis* causes plague. Wild rodents and their fleas are the normal hosts for plague, and involvement in humans is incidental and has caused epidemics. In the Middle Ages this disease resulted in the death of one-quarter of the population in Europe. It still exists today, with about 16,000 cases and 1700 deaths worldwide over the past 15 years, including a few cases in the United States.[72] Infection is by direct inoculation by flea bites or by oropharyngeal or pulmonary routes. Diagnosis is made by culturing the blood, stools, pharynx, sputum, or aspirates from the buboes or by serology.

Clinical Features Plague infections in humans vary from mild to severe. Patients may develop fever, malaise, regional adenopathy (bubonic plague), pneumonia (pneumonic plague), septicemia, meningitis, pharyngitis, and shock. Pustules or carbuncles may form at the site of bites or near buboes, sometimes with centrifugal vesicles. Der-

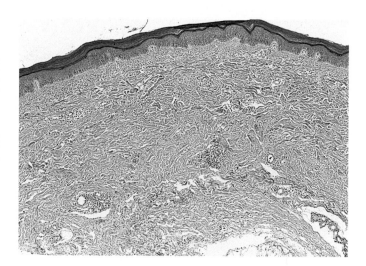

FIGURE 19-21 Indeterminant leprosy. Perivascular lymphohistiocytic infiltrate. The pattern is nonspecific unless acid-fast bacilli are found.

matologic manifestations of systemic infection range from generalized macular erythema to petechiae and purpura.

Yersinia enterocolitica and *Y. pseudotuberculosis* mostly cause fever and gastrointestinal disease, and 10 to 30 percent develop a reactive polyarthritis. About 30 percent of patients develop skin lesions, usually involving the trunk or legs, and often resembling erythema nodosum.[73–75]

Histopathological Features Histologic changes in the skin generally are not diagnostic and vary according to the type of lesion biopsied. The purpuric and petechial lesions may show microthrombi, hemorrhage, and other signs of disseminated intravascular coagulation.

Differential Diagnosis Yersiniosis can mimic many infectious diseases, and only definitive serology or cultures allow a specific diagnosis.

GRANULOMA INGUINALE

Granuloma inguinale (GI, donovanosis) is an uncommon venereal disease caused by the Gram-negative *Calymmatobacterium* (formerly *Donovania*) *granulomatis*.[76–78] The diagnosis usually is made from smears rather than cultures.

Clinical Features Asymptomatic genital or perianal ulcers tend to develop abundant friable granulation tissue, spreading in a serpiginous pattern (Table 19-12). When these ulcers become large, considerable local destruction may occur. Fibrotic vegetating ulcers may cause considerable destruction (esthiomene). Adenopathy usually is not prominent. Dissemination beyond the genital and inguinal region to the liver and other organs eventually may occur in neglected cases.

Histopathological Features The ulcerations show considerable granulation tissue, with a suppurative granulomatous infiltrate of macrophages (histiocytes), plasma cells, and neutrophils. Lymphocytes are few in number. The borders of the ulcers may exhibit acanthosis or pseudoepitheliomatous hyperplasia. Very large macrophages, up to 20 μm in diameter, may contain the 1- to 2-μm organisms (Donovan bodies),

which have a safety pin appearance when stained with Warthin-Starry or Giemsa (bipolar staining surrounded by a vacuole). Smears made from crushed biopsies stained with Wright or Giemsa stains are better for demonstrating the organisms than tissue sections. Semithin 1-μm sections prepared for electron microscopy and stained with toluidine blue also may be used to identify the organisms.

Differential Diagnosis Chancroid, syphilis, herpes simplex, and lymphogranuloma venereum also commonly produce genital ulcerations. (See the discussion that follows for the differential diagnosis of chancroid.) Pseudoepitheliomatous hyperplasia seen with GI may cause confusion with squamous cell carcinoma. Parasitized macrophages also are noted with rhinoscleroma, histoplasmosis, and leishmaniasis, but the staining and culture characteristics, clinical presentation, and location of the lesions usually easily allow a distinction.

CHANCROID

Chancroid is an uncommon venereal disease caused by *Haemophilus ducreyi*.[76–79]

Clinical Features The typical presentation is solitary, painful, nonindurated ulcers on the genitals after sexual contact (Table 19-13). The disease occurs in clustered outbreaks, usually in selected large cities. Prominent regional lymphadenopathy may be present.

Histopathological Features Ulcers may have acanthosis at the edge. The literature has stressed the three characteristic zones of inflammation, but this is not as specific as often implied.[80] Classically the ulcers have a surface of fibrin, neutrophils, and red cells. The middle zone consists of granulation tissue, swollen endothelial cells, and vessels that may contain thrombi. The deepest dermis contains a dense infiltrate of plasma cells and lymphocytes.

The coccobacilli (1.5 × 0.2 μm) are more readily demonstrated on smears than in tissue sections. They stain with Giemsa and are Gram-negative.

Differential Diagnosis Ulcers of secondary syphilis are clinically less painful and tend to be more indurated. The diagnosis rests on positive

---

TABLE 19-12

Granuloma Inguinale

Clinical Features

Genital ulcers with characteristic beefy red granulation tissue
Prominent lymphadenopathy (buboes) common

Histopathological Features

Ulceration, sometimes with epithelial hyperplasia at edge
Dermal mixed infiltrate of histiocytes, plasma cells, and few
  lymphocytes, with small neutrophilic microabscesses
Donovan bodies (1–2 μm Gram-negative organisms, Giemsa- and
  Warthin-Starry-positive) best seen on smear rather than in
  tissue sections

Differential Diagnosis

Other venereal ulcers, such as
  Syphilis
  Chancroid
  Lymphogranuloma venereum
  Herpes

TABLE 19-13

Chancroid

Clinical Features

Nonindurated painful solitary genital ulcer

Histopathological Features

Ulcer with three typical zones
  Surface neutrophils, erythrocytes, fibrin
  Middle zone of granulation tissue
  Deepest zone of dense plasma cells and lymphocytes
Gram-negative, Giemsa-positive bacilli in "school of fish" pattern,
  mainly in smears

Differential Diagnosis

Other venereal ulcers
  Syphilis
  Herpes simplex
  Lymphogranuloma venereum
  Granuloma inguinale

serology (RPR or VDRL, which may be negative initially), positive dark-field exam for spirochetes, or positive Warthin-Starry stains. Syphilis, like any ulcer on mucous membranes or genital skin, also tends to exhibit plasma cells, but the three zones of inflammation tend to be more distinct in chancroid. Granuloma inguinale also tends to lack the three zones. Plasma cells and granulation tissue again often are prominent. Macrophages containing Gram-negative and Giemsa- and Warthin-Starry-positive bacilli, clumped into collections of 10 to 20 organisms (Donovan bodies), are found. Lymphogranuloma venereum tends to produce multiple small painless ulcers. The histological changes of lymphogranuloma venereum are nonspecific, and the *Chlamydia* are difficult to identify with Giemsa stain. The diagnosis usually rests on serology or cultures. Herpes simplex ulcers tend to show the characteristic herpetic cytopathic epithelial changes (nuclear molding, steel-gray nuclei with margination of chromatin), multinucleated epithelial giant cell formation, and eosinophilic intranuclear inclusions.

RHINOSCLEROMA

Rhinoscleroma is sometimes called scleroma, because it may involve other portions of the respiratory tract besides the most frequent site, the nose. It is caused by *Klebsiella rhinoscleromatis*, a Gram-negative coccobacillus.[81] The disease is mainly found in Central America, Indonesia, and Egypt. Poor hygiene, malnutrition, and crowded living conditions contribute to the infection.

Clinical Features   In early stages, there is nasal congestion and non-specific symptoms. Later, tremendous deforming tissue proliferation occurs, followed by indurated scarring.

Histopathological Features   There is a dense diffuse infiltration of the tissue by many macrophages and plasma cells. Some of the larger macrophages (histiocytes called Mikulicz cells) contain many of the Frisch bacilli. They are visible with H&E but are best seen with Giemsa or PAS. The prominent plasma cell infiltrate may exhibit many Russell bodies, which are eosinophilic blobs resulting from considerable immunoglobulin synthesis. Russell bodies can be seen in any plasma cell–rich infiltrate from any cause.

Differential Diagnosis   Parasitized histiocytes with organisms about the same size occur with leishmaniasis, histoplasmosis, and granuloma inguinale. Rhinoscleroma exhibits more plasma cells and Russell bodies. (See Table 19-1 for a list of other diseases with many plasma cells.) Cultures or electron microscopy may be needed for definitive diagnosis of difficult cases. Rhinosporidiosis may also infect the nose, but it tends to be more polypoid clinically, and the histologic findings are much different.

TULAREMIA

This infection is caused by *Francisella tularensis*, a Gram-negative coccobacillus.[82] Since cultures may be hazardous, the diagnosis most commonly is made serologically. Antibodies may cross-react with those of brucellosis. Infection usually occurs after skin contact with infected wild rabbits, deer flies, or tick feces, but infection also may be acquired after contact with a wide variety of other animals.

Clinical Features   About 80 percent of cases are ulceroglandular tularemia, occurring after direct inoculation of the skin, usually the finger or hand. An erythematous papule eventually ulcerates, often forming a black eschar. Prominent adenopathy usually develops. Other

forms of tularemia of less interest in dermatopathology include oculoglandular, oropharyngeal, gastrointestinal, pulmonary, and typhoidal.

Histopathological Features   Biopsies typically reveal ulceration and necrosis surrounded by neutrophils. Suppurative granuloma formation eventually develops, sometimes with caseation. Organisms rarely are demonstrated with the Gram stain. The modified Dieterle silver stain, or a fluorescent antibody stain, is said to be more sucessful.

Differential Diagnosis   Usually the clinical history and physical findings easily point toward the diagnosis. Some other considerations for hand infections are considered under the topic of erysipeloid. Atypical mycobacterial infection and sporotrichosis may resemble tularemia clinically and histologically, except that the causative agents are different, as demonstrated by cultures and special stains. Prominent lymphadenitis also develops in cat-scratch disease, but the localized skin lesions usually are much less impressive.

CAT-SCRATCH DISEASE

The etiologic agent of this disease is now thought to be a Gram-negative bacillus identical to or similar to that of bacillary angiomatosis, described in the following.[72] *Bartonella* (formerly *Rochalimaea*) *henselae* has most recently been thought to be the cause in most cases. It is closely related to *Bartonella quintana*, the etiologic agent of louse-borne trench fever. *Afipia felis*, an unrelated organism, has also been implicated in cat-scratch disease, but current thinking favors *B. henselae*.[83,84] The diagnosis may be established by the cat-scratch skin test (Hanger-Rose test). Although it is not readily available and is unstandardized, the skin test is reliable when done 1 week after infection. The organism is extremely difficult to culture. Polymerase chain reaction (PCR) has been used to identify it in research situations.

Clinical Features   The primary lesion begins at the site of a cat scratch or bite, most commonly in children. Sometimes injuries from other animals or inanimate objects also have been implicated. The lesion resembles an insect bite, but does not itch, and may present as a macule, papule, vesicle, pustule, or erosion. The lesions may be solitary or multiple, usually smaller than 5 mm, and most commonly occur on the hand or forearm, healing uneventfully within 2 weeks. The cats themselves are not ill. Many human infections are subclinical and perhaps unnoticed. About a third of the patients develop fever or constitutional symptoms. Rarely, various morbilliform rashes, other skin eruptions, or internal organ involvement occurs. The diagnosis usually become suspected when tender regional adenopathy develops several weeks later. This usually is the chief complaint. There usually is no lymphangitis extending from the primary lesion, but the node may eventually suppurate. Involvement of the conjunctiva and preauricular lymphadenopathy is known as Parinaud's oculoglandular syndrome.

Histopathological Features   Biopsies of some skin lesions may show palisading granulomas around necrobiotic foci (Fig. 19-24). Lymphocytes and eosinophils may surround the macrophages and multinucleated giant cells. Sometimes there is ulceration or epithelial hyperplasia. Other skin lesions show only nonspecific perivascular or lichenoid lymphoplasmacytic or neutrophilic infiltrates. The Warthin-Starry stain occasionally will demonstrate the thin 0.2- to 2.5-μm rods.[3] The more commonly biopsied lymph nodes show characteristic stellate microabscesses around subcapsular foci of necrosis.[85] The necrosis becomes more extensive in older lymph nodes, and this becomes surrounded by a more granulomatous infiltrate. The nodes have also yielded positive Warthin-Starry stains in some cases.

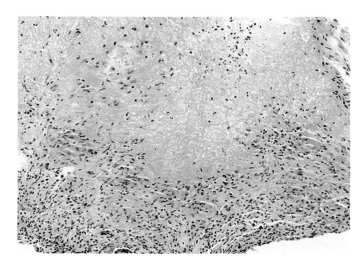

FIGURE 19-24   Cat-scratch disease. Palisading granuloma in the dermis, surrounding a necrotic focus at site of scratch.

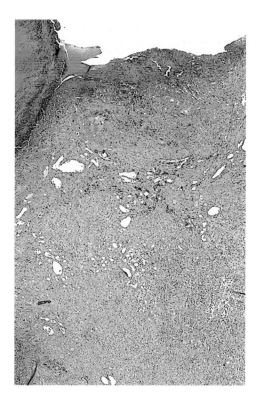

FIGURE 19-25   Bacillary angiomatosis. Ulcerated pyogenic granuloma–like nodule, with amphophilic smudgy stroma containing the bacilli.

Differential Diagnosis   The palisading granulomas in the skin lesions of cat-scratch disease may be confused with granuloma annulare, necrobiosis lipoidica, rheumatoid nodules, rheumatic fever nodules, foreign body granuloma, and caseating granulomatous infections such as mycobacterial and deep fungal infections. However, the clinical presentation and a careful history usually will help make a distinction, even if the cultures and special stains are negative and the skin test is not available. The suppurative granulomatous inflammation in the nodes may be confused with a wide variety of infectious diseases, especially tularemia, brucellosis, mycobacterial infections, infectious mononucleosis, yersiniosis, lymphogranuloma venereum, streptococcal and staphylococcal infections, sporotrichosis, Kawasaki's disease, and even lymphoma. Mononucleosis and lymphomas tend to be bilateral. Demonstration of the organisms with Warthin-Starry silver stains is critical.

BACILLARY ANGIOMATOSIS

This is an infection of immunocompromised patients, such as those with AIDS, with a Gram-negative bacillus, most recently designated *Bartonella henselae*. Some cases seem to involve *Bartonella quintana*.[86] Our knowledge of this condition is rapidly increasing, and the naming of the infectious agents is in a state of flux.[72] The organisms are related to the bacilli that cause cat-scratch disease, and this disease is discussed in the preceding. Despite infection by apparently the same or similar organisms, the lesions of bacillary angiomatosis are quite different from cat-scratch disease. The term bacillary angiomatosis refers to pyogenic granulomalike vasoproliferative papules and nodules of the skin, which contain colonies of numerous organisms. The term bacillary peliosis is used when the liver or spleen are involved. The lesions of bacillary angiomatosis have some similarity to the nodules of verruga peruana, which are a manifestation of infection with another similar organism found in the Andes Mountains, known as *Bartonella bacilliformis*, which also causes bartonellosis (Carrion's disease, Oroya fever).

Clinical Features   Friable grouped nodules or papules resembling pyogenic granulomas develop on the skin, sometimes after a history of a cat scratch. The cat flea (*Ctenocephalides felis*) has been implicated as a potential vector.[86] Some patients have presented with subcutaneous nodules, fungating masses, or hyperpigmented indurated plaques.[87]

Systemic dissemination may occur. This disease usually responds well to erythromycin and other antibiotics if treated in the early stages.

Histopathological Features   Nodules have the low-power appearance of a pyogenic granuloma or granulation tissue, with many blood vessels and plump endothelial cells proliferating in a pale edematous stroma (Figs. 19-25 and 19-26).[85,88] There are collections of neutrophils and pale smudgy amphophilic areas that contain the organisms. The bacilli usually are numerous and easily seen with the Warthin-Starry stain or by electron microscopy.

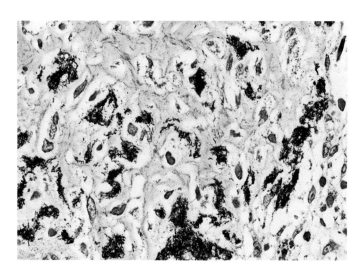

FIGURE 19-26   Bacillary angiomatosis. Warthin-Starry stain of numerous black clumped bacilli.

Differential Diagnosis   It is important to distinguish bacillary angiomatosis from Kaposi's sarcoma, which may occur in the same immunosuppressed population. A valuable clue is that the H&E sections of bacillary angiomatosis usually contain smudgy amphophilic areas that contain the organisms, which later are easily demonstrated by the Warthin-Starry stain. Pyogenic granulomas, ordinary granulation tissue, and other vascular neoplasms may cause some confusion, but these are easily excluded as long as the index of suspicion is high enough to do the stain for organisms.

MALAKOPLAKIA

Malakoplakia (meaning soft plaque) affects the gastrointestinal and urinary tracts and other organs more commonly than the skin.[89,90] The disease results from an inability of macrophages to phagocytize bacteria adequately. Some of the patients are on immunosuppressive therapy for lymphomas or renal transplantation. Others have underlying cancer or rheumatologic diseases. *Escherichia coli* is the most common offending organism, but *Staphylococcus aureus*, *Pseudomonas*, and others also have been cultured.

Clinical Features   Patients present with furuncular tender red nodules or papules, fluctuant abscesses or sinus tracts, or ulcers, most commonly in the groin.

Histopathological Features   There is a diffuse infiltrate of macrophages containing fine eosinophilic granules in their cytoplasm (von Hansemann cells) and small eccentric nuclei. Larger (5 to 15 μm) basophilic ovoid to round phagolysosomes also are present (Michaelis-Gutmann bodies). These inclusions are positive with PAS, von Kossa, and Perl's stains, since they contain calcium and iron. The Gram stain may also stain bacteria within the cytoplasm of the macrophages. Partially digested bacteria may also be found in the phagolysosomes, seen best with electron microscopy. Neutrophils, lymphocytes, and plasma cells may also be present in the infiltrate.

Differential Diagnosis   The macrophages of malakoplakia may be confused with macrophages that are digesting any nonspecific material. Parasitized macrophages are also seen with rhinoscleroma, granuloma inguinale, and histoplasmosis. Malakoplakia has also been confused with lymphoma.

PSITTACOSIS

Psittacosis (ornithosis) is an infection of birds caused by *Chlamydia psittaci*. It affects parrots (psittacines) as well as other birds. Occasionally it can be transmitted to humans by the respiratory route, usually resulting in a fever, pneumonitis, and systemic disease. About 85 percent of the humans have a history of contact with birds, but the birds themselves may be asymptomatic. The diagnosis is difficult to make, and is most often confirmed serologically, as the organism is difficult to culture. Bronchoalveolar lavage with PCR analysis has been used in some cases.

Clinical Features   The severity of illness varies greatly from mild to severe, and may result in death. Symptoms and signs include fever, severe headache, cough, chest pain, pleurisy, pericarditis, myocarditis, epistaxis, myalgia, malaise, and hepatosplenomegaly. Cutaneous lesions are faint red macules (Horder's spots), similar to the rose spots of typhoid fever. Other lesions may resemble urticaria, erythema multiforme, erythema nodosum, and purpura of disseminated intravascular coagulation.

Histopathological Features   The histology of skin biopsies has been poorly documented in the literature. Most likely this varies depending greatly on the type of lesion biopsied, as described in the clinical features. The rose spots apparently show perivascular lymphoid infiltrates as with any reactive erythema. Skin biopsies generally have not been used to make this diagnosis.

Differential Diagnosis   A wide variety of infectious diseases that cause pulmonary disease might be considered, such as mycoplasma pneumonia, Q fever, legionellosis, coccidioidomycosis, tuberculosis, and the more common bacterial and viral pneumonias.

LYMPHOGRANULOMA VENEREUM

Lymphogranuloma venereum (LGV) is an uncommon venereal disease caused by *Chlamydia trachomatis*.[76–78] It is five times more common in blacks, and is more common in warmer climates. The diagnosis may be made by culture or serology. The Frei intradermal skin test is no longer in general use.

Clinical Features   The primary genital lesions are 2- to 3-mm papules or small erosions, often becoming grouped herpetiform ulcers (Table 19-14). Nonspecific urethritis may occur. Subsequent spread through the lymphatics results in very prominent inguinal lymphadenopathy (buboes), resulting in the "groove sign" when the lymph nodes are enlarged on both sides of Poupart's ligament, especially in men. These nodes may eventually suppurate and drain, often subsiding in 3 months. Fibrosis of the lymphatics may cause obstruction, resulting in genital elephantiasis, rectal strictures, or fibrotic vegetating ulcerations of the pudenda ("esthiomene," which is Greek for "eating away"). This may be the initial presentation in women, in whom the primary skin lesions and inguinal buboes are less commonly seen. Rectovaginal fistulas in women may cause a "watering can perineum."

Histopathological Features   Early skin papules are nonspecific. Cutaneous ulcers are granulomatous, with many plasma cells and endothelial swelling. Occasionally Giemsa stain may reveal the *Chlamydia*, but usually it is difficult to interpret.

   The histology of the lymph nodes are more characteristic than the skin lesions. Stellate microabscesses are seen, later surrounded by granulomatous inflammation with many plasma cells. Similar changes can be seen in cat-scratch disease, tularemia, and certain deep fungal diseases. However, these conditions are not as common in the genital area. They become granulomatous in later stages.

TABLE 19-14

Lymphogranuloma Venereum

Clinical Features

   Multiple herpetiform genital ulcers
   Prominent regional lymphadenopathy

Histopathological Features

   Epidermis normal or ulcerated
   Diffuse mixed suppurative granulomatous infiltrate

Differential Diagnosis

   Other granulomatous diseases (see Table 19-1)
   Other genital ulcers
   Herpes simplex

Differential Diagnosis Chancroid usually results in larger, more painful ulcers, but buboes are common in both disorders. They may be distinguished by positive *Chlamydia* cultures or serology in LGV, and positive cultures or smears for *Hemophilus ducreyi* in chancroid. Granuloma inguinale also results in larger ulcers, which tend to develop considerable granulation tissue, without inguinal adenitis. Esthiomene may also occur in granuloma inguinale, but the demonstration of Donovan bodies with the Giemsa stain is the definitive test.

REFERENCES

1. Rapini RP: Practical evaluation of skin lesions in immunosuppressed patients. *Cutis* 42:125–128, 1988.
2. Chren M-M, Lazarus HM, Salata RA, Landefeld CS: Cultures of skin biopsy tissue from immunocompromised patients with cancer and rashes. *Arch Dermatol* 131:552–555, 1995.
3. Northcutt AD, Tschen JA: New ways to demonstrate pathogenic organisms. *Clin Dermatol* 9:205–215, 1991.
4. Rapini RP (ed): Use of the laboratory in dermatology. *Dermatol Clin* 12:1–212, 1994.
5. Rapini RP (ed): Special dermatopathology techniques. *Clin Dermatol* 9:115–272, 1991.
6. Rapini RP, Jordon RE: *Atlas of Dermatopathology.* Chicago, Year Book Medical Publishers, 1988.
7. Ackerman AB, Ragaz A: *The Lives of Lesions.* New York, Masson Publishing, 1984.
8. Barnett BO, Frieden IJ: Streptococcal skin diseases in children. *Semin Dermatol* 11:3–10, 1992.
9. Kobayashi S, Ikeda T, Okada H, et al: Endemic occurrence of glomerulonephritis associated with streptococcal impetigo. *Am J Nephrol* 15:356–360, 1995.
10. Shriner DL, Schwartz RA, Janniger CK: Impetigo. *Cutis* 56:30–32, 1995.
11. Darmstadt GL, Lane AT: Impetigo: An overview. *Pediatric Dermatol* 11:293–303, 1994.
12. Williams RE, MacKie RM: The staphylococci: Importance of their control in the management of skin disease. *Dermatol Clin* 11:201–206, 1993.
13. Sevinsky LD, Viecens C, Ballesteros DO, Stengel F: Ecthyma gangrenosum: A cutaneous manifestation of *Pseudomonas aeruginosa* sepsis. *J Am Acad Dermatol* 29:104–106, 1993.
14. Agger WA, Mardan A: *Pseudomonas aeruginosa* infections of intact skin. *Clin Infect Dis* 20:301–308, 1995.
15. Gemmell CG: Staphylococcal scalded skin syndrome. *J Med Microbiol* 43:318–327, 1995.
16. Cribier B, Piemont Y, Grosshans E: Staphylococcal scalded skin syndrome in adults: A clinical review illustrated with a new case. *J Am Acad Dermatol* 30:319–324, 1994.
17. Hardwick N, Parry CM, Sharpe GR: Staphylococcal scalded skin syndrome in an adult: Influence of immune and renal factors. *Br J Dermatol* 132:468–471, 1995.
18. Resnick SD: Staphylococcal toxin-mediated syndromes in childhood. *Semin Dermatol* 11:11–18, 1992.
19. Tierno PM Jr: Comparison of cotton and rayon/cotton tampons for efficacy of toxic shock syndrome toxin-1 production. *J Infect Dis* 173:1289–1291, 1996
20. Garland SM, Peel MM: Tampons and toxic shock syndrome. *Med J Aust* 163:8–9, 1995.
21. Gutierrez Rodero F, Ortiz de la Tabla V, Martinez C: Staphylococcal toxic shock syndrome associated with human immunodeficiency virus infection: Report of a case with bacteremia. *Clin Infect Dis* 22:875–876, 1996.
22. Chelsom J, Halstensen A, Haga T, Hoiby EA: Necrotizing fasciitis due to group A streptococci in Western Norway: Incidence and clinical features. *Lancet* 344:1111–1115, 1994.
23. Forni AL, Kaplan EL, Schlievert PM, Roberts RB: Clinical and microbiological characteristics of severe group A streptococcus infections and streptococcal toxic shock syndrome. *Clin Infect Dis* 21:333–340, 1995.
24. Reichardt W, Muller-Alouf H, Kohler W: Erythrogenic toxin type A (ETA): Epidemiological analysis of gene distribution and protein formation in clinical *Streptococcus pyogenes* strains causing scarlet fever and the streptococcal toxic shock-like syndrome (TSLS). *Int J Med Microbiol, Virol, Parasitol, Infect Dis* 279:283–293, 1993.
25. Stevens DL, Bryant AE, Hackett SP, et al: Group A streptococcal bacteremia: The role of tumor necrosis factor in shock and organ failure. *J Infect Dis* 173:619–626, 1996.
26. McHugh D, Fison PN: Ocular erysipelas. *Arch Ophthalmol* 110:1315, 1992.
27. Bratton RL, Nesse RE: St. Anthony's fire: Diagnosis and management of erysipelas. *Am Fam Phys* 51:401–404, 1995.
28. Gorby GL, et al: *Erysipelothrix rhusiopathiae* endocarditis: Microbiologic, epidemiologic, and clinical features of an occupational disease. *Rev Infect Dis* 10:317, 1988.
29. Norcross MC Jr, Mitchell DF: Blistering distal dactylitis caused by *Staphylococcus aureus*. *Cutis* 51:353–354, 1993.
30. Zemtsov A, Veitschegger M: *Staphylococcus aureus*–induced blistering distal dactylitis in an adult immunosuppressed patient. *J Am Acad Dermatol* 26:784–785, 1992.
31. Canoso JJ, Barza M: Soft tissue infections. *Rheum Dis Clin N Am* 19:293–309, 1993.
32. Green RJ, Dafoe DC, Raffin TA: Necrotizing fasciitis. *Chest* 110:219–229, 1996.
33. Brook I, Frazier EH: Clinical and microbiological features of necrotizing fasciitis. *J Clin Microbiol* 33:2382–2387, 1995.
34. Kotrappa KS, Bansal RS, Amin NM: Necrotizing fasciitis. *Am Fam Phys* 53:1691–1697, 1996.
35. Morantes MC, Lipsky BA: "Flesh-eating bacteria": Return of an old nemesis. *Int J Dermatol* 34:461–463, 1995.
36. Lille ST, Sato TT, Engrav LH, et al: Necrotizing soft tissue infections: Obstacles in diagnosis. *J Am College Surg* 182:7–11, 1996.
37. Brogan TV, Nizet V, Waldhausen JH: Streptococcal skin infections. *N Engl J Med* 334:1478, 1996.
38. Saiag P, Le Breton C, Pavlovic M, et al: Magnetic resonance imaging in adults presenting with severe acute infectious cellulitis. *Arch Dermatol* 130:1150–1158, 1994.
39. Schnetter D, Haneke E: Pyoderma gangrenosum vegetans. *Hautarzt* 45:635–638, 1994.
40. Su WPD, Duncan SC, Perry HO: Blastomycosis-like pyoderma. *Arch Dermatol* 115:170–173, 1979.
41. Anonymous: A case of cutaneous diphtheria. *Commun Dis Rep CDR Wkly* 2:111, 1992.
42. Harnish JP, et al: Diphtheria among alcoholic urban adults: A decade of experience in Seattle. *Ann Intern Med* 111:71, 1989.
43. Sarkany I, Taplin D, Blank H: Incidence and bacteriology of erythrasma. *Arch Dermatol* 85:578–582, 1962.
44. Dellion S, Morel P, Vignon-Pennamen D, Felten A: Erythrasma owing to an unusual pathogen. *Arch Dermatol* 132:716–717, 1996.
45. Montes LF, Black SH, McBride ME: Bacterial invasion of the stratum corneum in erythrasma: Ultrastructural evidence for a keratolytic action exerted by *Corynebacterium minutissimum*. *J Invest Dermatol* 49:474–485, 1967.
46. Wilson C, Dawber R: Trichomycosis axillaris: A different view. *J Am Acad Dermatol* 21:325–326, 1989.
47. Holland KT, Marshall J, Taylor D: The effect of dilution rate and pH on biomass and proteinase production by *Micrococcus sedentarius* grown in continuous culture. *J Applied Bacteriol* 72:429–434, 1992.
48. Shah AS, Kamino H, Prose NS: Painful, plaque-like, pitted keratolysis occurring in childhood. *Pediatr Dermatol* 9:251–254, 1992.
49. Neveling U, Kaschula RO: Fatal meningococcal disease in childhood: An autopsy study of 86 cases. *Ann Trop Pediatr* 13:147–152, 1993.
50. Gregory B, Tron V, Ho VC: Cyclic fever and rash in a 66-year-old woman: Chronic meningococcemia. *Arch Dermatol* 128:1645, 1648, 1992.
51. Assier H, Chosidow O, Rekacewicz I, et al: Chronic meningococcemia in acquired immunodeficiency infection. *J Am Acad Dermatol* 29:793–794, 1993.
52. Buntin DM, Rosen T, Lesher JL Jr, et al: Sexually transmitted diseases: Bacterial infections. *J Am Acad Dermatol* 25:287–299, 1991.
53. Steidl M, Neubert U, Volkenandt M, et al: Lupus vulgaris confirmed by polymerase-chain reaction. *Br J Dermatol* 129:314–318, 1993.
54. Degitz K: Detection of mycobacterial DNA in the skin: Etiologic insights and diagnostic perspectives. *Arch Dermatol* 132:71–75, 1996.
55. Chong LY, Lo KK: Cutaneous tuberculosis in Hong Kong: A 10-year retrospective study. *Int J Dermatol* 34:26–29, 1995.
56. Moiin A, Downham TF Jr: A slow growing lesion on the face: Lupus vulgaris. *Arch Dermatol* 132:83, 86, 1996.
57. Munn SE, Basarab T, Russell Jones R: Lupus vulgaris: A case report. *Clin Exp Dermatol* 20:56–57, 1995.
58. Tur E, Brenner S, Meiron Y: Scrofuloderma (tuberculosis colliquativa cutis). *Br J Dermatol* 134:350–352, 1996.
59. Arianayagam AV, Ash S, Jones RR: Lichen scrofulosorum in a patient with AIDS. *Clin Exp Dermatol* 19:74–76, 1994.
60. Jordaan HF, Schneider JW, Schaaf HS, et al: Papulonecrotic tuberculid in children: A report of eight patients. *Am J Dermatopathol* 18:172–185, 1996.
61. Farina MC, Gegundez MI, Pique E, et al: Cutaneous tuberculosis: A clinical, histopathologic, and bacteriologic study. *J Am Acad Dermatol* 33:433–440, 1995.
62. Gluckman SJ: *Mycobacterium marinum*. *Clin Dermatol* 13:273–276, 1995.
63. Sastry V, Brennan PJ: Cutaneous infections with rapidly growing mycobacteria. *Clin Dermatol* 13:266–271, 1995.
64. Zanelli G, Webster GF: Mucocutaneous atypical mycobacterial infections in acquired immunodeficiency syndrome. *Clin Dermatol* 13:281–288, 1995.
65. Cook SM, Bartos RE, Pierson CL, Frank TS: Detection and characterization of atypical mycobacteria by the polymerase chain reaction. *Diag Mol Pathol* 3:53–58, 1994.
66. Cree IA, Coghill G, Subedi AM, et al: Effects of treatment on the histopathology of leprosy. *J Clin Pathol* 48:304–307, 1995.
67. Porichha D, Misra AK, Dhariwal AC, et al: Ambiguities in leprosy histopathology. *Int J Lepr* 61:428–432, 1993.
68. Sehgal VN, Jain S: Clinico-pathological correlation across the leprosy spectrum: Relevance in current context. *Int J Lepr* 62:441–442, 1994.
69. Singh S, Sridhar MS, Sekhar PC, Bhaskar CJ: Cutaneous anthrax: A report of ten cases. *J Assoc Phys India* 40:46–49, 1992.
70. Burnett JW: Brucellosis. *Cutis* 56:28, 1995.
71. Zuckerman E, Naschitz JE, Yeshurun D, et al: Fasciitis-panniculitis in acute brucellosis. *Int J Dermatol* 33:57–59, 1994.

72. Walker DH, Barbour AG, Oliver JH, et al: Emerging bacterial zoonotic and vector-borne diseases: Ecological and epidemiological factors. *JAMA* 275:463–469, 1996.

73. Ikeya T, Mizuno E, Takama H: Three cases of erythema nodosum associated with *Yersinia enterocolitica* infection. *J Dermatol* 13:147, 1986.

74. Butler T: Yersinia infections: Centennial of the discovery of the plague bacillus. *Clin Infect Dis* 19:655–661, 1994.

75. Straley SC, Skrzypek E, Plano GV, Bliska JB: Yops of *Yersinia* spp: Pathogenic for humans. *Infect Immun* 61:3105–3110, 1993.

76. Joseph AK, Rosen T: Laboratory techniques used in the diagnosis of chancroid, granuloma inguinale, and lymphogranuloma venereum. *Dermatol Clinics* 12:1–8, 1994.

77. Goens JL, Schwartz RA, DeWolf K: Mucocutaneous manifestations of chancroid, lymphogranuloma venereum and granuloma inguinale. *Am Fam Phys* 49:415–418, 423–425, 1994.

78. Van Dyck E, Piot P: Laboratory techniques in the investigation of chancroid, lymphogranuloma venereum and donovanosis. *Gen Med* 68:130–133, 1992.

79. Martin DH, Sargent SJ, Wendel GD Jr, et al: Comparison of azithromycin and ceftriaxone for the treatment of chancroid. *Clin Infect Dis* 21:409–414, 1995.

80. King R, Gough J, Ronald A, et al: An immunohistochemical analysis of naturally occurring chancroid. *J Infect Dis* 174:427–430, 1996.

81. Batsakis JG, el-Naggar AK: Rhinoscleroma and rhinosporidiosis. *Ann Otol, Rhinol, Laryngol* 101:879–882, 1992.

82. Kodama BF, Fitzpatrick JE, Gentry RH: Tularemia. *Cutis* 54:279–280, 1994.

83. Bogle MS, Matich MD, French MA, Matz LR: Test and teach: Number seventy-two. Diagnosis: Bacillary angiomatosis. *Pathology* 25:253,319–320, 1993.

84. Hnatuk LAP, Brown DH, Snell GED: Bacillary angiomatosis: A new entity in acquired immunodeficiency syndrome. *J Otolaryngol* 23:216–220, 1994.

85. Batsakis JG, Ro JY, Frauenhoffer EE: Pathology consultation: Bacillary angiomatosis. *Ann Otol Rhinol Laryngol* 104:668–672, 1995.

86. Fagan WA, DeCamp NC, Kraus EW, Pulitzer DR: Widespread cutaneous bacillary angiomatosis and a large fungating mass in an HIV-positive man. *J Am Acad Dermatol* 35:285–287, 1996.

87. Webster GF, Cockerell CJ, Friedman-Kien AE: The clinical spectrum of bacillary antiomatosis. *Br J Dermatol* 126:535–541, 1992.

88. Granter SR, Barnhill RL: Bacillary angiomatosis. *Adv Pathol Lab Med* 6:491–504, 1993.

89. Palou J, Torras H, Baradad M, et al: Cutaneous malakoplakia. *Dermatologica* 176:288–292, 1988.

90. Palazzo JP, Ellison DJ, Garcia IE, et al: Cutaneous malakoplakia simulating relapsing malignant lymphoma. *J Cutan Pathol* 17:171–175, 1990.

91. Verweij PE, Meis JF, Eijk R, et al: Severe human psittacosis requiring artificial ventilation: Case report and review. *Clin Infect Dis* 20:440–442, 1995.

92. Crosse BA: Psittacosis: A clinical review. *J Infection* 21:251–259, 1990.

93. Grayston JT, Thom DH: The chlamydial pneumonias. *Curr Clin Topics Infect Dis* 11:1–18, 1991.

94. Green ST, Hamlet NW, Willocks L, et al: Psittacosis presenting with erythema-marginatum-like lesions: A case report and a historical review. *Clin Exp Dermatol* 15:225–227, 1990.

CHAPTER 20

THE TREPONEMAL AND RICKETTSIAL DISEASES

A. Neil Crowson / Cynthia M. Magro / Stephen Dumler /
Grace F. Kao / Raymond L. Barnhill

Infections with treponemes and rickettsial organisms can produce a broad array of clinical manifestations ranging from seemingly trivial virallike illnesses to fulminant progressive disease. Recognition of these infections often requires correlation of a comprehensive travel and medical history with a detailed knowledge of the clinical and pathological features.

TREPONEMAL DISEASES

The treponemal diseases are caused by bacteria of the family Spirochaetaceae. The pathogenic treponemes measure 6 to 20 by 0.10 to 0.18 µm, are coiled, and react with silver stains in dark-field and biopsy material[1] (Fig. 20-1). The nonvenereal treponematoses are endemic syphilis, yaws, and pinta.

Venereal Syphilis

Clinical Features   Venereal syphilis, caused by *Treponema pallidum*, was a significant cause of morbidity and mortality in the early twentieth century, although its incidence in the developed world has so diminished that many physicians are now unfamiliar with its manifestations.[1] The incidence of acquired syphilis has recently increased to 20 per 100,000 in North America.[1] Spread of *T. pallidum* is usually via contact between an infectious lesion and disrupted epithelium either at sites of trauma incurred during sexual intercourse or at sites of concurrent chancroid and other genital sores.[2,3] Coinfection with human immunodeficiency virus infection is not uncommon,[2] particularly in parts of Africa where the incidence is up to 360 per 100,000[2,4] and the transmission rate up to 60 percent.

The initial lesion of *primary syphilis*, the chancre, presents 21 days after exposure at the inoculation site as a painless, brown-red, indurated papule, nodule, or plaque up to 2 cm in diameter in which organisms are identifiable. Multiple lesions or regional lymph node enlargement may be seen. Following hematogenous dissemination of organisms, *secondary syphilis* occurs, resulting in widespread disease with constitutional symptoms such as fever and malaise,[1,4] generalized lymphadenopathy,[1,5] and a disseminated eruption of red-brown macules, papules, papulosquamous lesions resembling guttate psoriasis, and, rarely, pustules.[6] Follicular-based annular or serpiginous lesions may be seen, particularly in recurrent attacks. Alopecia, condyloma lata comprising confluent gray papules in anogenital areas, pitted hyperkeratotic palmoplantar papules (*syphilis cornee*), or, in severe cases, ulcerative lesions of *lues maligna* may develop. Shallow, painless ulcers are sometimes seen in mucosae. Primary- and secondary-stage lesions which resolve without therapy may herald evolution into a latent phase, comprising an early and late stage, defined by an infection of less than or more than 1-year's duration.[4] Following a variable latent period, the patient enters the tertiary stage. *Tertiary syphilis* encompasses gummatous skin and mucosal lesions termed *benign tertiary syphilis* and cardiovascular and neurologic manifestations. Skin lesions are solitary or multiple and comprise superficial nodular and deep gummatous subtypes, the former having smooth, atrophic centers with raised, serpiginous borders, and the latter manifesting as ulcerative subcutaneous swellings.[7] (See Tables 20-1 and 20-2.)

Congenital syphilis represents transplacental infection and affects over 50 percent of infants born to mothers with primary or secondary syphilis.[8] The diagnosis is made when organisms are seen by dark-field, fluorescent antibody, or conventional histochemical methods.[8] A presumptive case represents an infant born to a mother whose syphilis was inadequately treated or untreated at time of birth, or when an infant or child with a reactive treponemal test has any evidence of congenital syphilis: physical signs, long-bone involvement radiologically, a reactive cerebrospinal fluid (CSF) VDRL (Venereal Disease Research Laboratories test), an elevated CSF protein or white blood cell count, or quantitative treponemal titers four times higher than the mother's.[7,8,9] Clinical signs are rhinitis, chancres, or a desquamative maculopapular rash.[8,9]

Histopathological Features   Cutaneous syphilis manifests as a perivascular infiltrate composed of lymphoid cells and often plasma cells. The late secondary and tertiary stages also show infiltrates of epithelioid histiocytes and giant cells. In all stages, endothelial swelling and proliferation are apparent.

PRIMARY SYPHILIS

The primary syphilitic chancre manifests a variable histopathology depending upon whether the center or edge is biopsied; the center is often ulcerated whereas the edges show acanthosis, spongiosis, and exocytosis of lymphocytes and neutrophils (Fig. 20-2). The papillary dermis is edematous, and a dense dermal perivascular and interstitial lymphohistiocytic and plasmacellular infiltrate is present, often accompanied by neutrophils. An obliterative endarteritis characterized by endothelial swelling and mural edema (Fig. 20-3) completes the picture.

By silver (i.e., Steiner) stains or by immunofluorescent techniques, spirochetes are usually seen within and around blood vessels and along the dermoepidermal junction.[10] In their full length, the spirochetes show 8 to 12 spiral convolutions, each roughly 1 µm in length (Fig. 20-1). Silver stains also decorate melanin and reticulin fibers, which need to be differentiated based on recognition that melanin in the

TABLE 20-1

Primary Syphilis

Clinical Features

Painless papulonodular lesion
Develops 21 days after exposure
Lymphadenopathy in some cases

Histopathological Features

Frequent central ulceration
Lateral psoriasiform hyperplasia
Dense lymphoplasmacellular infiltrate
Obliterative endovasculopathy

Differential Diagnosis

Chancroid
Zoon's balanitis
Insect-bite reaction
Granuloma inguinale

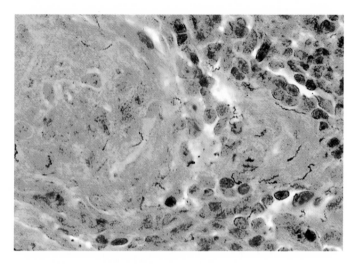

FIGURE 20-1   Primary syphilitic chancre. A silver stain (Steiner) reveals elongated coiled spirochetes from 8 to 12 μm in length in a perivascular disposition.

TABLE 20-2

Secondary and Tertiary Syphilis

Clinical Features

Secondary
  Fever
    Generalized lymphadenopathy
    Disseminated macular or papulosquamous eruption
    Occasionally alopecia, pustules, hyperkeratotic palmoplantar
      pits, ulcers
Tertiary
  Gummatous skin and mucosal lesions
    Solitary or multiple nodules
    Ulcerative subcutaneous lesions
  Cardiovascular disease
    Syphilitic large-vessel aneurysms
  Neurologic disease
    Tabes dorsalis
    Meningoencephalitis

Histopathological Features

Psoriasiform hyperplasia
Rare spongiform pustulation
Vacuolar or lichenoid interface injury pattern
Mixed lymphohistiocytic and plasmacellular infiltrate
Granulomata
Obliterative endovasculopathy

Differential Diagnosis

Lichenoid dermatitides
Psoriasiform dermatitides
Tuberculoid leprosy
Sarcoidal granulomatous dermatitides

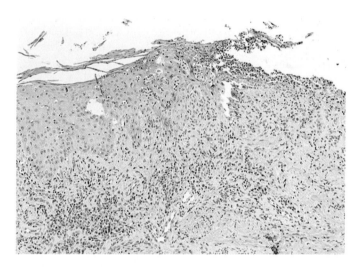

FIGURE 20-2   Primary syphilitic chancre. The epithelium is eroded, with a neutrophilic infiltrate centrally and psoriasiform hyperplasia laterally. The corium contains a dense plasma cell–rich infiltrate.

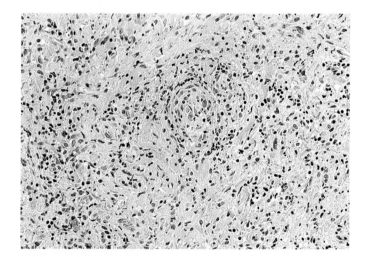

FIGURE 20-3   Primary syphilitic chancre. Endarteritis obliterans is manifested by endothelial cell swelling, endothelial hyperplasia and expansion of vessel walls by edema, and a lymphohistiocytic infiltrate with lumenal attenuation. A plasma cell–rich infiltrate is present.

dendritic processes of melanocytes has a granular appearance[11] and that reticulin fibers, although wavy, do not have a spiral architecture. Correlation with serology is prudent.

Differential Diagnosis   Chancroid, due to infection with *Haemophilus ducreyi*, is difficult to distinguish clinically from the syphilitic chancre. Chancroid lesions manifest dense lymphohistiocytic infiltrates with a paucity of plasma cells, a granulomatous vasculitis, and an epidermal reaction pattern similar to the syphilitic chancre by virtue of psoriasiform epidermal hyperplasia and spongiform pustulation.[2] A Giemsa or alcian-blue stain reveals coccobacillary forms between keratinocytes and along the dermoepidermal junction. Spirochetes may coinfect chancroid lesions.[2] Zoon's balanitis may mimic those chancres manifesting a lichenoid pattern of inflammation, whereas an insect bite reaction may resemble the ulcerative lesions of primary syphilis; obviously, neither will show spirochetes, however. Granuloma inguinale is distinctive by virtue of manifesting Donovan bodies.

SECONDARY SYPHILIS

In secondary syphilis, skin biopsies generally reveal variable epithelial alterations in the macular, papular, and papulosquamous eruptions, the latter showing the most pronounced psoriasiform epidermal hyperplasia. All may show spongiosis and basilar vacuolar alteration, sometimes with colloid body formation, exocytosis of lymphocytes, spongiform pustulation, and parakeratosis.[11,12] There may be patchy or confluent parakeratosis, sometimes accompanied by intracorneal neutrophilic abscesses, the latter mimicking psoriasis but lacking attenuation of the suprapapillary plates. Ulceration is not a feature except in lues maligna. Dermal changes include papillary dermal edema and perivascular and periadnexal lymphocyte- or histiocyte-predominant infiltrates which may be frankly granulomatous in nature in lesions over 4 months of age. Infiltrates are of greatest intensity in the papillary dermis and diminish in the reticular dermis. The pattern of papillary dermal infiltration may be lichenoid in character (Fig. 20-4), obscuring the superficial vasculature, or a cell-poor injury pattern may predominate. Atypical lymphoid forms, representing a type of lymphomatoid hypersensitivity, may suggest the possibility of mycosis fungoides[13] or non-Hodgkin's lymphoma. A neutrophilic eccrine hidradenitis may be seen.[11] Plasma cells are inconspicuous or absent in 25 percent of cases.[12] Eosinophils are usually absent. Endothelial swelling and mural edema are seen in only half of cases,[12] and mural necrosis is rare. Silver stains show spirochetes, best visualized within the epidermis and around the superficial blood vessels, in only one-third of cases[14]; by immunofluorescent microscopy, however, all cases are positive. Histologic variants of secondary syphilis include condylomata lata, lues maligna, syphilis cornee, syphilitic alopecia, and pustular and bullous lesions.[4] Condylomata lata show the aforementioned features of secondary syphilis; although epithelial hyperplasia is more pronounced, intraepithelial microabscesses are observed,[11,15] and treponemes are more numerous.[14] Lues maligna is an ulcerative form comprising endarteritis obliterans of deep vessels at the dermal-subcutaneous junction with attendant ischemic necrosis and a dense plasmacellular and histiocytic infiltrate. Defective cell-mediated immunity may play an integral role,[16,17] as suggested by the occurrence of lues maligna in the setting of HIV disease, where oral involvement may be a prominent manifestation.[4] The histopathology of syphilis cornee/keratoderma punctatum includes an epidermal invagination with a plug of laminated parakeratin, loss of the adjacent granular cell layer, thinning of the stratum spinosum,[18] and a moderately dense perivascular plasmacellular infiltrate with capillary wall thickening. Syphilitic alopecia manifests a superficial and deep perivascular and perifollicular lymphocytic and plasmacellular infiltrate with permeation

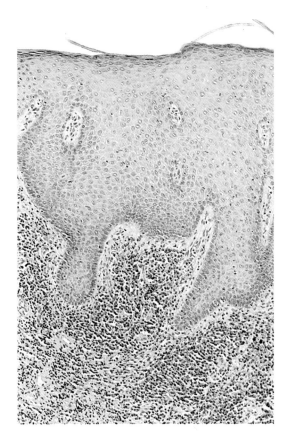

FIGURE 20-4 Secondary syphilis. Psoriasiform epidermal hyperplasia is accompanied by intracellular edema and exocytosis of lymphocytes. A bandlike lymphoplasmacellular dermal infiltrate is present.

of outer root sheath epithelium, perifollicular fibrosis,[11] an involutional tendancy with increased numbers of telogen hairs, and, in some cases, a necrotizing pustular follicular reaction.[6] A necrotizing pustular follicular reaction with nonnecrotizing granulomata and a perivascular lymphoplasmacellular infiltrate characterizes the rare entity of pustular secondary syphilis.[6] A bullous variant of secondary syphilis is described.[19] There is considerable overlap between cases of secondary and tertiary syphilis, as small, sarcoidal granulomata in papular lesions of secondary syphilis may progress to extensive lymphoplasmacellular and histiocytic infiltrates resembling nodular tertiary syphilis, whereas lesions of early tertiary syphilis may lack granulomata.[20,21,22]

Differential Diagnosis   Other causes of lichenoid dermatitis, namely, lichen planus, lichenoid hypersensitivity reactions, pityriasis lichenoides and connective tissue disease, sarcoidosis, psoriasis, and psoriasiform drug eruptions,[11] may all resemble syphilis. Prominent spongiosis, suprabasilar dyskeratosis, deep perivascular inflammation, and plasma cells are not characteristic of lichen planus or psoriasis. A middermal perivascular infiltrate, keratinocyte necrosis, and pronounced lymphocytic exocytosis characterize pityriasis lichenoides, but the infiltrate is purely lymphocytic, and spongiform pustulation is not seen. Tissue eosinophilia and plasma cell infiltrates are often noted in lichenoid hypersensitivity reactions and psoriasiform drug reactions.

TERTIARY SYPHILIS

Tertiary syphilis includes nodular tertiary syphilis confined to skin; benign gummatous syphilis principally affecting skin, bone, and liver; cardiovascular syphilis; neurosyphilis; and syphilitic hepatic cirrhosis.

In nodular tertiary syphilis, granulomas are small and limited to the dermis, where scattered nested epithelioid cells are intermingled with a few multinucleated giant cells and lymphoid and plasma cells. Granulomata may be absent,[22] and necrosis is not conspicuous. The vessels may show endothelial swelling.[17] Benign gummatous syphilis manifests granulomatous inflammation with central zones of acellular necrosis in involved organs, whereas in the skin, blood vessels throughout the dermis and subcutis manifest endarteritis obliterans with variable angiocentric plasmacellular infiltrates.[4]

The Nonvenereal Treponematoses

YAWS (FRAMBESIA TROPICA)

Yaws, caused by *T. pallidum pertenue*, is spread by casual contact between primary or secondary lesions and abraded skin, classically affects the buttocks, legs, and feet of children, and is most prevalent in warm, moist tropical climates. Seropositivity rates up to 95 percent are seen in areas of Ecuador.[23] *T. pallidum pertenue* is indistinguishable microscopically from *T. pallidum pallidum* but is distinctive by Southern blot analysis,[24] where a single substituted nucleotide is demonstrable.

Primary yaws
An erythematous papule, or *mother yaw*, is seen roughly 21 days after inoculation and enlarges peripherally to form a 1- to 5-cm nodule with an amber crust and adjacent satellite pustules. Lesions heal as pitted, hypopigmented scars. Fever, arthralgia, or lymphadenopathy may coexist.[25]

Secondary yaws
Progression to the secondary stage is characterized by involvement of skin, bones, joints, and cerebrospinal fluid. Skin lesions, or *daughter yaws*, resemble the mother yaw but are smaller and more numerous. Although periorificial lesions may resemble venereal syphilis, a circinate appearance may mimic fungal infection, hence the designation *tinea yaws*. A morbilliform eruption may occur, as may condylomatous vegetations involving axillae and groin. Macular, hyperkeratotic, and papillomatous lesions may be seen on palmoplantar surfaces and may cause the patient to walk with a painful, crablike gait, designated *crab yaws*.[25] *Pianic onychia* are papillomatous nail fold lesions.[25] Relapsing cutaneous disease occurs for up to 5 years and tends to involve periorificial and periaxillary sites.

Tertiary yaws
In tertiary yaws, skin manifestations include subcutaneous abscesses, coalescing serpiginous ulcers, keloids, keratoderma, and palmoplantar hyperkeratosis. The bone and joint manifestations include osteomyelitis, hypertrophic or gummatous periostitis, and chronic tibial osteitis. Obstructive hypertrophy of the nasal maxillary processes produces the rare but characteristic *goundou*.[25] Another otorhinolaryngologic complication termed *gangosa* comprises nasal septal or palatal perforation. Macular atrophy and culture-positive aqueous humor suggest that yaws may exhibit neurophthalmologic manifestations. In lower-prevalence areas, a less virulent form of the disease termed *attenuated yaws* manifests as greasy gray lesions in the skin folds.[4,25]

Histopathological Features   Primary lesions manifest epidermal acanthosis, papillomatosis, spongiosis, and neutrophilic exocytosis with microabscesses. A diffuse, dermal infiltrate of plasma cells, lymphocytes, histiocytes, and granulocytes is seen, which, unlike syphilis, is associated with little or no endothelial proliferation[26,27] (Fig. 20-5). A similar histopathology characterizes secondary lesions, which resemble

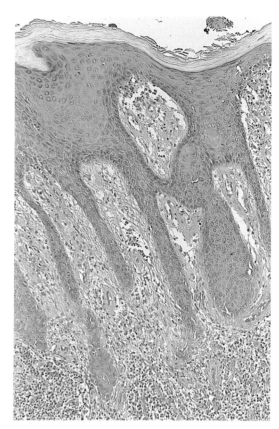

FIGURE 20-5   Yaws, the primary lesion. The biopsy shows psoriasiform epidermal hyperplasia with an intense lymphohistiocytic and plasmacellular infiltrate in the corium.

condylomata lata in their epidermal changes but differ by virtue of a diffuse, as opposed to a perivascular, dermal infiltrate (Fig. 20-6). The ulcerative lesions of tertiary yaws histologically resemble those of late syphilis.[26] Spirochetes are demonstrated in primary and secondary lesions by dark-field examination and between keratinocytes in silver stains, although, unlike *T. pallidum*, which is also found in the dermis, *T. pertenue* is almost entirely epidermotropic.[27]

Differential Diagnosis   The distinction of yaws from syphilis is based upon clinical features,[28] although localization of the organism in a skin biopsy may be helpful.

PINTA

Involvement in pinta, caused by *T. carateum*, is restricted to the skin[29] with hypopigmentation being the only significant sequela. Endemic to Central America, pinta is not observed outside the Western Hemisphere, affects no age group preferentially, is the mildest of the treponematoses, and is declining precipitously in incidence for reasons unkown. Transmission appears to be from lesion to skin, usually between family members.[29]

The primary lesion, an erythematous papule surrounded by a halo, occurs 1 to 8 weeks after inoculation and may expand by direct extension or through fusion of satellites to form an ill-defined plaque up to 12 cm in diameter on the legs or other exposed sites. The primary lesion in infants classically occurs where the baby was closely held by the affected mother. The secondary lesions, which bear the unfortunate and misleading appellation *pintids*, manifest months after inoculation as small, erythematous, scaly papules and psoriasiform plaques and are, like the primary lesions, highly infectious. In the tertiary stage, hypo-

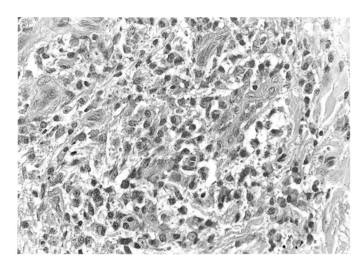

FIGURE 20-6   Yaws, the primary lesion. The biopsy shows an intense angiocentric and diffuse lymphohistiocytic and plasmacellular infiltrate.

pigmented macules are present over bony prominences, wrists, ankles, and elbows. Symmetric areas of achromia alternate with areas of normal or hyperpigmented, atrophic, or hyperkeratotic skin.

Histopathological Features   The features of primary and secondary lesions are similar, showing acanthosis, spongiosis, and a sparse dermal infiltrate of lymphocytes, plasma cells, and neutrophils disposed about dilated blood vessels which do not manifest endothelial swelling.[30] Lichenoid inflammation with attendant hyperkeratosis, hypergranulosis, basal layer vacuolopathy, and pigmentary incontinence may be seen. Tertiary stage lesions show either postinflammatory hyperpigmentation or are depigmented, manifesting complete absence of epidermal melanin; epidermal atrophy and perivascular lymphocytic infiltrates are seen in both. Organisms are seen in all but long-standing lesions.

ENDEMIC SYPHILIS (BEJEL)

Caused by *T. pallidum endemicum*, bejel is largely confined to the arid Arabian peninsula and the southern border of the Sahara desert,[29] where children are the principal reservoir for a disease spread by skin-to-skin contact or via fomites such as communal pipes or drinking vessels. The rare primary stage skin lesions comprise erythematous papules or ulcers of the oropharyngeal mucosa or the skin of the nipple of an uninfected mother nursing an infected infant. The more common initial manifestations are secondary stage lesions: multiple shallow, painless ulcers involving lips, buccal mucosa, tongue, fauces, or tonsils. Such lesions may be accompanied by hoarseness due to treponemal laryngitis, regional lymphadenopathy, condylomata lata involving the axillae and anogenital areas. Rarely the initial presentation may include erythematous, crusted papules, macules, or annular papulosquamous lesions accompanied in some patients by generalized lymphadenopathy or periostitis. The tertiary stage manifests as gummatous lesions of nasopharynx, larynx, skin, and bone which may progress to ulcers which heal as depigmented, sometimes geographic, scars with peripheral hyperpigmentation. Bone and joint involvement manifests as tibial periostitis mimicking yaws or as destructive lesions of the nasal septum and palate.[4,29] Ophthalmologic complications include uveitis, chorioretinitis, choroiditis, and optic atrophy.

Histopathological Features   The pathology of early lesions of endemic syphilis is not well described, although late lesions are said to show parakeratosis, acanthosis, spongiosis, pigmentary incontinence, and a dermal lymphohistiocytic and plasmacellular infiltrate.

LYME DISEASE

Named after the town of Lyme, Connecticut, where it was first encountered in 1975,[31] Lyme disease is caused by the the spirochete *Borrelia burgdorferi* and transmitted by *Ornithodorus*[32] ticks, with *Ixodes dammini* being the prototypic vector.[32,33] The index patients manifested inflammatory arthritis and central nervous system and cardiac symptoms[34] preceded by cutaneous erythema. Lyme disease, the most common tick-borne disease in the United States, has also been reported in Europe, Africa, and Asia.[35] Stage I (early) Lyme disease occurs when hematogenous dissemination from skin lesions of erythema chronicum migrans causes self-limited orchitis, splenomegaly, lymphadenopathy, and mild pneumonitis.[36] Neural and cardiac involvement, the former manifesting a classic triad of meningitis, cranial neuritis, and radiculoneuritis, and the latter manifesting as tachycardia and heart blocks due to an epi- and transmyocarditis, characterize stage II.[35,36] Stage III Lyme disease represents chronic disease at sites where spirochetes persist, namely, the skin, nervous system, and the musculoskeletal system. The latter encompasses findings typical for any reactive arthropathy syndrome, specifically synovitis and migratory oligoarthritis involving the knee, shoulder, wrist, and temporomandibular and ankle joints.[35,36]

Stage I Lyme Disease—Erythema Chronicum Migrans

Erythema chronicum migrans, the distinctive cutaneous manifestation of stage I Lyme disease,[37,38] represents the site of inoculation, although patients are often not aware of having suffered a tick bite. Beginning as an area of scaly erythema or a red papule 3 to 30 days after the tick bite, lesions spread peripherally, showing central clearing and occasionally reaching a diameter of 25 cm.[39] Presentations may be atypical by virtue of showing purpuric, vesicular, or linear lesions. Although lesions typically last for 4 weeks, they may persist for up to 1 year, and may be solitary or multiple, the latter reflecting hematogenous dissemination of the spirochete, often with concomitant fever, fatigue, headache, cough, and arthralgia.[32]

Histopathological Features   Skin biopsies show superficial and deep angiocentric, neurotropic, and eccrinotropic lymphocytic infiltrates, often accompanied by plasma cells and eosinophils, the former at the periphery and the latter in the center of the lesions.[38] The dermal alterations may be accompanied by spongiotic epithelial changes (Fig. 20-7), and some cases show edema of blood vessels, transmural migration of lymphocytes and plasma cells, granulomatous vasculitis with luminal thrombosis, lymphohistiocytic neuritis, and interstitial reticular dermal infiltrates with an associated sclerosing reaction.[4] The histomorphology varies according to the part of the lesion biopsied; a florid inflammatory cell infiltrate with granulomatous vasculitis and neuritis will be seen at the tick bite punctum, whereas a biopsy taken within 1 cm of the outermost edge will show a pauci-inflammatory process with only sparse mononuclear cells, no eosinophils or plasma cells, and a characteristic vasculopathy comprising endothelial swelling and hyperplasia and mural edema accompanied by mucinosis (Fig. 20-8).[40] Biopsies taken between these two sites show the characteristic superficial and deep perivascular lymphocytic, plasmacellular, and eosinophilic infiltrate with variable eczematous alterations described in most histopathology textbooks.[4] Although spirochetes have been identified, primarily from the lesional border, in only 40% of cases,[38] most patients manifest elevated IgM antibody titers,[37] and one should rely heavily upon serology in making the diagnosis.

Differential Diagnosis   The differential diagnosis includes other arthropod assaults, drug hypersensitivity, contact reactions, and connective tissue diseases such as lupus erythematosus, scleroderma, morphea, Sjogren's syndrome, mixed connective tissue disease, and relapsing polychondritis. Although tissue eosinophilia and epidermal changes

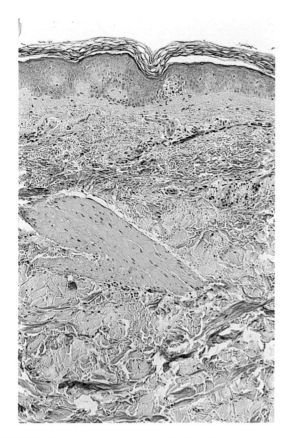

FIGURE 20-7   Erythema chronica migrans. Epidermal spongiosis with vesicle formation overlies a dermis showing a sparse nonspecific perivascular lymphocytic infiltrate.

help to discriminate Lyme disease from connective tissue disease, differentiation from erythema annulare centrifugum may be impossible.

Stage III Lyme Disease—Dermal atrophying and sclerosing lesions
Acrodermatitis chronica atrophicans often manifests as diffuse or localized erythema on one extremity with a "doughy" consistency of the dermis which progresses over months to atrophy; vessels and subcutaneous tissue may become visible to the naked eye.[41] Appendage structures

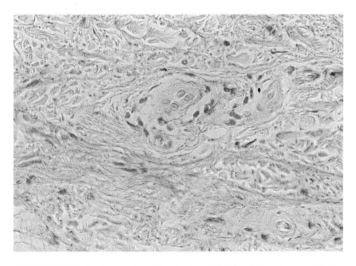

FIGURE 20-8   Erythema chronica migrans. A biopsy taken 1 cm inside the advancing lesional rim shows endothelial swelling and dermal mucinosis with a nonspecific, sparse perivascular lymphocytic infiltrate (alcian blue).

may disappear, causing hair loss and hypohidrosis. Located mainly near joints of the upper and lower extremities, sparing the palms, soles, face, and trunk,[42] late-stage lesions may manifest sclerosis in the form of pseudosclerodermatous plaques over the dorsa of feet, as linear fibrotic bands over ulnar and tibial surfaces, or as localized fibromas termed *juxtarticular nodes* overlying joints.[4,41] Serology is uniformly positive at this stage, and patients often manifest an elevated erythrocyte sedimentation rate (ESR) or hypergammaglobulinemia. Other atrophying and sclerosing disorders associated with Lyme disease include anetoderma, atrophoderma of Pasini and Pierini, facial hemiatrophy of Perry-Romberg, lichen sclerosus et atrophicus, eosinophilic fasciitis, and morphea.[4,43,44] In facial hemiatrophy, skeletal muscle becomes atrophic with loss of striations, edema, and vacuolation, and ocular and neurologic complications may include iritis, keratitis, optic nerve atrophy, trigeminal neuralgia, and facial palsy.[35]

Histopathological Features   The epidermis appears atrophic with loss of retia and diminution of a granular layer often surmounted by a keratotic scale. A cell-poor lymphocytic interface dermatitis with vacuolar basal layer degeneration and variable postinflammatory pigmentary alterations ranging from leukoderma to hyperpigmentation is noted in one-half of cases. The papillary dermis manifests edema which progresses to eosinophilic homogenization,[43,45] accompanied in some cases by a band-like lymphocytic infiltrate which may obscure the dermoepidermal junction in a lichenoid fashion, or may manifest an angiocentric and adnexotropic disposition extending through the dermis to involve the subcutis.[46] Eosinophils, neutrophils, and plasma cells may contribute to the inflammatory process.[46] Blood vessels, collagen fibers, and elastic tissue may be effaced.[46] End-stage lesions show telangiectasia, adnexal atrophy, degenerated or eosinophilic collagen, basophilic fragmented elastic fibers,[46] and lipoid phanerosis.[45] With respect to the other atrophying disorders, all manifest a variable sclerodermoid tissue reaction with adnexal atrophy and subcutaneous fibrosis. The histopathology of anetoderma, an elastolytic disorder, is discussed elsewhere.

Lymphocytoma cutis and malignant lymphoma
Lymphocytoma cutis is a benign cutaneous lymphoid hyperplasia ascribed to triggering factors, including drugs, contactants, and infections, implicating an excessive immune response to antigen as its etiologic basis. The demonstration of spirochetelike structures in patients with lymphocytoma cutis seropositive for antibodies to *Borrelia* subspecies is presumptive evidence of a causal relationship[47]; lesions are designated *borreliomas* and manifest clinically as solitary or multiple violaceous nodules and infiltrative plaques with a predilection for the earlobes, nipple, and areolae. Lesions may occur at sites of erythema chronicum migrans or in patients with stage II Lyme disease.[4] Malignant lymphoma has also been described.[48]

Histopathological Features   A dense nodular or diffuse folliculotropic, eccrinotropic, and neurotropic pandermal infiltrate of small lymphocytes with a variable admixture of immunoblasts, eosinophils, and plasma cells is seen (Fig. 20-9). Germinal centers may be observed, and a grenz zone of papillary dermal sparing is characteristic.

Differential Diagnosis   Other infections, particularly those due to herpes or mycobacteria, and reactions to insect bites, drugs,[49] and contactants mimic nodular Borrelial lymphocytoma cutis, whereas well-differentiated lymphocytic lymphoma and chronic lymphocytic leukemia mimic the diffuse variant. The presence of eosinophils, plasma cells, and germinal centers enable distinction from malignant lymphoma in some cases, with two notable caveats being the proliferation centers of low-grade lymphoproliferative disease, which mimic germinal centers at low-power microscopy, and the presence of a superficial lymphocytoma cutis pattern overlying an area of malignant lymphoma.

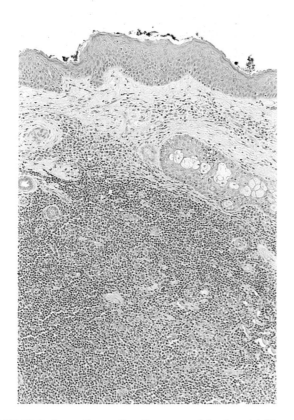

FIGURE 20-9 Lyme disease. Borrelioma—a nodular dermal infiltrate predominated by small lymphoid forms.

RICKETTSIAL INFECTIONS

Rickettsial infections include Rocky Mountain spotted fever, rickettsialpox, typhus, scrub typhus, and ehrlichioses. *Rickettsiae* are obligate intracellular bacteria that are transmitted to humans from infected arthropods.[50] Three genera contain significant pathogens, *Rickettsia*, *Orientia*, and *Ehrlichia*. Members of the *Rickettsia* genus include *Rickettsia rickettsii*, which causes Rocky Mountain spotted fever (RMSF); *Rickettsia conorii*, which causes Mediterranean spotted fever or boutonneuse fever; *Rickettsia akari*, which causes rickettsialpox, *Rickettsia typhi*, which causes murine or endemic typhus; and *Rickettsia prowazekii*, which causes epidemic typhus. *Rickettsia* species infect and damage endothelial cells which leads to cutaneous and systemic lymphohistiocytic vasculitis, the hallmark and major pathogenetic lesion of the vasculotropic rickettsioses. The rickettsial disease of greatest importance in the United States is Rocky Mountain spotted fever,[51] which is acquired after the bite of infected *Dermacentor* subspecies ticks. The next most prevalent vasculotropic rickettsiosis in the United States is the flea-borne murine typhus.[52]

Orientia (previously *Rickettsia*) *tsutsugamushi* is the etiologic agent of scrub typhus, another vasculotropic rickettsiosis that occurs predominantly in the Far East and is transmitted by larval mites. *Ehrlichia* species that are human pathogens infrequently cause reproducible and characteristic skin lesions; the cutaneous pathology and pathogenesis of *Ehrlichia* infections is unclear.

Clinical Features   The vasculotropic rickettsioses share many clinical features. RMSF is a severe febrile illness usually associated with headaches and rash that occurs after tick bite.[51] The predominant early lesions are blanching macules and papules that may develop into nonblanching petechiae or purpura as the illness progresses (Table 20-3).

Clinical Features

Fever
Headache
History of tick bite or exposure
Macular, maculopapular, or petechial rash may be focal or diffuse
Rash occurs approximately 3 to 7 days after onset of fever

Histopathological Features

Early—mixed lymphohistiocytic perivascular infiltrates around dermal vessels
Late—leukocytoclastic vasculitis with karyorrhexis and occasional fibrin thrombi
Early and late—endothelial cell swelling and loss, erythrocyte extravasation, edema

Differential Diagnosis

Insect-bite reaction
Drug reaction
Septic vasculitis
"Autoimmune" vasculitides

The eruption typically occurs between the third and fifth days of illness. These lesions may occur on any cutaneous surface, including the palms and soles, but are most frequently observed on the extremities and trunk, respectively. The degree of cutaneous involvement is highly variable, sometimes transient, and approximately 10 to 15 percent of infected patients will not develop any rash.[53] When present, the lesions may measure from less than 1 mm in diameter to large and irregular confluent purpuric lesions many centimeters in size. Rickettsialpox is associated with papulovesicles, but, frequently, infected patients also present with macules and papules as above. Petechial and purpuric lesions are less frequent with rickettsialpox and murine typhus than with RMSF.[52,54] The site of vector bite is rarely identified in RMSF and is frequently identified in Mediterranean spotted fever, rickettsialpox, and scrub typhus. The site often develops into a dark necrotic eschar between several millimeters and 1 cm in diameter.[50,54–56]

Histopathological Features   The histopathologic features are similar among the vasculotropic rickettsioses.[50] Thus, the specific changes of RMSF will be discussed (Table 20-3). Significant findings are mostly confined within the dermis.[55,57] The early (3 to 4 days) changes include a mild to moderate mixed lymphohistiocytic infiltrate that forms tight cuffs surrounding and penetrating into the walls of the superficial, middle, and lower dermal capillaries and venules; erythrocyte extravasation; endothelial swelling; and edema. The infiltrate may extend into the perivascular interstitium or may concentrate adjacent to adnexal structures such as eccrine units. Later (after 6 days), accrued vascular damage frequently yields leukocytoclastic vasculitis that is predominantly lymphohistiocytic with some neutrophilic infiltrates and karyorrhectic nuclear debris (Fig. 20-10). These later lesions are often clinically associated with palpable, nonblanching petechiae, or a hemorrhagic, purpuric rash. Less than half of these lesions will contain focal fibrin thrombi and well-defined vessel wall necrosis. Endothelial cell swelling and loss are frequent occurrences. The dermal infiltrate sometimes contains plasma cells or eosinophils. Infrequent findings include neutrophilic hidradenitis, perineural lymphocytic infiltration, and neutrophilic lobular panniculitis. Epidermal findings are usually associated with leukocytoclastic vasculitis, probably resulting from underlying vascular

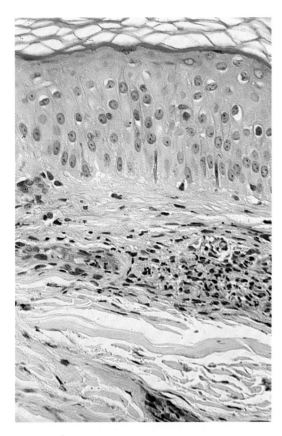

FIGURE 20-10   Rocky Mountain spotted fever. Leukocytoclastic vasculitis in Rocky Mountain spotted fever (RMSF) (*Rickettsia rickettsii* infection). One superficial dermal venule is completely obliterated by the necrotizing inflammatory vasculitis and thrombus, whereas an adjacent venule is relatively spared owing to the focality of the rickettsial infection. Thrombosis such as illustrated here is seen in less than half of all diagnostic biopsies from patients with RMSF. The pattern of leukocytoclastic vasculitis is most often recognized in patients with clinical illness exceeding 6 days.

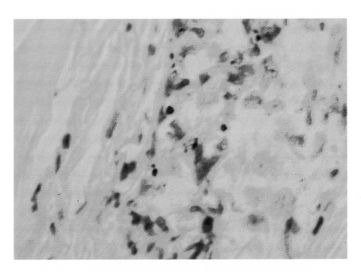

FIGURE 20-11   Rocky Mountain spotted fever. Immunohistologic demonstration of *Rickettsia rickettsii* in infected superficial dermal venule in a patient with Rocky Mountain spotted fever. Note that the rickettsiae are intimately associated with the endothelium, reflecting the intracellular niche of these bacteria. Because of focal infection, several step sections stained by an immunohistologic method such as immunoperoxidase or immunofluorescence are recommended. (Immunoperoxidase stain with rabbit anti–*R. rickettsii*, aminoethylcarbazol substrate, hematoxylin counterstain.)

compromise, and may include interface dermatitis with basal vacuolar degeneration and mild dermoepidermal interface lymphocytic exocytosis. Apoptotic keratinocytes are infrequently present. In rickettsialpox, the papulovesicular lesions result from a subepidermal separation.[54] When present, and especially with Mediterranean spotted fever and rickettsialpox, the site of vector bite may form into an eschar that includes severe lymphohistiocytic and neutrophilic infiltrates; endothelial cell proliferation; vascular, dermal, and epidermal necrosis; and extensive deposition of nuclear debris that results from the intense inflammation and local proliferation of rickettsiae.[54,56]

Characteristic spotted fever or typhus group rickettsiae may be visualized using specific antibody reagents and immunohistologic methods such as immunofluorescence or immunoperoxidase (Fig. 20-11)[54,55,58]; nonspecific staining methods such as Gram or Giemsa stains are nonrevealing and occasionally misleading. Rickettsiae are most often observed in endothelial cells in clusters or "colonies" at sites of severe vasculitis; however, rickettsiae are also observed in adjacent noninflamed vessels. The involvement of a vessel may be eccentric, with inflammation and rickettsiae present only in one wall. Characteristic lesions should be sampled, and multiple leveled sections should be examined because of the focality of the infection. Prior therapy with tetracycline antibiotics will abrogate the ability to detect rickettsiae in the biopsy tissue by immunohistologic methods. Immunohistology may

be performed rapidly by frozen section or on paraffin-embedded, formalin-fixed tissues with equal sensitivity. The additional histologic details discerned with the immunoenzymatic light-microscopic methods are confirmatory because of the colocalization of the intracellular rickettsiae and vascular inflammatory reaction. The sensitivity of immunohistology is approximately 70 percent, and specificity is nearly 100 percent when diagnosis is rendered by those skilled in the interpretation of rickettsial immunohistology. Polymerase chain reaction on acute phase blood has not increased sensitivity beyond that determined for immunohistology, and specific rickettsial antibodies are not usually detected by any method during the acute illness.

Differential Diagnosis   The histologic differential diagnosis includes diseases associated with vascular or capillary inflammation (Table 20-3): insect-bite reaction, drug reaction, septic vasculitis secondary to disseminated intravascular coagulation (DIC), other specific infectious agents, other physical or chemical agents, collagen vascular diseases, mixed cryoglobulinemia, Henoch-Shoenlein purpura, serum sickness, urticarial vasculitis, and vasculitis that occurs secondary to malignancy. Many of the lesions can be differentiated by other laboratory or histologic methods, including culture or special stains for specific infectious agents. Other laboratory and clinical findings will often aid in differentiation. In patients with DIC or sepsis, leukocytoclastic vasculitis with prominent fibrin thrombi are often identified, and most will have marked abnormalities in coagulation profiles, including prolongations in prothrombin and activated partial thromboplastin times, and fibrin split products or D-dimer tests are positive. Patients with RMSF infrequently have true DIC, and coagulation studies are only infrequently and mildly altered.

REFERENCES

1. Hook EW, Marra CM: Acquired syphilis in adults. *N Engl J Med* 326:1060–1069, 1992.
2. Magro CM, Crowson AN, Alfa M, et al: A morphological study of penile chancroid lesions in human immunodeficiency virus (HIV)-positive and -negative African men with a hypothesis concerning the role of chancroid in HIV transmission. *Hum Pathol* 27:1066–1070, 1996.

3. Greenblatt RM, Lukehart AA, Plummer FA, et al: Genital ulceration as a risk factor for human immunodeficiency virus infection. *AIDS* 2:47–50, 1988.

4. Crowson AN, Magro CM, Mihm MC: Treponemal diseases, in Elder DE, Johnson BE, Jaworsky C, Elenitsas R (eds): *Lever's Histopathology of the Skin*, 8th ed. Philadelphia, Lippincott, 503–516, 1997.

5. Hartsock RJ, Halling LW, King FM: Luetic lymphadenitis. *Am J Clin Pathol* 53:304–314, 1970.

6. Noppakun N, Dinerart SM, Solomon AR: Pustular secondary syphilis. *Int J Dermatol* 26:112–114,1987.

7. Tanabe JL, Huntley AC: Granulomatous tertiary syphilis. *J Am Acad Dermatol* 15:341–344, 1986.

8. Sanchez PJ: Congenital syphilis. *Adv Ped Inf Dis* 7:161–180, 1992.

9. Johnson PC, Farnie MA: Testing for syphilis. *Dermatol Clin* 12:9–17, 1994.

10. Sykes JA, Miller JN, Kalan AJ: *Treponema pallidum* within cells of a primary chancre from a human female. *Br J Vener Dis* 50:40–44, 1974.

11. Jeerapaet P, Ackerman AS: Histologic patterns of secondary syphilis. *Arch Dermatol* 107:373–377, 1973.

12. Abell E, Marks R, Wilson Jones E: Secondary syphilis: A clinicopathological review. *Br J Dermatol* 93:53–61, 1975.

13. Cochran RIE, Thomson J, Fleming KA, et al: Histology simulating reticulosis in secondary syphilis. *Br J Dermatol* 95:251–254, 1976.

14. Poulsen A, Kobayasi T, Secher L, et al: Treponema pallidum in macular and papular secondary syphilis skin eruptions. *Acta Derm Venereol (Stockh)* 66:251–258, 1986.

15. Montgomery H: *Dermatopathology*. New York, Harper and Row, 417–426, 1967.

16. Fisher DA, Chang LW, Tuffanelli DL: Lues maligna. *Arch Dermatol* 99:70-73, 1979.

17. Petrozzi JW, Lockshin NA, Berger RI: Malignant syphilis. *Arch Dermatol* 109:387–389, 1974.

18. Kerdel-Vegas F, Kopf AW, Tolmach JA: Keratoderma punctatum syphiliticum: Report of a case. *Br J Dermatol* 66:449–454, 1954.

19. Lawrence T, Saxe N: Bullous secondary syphilis. *Clin Exp Dermatol* 17:44–46, 1992.

20. Kahn LE, Gordon W: Sarcoid-like granulomas in secondary syphilis. *Arch Pathol* 92:334–337, 1971.

21. Lantis LR, Petrozzi JW, Hurley HJ: Sarcoid granuloma in secondary syphilis. *Arch Dermatol* 99:748–752, 1969.

22. Matsuda-John SS, McElgunn PST, Ellis CN: Nodular late syphilis. *J Am Acad Dermatol* 9:269–272, 1983.

23. Guderian RH, Guzman JR, Calvopina M, Cooper P: Studies on a focus of yaws in the Santiago Basin, province of Esmeraldas, Ecuador. *Trop Geogr Med* 43:142–147, 1991.

24. Noordhoek GT, Hermans PWM, Paul AN, et al: *Treponema pallidum* subspecies *pallidum* (Nichols) and *Treponema pallidum* subspecies *pertenue* (CDC 2575) differ in at least one nucleotide: Comparison of two homologous antigens. *Microb Pathog* 6:29–42, 1989.

25. Engelkens HJH, Judanarso J, Oranje AP, et al: Endemic treponematoses: I. Yaws. *Int J Dermatol* 30:77–83, 1992.

26. Williams HU: Pathology of yaws. *Arch Pathol* 20:596–630, 1935.

27. Hasselmann CM: Comparative studies on the histopathology of syphilis, yaws and pinta. *Br J Vener Dis* 33:5–23, 1957.

28. Greene CA, Harman RRM: Yaws truly—a survey of patients indexed under "Yaws" and a review of the clinical and laboratory problems of diagnosis. *Clin Exp Dermatol* 11:41–48, 1986.

29. Engelkens HJH, Niemel PLA, van der Sluis JL, et al: Endemic treponematoses: II. Pinta and endemic syphilis. *Int J Dermatol* 30:231–238, 1991.

30. Pardo-Castello V, Ferrer I: Pinta. *Arch Dermatol Syph* 45:843–864, 1942.

31. Steere AC, Grodzicki RL, Kornblatt AN, et al: The spirochetal etiology of Lyme disease. *N Engl J Med* 308:733–740, 1983.

32. Duray PH: Histopathology of clinical phases of human Lyme disease. *Rheum Dis Clin North Am* 15:691–725, 1989.

33. Benach JL, Bosler EM, Hanrahan JP, et al: Spirochetes isolated from the blood of two patients with Lyme disease. *N Engl J Med* 308:740–742, 1983.

34. Steere AC, Malawista SE, Snydman DR, et al: Lyme arthritis: An epidemic of oligoarticular arthritis in children and adults in three Connecticut communities. *Arthritis Rheum* 20:7–17, 1977.

35. Abele DC, Anders KH: The many faces and phases of borreliosis: I. Lyme disease. *J Am Acad Dermatol* 23:167–186, 1990.

36. Sigel LH, Curran AS: Lyme disease: A multifocal worldwide disease. *Annu Rev Publ Health* 12:85–109, 1991.

37. Asbrink E, Hovmark A: Cutaneous manifestations in *Ixodes*-borne Borrelia spirochetosis. *Int J Dermatol* 26:215–223, 1987.

38. Berger BW: Erythema chronicum migrans of Lyme disease. *Arch Dermatol* 120:1017–1021, 1984.

39. Cote J: Lyme disease. *Int J Dermatol* 30: 500–501, 1991.

40. Shulman KJ, Melski JW, Reed KD, et al: The characteristic histologic features of erythema chronicum migrans (abstract). *Lab Invest* 74:1996, p. 46A..

41. Burgdorf WHS, Woret WI, Schultes O: Acrodermatitis chronica atrophicans. *Int J Dermatol* 18:595–601, 1979.

42. Kaufman L, Gruber BL, Philips ME, Benach JL: Late cutaneous Lyme disease: Acrodermatitis chronica atrophicans. *Am J Med* 86:828–830, 1989.

43. Aberer E, Klade H, Stanek G, Gebhart W: *Borrelia burgdorferi* and different types of morphea. *Dermatologica* 182:145–154, 1991.

44. Aberer E, Stanek G, Ertl M, Neumann R: Evidence for spirochetal origin of circumscribed scleroderma (morphea). *Acta Derm Venereol (Stockh)* 67:225–231, 1987.

45. Montgomery H: *Dermatopathology*. New York, Harper and Row, 766–769, 1967.

46. Aberer E, Klade H, Hobisch G: A clinical, histological, and immunohistochemical comparison of acrodermatitis chronica atrophicans and morphea. *Am J Dermatopathol* 13:334–341, 1991.

47. Hovmark A, Asbrink E, Olsson I: The spirochetal etiology of lymphadenosis benign cutis solitaria. *Acta Derm Venereol (Stockh)* 66: 479–484, 1986.

48. Garbe C, Stein H, Dienemann D, Orfanos CD: *Borrelia burgdorferi*-associated cutaneous B-cell lymphoma: Clinical and immunohistologic characterization of four cases. *J Am Acad Dermatol* 24:584–590, 1991.

49. Magro CM, Crowson AN: Drug-induced immune dysregulation as a cause of atypical cutaneous lymphoid infiltrates: A hypothesis. *Hum Pathol* 27:125–132, 1996.

50. Dumler JS, Walker DH: Diagnostic tests for Rocky Mountain spotted fever and other rickettsial diseases. *Derm Clin* 12:25–36, 1994.

51. Walker DH: Rocky Mountain spotted fever: A seasonal alert. *Clin Infect Dis* 20:1111–1117, 1995.

52. Dumler JS, Taylor JP, Walker DH: Clinical and laboratory features of murine typhus in south Texas, 1980 through 1987. *JAMA* 266:1365–1370, 1991.

53. Sexton DJ, Corey GR: Rocky Mountain "spotless" and "almost spotless" fever: A wolf in sheep's clothing. *Clin Infect Dis* 15:439–448, 1992.

54. Kass EM, Szaniawski WK, Levy H, et al: Rickettsialpox in a New York City hospital, 1980 to 1989. *N Engl J Med* 331:1612–1617, 1994.

55. Walker DH: Diagnosis of rickettsial diseases. *Path Annu* 23:69–96, 1988.

56. Walker DH, Occhino C, Tringali GR, et al: Pathogenesis of rickettsial eschars: The tache noire of boutonneuse fever. *Hum Pathol* 19:1449–1454, 1988.

57. Kao GF, Ioffe O, Evancho CD, et al: Cutaneous histopathology of Rocky Mountain spotted fever (abstract). *J Cutan Pathol* 23:53, 1996.

58. Dumler JS, Gage WR, Pettis GL, et al: Rapid immunoperoxidase demonstration of *Rickettsia rickettsii* in fixed cutaneous specimens from patients with Rocky Mountain spotted fever. *Am J Clin Pathol* 93:410–414, 1990.

CHAPTER 21

FUNGAL INFECTIONS

Catharine Lisa Kauffman / Victoria Hobbs Hamet / Steven Tahan / Klaus Busam / Raymond L. Barnhill

Fungi are nonmotile eucaryotic organisms composed of cells enclosed by a rigid cell wall containing ergosterol and chitin or other polysaccharides but usually not cellulose. The organisms may be unicellular, such as yeasts, or multicellular, forming long filaments known as hyphae. Hyphae are divided into cells by septa. Various reproductive structures such as conidia and spores develop on hyphae; the morphology of these structures provides the basis for taxonomy. Some genera have the capacity to form either yeast or hyphal forms, or both depending on environmental conditions, a characteristic known as dimorphism.

Asexual reproduction is the primary means of propagation for many fungi. Sexual reproduction involves the fusion of two haploid nuclei followed by meiosis. The diploid state is transient and is called the perfect state. Fungi that have the capacity for sexual reproduction are classified under the phyla Zygomycota (e.g., mucormycotic organisms), Basidiomycota (e.g., mushrooms, toadstools, and plant pathogens), and Ascomycota. Ascomycota includes the order Onygenales, which in turn includes the genus *Arthroderma*.[1] Deuteromycota, or Fungi Imperfecti, is the form-phylum containing fungi with no known sexual reproduction; most of the pathogenic fungi were classified into this group until research during the past several decades demonstrated the sexual or so-called teleomorphic stage of many species, which were reclassified into other phyla.[2–6] The majority of the medically important species are now classified in the order Onygenales of the phylum Ascomycota; representative members include the dermatophytes and the causative agents of histoplasmosis and blastomycosis. As a matter of convenience, in this chapter, the anamorphic (asexual) classifications will be used.

Owing to their relatively small size and frequent absence of pigment, fungi are often difficult to discern on hematoxylin-eosin stained sections. Histopathological clues to the presence of a superficial fungal infection include (1) neutrophils within the stratum corneum; (2) foci of parakeratosis; and (3) variation in the thickness and appearance of the stratum corneum. Signs of a deeper fungal infection may include (1) pseudoepitheliomatous hyperplasia; (2) neutrophilic microabcesses or suppurative granulomas within the epidermis and dermis; (3) multinucleated giant cells within a dermal infiltrate; (4) empty spaces within multinucleated giant cells: (5) necrosis; and (6) vascular occlusion. The histological appearance of various fungi in tissue is summarized in Table 21-1.

SUPERFICIAL FILAMENTOUS INFECTIONS

Dermatophytoses

Superficial cutaneous fungal infections, referred to as ringworm or tinea, are among the most common infections in humans. The majority of these infections are caused by the anamorphic (asexual) genera *Epidermophyton*, *Microsporum*, and *Trichophyton*; teleomorphic or

sexual dermatophytes are placed into the genus *Arthroderma* of the order Onygenales. An important characteristic of dermatophytes is that their ability to parasitize is restricted to dead keratinized tissue. Dermatophytes are found only within the stratum corneum, the fully keratinized hair shaft, and the nail plate and bed.

Distinctive features seen only in culture, particularly of the macroconidia, provide the basis for identification. *Epidermophyton floccosum*, the pathogenic species of this genus, has snowshoe-shaped macroconidia occurring singly or in clusters of two to three cells with smooth, thin to moderately thick walls and one to nine septa. The macroconidia of *Microsporum* classically are spindle-shaped, appear rough, and have thick walls with one to 15 septa. *Trichophyton tonsurans* has macroconidia with thin, smooth walls and one to 12 septa. Macroconidia vary widely in shape and include clavate, cylindrical, and fusiform morphologies.[2]

Dermatophytes are divided into three catagories based on their natural habitat and usual host.[7–8] Anthropophilic dermatophytes typically infect only humans. Zoophilic dermatophytes usually are associated with animals but can infect humans, whereas geophilic dermatophytes are saprophytes that thrive on keratinous materials found in soil and also may invade keratinous tissues in animals or humans; however, some overlap has been observed between zoophilic and geophilic species.[9] Anthropophilic dermatophytes generally produce less inflammation than the zoophilic and geophilic species.[2] Dermatophyte species are distributed geographically; some species are ubiquitous, whereas others are highly restricted.[10,11]

TINEA CAPITIS

Dermatophytic infection of the scalp, eyebrows, and eyelashes is called tinea capitis. The most common etiologic agents are *Trichophyton* and *Microsporum* species. *T. tonsurans* has now superseded *M. audouinii* and *M. canis* as the primary cause of this condition in the United States as well as in most of North, Central, and South America.[12,13]

Clinical Features Infection occurs via direct or indirect person-to-person contact. Unlike *Microsporum* infections, childhood *T. tonsurans* infections do not always resolve at puberty.[11] Also, unlike *M. canis*, *M. audouinii*, and *M. ferrugineum*, which show green fluorescence with Wood's lamp; *T. tonsurans* does not fluoresce. *T. schoenleinii*, the etiologic agent of tinea favosa, shows a green-grey fluorescence with the Wood's lamp.

Tinea capitis infections may be small-spore ectothrix, large-spore ectothrix, large-spore endothrix, or tinea favosa. (Table 21-2) Small-spore ectothrix is caused by *Microsporum* species. Infection begins with hyphal invasion of the hair follicles. Hyphae grow within the hair shaft toward the hair bulb. As the hair emerges from the follicle, it is covered

TABLE 21-1

Histological Appearance of Fungi in Tissue

Disease	Spore Size and Location	Histological Findings	Fungal Budding
Candidiasis	3–7 μm yeast cells; hyphae 3–5 μm wide Skin vagina, mouth, larynx, esophagus—in superficial layers Esophagus and GI ulcers—in submucosa. Disseminated—often in foci near blood vessels.	Subcorneal pustules Spongioform pustules Variable acute and chronic dermal infiltrate that may be granulomatous	Blastospores, globose to oval
Pityriasis versicolor M. furfur	3–8 μm yeast cells; short, curved, rarely branching hyphae 2–4 μm diameter. In stratum corneum and in follicles.	Hyperkeratosis Possibly slight epidermal hyperplasia.	Unipolar globose budding. cells up to 8 μm Collarettes
Black piedra White piedra- T. beigelii	4–8 μm on hair surface, rectangular 2–4 μm, up to 8 μm, crowded in hair shaft. Appear polygonal 2° to crowding		Asci and Ascospores Arthroconidia along hair shaft only
Cryptococcosis	3–15 μm; Gelatinous: spores lie in pools of mucin. Granulomatous: Few spores, present in giant cells and macrophages	Epidermal hyperplasia Suppurative granulomas	Narrow, unequal
North American blastomycosis	5–15 μm Thick double wall Free in tissue, in giant cells	Pseudoepitheliomatous hyperplasia Suppurative granulomas with necrosis	Single, equal, broad-based
Coccidiomycosis	30–60 μm sporangia 4 μm endospores Free in tissue, in giant cells	Epidermal hyperplasia Suppurative granulomas	Endospores in spherules
Paracoccidioidomycosis	4–40 μm thick-walled yeast forms intra- and extracellular	Pseudoepitheliomatous hyperplasia Suppurative granulomas	Multiple/external budding in "ship's wheel" arrangement
Histoplasmosis	2–4 μm pseudocapsule, intra- and extracellular	Diverse types of granuloma or diffuse intracellular forms	Narrow, unequal budding
Sporotrichosis	4–6 μm round to oval bodies; up to 8 μm cigar-shaped bodies. Rare branching, nonseptate hyphae	Suppurative granulomas with neutrophilic microabscess surrounded by epithelioid and multinucleated histiocytes and an outer rim of lymphocytes.	Single or occasionally multiple buds
Chromoblastomycosis	6–12 μm round to oval muriform bronze-colored forms with central septation (sclerotic bodies)	Pseudoepitheliomatous hyperplasia Suppurative granulomas	Broad based equal budding
Phaeohyphomycosis	2–6 μm spores; may be septate hyphae, possibly branching; spores in chains; pseudohyphae; usually but not always pigmented.	Dermal or subcutaneous suppurative granulomas often encapsulated by fibrous wall resembling a cyst	Sprouting hyphal forms
Mycetoma (eumycetoma)	Up to 5 μm septate hyphal elements in grains that are brown or black; filamentous bacteria present in grains of actinomycetoma	Neutrophilic abscesses containing grains; granulation tissue; sinus tracts	
Nocardia	Filamentous branching Gram-positive, weakly acid-fast bacteria	Neutrophilic abscesses; tuberculoid granulomas on occasion (Nocardia brasiliensis)	
Actinomycosis	Filamentous branching Gram-positive bacteria, not acid fast, in granules.	Neutrophilic abscesses containing "sulfur granules"; sinus tracts; granulation tissue.	
Botryomycosis	Gram-positive or -negative cocci or rods in granules.	Neutrophilic abscesses containing granules	
Mucormycosis	20–30 μm, lack septa, 90° branching	Necrosis, thrombosis, infarction	
Aspergillosis	2–4 μm septate hyphae; 45° dichotomous branching; extracellular and intravascular	Thrombosis, infarction granulomatous	
Lobomycosis	10 μm; thick double wall	Histiocytic nodules with numerous intracellular organisms and fibroblastic proliferation	Short thick tube-like structures
Rhinosporidiosis	In submucosa, up to 350 μm sporangia; endospores 7–9 μm or more in diameter. Free in tissue, in giant cells	Pseudoepitheliomatous hyperplasia, erosions. Acute and chronic infiltrate in submucosa, hemorrhage.	Endospores in sporangia

TABLE 21-2

Dermatophytoses

Disease	Organism
Tinea capitis	
Small spore ectothrix	*Microsporum audouinii,*[a] *M. canis,*[z] *M. gypseum,*[g] *M. fulvum,*[g] *M. ferrugineum*[a]
Large spore endothrix	*Trichophyton tonsurans,*[a] *T. violaceum,*[a] *T. soudanense,*[a] *T. gourvilii,*[a] *T. yaoundei*[a]
Large spore ectothrix	*T. mentagrophytes* var. *interdigitale,*[a] *T. mentagrophytes* var. *mentagrophytes,*[z] *T. verrucosum,*[z] *T. megninii*[a]
Tinea favosa	*T. schoenleinii*[a] (*T. violaceum, M. gypseum* rare)
Tinea corporis	*T. rubrum,*[a] *T. mentagrophytes,*[z] *M. canis,* others
Tinea faciei	*T. mentagrophytes, T. rubrum*[a]
Tinea barbae	*T. mentagrophytes,*[z] *T. verrucosum,*[z] *T. rubrum,*[a] *T. violaceum,*[a] *T. megninii,*[a] *M. canis*[z]
Tinea cruris	*T. rubrum,*[a] *E. floccosum,*[a] *T. mentagrophytes*[a]
Tinea pedis	*T. rubrum,*[a] *T. mentagrophytes,*[a] *E. floccosum*[a]
Tinea manuum	*T. rubrum,*[a] *E. floccosum,*[a] *T. mentagrophytes*[a]
Tinea unguium	*T. rubrum,*[a] *T. mentagrophytes,*[a,z] (*E. floccosum,*[a] *T. violaceum,*[a] *T. schoenleinii,*[a] *T. tonsurans*[a] rare)

Key: [a] = Anthropophilic; [g] = Geophilic; [z] = Zoophilic.

with a mass of small arthrospores 2 to 5 μm in diameter. Clinical manifestations vary from mild inflammation, as seen in anthropophilic *Microsporum* species, to severe inflammatory reactions caused by the zoophilic and geophilic *Microsporum* species.

"Grey patch ringworm," typical of *M. audouinii* infection, is characterized by patches of dull bristles of hair with slight erythema and mild scaling. All hairs in a given area are affected, and lesions spread in a characteristic ring formation. *M. canis, M. gypseum,* and *M. fulvum,* the zoophilic and geophilic species, cause more host response, often leading to suppurative folliculitis or to kerion formation, characterized by intense inflammation, pus, crusting, and matting of hairs.

Large-spore endothrix is caused by *T. tonsurans* and *T. violaceum* in the United States. In Africa, *T. gourvilii, T. soudanense,* and *T. yaoundei* are common etiologic agents. These anthropophilic species produce "black dot ringworm," caused by intrafollicular hyphae that fragment into 5- to 8-μm wide arthrospores within the shaft, often resulting in breakage at the level of the follicular ostium. The alopetic patches are smaller than in grey patch ringworm, and not all hairs in the area are affected. Infections caused by *Trichophyton* species tend to be more inflammatory than those caused by *Microsporum* species, and kerion formation is often seen in association with *T. violaceum.*

Large-spore ectothrix infections are caused by *Trichophyton mentagrophytes* var. *mentagrophytes* and *T. verrucosum.* Arthroconidia 5 to 8 μm in diameter are arranged in straight chains along the external surface of the hair.[14] These organisms often cause suppurative folliculitis with subsequent atrophy of hair follicles, scarring, and patchy permanent alopecia.

Tinea favosa (also called favus) is usually caused by *T. schoenleinii* or rarely by *T. violaceum* and *M. gypseum,* and occurs most often in Eurasia and Africa.[2] Broad hyphae and air spaces develop within the hair shaft without arthrospores. Areas of scales, crusty debris, and masses of mycelium form cup-shaped scutula over the scalp.[2]

Histopathological Features   Fungal elements are seen in the stratum corneum, and hyphae invade the hair follicles and grow down the hair shaft toward the keratinizing cells (Table 21-2). Hyphal growth and arthroconidia formation occur either on the surface of the hair (ectothrix) or within the hair shaft (endothrix). In tinea favosa, hyphae are present within the stratum corneum, in hair shafts, and in scutula, which consist of tangled mycelial elements, sebum, debris, and scales forming a characteristic cup-shaped lesion. There is follicular atrophy and a chronic dermal inflammatory infiltrate. Histologic examination of a kerion reveals a dense perifollicular and perivascular infiltrate of lymphocytes, neutrophils, plasma cells, and eosinophils in the dermis.[2]

Differential Diagnosis   Seborrheic dermatitis, psoriasis, trichotillomania, alopecia areata, bacterial infection, "tinea" amiantacea, Langerhan's cell histiocytosis, lupus erythematosus, pseudopelade, impetigo, folliculitis decalvans, pyoderma, and secondary syphilis may be associated with variable crusting, scaling, perifollicular inflammation and hair loss and enter into the differential diagnosis of tinea capitis.[14,15]

TINEA CORPORIS

Clinical Features   Ringworm of the glabrous skin is called tinea corporis; it results from proliferation of fungi in the stratum corneum and may be caused by infection by any dermatophyte, with regional differences dictating the prevailing dermatophytic flora.[2] Infection of the skin at the site of inoculation spreads centrifugally followed by a secondary tissue response. The central area may clear as fungus is eliminated, with active proliferation continuing at the periphery resulting in characteristic annular, scaly patches with raised erythematous or vesicular margins.[2] The natural history varies depending on the attributes of the fungal species and the host. Special expressions of tinea corporis have been recognized. For example, *T. rubrum* commonly causes extensive eruptions, sometimes with psoriasiform lichenified plaques and nodular granulomatous perifolliculitis (Majocchi's granuloma).[16]

Histopathological Features   Dermatophytic infections can display a spectrum of histological patterns depending on the causative agent and the host response. For example, dry scaly patches and plaques, often caused by anthropophilic dermatophytes (Table 21-2), show hyperkeratosis (Fig. 21-1). Compact orthokeratosis, the presence of neutrophils within the stratum corneum, and "the sandwich sign" also may be clues to a dermatophyte infection.[17] "The sandwich sign" denotes hyphae "sandwiched in" between a superficial normal-appearing basket-weave pattern of orthokeratosis in the stratum corneum and a deeper layer of abnormal stratum corneum showing either parakeratosis or compact hyperkeratosis (Fig. 21-2).

Variable spongiosis and occasional subcorneal or intraepidermal pustule formation may be seen. The dermis contains a mild perivascular inflammatory infiltrate consisting of lymphocytes, histiocytes, eosinophils, and neutrophils. Zoophilic dermatophyte infections tend to be more inflammatory with vesicle formation. Hyphae within the stratum corneum may be visible even with hematoxylin and eosin if they are numerous, but are more easily seen with PAS or methenamine silver staining.

In Majocchi's granuloma owing to *T. rubrum,* arthroconidia and mycelia are seen in follicles, and there is a dermal infiltrate of lympho-

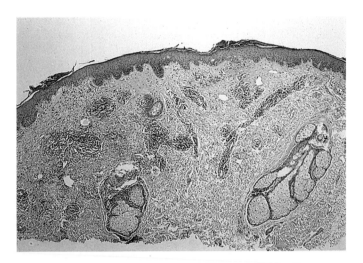

FIGURE 21-1 Dermatophyte infection. Scanning magnification discloses a nonspecific subacute dermatitis with hyperkeratosis.

cytes, histiocytes, epithelioid cells, and often foreign body giant cells. Rupture of the follicular wall releases conidia and mycelia, stimulating granuloma formation.[14,16]

Differential Diagnosis   In cases where the inflammation is minimal and hyphae are not visualized with routine staining, biopsy of tinea corporis may resemble that of normal skin. Lesions with hyperkeratosis, spongiosis, and mild inflammation may mimic subacute spongiotic dermatitis such as nummular eczema, seborrheic dermatitis, contact dermatitis, and pityriasis rosea. Zoophilic dermatophytic infections may be confused with impetigo, cellulitis, folliculitis decalvans, or other pustular infections.[14] Potassium hydroxide preparations usually reveal fungal elements in skin scrapings from tinea corporis. Cultures should be routinely obtained, and are positive in five to 15 percent of KOH-negative cases.[1]

TINEA BARBAE

Clinical Features   Tinea barbae, or ringworm of the beard and mustache, is a disease of adult males and is characterized by invasion of ter-

minal hairs of the face and neck. Most cases occur in farm workers infected by the zoophilic species *T. verrucosum* and *T. mentagrophytes*.[14] Clinical manifestations are similar to those of tinea capitis, with patches of erythema, scaling, and dull, fragile hairs. These organisms produce large-spore ectothrix invasion with spores in chains, often resulting in pustular folliculitis resembling kerion.[18]

Histopathological Features   Fungal elements often are visible within hair follicles and shafts, with arthroconidia along the shaft and free within the tissues. The cellular reaction is similar to that seen with pustular forms of tinea capitis.

Differential Diagnosis   Entities that must be differentiated from tinea barbae include acne, rosacea, papular syphilis, seborrheic dermatitis, and bacterial folliculitis. PAS and methenamine silver stains facilitate visualization of the hyphae.

TINEA CRURIS

Clinical Features   Tinea cruris refers to dermatophyte infection of the groin; the most common etiologic agents are *E. floccosum* and *T. rubrum*, with a minority of cases attributed to *T. interdigitale*.[2] It is more common in men and involves the perineum, scrotum, perianal area, and frequently the medial aspect of the buttocks. Intertriginous erythema is common and vesicles may be present. The borders are sharply demarcated, unlike plaques in these areas caused by *Candida*. Lesions are pruritic and often painful.[1]

Histopathological Features   Fungi are usually few in number and stain with the PAS reaction or methenamine silver nitrate. Chains of spores, as in *Epidermophyton* infections, or hyphae, as in *Trichophyton* infections, are present in the stratum corneum, which is variably parakeratotic and crusted.[19] The underlying dermis may contain a scant lymphohistiocytic infiltrate.

Differential Diagnosis   The differential diagnosis includes psoriasis, contact dermatitis, and seborrheic dermatitis. *Candida* intertrigo, which also is in the differential diagnosis, may be diagnosed by the presence of spores and pseudohyphae.

TINEA PEDIS

Clinical Features   Tinea pedis ("athlete's foot") is the most common form of dermatophytosis.[20,21] Occlusion of the feet and, in particular, the digital webspaces is the single most important factor influencing the severity, incidence, and prevalence of the disease.[12,22] There are three clinical varieties. Plantar moccasin-like disease, the most common type, affects the plantar surfaces and is associated with mild erythema, fine scaling, and pruritus.[20] *T. rubrum* is the usual etiologic agent.[20] Nail involvement is common, and there is often a history of atopy. Interdigital infection, characterized by maceration and erosion between toes, is related to a combination of dermatophytes (*T. rubrum* and *T. mentagrophytes*) and bacteria.[21] Vesiculobullous tinea pedis is caused by *T. mentagrophytes*, and is characterized by episodes of intense inflammation along the arch and sides of the foot, with scaling between episodes.[21]

Histopathological Features   Biopsies of tinea pedis are rarely done unless the infections are complicated or unusually severe. In acute tinea pedis, parakeratosis and spongiosis with intraepidermal vesicle formation are seen. A superficial acute and chronic infiltrate with focal exocytosis also may be observed. In chronic tinea pedis, hyperkeratosis and

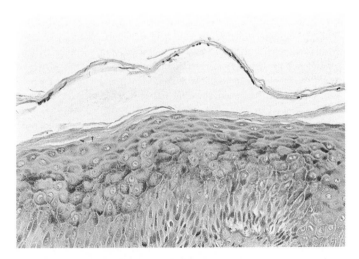

FIGURE 21-2 Dermatophyte infection. PAS with diastase stain shows hyphal elements in stratum corneum.

acanthosis are prominent. The dermis may contain a superficial lymphohistiocytic infiltrate.[14,19]

Differential Diagnosis   Other conditions that may mimic tinea pedis are contact dermatitis, dyshidrosis, pustular psoriasis, secondary syphilis, arsenical keratosis, fixed drug eruption, dermatitis repens, erysipelas, pyoderma, and idiopathic hyperkeratosis.[14] Infection with *Candida* and with bacteria such as *Brevibacterium epidermidis*, *Micrococcus sedantarius*, and several Gram-negative bacterial species may complicate the presentation.[21] A similar hyperkeratotic condition caused by the soil molds *Hendersonula toruloidea* and *Scytalidium hyalinum*, occurring mainly in West Africa, the Caribbean, India, and the Pacific, has been described.[23]

TINEA MANUUM

Clinical Features   Tinea manuum refers to a dermatophyte infection of the palmar or interdigital surfaces of the hand. Most cases are caused by *T. rubrum*, although some are owing to *T. mentagrophytes* or *E. floccosum*. Tinea pedis often is coexistent. The usual presentation is unilateral diffuse hyperkeratosis with prominent flexural creases.[2] Other presentations include crescentic exfoliating lesions, vesicular lesions, red papular and follicular patches, and erythematous scaly patches on the dorsum of the hand.[14]

Histopathological Features   The histopathology of tinea manuum is similar to that of tinea corporis: Fungi are noted in the stratum corneum, which is often hyperkeratotic. Spongiosis may be observed if blisters are present clinically.

Differential Diagnosis   Psoriasis, candidal infection, chronic pyoderma, contact dermatitis, lichen simplex chronicus, and secondary syphilis resemble tinea manuum. The "id," or dermatophytid reaction, is an allergic response occurring on the hand as a result of dermatophytic infection of the feet or other parts of the body. It may mimic tinea manuum or dyshidrotic pompholyx.

TINEA UNGUIUM

Clinical Features   Onychomycosis is a fungal infection of the nail and is caused by dermatophytes, yeasts, and molds. Tinea unguium is defined as invasion of the nail plate by dermatophytic species. Nail infections caused by *T. rubrum*, *T. mentagrophytes* var. *interdigital*, and *E. floccosum* often involve both the hands and feet, whereas those by *T. tonsurans*, *T. violaceum*, *T. schoenleinii*, and *T. megninii* are associated with scalp infections. The site of infection on the nail determines the clinical presentation.[24] The most common form is distal subungual onychomycosis, in which the hyponychium is infected. Subungual hyperkeratosis and the formation of a yellowish-grey mass lift the nail plate off the nail bed. The advanced form is called total onychomycosis and is characterized by progressive destruction of the entire nailbed and nailplate. Lateral onychomycosis is another common presentation; in this variant, infection begins in the lateral groove, often causing onycholysis and lateral pachyonychia.[24] White superficial onychomycosis (mycotic leukonychia) involves infection of only the superficial layers of the nail plate. Although rare in fingernails of the normal population, where it is usually caused by *T. mentagrophytes*, it is not uncommon in AIDS patients in whom it is usually caused by *T. rubrum*.[25,26] Also in AIDS patients, the nail plate can be invaded from the upper surface at the posterior nail fold, producing a distinctive pattern known as proximal white subungual onychomycosis.[25]

Histopathological Features   In the subungual invasive type, hyphal filaments and arthroconidia grow between lamellae of the nailplate, separating them mechanically. There is little to no inflammatory response in the surrounding soft tissue. Fungal concentrations in nail sections are variable, making diagnosis somewhat difficult.[14] In white superficial onychomycosis, hyphae and arthroconidia are present only in the superficial layers of the nail.

Differential Diagnosis   Onychomycosis is often caused by *Candida*, and may also be caused by molds such as *Scopulariopsis brevicaulis*, *Aspergillus* species, and *Hendersonula toruloidea*. Bacterial paronychia, psoriasis, eczema, Darier's disease, pityriasis rubra pilaris, peripheral circulatory problems, and endocrine disturbances may produce hyperkeratotic nails. Congenital abnormalities such as clubbing, Beau's lines, pachyonychia congenita, and nonmycotic leukonychia as well as drugs, trauma, and chemical irritants should be excluded.[24]

Dermatomycoses

Dermatomycosis denotes a non–dermatophytic fungal infection of hair, skin, and nails. Dermatomycoses other than candidiasis, piedra, and tinea versicolor, which are discussed later in this chapter, may be caused by a variety of soil organisms. *Hendersonula toruloidea* has been implicated in several reports of skin and nail infections as well as in a verrucous disease in an immunocompromised patient in Algeria.[27] The organism appears to be geographically limited to West Africa, the Caribbean, India, and the Pacific. *Scytalidium hyalinum* has been involved in skin and nail infections in patients from the Caribbean or West Africa. The clinical manifestations of these two infections resemble dry, scaly dermatophytic infections.[23] Cycloheximide, a usual component of culture media, prevents the growth of these organisms in routine cultures.[14] The soil molds *Scopulariopsis brevicaulis* and *Aspergillus* species have been implicated in onychomycosis, especially of the feet.[24]

Histopathological Features   Histological examination of dermatomycosis reveals hyphal elements that may be indistinguishable from dermatophyte infections.[28–30] Culture is necessary for definitive diagnosis.

YEAST INFECTIONS

Synonyms: Moniliasis; thrush; candidiasis; vulvovaginitis; muguet

Candidiasis

Candidiasis is caused by the dimorphic yeast-like fungus *Candida albicans*, or by other *Candida* species, including *C. tropicalis*, *C. krusei*, *C. glabrata*, *C. parapsilosis*, *C. lusitaniae*, *C. guilliermondii*, *C. kefyr* (*C. pseudotropicalis*), and *C. stellatoidea* (considered a variant of *C. albicans*).[31] As opportunistic organisms, they depend on a change in host physiology, defenses, or normal flora in order to colonize, invade, and cause disease. The degree of virulence among species varies greatly, with *C. albicans* and *C. tropicalis* being the most virulent.[31,32] Less virulent species require greater host debilitation to cause disease. *Candida* species that are rarely virulent include *C. ciferrii*, *C. haemulonii*, *C. catenulata*, *C. lipolytica*, *C. norvegensis*, *C. pulcherrima*, *C. rugosa*, *C. utilis*, *C. zeylanoides*, and *C. viswanathii*.[14,31,33]

   C. albicans is part of the normal flora of the gastrointestinal tract, oral cavity, and vagina.[31] *C. albicans* grows as a budding yeast; hyphal forms are hallmarks of tissue invasion, whereas blastoconidia are thought to be involved in hematogenous dissemination.[34] In oral lesions, the finding of mycelia is useful in differentiating a pathogenic infection.

Clinical Features The expression of candidal infection may be divided into acute mucocutaneous forms, chronic mucocutaneous forms, and disseminated disease.[35] In addition, cutaneous infection may result in intertriginous candidiasis, paronychia, onychomycosis, diaper candidiasis, and candidal granuloma.[14] Cutaneous candidal infections generally produce erythema with moist exudates having irregular edges and satellite papules. Subcorneal pustules lead to superficial erosions and peeling.

Acute mucocutaneous candidiasis may present as oral thrush, which occurs most often in infants, the elderly, and patients with terminal or chronic illnesses (Table 21-3).[36] It is characterized by friable white plaques on oral mucosa; unlike plaques of leukoplakia, they can be scraped off easily, revealing an erythematous base.[36] Acute atrophic candidiasis presents as a painful erythematous stomatitis. Chronic atrophic candidiasis, common among denture wearers, is characterized by asymptomatic erythema of the mucosa that bears the denture.[36,37] Inhaled corticosteroids and HIV infection are also associated with chronic oral candidiasis.[38] Other conditions involving the oral mucosa such as perlèche (angular cheilitis), leukoplakia, HIV-associated oral hairy leukoplakia, and median rhomboid glossitis may predispose the affected individual to mucosal invasion by *Candida* species.

Vulvovaginitis is characterized by itching, soreness, and a thick white exudate. Balanitis, more commonly seen in the uncircumcized, produces white pustules or vesicles on the glans penis. Other acute mucocutaneous forms include infections of the gastrointestinal tract, including esophagitis, gastritis, and peritonitis.

Chronic mucocutaneous candidiasis is a disorder of chronic, recurrent *Candida* infections of the skin, mucous membranes, and nails in patients with underlying defects in cell-mediated immunity (Table 21-3).[35] Lethal immune deficiencies involving dysgenesis of the thymus (Nezeloff syndrome, DiGeorge syndrome, and the "Swiss" type of agammaglobulinemia) may present in childhood with mild candidiasis

often limited to the oral cavity; death usually occurs prior to the age of 2 years from other infections.[19] Non-lethal immune deficiencies also present early in life and include endocrinopathy, which is associated with candidiasis of the oral cavity, skin, and nails and appears to be genetically transmitted, and a rare variant called candidal granuloma, which presents with multiple hyperkeratotic, crusted plaques.[38–41] Late-onset chronic mucocutaneous candidiasis is associated with thymoma and may accompany myasthenia gravis.[19,38] AIDS is often associated with chronic mucocutaneous candidiasis and frequently involves the oral cavity and esophagus.[42]

Systemic candidiasis is the most common invasive fungal infection in patients with cancer, burns, AIDS, or those undergoing organ transplantation. The mortality rate is about 40 percent, down from 80 percent in the 1970s; this decrease is attributed to early empiric antifungal and improved prophylactic treatment.[43] In a recent review, *Candida albicans* and *C. tropicalis* caused 54 and 25 percent, respectively, of cases of disseminated candidiasis in cancer patients.[32] Disseminated candidiasis is associated with cutaneous manifestations in 10 to 13 percent of patients (Table 21-4).[34,44,45] These manifestations are highly variable, ranging from very few to numerous erythematous macules, papules, and nodules that may be associated with purpura, necrotic eschars, subcutaneous abscesses, ecthyma gangrenosum-like ulcers, and nodular folliculitis in heroin users.[45–49] Systemic candidiasis with skin manifestations was caused by *Candida tropicalis* in 64 percent of cases.[45] The triad of high fever, papular erythematous rash, and diffuse severe myalgias in neutropenic patients suggests disseminated disease.[50]

Histopathological Features The vesicles and pustules of mucocutaneous candidiasis are characterized histologically by a subcorneal collection of lymphocytes and necrotic debris, with hyphae, pseudohyphae, and yeast cells confined to the stratum corneum (Figs. 21-3 and 21-4). Pseudohyphae are chains of cells formed by the repeated budding of blastoconidia; although they are separated by septa, mother and daughter cells remain physically attached. Although *C. glabrata* occurs as yeasts only, other species show numerous hyphae measuring 2 to 4 μm in diameter and a few spores that may show budding and measure 3 to 6 μm in diameter.[14,19] The organisms stain well with PAS, methenamine silver, Gridley, and Gram stains.[14,34]

TABLE 21-3

Mucocutaneous Candidiasis

Clinical Features

Various acute forms more common in infants, elderly, pregnant, or diabetic patients
Chronic mucocutaneous candidiasis
　Often associated with cell-mediated immune defect
　May involve genetic transmission
　Candidal granuloma (rare)
Chronic atrophic candidiasis in denture wearers
Erythema with irregular margins, moist exudates, and satellite papules
Oral friable white plaques that can be scraped off easily

Histopathological Features

Spores (3–6 μm), pseudohyphae, and hyphae seen in stratum corneum
Subcorneal pustules and vesicles
Candidal granuloma
　Prominent hyperkeratosis and papillomatosis
　Dense dermal infiltrate with giant cells

Differential Diagnosis

Dermatophyte infection
Impetigo
Subcorneal pustular dermatitis
Pustular psoriasis

TABLE 21-4

Disseminated Candidiasis

Clinical Features

Cutaneous findings in 10 to 13% of patients
Variable skin manifestations
C. tropicalis in 64% of cases with skin manifestations
Triad of fever, papular erythematous rash, and diffuse severe myalgias in neutropenic patients highly suggestive

Histopathological Features

Pseudohyphae, hyphae, and spores (3–6 μm) in dermis often near blood vessels
Spores may show budding
Perivascular inflammatory infiltrate
Leukocytoclastic vasculitis

Differential Diagnosis

Aspergillus fumigatus
Histoplasma capsulatum
　May be confused with *C. glabrata*, which forms spores only

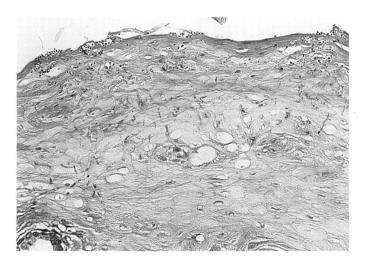

FIGURE 21-3 Candidiasis. Pale squamous epithelium demonstrates spongioform pustule formation with associated mycelial elements.

In candidal granuloma, hyperkeratosis and papillomatosis are prominent; parakeratosis and acanthosis may be noted.[41] A dense chronic inflammatory infiltrate with multinucleated giant cells may be found in the dermis and may extend into the subcutis.[19,40]

The histologic examination of disseminated candidiasis reveals *Candida* pseudohyphae and yeast cells within the dermis, often near or within blood vessels. Perivascular tissues and blood vessel walls may show edema.[44] The epidermis is intact, and small foci of hemorrhage and fibrin exudate may be seen in the middle and lower dermis. The tissue response varies from a perivascular chronic inflammatory infiltrate to a leukocytoclastic vasculitis characterized by groups of neutrophils, nuclear debris, and necrosis in and around blood vessels.[44,45]

Differential Diagnosis   Oral candidiasis resembles or may co-exist with leukoplakia, squamous cell carcinoma, or herpes simplex.[36] Esophageal infection may mimic CMV, herpes simplex, or peptic ulcer esophagitis. The differential diagnosis for a subcorneal pustule secondary to Candida includes dermatophytic infection, impetigo, subcorneal pustular dermatitis, and pustular psoriasis. Candidiasis may be differentiated from dermatophytic infection by the presence of spores and pseudohy-

phae. The best diagnostic test is the demonstration of pseudohyphal invasion on microscopic examination of mucocutaneous lesions. A positive culture may lend support but is not by itself diagnostic.[1]

The necrotic pustules and ulcerative plaques of ecthyma gangrenosum, characteristic of *Pseudomonas* septicemia, resemble the cutaneous findings of disseminated candidiasis.[48] Although skin manifestations are relatively uncommon in disseminated candidiasis, biopsy of skin lesions is important since blood cultures are positive in only 25 percent of cases.[51] When blastospores are not seen, *Candida* pseudohyphae may be confused with *Aspergillus* hyphae; however, the latter are Gram-negative. *C. glabrata*, which does not form pseudohyphae, may resemble *Histoplasma capsulatum*, although the latter usually elicits a granulomatous rather than a pyogenic response.[1]

Pityriasis Versicolor

Synonyms: Tinea versicolor; tinea flava; dermatomycosis furfuracea; chromophytosis[14]

Pityriasis (tinea) versicolor is caused by the lipophilic yeast *Malassezia furfur*, an organism also known in the literature as *Pityrosporum orbiculare*. *M. ovalis*, also known as *P. ovale*, is considered an in vitro variant of *M. furfur*.[14,52] The two morphologic forms may represent oval and round forms of a different phase of the yeast cycle.[53,54] For historical reasons, *M. furfur* is considered the preferred name.[1,19]

Clinical Features   Pityriasis versicolor occurs worldwide but has an increased prevalence, up to 40 percent, in tropical areas owing to high temperature and humidity (Table 21-5).[55] In temperate zones, the incidence is higher during the warmer months of the year.[56] The infection does not appear to be contagious and occurs under conditions permitting overgrowth of the fungus such as warm weather and continual perspiration.[1,57]

Small red or light brown scaly macules occur most commonly on the chest, upper back, shoulders, upper arms, and abdomen.[56] The macules enlarge and may become either hypopigmented or hyperpigmented depending on natural skin color and sun exposure. Depigmentation has been attributed to the production by the yeasts of dicarboxylic acids, such as azelaic acid, which competitively inhibit tyrosinase and that may have a direct toxic effect on melanocytes.[58] Hyperpigmentation appears to be related to an increase in melanosome size.[59] Although most cases are asymptomatic, the major complaint is cosmetic, as the

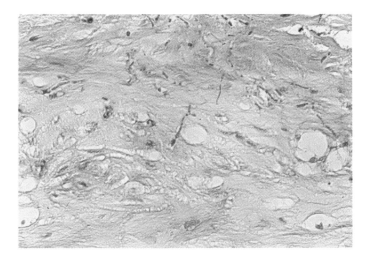

FIGURE 21-4 Candidiasis. Higher magnification illustrating pseudohyphae with branching.

TABLE 21-5
Pityriasis Versicolor

Clinical Features

   Caused by *Malassezia furfur* or *M. ovalis*
   Occurs in tropics and warm months of temperate zones
   Age of onset usually in early twenties in temperate zones
   Pale to brown, slightly scaling macules with over upper trunk

Histopathological Features

   Hyperkeratosis and slight acanthosis
   Superficial dermal lymphohistiocytic infiltrate
   Hyphae and spores seen in stratum corneum

Differential Diagnosis

   Tinea corporis
   Candidiasis
   Spongiotic dermatitis

fungus causes uneven tanning by filtering out ultraviolet radiation. Yellow fluorescence is seen with Wood's lamp examination.[57]

Histopathological Features   Most commonly one observes hyperkeratosis, slight acanthosis, spotty pigmentation of the epidermal basal layer, and a superficial perivascular lymphohistiocytic infiltrate.[1,59] PAS stain reveals numerous short hyphae and spores (so-called "spaghetti and meatballs") within the stratum corneum (Figs. 21-5 and 21-6; Table 21-5).

Differential Diagnosis   Spongiotic dermatitis, as in eczema, the "id" reaction, or infection by dermatophytes or *Candida* species, may be confused with pityriasis versicolor if fungal stains are not obtained.

Pityrosporum Folliculitis

Pityrosporum folliculitis is also known as *Malassezia* folliculitis.[60] The exact pathogenesis of this disease remains controversial.[1,61] The initiating event may be follicular occlusion followed by overgrowth of the organism rather than direct invasion of the follicle. Predisposing factors appear to include occlusion and greasy skin.[62]

Clinical Features   The typical patient is a young to middle-aged adult with pruritic papules on the trunk, shoulders, and occasionally the face (Table 21-6). Pustules, cysts, and "molluscoid" papules, which have a central depression similar to the papules of molluscum contagiosum, may be seen.[63]

Histopathological Features   Most cases show numerous spores inside the hair follicles that appear widely dilated and are plugged with keratinous material (Table 21-6). Occasional hyphae have been noted within distended follicles.[62] A perifollicular inflammatory cell infiltrate con-

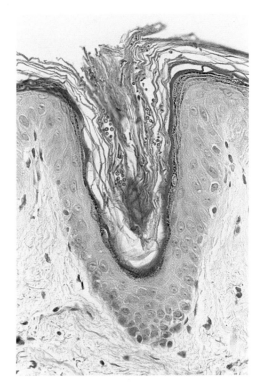

FIGURE 21-6   Tinea versicolor. Hyphae and spores in follicular orifice.

sisting of neutrophils, lymphocytes, and histiocytes is present in the intrafollicular and perifollicular regions, and pools of mucin, which may be confirmed by a colloidal iron stain, may be seen both within and around follicles.[53] A foreign body-type granulomatous reaction near a ruptured follicular wall has been reported.[63] The Splendore-Hoeppli phenomenon, characterized by a homogeneous, partially laminated core containing *Pityrosporum* spores surrounded by a thin layer of darkly stained filaments, occasionally may be seen within the follicle.[64]

Differential Diagnosis   The differential diagnosis includes acneiform drug eruptions, dermatophytic or bacterial folliculitis, follicular mucinosis, and acne vulgaris.[60]

Piedra and Trichosporonosis

Synonyms: Tinea nodosa; trichomycosis; molestia de Beigel; trichomycosis nodularis; trichomycosis nodosa; Beigel's disease; Chignon disease

Piedra, a superficial fungal infection of hair, produces firm nodules along the hair shaft. Two varieties, caused by unrelated fungal species, have been described.

Black piedra is caused by *Piedraia hortae*, an ascomycete that appears to be related to the family Piedraiaceae.[14] The teleomorphic reproductive propagule of the Ascomycota is the ascospore; these are produced in sacs called asci and are formed by the condensation of cytoplasm around the nucleus after meiosis.[14]

White piedra is caused by *Trichosporon beigelii*, a yeast-like fungus that is related to Basidiomycetes and that is found in soil and occasionally in normal skin.[1,65,66] Disseminated infection, called trichosporonosis, can occur in immunocompromised patients, particularly those receiving chemotherapy or with AIDS.[66]

Clinical Features   Black piedra occurs worldwide with increased frequency in tropical areas, particularly in South America, Southeast Asia,

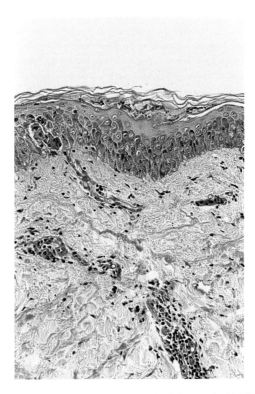

FIGURE 21-5   Tinea versicolor. PAS with diastase stain highlights short hyphae and spores (so-called "spaghetti and meatballs") in stratum corneum.

TABLE 21-6

Malassezia (Pityrosporum) Folliculitis

Clinical Features

Caused by *Malassezia furfur* or *M. ovalis*
Occurs in young to middle-aged adults
Pruritic papules on trunk, shoulders, and occasionally the face
Occlusion and greasy skin may predispose to infection

Histopathological Features

Numerous spores within dilated, plugged hair follicles
Neutrophils, lymphocytes, and histiocytes within follicles and in
   perifollicular regions
Foreign-body reaction near ruptured follicles
Pools of mucin may be seen within follicles

Differential Diagnosis

Acneiform drug eruption
Dermatophytic or bacterial folliculitis
Follicular mucinosis
Acne vulgaris

and Africa (Table 21-7).[1,67] Although scalp hair is the most common site of infection, the beard, mustache, and pubic hair also may be affected.[67]

Affected individuals have hard, dark brown to black nodules firmly adherent to their hair shafts. The nodules, measuring up to a few mm in length and up to 150 μm in thickness, are typically thickest in the center or on one end. The thin areas consist of a layer of aligned hyphae and arthrospores, which are spores resulting from hyphal fragmentation along septa; the thick area is composed of fungal cells cemented together.[1] Although unable to penetrate the cortex, the fungal infection begins under the cuticle, disrupting it and growing along the outer surface of the hair.[68] Hair follicles and skin are unaffected, and hair breakage is rare.

TABLE 21-7

Black Piedra

Clinical Features

Caused by *Piedra hortae*
Occurs in tropics
Usually involves scalp hairs
Hard, dark firmly adherent nodules
Hair breakage is rare
Skin and hair follicles are normal

Histopathological Features

Dark nodules, thicker in center or on one end
Tightly packed, dark hyphae fragmenting into arthrospores
Rectangular arthrospores (4–8 μm in diameter)
Asci containing ascospores within nodules

Differential Diagnosis

Pediculosis
Trichomycosis axillaris (hyphae 1 μm or less)
Trichorrhexis nodosa
Monilethrix trichoptilosis

White piedra occurs most commonly in semitropical and temperate areas and rarely in the southeastern United States (Table 21-8). The beard, axillary, and groin hairs are most frequently involved, although the fungus may also affect the scalp hair, eyelashes, and eyebrows. Familial spread may occur.[67] Genital white piedra has been reported to be caused by a synergistic infection by coryneform bacteria and *T. beigelii*.[65]

White piedra is characterized by soft, white, red, green, or light brown nodules along the hair shaft. The nodules may be scraped off easily.[67] Fungal infection begins under the cuticle and the growth is often intrapilar, causing weakness and breakage of hair at fungal nodules.[14] The cuticle usually is not disrupted significantly. Hair follicles and skin appear normal.

Disseminated infection by *T. beigelii* is called trichosporonosis and, in approximately 30 percent of patients, affects the skin.[69] Cutaneous involvement is characterized by purpuric papules and centrally necrotic or ulcerating nodules, typically present on the trunk, arms, and face.[66]

Histopathological Features   In KOH preparations, black piedra is characterized by dark, firmly adherent nodules consisting of tightly packed darkly pigmented hyphae that are segmented into rectangular arthrospores 4 to 8 μm in diameter.[1] Asci, containing ascospores, are visible within the nodules.

In white piedra, a loosely adherent, transparent green, red, white, or tan sheath may been seen on the hair shaft. This sheath is composed of disorganized, loosely packed mycelia often arranged at right angles to the hair shaft. Blastoconidia and arthroconidia measuring 2 to 4 μm and occasionally up to 8 μm in diameter are seen, whereas asci are not. Bacteria may be seen mixed among the fungal elements.[14]

In disseminated *T. beigelii* infections, pseudohyphae, numerous rectangular arthroconidia, and small numbers of blastoconidia are seen in the dermis.[66] Vasculitis and vascular thrombosis have been observed.[66]

Differential Diagnosis   Other conditions that may lead to perifollicular concretions include pediculosis, trichomycosis axillaris, and trichorrhexis nodosa; additionally, monilethrix trichoptilosis has focal node-like swellings along the follicle. The hyphae of trichomycosis axillaris are 1 μm or less in diameter, compared to 2 to 4 μm in white piedra.

TABLE 21-8

White Piedra

Clinical Features

Caused by *Trichosporon beigelii*
Occurs in semitropical and temperate areas
Usually involves the beard, axillary, or groin hairs
Soft, lightly colored nodules on hair; nodules may be scraped
   off easily
Hair breakage occurs near nodules
Normal skin and hair follicles

Histopathological Features

Loosely adherent, transparent sheath of variable color on shaft
Sheath composed of loosely arranged mycelia
Mycelia often perpendicular to hair shaft
Blastoconidia and arthroconidia (2–4 μm), up to 8 μm
No asci

Differential Diagnosis

Same as for black piedra

SYSTEMIC MYCOSES

Fungal infections acquired through the respiratory route can disseminate by progressive pulmonary infection with systemic spread following failure of the normal cell-mediated immune response or by reactivation of dormant sites of infection with secondary systemic dissemination. Mucocutaneous lesions, which occur in approximately 10 percent of patients having disseminated disease, sometimes represent the initial presenting sign of disseminated infection. In the majority of cases of cryptococcosis, coccidioidomycosis, and histoplasmosis, the development of skin lesions is essentially diagnostic of systemic disease since primary cutaneous infection is exceedingly rare. For this reason, cryptococcosis will be discussed in this section although it is a yeast.

Cryptococcosis

Synonyms: Torulosis; Busse-Buschke's disease; European blastomycosis

Clinical Features   Cryptococcosis is a common infection, with worldwide distribution, caused by *Cryptococcus neoformans*, a saprophyte found in soil enriched by bird droppings (Table 21-9).[70,71] *Cryptococcus* is unencapsulated in nature; its smallest forms measure less than 2 μm and thus it lodges in alveolar spaces following inhalation.[71] Encapsulation occurs in the lung and is associated with increased virulence because phagocytosis is impaired by concealment by opsonic antibodies.[72] The disease occurs more frequently but not exclusively in adults whose susceptibility is increased by immunosuppressive disorders such as lymphoma, carcinoma, sarcoidosis, collagen vascular disease, AIDS, or transplantation-related immunosuppressive treat-

ment.[73,74] Two varieties and five serotypes of *Cryptococcus neoformans* have been recognized based on capsular polysaccharides: *C. neoformans* var. *neoformans* (serotypes A, D, and AD) and var. *gattii* (serotypes B and C).[75] *C. neoformans* var. *neoformans* type A is the most common serotype of pathogenic *Cryptococcus* in the United States and in AIDS patients worldwide, including in Africa, where var. *gattii* usually is the more common pathogen.[75,76] In AIDS patients, cryptococcosis recently has been the most frequent systemic fungal infection.[77-79]

Primary cutaneous cryptococcosis is a very rare event that occurs following direct inoculation.[75] Pulmonary infection often is transient or asymptomatic, and in most instances cryptococcosis presents as a disseminated or a central nervous system infection, that is, as a chronic meningitis or a focal brain lesion resembling a tumor. Cutaneous lesions may appear as erythematous swellings, nodular firm, cystic-appearing excrescences, acneiform papules or pustules, crusted or infiltrating plaques, or cellulitis.[80] Any of these lesions may ulcerate.[77] In AIDS patients, numerous nodules resembling giant molluscum lesions are common.[81] Serum latex agglutination is valuable in diagnosis of active disease or to exclude such disease.[76]

Histopathological Features   In the past, two distinct histological patterns were described, a granulomatous pattern consisting of a dense mixed infiltrate with few organisms, and a gelatinous pattern, comprised of little inflammation and large numbers of spores (Figs. 21-7 and 21-8; Table 21-9). However, they can both be present and are not of recognizable clinical significance.[77,82] The characteristic feature includes aggregates of encapsulated yeasts, often but not always with a granulomatous response and sometimes with necrosis.[77,80] The yeast cells range from 2 to 15 μm in diameter and show narrow-based, unequal budding.[82] The yeast cytoplasm stains with PAS or methenamine silver and the capsule with Alcian blue or mucicarmine. A combination of PAS and Alcian blue stains highlights the yeast cyto-

---

TABLE 21-9

Cryptococcosis

Clinical Features

Caused by *Cryptococcus neoformans* var. *neoformans* in >80% of cases

C. neoformans is found in soil contaminated with bird and bat excreta

Usually inhaled, can disseminate to brain, meninges and cerebrospinal fluid

Skin involvement variable—papules, pustules, nodules, plaques, cellulitis

Most common systemic fungal infection in AIDS patients

Serum latex agglutination valuable in diagnosis of active disease

Histopathological Features

Large aggregates of encapsulated, budding, refractile yeast, 5–15 μm in diameter

Variable granulomatous infiltrate of lymphocytes, histiocytes, multinucleated giant cells and neutrophils

If infiltrate is dense, few organisms are seen. Those present are smaller and may lie within macrophages

Yeast stains with PAS, methenamine silver and Fontana-Masson

Capsule stains with Alcian blue and mucicarmine

Differential Diagnosis

Blastomycosis
Histoplasmosis
Lobomycosis

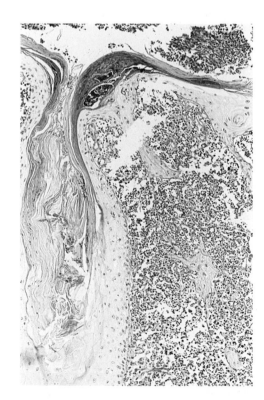

FIGURE 21-7   Cryptococcosis. A sheet of spores in the gelatinous form of cryptococcosis fills the papillary dermis with little inflammatory reaction.

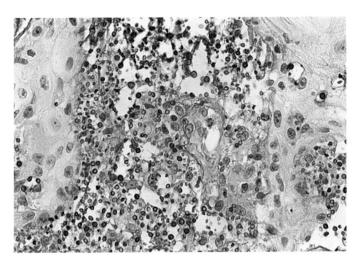

FIGURE 21-8 Cryptococcosis. Higher magnification discloses PAS plus distase-positive spores with surrounding clear halo characteristic of this organism.

plasm in red and the capsule in blue. *C. neoformans* stains black with the Fontana-Masson stain, a valuable feature in patients with AIDS infected with strains of low virulence and relatively little capsular material.[83] Variable acanthosis or ulceration of the overlying skin may be present.[83]

Differential Diagnosis The differential diagnosis between *C. neoformans, B. dermatitidis, H. capsulatum*, and lobomycosis may be aided by the Fontana-Masson stain that stains cryptococci alone black.[83]

North American Blastomycosis

Synonyms: Blastomycosis; Gilchrist's disease; Chicago disease

In contrast to fungal infections that preferentially develop in the immunosuppressed, blastomycosis, like coccidioidomycosis, paracoccidioidomycosis and histoplasmosis, is endemic and can infect healthy individuals.[84] First described in 1894 by Gilchrist, it is caused by *Blastomyces dermatitidis*, a dimorphic fungus.[85] Although called North American blastomycosis because the original cases clustered around states crossed by the Mississippi and Ohio rivers, it has also been reported in South America, Europe, and Africa.[86,87] B. dermatitidis is found in the acidic soil of wooded areas. The typical patient is a man between 25 and 50 years of age with occupational or recreational exposure to the outdoors. Blastomycosis also occurs in dogs.

Clinical Features Primary cutaneous blastomycosis is a rare event that has been described following accidental inoculation in the laboratory or during an autopsy. An ulcerated verrucous plaque arises at the inoculation site, followed by lymphangitis and nodules spreading in a sporotrichoid distribution. Spontaneous healing occurs in the ensuing months.

The more common clinical forms of blastomycosis are the primary pulmonary, chronic cutaneous, and disseminated (Table 21-10). Infection with *B. dermatitidis* begins with inhalation of conidia. If not cleared by bronchopulmonary macrophages, these will transform into yeast forms and multiply in the lung parenchyma, although pulmonary blastomycosis can heal spontaneously.[85] Subsequent hematogenous dissemination can occur. The clinical spectrum of pulmonary blastomycosis thus ranges from no symptoms whatsoever in up to 50 percent of those who have inhaled blastomycosis conidia or spores to an acute or chronic pneumonia Erythema nodosum may occur during the resolving phase of the acute pneumonia. Patients with acute pneumonia may

---

TABLE 21-10

North American Blastomycosis

Clinical Features

Caused by *Blastomyces dermatitidis*
Dimorphic fungus, found in acid soil of wooded areas
Endemic in South Central and Southeastern United States
More common in men with a history of outdoor exposure
Age 25–50 years
Cutaneous involvement in 70% of patients with disseminated disease
    Verrucous plaques with peripheral pustules—face, mucosa
    Occasional ulcers
    Erythema nodosum associated with pulmonary blastomycosis
Usually inhaled, can disseminate to bones and central nervous system

Histopathological Features

Pseudoepitheliomatous hyperplasia
Intraepidermal and dermal neutrophilic microabscesses
Suppurative granulomatous infiltrate with giant cells
Spores are thick-walled and 5–15 μm in diameter
    Present extracellularly, within giant cells, epidermal and dermal abscesses, and granulomas
    Buds are single and broad-based

Differential Diagnosis

Coccidioidomycosis
Tuberculosis
Paracoccidioidomycosis
Chromoblastomycosis
Blastomycosis-like pyoderma
Pyoderma gangrenosum
Halogenoderma

---

appear to recover but then return months later with disseminated infection. Chronic pulmonary blastomycosis often is associated with weight loss, fever, night sweats, chest pain, and hemoptysis.[84] Chest X-rays are non-diagnostic and may reveal masses in 32 percent and alveolar infiltrates in 48 percent of patients as well as cavitation, plural fibrosis, and hilar adenopathy simulating tuberculosis.[84,85]

Cutaneous blastomycosis occurs from hematogenous spread in 70 percent of patients with disseminated blastomycosis.[76] These patients develop verrucous plaques with peripheral pustules and occasional ulcerations on the face, mucous membranes, and arms. If cutaneous blastomycosis is present and there is no pulmonary disease, the latter is thought to have spontaneously resolved.[85]

Osteomyelitis occurs in 25 percent of patients with disseminated disease, most commonly affecting the spine, pelvis, skull, ribs, and long bones.[76,84] Granulomas, suppuration, or necrosis can be contiguous between bone and adjacent soft tissues, leading to subcutaneous abscesses. CNS infections occurs in less than 10 percent of patients and may be associated with meningitis and brain abscess formation.[76,85] Infection may also involve the genitourinary tract.[76]

Serological tests are of limited value at present because of a high rate of false positives and negatives. Although a positive immunodiffusion test is diagnostic, this test is negative in 10 percent of patients with disseminated infection and 60 percent of patients with localized infection.[76] Diagnosis is made by histologic examination and fungal culture.

Histopathological Features Biopsy of the active border of a plaque or of an ulcer reveals pseudoepitheliomatous hyperplasia. Intraepidermal and dermal neutrophilic abscesses also are seen. The dermis contains a granulomatous infiltrate consisting of lymphocytes, histiocytes, plasma cells, neutrophils, and multinucleated giant cells. *B. dermatitidis* spores are seen free in the tissue or in giant cells that are within the suppurative granulomas or surrounded by the pseudoepitheliomatous hyperplasia. *B. dermatitidis* spores measure 5 to 15 μm and have a thick wall consisting of the exterior and interior cell surfaces. An occasional single broad-based equal-sized bud is characteristic. Spores can be identified as an empty round space within the cytoplasm of giant cells using hematoxylin and eosin stain; however, their visualization is enhanced with PAS or methenamine silver stains (Fig. 21-9).[76,86]

Differential Diagnosis Blastomycosis may be distinguished from coccidioidomycosis by the greater number of intraepidermal microabcesses and the much smaller size of the spores (5–15 μm) compared to the sporangia of *C. immitis*. The etiologic agent of paracoccidioidomycosis has multiple buds with a narrow base, as opposed to the broad-based buds of *B. dermatitidis*. The dematiaceous fungi of chromoblastomycosis appear dark brown on hematoxylin and eosin stained sections, whereas *B. dermatitidis* appears as an empty space within giant cells.

Coccidioidomycosis

Synonyms: Posada's disease; coccidioidal granuloma; desert rheumatism; San Joaquin Valley fever; California disease

Coccidioidomycosis is a disease of the arid regions of the Southwestern United States, Mexico, and South America. *C. immitis* is found in the soil, and pulmonary disease is caused by inhalation of contaminated dust. Coccidioidomycosis can occur in cattle, primates, dogs, rodents, and humans in endemic areas.[88–91] *C. immitis* is a rapidly growing dimorphic organism that grows in less than a week on Sabouraud's agar. However, cultures must be carried out under strict precautions since the aleuriospores are highly infectious.

Clinical Features Three types of coccidioidomycosis have been described: pulmonary, cutaneous inoculation, and systemic (Table 21-11). Primary pulmonary coccidioidomycosis, by far the most common form, occurs in about 40 percent of individuals exposed to *C. immitis*, and manifests itself 10 to 14 days following exposure, with fever, chest

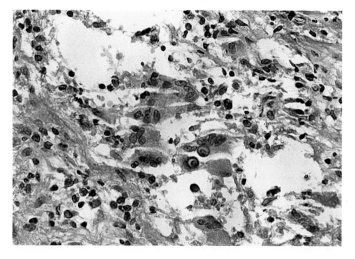

FIGURE 21-9 North American blastomycosis. Large spores with surrounding granulomatous inflammation demonstrated by PAS with diastase. Note halo around cytoplasm of the fungal cell owing to retraction because of shrinkage during processing.

TABLE 21-11

Coccidioidomycosis

Clinical Features

Caused by *Coccidioides immitis*
Endemic in arid regions of Southwestern United States, Mexico, and South America
Dimorphic soil fungus, inhaled with dust
Frequency of systemic disease: <0.5% of patients with pulmonary disease develop systemic disease.
Incidence
    Filipinos > African Americans > Mexicans > Caucasians
    20% Cutaneous involvement with disseminated disease
        Granulomatous plaques, pustules and nodules
        Erythema nodosum, erythema multiforme
Coccidioidin skin test converts weeks following exposure, remains positive for years

Histopathological Features

Acanthosis, intraepidermal microabscesses
Granulomatous infiltrate
    Lymphocytes, histiocytes, neutrophils, giant cells
    Eosinophils
    Variable abscess formation and necrosis
Sporangia are rare but large, up to 80 μm in diameter
    Numerous 1–4 μm endospores in sporangia
    Present in giant cells or extracellularly

Differential Diagnosis

North American Blastomycosis
Tuberculosis verrucosa cutis
Halogenoderma
Pemphigus vegetans

---

pain, headache, and cough. Chest X-rays may show cavitary pulmonary lesions that usually spontaneously resolve in 3 to 4 months. Simultaneously, or in the weeks following pulmonary infection, erythema nodosum and erythema multiforme may occur.[88]

Only 0.1 to 0.5 percent of patients with pulmonary coccidioidomycosis go on to develop systemic disease that can involve skin, central nervous, and musculoskeletal systems.[88]

Systemic coccidioidomycosis is associated with skin changes in about 20 percent of cases. These include granulomatous plaques, pustules, and nodules.[91] Systemic disease is more common in Filipinos, African Americans, and Mexicans, and affects men more often than women, with the exception of pregnant women. An immunosupressed state or immunosuppressive therapy can activate a latent pulmonary infection and result in systemic disease. Primary cutaneous coccidioidomycosis is quite rare; lesions resemble the verrucous plaques of primary cutaneous tuberculosis and often are associated with lymphangitis and lymphadenitis 2 to 3 weeks following accidental inoculation.[90]

If a patient has traveled to an endemic area and coccidioidomycosis is suspected, a chest X-ray and a coccidioidin skin test should be performed. The coccidioidin skin test becomes reactive 2 to 6 weeks following infection and remains positive for years; however, a negative test does not rule out disease in immunosuppressed patients.[76] Peripheral eosinophilia and eosinophilia of cerebrospinal fluid, lung, and other tissues may be seen in disseminated infection, most likely owing to increased interleukin-5 production.[89] The presence of complement-fixing antibodies correlates strongly with systemic disease.

Histopathological Features Examination of the verrucous plaques of primary inoculation coccidioidomycosis reveals acanthosis and a diffuse, dense, dermal infiltrate of neutrophils, lymphocytes, histiocytes, plasma cells, eosinophils, and giant cells. Spores are found within the giant cells and free in the tissue (Table 21-11).[90]

In the verrucous plaques and papulonodules of systemic coccidioidomycosis, there is acanthosis and formation of intraepidermal microabcesses, although to a lesser degree than in blastomycosis. Endothelial cell proliferation and a perivascular, acute and chronic inflammatory infiltrate are seen. In addition to perivascular inflammation, the dermis may contain a granulomatous infiltrate consisting of neutrophils, lymphocytes, histiocytes, plasma cells, eosinophils, and multinucleated giant cells. Within the granulomas, one observes abscess formation and necrosis, both in the verrucous plaques and in the subcutaneous abscesses noted clinically. The sporangia of *C. immitis* are usually few in tissue sections, but when present are quite large and thick-walled, measuring up to 80 μm (Fig. 21-10). They contain numerous endospores measuring 1 to 4 μm and are present within the giant cells or free in the tissue. Although they may be seen with hematoxylin- and eosin-stained sections, PAS and methenamine silver highlight the endospores.[88]

Differential Diagnosis The differential diagnosis includes both infectious and noninfectious processes that exhibit pseudoepitheliomatous hyperplasia, intraepidermal microabscesses, and suppurative granulomas in the dermis and subcutis. The verrucous plaques may resemble those seen in North American blastomycosis but have fewer microabcesses. Methenamine silver and PAS stains performed on multiple tissue sections should enable recognition of sporangia, which are not seen in North American blastomycosis, tuberculosis verrucosa cutis, halogenoderma, and pemphigus vegetans.

Paracoccidioidomycosis

Synonyms: South American blastomycosis; Lutz-Splendore-Almeida's disease

Paracoccidioidomycosis is endemic in the subtropical mountain forests of South and Central America and has also been reported in individuals who have previously spent time in these regions.[76] It is the most common systemic mycosis in Latin America, with 10 million individuals or about 10 percent of the endemic area's population presently infected.[92–94]

Clinical Features Like North American blastomycosis, coccidioidomycosis, and histoplasmosis, paracoccidioidomycosis usually is acquired by the respiratory route and is caused by a dimorphic fungus found in the soil.[93] Infection follows inhalation of the mycelia or conidia of *Paracoccidioides brasiliensis*, the causative agent (Table 21-12).[94] Infection rates are highest in the 30- to 50-year-old age group, and there is a striking male predominance of up to 48:1, most likely owing to inhibition by estrogens of conidium- and mycelium-to-yeast transformation.[78,79]

Pulmonary paracoccidioidomycosis is characterized by cough, fever, night sweats, and anorexia.[76] In some cases it resolves without dissemination; however, it may become latent, with possible reactivation years later.[78,79] Bilateral infiltrates, fibrosis, and cavitation may be seen on chest X-rays.[76,93]

Mucosal and skin involvement is common in progressive disease, occurring in 60 percent of patients.[92] This high prevalence has led to the hypothesis that it results from direct implantation in the oral-nasal mucosa.[76] Progressive painful ulcers develop on the gingivae, tongue, lips, and palate and may lead to perforation of the palate or nasal septum.[76] Cutaneous manifestations of paracoccidioidomycosis usually involve the face but may be disseminated. Acneiform papules or nodules slowly develop into crusted plaques with a well-defined, raised border.[92] Complications including difficulty speaking, swallowing, and breathing, and scarring fibrosis and draining sinus tracts may be seen in late stages of the disease.[82,91–94]

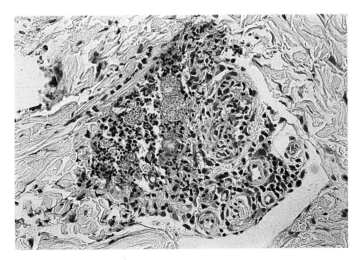

FIGURE 21-10 Coccidioidomycosis. Note large characteristic spherules containing endospores. (Courtesy Dr. D. Mehregan.)

TABLE 21-12

Paracoccidioidomycosis

Clinical Features

Caused by *Paracoccidiodes brasiliensis*
Dimorphic soil fungus of subtropical South and Central America
Infection occurs predominently in men
Pulmonary infection characterized by fever and weight loss
Mucocutaneous involvement in 60% of cases
  Ulcers of lip, tongue, palate
  Verrucous plaques, usually head and neck
  Cervical and submandibular adenopathy
  Difficulty eating, speaking, breathing

Histopathological Features

Ulceration, pseudoepitheliomatous hyperplasia
Granulomatous infiltrate
  Lymphocytes, histiocytes, neutrophils, giant cells
  Occasional necrosis, abscess formation
Yeast seen intra- and extracellularly, and in giant cells
Thick-walled, refractile, variably sized yeast measure 4–40 μm
  in diameter
Yeast occur singly, in chains or as a "captain's wheel" with
  multiple buds

Differential Diagnosis

North American Blastomycosis
Lobomycosis
Histoplasmosis
Leishmaniasis

Lymphadenopathy, most often in the cervical and submandibular nodes, may occur in disseminated disease. Hematogenous spread can lead to multiple organ involvement, including adrenal gland destruction, osteomyelitis, and central nervous system involvement.[92]

High titers (>1:1024) of complement-fixing antibodies to paracoccidioidin imply active disease. However, cross-reactivity to *H. capsulatum*, *B. dermatitidis*, and other fungal pathogens may make interpretation difficult. Some patients experience impaired delayed hypersensitivity.[95,96] Immunodiffusion tests are positive in 80 percent of patients with disease; however, cross-reactivity remains a problem. A recently developed PCR assay using the specific nucleotide sequence of P. brasiliensis DNA may provide a useful diagnostic marker.[97]

Histopathological Features Ulceration is commonly observed, both in mucosal lesions and at the center of the verrucous crusted plaques (Table 21-12). Pseudoepitheliomatous hyperplasia as well as a variable dermal granulomatous infiltrate consisting of lymphocytes, histiocytes, neutrophils, and multinucleated giant cells characterize longstanding plaques. Necrosis and abscess formation may be seen. T-cell subsets may play a role in immunoregulation, as the majority of cells in the granulomas are CD4-positive.[98]

P. brasiliensis yeast are readily present in hematoxylin-eosin, methenamine silver, or PAS-stained sections, and may be seen intra- or extracellularly, or within giant cells.[82] *P. brasiliensis* are thick-walled, refractile yeasts of variable size, 4 to 30 μm in diameter (Fig. 21-11). They may be observed singly, in chains, or budding in the distinctive "captain's-wheel" pattern with multiple, small, narrow-based buds concentrically rimming a central large yeast.[76,82]

Differential Diagnosis If the yeasts occur singly or in chains, it may be difficult to distinguish the etiologic agent of paracoccidioidomycosis from those of North American blastomycosis, lobomycosis, and histoplasmosis. Diligent search for the characteristic "captain's wheel" is helpful. The agent of North American blastomycosis has a single broad-based bud as opposed to the narrow budding pattern of *P. brasiliensis* and *Loboa loboi*. *H. capsulatum* buds are generally smaller (2–4 μm) than those of *P. brasiliensis*.

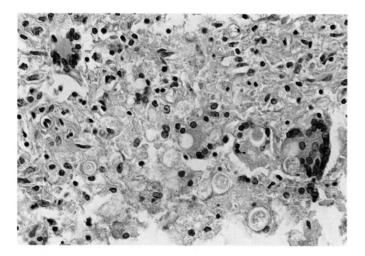

FIGURE 21-11 South American blastomycosis. There are large spores with narrow-based budding.

Classic Histoplasmosis

Synonyms: Darling's disease; cave disease; Ohio Valley disease

Histoplasmosis is caused by two strains of the dimorphic fungus *H. capsulatum*: var. "*capsulatum*" and var. "*duboisii*" (associated with African histoplasmosis).[99] The reservoir of infection is worldwide, particularly in soil contaminated by bird and bat excreta.[76] Despite the distinct clinical and histologic appearance of African histoplasmosis, H. capsulatum var. capsulatum and var. duboisii are variants of the same species since their yeast forms appear identical after prolonged growth at 37°C.[100]

Clinical Features Classic histoplasmosis is endemic in the southeastern and midwestern United States, with a positive histoplasmin skin test seen in up to 80 percent of the population.[101] It occurs in four forms: primary cutaneous inoculation, acute pulmonary infection, chronic pulmonary infection, and disseminated disease (Table 21-13). Prior to the advent of AIDS, disseminated histoplasmosis was a rare event, occurring in 1:100,000 to 1:500,000 of infected patients per year.[102] In endemic areas, disseminated histoplasmosis may affect 10 percent of the AIDS patients and, for three-quarters of these, this will be their first manifestation of HIV infection.[103–105]

Primary cutaneous histoplasmosis is extremely rare and results from direct inoculation. It presents as a chancriform ulcer with associated regional lymphadenopathy. Its course may be self-limited or it may progress to disseminated disease in the immunocompromised.[106]

The vast majority of individuals who inhale *H. capsulatum* spores remain asymptomatic. A minority, after an incubation period of 3 weeks, develop flu-like symptoms. Erythema nodosum or erythema multiforme may occur during the recovery phase.[107] Chest X-rays

TABLE 21-13

Classic Histoplasmosis

Clinical Features

Occurs worldwide in soil containing bird excreta
Common in Southeastern and Midwestern US where 80% of population may have a positive histoplasmin test
Pulmonary infection is portal of entry, asymptomatic in vast majority of cases
Disseminated disease, characterized by
  Mucosal ulcers
  Cutaneous nodules, plaques, ulcers, pustules, panniculitis
  Hepatosplenomegaly
  Anemia, meningitis
  Adrenal destruction

Histopathological Features

H. capsulatum var. capsulatum, 2–4 μm in diameter, argyrophilic, with pseudocapsule
Leukocytoclastic vasculitis, granulomatous infiltrate, panniculitis, ulceration
Yeast present in histiocytes, giant cells and yeast, and extracellularly

Differential Features

Rhinoscleroma
Granuloma Inguinale
Leishmaniasis
Cryptococcosis

reveal hilar lymphadenopathy and small scattered nodules that may heal with calcification.[102]

Chronic pulmonary histoplasmosis occurs in older men who have a history of chronic obstructive pulmonary disease, and is associated with fever, hemoptysis, and weight loss. Segmental interstitial infiltrates may progress to extensive fibrosis, cavitation, and destruction of lung tissue.[102]

Disseminated histoplasmosis may develop in infants or in the immunocompromised and can manifest as an indolent chronic illness or as a rapidly fatal one if left untreated.[108,109] Hepatosplenomegaly, anemia, and fever may be the presenting signs of acute disseminated histoplasmosis. In later stages, endocarditis, meningitis, and adrenal gland destruction may be seen.[102]

Mucosal ulcerations occur in 60 percent of patients with disseminated disease and may involve the oral, nasal, gastrointestinal, or genital mucosae.[102] In contrast, cutaneous manifestations of disseminated histoplasmosis are present in less than 25 percent of patients.[104] They range from exfoliative erythroderma to nodules, papules, ulcers, acneiform pustules, erythema multiforme, erythema nodosum panniculitis, and diffuse hyperpigmentation from Addison's disease.[99,104,107,110]

Histopathological Features   H. capsulatum is a small, 2- to 4-μm diameter yeast that divides with narrow-based, unequal buds (Table 21-13). Although it is called *"capsulatum,"* it lacks a true capsule, but its cell wall stains strongly with methenamine silver (Fig. 21-12). It usually is seen within the cytoplasm of histiocytes, although it may be seen extracellularly or within giant cells. A halolike clear space is sometimes seen separating the yeast wall from the macrophage cytoplasm.[111]

Biopsies of lesions from patients having primary cutaneous histoplasmosis, and of the ulcers of disseminated histoplasmosis, reveal an underlying lymphohistiocytic infiltrate with H. capsulatum within histiocytes faintly visible with hematoxylin and eosin but strongly visible with the methenamine silver stain. The pattern of inflammation in disseminated disease is variable and depends on the clinical presentation. Histologic examination of cutaneous papules and plaques reveals leukocytoclastic vasculitis consisting of a granulomatous infiltrate with multinucleated giant cells and variable foci of necrosis.[103,112] In Histoplasma panniculitis, the dermal infiltrate extends into the subcutaneous fat where the organisms may be seen.[110] The diagnostic benchmark of all biopsies from histoplasmosis patients is the presence of numerous spores.

Differential Diagnosis   The differential diagnosis for parasitized histiocytes includes rhinoscleroma, granuloma inguinale, and leishmaniasis.[19] Rhinoscleroma is associated with a plasma-cell rich infiltrate, and the Donovan bodies of granuloma inguinale do not stain with silver or PAS stains. Also, H. capsulatum lacks the kinetoplast of leishmania. Extracellular H. capsulatum can be distinguished from extracellular C. neoformans by the Fontana-Masson stain, which stains C. neoformans but not H. capsulatum.[83] Unlike the yeast forms of Candida glabrata, which are of similar size, the yeast forms of H. capsulatum stain only weakly or not at all with the Gram stain.

African Histoplasmosis

Clinical Features   African histoplasmosis caused by H. capsulatum var. duboisii occurs in two forms: localized and disseminated. The localized form is a chronic illness involving skin, bone, and lymph nodes. Variable numbers of cutaneous papules and plaques may ulcerate, and purulent bone lesions can extend into adjacent soft tissue, causing a subcutaneous abscess or a draining sinus tract.[100] The disseminated form involves liver, spleen, and other organs in addition to the features of the localized form, and often is fatal.[113,114]

Histopathological Features   Biopsies of cutaneous plaques reveal a granulomatous infiltrate consisting of lymphocytes, histiocytes, neutrophils, and giant cells. Numerous organisms measuring 8 to 15 μm are present, mostly within the giant cells and histiocytes (Fig. 21-13).[100,113,114]

INFECTIONS BY DEMATIACEOUS FUNGI

Dematiaceous fungi are pigment-producing organisms. Several different fungal infections can produce pigment: sporotrichosis, chromoblastomycosis, phaeohyphomycosis, tinea nigra, and alternaria.

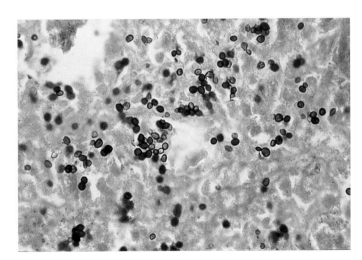

FIGURE 21-12   Histoplasmosis. Spores in clusters and chains are stained with Gomori methenamine silver (GMS) technique and show narrow-based budding. They are usually intracellular. (Courtesy Dr. F. von Lichtenberg.)

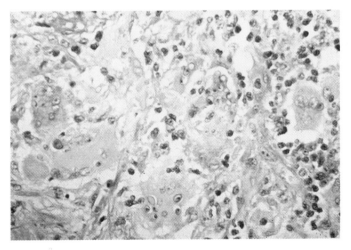

FIGURE 21-13   African histoplasmosis. Large yeast forms within cells are demonstrated by PAS with diastase, mostly within giant cells. (Courtesy Dr. J. R. Nethercott.)

Sporotrichosis

In 1898 Schenck described a case in Baltimore, where an organism was isolated from the arm and index finger of a patient.[115] The fungus was sent to EF Smith at the U.S. Department of Agriculture for further identification and was termed "sporotricha." Hoetken and Perkins reported a second case and named the organism Sporothrix schenckii. Although there were many reports of sporotrichosis in Europe at the beginning of the twentieth century, they have become rare and most cases are now reported in the United States, Central and South America, Australia, Asia, and South Africa. A major outbreak in the gold mines of Witwatersrand in South Africa in the 1940s allowed for an extensive study of the ecology and distribution of the organism.

Clinical Features   Three major clinical forms are recognized: lymphocutaneous, fixed cutaneous and disseminated.[115]

The lymphocutaneous form is the most common disease pattern seen with sporotrichosis. A hard nodule develops weeks to months after the infection at the site of inoculation. This nodule may drain seropurulent fluid and become ulcerated. Other lesions may follow along the lymphatic drainage system and there is associated lymphadenopathy. The initial lesion may remain for several weeks and ultimately heals with scarring. This form of infection may become chronic if not treated. The clinical differential diagnosis includes mainly leishmaniasis, nocardia, and other fungal infections and pyoderma gangrenosum.

Fixed cutaneous disease refers to localized skin lesions without lymphatic involvement. These lesions rarely lead to systemic disease. They are more difficult to diagnose and their clinical appearance may vary from ulcerative, verrucous to acneiform or erythematous. Clinically, many other lesions may need to be considered in the differential diagnosis, most importantly syphilis and cutaneous leishmaniasis.

The disseminated form of the disease can occur because of hematogenous or lymphatic spread. It may involve bone and joints, the lung, the CNS, the kidneys, and other visceral sites.[116]

Histopathological Features   The most important diagnostic use of a biopsy is for microbiological cultures, since the organism is rarely identified histologically. It is a fast growing fungus: Characteristic colonies become apparent within 3 to 5 days. The colony is typically lobated, smooth, or verrucous and becomes brown to black with age. The histological findings are by and large non-specific, but typically include a suppurative and/or granulomatous tissue reaction.[115,116] Lurie and Still classified the patterns as sporotrichotic, tuberculoid, and foreign body. In a later stage of the lesions, a fairly common granulomatous pattern is that of a central microabscess, surrounded by epithelioid histiocytes, which itself is surrounded by plasma cells and lymphocytes (Table 21-14; Fig. 21-14). If organisms are present, a fungal stain may reveal asteroid bodies or round to oval spores measuring 4-6 μm in diameter (Fig. 21-15). Cigar-shaped bodies measuring up to 8 μm are observed much less commonly. There may be single or multiple buds. No capsule is present.

Differential Diagnosis   The histologic differential diagnosis includes conditions with pseudoepitheliomatous hyperplasia and other granulomatous tissue reactions, in particular, other fungal and mycobacterial infections, tularemia, and cat-scratch disease.

Chromoblastomycosis

Synonyms: Chromomycosis; verrucous dermatitis; Pedroso's disease; Fonseca's disease; Gome's disease

Pedroso described the first case in Brazil in 1911 (published in 1920). Rudolph published the first clinical characterization of the dis-

TABLE 21-14

Sporotrichosis

Clinical Features

Caused by sporothrix schenckii
Inoculation into skin with trauma
Cutaneous and subcutaneous nodules
Frequent involvement of lymphatics
Three forms:
    Lymphocutaneous
    Fixed cutaneous
    Disseminated

Histopathological Features

Early
    Nonspecific infiltrate of lymphocytes, neutrophils, plasma cells
Established
    Pseudoepitheliomatous hyperplasia common
    Suppurative granulomas with concentric zones:
        Neutrophilic microabscess centrally
        Cuff of epithelioid and multinucleated histiocytes
        Outer cuff of lymphocytes and plasma cells
Organisms difficult to find in tissue
    4–6 μm Round or oval forms or up to 8 μm cigar-shaped forms; single or uncommon multiple buds
    Asteroid bodies may be present
    Rare branching, nonseptate hyphae

Differential Diagnosis

Other infectious agents
    Deep fungi
    Atypical mycobacteria
    Blastomycosis-like pyoderma
Halogenoderma
Pyoderma gangrenosum
Systemic vasculitis such as Wegener's granulomatosis

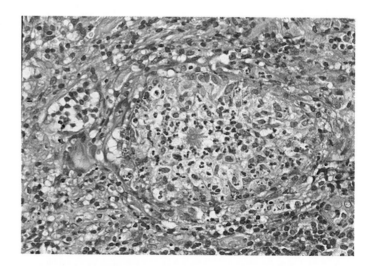

FIGURE 21-14 Sporotrichosis. Suppurative granuloma containing an asteroid body. (Courtesy Dr. S. Seopela.)

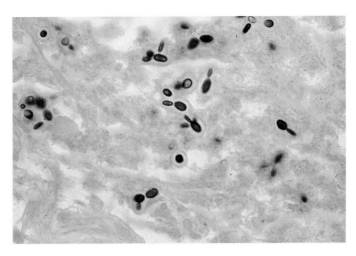

FIGURE 21-15 Sporotrichosis. Round to oval spore forms with budding demonstrated with GMS stain. (Courtesy Dr. F. von Lichtenberg.)

TABLE 21-15

Chromoblastomycosis

Clinical Features

> Caused by: Fonsecaea pedrosoi, Fonsecaea compactum, Cladosporium carrionii, Phialophora verrucosa, Rhinocladella acquaspersa most common
> Primary innoculation into skin, however extremities most frequent site, often distal
> Verucous plaques, nodules, tumors
> Scarring, central clearing

Histopathological Features

> Pseudoepitheliomatous hyperplasia
> Suppurative granulomas
> Organisms do not require special stain
>> Pigmented ("chestnut brown")
>> Sclerotic (septate) bodies
>> (Medlar bodies, "copper pennies")

Differential Diagnosis

> Other infectious processes
>> Phaeohyphomycosis
>> Other deep fungi
>> Mycobacteria and atypical mycobacteria
> Halogenoderma
> Pyoderma gangrenosum

---

ease in 1914. Chromoblastomycosis is primarily a disease of tropical and subtropical regions, but may occur in temperate climates.[117] Its inoculation typically is related to penetrating wounds, splinters, and thorns, and is associated with outdoor activity or agricultural work. A number of distinct organisms can cause chromoblastomycosis, including Fonsecaea pedrosi (most common), Fonsecaea compactum, Cladosporium carrionii, Phialophora verrucosa, and Rhinocladella aquaspera. Cultures of each of these organisms yields slow-growing green to black colonies, which are distinguished from each other by the microscopic appearance of the fungi. These organisms have been isolated from decaying wood or soil.

Clinical Features The initial lesion is an erythematous papule that subsequently develops into one or multiple coalescing warty papules or plaques. Carrion described five clinical presentations: nodules, tumors, plaques, warty lesions, and scarring lesions.[118] They typically occur on an extremity. The patients usually are otherwise well. There is frequently associated pruritus and scratching may lead to satellite lesions. The disease rarely spreads to non-cutaneous sites. A potential cutaneous complication is the development of squamous cell carcinoma in a long-standing lesion. KOH preparations may be diagnostic by revealing pigmented sclerotic bodies. The clinical differential diagnosis includes other fungal or mycobacterial infections, in particular tuberculosis, leprosy, blastomycosis, leishmaniasis, botryomycosis, and tertiary syphilis.

Histopathological Features A biopsy of a typical lesion usually shows hyperkeratosis, epidermal hyperplasia often with a pseudoepitheliomatous pattern, overlying a suppurative and granulomatous dermatitis (Table 21-15; Fig. 21-16).[119] The organisms may vary in number, but can easily be recognized on routine H&E-stained sections. The spores may be present free in tissue or located within giant cells. They are round to oval and bronze-colored measuring 6 to 12 μm in diameter, usually with a central septation. They have been called Medlar bodies, sclerotic bodies, or descriptively "copper pennies."

Differential Diagnosis When septation is present within a dividing sclerotic body, the findings are diagnostic and distinguish chromoblastomycosis from phaeohyphomycosis, in which budding occurs and the characteristic septations are not found. Phaeohyphomycosis also may exhibit septate hyphae, pseudohyphae, branching hyphae, and spores in chains. Pigmentation is not always present in the latter organisms.

Phaeohyphomycosis

Ajello coined the term phaeohyphomycosis in 1974 to encompass infections caused by dematiacious fungi that have hyphal elements and grow by budding. The most common fungi in this group are Exophiala jeanselmei and Wangiella dermatitidis.[120]

Clinical Features The spectrum of clinical presentations is broad, including subcutaneous pseudocysts and ulcerated and verrucous lesions. In the immunocompromised patient, dissemination may occur. E. jeanselmei typically is present in pheomycotic cysts, whereas W.

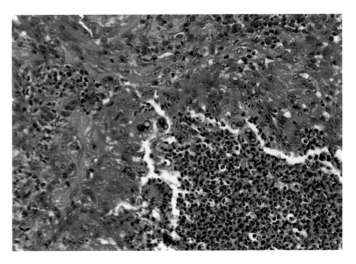

FIGURE 21-16 Chromoblastomycosis. Suppurative granuloma with pigmented sclerotic (Medlar) bodies.

dermatitidis is more often associated with ulcerating and verrucous lesions.[121]

Histopathological Features This histologic reaction pattern is that of a suppurative or mixed inflammatory cell infiltrate with a granulomatous tissue reaction (Table 21-16). There may be fibrous encapsulation of "cyst-like" lesions (phaeomycotic cyst) (Fig. 21-17). Foreign material such as vegetable matter or a splinter occasionally may be observed. Epidermal hyperplasia is only seen in verrucous lesions. Fungi are typically abundant and often located in or near suppurative foci. They are brown-colored and measure 2 to 6 μm, but may be larger (Fig. 21-18). The fungi in phaeohyphomycosis are budding spores often producing chains and have abundant hyphal elements that may be septate, branching, or exhibit pseudohyphae. Pigmentation may not always be obvious, and a Fontana-Masson stain may be needed to demonstrate melanin.

Differential Diagnosis Phaeohyphomycosis must be distinguished from chromoblastomycosis. In contrast to chromoblastomycosis, the fungi in phaeohyphomycosis are budding spores producing chains and have more abundant hyphal elements. True sclerotic bodies with thick walls and septae are absent. The differential diagnosis includes also hyalohyphomycosis, which lacks pigment, and other dematiaceous eumycotic mycetomas, in which fungal elements are clumped together like grains.

Tinea Nigra

Alexandre Cerqueira provided the first description of this disease in Brazil in 1891. The fungus was named Cladosporium werneckii. The fungus produces pigment and is most common in tropical regions. It is not a dermatophyte.[122]

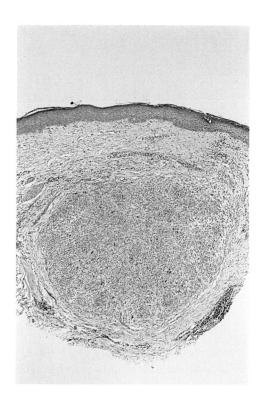

FIGURE 21-17 Phaeohyphomycosis. Well-circumscribed cyst-like lesion in deep dermis.

Clinical Features The lesions are typically asymptomatic and present as brown macules with minimal scale. They tend to expand slowly and almost always affect the palms. The major clinical differential diagnosis is melanoma of acral skin.[123]

Histopathological Features Usually abundant branching brown hyphal elements are present in the upper stratum corneum (Fig. 21-19). There tends to be associated parakeratosis and a mild superficial dermal perivascular inflammatory cell infiltrate. Deep dermal lesions are not

TABLE 21-16

Subcutaneous Phaeohyphomycosis

Clinical Features

Caused by Exophiala and Phialophora species most commonly
Inoculation into skin
Extremities, particularly fingers, wrists, knee, ankle
Usually solitary nodule

Histopathological Features

Usually circumscribed, encapsulated "phaeomycotic cyst"
Suppurative granuloma within "cyst"
Epidermis and dermis may be unaffected
Organisms
    Usually pigmented but not always
Morphological spectrum
    Budding yeast forms
    Pseudohyphae
    Candida-like hyphae with branching, septa, and in chains

Differential Diagnosis

Chromoblastomycosis
Mycetoma and related conditions
Candida

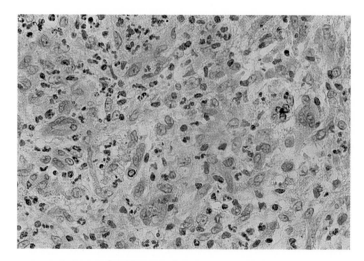

FIGURE 21-18 Phaeohyphomycosis. Neutrophilic and granulomatous infiltrates with pigmented budding yeast forms.

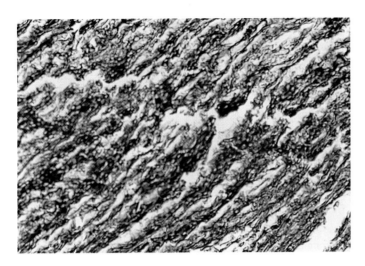

FIGURE 21-19   Tinea nigra. Confluent mass of pigmented hyphal elements from skin surface.

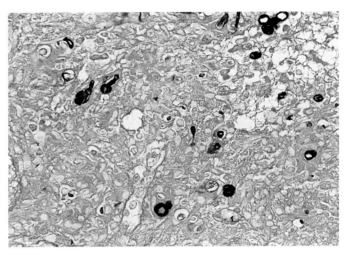

FIGURE 21-20   Alternaria. Budding spores demonstrated with GMS stain.

known to occur with the agent of tinea nigra, which distinguishes this disease from other dematiaceous mycoses.

Alternariosis

Alternaria species are saprophytic fungi whose natural habitat is soil and plants. It is one of the most ubiquitous fungi in indoor and outdoor environments. Workers exposed to logs and wood dust are at highest risk for infection.

Clinical Features   Exogenous and endogenous forms of alternariosis can occur in humans, for which alternaria usually is non-pathogenic. In the exogenous form, organisms are directly inoculated by trauma, such as a wood splinter. Skin manifestations include ulcers, warty and granulomatous lesions. Onychomycoses and keratomycoses as well as combinations of the two have been reported.[124] Most patients with the endogenous form of alternariosis are immunocompromised. In the endogenous form, infection occurs via the lungs by inhalation. Skin lesions develop subsequent to hematogenous spread. The organisms often involve the deep dermis and subcutis.[125] However, alternaria may also colonize superficial, pre-existing lesions. They tend to be indolent in their presentation, but are often difficult to cure. Unlike other common opportunistic infections, alternaria infections show little propensity to disseminate. Extracutaneous lesions have been reported to involve eyes, sinonasal region, bones, and peritoneum. The respiratory tract is the main site of allergic reactions to alternaria.

Histopathological Features   The reaction pattern is that of a suppurative and granulomatous dermatitis or panniculitis. In onychomycosis or keratomycoses fungal elements may be present in thickened layers of keratin without much associated inflammation. The organisms are brown and present as broad, branching septate hyphae, 5 to 7 μm thick, and round to oval spores, often doubly contoured measuring 3 to 10 μm (Fig. 21-20). They tend to be clustered. The spores may be free in tissue or within macrophages.

Differential Diagnosis   Alternaria infections must be distinguished from the other phaeohyphomycoses. It is also important to consider alternaria in onychomycoses so that non-dermatophytic pathogens of nail infections are not overlooked.[126]

MYCETOMA AND CLINICALLY SIMILAR CONDITIONS

Mycetoma is a chronic infectious disease localized to the skin and/or subcutaneous tissue. This disease is characterized by tumefaction, draining sinuses, and the presence of aggregates (grains) of microorganisms. It may be caused by either a fungus or an aerobic actinomycete and is typically initiated by trauma. Mycetomas have been classified into three different groups based on the micromorphology of its grains: botryomycosis (cocci or short rods), actinomycetoma (thin, branching, intertwined filaments), and eumycetoma (thick, branching, intertwined filaments).

Mycetoma (Eumycetoma)

Eumycetoma typically is caused by a fungus. The grains of fungi may be non-pigmented or pigmented (dematiaceous fungus). The most prevalent dematiaceous fungal agent of mycetomata is Madurella mycetomatis. A common non-pigmented etiologic agent of eumycetoma is Pseudallescheria boydii.

Clinical Features   Most patients affected live in tropical or subtropical regions.[127] The etiologic agents of mycetoma usually are associated with woody plants and soil. After the initial trauma, a small nodule develops, which subsequently expands and frequently drains into a sinus tract. Sinuses rarely occur prior to 3 months' duration. Sinuses may close and organisms may be discharged with subsequent healing. Many times new nodules form after the initial one has healed. With time, the lesions may extend deeply and involve bone forming cavities. Fungus may ultimately even spread via the lymphatics to visceral sites. Seventy percent of all mycetomas involve the foot.

Histopathological Features   The typical finding includes an aggregate of microorganisms (grain) in a microabscess surrounded by granulation tissue and fibrosis (Table 21-17; Fig. 21-21). Neutrophils are often numerous and a granulomatous tissue reaction is common. Eumycotic grains or granules (also known as sclerotia) are poorly organized collections of about 5-μm thick septate hyphal elements, which in the case of dematiaceous fungi are brown or black.[128] The micromorphology of

TABLE 21-17

Mycetoma and Related Conditions

Clinical Features

Caused by
   True fungus (eumycetoma, maduromycosis)
   Aerobic actinomycete (actinomycetoma or pseudomycetoma)
Inoculation into skin following trauma
Localized infection of skin, subcutis, fascia, bone
Tumefactive nodules
Ulceration
Draining sinuses with extrusion of sclerotia (grains, granules) in
   exudates
Bone involvement often extensive

Histopathological Features

Neutrophilic abscesses contain sclerotia (grains, granules)
Surrounding granulation tissue
Granulomatous inflammation
Sinus tracts
Organisms in sclerotia:
   Circumscribed mass of hyphae with or without associated host
      tissue and/or soil
   Distinction of organisms based on color, texture, shape, internal
      architecture
   True fungi
   Often filaments in granules from actinomycosis, usually without
      pigment

Differential Diagnosis

Other infections characterized by ulceration, tumefaction, draining
   sinuses
   Chromobastomycosis
   Botryomycosis
   Dermatophyte infection
   Actinomycosis

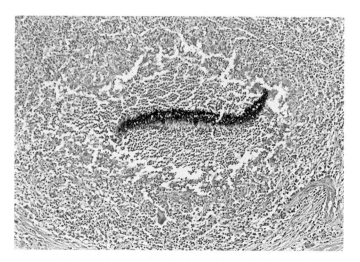

FIGURE 21-21 Mycetoma. Pigmented granule within abscess.

TABLE 21-18

Organisms Causing Mycetoma

Acremonium falciforme	Fusarium solani var. minus
Acremonium kiliensis	Hormonema sp.
Acremonium recifei	Leptosphaeria senegalensis
Aspergillus flavus	Leptosphaeria tompkinsii
Aspergillus nidulans	Madurella grisea
Corynespora cassicola	Madurella mycetomatis
Curvularia geniculata	Neotestudina rosatiii
Curvularia lunata	Phialophora verrucosa
Cylindrocarpon cyanescens	Plenodomus avramii
Cylindrocarpon destructans	Ploycytella hominis
Exophiala jeanselmei	Pseudallescheria boydii
Fusarium spp.	Pseudochaetosphaeronema larense
Fusarium moniliforme	Pyrenochaeta mackinnonii
Fusarium oxysprum	Pyrenochaeta romeroi
Fusarium solani	Scopulariopsis brumptii
Fusarium solani var. coeruleum	

the grains helps to distinguish eumycetomata from actinomycetomata and botryomycosis (see the following) (Tables 21-18 and 21-19).

Differential Diagnosis   The differential diagnosis includes other infectious causes of tumefactive lesions exhibiting ulceration and draining sinuses, such as chromoblastomycosis, botryomycosis, actinomycosis, and pseudomycetomas owing to dermatophytes. In general the presence of granules and their characteristic features allow separation of eumycetoma from the latter entities. For example, neither chromoblastomycosis nor dermatophyte infection are associated with the formation of true grains. Botryomycosis and actinomycosis are characterized by grains that contain bacteria rather the hyphae found in eumycetoma.

Nocardiosis

Nocardia and streptomyces spp. are free-living soil organisms. They are Gram-positive, aerobic, filamentous bacteria, which frequently are acid-fast. The predominant pathogenic species in humans are N. asteroides, N. brasiliensis, and N. otitidis-cavarum.

Clinical Features   Different clinical presentations have been described: actinomycetoma, disease limited to skin or limited to the lungs or CNS, a lymphocutaneous form, and a systemic form.[129] Skin involvement can occur via dissemination from another site, typically in an immunocompromised host.[130] Primary cutaneous nocardiosis usually is the result of traumatic inoculation from subsequent abscess for-

TABLE 21-19

Color of Grains in Actinomycetoma (Pseudomycetoma)

Organism	Grain Color
Nocardia brasiliensis	White
Nocardia asteroides	White (when present)
Nocardia otitidiscaviarum	White to yellow
Actinomadura madurae	Pink or cream
Streptomyces somaliensis	Yellow or brown
Actinomadura pelletieri	Red

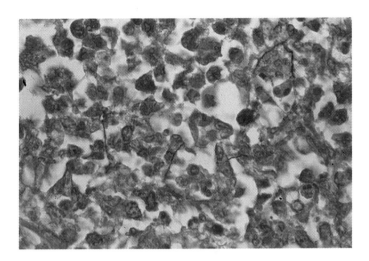

FIGURE 21-22 Nocardiosis. Filamentous bacteria stained with Fite-Faraco reaction. (Courtesy Drs. S. Lucas and F. von Lichtenberg.)

mation and drainage. Lymphocutaneous nocardiosis may be difficult to distinguish clinically from sporotrichosis. Thus, cultures are important in defining the disease.

Histopathological Features Basophilic Gram-positive filamentous structures (1 μm in diameter) stainable with modified acid fast methods are present usually in aggregates (Fig. 21-22). In visceral nocardiosis, in contrast to the "sulfur granules" of actinomyces (see below), the filaments in nocardia tend to break up into short bacillary segments like M. tuberculosis (Table 21-20). However, in mycetomas grains similar to the sulfur granules of Actinomyces may be formed. The inflammatory tissue reaction is usually that of a suppurative and granulomatous dermatitis. In localized cutaneous nocardiosis, an abscess is usually present. In the diagnostic work-up, pus, exudate, or abscess drainage material may be submitted for cultures. Tissue biopsies should also include a sample for microbiology. It is important to indicate on the laboratory requisition sheet that nocardia is suspected to guarantee adequate recovery of the organisms. Colonies can usually be detected in 10 days to 2 weeks.

Differential Diagnosis Nocardia must be distinguished from other infective agents producing suppurative granulomas. Special stains and cultures are essential for diagnosis. Nocardia are weakly acid fast, that is, Ziehl Neelsen-negative, but Fite-Faraco-positive. On Gram stain, they show a similar beaded and filamentous pattern similar to that of Actinomyces.

Actinomycosis

Actinomyces is a chronic suppurative infection noted for the production of "sulfur granules" (see the following). The disease is caused by several members of the order of Actinomycetales, most commonly by Actinomyces israelii.[131] They are saprophytic Gram-positive bacteria present in the normal floors of the mouth and gastrointestinal tract. Infection is often associated with mucosal trauma, such as from dental procedures or surgery.

Clinical Features Three major clinical presentations have been described: cervicofacial, thoracic, and abdominal.[131] The disease also may disseminate in immunocompromised patients. Cervicofacial actinomycosis accounts for more than half of the cases. It typically occurs in

TABLE 21-20

Nocardiosis

Clinical Features

Caused by *Nocardia asteroides, N. brasiliensis, N. otitidiscaviarum* most commonly
Men more commonly affected than women
Age 30–50 years most common
Immunosuppressed host more susceptible
Inoculation into skin following trauma common
Localized pyoderma, nodule
Lymphocutaneous form resembling sporotrichosis
Actinomycetoma
Other presentations
    Systemic
    Pulmonary
    Central nervous system
    Extrapulmonary

Histopathological Features

Neutrophilic abscess in dermis, subcutis
Occasional tuberculoid granulomas
Organism
    Filamentous, Gram-positive, acid-fast, obligate aerobe
Grains may be observed

Differential Diagnosis

Localized infection from bacteria, fungi, mycobacteria
Lymphocutaneous syndromes as from sporotrichosis, atypical mycobacteria
Mycetoma and actinomycetoma (pseudomycetoma)

the premandibular region as discrete slowly growing swelling. Subsequent abscess formation and drainage via sinus tracts are common. Potential complications include osteomyelitis. If infected oral material is aspirated pulmonary infection may develop (thoracic form: 15% of actinomycosis). Abdominal infection usually follows traumatic rupture of the intestine. Appendicitis with perforation is the most common precipitating event.

Histopathological Features The lesion typically begins as a cellulitis with subsequent abscess formation and fibrotic induration (Table 21-21). Discharge of the "sulfur granules" from sinus tracts is common. Histologically, these are aggregates of actinomyces organisms that appear as round to oval bodies up to 10 mm in diameter (Fig. 21-23). There is frequently an eosinophilic fringe (Splendore-Hoeppli phenomenon). At high magnification, the granules are composed of filamentous branching bacteria measuring less than 1 μm in diameter. In tissue, these structures typically are surrounded by macrophages.

Differential Diagnosis Actinomycosis needs to be distinguished from eumycetoma (branching filamentous hyphal structures > 1 μm) and botryomycosis (e.g., Gram-positive coccal forms or short Gram-negative rods).

Botryomycosis

Botryomycosis is a chronic bacterial infection usually caused by staphylococci and less commonly by other organisms such as Pseudomonas, Proteus, or E. coli.

TABLE 21-21

Actinomycosis

Clinical Features

Caused by Actinomyces israelii most commonly
Men more commonly affected than women
All ages but middle-aged men in particular
Inoculation into tissue following trauma
Painful cellulitis followed by
    Soft fluctuant lesions
    Draining sinuses
    Woody induration
Clinical presentations
    Oral-cervicofacial
    Thoracic
    Abdominal

Histopathological Features

Sinus tracts
Neutrophilic abscesses containing "sulfur granules"
Sulfur granules
    Round, oval or crescent-shaped forms that are basophilic
        centrally with an eosinophilic border (Splendore-Hoeppli
        material)
    Composed of Gram-positive, filamentous, branching bacteria
        (<1 μm in diameter)
    Positive for Gomori methenamine silver and Giemsa stains, in
        addition to Gram stain
    Not acid fast

Differential Diagnosis

Botryomycosis (Staphylococcus, Pseudomonas, Eschericheria,
    Proteus, etc.)
Nocardiosis
Other suppurative infections

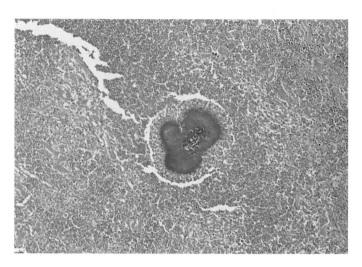

FIGURE 21-23 Actinomycosis. Note "sulfur granule" within abscess that is composed of branching filamentous bacteria.

demonstrates grains that are often (but not always) brown or black and contain true fungi, that is, filamentous hyphal elements.

ZYGOMYCOSES

The class zygomycetes is composed of three orders: the Mucorales, the Entomophthorales, and the Zoopogales.[14,136] Only the first two orders are known to cause infections in humans. The order Mucorales includes the genera Rhizopus, Absidia, Mucor, Cunninghamella, and Saksenaea.[136,137] Conidiobolus and Basidiobolus are the entomophthorales that may infect humans. The term "phycomycosis," which was formerly used interchangeably with mucormycosis or entomophthoramycosis, has fallen out of favor as a result of the reclassification of these fungi. Whereas the mucorales affect the immunocompromised, the entomophthorales can infect both normal and compromised individuals.[73]

Clinical Features   Lesions may affect not only skin, but also internal organs and bone. The skin lesions typically consist of small tender nodules with seropurulent discharge from draining sinuses.[132,133]

Histopathological Features   Common epidermal changes include hyperkeratosis, hyperplasia, and spongiosis. In the dermis, there is a mixed inflammatory cell infiltrate composed of neutrophils, lymphocytes, and histiocytes often with granulation tissue (Table 21-22).[134] Within the inflammatory infiltrate, there usually are granules of tightly clustered Gram-positive cocci (Fig. 21-24). Sometimes the granules are surrounded by amorphous eosinophilic material creating the so-called "Splendore-Hoeppli" phenomenon. This effect of seemingly radiating lateral projections gives the granules a striking similarity to actinomycotic granules.[135] The eosinophilic material has been found to contain immunoglobulins and is likely produced by the host's response to bacterial antigens. In some instances, Pseudomonas or Proteus may cause the same phenomenon, giving rise to granules mimicking actinomyces.[133] In those instances, the granules are composed of tight clusters of Gram-negative rods.

Differential Diagnosis   Botryomycosis must be discriminated from other infections associated with the formation of grains. Actinomycosis is typified by grains containing Gram-positive, filamentous, branching bacteria that are obligate aerobes and non-acid-fast. Eumycetoma

TABLE 21-22

Botryomycosis

Clinical Features

Caused by Staphylococci, pseudomonas, proteus, and E. coli
Tender nodules with draining sinuses
Internal organs and bones may be affected

Histopathological Features

Neutrophilic abscesses containing granules
Granules may exhibit Splendore-Hoeppli phenomenon
Granulation tissue
Sinus tracts
Granules contain
    Gram-positive or -negative cocci or rods without branching
        filaments

Differential Diagnosis

Actinomycosis
Mycetoma (eumycetoma and actinomycetoma)

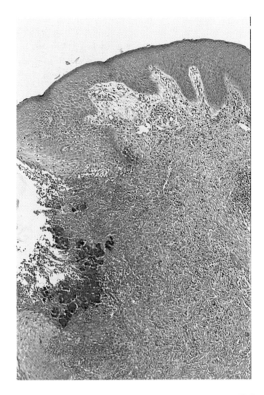

FIGURE 21-24   Botryomycosis. A group of basophilic granules lining an ulcer contains Gram-positive Staphylococci, surrounded by acute inflammation.

Mucormycosis

Synonyms: Zygomycosis; phycomycosis

Clinical Features   The mucorales are ubiquitous, saprophytic organisms found in soil and on decomposing organic material such as fruit and bread.[138] They can be cultured as normal flora from the feces and oral and nasal cavities of healthy individuals, but infection with tissue invasion occurs mainly in immunosuppressed patients.[139,140] Large numbers of sporangiospores are released into the air, and then inhaled, causing pulmonary and nasal sinus infection (Table 21-23).[141] Less commonly, ingestion or cutaneous inoculation may cause disease.[141] The most common risk factors are diabetes, leukemia, neutropenia, prior skin trauma, and the use of elasticized adhesive tape.[138,142]

Sporangiospores that have escaped host defense mechanisms can germinate into the hyphal form capable of invading blood vessels, which may lead to hematogenous dissemination or to infection and necrosis. Defects in macrophages or neutrophils increase susceptibility to systemic infection.[143] Macrophages prevent the transformation of *Rhizopus*, the most common etiological agent of mucormycosis, from its yeast to its hyphal form.[143] Neutrophils are able to damage the hyphal form.[144]

The clinical forms of mucormycosis are rhinocerebral, pulmonary, gastrointestinal, cutaneous, and disseminated. Rhinocerebral mucormycosis most commonly occurs in uncontrolled diabetics who rapidly develop fever, unilateral headache, periorbital or perinasal swelling, and drainage of discolored pus.[140–144]

If not treated with aggressive debridement and antifungal therapy, mucorales can invade brain tissue and bone, and cause death within days.[76] Pulmonary and gastrointestinal mucormycosis are the most common types that can progress to the disseminated form, which is 100 percent fatal if untreated and is associated with widespread abscess

formation and necrosis of multiple organs, including the brain, heart, and spleen.[142]

Two variants of cutaneous mucormycosis have been described: subacute and rapidly progressive. The subacute form occurs in an otherwise healthy host exposed to contaminated adhesive tape, and begins as vesicles and pustules that progress to eschars. The rapidly progressive form occurs in compromised patients and is characterized by an ecthyma-like necrotic black crust surrounded by cellulitis. If untreated, it may progress to disseminated disease.[138,145] Unfortunately, no serologic tests are yet available to detect mucormycosis.[76]

Histopathological Features   Extensive necrosis and vascular damage characterize the eschar. Only the hyphal form of the mucorales is seen in tissue. The hyphae are broad (up to 30 μm in diameter) with bulbous lateral protrusions. They often appear hollow, lack microscopically visible septa, branch at variable, up to 90 degree angles, and are visible with hematoxylin-eosin and with PAS and methenamine silver stains (Fig. 21-25).[138]

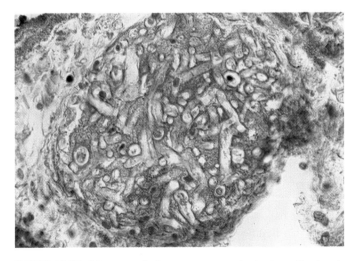

FIGURE 21-25   Mucormycosis. Large empty-appearing hyphae without septa show 90° branching.

Differential Diagnosis The hyphae of Aspergillus branch at an acute angle, show dichotomous branching, and often exhibit septa. Tissue culture is extremely helpful when hyphae are scarce or distorted in tissue.

Entomophthoramycoses

Conidiobolus and *Basidiobolus*, like the etiological agents of mucormycosis, are found in soil and plant detritus.[146,147] Both occur mainly in the tropical regions of Africa, South America, and Southeast Asia, and produce extensive soft tissue swelling without skin involvement.[148,149]

CONIDIOBOLUS

Clinical Features The pathogenic fungus *C. coronatus* typically infects men from 20 to 60 years of age involved in agricultural work.[147] Infection begins in the nasal mucosa and spreads to the nose, forehead, periorbital region, and cheeks, occasionally causing lymphedema.[76] Horses and mules can also develop nasal granulomas owing to *Conidiobolus*.[147]

Histopathological Features *Conidiobolus* causes a granulomatous tissue reaction consisting of lymphocytes, histiocytes, neutrophils, plasma cells, foreign body giant cells, and numerous eosinophils. Foci of necrosis may be seen within the granulomas that extend from the dermis to the subcutaneous tissue. Fungal hyphae may be observed within the giant cells and are thin-walled, broad (4-10 μm in diameter), and occasionally septate. They are rimmed by a thick eosinophilic sheath visible in hematoxylin-eosin or PAS-stained sections.[147]

BASIDIOBOLUS

Clinical Features Entomophthoramycosis caused by *Basidiobolus* is a childhood disease, with the majority of patients under 10 years of age.[146,148] It begins as a slowly growing, painless, rubbery nodule, usually on the lower extremities or buttocks. Gradually there is progressive subcutaneous swelling and additional nodules may appear.[149,150] The mode of transmission is unknown, although insect bites and direct contact with contaminated feces have been suggested as agents to transmit the etiologic agent.

Basidiobolus is a saprophyte and part of the normal flora of the gastrointestinal tract of reptiles and amphibians. It has been hypothesized that the practice of using toilet leaves (plants used in lieu of toilet paper) contaminated by *Basidiobolus* in soil and excreta is implicated in the perineal occurrence of disease.

Histopathological Features The dermis and subcutaneous tissues contain a mixed granulomatous and eosinophilic infiltrate, which may replace fat (similar to entomophthoramycosis caused by *Conidiobolus*). Septate, branching hyphae measuring 7 to 15 μm are seen within the granulomas, particularly toward the edge of the clinical lesion. The hyphae are surrounded by eosinophilic material (Splendore-Hoeppli phenomenon) a few microns thick.[146,150]

Differential Diagnosis In the tropics, filarial skin swellings must be considered in the differential diagnosis. *Basidiobolus* and *Conidiobolus* are similar histologically. Diagnosis is made on the basis of clinical presentation, typical histopathological findings, and tissue culture.

Aspergillosis

Aspergillus is a ubiquitous saprophyte found in soil, air, and decaying organic matter. Hospital renovations or construction sites producing contaminated dust have been implicated in outbreaks of aspergillosis.[82,151]

Clinical Features Aspergillosis is the second most common opportunistic infection in the immunocompromised host after candidiasis.[152] One important exception is AIDS patients, who develop cryptococcosis and histoplasmosis more often than aspergillosis.[153]

A. fumigatus is the most common human pathogen, followed by *A. flavus*, *A. niger*, and *A. terreus*. Aspergillus in Latin signifies "holy water sprinkler," thus named owing to the distinctive fruiting body shape of each *Aspergillus* species.[82]

The respiratory tract is the usual portal of entry. Localized lung disease can occur as allergic aspergillosis in atopic individuals, and as fungus balls (aspergillosis) or necrotizing pneumonia in patients with a prior history of lung disease such as sarcoidosis, tuberculosis, or pneumoconioses.

In acute invasive aspergillosis, widespread growth of *Aspergillus* in lung tissue leads to infarction. Predisposing conditions for this rapidly progressive and often fatal infection are neutropenia, hematologic malignancy, long-term immunosuppressive therapy for organ transplantation, or chronic granulomatous disease in children (Table 21-24).

TABLE 21-24

Aspergillosis

Clinical Features

Ubiquitous in decaying organic matter, soil, and dust
Caused by *Aspergillus flavus*, *A. niger*, and *A. fumigatus*
Predisposing conditions: neutropenia, hematologic malignancy, organ transplantation-associated immunosuppression, and chronic granulomatous disease
Primary cutaneous aspergillosis associated with burns, catheter sites, hospital construction dust, and adhesive tape
Primary cutaneous aspergillosis: ecthyma-like papule with central necrosis
Lungs are usually portal of entry heading to disseminated disease, metastases in 5–11% of patients—necrotizing plaques, subcutaneous granulomas or abscesses, maculopapular eruption, erythema
Hematogenous dissemination can involve central nervous system, liver, spleen, heart, kidneys, and eyes

Histopathological Features

Septate hyphae (2–4 μm diameter) that branch at a 45° angle, dichotomous
Variable granulomatous infiltrate: neutrophils, lymphocytes, histiocytes, and giant cells
In disseminated disease, hyphae may be intravascular and invade vessel walls

Differential Diagnosis

	Aspergillus	Mucor
Septae	present	absent
Diameter	2–4 μm	up to 30 μm
Angle of branching	45°	90°
	dichotomous	bulbous lateral protrusions

Hematogenous dissemination can affect multiple sites including the central nervous system, eye, heart, bone, kidney, liver, spleen, and skin.[152,153]

Cutaneous aspergillosis can arise as a primary infection or secondary to disseminated disease. Primary cutaneous aspergillosis generally occurs in immunocompromised hosts at sites where the skin is disrupted by catheter, burn, or trauma, or occluded by contaminated adhesive tape.[152–154] It begins as an erythematous macule, papule, or nodule that may develop a hemorrhagic bulla with subsequent ulceration, resulting in a centrally necrotic eschar. Potassium hydroxide preparations from the intermediate stage blister roof may reveal hyphae.[155] Cutaneous aspergillosis also may disseminate in the immunocompromised.[153]

In disseminated aspergillosis, cutaneous disease occurs in 5 to 11 percent of patients and presents as five main types: solitary necrotizing dermal plaque, subcutaneous granuloma or abscess, persistent maculopapular eruption with suppuration or necrobiosis, transient erythema or erythroderma, and progressive confluent granulomas.[156,157]

Histopathological Features   In both primary and disseminated cutaneous aspergillosis, histological examination of the dermis and subcutaneous fat reveals numerous septate hyphae (2 to 4 μm in diameter) that branch at a 45 degree angle and exhibit dichotomous branching (Fig. 21-26).[158] The hyphae are optimally visualized with methenamine silver or PAS stains (Table 21-24). Ulceration, necrosis, and a granulomatous infiltrate of neutrophils, lymphocytes, histiocytes, and giant cells may be seen.[152,154,158] In disseminated disease, hyphae may be seen within dermal vessels as well as invading vascular walls.[156]

Differential Diagnosis   Zygomycosis may also display vascular involvement. However, *Aspergillus* may be distinguished from *Mucor* by the hyphal width, the angle and pattern of dichotomous branching, and the visibilty of septa. In some instances, cultures may be necessary to make the latter distinction.

Hyalohyphomycoses

The term hyalohyphomycoses is used to denote opportunistic infections caused by colorless (hyaline) molds that are seen in tissue as septate, colorless hyphae and cause diseases other than aspergillosis, the most common hyalohyphomycosis that have not been previously discussed. The number of organisms causing hyalohyphomycosis continues to increase and includes *Fusarium, Paecilomyces, Acremonium, Penicillium marneffei,* and *Scopulariopsis.*[76,159]

Fusarium

Clinical Features   *Fusarium,* a common soil fungus, is a frequent cause of corneal and nail infections. Cutaneous infection may develop as a complication of ulcers, surgical trauma, and burns, especially in neutropenic patients. Disseminated *Fusarium* infection, like aspergillosis, may arise following pulmonary inhalation or as a result of spread of cutaneous disease.

Histopathological Features   The morphological findings are identical to aspergillosis.[73,76]

Penicillium Marneffei

Clinical Features   *P. marneffei,* the only known dimorphic *Penicillium,* produces infection in residents of or visitors to South China and Thailand. Infection begins with flu-like symptoms that progress to necrotic cutaneous ulcers and abscesses, generalized lymphadenopathy, hepatosplenomegaly, and death if not treated.[76,159]

Histopathological Features   The organism in tissue sections resembles *H. capsulatum,* except yeast cells multiply by fission rather than by budding.[159] The multiplying cells are elongated and have prominent cross walls.[76]

Acremonium and Paecilomyces

Acremonium is found in soil and may cause nail and corneal infections. In patients with severe medical conditions or predisposing factors, such as chronic granulomatous disease, cardiac valve prosthesis, or renal failure, both *Paecilomyces* and *Acremonium* may be associated with fatal infections of the lung, brain, heart, peritoneum, and bones.[160] *Paecilomyces,* also found in soil, has been implicated in outbreaks of corneal infection and endophthalmitis.[160,161]

Histopathological Features   Histological sections of cutaneous plaques or subcutaneous abscesses reveal septate, 2 to 4 μm diameter hyphae branching at an acute angle. Culture is required to further characterize the species causing hyalohyphomycosis.[160,161]

MISCELLANEOUS MYCOSES
Keloidal blastomycosis (Lobo's Disease)

Synonyms: Lobomycosis; Amazonian blastomycosis; leper of the Caiabi; pseudoleprosy; "miraip" and piraip ("that which burns" in Tupi language)[162,163]

Clinical Features   First described by Lobo in 1930, lobomycosis is characterized by slowly growing keloidal nodules and plaques on the body's cooler regions, that is, earlobes, extremities, and buttocks (Table 21-25).[162] Infection may be asymptomatic or associated with a burning sensation, and usually is preceded by trauma such as an animal or insect bite.[162–164] It occurs in tropical South America, especially among

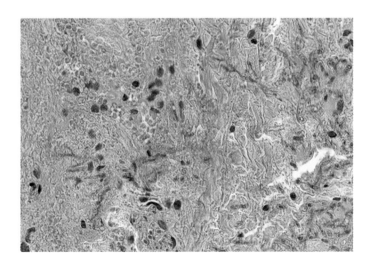

FIGURE 21-26   Aspergillosis. The hyphae are smaller than those observed in mucormycosis and exhibit 45-dichotomous branching.

TABLE 21-25

Lobomycosis

Clinical Features

Caused by *Loboa loboi* (*Paracoccidiodes loboi*)
Has not been grown in culture
Occurs in South America near Amazon/Orinoco rivers
Slow growing keloidal plaques and nodules
Also infects dolphins

Histopathological Features

Atrophic or acanthotic epidermis
Granulomatous infiltrate in lower dermis and subcutaneous tissues
Numerous uniform (10 μm) round *P. loboi* with transparent
   cytoplasm and thick double wall
P. loboi form beads joined by thin bridges

Differential Diagnosis

Leishmaniasis
Paracoccidioidomycosis
Cryptococcosis

Indians inhabiting the Amazon and Orinoco river basins.[162] Although the causative agent *Loboa loboi* has never been cultured, it has been hypothesized to be present in the water, plants, or soil of regions where disease has been reported.[162] Lobomycosis in dolphins, the only non-human hosts, has a similar clinical presentation to human disease: It involves the dermis and subcutaneous fat, rarely the lymph nodes, and spares other organs.[163]

Spontaneous remission with persistence of fungi in scar tissue may occur.[163] Affected individuals have defective cell-mediated immunity, which is also a predisposing factor for paracoccidioidomycosis.[165] Based on the observation that the morphology of *L. loboi* in tissue closely resembles that of *P. brasiliensis*, and that patients with Lobo's disease have serological cross-reactions in the test for paracoccidiomycosis, *L. loboi* is sometimes referred to by Brazilian scientists as *Paracoccidiodes loboi*. Infiltrating squamous cell carcinoma has been reported to develop in the longstanding plaques in a small number of (<1%) patients.[163,164]

Histopathological Features There is variable acanthosis and hyperkeratosis, with epidermal atrophy in some instances. The lower dermis and subcutaneous tissues contain a granulomatous infiltrate composed mainly of giant cells and macrophages. Large numbers of *P. loboi* are seen, mostly within the cytoplasm of giant cells and histiocytes but also extracellularly, surrounded by histiocytes.[164,165] Fibrosis, hyalinization, and loss of adnexal structures owing to inflammation are occasionally observed. *P. loboi* are fairly uniform in size, about 10 μm in diameter (Table 21-25). In hematoxylin and eosin-stained sections, the cytoplasm appears empty or contains a central pale nucleus, and is surrounded by a thick, double-contoured wall measuring 1 μm. Methenamine silver stain is better than PAS stain for demonstrating *P. loboi*, which typically form chains joined by thin bridges.[163,164]

Differential Diagnosis A granulomatous infiltrate with histiocytes also may be observed in leishmaniasis and lepromatous leprosy; however, the presence of numerous fungi can facilitate the distinction between lobomycosis, leishmaniasis and leprosy. More numerous organisms are seen in lobomycosis than in paracoccidioidomycosis or in cryptococcosis.

Rhinosporidiosis

Rhinosporidiosis is a chronic granulomatous infection of the mucocutaneous tissues. The etiologic agent is thought to be *Rhinosporidium seeberi*, an organism which has never been successfully cultured in a cell-free medium, isolated from nature, or transmitted to experimental animals.[1,14,166] *R. seeberi* is a fungus that occurs in tissues as very large spherules, called sporangia, which measure 250 to 350 μm in diameter and contain endospores.[1,14,167] Levy et al. (1986) reported in vitro cultivation in a human neoplastic epithelial cell culture line in which the epithelial cells developed polypoid excrescences suggesting elaboration of a growth factor by the organism.[168]

Clinical Features Rhinosporidiosis is characterized by large polypoid growths usually involving the nasal, ocular, or nasopharyngeal mucosa of patients 20 to 40 years of age. Eye infections may be more common in women.[14,169] Less commonly, this process may involve the skin, oropharynx, larynx, urethra, vagina, rectum, bone, and brain.[166] The disease affects both humans and animals and occurs most commonly in India, Sri Lanka, and other parts of south Asia, but it has occasionally been reported elsewhere, including the United States.[170,171] The modes of infection and transmission are unknown, although stagnant water and dust have been suspected as possible sources (Table 21-26).[169,172]

The most commonly affected site is the nose, accounting for approximately 70 percent of cases.[172] Presentation often involves unilateral obstruction or epistaxis, although bilateral involvement is not uncommon in later stages. A blood-tinged mucoid discharge, often containing spores and sporangia, may be noted, and local pruritus is sometimes

TABLE 21-26

Rhinosporidiosis

Clinical Features

Highest prevalence in India and Sri Lanka
Nasal area involved in 70% of cases
   Large polypoid, globoid, pedunculated, mottled nodules
Conjunctiva involved in 15% of cases, more in drier climates
   Sessile or stalked growth involving palpebral conjunctiva
Cutaneous infection rare
   Autoinoculation more common than primary cutaneous origin
   Papules evolve into verrucous nodules that may ulcerate
   Hematogenous dissemination very rare
      Numerous small (0.5–2 cm) nodules that may ulcerate
Other mucocutaneous sites in 8% of cases

Histopathological Features

Mild hyperkeratosis, hyperplasia, and areas of thinning near
   sporangia
Sporangia (30–350 μm) in submucosa
Endospores (7–9 μm) within sporangia, free in tissue, and inside
   giant cells
Submucosal infiltrate of neutrophils, lymphocytes, histiocytes,
   plasma cells, and multinucleated giant cells
Prominent vascularity, hemorrhage, and hemosiderin disposition

Differential Diagnosis

Midline lethal facial granuloma
Cryptococcus neoformans
Coccidioides immitis
   Spherules 30–60 μm, colorless, and flattened

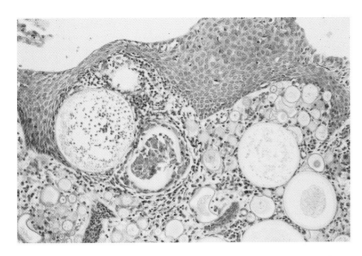

FIGURE 21-27 Rhinosporidiosis. Large sporangia are present in nasal submucosa. (Courtesy Dr. F. von Lichtenberg.)

reported.[172] Infection usually begins as a sessile tumor that may develop into a globoid pedunculated polyp weighing 20 g or more.[14] The color, ranging from pink to red, is caused by vascularization and free blood. Macroscopically visible whitish spherules or round bodies, representing bulging sporangia, impart a mottled appearance to the polyp, and give it a characteristic strawberry appearance.[14,172] Septal perforation is common.[172]

Histopathological Features The surface of the polypoid mass is stratified squamous or columnar epithelium with slight hyperkeratosis and hyperplasia, although there may be areas of thinning and erosion, particularly near mature sporangia (Table 21-26). Many endospores and sporangia in various developmental stages are noted in the submucosa, along with histiocytes, neutrophils, lymphocytes, and plasma cells; multinucleated giant cells, usually of the foreign-body type occasionally are seen (Fig. 21-27).[173] Spores usually range from 7 to 9 μm in diameter, whereas sporangia vary greatly in size from 30 to 300 μm; refractile spores may be noted free in tissue, often close to the surface, and within giant cells.[167,173] Release of spores from a spherule appears to incite a polymorphonuclear leukocyte response, and prominent vascularity, hemorrhage, and hemosiderin disposition often are seen.[14] In addition to the neovascularization, necrosis and neutrophilic microabcesses may be seen. The walls of the spherules and spores stain by GMS, Gridley, and PAS.

Differential Diagnosis Nasal and ocular disease may resemble midline, lethal facial granuloma because of the dense inflammatory infiltrate; however, cytologic atypia is not seen in rhinosporidiosis. Cryptococcosis may cause polypoid tumors that may be differentiated from rhinosporidiosis by microscopic examination of tissue.[14]

R. seeberi and *C. immitis* both produce spherules in the yeast tissue phase; however, on direct examination, *R. seeberi* spherules are globose, brown, and much larger than *C. immitis* spherules, which are colorless, not perfectly spherical, and measure 30 to 60 μm in diameter.[167]

REFERENCES

1. Kwon-Chung KJ, Bennett JE: *Medical Mycology*, Philadelphia, Lea & Febiger, 1992, chap. 1, pp. 3–34; chap. 6, pp. 105–161; chap. 8, pp. 170–182; chap. 9 pp. 183–190; chap. 13 pp. 280–336.
2. Weitzman I, Summerbell RC: The Dermatophytes. *Clin Microbiol Rev* 8:240–259, 1995.
3. Dawson CO, Gentles JC: The perfect states of *Keratinomyces ajello* Vanbreuseghem, *Trichophyton terrestre* Durie & Grey and *Microsporum nanum* Fuentes. *Sabouraudia* 1:49–57, 1961.
4. Griffin DN: The re-discovery of *Gymnoascus gypseum*, the perfect state of *Microsporum gypseum*, and a note on *Trichophyton terrestre. Trans Br Mycol Soc* 43:637–641, 1960.
5. Stockdale PM: *Nannizzia incurvata* gen. nov., sp. nov., a perfect state of *Microsporum gypseum* (Bodin) Guiart et Grigorakis. *Sabouraudia* 1:41–48, 1961.
6. Stockdale PM: *The Microsporum gypseum* complex (*Nannizzia incurvata* Stockd., *N. gypsea* (Nann.) comb. nov., *N. fulva* sp. nov.) *Sabouraudia* 3:114–126, 1963.
7. Ajello L: Present day concepts in the dermatophytes. *Mycopath Mycol Appl* 17:315–324, 1961.
8. Georg LK: Epidemiology of the dermatophytoses: sources of infection, modes of transmission and epidemicity. *Ann NY Acad Sci* 89:69–77, 1960.
9. Matsumoto T, Ajello L: Current taxonomic concepts pertaining to the dermatophytes and related fungi. *Int J Dermatol* 26:491–499, 1987.
10. Ajello L: Geographic distribution and prevalence of the dermatophytes. *Ann NY Acad Sci* 89:30–38, 1960.
11. Bronson DM, Desai DR, Barsky S, Foley SM: An epidemic of infection with *Trichophyton tonsurans* revealed in a 20-year survey of fungal infection in Chicago. *J Am Acad Dermatol* 8:322–329, 1983.
12. Aly, R: Ecology and epidemiology of dermatophyte infections. *J Am Acad Dermatol* 31:521–525, 1994.
13. Rippon JW: The changing epidemiology and emerging patterns of dermatophyte species. *Curr Top Med Mycol* 1:209–234, 1985.
14. Rippon JW: *Medical mycology. The Pathogenic Fungi and the Pathogenic Actinomycetes*, 3rd ed. Philadelphia: W.B. Saunders 1988, chap. 6, pp. 121–153; chap. 7, pp. 154–168; chap. 8, pp. 169–275; chap. 12, pp. 353–361, chap. 20, pp. 532–581.
15. Frieden IJ, Howard R: Tinea capitis: Epidemiology, diagnosis, treatment, and control. *J Am Acad Dermatol* 31:S42–S46, 1994.
16. Smith KJ, Neafie RC, et al: Majocchi's granuloma. *J Cutan Path* 18(1):28–35, 1991.
17. Gottlieb GJ, Ackerman AB: The "sandwich sign" of dermatophytosis. *Am J Dermatopathol* 8:347–350, 1986.
18. Birt AR, Wilt JC: Mycology, bacteriology, and histopathology of suppurative ringworm. *Arch Dermatol* 69:441–448. 1954.
19. Lever WF, Schaumburg-Lever G: *Histopathology of the Skin*, 7th ed. Philadelphia: JB Lippincott, 1990, chap. 19, pp. 364–389, chap. 20, pp. 394–398.
20. Odom R: Pathophysiology of dermatophyte infections. *J Am Acad Dermatol* 28:S2–S7, 1993.
21. Leyden JL: Tinea pedis pathophysiology and treatment. *J Am Acad Dermatol* 31:S31–S33, 1994.
22. Taplin D: Superficial mycosis. *J Invest Dermatol* 67:177–181, 1976.
23. Hay RJ, Reid S, Talwat E, Machamra K: Clinical features of superficial fungal infections caused by *Hendersonula toruloidea* and *Scytalidium hyalinum. Br J Dermatol* 110:677–683, 1984.
24. Andre J, Achten G: Onychomycosis. *Int J Dermatol* 26(8):481–490, 1987.
25. Daniel III CR, Lawrence AN, Scher RK: The spectrum of nail disease in patients with human immunodeficiency virus infection. *J Am Acad Dermatol* 27(1):93–97, 1992.
26. Dompmartin D, Dompmartin A, et al: Onychomycosis and AIDS. Clinical and laboratory findings in 62 patients. *Int J Dermatol* 29(5):337–339, 1990.
27. Mariat F, Liautaud B, et al: *Hendersonula toruloidea*, causative agent of a fungal verrucous dermatitis observed in Algeria. *Sabouraudia*, 16(2):133–140, 1978.
28. Campbell CK, Kurwa A, et al: Fungal infection of skin and nails by *Hendersonula toruloidea. Br J Dermatol* 89:45–52, 1973.
29. Peiris S, Moore MK, et al: *Scytalidium hyalinum* infection of skin and nails. *Br J Dermatol* 100:579–584, 1979.
30. Kurwa A, Campbell C: *Hendersonula toruloida* infection. *Br J Dermatol* 86:98–99, 1972.
31. Bodey, GP: *Candidiasis Pathogenesis, Diagnosis, and Treatment.* New York: Raven Press, Ltd, 1993.
32. Wingard JR: Importance of *Candida* species other than *C. albicans* as pathogens in oncology patients. *Clin Infect Dis* 20(1):115–125, 1995.
33. Barns SM, Lane DJ, Sogin ML, Bibeau C, Weisburg WG: Evolutionary relationships among pathogenic *Candida* species and relatives. *J Bacteriol* 173(7):2250–2255, 1991.
34. Ray TL: Systemic candidiases. *Dermatol Clin* 7: 259–268, 1989.
35. Maize JC, Lynch PJ: Chronic mucocutaneous candidiasis of the adult. *Arch Dermatol.* 105:96–98, 1972.
36. Lynch DP: Oral candidiasis. History, classification, and clinical presentation. *Oral Surg Oral Med Oral Pathol,* 78(2):189–193, 1994.
37. Budtz-Jorgensen E: Clinical aspects of *Candida* infection in denture wearers. *J Am Dent Assoc* 96:474–479, 1978.
38. Kirkpatrick CH: Chronic mucocutaneous candidiasis. *J Am Acad Dermatol* 31:3 Pt 2: S14–S17, 1994.
39. Aaltonen J, Komulainen J, Vikman A, et al: Autoimmune polyglandular disease type I: Exclusion map using amplifiable multiallelic markers in a microtiter well format. *Eur J Human Genet* 1:164–171, 1993.

40. Hauser FV, Rothman S: Monilial granuloma report of a case and review of the literature. *Arch Derm Syph* 61:297–310, 1950.

41. Kugelman TP, Cripps DF, et al: Candida granuloma with epidermophytosis. *Arch Dermatol* 88:86–93, 1963.

42. Odom RB: Common superficial fungal infections in immunosuppressed patients. *J Am Acad Dermatol* 31:S56–S59, 1994.

43. Meunier F: Die Therapie der invasiven candidosen. *Mycosis* 37 (Suppl 2):52–55, 1994.

44. Bodey GP, Luna M: Skin lesions associated with disseminated candidiasis. *JAMA* 229:1466–1468, 1974.

45. Grossman ME Silvers DN: Walther RR: Cutaneous manifestations of disseminated candidiasis. *J Am Acad Dermatol* 2:111–116, 1980.

46. File TM Jr, Marina OA, et al: Necrotic skin lesions associated with disseminated candidiasis. *Arch Dermatol* 115:214–215, 1979.

47. Benson PM, Roth RR, Hicks CB, et al: Nodular subcutaneous abscesses caused by *Candida tropicalis*. *J Am Acad Dermatol* 16:623–624, 1987.

48. Fine JD, Miller JA, et al: Cutaneous lesions in disseminated candidiasis mimicking ecthyma gangrenosum. *Am J Med* 70:1133–1135, 1981.

49. Collignon PJ, Sorrell TC: Disseminated candidiasis: Evidence of a distinctive syndrome in heroin abusers. *Br Med J* 287:861–862, 1983.

50. Jarowski CJ, Fialk MA, et al: Fever, rash, and muscle tenderness. A distinctive clinical presentation of disseminated candidiasis. *Arch Intern Med* 138(4):544–546, 1978.

51. Bodey GP: Fungal infections complicating acute leukemia. *J Chronic Dis* 19(6):667–687, 1966.

52. Yarrow D, Ahern DG: Discussion of the genera belonging to the imperfect yeasts: In Kreger-van Rij, NJW (Ed.): *The Yeasts: A Taxonomic Study*. Amsterdam: 1984, chap. V, genus 7, pp. 882–885.

53. Sina BC, Kauffman CL, Samorodin CS: Intrafollicular mucin deposits in *Pityrosporum* folliculitis. *J Am Acad Dermatol* 32:807–809, 1995.

54. Faergemann J, Fredriksson T: Experimental infections in rabbits and humans with *Pityrosporum orbiculare* and *P. ovale*. *J Invest Dermatol* 77:314–318, 1981.

55. Marples MJ: The incidence of certain skin diseases in western Samoa: a preliminary survey. *Trans Roy Soc Trop Med Hyg* 44:319–332, 1950.

56. Roberts SOB: Pityriasis: A clinical and mycological investigation. *Br J Dermatol* 81:315–326, 1969.

57. Borelli D, Jacobs PH, Nall L: Tinea versicolor: Epidemiologic, clinical, and therapeutic aspects. *J Am Acad of Dermatol* 25:300–303, 1991.

58. Nazzaro-Porro M, Passi S: Identification of tyrosinase inhibitors in cultures of *pityrosporum*. *J Invest Dermatol* 71:389–402, 1978.

59. Allen HB, Charles CR, et al: Hyperpigmented tinea versicolor. *Arch Dermatol* 112:1110–1112, 1972.

60. Abdel-Razek M, Fadaly G, et al: Pityrosporum (Malassezia) folliculitis in Saudi Arabia: Diagnosis and therapeutic trials. *Clin Exp Dermatol* 20:406–409, 1995.

61. Hill MK, Mark JD: Skin surface electron microscopy in *Pityrosporum* folliculitis. *Arch Dermatol* 126:181–184, 1990.

62. Back O, Faergemann J, Hornqvist R: *Pityrosporum* folliculitis: A common disease of the young and middle-aged. *J Am Acad Dermatol* 12:56–61, 1985.

63. Jacinto-Jamora S, Tamesis J, Katigbak ML: *Pityrosporum* folliculitis in the Philipines: diagnosis, prevalence, and management. *J Am Acad Dermatol* 24:693–696, 1991.

64. Clemmensen OJ, Hagdrup H: Splendore-Hoeppli phenomenon in *Pityrosporum* folliculitis (pseudoactinomycosis of the skin). *J Cutan Pathol* 18: 293–297, 1991.

65. Ellner KM, McBride ME, et al: White piedra: Evidence for a synergistic infection. *Br J Dermatol* 123:355–363, 1990.

66. Nahass GT, Rosenberg SP: Disseminated infection with *Trichosporon beigelii* report of a case and review of the cutaneous and histologic manifestations. *Arch Dermatol* 129:1020–1023, 1993.

67. Drake LA, Dinehart SM, et al: Guidelines of care for superficial mycotic infections of the skin: Piedra. *J Am Acad Dermatol* 34:122–124, 1996.

68. Chong KC, Adam BA: Morphology of *Piedraia hortae*. *Sabouraudia* 13:157–160, 1975.

69. Walsh TJ: Trichosporonosis. *Inf Dis Clin No Am* 3:43–52, 1989.

70. Levitz SM: The ecology of *Cryptococcus neoformans* and the epidemiology of cryptococcosis. *Rev Infect Dis* 13:1163–1169, 1991.

71. Hernandez AD: Cutaneous Cryptococcosis. *Dermatol Clin* 7:269–274, 1989.

72. Kozel TR, Gotschlich EC: The capsule of *Cryptococcus neoformans* passively inhibits phagocytosis of the yeast by macrophages. *J Immunol* 129:1982.

73. Warnock DW, Richardson MD: *Fungal Infection in the Immunocompromised Patient*, 2nd ed. Chichester: John Wiley & Sons, 1991, pp. 85–117 (cryptococcosis), pp. 154–182, (mucormycosis), pp. 162–166, (hyalohyphomycosis).

74. Haight DO, Esperanza LW, Greene JN, Sandin RL, DeGregorio R, Spiers A S.D: Case Report: Cutaneous manifestations of cryptococcosis. *Am Med Sci* 308:3,192—195, 1994.

75. Naka W, Masuda M, Konohana A, Shinoda T, Nishikawa T: Primary cutaneous cryptococcosis and *Cryptococcus neoformans* serotype D. *Clin Exp Dermatol* 20:221–225, 1995.

76. Richardson MD, Warnock DW: Fungal Infection. Diseases and Management. Oxford: Blackwell Scientific, 1993, pp. 115–122 (cryptococcosis), pp. 129–132 (blastomyco-

sis), pp. 134–140 (coccidiomycosis), pp 153–155 (paracoccidiomycosis), 123–127 (mucormycosis), pp. 159–160 (conidiobolomycosis), hyalohyphomycosis pp. 248–57.

77. Murakawa GJ, Kerschmann R, Berger T: Cutaneous *cryptococcus* infection with AIDS. Report of 12 cases and review of the literature. *Arch Dermatol* 132:545–548, 1996.

78. Goldani L, Sugar A: Paracoccidioidomycosis and AIDS: An overview. *Clin Infect Dis* 21:1275–1281, 1995.

79. Goldani LZ, Martinez R, Landell GAM, Machado AA, Coutinho V: Paracoccidioidomycosis in a patient with acquired immunodeficiency syndrome. *Mycopathologia* 105:71–74, 1989.

80. Anderson DJ, Schmidt C, Goodman J, Pomeroy C: Cryptococcal disease presenting as cellulitis. *Clin Infect Dis* 14:666–672, 1992.

81. Ghigliotti G, Carrega G, Farris A, Burroni A, Nigro A, Pagano G, et al: Cutaneous cryptococcosis resembling molluscum contagiosum in a homosexual man with AIDS. Report of a case and review of the literature. *Acta Derm Venereol* (Stockh) 72: 182–184, 1992.

82. Von Lichtenberg F: *Pathology of Infectious Diseases*. New York: Raven, 1991, pp. 201–248.

83. Ro JY, Lee SS, Ayala AG: Advantage of Fontana-Masson stain in capsule-deficient cryptococcal infection. *Arch Pathol Lab Med* 111:53–57, 1987.

84. Bradsher RW: Blastomycosis. *Clin Infect Dis* 14:(suppl 1):S82–S90, 1992.

85. Mercurio MG, Elewski BE: Cutaneous blastomycosis. *Cutis* 50:422–424, 1992.

86. Nouira R, Denguezli M, Skhiri S, Belajouzac C, Said M, Jarray M, et al: Blastomycoses cutaneo-pulmonaire. Ann dermoidal. *Venereology* 121:180–182, 1994.

87. Tosh FE, Hammerman KJ, Weeks RJ: Sarosiga: A common source epidemic of North American blastomycosis. *Am Rev Resp Dis* 109:525–529, 1974.

88. Quimby SR, Connolly SM, Winkelmann RK, Smilack JD: Clinicopathologic spectrum of specific cutaneous lesions of disseminated coccidioidomycosis. *J Am Acad Dermoidal* 26:79–85, 1992.

89. Harley WB, Blaser MJ: Disseminated coccidioidomycosis associated with extreme eosinophilia. *Clin Infect Dis* 18:627–629, 1994.

90. Trimble JR, Doucette J: Primary cutaneous coccidioidomycosis. Report of a case of a laboratory infection. *Arch Dermatol* 74:405–410, 1956.

91. Forbes W, Bestebreurtje AM: Coccidioidomycosis: A study of 95 cases of the disseminated type with special reference to the pathogenesis of the disease. *Milit Surg* 99:653–719, 1946.

92. Meyer RD: Cutaneous and mucosal manifestations of the deep mycotic infections. *Acta Derm Venereol* (Stockh) 121(suppl):57–72, 1986.

93. Kahanpaa A: Bronchopulmonary occurrence of fungi in adults. Acta Pathological et Microbiologica Scandinavica. Section B Supplement 227:16–38, 82–91, 1972.

94. Marques SA, Conterno LO, Sgarbi LP, Villagra AM, Sabongi VP, Bagatin E, et al: Paracoccidioidomycosis associated with acquired immunodeficiency syndrome. Report of seven cases. *Rev Inst Med Trop Sao Paulo* 37:261–265, 1995.

95. Mendes E, Raphael A: Impaired delayed hypersensitivity in patients with South American blastomycosis. *J Allerg* 47:17–22, 1971.

96. Mendes NF, Musatti CC, Leao RC, Mendes E, Naspitz CK: Lymphocyte cultures and skin allograft survival in patients with South American blastomycosis. *J Allergy Clin Immunol* 48:40–45, 1971.

97. Goldani LZ, Maia AL, Sugar AL: Cloning and nucleotide sequence of a specific DNA fragment from *Paracoccidioides brasiliensis*. *Clin Microbiol* 33:1652–1654, 1995.

98. Moscardi-Bacchi M, Soares A, Mendes R, Marques S, Franco M: In situ localization of T lymphocyte subsets in human paracoccidioidomycosis. *J Med Veter Mycol* 27: 149–158, 1989.

99. Dijkstra JW: Histoplasmosis. *Dermatol Clin* 7:251–258, 1989.

100. Nethercott JR, Schachter RK, Givan KF, Ryder DE: Histoplasmosis due to *Histoplasma capsulatum* var *duboisii* in a Canadian immigrant. *Arch Dermatol* 114: 595–598, 1978.

101. Chaker MB, Cockerell CJ: Concomitant psoriasis, seborrheic dermatitis, and disseminated cutaneous histoplasmosis in a patient infected with human immunodeficiency virus. *J Am Acad Dermatol* 29:311–313, 1993.

102. Goodwin RA, Loyd JE, Des Prez RM: Histoplasmosis in normal hosts. *Medicine* 60:231–266, 1981.

103. Eidbo J., Sanchez RL, Tschen JA, Ellner KM: Cutaneous manifestations of histoplasmosis in the acquired immune deficiency syndrome. *Am J Surg Pathol* 17(2):110–116, 1993.

104. Cohen PR, Bank DE, Silvers DN, Grossman ME: Cutaneous lesions of disseminated histoplasmosis in human immunodeficiency virus-infected patients. *J Am Acad Dermatol* 23:422–428, 1990.

105. Johnson PC, Khardori N, Najjar AF, Butt F, Mansell PWA: Progressive disseminated histoplasmosis in patients with acquired immunodeficiency syndrome. *Am J Med* 85:152–158, 1988.

106. Tesh RB, Schneidau JD: Primary cutaneous histoplasmosis. *N Engl J Med* 275(11): 597–599, 1966.

107. Medeiros AA, Marty SD, Tosh FE, Chin TDY: Erythema nodosum and erythema multiforme as clinical manifestations of histoplasmosis in a community outbreak. *N Engl J Med* 274(8):415–420, 1996.

108. Kauffman CA, Israel KS, Smith JW, White AC, Schwarz J, Brooks GF: Histoplasmosis in immunosuppressed patients. *Am J Med* 64:923–932, 1978.

109. Weinberg GA, Kleiman MB, Grosfeld JL, Weber TR, Wheat LJ: Unusual manifestations of histoplasmosis in childhood. *Pediatrics* 72:99–105, 1983.

110. Abildgaard WH, Hargrove RH, Kalivas J: Histoplasma Panniculitis. *Arch Dermatol* 121:914–916, 1985.

111. Petit N, Bonnet E, Chapel F, Bensa P, Gallais H, Lebreuil G: Cutaneous biopsies for diagnosis of histoplasmosis in an HIV patient. *Infection* 22(6):426–427, 1994.

112. Kalter DC, Tschen JA, Klima M: Maculopapular rash in a patient with acquired immunodeficiency syndrome. *Arch Dermatol* 121:1455–1456, 1458–1459, 1985.

113. Khalil M, Iwatt AR, Gugnani HC: African histoplasmosis masquerading as carcinoma of the colon. Report of a case and review of literature. *Dis Colon Rectum* 32:518–520, 1989.

114. Simon F, Chouc PY, Herve V, Branquet D, Jeandel P: Localisations osteo-articulaires de l'histoplasmose africaine (Histoplasma Duboisi). A propos d'un cas et revue de la littérature. *Rev. Rhum. [Ed. Fr.]* 61:829–838, 1994.

115. Davis BA: Sporotrichosis, in Thiers BH, Elgart M (eds): Cutaneous Mycology. *Dermatol Clin* 14:69–76, 1996.

116. Donabedian H, O'Donnell E, Olsewski C, et al: Disseminated cutaneous and meningeal sporotrichosis in an AIDS patient. *Diag Microbiol Dis* 12:111–115, 1994.

117. Binford CH, Connor DH: *Pathology of Tropical and Extraordinary Diseases*. Washington, DC: Armed Forces Institute of Pathology, 1976, pp. 585–586.

118. Carrion A: Chromoblastomycosis. *Ann NY Acad Sci* 50:1255–1282, 1950.

119. Elgart GW: Chromoblastomycosis, in Thiers BH, Elgart M (eds): Cutaneous Mycology. *Dermatol Clin* 14:77–83, 1996.

120. Ajello L, George LK, Steigbigel RT, Wange CJK: A case of phaeohyphomycosis caused by a new species of *Phialophora*. *Mycologia* 66:490–498, 1974.

121. Zeifer A, Connor DH: Phaemycotic cyst. A clinicopathologic study of 25 patients. *Am J Trop Med* 29:901–911, 1980.

122. Rippon JW: *Medical Mycology*. Philadelphia: W.B. Saunders, 1988.

123. Vaffee AS: Tinea nigra palmaris resembling malignant melanoma. *N Engl J Med* 283:1112, 1970.

124. Mitchel AJ, Solomon AR, Beneke ES, et al: Subcutaneous alternariosis. *J Am Acad Dermatol* 8:673–679, 1983.

125. Pedersen NB, Mardh PA, Hallber T, et al: Cutaneous alternariosis. *Br J Dermatol* 94:201–209, 1976.

126. Arrese JE, Pierard-Franchimont C, Peirard GE: Onychomycosis and keratomycocsis caused by alternaria sp. *Am J Dermatopathol* 18:611–613, 1966.

127. Khandara KC, Mahapatra LN, Seghal VN, et al: Black mycetoma of foot. *Arch Dermatol* 89:867–870, 1964.

128. McGinis MR Mycetoma, in Thiers BH, Elgart M (eds): Cutaneous Mycology. *Dermatol Clin* 14:97–104, 1996.

129. Boudoulas O, Camis C: Nocardia asteroides infection with dissemination to skin and joints. *Arch Dermatol* 121:898–900, 1985.

130. Warren NG: Actinomycosis, nocardiosis, and actinomycetoma, in Thiers BH, Elgart M (eds): Cutaneous Mycology. *Dermatol Clin* 14:85–95, 1996.

131. Bennhoff: Actinomycosis: Diagnostic and therapeutic considerations and a review of 32 cases. *Laryngoscope* 94:1198–1217, 1984.

132. Binford CH, Dooley JR: Botryomycosis, in Binford CH, Connor DH (eds): *Pathology of Tropical and Extraordinary Diseases*. Washington, DC: Armed Forces Institute of Pathology, 1970, pp. 561.

133. Bishop GF, Greer KE, Horwitz DA: Pseudomonas botryomycosis. *Arch Dermatol* 112:1568–1570, 1976.

134. Harman RRM, English MP, Halford M, et al: Botryomycosis. *Br J Dermatol* 102:215–222, 1990.

135. Waisman M: Staphylococcal actinophytosis (botryomycosis). *Arch Dermatol* 86:525–529, 1962.

136. Sanchez M, Ponge-Wilson I, Moy JA, Rosenthal S: Zygomycosis and HIV infection. *J Am Acad Dermatoid* 30:904–908, 1994.

137. Geller J, Peters M, and Su WP: Cutaneous mucormycosis resembling superficial granulomatous pyoderma in an immunocompetent host. *J Am Acad Dermatol* 29:462–465, 1993.

138. Wirth F, Perry R, Eskenazi A, Schwalbe R, Kao G: Cutaneous mucormycosis with subsequent visceral dissemination in a child with neutropenia: A case report and review of the pediatric literature. *J Am Acad Dermatol* 36:336–341, 1997.

139. Sugar AM: Agents of mucormycosis and related species. In: Mandell GL, Bennett JE, Dolin R, eds. *Principles and Practice of Infectious Diseases*. 4th ed. New York: Churchill Livingstone Inc., 1995:2311–2321.

140. Levy SA, Schmitt KW, Kaufman L: Systemic zygomycosis diagnosed by fine needle aspiration and confirmed with enzyme immunoassay. *Chest* 90(1):146–148, 1986.

141. Craig N, Lueder F, Pensler JM, Bean BS, Petrick ML, Thompson RB, et al: Disseminated rhizopus infection in a premature infant. *Pediatric Dermatol* 11:346–350, 1994.

142. Adam R, Hunter G, DiTomasso J, Comerci G: Mucormycosis: Emerging prominence of cutaneous infections. *Clin Infct Dis* 19:67–76, 1994.

143. Waldorf AR: Immunology of fungal diseases. *Immunol Ser* 47:243–271, 1989.

144. Diamond RD, Krzesicki R, Epstein B, Jao W: Damage to hyphal forms of fungi by human leukocytes in vitro. A possible host defense mechanism in aspergillosis and mucormycosis. *Am J Pathol* 91:313–328, 1978.

145. Lehrer RI, Howard DH, Sypherd PS, Edwards JE, Segal GP, Winston DJ: Mucormycosis. *Ann Intern Med* 93(1):93–108, 1980.

146. Vismer HF, De Beer HA, Dreyer L: Subcutaneous phycomycosis caused by *Basidiobolus haptosporus*. *S Afr Med J* 58:644–647, 1980.

147. Gugnani HC: Entomophthoramycosis due to Conidiobolus. *Eur J Epidemiol* 8:391–396, 1992.

148. Scholtens REM, Harrison SM: Subcutaneous phycomycosis. *Trop Geogr Med* 46:371–373, 1994.

149. Bittencourt AL, Araujo MG, Fontoura MS: Occurrence of subcutaneous zygomycosis (Entomophthoramycosis Basidiobolae) caused by *Basidiobolus haptosporus* with pulmonary involvement. *Mycopathologia* 71:155–158, 1980.

150. Antonelli M, Vignetti P, Dahir M, Mohamed MS, Favah A: Entomophthoramycosis due to *Basidiobolus* in Somalia. *Trans Roy Soc Trop Med Hyg* 81:1186–187, 1987.

151. Greenbaum RS, Roth JS, Grossman ME: Subcutaneous nodule in a cardiac transplant. Cutaneous aspergillosis. *Arch Dermatol* 129:1191–1194, 1993.

152. Stiller MJ, Teperman L, Rosenthal SA, Riordan A, Potter J, Shupack JL, et al: Primary cutaneous infection by *Aspergillus ustus* in a 62-year-old liver transplant recipient. *J Am Acad Dermatol* 31:344–347, 1994.

153. Hunt SJ, Nag C, Gross KG, Wrong DS, Mathes WC: Primary cutaneous aspergillosis near central venous catheters in patients with the acquired immunodeficiency syndrome. *Arch Dermatol* 128:1229–1232, 1992.

154. Mowad CH, Nguyen TV, Jaworsky C, Honig PJ: Primary cutaneous aspergillosis in an immunocompetent child. *J Am Acad Dermatol* 32:136–137, 1995.

155. Grossman ME, Fithian EC, Behrens C, Bissinger J, Fracaro M, Neu HC: Primary cutaneous aspergillosis in six leukemic children. *J Am Acad Dermatol* 12:313–318, 1985.

156. Skaria AM, Chavaz P, Hauser: Metastatische aspergillus-pannikulitis bei blastischer transformation eines myelodysplastischen syndromes und agranulozytose. *Hautarzt* 46:579–581, 1995.

157. Findlay GH, Roux HF, Simson IW: Skin manifestations in disseminated aspergillosis. *Br J Derm* 85(Supp 7):94, 1971.

158. Romero LS, Hunt SJ: Hickman catheter-associated primary cutaneous aspergillosis in a patient with the acquired immunodeficiency syndrome. *Int J Dermatol* 34:551–553, 1995.

159. Elgart ML, Warren NG, Elgart GW: *A Manual of Fungi for Dermatologists: Course Notes*. Washington, DC: November 1995.

160. Shing MM, Ip M, Li CK, Chik KW, Yuen PM: *Paecilomyces varioti* fungemia in a bone marrow transplant patient. *Bone Marrow Transpl* 17:281–283, 1996.

161. D Castro LC: Sporotrichosis-like lesions caused by a *Paecilomyces* genus fungus. *Int J Dermatol* 33:275–276, 1994.

162. Rodriguez-Toro G: Lobomycosis. *Internat J Dermatol* 32:324–332, 1993.

163. Rodriquez-Toro G, Tellez N: Lobomycosis in Colombian Amerindian patients. *Mycopathologia* 120:5–9, 1992.

164. Fuchs J, Milbradt R, Pecher SA: Lobomycosis (keloidal blastomycosis): Case reports and overview. *Cutis* 46:227–234, 1990.

165. Pecher SA, Fuchs J: Cellular immunity in lobomycosis (keloidal blastomycosis). *Allergol Immunopath* 16(6):413–415, 1998.

166. Azadeh B, Baghoumian N, et al: Rhinosporidiosis: Immunohistochemical and electron microscopic studies. *J Laryngol Otol* 108:1048–54, 1994.

167. Gori S, Scasso A: Cytologic and differential diagnosis of rhinosporidiosis. *Acta Cytologica* 38(3):361–366, 1994.

168. Levy MG, Meuten DJ, et al: In vitro cultivation of *rhinosporidium seeberi*: Interaction with epithelial cells. *Science* 234:474–476, 1986.

169. Thianprasit M, Thagerngpol K: Rhinosporidiosis. *Top Medical Mycol* 3:64–85, 1989.

170. Caldwell GT, Roberts JD: Rhinosporidiosis in United States: Report of a case originating in Texas. *JAMA* 110:1641, 1938.

171. Norman WB: Rhinosporidiosis in Texas. *Arch Otolaryngol* 72:361–363, 1960.

172. Karunaratne WAE: *Rhinosporidiosis in man*. University of London: The Athlone Press, 1964.

173. Thomas T, Gopinath N, et al: Rhinosporidiosis of the bronchus. *Br J Surg* 44:316–319, 1956.

CHAPTER 22

CUTANEOUS VIRAL INFECTIONS

Zafar M. Khan / Clay J. Cockerell

Viruses are the most prevalent of all infectious agents yet are the smallest, ranging in size from 20 to 300 nm in diameter. The term "filterable agent" was used to refer to viruses before they could be reliably visualized as they pass through 0.22-μm filters that retain other organisms. All viruses are obligate intracellular parasites and depend on the host cell's metabolism for replication. They are classified primarily by the nucleic acid content of their core, either DNA or RNA, as they contain only a single type of nucleic acid. They are also classified on the basis of the shape of their protein coat or capsid, which is either spherical or cylindrical.[1] Classification based on symptoms has proved useful to clinicians because certain viruses preferentially affect different organs such as the skin, the nervous system, or the respiratory tract. Skin changes often are prominent manifestations of human viral infections and the histopathologic changes associated with them vary from nonspecific features such as seen in viral exanthems to pathognomonic inclusion bodies in herpesvirus infection and cytomegalovirus infections.[1]

GENERAL PRINCIPLES OF VIRAL INFECTIONS

All viral infections are initiated by entry of the infectious particle, the virion, into the host cell by pinocytosis or phagocytosis. Viruses differ in the types of cells they infect, having tropisms for different tissues such as human papillomaviruses that have a tropism for epithelial cells. Viruses reach target cells through either inhalation, ingestion, or direct inoculation. After entry into the cell, enzymes remove the outer layer of the virus, the capsid, and viral nucleic acid is released into the cell. This may be followed either by active viral replication leading to an acute viral infection or, alternatively, viral nucleic acid may be incorporated into host nucleic acid leading to a latent infection. Different steps are required for viral replication depending on the agent in question. In some viruses such as enteroviruses, viral RNA acts as a messenger and is infectious itself, being immediately translated by host ribosomes into viral proteins. Other RNA viruses, such as influenza viruses, have noninfectious RNA that must first be transcribed into messenger RNA by a polymerase enzyme. Retroviruses, such as the human immunodeficiency viruses, are RNA viruses that contain reverse transcriptase, an enzyme that synthesizes DNA from viral RNA. DNA viruses generally are more complex and transcribe messenger RNA from their own DNA, using either host cell enzymes or intrinsic viral polymerases.

In active infections, nucleic acid replication occurs followed by the synthesis of proteins. In general, the time required for new virus production in acute infections is measured in hours, with thousands of new virions being formed in each cell. Newly formed virions are released from the infected cell, spreading to adjacent ones. During this process

the cell itself may be destroyed through lysis or may only be damaged and still survive.[2] Other viruses cause cell proliferation or neoplastic transformation such as warts or carcinomas caused by human papillomavirus (HPV).

Latent viral infections may be productive of virions or may remain silent. In some cases, latent infections become reactivated leading to the production of new virions, infection of adjacent cells, and active disease.

Viral exanthemata are produced primarily as a consequence of the host response to viruses present in the skin. Viral particles are disseminated through the bloodstream. Some have a direct tropism for endothelial cells such as togaviruses, and cause damage directly or by a type 3 (Arthus) reaction leading to infarcts. Most are recognized by the host as being foreign and incite antibody responses and cell-mediated immunity. Circulating immune complexes consisting of antibody and viral antigens may localize in dermal blood vessels, inciting an inflammatory reaction that leads to the development of a cutaneous eruption usually with a clinical appearance of erythematous macules and papules. In the case of most RNA viral infections, there is no replication of virus, and once the virus is cleared from the skin, the eruption resolves. This is the case with the echoviruses, Coxsackie A, most togaviruses, and rubella. Some RNA viruses are able to enter epidermal cells and replicate, leading to cytolysis and vesicles such as in the vesicular exanthem of some Coxsackie A viruses. Replication in epidermal cells is characteristic of many DNA viruses, however, which explains why these viruses are capable of replication after direct inoculation into the epidermis. Intraepidermal viral replication may lead to the formation of vesicles and pustules that develop as a consequence of focal necrosis and a secondary inflammatory response in which there may be spongiosis, ballooning degeneration, and/or acantholysis accompanied by an infiltrate of inflammatory cells consisting of lymphocytes, neutrophils, eosinophils, and plasma cells. Vesicular lesions are caused most commonly by poxviruses, herpes simplex, varicella zoster, and some Coxsackie viruses.

Antibody production is stimulated by cutaneous viral infection that may serve to prevent spread of infection through the bloodstream. However, the cell-mediated immune response is the major local inflammatory reaction that is induced and is the prime means of containing the infection as well as leading to its resolution. In immunocompromised hosts, however, there is an inability to halt the spread of the infection that often leads to serious consequences.

Factors affecting the distribution of eruptions in viral infections are poorly understood. Viruses tend to localize in areas that have been previously traumatized, in dependent areas, and at sites of preexisting inflammation that may explain the distribution in some cases. However, the reasons for the cephalocaudal progression in rubella or the centripetal distribution of varicella are unknown.

VIRAL EXANTHEMS

The term "viral exanthem" refers to a cutaneous eruption, usually widespread, that develops as a consequence of a viral illness (Table 22-1). They usually present as generalized eruptions of erythematous macules, papules, and vesicles often in association with fever. Individuals of any age may be affected, although they develop in children most commonly. The eruption may develop either as a consequence of direct viral infection of the skin or secondary to the host's immune response to the virus. Because viral exanthems may have subtle clinical and histopathological features that may not be easily recognized, definitive diagnosis may be difficult and often requires correlation of physical findings, laboratory data, epidemiologic data, and historical features.

Measles

Measles is caused by an RNA virus that is 120 to 140 nm in size that is classified as a paramyxovirus. It is in the same family as the virus that causes mumps. Measles is an acute contagious viral disease characterized by coryza, cough, conjunctivitis, and Koplik's spots that precedes the appearance of a generalized eruption of pink to red macules and papules. The disease has a worldwide distribution affecting primarily children between the ages of 3 and 6. It is a disease of winter and spring, with a peak incidence in March or April, and is spread via aerosolized respiratory droplets.[3]

Persons immunized with killed measles vaccine between the years 1961 and 1968 and subsequently exposed to wild measles virus are at risk for atypical measles.[4]

Clinical Features In typical, uncomplicated disease, there are three characteristic phases of the illness (Table 22-1). First, there is an asymptomatic incubation period of almost 9 to 10 days. This is followed by a prodromal stage with malaise, fever, coryza, and cough that lasts for 3 to 4 days. Finally, the cutaneous eruption develops that rarely lasts longer than 6 days. The typical Koplik's spots, originally described by Henry Koplik in New York, are pinpoint red dots with minute bluish-white specks located primarily on the soft palate and buccal mucosa, especially opposite the second molar. They usually precede the onset of skin changes by 1 to 2 days and may coalesce to involve the entire pharynx. Similar spots may appear on the conjunctiva and the mucosa of the gastrointestinal tract. The cutaneous eruption is characterized by discrete erythematous macules and papules that first appear on the face, especially behind the ears and forehead, and spread to involve the neck and trunk before finally involving the extremities. It usually takes approximately 3 days for the eruption to reach its maximum intensity before beginning to wane. Individual lesions are pinkish to red and may be petechial or hemorrhagic. With resolution, the lesions acquire a brownish color and desquamate with a fine, branny scale.

In some cases, there may be extensive capillaritis leading to marked hemorrhage with involvement of the respiratory and GI tract, so-called "black" measles. In rare cases, especially in tropical zones, there may be bullae.

Atypical measles differs from the usual form of the disease, as patients may be more severely ill experiencing high spiking fevers to 40°C with severe headache, prostration, nausea, and vomiting followed by sore throat, conjunctivitis, photophobia, and cough with pleuritic chest pain. On the third to fourth day of illness, an eruption begins on the distal extremities, manifesting first as edema of the hands and feet. An eruption of urticarial and erythematous macules and papules develops that may become purpuric or vesicular, often in an inverse photodistribution. Koplik's spots are not seen. The entire process usually lasts from 3 to 10 days.

Histopathological Features Skin biopsy specimens of fully developed lesions typically show slight psoriasiform hyperplasia of the epidermis, variable amounts of spongiosis with parakeratosis, and occasional dyskeratotic keratinocytes (Table 22-1). There is also a sparse infiltrate of lymphocytes surrounding the blood vessels in the superficial dermis associated with extravasation of erythrocytes. In some cases, especially in severe hemorrhagic and bullous forms, there may be true lymphocytic vasculitis of the small blood vessels. In the epidermis there are variable numbers of syncytial giant cells with multiple nuclei ranging from 3 to 20.[5] These are the "Warthin-Finkeldy" giant cells and represent the cutaneous equivalent to cells that are seen in visceral sites such as the lung. In addition, there are multinucleated lymphoid cells with intranuclear and sometimes cytoplasmic inclusions in the dermis. Koplik's spots have the same morphologic changes, but usually more giant cells are seen.

Atypical measles demonstrates similar histologic changes, although there may be more vascular involvement, as deposition of immune complexes are thought to play a role in the development of the eruption.

Differential Diagnosis Early in the course of infection when Koplik's spots are present, the clinical diagnosis is not difficult; however, in the absence of Koplik's spots, measles can be confused with other morbilliform eruptions, including Kawasaki's disease, rubella, scarlet fever, roseola, erythema infectiosum, infectious mononucleosis, and drug eruptions. The characteristic intracellular inclusions and the multinucleated giant cells are helpful in establishing the diagnosis.

Atypical measles must be distinguished from conditions such as erythema multiforme, Rocky Mountain spotted fever, infectious mononucleosis, and drug eruptions, as well as typical measles.

Rubella (German Measles)

Rubella is caused by a 50- to 85-nm RNA virus that is a member of the togavirus family. It is a disease of school-aged children and adolescents, although young children often escape the illness. Outbreaks commonly develop in isolated populations, such as on military bases and in schools. As with measles, there is a worldwide distribution with a peak incidence in the spring. Although it is spread by droplets from infected individuals, prolonged contact is required for transmission. The period of infectivity lasts from the end of the incubation period to the disappearance of the cutaneous eruption, which is usually between 16 to 18 days. If infection occurs during the first trimester of pregnancy, there may be severe fetal malformations.

Clinical Features Initially, there is a mild prodrome of 2 to 3 weeks duration characterized by fever and catarrh. An exanthem manifest as pinpoint petechiae may be seen on the soft palate in 20 percent of patients during this phase, which is known as Forsheimer's sign. Lymphadenopathy then develops, followed by a cutaneous eruption that begins on the face involving the malar area ("butterfly distribution") and spreads to involve the postauricular areas and eventually the trunk and extremities (Table 22-1). Although characteristic, the eruption may be absent in 25 percent of cases. There is centrifugal spread with coalescence on the trunk with concomitant fading on the face. The eruption is characterized by bright red, slightly raised macules and fine papules. A mild branny desquamation may be seen in the resolution phase. Cervical and occipital lymphadenopathy is highly characteristic and has been termed "Winterbottom's sign." Splenomegaly, arthralgia, thrombocytopenia, purpura, and testicular pain occasionally are noted.[6]

Rubella acquired during pregnancy is associated with a significant incidence of fetal abnormalities. The skin is involved in the fetal rubella syndrome in that it is a site of extramedullary hematopoiesis manifest

TABLE 22-1

Viral Exanthems

Diseases	Etiology	Clinical Features	Histopathological Features	Differential Diagnosis
Measles	Measles virus/RNA virus	Incubation period 9 to 10 days Erythematous macules and papules first on the face then spread to neck, trunk, and extremities Koplik's spots	Superficial psoriasiform spongiotic dermatitis with dyskeratotic keratinocytes Warthin-Finkeldy giant cells	Drug eruption, rubella, fifth disease, Kawasaki's disease, scarlet fever
Rubella (German measles)	Rubella virus/RNA virus	"Butterfly" facial rash, Forsheimer's spots, centrifugal spread, cervical and occipital lymphadenopathy (Winterbottom's sign)	Sparse superficial perivascular dermatitis with slight spongiosis, Turk cells (atypical lymphocytes) in peripheral blood and in skin infiltrate	Scarlet fever, infectious mononucleosis, fifth disease, typhus, Rocky Mountain spotted fever, secondary syphilis, and toxoplasmosis
Fifth disease (erythema infectiosum)	Parvovirus B19/DNA virus	Incubation period 2 weeks, "slapped cheeks" sparing circumoral areas, reticulated erythematous eruption on extensor extremities	Sparse superficial perivascular dermatitis and focal spongiosis	Juvenile rheumatoid arthritis, erythema multiforme, rubella, bilateral facial erysipelas
Roseola (exanthem subitum)	Human herpes virus (HHV-6) DNA virus	Incubation period 4 to 7 days, rose-pink macules and papules on trunk sparing face	Sparse superficial perivascular dermatitis	Rubella, measles, fifth disease, scarlet fever, and morbilliform drug eruptions
Varicella (chickenpox) and herpes zoster	Varicella-zoster virus/DNA virus	Incubation period 11 to 20 days, vesicles 1 to 3 mm surrounded by red halo "dew drop on a rose petal" Herpes zoster, painful vesicles within a sensory dermatome	Steel-gray nuclei, margination of chromatin, multinucleated giant cells, acantholysis associated with leukocytoclastic vasculitis and inflammation of nerves	Miliaria crystallina, id reaction
Hand, foot, and mouth disease	Coxsackie virus A16, A5, A10, A7, A9, B1, B3, B5	Incubation period 3 to 6 days, papulovesicles, and ulceration of palate buccal mucosa "Football"-shaped vesicles on dorsa of fingers and toes	Spongiosis, ballooning, and epidermal necrosis with superficial perivascular dermatitis	Varicella, herpes simplex, erythema multiforme
Acute exanthem of HIV infection	HIV-1/RNA virus	Incubation period 3 to 6 weeks, morbilliform eruption involves trunk, chest, and upper arms	Superficial perivascular dermatitis, spongiosis, and necrotic keratinocytes	Drug eruption, CMV, infectious mononucleosis
Infectious mononucleosis	Epstein-Barr/DNA virus	Pharyngitis, fever and cervical adenopathy, splenomegaly, lymphocytosis, pinkish macules and papules on trunk and upper arms	Superficial perivascular dermatitis, spongiosis and parakeratosis, atypical lymphocytes in infiltrate	Drug eruption, CMV, toxoplasmosis
Acute exanthem of cytomegalovirus	CMV/DNA virus	Similar to EBV "mononucleosis syndrome"	Similar to other viral exanthemata with characteristic "owl's eye" inclusions in cytoplasm and nuclei of endothelial cells	Infectious mononucleosis, toxoplasmosis

clinically as bluish-purple papules in the skin. This finding has been termed the "blueberry muffin" baby syndrome.[7,8]

Patients who receive the live, attenuated rubella vaccine occasionally may develop mild symptoms of rubella with an eruption, lymphadenopathy, and arthralgias.

Histopathological Features   There is little published about the histopathology of the cutaneous eruption of rubella but in the few cases examined, a sparse infiltrate of lymphocytes around superficial blood vessels in the dermis associated with slight spongiosis has been observed (Table 22-1; Fig. 22-1). Atypical lymphocytes known as Turk cells may be present in the circulation and therefore would be expected to appear coincidentally in the inflammatory infiltrate in the skin.

Extramedullary hematopoiesis of fetal rubella syndrome is manifest histologically by a diffuse dermal infiltrate of hematopoietic precursors, especially of myeloid elements. As some of these cells may appear primitive and cytologically atypical, it is important to exclude this from leukemia cutis.

Differential Diagnosis   The exanthem of rubella may resemble that of rubeola, scarlet fever, erythema infectiosum, measles, eruptions caused by Coxsackie and echo viruses, infectious mononucleosis, scarlet fever, typhus, Rocky Mountain spotted fever, secondary syphilis, and toxoplasmosis. The butterfly facial eruption associated with occipital lymphadenopathy is highly suggestive. It is important that an accurate diagnosis be rendered so that pregnant women can be removed from possible exposure.

Erythema Infectiosum (Fifth Disease)

Erythema infectiosum, also known as fifth disease, is caused by parvovirus B19, an encapsulated single-stranded DNA virus. The disease is endemic and local outbreaks among school-aged children are common. The virus is spread by aerosolized droplets in individuals who come into close contact.[9,10] The disease has an incubation period of 2 weeks. Intrauterine infection may cause hydrops fetalis and death. The bone marrow is commonly affected by the infection, and transient bone marrow depression and even aplastic anemia have been observed, the latter in patients with sickle cell anemia and HIV infection.

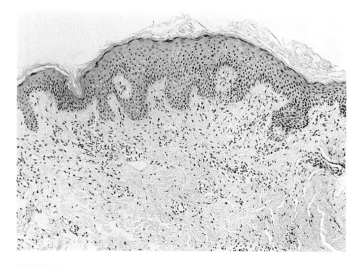

FIGURE 22-1   Viral exanthem. The lesion shows slight acanthosis of the epidermis and a nonspecific superficial perivascular lymphocytic infiltrate.

Clinical Features   Patients usually develop malaise, nausea, and low-grade fever for 1 to 2 days before the development of the distinctive cutaneous eruption that appears suddenly. There is a diffuse or figurate erythema that begins macular and becomes somewhat indurated, developing a well-defined border situated on the cheeks sparing the circumoral areas, resulting in a "slapped cheeks" appearance (Table 22-1). As the eruption of the face wanes, within days, a characteristic reticulated erythematous eruption of macules and papules appear on the extensor extremities and buttocks that may spread to the hands and feet. The exanthem disappears in 7 days, although erythema may persist for as long as 10 days. Recurrences of the eruption up to 21 days following its onset are not uncommon, especially following inciting stimuli such as sunlight, heat, cold, emotional excitement, bathing, or exercise.

A variant of the condition known as the petechial glove and sock syndrome caused by the same virus is manifest as acral pruritus, fever, edema, pain, petechiae, and erosions.

Histopathological Features   As with rubella, the histopathology of erythema infectiosum has been described only rarely. There is a superficial perivascular infiltrate of lymphocytes, and occasional histiocytes, with subtle dermal edema (Table 22-1). Slight spongiosis also may be seen.

Differential Diagnosis   Drug eruptions as well as exanthems of echovirus, enterovirus, measles, juvenile rheumatoid arthritis, scarlet fever, bilateral facial erysipelas, erythema multiforme, and rubella may give similar findings, but the typical reticulate pattern of the eruption on the arms coupled with the slapped cheeks appearance usually are distinct and allow the diagnosis to be rendered.

Roseola (Exanthem Subitum)

Roseola is a contagious self-limiting disease of infancy with short duration and usually lasts for 3 to 5 days. The etiologic agent is human herpesvirus (HHV-6), which is a member of the family *Herpesviridae*.[11,12] The virus is a double-stranded DNA, enveloped virus having a morphology similar to that of other herpesviruses.[13]

Clinical Features   Roseola most commonly infects infants, with a peak incidence of 2 years, up to 30 percent of whom may be affected. It is rare in infants under the age of 6 months, however. The virus is spread through aerosolized droplets, and after an incubation period of 4 to 7 days there is the sudden onset of high fever (to 103°F) (Table 22-1). Palpebral edema often is the first sign of the infection. Accompanying symptoms include hematuria, coryza, vomiting, restlessness, and an erythematous pharynx. Mild cervical and occipital adenopathy commonly develops. The fever subsides suddenly after 3 to 5 days, following which an eruption of rose-pink macules and papules up to 3.5 mm in diameter appears on the trunk and neck, often sparing the face. The eruption fades within 1 to 2 days without sequelae. There may be no eruption in some cases.

Histopathological Features   The histologic changes of roseola are similar to those of the other viral exanthemata described in the preceding, namely, a sparse perivascular infiltrate of lymphocytes in the dermis with minimal other changes. No specific findings are seen that allow the diagnosis to be made in the absence of clinical correlation.

Differential Diagnosis   Other viral exanthemata, including rubella, measles, fifth disease, infectious mononucleosis, scarlet fever, and morbilliform drug eruptions, should be considered in the differential diagnosis.

Dengue Fever

Dengue viruses are members of the Flaviviridae family in the Togavirus group and are all single-stranded RNA viruses that are transmitted by insect vectors, most commonly the *Aedes* mosquito.[14] The disease is endemic in the Americas, especially in the Caribbean basin, Mexico, and northern South America. There are pockets of disease in the United States as well as imported cases.[15]

Clinical Features   The incubation period is 2 to 8 days following the mosquito bite. The onset of the infection is heralded by the abrupt onset of chills, fever, headache, conjunctival injection, severe bone pain ("break bone fever"), arthralgias, myalgias, low back pain, and an exanthem. The exanthem is morbilliform in nature and is central in distribution. Petechiae may be seen with initial infections, although hemorrhagic manifestations (dengue hemorrhagic fever) are seen more commonly with secondary infections and represent manifestations of a hyperimmune state that develops on second exposure to the virus. Bleeding manifestations include petechiae, purpura, bleeding of the gums, nose, gastrointestinal tract, and in association with menses. Uncomplicated dengue resolves within 5 to 7 days, although it may recur. Hemorrhagic dengue may be fatal.

Histopathological Features   The morbilliform eruption appears similar to other exanthemata described in the preceding with the characteristic perivascular infiltrate of lymphocytes and slight spongiosis. Hemorrhagic dengue demonstrates numerous extravasated erythrocytes and may show changes of an immune complex–mediated leukocytoclastic vasculitis with marked thrombosis.

Differential Diagnosis   Depending on which type of infection is present, the differential diagnosis will vary. For the morbilliform eruption, scarlet fever, measles, rubella, toxoplasmosis, syphilis, drug eruption, and the acute HIV seroconversion reaction must all be distinguished. For hemorrhagic dengue, meningococcemia, Rocky Mountain spotted fever, and other forms of vasculitis must be distinguished.

Hand, Foot, and Mouth Disease

Hand, foot, and mouth disease (HFMD) is a mucocutaneous disorder that characteristically involves only a few localized sites and is caused by Coxsackie viruses, most commonly A16, but also A5, A10, A9, B2, and B5. The disease is most common in children and is highly contagious. Most outbreaks occur between the months of June and October.[16]

Clinical Features   The illness begins with fever up to 101°F with associated malaise, soreness of the throat and mouth, and refusal to eat. Cough, headache, diarrhea, and arthralgias may be present. Initially, small reddish macules appear on the oropharynx that evolve into small papulovesicles that are from 1 to 3 mm in size (Table 22-1). These ulcerate, developing a yellow-gray base with a red areola. Ulcerations are found most commonly on the palate, buccal mucosa, tongue, and gingiva. The limbs commonly are involved, especially the sides and dorsa of the fingers and toes. As with mucosal lesions, initially, there are reddish macules that evolve into oval or "football"-shaped vesicles with a surrounding red halo. Rarely, lesions may be disseminated, especially in patients with altered cutaneous barrier function, such as in atopics. The process usually resolves without incident after several days.

Histopathological Features   There is a variably intense inflammatory infiltrate in the superficial dermis consisting primarily of lymphocytes, but there may be variable numbers of neutrophils and eosinophils. The most prominent changes are in the epidermis in fully developed lesions where there is intracellular edema ("ballooning"), spongiosis, and localized epidermal necrosis. Usually, there is minimal epidermal hyperplasia. In time, there is confluent epidermal necrosis, crusting, and slough of degenerated epithelium with reepithelialization.[17]

Mucosal ulcers may appear quite similar to aphthous ulcers. There is a localized ulceration beneath which there is an infiltrate of lymphocytes, plasma cells, and neutrophils.

Differential Diagnosis   Other viral vesicular disorders that may be confused with hand, foot, and mouth disease include varicella, herpes simplex virus infection, and exanthems induced by other Coxsackie viruses as well as echoviruses. Erythema multiforme also may appear similar, especially when there is involvement of the palms and soles. Distinction of HFMD from the latter conditions is based on clinical features, balloon degeneration of keratinocytes, and absence of characteristic viral cytopathic changes as in herpes simplex.

Acute Exanthem of HIV Infection

Acquired immunodeficiency syndrome (AIDS) is caused by the human immunodeficiency virus-1 (HIV-1), which is a 100-nm lentivirus that contains single-stranded RNA. The virus contains the enzyme reverse transcriptase and thus is subclassified as a retrovirus following entry into target cells. Complementary DNA is formed from the RNA template by this enzyme in the production of infective virions, which is the opposite of the usual mechanism of transcription. The primary target cell is the helper (CD4+) T lymphocyte.[18] Infection leads to progressive deterioration of the cell-mediated arm of the immune system through continued destruction of target cells. Over time, opportunistic infections and neoplasms develop that eventually prove fatal to the host. Many of these conditions involve the skin and, although they may not be life-threatening, they cause significant morbidity.

The acute reaction associated with HIV seroconversion refers to an acute viral prodrome associated with a cutaneous eruption that corresponds to the acute infection with HIV-1. The infection is transmitted via exchange of blood or body fluids, specifically semen and vaginal secretions, so that sexual contact is of prime importance in its spread. HIV disease is most prevalent in homosexual men in the United States and in heterosexual populations in Central Africa. The incidence is increasing rapidly in the Far East, South America, and India. There are two main subtypes: One is more aggressive and is spread through male homosexual contact; the other strain is slowly progressive, has a greater tropism for epithelial cells, and is spread more readily by heterosexual contact. Following infection, there is an incubation period of 3 to 6 weeks, during which there is marked viremia with widespread dissemination of virus accompanied by an acute syndrome that develops in 70 to 80 percent of individuals. Within 1 to 3 months, there is a marked immune response to the virus that results in a dramatic decline in the viremia. A "latency" period follows in which there is a gradual but relentless decline in the CD4 cell number.[19]

Clinical Features   The acute HIV exanthem usually is characterized as a benign, often subclinical disorder (Table 22-1). Patients are highly infectious during this time. The incubation period ranges from 3 to 6 weeks and varies with the route of infection, being shorter for hematogenous transmission and with larger viral inocula. Patients develop a sensation of malaise and soon thereafter develop fever that can be as high as 102° F or occasionally higher. Night sweats, pharyngitis, fatigue, lymphadenopathy, and a fine morbilliform eruption that involves the trunk, chest, back, and upper arms develops within 1 to several days.[20] The eruption consists of pinkish macules and fine papules that may be urticarial and that develop on the trunk and spread to involve the proximal extremities, neck, and occasionally the face. Sometimes lesions may be more inflamed, and in one case, necrotizing lesions were observed. Most cases resolve without incident after 4 to 5 days, although a severe form of acute HIV infection may develop with persistent HIV p24 antigenemia, recurrent viremia, rapid decline in CD4+ cell numbers, and accelerated disease progression. Systemic manifestations include pneumonitis, esophagitis, meningitis, abdominal pain, and melena. Skin changes that may be seen include urticaria, perlèche, palatal and esophageal ulcers, enanthemata, and candidiasis.[21] Herpes infections also may supervene. The prognosis for patients with HIV infection who suffer from prolonged symptomatic primary HIV infection is significantly poorer than for those with asymptomatic or mild primary infection, with 78 percent progression to CDC group IV at 3 years compared to 10 percent, respectively.

The pathogenesis of the acute HIV exanthem has not been fully elucidated but is thought to correspond to widespread infection of cells with HIV. This most likely leads to release of cytokines and inflammatory mediators that result in expression of disease.[22]

Histopathological Features   Histologic evaluation of skin biopsies taken from the morbilliform eruption demonstrates an infiltrate consisting primarily of lymphocytes with occasional plasma cells around blood vessels of the superficial vascular plexus (Table 22-1). There is also slight spongiosis and occasional individually necrotic keratinocytes in the epidermis. These findings are similar to those observed in other viral exanthemata as well as in morbilliform drug eruptions. Although most cases in which skin biopsies have been performed have demonstrated these findings, one case in which there was a denser dermal infiltrate associated with epidermal necrosis has been reported. Immunocytochemistry has revealed that most of the infiltrating cells in skin lesions are CD4+ T cells with an admixture of CD8+ cells.[23]

Although no specific laboratory findings other than demonstration of specific evidence of HIV infection, such as the presence of HIV p24 antigen or antibodies directed to HIV, can be found, an elevated erythrocyte sedimentation rate, leukopenia, and cerebrospinal fluid lymphocytic pleocytosis may be observed. In the case of fulminant acute HIV infection, laboratory findings of profound immunosuppression, as alluded to herein, may be demonstrated.

Clinical Features of Cutaneous Manifestations of HIV Infection   The cutaneous manifestations that develop as a consequence of the immune deficiency induced by HIV can be divided into infections, neoplasms, pruritic conditions, papulosquamous and related inflammatory diseases of the skin, as well as changes in hair, nails, and mucosa (Table 22-2). Many of these appear similar to what is observed in affected immunocompetent hosts; however, because of the immunocompromised state of the patient, they may have unusual appearances or may be much more severe.

Herpesvirus infections, including herpes simplex, zoster, cytomegalovirus (CMV), and Epstein-Barr virus (EBV), are quite common in these patients.[24] Herpes simplex and zoster may lead to persistent necrotizing ulcers with extensive scarring.[25] Chronic, verrucous lesions may develop that may simulate other lesions of the skin with epithelial hyperplasia, including neoplasms and granulomatous infections. Cytomegalovirus may induce ulcers or may cause purpuric papules that simulate leukocytoclastic vasculitis. Epstein-Barr virus infection in patients with AIDS leads to oral hairy leukoplakia, which manifests as white, verrucous plaques on the sides of the tongue.[26] Human papillomavirus infections also are common and produce similar findings to those discussed in the following. Molluscum contagiosum very commonly affects HIV-infected patients, especially those with CD4+

TABLE 22-2

Cutaneous Manifestations of Human Immunodeficiency Virus

Infections
  Other viral infections
    Herpes simplex
    Cytomegalovirus
    Epstein-Barr virus
    Molluscum contagiosum
  Bacterial infections
    Bacterial folliculitis
    Impetigo
    Bacillary angiomatosis
    Botryomycosis
    Mycobacterial infections
    Syphilis
  Parasitic infections
  Ectoparasitic infestations
  Fungal infections
    Blastomycosis
    Candidiasis
    Coccidioidomycosis
    Cryptococcosis
    Histoplasmosis
    Paracoccidioidomycosis
    Sporotrichosis
Neoplasms
  Kaposi's sarcoma
  Lymphoma
Inflammatory conditions
  Psoriasis
  Seborrheic dermatitis
  Eosinophilic folliculitis
  Papular eruption of AIDS
  Many others

counts below 250 cells/dL. There are characteristically waxy, translucent umbilicated papules that may be widespread, commonly involving the face but also the trunk and genitalia. In some cases, these may become quite large and simulate neoplasms, especially keratoacanthoma.[27]

Bacterial infections also are commonly encountered in these patients.[28] Bacterial folliculitis, impetigo, bacillary angiomatosis, botryomycosis, pseudomonas infections, streptococcal axillary lymphadenitis, mycobacterial infections, syphilis, and other venereal diseases all may be seen. These disorders may be localized or may be widespread, involving many organs. Most banal bacterial infections, such as folliculitis and impetigo, are caused by staphylococcus and streptococcus, organisms commonly encountered in immunocompetent hosts. *Staphylococcus aureus* is the most common cutaneous and systemic bacterial pathogen in HIV-infected adults. Folliculitis is generally manifest as widely distributed acneiform papules and pustules. In some cases the bacterial density may increase significantly as a consequence of immunodepression, leading to botryomycosis or ecthyma.[29] These disorders appear as nondescript verrucous papules or as necrotizing ulcerations, respectively. Soft tissue and deeply seated bacterial infections, such as cellulitis, pyomyositis, deep soft tissue abscesses, and necrotizing fasciitis, also may develop. These generally are manifest as diffuse, red, warm tender areas in the skin. Although impetigo is seen most commonly on the face and shoulders, in patients with HIV infection it is seen more often in the axillary, inguinal, and other intertriginous locations. The infection usually begins with painful red macules that may develop superficial vesicles that rupture oozing serous and purulent fluid. Botryomycosis is most commonly caused by *S. aureus* and represents a manifestation of extension of staphylococcal folliculitis with the formation of bacterial colonies in the dermis. Clinically, this is often manifest as a nondescript papule or plaque in the skin that may be surrounded by pustules on the trunk, neck, or extremities. An atypical plaquelike staphylococcal folliculitis has been described in patients with HIV infection. These appear as violaceous plaques up to 10 cm in diameter with superficial pustules and crusts occurring in the groin, axilla, or scalp. Infection with *Pseudomonas* spp. also is seen in patients who are HIV infected, and up to 8 percent of all cases of bacteremia in patients with AIDS are caused by these organisms.[30]

Virtually any of the mycobacteria, especially *Mycobacterium haemophilum* and *M. avium-intracellulare*, may induce skin lesions in up to 10 percent of patients with systemic mycobacterial infections.[31] Infection with *M. bovis* following bacille Calmette-Guerin (BCG) vaccination in a patient with HIV infection also has been reported. Mycobacterial skin lesions may assume a number of different appearances, including small papules and pustules that resemble folliculitis, atopic dermatitis–like eruptions, localized cutaneous abscesses, suppurative lymphadenitis, nonspecific ulcerations, palmar and plantar hyperkeratoses, and sporotrichoid nodules.

Syphilis is common in patients with HIV infection and of all reported cases of syphilis, 25 percent develop in HIV-infected hosts.[32] It may assume a number of forms in these patients ranging from classic papulosquamous forms with involvement of the palms, soles, and mucous membranes to unusual manifestations, including rapid progression from the primary chancre to gummatous tertiary lues in a matter of months, lues maligna (syphilis with vasculitis), sclerodermiform lesions, rupial verrucous plaques, extensive oral ulcerations, keratoderma, deep cutaneous nodules, rubeoliform eruptions, and widespread gummata.

Over 50 cases of bacillary angiomatosis, a condition caused by rickettsialike organisms *Bartonella* (formerly *Rochalimaea*) *henselae* and *B. quintana*, have been reported.[33] There are a number of different clinical manifestations of this disorder, many of which are visceral. Cutaneous vascular lesions are the most common and of these, small pinpoint reddish to purple papules are the earliest lesions. These may assume an appearance similar to pyogenic granulomata and are seen in two-thirds of patients with cutaneous disease. They range in number from one to several thousand and in size from 1 mm to several centimeters. Lesions may ulcerate and/or be covered by a crust. The second most common skin lesion is the subcutaneous nodule that occurs in approximately 50 percent of patients with skin lesions. They may be located deeply in the subcutis, extending to involve soft tissue and bone. Two cases of deeply seated skeletal muscle pyomyositis have been reported. When bone is involved, lesions are generally osteolytic in nature. Nondescript crusted ulcerations, plaques, and cellulitis may also be seen in 5 to 10 percent of patients. Viscera may be involved either as disseminated vascular lesions or as bacillary peliosis hepatis of the liver. Although virtually every organ system may be affected, the liver and spleen are the most common sites of involvement.

In addition to bacterial and fungal infections, a number of parasitic infections and ectoparasitic infestations may be encountered in patients with HIV infection. Some of these include scabies, both classical and crusted types, demodicidosis, *Pneumocystis carinii* infection, acanthamebiasis, and leishmaniasis, as well as toxoplasmosis. Just as in the case of other infections, these may occur either as localized conditions or as multiorgan visceral disease. As with other infectious disorders in HIV-infected patients, clinical morphologies may be unusual so that skin biopsies and cultures often are necessary to establish an accurate diagnosis.

Scabies may have a number of different clinical manifestations in patients with HIV infection. Hyperkeratotic plaques on the palms, soles,

trunk, or extremities may develop, having an appearance similar to crusted scabies in other settings. In other patients, only scattered pruritic papules accompanied by slight scale of the trunk and extremities may be seen. A widespread papulosquamous eruption that may resemble atopic dermatitis as well as scalp and facial scaling that may mimic seborrheic dermatitis also have been reported. Characteristic burrows may be difficult to identify so that virtually any patient with a scaly persistent pruritic eruption should have skin lesions scraped and examined histologically in search of mites or scabies.

P. carinii in the skin may have several different clinical manifestations.[34] The most commonly reported form is that of friable reddish papules or nodules seen in the ear canal or the nares. Small translucent molluscum contagiosum–like papules, bluish cellulitic plaquelike lesions, and deeply seated abscesses also have been observed. Acanthamebiasis consists of painful nodular lesions with ulcerations usually on the trunk or extremities.

Blastomycosis, candidiasis, coccidioidomycosis, cryptococcosis, histoplasmosis, paracoccidioidomycosis, and sporotrichosis are some of the systemic fungal infections that occur in HIV-infected individuals.[35,36] Other rarer fungal infections also have been noted, including zycomycosis, aspergillosis, and disseminated dermatophytosis. As with the other conditions described herein, mucosal and cutaneous lesions may have many unusual clinical morphologies in these patients, many of which defy accurate clinical diagnosis.

In addition to infectious disorders, a number of noninfectious cutaneous signs and symptoms develop in these patients. Some of these include psoriasiform dermatoses such as seborrheic dermatitis, psoriasis, Reiter's disease, and pityriasis rubra pilaris; noninfectious papular, pruritic conditions such as eosinophilic pustular folliculitis, severe xerotic dermatitis, papular dermatitis of AIDS, papular urticaria, and atopic dermatitis; disorders of blood vessels including vasculitis, idiopathic thrombocytopenic purpura, hyperalgesic pseudothrombophlebitis, diffuse facial and truncal telangiectasia, and erythema elevatum diutinum; photoaggravated and photoinduced disorders, including chronic actinic dermatitis, porphyria cutanea tarda, photoexacerbated drug eruptions, and photoexacerbated rosacea; drug eruptions; and neoplasms, both epithelial and mesenchymal.[37,38] It is beyond the scope of this chapter to discuss each of these here.

Histopathological Features of Cutaneous Manifestations of HIV Infection Histopathologic findings of folliculitis generally include collections of neutrophils within infundibula of hair follicles and a mixed perifollicular inflammatory cell infiltrate. When rupture of follicles occurs, there is often a perifollicular granulomatous infiltrate with fibrosis. Botryomycosis is characterized by a diffuse inflammatory cell infiltrate in the dermis associated with colonies of Gram-positive bacteria forming grains in the skin. These generally appear bluish-purple on hematoxylin and eosin–stained sections. Ecthyma is manifested histologically as a deep ulcer that often extends to the subcutaneous fat with extensive degeneration of dermal collagen. There is a mixed inflammatory cell infiltrate of neutrophils, eosinophils, and histiocytes.

Histopathologic findings in bacillary angiomatosis are characterized by a lobular proliferation of capillaries associated with enlarged epithelioid-appearing endothelial cells. The background stroma usually is edematous in superficial lesions and more compact in deeper ones. Neutrophils and leukocytes are often seen in the interstitium between vessels. The presence of neutrophils in the body of lesions is a valuable finding that permits distinction from ulcerated pyogenic granulomata that may have similar histologic features, although neutrophils are present primarily under areas of ulceration. Granular amphophilic aggregates are characteristically seen adjacent to vessels, often in association with neutrophils, which represent masses of *Bartonella* organisms. These appear black after staining with the Warthin-Starry stain.

Electron microscopy is confirmatory. Although the diagnosis usually can be made on the basis of microscopic examination of routine hematoxylin and eosin–stained tissue sections, on occasion, atypia of endothelial cells may be marked, causing histologic confusion with angiosarcoma.

The histopathology of cutaneous syphilis usually is similar to that of immunocompetent hosts demonstrating the characteristic superficial and deep psoriasiform lichenoid pattern of inflammation associated with plasma cells and histiocytes. On the other hand, unusual histologic findings may be seen, including vasculitis as well as very sparse inflammatory infiltrates with minimal numbers of plasma cells and abundant spirochetes.

Cutaneous mycobacterial infections may assume classic patterns of suppurative granulomatous infiltrates in the dermis associated with pseudocarcinomatous hyperplasia, although other unusual patterns may be observed, including dense areas of suppuration with minimal granulomatous infiltrate.

In crusted scabies there is usually a superficial and mid- to deep perivascular and interstitial infiltrate of lymphocytes with numerous eosinophils. The epidermis is hyperplastic with prominent crusting and many mites visible in the cornified layer. In patients with post–scabetic "id" reactions, a spongiotic dermatitis may be noted, and in nodular scabies, a dense mixed inflammatory infiltrate with numerous eosinophils in a nodular configuration resembling a pseudolymphoma may be seen. In nodular scabies, the number of mites is few and it may be difficult to find them.

Demodicidosis characteristically shows abundant demodex mites within follicular infundibula associated with a mixed infiltrate of neutrophils and eosinophils within and around the infundibula of hair follicles.

P. carinii in the skin has an appearance similar to that in the lung, with a diffuse infiltrate of foamy appearing cells that, when stained with Gomori's methenamine silver or Steiner stains, highlight the microorganisms resulting in the "teacup and saucer" appearance.

Acanthamebiasis shows a diffuse infiltrate of amebic cysts and trophozoites throughout the skin, especially around blood vessels and in the subcutaneous fat. Careful inspection is required as these may appear similar to histiocytes or other normal-appearing structures in the skin. Erythrophagocytosis may be noted.

Noninfectious inflammatory skin diseases appear similar histologically to those seen in immunocompetent hosts with the exception that individually necrotic keratinocytes are present with greater frequency. Eosinophilic folliculitis differs from other forms of folliculitis in that there is a dense infiltrate of eosinophils within the follicular ostia of affected hair follicles in prototypical cases. In many cases, however, lesions are biopsied late in their evolution so that only perifollicular fibrosis and granulomatous inflammation may be seen.

Differential Diagnosis   The differential diagnosis includes other viral exanthemata, such as those caused by Epstein-Barr virus (EBV), parvovirus, measles, and rubella. Drug eruptions also must be excluded, especially as HIV-infected patients may be under treatment with numerous medications.

The diagnosis is based on the presence of a characteristic clinical picture in an individual with risk factors for the development of HIV infection. Blood tests that reveal either positive anti-HIV antibody titers by the ELISA method and Western blot assay or circulating p24 antigen are confirmatory. Other possible viral disorders should be excluded by obtaining acute and convalescent viral titers.

The differential diagnosis of cutaneous manifestations of HIV infection is vast. Histologic findings usually are characteristic of the disorder in question, especially in the case of infectious illnesses.

Infectious Mononucleosis

Infectious mononucleosis is caused by the Epstein-Barr virus, which is a member of the human herpesvirus family. It is an enveloped, icosahedral DNA virus that grows well in B lymphocytes, leading to their immortalization. Infections typically develop in teens and young adults between the ages of 17 and 25.[39] It occurs less commonly in young children and is rarely seen before the age of 1 or over the age of 40 years. There is a long incubation period of between 30 and 50 days.

Clinical Features   There is an initial prodrome of 3 to 5 days manifest as headache, malaise, myalgia, and fatigue. The classic clinical triad is pharyngitis, fever, and cervical adenopathy, which is seen in over 80 percent of patients. Fever may be as high as 39°C and may persist for 7 to 10 days. Other symptoms that may be encountered include nausea, anorexia, headache, muscle pain, weakness, arthralgias, rhinitis, and ocular pain. Tender, firm lymphadenopathy is seen in virtually all cases and may be generalized. Splenomegaly is quite common, being present in 50 to 60 percent of patients and may be accompanied by hepatomegaly. Either absolute or relative lymphocytosis sometimes up to 50,000 cells/dL develops, with up to 20 percent atypical lymphocytes.

Mucocutaneous findings include small petechiae at the junction of the hard and soft palate in 20 to 30 percent of cases. Eyelid petechiae and periorbital edema may also be seen. An exanthem develops in 10 to 15 percent of patients, usually on day 4 to 6 of the illness. There are pinkish macules and fine papules that appear first on the trunk and upper arms with spread to the face and forearms and occasionally to the thighs and legs (Table 22-1). The eruption may be either morbilliform, scarlatinaform, or urticarial and usually fades after 3 to 4 days.

Administration of ampicillin and, less commonly, penicillin, cephalosporins, or tetracycline leads to the development of an exanthematous eruption that is usually more widespread and erythematous than the primary eruption.[40] It usually develops 7 to 10 days following institution of the antibiotic. Periorbital edema is present in 25 to 30 percent of cases. Occasionally, jaundice, arthritis, and pneumonitis may be seen.

Histopathological Features   The pathology of the cutaneous exanthem is similar to that observed with other viral exanthemata described, namely, a sparse infiltrate of lymphocytes with slight spongiosis and parakeratosis (Table 22-1). Atypical lymphocytes may be present coincidentally in the infiltrate, a manifestation of the presence of circulating atypical cells. Biopsies of enlarged lymph nodes most commonly demonstrate reactive lymphoid hyperplasia, although marked immunoblastic proliferation with cytologic atypia of lymphocytes may simulate immunoblastic lymphoma or Hodgkin's disease.

Histologic findings in the ampicillin-associated eruption are more florid than those of the primary EBV-induced exanthem. In addition to the perivascular infiltrate of lymphocytes, there may be vacuolar interface changes as well as spongiosis. There is often a denser infiltrate of inflammatory cells in the dermis that may be accompanied by scattered neutrophils and eosinophils.

Differential Diagnosis   Cytomegalovirus, toxoplasmosis, streptococcal pharyngitis, tularemia, viral pharyngitis, diphtheria, acute leukemia, acute infectious lymphocytosis, infectious hepatitis, and drug eruptions must all be distinguished. Clinical findings coupled with serologic studies usually are adequate in establishing a definitive diagnosis.

Other Viral Exanthems

A number of other viruses may lead to the development of exanthems and should be kept in mind when evaluating the cause of a febrile illness associated with a cutaneous eruption. Some of these include the echoviruses 2, 4, 5, 6, 9, 11, 16, 18, 25, and 30; Coxsackie viruses A4, A5, A6, A9, A10, A16, B2, B3, and B5; adenovirus and reoviruses types 1 and 2; and most recently, the hepatitis viruses A, B, and C. These eruptions develop most commonly in younger children and infants. The viruses are distributed widely.

There are a wide variety of arthropod-borne viral illnesses that may have cutaneous findings, most of which are associated with the development of hemorrhagic fevers. Some of these may produce morbilliform eruptions, however. These include Togaviruses, such as Chikungunya, O'Nyong-Nyong, Sindbis, Ross River, and Bharma forest; Bunyaviruses; Arenaviruses, such as Lassa, Junin, and Machupo; Filoviruses, such as Marburg and Ebola; and Hantaviruses.

Clinical Features   The exanthem associated with Coxsackie virus A9 is prototypical and has been most well-studied. Typically, there is a prodrome with fever sometimes as high as 103°F with malaise, sore throat, and cervical adenopathy. After several days of fever, an eruption develops first on the face with spread to the neck and trunk, followed by the extremities and occasionally the palms and soles. There is minimal pruritus. Individual lesions are pinkish to red macules and small papules ranging in size from 2 to 13 mm in diameter. Small vesicles and petechiae may be seen. Other findings include conjunctivitis, muscle weakness, orchitis, hepatosplenomegaly, myocarditis, diarrhea (echovirus 4), pleurodynia (Coxsackie B2 and B5), and meningitis (Coxsackie virus A9 and echovirus 9).

Hepatitis A has been reported to cause a generalized morbilliform eruption similar to other viral exanthemata. Hepatitis B, however, has been associated with both a directly induced urticarial eruption as well as a secondary chronic urticaria that occasionally may be associated with lupus erythematosus.[41] Polyarteritis nodosa has also been associated with hepatitis B.[42] Hepatitis C may be associated with porphyria cutanea tarda as well as small- and medium-sized vessel vasculitis that may be thrombotic in nature secondary to elevated levels of circulating cryoglobulins or may be immune complex–mediated leading to a typical appearance of leukocytoclastic vasculitis with purpuric papules.[43]

Viral hemorrhagic fevers are manifest by eruptions of erythematous macules, petechiae, purpura, and widespread intracutaneous and visceral hemorrhage. These manifestations are a consequence of thrombocytopenia, diminished coagulation factors, platelet dysfunction, disseminated intravascular coagulation, and direct vascular injury.

Histopathological Features   The findings are similar to those described in the preceding and are not specific for any infection. The histologic features of disorders induced by hepatitis viruses are similar to those induced on other bases and are discussed elsewhere. Viral hemorrhagic fevers are associated with abundant intradermal hemorrhage and, in the case of disseminated intravascular coagulation, marked thrombosis of vessels with secondary ischemic necrosis is seen.

Differential Diagnosis   The differential diagnosis is similar to that for other viral exanthems described. In many cases, because acute and convalescent viral titers are not determined, the diagnosis is never confirmed. Nevertheless, the diagnosis of a viral exanthem should be considered in any instance in which a patient develops an acute febrile illness associated with a cutaneous eruption.

HERPES SIMPLEX

Infection with human herpesvirus hominis is one of the most common mucocutaneous viral infections of humans. There are eight herpes-

viruses that have now been defined. For the purposes of this discussion, only types 1 and 2 will be discussed.

Clinical Features   Herpes simplex is characterized by an acute eruption of tense, umbilicated, grouped vesicles on an erythematous base usually at or near a mucocutaneous junction (Table 22-3). The onset usually is preceded by a prodrome of burning and itching a few hours before the eruption. The vesicles appear in groups and are of pinhead size, which later become seropurulent. Primary genital herpes simplex infection (HSV-2) occurs most commonly in young adults. It is transmitted through sexual contact and present as painful, erosive balanitis, vulvitis, or vaginitis. Individuals who have a primary attack are prone to recurrent attacks that may have their onset shortly after the primary infection or it may be delayed for months to years. There may be a variable duration between recurrences in the "latency" period. A complication of recurrent HSV is the secondary development of erythema multiforme.

HSV also commonly occurs as a folliculitis (see Chap. 10), may involve distinctive sites such as the fingers or hands (herpetic whitlow),

---

TABLE 22-3

Herpes Simplex

Clinical Features

Localized clusters of vesicles usually on the lip (type 1) or genital mucosa (type 2)
Prodrome of burning a few hours before eruption
Primary and recurrent lesions
HSV type 1 usually above the waistline; HSV type 2 usually below waist
Herpetic folliculitis
Herpetic whitlow (involvement of fingers)
Generalized and chronic localized herpes, often in immunocompromised hosts

Histopathological Features

"Steel-gray" nuclei of keratinocytes
Margination of chromatin and multinucleated epithelial giant cells
Eosinophilic intranuclear inclusions with clear halo
Intracellular edema and ballooning degeneration
Reticular degeneration and rupture of cell walls of epithelial cells
Acantholysis
Multiloculated intraepidermal vesicle formation
Lymphoid infiltrates, often rather dense in dermis
Infiltration of nerve twigs by infiltrate
Occasional lymphocytic and leukocytoclastic vasculitis

Differential Diagnosis

Other viral exanthems
Erythema multiforme
Drug eruptions
Pityriasis lichenoides
Graft-versus-host reaction
Radiation dermatitis
Impetigo
Syphilitic chancre
Chancroid
Aphthae
Traumatic ulcerations

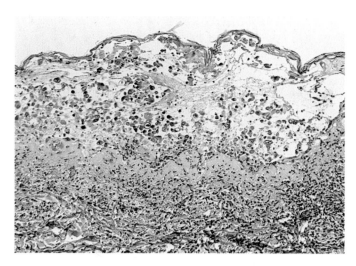

FIGURE 22-2   Herpes simplex infection. Scanning magnification shows a multiloculated intraepidermal vesicle.

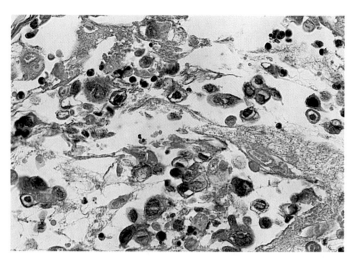

FIGURE 22-4   Herpes simplex infection. An intraepidermal vesicle shows prominent intracellular edema of keratinocytes, acantholysis, reticular degeneration, and occasional eosinophilic inclusion bodies within nuclei. The inclusion bodies are surrounded by a clear halo.

the cervix of the female genital tract (herpes cervicitis), the cornea and conjunctiva (herpes keratoconjunctivitis), the low back and buttocks (recurrent lumbosacral herpes), and may become generalized or chronic at a local site (chronic ulcerative herpes), particularly in immunocompromised individuals.

Kaposi's varicelliform eruption or eczema herpeticum refers to secondary usually widespread involvement of a primary dermatosis, such as atopic dermatitis, Darier's disease, pemphigus foliaceus, or other dermtitides by HSV. Lesional skin or skin previously involved by the dermatitis is preferentially affected by typical vesicles of HSV.

Histopathological Features   The earliest change occurs in the epidermis in which there is pallor and swelling of the cytoplasm of keratinocytes, imparting a "steel-gray" appearance of nuclei (Figs. 22-2 to 22-4). The nuclei also show margination of chromatin (Table 22-3). Infected keratinocytes may fuse, forming characteristic multinucleated epithelial giant cells (Fig. 22-5). Eosinophilic inclusion bodies usually surrounded by a clear halo may be observed in the nuclei of infected cells. Spongiosis and intracellular edema also are present in the epidermis and the epithelium of hair follicles. Infected keratinocytes characteristically develop intracellular edema, leading to ballooning degeneration, which is a feature of viral vesicles. Epithelial cells showing ballooning degeneration lose intercellular adhesions and thus become acantholytic. Intracellular edema also results in reticular degeneration and the rupture of cell walls. The latter phenomenon and acantholysis eventuate in multiloculated intraepidermal vesicles. In time, keratinocytes become necrotic and develop pyknotic nuclei and dense eosinophilic cytoplasm.

There is a variably dense inflammatory infiltrate in the dermis consisting of lymphocytes, neutrophils, and eosinophils. There often is associated lymphocytic or leukocytoclastic vasculitis and inflammation within and around nerve twigs.

VARICELLA (CHICKENPOX) AND HERPES ZOSTER

Varicella is one of the most common childhood infections. The disease is caused by the varicella-zoster virus, which is a double-stranded DNA virus and is a member of the family Herpesviridae. Airborne droplet infection is the usual route of transmission, although direct contact is another mode of spread. It is one of the most contagious of all infections. Herpes zoster represents reactivation of latent varicella infection that resides in sensory ganglia.[44]

Clinical Features   The incubation period ranges from 11 to 20 days and is followed by a prodrome of mild fever and malaise often accompanied by photophobia (Table 22-4). The eruption is characterized by crops of erythematous macules and papules on the trunk and face that rapidly evolve into vesicles of 1- to 3-mm size with clear serous fluid surrounded by narrow red halo. "Dew drops on a rose petal" is a description that has been given to the vesicular eruption. The number of vesicles varies, ranging from only a few to several hundred. Older lesions crust and begin to heal usually within 1 week to 10 days.

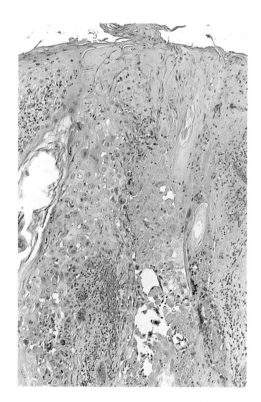

FIGURE 22-3   Herpes folliculitis. There is edema and ballooning degeneration of follicular epithelial cells with vesicle formation.

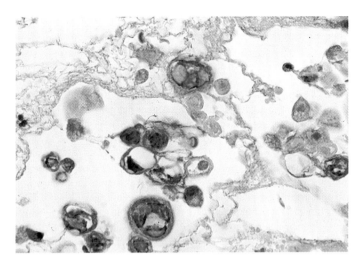

FIGURE 22-5   Herpesvirus infection. The intraepidermal vesicle shows striking multinucleated giant cells. The nuclei within these giant cells exhibit molding and a prominent ground-glass appearance of chromatin. There is also prominent reticular degeneration resulting in the intraepidermal vesicle.

Herpes zoster is manifest as a painful eruption of vesicles on erythematous bases that develops within a sensory dermatome, usually on the trunk but in some cases the face, neck, or scalp may be involved (Table 22-5). Usually, older individuals are affected, although patients with immunocompromise such as those with HIV infection also commonly develop the condition. Zoster in HIV-infected patients may assume a number of unusual manifestations, especially persistent crusted, verrucous lesions.[45]

Histopathological Features   As in the case of herpes simplex, the changes are within the epidermis with steel-gray nuclei, margination of chromatin, multinucleated giant cells, acantholysis, and intraepidermal vesiculation (Table 22-3). No significant differences have been observed between zoster and varicella, although biopsy specimens from immunocompromised patients with zoster often demonstrate extensive infection of the epidermis with marked necrosis and involvement of cutaneous adnexal structures, such as hair follicles, sebaceous glands, and eccrine sweat units.

Differential Diagnosis   Herpes simplex may appear identical histopathologically and can only be distinguished on the basis of clinical findings and the results of viral cultures. Most cases of herpes simplex

---

TABLE 22-4

Varicella (Chickenpox)

Clinical Features

Incubation period of 11 to 20 days
Mild fever, photophobia
"Dew drops on rose petal" vesicular eruption on face and trunk

Histopathological Features

Same as herpes simplex

Differential Diagnosis

Miliaria crystallina
"Id" reaction
Other viral exanthems

TABLE 22-5

Herpes Zoster

Clinical Features

Unilateral painful eruption of vesicles within a sensory dermatome
Ophthalmic branch of trigeminal nerve commonly involved
May be disseminated in immunocompromised patients

Histopathological Features

Same as herpes simplex

Differential Diagnosis

Same as herpes simplex
Dermatomal herpes simplex
Angina pectoris
Early glaucoma

---

appear as localized clusters of vesicles on erythematous bases, usually on the lip or a mucosal surface. Occasionally, a zosteriform distribution may be observed, which is of most importance in cases involving the maxillary branch of the facial nerve, as treatment of the two diseases differs significantly. Late-stage necrotizing ulcers in immunocompromised patients must be distinguished from other causes of ulcers, including serious opportunistic infections caused by other viruses, fungi, or bacteria. Verrucous herpesvirus infections may simulate neoplastic disorders as well as other infections. Biopsies may be required to define the nature of these lesions. Relatively few widespread vesicular eruptions should be confused with varicella, although miliaria crystallina and widespread spongiotic dermatitis, such as an id reaction, could conceivably appear similar.

The differential diagnosis of herpesvirus infection in general includes other viral infections/exanthems, erythema multiforme, drug reactions, graft-versus-host reaction, pityriasis lichenoides, radiation dermatitis, and connective tissue disease. Identification of the characteristic viral cytopathic changes, culture, immunostaining for the virus, or use of other techiques is necessary to distinguish herpes from the other entities listed in the preceding.

HUMAN PAPILLOMAVIRUS INFECTIONS

Human papillomavirus (HPV) infection is an extremely prevalent disorder and is one of the most common viral infections of humans.[49] The causative agents are small double-stranded DNA viruses that are 50 to 55 nm in diameter. Over 70 different strains now have been described (Table 22-6). HPV is transmitted by close, repeated contact that is often sexual in nature, although patients may inoculate themselves from spreading lesions from one body site to another. These viruses all have a tropism for epithelial cells. Following internalization, the virus enters the nucleus, where it leads to either productive infection or undergoes latency. Once infected, the host virtually always remains infected for life, whether or not clinical lesions develop. In active infections, transcription of HPV takes place primarily in basal cells, whereas virion production occurs in more differentiated layers of the epithelium. Thus, only the surface epithelium contains infectious viral particles.

In addition to causing verrucae and papillomata, HPV infection may lead to carcinoma. Proteins produced by the oncogenic HPVs bind p53, a tumor suppressor gene product, which leads to unregulated cell growth and neoplasia. Different HPV types tend to cause different clinical lesions; however, there is significant overlap. Types 6 and 11 gen-

TABLE 22-6

Human Papillomavirus

Condyloma acuminatum HPV-6, 8, 11, 16, and 18
Verruca vulgaris HPV-1, 2, 3, and 4
Verruca plana HPV-3
Verruca plantaris and palmaris HPV-2
Epidermodysplasia verruciformis HPV-3, 5, 12, 17, 19–29
Bowenoid papulosis HPV-16, 18
Verrucous carcinoma HPV-61,11

erally induce benign lesions, whereas types 16, 18, 31, and 33 are associated with potential for malignancy, especially types 16 and 18.

Clinical Features   Condyloma acuminatum, also known as "venereal wart," is the most common venereal disease in the United States and poses a public health problem of major magnitude (Table 22-7). The annual incidence of this disorder has been reported to be as high as 106.5 per 100,000 or about 0.1 percent of the entire population. The

incubation period varies from 3 weeks to 8 months, averaging 2.8 months. Men and women are affected similarly, and the median age of infection with anogenital HPV is 22 to 25 years. In men the most common sites of involvement are the penis, urethra, scrotum, perianal, anal, and rectal area.[50] HPV types 6, 8, 16, and 18 are the most common viral isolates from anogenital condylomata. Clinically, lesions usually are manifest as soft, sessile tumors with surfaces that may be either smooth or markedly digitated with numerous fingerlike projections. Penile condylomata are usually 3 to 5 mm in diameter and often occur in groups of three to four.

In women, the spectrum of clinical disease induced by HPV may be quite broad.[51] Classic exophytic lesions of the external genitalia generally are readily recognized, although detection of other forms of HPV infection requires colposcopic and sigmoidoscopic examination. Vulvar condylomata acuminata appear as soft, whitish, sessile tumors with papillae or fine, fingerlike projections seen most commonly in moist areas such as the introitus and labia. Cervical condylomata occur in 20 percent of women with HPV infection of other areas of the genital tract. These usually appear as papillary epithelial projections at the cervical transformation zone and involve the squamous epithelium on colposcopic examination.

TABLE 22-7

Human Papillomavirus Infection

Clinical Features	Histopathological Features	Differential Diagnosis
Condyloma acuminata	*Condyloma acuminata*	*Condyloma acuminata*
Anogenital areas	Polypoid configuration	Bowenoid papulosis
Soft sessile lesions	Epidermal hyperplasia	Squamous papilloma
smooth or digitated surface 3–5 mm	Focal parakeratosis in invaginations of epidermis	Verrucous carcinoma
Often multiple	Koilocytes	
	Dyskeratosis	
Verruca vulgaris	*Verruca vulgaris*	*Verruca vulgaris*
Exposed skin	Hyperkeratosis	Epidermal nevus
Fingers, hands, dorsal aspects; face	Focal parakeratosis overlying epidermal papillomatosis	Seborrheic keratosis
Hyperkeratotic papules, plaques	Digitated epidermal hyperplasia	
Solitary or grouped lesions	Hypergranulosis	
Filiform variants on face	Vacuolization of upper Malpighian layer with prominent keratohyaline granules	
Mosaic variants on palms and soles	Dilated vessels in dermal papillae	
Verruca plana	*Verruca plana*	*Verruca plana*
Face, extremities	Basket-weave hyperkeratosis	Seborrheic keratosis
Skin-colored or brown, slightly elevated papules	Often absence of parakeratosis	Stucco keratosis
Barely palpable 1–3 mm	Slight or no papillomatosis	
Usually multiple or numerous	Hypergranulosis	
	Vacuolated keratinocytes (Bird's eye cells) in upper Malpighian layer	
Verruca plantaris	*Verruca plantaris*	*Verruca plantaris*
Soles, particularly ball of foot	Hyperkeratosis	Punctate keratosis
Solitary often	Prominent papillomatosis	Verrucous carcinoma
Firm papules or plaques	Vacuolization of keratinocytes	
Often marked hyperkeratosis	Prominent eosinophilic cytoplasmic inclusions at periphery of cell	
	Rounded deeply basophilic nuclei	

Verrucae vulgares or common warts are the most common manifestation of HPV infection, occurring most frequently on the dorsal aspects of the fingers and hands (Table 22-7). Clinically they are manifest as circumscribed firm papules or plaques with a rough surface. They may occur singly or in groups and are caused most commonly by HPV types 1, 2, 3, and 4. Filiform warts are variants that are more slender and elongated. They are commonly situated on the eyelids and beard region.

Verruca plana or flat warts often present as 1- to 3-mm slightly elevated, skin-colored, or slightly brownish papules. They usually are well-demarcated and exhibit a minimally hyperkeratotic surface. They often are multiple and commonly involve the face or extremities.

Warts on the soles (verruca plantaris) are variants of verrucae vulgares and can present in a number of different forms. Most commonly, these are solitary lesions on the ball of the foot with a markedly thickened cornified layer. Mosaic warts represent coalesced clusters of warts that occur on the sole but are not generally as elevated as other plantar verrucae, possibly because of the constant pressure exerted by the weight of the body. They tend to recur following removal, and because of the massive number of viral particles being shed from them, they tend to be more contagious than other verrucae. Plantar warts may lead to severe pain on walking and often pose a difficult therapeutic problem.

Bowenoid papulosis refers to a localized form of squamous cell carcinoma in situ that develops as a consequence of infection by oncogenic HPVs, especially types 16 and 18. They may appear identical to condylomata acuminata but usually are manifest as small, brown, flat-topped papules involving the genital and perigenital area. The condition is seen in both sexes but is more common in men. Lesions may become confluent and hyperplastic, and in some cases, they may progress to fully developed squamous cell carcinoma.[52] The shaft of the penis is involved more commonly than the glans.

Giant HPV-induced verrucous carcinoma are manifest as large, vegetating tumors present most commonly in the genital and perigenital areas. These lesions are similar clinically to the Buschke-Lowenstein variant of verrucous carcinoma. Epidermodysplasia verruciformis may clinically simulate widespread warts or, in some cases, other forms of erythroderma or widespread erythematous scaly dermatoses.

Epidermodysplasia verruciformis refers to a cutaneous eruption caused by specific subtypes of HPV, especially types 3 and 5, in which patients inherit an abnormal propensity to develop cutaneous squamous cell carcinoma following ultraviolet irradiation in an autosomal dominant fashion. Skin lesions are manifested as widespread papules that are usually red, flat, or skin-colored, and wartlike on the sun-exposed surfaces. Malignant transformation is common.

Histopathological Features Infection with HPV characteristically causes squamous epithelial proliferation. Histologically, condyloma accuminatum is manifest as a papular or nodular lesion with prominent acanthosis and, often, koilocytosis (Table 22-7). Lesions are usually gently papillated (Fig. 22-6), although they may be digitated. The epithelial retia are bulbous and branching and may simulate pseudocarcinomatous hyperplasia in some cases. The cells of the upper portion of the epithelium have perinuclear vacuolization and round hyperchromatic nuclei (Fig. 22-7). In many cases, an increase in the number of mitoses is observed. The dermis or lamina propria appears edematous with dilated blood vessels and a variably intense lymphocytic infiltrate.

Verrucae vulgares generally show epidermal hyperplasia with acanthosis, papillomatosis, dilated blood vessels in the papillary dermis, intraepidermal hemorrhage, and parakeratosis (Fig. 22-8). The koilocytes of verrucae contain enlarged, clumped keratohyaline granules that appear intensely basophilic. Vertical columns of parakeratosis also are present at the tips of individual digitations. There is often hemorrhage within the cornified layer at the tips of individual digitations. These

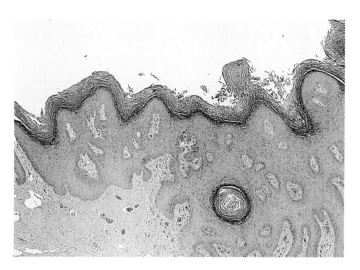

FIGURE 22-6   Condyloma acuminatum. The lesion shows hyperkeratosis and a polypoid configuration and slight papillomatosis.

changes are more pronounced in relatively early well-developed lesions; however, involuted or the older lesions often lack these characteristic features, demonstrating compact ortho- and parakeratosis with wedge-shaped hypergranulosis, slight papillomatosis, and acanthosis.

Verrucae plana are only slightly elevated and show less pronounced or no papillomatosis compared to common verruca (Fig. 22-9). In general, the stratum corneum has a basket-weave pattern of hyperkeratosis without parakeratosis. Perhaps the most striking finding is the presence of vacuolated koilocytes (so-called bird's eye cells) in the superficial malpighian layer of the epidermis.

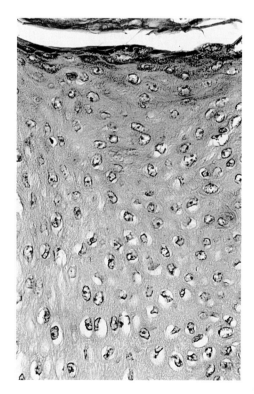

FIGURE 22-7   Condyloma acuminatum. This field shows koilocytes with the characteristic distortion of nuclear outlines.

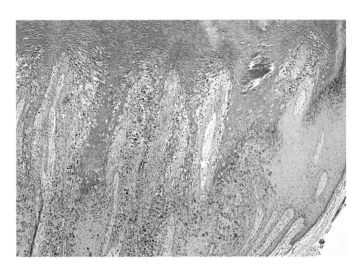

FIGURE 22-8 Verruca vulgaris. The epidermis shows striking papillomatosis with overlying hyperkeratosis. Hypergranulosis and vacuolization of keratinocytes also can be observed.

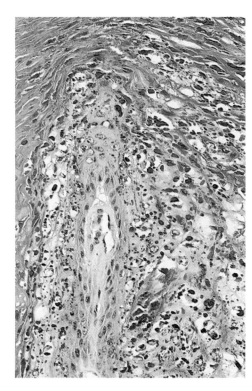

FIGURE 22-10 Verruca plantaris. The lesion exhibits hypergranulosis with prominent vacuolization of keratinocytes, many of which contain large keratohyaline granules.

Histologically, plantar verrucae show features similar to verruca vugaris, although there is minimal papillomatosis as lesions tend to be endophytic. Parakeratosis is minimal with the cornified layer having a basket-weave appearance beneath which there is a markedly thickened granular layer (Fig. 22-10). Koilocytic cells, if present, are located in the upper portion of the epidermis, especially the granular layer.

Bowenoid papulosis demonstrates architectural features similar to condyloma acuminatum, but cytolocially, changes of atypical keratinocytic proliferation and features of squamous cell carcinoma in situ are seen (Figs. 22-11 and 22-12). Individual keratinocytes are large, hyperchromatic, pleomorphic, closely crowded together, and fail to demonstrate normal maturation from basal cell layer to the granular cell layer. Epidermodysplasia verruciformis is manifest histologically by papillomatosis, large vacuolated cells in the epidermis, and variable keratinocytic atypia. In some cases, there is an unusual form of dyskeratosis with corps rond–like bodies in the basket-weave stratum corneum.

Differential Diagnosis Condylomata accuminata may be confused with hymenal papillomatosis in women as well as pearly penile papules in men. Seborrheic keratoses also may appear similar. These must be distinguished from Bowenoid papulosis, the malignant counterpart of condylomata that in some cases can only be done on the basis of histologic evaluation. Verrucae may appear similar to seborrheic keratoses as well as keratoacanthoma, solar keratosis, and squamous cell carcinoma, in some cases. Plantar verrucae appear similar to clavi and must be distinguished from carcinoma cuniculatum, a variant of verrucous squamous cell carcinoma, if lesions persist. Epidermodysplasia verruci-

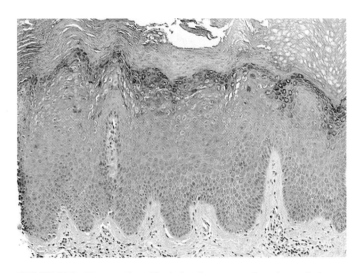

FIGURE 22-9 Verruca plana. The lesion demonstrates hyperkeratosis, hypergranulosis, slight acanthosis, and the characteristic vacuolated or "bird's eye" cells in the upper spinous layer.

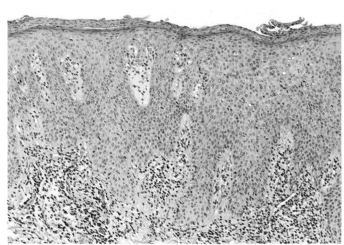

FIGURE 22-11 Bowenoid papulosis. The proliferative epidermis shows full-thickness atypia of keratinocytes.

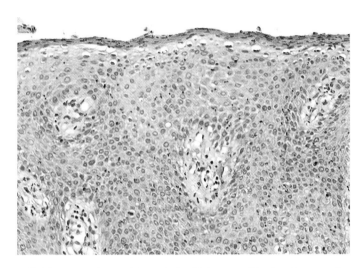

FIGURE 22-12 Bowenoid papulosis. Higher magnification demonstrating parakeratosis, absence of granular layer, and atypia of keratinocytes in the spinous layer.

formis may simulate morbilliform exanthemata in some cases.[53] With all of these conditions, histologic evaluation should allow for easy distinction.

CYTOMEGALOVIRUS

CMV is an enveloped, DNA virus measuring 110 nm in diameter that is a member of the herpesvirus group. The virus is widespread and subclinical infections are prevalent, as most of the population at large demonstrates some CMV antibody. Transmission is via body fluids, including saliva, blood, urine, semen, breast milk, and cervical secretions. Viral secretion may persist for years. Patients at risk for clinical infections are those immunocompromised for one reason or another, such as HIV-infected patients, transplant recipients, chemotherapy patients, and pregnant women.[54]

Clinical Features   Although most cases are subclinical, a "mononucleosis syndrome" that is similar to that caused by Epstein-Barr virus may develop (Table 22-8). Affected patients develop a sore throat without exudate, fever, malaise, myalgias, lymphadenopathy, and hepatosplenomegaly. An exanthem manifest by an eruption of erythematous macules and papules that may be either urticarial or petechial may develop. The eruption may be precipitated by administration of ampicillin as with infectious mononucleosis. A vasculitis with palpable purpura has also been reported.[55]

In patients with AIDS, CMV may cause chronic perineal and lower extremity ulcerations, chorioretinitis, gastroenteritis, pneumonia, as well as other visceral involvement.[56]

Fetal infection with CMV results in significant, often fatal, developmental abnormalities. As with congenital rubella, extramedullary hematopoiesis may be seen in the skin as purplish papules and nodules.

Histopathological Features   The acute exanthem of CMV infection generally appears histologically similar to other viral exanthemata with the possible exception of scattered enlarged fibroblasts and/or endothelial cells in the dermis. There is characteristically a sparse infiltrate of lymphocytes around blood vessels in the upper dermis with slight spongiosis. CMV does not infect keratinocytes so that epidermal changes

usually are minimal. Virally infected cells in the dermis are characteristically enlarged one- to three-fold and contain purplish, crystalline inclusions in the cytoplasm and the nuclei. These latter inclusions result in the characteristic "owl's eye" appearance of the cells.

CMV vasculitis is a manifestation of endothelial cell infection with swelling, inflammation, and secondary vascular compromise. Ulcerations in immunocompromised hosts are usually not caused by CMV itself but by another agent such as herpesvirus with secondary colonization.

Differential Diagnosis   Infectious mononucleosis, toxoplasmosis, listeriosis, other viral exanthemata, infectious hepatitis, and drug eruptions all must be excluded. CMV vasculitis appears similar to other forms of vasculitis and must be excluded on the basis of clinical and serologic grounds. Histologic visualization of infected cells is diagnostic.

POXVIRUS INFECTIONS

Poxviruses are the largest animal viruses and are the only viruses that are visible by light microscopy (Table 22-9). Three groups affect humans: orthopoxviruses such as variola and vaccinia, which are ovoid and 300 × 250 nm in diameter; parapoxviruses such as those that cause orf and milker's nodule, which are cylindrical and 260 × 160 nm in diameter; and the molluscum contagiosum virus, which has an oval, bullet-shape and is 275 × 200 nm in diameter. Humans may also be affected by tanapox, which is somewhat similar to the parapoxviruses.

TABLE 22-8

Cytomegalovirus Infection

Clinical Features

"Mononucleosis syndrome" similar to that caused by Epstein-Barr virus
Exanthem of macules and papules

Histopathological Features

Sparse spongiotic perivascular dermatitis
Characteristic "owl's eye" viral inclusion in endothelial cells
Vasculitis

Differential Diagnosis

Toxoplasmosis
Infectious mononucleosis
Listeriosis
Other viral exanthemata

TABLE 22-9

Poxvirus Infections

Orthopoxviruses
  Variola
  Vaccinia
  Cowpox
Parapoxviruses
  Orf
  Milker's nodule
  Tanapox
Virus of molluscum contagiosum

These are complex DNA viruses that replicate in the cytoplasm and are adapted to proliferation in keratinocytes. Spread is primarily by direct contact with infectious material from an infected individual or animal or via fomites, although variola is spread via aerosolized droplets.

Clinical Features   All of the poxvirus infections have prominent cutaneous manifestations. Although smallpox vaccination is no longer routine except in military settings, occasional infections with vaccinia are encountered. The most important manifestation is eczema vaccinatum, which represents a widespread eruption of edematous, inflamed lesions in individuals with altered cutaneous barrier function, such as those with atopic dermatitis who are exposed to the virus. There is usually high fever and lymphadenopathy. The condition may be fatal and there is a 5 percent mortality rate.

Animal poxviruses may affect humans. Human monkeypox is clinically indistinguishable from smallpox, although there is more marked lymphadenopathy.[57] Cowpox is primarily a disease of cattle, although humans may be infected on occasion. After an incubation period of 5 to 7 days, a papule develops that vesiculates, becomes pustular, and then ulcerates. The pustule, which is often umbilicated, is surrounded by a zone of erythema and edema. There is characteristically lymphangitis and lymphadenitis with fever, myalgia, and constitutional symptoms. Lesions heal over 3 to 4 weeks. Lesions are present on the hands, arms, or face most commonly and may be multiple.[58]

Orf is caused by a parapoxvirus that is widespread in sheep and goats, affecting mainly lambs and kids. Human lesions are caused by direct inoculation of infected material and are common among shepherds, veterinarians, surgeons, and other individuals with exposure to these animals.[59] There is an incubation period of 5 to 6 days, following which a small, firm, red or reddish-blue papule enlarges to form an umbilicated hemorrhagic pustule or bulla. The lesion enlarges to up to 3 to 5 cm in diameter and becomes crusted. There is a grayish to violaceous ring that is surrounded by a zone of redness and warmth. The lesions usually are solitary or few in number and are located most commonly on the fingers, hands, or forearms. There may be tenderness and associated lymphangitis and regional adenitis with mild fever. Spontaneous recovery is usual by 3 to 6 weeks.

Milker's nodule also is caused by a parapoxvirus that most commonly leads to infection of the teats and mouths of cattle, so that milkers, farmers, and veterinarians are accidental hosts. The infection may be transmitted by contaminated fomites in some cases. There is an incubation period of 5 days to 2 weeks, following which a small, red papule develops that enlarges and becomes violaceous, firm, and slightly tender over the course of 1 week.[60] The epidermis becomes opaque and grayish, and soon after a crust develops centrally. As with other poxvirus infections, there is usually central umbilication. There is a surrounding zone of erythema and there may be lymphangitis. Lesions resolve over 4 to 6 weeks without scar. In contrast to orf, lesions usually are not solitary and number between two and five, but may be more numerous. The most common sites of involvement are the hands and fingers. Rarely, a more widespread papulovesicular eruption of the hands, arms, legs, and neck may be associated.

Tanapox is an acute febrile illness associated with a localized nodular skin lesion caused by an unclassified poxvirus.[61] The infection was first seen in the Tana River area in Kenya and is probably widely distributed in tropical Africa. The virus affects monkeys and humans and is acquired by inoculation through abraded skin. There is mild preeruptive fever accompanied by headache and backache. The lesion begins as a localized zone of erythema and induration that develops into a nodule over the course of 2 weeks. The limbs are most commonly involved. There is usually accompanying localized lymphadenopathy that is often painful. The nodule ulcerates in the third week and heals slowly with a scar over 6 weeks. Most cases are characterized by a solitary lesion, although they may be multiple.

Molluscum contagiosum is the most common human disease induced by poxviruses. Infection follows contact with infected individuals and fomites. It is common in childhood, although it is rare under the age of 1 year. In children, the face, limbs, and trunk are commonly involved. A second peak occurs in young adults as a result of sexual transmission, with involvement of the genital and perineal skin. The face is commonly involved in HIV-infected patients. Any body site may be involved, including the mucous membranes. The incubation period ranges from 14 days to 6 months. The individual lesion is a translucent, skin-colored to whitish dome-shaped papule that is characteristically umbilicated with a central pore. Lesions range from 1 to 10 mm and may be significantly larger, sometimes assuming features similar to keratoacanthoma, especially in immunocompromised hosts. Small lesions may coalesce to form plaques. In time, lesions may become inflamed, suppurate, and become crusted, leading to the eventual resolution. Most cases are self-limited and resolve within 6 to 9 months, although some may persist for as long as 3 or 4 years.

Histopathological Features   The acute, inflammatory poxviral infections all have similar histologic features and are all manifest by prominent spongiosis, ballooning degeneration, dermal edema, and acute inflammation. Individual lesions demonstrate changes that are distinct and permit differentiation in many cases. In vaccinia and cowpox, there is proliferation of the basal layer of the epidermis that contains large, eosinophilic cytoplasmic inclusions. There is necrosis of the epithelium with spongiosis, pallor of keratinocytes, and a dense infiltrate consisting mostly of neutrophils, lymphocytes, and some eosinophils. Also, there are extravasated erythrocytes in the dermis with prominent papillary dermal edema.

Orf demonstrates marked inter- and intracellular edema, vacuolization, and ballooning degeneration (Fig. 22-13). There is a dense infiltrate in the dermis, which has a characteristic architecture, consisting mainly of histiocytes and macrophages centrally with lymphocytes and

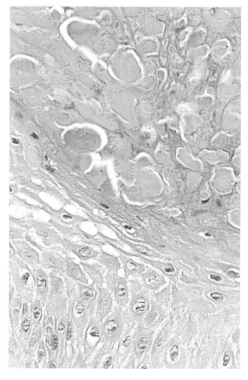

FIGURE 22-13 Orf. High magnification shows spongiosis and intracellular edema of the keratinocytes. Eosinophilic inclusions are noted in the cornified layer.

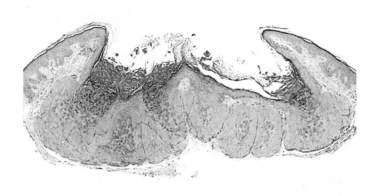

FIGURE 22-14 Molluscum contagiosum. Scanning magnification shows the characteristic lobular architecture of epithelium infected by molluscum contagiosum.

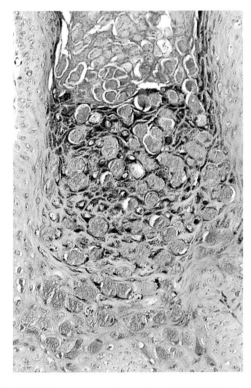

FIGURE 22-15 Molluscum contagiosum. The epithelial cells contain the characteristic eosinophilic cytoplasmic inclusion bodies. The nuclei are pushed to the periphery of the cell by the inclusion body.

plasma cells at the periphery. Characteristically, there are very few neutrophils. There is also prominent vascularity with an increased number of small blood vessels, many of which show swelling and proliferation of endothelial cells. Ultrastructural studies show viral particles within the cytoplasm of degenerating epidermal cells.

Milker's nodule is characterized by multilocular vesicle formation in the epidermis that is strikingly acanthotic. There is characteristically less ballooning degeneration than in orf. There is often marked parakeratosis, and eosinophilic cytoplasmic and intranuclear inclusions commonly are visualized. The dermis is edematous and there is an infiltrate of mononuclear cells that may be granulomatous.

The molluscum contagiosum virus initially enters basal keratinocytes and is accompanied by an increase in cell turnover leading to epidermal proliferation (Figs. 22-14 and 22-15). The basal layer remains intact, whereas cells at the core of the lesion become enlarged as a consequence of the accumulation of masses of viral material and appear as large purplish-red bodies (molluscum bodies) that are up to 25 μm in diameter. There is a distinct lobulated character to the proliferation that coalesces, forming a central crater that corresponds to the central umbilication seen clinically. Lesions typically have an exo-endophytic appearance. Inflammatory changes in the dermis usually are minimal, but may be pronounced when lesions rupture and discharge their contents into the dermis.

Differential Diagnosis Each of the inflammatory poxviral illnesses must be distinguished from one another on the basis of clinical setting, number of lesions, histologic findings, and electron microscopy. Other acute inflammatory infections must be excluded, including primary tuberculosis and sporotrichosis. Acute foreign body granulomatous reactions, pyogenic granulomata, as well as other processes associated with pronounced inflammatory reactions and dermal edema, such as Sweet's syndrome and polymorphous light eruption, must be excluded on both clinical and histologic grounds.

REFERENCES

1. White DO, Femer FJ: *Medical Virology*, 3rd ed., London, Academic, 1986.
2. Mandell GL, Douglas RG, Bennett JE (eds): *Principles and Practice of Infectious Diseases*, 3rd ed. New York, Churchill Livingstone, 1990.
3. Fraser KB, Martin SJ: *Measles Virus and Its Biology*. New York, Academic Press, 1978.
4. McNair Scott TF, Bonanno DE: Reactions to live measles virus vaccine in children previously inoculated with killed virus vaccine. *N Engl J Med* 277:248–250, 1967.
5. Ackerman AB, Suringa DWR: Multinucleate epidermal cells in measles: A histologic study. *Arch Dermatol* 103:180–184, 1971.
6. Cooper LZ, Ziring PR, Ockerse AB, et al: Rubella: Clinical manifestations and management. *Am J Dis Child* 118:18–29, 1969.
7. Castrow FF, De Beukelaer M: Congenital rubella syndrome: Unusual cutaneous manifestations. *Arch Dermatol* 98:260–262, 1968.
8. Miller E, Cradock-Watson JE, Pollock TM: Consequences of confirmed maternal rubella at successive stages of pregnancy. *Lancet* ii:781–784, 1982.
9. Anderson MJ, Lewis E, Kidd IM, et al: An outbreak of erythema infectiosum associated with human parvovirus infection. *J Hyg* 93:85–93, 1984.
10. Ager EA, Chin TDY, Poland JD: Epidemic erythema infectiosum. *N Engl J Med* 275:1326–1331, 1966.
11. Berenberg W, Wright S, Janeway CA: Roseola infantum (exanthem subitum). *N Engl J Med* 241:253–259, 1949.
12. Irving WL, Cunningham AL: Serological diagnosis of infection with human herpesvirus type 6. *Br Med J* 300:156–159, 1990.
13. Yamanishi K, Okuno T, Shiraki K, et al: Identification of human herpesvirus-6 as a causal agent for exanthem subitum. *Lancet* i:1065–1067, 1988.
14. Halstead SB: The pathogenesis of dengue. *Am J Epidemiol* 114:632–648, 1981.
15. Halstead SB: Observations related to pathogenesis of dengue hemorrhagic fever. *Yale J Biol Med* 42:350–362, 1970.
16. Cawson RA, McSwiggan DA: An outbreak of hand, foot and mouth disease in a dental hospital. *Oral Surg Oral Med Oral Pathol* 27:451–459, 1969.
17. Parra CA: Hand, foot, and mouth disease: Light and electron microscopic observations. *Arch Dermatol Forsch* 245:147, 1972.
18. Coffin JM: Retroviraidae and their replication, in Fields B, Knipe D, Chanock R (eds): *Virology*, 2nd ed. New York, Raven, 1990, pp. 1437–1500.
19. Tindall B, Barker S, Donovan B, et al: Characterization of the acute clinical illness associated with human immunodeficiency virus infection. *Arch Intern Med* 148:945–949, 1988.
20. Sinicco A, Palestro G, Caramello P, et al: Acute HIV-1 infection: Clinical and biologic study of twelve patients. *J Ac Immun Def Syndr* 3:260–265, 1990.
21. Gaines H: Primary HIV infection: Clinical and diagnostic aspects. *J Infect Dis* (suppl) 61:1–46, 1989.
22. Ho DD, Sarngadharan MG, Reznick, L, et al: Primary human T-lymphocyte virus type III infection. *Ann Int Med* 103:880–883, 1985.
23. McMillan A, Bishop PE, Aw D, Peutherer JF: Immunohistology of the skin rash associated with acute HIV infection. *AIDS* 3:309–312, 1989.
24. Safran S, Ashley R, Houlihan C, et al: Clinical and serologic features of herpes simplex virus infection in patients with AIDS. *AIDS* 5:1107–1110, 1991.

25. Gilson IH, Barnett JH, Conans MA, et al: Disseminated ecthymatous varicella-zoster virus infection in patients with acquired immunodeficiency syndrome. *J Am Acad Dermatol* 20:637–642, 1989.

26. Reichart PSA, Langford A, Gelderblom HR, et al: Oral hairy leukoplakia: Observations in 95 cases and review of the literature. *J Oral Pathol Med* 18:410–415, 1989.

27. Cockerell CJ: Mucocutaneous signs of AIDS other than Kaposi's sarcoma, in Friedman-Kien AE, Cockerell CJ (eds): *Color Atlas of AIDS*, 2nd ed. Philadelphia, Saunders, 1996.

28. Berger TG, Greene I: Bacterial, viral, fungal and parasitic infections in HIV disease and AIDS. *Dermatol Clin* 3:465–492, 1991.

29. Patterson JW, Kitces EN, Neafie RC: Cutaneous botryomycosis in a patient with acquired immunodeficiency syndrome. *J Am Acad Dermatol* 16:238–242, 1987.

30. Sangeorzan JA, Bradley SF, Kaufman CA: Cutaneous manifestation of *Pseudomonas* infection in the acquired immune deficiency syndrome. *Arch Dermatol* 126:832–833, 1990.

31. Barbaro DJ, Orcutt VL, Colder BM: *Mycobacterium avium-intracellulare* infection limited to the skin and lymph nodes in patients with AIDS. *Rev Infect Dis* 11:625–628, 1989.

32. Glover RA, Piaquadio DJ, Kern S, Cockerell CJ: An unusual presentation of secondary syphilis in a patient with human immunodeficiency virus infection: A case report and review of the literature. *Arch Dermatol* 128:530–534, 1992.

33. Cockerell CJ, LeBoit PE: Bacillary angiomatosis: A novel pseudoneoplastic, infectious vascular disorder. *J Am Acad Dermatol* 22:501–519, 1990.

34. Hennessey NP, Parro EL, Cockerell CJ: Cutaneous *Pneumocystis carinii* infection in patients with acquired immunodeficiency syndrome. *Arch Dermatol* 127:1699–1701, 1991.

35. Manrique P, Mayo J, Alvarez JA, et al: Polymorphous cutaneous cryptococcosis: Nodular, herpes-like, and molluscum-like lesions in a patient with the acquired immunodeficiency syndrome. *J Am Acad Dermatol* 26:122–124, 1992.

36. Cohen PR, Bank DE, Silvers DN, Grossman ME: Cutaneous lesions of disseminated histoplasmosis in human immunodeficiency virus–infected patients. *J Am Acad Dermatol* 23:422–428, 1990.

37. Chaker MB, Cockerell CJ: Concomitant psoriasis, seborrheic dermatitis and disseminated cutaneous histoplasmosis in a patient infected with human immunodeficiency virus. *J Am Acad Dermatol* 29:311–313, 1993.

38. Rosenthal D, LeBoit PE, Klumpp L, Berger TG: Human immunodeficiency virus–associated eosinophilic folliculitis: A unique dermatitis associated with advanced human immunodeficiency virus infection. *Arch Dermatol* 127:206–209, 1991.

39. Andiman WA: The Epstein-Barr virus and EB virus infections in childhood. *J Pediatr* 95:171–182, 1979.

40. Pullen H, Wright N, Murdoch J McC: Hypersensitivity reactions to antibacterial drugs in infectious mononucleosis. *Lancet* ii:1176–1178, 1967.

41. McElgunn PSJ: Dermatologic manifestations of hepatitis B virus infection. *J Am Acad Dermatol* 8:539–548, 1983.

42. Michalak T: Immune complexes of hepatitis B surface antigen in the pathogensis of periarteritis nodosa: A study of seven necropsy cases. *Am J Pathol* 90:619–632, 1987.

43. Caroli J: Serum sickness–like prodromata in viral hepatitis: Caroli's triad. *Lancet* I: 964–965, 1972.

44. Juel-Jensen BE, MacCallum FO: *Herpes Simplex, Varicella* and *Zoster*. London, Heinemann, 1972.

45. Gilson IH, Banett JH, Conant MA, et al: Disseminated ecthymatous herpes varicella-zoster virus infection in patients with acquired immunodeficiency syndrome. *J Am Acad Dermatol* 20:637–642, 1989.

46. Peto TEA, Juel-Jensen BE: Varicella zoster virus disease in Monk BE, Graham-Brown RAC, Sarkany I (eds): *Skin Disorders in the Elderly*. Oxford, Blackwell, 1988, pp. 80–96.

47. Nahmias AJ, Keyserling HL, Kerrick GM: Herpes simplex, in Remington JS, Klein JO (eds): *Infectious Diseases of the Fetus and Newborn Infant*, 2nd ed. Philadelphia, WB Saunders, 1983, p. 636.

48. Corey L: First-episode, recurrent and asymptomatic herpes simplex infections. *J Am Acad Dermatol* 18:169–172, 1988a.

49. Beutner KR, Becker TM, Stone KM: Epidemiology of HPV infections. *Dermatol Clin* 9:211–218, 1991.

50. Syrjanen SM, von Krogh G, Syrjanen KJ: Anal condylomas in men: 1. Histopathological and virological assessment. *Genito Med* 65:216–224, 1989.

51. Campion MJ: Clinical manifestations and natural history of genital human papillomavirus infection. *Obstet Gynecol Clin N Am* 14:363–388, 1987.

52. Rütlinger R, Buchmann P: HPV 16: Positive bowenoid papulosis and squamous cell carcinoma in an HIV-positive man. *Dis Colon Rect* 32:1042–1045, 1989.

53. Berger G, Sawchuk WS, Leonardi C, et al: Epidermodysplasia verruciformis–associated papillomavirus infection complicating human immunodeficiency virus disease. *Br J Dermatol* 126:79–83, 1991.

54. Jacobson MA, Mills J: Serious cytomegalovirus disease in the acquired immunodeficiency syndrome (AIDS). *Ann Intern Med* 108:585–594, 1988.

55. Lin CS, Pinha PD, Krishnan MN, et al: Cytomegalic inclusion disease of the skin. *Arch Dermatol* 117:282–284, 1981.

56. Feldman PS, Walker AN, Baker R: Cutaneous lesions heralding disseminated cytomegalovirus infections. *J Am Acad Dermatol* 7:545–548, 1982.

57. Jezek Z, Szczeniowski M, Paluku KM, et al: Human monkeypox: Clinical features of 282 patients. *J Infect Dis* 156:293–298, 1987.

58. Casemore DP, Emslie ES, Whyler DK, et al: Cowpox in a child, acquired from a cat. *Clin Exp Dermatol* 12:286–287, 1987.

59. Gill MJ, Arlette J, Buchan KA, et al: Human orf. *Arch Dermatol* 126:356–358, 1990.

60. Leavell UW, Phillips IA: Milker's nodules. *Arch Dermatol* 111:1307–1311, 1975.

61. Jezek Z, Arita I, Szczeniowski M, et al: Human tanapox in Zaire: Clinical and epidemiological observations on cases confirmed by laboratory studies. *Bull WHO* 63: 1027–1035, 1985.

62. Kwittken J: Molluscum contagiosum: Some new histologic observations. *Mt Sinai J Med* 47:583–588, 1980.

CHAPTER 23

PROTOZOAL AND ALGAL INFECTIONS OF THE SKIN

Ann Marie Nelson / Freddye Lemons-Estes

Protozoa are unicellular parasites that infect hundreds of millions of people each year. Infections are often latent but may progress to active disease when the host-parasite balance shifts in favor of the parasite. Numbers of parasites (at initial infection or later), host immunity, and other factors may influence this balance. International travel, extension of vector habitats, and increased numbers of immunocompromised hosts (chemotherapy, transplants, human immunodeficiency virus infection) have increased the pool of susceptible hosts.

Protozoa may cause cutaneous lesions as the primary target or as a secondary or incidental site. Leishmaniasis, the most common form of protozoal dermatitis, affects millions of people in the tropical and subtropical belts of the world. As many as a billion people carry *Entamoeba histolytica*, but cutaneous lesions are rare and occur as secondary complications of chronic diarrhea or fistulas. Lesions may develop at the inoculation site of visceral infections, i.e., kala-azar or Chagas disease. Iatrogenic and HIV-associated immunocompromise have resulted in an increase in acanthamebiasis and toxoplasmosis. Cutaneous lesions in these patients often represent a manifestation of disseminated disease. Many protozoal diseases cause cutaneous immune reactions in the absence of cutaneous organisms.

Algae, both chlorophyllic and achlorophyllic, cause infections in wild and domestic animals and may rarely cause disease in humans.

LEISHMANIASIS

Leishmaniasis is a spectrum of diseases caused by various species of the dimorphis protozoa *Leishmania* and is prevalent throughout Asia, Africa, the Americas, and the Mediterranean with up to 1.5 million new cases each year. Dogs, cats, and rodents typically serve as reservoirs. Humans acquire the infection from the bite of infected female sandflies carrying the flagellated metacyclic promastigote forms in their gastrointestinal tract. The infective promastigotes enter at the inoculation (bite) site and invade reticuloendothelial cells. There, they transform into aflagellate amastigotes and proliferate intracellularly until the cell ruptures. The incubation period for cutaneous leishmaniasis varies from 2 to 8 weeks but may be several months or years depending on the size of the inoculum and the immunologic status of the host.[1]

Three serologically and biochemically distinct species of *Leishmania*, *L. tropica*, *L. aethiopica*, and *L. major* are responsible for Old World leishmaniasis. They are transmitted by sandflies of the genus *Phlebotomus*. New World leishmaniasis with purely cutaneous involvement is caused by *L. braziliensis peruviana*, *L. braziliensis guyanensis*, and *L. mexicana*, all of which are transmitted by sandflies of the genus

Lutzomyia. *L. braziliensis braziliensis* is the etiologic agent of mucocutaneous leishmaniasis and is transmitted by the genera *Lutzomyia* and *Psychodopygus*. Visceral leishmaniasis is caused by three distinct subspecies of *Leishmania donovani*, *L. donovani donovani*, *L. donovani infantum*, and *L. donovani chagasi*. *L. donovani donovani* and *L. donovani infantum* are transmitted by the genus *Phlebotomus*, whereas *L. donovani chagasi* is transmitted by the genus *Lutzomyia*. New isolation and identification techniques continue to distinguish new subspecies of *Leishmania*.

Clinical Features Old World leishmaniasis (e.g., Baghdad boil, Biskra button, *Leishmania* tropica, Lahore sore, *bouton d' orient*) is characterized by two types of lesions, moist (rural) and dry (urban) (see Table 23-1). Moist lesions present as a slowly growing indurated red papule that may be intensely pruritic; multiple lesions are common. The papules enlarge in a few months to form nodules with an indurated border and dusky discoloration. These nodules tend to ulcerate within a few weeks, forming ulcers up to 5 cm in diameter with depressed granulating centers and raised indurated margins. Secondary bacterial infection is fairly common after ulceration. Spontaneous healing usually occurs within 6 months, leaving a characteristic depressed flattened white or pink cribriform scar. Dry lesions have a similar presentation but follow a more protracted course. Lesions are often single and occur primarily on the face. The progression to the nodular form occurs; however, the lesions do not ulcerate for several months. Healing may be delayed up to 2 years.[2]

New World leishmaniasis encompasses several clinical entities. The "Bay" sore typically occurs on the face as one or occasionally multiple erythematous plaques that typically do not ulcerate. "Apple-jelly" nodules resembling lupus vulgaris are sometimes seen. The "Chiclero" ulcer is similar but is more often a single erythematous plaque that ulcerates; it affects the ear in 40 percent of cases and can be quite destructive of the cartilage. "Uta" presents as one or several papules on exposed sites; lesions usually ulcerate and are self-healing. In "pian bois" there is a single skin ulcer. Lymphatic spread may occur and result in widespread ulceration; however, mucocutaneous involvement is extremely uncommon.

Leishmaniasis recidivans (lupoid leishmaniasis) is a relapsing form of the disease that may occur with any of the cutaneous leishmaniases but is usually secondary to *L. tropica* infection. Most cases are in Iran and Iraq. Typically arising months to years after the primary lesion has healed, the disease presents as erythematous sometimes circinate papules with a whitish scale.[3] Lesions begin on the face, often at the edge of healed scars, and spread on an erythematous base. Patients are

TABLE 23-1

Leishmaniasis

Clinical Features

Spectrum of disease caused by multiple species of *Leishmania*
Old World cutaneous (*L. tropica, L. major, L aethiopica*)
   Middle East, Africa, Asia, Mediterranean
     Rural (moist), multiple, progress from papules to ulcer with
       spontaneous healing in 6 months
     Urban (dry), single, on face, protracted course of up to 2 years
       or more
New World cutaneous and mucocutaneous (*L. braziliensis, L. tropica*)
   Bay sore usually visceral (*L. donovani*)

Histopathological Features

Ulceration often
Histiocytic infiltrates with varying admixtures of lymphocytes, neutrophils, and plasma cells
Epithelioid granulomas on occasion (with greater immunity)
Intracellular organisms (amastigote forms—Leishman-Donovan
   bodies) varied in number depending on age of lesion and immunologic status of host
Amastigotes with round basophilic nucleus and small basophilic
   rodlike kinetoplast
Giemsa stain—nucleus purple and kinetoplast intense red or reddish
   purple

Laboratory Evaluation

Giemsa, PAS, silver stains
Culture on Novy-MacNeal-Nicolle (NNN) or Schneider's *Drosophila*
   medium

Differential Diagnosis

American trypanosomiasis
Histoplasmosis
Rhinoscleroma
Granuloma inguinale
Leprosy
Atypical mycobacteriosis

Visceral leishmaniasis (kala-azar) infrequently presents with cuta-neous lesions. The reticuloendothelial system is the primary target of the parasite, and disease is generally characterized by fever, weight loss, hepatosplenomegaly, and pancytopenia. On rare occasions, an initial papule or nodule (leishmanoma) arises at the site of the infecting bite. Later in the course of the disease melanin deposition may result in hy-perpigmented patches on the forehead, over the temples, periorally, and on the midabdomen.

Post-kala-azar dermal leishmaniasis (dermal leishmanoid) occurs predominantly in India but may also be seen in Africa. Approximately 2 percent of patients in Africa develop the syndrome shortly after treat-ment, whereas 20 percent in India will develop lesions up to 10 years after treatment. The disease may present as hypopigmented or hyper-pigmented macules predominantly on the face (often in a butterfly dis-tribution) or as warty papules or nodules. The nodules are rarely greater than 1 cm and are found primarily on the face (especially around the mouth and nose) and to a lesser extent on the trunk and extremities. The lesions are chronic and may occur as a single type or in combination.

Histopathological Features   The diagnosis of leishmaniasis ultimately depends on the isolation or identification of the organism from tissue. Common to all leishmanial lesions are dermal infiltrates of large histio-cytes and varying numbers of organisms. The histiocytes range from 20 to 30 μm in diameter and have abundant cytoplasm. Organisms vary in number depending upon the age of the lesion and the immunologic sta-tus of the host. They are more numerous in early lesions and those aris-ing in the immunocompromised host. Amastigote forms (Leishman-Donovan bodies) are generally found intracellularly—singularly or in great numbers. In routine hematoxylin and eosin stained sections, amastigotes are 1 to 3 μm in diameter, round to oval, and nonencapsu-lated with a distinct cytoplasmic membrane (Fig. 23-1). Amastigotes have a round basophilic nucleus approximately 1 μm in diameter and a small basophilic rodlike kinetoplast. In Giemsa-stained sections the nucleus is purple and the kinetoplast an intense red or reddish purple. Various admixtures of lymphocytes, neutrophils, and plasma cells are also present. Areas of ulceration may have pseudoepithelial hyperplasia (PEH) at the edge of the ulcer and show predominantly nonspecific inflammatory infiltrates (Fig. 23-2). As the lesions age, there tends to be gradual reduction in the number of organisms[5] and histiocytes with

hypersensitive with good humoral and cellular immune (skin test) responses but are unable to completely eliminate the parasites. As the central lesion heals, active peripheral ones continue to form. The course is chronic and often relentless, lasting 20 to 40 years in some cases.

Disseminated cutaneous leishmaniasis presents as a single ulcer, nodule, or plaque on the face and other exposed areas. Nodular or plaquelike satellite lesions develop from the primary lesion and may disseminate over the entire body. Patients are anergic to leishmanial antigens and do not mount a specific cellular immune response to the infection. The organisms proliferate indefinitely, forming many lesions teeming with parasites.[4]

The ulcerative cutaneous lesions of mucocutaneous leishmaniasis develop exactly as those seen in Old World leishmaniasis but are more frequently multiple and tend to become extremely large. Cutaneous lesions may extend to involve mucosal surfaces, but lymphatic and hematogenous spread of parasites are the usual routes for mucosal involvement. Mucocutaneous leishmaniasis tends to occur in patients with untreated or poorly healing primary lesions. Although mucosal membrane involvement is uncommon in Central America, it is present in up to 80 percent of affected persons in Brazil and has a predilection for the nasopharynx.

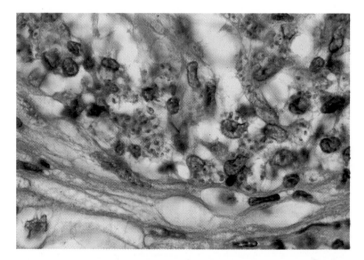

FIGURE 23-1   Cutaneous leishmaniasis. Skin biopsy showing numerous round to oval amastigotes in histiocytes. The nucleus is easily seen in most organisms; the smaller rodlike kinetoplasts are more difficult to identify.

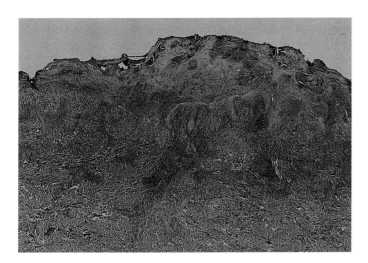

FIGURE 23-2 Cutaneous leishmaniasis. Skin biopsy showing diffuse, acute, and chronic inflammation with ulceration. There is an admixture of lymphocytes, plasma cells, histiocytes, and neutrophils extending into the deep dermis.

presence of yeast cells of *Histoplasma capsulatum* within histiocytes and occasionally within giant cells. In sections stained with hematoxylin and eosin, spores appear as 2- to 4-μm round to oval bodies surrounded by clear spaces. Spores are better visualized with methenamine silver stain. They also stain deeply basophilic with Giemsa or Gram's stain and are periodic acid–Schiff (PAS)-positive. In rhinoscleroma, the histiocytes (Mikulicz cells) range from 10 to 100 μm in diameter and have pale vacuolated cytoplasm containing the bacilli *Klebsiella rhinoscleromatis*. The bacilli are 2 to 3 μm in length and appear round to oval in cross section with routine hematoxylin and eosin staining. The organisms may be better visualized with Giemsa, PAS, or silver stains. The inflammatory infiltrate is rich in plasma cells with prominent Russell bodies. The intracytoplasmic inclusions (Donovan bodies) seen within the cytoplasm of histiocytes in granuloma inguinale are small, oval, and 1 to 2 μm in diameter. The multivacuolated histiocytes may be 20 μm or more in diameter. Each vacuole, also known as a *capsule*, contains a small Donovan body. They are better seen in Giemsa-stained sections which demonstrate bipolar staining of the inclusions surrounded by a paler-staining vacuole or capsule. The accompanying inflammatory infiltrate is rich in plasma cells with few lymphocytes and scattered microabscesses.

The histologic spectrum seen in leprosy varies with the type of disease. Histiocytes have abundant foamy or vacuolated cytoplasm and may be separated from the epidermis by a narrow grenz zone and may be scattered amongst other inflammatory cells in the dermis or form granulomata. The granulomata tend to be elongated and course along nerves. Epithelioid histiocytes may also be seen. Organisms are best seen with a Fite acid-fast stain and appear as red-staining bacilli measuring approximately 0.5 by 5 μm, primarily within histiocytes. Atypical mycobacteriosis also has a varied histologic appearance. Earlier lesions may show dermal infiltrates of histiocytes, lymphocytes, and neutrophils with occasional microabscess formation. As the lesions age, epithelioid and tuberculoid type granulomata as well as Langhans' giant cells are noted. Epithelial hyperplasia and hyperkeratosis may also be present. Variable numbers of organisms primarily within histiocytes are seen in acid-fast-stained sections.

development of a granulomatous infiltrate containing epithelioid cells and multinucleated giant cells. Caseous necrosis is notably absent.[6]

The pigmented lesions show varying amounts of melanin deposition, admixtures of lymphocytes, histiocytes, and plasma cells in the upper dermis. Organisms are sparse and may not be found in some lesions. Erythematous macular lesions tend to have a more cellular dermal infiltrate with a prominent plasma cell component. Organisms are generally more prevalent in these lesions than the pigmented variety. Nodular and warty lesions show varying degrees of epithelial hyperplasia and a dense dermal infiltrate of histiocytes and epithelioid cells admixed with lymphocytes and plasma cells that extends into the subcutaneous fat. A narrow grenz zone may separate the infiltrate from the epidermis. Organisms are abundant in some lesions and difficult to find in others. Ulcerated mucosal lesions show nonspecific inflammatory infiltrates in areas of ulceration, varying degrees of epithelial hyperplasia, and a dense dermal infiltrate of histiocytes, lymphocytes, and plasma cells. New lesions may have neutrophils admixed. Tubercle-type granulomata and Langhans'-type giant cells may also be observed.

Lesions in which organisms cannot be identified in histologic sections require culture of an aspirate from the edge of an ulcer or from a homogenate of tissue from the lesion using Novy-MacNeal-Nicolle (NNN) medium or Schneider's *Drosophila* medium for a specific diagnosis. The spindled flagellated promastigotes, which measure 10 to 15 μm, usually grow in 1 to 2 weeks; however, cultures should not be considered negative for 4 weeks. Direct smears of material obtained from the edge of an ulcer and stained with Giemsa may reveal organisms that are somewhat larger (2 to 4 μm) than those seen in fixed tissue.[7]

Differential Diagnosis The histopathological differential diagnosis includes American trypanosomiasis, histoplasmosis, rhinoscleroma, granuloma inguinale, leprosy, and atypical mycobacteriosis. Each of these entities is characterized by an infiltrate or parasitized histiocytes admixed with chronic inflammatory cells. However, *Leishmania* amastigotes can generally be differentiated histologically from other organisms.

Differentiation of *Leishmania* amastigotes from those of *Trypanosoma cruzi* may be quite difficult. *T. cruzi* amastigotes are larger (3 to 5 μm), round to oval with a distinct cytoplasmic membrane, a round nucleus, and a basophilic kinetoplast that is larger than that typically seen in *Leishmania*.[8] The diagnostic feature of histoplasmosis is the

TRYPANOSOMIASIS

Trypanosomiasis in humans is caused by two distinctly different species of the genus *Trypanosoma*. *T. brucei gambiense* and *T. brucei rhodesiense* are the etiologic agents of African sleeping sickness in western, eastern, and central Africa. *T. cruzi* is responsible for American trypanosomiasis (Chagas disease) and extends from the southern parts of the United States through Mexico, Central America, and as far south as Argentina. The highest prevalence is in Brazil. African trypanosomiasis is transmitted by the bites of male and female tsetse flies of the genus *Glossina*. *Glossina palpalis* and *G. tachinoides* most frequently transmit *T. brucei gambiense*; *G. pallidipes* and *G. morsitans* are the usual vectors for transmission of *T. brucei rhodesiense*. *Trypanosoma brucei gambiense* is limited by the habitat of its vectors to forest belts, especially along rivers in tropical west and central Africa and has no known animal reservoirs. The vectors of *T. brucei rhodesiense* are game-feeding tsetse that breed along lightly covered brush. The Rhodesian disease is typically confined to eastern Africa in the savanna areas where cattle are raised. *T. brucei rhodesiense* has several animal reservoirs (bushbuck, hartebeest, domestic ox, sheep). Humans are incidentally infected.

In the African forms of the disease, trypanosomes ingested by the fly during a blood meal reproduce in the midgut. Infective trypomastigotes are passed into the bite wound, when the fly feeds, and proliferate locally in the interstitium.[9] From there they enter the dermal lymphatics or general circulation. *T. brucei gambiense* and *T. brucei rhodesiense* do not directly invade most tissue cells but produce injurious effects on almost every tissue and organ in the body. American trypanosomiasis is transmitted by various species of the triatomid bugs (reduviid bug, "kissing bug," or "assassin bug"). A variety of mammalian hosts including domestic animals (especially dogs and cats), rodents, armadillos, bats, and raccoons serve as reservoirs. The reduviid bug ingests trypomastigotes while feeding on an infected animal. The parasite multiplies and matures in the gastrointestinal tract of the insect. The infective trypomastigotes are located in the hindgut and are passed in the feces that are stimulated as the insect feeds. The infective feces contaminate the insect's bite site, conjunctivae, mucous membranes, or breaks in skin. Trypomastigotes are engulfed by histiocytes or actively invade histiocytes, adipose cells, and muscle cells immediately below the inoculation site. Intracellularly they transform into aflagellate amastigotes and proliferate until the host cells rupture. Parasites are released to invade other cells and to enter the lymphatics or bloodstream to travel to distant sites.[10]

Congenital transmission may occur in both African and American trypanosomiasis but is extremely uncommon at any stage in the African forms of disease. Transmission of disease by contaminated blood products[11,12] and laboratory accidents also occurs.

Clinical Features   There are two distinct clinical forms of African trypanosomiasis (see Table 23-2). Gambian disease is characterized by prominent lymph node involvement, late invasion of the central nervous system, and a chronic progressive course that may last years before death ensues. Rhodesian disease is usually acute with chancre, fever, involvement of the central nervous system within 3 to 4 weeks, prominent cardiac symptoms, and death within 3 to 6 months if untreated. The incubation period in Gambian disease is asymptomatic and varies from a few days to several months in Africans. It is typically short in Rhodesian disease and in cases involving non-Africans.

A primary lesion, the trypanosomal chancre may appear at the bite site within 5 to 15 days. It is more common in Rhodesian disease and in non-Africans.[13] The painful chancre appears as a red-purple nodule 2 to 5 cm in diameter. It is well circumscribed and indurated and may have a surrounding white halo; ulceration may occur. The lesion persists for 2 to 3 weeks and spontaneously subsides. Trypanosomes may be in aspirates from the chancre and are seen in blood films at the end of the incubation period. The infection may be abortive and terminate without development of symptoms, or parasites may invade lymphatic tissues with accompanying febrile attacks. Generalized lymphadenopathy, which occurs as the disease progresses in both Gambian and Rhodesian disease, is much less pronounced in the latter. Prominent enlargement of the posterior cervical nodes is characteristic of Gambian disease and is known as *Winterbottom's sign*. It may not develop in Rhodesian disease. Trypanosomes are in aspirates from enlarged lymph nodes.

Cutaneous signs are more commonly associated with Rhodesian disease. An irregular, circinate, evanescent rash resembling erythema multiforme appears in up to 50 percent of all cases. It is commonly seen in non-Africans and is typically associated with fevers. The lesions occur primarily on the trunk, shoulders, and thighs. The rash is fairly transient, lasting only a few hours, and may be associated with underlying edema and pruritus. The rash is thought to represent a type III hypersensitivity reaction. Other less common lesions include urticaria, erythema nodosum, and transient painful edemas of hands, feet, and eyelids. Deep hyperesthesias (Kerandel's sign) are reported in 20 percent of Europeans but are uncommon in Africans.[4]

The incubation period for American trypanosomiasis or Chagas disease is approximately 5 to 17 days. Organisms proliferate at the site of the infecting bite and typically produce a single primary lesion or *chagoma,* but hematogenous dissemination may result in multiple lesions on the trunk and extremities.[4] The chagoma is an erythematous

TABLE 23-2

Trypanosomiasis

Clinical Features

Caused by *Trypanosoma gambiense* and *Trypanosoma rhodesiense*:
African forms of the disease (Gambian and Rhodesian forms)
   Trypanosomal chancre—painful red-purple nodule 2 to 5 cm at site of bites of tsetse flies
   Evanescent circinate eruption resembling erythema multiforme
   Urticaria, erythema nodosum, painful edemas
   Lymphadenopathy
Caused by *Trypanosoma cruzi*: American forms of the disease (Chagas disease)
   Chagoma—erythematous indurated nodule at site of bite of reduviid bug
   Acute, subacute, or chronic course
   Fever, malaise, edema of face and extremities

Histopathological Features

Trypanosomal chancre and chagoma
   Epidermal ulceration and hyperplasia
   Infiltrate of histiocytes, plasma cells, and lymphocytes
   Vasculitis
Trypomastigotes with nucleus and kinetoplast that stain with Giemsa
   Multiply in interstitium in chancre and intracellularly in chagoma

Laboratory Evaluation

Giemsa, Wright, Romanovsky stains
Culture *T. brucei gambiense* and *T. brucei rhodesiense* on Tobie and Weinnan media or *T. cruzi* on Novy-MacNeal-Nicolle (NNN) medium

Differential Diagnosis

Trypanosomal chancre
   Syphilis
Chagas disease
   Leishmaniasis
   Histoplasmosis
   Rhinoscleroma
   Granuloma inguinale

indurated nodule with a scale that eventually ulcerates. It attains a size of several centimeters within a few days and becomes very painful. Trypomastigotes or amastigotes may be aspirated from the chagoma in the early stages of disease. The lesion gradually subsides spontaneously over 2 to 3 months. Infections may occur via the conjunctival route resulting in unilateral lacrimal sac inflammation, conjunctivitis, edema, and erythema (Romaña's sign). Occuloglandular syndrome may also develop.

Chagas disease may pursue an acute, subacute, or chronic course. Acute disease is usually a mild febrile illness characterized by malaise, edema of the face and lower extremities, and generalized adenopathy. Amastigotes may be found in any enlarged lymph node and are most abundant in the regional nodes draining the chagoma. The acute phase resolves in 4 to 8 weeks followed by a latent or subacute phase of variable duration which is characterized by parasitemia and antibodies to many antigens of *T. cruzi*. Years to decades later 10 to 30 percent of infected individuals will develop the cardiac and/or gastrointestinal symptoms of chronic Chagas disease.[14] *T. cruzi* can also invade the central nervous system and in rare cases cause meningoencephalitis.

Histopathological Features   Definitive diagnosis of both African and American trypanosomiasis depends on the demonstration of the organism in blood or tissue (biopsy or aspiration material from bone marrow, enlarged lymph nodes, and primary skin lesions). Centrifuged cerebral spinal fluid is also a source of organisms when the central nervous system is affected. Trypomastigotes of *T. brucei gambiense* and *T. brucei rhodesiense* are morphologically identical and exhibit pleomorphism in human blood and spinal fluid. Typical slender flagellates (15 to 30 μm by 1.5 to 3.5 μm) with a pointed anterior end and blunted posterior exhibit a large central nucleus, small discrete subterminal kinetoplast, and an 8- to 30-μm flagellum which passes along the edge of an undulating membrane and projects from the anterior end. Their cytoplasm is pale and usually contains minute refractile volutin granules. Short or stumpy forms approximately 20 μm by 3.5 μm with or without a flagellum are also noted. The nucleus and kinetoplast stain dark and cytoplasm pale with Giemsa, Wright, and Romanovsky stains.[8]

The trypanosomal chancre is characterized histologically by an intense inflammatory infiltrate of histiocytes, plasma cells, and lymphocytes with marked interstitial edema and tissue damage. Typically there is vasculitis with endothelial cell proliferation, vasodilation, perivascular mononuclear cell infiltrate with prominent plasma cells, and fibrosis. Trypomastigotes multiply within the interstitium but are difficult to visualize in routine sections stained with hematoxylin and eosin.[15] Over-stained Giemsa sections are the preferred means of identification. Varying degrees of epithelial hyperplasia and ulceration with associated acute inflammatory changes may also be seen.

Histologic examination of enlarged lymph nodes show follicular hyperplasia with sinus histiocytosis and infiltration by plasma cells, lymphocytes, and pale-staining mononuclear cells. Trypomastigotes are generally quite prevalent and develop antigenic characteristics quite different from those organisms seen in blood. Lymphocyte depletion occurs as the infection progresses.[15]

T. cruzi appears in blood as trypomastigotes approximately 10 days after onset of infection and in tissue as amastigotes. The pleomorphic trypomastigotes range from 15 to 22 μm in length. They are characteristically C or S in shape. The nucleus is usually centrally located and a large oval kinetoplast is located at the extreme posterior end. The flagellum arises near the kinetoplast and passes through the margin of a delicate undulating membrane and proceeds anteriorly for approximately a third of the body length. Amastigotes of *T. cruzi* are small oval bodies 3 to 5 μm in diameter. They have a discrete cytoplasmic membrane, a round to oval nucleus, and a small rod-shaped kinetoplast. Amastigotes are predominantly intracellular and have a predilection for cells of mesenchymal origin; however, practically every organ of the body may be invaded.

Histologically, the chagoma consists of an intense inflammatory reaction with invasion of histiocytes, adipose cells, and adjacent muscle cells by amastigotes proliferating at the inoculation site. Varying amounts of epithelial hyperplasia and ulceration may also be seen. As the parasitized host cells rupture, there is an infiltrate of neutrophils and mononuclear cells, predominantly histiocytes. A lipogranuloma eventually forms but not prior to the spread of organisms to regional nodes. The lymph nodes show reactive follicular hyperplasia, sinus histiocytosis, and infiltrates of plasma cells, lymphocytes, and mononuclear cells.

Organisms may be difficult to find in blood, spinal fluid, and tissue in both African and American trypanosomiasis. *T. cruzi* may be cultivated on NNN medium and *T. brucei gambiense* and *T. brucei rhodesiense* on Tobie and Weinnan media. Diagnosis may also be made by inoculation of laboratory animals and xenodiagnosis. Note that small laboratory animals are less susceptible to *T. brucei gambiense*. Serologic techniques are available for detection of disease and have variable sensitivities and specificities.[16]

Differential Diagnosis   The vascular changes seen in the trypanosomal chancre resemble those in secondary syphilis.[17] Endothelial proliferation, vasodilation, and prevalent plasma cells in the perivascular infiltrate are seen in both diseases. Organisms may also be difficult to see in both and require special stains. A Giemsa stain will help identify trypanosomes and a Warthin-Starry silver impregnation will aid in the identification of spirochetes.

The differential diagnosis for American trypanosomiasis includes leishmaniasis, histoplasmosis, rhinoscleroma, and granuloma inguinale. The special features of each of these entities have already been discussed. The presence of a kinetoplast distinguishes *T. cruzi* from organisms lacking this structure. Differentiating American trypanosomiasis from leishmaniasis may be quite difficult but the kinetoplast of *T. cruzi* is larger than that of *Leishmania* species.

TOXOPLASMOSIS

Toxoplasma gondii is an obligate intracellular coccidian parasite that is transmitted to humans as infective oocysts from feline feces or by ingesting the undercooked meat of infected animals.[18] See Table 23-3. It is estimated that up to 50% of the population in the United States are infected; thus, reactivation rather than newly acquired infections is the major source of disease.[19] In immunocompetent hosts, the infection is usually arrested in the cyst stage, but these cysts may persist for life. Infection can progress to active disease in immunocompromised patients (e.g., HIV infection, chemotherapy, after transplantation).

TABLE 23-3

Toxoplasmosis

Clinical Features

Caused by *Toxoplasma gondii*
Cutaneous manifestations in <10% of acute infections, increased in immunocompromised
Recurrent infections rarely presenting as cutaneous dissemination
Most common presentation a maculopapular, erythematous rash over the trunk
Case reports of nodular, pustular, lichenoid, vegetative forms

Histopathological Features

Nonspecific, perivascular lymphoid infiltrates
Necrosis and hemorrhage variable
Organisms cannot be identified in 50% or more cases
Diagnostic forms include:
   Tachyzoites, round to crescentic, 4 to 8 μm, intra- or extracellular
   Pseudocysts, intracellular
   Cysts, spherical, filled with bradyzoites (PAS-positive)

Laboratory Evaluation

IgG and IgM, toxoplasma titers (Sabin-Feldman, IFA, agglutination, etc.)

Differential Diagnosis

Other causes of mononucleosislike syndromes (e.g., Epstein-Barr, cytomegalovirus)
Leishmaniasis and cutaneous trypanosomiasis (reaction, lack of kinetoplast in *T. gondii*)
Histoplasmosis (staining characteristics)

Clinical Features   Acute infection is often asymptomatic or mild. Symptoms vary, but most patients have fever and lymphadenopathy. Cutaneous lesions are less common but have been reported in up to 10 percent of patients. The frequency is higher in severe or disseminated cases or those in the immunocompromised host.[19–21] Approximately 1 percent of cases of acute mononucleosislike syndrome are due to acute toxoplasmosis. Cutaneous lesions also occur in reactivation cases. The most common manifestation is a maculopapular, erythematous rash involving the trunk. When extremities are involved, the palms and soles are usually spared.[22] Other lesions described in documented cases include nodular, papulopustular, lichenoid, vegetative, and erythema multiforme–like dermatitis.[22] Dermatomyositis and polymyositis are serologically linked to toxoplasmosis.

Histopathological Features   The histologic features vary with the clinical presentation.[18,20] Findings in the maculopapular rash are nonspecific, consisting of a perivascular lymphocytic infiltrate; vasculitis with necrosis and hemorrhage are reported in isolated cases. Definitive diagnosis requires visualization of the characteristic tachyzoites, pseudocysts, or cysts in tissue; hematoxylin and eosin staining is usually adequate. Tachyzoites actively enter cells, especially those of the reticuloendothelial system, and are found intracellularly or in areas of necrosis. They measure 4 to 8 by 2 to 3 μm on touch preparations but are smaller and more rounded in fixed tissue. Tachyzoites are only weakly PAS-positive and are not argyrophilic. Pseudocysts are intracellular colonies of zoites; they fit the contour of the parasitized cell, giving them an irregular shape. Pseudocysts measure from 8 to 30 μm in greatest dimension. True cysts are spherical in most tissue but elongate in muscle. They contain hundreds of tightly packed bradyzoites; the cyst membrane is thin, slightly eosinophilic, and argyrophilic. Bradyzoites appear as small, blue structures with little visible cytoplasm; they are strongly PAS-positive. Diagnostic forms of *Toxoplasma gondii* are detectable in fewer than half of the cutaneous biopsies, even by immunohistochemistry. The diagnosis in these cases is frequently based on identification of organisms from other sites such as brain (most common site of infection), bone marrow, or lung.

Differential Diagnosis   Clinically, cutaneous lesions of toxoplasmosis must be differentiated from the myriad other maculopapular rashes of various etiologies. Acute seroconversion, positive titers indicative of recrudescence, and/or identification of diagnostic organisms in other tissues is supportive of the diagnosis of toxoplasmosis[21] in the appropriate clinical setting. Histologic findings in most cases are also nonspecific. When organisms are identified, they must be differentiated from other protozoa (*Leishmania* or *Trypanosoma species*). The host response in leishmaniasis and trypanosomiasis is sufficiently different to eliminate misdiagnosis in most cases (see above); the zoites of *T. gondii* also lack kinetoplasts. *Histoplasma capsulatum* has a similar size and infects reticuloendothelial cells but, unlike *T. gondii*, usually elicits a granulomatous reaction in immunocompetent hosts. Yeast forms of *H. capsulatum* are surrounded by a small halo (shrinkage artifact) and silver with Grocott methenamine silver, features not seen in toxoplasmosis. Intracytoplasmic inclusions of cytomegalovirus (CMV) can mimic pseudocysts; if diagnostic intranuclear inclusions of CMV are not seen, immunohistochemical stains can be used for differential diagnosis. CMV inclusions are argyrophilic. Immunohistochemical studies increase sensitivity and specificity of diagnosis, but antibody may vary by lot or manufacturer. Polymerase chain reaction (PCR) techniques are now available.[23,24]

ACANTHAMEBIASIS

Acanthamoeba species (e.g., *A. castellani, A. culbertsoni, A. rhisodes, A. polyphaga*) and leptomixids (e.g., *Balamuthia mandrillaris*) are free-living amoebae found in soil and water throughout the world. Species that are able to tolerate temperatures above 37°C are most likely to cause human disease.[18,25–27] Multiplication occurs in the trophozoite stage by binary fission. Both cyst and trophozoite stages exist in nature and are identifiable in tissue sections. Transmission may occur via respiratory mucosa or contaminated skin lesions; spread is hematogenous. *Acanthamoeba* and *Balamuthia* infections are increased in contact lens wearers and in the immunocompromised host.

Clinical Features   Although granulomatous meningoencephalitis and keratoconjunctivitis are the classic clinical presentations, chronic skin lesions occur prior to or coincidental with CNS disease in a significant percentage of cases (Table 23-4).[28–31] Infections have been limited to skin in patients with AIDS. Skin lesions start as papules and nodules (cutaneous and subcutaneous), are usually multiple as well as multifocal, and may appear in crops. Lesions may be painful or nontender, indurated, and violaceous to erythematous and may progress to draining pustules and ulcers. The ulcers are poorly demarcated, have elevated borders, and eventually heal. Reported sites have included trunk, face, and extremities; several cases were disseminated. Secondary bacterial infection is also reported.

TABLE 23-4

Acanthamebiasis

Clinical Features

Caused by *Acanthamoeba* species and leptomixids (*Balamuthia mandrillaris*)
Most cases in immunocompromised (HIV-infected) hosts
Papules, ulcers, and nodules (cutaneous and subcutaneous)
Variably painful
Hematogenous dissemination with multiple, sometimes generalized eruptions
Can involve trunk, face, and extremities

Histopathological Features

Granulomatous inflammation and/or ulcers and abscesses
Vasculitis, sometimes leukocytoclastic
Trophozoites measure 8 to 25 μm, have characteristic "bull's-eye" karyosome
Cysts have wrinkled ectocyst (argyrophilic)
Immunohistochemical and electron microscopy aid in identification of species

Laboratory Evaluation

Culture on nonnutrient agar
Smears and aspirates can be used for wet-mount examination

Differential Diagnosis

Granulomatous and ulcerative infections in the immunocompromised host
Blastomyces dermatitidis infection
Other amebic infections

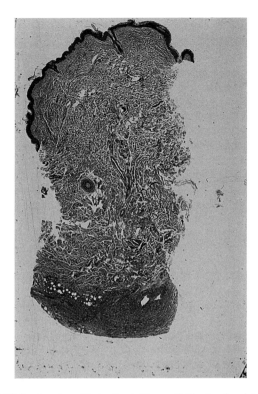

FIGURE 23-3 Acanthamebiasis. Punch biopsy of skin showing deep perivascular inflammation with abscess formation.

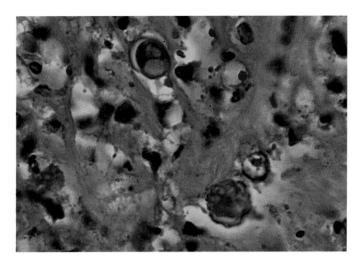

FIGURE 23-4 Acanthamebiasis. Trophozoites and cysts are present. Note the wrinkled ectocyst and the prominent nuclear karyosome.

Histopathological Features Histology shows granulomata with a marked cellular response consisting of histiocytes, lymphocytes, and plasma cells (Table 23-4).[28,32,33] A neutrophilic infiltrate may be present in pustules and acute ulcers and in cases of abscess formation (Fig. 23-3). Leukocytoclastic vasculitis has been reported.[29] Skin lesion in the immunocompromised host may show an altered response with lack of giant cells and only poorly formed granulomata. Variable numbers of organisms are throughout the lesion and may surround dermal vessels. Acanthamoeba trophozoites measure 8 to 12 μm in tissue; the leptomixids are somewhat larger, 15 to 25 μm. Both trophozoites and cysts are seen on hematoxylin and eosin. Cysts have a double-contoured wall, or ectocyst, that is wrinkled after fixation (Fig. 23-4). The ectocyst is best seen with silver impregnation, periodic acid–Schiff, or calcofluor white. Acanthamoebae have a single large nucleus with a large central karyosome (nucleolus) that has a "bull's-eye" appearance. *Balamuthia* may have double nuclei; the karyosome is less prominent than those of *Acanthamoeba*. The species usually cannot be determined by morphologic features; immunohistochemical stains, electron microscopy, or culture are required.

Differential Diagnosis Acanthamoeba infection must be differentiated from other papulonodular and ulcerative lesions in the immunocompromised host, including many parasitic, fungal, bacterial, and viral infections. Most of these can be ruled out by biopsy, direct examination of material, or culture. Cysts can be confused with *Blastomyces dermatitidis*; the yeast are slightly smaller and have broad-based budding and multiple nuclei and lack the prominent karyosome of the amoebae. Other parasites can be ruled out based on size and morphology. Macrophages may be confused with trophozoites; nuclear morphology or immunohistochemical stains can be used as diagnostic aids.

AMEBIASIS

Entamoeba histolytica is a pathogenic intestinal amoeba that is usually acquired via the fecal-oral route through ingestion of cysts.[18,34,35] Prevalence rates are highest in areas where sanitation is poor, such as developing countries. Most infected individuals are asymptomatic cyst passers; the parasite resides in the colon but does not invade mucosal tissues.[36] In most symptomatic patients, *E. histolytica* causes colitis or proctitis, but severe cases may spread to liver, lung, skin, or subcutaneous tissue. Cutaneous involvement results from several mechanisms: direct extension of a bowel infection to the anogenital region; at sites of perforation of fistulization of hepatic, pleural, or enteric abscesses; and as a consequence of surgical interventions. Genital (cervical, vulvovaginal, or penile) ulcers can occur, especially in patients who practice anal receptive intercourse or have poor hygiene. Rare cases of primary inoculation of the skin of the orbit, face, and legs are reported from contact with contaminated material.

Clinical Features Anogenital lesions present as serpiginous or spreading ulcers with well-demarcated, raised borders that are frequently undermined (Table 23-5). The ulcer crater contains necrotic slough, a sanguinopurulent exudate, and granulation tissue. Ulcers are often painful and have a variable course (weeks to years). Rapid, fatal spread has been reported in young patients or those with compromised immune status. Some patients develop granulomata (amebomas) or marked PEH resembling a condyloma (which may be clinically mistaken for carcinoma). Infection and malignancy may coexist, and secondary bacterial infection occurs. Either an ulcer or granuloma may form at the site of perforation.

Histopathological Features The lesions themselves are nonspecific. The ulcer has a necrotic base with acute and chronic inflammation, granulation tissue, and edema (Table 23-5). In chronic lesions granulomata and fibrosis may be prominent. Varying degrees of acanthosis and papillomatosis occur at the epithelial margin; pseudoepitheliomatous hyperplasia is common. Trophozoites are in the areas of inflammation or at the interface between necrotic and viable tissue. They measure 15 to 25 μm, have fine granular cytoplasm and phagocytized erythrocytes, and are usually isolated from the surrounding tissue by a small space

TABLE 23-5

Entamebiasis

Clinical Features

Caused by *Entamoeba histolytica*

Increased frequency in patients with poor hygiene, severe dysentery, or immunosuppression

Due to direct extension of invasive intestinal disease (most common), rupture or fistulization of hepatic or pleural abscesses, direct contamination (rare)

Painful, necrotic ulcers

Epithelial hyperplasia common

Histopathological Features

Ulcerative dermatitis with acute and chronic inflammation

Granulomata, marked pseudoepitheliomatous hyperplasia may be present

Trophozoites easily identified in tissues, 15 to 25 μm or greater

Typical nuclear structure with smooth rim of chromatin on nuclear membrane

Laboratory Evaluation

Direct smears stained with iron-hematoxylin or trichrome

Serologic tests are often nondiagnostic

Differential Diagnosis

Genital ulcer diseases

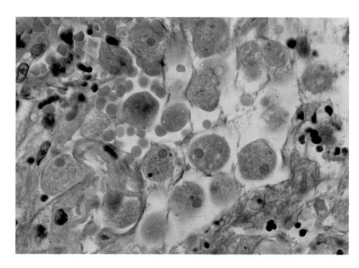

FIGURE 23-5   *Entamoeba histolytica.* On oil immersion multiple trophozoites can be seen. Note the lack of cohesion, the thin rim of nuclear chromatin, and the erythrophagocytosis.

(shrinkage artifact). The nucleus is small and round with a uniform, blue ring of chromatin along the nuclear membrane; it may not be visible in all sections. For the experienced observer, the organisms are easily seen on hematoxylin and eosin (Fig. 23-5) but may be easier to locate using periodic acid–Schiff stain. Material from the ulcer edge can also be examined directly, using iron hematoxylin or trichrome stains.

Differential Diagnosis   Clinically, the ulcers must be differentiated from other anogenital or cutaneous ulcers (e.g., syphilis, chancroid, or viral) by biopsy or direct smear. Pseudoepitheliomatous lesions should be differentiated from carcinomas or condylomas. Trophozoites of *E. histolytica* can be differentiated from macrophages by their nuclear configuration; the nuclei of macrophages are convoluted and have an irregular distribution of chromatin.

PROTOTHECOSIS AND CHLORELLOSIS

Protothecosis is a rare exogenous, nontransmissible infection caused by the achlorophyllic algae *Prototheca wickerhamii* and *P. zopfii*.[37,38] Both species are ubiquitous in soil, contaminated water, and vegetation. The index case of human protothecosis was reported in a rice farmer from Sierra Leone in 1964.[39] There are now more than 60 cases recorded in the world literature[40,41]; they have come from almost all continents in both tropical and temperate climates. Cases have recently been reported in HIV-infected individuals.[41–43] *Chlorella* species are chlorophyllic or green algae. Although chlorellosis has been described in several animals, there is only one published report involving a human.[40]

Clinical Features   There are two clinical syndromes associated with *Prototheca* infection: a localized infection of the olecranon bursa in patients with normal immunity and an eczematoid dermatitis in immunocompromised individuals (Table 23-6).[40,44,45] Infections have also

involved subcutaneous tissue, lymph nodes, and deep organs, and there is a recent report of meningitis in an HIV-infected individual.[43] Many infections have been associated with trauma and/or contact with contaminated water, but the source of the infection is often unknown.

Protothecosis of the olecranon bursa develops several weeks after injury to the elbow. There is local swelling or thickening of the bursa, development of draining sinuses, and epithelial hyperplasia. Systemic symptoms are not reported. In the cutaneous and subcutaneous forms there are single or multiple lesions, usually over an exposed surface of the body such as the face or limbs. The lesions develop slowly, spread centrifugally, and do not resolve. Typical lesions are indurated and maculopapular with an overlying crust and may have focal ulceration.

Histopathological Features   In olecranon bursitis, histopathologic changes include areas of caseation necrosis surrounded by granulation tissue, Langhans' giant cells, and fibrosis (Table 23-6). *Prototheca* organisms are scattered throughout the areas of caseation. In the cutaneous lesions, the inflammatory response varies from minimal to necrotizing granulomata and appears related to the depth of the invasion. The organisms may be in any or all layers of the skin and may be single or in clusters, extracellular or within giant cells. Although the organisms are usually apparent on routine staining by hematoxylin and eosin (H&E), they are much better seen with fungal stains such as Gomori methenamine-silver (GMS), PAS, and Gridley fungus (GF). These spherical, unicellular organisms with hyaline sporangia reproduce asexually by internal septation and cytoplasmic cleavage. *P. wickerhamii* is smaller and measures from 2 to 12 μm in diameter; *P. zopfii* measures from 10 to 25 μm. *P. wickerhamii* divides to form characteristic morulas (Fig. 23-6), a form usually not produced by *P. zopfii*.[37,40] Fluorescent immunoassay aids in determining the species; specific antisera for each of the *Prototheca* species are available and can be used on either fresh or formalin-fixed tissue. *Chlorella* are similar to *Prototheca* and must be differentiated in tissue sections by immunohistochemical staining or electron microscopy.[37] Material from skin scrapings, biopsy, and aspirates can be cultured on Sabouraud's medium and require 1 to 2 days for growth. Differentiation is done by sugar assimilation tests.[37,46]

Differential Diagnosis   Protothecosis of the olecranon bursa is quite specific clinically and can be confirmed by biopsy, wet mount, or culture. Cutaneous protothecosis must be differentiated from other granu-

TABLE 23-6

Prototheosis and Chlorellosis

Clinical Features

Caused by *Prototheca wickerhamii* or *Prototheca zopfii*
Rare, < 100 reported cases worldwide
Majority of cases in adults, Men slightly > women
Associated with contaminated water or soil
Two syndromes:
    Olecranon bursitis in immunocompromised host
    Chronic eczematoid dermatitis

Histopathological Features

Granulomatous inflammation, may have caseous necrosis in bursa
Severity of skin lesions related to depth of invasion
Organisms in areas of necrosis
Diagnostic features include
    Size (*P. wickerhamii*, 2–12 μm; *P. zopfii* 10–25 μm)
    Septation and morula formation
    Stain well with fungal stains
Species identification by immunofluorescence
Confirmation by electron microscopy

Laboratory Evaluation

Culture on Sabouraud's medium
Sugar assimilation

Differential Diagnosis

Olecranon bursitis is clinically unique
Granulomatous dermatitides (fungal, mycobacterial, etc.)
Chromomycosis

---

lomatous diseases; biopsy or culture is required. *Prototheca* species are distinguished from *Cryptococcus neoformans*, *Coccidiodes immitis*, *Blastomyces dermatitidis*, and other fungi by the type of division. In rare cases mimicking chromomycosis,[47] or if typical morula or septate forms are not seen, immunofluorescence studies can be performed.

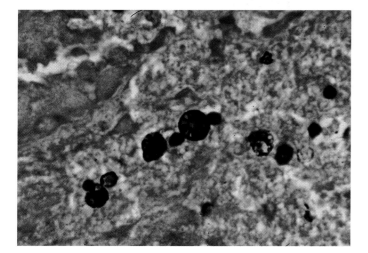

FIGURE 23-6 *Prototheca wickerhamii.* Grocott methenamine silver impregnation of olecranon bursa biopsy reveals the pleomorphic organisms; note the classic morula or "daisy" form.

REFERENCES

1. Kubba R, Al-Gindan Y, El-Hassan AM, et al: Clinical diagnosis of cutaneous leishmaniasis (oriental sore). *J Am Acad Dermatol* 16:1183–1189, 1987.
2. Kubba R, Al-Gindan Y: Leishmaniasis. *Dermatol Clin North Am* 7:331–351, 1989.
3. Norton SA, Frankenburg S, Klaus SN: Cutaneous leishmaniasis acquired during military service in the Middle East. *Arch Dermatol* 128:83–87, 1992.
4. Mackey S, Wagner K: Dermatologic manifestations of parasitic diseases. *Infect Dis Clin North Am* 8(3):713–743, 1994.
5. Herwaldt BL, Arana BA, Navin TR: The natural history of cutaneous leishmaniasis in Guatemala. *J Infect Dis* 165:518–527, 1992.
6. Ridley DS, Ridley MJ: The evolution of the lesion in cutaneous leishmaniasis. *J Pathol* 141:83–96, 1983.
7. Evans TG: Leishmaniasis. *Infect Dis Clin North Am* 7:3:527–546, 1993.
8. Conner DH, Neafie RC, Dooley JR: African trypanosomiasis, in Binford CH, Connor DH (eds): *Pathology of Tropical and Extraordinary Diseases*. Washington, DC, Armed Forces Institute of Pathology, 1976, pp 252–257.
9. Bales JD: African trypanosomiasis, in Strictland GT (ed): *Hunter's Tropical Medicine*, 7th ed. Philadelphia, WB Saunders, 1991, pp 617–628.
10. Tulio M, Garcia-Zapata A, McGreevy PB, et al: American trypanosomiasis, in Strictland GT (ed): *Hunter's Tropical Medicine*, 7th ed. Philadelphia, WB Saunders, 1991, 628–638.
11. Grant H, Gold JWM, Wittner M, et al: Transfusion-associated acute Chagas disease acquired in the United States. *Ann Intern Med* 111:849–850, 1989.
12. Nickerson P, Orr P, Schroeder ML, et al: Transfusion-associated *Trypanosoma cruzi* infection in a non-endemic area. *Ann Int Med* 111:851–853, 1989.
13. Duggan AJ, Hutchinson MP: Sleeping sickness in Europeans: A review of 109 cases. *J Trop Med Hyg* 69:124–131, 1966.
14. Kirchoff LV: Chagas disease. *Infect Dis Clin North Am* 7(3):487–502, 1993.
15. Gutierrez Y: Blood and tissue flagellates, in Gutierrez Y (ed): *Diagnostic Pathology of Parasitic Infections with Clinical Correlations*. Philadelphia, Lea & Febiger, 1990, pp 20–54.
16. Cattland P, de Raadt P: Laboratory diagnosis of trypanosomiasis. *Clin Lab Med* 11:899–908, 1991.
17. Cochran R, Rosen T: African trypanosomiasis in the United States. *Arch Dermatol* 119:670–674, 1983.
18. Orihel TC, Ash LR: Protozoa, in *Parasites in Human Tissues*. Chicago, American Society of Clinical Pathologists, 1995, pp 2–69.
19. Dover JS, Johnson RA: Cutaneous manifestations of human immunodeficiency virus infection. *Arch Dermatol* 127:1549–1559, 1991.
20. Gutierrez Y: The tissue apicomplexa, in Gutierrez Y (ed): *Sarcocystis lindemanni* and *Toxoplasma gondii*, in *Diagnostic Pathology of Parasitic Infections with Clinical Correlations*. Philadelphia, Lea & Febiger, 1990, pp 108–135.
21. Frenkel JK: Toxoplasmosis, in Strickland GT (ed): *Hunter's Tropical Medicine*, 7th ed. Philadelphia, WB Saunders, 1991, pp 658–669.
22. Mawhorter SD, Effron D, Blinkhorn R, Spagnuolo PJ: Cutaneous manifestations of toxoplasmosis. *Clin Infect Dis* 14:1084–1088, 1992.
23. Beaman MH, McCabe RE, Wong SY, et al: *Toxoplasma gondii*, in Mandell GL, Bennett JE, Dolin R (eds): *Mandell, Douglas, and Bennett's Principles and Practice of Infectious Diseases*, 4th ed, vol 2. New York, Churchill Livingstone, 1995, pp 2455–2475.
24. Woods GL, Gutierrez Y: *Diagnostic Pathology of Infectious Diseases*. Philadelphia, Lea & Febiger, 1993, pp 503–505.
25. Visvesvara GS, Stehr-Green JK: Epidemiology of free-living ameba infections. *J Protozool* 37:25S–33S, 1990.
26. Culbertson CG: Amebic meningoencephalitides, in Binford CH, Connor DH (eds): *Pathology of Tropical and Extraordinary Diseases: An Atlas*. Washington, DC, Armed Forces Institute of Pathology, 1976, pp 317–324.
27. Ma P, Visvesvara S, Martinez A, et al: *Naegleria* and *Acanthamoeba* infections: Review. *Rev Infect Dis* 12:506–509, 1990.
28. Gutierrez Y: The free-living amebae: *Naegleria* and *Acanthamoeba*, in Gutierrez Y (ed): *Diagnostic Pathology of Parasitic Infections with Clinical Correlations*. Philadelphia, Lea & Febiger, 1990, pp 80–93.
29. Helton J, Loveless M, White CR Jr: Cutaneous *Acanthamoeba* infection associated with leukocytoclastic vasculitis in an AIDS patient. *Am J Dermatopathol* 15:146–149, 1993.
30. Tan B, Linne-Weldon M, Rhone DP, et al: *Acanthamoeba* infection presenting as skin lesions in patients with the acquired immunodeficiency syndrome. *Arch Pathol Lab Med* 117:1043–1046, 1993.
31. May L, Sidhu G, Buchness M: Diagnosis of *Acanthamoeba* infection by cutaneous manifestations in a man seropositive to HIV. *J Am Acad Dermatol* 26:352–355, 1992.
32. Von Lichtenberg F: Protozoal infections, in *Pathology of Infectious Diseases*. New York, Raven Press, 1991, pp 243–295.
33. Lever WF, Schaumburg-Lever G: Diseases caused by protozoa, in *Histopathology of the Skin*, 6th ed. Philadelphia, JB Lippincott Company, pp 356–359.
34. Connor DH, Neafie RC, Meyers WM: Amebiasis, in Binford CH, Connor DH (eds): *Pathology of Tropical and Extraordinary Diseases: An Atlas*. Washington, DC, Armed Forces Institute of Pathology, 1976, pp 308–316.

35. Wolfe MS: Amebiasis, in Strickland GT (ed): *Hunter's Tropical Medicine*, 7th ed. Philadelphia, WB Saunders Company, 1991, pp 550–565.

36. Gutierrez Y: The intestinal amebae, in *Diagnostic Pathology of Parasitic Infections with Clinical Correlations*. Philadelphia, Lea & Febiger, 1990, pp 55–79.

37. Chandler FW, Watts JC: Protothecosis and infections caused by green algae, in *Pathologic Diagnosis of Fungal Infections*, 2d ed. Chicago, American Society of Clinical Pathologists, 1987, pp 43–53.

38. Naryshkin S, Frank I, Nachamkin I: *Prototheca zopfii* isolated from a patient with olecranon bursitis. *Diagn Microbiol Infect Dis* 6:171–174, 1987.

39. Davies RB, Spencer H, Wakelin PV: A case of human protothecosis. *Trans Roy Soc Trop Med Hyg* 1964, 58:448–451.

40. Nelson AM, Neafie RC, Connor DH: Cutaneous protothecosis and other extraordinary "aquatic-borne" cutaneous infections, in Mandojano RM (ed): *Clinical Dermatology (Aquatic Dermatology)*. Philadelphia, JB Lippincott Company, 1987, pp 76–87.

41. Woolrich A, Koestenblatt E, Don P, Szaniawski W: Cutaneous protothecosis and AIDS. *J Am Acad Dermatol* 31:920–924, 1994.

42. Laeng RH, Egger C, Schaffner T, et al: Protothecosis in an HIV-positive patient. *Am J Surg Pathol* 18(12):1261–1264, 1994.

43. Kaminaski ZC, Kapila R, Sharer LR, et al: Meningitis due to *Prototheca wickerhamii* in a patient with AIDS. *Clin Infest Dis* 15:704–706, 1992.

44. Connor DH, Gibson DW, Ziefer AM: Diagnostic features of three unusual infections: Micronemiasis, phaeomycotic cyst, and protothecosis, in Majno G, Cotran RS (eds): *Current Topics in Inflammation and Infection*. Baltimore, William and Wilkins, 1982, pp 205–239.

45. Tyrin SK, Lee PC, Walsh P, et al: Papular protothecosis of the chest: Immunologic evaluation and treatment with a combination of oral tetracycline and topical amphotericin B. *Arch Dermatol* 125:1249–1252, 1989.

46. Kuo TT, Hsueh S, Wu JL, Wang AM: Cutaneous protothecosis: A clinicopathologic study. *Arch Pathol Lab Med* 111:737–740, 1987.

47. McAnally T, Parry EL: Cutaneous protothecosis presenting as recurrent chromomycosis. *Arch Dermatol* 121:1066–1069, 1985.

CHAPTER 24

HELMINTHIC DISEASES
OF THE SKIN

Franz von Lichtenberg

Skin lesions caused by endemic worm infections continue to plague millions of people in tropical rural regions, but multinational efforts to eradicate guinea worm disease[1] and to prevent African river blindness caused by *Onchocerca volvulus*[2] are now well under way. With improving hygiene and antibiotic use, elephantiasis caused by lymph-dwelling filariae has also been fading slowly. Skin lesions caused by helminth species domestic to the United States and Europe have always been uncommon but do crop up occasionally as do imported cases. Although when biopsied, such specimens are usually sent to a helminthologist for consultation, any knowledgeable pathologist should be able to arrive at a precise, etiologic diagnosis with a small set of specific morphologic criteria and with information on patient exposure or travel. The life cycles of parasitic worms may be complex and varied, but humans can only be infected in three manners: ingestion of eggs or larvae (see *cysticercosis*); skin penetration of larvae (see *strongyloidiasis*); or bite or sting of an insect vector (see *bancroftian filariasis*). Many vector-borne helminths are linked to a specific environment or geographic area (see *snail-borne Schistosoma haematobium*); other helminths are obligate parasites of nonhuman hosts which act as their reservoirs (see *larva migrans*). Therefore, helminth-infected patients should always be asked three questions: (1) Where have you been ("Unde venis")?; (2) What have you eaten ("Quod edisti")?; and (3) What contacts have you had with vectors and wild or domestic animals ("Quod tetigisti")? At a minimum, these questions should help to clarify whether a given helminth infection is likely to have been acquired in a temperate zone or in the tropics.

When a suspected helminth structure is seen microscopically, whether intact or damaged, one should first exclude the possibility of confusion with insect or plant material (see algorithm, Fig. 24-1). Plant cells can easily be recognized by their stiff, refringent angular cell walls and prominent glycogen granules; insect cuticles are chitinous, thick, and pigmented and may show elaborate appendages, e.g., legs or mandibles; nevertheless, distinction between a partially destroyed worm or helminth egg and other kinds of partly digested foreign body material can sometimes be difficult. Both may appear fragmented and birefringent under polarized light and therefore distinguishable only by virtue of their microscopic contour.

The most critical decision to be made regarding helminth structures in the skin concerns taxonomy, i.e., whether a given nematode structure belongs to the order of roundworms (nematodes), tapeworms (cestodes), or flukes (trematodes) (Fig. 24-1). In dermatopathology, that decision is relatively simple, since adult tapeworms and their eggs are restricted to the gut lumen, and the only cestode life stage found in the human skin is thus a cystic larva. In addition, all roundworm (nematode) species whose adult specimens are able to dwell in cutaneous tissue are viviparous, i.e., spawn larvae but not eggs. By the same token, when noncystic helminth larvae are found in the skin, they most likely belong

to a roundworm (nematode). The only skin lesion caused by trematode larvae is a transitory and rarely biopsied rash known as *swimmer's itch*. Finally, adult trematodes have short life spans in ectopic sites, such as subcutaneous tissue, and therefore seldom are found intact; instead, they can usually be identified by the characteristics of their residual eggs (see *paragonimiasis*). The following histologic criteria are useful for assigning specimens to each of the three helminth orders:

1. *Adult nematodes* in the skin can range in length from a barely visible 2 mm to 35 cm and are round and slender in contour; they have a nonsegmented body with a true collagenous epicuticle surrounding a coelomic cavity which contains their sexually differentiated reproductive organs as well as a digestive tract with a distinct, proximal esophageal segment (Fig. 24-2) and with both buccal and anal openings. *Invasive nematode* larvae are at least one order of magnitude smaller than their corresponding adults, measuring up to 500 μm in length but no more than 10 to 30 μm in cross section (see *strongyloidiasis*). They lack sexual differentiation and show tiny, basophilic, dotlike nuclei (Fig. 24-3).

2. *Tapeworm larvae* in the skin range in size from 1 to 10 cm. They form rounded cysts bound by a hyaline wall and contain an inwardly protruding embryo lined by a noncollagenous syncytial absorptive tegument with a brush border (*gastrodermis*). When a scolex or scolices are present (Fig. 24-4), they possess arrays of sucker plates and rostella studded with sharktooth-shaped hooklets.

3. *Adult trematodes* (*flukes*) found in the skin are leaf-shaped. They are nonsegmented worms with a syncytial, noncollagenous tegument showing specializations, e.g., spines or tubercles, ventral sucker plates, a primitive gut ending in two blind bifurcations (ceca), and either hermaphroditic or sexually dimorphic reproductive organs, with prominently granulated vitellaria (Fig. 24-5). *Trematode eggs* can have round or elliptic shells and can measure up to 140 μm in greatest diameter. Fragmented or calcified eggs are of course smaller. Skin-penetrating *trematode larvae*, like those of nematodes, are of microscopic size but instead of a true cuticle they have a syncytial, noncollagenous tegument, and their nuclei are larger and more distinct than those of roundworm larvae (Fig. 24-6).

By following the algorithmic sequence outlined in Fig. 24-1, i.e., the successive definition of helminth life stage, taxonomic order, and likely site of patient exposure, the differential diagnosis of parasitic helminths can be narrowed down to a small number of possibilities from which the definitive diagnosis is then chosen by applying species-specific criteria (outlined below). If the characteristics of the parasite differ from those of any listed species, consultation is advised, since rare and new helminthic infections of humans are discovered from time to time and should by all means be reported.[3]

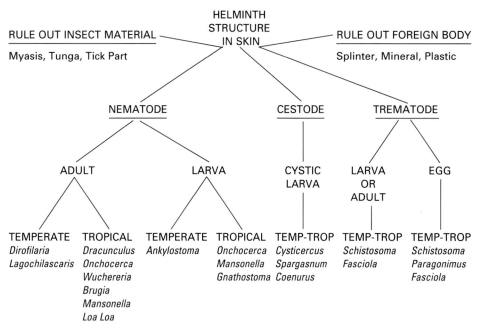

FIGURE 24-1 Algorithm proposed for speciating helminth material found in tissue sections.

NEMATODE INFECTIONS

Onchocerciasis (Oncocerciasis, River Blindness, Sowda)

Onchocerciasis is a chronic dermatitis, accompanied by progressive keratitis, uveitis, and loss of sight ("river blindness") caused by the filarial nematode *Onchocerca volvulus*, which is transmitted by the bite of black flies (*Simulium* subspecies). Onchocerciasis is endemic in the savannahs and rain forests of subequatorial Africa, and in Yemen, central America, and the Amazon basin of South America. The skin and eye lesions are elicited by numerous tissue-invading microfilariae spawned by relatively few adult worms dwelling in scattered subcutaneous inflammatory nodules which are walled off by dense fibrous tissue.

Clinical Features Onchocercal nodules are discrete, movable, up to 5 cm across, and often located close to bony prominences. Endemic onchocercal dermatitis is intensely itchy, predominantly papular and lichenoid, and, if severe and untreated, can lead to cachexia and death from intercurrent infection. Lesions are most often generalized; less frequently, especially in Yemen and in the savannah regions of Africa, lesions are limited to a single extremity (Sowda).[4] Depending on their duration, the lesions can be spottily depigmented (*leopard skin*), scaly and atrophic (*lizard skin*), or thickened and hyperkeratotic (*elephant skin*). In advanced disease there may be lymphedema of the groin (*hanging groin*). Onchocerciasis acquired by travelers to endemic regions is seen up to 2 years later as an itchy rash with marked peripheral eosinophilia, sometimes affecting one extremity only (as in Sowda).

Histopathological Features Onchocercal nodules contain several long, tangled, and coiled worms of both sexes. In cross section they measure up to 450 μm in diameter—one of the largest human parasitic filariae (Fig. 24-7). The female worms show prominent bicornual uteri

containing maturing microfilariae which are unsheathed, measuring up to 350 μm in length by 9 μm in width. In patients treated with ivermectin or diethyl carbamazine (DEC), adult worms appear largely intact, but their uteri are empty of microfilariae. Adult worms are embedded in dense granulation tissue and in mixed inflammatory cells including macrophages and multinuclear giant cells of the foreign-body type. These aggregates, in turn, are surrounded by thick layers of collagen bundles encapsulating the nodules. Microfilariae in transit toward the epidermis and cornea can be spotted insinuating themselves between collagen fibers. Because of their slender width, microfilariae seen in cross section can be confused with host cell nuclei.

Early epidermal changes in onchocerciasis may be minimal with variable numbers of microfilariae, concentrated in the papillary dermis, and with clusters of macrophages, plasma cells, and eosinophils surrounding vessels and adnexa. Little or no inflammation is seen around intact microfilariae (Fig. 24-8), but degenerate larvae can evoke focal microabscesses followed by granuloma formation as the dead microfilariae are broken down. Treatment with DEC results in epidermotropism and synchronized death of microfilariae and a marked systemic flareup of the skin and eye lesions ("Mazzotti reaction") with eosinophilic microabscesses forming around the dying larvae. In advanced stages of onchocerciasis, secondary skin changes appear, e.g., acanthosis, parakeratosis, depigmentation, and pigment phagocytosis. Finally, progressive scarring of the dermis may ensue with deposition of hyaline collagen and with concomitant epidermal atrophy.

Differential Diagnosis In endemic West Africa, *Mansonella streptocerca* can cause epidermal lesions closely mimicking those of onchocerciasis. Indeed, *Mansonella* microfilariae, like those of *Onchocerca* are unsheathed and are found in the skin rather than the blood, but adult *Mansonella* worms are smaller (40 to 85 μm across) and are found singly or in pairs in nonencapsulated inflammatory foci in the reticular dermis, smaller than the prominent nodules found in onchocerciasis.[5] The *Calabar swellings* of loiasis are itchy, are localized to the extremities, and show intense eosinophil infiltration but little epidermal change and are fleeting in duration; moreover, seldom can microfilariae be detected histologically in these lesions. Serodiagnosis can be useful in travelers returned from endemic areas for differentiating early onchocerciasis from nonparasitic dermatoses associated with eosinophilia. Currently, the CDC uses an ELISA test for IgG4 antibodies followed by Western blotting against a cocktail of recombinant onchocerca antigens.[6]

Lymphatic Filariasis (Bancroftian Filariasis; Malayan Filariasis)

Lymphatic filariasis is defined as infection by any of the mosquito-borne filarial species—*Wuchereria bancrofti, Brugia malayi, Brugia pahangi,* or *Brugia timori*—whose long and threadlike adult worms dwell inside human lymph vessels and/or nodes while their microfilariae circulate in the bloodstream. The skin lesions caused by these

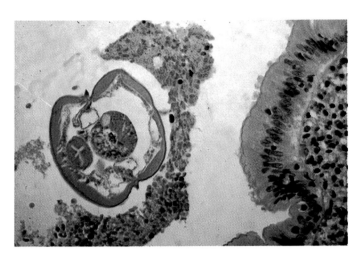

FIGURE 24-2 Cross section of an adult nematode (*Enterobius vermicularis*). Note thick collagenous epicuticle (with paired alae), empty-appearing coelomic cavity, and prominent esophageal bulb [hematoxylin and eosin (H&E) stain].

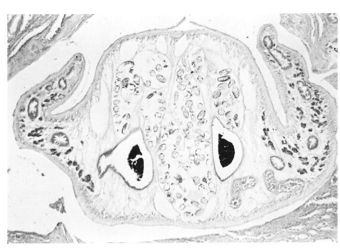

FIGURE 24-5 Adult trematode (*Fasciola hepatica*). Note syncytial tegument and paired, pigment-containing ceca plus egg-filled uteri (H&E). (*Courtesy of Dr. H. Zaiman, with permission.*)

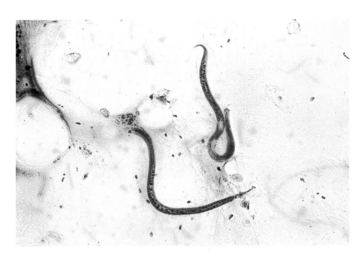

FIGURE 24-3 Larvae of a nematode (*Strongyloides stercoralis*) stained with Fuchsin, as seen in a bronchial washing (Ziehl-Neelson).

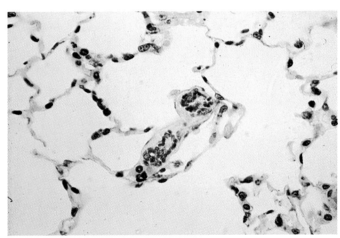

FIGURE 24-6 Trematode larva (schistosomulum of *Schistosoma mansoni*) during lung passage. Note prominent, patterned nuclei and delicate syncytial tegument (H&E).

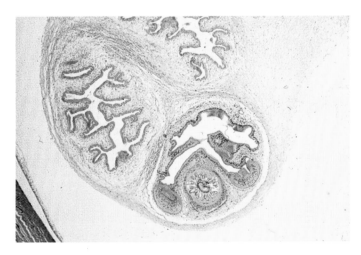

FIGURE 24-4 Cystic cestode larva (*Cysticercus cellulosae*) showing scolex with hooklet-bearing rostellum and internal gastrodermis (H&E).

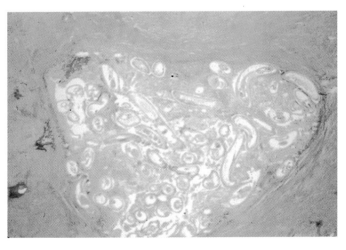

FIGURE 24-7 Section of subcutaneous nodule containing several coiled adult *Onchocerca volvulus* worms which appear empty following treatment with ivermectin. Note broad collagenous capsule (H&E).

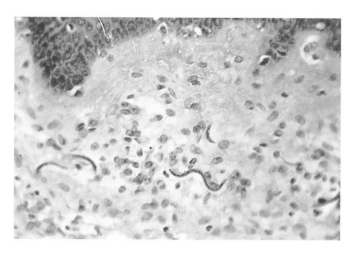

FIGURE 24-8 Intact *O. volvulus* microfilariae in human dermis accompanied by sparse inflammatory infiltrate and mild edema (H&E). (*Courtesy of Dr. H. Zaiman, with permission.*)

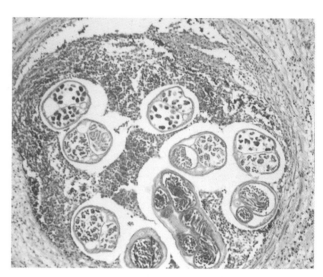

FIGURE 24-9 Intact female *Wuchereria bancrofti* in an inguinal lymphatic vessel. Note the maturing intrauterine microfilariae and the surrounding, eosinophil-enriched inflammatory exudate (H&E).

filariae can result from (1) focal inflammation around adult worms located in dermal lymphatics (*filarial abscess* and/or *granuloma*), (2) lymph stasis and edema elicited by these worms or their antigens, with or without bacterial or fungal superinfection (*filarial lymphedema, elephantiasis*), or (3) systemic allergic responses to worm or microfilarial antigens (*tropical eosinophilia, occult filariasis*). Of the four lymphatic filariae, *W. bancrofti* is most widely distributed throughout the wet tropics with multiple strains of varying diurnal or nocturnal microfilarial periodicity; the other three species are focalized to the Western Pacific and Far East. Lymphatic filariae are well-adapted human parasites, and many endemic infections are subclinical with or without microfilaremia. Only a minority of heavily and repeatedly infected individuals manifest the skin pathology described below.

Clinical Features   Sterile abscesses elicited by filariae are localized in the subcutis along the lymphatics draining the extremities or genitals and may be red, hot, and painful and may erupt through the skin much like bacterial abscesses. Episodes of acute lymphedema may be accompanied by fever, peripheral eosinophilia, and patient anxiety or depression; filarial fevers are fleeting but tend to recur, with lymphedema or hydrocele eventually turning chronic. Unless hygienic precautions are taken, chronic filarial lymphedema can then become superinfected by bacteria or fungi, resulting in marked enlargement of the extremity with verrucous epidermal change, hyperkeratosis, and thickened fibrotic dermis, a condition known as *elephantiasis*. Filarial skin lesions tend to be bilateral but asymmetric; the external genitalia and lower extremities are most often affected, except in Pacific foci where lymphedema of the arm and mammary region are frequent. Treatment with diethyl carbamazine may cause an attack of generalized hives or eczema. In occult filariasis, subcutaneous lymph node swelling mimicking lymphoma may occur, together with or without asthmalike symptoms.

Histopathological Features   Biopsies of subcutaneous filarial abscesses or granulomas are rarely taken and only about half or fewer show intact worms; when present, coiled segments of *W. bancrofti* measure up to 150 μm in diameter, those of Far Eastern filariae less than 100 μm. Intact gravid females contain bicornual uteri packed with

microfilarial progeny in various stages of development (Fig. 24-9). However, only fragments of partly or totally destroyed worms may be found after serial sectioning. These are typically birefringent and strongly periodic-acid-Schiff (PAS)–positive; occasionally, both intact and disintegrating worm segments may coexist. Microfilariae must be diligently searched for, especially when adult worms cannot be found; their number is usually small and their profile in cross section can be as narrow as 7 μm. Indeed, their minute, speckled nuclei do mimic host nuclear chromatin. Microfilariae are only rarely found outside small vessels and can also be seen scattered in the lumens of venules in the skin of asymptomatic individuals, without any host inflammatory reaction.

If a skin lesion shows neither macro- nor microfilariae detectable by histology, certain features can still suggest filarial infection, e.g., presence of 20 percent or more eosinophils with Charcot-Leyden crystals in an abscess or granuloma surrounded by a wide halo of inflammatory edema and by lymph vessels showing either extensive ectasia or endolymphangitis of the polypoid or occlusive type (Fig. 24-10).[7] However, older filarial lesions evolving toward healing and scarring may show few or no distinctive histologic markers even when clinical evidence clearly points to filariasis.

In essence, the histologic features mentioned in the few existing descriptions of chronic filarial lymphedema and elephantiasis are similar to those of nonfilarial lymphedema and elephantiasis. There is lymphangiectasia and tortuosity of lymph vessels, sparse chronic inflammation with lymphocytic predominance, and various degrees of epidermal acanthosis, hyperplasia, and hyper- and parakeratosis. The distinctive form of polypoid endolymphangitis seen in early filariasis may persist in chronic lesions, but filarial worms are rarely found, since most are located upstream from edematous skin, close to the groin or to axillary lymph nodes. Recent studies indicate that the cells infiltrating skin with significant filarial lymphedema are predominantly CD-3, CD-8+ T lymphocytes.[7]

The landmark lesion of occult filariasis or tropical eosinophilia is the *Meyers-Kouvenaar (M-K) body*, i.e., a nonviable or degenerate microfilaria enveloped by a sunburstlike, eosinophilic semihyaline precipitate, surrounded in turn by a small eosinophilic abscess or eosinophil-enriched epithelioid cell granuloma (Fig. 24-11). M-K bodies are usu-

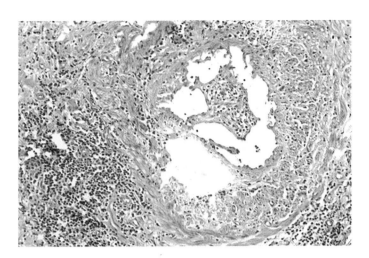

FIGURE 24-10   Polypoid endolymphangitis distal to a degenerating filarial worm. The infiltrate is rich in lymphoid cells and eosinophils (H&E).

ally found in lymph nodes or in lung tissue rather than in the skin, accompanied by high peripheral eosinophilia and sometimes by asthma or by a transient eczematoid skin rash.[8]

Differential Diagnosis   In areas endemic for multiple filarial species, onchocercal hanging groin can mimic filarial lymphedema but is always accompanied by systemic dermatitis and/or eye lesions. Also, in contrast to *O. volvulus* microfilariae, those of *W. bancrofti* and *B. malayi* are sheathed and blood-borne. The Calabar swellings of loiasis typically occur in expatriates and tourists rather than in residents of the tropics. These swellings may be accompanied by systemic symptoms and eosinophilia and can mimic fevers caused by lymphatic filariae. *L. Loa* microfilariae, like those of *W. bancrofti*, circulate in the bloodstream and are sheathed, but the two species can be distinguished by the number of nuclei in their tail ends. In addition, migration of adult filariae to serosal cavities and/or to the cornea of the eye is typical of loiasis, but extremely rare in lymphatic filariasis.

Conversely, in the absence of geographic and clinical information, involuting filarial granulomas of the subcutis or lymph nodes without detectable cuticular residua can mimic mycobacterial or fungal infection. Also, testing for microfilaremia may not reliably distinguish chronic filarial from nonfilarial lymphedema, since false negatives are common in the late stages of infection; in such cases, an IgG4-antibody ELISA can be helpful. For current information on medical and/or surgical treatment, a recent monograph should be consulted.[9]

Cutaneous Dirofilariasis (Zoonotic Filariasis, *Dirofilaria conjunctivae* Infection)

Dirofilariasis of the skin is distinct from lung infection caused by the dog heartworm, *D. immitis*. In Florida and adjacent southeastern United States, the causal agent of cutaneous dirofilariasis is *D. tenuis*,[10] a natural parasite of raccoons; on the eastern seaboard, it is *D. ursi*, a parasite of bears; in Europe it is *D. repens* whose reservoirs are domestic dogs and cats. All three species are transmitted by unknown mosquito vectors. Since a human is an accidental, nonpermissive host for dirofilariae, worms do not reach sexual maturity, and microfilariae are not generated. By the same token, skin lesions are limited to a solitary inflammatory nodule surrounding a fourth-stage (larval) to fifth-stage (adult) worm.

Clinical Features   The usual history is the finding of a small, newly arisen subcutaneous nodule anywhere on the body, including the extremities, eyes, or genitals, nonpainful at first, but later becoming inflamed with further growth over several weeks but without any systemic symptoms. Eosinophilia, if present, is usually mild. The nodule, labeled with miscellaneous diagnoses, is eventually excised, resulting in permanent cure.

Histopathological Features   An eosinophil-enriched abscess is seen, surrounding multiple cross sections of a coiled filarial worm measuring about 200 to 350 μm across. The worm is more often degenerate than intact and has a thick, laminated cuticle with prominent bilateral internal ridges, characteristic of the *Dirofilaria* genus (Fig. 24-12). Females show paired uteri, males a sex tube adjacent to the gut, but there are never mature oocytes or sperm. The abscess cavity containing the worm is walled off by granulation tissue rich in eosinophils and, in older lesions, by fibrosis, giant cells, and granulomas.

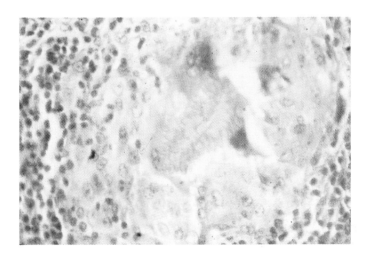

FIGURE 24-11   Meyers-Kouvenaar body in a cervical lymph node consisting of a degenerating microfilaria with stellate eosinophilic fringe engulfed by a small granuloma. Case of occult filariasis (H&E).

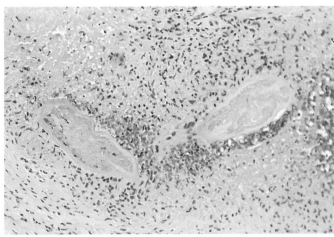

FIGURE 24-12   Segments of a fifth-stage *Dirofilaria tenuis* embedded in an eosinophil-enriched subcutaneous abscess. Note inner cuticular ridges (H&E).

Differential Diagnosis   Prior to biopsy, dirofilariasis is diagnosed only if the worm is visible beneath the conjunctiva,[10] but, once the microscope shows a filaria with internal cuticular ridges, the diagnosis cannot be missed. Of the few adult nematodes known to infect the skin in nontropical countries, only *Lagochilascaris* is of comparable size, but its lesions contain multiple worms and are large and fistulizing. For the differential diagnosis of other migratory cutaneous larvae, see below.

Dracontiasis (Guinea Worm Diseases, *Dracunculus* Infection)

Dracontiasis is a chronic subcutaneous inflammatory lesion caused by the stringlike but nonfilarial nematode *Dracunculus medinesis*. Adult guinea worms shed larvae into water by emerging through a hole in the skin; the larvae enter crustaceans of the genus *Cyclops*, in whom they mature to their infective stage. A human drinks the cyclops-infested water, completing the infectious cycle. Provision of a safe communal water source breaks the cycle and is the cornerstone of an increasingly successful, worldwide eradication campaign against the guinea worm. Formerly a disease of many millions, today it is much reduced even in subequatorial Africa and has nearly been eradicated on the Indian subcontinent.[1]

Clinical Features   After year-long incubation, lesions start as a single, localized reddish swelling on the leg, especially the ankle or foot; they then blister and open, permitting the head of the 15-cm-long worm to protrude. The abscess underlying the swelling is painful and incapacitating. If the worm is not removed by gradually rolling it onto a wooden stick (the *caduceus*), it eventually dies and calcifies, thus perpetuating the inflammation and scarring. Treatment with metronidazole can facilitate worm extraction while also reducing local inflammation.[11]

Histopathological Features and Differential Diagnosis   When guinea worm lesions have matured, their gross appearance is pathognomonic, and biopsies are rarely taken, except to document ectopic locations. Centrally, collections of neutrophils and eosinophils form abscesses surrounded by granulation tissue and inflamed scar tissue. Worm segments, when present, can measure up to 2 mm in diameter.

Cutaneous Larva Migrans (Creeping Eruption, Zoonotic Hookworm Infection)

Cutaneous larva migrans is distinct from visceral larva migrans, a systemic childhood disease caused by *Toxocara*, which infects dogs and cats. Narrowly defined, cutaneous larva migrans is an acute, linear, wavy, inflammatory skin track left behind by the penetration and burrowing of larvae of the animal hookworm *Ancylostoma caninum* or *A. braziliense*, natural parasites of dogs and cats, respectively. Note, however, that similar streaky skin eruptions can also be caused by other larval nematodes and even by insect larvae (see below).

Clinical Features   The condition occurs worldwide after skin exposure to pet excreta, often on summer beaches. Although the feet are the commonest site, any part of the body can be affected. A single raised, itchy, erythematous track of 10 or more cm in length is the norm, advancing at a rate of 3.5 to 5 cm per 24 h, sometimes disappearing and reappearing but ultimately destined to fade away after a couple of weeks.

Histopathological Features   There is no need to take a biopsy. Animal hookworm larvae migrate between the basal and spinous epithelial layers in the uninflamed part of the epidermis, far ahead of the inflamed portion of the track from which biopsies are usually taken. One there-

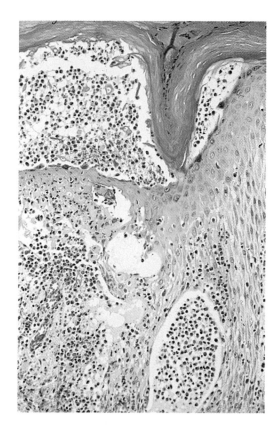

FIGURE 24-13   Histologic section of a larva migrans tract. A mixed acute inflammatory exudate percolates into the tract left behind by the larva.

fore usually visualizes only an empty intraepidermal space containing sparse exudate and surrounded by a rich neutrophilic and eosinophilic infiltrate (Fig. 24-13). Scratching of the lesion and bacterial superinfection can, of course, markedly worsen the histologic picture.

Differential Diagnosis   Cutaneous larva migrans, due to animal hookworms, is a self-healing condition and should be differentiated from helminthic diseases with chronic and/or systemic manifestations requiring treatment, including (1) invasion of the skin by human hookworm larvae in an infected, hypersensitive host; (2) *larva currens*, i.e., skin burrowing of invasive *Strongyloides* larvae during chronic infection or hyperinfection; and (3) skin manifestations of *Gnathostoma spinigerum*, a nematode endemic in eastern Asian countries. Differential diagnostic tests should include a search for ova and larvae in excreta and the use of appropriate serologic tests. Botfly larvae invading the skin are relatively large and are usually in a superficial location and can therefore often be directly visualized and/or extracted. As a general rule, any larva found in the skin is best preserved for identification intact, rather than embedded and sectioned. Streaky intraepidermal tunnels with eosinophilia can also be seen in early incontinentia pigmenti, but that condition occurs almost exclusively in newborns.

Other Nematode Skin Lesions: Cutaneous Strongyloidiasis (Larva Currens), Gnathostomiasis, Lagochilascariasis

Chronic strongyloidiasis is widespread in many developing countries. In its course, the skin is occasionally invaded by filaroid larvae entering via the perianal zone. This results in a streaky dermatitis named *larva currens* characterized by serpiginous, itchy tracts which resemble those caused by animal hookworms (see larva migrans) except for the greater speed of *Strongyloides* larvae (up to 5 cm/h). Patients with larva currens are at risk for strongyloides hyperinfection; careful and repeated stool examination for larvae is therefore indicated, followed by treatment with thiabendazole. Rare instances of skin lesions due to other strongylid soil nematodes and animal parasites have also been reported.[12,13]

In *gnathostomiasis*, the spirurid worm *Gnathostoma spinigerum* parasitizes the stomach wall of various mammals; its larvae inhabit freshwater fish. Human infection is therefore found principally in Far Eastern countries, where uncooked or undercooked fish dishes are customarily eaten. *Gnathostoma* larvae measure up to 12.5 mm in length by 1.2 mm wide; after penetrating the stomach wall, they can migrate anywhere in the human body, including the CNS, causing inflammation with sometimes severe or even fatal consequences. Skin larvae induce a localized pruritic and erythematous subcutaneous induration known in China as *Yangtze river edema*; the swelling usually disappears spontaneously after 2 weeks but may recur in a different location. Other, more superficial lesions may resemble the tracts of larva migrans,[14] but *Gnathostoma* larvae, when seen or excised, are considerably larger than those of hookworms. Histologically, the lesions show extensive edema with fibrinous and granulocytic exudation. Intact larvae are identifiable by their quadruple rows of pointed anterior hooklets, but classification based on histologic sections is difficult; any nematode wider than 250 μm in diameter found in the skin of a patient with a history of having ingested uncooked fish can be assumed to be *G. spinigerum* (Fig. 24-14), and any such patient should be given a complete diagnostic workup in anticipation of surgery to remove the worm(s) if necessary.

Lagochilascaris minor is a rare cause of human infection, reported mainly from Mexico, South America, and the Caribbean. The natural host of *L. minor* is the opossum; human infections present in the neck of a young person as chronic skin swellings with tunnelling pockets of suppuration. The abscesses contain multiple immature and/or mature ascarid nematodes measuring up to 0.5 mm across which may extrude to the surface through fistulous openings. Without treatment, the suppuration continues with periodic exacerbations and bacterial superinfections, ultimately resulting in scarring and deformity.[15] Clinical diag-

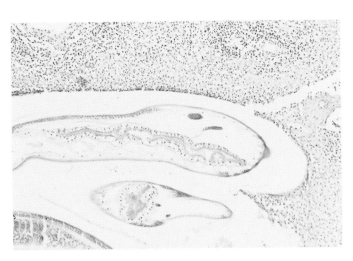

FIGURE 24-15 Two adult *Lagochilascaris minor* worms in a fistulous tract, shown in oblique section, surrounded by purulent exudate. Note the paired cuticular alae (H&E).

nosis is confirmed by finding prominent lateral alae on the worms' cuticle (Fig. 24-15) or by visualizing eggs with a characteristic, pitted surface, either in utero or free in the exudate.

CESTODE INFECTIONS

Cutaneous Cysticercosis (*Taenia solium* Cystic Larvae, "Bladder Worm")

Cysticerci are the cystic larvae of the tapeworm *Taenia solium*. Normally, adult *T. solium* inhabits the gut of humans, its definitive host, whereas cysticerci infect the tissues of its intermediate host, the pig. Humans acquire cysticercosis by accidentally ingesting *T. solium* eggs in uncooked food. Both intestinal tapeworm infection and cysticercosis are common in the developing world wherever pigs are raised, but the main target of cysticerci is the central nervous system, and localizations in the skin occur in only about 6 percent of cases. Therefore, when cysticerci are found in the skin or muscle, they are likely to be found also in the brain, but not vice versa. Cysticercosis has a long incubation period; it can also remain asymptomatic for years, and its clinical presentation and outcome are varied and hard to predict.

Clinical Features Cysticerci of the skin occur in patients with or without neurologic symptoms and may be single or multiple. They appear as rounded nodules underlying normal epidermis anywhere on the body and are firm, elastic to the touch, and movable by lateral pressure but do not seem obviously cystic by palpation; indeed, they are sometimes confused with small benign tumors, e.g., schwannomas or fibrolipomas, but their cystic nature declares itself as soon as the overlying skin is incised. Dermal cysticerci can remain asymptomatic for many years or elicit an inflammatory flareup when the cyst degenerates and begins to leak. When treated with Albendazole or with Praziquantel, dermal cysts become inflamed, followed by shrinkage and virtual disappearance after a couple of weeks.

Histopathological Features Intact, viable cysticerci elicit remarkably little inflammation. The cyst lining is a relatively thin and flat syncytial tegument with underlying mesenchyme containing myocytes and excretory ducts. The inverted scolex ends in a rostellum bearing a row of delicate, birefringent hooklets, flanked by two pairs of sucker caps. The inner epithelial lining of its neck is destined to become the adult tape-

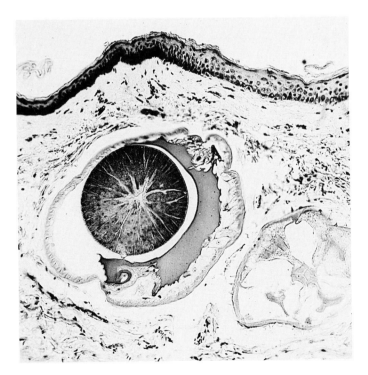

FIGURE 24-14 *Gnathostoma spinigerum* larva located in the upper dermis. (*AFIP accession #75-8589-3, Atlas Fig. 9-14-11, p. 474, with permission.*)

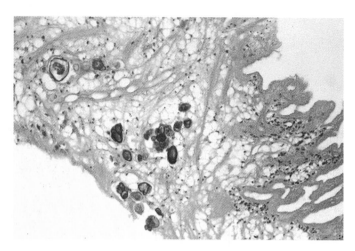

FIGURE 24-16 Degenerating cysticercus scolex. Note purplish calcareous bodies (H&E).

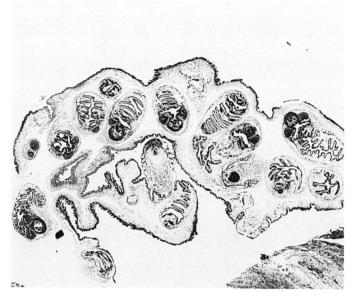

FIGURE 24-17 Cross section of a *Coenurus* showing multiple scolices (H&E). (*AFIP accession #69-4736, Atlas Fig. 11-4-2, p. 544, with permission.*)

worm's absorptive surface (*gastrodermis*). It is taller than the bladder wall, hyaline in appearance, and has microvilli forming a brush border (Fig. 24-4). The worm's mesenchyme is speckled with ovoid concretions containing central purplish dots, named *calcareous bodies*, which are found as well in cestodes of other species. In degenerating and dead cysticerci, all these features are faded or totally obliterated, and the carcass of the scolex may be calcified, but hooklets and calcareous bodies persist for a long time and usually can be found if searched for (Fig. 24-16). As cysticerci degenerate and leak, they may elicit considerable inflammation of the surrounding subcutaneous tissue with infiltration of neutrophils and eosinophils later shading into a granulomatous pattern. The final result is a centrally calcified scar.

Differential Diagnosis A cystic subcutaneous tapeworm larva of 1 to 4 cm bearing a single scolex is considered to be a cysticercus unless otherwise proven. The rare racemose form found in the CNS has not been reported in skin. Larger cysts with either multiple scolices or none at all should raise the possibility of coenuriasis or sparganosis, respectively (see below).

Coenuriasis (Dog Tapeworm Larva)

About 50 cases of coenuriasis of the human central nervous system or skin have been reported to date. The majority represent the intermediate stage of *Taenia multiceps*, a dog tapeworm, or of related wild animal parasites.[16] As in cysticercosis, humans acquire the infection by accidentally ingesting eggs, and the clinical and pathologic features also closely resemble those of cysticercosis except that the cysts are larger, up to 10 cm in diameter, and contain multiple (up to 100) scolices rather than a single scolex. In addition, daughter cysts may be present, either swimming in the cyst fluid or budding off in grapelike fashion from the main cyst (Fig. 24-17).

Sparganosis (Spargana, Plerocercoid Tapeworm Larvae)

Spargana are the second-stage (plerocercoid) larvae of tapeworms of the *Spirometra* genus whose adult worms parasitize dogs or cats. Human sparganosis is acquired by ingesting water infested with small crustaceans, which function as hosts of first-stage (procercoid) larvae, by

ingesting uncooked reptile or fish meat already infected with pleurocercoids, or by applying such meat to the skin for medicinal purposes, as is customary in some Asian countries. Consequently, in some eastern countries, sparganosis is far more common than coenuriasis (see above) but is still a rarity in the United States.[17] Subcutaneous spargana are the most frequent, followed by CNS localizations.

Clinical Features Spargana are nonsegmented, ribbonlike worms up to 40 cm long but only 3 mm wide, and they are actively motile. Subcutaneous nodules rarely exceed 3 cm in width and may disappear and reappear. As long as worms are intact, there is little reaction, but eventually death occurs, causing significant local inflammation and pain, and motivating surgical intervention.

Histopathological Features and Differential Diagnosis On histology, several segments of the plerocercoid may be seen, composed of parvicellular mesenchyma covered by a simple tegument analogous to that lining a cysticercus wall. However, there is no formed scolex, other than a vestigial tegumental duplication at the anterior end of the primitive larva (Fig. 24-18). The host inflammatory changes surrounding the larva vary with the state of the larva and resemble those already described in the section on cysticerci.

TREMATODE INFECTIONS

Paragonimiasis (Lung Fluke Infection)

Human paragonimiasis is most frequently caused by *P. westermani*, the oriental lung fluke, but at least seven additional species are known to infect humans or animals in the Far East, Africa, and Latin America. Paragonimi are leaf-shaped, hermaphroditic flukes whose life cycle passes from eggs through successive larval stages in fresh water snails, in snail-eating crustaceans, and in crustacean-eating mammals in which larvae either reach maturity or, if the host is nonpermissive, remain indefinitely dormant. After migrating toward their host target sites, mature worms embed themselves in the lung, brain, liver, or bone, forming cystic cavities, in which they nest and lay eggs over long periods.

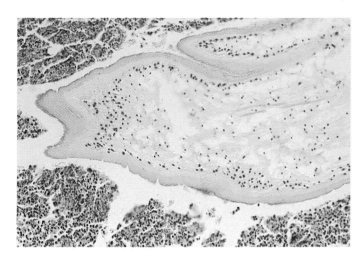

FIGURE 24-18 Subcutaneous plerocercoid of *Spirometra mansonoides* (Sparganum). Note simple tegument and mesenchyme without scolex formation. The larva is surrounded by eosinophil-enriched exudate (H&E).

Worms retained in ectopic sites from which eggs cannot be excreted, such as the skin, tend to die earlier, with formation of an abscess and, eventually, a calcified nodule. Whether active or calcified, cutaneous paragonimiasis therefore denotes the likelihood of visceral involvement and the need for systemic clinical and parasitologic patient evaluation.

Clinical and Histopathological Features   Early stages of skin involvement, as seen in China, are said to resemble the creeping eruption of cutaneous larva migrans (see above). Later skin lesions present' as inflammatory or calcified subcutaneous nodule, 2 to 4 cm in diameter, most often in an abdominal site. Histologically, lesions show variable mixtures of eosinophilia, abscess formation, necrosis, and focal calcification. Intact trematodes are seldom found in these lesions, but there may be residual eggs which are thin-shelled, birefringent, and operculated and measure 80 to 118 μm in greatest diameter (Fig. 24-19).

Differential Diagnosis   Skin nodules caused by *Paragonimus* can be differentiated from those caused by *Fasciola* based on the larger egg size of the latter. Skin nodules caused by cestode larvae do not contain any eggs at all. Old *Paragonimus* nodules may be mistaken for mycobacterial lesions if eggs are not searched for carefully in multiple sections.[18]

Fascioliasis (Liver Fluke Infection)

Fasciola hepatica, the common liver fluke, has a cosmopolitan distribution and infects sheep, goats, and other herbivores who consume plants on which metacercariae have been deposited by a snail intermediate host. Humans are accidental hosts, most often acquiring the infection from field-collected herbs, such as watercress. During its early migration from the gut to the liver, *F. hepatica* can track through many sites including the skin, thus giving rise to ectopic lesions before settling into the lumen of a large bile duct or gallbladder. Similar pathology is caused by *F. gigantica*, a closely related but larger fluke found mainly in the tropics.

Clinical Features   Early fascioliasis may be accompanied by fever, abdominal pain, urticarial rash, and high peripheral eosinophilia. Itchy skin tracks resembling those of cutaneous larva migrans or paragonimiasis (see above) may accompany this syndrome. Late disease may resemble chronic calculous cholecystitis or cholangitis, sometimes with painful subcutaneous nodules persisting, mostly on the abdomen, up to 6 cm in diameter.

Histopathological Features and Differential Diagnosis   Fasciolae seen in biopsies of early tracks are immature, lacking vitellaria glands, but show the spined, syncytial tegument typical of trematodes as well as branched ceca (Fig. 24-20). The surrounding tissue may show massive eosinophilia and Charcot-Leyden crystals. In chronic lesions, there is a mix of necrosis, granulomatous inflammation, and calcification. Similar to paragonimiasis, worms are likely to be degenerate or absent, but eggs may persist; they are thin-walled, operculated, and measure 140 by 90 μm, among the largest helminth eggs found in humans. The larger egg size distinguishes fascioliasis from paragonimiasis, and the absence of a spine differentiates its eggs from those of the schistosomes. This distinction is important because each trematode parasite requires different therapy.

Schistosomiasis (Swimmer's Itch, Bilharziosis)

Schistosomiasis is a widespread chronic endemic infection spread by sexually dimorphic trematodes which mate and lay eggs inside the vein lumen of their definitive host and whose invasive larval forms, named *cercariae*, develop in aquatic snails. Human skin lesions can be caused (1) by schistosomes adapted to animals or birds which cause an abortive infection in humans or (2) by one of the tropical, human-adapted schis-

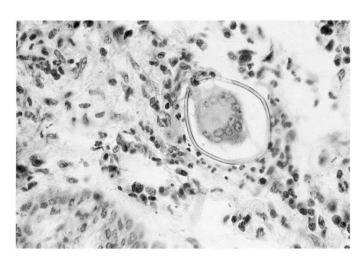

FIGURE 24-19 Egg shell of *Metagonymus yokogawai* containing a foreign-body giant cell (H&E).

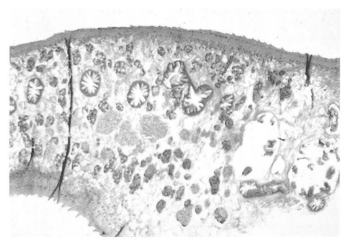

FIGURE 24-20 Section through lateral portion of *Fasciola hepatica* showing complex branching of ceca and spined tegument (H&E).

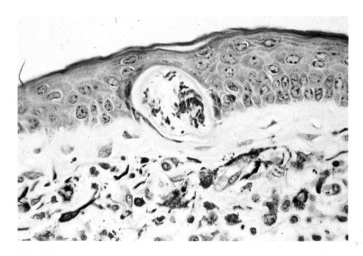

FIGURE 24-21   Schistosomulum of *Schistosoma mansoni* entering the dermis. Note degranulating mast cells (Dominici stain).

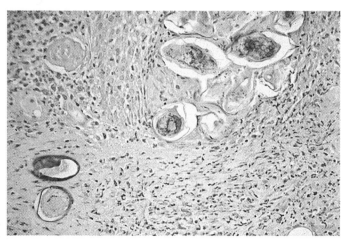

FIGURE 24-22   Two acid-fast-positive eggs of *Schistosoma mansoni* and a convoy of seven acid-fast-negative eggs of *S. haematobium* in a single histologic field (Ziehl-Neelsen).

tosome species, most commonly *S. mansoni, S. haematobium,* or *S. japonicum,* which can cause chronic, potentially severe systemic human disease and are known to infect millions of people in their endemic tropical countries.

A papular erythematous skin rash named *swimmer's itch* follows penetration of the human skin by cercarial larvae of bird or animal schistosomes of various species found in snail-infested lakes and ponds, worldwide. This rash is self-healing within hours or days, since animal schistosomes exposed to human tissue always die at an early developmental stage.

More rarely, a similar rash occurs soon after exposure to cercariae of any of the major human-adapted schistosomes. This rash is usually mild and is more frequently seen in adult travelers to the tropics than in residents of the endemic zone who have been exposed to infection from childhood.[19] However, skin penetration by the major human schistosomes is followed within a few weeks by full-scale systemic infection and should therefore be recognized and treated. During its early, prepatent stage, schistosomiasis is diagnosable only by serology. ELISA and Western blotting should be used in combination,[20] and inquiry about patient travel and water contact should be made.

Skin lesions, due to ectopic egg laying by established schistosome worms during the chronic phase of infection, have also been reported, but are truly exceptional, rarer than CNS lesions. Most have been seen in the perianal and scrotal region, but an occasional one has been periumbilical. There is even a solitary report of a nasal skin lesion.

Clinical and Histopathological Features   Cercarial skin rashes, whether of the swimmer's itch or the tropical variety, are more often localized than generalized; are erythematous, maculopapular, and intensely pruritic; occur within hours of water contact; and fade within days. Only two biopsy studies of these lesions have been published.[19] Similar to animal models, these studies showed vasodilation and edema of the reticular dermis, basophil degranulation, and perivascular infiltration by sparse neutrophils and eosinophils (Fig. 24-21). Around dying schistosomula there was exocytosis and formation of eosinophil-enriched microabscesses.

Dermal schistosome egg deposits present as mildly inflamed subcutaneous nodules or tumorlike masses, tender but not painful with little or no erythema. On histology, they show granulomas of various stages

of activity or involution formed around schistosome eggs. These eggs measure up to 120 μm in length. In paraffin sections they are too distorted to discern the spines which characterize each species; however, *S. mansoni* and *S. japonicum* eggs are acid-fast by the Ziehl-Neelsen method, whereas *S. haematobium* eggs are negative (Fig. 24-22).

Differential Diagnosis   Differentiation of acute cercarial dermatitis from other allergic and pruritic dermatoses must be made on clinical and serologic grounds. Patients with chronic schistosome egg lesions of the skin usually also excrete eggs in the feces or urine or present with clinical evidence of urinary or hepatointestinal schistosome pathology. The only helminth eggs larger in size than those of schistosomes are the operculated ones of *Fasciola.*

REFERENCES

1. Hopkins DR, Ruiz-Tiben E, Ruebush T II, et al: Dracunculiasis eradication: March 1994 update. *Am J Trop Med Hyg* 52:14–20, 1995.
2. Samba EM: The onchocerciasis control programme in west Africa. An example of effective public health management. WHO Distribution and Sales, Geneva, 1994.
3. Gutierrez Y: Introduction to Nematodes, in *Diagnostic Pathology of Parasitic Infections with Clinical Correlations.* Philadelphia, Lea & Fibiger, pp. 177–183, 1990.
4. Connor DH, Gibson DW, Neafie RC, et al: Sowda—onchocerciasis in North Yemen. A clinicopathologic study of 18 patients. *Am J Trop Med Hyg* 32:123–137, 1983.
5. Meyers WM, Connor DH, Harman LE, et al: Human streptocerciasis. A clinicopathologic study of 40 Africans (Zairians) including identification of the adult filaria. *Am J Trop Med Hyg* 21:528–545, 1972.
6. Ramachandran CP: Report on a multicenter effort to develop improved immunodiagnostic tests to monitor onchocerciasis programs. *Parasitol Today* 9:76–79, 1993.
7. Von Lichtenberg F: Inflammatory responses to filarial connective tissue parasites. *Parasitology* 94:S101–S122, 1987.
8. Friedman DO, Horn TD, Silva CME, et al: Predominant Cd-8 infiltrate in limb biopsies of individuals with filarial lymphedema and elephantiasis. *Am J Trop Med Hyg* 53: 633–638, 1995.
9. Ottesen E: Filarial infections. *Infect Dis Clin North Am* 7(3):619–633, 1993.
10. Orihel TC, Beaver PC: Morphology and relationship of *Dirofilaria tenuis* and *Dirofilaria conjunctivae. Am J Trop Med Hyg* 14:1030–1043, 1964.
11. Muller R: Guinea worm disease: Epidemiology, control and treatment. *Bull WHO* 57: 683–689, 1979.
12. Ginsburg B, Beaver PC, Wilson ER, et al: Dermatitis due to larvae of the soil nematode, *Pelodera strongyloides. Pediatr Dermatol* 2:33–37, 1984.
13. Little MD: Dermatitis in a human volunteer infected with *Strongyloides* of the nutria and raccoon. *Am J Trop Med Hyg* 14:1007–1009, 1965.

14. Bhaibulaya M, Charoenlarp P: Creeping eruption caused by *Gnathostoma spinigerum*. *Southeast Asian J Trop Med Publ Health* 14:266–268, 1983.

15. Botero D, Little MD: Two cases of human lagochilascariasis infection in Columbia. *Am J Trop Med Hyg* 33:381–386, 1984.

16. Kurtycz DFI, Alt B, Mack E: Incidental coenurosis: Larval cestode presenting as an axillary mass. *Am J Clin Path* 80:735–738, 1983.

17. Sparks AK, Neafie RC, Connor DH: Sparganosis, in Binford CH, Connor DH (eds): *Pathology of Tropical and Extraordinary Diseases*. Washington D.C., AFIP, 1976, pp 534–538.

18. Yokogawa M: *Paragonimus* and paragonimiasis. *Adv Parasitol* 3:99–158, 1965.

19. Gonzalez E: Schistosomiasis, cercarial dermatitis, and marine dermatitis. *Dermatol Clin* 7:291–300, 1984.

20. Tsang VL, Wilkins PP: Immunodiagnosis of schistosomiasis. Screen with FAST-ELISA and confirm with immunoblot. *Clin Lab Med* 11:1029–1039, 1991.

PART FOUR

PROLIFERATIONS— HAMARTOMAS, HYPERPLASIAS, NEOPLASIAS

CHAPTER 25

CUTANEOUS CYSTS AND RELATED LESIONS

Glynis A. Scott

Cysts are one of the most common specimens received by the pathologist. A cyst is any cavity which is lined by an epithelium. Cysts may be found in virtually any organ in the body and are often lined by epithelium which is native to that particular organ. Although cysts may be classified on the basis of several different criteria, the *diagnosis* of cutaneous cysts is predominantly based on the nature of the epithelial lining. Recognition of the nature of the epithelial cyst wall lining is also important for understanding the histopathogenesis of these lesions, which usually arise from normal counterparts in the skin, predominantly adnexal structures.

Classification of cutaneous cysts may be approached in a variety of ways. One may classify them based on their presumed appendage of origin, whether it be hair, eccrine gland, apocrine gland, or salivary gland, or based on whether they are developmentally or nondevelopmentally derived. There is considerable overlap between what one might consider to be a cyst and what one might consider to be an appendageal tumor. For example, several authors classify apocrine and eccrine hidrocystomas as appendageal tumors,[1] because they arise from apocrine and eccrine glands, respectively. Some authors consider endometriosis and endosalpingiosis to be cutaneous cysts even though they represent heterotopic rests of normal tissue which have implanted at distant sites. Because of the extensive overlap between classification schemes of cutaneous cysts, a simple algorithm for the diagnosis of cutaneous cysts based on the nature of their epithelial lining is presented (Fig. 25-1). Clinical and histologic features of cutaneous cysts are summarized in Tables 25-1 to 25-5.

CYSTS LINED BY STRATIFIED SQUAMOUS EPITHELIUM

Cysts lined by stratified squamous epithelium can be conveniently divided into those which contain other structures within the cyst wall, such as steatocystoma, dermoid cysts, and thymic cysts, and those which lack additional structures within the cyst wall, including epidermoid cysts, pilar cysts, vellus hair cysts, milia, follicular hybrid cysts, pigmented follicular cysts, and proliferating epithelial cysts.

Epidermoid Cysts

Epidermoid cysts (ECs) are by far the most common cyst received in the pathology laboratory. They present predominantly on the face, neck, and torso, although ECs of the palms and soles have been reported. ECs have also been termed *infundibular cysts*, reflecting the belief that they arise from the infundibular portion of the hair follicle. Cysts which arise on acral surfaces of the skin are believed to arise from implantation of epidermis into the dermis through trauma, whereas the more commonly

observed cysts on nonacral skin are thought to arise from inflammation of the hair follicle. An EC arising from an eccrine duct has been reported.[2] Recently described variants of EC include ECs with associated basal cell carcinoma[3] and plantar ECs with associated human papilloma virus infection.[4] Proliferating epithelial cyst,[5] a variant of EC, is discussed in detail under "Newly Described Entities" at the end of the chapter.

Histopathological Features   ECs are located predominantly in the dermis and contain abundant laminated orthokeratin in the cyst cavity. The cyst wall consists of a stratified squamous epithelium with a variably thick granular layer (Fig. 25-2). Rupture of the cyst results in an intense foreign-body giant cell reaction, with lymphocytes, neutrophils, and eventually scar formation. Fragments of keratin may be identified within giant cells in ruptured ECs.

Differential Diagnosis   ECs can be distinguished from pilar cysts by the presence of a granular layer; the nature of the keratin, which is loose and flaky in ECs and compact and homogeneous in pilar cysts; and the absence of palisading of nuclei in the basal layer. Calcification, commonly present in pilar cysts, is usually absent in ECs. Pilar sheath acanthoma and Pore of Winer are also lined by a keratinizing stratified squamous epithelium and are distinguished from ECs by the lack of communication with the skin surface in ECs and the nature of the epithelial lining, which is acanthotic and displays platelike extensions and budding in pilar sheath acanthoma and in Pore of Winer.

Pilar Cysts

Pilar cysts, originally termed *sebaceous cysts*, are also known as *trichilemmal cysts* or *isthmus-catagen* cysts.[6] They occur predominantly on the scalp (90 percent), but otherwise share clinical features with ECs. There is a strong female preponderance, and pilar cysts are usually solitary, but multiple pilar cysts may occur. Pilar cysts arise from the isthmus of anagen hairs or from the sac surrounding catagen and telogen hairs, areas in which the inner root sheath is lacking. Proliferating pilar cysts (proliferating trichilemmal tumor) arise from irritation of pilar cysts and may also be considered an adnexal tumor. Although rare, trichilemmal carcinoma[7] has been reported to occur in association with pilar cysts.

Histopathological Features   Pilar cysts are usually located in the middle to deep reticular dermis and are characterized by a 3- to 4-layer-thick lining of keratinocytes which exhibit abrupt keratinization into compact homogenous keratin (Fig. 25-3). A characteristic feature of pilar cysts is the apparent absence of intercellular bridges between the keratinocytes and peripheral palisading of nuclei. The cells closest to

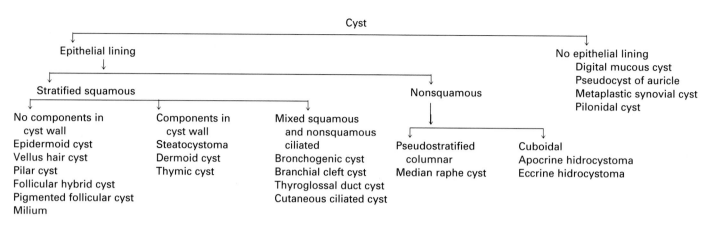

FIGURE 25-1 Algorithm for diagnosis of cutaneous cysts.

the cyst cavity are pale and show abrupt transition to homogeneous keratin. Occasional cholesterol clefts can be observed in the keratinous material. When ruptured, a foreign-body giant cell reaction is observed along with calcification and occasionally ossification. It is not uncommon to observe some areas of the cyst which contain a granular layer (so-called pseudohybrid cyst), but the predominantly trichilemmal type of keratinization establishes the true nature of the cyst.

Proliferating Trichilemmal Cyst (Tumor) and Trichilemmal Carcinoma

Proliferating pilar tumors arise from pilar cysts which have been irritated and are predominantly located on the scalp of elderly women. The size varies from 0.2 to 10.0 cm, but larger sizes have been reported (up to 25 cm). These lesions exhibit lobules and sometimes sheets of cells with areas of trichilemmal keratinization evident throughout the tumor. Squamous eddies are usually easily identified.[8] Proliferating pilar cysts usually fill the dermis and may extend into the subcutis. They often contain abundant compact keratin which fills the cyst cavity. As in pilar cysts, a foreign-body giant cell reaction may be observed at the periphery of the lesion.

Trichilemmal carcinoma is extremely rare. Patients are middle-aged to elderly, and lesions present as solitary nodules, papules, or plaques on sun-exposed areas of the body. Characteristic histologic features include a solid growth pattern of highly atypical keratinocytes with easily identifiable mitotic figures as well as lobular and trabecular growth patterns. Lesions are usually confined to the dermis; however, extension into the subcutis may be seen, and ulceration may be present. In some cases, continuity of the tumor with hair follicle epithelium may be observed. Tumor cells are characterized by abundant clear cytoplasm, some containing intracytoplasmic eosinophilic globules.[8] Microcysts with keratohyaline plugs may be seen, and tumor lobules are surrounded by stratified squamous epithelium with an outer layer of clear cells with palisading nuclei and subnuclear vacuolization, simulating outer root sheath differentiation.[8]

Differential Diagnosis Well-differentiated squamous cell carcinoma (SCC) may be confused with proliferating pilar tumor, but the well-demarcated nature of the lobules, the noninfiltrative borders, and the absence of significant atypia help to distinguish proliferating pilar tumors from squamous cell carcinoma. In addition, the presence of clear cells with palisading at the periphery is also a useful distinguishing feature of proliferating pilar tumors. Trichilemmal carcinoma may be indistinguishable from SCC; however, the presence of areas of trichilemmal keratinization and absence of overlying in situ carcinoma help to establish the diagnosis. In addition, careful inspection may reveal residual areas of benign proliferating pilar tumor.

TABLE 25-1

Classification of Cutaneous Cysts

Epithelial-lined cysts
  Stratified squamous
    Epidermoid cyst (infundibular cyst)*
    Pilar cyst (trichilemmal cyst)
    Vellus hair cyst*
    Milia*
    Follicular hybrid cyst*
    Pigmented follicular cyst*
  Stratified squamous with components in cyst wall
    Steatocystoma (simplex and multiplex)
    Dermoid cyst
    Thymic cyst
  Cuboidal†
    Eccrine hidrocystoma
    Apocrine hidrocystoma
  Mixed squamous and nonsquamous ciliated
    Bronchogenic cyst
    Branchial cleft cyst
    Thyroglossal duct cyst
    Cutaneous ciliated cyst
    Ciliated cyst of vulva
    Omphalomesenteric cyst†
  Pseudostratified columnar
    Median raphe cyst
Cysts not lined by an epithelium
  Digital mucous cyst
  Mucocele
  Metaplastic synovial cyst
  Pilonidal cyst
  Pseudocyst of auricle
New entities
  Proliferating epithelial cyst

*These cysts arise from the infundibular portion of the hair follicle.
†These are discussed in detail in Chap. 18.

TABLE 25-2

Clinical and Histologic Features of Cysts Lined by Stratified Squamous Epithelium

Cyst	Clinical Features	Histopathological Features	Other Features
Epidermoid inclusion (infundibular cyst)	Solitary or multiple, face, neck, torso; occasionally palms and soles	Stratified squamous lining with variably thick granular layer, loose, abundant laminated orthokeratin	Rupture associated with foreign-body giant cell reaction, inflammation, and scarring
Pilar (trichilemmal)	Usually solitary, may be multiple, head and scalp	Stratified squamous lining of keratinocytes with poorly defined intercellular bridges; Abrupt keratinization to compact keratin; No or attenuated granular layer	Proliferating pilar tumor arises from the benign cystic counterpart
Vellus hair	Multiple, autosomal dominant or sporadic, trunk, chest, and extremities, small and may be pigmented	Small, dermally located, thin stratified squamous lining; Characteristic presence of multiple vellus hairs in cyst lumen	Connection to a vellus hair may be identified
Milium	Small, 1- to 2-mm papules, primary or associated with blistering disorders	Small cysts arising from infundibulum of vellus hairs, lined by thin stratified squamous lining	Milia secondary to scarring or bullous disease probably arise from eccrine ducts
Pigmented follicular	Solitary lesions on the face, M>>>F, deeply pigmented	Stratified squamous epithelium with numerous pigmented hair shafts in lumen	Connection to the surface of the epidermis usually observed
Hybrid	Rare, scalp or face, wide age range	Superior portion of cyst lined by stratified squamous epithelium, like an EC; sharp transition to lower portion showing trichilemmal keratinization	Hybrid cyst consisting of other combinations of hair follicle derivation may be seen
Proliferating epithelial cyst	Rare, 1:1.8 F/M ratio, pelvic, anogenital area, scalp, upper extremities, trunk	Acanthotic papillomatous or verrucous stratified squamous lining, atypia, mitotic figures may be present	Carcinomatous change may be seen, local recurrence relatively common, frequent connection with epidermis

Abbreviations: F = female; M = male; EC = epidermoid cyst.

Vellus Hair Cysts

Vellus hair cysts most commonly present as multiple lesions as part of an autosomal dominant disease termed *eruptive vellus hair cysts* (EVHC) or as solitary lesions in a nonheritable form.[9–12] In sporadic cases, lesions appear abruptly in the first or second decade, but cases appearing in adults have also been reported. Familial cases appear at an earlier age (birth or infancy). Eruptive vellus hair cysts may be associated with other cutaneous lesions such as steatocystoma multiplex,[13–15]

trichostasis spinulosa,[16] or other heritable disorders, such as pachyonychia congenita, and neurologic disorders.[14,17] Lesions are small (1 to 3 mm) and may be pigmented with red, brown, gray, and black colors. Preferred locations include the anterior chest, abdomen, and extremities; however, face, groin, and neck may also be affected. The pathogenetic mechanism of vellus hair cysts is unknown; however, faulty development of vellus hair infundibulum, evolution from blocked terminal hair follicles, and hamartomatous differentiation toward vellus hair follicles have been postulated.

TABLE 25-3

Clinical and Histologic Features of Cysts Lined by Stratified Squamous Epithelium and Containing Elements within the Cyst Wall

Cyst	Clinical Features	Histopathological Features	Other Features
Steatocystoma	Simplex (solitary) or multiplex (hereditary), axilla, groin, chest	Ruggated wall lined by very thin stratified squamous lining with glassy pink cuticle overlying the internal surface	Sebaceous glands arranged within the outer wall of the cyst
Dermoid	Infants and children, periocular, congenital, firm nodules, 1–4 cm	Unilocular cyst with stratified squamous lining, wall contains various appendageal elements such as hair follicles, sebaceous glands, eccrine glands	
Thymic cyst	Neck or anterior mediastinum	Unilocular or multilocular, cuboidal epithelium or stratified squamous, occasional ciliated cells	Thymic tissue may be identified in wall Pseudoepitheliomatous hyperplasia or even malignant transformation may occur, though rare

TABLE 25-4

Clinical and Histologic Features of Cysts Lined by Mixed Squamous and Nonsquamous Ciliated Epithelium

Cyst	Clinical Features	Histopathological Features	Other Features
Bronchogenic	Neck, but may occur on face, back, shoulder, abdomen	Ciliated lining with goblet cells, stratified squamous lining in some areas due to metaplasia	Wall may contain smooth muscle or cartilage
Branchial cleft	Jaw and preauricular area in areas of lymph nodes	Pseudostratified columnar epithelium with cilia and areas of stratified squamous epithelium	Lymphoid follicles are abundant and may be the predominant component
Ciliated (mucinous) cyst of vulva	Labia minoris	Mucin-containing cells with some cilia	Mullerian origin
Cutaneous ciliated	Buttocks, LE,* women	Cuboidal/columnar single layer of ciliated cells	Same origin as ciliated cyst of vulva
Thyroglossal duct	Midline of neck	Cuboidal ciliated epithelium admixed with stratified squamous epithelium	Characteristic presence of thyroid follicles in cyst wall

*LE = lower extremities

TABLE 25-5

Clinical and Histologic Features of Cysts Not Lined by an Epithelium

Cyst	Clinical Features	Histopathological Features	Other Features
Digital mucous cyst	Dorsum of finger	Collagenous wall, lumen which contains acid mucopolysaccharides	Connected to the interphalangeal joint
Pseudocyst of auricle	Asymptomatic swelling of upper pinna of the ear	Cystic space within the cartilage associated with some degenerative changes	Most likely represents developmental defect in ear formation exacerbated by trauma
Metaplastic synovial cyst	Occur in areas of trauma or surgical sites	Villous projections into cystic cavity, lined by fibrinous exudate, epithelioid cells, inflammation	Immunocytochemically and histologically similar or identical with synovium
Pilonidal cyst	Sacrococcygeal area, but any area may be affected	Acute and chronic inflammation surrounding sinus tract or cystic cavity, hair shafts often identified	May rarely progress to squamous cell carcinoma

Histopathological Features   Vellus hair cysts are typically located in the middle to upper dermis and consist of a thin-walled cyst lined by stratified squamous epithelium with an attenuated granular layer (Fig. 25-4). Like ECs, vellus hair cysts arise from the infundibular portion of the hair follicle. The cyst wall may contain telogenlike hair follicle structures. Their most characteristic feature, however, is the presence of multiple vellus hairs cut in cross section in the cyst cavity along with keratin fragments. While it is unusual to observe other structures within the cyst wall, small arrector pili muscles have been observed attached to the outer cyst wall. Ultrastructural examination of EVHC[18] reveals in-fundibular type of keratinization. Melanocytes and Langerhans' cells may also be seen within the cyst wall.[18]

Differential Diagnosis   Steatocystoma is in the differential diagnosis of vellus hair cysts, because these two cystic lesions share a similar epithelial lining. In contrast with vellus hair cysts, however, which do not usually contain components within its cyst wall, steatocystoma typically has readily identifiable sebaceous glands in the cyst wall, as well as a pink cuticle on the luminal aspect of the epithelial lining.

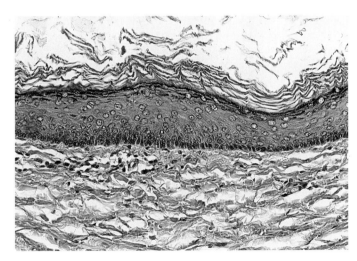

FIGURE 25-2   Epidermoid cyst. The cyst is notable for laminated keratin, the presence of a granular layer, and squamous epithelium resembling the epidermis.

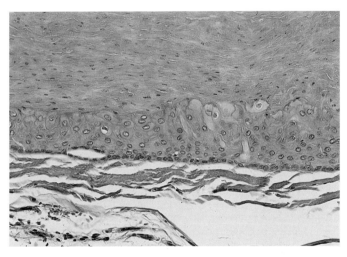

FIGURE 25-3   Trichilemmal (pilar) cyst. The epithelial lining resembles the isthmus of the hair follicle and is remarkable for the formation of amorphous keratin, the absence of a granular layer, and peripheral palisading of nuclei.

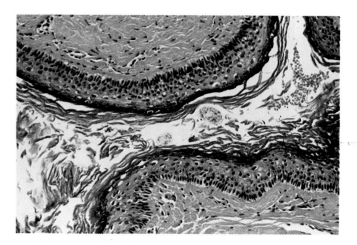

FIGURE 25-4 Vellus hair cyst. The cyst lining resembles an epidermoid cyst but contains fragments of hair shaft.

Milia

Milia present as multiple small superficially located lesions that range from 1 to 2 mm in diameter. They may be primary, usually arising on the face, or secondary to bullous disorders such as porphyria, epidermolysis bullosa, and pemphigoid or secondary to trauma such as dermabrasion.

Histopathological Features Milia are a miniature version of an epidermoid cyst but arise from the infundibular portion of vellus hairs rather than terminal hairs. Their lining is a stratified squamous epithelium and contains a granular layer, and the cyst cavity is filled with keratinous debris. Unlike vellus hair cysts, multiple cross sections of hair shafts in the cyst cavity are not seen. Often the cyst wall can be seen arising from a vellus hair. In contrast with primary milia, secondary milia arise from eccrine ducts. In cases in which a connection to a hair or eccrine appendage cannot be demonstrated, implantation of epidermis in scar tissue is the probable histogenetic mechanism.

Differential Diagnosis Milia can be distinguished from vellus hair cysts by the lack of hair shafts in the cyst cavity and from steatocystoma by the lack of sebaceous glands in the cyst wall and lack of a pink cuticle.

Follicular Hybrid Cysts

Follicular hybrid cysts, first described by Brownstein in 1983,[19] are rare mixed types of cysts in which infundibular keratinization is observed in the upper portion of the cyst and trichilemmal keratinization is seen in the lower portion of the cyst. Face and scalp are the primary sites, and any age may be affected. Requena and Yus[20] have expanded this concept to include cysts that combine features of both infundibular and pilomatric differentiation, trichilemmal and pilomatric differentiation, and vellus hair cyst and steatocystoma.

Histopathological Features The originally described hybrid cyst combines infundibular keratinization in the upper portion of the cyst wall with trichilemmal keratinization in the lower portion of the cyst wall. Occasional connection with the overlying epidermis may be observed. To fulfill the requirements of a true hybrid cyst, an abrupt transition from infundibular to trichilemmal keratinization must be observed.

Differential Diagnosis Follicular hybrid cysts can be distinguished from the more common ECs and pilar cysts by the presence of two types of keratinization.

Pigmented Follicular Cyst

Pigmented follicular cysts are rare and were first described by Mehregan and Medenica[21] and are solitary lesions located predominantly on the head and neck, ranging in size from 0.4 cm to 1.5 cm. Patients range in age from 20 to 60 years of age, and there is a strong male predominance. In 5 of 7 cases reported, the lesions were deeply pigmented.

Histopathological Features The cysts open to the epidermis and are lined by a stratified squamous epithelium in which the keratinocytes closest to the cyst cavity contain keratohyalin granules. The cyst lining shows rete ridge–like areas, and the lumen is filled with numerous thick pigmented hair shafts cut on cross section.

Differential Diagnosis Pigmented follicular cysts may be confused with vellus hair cysts, but the presence of pigmented hair shafts and connection with the epidermis in pigmented follicular cysts help to distinguish these two entities.

CYSTS WITH STRATIFIED SQUAMOUS EPITHELIAL LINING AND COMPONENTS WITHIN THE CYST WALL

Steatocystoma

Steatocystoma may occur as solitary noninherited tumors in adults, referred to as *steatocystoma simplex*, or as multiple lesions inherited as an autosomal dominant disease. In the heritable form, numerous small white or yellowish lesions distributed in the axillae, groin, or chest are noted, although other areas of the body may be affected.[22] The lesions usually occur at puberty, suggesting some androgenic control. Some authors regard steatocystomas as retention cysts, whereas others consider them to represent a variant of dermoid cysts. The histogenesis of these cysts is now thought to represent a nevoid or hamartomatous condition of the pilar-sebaceous junction.

Histopathological Features Steatocystoma simplex and multiplex share histologic features consisting of a thin-walled cyst lined by stratified squamous epithelium which tends to be very ruggated and contains a pink crenulated eosinophilic cuticle on its surface (Figs. 25-5 and 25-6). Characteristic features of this cyst include the presence of sebaceous glands arising from or adjacent to the cyst wall, as well as occasional hairs.

Differential Diagnosis Steatocystomas may be distinguished from ECs by the thinner cyst wall lining of steatocystoma, as well as the presence of sebaceous glands within the wall, and the pink cuticle. Similarly, milia and vellus hair cysts, which are similar in size as steatocystoma, lack the cuticle, as well as the sebaceous glands in the wall.

Dermoid Cysts

The typical dermoid cyst is a well-defined, hard, rubbery, raised, yellow-to-pink lesion with fine hairs on its surface, varying from 1 to 4 cm in size. Dermoid tumors, the solid counterparts of dermoid cysts, also

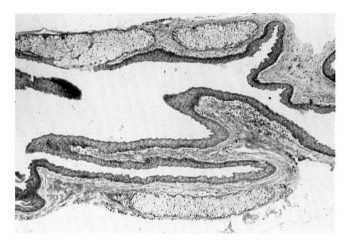

FIGURE 25-5 Steatocystoma. The cyst has a serpiginous configuration and sebaceous elements are present in the wall.

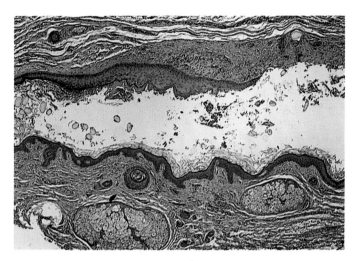

FIGURE 25-7 Dermoid cyst. The cyst resembles an epidermoid cyst but contains hair fragments within the lumen. In addition, there are hair follicles and sebaceous glands associated with the epithelial lining.

called *choristomas*, are benign, congenital overgrowths of tissue located in an abnormal location.[23] Dermoid cysts are located in the dermis or subcutis, are usually present at birth, and are predominantly located around the eyes and in the midline area of the face.

Histopathological Features Dermoid cysts are generally rather large, are lined by a stratified squamous epithelium, and contain mature epidermal appendages within their wall (Fig. 25-7). The presence of hairs projecting into the cyst wall is not uncommon. In the dermis surrounding the cyst wall, eccrine glands, sebaceous glands, and occasionally apocrine glands may be observed.

Differential Diagnosis Dermoid cysts differ from ECs by the presence of adnexal structures in their wall, and from steatocystoma by their thicker lining, lack of a cuticle, and greater number and types of adnexal structures in the cyst wall.

Thymic Cysts

Thymic cysts are unusual lesions which may be either developmental or acquired and almost invariably occur in the neck or anterior mediastinum.[24] Thymic cysts are usually asymptomatic; however, a small proportion of patients may experience hoarseness, dysphagia, and stridor, due to compression of pharyngeal tissue by the cyst. Although rare, malignant transformation of thymic cysts has been reported.[25] Some thymic cysts may arise from persistent embryonal thymic remnants; however, a larger proportion probably arise as acquired lesions due to inflammation, ulceration, and reactive lymphoid hyperplasia.[26]

Histopathological Features Thymic cysts may be unilocular or multilocular (Fig. 25-8).[27] The lining is composed of a thin layer of flattened or cuboidal epithelium or a stratified squamous epithelium with occasional ciliated cells. Some thymic cysts lack a lining completely.

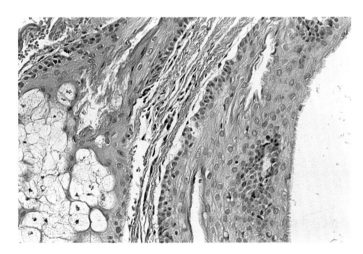

FIGURE 25-6 Steatocystoma. The cyst is lined by an irregular eosinophilic cuticle and there are sebaceous elements in the wall.

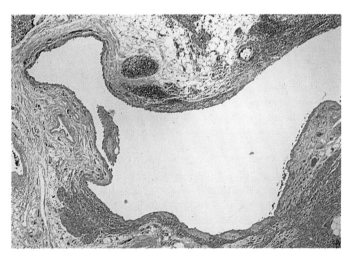

FIGURE 25-8 Thymic cyst. A large unilocular cyst is lined by cuboidal epithelium and associated thymic tissue. The latter contains lymphoid infiltrates with Hassle's corpuscles.

Ulceration and inflammation of the cyst wall may be observed, and a connection with Hassle's corpuscles may be identified. Although uncommon, pseudoepitheliomatous hyperplasia of the lining of the cyst may be observed.[26] The cyst wall is composed of fibrovascular tissue with scattered islands of thymic epithelium around it. Thymic tissue consists of abundant lymphoid cells with Hassle's corpuscles and associated cholesterol granulomas.

Differential Diagnosis   Because thymic cysts often contain a dense infiltrate of lymphocytes, a cutaneous lymph node is in the differential diagnosis. However, the presence of scattered Hassle's corpuscles and the presence of a cyst wall help distinguish thymic cysts from lymph nodes. The presence of Hassle' corpuscles distinguishes thymic cysts from other cysts which contain ciliated epithelium in their lining, such as bronchogenic cysts and branchial cleft cysts.

CYSTS LINED BY MIXED SQUAMOUS AND NONSQUAMOUS AND CILIATED EPITHELIUM

Bronchogenic Cysts

Bronchogenic cysts are most commonly located on the neck and within the thoracic cage in the vicinity of the bronchial trees but may be present on the back, shoulder, abdomen, or face. These cysts are usually located in the subcutis and occasionally may drain through fistulas to the surface of the skin. The pathophysiology of bronchogenic cysts is due to sequestration of respiratory epithelium from the tracheal bronchial tree during embryonic development. Localization outside the areas of development of the tracheal bronchial tree is due to migration of the tissue to ectopic sites.

Histopathological Features   Bronchogenic cysts are characterized by a lining which is respiratory, consisting of goblet cells filled with mucin, as well as ciliated pseudostratified columnar epithelium (Figs. 25-9 and 25-10). Squamous metaplasia of the cyst wall may occur, resulting in both stratified squamous as well as ciliated columnar cells and goblet cells.[28] The wall of the cyst may contain strands of smooth muscle and rarely cartilage.

Differential Diagnosis   Bronchogenic cysts may be distinguished from branchial cleft cysts and cutaneous ciliated cysts by the absence of lymphoid follicles in the former and the clinical presentation in the latter.

Branchial Cleft Cysts

Branchial cleft cysts are most commonly located in the jaw and preauricular area of the face, nestled among lymph node groups in the head and neck. They arise from branchial cleft remnants whose migration was arrested during embryologic development. Alternatively, branchial cleft cysts may represent inclusion of branchial-type epithelium within lymph nodes.

Histopathological Features   The cysts are lined by a stratified squamous or pseudostratified ciliated columnar epithelium (Fig. 25-11). The most characteristic feature, however, is the presence of abundant lymphoid tissue within and surrounding the cyst wall.

Differential Diagnosis   Like thymic cysts, the abundant lymphoid tissue may suggest a cutaneous lymph node. However, careful inspection will reveal a cystic space lined by squamous or pseudostratified ciliated epithelium in branchial cleft cysts.

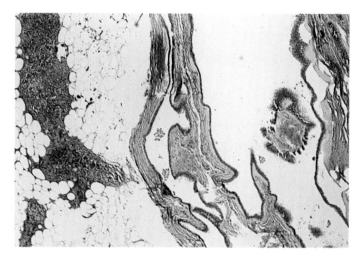

FIGURE 25-9   Bronchogenic cyst. The cyst is lined by respiratory epithelium and ciliated pseudostratified columnar epithelium.

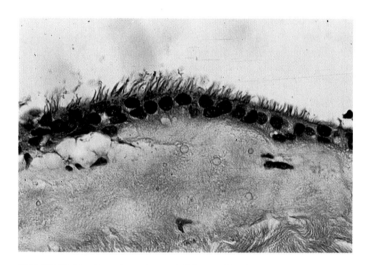

FIGURE 25-10   Bronchogenic cyst. High magnification shows ciliated epithelium lining the cyst.

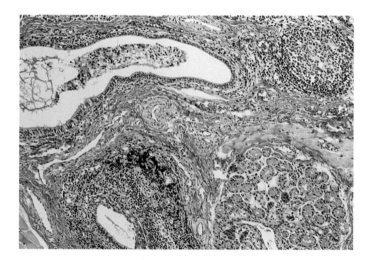

FIGURE 25-11   Branchial cleft cyst. Note lymphoid tissue surrounding cyst wall.

Thyroglossal Duct Cysts

Thyroglossal duct cysts are usually observed in midline areas of the neck and are detected in childhood or young adulthood. They represent remnants of the thyroglossal duct which have failed to migrate. A characteristic clinical feature is the movement of the cyst with deglutition.

Histopathological Features   Thyroglossal duct cysts are lined by a simple cuboidal or columnar epithelium or stratified squamous epithelium which may contain some ciliated columnar cells (Fig. 25-12). In addition, a pseudostratified columnar ciliated lining may be observed. A tract connecting it to the hyoid bone is frequently present. The most characteristic feature of thyroglossal duct cysts, however, is the presence of thyroid follicles within the wall of the cyst. These are characterized by low cuboidal cells which surround homogeneous pink material.

Differential Diagnosis   While thyroglossal duct cysts share features with other cysts, such as the presence of a stratified squamous or columnar lining, the presence of thyroid epithelium distinguishes this cyst from all others.

Cutaneous Ciliated Cysts

Cutaneous ciliated cysts are uncommon lesions. They usually occur as solitary lesions on the buttocks and lower extremities in women in their teen years to young adulthood, with only two reported cases occurring in men.[29,30] Other sites include one case on the shoulder, which may represent a bronchogenic cyst, and one case on the scalp.[31] Kurban and Bhawan[1] suggest that these cysts should be renamed *cutaneous mullerian cysts* to reflect their presumed mullerian duct origin. Others, however, citing the occasional occurrence of these lesions in men too, suggest that these lesions arise from eccrine glands which have undergone ciliated metaplasia.[29,30]

Histopathological Features   Cutaneous ciliated cysts may be located in either the subcutis or deep dermis and are both unilocular or multilocular. A common feature is the presence of papillary projections into the lumen of the cyst. The lining of the cyst is a simple cuboidal to columnar ciliated epithelium, with some areas of pseudostratified cili-

ated epithelium. Foci of squamous metaplasia may be seen. The tissues surrounding the cyst are free of skin appendages, glandular elements, or muscle fibers.[32]

Differential Diagnosis   Other cysts which contain a ciliated lining epithelium may be confused with cutaneous ciliated cyst; however, the absence of associated lymphoid tissue (which would be present in bronchogenic cysts) or associated structures such as thymic tissue or thyroid glands helps to establish the diagnosis. Apocrine hidrocystoma is in the histologic differential diagnosis; however, cutaneous ciliated cysts lack decapitation secretion seen in apocrine hidrocystoma.

Ciliated Cyst of Vulva

Ciliated cysts of the vulva (also called *paramesonephric mucinous cysts of the vulva*) are uncommon developmental anomalies which represent heterotopic rests of mullerian epithelium,[33,34] share many histologic features with cutaneous ciliated cysts, and are considered the same entity by some authors.[1] The cysts arise in multiparous young women and may be related to pregnancy or use of exogenous progesterone. The cysts are usually located on the superior portion of the labium minus and range in size from 1.0 to 3.0 cm and may be painful and discharge fluid. Malignant transformation has not been reported, and excision is curative.

Histopathological Features   The cyst wall is lined by tall columnar or cuboidal clear cells which exhibit cilia on the luminal aspect, and in some cases small papillary projections are present (Fig. 25-13). Squamous metaplasia of the lining may be observed. Nuclei are basally located and cells rest on a fibrous connective tissue lining. The cells contain neutral mucins, as demonstrated by mucicarmine and PAS stains.

Differential Diagnosis   The close similarity between the lining of the ciliated cyst of the vulva with that of the endocervix may suggest a diagnosis of metastatic endocervical adenocarcinoma; however, the lack of atypia in vulvar ciliated cyst differentiates the two lesions. Mesonephric cysts are more common and can be differentiated from ciliated cysts of the vulva by the nature of the epithelial lining, which is low-columnar and flattened in mesonephric cysts and does not contain mucin.

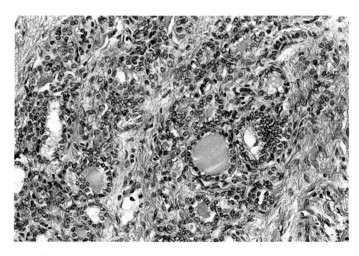

FIGURE 25-12   Thyroglossal duct cyst. Thyroid follicles are present near the wall of the cyst.

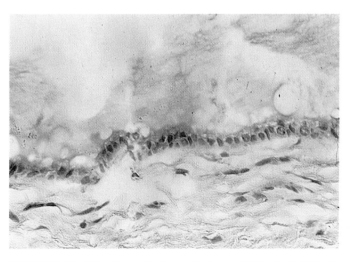

FIGURE 25-13   Ciliated cyst of vulva. A single row of ciliated cuboidal cells lines the cyst.

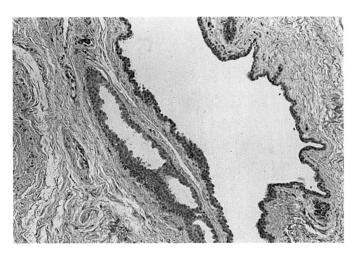

FIGURE 25-14 Median raphe cyst. The cyst is lined by pseudostratified columnar epithelium.

CYSTS LINED BY PSEUDOSTRATIFIED COLUMNAR EPITHELIUM

Median Raphe Cysts

Median raphe cysts are located exclusively on the ventral aspect of the penis, occur in young men, and are usually solitary and small, measuring only a few millimeters in diameter.[35] Previous reports of apocrine cystadenoma arising on the penis most likely represent median raphe cysts. Median raphe cysts arise due to defects in embryologic development of male genitalia, either from incomplete closure of the urethral or genital folds or from outgrowths of embryologic epithelium after primary closure of the folds. Median raphe cysts do not communicate with the urethra.

Histopathological Features   Irregularly shaped unilocular cystic spaces without connection to the overlying epidermis characterize these lesions (Fig. 25-14). Median raphe cysts are lined by a pseudostratified columnar epithelium which varies in thickness, although it usually does not exceed four to five cell layers. In some areas a single layer may be observed consisting of fusiform cells. Occasional mucin-containing cells may also be seen.[35]

Differential Diagnosis   The characteristic location of these cysts, along with the nature of the lining, usually makes the diagnosis obvious.

CYSTS WITHOUT AN EPITHELIAL LINING

Digital Mucous Cysts

Digital mucous cysts are usually located on the dorsum of the finger next to the distal interphalangeal joint and are also called *ganglions*. They communicate with the adjacent joint space, to which they are attached by a pedicle.

Histopathological Features   Digital mucous cyst consists of a compressed collagenous fibrous wall, which contains acid mucopolysaccharides which stain positively with alcian blue and colloidal iron stains. Occasionally a thin attenuated single epithelial lining may be observed, reflecting the origin from the synovial lining of the adjacent joint space.

Differential Diagnosis   Other lesions in which mucin is a prominent feature, such as focal papular mucinosis and myxedema, may be confused with digital mucous cyst. However, the characteristic location of digital mucous cysts and the sharply localized distribution of the mucin help to distinguish digital mucous cyst from these other lesions.

Pilonidal Sinus

Pilonidal cysts (or sinus) most commonly, but not exclusively, arise in the sacrococcygeal region and are more common in men. They may be congenital or acquired, and two theories of origin have been proposed. One school of thought is that pilonidal cysts are developmental abnormalities,[6] whereas others believe the cysts are acquired and result from penetration of hairs into the skin which induces the formation of a sinus or cyst.[36] Inflammation and infection are commonly associated with pilonidal cysts, and, although rare, development of squamous cell carcinoma has been reported.[37–39] Squamous cell carcinoma arising in pilonidal sinus is usually well-differentiated, but its clinical course is aggressive.

Histopathological Features   The sinus tract or cyst wall is located in the deep dermis or subcutis and is associated with a dense neutrophilic and lymphohistiocytic infiltrate. The cyst wall is lined by a stratified squamous epithelium, but the associated inflammatory infiltrate may obliterate or obscure the lining, and, in some cases, only a fibrous wall can be identified. A diagnostic feature of pilonidal cyst is the presence of hair shafts within the cyst or embedded in the inflammatory infiltrate. A connection with the epidermis is frequently but not invariably identified.

Differential Diagnosis   The characteristic clinical presentation, in association with the histologic features described above, usually makes the diagnosis of pilonidal cyst straightforward. However, entities such as Crohn's disease, which may display inflamed fistulas extending from the large bowel to the skin in that region, and deep-seated infection should be considered in the histologic differential diagnosis. Crohn's disease lacks the epithelial lining and embedded hair shafts of pilonidal sinus and will display noncaseating granulomas. In the absence of a clear cyst or cyst lining, a deep-seated abscess should be excluded with appropriate stains for organisms.

Pseudocyst of Auricle

Pseudocyst of the auricle (PCA), also known as *endochondral pseudocyst, cystic chondromalacia,* or *intracartilaginous cyst,* is an uncommon lesion arising in the upper anterior portion of the auricle. The majority of cases arise in males, and all ages are involved[40] with the majority of patients presenting during middle age. PCAs are usually unilateral but may be bilateral.[40] They are asymptomatic and arise over the course of several weeks and present with cystic swelling of the anterior auricle. The etiology is unclear but may be due to embryologic malformation of the pinna in association with ischemic necrosis and trauma.

Histopathological Features   A cyst is present within the cartilage and lacks an epithelial lining. Inflammation is absent, and the overlying epidermis is normal. The cyst contains a straw-colored sterile fluid, which is rich in albumin.[41] The cavity may be filled with fibrous tissue and granulation tissue,[42] and degenerative changes in the cartilage may be observed.

Differential Diagnosis   Entities to be considered in the differential diagnosis of PCA include subperichondral hematoma and relapsing polychondritis. Subperichondral hematoma will display large collections of blood within the cartilage, and a prior history of trauma can usually be elicited. Relapsing polychondritis may present with a similar clinical appearance, but PCA and relapsing polychondritis may be distinguished by the presence of perichondral inflammation in relapsing polychondritis and the presence of a cyst in PCA.

Metaplastic Synovial Cysts

Metaplastic synovial cysts (MSCs) may arise in any site which has undergone trauma or disruption, including after injection of air into tissue,[43] within scars after surgery,[44,45] or following a puncture wound.[46] Although usually located in the dermis, MSC frequently communicates with the overlying epidermis through fistulous tracts. The clinical impression most frequently includes suture granuloma, but other lesions, including leiomyoma and basal cell carcinoma, have also been included in the clinical differential diagnosis.[46]

Histopathological Features   Metaplastic synovial cysts are located in the dermis and contain broad villous projections which project into the cyst cavity (Fig. 25-15). The villous projections are lined by inflammatory cells, reactive cuboidal or epithelioid cells, and a fibrinous exudate. Mitotic figures and binucleated lining cells may be observed. The lining is strikingly reminiscent of inflamed synovium, simulating the appearance of villous synovitis. The core of the villous structure consists of loose connective tissue which contains spindled fibroblastlike cells aligned perpendicularly to the surface of the villi, and a scar can usually be identified at the base of the villous structure. Immunocytochemistry is strongly positive for vimentin in the spindled cells of the villi and in the epithelioidlike lining cells[45,46] and is negative for epithelial markers. In some cases, the lining cells are weakly positive for alpha-1-antichymotrypsin and lysozyme.[45]

Differential Diagnosis   The histologic differential diagnosis includes other cysts which lack a true epithelial lining, including digital mucous cyst and pilonidal sinus. However, digital mucous cyst lacks villous structures and will display mucin within the cyst cavity. Pilonidal sinus will contain an intense inflammatory cell infiltrate, and usually fragments of hair can be identified.

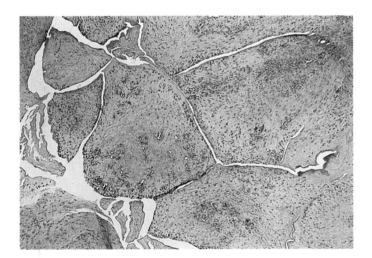

FIGURE 25-15   Metaplastic synovial cyst. There are bulbous projections lined by cuboidal cells reminiscent of inflamed synovium.

RECENTLY DESCRIBED ENTITIES

Proliferating Epithelial Cysts

Proliferating epithelial cysts (PECs) were first described by Sau and colleagues[5] in 1995 in which 33 examples were presented. The male-to-female ratio is approximately 1:2, and PECs occur in patients from 21 to 88 years of age. PECs show epidermal-type keratinization and arise in ECs. Unlike proliferating pilar cysts, PECs are widely distributed, with over 79 percent arising in areas other than the scalp. Simple excision of PECs may be followed by recurrence of the lesions, with 20 percent of the patients in this series showing recurrence from 5 months to 3 years after initial excision, and three patients having multiple local recurrences. One patient died 2 years after surgery because of intractable local spread. No metastatic cases were observed.

Histopathological Features   PECs are subepidermal cystic tumors; however, a significant proportion (45 percent) show a connection to the overlying epidermis. The cyst wall lining is similar to a more typical epidermoid cyst; however, in areas there is abundant proliferation of cells in which the cells acquire pale eosinophilic cytoplasm and sharp cytoplasmic borders. Other areas show a prominent granular layer adjacent to areas of loose laminated keratin. The epithelium shows various degrees of acanthosis, papillomatosis, hypergranuloses, parakeratosis, and hyperkeratosis. Cellularity and atypia are quite variable and approximately 6 percent of the tumors show marked epithelial proliferation. Cytologic atypia may be observed, particularly in the more cellular lesions. Mitotic figures may be observed, and in some cases may be frequent.

Differential Diagnosis   Squamous cell carcinoma (SCC) is the most difficult lesion to distinguish from PEC. This is because focal areas of PEC will show marked cytologic atypia, making the distinction from SCC extremely difficult. Features in favor of PEC include a tendency to keratinize centrally, sharp circumscription, and evidence of a preexisting EC. Absence of overlying in situ carcinoma also helps to differentiate between SCC and PEC. Pilomatricoma can be distinguished from PEC by the absence of sheets of basaloid cells, which are seen in pilomatricoma, and by the presence of trichilemmal keratinization in PEC.

REFERENCES

1. Kurban RS, Bhawan J: Cutaneous cysts lined by nonsquamous epithelium. *Am J Dermatopathol* 13:509–517, 1991.
2. Egawa K, Honda Y, Ono T: Epidermoid cyst with sweat ducts on the torso. *Am J Dermatopathol* 17:71–74, 1995.
3. Mehregan DA, Al-Sabah HY, Mehregan AH: Basal cell epithelioma arising from epidermoid cyst. *J Dermpathol Surg Oncol* 20:405–406, 1994.
4. Kato N, Ueno H: Two cases of plantar epidermal cyst associated with human papillomavirus. *Clin Exp Dermatol* 17:252–256, 1992.
5. Sau P, Graham JH, Helwig EB: Proliferating epithelial cysts: Clinicopathological analysis of 96 cases. *J Cutan Pathol* 22:394–406, 1995.
6. Pinkus, H: Sebaceous cysts are trichilemmal cysts. *Arch Dermatol* 99: 544–555, 1969.
7. Wong T-Y, Suster S: Trichilemmal carcinoma: A clinicopathologic study of 13 cases. *Am J Dermatopathol* 16:463–473, 1994.
8. Brownstein MH, Arluk DJ: Proliferating trichilemmal cyst: A simulant of squamous cell carcinoma. *Cancer* 48:1207–1214, 1981.
9. Esterly NB, Fretzin DF, Pinkus H: Eruptive vellus hair cysts. *Arch Dermatol* 113:500–503, 1977.
10. Stiefler RE, Bergfeld WF: Eruptive vellus hair cysts: An inherited disorder. *J Am Acad Dermatol* 3:425–429, 1980.
11. Binham JQ, Gross AS, Onadeko OO, et al: Acneiform eruption due to eruptive vellus hair cysts. *South Med J* 85:322–325, 1992.
12. Grimalt R, Gelmetti C: Eruptive vellus hair cysts: Case report and review of the literature. *Pediatr Dermatol* 9:98–102, 1992.

13. Ohtake N, Kubota Y, Takayama O, et al: Relationship between steatocystoma multiplex and eruptive vellus hair cysts. *J Am Acad Dermatol* 26:876–878, 1992.

14. Moon SE, Lee YS, Youn JI: Eruptive vellus hair cyst and steatocystoma multiplex in a patient with pachyonychia congenita. *J Am Acad Dermatol* 30:275–276, 1994.

15. Nogita T, Chi H-I, Nakagawa H, et al: Eruptive vellus hair cysts with sebaceous glands. *Br J Dermatol* 125:475–476, 1991.

16. Amichai B, Cagnano M, Halevy S: Coexistence of trichostasis spinulosa and eruptive vellus hair cysts. *Int J Dermatol* 33:858–859, 1994.

17. Morgan MB, Kouseff BG, Silver A, et al: Eruptive vellus hair cysts and neurologic abnormalities: Two related conditions? *Cutis* 47:413–415, 1991.

18. Kumakiri M, Takashima T, Iju M, et al: Eruptive vellus hair cysts—a facial variant. *J Am Acad Dermatol* 7:461–467, 1982.

19. Brownstein MH: Hybrid cyst: A combined epidermoid and trichilemmal cyst. *J Am Acad Dermatol* 9:872–875, 1983.

20. Requena L, Yus ES: Follicular hybrid cysts: An expanded spectrum. *Am J Dermatopathol* 13:228–233, 1991.

21. Mehregan AH, Medenica M: Pigmented follicular cysts. *J Cutan Pathol* 9:423–427, 1982.

22. Requena L, Martin L, Renedo G, et al: A facial variant of steatocystoma multiplex. *Cutis* 51:449–452, 1993.

23. Oakman JH, Lambert SR, Grossniklaus HE: Corneal dermoid: Case report and review of classification. *J Pediatr Opthamol Strabismus* 30:388–391, 1993.

24. Miller MB, DeVito MA: Cervical thymic cyst. *Otolaryngol Head Neck Surg* 112:586–588, 1995.

25. Babu MK, Nirmala Y: Thymic carcinoma with glandular differentiation arising in a congenital thymic cyst. *J Surg Oncol* 57:277–279, 1994.

26. Suster S, Barbuto D, Carlson G, et al: Multilocular thymic cysts with pseudoepitheliomatous hyperplasia. *Hum Pathol* 22:455–460, 1991.

27. Mishalani SH, Lones MA, Said JW: Multilocular thymic cyst. *Arch Pathol Lab Med* 119:467–470, 1995.

28. Van der Putte SCJ, Toonstra J: Cutaneous "bronchogenic" cyst. *J Cutan Pathol* 12:404–409, 1985.

29. Leunforte JF: Cutaneous ciliated cystadenoma in a man. *Arch Dermatol* 118:1010–1012, 1982.

30. Ashton MA: Cutaneous ciliated cyst of the lower limb in a male. *Histopathology* 26:467–469, 1995.

31. Sickel JZ: Cutaneous ciliated cyst of the scalp: A case report with immunocytochemical evidence for estrogen and progesterone receptors. *Am J Dermatopathol* 16:76–79, 1994.

32. Farmer ER, Helwig EB: Cutaneous ciliated cysts. *Arch Dermatol* 114:70–73, 1978.

33. True L, Golitz LE: Ciliated plantar cyst. *Arch Dermatol* 116:1066–1067, 1980.

34. Hart W: Paramesonephric mucinous cysts of the vulva. *Am J Obstet Gynecol* 107:1079–1083, 1970.

35. Asarch RG, Golitz LE, Sausker WF: Median raphe cysts of the penis. *Arch Dermatol* 115:1084–1086, 1979.

36. Yabe T, Furukawa M: The origin of pilonidal sinus: A case report. *J Dermatol* 22:696–699, 1995.

37. Davis KA, Mock CN, Versaci A, Lentrichia P: Malignant degeneration of pilonidal cysts. *Am Surg* 60:200–204, 1994.

38. Kim YA, Thomas I: Metastatic squamous cell carcinoma arising in a pilonidal sinus. *J Am Acad Dermatol* 29:272–274, 1993.

39. Jeddy TA, Vowles RH, Southam JA: Squamous cell carcinoma in a chronic pilonidal sinus. *Br J Clin Prac* 48:160–161, 1994.

40. Santos AD, Kelley PE: Bilateral pseudocyst of the auricle in an infant girl. *Pediatr Dermatol* 12:152–155, 1995.

41. Fukamizu H, Imaizumi S: Bilateral pseudocysts of the auricles. *Arch Dermatol* 120:1238–1239, 1984.

42. Engel D: Pseudocysts of the auricle in Chinese. *Arch Otolaryngol* 83:197–202, 1966.

43. Selye H: On the mechanism through which hydrocortisone affects the resistance of tissues to injury: An experimental study of the granuloma pouch technique. *J Am Acad Dermatol* 152:1207–1213, 1953.

44. Gonzalez JG, Ghiselli RW, Santa Cruz DJ: Synovial metaplasia of the skin. *Am J Surg Pathol* 11:343–350, 1987.

45. Stern DR, Sexton FM: Metaplastic synovial cyst after partial excision of nevus sebaceus. *Am J Dermatol* 10:531–535, 1988.

46. Bhawan J, Dayal Y, Gonzalez-Serva A, Eisen R: Cutaneous metaplastic synovial cyst. *J Cutan Pathol* 17:22–26, 1990.

CHAPTER 26

TUMORS OF THE EPIDERMIS

Alan S. Boyd

Many cutaneous biopsies are performed to evaluate a lesion's malignant potential. Fortunately, most of these tumors are benign. The distinction is important, however, since significant surgical procedures may be needed for some tumors but are inappropriate for others. Further, some of these lesions may indicate underlying conditions that require additional evaluation and treatment. For these, as well as other reasons, it is imperative that dermatopathologists seek to accurately classify those epidermal tumors that they are called on to evaluate.

EPIDERMAL NEVI AND RELATED PROCESSES

Epidermal Nevus

Epidermal nevi are proliferations of the epithelium that may be associated with different syndromes. Most tumors are isolated lesions that are present at birth or arise within the first few years of life. Others are associated with what is termed the "epidermal nevus syndrome." These patients demonstrate defects of the central nervous system (epilepsy, mental retardation), skeletal system (bone anomalies, cysts, deformities), eyes (colobomas, cataracts, choristomas), and oral cavity (absent or malformed teeth).[1] The most impressive variant is nevus unius lateris, which is characterized by epidermal nevi arranged in a whorled fashion on the trunk or extremities in the pattern of Blaschko's lines. Greater and more systematized involvement typifies ichthyosis hystrix. The term epidermal nevus syndrome has been applied solely to five conditions—Schimmelpenning syndrome, nevus comedonicus syndrome, pigmented hair epidermal nevus syndrome, Proteus syndrome, and the CHILD syndrome.[2] Chromosomal breakpoints, indicating genetic mosaicism, have been found on some cell lines in affected patients.[3]

Clinical Features Epidermal nevi present as papules, nodules, and patches of verrucous epidermal hyperkeratosis (Table 26-1). They may be isolated, linear, zosteriform, or whorled.[4] Most lesions exhibit different shades of brown but may also be grey, black, or flesh-colored. Inflammation or irritation usually are confined to traumatized epidermal nevi. Most lesions are asymptomatic but mild pruritus may occur.

Histopathological Features There are several different variants of epidermal nevi.[5] The most common demonstrates sharply demarcated hyperkeratosis with papillomatosis (Table 26-1). The epidermis is acanthotic with a focally thickened granular layer and columns of parakeratosis.[1] The basal layer is frequently hyperpigmented.[6] A second type shows features reminiscent of acrokeratosis verruciformis with a "church spire" type of papillomatosis. There is significant hyperkeratosis, acanthosis, and an exaggerated granular layer. Epidermolytic hyperkeratosis is seen in some specimens.[1] These lesions demonstrate irregularly shaped keratohyalin granules, perinuclear vacuolization, and

moderate to marked hyperkeratosis. Finally, the verruca vulgaris variant demonstrates vacuolated cells with orthohyperkeratosis, parakeratosis, papillomatosis, and an increased number of keratohyalin granules. Other variants resemble a seborrheic keratosis or porokeratosis.[5] Psoriasiform changes also may be seen but are more common in an inflamed linear verrucous epidermal nevus (ILVEN). Acantholysis is present in some lesions and may represent a mosaic form of Darier's disease.[7] The dermis typically is not involved; however, a lichenoid or perivascular inflammatory infiltrate may be present. Pigment incontinence also may be found. Squamous cell carcinoma, basal cell carcinoma, and keratoacanthoma have been described in association with epidermal nevi.[8]

Differential Diagnosis Epidermal nevi must be differentiated from seborrheic keratoses, warts, and acrokeratosis verruciformis. Seborrheic keratoses have horn pseudocysts and a "flat bottom" epidermal acanthosis. Papillomatous variants are more regularly arrayed than are epidermal nevi. Verrucae have koilocytic changes and hypergranulosis. Additionally, prominent vascular structures and occasional ectasia may be seen in the papillary dermis. These changes are not present in epidermal nevi. Epidermolytic hyperkeratosis is present in numerous lesions and is typically an unexplained finding. Bullous ichthyosiform erythroderma shows the typical changes of epidermolytic hyperkeratosis but involves the entire epidermis. In epidermal nevi with epidermolytic hyperkeratosis, the process usually is intermittent. Acrokeratosis verruciformis is papillomatous and hyperkeratotic but regular and symmetrical. Clinical information may be required to differentiate among these entities.

Dowling-Degos Disease

Synonyms: reticulate pigmented anomaly of the flexures

Dowling-Dego's disease (DDD) is believed to be part of a disease spectrum that includes Haber's syndrome, reticulate acropigmentation of Kitamura (RAPK), pigmentation reticularis faciei et colli with epithelial cystomatosis, and familial multiple follicular hamartoma.[9–13] It is inherited as an autosomal dominant trait and is more common in women than men.[9,13] An association with mild mental retardation has been described.[10]

Clinical Features Affected patients have reticulate flexural pigmentation and pitted scars around the mouth that may extend onto the face (Table 26-2).[12] Comedo-like lesions also have been described, and this condition has been confused with chloracne.[10,12–14] RAPK shows symmetrical atrophic freckle-like lesions and pitting on the dorsal hands, feet, and sides of the neck.[13] Slow progressive hyperpigmentation of

---

TABLE 26-1

Epidermal Nevus

Clinical Features

Verrucous brown papules and patches in an isolated or linear array
Slight scaling and hyperkeratosis
Few symptoms

Histopathological Features

Irregular epidermal hyperkeratosis, papillomatosis, hypergranulosis
Occasional parakeratosis and epidermolytic hyperkeratosis
Basal layer hyperpigmentation
Scant perivascular lymphohistiocytic inflammatory infiltrate

Differential Diagnosis

Seborrheic keratosis
Wart
Epidermolytic hyperkeratosis
Acrokeratosis verruciformis

---

atrophic macules begins in adolescence. These lesions eventually may become grey-blue to black. Pigmented scars are found at the angles of the mouth with comedone-like lesions on the neck.[12]

Histopathological Features The epidermis is slightly thinned or atrophic (Table 26-2).[15] The stratum corneum may be slightly hyperkeratotic but is largely unremarkable. Slightly branching club shaped rete ridges project into the dermis. These rete ridges are hyperpigmented, occasionally in a patchy manner, and two to four cells in width. Their branching has been likened to an "antler."[10,16] This epidermal proliferation also is present along the infundibulum of hair follicles.[11] Melanin is present in basal keratinocytes as finely dispersed granules scattered uniformly within the cytoplasm.[16] Small intraepidermal keratin cysts may be seen, and plugging of the follicular infundibulum is present.[16] The dermis has a nonspecific perivascular lymphohistiocytic infiltrate and pigment-laden macrophages.

Differential Diagnosis Dowling-Dego's disease should be differentiated from an adenoid seborrheic keratosis, a solar lentigo, and acanthosis nigricans. Adenoid seborrheic keratoses usually are much more proliferative lesions extending in a glandlike array well into and usually through the papillary dermis. The epidermal rete ridges in DDD are unlikely to be as extensive as in adenoid seborrheic keratoses, and horn pseudocyst production is limited. Solar lentigos rarely demonstrate horn pseudocysts and usually are more pigmented than DDD. Acanthosis nigricans shows a more regular papillomatosis without downward projections of rete ridges, greater hyperkeratosis, and minimal basal layer hyperpigmentation.

Acanthosis Nigricans

This condition was initially reported by Pollitzer in 1890.[17] It is divided into four clinical categories—benign, malignant, syndromic and obesity-associated.[18] Associated syndromes include the type A (HAIR-AN) and type B syndrome, both of which are characterized by insulin-resistant diabetes mellitus.[19,20] Other syndromes include the Hirschowitz syndrome, the Lawrence-Seip syndrome, and leprechaunism.[20–22] Certain drugs induce acanthosis nigricans including nicotinic acid, estrogens, systemic corticosteroids, insulin, pituitary extract, oral contraceptives, fusidic acid, and methyltestosterone.[19] The cutaneous changes of acanthosis nigricans are believed to result from prolonged growth factor stimulation of keratinocytes and dermal fibroblasts.[19]

Clinical Features Acanthosis nigricans is seen in all races, but is more common in African Americans and Hispanics.[19] Obesity is a predisposing factor. It is found at all ages, including birth, but is most common in young patients (Table 26-3).[19] The earliest changes include an ill-defined darkening or hyperpigmentation of the skin, accompanied by dryness and a rough texture. As the disease progresses, the affected skin becomes darker and thicker, eventually assuming a velvet texture. Patches may become yellow, brown, grey, or black.[19] Skin lines are accentuated as furrowing occurs. Small papillomatous projections are seen in early disease and grow as the process proceeds.[20,24] The axillae and sides of the neck are most commonly involved, but almost any cutaneous surface may be affected. Mucosal involvement is present, partic-

---

TABLE 26-2

Dowling-Dego's Disease

Clinical Features

Reticulate pigmentation of the flexures
Pitted perioral scars
Comedo-like lesions

Histopathological Features

Mild hyperkeratosis
Slightly thinned epidermis
Downward projection of the epidermal rete ridges
Basal layer hyperpigmentation
Occasional small horn pseudocysts

Differential Diagnosis

Adenoid seborrheic keratosis
Solar lentigo
Acanthosis nigricans

TABLE 26-3

Acanthosis Nigricans

Clinical Features

All ages affected
Velvety plaques involving the axillae and neck
Mucosal lesions seen
Associated with obesity, underlying malignancy, various syndromes, and drug-intake

Histopathological Features

Papillomatosis, moderate hyperkeratosis, and a mildly thinned epidermis
Minimal basal layer hyperpigmentation and rare horn pseudocyst formation
Mild perivascular inflammation

Differential Diagnosis

Seborrheic keratoses (including stucco keratoses)
Epidermal nevi
Confluent and reticulate papillomatosis

ularly in persons affected with associated malignancy. Mucosal surfaces are hyperpigmented but not velvety.

Histopathological Features   Fully developed lesions show regular papillomatosis, mild acanthosis, and hyperkeratosis (Table 26-3).[19,20] Parakeratosis is uncommon. Intermittent areas of epidermal atrophy may be present and may be accentuated, depending on the patient's overall health. Horn pseudocysts are rare. There is mild hyperpigmentation along the basal layer and in the epidermis. The papillomatosis is believed to derive from an upward projection of the dermal papillae into an already thinned epidermis.[24,25] Usually there is a scant perivascular lymphohistiocytic infiltrate and mild pigment incontinence. Mucin deposition has been described.[19] Mucosal disease demonstrates epithelial hyperplasia with parakeratosis. Papillomatosis also may be seen with little or no hyperpigmentation and pigment incontinence.[25] An infiltrate of lymphocytes, plasma cells, and occasional neutrophils is present.

Differential Diagnosis   The differential diagnosis for acanthosis nigricans includes seborrheic keratoses, epidermal nevi, and confluent and reticulate papillomatosis. Seborrheic keratoses usually have a greater number of horn pseudocysts, occasional parakeratosis, and "flattening out" along the base of the epidermal proliferation. However, stucco keratoses, a variant of seborrheic keratoses, may be particularly difficult to differentiate from acanthosis nigricans. Epidermal nevi have a more broad and "rough" papillomatosis with greater amounts of hyperkeratosis. Epidermal atrophy is unusual in these lesions. Confluent and reticulate papillomatosis shows intermittent parakeratosis, a greater degree of basal layer hyperpigmentation, and elastic fiber fragmentation.

Confluent and Reticulate Papillomatosis of Gougerot and Carteaud

Confluent and reticulate papillomatosis was initially described in 1927 by Gougerot and Carteaud.[26] This disorder may represent an imbalance of the endocrine system, a variant of amyloidosis, or an abnormal host response to colonization by *Pityosporum* organisms.[27,28] It is currently believed to be a disorder of keratinization.

Clinical Features   This eruption occurs around adolescence (Table 26-4).[27,28] It affects women more than men and African Americans

---

TABLE 26-4

Confluent and Reticulate Papillomatosis

Clinical Features

  Begins around adolescence
  Women > men; African Americans > Caucasians
  Small (4–5 mm) patches of hyperpigmentation arising on the chest
    and back
  Confluence of the lesions toward the midline

Histopathological Features

  Papillomatosis, hyperkeratosis, parakeratosis, and acanthosis
  Increased basal layer pigmentation
  Epidermal downgrowths from between the rete ridges

Differential Diagnosis

  Acanthosis nigricans
  Dowling-Dego's disease
  Seborrheic keratoses

---

more than Caucasians.[27,29,30] It is considered non-hereditary; however, familial cases have been reported.[31] Summertime aggravation has been reported.[28] The chest, upper arms, back, and neck are most commonly affected. One- to 2-mm papules emerge and enlarge to 4- to 5-mm. The eruption becomes confluent around the midline and more reticulated as it expands peripherally. Axillary lesions are slightly verrucous.[30] Lesions initially are red to brown and become darker and more grey as they age. A true scale is not present but scraping the lesions may yield a small amount of keratogenous debris. Patients experience no symptoms and mucosal involvement does not occur. Once the eruption has reached its full expansion it tends to remain unchanged.[28]

Histopathological Features   The epidermis is hyperkeratotic with papillomatosis and parakeratosis (Table 26-4). Some follicular plugging with laminated keratin may be seen.[30] Downgrowths of the epidermis may occur between the papillomatous rete ridges. Acanthosis as well as atrophy of the stratum malpighii have been described.[28,30] The granular layer is normal or slightly decreased. There is a mild increase or decrease of basal layer pigmentation. Blood vessels in the dermis are slightly dilated and demonstrate a minimal perivascular lymphohistiocytic infiltrate.[28] Fragmentation of the elastic fibers in the upper and lower dermis have been described.[28,30] Mild papillary dermal edema may be present.[28]

Differential Diagnosis   Confluent and reticulate papillomatosis must be differentiated from acanthosis nigricans, Dowling-Degos disease, and seborrheic keratoses. Acanthosis nigricans shows less basal layer hyperpigmentation, few dermal changes, and no parakeratosis. Additionally, endophytic epidermal proliferations are not seen with this disease. Dowling-Dego's disease demonstrates greater pigment deposition along the basal layer and the occasional presence of a horn pseudocyst. Seborrheic keratoses usually are more hyperkeratotic, possess horn pseudocysts, and are more likely to show epidermal acanthosis. Inflammation is also much more likely with these lesions.

Inflammatory Linear Verrucous Epidermal Nevus

The inflammatory linear verrucous epidermal nevus (ILVEN) is believed to be a variant of an epidermal nevus and was first reported by Unna in 1896.[32] An initial series of 25 cases was presented in 1971.[33]

Clinical Features   These lesions have their onset early in life, half by 6 months of age.[5,33–35] The legs and thighs are most commonly involved, but they may also be seen on the arms, buttocks, groin, and genitalia. Females are more often affected than males.[36] Intense pruritus is common.

    Inflammatory linear verrucous epidermal nevi begin as flesh-colored to red papules that arise in a linear fashion. The papules become dark red to brown with scaling and crusting. They may clinically resemble eczematous dermatitis or psoriasis and may develop a lichenoid appearance.[5,33]

Histopathological Features   The epidermis shows exaggerated rete ridges with hyperkeratosis and parakeratosis (Fig. 26-1). There may be a sharp demarcation between the areas of parakeratosis with a decreased to absent granular layer and orthohyperkeratosis with an intact or accentuated granular layer.[35,37] This alternating type of pattern is characteristic of ILVEN. There is acanthosis with psoriasiform changes, mild to moderate papillomatosis, and an even elongation of the rete ridges. Mitotic activity may be brisk but atypical mitotic figures are not seen.[33] Exocytosis is present in some specimens and microabscesses may form.[34,35,37] There may be slightly increased dermal vascularity.[33] The dermis contains a perivascular and interface inflammatory infiltrate that

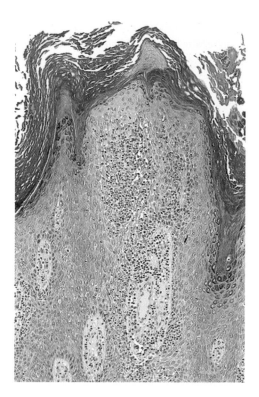

FIGURE 26-1 Inflammatory linear verrucous epidermal nevus. The epidermis is hyperkeratotic and papillomatous with interface inflammation.

may be quite brisk at times.[33,34] The lymphocytes are primarily T cells.[35]

Differential Diagnosis   It is important to differentiate ILVEN from psoriasis, contact dermatitis, eczematous dermatitis, resolving warts, and lichen striatus. Psoriasis vulgaris does not show the typical alternating parakeratosis and orthohyperkeratosis seen in ILVEN. Additionally, the dilated papillary dermal vessels, infiltrating neutrophils, neutrophil rich Munro's microabscesses and thinned suprapapillary plates favor a diagnosis of psoriasis. Chronic eczematous and contact dermatitis are psoriasiform with mild spongiosis and exocytosis but do not show the parakeratosis seen with ILVENs and have infiltrating eosinophils.[33] Senescent warts often demonstrate papillomatosis but usually do not have psoriasiform changes and show parakeratosis emanating from the tips of the papillomatous projections.

Lichen striatus differs from ILVEN by showing either a lichenoid tissue reaction with features of lichen planus or lichen niditus, or spongiotic dermatitis with dyskeratosis rather than the alternating pattern of ortho- and parakeratosis typical of ILVEN.

Nevus Comedonicus

Nevus comedonicus is a linear lesion characterized by a proliferation of keratin filled comedones and was initially described by Kofmann in 1895.[39] It is a rare condition with no suggestion of a heritable pattern or sex preference.[40,41] It has been primarily described in Caucasians but may be seen in all races. Most lesions are present at birth but some develop during adolescence or adulthood. Although it is usually an isolated lesion it may be associated with skeletal defects, CNS abnormalities, ocular pathology, and other cutaneous diseases such as ichthyosis, furunculosis, Becker's nevus, basal cell carcinoma, eccrine nevus, and trichilemmal cysts.[41–44] Nevus comedonicus has arisen following blunt trauma, herpes zoster, lichen planus, smallpox vaccination, and pyo-

TABLE 26-5

Nevus Comedonicus

Clinical Features

Close set or grouped aggregate of dark papules with keratin-filled plugs, usually unilateral and linear, found mostly on face, neck, and trunk

Occasionally arise following a traumatic event

May be associated with rupture, inflammation, abscesses, and scarring

Histopathological Features

Epidermal invagination filled with compact and lamellated keratin

Slight papillomatous proliferation into surrounding dermis

Atrophic sebaceous glands and rudimentary hair bulbs present

Granulomatous inflammation and scarring with comedo rupture

Differential Diagnosis

Dilate pore of Winer

Trichofolliculoma

Pilar sheath acanthoma

Infundibular cyst

Porokeratotic eccrine ostial and dermal duct nevus

derma.[40,41,44] Lesions are believed to represent rudimentary hair follicles with some type of developmental anomaly.[42,43]

Clinical Features   Nevus comedonicus usually is unilateral and linear or zosteriform (Table 26-5). There is some suggestion that these tumors follow the lines of Blaschko.[41] Bilateral and symmetric involvement has been described.[42] They involve the face, neck, thorax, and abdomen.[40,41] Lesions consist of slightly raised papules containing a firm, dark hyperkeratotic plug that resembles a comedo.[40,43,45] The skin has a rough texture and is hypo- or hyperpigmented between comedos.[41] The keratin plugs are adherent and not easily removed. There may be a slight burning sensation to the lesion but most are without symptoms. Some lesions become chronically inflamed and suppurative. Fistulas, scarring, and abscesses may result.[40,41]

Histopathological Features   Epithelium lined invaginations are present and may be normal or decreased in thickness (Fig. 26-2) (Table 26-5). Irregular papillomatous projections proliferate into the surrounding dermis. Epidermolytic hyperkeratosis has been described.[41,43] Atrophic or abortive hair follicles and rudimentary sebaceous glands may be seen.[40,41,43] The epithelial lining forms a compact, lamellated keratin plug. Parakeratosis is absent.[43] The interfollicular epidermis appears normal.[40] The surrounding dermis is largely unremarkable unless one of the comedos has ruptured.

A similar lesion, the dilated pore nevus, has been described as a hamartoma of the dilated pore of Winer and clinically and histologically resembles a nevus comedonicus.[46] The former lesion shows a more prominent granular layer and a greater degree of epithelial proliferation. It appears likely that nevus comedonicus may represent a spectrum of pilosebaceous malformations with the dilated pore nevus representing one end of that spectrum.

Differential Diagnosis   Nevus comedonicus must be differentiated from a dilated pore of Winer, a trichofolliculoma, a pilar sheath acanthoma, the upper portion of an infundibular (epidermoid) cyst and a porokeratotic eccrine ostial and dermal duct nevus.[42,46] A dilated pore of Winer is a solitary lesion and shows a more proliferative and hyper-

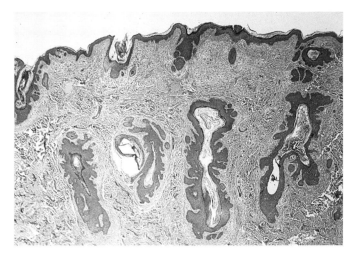

FIGURE 26-2 Nevus comedonicus. The epithelium lined invaginations show small papillary projections into the surrounding dermis.

plastic epithelium as is expands into the surrounding dermis. Association with sebaceous glands is rare. A trichofolliculoma is a solitary proliferation of incompletely differentiated hair follicles inserting into a single dilated infundibulum. This infundibulum is filled with keratogenous debris and small hair shafts. Pilar sheath acanthomas are proliferations of the sebaceous duct and demonstrate a diminished to absent granular layer and pink-staining keratinocytes. Infundibular cysts occasionally demonstrate a connecting infundibulum with features typical for a nevus comedonicus. However, there usually is a single structure and the epithelial lining is not proliferative. Finally, the porokeratotic eccrine ostial and dermal duct nevus usually is found on acral skin and demonstrates a coronoid lamella.

Familial Dyskeratotic Comedones

This entity was initially described in 1972.[47] To date, fewer than 20 cases have been reported. The condition is believed to be inherited as an autosomal dominant trait.[48–50] The patients' health is otherwise normal.

Clinical Features   Lesions appear in childhood or adolescence as open comedones and small hyperkeratotic papules.[48,50] These papules may appear as cutaneous horns. The eruption is generalized but spares the palms, soles, and mucous membranes. Nails and hair are normal.[50] The papules occasionally have a pruritic or burning sensation. Inflammation may be noted if the comedones rupture.

Histopathological Features   Epithelium lined invaginations are present and are filled with laminated keratinous material.[48–50] There are focal areas of acantholysis and dyskeratosis particularly at the base of the invagination. Grains, corps ronds, and suprabasilar clefts are appreciated but hair shafts and other pilosebaceous structures are generally absent. Proliferation of epidermal "villi" into the surrounding dermis is not seen. Electron microscopy reveals decreased desmosomal attachments.[50] Acantholytic cells and grains possess a dense perinuclear tonofilament and keratohyalin aggregation similar to that in other acantholytic diseases.

Differential Diagnosis   The differential diagnosis for familial dyskeratotic comedones includes Darier's disease, warty dyskeratoma and comedones or nevus comedonicus.[50] Darier's disease does not demonstrate formation of comedones and usually has a much greater degree of

acantholysis and corps rond formation. Warty dyskeratomas tend to be larger, "flask"-shaped, more acantholytic, and more villous. Comedones as seen in isolated lesions or nevus comedonicus may have pilosebaceous structures associated with the lesions but do not demonstrate acantholysis or dyskeratotic keratinocytes.

Granuloma (Acanthoma) Fissuratum

This condition was initially described in 1932 by Sutton as occurring in the mouth.[52] Granuloma fissuratum may arise from poorly fitting dentures and accumulation of food particles with maceration. In 1965 Epstein reported it's occurrence behind the superior pole of the ear and proposed a relationship to poorly fitting spectacles.[53] It is also believed to arise on the nose from similar factors.[54] Glass frames constructed with nitrate and cellulose acetate result in rough matt finishes and prolonged skin contact may provoke these lesions.[55] The weight of the glasses, concomitant skin disease, maceration, and abnormal anatomy also play a role.[56,57] Some authors believe this condition is a variant of prurigo nodularis. Resolution of the disease occurs in 1 to 6 months if the glasses are repaired or replaced. This disease is also known as acanthoma fissuratum and "spectacle-frame acanthoma."[56,57]

Clinical Features   Lesions appear as smooth to fissured growths on the nasal bridge and behind the ears, usually at the upper pole of the sulcus (Table 26-6).[58] A shallow to deep longitudinal fissure is present. Most cases are unilateral but bilateral cases have been described.[57] Lesions are flesh-colored to red and are firm. Symptoms are uncommon. Perilesional inflammation may be present. The overlying skin is usually intact and ulceration is rare.[57]

Histopathological Features   The epidermis shows acanthosis and hyperkeratosis with mild to moderate parakeratosis (Table 26-6). The granular layer is present and may be accentuated. Spongiosis is variably present.[56,58] The epidermis forms a central depression corresponding to the longitudinal fissure seen clinically. This depression may be filled with keratogenous debris and inflammatory cells.[56] Elongation and broadening of the rete ridges have been described.[58] Blood vessels in the papillary dermis may be dilated. The perivascular inflammatory infiltrate consists of lymphocytes, plasma cells, and eosinophils. Mild dermal fibrosis may be present.[57]

TABLE 26-6
Granuloma (Acanthoma) Fissuratum

Clinical Features

    Smooth flesh-colored to red nodules at the upper pole of the post-auricular sulcus and on nasal bridge

    Provoked by improperly fitting spectacle frames

Histopathological Features

    Longitudinal epidermal depression-filled with hyperkeratotic and inflammatory debris

    Acanthosis, hyperkeratosis, and parakeratosis

    Perivascular inflammatory infiltrate of lymphocytes, plasma cells, eosinophils

    Mild dermal fibrosis

Differential Diagnosis

    Lichen simplex chronicus

    Prurigo nodule

    Chronic eczematous/contact dermatitis

Differential Diagnosis   Granuloma fissuratum must be differentiated from lichen simplex chronicus, prurigo nodules, and chronic eczematous/contact dermatitis. Lichen simplex chronicus and prurigo nodules generally show little or no spongiosis and a very prominent granular layer. Dermal fibrosis usually is present with "collagen streaking" between the rete ridges and mild pseudoepitheliomatous or psoriasiform epidermal hyperplasia. Additionally, a longitudinal depression is not found in these conditions. Similarly, with chronic eczematous or contact dermatitis the granular layer is well-formed and a psoriasiform hyperplasia is common. Eosinophils may be numerous and again, a longitudinal depression is not appreciated.

Prurigo Nodularis

Prurigo nodularis results when a focal proliferative epidermal response occurs secondary to repeated trauma. It was initially described in 1909 by Hyde as an eruption with recalcitrant pruritus and typically involved the extremities of women.[59] Neural hyperplasia was noted and the disease has been termed "Pautrier neuroma."[24] Different etiologies have been proposed for this disease, including a Merkel cell disorder, arthropod assaults, protracted folliculitis, trauma, deposition of eosinophil granules, and underlying eczematous dermatosis.[60–62] Prurigo nodularis is found is association with hypertension, obesity, renal dysfunction, anemia, hepatic disease, and associated psychiatric disorders such as anxiety or depression.[60] Most patients have an elevated IgE count.[60]

Clinical Features   Lesions present as small nodules on the extensor surfaces of the lower extremities (Table 26-7).[60,63] The arms and trunk may be involved, but areas that cannot be reached are free of disease. No part of the body is exempt from involvement, including the face. Proximal lesions are common. Prurigo nodules are dark, lichenified, verrucous, firm, and may possess overlying scale crust.[64] Excoriation is not uncommon. A halo of post-inflammatory pigmentation may be present.[60] Pruritus usually is described as profound and is provoked by stress and heat.[64] Middle-aged women are most commonly affected. The condition is rare in children.

Histopathological Features   The epidermis shows the typical changes of long standing and repeated trauma—orthohyperkeratosis, a thickened granular layer, and acanthosis with occasional mild spongiosis (Table 26-7).[63] The epidermal proliferation may be psoriasiform (Fig. 26-3). The tumors are symmetrical and usually well-circumscribed. Careful inspection may reveal the underlying etiology, such as chronic eczematous or contact dermatitis. If particularly proliferative, the epidermis may demonstrate pseudoepitheliomatous hyperplasia, that is, the proliferation of a mildly eosinophilic and pale epidermis with asymmetric, bulbous epithelial acanthosis.

In the dermis is a mild to moderate perivascular inflammatory infiltrate composed of lymphocytes, histiocytes, and occasional eosinophils.[64] If the lesions are chronic, plasma cells may be present. Mast cells are normal in number and Merkel cells are increased.[62,64] Occasional neutrophils are present.[61] The papillary dermis shows mild fibrosis between the downgrowing rete ridges.[63] Fibroblasts may be abundant. Blood vessels are increased and subepidermal fibrin is deposited.[60] Nerve counts in affected tissues are greater than controls; however, the previously reported phenomenon of neural hyperplasia has been disproven.[60,64] Ultrastructural findings include abnormalities in neural axons and surrounding Schwann cells.[63] Schwann cells demonstrate absent endoplasmic reticulum, diminished numbers of mitochondria, and a few asymmetric, membrane-bound vacuoles.

Differential Diagnosis   The differential diagnosis for prurigo nodularis includes lichen simplex chronicus, keratoacanthoma, and pseudoepitheliomatous hyperplasia associated with other disorders. Lichen simplex chronicus is not a nodule but rather a patch or plaque. As such the symmetry and circumscription seen with prurigo nodularis is lacking. Additionally, the epidermal hyperplasia is not as pronounced and tends to be more regular or psoriasiform. Keratoacanthomas commonly demonstrate the proliferative epidermal characteristics seen in prurigo nodularis. However, the keratogenous plug, epidermal atypia, and intraepidermal neutrophilic microabscesses are not present in prurigo nodularis. Pseudoepitheliomatous hyperplasia is a pathologic reaction pattern that arises following trauma or irritation from a variety of causes. Deep fungal infections, Spitz nevi, granular cell tumors, and halogenodermas may demonstrate this reaction pattern. Special stains for microorganisms and different cell types may help differentiate these diseases from prurigo nodularis.

TABLE 26-7

Prurigo Nodularis

Clinical Features

Nodules with lichenification and excoriation
Very pruritic
Occur preferentially on the proximal extremities in middle-aged women

Histopathological Features

Extensive hyperkeratosis with hypergranulosis in a psoriasiform or pseudoepitheliomatous pattern
Occasional mild spongiosis and parakeratosis
Perivascular inflammation with occasional eosinophils and plasma cells
Mild papillary dermal fibrosis

Differential Diagnosis

Lichen simplex chronicus
Keratoacanthomas
Pseudoepitheliomatous hyperplasia (deep fungal infections, Spitz nevi, granular cell tumors, etc.)

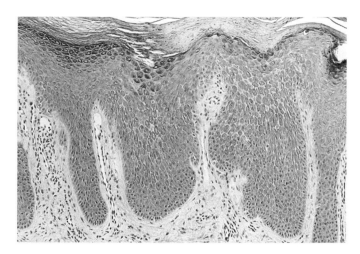

FIGURE 26-3   Prurigo nodularis. The epidermis proliferates with psoriasiform features, hypergranulosis, and hyperkeratosis.

ACANTHOMAS/KERATOSES

Epidermolytic Acanthoma

Shapiro and Baraf initially described epidermolytic acanthomas in 1970.[65] These tumors present as isolated or disseminated lesions.[66] The epidermolysis may represent an increased metabolic activity of the corneocytes or a neoplastic recapitulation of a developmental anomaly.[67] HPV infection has not been found using PCR testing.[68]

Clinical Features   Most patients are middle-aged (Table 26-8). Lesions are found on almost all body sites and are more common in men than women.[69] Epidermolytic acanthomas are 2- to 5-mm slightly raised papules with verrucoid features. Some are smooth surfaced and others are mildly scaly. Tumors are flesh colored to slightly grey.

Histopathological Features   The stratum corneum is compact or loosely laminated and is moderately to markedly hyperkeratotic (Table 26-8).[67,69,70] Some parakeratosis may be present.[66,69,70] Eosinophilic anuclear bodies may be present and represent individually keratinized cells that have been retained in the stratum corneum. The basal layer is involved, but the remainder of the stratum malpighii is abnormal.[69,70] The granular layer is most affected and demonstrates thickening with coarse, enlarged keratohyaline granules (Fig. 26-4).[66,67] Vacuolar changes are prominent. The spinous layer demonstrates similar changes and eosinophilic granules.[66,67] Eosinophilic material arranged in strands is present in the spinous and granular layers. The cell layer immediately above the stratum basale demonstrates clear-cell changes and prematurely cornified keratinocytes.[69] There is a non-specific perivascular lymphohistiocytic infiltrate in the dermis.[67]

On electron microscopy the basal cells appear normal aside from some increased numbers of mitochondria and endoplasmic ribosomes.[66,67] Suprabasal cells demonstrate abnormal tonofilament aggregation around the nucleus. This pattern is accentuated in upper levels of the epidermis. Desmosomes are normal.[67] The eosinophilic strands in the stratum spinosum are also abnormal tonofilaments set in a whirling pattern. Intracellular edema begins in the upper spinous layer and is seen throughout the granular layer. Cells of the stratum corneum do not appear to cornify uniformly.

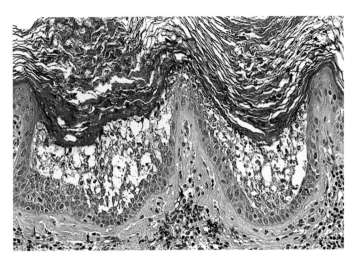

FIGURE 26-4   Epidermolytic acanthoma. The spinous and granular layers are vacuolated with enlarged keratohyaline granules. Hyperkeratosis also is present.

Differential Diagnosis   Epidermolytic hyperkeratosis may be seen in numerous skin diseases including bullous ichthyosiform erythroderma, ichthyosis hystrix, keratoderma palmaris et plantaris, nevus unis lateris, epidermolytic leukoplakia, and acrosyringeal epidermolytic papulosis neviformis.[45] Small biopsies of these entities may not be discernible from an epidermolytic acanthoma without clinical information. Epidermolytic hyperkeratosis is also present in a number of isolated skin lesions such as infundibular cysts, seborrheic keratoses, and actinic keratoses.[67] It is important to differentiate epidermolytic acanthomas from warts. The endophytic palmoplantar warts (myrmecia warts) typically show perinuclear vacuolization and numerous keratohyaline granules. However, these granules are usually more eosinophilic than those appearing in epidermolytic hyperkeratosis. Additionally, vascular dilatation in the dermal papillae and prominent papillomatosis are seen.

Warty Dyskeratoma

Warty dyskeratoma was originally described by Helwig and Allen, but the term was coined by Syzmanski in 1957.[71–73] These lesions are believed to arise from pilosebaceous structures; however, this view has been criticized.[74] Serial sectioning through some lesions has failed to show evidence of follicular derivation. Additionally, oral warty dyskeratomas have not been found in a distribution similar to that of ectopic sebaceous glands. Some investigators believe warty dyskeratomas are isolated variants of Darier's disease.[75] Oral lesions may arise secondary to irritation and trauma. The use of tobacco and other chemical carcinogens has been implicated in their etiology.[75–77] Glaborous lesions arise on sun exposed areas perhaps because of prolonged ultraviolet light exposure.[75] Infectious etiologies have been ruled out.[78] Circulating antibody-induced acantholysis, as seen in pemphigus, has been suspect.

Clinical Features   Glaborous lesions generally are single and slow-growing, and are found predominantly on the head, neck, and extremities (Table 26-9).[75,76] Tumors appear primarily on patients in the fourth to fifth decades, and more often in men than women.[73,75,78,79] Multiple warty dyskeratomas have been described.[70,74,78] Tumors are flesh-colored to brown papules with a rolled, smooth edge and a central, hyperkeratotic plug. Foul-smelling cheesy material may drain from these lesions.[76,78] Pruritus and bleeding may occur, but most papules are without symptoms. The diagnosis is rarely made clinically.[78] Malignant degeneration has not been described.[16]

TABLE 26-8

Epidermolytic Acanthoma

Clinical Features

Small flat or verrucous papules
Most common on the extremities
Occur in middle-aged persons, men more than women

Histopathological Features

Hyperkeratosis with dense and loosely packed keratinocytes
Large, coarse basophilic granules in the granular layer with vacuolated keratinocytes
Fine eosinophilic granules and strands in the spinous and granular layers
Normal basal layer

Differential Diagnosis

Epidermolytic hyperkeratosis seen in different cutaneous tumors and diseases
Warts, particularly the palmoplantar type

TABLE 26-9

Warty Dyskeratoma

Clinical Features

Isolated lesions on the sun-damaged skin of middle-aged persons
Also seen on oral mucosa
Papulo-nodule with central pore or umbilication
May discharge foul-smelling material

Histopathological Features

Flask-shaped cystic invagination involving a pilosebaceous structure
Parakeratotic and hyperkeratotic material in infundibulum
Suprabasal acantholysis with villi and acantholysis
Dyskeratosis, corps ronds, and grains are present

Differential Diagnosis

Darier's disease
Hailey-Hailey disease
Pemphigus vegetans
Syringocystadenoma papilliferum

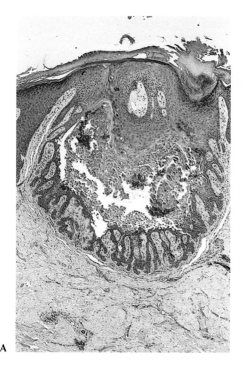

A

Oral lesions are rare but are similar to glaborous tumors. They usually are not painful and are found on keratinizing surfaces exposed to trauma.[75,76] Like their glaborous counterparts, they are small papules or nodules with a central crater. They may assume a papillomatous appearance and are flesh-colored to white.

Histopathological Features Glaborous lesions usually are associated with pilosebaceous structures and early changes are limited to the upper portion of the follicular infundibulum (Table 26-9).[79] Single follicles usually are involved, but multiple follicle involvement has been described.[79] Adjacent sebaceous glands are present in some specimens. The epithelium surrounding the follicular ostia may form a collarette with hypergranulosis and acanthosis.[80] The follicles become cystic, enlarged, and flask-shaped (Fig. 26-5).[73,75] They extend deep into the reticular dermis and are filled with parakeratotic and hyperkeratotic debris.[70,73,78] The papillomatous epithelial wall lining extends into the surrounding dermis. There is acantholysis and dyskeratosis of involved keratinocytes. Corps ronds and grains are formed. These features are similar to those seen in Darier's disease. Suprabasal lacunae are present and keratin pearl-like structures may be seen in lesions of long standing. Villi are covered by a single layer of epithelial cells and extend into the cystic cavity. The basement membrane zone demonstrates a loss of fine elastic twigs.[80] The cystic structure is surrounded by a sheath of fibrovascular connective tissue.[79] There is a moderate perivascular inflammatory infiltrate in the dermis consisting of lymphocytes, histiocytes, rare eosinophils, and occasional plasma cells. Postinflammatory pigment incontinence has been described.[73,79]

Oral lesions are similar to those from glaborous skin.[73,76,77] Corps ronds and grains are not as well developed in mucosal lesions. Ongoing mechanical trauma in these areas may dislodge the keratotic plug.[76]

Ultrastructurally, the dyskeratotic and acantholytic cells are similar to those in Darier's disease.[75] The cytoplasm contains dense, perinuclear bands of tonofilaments. Numerous ribosomes and polyribosomes are present.[77] Acantholysis may result from poor desmosome–tonofilament complexes between cells.

Differential Diagnosis Warty dyskeratomas must be differentiated from other acantholytic diseases, such as Darier's disease (the hypertrophic variant), Hailey-Hailey disease, and pemphigus vegetans.[79]

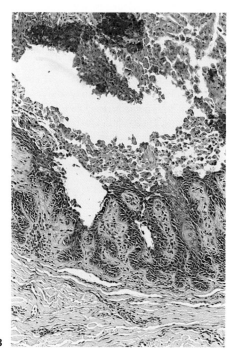

B

FIGURE 26-5 Warty dyskeratoma. *A.* Note proliferative nodule containing cystic cavity and keratinous material. *B.* The lining epidermis shows dyskeratosis and acantholysis.

None of these diseases forms the typical flask-shaped invagination seen in warty dyskeratoma. Additionally, the acantholysis is probably less than with Hailey-Hailey disease and pemphigus vegetans. Pemphigus vegetans demonstrates numerous infiltrating eosinophils and may be ruled out using direct immunofluorescence testing. Darier's disease usually shows more dyskeratosis and corps ronds and grains formation than warty dyskeratoma. Syringocystadenoma papilliferum may show villi formation similar to that seen in warty dyskeratomas and should be differentiated from these tumors. However, the epidermis is often eroded, plasma cells are generally abundant, and no keratogenous plug is present.[70,73]

Acantholytic Acanthoma

Acantholytic acanthoma was originally described by Brownstein in 1988.[81] These are isolated lesions without a relationship to other disorders.[82] It is termed an acanthoma because the growths are composed of proliferating benign keratinocytes. They are known to proliferate in the face of diminished immune surveillance and immunosuppression may be causative.[82]

Clinical Features   Lesions usually are isolated and present on the trunk or extremities (Table 26-10).[81,82] The mucous membranes, face, soles, and palms are spared.[83] They are 5 to 15 mm in diameter and are erythematous to dark. Most patients are elderly men.[82,83] The lesions usually are asymptomatic, but itching has been noted.[82,83]

Histopathological Features   The epidermis demonstrates hyperkeratosis, parakeratosis, and irregular hyperplasia (Table 26-10).[81,82,84] The lesions are symmetrical and well-circumscribed. Some papillomatosis occasionally is present, and focal crusting and spongiosis may be appreciated. Acantholysis is present throughout most of the epidermis and is accentuated in the granular or suprabasalar layers.[83] Dyskeratotic cells and grains occasionally are present.[83,84] Atypia is absent. There is a nonspecific perivascular lymphohistiocytic infiltrate in the underlying dermis. Occasional eosinophils are seen.[81,83]

Differential Diagnosis   Focal and limited biopsies of acantholytic disorders such as pemphigus vulgaris, pemphigus vegetans, Hailey-Hailey, and Grover's disease may mimic an acantholytic acanthoma.[82] These disorders, however, are eruptions with widespread involvement and would not be symmetrical and well-circumscribed. Eosinophils are prominent in pemphigus, and it is useful to differentiate them with immunofluorescent techniques. The acantholysis of Hailey-Hailey is commonly very extensive and Grover's disease may demonstrate numerous dyskeratotic cells with grains. Seborrheic keratoses may have sporadic acantholysis, but usually contain hyperpigmentation along the basal layer, horn pseudocysts, and a "flat bottom." Acantholytic actinic

keratoses show keratinocyte atypia, and warty dyskeratomas are "flask-shaped" with a parakeratotic plug.

Seborrheic Keratosis

Seborrheic keratoses are among the most common human neoplasms, occurring in about 20 percent of the elderly.[85] About 20 percent of the elderly have these lesions. The histologic features of seborrheic keratoses were described in 1926 by Freudenthal.[86]

These neoplasms arise in most persons as incidental tumors. One subset of patients may develop seborrheic keratoses when afflicted by underlying malignancies. The sign of Leser-Trelat is a sudden eruption of seborrheic keratoses in persons with concomitant cancers, most commonly an adenocarcinoma of the gastrointestinal tract.[70] This sign was originally described separately by Edmund Leser and Ulysse Trelat in the late nineteenth century.[87] It is a rare phenomenon and may be associated with the development of acanthosis nigricans, acquired ichthyosis, and hypertrichosis lanuginosa.[88] The seborrheic keratoses are indistinguishable clinically and histologically from those occurring in healthy patients, but arise rapidly on the chest and back. They may demonstrate a "Christmas tree" or "splash" pattern.[88] Pruritus is common and portends a poor prognosis. This phenomenon is believed to arise from tumor secreted growth factors.[87] Seborrheic keratoses in persons with colon cancer have been described as demonstrating a "halo" effect. Numerous lesions also are a part of the Weary-Kindler syndrome.[89]

Clinical Features   Seborrheic keratoses have a "stuck-on" appearance (Table 26-11).[70] They are flesh-colored to dark black and range in size from a millimeter or two to several centimeters in diameter. They may be found anywhere except the palm and soles, but there is a predilection for the head, neck, and trunk. A variant of seborrheic keratoses termed stucco keratoses arise as warty 1- to 3-mm verrucous papules with a propensity for the distal extremities.

TABLE 26-10

Acantholytic Acanthoma

Clinical Features

Solitary, asymptomatic papule or nodule on the trunk
5 to 15 mm in diameter and hyperkeratotic
Most common in middle-aged men

Histopathological Features

Acantholysis throughout most of the epidermis
Hyperkeratosis, parakeratosis, and acanthosis
Symmetrical and circumscribed

Differential Diagnosis

Pemphigus vulgaris
Pemphigus vegetans
Hailey-Hailey disease
Grover's disease
Acantholytic changes of seborrheic keratoses or actinic keratoses
Warty dyskeratoma

TABLE 26-11

Seborrheic Keratosis

Clinical Features

Middle-aged and older patients on the head, neck, and trunk
Flesh-colored to dark black papules with a "stuck on" appearance
1 millimeter to several centimeters in diameter and sharply demarcated
Smooth to warty with a crumbly texture

Histopathological Features

Benign squamoid and basaloid proliferation with acanthosis, hyperkeratosis, papillomatosis, reticulation, and horn pseudocysts
Basal layer hyperpigmentation
Infiltrating lymphocytes in the dermis and epidermis

Differential Diagnosis

Hidroacanthoma simplex/eccrine poroma
Basal cell carcinoma
Fibroepithelioma of Pinkus
Epidermal nevus (particularly the inflammatory linear verrucous variant)
Acantholytic changes of isolated lesions

Histopathological Features There are several different histologic variants of seborrheic keratoses (Table 26-11). These have been designated as acanthotic, hyperkeratotic or papillomatous, adenoidal (reticulated), clonal, macular or incipient, pedunculated, and irritated or inflamed. These variants demonstrate a characteristic pattern of growth; basal and squamous proliferation with hyperkeratosis, papillomatosis, and horn pseudocyst production.[90] Spongiosis is present in some lesions, particularly those that have been irritated, but atypia is unusual.[91] Mitotic figures may be seen and are normal in configuration.[91] Squamous eddies may be observed as well and are not necessarily restricted to irritated or inflamed lesions.[70,91,92] Additional features include clear-cell changes, sebaceous differentiation, and trichilemmal differentiation.[70,93] Regression and atrophy of seborrheic keratoses have been described and peritumoral amyloid deposition is present in up to 18 percent of lesions.[70,94–96]

Acanthotic

This is one of the most common variants of seborrheic keratosis. On low power the lesions have a smooth dome shape of surface.[95] The epidermis is broad and composed of basaloid cells (Fig. 26-6 A,B). Horn pseudocysts are present and may be very large. Hyperkeratosis is minimal and papillomatosis essentially is absent.[70] The base of the lesion demonstrates a "flat bottom." Hyperpigmentation usually is visible along the basal layer, but may involve the upper cell layers as well.

Hyperkeratotic (Papillomatous)

The epidermis shows a papillomatous, "church spire" proliferation. There is orthokeratotic and parakeratotic hyperkeratosis. The rest of the stratum malpighii is acanthotic with basaloid and squamous cell proliferation. The stratum corneum is loosely laminated and interdigitated.[70] The base of the lesion is flat. There usually is some hyperpigmentation

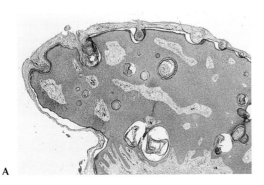

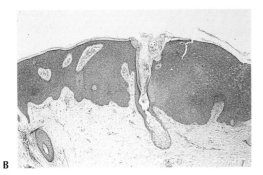

FIGURE 26-6 Seborrheic keratosis. *A*. The epithelium is acanthotic with horn pseudocysts and minimal hyperkeratosis. *B*. Acanthosis and a "flat bottom" are present in this lesion.

along the basal layer. Stucco keratoses are probably variants of hyperkeratotic seborrheic keratoses. These lesions demonstrate a regular, sharp-pointed papillomatosis. Pigment deposition is minimal. They may be indistinguishable from acrokeratosis verruciformis of Hopf.

Adenoidal (Reticulated)

In this variant the epithelium is elongated and reticulated with moderate to prominent pigment deposition. Small-horn pseudocysts are present. Epithelial anastomosis is common and surrounds some horn pseudocysts. The pattern is reminiscent of a proliferative solar lentigo and some investigators believe that these tumors are identical.[95,97]

Clonal

Clonal seborrheic keratoses demonstrate a nesting pattern.[95] The epidermis is mildly hyperkeratotic with acanthosis. Within the acanthotic epidermis are "clones" of basaloid epidermal cells surrounded by otherwise unremarkable keratinocytes. This pattern is termed the Borst-Jadassohn phenomenon and may be seen in other cutaneous tumors.

Macular

Also known as an "incipient" seborrheic keratosis, the macular variant demonstrates subtle changes.[70] The epidermis is minimally acanthotic and hyperkeratotic. Epidermal proliferation is flat and even across the bottom. There may be increased basal layer pigmentation, but it is generally minimal and difficult to discern.

Pedunculated (Sessile)

These typically arise on the eyelids, neck, and in the axillae.[70,95] There is attenuated collagen in the dermis with dilated blood vessels that often contain inspissated erythrocytes. The epidermis generally is acanthotic, hyperpigmented, and similar to that seen with an acanthotic seborrheic keratosis.

Irritated (Inflamed)

This is a common designation and often is applied to one of the previously mentioned variants that displays exocytosis, apoptosis, acantholysis, scale-crust formation, spongiosis, and trichilemmal keratinization.[70,91,98] Basaloid cells undergo conversion into squamoid cells by acceleration of cellular maturation.[95] The papillary dermis contains a perivascular and interface inflammatory infiltrate composed of lymphocytes and mononuclear-cells. A purely lichenoid infiltrate is not believed to be associated with externally irritated lesions.[99] Neutrophilic microabscesses may be present but eosinophils are rare and raise the possibility of a secondary contact dermatitis from topically applied medicaments.[98] Plasma cells are not common but are seen with lesions of long standing. Some extravasation and exocytosis of erythrocytes may be observed.[91] Dermal papillae may be hyalinized with necrotic adjacent epithelium.[99] Seborrheic keratoses that have been traumatized by rubbing have demonstrated hair germ buds.[99]

Seborrheic keratoses have been found in association with benign and malignant lesions. Keratotic compound nevi have features of an adenoidal seborrheic keratosis and compound nevus.[100,101] These typically are found on the trunk of young women. Trichostasis spinulosa has been noticed in some lesions and seborrheic keratosis-like changes have been reported in the lining of infundibular (epidermoid) cysts.[102] Basal cell carcinoma, squamous cell carcinoma, malignant melanoma, keratoacanthoma, adenocarcinoma, Bowen's disease and bowenoid transformation have been described in association with seborrheic keratoses.[85,90,97,103–107] A nonmelanoma skin carcinoma was found associated with 4.6 percent of seborrheic keratoses.[97] In persons with widespread cutaneous diseases such as psoriasis or cutaneous T-cell lymphoma seborrheic keratoses taken from involved skin may demonstrate histopathologic changes of these dermatoses.[70]

Human papillomaviruses have been found in some seborrheic keratoses but are not believed to be causative.[108,109] HPV type 5 is found in cutaneous seborrheic keratoses from persons with epidermodysplasia verruciformis, and 42 percent of lesions from the groin were found to contain HPV types 6, 11, and 16.[109,110] Involved keratinocytes demonstrate pale staining and clumping of keratohyaline granules in the upper stratum malpighii. HPV particles were found on electron microscopy in all four cases studied.[108] Increased melanin production in infected cells also has been described.[108]

Differential Diagnosis   The differential diagnosis for seborrheic keratosis varies depending on the histologic type. Hidroacanthoma simplex/eccrine poroma, basal cell carcinoma, fibroepithelioma of Pinkus, epidermal nevi (particularly the inflammatory linear verrucous variant), and epidermal acantholysis should be differentiated from seborrheic keratoses.[70,91] Hidroacanthoma simplex and eccrine poromas have very bland proliferating cells with a "clonal" pattern of growth. Ductal differentiation may be seen and the lesions are endophytic rather than exophytic or papillomatous. Basal cell carcinomas have the epidermal acanthosis and hyperpigmentation seen in acanthotic seborrheic keratoses. However, atypia, apoptosis, stromal retraction, peripheral palisading, and mucin production are much more common in basal cell carcinomas. Similarly, the fibroepithelioma of Pinkus is a reticulated variant of basal cell carcinoma but does not demonstrate horn pseudocyst production and shows a surrounding fibromucinous stroma. Epidermal nevi may be very difficult to differentiate from inflamed seborrheic keratoses. Both lesions are papillomatous, hyperkeratotic, and acanthotic. However, the regular acanthosis which results in the "flat bottom" of seborrheic keratoses generally is absent from epidermal nevi. Additionally, horn pseudocysts are not present in these latter lesions. Acantholysis may be found in various inflamed and benign processes, including acantholytic acanthoma, acantholytic actinic keratosis, and Darier's disease. Epidermal hyperpigmentation and horn pseudocyst production favor a diagnosis of seborrheic keratosis.

Dermatosis Papulosa Nigra

This disorder was first described in 1925 by Castellani.[111] It occurs almost exclusively in African Americans, Filipinos, Mexicans, Vietnamese, and Native Americans.[111,112] Caucasians have been described with dermatosis papulosa nigra, but it is uncommon.[111] Women are more commonly afflicted than men, and there seems to be a genetic component to this disease.[111]

Clinical Features   These lesions are primarily localized to the face (Table 26-12).[70,111] They are well-demarcated, are 1 to 5 mm in diameter, and have a pedunculated appearance. Most are hyperpigmented, but some may be flesh-colored. They are rarely pruritic.

Histopathological Features   The pathologic features essentially are identical to those of seborrheic keratoses (Table 26-12).[3,111] Mild hyperkeratosis with parakeratosis, acanthosis, and basal layer hyperpigmentation are present. Some specimens demonstrate reticulated epidermal proliferation and horn pseudocysts. The dermis shows mildly attenuated collagen, giving the lesions a fibroepithelial polyp-like appearance. Immature pilosebaceous structures may be appreciated.[111] Inflamed lesions are similar to inflamed seborrheic keratoses and show spongiosis, perivascular lymphocytes, scale-crust formation, and exocytosis.

Differential Diagnosis   These lesions should be differentiated from fibroepithelial polyps and seborrheic keratoses, particularly the pedunculated variant. Fibroepithelial polyps typically have very attenuated collagen and dilated vascular spaces with inspissated erythrocytes. These features generally are lacking in dermatosis papulosa nigra. Dermatosis papulosa nigra usually are smaller than seborrheic keratoses and may show a completely circumscribed and symmetrical lesion despite a small biopsy specimen. The pedunculated variant of a seborrheic keratosis may be identical to dermatosis papulosa nigra.

Melanoacanthoma

Melanoacanthoma initially was described by Bloch in 1927 and named in 1960 by Mishima and Pinkus.[113,114] Cutaneous lesions are almost exclusively restricted to Caucasians, whereas oral melanoacanthomas are present mostly in African-American women.[115,116] Glaborous lesions are present in persons over 55 years of age with no gender preferences and develop slowly.[115–117] Oral lesions are most common in young adults.[116] They usually are solitary and develop over weeks to months.[117] The pathophysiology of melanoacanthomas is unclear but may involve a block in the transfer of melanin from melanocytes to

---

TABLE 26-12

Dermatosis Papulosa Nigra

Clinical Features

Small dark pedunculated papules on the face
Restricted to African Americans, Hispanics, Vietnamese, Native Americans, and Filipinos

Histopathological Features

Epidermal acanthosis or reticulation with basal layer hyperpigmentation
Polypoid appearance
Inflamed lesions with spongiosis, exocytosis, and perivascular lymphocytes

Differential Diagnosis

Fibroepithelial polyp
Seborrheic keratosis, particularly the pedunculated variant

TABLE 26-13

Melanoacanthoma

Clinical Features

Glaborous lesions arise on the head, neck, and abdomen of older patients
Oral lesions are seen in younger patients, particularly African-American females
Tumors are slightly raised, very dark, and several centimeters in diameter

Histopathological Features

The epidermis is acanthotic, well-demarcated, and usually symmetrical
Pigmentation is prominent and restricted to the melanocytes and dermal melanophages

Differential Diagnosis

Seborrheic keratosis, particularly the acanthotic and hyperpigmented variant

epithelial cells.[116] Pigment retention by secondarily stimulated melanocytes may result from trauma. These lesions probably are reactive rather than neoplastic.

Clinical Features   Melanoacanthomas are well-demarcated, slightly raised, usually solitary and arise on the head, neck, abdomen, and extremities (Table 26-13).[115,116] They are up to several centimeters in diameter and are very dark. These lesions are similar to a heavily pigmented seborrheic keratosis.[70] Oral melanoacanthomas also are dark and solitary. They are most common on the buccal or labial mucosa.

Histopathological Features   Histopathologic features essentially are identical for glabrous and mucosal lesions. The epidermis is acanthotic and mildly hyperkeratotic.[115,116] Some elongation and fusion of rete ridges is seen. Spongiosis is greater in oral melanoacanthomas.[117] Large dendritic melanocytes contain considerable pigment. Pigment incontinence is prominent with uptake by dermal melanophages.[116] Mitotic activity and epidermal atypia are not appreciated. S-100 stains reveal intraepidermal melanocytes with large dendrites.

Oral lesions may have mildly increased vascularity and occasional eosinophils.[115,116] Ultrastructurally, large dendritic melanocytes are seen in the basal and spinous layers of the epidermis.[116] Visible melanin is restricted to melanocytes.

Differential Diagnosis   Melanoacanthomas may be difficult to differentiate from heavily pigmented seborrheic keratoses, particularly the acanthotic variant. Most pigmented seborrheic keratoses demonstrate horn pseudocysts, pigmented keratinocytes, and mild to moderate hyperkeratosis.

Clear-cell Acanthoma

These lesions, also known as pale cell acanthomas, were first described in 1962 by Degos et al.[70,118] They were previously thought to be a variant of a seborrheic keratosis.[119] The profile of composite keratins is different from that of the acrosyringium but similar to those found in normal skin.[119]

TABLE 26-14

Clear-cell Acanthoma

Clinical Features

Found on the lower extremity or foot in older patients
Lesions are well demarcated, erythematous, and have a moist
    surface
A peripheral collarette of scale may be appreciated

Histopathological Features

Acanthosis with clear-cell changes is present and is well-
    demarcated from normal epithelium
Psoriasiform-like hyperplasia with some fusion of rete ridges
Infiltrating neutrophils in the epidermis
Clear cells are PAS-positive and diastase-resistant
Epidermal melanin absent

Differential Diagnosis

Seborrheic keratosis with clear-cell changes
Eccrine poroma
Psoriasis vulgaris

Clinical Features   Patients usually are middle-aged or older and most are Caucasians (Table 26-14). Men and women are affected equally.[55] Lesions are single and are present on the lower legs and feet.[120,121] Tumors are moist and smooth with a well-circumscribed border. A "stuck-on" appearance is present in some lesions. They are brown to erythematous in color and may have a vascular appearance. Clear-cell acanthomas may blanch when pressure is applied.[70] Some lesions are scaly or crusted and appear eczematous in nature.[70] Tumors are about 10 mm in diameter and are asymptomatic. Polypoid and giant variants have been described.[120,122]

Histopathological Features   The epidermis is acanthotic with clear-cell changes that are readily demarcated from adjacent normal epidermis (Table 26-14) (Fig. 26-7 A,B).[70,120,121,123] Pale cells are polyhedral and larger than normal keratinocytes. They are also PAS-positive and diastase sensitive indicating the presence of glycogen.[57,90] Mitoses are few and significant atypia is uncommon.[121] Spongiosis is present. Rete ridges are elongated, occasionally in a psoriasiform manner and may show fusion. A collarette is appreciated at the sharply demarcated margins of the lesion. The granular layer is absent and infiltrating neutrophils are seen (Fig. 26-7 C).[23] Neutrophilic microabscesses have been reported.[121] The stratum corneum may be parakeratotic with serous exudate.[121] Melanin is present in dermal melanophages but often is absent in the epidermis and along the basal layer.[70] A pigmented variant has been described and demonstrates impressive numbers of melanocytes with elongated dendrites containing melanin granules.[124] A cystic variant also has been reported.[23] Follicular and acrosyringeal structures are present.[121,123] Blood vessels may be present in increased numbers and are slightly dilated. A perivascular lymphohistiocytic infiltrate is appreciated.[70,120] Occasional neutrophils may be present. Sweat glands may be dilated and hyperplastic, indicating sweat retention.[120]

Ultrastructurally, the affected keratinocytes show increased glycogen.[120] The nuclei and cytoplasmic organelles otherwise are normal. The pigmented variant of clear-cell acanthoma shows increased melanosomes within dendritic cells.[124]

Differential Diagnosis   The differential diagnosis for clear-cell acanthoma includes seborrheic keratosis, eccrine poroma, and psoriasis. Seborrheic keratoses may have an increase in intracellular glycogen but lack the sharply demarcated pale cell changes in adjacent epidermis. Additionally, horn pseudocysts and the "flat bottom" appearance of seborrheic keratoses usually are lacking. Eccrine poromas do not have clear-cell changes and demonstrate ductal differentiation. Psoriasis vulgaris demonstrates regular psoriasiform hyperplasia, prominent parakeratosis, and neutrophilic microabscesses. Clear cells are absent.

Large-Cell Acanthoma

Large-cell acanthoma was initially described in 1967 by Pinkus.[125] It is likely induced by prolonged sun exposure since it arises in areas of solar damage on elderly patients.[126] These tumors may be a variant of an actinic keratosis or a solar lentigo.[126,127] DNA analysis has shown that the cells are aneuploid or tetraploid and that abnormal clones are present.[128,129] Most cases are single but multiple lesions have been described.[126] Large-cell acanthomas have a benign and indolent clinical course.[129] Some investigators believe that women are more commonly affected than men, whereas others have found an equal incidence between the sexes.[126,127,129]

Clinical Features   Large-cell acanthomas usually are less than 1 centimeter in diameter (Table 26-15).[70,130] They arise on sun damaged skin and are dry and smooth. Lesions are slightly hyperpigmented and occasionally hyperkeratotic.[126,128,130]

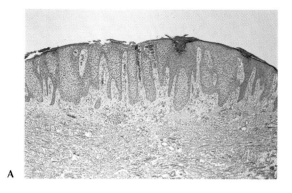

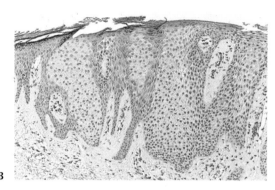

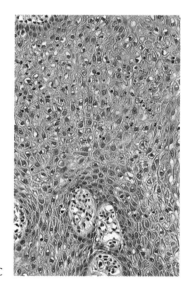

FIGURE 26-7 Clear-cell acanthoma. *A*. The epidermis is psoriasiform with areas of clear-cell proliferation. *B*. Clear-cell changes are well demarcated from adjacent epidermis. *C*. Mild spongiosis and exocytosis by neutrophils are appreciated.

Histopathological Features The pathologic features are believed to be pathognomonic.[130] Lesions are well circumscribed with a clear demarcation between affected and uninvolved epidermis (Table 26-15).[126,130] Keratinocytes are enlarged with proportionally larger nuclei (Fig. 26-8). These nuclei are pleomorphic but not hyperchromatic.[127,130] Mitotic activity is not prominent and adnexal structures within the epidermis are not involved (acrosyringium).[126] Rete ridges are bulbous.[131] Ortho-hyperkeratosis is appreciated and the granular layer may be enhanced or reduced. The basal layer shows modest hyperpigmentation but the number of melanocytes is not increased.[130,131] Solar elastosis and telangiectasias are present in the dermis.[126,127,129,130] Perivascular inflammation may be present but usually is mild. Three types of large cell

TABLE 26-15

Large-cell Acanthoma

Clinical Features

  Arise on the sun-damaged skin of elderly patients
  Lesions are slightly hyperpigmented, flat, and mildly hyperkeratotic
  Less than 1 cm in diameter

Histopathological Features

  Well-demarcated enlarged keratinocytes and nuclei
  Rare mitotic figures
  Slight hyperkeratosis without parakeratosis
  Bulbous rete ridges with mild hyperpigmentation along the basal
    layer
  Solar elastosis and telangiectasias

Differential Diagnosis

  Actinic keratosis
  Seborrheic keratosis
  Solar lentigo
  Acrokeratosis verruciformis
  Stucco keratosis

acanthoma have been described—the classic lesion, one with verrucous hyperkeratosis (much like an acrokeratosis verruciformis of Hopf), and a flat hyperkeratotic variant.[131]

Differential Diagnosis Large-cell acanthomas (LCA) must be differentiated from actinic keratoses, seborrheic keratoses, and solar lentigo.[130] It must be acknowledged that LCA may show some overlap with seborrheic keratoses, solar lentigines, and lichenoid keratoses since these are all related lesions. Actinic keratoses usually demonstrate a loss of the granular layer, parakeratosis, and cytologic atypia with mitotic activity. Seborrheic keratoses have horn pseudocysts but are not well-demarcated at the lateral aspects of the lesion and do not show enlarged nuclei and keratinocytes. Solar lentigines have a more lentiginous proliferation of rete ridges with prominent hyperpigmentation. Additionally, cellular and nuclear enlargement are not present.

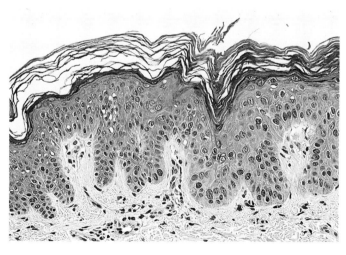

FIGURE 26-8 Large-cell acanthoma. Keratinocyte nuclei are enlarged and slightly pleomorphic.

KERATINOCYTIC DYSPLASIA

Actinic Keratosis

Synonym: solar keratosis

In 1926 Freudenthal described what are now known as actinic keratoses.[132] These precancerous changes of the skin are found in 11 to 25 percent of the population and are most common on the sun-exposed skin of elderly patients.[133] Some clinicians consider them to be equivalent with squamous cell carcinoma in situ.[134] Surrounding "normal" skin shows this atypia, suggesting that there exists a stepwise progression of keratinocyte atypia from the subclinical to overt squamous cell carcinoma.[135] There is concern that these lesions will eventually convert to a frank cutaneous malignancy. Among untreated lesions this risk is approximately 1 per 1000 per year.[134] Thick, hyperkeratotic, and ulcerative lesions are most at risk. About 20 to 25 percent of patients with actinic keratoses will eventually develop a squamous-cell carcinoma.[135]

Clinical Features   Typical actinic keratoses are small, hyperkeratotic growths on sun-exposed surfaces in middle-aged and older patients (Table 26-16).[134] They are well-demarcated from surrounding skin and are slightly red. The overlying scale is white to grey or yellow.[136] Most lesions are stable and less than a centimeter in size.[137] Affected patients usually have a history of prolonged sun exposure or who tan poorly and freckle easily.[134] Lesions usually are asymptomatic, but mild pruritus or tenderness may be present.

The spreading pigmented actinic keratosis is a variant of actinic keratosis, which is larger and more deeply pigmented.[136,138] Lesions are 1 centimeter or greater in diameter and spread in a centrifugal manner. The base is erythematous with adherent scales. The face is most often involved.[139] The transfer of pigment from melanocytes to keratinocytes may be impaired.[136] The hyperpigmentation may be a protective mechanism to prevent further solar damage.

Other variants of actinic keratosis have been described. Lichenoid actinic keratoses are likely to be slightly larger than most lesions and to arise on the chest.[140] Hypertrophic actinic keratoses are more commonly seen on the distal upper extremity.[141] A proliferative variant of actinic keratosis has been described.[137] These are red, scaly macules or patches without well-defined borders or symptoms. They are poorly circumscribed and may reach 3 to 4 cm in diameter. Scarring from previous therapy is common since these lesions respond poorly to routine methods of eradication.

Histopathological Features   Actinic keratoses demonstrate atypical epidermal proliferation (Table 26-16). There is hyperkeratosis with parakeratosis and usually a loss of the underlying granular layer. The parakeratotic nuclei may be large with oval or circular features. The basal layer becomes proliferative with slight budding into the dermis.[142] Mild spongiosis above the atypical basal cells is common. The keratinocytes show increased mitotic activity.[38,142] Some liquefactive degeneration of the basal layer also may be present.[142] Acantholysis is seen as a focal occurrence or as a dominant process. Adnexal structures usually are spared. The dermis demonstrates a mild superficial perivascular inflammatory infiltrate.[134]

There are different histopathologic variants of actinic keratoses. Hypertrophic actinic keratoses have thickened, acanthotic epidermis (Fig. 26-9). Atypia is common along the basal layer but may be minimal. An overall irregular, psoriasiform hyperplasia may be seen. Papillomatous proliferation is more common in acral lesions.[141] The papillary dermis may show mild fibrosis with elongation of dermal capillaries.

Atrophic actinic keratoses show a thinned and atrophic stratum malpighii.[141] Atypical cells are found predominantly along the basal layer. Acantholytic actinic keratoses demonstrate widespread keratinocyte acantholysis.[142] Dyskeratotic cells may be seen. Actinic keratoses with prominent epidermolysis are known as epidermolytic actinic keratoses.[142] Bowenoid actinic keratoses display prominent bowenoid features (Fig. 26-10).[137] Full-thickness atypia, dyskeratotic cells, and mild parakeratosis are prominent. The infundibulum of hair follicles may be involved by this atypia, but the outer root sheath is spared. Biopsies should demonstrate complete excision of the lesion to differentiate these lesions from squamous cell carcinoma in situ. Pigmented actinic keratoses display moderate pigment incontinence and hyperpigmentation along the basal layer.[142] Distinct nests of melanocytes are not present. Actinic keratoses with an interface inflammatory infiltrate are known as lichenoid actinic keratoses (Fig. 26-11).[140] Proliferative actinic keratoses demonstrate keratinocyte atypia extending to the level of the sebaceous glands.[137]

The spreading pigmented variant of actinic keratosis is hyperkeratotic and parakeratotic with occasional dyskeratosis.[136,139] The epi-

---

TABLE 26-16

Actinic Keratosis

Clinical Features

Small, erythematous keratotic lesions on the sun-damaged skin of elderly patients
Scale may be white to yellow-brown
Borders are sharply demarcated
Typically asymptomatic but itching or tenderness may occur

Histopathological Features

Hyperkeratosis with intermittent large parakeratotic nuclei
Parakeratosis spares adnexal structures
Keratinocyte atypia is prominent along the basal layer
Spongiosis in the immediate suprabasalar layer
Budding of basal layer keratinocytes into the dermis
Perivascular inflammation and solar elastosis

Differential Diagnosis

Squamous-cell carcinoma in situ
Bowenoid papulosis
Spongiotic dermatoses

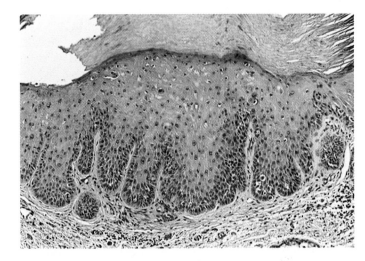

FIGURE 26-9 Hypertrophic actinic keratosis. The epidermis is acanthotic and variably atypical. Hyperkeratosis may be minimal or significant.

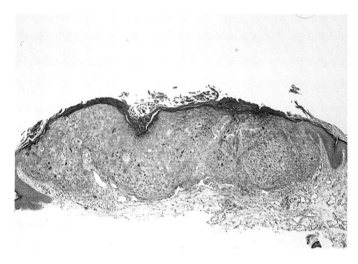

FIGURE 26-10   Bowenoid actinic keratosis. Epidermal atypia is full thickness and resembles Bowen's disease.

dermis is atypical and buds slightly into the underlying dermis. Acantholysis with basal layer clefting is present.[139] The epidermal pigmentation begins abruptly with the onset of keratinocyte atypia. Melanin is seen in all layers of the epidermis, including the parakeratotic stratum corneum. Pigment incontinence and solar elastosis are prominent in the dermis.[136,139] Ultrastructurally, spreading pigmented actinic keratoses have a normal number of melanocytes with types II–IV melanosomes. These melanosomes typically are single and may be present in both keratinocytes and Langerhans cells.

Differential Diagnosis   The differential diagnosis for actinic keratoses depends in large part on which variant is being evaluated. For routine actinic keratoses considerations include squamous cell carcinoma in situ, spongiotic dermatoses, and bowenoid papulosis. Squamous-cell carcinoma in situ and bowenoid papulosis demonstrate full thickness atypia with dyskeratotic cells, whereas actinic keratoses have atypia restricted to the basal layer or the lower-cell layers of the spinous layer. Additionally, there are few dyskeratotic cells present in actinic keratoses. Spongiotic dermatoses must also be ruled out since some actinic keratoses demonstrate minimal keratinocyte atypia and mild spongiosis, particularly if they have been irritated. The presence of different types

of inflammatory cells in the dermis may aid in differentiation. Hypertrophic actinic keratoses must be differentiated from inflamed seborrheic keratoses since both lesions will show acanthosis and may have minimal atypia. The presence of horn pseudocysts, papillomatosis, and exocytosis by inflammatory cells supports a diagnosis of an inflamed seborrheic keratosis. Pigmented actinic keratoses and the spreading pigmented actinic keratosis must be differentiated from solar lentigines and minimally acanthotic seborrheic keratoses. Keratinocyte atypia and the lack of lentiginous proliferation supports a diagnosis of actinic keratosis. Acantholysis and epidermolysis may be seen in various dermatoses and in lesions such as acantholytic and epidermolytic acanthomas. These neoplasms however do not demonstrate keratinocyte atypia and normally fail to show proliferation of the basal layer. Finally, lichenoid actinic keratoses should be distinguished from benign lichenoid keratoses and inflamed seborrheic keratoses.[140] Given the nature of the inflammatory infiltrate this may be difficult since the interface may be obscured. Clear-cut keratinocyte atypia is a key feature and must be distinguished from reactive "atypia," which is not always possible. Benign lichenoid keratoses demonstrate more keratinocyte dyskeratosis and the presence of colloid bodies in the papillary dermis. They are also more expansive than lichenoid actinic keratoses.

Actinic Cheilitis

Actinic cheilitis is also known as cheilitis exfoliativa, solar cheilosis, or actinic keratosis of the lip.[143] Initial studies suggested an association between this condition and prolonged sun exposure.[144] Other potential etiologies include smoking, poor dentition, HSV infection, and syphilis.[143,145] This condition is largely restricted to persons with considerable ultraviolet light exposure.[145,146] Persons with fair skin are more at risk and, although it has been described in African Americans, it is rare.[143,145] Lesions typically arise on the lower lip either because this site is unprotected from solar rays or the angle at which these rays strike the vermilion surface.[146] Evolving squamous-cell carcinoma has a greater potential for lymphatic spread than does squamous-cell carcinoma of the glaborous skin.

Clinical Features   Actinic cheilitis is almost universally restricted to older persons with significant actinic damage (Table 26-17). The lip displays a generalized atrophy with scaling, dryness, and erosions.[143,146] There is a mottled appearance with an indistinct vermilion border. The

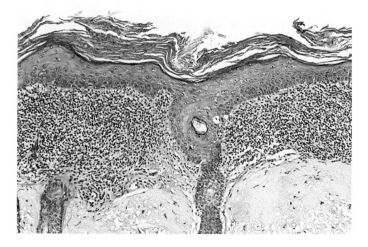

FIGURE 26-11   Lichenoid actinic keratosis. The epidermis shows keratinocyte atypia with a lichenoid inflammatory infiltrate in the papillary dermis.

TABLE 26-17
Actinic Cheilitis

Clinical Features

   Lower lip involved in patients with extensive sun exposure
   Scaling, crusting, and erosions are seen
   Loss of elasticity, dryness, and atrophy

Histopathological Features

   Epidermis with acanthosis, hyperkeratosis, and parakeratosis
   Keratinocyte atypia is mild to moderate
   Solar elastosis and telangiectasias in the dermis

Differential Diagnosis

   Contact cheilitis
   Plasma cell cheilitis

lip is pale white to pink or brown. Linear striations, thickened keratoses, and crusting may be apparent.[145] The lip tends to lose its plasticity. A recurrent cycle of crusting and healing may be described. Prolonged ulceration is worrisome for a squamous-cell carcinoma. An acute form of actinic cheilitis has been described that is less common in the elderly.[143] It occurs predominantly in the summer months after sunlight exposure. The lip becomes red and swollen with severe congestion, fissuring, and ulceration. Blisters may also be appreciated.

Histopathological Features   The epithelium is thickened, acanthotic, and hyperkeratotic (Table 26-17).[143] Parakeratosis is present. The keratinocytes display mild to moderate atypia but early lesions may demonstrate little or no atypia.[145] Mitotic activity is present. The dermis shows moderate to severe solar elastosis and a nonspecific perivascular inflammatory infiltrate. Scattered plasma cells are seen.[143] Dilated blood vessels are common.

Differential Diagnosis   The differential diagnosis includes contact cheilitis and plasma cell cheilitis. Contact cheilitis is much like contact dermatitis elsewhere in that spongiosis, lymphocytes, and eosinophils are prominent. Keratinocyte atypia is not appreciated and the parakeratosis is not as prominent as in contact cheilitis. Plasma cell cheilitis demonstrates large masses of plasma cells without keratinocyte atypia.

Arsenical Keratosis

Precancerous keratoses have been described in patients exposed to arsenic containing substances such as medications (Fowler's solution), mining/smelting products, well water, industrial compounds, and pesticides or fungicides.[147] An association between arsenic exposure and Bowen's disease also is well known.[148–150]

Clinical Features   Lesions begin as small papules with dense hyperkeratosis (Table 26-18).[147,150] They are yellow but may be slightly brown or dark. The palms and soles are primarily affected and a mild keratoderma sometimes is present. The thenar and lateral borders of the palms and roots of the fingers are most commonly affected.[149] Keratoses may coalesce to form plaques. Similar lesions are found elsewhere on the body. Keratoses begin as soon as 4 years after exposure but usually take 20 to 30 years to manifest.[148]

Histopathological Features   The stratum corneum is hyperkeratotic and compact (Table 26-18). Mild papillomatosis may also be present. The granular layer usually is accentuated but may be thinned or absent.[148] Keratinocyte atypia is present particularly along the basal layer.[147] Cytologic atypia may be so mild as to be almost nonexistent or as profound as Bowen's disease.[149] Budding into the dermis may be seen. These lesions are divided into type A (benign) and type B (bowenoid or malignant).[149] The dermis shows some perivascular inflammatory cells but the typical solar elastosis seen in actinic keratoses is absent. Adjacent epithelium is slightly thinned with absent or atrophic adnexal structures.[149] Transformation into a basal-cell carcinoma or squamous-cell carcinoma has been described.[147] Some areas demonstrate seborrheic keratosislike changes.

Differential Diagnosis   Arsenical keratoses must be distinguished from actinic keratoses, warts, or Bowen's disease.[148] Actinic keratoses usually show a less compact hyperkeratosis, mild suprabasal spongiosis, and solar elastosis. Warts are more papillomatous than arsenical keratoses, typically have columns of parakeratosis, may possess large keratohyaline masses, and usually show dilated capillaries in the uppermost papillary dermis. Additionally, warts show no significant keratinocyte atypia. Bowen's disease has "full thickness" atypia involving all the layers of the epidermis except the stratum corneum, whereas arsenical keratoses demonstrate such features less commonly. Additionally, Bowen's disease has dyskeratotic keratinocytes and a less compact stratum corneum.

INTRAEPIDERMAL CARCINOMAS

Bowen's Disease

Bowen's disease was originally described by Bowen in 1912 and is believed by most authors to be squamous cell carcinoma in situ.[151] These lesions are associated with chronic solar damage, radiation therapy, and arsenic or paraquat exposure.[147,152,153] This disease (erythroplasia of Queyrat) may also be more common in uncircumcised males.[154] Recently, human papillomavirus (HPV) infection has been

---

TABLE 26-18

Arsenical Keratosis

Clinical Features

Hyperkeratotic papules on the palms and soles in persons exposed to arsenic
Lesions are compact with a yellow to brown color

Histopathological Features

Compact hyperkeratotic stratum corneum
Mild to moderate keratinocyte atypia
Transformation to basal-cell carcinoma or squamous-cell carcinoma occurs
Perivascular dermal inflammation is present but solar elastosis is not

Differential Diagnosis

Actinic keratosis
Verruca vulgaris
Bowen's disease

TABLE 26-19

Bowen's Disease

Clinical Features

Glaborous and anogenital patches a few centimeters in diameter
Well-demarcated and scaling with mild erythema
Patients usually are older and lesions arise in sun-damaged areas
Women more often affected than men

Histopathological Features

Epidermis demonstrates acanthosis and hyperkeratosis
Mild to moderate psoriasiform hyperplasia
Full thickness epidermal atypia with dyskeratotic cells and atypical mitoses
Loss of epidermal polarity
Frequent involvement of adnexal structures

Differential Diagnosis

Bowenoid actinic keratoses and bowenoid papulosis
Extramammary Paget's disease
Epidermotropic carcinoma metastatic to the skin
Erythroplasia of Queyrat
Podophyllin treated condylomata acuminata

described in Bowen's disease. HPV type 2 has been found with extra-genital disease and type 16 has been reported with genital involvement.[153,155] HPV associated extragenital disease is linked to African-American race, an acral location, youth, and a hyperkeratotic or verrucous appearance.[156] It was originally believed that Bowen's disease was a marker for internal malignancy and that cancers were more common in this population.[153,157] However, recent data casts doubt on this assertion.[153,158,159]

Clinical Features   There are two clinical variants of Bowen's disease—that involving the anogenital area and that of glaborous skin. Anogenital disease involves the mucous membranes but mucosal sites such as the oral cavity and conjunctiva are also involved.[153] Glaborous lesions appear as slowly enlarging, well-demarcated patches, or plaques.[152,153,156] Some are large and poorly defined.[152] Tumors display mild scaling or crusting. Verrucous and hyperkeratotic variants are seen. Presentation as a cutaneous horn and within a lesion of porokeratosis also have been described.[160,161] Most are flesh-colored to erythematous. A pigmented variant is seen in anogenital lesions. Normal appearing skin is seen within some plaques.[162] Most patches of Bowen's disease are a few millimeters to a few centimeters in diameter.[163] Lesions are most common on sun-exposed sites particularly the lower extremities in women.[152,164] Lesions on the face are also more common in female patients. Terminal hair follicles may protect against this disease but vellus follicles are more often involved. Patients usually are in the sixth to eighth decade.[153] Bowen's disease pursues a relatively benign course but may progress to invasive squamous-cell carcinoma.[156]

Histopathological Features   The stratum corneum is hyperkeratotic and usually parakeratotic (Table 26-19).[153,165,166] The parakeratosis may be extensive and plate-like. The rest of the epidermis is acanthotic with occasional psoriasiform hyperplasia (Fig. 26-12 A). The cells display "full-thickness" atypia with a "windblown" appearance.[153,167] There is a loss of epidermal polarity in that normal and progressive keratinocyte maturation has ceased.[165] Keratinocytes are enlarged and have atypical nuclei with frequent mitoses (Fig. 26-12 B). Dyskeratosis is variable but usually is prominent. Keratinocytes may be multinucleated and are slightly eosinophilic is some sections.[166] Importantly, involvement of the adnexa, particularly pilosebaceous structures, may be present.[153] The infundibulum, sebaceous glands, and external root sheath may be replaced by tumor cells.[152] Hyperpigmentation along the basal layer and dermal melanophage proliferation is accentuated in pigmented variants. Dermal invasion occurs in three to five percent of cases.[167] A perivascular inflammatory infiltrate often is present and eosinophils are seen particularly when topical medicaments have been applied.[153,162] Some increased vascularity may be appreciated.[162] Regression with fibrosis and scarring of the papillary dermis has been described.[162] Amyloid deposition is present in both lesional and interlesional skin. This may result from cytokeratin degradation from dyskeratotic keratinocytes.[162] Differentiation towards a sebaceous carcinoma and eccrine sweat gland carcinoma have been described.[167,168]

Differential Diagnosis   Bowenoid actinic keratoses, bowenoid papulosis, extramammary Paget's disease, epidermotropic carcinoma metastatic to the skin, erythroplasia of Queyrat, and podophyllin treated condylomata acuminata must be differentiated from Bowen's disease.[153,154,165,167] Bowenoid actinic keratoses and bowenoid papulosis are identical to Bowen's disease. However, these tumors are smaller and usually have been completely removed by the biopsy. Extramammary Paget's disease usually shows pale cells that stain for PAS, gross cystic disease fluid protein, Cam 5.2, and carcinoembryonic antigen. The use of murine monoclonal antibodies have been used to distinguish between these two diseases.[169] Epidermotropic carcinoma metastatic to the skin

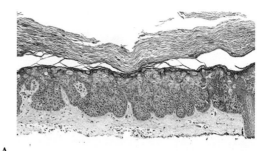

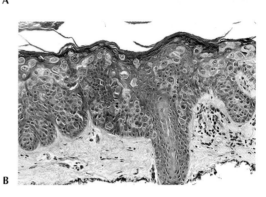

FIGURE 26-12   Bowen's disease. *A*. The epidermis is psoriasiform and slightly hyperkeratotic. *B*. Keratinocytes demonstrate "full-thickness" atypia with increased mitotic activity and dyskeratosis.

such as eccrine porocarcinoma demonstrates atypical cells within the epidermis but usually in a pagetoid pattern. Dyskeratotic cells are also more prevalent in Bowen's disease. Erythroplasia of Queyrat may be Bowen's disease of the glans penis and as such cannot be consistently distinguished from the latter. Finally, podophyllin-treated condyloma acuminata demonstrate dyskeratotic cells with large, atypical mitotic figures and may be mistaken for Bowen's disease. However, the atypia is usually not full thickness, epidermal changes consists of "knuckling" rather than a psoriasiform pattern and koilocytic cells may be present.

Erythroplasia of Queyrat

This disorder was initially described by Tarnovsky in 1891 but named after Queyrat in 1911.[163,170] Many investigators consider it to be identical to Bowen's disease; however, some differences do exist between the two conditions.[163,171] Erythroplasia of Queyrat is not associated with internal malignancies or arsenic exposure and dermal invasion with metastatic spread is more likely.[171] Trauma, friction, poor hygiene, smegma irritation, concomitant syphilis, and other sources of inflammation are believed to incite this disease.[171,172] Lesions have been present an average of 2 years prior to diagnosis.[154] Twenty percent of invasive lesions will demonstrate nodal spread, but only about five percent of such lesions result in the patient's death.[172]

Clinical Features   Lesions typically are present in uncircumcised men in the third to sixth decade of life (Table 26-20).[172] They are most common on the glans but may also be present on the urethral meatus, corona, sulcus, and prepuce (Table 26-20).[154] Erythroplasia of Queyrat is usually a single lesion but multiple tumors have been described. They are smooth, red velvety plaques with minimal induration.[154,163,171,173] The surface may be moist and glistening or hyperkeratotic and scaling.[163,172] The margins are well-demarcated. Symptoms are few but some mild itching or bleeding may be present.[172]

TABLE 26-20

TABLE 26-20

Erythroplasia of Queyrat

Clinical Features

> Well-demarcated, red velvety plaques on the glans penis in uncircumcised men
> Usually asymptomatic but may demonstrate mild itching or bleeding
> May involve other areas of the penis, vulva, or other mucosal surfaces

Histopathological Features

> Full thickness epidermal atypia with abnormal mitoses and dyskeratotic keratinocytes
> Loss of epidermal polarity
> Plasma cells in the dermis

Differential Diagnosis

> Bowenoid papulosis

Histopathological Features   The histologic changes are those of squamous cell carcinoma in situ (Table 26-20). The epidermis is irregularly acanthotic with occasional psoriasiform changes and shows a loss of polarity.[172,173] Dyskeratotic cells are present.[171-173] The nuclei are atypical and hyperchromatic and multinucleated cells may be present. Ten percent of cases demonstrate dermal invasion (squamous cell carcinoma).[172] The dermis contains a perivascular inflammatory infiltrate with a variable number of plasma cells.

Differential Diagnosis   Bowenoid papulosis may be indistinguishable from erythroplasia of Queyrat.[154] The epidermis may show the appearance of papule on low power. Frank koilocytosis is uncommon; however, small basophilic bodies with a surrounding halo may be present in the stratum granulosum and stratum corneum.[174]

Intraepithelial Epithelioma

Synonyms: Intraepithelial epithelioma of Borst-Jadassohn

The intraepithelial epithelioma (IEE) is a controversial lesion. The presence of an intraepithelial spread of atypical keratinocytes initially was described by Borst in 1904 and Jadassohn 22 years later.[175] Borst most likely described the intraepidermal spread of a squamous cell carcinoma, whereas Jadassohn was probably reporting the same phenomenon occurring in a basal cell carcinoma. Montgomery first coined the term "intraepithelial epithelioma of Borst-Jadassohn" in 1929.[176] The IEE probably constitutes the intraepidermal spread of keratinocytes with varying degrees of atypia. Some authors believe that most cases have included a variety of lesions, such as irritated seborrheic keratoses, squamous cell carcinomas (or Bowens's disease), hidroacanthoma simplex, epidermal nevi, or clear-cell acanthomas.[175,177] The names Borst and Jadassohn are probably best discarded when discussing IEE since these descriptions simply refer to a histologic phenomenon rather than a distinct clinical lesion.[178] Thus, if IEE exists, it is a diagnosis of exclusion, that is, one may apply the term only after ruling out clonal seborrheic keratosis, hidroacanthoma simplex, squamous cell carcinoma in situ, and so on. The tumor may represent an incipient keratinocytic dysplasia and an acrosyringeal derivation has been proposed.[179] However, further study is needed to clearly confirm that IEE is a legitimate entity rather than one of the conditions mentioned earlier.

INTERMEDIATE LESIONS

Keratoacanthoma

Synonyms: Molluscum sebaceum

Keratoacanthomas (KA) are rapidly growing cutaneous tumors with atypical histologic features that resolve, leaving an atrophic scar. They were initially described in 1889 by Sir Jonathan Hutchinson as a "crateriform ulcer of the face" and today are believed to be a squamoproliferative lesion with keratinocytic atypia ranging from none to frank squamous cell carcinoma.[180] Most keratoacanthomas arise as solitary lesions in sun-exposed sites; however, different clinical syndromes are associated with these tumors.[181] Multiple KAs of Ferguson Smith is an autosomal dominant disorder that begins in childhood to early adulthood. Numerous lesions arise and disperse over the years. This disorder must be differentiated from the generalized eruptive keratoacanthomas of Grzybowski. In this disease the erupting keratoacanthomas are smaller, 2 to 3 mm in diameter, and may number in the hundreds or thousands. Familial inheritance is not present and pruritus is common. Another condition, multiple persistent keratoacanthomas, occurs sporadically and consists of slow healing tumors. Three syndromes—Muir-Torre, xeroderma pigmentosum, and Cowden's—demonstrate an increased incidence of tumor formation. Keratoacanthomas have been found in association with numerous benign and malignant lesions, including nevus sebaceous of Jadassohn, scar, vaccination site, melanoma, basal cell carcinoma, arterial puncture site, linear epidermal nevus, nevomelanocytic nevus, and miliaria.[8,181-185] They have also arisen in *Herpes simplex* infections, radiodermatitis, pustular psoriasis, seborrheic dermatitis, discoid lupus erythematosus, lichen planus, lichen simplex chronicus, folliculitis, weather beaten skin, erythema multiforme, PUVA-treated skin, eczematous dermatitis, and drug eruptions.[181,183,186] Keratoacanthomas also are known to occur following cutaneous trauma.[181]

TABLE 26-21

Keratoacanthoma

Clinical Features

> Flesh-colored to erythematous nodules with a central keratin plug
> Typically present on older patients in sun-exposed sites
> Resolving lesions are scarred and atrophic
> Lesions may exist at previous sites of trauma or with various dermatoses

Histopathological Features

> Overlying epithelium forms "lips" with adjacent hypergranulosis and hyperkeratosis
> Cutaneous plug is eosinophilic and parakeratotic
> Infiltrating epithelium is eosinophilic and may be atypical with increased mitotic activity
> Entrapped collagen and elastic fibers are seen
> Horn pearls and neutrophilic or eosinophilic microabscesses are present

Differential Diagnosis

> Squamous-cell carcinoma
> Dilated pore or infundibular cyst
> Resolving inflamed wart
> Prurigo nodularis
> Perforating disorder

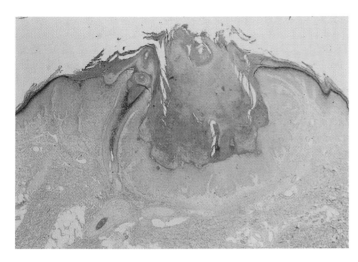

FIGURE 26-13 Keratoacanthoma. The typical keratoacanthoma shows a keratotic plug with surrounding "lips" of epidermis.

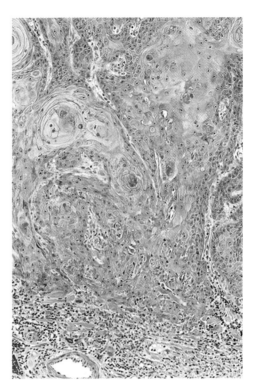

FIGURE 26-14 Keratoacanthoma. Proliferating cells of keratoacanthomas are eosinophilic and variably atypical.

These tumors are believed to arise secondary to long–standing solar damage since they originate in sun-exposed areas and their occurrence parallels increased ultraviolet exposure.[181] However, chemical tumorigenesis has been demonstrated in animals and human tumors have developed following exposure to tar, pitch, and podophyllin.[181,183] Viral causes also have been postulated and HPV type 25 has been found in some lesions.[181,187] There appears to be a genetic predisposition to develop keratoacanthomas.[181] A proportion of KA is thought to begin in hair follicles.[181]

Clinical Features   Keratoacanthomas typically arise on the sun-exposed skin of older persons (Table 26-21).[181] The peak incidence begins in the sixth decade and lesions are commonly found on the face, hands, and forearms in men and on the face and legs of women.[181] Males are more commonly affected than females. Lesions pass through several stages of development.[181] The initial or proliferative phase consists of a smooth, hemispheric nodule that enlarges rapidly over a 2- to 4-week period. These are flesh-colored to slightly erythematous and asymptomatic. The next stage, the mature form, demonstrates a dome or berry shaped nodule with a central crater containing a plug of compact keratin. This stage lasts several weeks or months. The final phase is that of a resolving lesion. These keratoacanthomas resorb and expel the keratogenous core. Over weeks to months they become progressively more depressed and eventuate into a scar with variable atrophy.

Several clinical scenarios are seen with keratoacanthomas.[181] In the agglomerate type several nodules coalesce to form a large keratotic plaque. The giant keratoacanthoma is a particularly large lesion, up to 9 cm in diameter. Keratoacanthoma centifugum (coral reef KA, nodul-vegetating KA, aggregated KA) shows expansive growth occasionally to 20 cm in diameter. As the lesion is expanding the central area heals with scarring and atrophy. Subungual keratoacanthomas are painful, persistent lesions that arise under the nails, usually on the fingers. The thumb and fifth finger are most commonly involved and bony destruction may take place. Mucosal keratoacanthomas may develop in the mouth and on other mucous membranes, including the bulbar conjunctiva, nasal mucosa, and genitalia.

Histopathological Features   Lesions in the first or initial phase demonstrate an invaginating epidermis with a keratin-filled crater (Fig. 26-13) (Table 26-21). Adjacent epithelium shows acanthosis, hypergranulosis, and premature cornification.[181] Parakeratosis may be present but orthohyperkeratosis is the rule. Invaginating strands of epithelium may be carcinoma like (pseudoepitheliomatous) and typically possess an eosinophilic or "glassy" appearance (Fig. 26-14).[181,188] Some acantholysis may be present. Fully developed keratoacanthomas have similar features that are more exaggerated. The overlying epidermis develops "lips" surrounding the crateriform plug that has expanded and consists of parakeratotic material. Epidermal proliferations become more exaggerated as they invade the dermis. Mitotic activity and atypical mitotic figures are more common, particularly at the edges of the epithelial proliferation. Intraepidermal neutrophilic and eosinophilic microabscesses are present. Horn pearls are seen.[181] Within the epidermis are occasional fragments of entrapped collagen and elastin fiber fragments.[181]

The second or established phase is characterized by a lichenoid inflammatory infiltrate, composed largely of lymphocytes but eosinophils may also be prominent.[189] Neutrophils and plasma cells often are present. The stroma may be granulomatous if epithelium has ruptured into the dermis and is being resorbed. Atypical eccrine sweat duct hyperplasia also may be present. Melanocyte proliferation with increased dendricity has been described in proliferative epithelium.[190]

Lesions in the third or involuting phase take on a flattened, less crateriform appearance.[191] The epidermis becomes variably acanthotic and hypergranulotic with sharp, jagged rete ridges. Dyskeratotic keratinocytes are seen. Atypia is diminished. The eosinophilic quality of invading epithelium is diminished. Small keratin-filled cystic structures may be appreciated in the papillary dermis.[191] Dermal vascularity is increased and fibrosis is variably prominent in the papillary dermis. Granulation tissue in the deep aspects of the tumor may be observed.[181] The inflammatory infiltrate becomes largely lichenoid with giant cells, plasma cells, and neutrophils. This involutional phase is believed to be immunologically mediated.[191] Infiltrating inflammatory cells invade the tumor and ameliorate the proliferative state of the tumor.

Like most neoplastic processes, perineural and vascular invasion have been described.[192,193] Perineural invasion is more common with head and neck lesions. These tumors tend to be large and deeply infiltrating. However, although prognosis has been reported not to be adversely affected by this process, such lesions should be considered to be squamous-cell carcinoma.[192] Vascular invasion has not been associated with metastatic disease. It appears likely that involvement of vessel walls by tumor cells is more of a passive phenomenon dictated by the proximity of large vessels than one of malignant invasion.[193] Atypical and tripolar mitotic figures have also been described but are not associated with an increased incidence of recurrence.[194,195] Aneuploidy is present in some keratoacanthomas although to a lesser extent than in well differentiated squamous cell carcinoma.[181]

Ultrastructurally, keratoacanthomas demonstrate an increased number of desmosomes compared to normal skin.[181] Intranuclear inclusions have been described.

There has been considerable discussion regarding the biological nature of keratoacanthomas.[188,196–199] Metastatic spread of lesions, considered by some the sine qua none of malignancy, has been described in some keratoacanthomas.[188,196,199] It is debatable as to how all KA should be categorized but currently they may be thought of as a continuum of squamous proliferations ranging from benign to low-grade squamous-cell carcinomas with some potential for metastasis.

Differential Diagnosis Keratoacanthomas must be distinguished from squamous cell carcinomas, dilated pores, infundibular cysts, or resolving inflamed warts.[181,191] Since keratoacanthomas probably represent a biological spectrum of lesions, distinction of KA from squamous-cell carcinoma is often not possible for a subset of tumors.

Criteria utilized for this discrimination include architecture, that is, overall symmetry and circumscription of the lesion, degree of cytological atypia (none or slight to moderate atypia favoring keratoacanthoma and marked atypia squamous cell carcinoma), and evidence of involution (favoring KA). Atypical eccrine ductal hyperplasia, intraepidermal microabscesses, tissue eosinophilia, and intraepithelial elastic fibers are more commonly found in keratoacanthomas than squamous cell carcinomas.[181,200]

Dilated pores and infundibular cysts demonstrate aggregations of keratin but usually without inflammation or parakeratosis. The epithelial lining also is benign without the typical eosinophilic changes seen in keratoacanthomas. Resolving inflamed warts may be endophytic but typically are exophytic as well. The "lips" or buttressing commonly present in keratoacanthomas will be absent from these lesions as will the eosinophilic features of the proliferating epithelium, the neutrophilic microabscesses, and the infiltrating eosinophils.

MALIGNANT TUMORS

Basal-cell Carcinoma

Basal cell carcinoma is the most common malignant disease in humans.[201] This tumor was originally described by Jacob in 1927.[202] Between 1971 and 1977 the incidence of basal cell carcinoma rose 18 percent.[203] Each year there are 750,000 to 930,000 new cases diagnosed.[204] Basal cell carcinomas typically begin after age 30 and peak at age 70.[205] Childhood disease is rare in immunocompetent patients.[206] Persons with blue or green eyes, easy freckling, blond or red hair, and significant outdoor exposure are at increased risk for these tumors.[205] Anatomic areas with increased sebaceous gland concentration are more likely to be involved.[203]

Risk factors for basal-cell carcinoma include exposure to arsenic, x-irradiation, coal-tar derivatives, and ultraviolet light.[147,203,205,207–210] Tumors may arise in scars, thermal burns, and chronic inflammation (draining sinuses, leg ulcers, hidradenitis, etc.).[207,208,210] Immuno-

compromised patients are at increased risk for basal-cell carcinoma perhaps because of impaired cell-mediated immunity and an increased susceptibility to oncogenic viruses.[211] Certain genodermatoses including albinism, xeroderma pigmentosa, Rasmussen syndrome, Rombo syndrome, Bazex syndrome, and Darier's disease have an increased incidence of basal-cell carcinoma.[203,210,212]

Different tumors have been associated with basal cell carcinoma. These may be little more than coincidence but in some instances the cutaneous malignancy may have arisen from prolonged irritation and inflammation. Warts, porokeratomas, varicella scars, neurofibromas, keratoacanthomas, lesions of lupus vulgaris, nevi sebaceus, linear epidermal nevi, seborrheic keratoses, nevomelanocytic nevi, condyloma acuminata, infundibular cysts, hemangiomas and pilomatricomas have all been associated with a basal cell carcinoma.[207,210,212–215] Basal cell proliferation with peripheral cell palisading and stromal retraction occasionally is seen in the epidermis overlying a dermatofibroma. These changes may represent follicle induction by underlying stroma;, however, recent evidence has shown that these proliferating cells are more likely epidermal basal cells than follicular keratinocytes.[216] Basal cell carcinomas may also be found with malignant tumors such as melanomas, squamous cell carcinomas and keratoacanthomas.[210,213]

Basal-cell carcinomas are believed to derive from the epidermis, specifically the basal cell layer and the outer root sheath of the hair follicle.[207,217] The cells of origin are likely pleuripotential and may be progenitor epithelial cells in the case of adults or primary epithelial germ cells in the case of linear unilateral basal cell nevi. Anti-keratin antibodies have shown that basal cell carcinomas possess a keratin component not normally found in the basal layer and stain similarly to the lower part of the hair follicle epithelium.[218]

A patient's immune system affects the pathogenesis and eventual outcome of these tumors. Environmental carcinogens, such as oncogenic viruses, may be potentiated by concomitant immunosuppression.[211] Basal cell carcinomas are ten times more common in persons who have undergone a solid organ transplant and herpes-virus like DNA sequences have been found in these lesions.[219,220] Tumors may be more aggressive with an increased tendency to recur or metastasize.[221] Certain histologic types may also be more prevalent among immunosuppressed patients. Infiltrative basal cell carcinomas are more common compared to nodular tumors in immunocompromised patients.[211] Superficial basal-cell carcinomas predominate in persons with diabetes mellitus and/or chronic renal failure and are the predominant pattern among persons with HIV.[211]

Basal-cell carcinoma arises on the sun-exposed cutaneous surfaces primarily in persons beginning in middle age. Just over half of all patients are men and about 85 percent appear on the head and neck.[201,222] Only about 10-15% of tumors develop on sun protected skin.[210] Twenty to 30 percent occur on the nose alone making it the most commonly involved site.[104] Basal-cell carcinomas are most prevalent among Caucasians. African Americans and Hispanics also are affected but to a lesser extent.[223] Among African Americans, women are more likely to be affected. As with Caucasians, most lesions in African Americans arise on the head and neck; however, the nose is less often involved. The high melanin content in African American skin may protect against tumor development.[224] The histologic subtypes are similar between the races.[224]

Clinical Features Typical lesions are flesh-colored or translucent to slightly erythematous papules and nodules with raised, rolled borders (Table 26-22). Bleeding and crusting occasionally are seen. Telangiectasias may be present, particularly at the borders. Some lesions ulcerate but significant scaling is unusual. Large tumors destroy structures such as ears, eyes, and nasal passages. Different variants may have different clinical presentations. The cicatricial or scarring basal-cell car-

TABLE 26-22

Basal-cell Carcinoma

Clinical Features

Flesh-colored to pearly raised papules and nodules on sun-exposed
sites
May bleed or ulcerate and occasionally destroy contiguous
structures
Indurated plaques are seen
Superficial variant with erythema, scaling, and some epidermal
breakdown
Pigmented variant with hyperpigmentation, at times very black

Histopathological Features

Nodular
Small to large aggregates of basaloid cells emanating from the
epidermis or follicular structures
Peripheral palisading, stromal retraction, and mitoses are present
Necrosis, apoptosis, calcification, and mucin production are
variable
Superficial
Small, discrete islands of basaloid cells present intermittently
along the basal layer
Prominent peripheral palisading and stromal retraction
Peritumoral mucin production
Keratotic, infundibulocystic
Keratin-filled cysts with features suggesting follicle derivation
Reticulated basaloid cells with some mitotic activity and mucin
production
Stromal retraction is unusual
Infiltrative, morpheaform
Small islands of basaloid cells with an angulated and "spiky"
configuration
Poor peripheral palisading and minimal stromal retraction
Fibrotic and variably mucinous stroma
Deep infiltration and poor circumscription
Adenoid, fibroepithelioma of Pinkus
Aggregates of basaloid cells in the uppermost dermis
Extension into the dermis of elongated strands of palisading basa-
loid cells
Mucin in the dermis and stromal fibromucinous changes
"Glandular" appearance to the tumor at low power

Clear cell
Islands of clear cells without peripheral palisading
Typical aggregates of nodular basal-cell carcinoma
Minimal nuclear atypia
Metatypical
Tumor nests with more eosinophilic characteristics
Poor peripheral palisading and stromal retraction
Keratin pearls, increased mitotic activity and premature
cornification

Differential Diagnosis

Nodular, micronodular
Eccrine spiradenoma
Nodular hidradenoma
Trichoepithelioma/trichoblastoma.
Superficial
Actinic keratosis
Seborrheic keratosis
Keratotic, infundibulocystic
Trichoepithelioma/trichoblastoma
Basaloid follicular hamartoma
Reticulated seborrheic keratosis
Infiltrative, morpheaform
Microcystic adnexal carcinoma
Desmoplastic trichoepithelioma
Adenoid, fibroepithelioma of Pinkus
Primary cutaneous adenoid cystic carcinoma
Malignant mixed tumor of the skin (malignant chondroid
syringoma)
Aggressive digital papillary adenocarcinoma
Clear cell
Sebaceous adenoma
Tricholemmoma
Clear-cell hidradenoma
Clear-cell acanthoma
Balloon-cell nevus and balloon-cell melanoma
Metatypical
Squamous-cell carcinoma

---

cinoma has an actively spreading indurated border with an atrophic or scar-like border.[210] Halo basal cell carcinomas are 1- to 2-mm erythematous papules on sun-exposed sites with surrounding hypergmentation.[210] Multicentric (multifocal, "field-fire") basal-cell carcinoma shows grouped tumors arising close to one another.[210] Finally, the linear variant demonstrates a longitudinal arrangement of tumor perhaps propagated by the Koebner phenomenon.[225]

Basal-cell carcinoma rarely invokes significant symptoms. Burning, stinging, or shooting pain is uncommon but may indicate perineural invasion.[226] This complication is present in 0.1 to 1.0 percent of cases and may be seen with recurrent lesions or those previously treated with radiotherapy. Motor symptoms from neural involvement also have been described. Lesions of the preauricular and cheek area are most commonly involved.[226] Tumor spreads proximally along perineural tissue planes and may be the only symptoms prior to clinical evidence of recurrence.

Metastases are rare in basal cell carcinoma.[201] Metastatic spread is most closely linked to the size of the original lesion and the depth of tumor invasion but less so to the histologic subtype.[222,227,228] A history of previous radiotherapy to the neoplasm also may be associated with metastatic spread.[228] Tumors larger than 3 cm in diameter have a 2 percent incidence of metastases and/or death. At 5 cm in diameter this rate is 25 percent and with lesions 10 cm in diameter the metastatic and/or death rate is 50 percent.[229] Tumors larger than 100 cm^2 have almost universally resulted in metastatic disease or death.[209] "Giant" basal-cell carcinomas are greater than 5 cm in diameter.[209,222] Basal-cell carcinomas arising in persons younger than 35 years may demonstrate rapid and aggressive growth patterns.[228]

Histopathological Features   Basal-cell carcinomas exhibit several histological patterns (Table 26-22). It is inappropriate in most instances, to simply render the diagnosis of "basal-cell carcinoma" histologically, since different variants behave differently and with variable outcomes and prognoses.[230] Nonetheless, it must be emphasized that many BCC exhibit two or more histological patterns, making subclassification difficult. The predominant histological pattern should guide classification of BCCs.

Nodular

More than half of all basal-cell carcinomas are of the nodular type (also known as nodulo-cystic).[201] Clinically, these are the typical slow-growing pearly nodules with rolled borders and telangiectasias.[201] Histologically, the tumors demonstrate aggregates of basophilic staining neoplastic cells with well-defined contours.[230] Palisading of the peripheral row of cells usually is obvious and retraction from surrounding stroma is seen (Fig. 26-15). Aggregates of cells that have become particularly large may demonstrate central necrosis with eosinophilic, granular features presumably owing to an outstripping of the growing nodule's blood supply. Mucin may be present within the aggregates of neoplastic cells and when exaggerated form large pools giving the tumor a "cystic" structure." The surrounding stroma tends to be myxoid and slightly fibrotic. Calcification may be present particularly in lesions of long standing. Mitotic activity and keratinocyte dyskeratosis usually are mild but may be marked in more aggressive lesions.

A "mixed" basal-cell carcinoma is a hybrid between a nodular and micronodular tumor with approximately equal portions of each type of lesion.[230] This pattern is not uncommonly observed but the designation is infrequently used.

Superficial

This variant previously has been called superficial multicentric. This term has lost popularity since it is believed that the individual nests of tumor cells arise not from multiple sites (multicentric) but rather from a single site and serpiginously wind through the epidermis as they proliferate. Nests of basaloid cells extend from the epidermis and hair follicle epithelium.[230] Tumor islands are relatively small and tend to have a broad base of attachment to the epidermis (Fig. 26-16). Neoplastic cells resemble primordial germ cells.[230] Peripheral palisading usually is prominent and the surrounding stroma is somewhat blanched because of the presence of mucin. Tumor lobules have a rounded and well-defined peripheral contour. Retraction spaces usually are prominent but are not typically filled with mucin. Mitotic activity is present but is rarely sig-

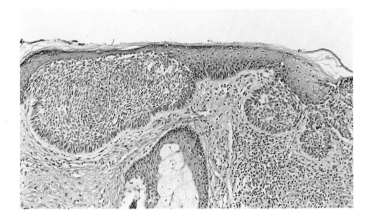

FIGURE 26-16 Superficial basal cell carcinoma. Atypical basaloid cells show stromal retraction and a broad attachment to the overlying epidermis.

nificant. Clinically, the lesions appear as erythematous patches or plaques with mild to moderate scaling, superficial ulcerations, and well-defined borders.[205] They are typically round or oval but may be irregular in shape. Tumors larger than 1.5 cm in diameter commonly have an infiltrating component.

Micronodular

These tumors are plaque-like, indurated, firm, and poorly defined.[231] Typically, they are difficult to remove and have an increased incidence of recurrence. Histologically, micronodular basal-cell carcinomas demonstrates small rounded nodules of tumor similar to the nodular variant but smaller. They are approximately the size of hair bulbs and display minimal palisading.[231] Tumor nodules are widely dispersed in an asymmetric pattern (Fig. 26-17). Retraction spaces are uncommon. The surrounding stroma is collagenous and slightly myxoid particularly adjacent to the tumor nodules.[230,231]

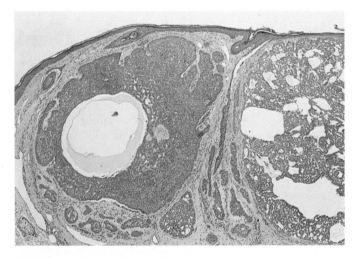

FIGURE 26-15 Nodular basal cell carcinoma. These tumors are composed of nodular aggregates of atypical basaloid cells with peripheral palisading and stromal retraction.

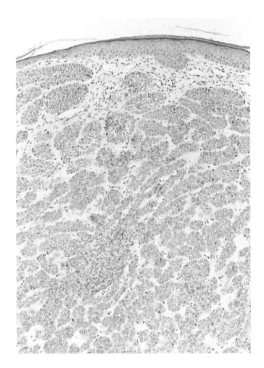

FIGURE 26-17 Micronodular basal cell carcinoma. Small nests of atypical basaloid cells typify the tumor.

Pigmented

Pigmented basal-cell carcinomas are more common in African Americans and Hispanics.[232] They resemble nodular tumors but are variably pigmented and may simulate melanocyte tumors. The hyperpigmentation may be light brown to dark black and involve all or only parts of the lesion. The histologic features are essentially identical to nodular basal- cell carcinomas. Pigment is present in the tumor aggregates or the surrounding stroma within melanophages (Fig. 26-18).[233]

Adamantinoid

This variant is histologically similar to the dental ameloblastoma or adamantinoma.[234] Tumor masses have a surrounding layer of cells with palisading nuclei.[234,235] These cells have stellate cytoplasm with elongated nuclei. The row of cells immediately adjacent to the outer row develop thin connecting bridges across empty spaces that give these tumors their adamantinoid features.[235] Ultrastructurally, these cells demonstrate moth-eaten cytoplasmic features.[235] Basaloid cells within the interior of these lobules are unremarkable without abnormally enlarged or multilobulated nuclei or increased mitotic activity. Hyaluronic acid, chondroitin sulfate, and glycogen are prevalent.[234,235] The presence of these glycosaminoglycans may result from active fibroblast production rather than degenerative processes.

A tumor termed the granular cell basal-cell carcinoma may be a variant of the adamantinoid basal cell carcinoma.[236] In these tumors the lobules have granular features and large cytoplasmic inclusions.[236] Nodular basal cell carcinoma merges with granular lobules.[210] Nuclei are bland to vesicular with little mitotic activity and are occasionally eccentric. The cytoplasm is eosinophilic and granular. The granules measure up to 15 m in diameter and may have halos around them. Ultrastructurally the granules appear like lysosomes.[210,236] Smaller granules fuse to form larger ones. Tonofilaments and desmosomes are present. Unlike the cells of granular cell tumors, these neoplasms are clearly of epidermal origin.

Clear-cell

Clear-cell basal cell carcinomas demonstrate variable numbers of transparent tumor cells (Fig. 26-19). Most tumors have the overall configuration of a nodular basal-cell carcinoma and aggregates of typical basaloid cells are usually present. Clear-cell changes may be present only at the periphery of a tumor lobule or may involve the whole of the lobule.[237,238] The affected cells are typically round to polyhedral and have pale, eosinophilic, vacuolated, or finely granular cytoplasm.[238] Palisading is usually minimal to absent. Nuclei are eccentrically placed and are atypical but not profoundly so.[237,238] PAS staining for glycogen is variably positive but mild deposition of sulfated mucin is observed.[237,238] Electron microscopy shows numerous vacuoles occupying almost the entirety of the cytoplasm and indenting the nuclei.[238] The vacuoles do not have a limiting membrane and appear empty. They are believed to be end-stage mitochondria or lysosomal degeneration.[210,238]

Signet-ring Cell

These tumors derive their name from the signet-ring or crescent shape the nuclei assume.[210,231] Tumor cells contain large, hyalinized intracytoplasmic aggregations that distort the nuclei. These inclusions stain for high and low molecular weight cytokeratin but not actin or vimentin.[239] The inclusions are believed to represent an aberrant form of keratinization in which intermediate filaments aggregate at the cell periphery. The overall architecture of signet-ring cell basal-cell carcinomas is similar to the nodular variant.

Adenoid

The adenoid basal-cell carcinoma is likely a variant of nodular basal-cell carcinoma since areas of this latter subtype commonly are present. Tumors show reticulated basaloid cells extending into the dermis. The strands are several cells wide and may show significant peripheral palisading and stromal retraction. Mucin deposition is often quite prominent. Lumina may be present and are often filled with colloidal or amorphous granular material. Connections with the overlying epidermis may not be readily visible but usually are established by cutting additional tissue sections.

Infiltrating (Infiltrative)

Infiltrating basal-cell carcinomas tend to fall somewhere between the nodular and morpheaform variants both histologically and clinically. These tumors are composed of atypical basaloid cells in varying sized

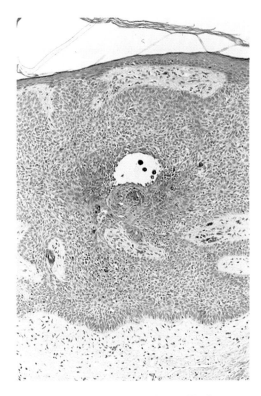

FIGURE 26-18 Pigmented basal cell carcinoma. The features are similar to those of a nodular basal cell carcinoma. Melanin is present within basaloid cells and tissue macrophages.

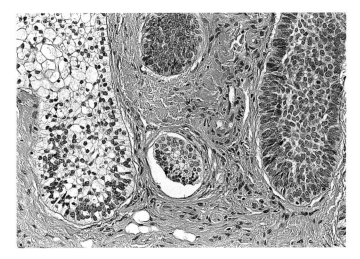

FIGURE 26-19 Clear-cell basal cell carcinoma. Collections of atypical clearcells are seen in association with lobules of nodular basal cell carcinoma.

nodules and islands with irregular, jagged peripheral contours (Fig. 26-20).[217,230] Elongated strands four to eight cells wide invade the deeper dermis.[217] The surrounding stroma is fibrous but minimally mucinous. Peripheral palisading and stromal retraction are rare.[230] The tumor is poorly circumscribed.[217] Invasion of the subcutis and muscle are occasionally appreciated. Inflammation is minimal. This tumor is more aggressive, more difficult to eradicate, and is capable of greater destruction than nodular variants. Clinically, infiltrative basal-cell carcinomas are yellow-white in color without a sharply defined or rolled border.[217] Tumors blend imperceptibly with surrounding skin.

Sclerosing (Morpheaform)

Sclerosing basal-cell carcinomas also are known as morpheaform (morphemic), fibrosing, scirrhous, or desmoplastic and comprise up to 5 percent of all lesions.[240] Tumors are white or yellow and are fibrotic. They are usually macular and rarely ulcerate or bleed.[205] No particular anatomic site is preferred.[241] Tumor islands are small, thin, and elongated (Fig. 26-21). They tend to be less than five cells in width and possess sharp, angulated ends.[230] Peripheral palisading is absent and stromal retraction is rare. Mitotic activity usually is present but is not marked. The surrounding dermis is fibrous and dense to the point of sclerosis. Tumors are usually poorly circumscribed and may invade deeply into muscle and fat.

Keratotic

Keratotic basal cell carcinomas are also known as "pilar" basal-cell carcinomas since they appear to be differentiating along pilosebaceous lines. These tumors probably are a subtype of nodular basal-cell carcinoma. Basaloid cells appear squamous with amphophilic cytoplasm.[242] Tumor nodules contain cysts that lack a granular cell layer and are filled with keratin and parakeratotic material. These cysts possibly are attempts at hair shaft formation. Calcification is occasionally present and palisading may be seen. Stroma is usually not abundant. Mitotic

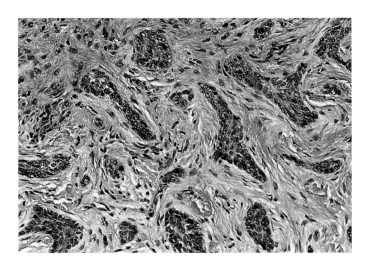

FIGURE 26-21   Sclerosing basal cell carcinoma. Aggregates of tumor cells are thin, hyperchromatic and set in a fibrotic stroma.

activity is minimal.[242] Unlike follicular basal cell carcinomas, keratotic basal-cell carcinomas are not usually well-circumscribed.

Pleomorphic

Pleomorphic basal-cell carcinomas also have been called basal-cell epithelioma with monster cells.[243] These tumors have features of a typical nodular basal-cell carcinoma.[243,244] Growth usually is well-circumscribed and solid but occasionally with adenoid or cystic features. Scattered throughout the tumor are enlarged mononuclear and/or multinucleated tumor cells (Fig. 26-22).[244] The nuclei are hyperchromatic and irregularly outlined with a vesicular appearance. Prominent nucleoli also are seen occasionally. Mitoses are seen but are not necessarily atypical.[243,244] All cases evaluated have been aneuploid.[244]

Metatypical

This subtype of basal-cell carcinoma has been the source of some confusion regarding its histologic features.[242,245] It is probably best to use this designation when evaluating a basal cell carcinoma with features intermittent between a nodular basal cell carcinoma and a squamous cell

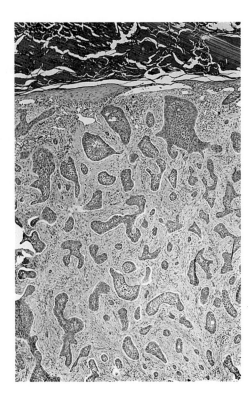

FIGURE 26-20   Infiltrating basal cell carcinoma. Tumor lobules are angulated and jagged with poor palisading and stromal retraction.

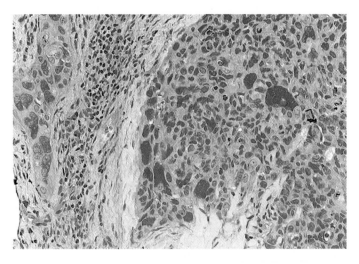

FIGURE 26-22   Pleomorphic basal cell carcinoma. Enlarged nuclei and giant cells are present within lobules of nodular basal cell carcinoma.

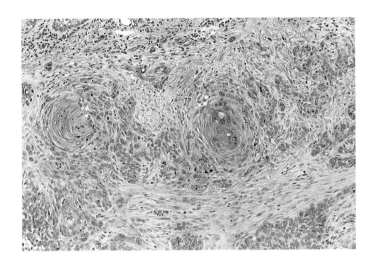

FIGURE 26-23 Metatypical basal cell carcinoma. Tumor islands are slightly basaloid with absent palisading and stromal retraction. Dyskeratosis and keratin pearl formation are seen.

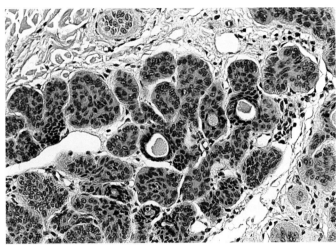

FIGURE 26-24 Basal cell carcinoma with eccrine differentiation. Typical lobules of nodular basal cell carcinoma show ductal differentiation containing sudiforous material.

carcinoma. These tumors have basaloid cells with variable eosinophilic features, prominent mitotic activity, and numerous apoptotic cells (Fig. 26-23). Peripheral palisading and stromal retraction are rare to absent. Nuclei are enlarged and some spindling of cells may be appreciated. Premature cornification is common. Keratin pearls occasionally are seen.[242] These tumors tend to be more aggressive with a greater incidence of perineural and lymphatic spread.[242] They may grow with the speed of squamous-cell carcinomas and have clinical features of both tumor types.[205]

Basosquamous

The diagnosis of basosquamous basal cell carcinoma is most appropriately used when evaluating a tumor with contiguous areas of basal-cell carcinoma and squamous-cell carcinoma.[205] The typical features of both tumor types are present with a minimal intermediate area of blending between the two.[242] The term "mixed carcinoma of the skin" has been used when no intermediate tumor cells are present.[242] Some authors have applied this term to so-called "collision" tumors, that is, basal-cell carcinoma colliding with squamous-cell carcinoma. The term has also been used perhaps in a similar way for metatypical BCC, to identify tumors intermediate to BCC and SCC throughout the neoplasm. Given the disparate uses of this term it is perhaps best that it be abandoned or strictly defined.

Basal Cell Carcinoma with Adnexal Differentiation

The presence of eccrine differentiation among otherwise unremarkable basal-cell carcinomas has been reported.[247–251] Within tumor aggregates are found collections of cells similar to the intra-epidermal portion of embryonic eccrine ducts (Fig. 26-24). Staining for CEA is positive 0within these ductal structures.

Sebaceous differentiation of basaloid cells may also be present. These cells arise in a typical nodular basal-cell carcinoma and possess a "lipidized" cytoplasm (Fig 26-25). They may be difficult to differentiate from sebaceous neoplasms.

Infundibulocystic

Proliferating basaloid cells show continuity with the overlying epidermis.[252] Bud-like structures are seen. There is some solid and reticulated pattern of growth with few mitotic figures (Fig. 26-26). Cysts with an infundibular lining are present and contain cornified cells. Cells within

these cysts demonstrate a transition in character from outer basaloid to inner squamous. Follicular bulbs and dermal papillae are lacking and other features of follicular differentiation are absent. The surrounding stroma is minimally fibrotic or mucinous.[251] These tumors are believed to be differentiating toward the upper infundibular structures of hair follicles.[252]

Follicular

Follicular basal-cell carcinomas demonstrate matrical proliferation.[253,254] Shadow cells are present adjacent to islands of basaloid cell proliferation. These cells possess a central unstained area compatible with the shadow of a lost nucleus. Calcification may be present.[254] Mitotic activity is minimal and tumor cells are not excessively anaplastic.[253] These lesions must be differentiated from a pilomatricoma.[253]

Fibroepithelioma of Pinkus

This tumor was described by Pinkus in 1953.[255] They typically arise on the lumbosacral regions as pink to flesh-colored nodules with a constricted base and may suggest fibroepithelial polyp or seborrheic

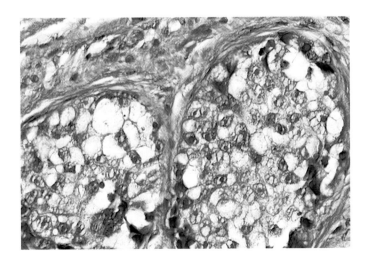

FIGURE 26-25 Basal cell carcinoma with sebaceous differentiation. Aggregates of nodular basal cell carcinoma show sebaceous differentiation.

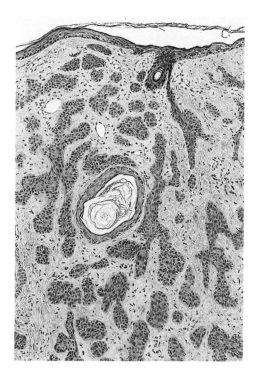

FIGURE 26-26 Infundibulocystic basal cell carcinoma. Connection to the epidermis is seen. Basaloid cells proliferate in a reticulated manner and form small cysts.

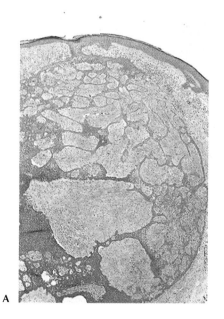

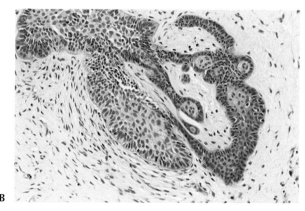

FIGURE 26-27 Fibroepithelioma of Pinkus. *A*. The tumor proliferates symmetrically as reticulated strands of basaloid cells surrounding fibromucinous stroma. *B*. Ductal differentiation is present in some areas.

keratosis.[241,256] Elongated, branched, and trabecular strands of basaloid cells extend deep into the dermis and proliferate symmetrically (Fig. 26-27 A). Horn cysts may be present and palisading is seen. Stromal retraction is uncommon. The surrounding stroma is fibromucinous and stromal–stromal separation may be present. Eccrine ducts are appreciated within some strands of basaloid cells (Fig 26-27 B).[257] This finding suggests that the tumor arises as a replacement of eccrine sweat ducts by infiltrating basaloid cells. A cystic variant of the fibroepithelioma has been described.[256]

Basal-cell Carcinoma with Myoepithelial Differentiation

This newly described variant has some features of a nodular basal cell carcinoma.[258] In the papillary dermis the tumor nodules are unremarkable. Deeper in the dermis the basaloid cells become oval to spindled and develop eccentric nuclei with homogenous ground-glass eosinophilic cytoplasm.[258] Scattered cells with signet ring formation are seen and the surrounding stroma is chondromyxoid. Tumor cells stain positively for CAM 5.2 (a keratin stain) and muscle specific actin. Additional stains for cytokeratins (AE1/AE3), vimentin, fibrillary acid protein, and S-100 are variably positive. This staining pattern is nonspecific but is compatible with myoepithelial cells.

Recurrent Basal-cell Carcinoma

Basal cell carcinomas that reappear after previous treatment are considered recurrent lesions. This occurs in about nine percent of conventionally treated lesions and one percent of those removed using Mohs micrographic surgery.[201] Lesions of the nose and ears are most prone to recurrence.[201,222] Most recurrences occur within 3 years but about 20 percent do so between the sixth and tenth year postoperatively.[222] There is a 40 percent recurrence rate when treating recurrent lesions. Recurrences may be difficult to discern clinically since the tumor may be intermingled with repair reaction and scarring.[205] Hemorrhage, erythema, and ulceration are indications of recurrence. Aggressive variants recur more often than nodular lesions.[201,230,259] There is a significant association between tumor recurrence and the measured distance to the closest free tissue margin, an aggressive tumor growth pattern, "spiked" shape of tumor nodules, poor peripheral palisading, nuclear pleomorphism, and an infiltrating invading edge.[204]

Host Response

Basal-cell carcinomas have varying degrees of inflammation. Most inflammatory cells are lymphocytes and most of these are T cells.[207,261] The helper/suppressor ratio ranges from 1.0 to 2.2.[207,261] Natural killer cells and B cells are present but rare.[207] Plasma cells are prominent around lesions that have ulcerated but otherwise are uncommon. Thirty to 50 percent of infiltrating T cells express activation antigens on their cell surfaces.[207] Monocytes and macrophages comprise one to 25 percent of infiltrating cells and most express HLA-DR antigens.[207,261] Langerhans cells make up four to 15 percent of the inflammatory infiltrate.[207] Mast cells may play a significant role in the biology of these tumors.[207,262] An increased number of these cells is present around tumor islands. Mast cells are prevalent around fibrotic tumors and this increased fibrosis may result from cell degranulation. Patients who are immunosuppressed and have diminished T-cell counts have a corresponding decrease in the number of peritumoral inflammatory cells.[211] The increased proclivity for tumors in these patients to invade deeper, recur, and metastasize could be related to diminished immune surveillance.

Amyloid deposition is found in 50 to 75 percent of basal-cell carcinomas and is more common in cystic, adenoid, and nodular subtypes.[263,264] Host and tumor location do not influence amyloid deposition. This substance is believed to derive from degenerating epithelial cells via filamentous degeneration or apoptosis.[263] Mucin deposition is common among basal-cell carcinomas. This contributes to peritumoral blanching. Mucin is composed of hyaluronic acid and dermatan sulfate and is produced by tumor cells.[201] Sclerosing basal-cell carcinomas produce a cytokine that stimulates fibroblast production of mucin.[201] Hyaline inclusions have also been described in some basal-cell carcinomas.[260] These inclusions are composed of various types of intermediate filaments and stain for vimentin, keratin, and smooth-muscle myosin.[260] Collagenous crystalloids have been described in the collagen surrounding some basal-cell carcinomas.[265] These structures consist of radially arranged clusters of eosinophilic needle-shaped fibers. The stain for types I and I collagen are slightly birefringent and measure 20 to 40 meters in diameter. They are believed to derive from degenerative processes of the extracellular matrix.

Some basal cell carcinomas, particularly fibrotic variants, may demonstrate regression.[210,266] New collagen is deposited with decreased skin appendages and increased vascularity. Tumor islands lose their peripheral palisading and undergo apoptosis. Infiltrating inflammatory cells are CD3- and CD4-positive lymphocytes and occasional plasma cells. T-helper cells (CD4) may induce this regression by cytokine production.[266]

Immunohistochemistry

Basal-cell carcinomas take up cytokeratin stains. These proteins are intermediate filaments that are produced by epithelial cells.[201] Tumors express primarily types 5 and 14, which is consistent with tumors of a "basaloid" origin. These tumors also stain for alpha-2 and β1 integrins but are negative for intercellular adhesion molecule 1 (ICAM-1), leukocyte function antigen 1 α (LFA-1α) and vascular cell adhesion molecule 1 (VCAM-1).[267] There is no association between integrin staining and tumor subtype. HLA-DR antigens are present on some tumor cells, particularly when they are in close proximity to HLA-DR+ infiltrating lymphocytes.[261] p53 Protein expression has been found on most basal-cell carcinomas.[268] This protein is preferentially expressed on more aggressive tumors.[269]

Electron Microscopy

Ultrastructurally, basal-cell carcinomas have enlarged nuclei with small nucleoli and numerous chromatin aggregations.[201] Nodular islands of tumor demonstrate a continuous band of types IV and V collagen and laminin, indicating the presence of a basement membrane. These basement membranes are intermittently discontinuous. Morpheaform and basosquamous variants do not possess a basement membrane, perhaps contributing to their aggressive behavior. Tumors that are able to dissolve basement membranes potentiate their invasive behavior by cell movement across physiologic barriers.[270] Increased collagenase production by peritumoral fibroblasts decreases anchoring fibrils and collagen content.[201] Desmosomes are present, however, their numbers are diminished.[201] This likely accounts for tumor friability seen clinically. Hemidesmosomes are decreased in number and are responsible for the retraction spaces between tumor nodules and surrounding stroma.[201] Microfilaments of the cellular cytoskeleton are uncommon in normal epithelium but are found in basal-cell carcinoma cells.[271] These are more prevalent in invasive subtypes.

Differential Diagnosis   The differential diagnosis for basal cell carcinomas depends on the different subtypes that are being evaluated. Nodular basal-cell carcinomas must be differentiated from benign adnexal proliferations such as eccrine spiradenoma, nodular hidradenoma, and trichoepithelioma or trichoblastoma. Eccrine spiradenomas are well demarcated intradermal nodules with no connection with the overlying epidermis. Tumor nodules are composed of cells with small dark nuclei and larger cells with pale staining nuclei. Mitosis and dyskeratosis are uncommon. Nodular hidradenomas and other tumors of the acrosyringium do not necessarily have a connection with the epidermis and have few mitoses. Differentiation towards eccrine ducts may be present. These tumors invade deeper than most nodular basal-cell carcinomas, do not commonly undergo necrosis and demonstrate no peripheral cell palisading or mucin deposition. Trichoepitheliomas and trichoblastomas may be the most difficult tumors to distinguish from nodular basal-cell carcinoma and the infundibulocystic or keratotic variants and in fact may be part of a histological continuum with basal-cell carcinoma. These former tumors may have connections to overlying epidermis as well as occasional foci of calcification. Small keratin cysts are seen but the proliferation of basaloid cells does not typically palisade and is rarely associated with mucin production. Mitotic activity and apoptosis also are diminished. Trichoepitheliomas produce papillary mesenchymal bodies.[272] These bodies are fibroblastic proliferations representing abortive attempts to construct papillary mesenchyme. Trichoepitheliomas and trichoblastomas typically induce a mild to moderate fibrosis to the surrounding dermis. This stromal change is usually prominently demarcated from otherwise normal dermis. Stromal-stromal separation is seen. The stroma of trichoepitheliomas is CD34 positive, whereas that around basal-cell carcinomas is negative.[253] Keratotic and infundibulocystic basal cell carcinomas must also be distinguished from basaloid follicular hamartomas and reticulated seborrheic keratoses.[253,273] Basaloid follicular hamartomas are composed of thin anastomosing cords of cells with squamoid and basaloid features. Surrounding stroma is scant and mildly fibrotic but may occasionally separate from surrounding dermis (stromal–stromal separation). Reticulated seborrheic keratoses typically have prominent pigmentation along the basal layer, a flat bottom, horn pseudocysts, and banal basaloid cells.

Infiltrative or morpheaform basal-cell carcinoma must be differentiated from microcystic adnexal carcinoma and desmoplastic trichoepithelioma. Microcystic adnexal carcinoma demonstrates rare mitotic activity and ductal differentiation in deeper tissues. Necrosis is uncommon. CEA and S-100 staining occasionally are positive.[274] Desmoplastic trichoepitheliomas show an invagination of the epidermis consistent with the "dell" present in the lesions clinically. Proliferating cells are basaloid and keratin cysts are seen. Mitoses are very rare and mucin, calcification, and apoptosis are absent.

Superficial basal-cell carcinomas appear similar to actinic keratoses and seborrheic keratoses. Proliferative actinic keratoses show aggregation and palisading of atypical basal cells. However, mucin deposition in the papillary dermis and stromal retraction are absent. Seborrheic keratoses may have basaloid cell proliferation. Mitotic activity and peripheral palisading, however, are not seen and horn pseudocysts usually are present.

Basal-cell carcinomas with a glandular appearance (adenoid, fibroepithelioma of Pinkus, eccrine epithelioma) demonstrate ductal structures and must be distinguished from sweat gland carcinomas such as primary cutaneous adenoid cystic carcinoma, malignant mixed tumor of the skin, and aggressive digital papillary adenocarcinoma.[275] Primary cutaneous adenoid cystic carcinomas have a cribiform or "punched out" configuration with rare attachment to the epidermis or hair follicles. Mitotic activity is rare and peripheral palisading is uncommon. CEA staining is variably positive. Malignant mixed tumor of the skin (malignant chondroid syringoma) demonstrates a proliferation of ducts and invades deeply. This proliferation is not well-demarcated and tends to be in the deeper dermis. Islands of cells and trabeculae are seen. Atypia is subtle. The surrounding matrix is largely mucinous or chondroid. Basaloid cells are CEA positive. Aggressive digital papillary adenocarcinomas show little involvement with the epidermis and extend deep into subcutaneous tissues and bone. These tumors are poorly circumscribed. Papillary projections are seen along with significant mitotic activity and tumor necrosis.

Clear-cell basal-cell carcinomas must be differentiated from other clear-cell neoplasms, such as sebaceous adenomas, tricholemmomas, clear-cell hidradenomas, and clear-cell acanthoma.[237] Balloon cell nevus (and balloon cell melanoma) and metastases of renal cell carcinoma also must be distinguished from these tumors.[238] Sebaceous adenomas have clear cells and basaloid cells but do not demonstrate atypia or mucin production. Evidence of sebaceous differentiation also usually is visible. Tricholemmomas do not have significant mitotic activity and may show areas of hypergranulosis. Clear-cell hidradenomas demonstrate ductal differentiation with few mitoses and no mucin production or stromal retraction. Clear-cell acanthomas only involve the epidermis and show infiltrating neutrophils but no atypia. Balloon cell melanocytic proliferations have no stromal retraction or mucin deposition. Malignant variants may show pagetoid spread. These tumors are S-100 positive and cytokeratin negative in distinction to clear-cell basal-cell carcinomas. Metastatic renal-cell carcinoma typically has numerous extravasated erythrocytes and minimal connection to the epidermis. Basaloid cells also are absent.

Finally, some basal-cell carcinomas lack typical basaloid staining and appear eosinophilic. Tumors such as metatypical basal-cell carcinomas may be confused with squamous cell carcinomas. This distinction may be an academic one since squamous-cell carcinomas and metatypical basal-cell carcinomas behave similarly; however, with more nodular lesions a definitive diagnosis may be important. Staining with Ber EP4 has been used to distinguish between the two types of malignancy.[276] Basal cell carcinomas may take up the stain but squamous cell carcinomas do not.

Nevoid Basal-cell Carcinoma Syndrome

This syndrome was initially described by Howell and Caro in 1959.[277] It is also known as the Gorlin syndrome, the basal-cell nevus syndrome and the Gherkin-Goltz syndrome.[278,279] This complex of symptoms is inherited as an autosomal dominant trait but about 35 to 50 percent of affected patients represent new mutations.[278,279] The disease usually begins between 17 and 35 years of age but has been described in children as young as 2 years.[280] Disease activity is increased at puberty.[279,280] The prevalence is approximately one in 56,000.[208] Because of the relatively young age of affected patients there is not a strong association between cumulative sun exposure and tumor development. However, in susceptible persons sun exposure does exacerbate the development of basal-cell carcinomas.[208] A malfunctioning tumor suppressor gene on chromosome 9q22-q31 is believed to cause this condition.[281]

Clinical Features   The features of the nevoid basal-cell carcinoma syndrome are divided into five major categories.[279–281] The first is the presence of numerous basal-cell carcinomas (Table 26-23). These may range from a few to a thousand and are similar to routine basal-cell carcinomas.[281] They may be very small and flesh-colored to brown. Tumors appear as dome-shaped papules to soft nodular or flat plaques on the face and trunk. Lesions vary from 1 to 10 mm and may be mistaken for skin tags, nevi, molluscum contagiosum or hemangio-

TABLE 26-23

Nevoid Basal-cell Carcinoma

Clinical Features

Numerous flesh-colored to brown papules 1 to 10 mm in diameter
Develop on the face and trunk beginning around puberty
Autosomal dominant inheritance
Jaw and cutaneous cysts, skeletal anomalies (particularly bifid ribs), ectopic CNS calcification, and palmar/plantar pitting

Histopathological Features

Basal-cell Carcinomas
    Essentially identical to those found idiopathically
    Most commonly nodular and superficial variants
    Calcification and pigment deposition are more common
Jaw and Cutaneous Cysts
    Epithelial lining with granular layer similar to infundibular cysts
    Epithelial lining with corrugated, compact lining similar to steatocystomas
Cutaneous Pits
    Sharply defined absence of keratin and thinned epidermis at base of pit
    Diminished or absent granular layer

Differential Diagnosis

Basal-cell Carcinomas
    Eccrine spiradenoma
    Nodular hidradenoma
    Trichoepithelioma/trichoblastoma.
Jaw and Cutaneous Cysts
    Dilated pore
    Dermoid cyst
Cutaneous Pits
    Pitted keratolysis

mas.[279,280] These tumors may be aggressive, particularly when they involve the embryonic clefts of the face.[282]

The second feature is the development of numerous cysts particularly epithelium lined jaw cysts. These lesions begin to develop after age 7 and may cause pain, tooth shifting, drainage, and jaw swelling.[279,280] Cutaneous cysts may also be present and arise on the trunk and limbs in about half of affected patients.[279] These cysts contain thick, discolored liquid with features similar to steatocystomas.[284] Intermittent milial cysts are present in 35 to 50 percent of patients.[279]

Skeletal anomalies are prevalent in this syndrome and include bifid ribs, frontal bossing of the skull, bridging of the sella turcica, and spinal deformities.[280] Intracranial calcification, particularly of the falx cerebri, is seen.[208,279] Finally, pitting of the palms and soles is appreciated.[284] These pits are 1 to 3 mm in depth and 2 to 3 mm in diameter. They develop during the second decade of life.[280]

Additional features include neuropsychiatric defects such as schizophrenia, electroencephalographic abnormalities, mental retardation, and cerebellar degeneration.[280,282] Tumors and abnormalities of the reproductive system also may occur.

Histopathological Features   Histologically, the basal-cell carcinomas are identical to those found in patients without this syndrome (Table 26-23).[280] Tumors are most commonly of the nodular and superficial subtype with morpheaform, adenoid, and fibroepithelial variants less likely. Calcification and pigment deposition may be increased.[285]

The cutaneous cysts are similar to infundibular cysts.[283] These tumors have an epithelial lining with a distinct granular layer and produce keratin. Some cysts, however, resemble keratinous jaw cysts. These lesions show a festooned or corrugated epithelium two to five cells thick that lacks a granular layer. These features are similar to those of steatocystomas, but sebaceous glands are absent.[283]

Cutaneous pits demonstrate a sharply defined absence of keratin. The epidermis is thinned at the base and the rete ridges proliferate irregularly. The granular layer is diminished.[284] These pits are believed to result from premature desquamation of the keratinocytes.

Differential Diagnosis   The differential diagnosis for these tumors is the same as for idiopathic basal-cell carcinomas. The cutaneous cysts in this syndrome are similar to infundibular cysts and steatocystomas. Infundibular cysts may appear similar to dilated pores since both possess a lining containing a granular layer. Steatocystomas usually have sebaceous glands in the lining wall and may contain small hair shaft fragments. These may also be confused with dermoid cysts that show more pilosebaceous differentiation and the presence of eccrine or apocrine glands.

Cutaneous pits may be seen in pitted keratolysis but in this disease gram positive filamentous or coccoidal bacteria are present.

Squamous-cell Carcinoma

Squamous-cell carcinomas are the second most common cutaneous malignancy.[286] They account for about 20 percent of all skin cancers and are the most prevalent skin cancer in blacks.[210,287] Approximately 100,000 new cases of squamous-cell carcinoma occur annually.[288] The lifetime risk of developing one of these tumors is between four and 14 percent.[289] This incidence has been steadily increasing about four to eight percent per year since the 1960's with a three- to four-fold increase over the past 20 to 30 years.[286,288] The case fatality rate for cutaneous squamous cell carcinomas is approximately seven per 1000.[290] Between 2000 and 2500 deaths annually are attributed to these neoplasms.[286] The death rate for squamous-cell carcinomas of the skin is decreasing in most countries but increasing in some. Risk factors for developing a squamous-cell carcinoma include increased age, light skin pigmentation, immunosuppression, and genetic disorders such as xeroderma pigmentosum.[287]

The most common inciting cause of cutaneous squamous-cell carcinomas is cumulative ultraviolet radiation (UVR) exposure.[286] Sunlight is the greatest source of UVR with UVB being the most damaging factor.[290] A depletion of the ozone layer may play a role in this susceptibility.[289] Other etiologic factors include ionizing radiation exposure, ultraviolet light treatment including PUVA therapy, human papillo-

---

TABLE 26-24

Squamous-cell Carcinoma

Clinical Features

Most commonly affect the head and neck of elderly patients
Quickly growing flesh colored to red nodules on sun-exposed skin
Overlying scale or crusting
Lip lesions with atrophy, crusting, and ulceration
Usually asymptomatic unless perineural invasion is present
Ulcerating, papillomatous, and subcutaneous variants

Histopathological Features

Conventional
   Aggregates of atypical epithelial cells invading the dermis
   May derive from an actinic keratosis or Bowen's disease
   Variable mitotic activity, keratin pearl formation, premature
      cornification
   Focal acantholysis and/or spindle-cell proliferation
   Nonspecific inflammatory infiltrate with lymphocytes and plasma
      cells
Spindle cell
   Spindle cells emanating from the basal layer and invading the
      dermis
   Mitotic activity and atypia are present
   Pleomorphic giant cells occasionally are seen
   Cells are cytokeratin positive and occasionally vimentin-positive
Acantholytic
   Lobules and nests of atypical, acantholytic keratinocytes
   Premature cornification with free-floating neoplastic ker-
      atinocytes
Signet ring
   Atypical nuclei are displaced yielding a signet ring appearance
   Paranuclear clear zone or nuclear displacement by eosinophilic
      globule
   Strong staining for glycogen
Pseudovascular
   Proliferation of pleomorphic, atypical cells with "hobnail"
      appearance

   Cellular aggregates with vascular appearance
   Erythrocytes contained in pseudovascular spaces
   Moderate to marked mitotic activity
Subcutaneous
   Intradermal aggregates of atypical, epithelioid cells
   Mitotic activity and premature cornification variable
   Atypical mitoses occasionally seen
   Connection to epidermis or adnexal structures present on deeper
      sectioning

Differential Diagnosis

Conventional
   Pseudocarcinomatous hyperplasia
   Inflamed seborrheic keratosis
   Metatypical basal cell carcinoma
   Inflamed wart
Spindle cell
   Spindle-cell malignant melanoma
   Atypical fibroxanthoma
Acantholytic
   Acantholytic dermatoses (Hailey-Hailey disease, pemphigus vul-
      garis, transient acantholytic dermatosis)
   Angiosarcoma
Signet ring
   Metastatic gastric or colon carcinoma
   Paget's disease
   Signet ring cell basal-cell carcinoma
   Myxoid liposarcoma
Pseudovascular
   Angiosarcoma
Subcutaneous nodular
   Metastatic squamous-cell carcinoma

mavirus infection (particularly type 16), arsenic ingestion, polycyclic aromatic hydrocarbon exposure, immunosuppression, preexisting chronic dermatoses and ulcer/sinus tract formation.[147,286,291] Squamous-cell carcinoma of the lip is associated with smoking and tobacco chewing.[287,289]

Cutaneous conditions associated with the development of squamous-cell carcinoma include porokeratosis, lupus erythematosus, lichen planus, lichen sclerosus, epidermolysis bullosa, erythema ab igne, acrodermatitis chronic atrophicans, dissecting cellulitis of the scalp, chromoblastomycosis, nevus sebaceous, linear epidermal nevus, granuloma inguinale, acne conglobata, and lymphogranuloma venereum.[286]

Two specific types of squamous-cell carcinoma deserve comment. Marjolin's ulcers are squamous-cell carcinomas developing in scar tissue or chronic wounds. These include fistulas, venous ulcers, draining sinuses of osteomyelitis, pressure ulcers, vaccination sites, chronic hidradenitis suppurativa, discoid lupus erythematosus, frostbite, burn sites, and donor sites of skin grafts.[289] The lesions present as shallow ulcerations with a nodular surface and well-defined peripheral margins. Exophytic nodular excrescences with granulation tissue also may be seen. These tumors have a 30 percent incidence of metastatic disease.

Most squamous cell carcinomas arise on the head and neck.[290] The extremities, particularly the hands, are also frequently affected but the trunk is not commonly involved.[286] Men are more often affected than women.[288] Deeper skin invasion is associated with an increased metastatic disease and recurrence rates.[288] Tumors greater than 2 cm in diameter are twice as likely to recur and three times as likely to metastasize.[289] Tumor thickness may be measured in millimeters similar to that for melanomas.[289]

Perineural invasion may be present and lowers the 5-year survival rate.[287] These tumors are larger at presentation (most > 2 cm in diameter), less well-differentiated and associated with lymphadenopathy.[292] Forehead location and a history of previous treatment also are more common.[293] Perineural invasion affects 2.4 to 14 percent of cutaneous squamous cell carcinomas.[289] Lesions are initially painful and later anesthetic.[290,292] Muscle weakness is uncommon but is seen in late stages. Cranial nerves VII and VI (mandibular and maxillary divisions) are most commonly involved.[288,289] Extensive perineural invasion may eventuate in direct intracranial extension and death.[286] The survival rate of affected persons is usually less than 30 percent.[293]

Metastatic disease is uncommon. The overall rate approximately two percent but is between 10 and 15 percent for lesions on the lips and ears.[294] Metastases are more prevalent in tumors that are poorly differentiated, of long standing duration, and inadequately treated.[288,295] Eighty-five percent of metastases affect only the lymph nodes but involvement of lungs, liver, bones, brain, and mediastinum also may occur.[288,290]

Forty percent of persons who have undergone an organ transplant develop a cutaneous malignancy.[289] This risk is approximately 250 times normal and the incidence increases by four percent each year after transplantation.[219,289] Squamous-cell carcinomas outnumber basal-cell carcinomas. These cancers are potentially more aggressive with a higher rate of metastasis and death.[289] Aggressive lesions are seen more commonly in the elderly, on the head, in recurrent tumors, and with a deeper degree of invasion. These tumors are likely induced by the degree of immunosuppression and the presence of human papillomavirus infection. HPV types 5 and 8 are found in some specimens.[296] Herpes-virus-like DNA sequences have also been detected in transplant patients.[220] Since most lesions arise on sun-exposed skin cumulative ultraviolet light exposure, particularly prior to age 30, also is an important factor.[219]

Clinical Features Squamous-cell carcinomas may have a number of different clinical presentations (Table 26-24). Most tumors are nodules

with overlying scale or scale-crust.[290] Lesions are skin-colored but some may be red to brown and telangiectasias are present. Exophytic cauliflower-shaped lesions, indurated crusted plaques, ulceration, and subcutaneous nodules also may be seen. Different histologic types may have more specific clinical features. The surrounding skin usually demonstrates moderate to severe dermatoheliosis. Squamous-cell carcinomas of the lip present as rough, scaling papules on the lower lip with frequent ulceration in middle-aged to elderly males.[289] The lip mucosa is typically dry and atrophic with leukoplakia and variable pigmentation. Patients' lips may be chapped or crusted. A history of smoking and/or tobacco chewing is common and metastatic disease is more frequent.

Histopathological Features Squamous-cell carcinoma has been classified into four histologic categories—conventional, spindle cell, acantholytic, and verrucous (Table 26-24).[286] This is a useful paradigm for purposes of classification but other histologic subtypes also exist. The Broders classification considers the degree of tumor differentiation.[298] Grade 1 tumors are composed of less than 25 percent undifferentiated cells, grade II are less than 50 percent undifferentiated, grade III are less than 75 percent undifferentiated and grade IV are greater than 75 percent undifferentiated. Use of this scale for tumor classification is no longer popular. Squamous-cell carcinomas arise from precursor lesions, including actinic keratoses, thermal keratoses, arsenical keratoses, chronic radiation keratoses, erythroplasia of Queyrat, epidermodysplasia verruciformis, and Bowen's disease.[286]

In conventional squamous cell carcinoma atypical, slightly epithelioid cells emanate from the epidermis and spread into the dermis (Fig. 26-28 A). Nuclei are enlarged and pleomorphic (Fig. 26-28 B). Mitotic activity is variable but usually is greater than basal-cell carcinomas. Atypical mitotic figures and keratin pearls are present. Dyskeratotic and prematurely cornifying cells are seen. The depth of dermal invasion is variable. If deep enough the tumor may show lateral spread on reaching the fascial or capsular plane, muscle, periosteum, or perichondrium.[289] Perineural invasion shows invasion of the perineurium by atypical squamous cells.[290] Involvement of the nerves is suspect in specimens showing inflammatory cells around cutaneous nerve twigs.[292] Small foci of acantholysis or spindling may be present. Inflammation is observed in ulcerating tumors and typically consists of lymphocytes, plasma cells, and neutrophils.[298] Eosinophils are also frequently present.[189] These cells do not seem to influence prognosis and are unrelated to the etiology, duration, site of the tumor, or age of the patient. Staining with anticytokeratin antibodies is positive for mostly high and (but less frequently) low molecular weight cytokeratins.[299] Vimentin may also be positive in poorly differentiated lesions.[300]

SPINDLE-CELL

Spindle-cell squamous-cell carcinomas (SCSCCs) may be associated with previous trauma and/or radiotherapy.[289] They are commonly ulcerated.[300] Histologically, atypical spindle cells are seen emanating from the epidermis and intermingle with strands of collagen in a whorled fashion.[290] They are arranged into intertwining fascicles and bundles (Fig. 26-29).[300] Surrounding stroma may be myxoid and pleomorphic giant cells may be appreciated.[289] Individual tumor cells are eosinophilic with hyperchromatic, elongated nuclei, and multiple nucleoli.[289,300] Nuclei also may be pleomorphic and vesicular. Mitotic activity with occasional atypical figures is present.[300] Ultrastructurally, myofilaments and tonofilament associated desmosomes have been noted.[289,300,301] Many SCSCCs stain for both cytokeratin and Vimentin.[300] This gradient between the two tumors may be explained by a metaplastic change with more mesenchymal differentiation in the

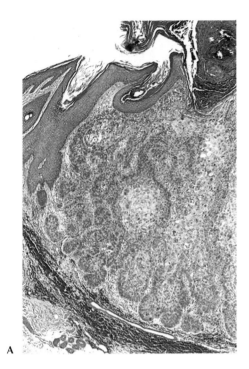

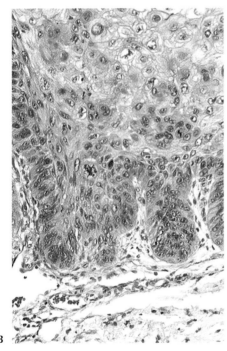

FIGURE 26-28   Squamous cell carcinoma. *A*. Atypical keratinocytes extend from the epidermis into the dermis. *B*. Tumor cells have enlarged, hyperchromatic nuclei with prominent mitotic activity.

spindle-cell squamous-cell carcinoma.[300] Previously, spindle-cell tumors taking up the vimentin stain were thought to be atypical fibroxanthomas and it is likely that many such tumors have been misdiagnosed.

ACANTHOLYTIC

These tumors also are called pseudoglandular, adenoid, carcinoma segregans, or adenoacanthoma.[286,302] Lesions typically arise on the head and neck as a nodule or ulcer in elderly men.[303] They have been associ-

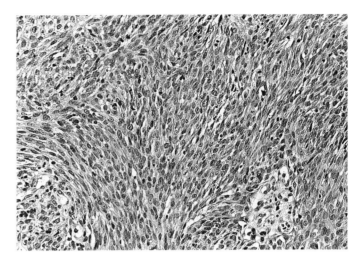

FIGURE 26-29   Spindle-cell squamous cell carcinoma. Tumor cells are atypical and spindled in a slightly whorled fashion. Mitotic activity is brisk.

ated with recurrent tumors following radiation therapy and portend a better prognosis.[289,304] Similar lesions have been described in the oropharynx, lung, larynx, vulva, and breast.[302] The acantholysis is likely an accentuation of the same process seen in actinic keratoses. The tumor is arranged in cords and nests in a glandular (pseudoglandular) or adenoid pattern (Fig. 26-30 A). Polygonal cells surround lumen-like spaces containing free-floating, neoplastic keratinocytes (Fig. 26-30 B).[302] Dyskeratotic cells may be few or abundant and are single or grouped.[289] PAS staining may demonstrate abundant glycogen.

The signet ring cell squamous-cell carcinoma is probably a variant of the acantholytic subtype.[305] Tumor cells demonstrate a paranuclear clear zone similar to other signet ring cell malignancies (Fig. 26-31). A second type shows nuclear displacement by a deeply eosinophilic globule resembling the cytoplasm of dyskeratotic cells.[305] The clear zone around the nucleus stains positively for glycogen, whereas the eosinophilic globule is PAS+ but diastase resistant. Keratin stains are strongly positive in concentric rings at the periphery of these cells. These tumors may have a more aggressive clinical course.

PSEUDOVASCULAR ADENOID

This squamous-cell carcinoma may be a subtype of the acantholytic variant but tends to show much less acantholysis and more of a glandular appearance.[298,302] These tumors are most common in elderly males. They are crusted, heaped up nodules or ulcers with a prominent advancing margin. Metastatic disease and death are common. Histologically, the tumor shows an interanastomosing array of tumor cells displaying pseudovascular lumen-like features with connection to the overlying epidermis. Tumor cells dissect through dermal collagen and around adnexal structures. The channels and cystic spaces are lined by plump neoplastic cells. Tumor cells are round or polygonal with moderately abundant cytoplasm and "hobnail" features. Nuclei are pleomorphic and hyperchromatic with prominent nucleoli.[298] Intracytoplasmic vacuoles mimic primitive vascular lumina. The pseudoglandular spaces are largely empty but contain occasional erythrocytes or detached tumor cells. Mitotic activity may be moderate to marked and atypical mitoses are seen. Inflammation and peritumoral fibrosis are present. Continuity with dermal blood vessels may be seen.[302] Hyaluronic acid is present in many of the pseudovascular structures. The tumors stain for cytokeratin and epithelial membrane antigens.[298,302] Factor VIII, CD31, and CD34 are negative. Vimentin uptake is present in some lesions. Ultrastructurally, tonofibrils are present but Weibel-Pelade bodies and other evidence of vascular derivation are not seen.[298]

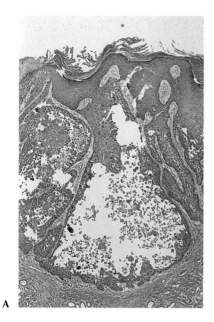

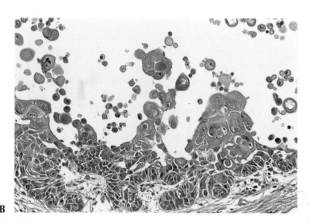

FIGURE 26-30 Acantholytic squamous cell carcinoma. *A.* Aggregates of invading atypical keratinocytes demonstrate acantholysis. *B.* Enlarged, free-floating keratinocytes are present.

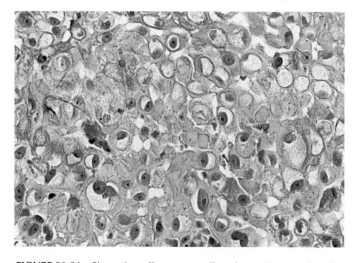

FIGURE 26-31 Signet ring cell squamous cell carcinoma. A paranuclear clear zone has pushed the nuclei aside forming a "signet ring" appearance.

SUBCUTANEOUS

These tumors present as asymptomatic subcutaneous nodules on the head and neck.[306] Overlying skin is unremarkable. Subcutaneous squamous cell carcinomas show an intradermal collection of atypical epithelioid cells with mitoses, premature cornification, and squamous eddies. Connection to the overlying epidermis is not immediately appreciated but may be found if additional sections are obtained. These tumors have a high incidence of perineural invasion.[306] Subcutaneous squamous cell carcinoma is believed to arise as a microscopic focus of epidermal atypia that quickly invades the dermis tethered by a thin stalk.[288] This epidermal connection is soon lost and the tumor appears to be solely confined to the dermis. Some tumors may arise from adnexal epithelium.[306] Differentiation from metastatic squamous-cell carcinoma may be difficult.

PAPILLARY

Papillary squamous-cell carcinomas are more common in elderly women but may also be present in immunosuppressed patients.[307] They are rapidly growing tumors with red to tan features and are exophytic. Atypical cells arise atop a fibrovascular stalk with invasion of the underlying dermis.[307] Mitoses are widespread and HPV DNA evaluation has been negative.

Differential Diagnosis The differential diagnosis for squamous-cell carcinoma depends on the subtype being considered. Conventional squamous-cell carcinoma must be distinguished from pseudocarcinomatous proliferation, metatypical basal-cell carcinoma, inflamed seborrheic keratosis, and inflamed wart. Pseudocarcinomatous hyperplasia demonstrates an irregular invasion of the dermis by strands of epithelial cells. These may be tapered and proliferate in a poorly circumscribed manner. The cells are typically (but uncommonly) well differentiated and mitotic activity and nuclear hyperchromasia are lacking. Inflammatory cell infiltration may also be present. Distinguishing these two entities in some instances may be impossible. Inflamed seborrheic keratoses typically do not have a significant mitotic activity. Nuclei also are not usually pleomorphic or hyperchromatic. The overall configuration may show the outline of a seborrheic keratosis with acanthosis, spongiosis, and vague papillomatous proliferation. Hyperkeratosis is common and may contain aggregates of serum with inspissated erythrocytes. The typical "flat bottom" of a seborrheic keratosis also may be present and significant numbers of inflammatory cells may be seen. Metatypical basal-cell carcinomas have features intermediate between squamous-cell carcinoma and basal-cell carcinoma.[205,307] Cells are predominantly basaloid but with some epithelioid features. Slight spindling may be seen along with apoptosis, a moderate mitotic rate, and keratin pearls. Some peripheral palisading and mucinous changes in the surrounding stroma occasionally are present but stromal retraction is rare. Finally, inflamed and/or resolving warts may be similar to squamous-cell carcinomas. Inflamed warts may have increased numbers of mitoses and nuclear enlargement. However, these lesions are not typically endophytic, usually lack nuclear hyperchromatism, are papillomatous, and demonstrate focal areas of hypergranulosis. Additionally, warts have dilated capillaries in the superficial dermis.

Spindle-cell squamous-cell carcinomas (SCSCCs) are easily confused with two other spindle-cell malignancies of the skin, spindle-cell melanoma, and atypical fibroxanthoma (AFX).[286,289] Superficial malignant fibrohistiocytomas, sarcomas, and cutaneous metastases also may show similar changes. Spindle-cell melanomas usually derive from lentiginous melanomas of sun-exposed skin and may have pagetoid spread of atypical melanocytes. Pigment deposition, a comparatively reduced mitotic rate, and nuclear pseudoinclusions may also be present.

These tumors usually are Vimentin and S-100 positive but cytokeratin negative, whereas SCSCCs are cytokeratin positive and S-100 negative. Vimentin may be positive in some SCSCCs.[300] Atypical fibroxanthomas have scattered giant cells with atypical nuclei and bizarre mitotic figures. These tumors are vimentin-positive and cytokeratin-negative. Electron microscopy analysis for the presence of tonofilaments will help distinguish SCSCCs.

Acantholytic squamous cell carcinomas usually are easily distinguished from other acantholytic disorders (Hailey-Hailey disease, pemphigus vulgaris, transient acantholytic dermatosis, etc.) since the acantholysis involves atypical cells and extends deep into the dermis. However, angiosarcoma may be difficult to differentiate from this squamous-cell variant. Red blood cell entrapment in some pseudolumina occasionally is present. Immunostaining for cytokeratin and epithelial membrane antigen will be positive in acantholytic squamous-cell carcinoma but negative in angiosarcomas. The signet ring cell variant of acantholytic squamous-cell carcinoma must be differentiated from metastatic gastric and colon cancer. Benign lipoblastoma, Paget's disease, signet ring cell basal-cell carcinoma, myxoid liposarcoma, and round-cell liposarcoma also may demonstrate signet ring cells.

Angiosarcoma is in the differential diagnosis for pseudovascular adenoid squamous-cell carcinoma. The lining cells in both disorders show "hobnailing" and atypia. Immunostaining is helpful in distinguishing between the two tumors since angiosarcomas are cytokeratin negative but vimentin, *Ulex*, CD31, and CD34-positive.

Subcutaneous squamous-cell carcinomas must be differentiated from metastatic disease. Step sectioning the tissues to search for a connection to the epidermis or adnexal epithelium is useful.

Verrucous Carcinoma

Verrucous carcinoma is composed of three entities—oral verrucous carcinoma, plantar verrucous carcinoma, and the Buschke-Loewenstein tumor.[308] Oral verrucous carcinoma is also known as panoral verrucous carcinoma or oral florid papillomatosis and was described in 1948.[309,310] It is rare and comprises only four to nine percent of oral squamous malignancies.[311] Tobacco use (especially chewing), betel nut/leaf use, poor oral hygiene, and malfitting dentures may induce this tumor.[311] Plantar verrucous carcinoma is a distinct type of squamous-cell carcinoma of the sole.[312] This neoplasm is also is known as epithelioma cuniculatum, papillomatosis cutis, papillomatosis cutis carcinoides, plantar verrucous carcinoma, and carcinoma cuniculatum.[313] "Cuniculatum" means "rabbit burrow" or "rabbit warren," indicative of the numerous openings these tumors have to the cutaneous surface.[310,313] Abundant crypts and sinuses are present. This tumor is slow growing and rarely metastasizes but may display locally aggressive features.[310] Plantar verrucous carcinoma has not been linked with human papillomavirus infection but proliferating cell nuclear antigen studies have suggested that the cells resemble large warts or condylomata.[313,314] Most clinicians consider these tumors to be low grade and highly keratinizing squamous-cell carcinomas. Low dose radiotherapy and chronic infection or inflammation may be responsible for these lesions.[315] Buschke-Loewenstein tumors appear as large or giant condyloma acuminata involving the anogenital mucosa. They were initially described in 1925 and also have been termed giant malignant condyloma, verrucous carcinoma of the anogenital mucosa, and carcinoma like condyloma.[316,317] Most cases are owing to infection with HPV type 6 or 11.[318] These tumors compose five to 25 percent of all penile malignancies.[317]

Clinical Features Oral verrucous carcinoma presents as a slowly enlarging white to grey growth on the buccal mucosa of older males (Table 26-25).[311] The gingiva also may be involved. The average age of

TABLE 26-25

Verrucous Carcinoma

Clinical Features

Oral verrucous carcinoma
  Grey or white warty growth on buccal or gingival mucosa
  More common in older men
Plantar verrucous carcinoma
  Painful, exophytic, verrucous mass on the heel, toe, or ball of foot
  Extrude foul-smelling keratogenous material
Buschke-Loewenstein tumor
  Polypoid mass on the glans penis in uncircumcised males
  May ulcerate or form sinus tracts
  May occlude structures such as the urethra

Histopathological Features

Oral verrucous carcinoma
  Hyperkeratosis with orthokeratosis
  Rete pegs with pushing well polarized base
  Large cells with scattered mitoses
Plantar verrucous carcinoma
  Exophytic and endophytic epithelial proliferation forming crypts and sinuses
  Hyperkeratosis and parakeratosis
  Infrequent mitoses
Buschke-Loewenstein tumor
  Hyperplastic, exophytic epithelial proliferation with infrequent mitoses
  Well-differentiated epidermal proliferation forming crypts and sinuses
  Hypergranulosis with koilocyte-like changes

Differential Diagnosis

Low-grade squamous-cell carcinoma
Warts or condyloma acuminata
Pseudoepitheliomatous hyperplasia

affected patients is 65 years.[311] Invasion into the cheek and/or mandible may be seen.[311]

Plantar verrucous carcinoma is a slow-growing, exophytic, or polypoid tumor. It is most common on the heel or ball of the foot but has been described on the toes, toe web spaces, leg, knee, wrist, finger, hand, abdominal wall, buttocks, nose, and scalp.[313] Lesions are typically tender, pink to flesh-colored, and well circumscribed at their borders.[315] Most tumors have been treated as recalcitrant warts or corns for some time.[313,315] Plantar verrucous carcinoma is more common in middle-aged to older males.[315] Foul-smelling keratogenous material is excreted through multiple sinus openings. Penetration of the tumor to the dorsum of the foot and involvement of the metatarsal bones have been described.[312] Metastases are rare.[315]

The Buschke-Loewenstein tumor is a cauliflower-like polypoid excrescence that arises on the glans penis in uncircumcised men between the ages of 18 and 86 years.[317] The prepuce, coronal sulcus, and perianal mucosa also may be involved. Lesions may ulcerate and form fistulous tracts.[308,319] A foul smell is common. Compression of the urethra and other structures may occur. These tumors may involve the genitalia, perineum, and urethra. Perianal tumors have a higher degree of malignant degeneration but no increased mortality.[318] Activities such as walking and defecation may become difficult.[320] Buschke-Loewenstein tumors have a similar appearance in women.[317]

Histopathological Features   The epithelium of the oral verrucous carcinoma mimics a low-grade mucosal squamous cell carcinoma. It is moderately verrucous or papillomatous (Table 26-25) (Fig. 26-32 A).[311] There is hyperkeratosis and parakeratosis overlying bulbous rete pegs which invade the dermis in a "pushing" rather than an infiltrating manner (Fig. 26-32 B). These rete pegs are blunt and well polarized. Keratin-lined clefts are seen. Cells are large with prominent cytoplasm and frequent keratinization. Nuclei and nucleoli are enlarged but significant cytological atypia is usually not evident. Mitotic activity is present but is scattered. Parabasal mitoses are common.[311] Formation of keratin pearls is infrequent. An inflammatory infiltrate is seen and may be abundant if the keratin has been extruded into the dermis.[311]

Plantar verrucous carcinomas show hyperkeratosis with papillomatosis, parakeratosis, and acanthosis.[310] There is an exophytic and endophytic component to this epidermal proliferation.[315] Epithelium-lined crypts are filled with orthokeratotic and parakeratotic material.[313,315] The endophytic epithelium forms broad columns and shows minimal atypia with few mitotic figures. Keratogenous cysts and microabscesses are seen.[310] Infiltration between bones and muscles may be appreciated. The inflammatory infiltrate is composed of lymphocytes, histiocytes, plasma cells, and rare eosinophils. The stroma is variably edematous with some abscesses.[315]

Buschke-Loewenstein tumors are hyperplastic and exophytic.[317] They have a configuration much like that of a condyloma accuminatum and demonstrate koilocytic changes. These may be indistinguishable from those present in condyloma acuminata.[320] Hyperkeratosis with parakeratosis and a very prominent granular layer are seen.[308,317,320] The epithelium extends broadly into the dermis as blunt-shaped masses forming sinuses and keratin-filled cysts.[317] The keratinocytes are well-differentiated squamous cells with little cytologic atypia. Nuclei are enlarged and have prominent nucleoli; however, mitotic activity is infrequent.[308,320] Horn pearls, apoptotic cells, and multinucleated keratinocytes are uncommon.[317,320] Vascular and lymphatic invasion are not present. An inflammatory infiltrate is present and is identical to that

seen in plantar verrucous carcinomas. Foci of frank squamous-cell carcinoma occasionally may be seen in some tumors and are associated with an increased incidence of nodal involvement and recurrence.[317] Consequently, step sectioning through the tumor is important.

Differential Diagnosis   The differential diagnoses for these three entities are essentially identical. They must be distinguished from low-grade squamous-cell carcinomas, warts, and pseudocarcinomatous hyperplasia.[313,317] Squamous-cell carcinomas typically have a substantial amount of apoptosis, premature cornification, squamous eddy formation, mitotic activity, and cytological atypia. These are absent in most examples of verrucous carcinoma with the exception of those Buschke-Loewenstein tumors with foci of frank squamous-cell carcinoma. The presence of atypical mitoses suggests a squamous-cell carcinoma. Condyloma acuminata and verruca vulgares may demonstrate the papillomatosis present in tumors of Buschke-Loewenstein and plantar verrucous carcinoma. Koilocytic changes also may be seen. However warts typically are not endophytic with broad columns of epidermis and do not usually show the same degree of mitotic activity. It is important to inquire about recent application of topical podophyllin since this medication may produce atypical mitotic features similar to a squamous-cell carcinoma. Pseudoepitheliomatous hyperplasia demonstrates asymmetric epithelial proliferation with a prominent granular layer and minimal if any atypia. The invading epithelium is also more "pointed" than blunt.

Adenosquamous Carcinoma

Adenosquamous carcinoma is a rare tumor that arises in the skin, lung, female genital tract, salivary gland, and submucosal glands of the head and neck.[321,322] These tumors are of sweat gland origin and arise from the pleuripotential cells in or around the acrosyringium.[321] Affected patients have a prognosis with low 5-year survival rates.[323]

Clinical Features   These neoplasms present as asymptomatic nodules on the head and neck of elderly men (Table 26-26).[321] Tumors arising on the vulva have poor survival rates.[322]

Histopathological Features   Adenosquamous carcinomas are composed of nests and islands of atypical squamous cells infiltrating the der-

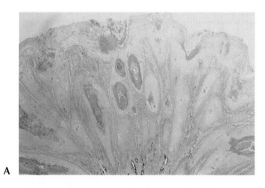

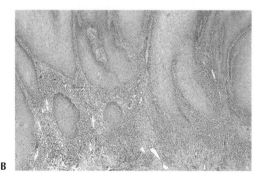

FIGURE 26-32   Oral verrucous carcinoma. *A*. The epidermis is verrucous and hyperkeratotic. *B*. Rete pegs with atypia "push" into the dermis.

TABLE 26-26

Adenosquamous Carcinoma

Clinical Features

   Asymptomatic nodules on the head and neck in elderly men

Histopathological Features

   Atypical keratinizing squamous cells with proliferating glandular structures
   Alcian blue positive mucin formation within the glands and cystic spaces
   No goblet cells or signet ring cells

Differential Diagnosis

   Adenosquamous carcinoma from other sites (salivary gland, submucosal gland, etc.)
   Eccrine epithelioma
   Microcystic adnexal carcinoma
   Sebaceous carcinoma

mis (Table 26-26). The tumors form glandular and cystic spaces lined by mucin-secreting epithelium.[322] Some islands of cells undergo keratinization.[321] Goblet and signet ring cells are not appreciated. The mucin stains with PAS, mucicarmine, and alcian blue.[321,322] It is hyaluronidase-resistant and sialidase-sensitive, meaning that it is an epithelial mucin.[321] Areas of glandular differentiation stain for CEA.[321,322]

Differential Diagnosis   Adenosquamous carcinomas must be differentiated from adenosquamous carcinomas arising in other sites, such as the salivary glands. Other carcinomas, such as eccrine epithelioma, microcystic adnexal carcinoma, and sebaceous carcinoma, should be distinguished as well. Eccrine epitheliomas also show cystic spaces with alcian blue positive mucin deposition. However, the tumor cells are not squamous appearing, the stroma is more fibrous, and the glandular elements are not as prominent but more tubular or ductal. Microcystic adnexal carcinomas have a more tubular or ductal appearance but no mucin deposition. Sebaceous carcinomas are formed by proliferation of cells with sebaceous differentiation. The glandular appearance is less prominent and pagetoid spread of atypical epithelial cells is seen.

Mucoepidermoid Carcinoma

These tumors are identical to those arising in the major salivary glands.[323] Metastatic disease should be considered when encountering these tumors.

Clinical Features   Mucoepidermoid carcinomas do not have characteristic clinical features.[323] Most lesions have arisen as skin-colored nodules with occasional ulceration on the sun-exposed surfaces of elderly patients (Table 26-27).

Histopathological Features   The tumor is composed of two different populations of cells (Table 26-27). The first is that of large polygonal squamous cells with vesicular, hyperchromatic nuclei that have been shifted to the periphery of the cell. The mitotic activity is variable. The second group of cells is that of the goblet cells. These demonstrate vacuolated cytoplasm and are located at the periphery of tumor lobules. Occasional mitoses are present. The goblet cells contain mucin that stains for PAS, mucicarmine, and alcian blue.[323] Tumor lobules are surrounded by a non-specific lymphohistiocytic inflammatory infiltrate. Keratinocyte atypia is present in some acrosyringium, suggesting that

these tumors differentiate from sweat gland structures. Connection to the epidermis and adnexal structures may be seen in some foci.

Differential Diagnosis   Mucoepidermoid carcinoma must be differentiated from sebaceous carcinomas and adenosquamous carcinomas. Sebaceous carcinomas typically show aggregates of basaloid cells with clear features. However, pagetoid spread and evidence of sebaceous differentiation are seen with these tumors. Adenosquamous carcinomas form tumor islands and nests and do not have goblet cells.

Carcinosarcoma

Carcinosarcomas are rare tumors with both malignant epithelial and mesenchymal elements.[324] They may occur in many sites, including the skin, bladder, breast, kidney, cervix, and gall bladder.[324] These neoplasms may be sarcomatoid carcinomas with variable degrees of differentiation.[324] Metaplastic changes in malignant epithelial cells may form the neoplastic mesenchymal cells.[325]

Clinical Features   Tumors appear as eroding and ulcerating nodules on the skin of older patients (Table 26-28). Death from metastatic spread has been reported.[326]

Histopathological Features   Basaloid and squamoid cells with stromal retraction, peripheral palisading, and mucin deposition form the superficial aspects of these tumors (Table 26-28).[324] In the deeper dermis sarcomatous changes appear and consist of spindled cells with nuclear atypia and mitotic activity.[324] These two cell populations usually are easily distinguished. The basaloid and squamoid cells are cytokeratin-positive but the sarcomatous cells may stain less intensely or are not at all. Similarly, sarcomatous cells are vimentin-positive but epithelial cells are negative.[326] Basal-cell carcinomas, squamous-cell carcinoma, and malignant eccrine spiradenoma have been described in carcinosarcoma.[326] Reported mesenchymal tumors have included malignant fibrous histiocytoma-like, osteogenic, rhabdomyoblastic, cartilaginous, and fibrosarcomatous elements.[326]

Differential Diagnosis   Carcinosarcomas must be differentiated from malignant mixed tumors of the skin and malignant fibrous histiocytomas. Malignant mixed tumors of the skin show deposition of mucoid and cartilaginous stroma with proliferating ducts and tubules. These epithelial elements may be atypical with mitotic activity.[324] Lobular

---

TABLE 26-27

Mucoepidermoid Carcinoma

Clinical Features

   Flesh-colored nodules on sun-exposed skin in older patients

Histopathological Features

   Tumors with two cell types; polygonal squamous cells and goblet cells
   Atypia is seen with occasional mitoses
   Connection to the epidermis and adnexal structures is present

Differential Diagnosis

   Sebaceous carcinoma
   Adenosquamous carcinoma

TABLE 26-28

Carcinosarcoma

Clinical Features

   Solitary nodules with epidermal ulceration and breakdown on the skin of elderly patients

Histopathological Features

   Two types of cellular proliferation—basaloid or squamoid cells with palisading, retraction, and surrounding fibromucinous stroma (cytokeratin+/vimentin−)
   Second cell type composed of atypical spindle-shaped cells (cytokeratin−/vimentin+)

Differential Diagnosis

   Malignant mixed tumor of the skin
   Malignant fibrous histiocytoma

growth is also present but the proliferating atypical spindle cells are not seen. Malignant fibrous histiocytomas do not involve the upper dermis and show no basaloid or squamoid proliferation. However, they may stain for both vimentin and cytokeratin, potentially causing some confusion.

Lymphoepithelioma-like Carcinoma

This tumor was first described by Swanson et al. and is similar to lymphoepitheliomas occurring in the nasopharyngeal region.[327] These neoplasms may also be found in the salivary gland, larynx, thymus, lung, tonsil, and the uterine cervix.[328,329] They are called "lymphoepithelioma-like" since lymphoepitheliomas are associated with Epstein-Barr virus infection, whereas the former have consistently been EBV negative.[330,331] These tumors are believed to differentiate from adnexal, particularly follicular, epithelium, since sebocytes have been found in some tumors.[330]

Clinical Features   Tumors are typically on the face and scalp in older patients (Table 26-29).[330,331] They are flesh-colored dome-shaped nodules of long standing. The lesions may metastasize and fatalities have been reported.[330]

Histopathological Features   The tumor masses have minimal if any connection to the epidermis or follicular epithelium and appear as nodules in the reticular dermis (Table 26-29).[330] They are asymmetric, poorly circumscribed and form a somewhat "follicular" pattern. Tumor cells are epithelioid and of moderate size with vacuolated cytoplasm. The nuclei are vesicular and contain prominent, eosinophilic nucleoli. There is a high nuclear to cytoplasm ratio to these cells.[329] Mitoses are present and may be atypical.[329,330] Tumor nodules are surrounded by enveloping masses of T cells and occasional plasma cells.[328–332] Eosinophils also may be present. The tumor cells are cytokeratin and epithelial membrane antigen positive but S-100, carcinoembryonic antigen, Factor XIIIa, and leukocyte common antigen negative.[328–330,332] Epstein-Barr virus evaluations have been negative.[329–332]

Differential Diagnosis   Lymphoepithelioma-like carcinomas should be differentiated from lymphomas, pseudolymphomas, cutaneous lymphadenomas, and metastatic lymphoepithelioma.[329,330,333] Cutaneous lymphomas may show a follicular proliferation but tumor cells are not typically this vesicular or large and are not cytokeratin positive.

Analysis for lymphocyte antigens such as UCHL-1 and L26 are positive in cutaneous lymphomas. Likewise, pseudolymphomas may have plasma cells, eosinophils, and a follicular proliferation but do not stain for cytokeratin and epithelial membrane antigen. Cutaneous lymphadenomas are intradermal lobular proliferations of cytokeratin-positive cells with infiltrating lymphocytes and a stromal reaction. However, they have a basaloid appearance with peripheral palisading and lack investing lymphocytes and plasma cells. Finally, metastatic disease from distant lymphoepitheliomas, most likely otorhinolaryngologic, must be ruled out as well.

MISCELLANEOUS "TUMORS"

Cutaneous Horn

Synonym: Cornu cutaneum

The term cutaneous horn refers to a cohesive mass of cornified material which protrudes from the cutaneous surfaces with a height at least half that of their width irrespective of underlying etiology.[160,334]

Clinical Features   Cutaneous horns present as a yellow to grey protrusions of keratinized material that is organized in the shape of a horn or spike (Table 26-30).[160,334] They are more common in women than men but men are more likely to have a malignant cause for their tumors. Larger lesions and those arising on older patients are also more likely to be malignant. Cutaneous horns are most common on the face, ears, dorsum of the hands, and scalp.

Histopathological Features   The stratum corneum is compact and exaggerated (Table 26-30) (Fig. 26-33). It may be lamellated or composed of parakeratotic squames. This parakeratosis may be intermittent forming a vertical "skip" pattern. Cutaneous horns arising from tricholemmomas show a trichilemmal form of keratinization rather than epidermal. The most common causes of cutaneous horns are actinic keratoses (37%), verrucas (23%), squamous cell carcinomas (18%), and seborrheic keratoses (16%).[160] Other tumors that cause these lesions include trichilemmal cyst, keratoacanthoma, Bowen's disease, molluscum contagiosum, benign lichenoid keratosis, infundibular cyst, sebaceous adenoma, dermatofibroma, angiokeratoma, epidermolytic acanthoma, pyogenic granuloma, subepidermal calcified nodule, basal cell carcinoma, arsenical keratosis, verrucous epidermal nevus, sebaceous carcinoma, and penile verrucous carcinoma.[160,334–336]

TABLE 26-29

Lymphoepithelioma-like Carcinoma

Clinical Features

Flesh-colored nodules on the face and scalp of elderly patients

Histopathological Features

Intradermal nodules of epithelioid cells with vesicular nuclei and vacuolated cytoplasm
Mitotic activity and prominent nucleoli are seen
Tumor cells are cytokeratin-positive and leukocyte common antigen-negative
Surrounding lymphocytes and plasma cells are present

Differential Diagnosis

Cutaneous lymphomas/pseudolymphomas
Cutaneous lymphadenoma
Metastatic lymphoepithelioma

TABLE 26-30

Cutaneous Horn

Clinical Features

Hyperkeratotic grey to yellow masses on the face, scalp, hands, and ears
The lesion's height is at least half the diameter of the base

Histopathological Features

Compact stratum corneum in a conical formation
Lamellated with occasional parakeratosis
Underlying lesions are typically actinic keratoses, verrucas, squamous cell carcinomas, or seborrheic keratoses

Differential Diagnosis

Wart
Inflamed seborrheic keratosis

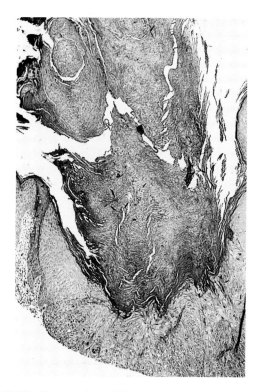

FIGURE 26-33 Cutaneous horn. This cutaneous horn demonstrates compact and exaggerated hyperkeratosis with underlying atypia.

Differential Diagnosis Hyperkeratotic lesions with compact keratinization must be distinguished from cutaneous horns. These include warts and inflamed seborrheic keratoses. Warts are typically hyperkeratotic with intermittent parakeratosis but the keratin usually is not compact or conical and is limited in scope. Inflamed seborrheic keratoses may demonstrate hyperkeratosis with parakeratosis. These tumors, however, show intermittent serum deposition within the stratum corneum and infiltrating inflammatory cells.

Stucco Keratosis

Synonym: Verruca dorsi manus et pedis

Stucco keratoses were initially described by Kocsard in 1958.[337,338] Similar lesions have been reported in pitch and tar workers.[337] Their etiology is unclear but may be owing to heat or chemical exposure.[339] They are more common in Australia than England, perhaps because of the amount of sun exposure in these countries.[340]

Clinical Features Stucco keratoses are typically multiple and involve the lower extremities below the knee (Table 26-31).[337] They may also affect the upper extremities but spare the palms and soles. Symptoms are rare. They are discrete grey to white keratotic papules 1 to 4 mm in diameter with a "stuck on" appearance.[337,339] They have a flat or convex surface and are dry and rough in texture. Most patients are older and males are affected more than females.[340] Approximately 20 percent of the populace develop these lesions.

Histopathological Features The epidermis has a "church spire" configuration with papillomatosis and loose hyperkeratosis (Table 26-31).[337,339,340] Modest acanthosis is seen but parakeratosis and horn pseudocysts are absent. The granular layer is thickened and the base of the tumor is evenly flat. Atypia is not appreciated. Perivascular inflammation may be present but is minimal.[337]

<table>
<tr><td colspan="1">TABLE 26-31</td></tr>
<tr><td>Stucco Keratosis</td></tr>
</table>

Clinical Features

White to grey keratoses with a "stuck on" appearance arising on the extremities
Most patients are middle-aged to older

Histopathological Features

Regular, even papillomatosis with hyperkeratosis
Parakeratosis, horn pseudocysts, basal layer hyperpigmentation, and atypia are absent

Differential Diagnosis

Papillomatous seborrheic keratosis
Actinic keratosis
Large-cell acanthoma

Differential Diagnosis Stucco keratoses must be differentiated from seborrheic keratoses, actinic keratoses, and large-cell acanthomas.[337] The tumor known as acrokeratosis verruciformis of Hopf essentially is indistinguishable from stucco keratoses. Seborrheic keratoses, particularly the papillomatous variant, are hyperkeratotic with papillomatosis. Unlike stucco keratoses, however, they may show parakeratosis, horn pseudocysts, and basal layer hyperpigmentation. Actinic keratoses have atypical cells with mitotic activity and are rarely papillomatous. Large-cell acanthomas, which some investigators believe are variants of actinic keratoses, may appear similar to stucco keratoses but demonstrate large nuclei with occasional mitotic activity.[337]

Clavus (Corn)

Clavi (corns) are hyperkeratotic lesions of the feet and are seen only in races that wear shoes.[341] They are a consequence of persistent frictional injury and are typically painful.[342] Women are affected more often than men. Underlying bony prominences and other orthopedic abnormalities exert pressure through the skin.

<table>
<tr><td colspan="1">TABLE 26-32</td></tr>
<tr><td>Clavus (Corn)</td></tr>
</table>

Clinical Features

Yellow to brown hyperkeratotic lesion on the feet
May be hard with a smooth surface (hard corn) or macerated and sodden (soft corn)
Women more commonly affected

Histopathological Features

Concave, cup-shaped depression with hyperkeratosis and parakeratosis
Spinous and granular layer decreased

Differential Diagnosis

Verruca
Callus
Porokeratoma

Clinical Features   Lesions are yellow to brown with a central core.[341] Hard corns are burnished with a smooth surface (Table 26-32). Soft corns are macerated and sodden.

Histopathological Features   Tumors are endophytic with a cup-shaped depression (Table 26-32). A thick parakeratotic plug is seen. The spinous and granular layers are decreased.

Differential Diagnosis   These tumors should be differentiated from verrucas, calluses, and porokeratosis. Warts may show a concave depression but the granular layer is usually accentuated not diminished. Calluses also demonstrate concave depression and typically show less parakeratosis. Porokeratomas are hyperkeratotic with coronoid lamellae. However, these lesions are not endophytic and demonstrate focal areas of dyskeratotic keratinocytes.

Callus

These are hyperkeratotic lesions caused by chronic friction or pressure.[343] They may be seen on the palms and soles but are more common on the feet. They result from poorly fitting shoes or clothes and bony deformities. Calluses affect persons of all ages but are most typical on persons whose skin is exposed to consistent and constant friction.[343]

Clinical Features   Calluses may be preceded by blisters and inflammation.[343] Fully developed lesions are yellow to brown or flesh-colored (Table 26-33). They are typically hard and dry but rarely painful. They do not possess a central core. The overlying skin markings may be accentuated.

Histopathological Features   The stratum corneum is compact, hyperkeratotic, and variably parakeratotic (Table 26-33).[343] The granular and spinous layer are accentuated. Tumors may be concave with a cup-shaped depression. Perivascular inflammation is present but is not abundant.

Differential Diagnosis   Calluses must be distinguished from clavi (corns) and verrucas. Clavi also show a concave depression but a diminished granular layer and more parakeratosis. Warts are also concave with a prominent granular layer but may have koilocytic change and increased vascularity.

Punctate (Mechanical) Keratoses

Synonyms: Keratosis punctata palmaris et plantaris; punctate keratosis of the palm and soles.

This condition is inherited as an autosomal dominant trait. Eleven percent of the population is affected.[344,345] Lesions usually appear in adolescence and there is an association with atopy.[344,346] There is a sub category of this disease affecting African-American males in which the lesions are confined to the palmar creases.[247–249]

Clinical Features   Punctate keratoses are small, hyperkeratotic papules 2 to 10 mm in diameter (Table 26-34).[344] They are firm and round to oval.[349] Lesions appear on the palms and soles particularly the medial aspects.[346] The keratotic plug may be removed leaving a small pit behind. Punctate keratoses usually are asymptomatic but may occasionally be painful.[344,346]

Histopathological Features   The epidermis shows a small cup-shaped depression filled with hyperkeratotic stratum corneum (Table 26-34).[344,347–351] This plug of hyperkeratotic material is conical or wedge-shaped with its apex at the depth of the depression.[349] Parakeratosis usually is absent but may be seen in small amounts in a vertical configuration. The surrounding rim of normal epidermis is also hyperkeratotic. The epidermis beneath the keratin plug may be compressed. The granular layer is accentuated in some cases and thinned in others.[345,349] Mild spongiosis may be present. Occasional acantholysis and dyskeratosis have been described.[350] There may be a mild perivascular inflammatory infiltrate in the dermis.[344,349] Blood vessels may be slightly dilated with mild dermal edema. Occluded blood and lymph vessels have been reported.[345] Ultrastructurally, keratohyaline granules, membrane coating granules, and desmosomes appear normal.[344] Membrane coating granules are also normal but may be present in diminished numbers. This scarcity may prevent normal keratinocyte desquamation.[349]

Differential Diagnosis   Punctate keratoses must be differentiated from punctate porokeratosis, perforating diseases, calluses, and verrucas. Porokeratomas, particularly the punctate variant, are hyperkeratotic with columns of parakeratosis (coronoid lamellae). These tumors have dyskeratotic cells underlying the coronoid lamellae. Perforating dis-

---

TABLE 26-33

Callus

Clinical Features

Flesh-colored to yellow/brown hyperkeratotic lesions on the palms and soles
Elevated, hard, and dry and usually asymptomatic

Histopathological Features

Hyperkeratotic stratum corneum with variable parakeratosis
Cup-shaped depression with hypergranulosis and accentuated spinous layer

Differential Diagnosis

Clavus
Verruca

TABLE 26-34

Punctate (Mechanical) Keratosis

Clinical Features

Onset in childhood or adolescence in persons with an atopic diathesis
Multiple, hard, hyperkeratotic papules on the palms and soles
Crateriform pits when the hyperkeratotic mass is removed

Histopathological Features

Wedge-shaped hyperkeratotic plug depressing the epidermis
Parakeratosis and width of the granular layer are variable
Perivascular inflammation and vascular dilatation are present

Differential Diagnosis

Punctate porokeratosis
Perforating disorders
Callus
Verruca

eases may show a conical shaped mass of hyperkeratotic material but this mass is basophilic and contains inflammatory cells. The dermis is inflamed and fibrotic. Calluses are also parakeratotic endophytic lesions. These may be differentiated from punctate keratoses, however, by the relative confluence of the parakeratosis (not columnar), the lack of a conical configuration to the hyperkeratotic mass, and the increased granular layer. Punctate keratoses may suggest endophytic verrucas but lack significant papillomatosis and viral cytopathic alterations that are generally present in verrucas.

REFERENCES

1. Hodge JA, Ray MC, Flynn KJ: The epidermal nevus syndrome. *Int J Dermatol* 30:91–98, 1991.
2. Happle R: Epidermal nevus syndromes. *Sem Dermatol* 14:111–121, 1995.
3. Stosiek N, Ulmer R, von den Driesch P, et al: Chromosomal mosaicism in two patients with epidermal verrucous nevus. *J Am Acad Dermatol* 30:622–625, 1994.
4. Submoke S, Piamphongsant T: Clinico-histopathological study of epidermal nevi. *Aust J Dermatol* 24:130–136, 1983.
5. Su WPD: Histopathologic varieties of epidermal nevus. *Am J Dermatopathol* 4:161–170, 1982.
6. Talanin N, Aklovbyan V, Tukhvatulina Z: Two cases of unilateral verrucous nevus. *Cutis* 49:443–446, 1992.
7. Cambiaghi S, Brusasco A, Grimalt R, et al: Acantholytic dyskeratotic epidermal nevus as a mosaic form of Darier's disease. *J Am Acad Dermatol* 32:284–286, 1995.
8. Rosen T: Keratoacanthomas arising within a linear epidermal nevus. *J Dermatol Surg Oncol* 8:878–880, 1982.
9. Crovato F, Desirello G, Rebora A: Is Dowling-Desog disease the same disease as Kitamura's reticulate acropigmentation? *Br J Dermatol* 109:105–110, 1983.
10. Rebora A, Crovato F: The spectrum of Dowling-Degos disease. *Br J Dermatol* 110:627–630, 1984.
11. Cox NH, Long E: Dowling-Degos disease and Kitamura's reticulate acropigmentation: support for the concept of a single disease. *Br J Dermatol* 125:169–171, 1991.
12. Kershenovich J, Langenberg A, Odom RB, et al: Dowling-Degos' disease mimicking chloracne. *J Am Acad Dermatol* 27:345–348, 1992.
13. Ostlere L, Holden CA: Dowling-Degos disease associated with Kitamura's reticulate acropigmentation. *Clin Exp Dermatol* 19:492–495, 1994.
14. Kikuchi I, Crovato F, Rebora A: Haber's syndrome and Dowling-Degos disease. *Int J Dermatol* 27:96–97, 1988.
15. Erel A, Gurer MA, Edali N: Reticulate acropigmentation of Kitamura: Two case reports. *Int J Dermatol* 32:726–727, 1993.
16. Wilson-Jones E, Grice K: Reticulate pigmented anomaly of the flexures. *Arch Dermatol* 114:1150–1157, 1978.
17. Pollitzer S: Acanthosis nigricans, in Unna PG, Morris M, Besnier E, et al., (eds): *International Atlas of Rare Skin Diseases.* London: HK Lewis & Co., 1890, pp. 1–3.
18. Curth HO: The necessity of distinguishing four types of acanthosis nigricans, in Jadassohn W, Schirren CG, (eds): *XIII Congressus Internationalis Dermatologiae 31.7–5.8 1967 Munchen.* Berlin: Springer-Verlag, 1968, 557–558.
19. Schwartz RA: Acanthosis nigricans. *J Am Acad Dermatol* 31:1–19, 1994.
20. Esperanza LE, Fenske NA: Hyperandrogenism, insulin resistance, and acanthosis nigricans (HAIR-AN) syndrome: Spontaneous remission in a 15 year-old girl. *J Am Acad Dermatol* 34:892–897, 1996.
21. Potasman I, Stermer E, Levy N, et al: The Groll-Hirschowitz syndrome. *Clin Genet* 28:76–78, 1985.
22. Sasaki T, Ono H, Nakajima H, et al: Lipoatrophic diabetes. *J Dermatol* (Tokyo) 19:246–249, 1992.
23. Hamaguchi T, Penneys N: Cystic clear-cell acanthoma. *J Cutan Pathol* 22:188–190, 1995.
24. Schwartz RA, Janniger CK: Childhood acanthosis nigricans. *Cutis* 55:337–341, 1995.
25. Hall JM, Moreland A, Cox GJ, et al: Oral acanthosis nigricans-like lesions after local application of fusidic acid. *Am J Dermatopathol* 10:68–73, 1988.
26. Gougerot H, Carteaud A: Papillomatose pigmentes innominee. *Bull Soc Fr Dermatol Syphilol* 34:719–721, 1927.
27. El-Tonsy MH, El-Benhawi MO, Mehregan AH: Confluent and reticulated papillomatosis. *J Am Acad Dermatol* 16:893–894, 1987.
28. Lee SH, Choi EH, Lee WS, et al: Confluent and reticulated papillomatosis: A clinical, histopathological, and electron microscopic study. *J Dermatol* 18:725–730, 1991.
29. Atherton DJ, Wells RS: Confluent and reticulate papillomatosis. *Clin Exp Dermatol* 5:465–469, 1980.
30. Hamilton D, Tavafoghi V, Shafer JC, et al: Confluent and reticulated papillomatosis of Gougerot and Carteaud. *J Am Acad Dermatol* 2:401–410, 1980.
31. Sau P, Lupton GP: Reticulated truncal pigmentation. *Arch Dermatol* 124:1272–1275, 1988.
32. Unna PG: *The Histopathology of the Diseases of the Skin.* New York, Macmillan, 1896, p. 1148.
33. Altman J, Mehregan AH: Inflammatory linear verrucose epidermal nevus. *Arch Dermatol* 104:385–389, 1971.
34. Morag C, Metzker A: Inflammatory linear verrucous epidermal nevus: Report of seven new cases and review of the literature. *Ped Derm* 3:15–18, 1985.
35. de Jong EMGJ, Rulo HFC, de Kerkhof PCM: Inflammatory linear verrucous epidermal nevus (ILVEN) versus linear psoriasis. *Act Derm Venereol* (Stockh) 71:343–346, 1991.
36. Rulo HFC, van de Kerkhof PCM: Treatment of inflammatory linear verrucous epidermal nevus. *Dermatologica* 182:112–114, 1991.
37. Dupre A, Christol B: Inflammatory linear verrucose epidermal nevus. *Arch Dermatol* 113:767–769, 1977.
38. Sober AJ, Burstein JM: Precursors to skin cancer. *Cancer Suppl* 75:645–650, 1995.
39. Kofmann S: Ein fall von seltener lokalisation und verbreitung von komedonen. *Archs Derm Syph* 32:177–178, 1895.
40. Nabai H, Mehregan AH: Nevus comedonicus. *Acta Dermato Venereol* (Stockh) 53:71–74, 1973.
41. Cestari TF, Rubim M, Valentini BC: Nevus comedonicus: case report and brief review of the literature. *Ped Derm* 8:300–305, 1991.
42. Dudley K, Barr WG, Armin A, et al: Nevus comedonicus in association with widespread, well-differentiated follicular tumors. *J Am Acad Dermatol* 15:1123–1127, 1986.
43. Kim SC, Kang WH: Nevus comedonicus associated with epidermal nevus. *J Am Acad Dermatol* 21:1085–1088, 1989.
44. Grimalt R, Caputo R: Posttraumatic nevus comedonicus. *J Am Acad Dermatol* 28:273–274, 1993.
45. Aloi FG, Molinero A: Nevus comedonicus with epidermolytic hyperkeratosis. *Dermatologica* 174:140–143, 1987.
46. Resnik KS, Kantor GR, Howe NR, et al: Dilated pore nevus. *Am J Dermatopathol* 15:169–171, 1993.
47. Carneiro SJC, Dickson JE, Knox JM: Familial dyskeratotic comedones. *Arch Dermatol* 105:249–251, 1972.
48. Leppard BJ: Familial dyskeratotic comedones. *Clin Exp Dermatol* 7:329–332, 1982.
49. Price M, Jone RR: Familial dyskeratotic comedones. *Clin Exp Dermatol* 10:147–153, 1985.
50. Hall JR, Holder W, Knox JM, et al: Familial Dyskeratotic. *J Am Acad Dermatol* 17:808–814, 1987.
51. Schwartz RA, Rojas-Corona RR, Yu GSM, et al: Keratosis punctata of the palmar creases. *Cutis* 32:75–77, 1983.
52. Sutton RL: A fissured granulomatous lesion of the upper labioalveolar fold. *Arch Dermatol* 26:425–427, 1932.
53. Epstein EE: Granuloma fissuratum of the ears. *Arch Dermatol* 91:621–622, 1965.
54. Farrell WJ, Wilson JW: Granuloma fissuratum. *Arch Dermatol* 97:34–37, 1968.
55. Barnes HM, Calnan CD, Sarkany I: Spectacle from acanthoma. *Trans St. Johns Dermatol Soc* 60:99–102, 1974.
56. MacDonald DM, Martin SJ: Acanthoma fissuratum—spectacle frame acanthoma. *Acta Dermato Venereol* (Stockh) 55:485–488, 1975.
57. Cerroni L, Soyer HP, Chimenti S: Acanthoma fissuratum. *J Dermatol Surg Oncol* 14:1003–1005, 1988.
58. Fretzin DF: Granuloma fissuratum of the ears. *Arch Dermatol* 93:448–449, 1966.
59. Hyde W: *Diseases of the Skin,* 8th ed. New York: Lea & Febiger, 1909, pp. 174–175.
60. Payne CMER, Wilkinson JD, McKee PH, et al: Nodular prurigo: A clinicopathological study of 46 patients. *Br J Dermatol* 113:431–439, 1985.
61. Perez GL, Peters MS, Reda AM, et al: Mast cells, neutrophils and eosinophils in prurigo nodularis. *Arch Dermatol* 129:861–865, 1993.
62. Nahass GT, Penneys NS: Merkel cells and prurigo nodularis. *J Am Acad Dermatol* 31:86–88, 1994.
63. Feuerman EJ, Sandbank M: Prurigo nodularis: Histological and electron microscopical study. *Arch Dermatol* 111:1472–1477, 1975.
64. Lindley RP, Payne CMER: Neural hyperplasia is not a diagnostic prerequisite in nodular prurigo. *J Cutan Pathol* 16:14–18, 1989.
65. Shapiro L, Baraf CS: Isolated epidermolytic acanthoma. *Arch Dermatol* 101:220–223, 1970.
66. Hirone T, Fukushiro R: Disseminated epidermolytic acanthoma. *Acta Dermatol Venereol* (Stockh) 393–402, 1973.
67. Knipper JE, Hud JA, Cockerell CJ: Disseminated epidermolytic acanthoma. *Am J Dermatopathol* 15:70–72, 1993.
68. Leonardi C, Zhu W, Kinsey W, et al: Epidermolytic acanthoma does not contain human papillomavirus DNA. *J Cutan Pathol* 18:103–105, 1991.
69. Shapiro L, Baraf CS: Isolated epidermolytic acanthoma. *Arch Dermatol* 101:220–223, 1970.
70. Brownstein MH: The benign acanthomas. *J Cutan Pathol* 12:172–188, 1985.
71. Helwig EB: Proceedings of the 20th Seminar on Skin Neoplasms and Dermatoses, International Congress of Clinical Pathologists. Chicago, American Society of Clinical Pathologists, 1955, pp. 53–56.

72. Allen AC: *The Skin: A Clinicopathologic Treatise.* St Louis: CV Mosby Co, 1954, pp. 558–559.
73. Syzmanski FJ: Warty dyskeratoma. *Arch Dermatol* 75:567–572, 1957.
74. Azuma Y, Matsukawa A: Warty dyskeratoma with multiple lesions. *J Dermatol* 20:374–377, 1993.
75. Laskaris G, Sklavounou A: Warty dyskeratoma of the oral mucosa. *Br J Oral Maxil Surg* 23:371–375, 1985.
76. Harrist TJ, Murphy GF, Mihm MC: Oral warty dyskeratoma. *Arch Dermatol* 116:929–931, 1980.
77. Newland JR, Leventon GS: Warty dyskeratoma of the oral mucosa. *Oral Surg* 58:176–183, 1984.
78. Niren NM, Waldman GD, Barsky S: Warty dyskeratoma. *Cutis* 29:79–81, 94, 1982.
79. Tanay A, Mehregan AH: Warty dyskeratoma. *Dermatologica* 138:155–164, 1969.
80. Panja RK: Warty dyskeratoma. *J Cutan Pathol* 4:194–200, 1977.
81. Brownstein MH: Acantholytic acanthoma. *J Am Acad Dermatol* 19:783–786, 1988.
82. Megahead M, Scharffetter-Kochanek K: Acantholytic acanthoma. *Am J Dermatopathol* 15:283–285, 1993.
83. Barnette DJ, Cobb M: A solitary, erythematous, hyperkeratotic papule. *Arch Dermatol* 131:211, 212, 214, 215, 1995.
84. O'Connell BM, Nickoloff BJ: Solitary labial papular acantholytic dyskeratoma in an immunocompromised host. *Am J Dermatopathol* 9:339–342, 1987.
85. Baer RL, Garcia RL, Partsalidou V, et al: Papillated squamous cell carcinoma in situ arising in a seborrheic keratosis. *J Am Acad Dermatol* 5:561–565, 1981.
86. Freudenthal W: Verruca senilis und keratoma senile. *Arch Dermatol Syph* 152:505–528, 1926.
87. Schwartz RA: Sign of Leser-Trelat. *J Am Acad Dermatol* 35:88–95, 1996.
88. Czarnecki DB, Rotstein H, O'Brien TJ, et al: The sign of Leser-Trelat. *Australas J Dermatol* 24:93–99, 1983.
89. Kapasi Y, Khopkar U, Raj S, et al: Weary-Kindler syndrome with multiple seborrheic keratoses. *Int J Dermatol* 32:444–445, 1993.
90. Rao BK, Freeman RG, Poulos EG, et al: The relationship between basal cell epithelioma and seborrheic keratosis. *J Dermatol Surg Oncol* 20:761–764, 1994.
91. Chen M, Shinmori H, Takemiya M, et al: Acantholytic variant of seborrheic keratosis. *J Cutan Pathol* 17:27–31, 1990.
92. Lever WF: Inverted follicular keratosis is an irritated seborrheic keratosis. *Am J Dermatopathol* 5:474, 1983.
93. Nakayasu K, Nishimura A, Maruo M, et al: Trichilemmal differentiation in seborrheic keratosis. *J Cutan Pathol* 8:256–262, 1981.
94. Yamamoto H, Ito A, Yoshitatsu S: Seborrheic keratosis with possible central regression. *Cutis* 44:241–243, 1989.
95. Wade TR, Ackerman AB: The many faces of seborrheic keratoses. *J Dermatol Surg Oncol* 5:378–382, 1979.
96. Olsen KE, Westermark P: Amyloid in basal cell carcinoma and seborrheic keratosis. *Acta Derm Venereol* (Stockh) 74:273–275, 1994.
97. Maize JC, Snider RL: Nonmelanoma skin cancers in association with seborrheic keratoses. *Dermatol Surg* 21:960–962, 1995.
98. Berman A, Winkelmann RK: Inflammatory seborrheic keratoses with mononuclear-cell infiltration. *J Cutan Pathol* 5:353–360, 1978.
99. Berman A, Winkelmann RK: Histologic changes in seborrheic keratoses after rubbing. *J Cutan Pathol* 7:32–38, 1980.
100. Gurbuz O, Hurwitz RM: Keratotic melanocytic nevus. *Int J Dermatol* 29:713–715, 1990.
101. Wagner RF: Benign pigmented tumor with combined features of seborrheic keratosis and compound nevus. *Cutis* 48:463–464, 1991.
102. Chun SI, Im S: An epidermoid cyst with a seborrheic verruca-like cyst wall. *J Dermatol* 17:260–263, 1990.
103. Yakar JB, Sagi A, Mahler D, et al: Malignant melanoma appearing in seborrheic keratosis. *J Dermatol Surg Oncol* 10:382–383, 1984.
104. Kwittken J: Keratoacanthoma arising in seborrheic keratosis. *Cutis* 14:546–547, 1974.
105. Smith KJ, Skelton HG, Palominon NJ: Adenocarcinoma arising in a seborrheic keratosis. *Arch Dermatol* 127:1738–1739, 1991.
106. Monteagudo JC, Jordan E, Terencio C, et al: Squamous cell carcinoma in situ (Bowen's disease) arising in seborrheic keratosis: Three lesions in two patients. *J Cutan Pathol* 16:348–352, 1989.
107. Rahbari H: Bowenoid transformation of seborrhoeic verrucae (keratoses). *Br J Dermatol* 101:459–463, 1979.
108. Zhao Y, Lin Y, Luo R, et al: Human papillomavirus (HPV) infection in seborrheic keratosis. *Am J Dermatopathol* 11:209–212, 1989.
109. Leonardi CL, Zhu WY, Kinsey WH, et al: Seborrheic keratoses from the genital region may contain human papillomavirus DNA. *Arch Dermatol* 127:1203–1206, 1991.
110. Jacyk WK, Dreyer L, de Villiers EM: Seborrheic keratoses of black patients with epidermodysplasia verruciformis contain human papillomavirus DNA. *Am J Dermatopathol* 15:1–6, 1993.
111. Grimes PE, Arora S, Minus HR, et al: Dermatosis papulosa nigra. *Cutis* 32:385–386, 392, 1983.
112. van Dijk E: Dermatosis papulosa nigra. *Dermatologica* 136:441, 1968.
113. Bloch B: Ueber b enigne, nicht naevoide melanoepithliome der haut nebst bemerkungen ueber das wesen und die genese der dendritenzellen. *Arch Dermatol Syph* 158:20–40, 1926.
114. Mishima Y, Pinkus H: Benign mixed tumor of melanocytes and malpighian cells. *Arch Dermatol* 81:539–550, 1960.
115. Goode RK, Crawford BE, Callihan MD, et al: Oral melanoacanthoma. *Oral Surg Oral Med Oral Pathol* 56:622–628, 1983.
116. Tomich CE, Zunt SL: Melanoacanthosis (melanoacanthoma) of the oral mucosa. *J Dermatol Surg Oncol* 16:231–236, 1990.
117. Zemtsov A, Bergfeld WF: Oral melanoacanthoma with prominent spongiotic intraepithelial vesicles. *J Cutan Pathol* 16:365–369, 1989.
118. Degos R, Delort J, Civatte J, et al: Tumeur epidermique d'aspect particulier: acanthome a cellules claires. *Ann Dermatol Syphiligr* (Paris) 89:361–371, 1962.
119. Ohnishi T, Watanabe S: Immunohistochemical characterization of keratin expression in clear-cell acanthoma. *Br J Dermatol* 133:186–193, 1995.
120. Degos R, Civatte J: Clear-cell acanthoma. *Br J Dermatol* 83:248–254, 1970.
121. Brownstein MH, Fernando S, Shapiro L: Clear-cell acanthoma. *Am J Clin Pathol* 59:306–31, 1973.
122. Petzelbauer P, Konrad K: Polypous clear-cell acanthoma. *Am J Dermatopathol* 12:393–395, 1990.
123. Zak FG, Martinez M, Stasinger AL: Pale cell acanthoma. *Arch Dermatol* 93:674–678, 1966.
124. Langer K, Wuketich S, Konrad K: Pigmented clear-cell acanthoma. *Am J Dermatopathol* 16:134–139, 1994.
125. Pinkus H: Epidermal mosaic in benign and precancerous neoplasia (with special reference to large-cell acanthoma). *Acta Dermatol* 65:75–81, 1970.
126. Rabinowitz AD: Multiple large cell acanthomas. *J Am Acad Dermatol* 8:840–845, 1983.
127. Roewert HJ, Ackerman AB: Large-cell acanthoma is a solar lentigo. *Am J Dermatopathol* 14:122–132, 1992.
128. Rabinowitz AD, Inghirami G: Large-cell acanthoma. *Am J Dermatopathol* 14:136–138, 1992.
129. Argenyi ZB, Huston BM, Argenyi EE, et al: Large cell acanthoma of the skin. *Am J Dermatopathol* 16:140–144, 1994.
130. Rahbari H, Pinkus H: Large cell acanthoma. *Arch Dermatol* 114:49–52, 1978.
131. Sanchez Yus E, del Rio E, Requena L: Large-cell acanthoma is a distinctive condition. *Am J Dermatopathol* 14:140–147, 1992.
132. Freudenthal W: Verruca senilis und keratoma senile. *Arch Derm Syph* (Berl) 152:505–528, 1926.
133. Frost CA, Green AC: Epidemiology of solar keratoses. *Br J Dermatol* 131:455–464, 1994.
134. Biesterfeld S, Pennings K, Grussendorf-Conen EI, et al: Aneuploidy in actinic keratosis and Bowen's disease: Increased risk for invasive squamous cell carcinoma. *Br J Dermatol* 133:557–560, 1995.
135. Pearse AD, Marks R: Actinic keratoses and the epidermis on which they arise. *Br J Dermatol* 96:45–50, 1977.
136. Dinehart SM, Sanchez RL: Spreading pigmented actinic keratosis. *Arch Dermatol* 124:680–683, 1988.
137. Goldberg LH, Joseph AK, Tschen JA: Proliferative actinic keratosis. *Int J Dermatol* 33:341–345, 1994.
138. James MP, Wells GC, Whimster IW: Spreading pigmented actinic keratosis. *Br J Dermatol* 98:373–379, 1977.
139. Subrt P, Jorizzo JL, Apisarnthanarax P, et al: Spreading pigmented actinic keratosis. *J Am Acad Dermatol* 8:63–67, 1983.
140. Prieto VG, Casal M, McNutt NS: Immunohistochemistry detects differences between lichen planus-like keratosis, lichen planus and lichenoid actinic keratosis. *J Cutan Pathol* 20:143–147, 1993.
141. Billano RA, Little WP: Hypertrophic actinic keratosis. *J Am Acad Dermatol* 7:484–489, 1982.
142. Kiyokane K, Sakatani S, Kusakabe H, et al: A statistical study on histopathologic findings of solar keratosis. *J Med* 23:399–408, 1992.
143. Picascia DD, Robinson JK: Actinic cheilitis: A review of the etiology, differential diagnosis, and treatment. *J Am Acad Dermatol* 17:255–264, 1987.
144. Ayers S: Chronic actinic cheilitis. *JAMA* 81:1183–1186, 1923.
145. Girard KR, Hoffman BL: Actinic cheilitis. *Oral Med Oral Surg Oral Pathol* 50:21–24, 1980.
146. Robinson JK: Actinic cheilitis. *Arch Otolaryngol Head Neck Surg* 115:848–852, 1989.
147. Maloney ME: Arsenic in dermatology. *Dermatol Surg* 22:301–304, 1996.
148. Yeh S, Lin CS: Arsenical cancer of skin. *Cancer* 21:312–339, 1968.
149. Yeh S: Skin cancer in chronic arsenism. *Hum Pathol* 4:469–485, 1973.
150. Sharma SC, Simpson NB: Treatment of arsenical keratosis with etretinate. *Acta Dermato Venereol* (Stockh) 63:449–452, 1983.
151. Bowen JT: Precancerous dermatoses. *J Cutan Dis Incl Syph* 30:24, 1912.
152. Kossard S, Rosen R: Cutaneous Bowen's disease. *J Am Acad Dermatol* 27:406–410, 1992.
153. Lee MM, Wick MM: Bowen's disease. *Clin Dermatol* 11:43–46, 1993.

154. Gerber GS: Carcinoma in situ of the penis. *J Urol* 151:829–833, 1994.

155. Ikenberg H, Gissmann, L, Gross G, et al: Human papilloma virus type 16 related DNA in genital Bowen's disease and bowenoid papulosis. *Int J Cancer* 32:563–565, 1983.

156. Kettler AH, Rutledge M, Tschen JA, et al: Detection of human papillomavirus in non-genital Bowen's disease by in situ DNA hybridization. *Arch Dermatol* 126:777–781, 1990.

157. Peterka ES, Lynch FW, Goltz RW: An association between Bowen's disease and internal cancer. *Arch Dermatol* 84:623, 1961.

158. Reymann F, Ravnborg L, Schou G, et al: Bowen's disease and internal malignant diseases. A study of 581 patients. *Arch Dermatol* 124:677–679, 1988.

159. Arbesman H, Ransohoff DF: Is Bowen's disease a predictor for the development of internal malignancy? A methodological critique of the literature. *JAMA* 257:516–518, 1987.

160. Schosser RH, Hodge SJ, Gaba CR, et al: Cutaneous horns: a histopathologic study. *So Med J* 72:1129–1131, 1979.

161. Otsuka F, Huang J, Sawara K, et al: Disseminated porokeratosis accompanying multicentric Bowen's disease. *J Am Acad Dermatol* 23:355–359, 1990.

162. Murata Y, Kumano K, Sashikata T: Partial spontaneous regression of Bowen's disease. *Arch Dermatol* 132:429–432, 1996.

163. Kaye V, Zhang G, Dehner LP, et al: Carcinoma in situ of penis. *Urology* 36:479–481, 1990.

164. Cox NH: Body site distribution of Bowen's disease. *Br J Dermatol* 130:714–716, 1994.

165. Fitzpatrick JE: The histologic diagnosis of intraepithelial pagetoid neoplasms. *Clin Dermatol* 9:255–259, 1991.

166. Collina G, Rossi E, Bettelli S, et al: Detection of human papillomavirus in extragenital Bowen's disease using in situ hybridization and polymerase chain reaction. *Am J Dermatopathol* 17:236–241, 1995.

167. Saida T, Okabe Y, Uhara H: Bowen's disease with invasive carcinoma showing sweat gland differentiation. *J Cutan Pathol* 16:222–226, 1989.

168. Jacobs DM, Sandles LG, Leboit PE: Sebaceous carcinoma arising from Bowen's disease of the vulva. *Arch Dermatol* 122:1191–1193, 1986.

169. Reed W, Oppedal BR, Larsen TE: Immunohistology is valuable in distinguishing between Paget's disease, Bowen's disease and superficial spreading malignant melanoma. *Histopathology* 16:583–588, 1990.

170. Queyrat L: Erythroplasie du gland. *Bull Soc Fr Dermatol Syphiligr* 22:378–382, 1911.

171. Dixon RS, Mikhail GR: Erythroplasia (Queyrat) of conjunctiva. *J Am Acad Dermatol* 4:160–165, 1981.

172. Bernstein G, Forgaard DM, Miller JE: Carcinoma in situ of the glans penis and distal urethra. *J Dermatol Surg Oncol* 12:450–455, 1986.

173. Schellhammer PF, Jordan GH, Robey EL, et al: Premalignant lesions and nonsquamous malignancy of the penis and carcinoma of the scrotum. *Urol Clin No Am* 19:131–142, 1992.

174. Gross G, Hagedorn M, Ikenberg H, et al: Bowenoid papulosis. Presence of human papillomavirus (HPV) structural antigens and of HPV 16-related DNA sequences. *Arch Dermatol* 121:858–863, 1985.

175. Hodge SJ, Turner JE: Histopathologic concepts of intraepithelial epithelioma. *Int J Dermatol* 25:372–375, 1986.

176. Montgomery H: Superficial epitheliomatosis. *Arch Dermatol* 20:338–357, 1929.

177. Steffen CG, Ackerman AB: Intraepidermal epithelioma of Borst–Jasassohn. *Am J Dermatopathol* 7:5–24, 1985.

178. Berger T, Baughman R: Intra–epidermal epithelioma. *Br J Dermatol* 90:343–349, 1974.

179. Cook MG, Ridgway HA: The intra-epidermal epithelioma of Jadassohn: A distinct entity. *Br J Dermatol* 101:659–667, 1979.

180. Hutchinson J: Morbid growths and tumors. 1. The "crateriform ulcer of the face," a form of acute epithelial cancer. *Trans Pathol Soc London* 40:275–281, 1889.

181. Schwartz RA: Keratoacanthoma. *J Am Acad Dermatol* 30:1–19, 1994.

182. Bart RS, Lagin S: Keratoacanthoma following pneumococcal vaccination: A case report. *J Dermatol Surg Oncol* 9:381–382, 1983.

183. Sanchez Yus E, Requena L: Keratoacanthoma within a superficial spreading malignant melanoma in situ. *J Cutan Pathol* 18:288–292, 1991.

184. Bryant J: Basal cell carcinoma associated with keratoacanthoma. *J Dermatol Surg Oncol* 11:1230–1231, 1985.

185. Shellito JE, Samet JM: Keratoacanthoma as a complication of arterial puncture for blood gases. *Int J Dermatol* 21:349, 1982.

186. Sina B, Adrian RM: Multiple keratoacanthomas possibly induced by psoralens and ultraviolet A photochemotherapy. *J Am Acad Dermatol* 9:686–688, 1983.

187. Gassenmaier A, Pfister H, Hornstein OP: Human papillomavirus 25–related DNA in solitary keratoacanthoma. *Arch Dermatol Res* 279:73–76, 1986.

188. Hodak E, Jones RE, Ackerman AB: Solitary keratoacanthoma is a squamous-cell carcinoma: Three examples with metastases. *Am J Dermatopathol* 15:332–342, 1993.

189. Lowe D, Fletcher CDM, Shaw MP, et al: Eosinophil infiltration in keratoacanthoma and squamous cell carcinoma of the skin. *Histopathology* 8:619–825, 1984.

190. Sanchez–Yus, Gonzalez–Moran A: Proliferation of melanocytes in keratoacanthoma. *Arch Dermatol* 121:968–969, 1985.

191. Blessing K, Nafussi AA, Gordon PM: The regressing keratoacanthoma. *Histopathology* 24:381–384, 1994.

192. Lapins NA, Helwig EB: Perineural invasion by keratoacanthoma. *Arch Dermatol* 116:791–793, 1980.

193. Calonje E, Wilson Jones E: Intravascular spread of keratoacanthoma. *Am J Dermatopathol* 14:414–417, 1992.

194. Giltman LI: . Tripolar mitosis in a keratoacanthoma. *Acta Dermato Venereol* (Stockh) 61:362–363, 1981.

195. Giltman LI: Does the presence of atypical mitotic figures in keratoacanthomas indicate a more aggressive biologic behavior. *Dermatol Surg* 21:990–991, 1995.

196. Grant–Kels JM: Response of J.M. Grant–Kels. *Am J Dermatopathol* 15:343–345, 1993.

197. From L: Response of L. From. *Am J Dermatopathol* 15:346, 1993.

198. Reed RJ: Response of R.J. Reed. *Am J Dermatopathol* 15:347–351, 1993.

199. Jones RE: Response of R.E. Jones. *Am J Dermatopathol* 15:352, 1993.

200. Jordan RCK, Kahn HJ, From L, et al: Immunohistochemical demonstration of actinically damaged elastic fibers in keratoacanthomas: An aid in diagnosis. *J Cutan Pathol* 18:81–86, 1991.

201. Miller SJ: Biology of basal cell carcinoma (Part I). *J Am Acad Dermatol* 24:1–13, 1991.

202. Jacob A: Observations respecting an ulcer of peculiar character, which attacks the eyelids and other parts of the face. *Dublin Hospital Reports and Communications in Medicine and Surgery* 4:232–239, 1827.

203. Carter DM, Lin AN: Basal cell carcinoma, in Fitzpatrick TM, Eisen AZ, Wolff K, et al (eds): *Dermatology in General Medicine*, 4th ed. New York: McGraw-Hill, 1993, pp. 840–847.

204. Miller DL, Weinstock MA: Nonmelanoma skin cancer in the United States: incidence. *J Am Acad Dermatol* 30:774–778, 1994.

205. Goldberg LH: Basal cell carcinoma. *Lancet* 347:663–667, 1996.

206. Price MA, Goldberg LH, Levy ML: Juvenile basal cell carcinoma. *Ped Dermatol* 11:176–177, 1994.

207. Miller SJ: Biology of basal cell carcinoma (Part I). *J Am Acad Dermatol* 24:161–175, 1991.

208. Goldstein AM, Bale SJ, Peck GL, et al: Sun exposure and basal cell carcinoma in the nevoid basal cell carcinoma syndrome. *J Am Acad Dermatol* 29:34–41, 1993.

209. Sahl WJ, Snow SN, Levine NS: Giant basal cell carcinoma. *J Am Acad Dermatol* 30:856–859, 1994.

210. Johnson TM, Tschen J, Ho C, et al: Unusual basal cell carcinomas. *Cutis* 54:85–92, 1994.

211. Oram Y, Orengo I, Griego RD, et al: Histologic Patterns of basal cell carcinoma based upon patient immuostatus. *Dermatol Surg* 21:611–614, 1995.

212. Rao BK, Freeman RG, Poulos EG, et al: The relationship between basal cell epithelioma and seborrheic keratosis. *J Dermatol Surg Oncol* 20:761–764, 1994.

213. Coskey RJ, Mehregan AH: The association of basal cell carcinomas with other tumors. *J Dermatol Surg Oncol* 13:553–555, 1987.

214. Ikeda I, Ono T: Basal cell carcinoma originating from an epidermoid cyst. *J Dermatol* 17:643–646, 1990.

215. Boyd AS, Rapini RP: Cutaneous collision tumors. *Am J Dermatopathol* 16:253–257, 1994.

216. Fujisawa H, Matsushima Y, Hoshino M, et al: Differentiation of the basal cell epithelioma-like changes overlying dermatofibroma. *Acta Derm Venereol* (Stockh) 71: 354–356, 1991.

217. Siegle RJ, MacMillan J, Pollack SV: Infiltrative basal cell carcinoma: a nonsclerosing subtype. *J Dermatol Surg Oncol* 12:830–836, 1986.

218. Shimizu N, Ito M, Tazawa T, et al: Immunohistochemical study on keratin expression in certain cutaneous epithelial neoplasms. *Am J Dermatopathol* 11:534–540, 1989.

219. Bavinck JNB, de Boer A, Vermeer BJ, et al: Sunlight, keratotic skin lesions and skin cancer in renal transplant recipients. *Br J Dermatol* 129:242–249, 1993.

220. Rady RL, Yen A, Rollefson JL, et al: Herpesvirus–like DNA sequences in non–Kaposi's sarcoma skin lesions of transplant patients. *Lancet* 345:1339–1340, 1995.

221. Sitz KV, Keppen M, Johnson DF: Metastatic basal cell carcinoma in acquired immunodeficiency syndrome-related complex. *JAMA* 257:340–343, 1987.

222. Randle HW: Basal cell carcinoma: identification and treatment of the high-risk patient. *Dermatol Surg* 22:255–261, 1996.

223. Abreo F, Sanusi ID: Basal cell carcinoma in North American blacks. *J Am Acad Dermatol* 25:1005–1011, 1991.

224. Woods SG: Basal cell carcinoma in the black population. *Int J Dermatol* 34:517–518, 1995.

225. Peschen M, Lo JS, Snow SN, et al: Linear basal cell carcinoma. *Cutis* 51:287–289, 1993.

226. Niazi ZBM, Lamberty BGH: Perineural infiltration in basal cell carcinomas. *Br J Plast Surg* 6:156–157, 1993.

227. Lo JS, Snow SN, Reizner GT, et al: Metastatic basal cell carcinoma: Report of twelve cases with a review of the literature. *J Am Acad Dermatol* 24:715–719, 1991.

228. Sahl WJ:, Basal cell carcinoma: Iinfluence of tumor size on mortality and morbidity. *Int J Dermatol* 34:319–321, 1995.

229. Snow SN, Sahl WJ, Lo J, et al: Metastatic basal cell carcinoma: Report of 5 cases. *Cancer* 73:328–335, 1994.

230. Sexton M, Jones DB, Maloney ME: Histologic pattern analysis of basal cell carcinoma. *J Am Acad Dermatol* 23:1118–1126, 1990.

231. Hendrix JD, Parlette HL: Micronodular basal cell carcinoma: A deceptive histologic subtype with frequent clinically undetected tumor extension. *Arch Dermatol* 132:295–298, 1996.

232. Bigler C, Feldman J, Hall E, et al: Pigmented basal cell carcinoma in Hispanics. *J Am Acad Dermatol* 34:751–752, 1996.

233. Bleehen SS: Pigmented basal cell epithelioma. *Br J Dermatol* 93:361–370, 1975.

234. Lerchin E, Rahbari H: Adamantinoid basal cell epithelioma. *Arch Dermatol* 111:586–588, 1975.

235. Nishimura M, Hori Y: Adamantinoid basal cell carcinoma. *Arch Pathol Lab Med* 115:624–626, 1991.

236. Barr RJ, Graham JH: Granular cell basal cell carcinoma. *Arch Dermatol* 115:1064–1067, 1979.

237. Barr RJ, Williamson C: Clear-cell basal cell carcinoma. *Arch Dermatol* 120:1086 (abstr), 1984.

238. Starink TM, Blomjous CEM, Stoof TJ, et al: Clear-cell basal cell carcinoma. *Histopathology* 17:401–405, 1990.

239. White GM, Barr RJ, Liao SY: Signet ring cell basal cell carcinoma. *Am J Dermatopathol* 13:288–292, 1991.

240. Salasche SJ, Amonette RA: Morpheaform basal–cell epitheliomas. A study of subclinical extensions in a series of 51 cases. *J Dermatol Surg Oncol* 7:387–394, 1981.

241. Betti R, Inselvini E, Carducci M, et al: Age and site prevalence of histologic subtypes of basal cell carcinomas. *Int J Dermatol* 34:174–176, 1995.

242. de Faria JL: Basal cell carcinoma of the skin with areas of squamous cell carcinoma: A basosquamous cell carcinoma. *J Clin Pathol* 38:1273–1277, 1985.

243. Elston DM, Bergfeld WF, Petroff N: Basal cell carcinoma with monster cells. *J Cutan Pathol* 20:70–73, 1993.

244. Garcia CA, Cohen PR, Herzberg AJ, et al: Pleomorphic basal cell carcinoma. *J Am Acad Dermatol* 32:740–746, 1995.

245. Wick MR: Malignant tumors of the epidermis, in Farmer ER, Hood AF (eds): *Pathology of the Skin.* Norwalk, CT: Appleton & Lange, 1990, pp. 568–595.

246. Weber PJ, Gretzula JC, Garland LD, et al: Syringoid eccrine carcinoma. *J Dermatol Surg Oncol* 13:64–67, 1987.

247. Hanke CW, Temofeew RK: Basal cell carcinoma with eccrine differentiation (eccrine epithelioma). *J Dermatol Surg Oncol* 12:820–824, 1986.

248. Yus ES, Caballero LR, Salazar IG, et al: Clear-cell syringoid eccrine carcinoma. *Am J Dermatopathol* 9:225–231, 1987.

249. Moy RL, Rivkin JE, Lee H, et al: Syringoid eccrine carcinoma. *J Am Acad Dermatol* 24:864–867, 1991.

250. Heenan PJ, Bogle MS: Eccrine differentiation in basal cell carcinoma. *J Invest Dermatol* 100:295S–299S, 1993.

251. Kato N, Ueno H: Infundibulocystic basal cell carcinoma. *Am J Dermatopathol* 15:265–267, 1993.

252. Walsh N, Ackerman AB: Infundibulocystic basal cell carcinoma: A newly described variant. *Mod Pathol* 3:599–608, 1990.

253. Aloi FG, Molinero A, Pippione M: Basal cell carcinoma with matrical differentiation. *Am J Dermatopathol* 10:509–513, 1988.

254. Ambrojo P, Aguilar A, Simon P, et al: Basal cell carcinoma with matrical differentiation. *Am J Dermatopathol* 14:293–297, 1992.

255. Pinkus H: Premalignant fibroepithelial tumors of the skin. *Arch Dermatol* 67:598–603, 1953.

256. Jones CC, Ansari SJ, Tschen JA: Cystic fibroepithelioma of Pinkus. *J Cutan Pathol* 18:220–222, 1991.

257. Stern JB, Haupt HM, Smith RRL: Fibroepithelioma of Pinkus: Eccrine duct spread of basal cell carcinoma. *Am J Dermatopathol* 16:585–587, 1994.

258. Suster S, Cajal SR: Myoepithelial differentiation in basal cell carcinoma. *Am J Dermatopathol* 13:350–357, 1991.

259. Lang PG, Maize JC: Histologic evolution of recurrent basal cell carcinoma and treatment implications. *J Am Acad Dermatol* 14:186-196, 1986.

260. Sahin AA, Ro JY, Grignon DJ, et al: Basal cell carcinoma with hyaline inclusions. *Arch Pathol Lab Med* 113:1015–1018, 1989.

261. Kohchiyama A, Oka D, Ueki H: Expression of human lymphocyte antigen (HLA)—DR on tumor cells in basal cell carcinoma. *J Am Acad Dermatol* 16:833–838, 1987.

262. Cohen MS, Rogers GS: The significance of mast cells in basal cell carcinoma. *J Am Acad Dermatol* 33:514–517, 1995.

263. Satti MB, Azzopardi JG: Amyloid deposits in basal cell carcinoma of the skin. *J Am Acad Dermatol* 22:1082–1087, 1990.

264. Olsen KE, Westermark P: Amyloid in basal cell carcinoma and seborrheic keratosis. *Acta Derm Venereol* (Stockh) 74:273–275, 1994.

265. Zamecnik M, Skalova A, Michal M: Basal cell carcinoma with collagenous crystalloids. *Arch Pathol Lab Med* 120:581–582, 1996.

266. Hunt MJ, Halliday GM, Weedon D, et al: Regression in basal cell carcinoma: An immunohistochemical analysis. *Br J Dermatol* 130:1–8, 1994.

267. Pentel M, Helm KF, Maloney MM: Cell surface molecules in basal cell carcinomas. *Dermatol Surg* 21:858–861, 1995.

268. Shea CR, McNutt NS, Volkenandt M, et al: Overexpression of p53 protein in basal cell carcinomas of human skin. *Am J Pathol* 141:25–29, 1992.

269. De Rosa G, Saibano S, Barra E, et al: p53 protein in aggressive and non-aggressive basal cell carcinoma. *J Cutan Pathol* 20:429–434, 1993.

270. Kallioinen M, Autio–Harmainen A, Dammert K, et al: Discontinuity of the basement membrane in fibrosing basocellular carcinomas and basosquamous carcinomas of the skin: An immunohistochemical study with human laminin and type IV collagen antibodies. *J Invest Dermatol* 82:248–251, 1984.

271. Jones JCR, Steinman HK, Goldsmith BA: Hemidesmosomes, collagen VII, and intermediate filaments in basal cell carcinoma. *J Invest Dermatol* 93:662–671, 1989.

272. Brooke JD, Fitzpatrick JE, Golitz LE: Papillary mesenchymal bodies: A histologic finding useful in differentiating trichoepitheliomas from basal cell carcinomas. *J Am Acad Dermatol* 21:523–528, 1989.

273. Brownstein MH: Basaloid follicular hamartoma: Solitary and multiple types. *J Am Acad Dermatol* 27:237–240, 1992.

274. Sebastien TS, Nelson BR, Lowe L, et al: Microcystic adnexal carcinoma. *J Am Acad Dermatol* 29:840–845, 1993.

275. Boyd AS: Carcinomas of sweat gland origin, in Demis DJ, (ed): *Clinical Dermatology.* Philadelphia: Lippincott-Raven, 1995, in press.

276. Tellechea O, Reis JP, Domingues JC, et al: Monoclonal antibody Ber EP4 distinguishes basal-cell carcinoma from squamous-cell carcinoma of the skin. *Am J Dermatopathol* 15:452–455, 1993.

277. Howell JB, Caro MR: The basal cell nevus. *Arch Dermatol* 79:67–80, 1959.

278. Bale AE, Gailani MR, Leffell DJ: Nevoid basal cell carcinoma syndrome. *J Invest Dermatol* 103:126S–130S, 1994.

279. Gorlin RJ: Nevoid basal cell carcinoma syndrome. *Derm Clin No Am* 13:113–125, 1995.

280. Gutierrez MM, Mora RG: Nevoid basal cell carcinoma syndrome. *J Am Acad Dermatol* 15:1023–1030, 1986.

281. Shanley S, Ratcliffe J, Hockey A, et al: Nevoid basal cell carcinoma syndrome: review of 118 affected individuals. *Am J Med Gen* 50:282–290, 1994.

282. Pratt MD, Jackson R: Nevoid basal cell carcinoma syndrome. *J Am Acad Dermatol* 16:964–970, 1987.

283. Barr RJ, Headley JL, Jensen JL, et al: Cutaneous keratocysts of nevoid basal cell carcinoma syndrome. *J Am Acad Dermatol* 14:572–576, 1986.

284. Howell JB, Mehregan AH: Pursuit of the pits in nevoid basal cell carcinoma syndrome. *Arch Dermatol* 102:586–597, 1970.

285. Lindberg H, Jepsen FL: The nevoid basal cell carcinoma syndrome. *Histopathology* of the basal cell tumors. *J Cutan Pathol* 10:68–73, 1983.

286. Johnson TM, Rowe DE, Nelson BR: Squamous cell carcinoma of the skin (excluding lip and oral mucosa). *J Am Acad Dermatol* 26:467–484, 1992.

287. Kwa RE, Campana K, Moy RL: Biology of cutaneous squamous cell carcinoma. *J Am Acad Dermatol* 26:1–16, 1992.

288. Haydon RC: Cutaneous squamous carcinoma and related lesions. *Otolaryngol Clin No Am* 26:57–71, 1993.

289. Berstein SC, Lim KK, Brodland DG, et al: The many faces of squamous cell carcinoma. *Dermatol Surg* 22:243–254, 1996.

290. Marks R: Squamous cell carcinoma. *Lancet* 347:735–738, 1996.

291. Sanchez–Lanier M, Triplett C, Campion M: Possible role for human papillomavirus 16 in squamous cell carcinoma of the finger. *J Med Virol* 44:369–378, 1994.

292. Ampil FL, Hardin JC, Peskind SP, et al: Perineural invasion in skin cancer of the head and neck. *J Oral Maxillofac Surg* 53:34–38, 1995.

293. Lawrence N, Cottel WI: Squamous cell carcinoma of skin with perineural invasion. *J Am Acad Dermatol* 31:30–33, 1994.

294. Rowe DE, Carroll RJ, Day CL: Prognostic factors for local recurrence, metastasis and survival rates in squamous cell carcinoma of the skin, ear and lip. *J Am Acad Dermatol* 26:976–990, 1992.

295. Dinehart SM, Pollack SV: Metastases from squamous cell carcinoma of the skin and lip: an analysis of 27 cases. *J Am Acad Dermatol* 21:241– 248, 1989.

296. Barr B, McLoren K, Smith IN, et al: Human papillomavirus infection and skin cancer in renal allograft recipients. *Lancet* 124–128, 1989.

297. Broders AC: Practical points on the microscope grading of carcinoma. *N Y J Med* 32:667–671, 1932.

298. Banerjee SS, Eyden BP, Wells S, et al: Pseudoangiosarcomatous carcinoma: a clinicopathological study of seven cases. *Histopathology* 21:13–23, 1992.

299. Iyer PV, Leong ASY: Poorly differentiated squamous cell carcinomas of the skin can express vimentin. *J Cutan Pathol* 19:34–39, 1992.

300. Smith KJ, Skelton HG, Morgan AM, et al: Spindle cell neoplasms coexpressing cytokeratin and vimentin (metaplastic squamous cell carcinoma). *J Cutan Pathol* 19:286-293, 1992.

301. Harris M: Spindle cell squamous carcinoma: Ultrastructural observations. *Histopathology* 6:197–210, 1982.

302. Nappi O, Wick MR, Pettinato G, et al: Pseudovascular adenoid squamous cell carcinoma of the skin. *Am J Surg Pathol* 16:429–438, 1992.

303. Johnson WC, Helwig EB: Adenoid squamous cell carcinoma (adenoacanthoma): A clinicopathologic study of 155 patients. *Cancer* 19:1639–1650, 1966.

304. Caya JG, Hidayat AA, Weiner MJ: A clinicopathologic study of 21 cases of adenoid squamous cell carcinoma of the eyelid and periorbital region. *Am J Opthalmol* 99: 291–297, 1985.

305. Cramer SF, Heggeness LM: Signet–ring squamous cell carcinoma. *Am J Clin Pathol* 91:488–491, 1989.

306. Howe NR, Lange PG: Squamous cell carcinoma presenting as subcutaneous nodules. *J Dermatol Surg Oncol* 17:779–783, 1991.

307. Martin RW, Farmer ER, Rady PL, et al: Cutaneous papillary squamous cell carcinoma in an immunosuppressed host. *J Cutan Pathol* 21:476–477, 1994.

308. Sherman RN, Fung HK, Flynn KJ: Verrucous carcinoma (Buschke-Loewenstein tumor). *Int J Dermatol* 30:730–733, 1991.

309. Ackerman LV: Verrucous carcinoma of the oral cavity. *Surgery* 23:670–678, 1948.

310. Kathuria S, Reiker J, Jablokow VR, et al: Plantar verrucous carcinoma (epithelioma cuniculatum): Case report with review of the literature. *J Surg Oncol* 31:71–75, 1986.

311. Florin EH, Kolbusz RV, Goldberg LH: Verrucous carcinoma of the oral cavity. *Int J Dermatol* 33:618–622, 1994.

312. Aird I, Johnson HD, Lennox B, et al: Epithelioma cuniculatum. A variety of squamous carcinoma peculiar to the foot. *Br J Surg* 42:245-250, 1954.

313. Coldiron BM, Brown FC, Freeman RG: Epithelioma cuniculatum (carcinoma cuniculatum) of the thumb: A case report and literature review. *J Dermatol Surg Oncol* 12:1150–1155, 1986.

314. Noel JC, Heene M, Peney MO, et al: Proliferating cell nuclear antigen distribution in verrucous carcinoma of the skin. *Br J Dermatol* 133:868–873, 1995.

315. McKee PH, Wilkinson JD, Black MM, et al: Carcinoma (epithelioma) cuniculatum: A clinico-pathological study of nineteen cases and review of the literature. *Histopathology* 5:425–436, 1981.

316. Buschke A, Loewenstein L: Uber carcinomahnliche condylomata acuminata des penis. *Klin Wochenschr* 4:1726–1728, 1925.

317. Schwartz RA: Buschke-Loewenstein tumor: Verrucous carcinoma of the penis. *J Am Acad Dermatol* 23:723–727, 1990.

318. Seixas ALC, Ornellas AA, Marota A, et al: Verrucous carcinoma of the penis: Retrospective analysis of 32 cases. *J Urol* 152:1476–1479, 1994.

319. Chu QD, Vezeridis MP, Libbey NP, et al: Giant condyloma acuminatum (Buschke-Loewenstein tumor) of the anorectal and perianal regions. *Dis Colon Rectum* 37:950–957, 1994.

320. Schwartz RA, Nychay SG, Lyons M, et al: Buschke-Lowenstein tumor: verrucous carcinoma of the anogenitalia. *Cutis* 47:263–266, 1991.

321. Weidner N, Foucar E: Adenosquamous carcinoma of the skin. *Arch Dermatol* 121:775–779, 1985.

322. Friedman KJ: Low–grade primary cutaneous adenosquamous (mucoepidermoid) carcinoma. *Am J Dermatopathol* 11:43–50, 1989.

323. Landman Gilles, Farmer ER: Primary cutaneous mucoepidermoid carcinoma: Report of a case. *J Cutan Pathol* 18:56–59, 1991.

324. Leen EJ, Saunders MNP, Vollum DI, et al: Carcinosarcoma of the skin. *Histopathology* 26:367–371, 1995.

325. McKee PH, Fletcher CDM, Stavrinos P, et al: Carcinosarcoma arising in eccrine spiradenoma. *Am J Dermatopathol* 12:335–343, 1990.

326. Izaki S, Hirai A, Yoshizawa Y, et al: Carcinosarcoma of the skin: Immunohistochemical and electron microscopic observations. *J Cutan Pathol* 20:272–278, 1993.

327. Swanson SA, Cooper PH, Mills SE, et al: Lymphoepithelioma-like carcinoma of the skin. *Mod Pathol* 1:359–365, 1988.

328. Walker AN, Kent D, Mitchell AR: Lymphoepithelioma-like carcinoma in the skin. *J Am Acad Dermatol* 22:691–693, 1990.

329. Wick MR, Swanson PE, LeBoit PE, et al: Lymphoepithelioma-like carcinoma of the skin with adnexal differentiation. *J Cutan Pathol* 18:93–102, 1990.

330. Requena L, Sanchez Yus E, Jimenez E, et al: Lymphoepithelioma-like carcinoma of the skin: A light-microscopic and immunohistochemical study. *J Cutan Pathol* 21: 541–548, 1994.

331. Axelsen SM, Stamp IM: Lymphoepithelioma-like carcinoma of the vulvar region. *Histopathology* 27:281–283, 1995.

332. Carr KA, Bulengo S, Weiss LM, et al: Lymphepitheliomalike carcinoma of the skin. *Am J Surg Pathol* 16:909–913, 1992.

333. Santa Cruz DJ, Barr RJ, Headington JT: Cutaneous lymphadenoma. *Am J Surg Pathol* 15:101–110, 1991.

334. Yu RCH, Pryce DW, MacFarlane AW, Stewart TW: A histopathological study of 643 cutaneous horns. *Br J Dermatol* 124:449–452, 1991.

335. Thornton CM, Hunt SJ: Sebaceous adenoma with a cutaneous horn. *J Cutan Pathol* 22:185–187, 1995.

336. Schwartz JJ: HIV-related molluscum contagiosum presenting as a cutaneous horn. *Int J Dermatol* 31:142–144, 1992.

337. Willoughby C, Soter NA: Stucco keratosis. *Arch Dermatol* 105:859–861, 1972.

338. Kocsard E, Ofner F, Coles JF, et al: Senile changes in the skin and visible mucous membranes of the Australian male. *Australas J Dermatol* 4:216–223, 1958.

339. Shall L, Marks R: Stucco keratoses: A clinico-pathological study. *Acta Derm Venereol* (Stockh) 71:258–261, 1991.

340. Scott O, Ward J: Stucco keratosis. *Br J Dermatol* 64:376–379, 1971.

341. Waisman M: Clavus (corn), in Demis DJ (ed): *Clinical Dermatology*. Philadelphia: Lippincott-Raven, 1995.

342. Cure for the corn. *Br Med J* 1:113, 1976.

343. Waisman M: Callus, in Demis DJ (ed): *Clinical Dermatology*. Philadelphia: Lippincott-Raven, 1995.

344. Patterson J: Palmar and plantar hyperkeratosis, in Demis DJ (ed): *Clinical Dermatology*. Philadelphia: Lippincott-Raven, 1995.

345. Rustad OJ, Vance JC: Punctate keratoses of the palms and soles and keratotic pits of the palmar creases. *J Am Acad Dermatol* 22:468–476, 1990.

346. Anderson WA, Elam MD, Lambert WC: Keratosis punctata and atopy. *Arch Dermatol* 120:884–890, 1984.

347. Orget M, Sanchez-Conejo-Mir J, Quintana del Olmo J, et al: Keratosis punctata of the palmar creases. *J Cutan Pathol* 16:109–111, 1989.

348. Weiss RM, Rasmussen JE: Keratosis punctata of the palmar creases. *Arch Dermatol* 116:669–671, 1980.

349. Rubenstein DJ, Schwartz RA, Hansen RC, et al: Punctate hyperkeratosis of the palms and soles. *J Am Acad Dermatol* 3:43–49, 1980.

350. Caputo R, Carminati G, Ermacora E, et al: Keratosis punctata palmaris et plantaris as an expression of focal acantholytic dyskeratosis. *Am J Dermatopathol* 11:574–576, 1989.

CHAPTER 27

TUMORS OF MELANOCYTES

Raymond L. Barnhill

Melanocytic lesions continue to be one of the most significant problems faced by dermatopathologists and pathologists. The recognition of Spitz tumors, various atypical nevi, and cutaneous melanoma and their distinction from other melanocytic lesions remain a daunting challenge to all histopathologists who interpret skin biopsies. This chapter discusses the entire spectrum of melanocytic lesions occurring in the skin according to guidelines provided in Table 27-1.

CIRCUMSCRIBED PIGMENTED LESIONS COMPOSED OF BASILAR MELANOCYTES

Solar Lentigo

Synonyms: *Lentigo senilis, liverspot*

The solar lentigo occurs on sun-exposed skin (Table 27-2)[1-4] in more than 90 percent of the Caucasian population over the age of 60 years.[1] Solar lentigines are distinguished from common freckles by their persistence despite absence of sun exposure. Solar lentigines are prominent in xeroderma pigmentosum. The photochemotherapy-induced (PUVA) lentigo has been observed in patients receiving long-term methoxsalen photochemotherapy (PUVA) for psoriasis.[5-7]

Clinical Features   Solar lentigines are well-circumscribed round, oval, or irregularly bordered macules of yellow, tan, or brown color, varying in size from about 1 to 3 cm in diameter, with a tendency to confluency.[1-4] Solar lentigines occur on sun-exposed areas, predominantly the dorsal aspects of hands and forearms, the face, and upper chest and back. The "sunburn," hypermelanotic, or "ink spot" solar lentigo is characterized by a striking jet-black color and a stellate outline.[8] The PUVA lentigo has a close clinical resemblance to the solar lentigo, particularly the hypermelanotic type.[5-7]

Histopathological Features   In general, the solar lentigo is notable for elongated, club-shaped epidermal rete ridges, basal layer hyperpigmentation most prominent at the tips of the rete, and an increased frequency of basilar melanocytes; however, the melanocytes may not be increased in number (Table 27-2) (Fig. 27-1).[1,4] The epidermis between rete ridges is usually atrophic. On occasion, there is slight cytologic atypia of basilar melanocytes.[9] There may also be hyperkeratosis and rather prominent elongation and anastomosis of rete. Solar elastosis is almost always present.

The solar lentigo may show transitions to reticulated seborrheic keratosis, large cell acanthoma, and lichenoid keratosis.[10,11] Some solar lentigines develop an associated lichenoid dermatitis and hence are termed *lichenoid* or *lichen planus–like keratosis.*

Similar to solar lentigines, the PUVA lentigo exhibits lentiginous melanocytic hyperplasia, and low-grade cytologic atypia of melanocytes is occasionally noted.[5,6]

Differential Diagnosis   The differential diagnosis includes lentiginous melanocytic proliferation with atypia involving sun-exposed skin LMPS (so-called lentigo maligna) (Table 27-2) and pigmented actinic keratosis. In general, LMPS, particularly when present on the central face, is characterized by absence or diminution of the epidermal rete pattern in contrast to solar lentigo. In addition, there is usually a greater frequency of basilar melanocytes and prominent involvement of adnexal epithelium by the lentiginous proliferation of melanocytes in lentigo compared to solar lentigo. Finally, LMPS is characterized by a striking cytologic atypia of basilar melanocytes that should not be seen in solar lentigo. Nonetheless, on occasion, one may encounter lesions transitional between solar lentigo and LMPS.

LENTIGINES AND ACQUIRED MELANOCYTIC NEVI

Lentigines and melanocytic nevi are thought to represent progressive stages of melanocyte migration and proliferation in the skin (Table 27-1).[12-14] Melanoblasts or a related precursor cell are believed to migrate from the neural crest, taking residence in the epidermis early in development.[15,16] Proliferation of these cells in the basilar epidermis may give rise sequentially to lentigo and the three subsequent stages of the melanocytic nevus. The proliferation of melanocytes as clusters or nests within the epidermis defines the junctional nevus.[14,17,18] The term *nevus cell* describes the cells within these nests or clusters. These cells are closely related to melanocytes but are perhaps functionally somewhat altered by an aggregative pattern of growth.[19] These cells tend to lose the dendritic processes that are characteristic of solitary basilar melanocytes and to assume a more rounded morphology. In general, these cells have more abundant cytoplasm, somewhat larger nuclei, and somewhat more prominent nucleoli compared to the basilar melanocyte. Ultrastructurally, nevus cells contain single melanosomes in all stages of development similar to melanocytes.[19] Thus, many authors consider nevus cells to be melanocytes and dismiss the need for alternative nomenclature.

The presumptive natural history of melanocytic nevi includes proliferation within the epidermis as junctional nests, subsequent migration or "dropping off" of nevus cells into the papillary dermis, where proliferation results in nests of cells.[17] According to this hypothesis, eventually all intraepidermal proliferation of melanocytes ceases, and the nevi become entirely intradermal.[17,18] Nevus cells entering the dermis have a reduction in both proliferation and metabolic activity, except for the formation of melanosomes.[17,18,20] Thus, the cellularity of a nevus tends to decrease with age; because of this cessation of replication, the nevus cells are gradually replaced by mesenchymal elements—fibrous matrix, mucin, and fat.[18] Most dermal nevi are believed to undergo progressive involution, perhaps via acrochordons and eventual shedding.[21] This developmental sequence may be arrested at any point such that a lentigo, junctional nevus, or compound nevus may persist indefinitely.[14]

TABLE 27-1

Histological Criteria for the Classification of Melanocytic Nevi

Location of melanocytes in the skin (depth)
    Superficial
        Intraepidermal
        Papillary dermis
        Upper half of reticular dermis
    Deep
        Lower half of reticular dermis
        Subcutaneous
        Fascial
Disposition of melanocytes
    Intraepidermal
        Basilar melanocytes (single-cell pattern)
            Normal numbers
            Increased frequency
                With elongated rete (lentiginous)
                Without elongated rete
        Pagetoid pattern
        Nested pattern
            With lentiginous pattern
            Without lentiginous pattern
    Dermal
        Diffuse, interstitial
        Patchy perivascular, periadnexal, perineurial
        Wedge pattern (deep apex of nests, fascicles of melanocytes
            extend into reticular dermis or subcutaneous fat)
        Plexiform pattern (discrete nests, fascicles associated with
            neurovascular or adnexal structures of reticular dermis with
            intervening normal dermis)
        Bulbous aggregates, nodules (cellular nests or fascicles with
            rounded contours, usually extending into reticular dermis,
            subcutis)
        Alveolar pattern
        Maturation/differentiation
Stroma
    Desmoplasia, sclerosis
Cell type
    Small round or oval cells
    Fusiform/spindle cell
    Epithelioid cell (abundant cytoplasm, overall enlarged)
    Dendritic cell (lengthy, delicate cellular processes)
    Intermediate, difficult to classify cell types
    All with varying degrees of melaninization

Lentigo Simplex

Clinical and Histopathological Features   The simple lentigo, also called *nevoid lentigo*, is a regular, well-circumscribed macule measuring 1 to 5 mm in diameter and having a uniform light-brown, brown, or dark-brown color.[22] The simple lentigo may occur in a localized or in a widespread pattern as in lentiginosis profusa or in association with certain syndromes, as, for example, LEOPARD (multiple lentigines), LAMB, or Peutz-Jeghers syndrome.[22]

The simple lentigo is defined histologically by three features: (1) increased frequency of basilar melanocytes compared to adjacent normal skin, (2) elongated, club-shaped epidermal rete, and (3) basilar hyperpigmentation of the epidermis (Fig. 27-2), which may extend into the upper portion of the epidermis and stratum corneum.[12–14,23] There is increased melanin and an increased frequency of melanocytes at the tips

TABLE 27-2

Solar Lentigo and Lentigo Maligna

Solar lentigo	Atypical lentiginous melanocytic proliferations of sun-exposed skin (lentigo maligna)
Clinical Features	
Onset over age 30–40 years	Onset generally over age 50 years
Sun-exposed skin face, dorsal hands	Sun-exposed skin, cheek most common site
5- to 15-mm or larger macule	10- to 200-mm or larger macule
Medium to dark brown	Tan, brown, dark brown, black
Slightly rough surface	"Varnishlike" stain
Some variation in color	Often marked variegation
Some asymmetry	Prominent asymmetry
Regular or slightly irregular border	Irregular or notched border
Histopathological Features	
Usually well-circumscribed	Usually poorly circumscribed
Symmetry	Usually some asymmetry
Elongated, club-shaped rete ridges	Often effacement of epidermis
Increased number of basilar melanocytes often	Increased frequency of basilar melanocytes
Melanocytes more frequent on tips of rete	No particular affinity for rete ridges
Intraepidermal nests of melanocytes usually not present	Formation of intraepidermal nests with diminished cohesion
Basilar melanocytes usually not involving adnexae	Basilar melanocytes often involve adnexal epithelium
Occasional variable cytologic atypia of melanocytes	Greater cytologic atypia
	Melanocytes often slightly pleomorphic, with high nuclear-to-cytoplasmic ratio, spindle-shaped

of the elongated epidermal rete with diminished frequency proceeding upward along the sides and between the rete.

Differential Diagnosis   A simple lentigo must be discriminated from a freckle and a solar lentigo. A simple lentigo differs from a freckle because of elongated epidermal rete ridges and an increased frequency of basilar melanocytes. The simple lentigo does not usually have rete ridges as elongated and showing anastomosis or solar elastosis to the degree observed in solar lentigo. In addition, melanocytic hyperplasia may not be present in solar lentigo.

A common dilemma is differentiating a simple lentigo from a typical melanocytic nevus or dysplastic nevus. The melanocytic nevus is distinguished by the presence of junctional nests.[13]

Melanotic Macules and Lentigines of Mucocutaneous Sites

Certain pigmented macules may involve mucosal sites such as the conjunctiva, oral mucosa, the vermillion border of the lip, and genitalia.[24,25] Multiple lentigines may involve the oral mucosa and vermillion border as part of the Peutz-Jeghers syndrome.[26,27]

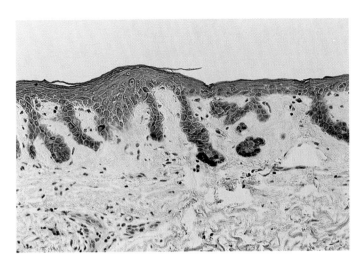

FIGURE 27-1   Solar lentigo. Note elongated club-shaped epidermal rete with basal layer hyperpigmentation.

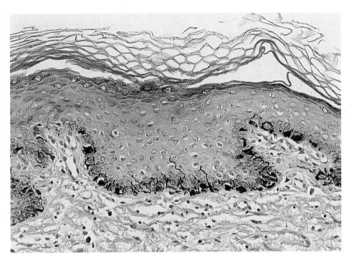

FIGURE 27-3   Penile lentigo. There are slightly increased numbers of basilar melanocytes.

Clinical Features   These lesions are usually solitary or multiple macules measuring 1 to 5 mm and are often characterized by uniform light- to dark-brown or black homogeneous color.[24,25] The borders are generally regular and well defined. Occasional lesions on the genitalia in particular are notable for a mottled appearance and large size, i.e., measuring up to 50 mm in greatest diameter.[24] The latter clinical appearance suggests melanoma, but such lesions generally do not show atypical changes histologically (see below) or eventuate in melanoma.[24]

Histopathological Features   The histologic spectrum of these lesions may vary from slight acanthosis of epithelium, presence or absence of club-shaped rete, and presence or absence of basilar melanocytic hyperplasia (Fig. 27-3). The lesions without melanocytic hyperplasia may be designated as a *melanotic macule* or *melanosis*. Lesions with melano-

cytic hyperplasia are best termed *lentigines*. As with other simple lentigines, there is hyperpigmentation of the basilar epithelium.

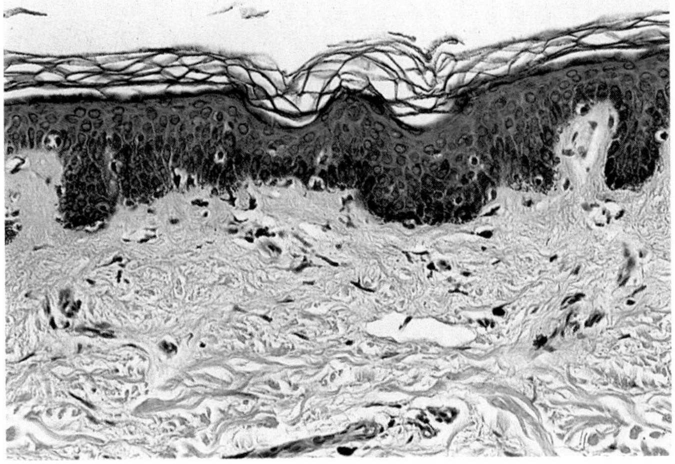

Differential Diagnosis   The differential diagnosis includes melanocytic nevi of mucosal sites, atypical melanocytic proliferations, and melanoma. In general, as with melanocytic lesions located on other sites, progressively greater clinical atypicality raises concern about atypical histologic changes and melanoma.

Histologically atypical melanocytic lesions and melanoma on mucosae are characterized by progressively greater frequency of basilar melanocytes and prominent cytologic atypia. In the case of melanoma, the basilar melanocytes often reach confluence along the basal layer in a lentiginous pattern. The melanocytes exhibit continuous marked cytologic atypia. Pagetoid spread is variable and may be absent, minimal, or prominent.

Common Acquired Melanocytic Nevi

Common acquired nevi range from small, well-circumscribed pigmented macules to raised, flesh-colored lesions, defined by the location of aggregations of *nevus cells* in the skin: Junctional nevi have intraepidermal collections of nevus cells, dermal (intradermal) nevi have nevus cells in the dermis, and compound nevi have nevus cells in both areas.[17,18]

The natural history of acquired melanocytic nevi is poorly documented.[14,17,18] The prevalence of nevi is related to age, race, and genetic and environmental factors.[28–34] Very few nevi are present in early childhood, but they increase in number, reaching a peak in the third decade of life, and tend thereafter to disappear with increasing age.[35] There is a period of particularly rapid development of nevi at puberty. In general, the greatest numbers of nevi are noted among individuals aged 20 to 29 years,[35] and there are no substantial differences between men and women.[35] Caucasians in general have greater numbers of nevi than darker-skinned groups, i.e., blacks and Asians.[36] Furthermore, a greater prevalence of nevi is associated with lighter skin color in Caucasians.[37] The frequency of melanocytic nevi on the palms and soles, nail beds, and conjunctivae is also related to race: nevi on these surfaces are more prevalent in blacks than in whites.[38]

FIGURE 27-2   Lentigo simplex. There are elongated epidermal rete and basal layer hyperpigmentation, most prominently involving the lower aspects of the rete.

TABLE 27-3

TABLE 27-3

Common Acquired Melanocytic Nevi

Clinical Features

Onset childhood, adolescence, third decade, or later
3- to 6-mm macule, papule (slight to clear elevation), often
   dome-shaped, globoid, polypoid, or papillomatous
Round, oval
Symmetric
Well-defined regular borders
Homogenous tan, brown, dark brown
Slight accentuation of skin cleavage lines with oblique lighting

Histopathological Features

Symmetry
Well-circumscribed
Regular arrangement of junctional nests of nevus cells, if present
Fairly uniform size, shape, position of nests
Nests usually at tips of epidermal rete
Cohesive nests usually
Generally no pagetoid spread
Nevus cells usually confined to papillary dermis or superficial
   reticular dermis
Usual transition or maturation from epithelioid to lymphocytoid
   to spindled nevus cells
Mitotic figures uncommon or rare in dermis
Usually only minimal nuclear pleomorphism

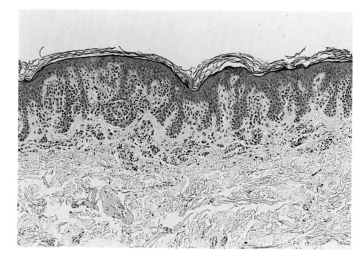

FIGURE 27-4   Lentiginous compound nevus. The epidermis shows lentiginous and junctional nested pattern of melanocytes.

Clinical Features   Melanocytic nevi are well-circumscribed round or ovoid lesions, generally measuring from 2 to 6 mm in diameter (Table 27-3).[22] Although many nevi display slight asymmetry, the borders are usually regular and well defined. The natural history is believed to be a progression from a junctional nevus to a compound nevus then to a dermal nevus and subsequent involution.[14,17,18,23] The junctional nevus is macular with slight accentuation of skin markings visible with side lighting. Junctional nevi display a uniform, medium- to dark-brown color. Compound nevi show variable elevation and in general somewhat lighter shades of brown than do junctional nevi. Dermal nevi are usually more elevated and show lighter shades of brown or even flesh tones compared to compound nevi. However, there is clinical overlap among all three types of nevi.[22] Dermal nevi and, to a lesser degree, compound nevi may be dome-shaped or papillomatous. Nevi may have a verrucous surface simulating that of seborrheic keratosis. Many nevi contain hairs that are coarse and dark compared to those in surrounding skin.

Histopathological Features   Melanocytic nevi are usually symmetric and well-circumscribed (Fig. 27-4). The junctional component as a general rule does not extend peripherally beyond a dermal component,[14] if present (see *dysplastic nevi*). The surface profile may vary from being flat to dome-shaped, polypoid, or papillomatous (Figs. 27-4 and 27-5)[23] and tends to correlate with type of nevus, e.g., junctional nevi are relatively flat, compound nevi are slightly raised, and dermal nevi are often dome-shaped, polypoid, or papillomatous. This surface configuration also correlates with anatomic location. Most nevi on acral sites are relatively flat or slightly raised, junctional or compound nevi.[13,17,18,23,39] In contrast, many nevi on the head and neck and, to a lesser extent, on the trunk are dome-shaped or polypoid.

The junctional nevus has nesting of nevus cells within the epidermis.[17,18,23] A junctional nest, or theque, contains five or more nevus cells in close apposition, cohesive, and usually above the basement membrane (Fig. 27-6).[13,39] The size, shape, location, and spacing of these nests tend to be regular.[23] The junctional nests are usually located on the tips of elongated rete rather than on the sides or between rete.

The compound nevus has nevus cells within the dermis as well as junctional nesting, whereas the dermal (or intradermal) nevus has no intraepidermal component (Fig. 27-5) (Table 27-3).[17] Most nevi are compound; on serial sectioning 80 percent of apparent dermal nevi will have junctional nests.[39] Common acquired nevi are generally confined to the adventitial dermis (the finely textured collagenous stroma comprising the papillary dermis and surrounding adnexal structures and blood vessels).[17] Dermal nevi mainly proliferate in and expand the papillary dermis, resulting in progressive elevation of nevus contours commensurate with the volume of nevus cells (Fig. 27-5).

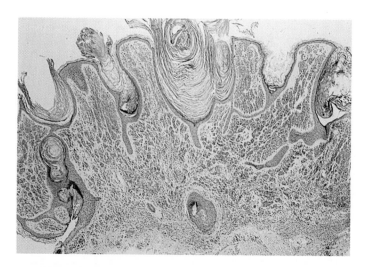

FIGURE 27-5   Papillomatous dermal nevus. The epidermal surface has a papillary topography.

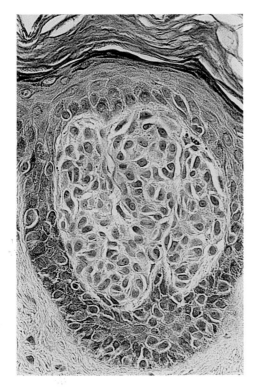

FIGURE 27-6   Junctional nevus. Cohesive nest of epithelioid (type A) nevus cells.

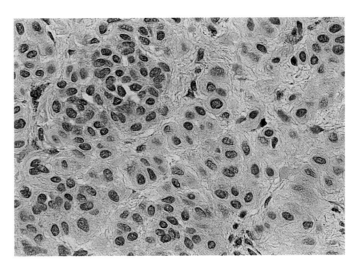

FIGURE 27-7   Dermal nevus. Type B (lymphocytoid) nevus cells in dermis. The cells contain minimal cytoplasm and uniform round or oval nuclei.

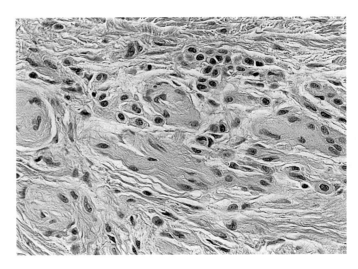

FIGURE 27-8   Dermal nevus. Type C (spindled) nevus cells. The cells resemble Schwann cells and are separated by delicate connective tissue.

MATURATIONAL SEQUENCE AND CYTOLOGY OF NEVUS CELLS

Nevus cells within junctional nests or the superficial dermis exhibit cohesive rounded nesting, a tendency to synthesis of melanin, and cytologic characteristics of epithelial cells and have been termed *epithelioid* or *type A cells* (Fig. 27-6).[14,17,18,20,23,40,41] The latter features refer to the abundant pinkish cytoplasm and the rounded or polygonal configuration of the cells. In general, the nuclei are slightly larger than those of basilar melanocytes.[19] The nuclei have a uniform dispersion of chromatin, generally with a ground-glass basophilic appearance and delicate nuclear membranes.[17,19,20,40] Small nucleoli may also be observed. Type B nevus cells in the papillary dermis usually subjacent to the type A cells resemble lymphocytes (Fig. 27-7).[20,40] This is due to a smaller amount of cytoplasm and the tendency to form more-compacted cords and nests of cells. Generally, the latter nevus cells do not synthesize melanin or form rounded nests.[17,19,20,40] The final stage of maturation is that of type C nevus cells with elongate or spindle-shaped morphology and separation by delicate fibrous tissue (Fig. 27-8).[17,19,20,40,42] The latter cells have considerable resemblance to fibroblasts or Schwann cells.

Giant cells are observed in melanocytic nevi and melanoma.[17] Nevus giant cells are principally of two types. One type contains tightly packed nuclei with scant cytoplasm and has been called a *mulberry*-type giant cell. The molding of nuclei may lead to misinterpretation as a bizarre, atypical nevus cell. This cell type is often in the dermal component of a nevus. The second type has a peripheral, wreathlike arrangement of nuclei with central pink or slightly bluish cytoplasm. The latter cell type may closely simulate or on occasion be identical to a Touton giant cell. This particular giant cell is commonly observed in junctional nests.

Another common feature, the pseudonuclear inclusion,[43] is an invagination of cytoplasm that on cross section seems to lie within the nucleus and has the same staining properties as the nevus cell cytoplasm, often a pale or "dusty" ground-glass appearance.

VARIANTS OF MELANOCYTIC NEVI

See Table 27-4.

Melanocytic Nevus of Acral Skin

Clinical and Histopathological Features   Acral nevi are usually macular or only slightly elevated, uniform brown or dark-brown lesions that are often indistinguishable from simple lentigines.[22] These are usually relatively small (less than 5 to 6 mm), well-circumscribed, and symmetric compound nevi. On occasion, the junctional nests are somewhat enlarged, but they usually have a fairly uniform round or oval shape and are similar in size and spacing. Lentiginous melanocytic proliferation (Fig. 27-9) and some degree of upward migration of melanocytes are commonly observed in acral nevi.[44–47]

TABLE 27-4

Uncommon Findings in or Presentations of Melanocytic Nevi

Agminated (speckled) lentiginous or melanocytic nevi[77]	Circumscribed grouping of hyperpigmented macules and/or papules equivalent to nevus spilus but with absence of background macule; hyperpigmented foci are lentigines, junctional or compound nevi
Amyloid deposition[78]	Degenerative nevus cells.
Angiomatous, pseudovascular pattern[79,80]	Nevus cell pattern resembles vascular or lymphatic spaces, possibly secondary to tissue shrinkage, processing
Cockarde (Cockade) nevus[81]	Peripheral pigmented halo (junctional nevus usually) with intervening nonpigmented annulus about central nevus (junctional or compound nevus)
Keratinous cyst rupture, folliculitis, abscess formation[82,83]	Enlargement, change in color suggesting melanoma
Meyerson's nevus[84,85]	Subacute eczematous epidermal changes associated with nevus, often forming eczematous halo
Nevus (osteonevus) of Nanta[86]	Bone formation in nevus (metaplastic ossification)
Perinevoid alopecia[87]	Hair loss associated with scalp nevi; inflammatory reaction resembling halo nevus but associated with hair follicles
Psammoma bodies[88]	Probably associated with degenerative nevus cells

Differential Diagnosis   Acral nevi must be distinguished from atypical or dysplastic nevi and melanoma. Both atypical nevi and melanoma demonstrate greater architectural and cytologic atypicality. In particular, an increased frequency of basilar melanocytes is an important feature of both atypical nevi and acral lentiginous melanoma. Irregular nesting patterns, discohesion of nests, prominent pagetoid spread, poor

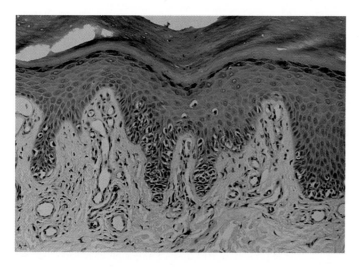

FIGURE 27-9 Compound nevus of acral skin. There is prominent lentiginous melanocytic proliferation.

lateral demarcation, and mononuclear cell infiltrates are also features of atypical acral (dysplastic) nevi.

The atypical basilar melanocytes in acral nevi and melanoma often have enlarged hyperchromatic nuclei with prominent pleomorphism. Such cells show a contiguous basilar disposition in acral lentiginous melanoma. The dendritic processes of such cells often extend throughout the epidermis and reach the granular layer.

Balloon Cell Nevus

Clinical and Histopathological Features   The balloon cell nevus is a rare variant of melanocytic nevus in which over half of the nevus cell population is composed of balloon nevus cells.[48–51] The balloon cells are admixed with typical nevus cells and cells transitional between ordinary nevus cells and balloon cells.[48–50] The balloon cells are enlarged with clear, foamy, or vacuolated cytoplasm[48] and contain relatively small centrally located, round nuclei with uniform basophilic chromatin. Multinucleate balloon giant cells are commonly observed.

Electron microscopy of balloon cells has demonstrated progressive vacuolization of melanocytes resulting from the enlargement and lysis of melanosomes.[50,51] The latter phenomenon is considered to be a degenerative process, but the pathogenesis for these changes has not been established.[50]

Differential Diagnosis   The primary entity to be distinguished from balloon cell nevus is balloon cell melanoma (BCM) (see below). In contrast to balloon cell nevus, BCM occurs in older patients and is histologically characterized by prominent cytologic atypia and mitotic activity.

Other entities entering into the differential diagnosis include xanthomas, granular cell tumors, and sebaceous neoplasms.[48,49]

Halo Nevus

Synonyms: *leukoderma acquisitum centrifugum, Sutton's nevus, perinevoid vitiligo,* or *perinevoid leukoderma*

The halo nevus is surrounded by a white (hypo- or depigmented) band or halo and histologically has a dense mononuclear cell infiltrate filling the papillary dermis.[52–56] The nevus is almost always acquired, but other types of nevi may develop halos.[52–57]

Halo nevi generally affect individuals under the age of 20,[55,56] and the overall incidence is probably less than 1 percent.[58] There is no difference in incidence between males and females.[55] Approximately 20 percent of individuals with halo nevi have vitiligo, and halo nevi have an association with melanoma and dysplastic nevi.[59]

The natural history of halo nevi has not been well documented. However, in general, the hypopigmentation is thought to develop over weeks to months.[54–56] The central nevus may persist, or more likely, undergoes involution over months to years.

The depigmentation has been ascribed to: (1) an immune response against antigenically altered (perhaps atypical) nevus cells[60,61] or (2) cell-mediated and/or humoral (antibody-mediated) reaction against nonspecifically altered melanocytes and possible cross-reactivity with melanocytes at a distant site or sites.[62]

Clinical Features   The central melanocytic nevus may be relatively flat or raised and dark brown to pink (Table 27-5)[22,54–56] and exhibits surface scale or crusting. The central nevus is surrounded by a well-circumscribed annulus of hypo- or depigmented skin, commonly measures 3 to 6 mm in longest diameter, has regular and well-defined borders and homogeneous coloration.[54–56] The subsequent course of a halo nevus is variable. Both the central nevus and the halo may persist or regress

TABLE 27-5

Halo Nevus and Malignant Melanoma

Halo nevus	Melanoma
Clinical Features	
Central nevus 3–6 mm in size	Usually > 6 mm
Symmetry of central nevus and halo	Asymmetry
Regular borders	Irregular borders
Uniform color of central nevus—tan, brown, or pink halo—hypo- or depigmentation	Haphazard or irregular color
Histopathological Features	
Symmetry	Asymmetry
Usually well circumscribed	Poorly circumscribed
Mononuclear cell infiltrate orderly with well-defined inferior margin	Often variation in pattern of infiltrate
Maturation/differentiation of nevus elements	Usually no maturation
Apoptosis of nevus cells common	Apoptosis may be observed
Rete ridges maintained	Effaced rete ridges common
Little or no cytologic atypia commonly	Prominent cytologic atypia
Few mitoses in dermal component	Mitoses in dermal component frequent
Atypical mitoses usually absent	Atypical mitoses may be observed

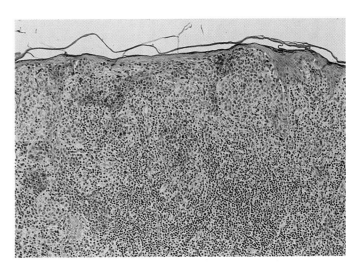

FIGURE 27-10 Halo nevus. Scanning magnification shows dense mononuclear cell infiltrate that obscures junctional and papillary dermal nests of nevus cells.

Most of the infiltrating cells in halo nevi are T lymphocytes and monocyte/macrophages.[59] There are approximately equal numbers of helper/inducer (CD4+) and cytotoxic/suppressor (CD8+) T cells. The nevus cells also express class I HLA antigens to a much greater extent than class II antigens. These findings suggest a specific cell-mediated immune response in halo nevi.[64]

Differential Diagnosis The halo nevus must be distinguished from melanoma. This distinction is not a significant problem for halo nevi showing little or no cytologic atypia (Table 27-5). Such halo nevi generally are small, i.e., less than 5 to 6 mm, symmetric, and have an orderly appearance compared to melanoma. Halo nevi are notable for

completely.[68–70] The central nevus may not change or may become irregularly pigmented or pink or red. Probably over half of all halo nevi undergo complete regression.[54] The period of time associated with nevus regression varies from months to as long as several years.

Halo nevi are most typically located on the upper back but may be found in any location.[54–56] Approximately 25 to 50 percent of affected individuals have two or more halo nevi.

Histopathological Features The halo nevus may be junctional, compound, or dermal.[54–56] In the fully evolved stages, the central nevus is associated with a well-circumscribed, dense, almost bandlike infiltrate of mononuclear cells, almost exclusively lymphocytes and histiocytes, that occupies the papillary dermis and permeates nests of nevus cells (Figs. 27-10 and 27-11) (Table 27-5). It is often difficult to distinguish nevus cells from surrounding mononuclear cells. Degenerating nevus cells can sometimes be identified in this zone. Homogeneous eosinophilic (apoptotic) bodies, representing degenerated cells, are often observed near the dermal-epidermal junction. Occasional nevus cells within the infiltrate show prominent eosinophilic cytoplasm and slightly enlarged nuclei. Although most halo nevi demonstrate no obviously atypical nevus cells, some display varying degrees of cytologic atypia.[24] The peripheral zones of the nevus, corresponding to the clinical halo, show diminished or absent basilar melanocytes and melanin in the basal layer.[56] The papillary dermis in this annulus may also demonstrate slight reparative alteration of the stroma, but usually no inflammatory cell infiltrates are found.[56]

With complete regression, all nevus cells are destroyed with resulting thickening of the papillary dermis, occasional delicate fibroplasia and frequent mucinous alteration, vascular ectasia, variable residual mononuclear cell infiltrates, and melanophages. There may be complete depigmentation of the epidermis. Occasional nevi with typical hypopigmented halos do not exhibit cellular infiltrates.[57–63]

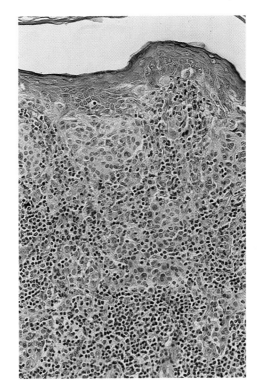

FIGURE 27-11 Halo nevus. Note maturation of nevus cells in dense infiltrate.

the symmetry and well-defined inferior margin of the mononuclear cell infiltrate contained in the papillary dermis. An important feature is the maturation of nevus cells. Although mitotic figures may be noted in the dermal component of any melanocytic lesion, more than a few mitoses, mitoses in the deepest dermal cells, and atypical mitoses are of particular concern.

Lentiginous Junctional Nevus (Nevoid Lentigo, "Jentigo"), Lentiginous Compound Nevus

These nevi show a prominent lentiginous pattern of the epidermis, i.e., elongated epidermal rete, lentiginous melanocytic hyperplasia, and basal layer hypermelanosis (Fig. 27-4).[23] The degree of junctional nesting may vary from almost none (nevoid lentigo) to prominent nesting.

Differential Diagnosis   Lentiginous nevi must be distinguished from dysplastic nevi and lentigo maligna. Lentiginous nevi lack the increased frequency of melanocytic proliferation and the cytologic atypia found in dysplastic nevi and lentigo maligna. In addition, lentigo maligna often exhibits an effacement of the epidermal rete and pronounced involvement of adnexal structures in contrast to lentiginous nevi.

Neural Nevus (Neurotized Nevus)

Neural nevus indicates complete or nearly complete neurotization (maturation to type C cells) of a dermal nevus (Fig. 27-8).[17,18,20,40] In some instances, it may not be possible to distinguish this lesion from a solitary cutaneous neurofibroma. However, nesting of cells suggests a nevus.

Nevus Spilus (Speckled Lentiginous Nevus)

The nevus spilus is a slightly hyperpigmented (tan) macular lesion that contains hyperpigmented foci or speckles that may be either flat or raised.[22,65–69] The nevus spilus may be congenital or acquired and often becomes more prominent after solar exposure.[65] There are several reports of melanoma arising in association with a nevus spilus.[70–72]

Clinical and Histopathological Features   The tan macular area commonly varies from under 1 cm to 10 or 20 cm in greatest diameter.[22,65–69] The hyperpigmented speckles are approximately 1 to 6 mm in greatest diameter and may be macular or papular. Large nevi spili may be unilateral, segmental, or zosteriform (speckled zosteriform lentiginous nevus).[22,68]

The tan macule or patch exhibits lentiginous melanocytic hyperplasia associated with elongated epidermal rete ridges. The hyperpigmented macular foci show lentiginous melanocytic hyperplasia, or junctional nevus, whereas the papular foci contain junctional or compound nevus elements. The histologic changes of spindle and epithelioid cell (Spitz) tumors have been noted in the raised speckled area. Varying degrees of architectural disorder and/or cytologic atypia may be observed in nevus spilus (see discussion of *dysplastic melanocytic nevi*).[70–72]

Differential Diagnosis   The histologic differential diagnosis includes large or congenital lentigo, congenital nevus, and dysplastic nevus. Unless the dark speckles which usually show junctional or compound nevus are present in the biopsy, the histology of nevus spilus may be indistinguishable from lentigo. The clinical features should enable one to recognize nevus spilus.

TABLE 27-6

Recurrent Melanocytic Nevus

Clinical Features

Onset ~ 6 weeks to 6 months after previous surgery
Macular pigmentation
Limited to scar
4–6 mm (usually < 1.5 cm)
Some irregularity of borders often

Histopathological Features

Effacement of epidermis
Dermal scar
Intraepidermal melanocytic proliferation limited to area above scar
Lentiginous or nested pattern of intraepidermal melanocytes
Variable cytologic atypia, usually low-grade

Differential Diagnosis

Dysplastic nevus
Melanoma

Recurrent Melanocytic Nevus

Synonyms: *pseudomelanoma, persistent/recurrent melanocytic nevus*

The recurrent melanocytic nevus shows pigmentation at the site of previous nevus removal or biopsy.[73,74] Most of the recurrences have followed a shave excision. Approximately half of cases recur within 6 months.[73,74] This phenomenon is thought to result from an intraepidermal proliferation of residual melanocytes, possibly from nearby sweat ducts, hair follicles, or intraepidermal melanocytes.[74]

Clinical Features   These lesions are characterized by circumscribed hyperpigmentation within a scar from the previous surgical procedure for nevus removal (Table 27-6).[22,73,74] The lesion is usually macular and exhibits variable irregularity of borders and pigment pattern.[73,74] Most recurrent nevi measure 4 to 6 mm in diameter and almost all are smaller than 1.5 cm.

Histopathological Features   Histologic examination usually reveals intraepidermal melanocytic proliferation confined to the area above a dermal scar (Fig. 27-12) (Table 27-6).[73,74] There is effacement of the epidermal rete ridge pattern and variable lentiginous and/or nested intraepidermal proliferation of melanocytes (Fig. 27-13). The melanocytes often contain abundant melanin and relatively uniform nuclei but occasionally exhibit low-grade cytologic atypia. Dysplastic nevi tend to recur with fairly similar grades of cytologic atypia, compared to the original lesion removed. Frequently, there are residual dermal nevus cells beneath the superficial dermal scar.

Differential Diagnosis   The differential diagnosis includes recurrent atypical (dysplastic) nevus, lentiginous melanocytic proliferations developing in melanoma scars, and recurrent melanoma. In general, the recurrent melanocytic nevus is usually but not always confined to the area of the surgical scar, appears within 6 months of surgery, and exhibits well-defined margins and a banal histologic picture. Recurrent dysplastic nevi may have greater cytologic atypia than conventional recurrent nevi. Clinical features suggesting melanoma include irregular pigmentation, recurrence beyond the confines of the surgical scar, and a longer interval to recurrence (greater than 6 months).

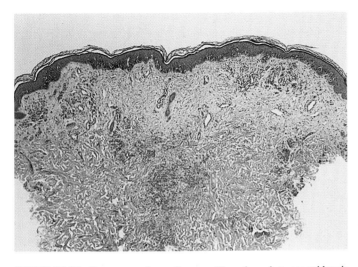

FIGURE 27-12   Recurrent melanocytic nevus. Dermal scar between epidermis and aggregates of residual dermal nevus cells (lower center of field).

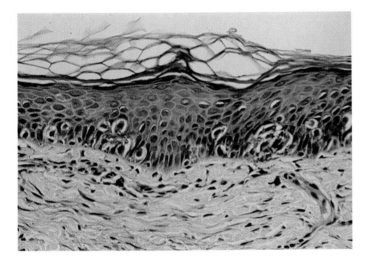

FIGURE 27-13   Recurrent melanocytic nevus. There is irregular intraepidermal melanocytic proliferation. However, significant atypia of melanocytes is not observed.

Review of the previous biopsy is mandatory to rule out an atypical proliferation, particularly melanoma. Reexcision of a recurrent nevus is not necessary unless abnormal features are present, e.g., extension of the lesion beyond the surgical scar or substantial cytologic atypia.

Unusual (or Atypical) Melanocytic Nevi of Genital (Vulvar) Skin

Particular melanocytic nevi occurring on the vulva and in other locations, such as the scrotum or umbilicus, are thought to have distinctive histopathologic features compared to most nevi from nongenital sites.[75,76] As with all melanocytic lesions, how such nevi are selected for removal may influence these observations. The significance of the histologic features of such nevi in terms of melanoma risk and association with an atypical nevus phenotype has not been elucidated and requires further study. Some of the unusual vulvar nevi previously reported exhibit features intermediate between ordinary nevi and melanoma, and thus, share features with dysplastic nevi.

TABLE 27-7

Unusual Genital (Vulvar) Melanocytic Nevi

Clinical Features

Occurrence in premenopausal women (range 14–40 years of age)
Often enlarged, up to 10 mm in diameter
Other features not well studied

Histopathological Features

Symmetric
Well-circumscribed usually
Enlarged junctional nests with diminished cohesion
Lentiginous melanocytic proliferation
Confluence of cells, nests along dermal-epidermal junction
Variation in size, shape, position of junctional nests
Extension of intraepidermal component along adnexal epithelium
Generally no pagetoid spread
Generally no lateral extension
Fibroplasia common, often lamellar
Lymphocytic infiltrates
Cytologic atypia, often slight to moderate
Somewhat enlarged intraepidermal melanocytes, often abundant
    cytoplasm
Multinucleate nevus giant cells
Maturation of nevus cells common

Differential Diagnosis

Vulvar melanoma
Spindle and epithelioid cell (Spitz) tumor
Dysplastic nevus

Clinical and Histopathological Features   Such nevi are often larger (up to 10 to 12 mm) than nongenital ordinary nevi, are often relatively flat but not necessarily so, generally have fairly regular borders, and often are a complex mahogany color, i.e., an admixture of tan, brown, and red (Table 27-7).

In general, these nevi possess an overall symmetry and are well-circumscribed (Table 27-7).[75,76] The most notable features are those shared with dysplastic nevi, namely prominent lentiginous melanocytic proliferation; enlarged junctional nests; variation in the size, shape, position, and reduced cohesion of junctional nests; confluence and bridging of nests; and often cytologic atypia of melanocytes, generally low-grade.[75,76] The intraepidermal melanocytes are often slightly enlarged with abundant cytoplasm, resembling the epithelioid cells in Spitz tumor (Figs. 27-14 and 27-15).

Differential Diagnosis   The differential diagnosis includes melanoma, spindle and epithelioid cell (Spitz) tumors, and dysplastic nevus. Although abnormal architecture and cytologic atypia may be present in these peculiar nevi, these features are not as developed as in melanoma. Melanoma usually demonstrates asymmetry, contiguous proliferation of basilar intraepidermal melanocytes, prominent pagetoid spread, poorly defined margins, greater cytologic atypia, and more developed host response. Vulvar melanoma tends to occur in older women (average age approximately 65 years) compared to these unusual genital nevi (Table 27-7). Spindle and epithelioid cell (Spitz) tumors are recognized by typical enlarged monomorphous epithelioid/fusiform cells. Although these unusual nevi are not considered dysplastic by many, this issue has not been settled. In a general sense, they may qualify as nevi exhibiting architectural disorder and cytologic atypia.

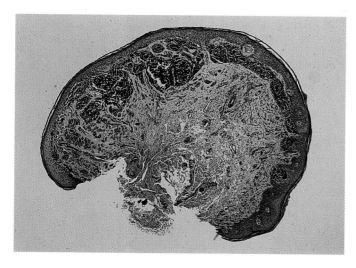

FIGURE 27-14 Vulvar nevus. Note large confluent nests of nevus cells along dermal-epidermal junction.

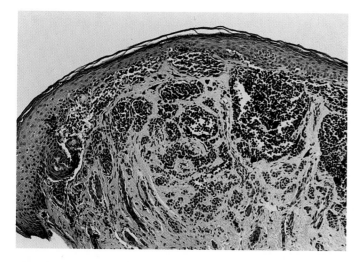

FIGURE 27-15 Vulvar nevus. Irregular, confluent, and bridging nests along dermal-epidermal junction.

CONGENITAL MELANOCYTIC NEVI AND ASSOCIATED NEOPLASMS, CONGENITAL AND CHILDHOOD MELANOMA

The term *congenital nevus* denotes presence at birth.[89,90] However, congenital melanocytic nevi (CMN) also frequently differ from common acquired nevi because of (1) overall size, (2) depth of involvement by nevus cells, (3) adnexal/vascular involvement, and (4) diversity of neurocristic differentiation.[91] Most melanocytic nevi greater than 1.5 cm in diameter are probably congenital.[89] However, smaller CMN may be indistinguishable from acquired nevi.[90,92–94]

Incidence and Melanoma Risk

The significance of CMN, particularly the larger varieties, relates to their risk for progression to melanoma and cosmetic disfigurement.[95–100] There is considerable controversy surrounding the melanoma risk and management of CMN. Accurate estimates of melanoma risk associated with CMN are difficult to obtain. The prevalence of relatively small CMN is approximately 1 percent, and thus these nevi are fairly common.[90,96] However, one particular problem associated with

estimating melanoma risk in these nevi is the lack of specificity of histologic features for CMN of this size.[93] At present, a general estimate of melanoma risk associated with small CMN is approximately 5 percent.[96] However, this may be an overestimate. Giant CMN are rare, with an incidence of approximately 1 in 20,000 births.[101] Very high estimates of melanoma risk associated with large/giant CMN are largely explained by referral bias. A lifetime risk of approximately 6.3 percent has been estimated from the Danish Birth Registry.[102,103]

Clinical Features   The clinical characteristics of CMN are related to size and age.[22,89,90,95,96] Small congenital nevi less than 1.5 cm in greatest diameter may be indistinguishable from common acquired nevi, and documentation at birth may be the only means of confirming a congenital origin.[96] In general, CMN in the range of 1.5 to 10 or 20 cm in diameter are well-circumscribed and have elongate or oval morphology and an orderly distribution of pigment (Table 27-8).[89] Most of these nevi are brown, but they range in color from tan to dark brown or black. A speckled or mottled appearance is also common, and many have coarse, terminal hair follicles.

Giant CMN often involve a large portion of the dorsal surface of the individual and are most commonly raised and exhibit a variably papular, lumpy, rugose, or even verrucous surface (Table 27-9). The skin surface may be shiny or contain numerous terminal hairs. Soft-tissue hypertrophy may mimic changes found in neurofibromatosis. The color is most often a dark brown or black, but considerable variegation of pigment is often noted. Giant CMN are also remarkable for scattered, smaller satellite nevi on the skin surface beyond the garment nevus.[95,96]

TABLE 27-8

Small- and Medium-Sized Congenital Nevi

Clinical Features

May occur anywhere but head and neck common
Symmetry
< 1.5 to 20 cm
Round, oval, elongate
Tan, brown, dark brown, often mahogany; or black
Slightly raised plaque
Pebbled or rugose surface
Coarse hairs often

Histopathological Features

Lentiginous melanocytic hyperplasia often
Junctional, compound or dermal
Small congenital nevi (< 1.5 cm)
   Involvement of upper half of reticular dermis common
     Interstitial pattern
     Perivascular, periadnexal pattern
Medium-sized congenital nevi (1.5 to 20 cm)
   Involvement of reticular dermis, particularly lower half
     Diffuse dermal involvement by nevus cells
     Interstitial pattern
     "Inflammatory" pattern
   Nevus cells within appendages, blood vessels, nerves

Differential Diagnosis

Becker's nevus
Dysplastic nevus
Epidermal nevus
Congenital lentigo
Melanoma

Large or Giant Congenital Nevi

Clinical Features

Symmetry
> 20 cm
Involvement of major anatomic area, segmental
Often dorsal involvement
Occasional congenital deformities
Well-defined borders
Brown, dark brown, black
"Animal pelt" features, rugose, doughy
Soft-tissue hypertrophy
Hypertrichosis
Scattered satellite nevi distant from giant nevus
Involvement of meninges common for head and neck nevi

Histopathological Features

Lentiginous melanocytic hyperplasia common
Usually compound or dermal
Reticular dermal involvement, superficial and deep, usually
    Diffuse
    Interstitial
    Perivascular, periadnexal
Subcutaneous involvement, septal > > lobular
Maturation
Neural differentiation, neuroid or neurofibromalike pattern,
    on occasion
Wagner-Meissner-like corpuscles
Fascial or muscle involvement
Cellular nodules in reticular dermis, on occasion
Blue nevus component, on occasion
Spindle and epithelioid cell tumor component, on occasion
Hamartomatous elements
    Cartilaginous differentiation
    Adipose differentiation

Differential Diagnosis

Becker's nevus
Neurofibromatosis
Melanoma
Peripheral nerve sheath tumors

Histopathological Features The histological characteristics observed in CMN are related to the size of the nevus primarily and to a lesser degree the age of the individual (Tables 27-8 and 27-9).[23,90,93,94,98,100,104,105] There is now evidence that the depth of nevus cell involvement throughout the dermis and subcutis is established early and remains for the most part unchanged.[96,105] However, the superficial (intraepidermal and superficial dermal) components of a CMN may mature in some instances. It is believed that immature disordered patterns such as pagetoid spread, large irregular nests, and cytologic atypia do diminish (or mature) with time.[105,106] However, the latter conclusion must be made with some circumspection because of the rather prominent morphologic heterogeneity throughout many CMN.[105]

Small CMN may display considerable heterogeneity.[90,92,93] Some may be entirely junctional and indistinguishable from acquired nevi.[90,105,107] Many small nevi, particularly those measuring less than 1.5 cm in diameter, also demonstrate what has been termed a superficial pattern,[94,105] i.e., junctional nests alone or a compound or entirely dermal pattern with aggregates of nevus cells extending to no greater depth

than the upper half of the reticular dermis. Such a pattern may be seen in a significant percentage of acquired nevi. Up to 28 percent of acquired nevi may also exhibit nevus cells extending into the lower two-thirds of the reticular dermis.[93]

Histologic features considered characteristic of CMN[89,93,94] include involvement of the lower third of the reticular dermis by nevus cells, and close association of nevus cells with or within appendageal and neurovascular structures at the midreticular dermal level or deeper (Figs. 27-16 to 27-18).[89] In contradistinction to acquired nevi, CMN are notable for nevus cells being disposed, "fanning out," or splaying collagen bundles of the reticular dermis as single cells, files, sheets, and cords of cells (two cells in tandem). CMN also show a typical pattern of maturation of nevus cells from superficial to deep dermis. Near the epidermal surface, nevus cells tend to be aggregated in nests and may exhibit epithelioid cell features.[89,105] With increasing depth, the nevus cells often demonstrate greater separation, i.e., splaying, and slightly diminished cellular and nuclear sizes. Extension of nevus cells into the subcutaneous fat is also a common feature, particularly in larger varieties of congenital nevi.[89,105]

With increasing sizes of CMN, there is greater tendency for deep dermal, appendageal, and neurovascular involvement.[93,94,100,105] However, even some congenital nevi less than 1.5 cm in diameter tend to involve eccrine and follicular units at the midreticular dermal level or deeper, much more commonly than acquired nevi.[96]

Because of histologic overlap between small CMN and acquired nevi, there are no features with 100 percent specificity and 100 percent sensitivity for recognition of small CMN.[93] Nonetheless, the presence of nevus cells in the lower half of the reticular dermis, in an appendageal/neurovascular pattern, or in both will enable one to detect a majority of small CMN.[93] Absence of the latter features does not preclude a congenital origin.[93,108]

Giant CMN, most medium-size CMN, and a small percentage of nevi less than 10 cm in diameter tend to exhibit distinctive features (Table 27-9).[93–95,100,104,105] Probably the most characteristic feature is the diffuse proliferation of nevus cells throughout the reticular dermis with frequent extension into the subcutaneous fat.[89,94,95,100,105] There is usually a grenz zone separating the epidermis from the dermal infiltration of nevus cells[100,108]; however, junctional nests may be noted. The nevus cells tend to infiltrate collagen in an orderly and uniform pattern. The nevus cells also often extend along the fibrous trabeculae of the subcutaneous fat and occasionally infiltrate fat lobules.[89,105] Aggregates

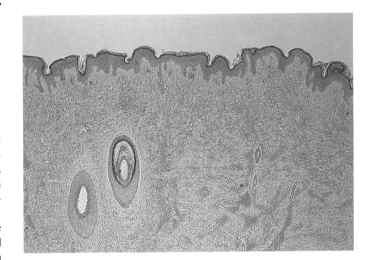

FIGURE 27-16 Small congenital nevus. There are aggregates of nevus cells in papillary dermis and distributed throughout reticular dermis in association with blood vessels and adnexal structures.

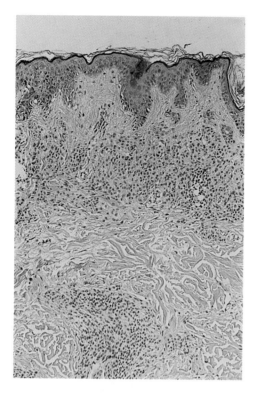

FIGURE 27-17 Small congenital nevus. Discrete nests of nevus cells in dermis.

of nevus cells also tend to cuff or infiltrate follicular epithelium, sebaceous glands, eccrine ducts and glands, the perineurium of nerve twigs, and the walls of vascular structures.[89,92,93,105] The perivascular and periadnexal cuffing by nevus cells may closely resemble an inflammatory process such as a gyrate erythema. Foci of hypercellularity are also sometimes noted within the dermal population of cells.[105]

A subset of large/giant CMN are also characterized by spindle cell or neuroidal differentiation resembling a neurofibroma (neuroid CMN).[95,109] The constituent cells have a wavy configuration and are embedded in a delicate stroma. Neural differentiation resembling neural tubules or pseudo-Meissnerian structures also may occur.[89,95,109] Such nevi may be associated with congenital anomalies such as clubfoot and spina bifida.[109]

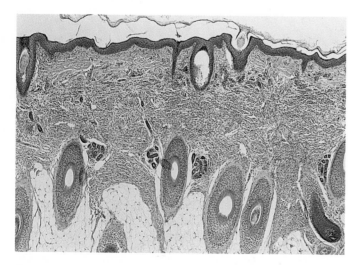

FIGURE 27-18 Giant congenital nevus. Nevus cells diffusely infiltrate dermis.

TABLE 27-10

Intraepidermal and Dermal Proliferations Developing in Large/Giant Congenital Nevi

Benign	Indeterminate/malignant
Epithelioid cell	
Intraepidermal	
Pagetoid spread in nevi	Pagetoid melanoma
Dermal	
Expansile nodule of epithelioid cells	Melanoma, epithelioid cell type
Epithelioid schwannoma	Malignant epithelioid schwannoma
Pigmented spindle cell	
Dermal	
Expansile nodule of spindle cells	Melanoma, pigmented spindle-cell type
Spindle cell with schwannian/ perineurial differentiation	
Dermal	
Neurofibromalike tumor	
Schwannoma	Malignant peripheral nerve sheath tumor
Small round cell	
Dermal	
Expansile nodule of small cells	Small cell melanoma ("lymphoblastic"-type melanoma)
Specific mesenchymal ("ectomesenchymal") differentiation	
Cartilage	
Lipoma	Rhabdomyosarcoma
Hemangioma	
Neuronal elements	
Ganglioneuroma	Ganglioneuroblastoma
Unclassified or undifferentiated neoplasms	Undifferentiated sarcoma

SOURCE: *Adapted from Hendrickson and Ross.*[110]

Large CMN may also show a variety of other patterns suggesting that they are indeed hamartomas of neural crest differentiation.[104] Such nevi may contain heterologous elements such as cartilage, bone, adipose tissue, vascular malformation, hemangioma, lymphangioma, mastocytoma, and schwannoma.[89,95,96,104,109] Foci suggesting blue nevus, cellular blue nevus, and spindle and epithelioid cell nevus are occasionally noted.

Congenital Nevi with Atypical Features

All varieties of congenital nevi may exhibit varying degrees of architectural and cytologic atypia of both the intraepidermal and dermal components (Table 27-10).[104,105] Perhaps one of the most common findings is lentiginous melanocytic proliferation, which may occur with or without variation in junctional nesting and/or cytologic atypia of the intraepidermal melanocytes.[105]

Intraepidermal Pagetoid Spread of Melanocytes

Another common finding, particularly in CMN in individuals under the age of 10 years and especially in the first year of life, is upward migration of intraepidermal melanocytes.[105,106,110-112] Although the latter changes may be alarming, the proliferation is usually orderly and often confined to the lower half of the epidermis, and cytologic atypia is absent or low-grade.[105] One may encounter a spectrum of atypicality within the intraepidermal component, ranging from little or no atypia to frank melanoma in situ.

Dermal Nodular Proliferations

Large/giant CMN may give rise to intradermal nodular melanocytic proliferations (Fig. 27-19) (Table 27-10). Such proliferations may occur in the superficial or deep reticular dermis and be composed of epithelioid, spindled, or small cells.[104,105,110–112] Varying degrees of cytologic atypia, mitotic activity, and occasionally necrosis may be observed. Most of these cellular aggregates tend to blend with the surrounding nevus. The vast majority of such proliferations, particularly in the neonatal period, are biologically benign, despite atypical histologic features. Small round cell tumors should be evaluated especially carefully for malignancy. Many of these nodular proliferations are composed of enlarged epithelioid or spindled cells containing granular cytoplasmic melanin. Usually the melanin does not have the finely divided ("dusty") character observed in melanoma cells. The nuclei also tend to be uniform, compared to the pleomorphism and clumped chromatin of melanoma cells.[105]

Melanoma Developing in Congenital Nevi

Conventional melanoma originating from an intraepidermal location occurs most commonly in relatively small CMN (Table 27-10).[100,110] Such melanomas are usually of the pagetoid or nodular type. However, such melanomas are uncommonly observed in large/giant CMN.[110,111] The great majority of melanomas developing in the latter setting are dermal and composed of epithelioid cells, spindle cells, or small round cells resembling malignant lymphoma (Figs. 27-20 and 27-21) (Table 27-10).[95,104,110–112] Some melanomas may have the characteristics of malignant blue nevus or malignant epithelioid schwan-

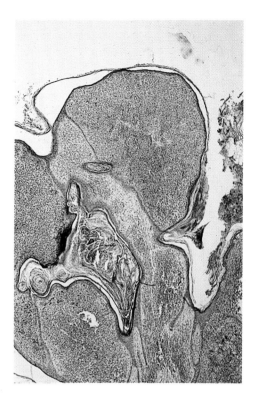

FIGURE 27-20   Small-cell (verrucous) melanoma. Diffuse sheet of small cells in dermis.

noma.[110,113] Such tumors usually manifest cohesive cellular nodules distinctly different from the surrounding nevus, substantial nuclear pleomorphism, necrotic cells, mitotic activity, and striking cellularity.[110–112] Interpretation of such tumors may be exceedingly difficult, and a final diagnosis of benign or malignant tumor may not be possible.

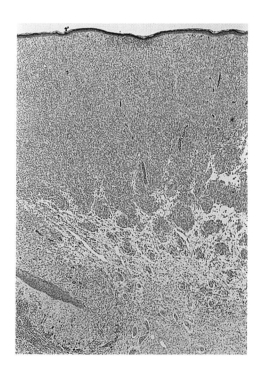

FIGURE 27-19   Atypical nodular spindle-cell proliferation in giant congenital nevus of newborn. Cellular nodules of relatively small spindle cells are present.

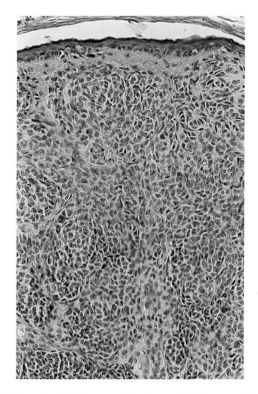

FIGURE 27-21   Small-cell (verrucous) melanoma. Uniform population of cells resembling lymphoma. The patient died of metastases.

Melanomas developing in newborns and infants under a year of age are extremely rare and such a diagnosis must always be seriously questioned.[111–112] Furthermore, the vast majority of epithelioid and spindle cell nodular proliferations developing in CMN, particularly in young individuals, are benign or not aggressive.[105,111,112] A prudent approach is to ensure complete surgical removal of such nodular lesions and to carefully monitor the patient for recurrence or metastasis. However, many of the true biologic melanomas arising in giant CMN are of the small-cell type.[95,104,110–112] The cells are disposed in sheets in a delicate myxoid stroma.[104,110] The cells are closely crowded, have minimal cytoplasm, and contain small round or slightly oval nuclei with dense, uniformly dispersed chromatin. The cells take on the appearance of lymphoblastic lymphoma or comparable "blastic" tumors. Mitotic figures and nuclear debris are also commonly observed.

Other Mesenchymal Tumors

Giant CMN may exhibit specific mesenchymal differentiation and rarely give rise to hamartomatous mesenchymal tumors containing cartilage, vascular channels, and other elements.[110] Rarely liposarcoma, rhabdomyosarcoma, ganglioneuroblastoma, and other primitive sarcomas have been reported to arise in giant congenital nevi.[104,110]

Leptomeningeal Melanocytosis (Neurocutaneous Melanosis)

CMN, not necessarily large or giant, involving the scalp, neck, or posterior midline may be associated with melanocytic proliferations localized to the cranial and/or spinal leptomeninges.[95,96,104] Histologically, aggregates of melanocytes are present in the basal subarachnoid cisterns. The latter lesion may be asymptomatic or result in hydrocephalus, either communicating or noncommunicating type; seizures; mental retardation; other neurologic signs; and leptomeningeal melanoma. Meningeal biopsy may be necessary to confirm a diagnosis of leptomeningeal melanocytosis.

Focal Melanocytic Aggregates in Skin, Placenta, and Lymph Nodes Associated with Large/Giant Congenital Nevi

Occasional reports have highlighted melanocytic lesions or satellites identified in the skin, placenta, and lymph nodes of patients with large/giant CMN.[114,115] Explanations for these peculiar lesions have included arrested or aberrant migration of neural crest elements during embryogenesis and benign metastases from the large CMN.

Differential Diagnosis   The differential diagnosis for small CMN less than 1.5 cm in diameter is primarily that of acquired melanocytic nevi and dysplastic nevi. Since there are no specific features for small CMN histologically, the distinction from acquired nevi often rests on documentation at birth. Acquired dysplastic nevi are superficial proliferations that often involve the papillary dermis, resulting in a compound nevus.

One particular problem associated with CMN is the presence of prominent upward migration of melanocytic cells throughout the epidermis in congenital nevi of children and particularly neonates. These proliferations suggest melanoma in situ or even invasive melanoma. However, in general, the pattern within the epidermis has an orderly character and many of the cells do not reach the granular layer. Furthermore, careful examination will reveal low-grade or no cytologic atypia of these cells. In our experience and in the experience of others, virtually all these proliferations are benign.

Another diagnostic difficulty is the distinction of tumoral dermal nodules in large CMN from melanoma. Relatively small nodules generally measuring less than 1 cm in greatest diameter are common in giant CMN. These nodules exhibit compact cellularity, and the constituent cells are usually larger and exhibit variable degrees of cytologic atypia. The distinction from melanoma relates to the gradual blending of the cellular nodule with the surrounding nevus. Necrotic cells, significant cytologic atypia, and easily found mitotic activity are also features suggesting melanoma. Age is a significant factor to be considered in the evaluation of these proliferations. A diagnosis of melanoma should be made with extreme caution in individuals under the age of 1 year.[105,111,112]

Congenital Melanoma

Melanoma at birth is exceedingly rare and may be classified into three varieties.[116–119] Only a few cases of the first type have been reported (reviewed in Trozak and coworkers), and this type is characterized by maternal melanoma metastatic to the fetus.[117–119] Neonates usually present at birth with widespread visceral metastases and are dead of disease within days to months. The placenta usually shows metastatic melanoma. Primary congenital melanoma may develop de novo or in association with a giant congenital nevus. Only a small number of cases of either type has been reported.[117–119]

Because of the extreme rarity of these lesions, a diagnosis of congenital or neonatal melanoma must be viewed with considerable skepticism.[105,111,112] Virtually all such lesions are biologically benign.

Childhood Melanoma

The incidence of melanoma increases with age but is exceptionally rare in prepubertal individuals (estimated incidence approximately 0.4 percent among all melanomas)[116–121] and uncommon under the age of 20 years (incidence approximately 2 percent).[118–120] With the realization that many cases of childhood melanoma in the past had been considered to be spindle and epithelioid cell (Spitz) tumors or atypical proliferations in CMN, it has become evident that melanoma is much less common and may have no better prognosis in children compared to adults.[116–122] Analysis of melanomas in individuals under the age of 20 seems to show fairly similar clinical and histologic features compared to melanomas in adults.[120] However, probably too few cases of melanoma have been reported in prepubescent children to make any definitive statements about melanomas in this age group. A recent study from Children's Hospital in Boston has described three variants of childhood melanoma: (1) adult variants, (2) small-cell variants, and (3) Spitz-like melanomas (including metastasizing Spitz tumors).[121] It will be necessary to obtain such information from multiple centers or through a central registry.

SPITZ TUMOR AND VARIANTS

Synonyms: *Spitz's nevus, spindle and epithelioid cell nevus, nevus of large spindle and/or epithelioid cells, spindle cell nevus, juvenile melanoma, benign juvenile melanoma*

The spindle and epithelioid cell tumor is a melanocytic, usually acquired, proliferation with a distinct histopathologic appearance. The characteristics that set this lesion apart from other nevi are large epithelioid and/or spindle cells in varying proportions.[123,124] The lesion is frequently misdiagnosed as melanoma.

TABLE 27-11

Spitz Tumor

Clinical Features

Configuration: plaque, papule, or nodule, often dome-shaped
Size: small (usually < 1 cm)
Profile: smooth surface topography
Color: pink/red; darker forms occur
Age: majority in children and adolescents
Location: face and extremities, most common
Number: usually solitary; rare multiple forms occur
Symptoms: commonly asymptomatic; rarely pruritic
History of growth: months; usually less than a year

Histopathological Features

Cytologic features
    Spindle and/or epithelioid cell type*
    Overall monomorphous population of cells*
    Occasional striking pleomorphism in a minority of cells
Architectural features
    Symmetry*
    Sharp lateral demarcation*
    Zonation in depth (e.g., "maturation")*
    Orderly nondisruptive infiltration of collagen by Spitz melanocytic*
        cells
Other helpful diagnostic features
    Absent or rare, but not atypical, mitoses in deep parts*
    Giant melanocytic cells
    Irregular contours of growth at deep margin*
    Kamino bodies
    Paucity or absence of single-cell upward spread
    Junctional clefts
    Loss of cohesion between cells (retraction spaces)
    Perivascular or diffuse inflammatory infiltrate
    Superficial distribution of pigmentation
    Telangiectasia and edema
    Epidermal hyperplasia

Differential Diagnosis

Melanocytic lesions
    Malignant melanoma
    Dysplastic nevi with features of Spitz tumor
    Variants of nevi with spindle and/or epithelioid cells
        Pigmented spindle cell tumor
        Desmoplastic Spitz tumor
        Plexiform spindle cell nevus/deep-penetrating nevus
        Cellular blue nevus
        Various "combined" nevi
Nonmelanocytic lesions
    Epithelioid cell histiocytoma
    Reticulohistiocytoma
    Cellular neurothekeoma

*Most helpful features

Clinical Features

Spitz tumors most often present as a solitary, asymptomatic, red/pink or flesh-colored, hairless, dome-shaped, smooth nodule measuring less than 1 cm in diameter (Table 27-11).[22,23,96,125–134] Some lesions may be tan, brown, or even black in color. Pedunculated and polypoid forms occur.[126] Spitz tumors may involve any site; however, they are more common on the face and the extremities. Spitz tumors may be slightly more common in females.

Multiple Spitz tumors may occur in either a grouped (agminate) or disseminated pattern.[96,135] The disseminated type is characterized by numerous (up to hundreds) Spitz tumors all over the body, typically sparing the palms, soles, and mucous membranes.

The vast majority of lesions with characteristics of Spitz tumors are benign. However, because of the histologic resemblance of Spitz tumors to some melanomas, the presence of atypical variants, and rare metastases from such lesions, there is some justification for the belief that uncommonly or rarely melanoma may develop in association with Spitz tumors. The exact nature and classification of these lesions awaits definitive study. An aggressive variant termed malignant Spitz tumor has been reported to result in regional lymph node metastases (see below).[136]

Histopathological Features

The majority of Spitz tumors (about two-thirds or more) are compound, 5 to 10 percent of the cases are junctional, and 12 to 20 percent are dermal (see Figs. 27-22 to 27-28).[96,132,133,137]

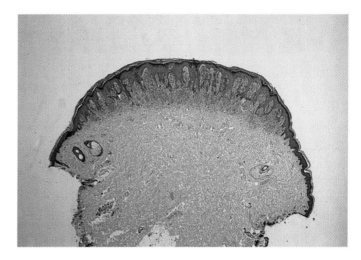

FIGURE 27-22   Spitz tumor. Note small size, dome-shaped morphology, striking symmetry, and sharp lateral demarcation.

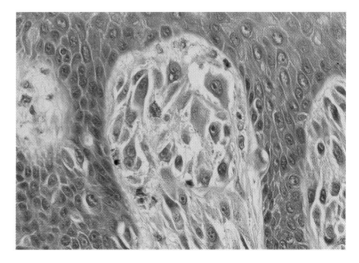

FIGURE 27-23   Spitz tumor. Large epithelioid cells and spindle cells in papillary dermis. Note angular contours of cells; some are triangular, rhomboidal, and polygonal in morphology. The cytoplasm is pink with a ground-glass appearance. Many nuclei contain prominent nucleoli.

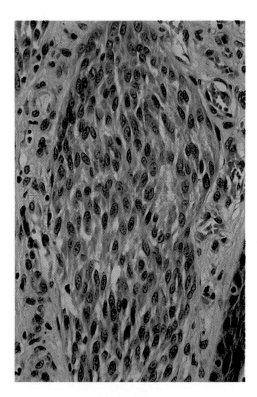

FIGURE 27-24   Spitz tumor. Fascicles of spindle cells with abundant cytoplasm. Note striking uniformity of spindle cells. The cells have abundant pink cytoplasm. Also note uniformity of nuclei with evenly dispersed chromatin.

The most distinctive histologic features and an absolute prerequisite for diagnosis are large spindle-shaped and/or epithelioid melanocytes (Figs. 27-23 and 27-24) (Table 27-11).[132] The *spindle cells* are elongated, fusiform, and often plump (Fig. 27-24) and may exhibit dendrites. The cells possess centrally located nuclei, comparable in size to or even larger than nuclei of keratinocytes (Fig. 27-24). Nuclear contours are typically smooth and regular. The chromatin pattern is usually finely dispersed or slightly vesicular. Typically, a distinct, single, centrally located, round eosinophilic or amphophilic nucleolus is present. The spindle cells are arranged in fascicles or elongated nests, characteristically in vertical orientation or concentric arrangements within nests.

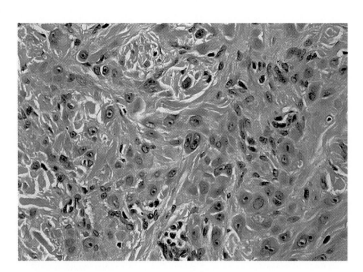

FIGURE 27-25   Spitz tumor. Base of Spitz tumor shows orderly infiltration of collagen by individual cells (maturation).

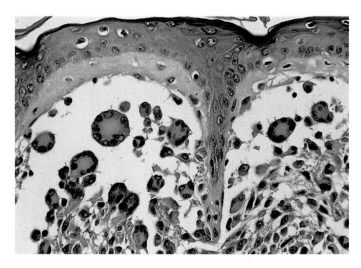

FIGURE 27-26   Spitz tumor. Nevus giant cells in papillary dermis. There is prominent discohesion.

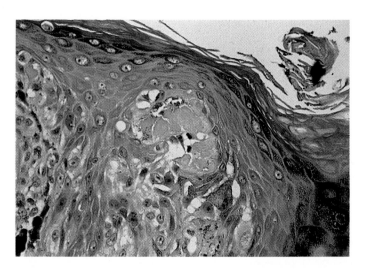

FIGURE 27-27   Spitz tumor. Within the epidermis above dermal papilla is a coalescent aggregate of eosinophilic globules (Kamino bodies).

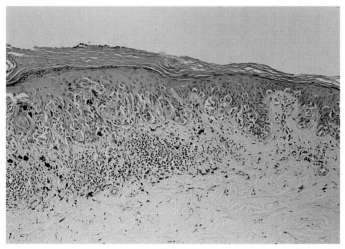

FIGURE 27-28   Spitz tumor with architectural disorder and cytologic atypia. The lesion demonstrates architectural disorder as indicated by lentiginous melanocytic proliferation and variation in junctional nesting pattern.

The *epithelioid cells* are large, round, oval, polygonal, rhomboidal, or polyangular cells with distinct cellular borders (Fig. 27-23) and nuclei that are similar to those in the spindle cells but also sometimes irregularly shaped or lobulated. Multinucleated cells are often seen when epithelioid forms constitute the predominant cell type (Fig. 27-26). The cytoplasm of the spindle and epithelioid cells is usually abundant with a homogeneous eosinophilic or bluish, sometimes "ground-glass," appearance. Melanin is typically absent or scarce.

The two cell types may be admixed in varying proportions, but either may occur alone. Regardless of the proportion of spindle or epithelioid cells, one of the most characteristic features of Spitz tumor is the uniformity of the cells and nuclei. From side to side in horizontal zones, the cells tend to show a strikingly uniform appearance and size. In all age groups, Spitz tumors with predominant spindle cell morphology are the most common type and are especially prevalent in adults.[128,129] Spitz tumors of the epithelioid cell type are observed mainly in childhood.

Whereas spindle and/or epithelioid cells are a prerequisite for diagnosis, they must appear in an appropriate architectural arrangement. The major architectural criteria include symmetry, sharp lateral demarcation, size (generally smaller than 1cm), maturation (zonation), lack of deep extension, and lack of significant pagetoid spread. These and other criteria, such as few or no deeply located mitoses and the lack of significant cytologic atypia, which are thought to reflect ordered growth, favor benignancy.[23]

MATURATION (ZONATION)

Maturation (zonation) refers to the appearance of layers of differing morphology from "top to bottom."[23] There is transition from larger nests at the dermal-epidermal junction to smaller nests and single cells near the deep margin of the nevus. With this transition from top to bottom, the cellular elements exhibit a nondisruptive insinuation among collagen bundles without induction of new stroma (Fig. 27-25). The distribution of pigment also may be zonal. If melanin is present in Spitz tumors, it is largely confined to cells immediately subjacent to the epidermis.[132] The cytologic features of the spindle and/or epithelioid cells may change from above downward, leading to a gradient in cell size and shape, such as from large plump cells at the top to smaller or slender cells at the bottom.

ABSENT OR RARE MITOSES IN DEEP PARTS

Mitoses are variable; they may be numerous, rare, or absent. Mitoses most commonly occur in the upper portion of the lesion and are usually bipolar. Although an occasional mitosis in the deeper parts of the lesion or a rare atypical mitosis may be observed, they should nonetheless prompt careful evaluation for melanoma.[23,134]

KAMINO BODIES

Eosinophilic amorphous globules, either singly or in aggregates, at the dermal-epidermal junction occur frequently in Spitz tumors (Fig. 27-27)[138] and are useful since they are found less frequently in melanoma. However, they are nonspecific.[132] Ultrastructurally, Kamino bodies are composed of amorphous masses and bundles of filaments.[139] Immunohistochemically, they contain basement membrane components, including collagen types IV and VII, as well as laminin.[140] Degenerate material derived from melanocytes and keratinocytes may also be present.[138]

PAGETOID SPREAD

Pagetoid spread of single melanocytes occurs less commonly in Spitz tumor than in melanoma.[23,132,134] Upward migration of melanocytes in Spitz tumor usually takes the form of transepidermal elimination of nests of two or more cells.

JUNCTIONAL CLEAVAGE

At the dermal-epidermal junction, the fascicles of spindle cells are often separated by a cleftlike retraction space from the adjacent epidermis, a result of tissue shrinkage during processing (Fig. 27-26).[132]

ADNEXAL INVOLVEMENT

Spitz tumors and its variants have a propensity to involve hair follicles and eccrine ducts. In most instances, intraepidermal fascicles of cells track along the adventitial sheaths of appendageal structures into the papillary dermis and often into the reticular dermis.

PERIVASCULAR OR DIFFUSE INFLAMMATORY INFILTRATE

The distribution of the inflammatory infiltrate tends to be perivascular but may also be diffuse in some Spitz tumors.[132]

EPIDERMAL HYPERPLASIA

Epidermal hyperplasia is a common finding in Spitz tumors.

Spitz Tumor with Architectural Disorder and Cytologic Atypia (Atypical Spitz Tumor)

Spitz tumors with atypical features are encountered not uncommonly, yet standardized criteria for recognizing or categorizing such lesions are not available.[23,134] In general, atypical features may be subdivided into those involving primarily the epidermis and/or the dermis/subcutis (Table 27-12).

Atypical Features of the Intraepidermal Component

Spitz tumors (and pigmented spindle cell tumors) may show morphologic features of conventional dysplastic nevi and thus may be considered to have architectural disorder and/or cytologic atypia (melanocytic dysplasia) (Table 27-12).[23,134,141] The essential criteria for diagnosis are (1) disordered architectural patterns of the intraepidermal component, i.e., lentiginous melanocytic proliferation and/or significant variation in junctional nesting (variation in size, shape, orientation, spacing of junctional nests; horizontal confluence and bridging of nests; diminished cellular cohesion of nests), and (2) cytologic atypia of melanocytes (Fig. 27-28). The features of such Spitz tumors are outlined in Table 27-12.

Intraepidermal or Mainly Intraepidermal Spitz Tumors with Prominent Pagetoid Spread (Pagetoid Spitz Tumor)

A distinctive variant is the mainly intraepidermal subtype with a prominent pagetoid pattern.[23,134,142] This variant may occur anywhere but is most commonly encountered on the lower extremities of young women. The most important reason for recognizing this lesion is its frequent

Spitz Tumor/Pigmented Spindle Cell Tumor with Architectural Disorder and Cytologic Atypia

Intraepidermal variant
  Architectural disorder
    Disordered intraepidermal melanocytic proliferation:*
      Lentiginous or single-cell pattern*
      Disordered junctional nesting*
        Variation in size, shape, orientation, spacing, cellular
          cohesion of nests
        Horizontal confluence and bridging of nests
      Pagetoid spread
    Asymmetry
    Poorly circumscribed
    Lateral extension of intraepidermal component ("shoulder
      phenomenon")
  Cytologic atypia*
    Nuclear pleomorphism
    Variation in nuclear chromatin patterns
    Nuclear enlargement
    Variation in nucleoli
  Host response
    Patchy to bandlike mononuclear infiltrates in papillary dermis
    Fibroplasia
Dermal variant
  Architectural disorder*
    Expansile nodules
    Increased cellularity
    Loss of cellular cohesion
    Asymmetry
    Deep extension
    Lack of maturation or orderly infiltration of collagen
    Ulceration
    Necrosis
  Cytologic atypia (as above)
  Mitotic activity
    Numerous mitoses
    Mitoses at base of lesion
    Atypical mitoses
  Host response
    Prominent mononuclear cell infiltrates
    Formation of tumor stroma

*Essential criteria for diagnosis

misdiagnosis as in situ or microinvasive melanoma. Most lesions measure less than 5 or 6 mm.[142]

Scanning magnification usually discloses a mainly intraepidermal proliferation of enlarged epithelioid cells usually devoid of melanin (Fig. 27-29) with an overall symmetry from side to side and reasonably well defined margins.[142] However, some lesions have ill-defined margins. Many of these lesions show a combination of both a single-cell and nested proliferation of epithelioid melanocytes. The single-cell proliferative pattern is often both basilar and pagetoid and commonly varies within the lesion. Typical junctional nests of epithelioid cells with associated clefting are also usually present and may be quite small in size. Nests of cells or single Spitz tumor cells may or may not be present in the papillary dermis. Often the degree of pagetoid spread is focal or limited; however, it may be prominent in some lesions, raising the possibility of melanoma in situ (Fig. 27-29).

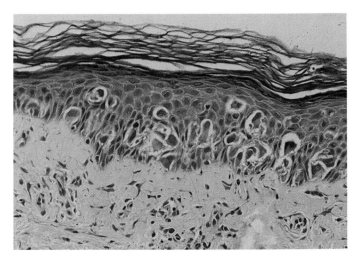

FIGURE 27-29 Pagetoid Spitz tumor. Pagetoid spread suggests melanoma in situ. Note characteristic cytologic details of Spitz tumor cells. The cells are polyangular, containing abundant ground-glass cytoplasm, and the nuclei have dispersed chromatin.

Atypical Features of the Dermal Component

Atypicality of the dermal component includes cohesive cellular nodules, increased cellularity, diminished cellular cohesion, asymmetry, deep extension into the lowermost dermis or subcutis, lack of maturation or orderly infiltration of collagen, cytologic atypia, mitotic activity especially deep, and mononuclear infiltrates (Fig. 27-30).[23,134] Because of the rarity of such lesions and the lack of sufficient follow-up in many instances, the significance of these various features has not been elucidated. There is little question that the presence of these various features in any given lesion is highly worrisome for melanoma and that as these features increase in number and severity, the likelihood of melanoma increases.

In evaluating such lesions, a number of factors should be weighed in the final interpretation (Table 27-13). Clinical factors such as the age of the patient, location of the tumor, clinical appearance, history of recent change in a long-standing stable lesion, size greater than 1 cm, and family history of melanoma should be carefully considered. The older the patient, especially individuals beyond the age of 30 years, the much greater the likelihood of malignancy. As a general rule, one's threshold for diagnosing melanoma in such lesions should correlate inversely with the age of the patient, i.e., a high threshold for very young individuals and a lower threshold for elderly individuals. The location of atypical tumors on sites less commonly involved by Spitz tumors, such as the back, is also another such factor suggesting careful scrutiny of the lesion for melanoma. If after weighing these various factors, one cannot make a clear-cut diagnosis of melanoma, a practical approach is to communicate this situation to the clinician and patient.

Differential Diagnosis   The intraepidermal or junctional variants of Spitz tumors must first of all be discriminated from in situ or early invasive melanoma. These intraepidermal Spitz tumors often show relatively small size, symmetry, evidence of growth control, and sharp circumscription compared to melanoma. Of particular importance are the cytologic characteristics of the epithelioid cells; they tend to be fairly monotypic with abundant pinkish cytoplasm that has a ground-glass appearance, rather than the granular cytoplasm often observed in melanoma cells. The nuclei of Spitz tumor cells are also fairly uniform with evenly dispersed chromatin versus the pleomorphism of melanoma cells.

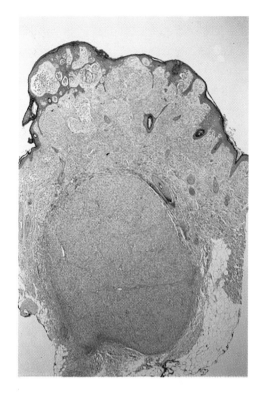

FIGURE 27-30   Atypical Spitz tumor. The lesion is dome-shaped and fairly symmetric but is characterized by an expansile cellular nodule with only slight maturation.

Compound and dermal Spitz tumors and their atypical variants must also be discriminated from invasive melanoma. The features outlined above and listed in Table 27-13 provide guidelines for this distinction. However, many Spitz lesions show atypical features. The absence or incomplete development of major diagnostic features, such as symmetry or sharply demarcated lateral borders, are of concern and should prompt a careful search for features of melanoma. Even if symmetry and sharp lateral demarcation are observed, the presence of extensive pagetoid spread, the lack of maturation in depth, prominent cellularity of the dermal component, nuclear pleomorphism of more than a small proportion of cells, cohesive cellular nodules in the dermis, or deeply located (albeit rare) mitoses are worrisome.

Detailed knowledge of diagnostic criteria and their relative weight are critical in the histologic assessment of such atypical lesions. When an atypical lesion is present, the author considers it appropriate to comment whether the lesion shows only slight atypicality or whether its features approach melanoma. Depending on the severity of the atypia, one should acknowledge that melanoma cannot completely be excluded. A diagnosis of malignancy should not be made unless there is sufficient histologic evidence, so that overtreatment and undue psychological burden for the patient can be avoided.

Nonmelanocytic lesions that need to be considered in the differential diagnosis include juvenile xanthogranuloma, cellular neurothekeoma, epithelioid cell histiocytoma, and reticulohistiocytoma.

Metastasizing Spitz Tumor

Melanocytic lesions classified as Spitz tumors have been reported to spread to regional lymph nodes.[124,126,136] These metastasizing melanocytic lesions, albeit resembling in many ways Spitz tumors, tend to be unusually large and deep or show other atypical features.[136,143]

TABLE 27-13

Comparison of Spitz Tumor, Atypical Spitz Tumor, and Melanoma

	Spitz tumor	*Spitz tumor with architectural disorder and cytologic atypia*	*Melanoma*
Size	Usually < 1 cm	Often > 1 cm	Usually > 1 cm
Symmetry	Symmetry	Often asymmetric	Asymmetric
Lateral borders	Sharply demarcated	Often poorly defined	Often poorly defined
Lateral extension	Uncommon	Common	Common
Lentiginous melanocytic proliferation	Uncommon	Variable	Common
Irregular nesting	Uncommon	Common	Frequent
Upward migration	Common in children, nests > single cells	Variable, prominent on occasion	Frequent, usually as single cells
Ulceration	Uncommon	Variable	Common
Kamino bodies	Common	Common	Uncommon
Cell type	Monomorphous	Monomorphous	Pleomorphic
Deep extension	Uncommon	Common	Variable
Expansile nodules	Uncommon	Common	Frequent
Maturation/zonation	Common	Uncommon	Uncommon
Deep border	Orderly infiltrating pattern	Often rounded, "pushing"	Irregular
Cellularity	Variable	Prominent	Prominent
Cytologic atypia	Uncommon	Common	Prominent
Cellular cohesion	Diminished	Diminished	Variable
Mitoses, deep	Uncommon	Common	Frequent
Atypical mitoses	Uncommon	Variable	Common
Mononuclear infiltrates	Perivascular	Patchy	Bandlike, patchy

TABLE 27-14

Desmoplastic Spitz Tumor

Clinical Features

Firm papule or nodule
Adults (peak incidence in third decade)
Most commonly located on extremities

Histopathological Features

Spindle and/or epithelioid cells
Predominantly intradermal location of melanocytes
Sometimes junctional component
Dermal stroma with increased collagen
Usually circumscribed, but with ill-defined borders
Often vaguely wedge-shaped
Usually diffuse distribution of cells with low cell density
Typically small nests and single melanocytes
Maturation often present
Mitoses absent or rare
Multinucleate giant cells not uncommon (usually superficial)
Melanin usually sparse or absent

Differential Diagnosis

Desmoplastic melanoma
Sclerosing blue nevus
Dermatofibroma

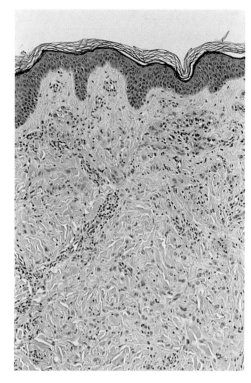

FIGURE 27-31 Desmoplastic Spitz tumor. The lesion is entirely intradermal and characterized by a nondescript appearance at this magnification. Nonetheless, the tumor exhibits symmetry and an orderly pattern.

Further studies are needed to clarify the nature of these tumors, i.e., whether they are unique or simply an unusual form of melanoma.

Desmoplastic Spitz Tumor

Clinical Features Although the desmoplastic Spitz tumor *(also known as sclerosing Spitz nevus, desmoplastic nevus)* is considered by many to be an unusual variant of Spitz tumor,[23,144] some authors maintain that this lesion is a distinct entity.[145] Desmoplastic Spitz tumor typically presents as a firm dome-shaped flesh-colored papule or nodule, measuring up to 1 cm in greatest diameter, is most often located on the extremities, and suggests a dermatofibroma (Table 27-14).[128,144] This variant of Spitz tumor primarily affects adults, with a peak incidence in the third decade.

Histopathological Features The desmoplastic Spitz tumor is a poorly circumscribed growth of large polygonal or elongated melanocytes in a collagen-rich stromal background (Table 27-14)(Figs. 27-31 and 27-32).[23,128,144] It is usually a wholly intradermal lesion. The desmoplastic changes in Spitz tumors may comprise the entire lesion or any portion of it. In the superficial dermis, melanocytes may be grouped in nests or aggregates, but in the deeper parts of the lesions they tend to infiltrate singly between typically thickened collagen bundles (Fig. 27-32). The latter phenomenon is maturation. Scattered multinucleated giant cells or large pleomorphic forms may be present. Cytologically, the melanocytes of desmoplastic Spitz tumors are characterized by nuclei that are often hyperchromatic with clumped or finely dispersed chromatin. Nucleoli are commonly inconspicuous but may be prominent, especially in larger cells. The size of the nuclei tends to diminish as melanocytes approach the base of the lesion, which is usually ill-defined. Mitoses are rare (usually fewer than 1 per 20 HPF).[143]

Differential Diagnosis The major differential diagnostic problem with desmoplastic Spitz tumor is its distinction from desmoplastic melanoma (Table 27-15). The desmoplastic Spitz tumor may present in a similar fashion to desmoplastic melanoma, i.e., an indurated amelanotic or slightly pigmented nodule. However, in other respects, the desmoplastic Spitz tumor is different from desmoplastic melanoma. This nevus is more commonly found on the extremities of young individuals versus the head and neck of elderly persons in desmoplastic melanoma. Histologically, desmoplastic Spitz tumors tend to be small, well-circumscribed, superficial lesions whereas desmoplastic melanomas are often larger, poorly demarcated, and characterized by deep involvement

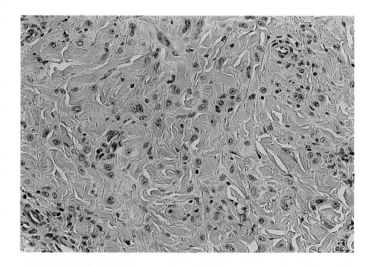

FIGURE 27-32 Desmoplastic Spitz tumor. Nests, cords, and individual cells dispersed in sclerotic dermis.

TABLE 27-15

Desmoplastic Spitz Tumor vs. Desmoplastic Melanoma

	Desmoplastic Spitz tumor	Desmoplastic melanoma
Preferred site	Extremities	Head and neck
Preferred age group	Early adulthood	Late adulthood
Melanocytic atypia		
Intraepidermal	Rare	Common
Dermal	Not uncommon, but usually slight	Common, often more than slight
Mitoses	Rare	Variable
Necrosis	Absent	Occasional
Maturation	Common	Uncommon

of the dermis or subcutis. The desmoplastic variant of Spitz tumor also shows maturation, i.e., isolation of individually smaller cells with increasing depth versus little or no such transition in desmoplastic melanoma. The cell types in the two processes tend to be rather different. Desmoplastic Spitz tumors contain typical large epithelioid or fusiform cells whereas desmoplastic melanoma is notable for pleomorphic spindle cells often with hyperchromatic nuclei.

Although the blue nevus may have pronounced sclerosing features, it is usually a more ill-defined melanocytic lesion than desmoplastic Spitz tumor and is composed of a more slender and more diffusely pigmented melanocytic population than the plumper cells of Spitz tumor.

Nonmelanocytic dermal spindle cell lesions that may share morphologic features of desmoplastic Spitz tumor are dermatofibroma, reticulohistiocytoma, and epithelioid cell histiocytoma (see above).

PIGMENTED SPINDLE CELL TUMOR

Synonym: *pigmented spindle cell nevus of Reed*

Clinical Features The pigmented spindle cell tumor (PSCT) is a distinctive clinicopathologic entity important to recognize because of its frequent confusion with melanoma (Table 27-16). PSCT usually presents as a symmetric, sharply circumscribed, dark-brown or black papule or nodule.[22,23,141,146–149] It is typically a small lesion, often measuring less than 0.6 cm in diameter. PSCT is commonly located on the extremities. It appears to affect women slightly more than men and there is often a history of recent onset.[141,147,148]

Histopathological Features These lesions are usually relatively small, strikingly well-circumscribed, and remarkable for a slightly elevated, flat-topped plaquelike appearance of the epidermis (Table 27-16) (Fig. 27-33).[23,141,146–149] Although the PSCT may be junctional or compound, many are almost entirely intraepidermal. If papillary dermal involvement occurs, the base of PSCT is typically broad with pushing borders.

The PSCT contains uniform, delicate, spindle cells present in tightly packed fascicles. These fascicles tend to have a fairly uniform and symmetric spacing and size within the epidermis and are often vertically oriented. The fusiform cells are often slightly more slender than the spindle cells of "classic" Spitz tumor (Fig. 27-34). Their nuclei are equal in size or smaller than the nuclei of adjacent keratinocytes.[147] Nucleoli are usually inconspicuous. Some PSCT, particularly in children, may show florid upward migration of single melanocytes, closely simulating

TABLE 27-16

Pigmented Spindle Cell Tumor

Clinical Features

Peak incidence in third decade
Most often located on extremities (especially thigh)
Women more often affected than men
Small (usually smaller than 0.6 cm)
Symmetric
Pigmented (usually evenly, often heavily)
Sharply circumscribed
Papule or nodule
History of recent onset

Histopathological Features

Junctional or compound tumor
Predominantly spindle cells, but occasional epithelioid cells
Spindle cells more slender and delicate than in Spitz tumors
Uniform population of cells from side to side
Symmetric configuration
Predominance of junctional nests or fascicles
Typically ovoid nests with fusiform cells oriented vertically
Often confluence of nests leading to irregular shapes
Sharp lateral borders, occasional lentiginous lateral spread
Usually abundant coarse melanin
Uniform nuclear features
Decrease in cell size from top to bottom ("maturation")
Mitoses not uncommon in intraepidermal component
Absent or rare dermal mitoses

Differential Diagnosis

Lentiginous melanoma
Pagetoid melanoma
Dysplastic nevus

melanoma in situ.[23,148] Also in contrast to ordinary Spitz tumor, melanocytes of PSCT contain variable amounts of granular melanin. Heavy pigmentation may also involve the adjacent keratinocytes, cornified layer, and papillary dermis.[23]

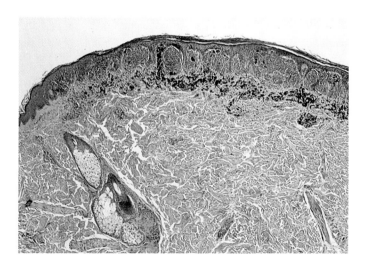

FIGURE 27-33 Pigmented spindle cell tumor. The lesion is small, symmetric, and well-circumscribed.

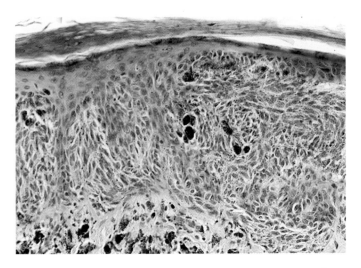

FIGURE 27-34   Pigmented spindle cell tumor. Fascicles of spindle cells are both vertically and horizontally disposed and seem to be part of the thickened epidermis. Note uniformity of spindle cells.

There is a histologic continuum of Spitz tumor and PSCT[23] (Table 27-16). One will encounter many nevi showing varying degrees of transition between these two poles of the spectrum. For example, some nevi may exhibit slender spindle cells typical of PSCT yet contain somewhat larger fusiform cells and epithelioid cells that are less heavily melaninized.

PIGMENTED SPINDLE CELL TUMOR WITH ARCHITECTURAL DISORDER AND CYTOLOGIC ATYPIA

The same discussion applies to the atypical variants of PSCT as for atypical forms of Spitz tumor[23,134,141] (Table 27-12). However, most atypical variants of PSCT are primarily intraepidermal. Substantial overlap may occur with conventional dysplastic nevi.

Differential Diagnosis   Pigmented spindle cell tumor and its atypical variants must be distinguished from in situ or microinvasive melanoma and from dysplastic nevus.

PSCT (particularly atypical forms of PSCT) and lentiginous melanocytic proliferations of sun-exposed skin (LMPS, lentigo maligna) may show considerable similarity on occasion.[23] Both are typically composed of pigmented spindle cells that may be arranged in junctional nests and may involve skin appendages. Discrimination of the two is based on clinical features, the usual small size, sharp circumscription, predominantly nested pattern, and uniformity of cell type in PSCT. LMPS, however, tends to be broader and poorly circumscribed and usually typified by a mainly basilar single-cell proliferation of pleomorphic melanocytes. Rare lesions may show such overlap that distinction may not be possible. Such lesions should be completely excised with a cuff of normal tissue, and the patients carefully monitored.

PSCT and atypical variants of PSCT are often confused with pagetoid variants of melanoma because of prominent pagetoid spread.[23,141] One must again rely on clinical factors, i.e., young age, anatomic site (e.g., the extremities), as well as the overall morphologic appearance. PSCT are typically small, well-demarcated, symmetric, and orderly. Even with striking pagetoid spread in some lesions, the latter features argue strongly in favor of a benign process, especially if present in a young individual and on a site such as the thigh. However, atypical forms of PSCT are extremely challenging, and all the clinical and histologic features must be carefully weighed. In many instances, a clear-cut diagnosis of melanoma cannot be made. Such lesions should be designated as pigmented spindle cell tumor (or melanocytic proliferation) with atypical features, and appropriate surgery and careful follow-up of the patient arranged. Recurrence of such lesions appears to be extremely rare.

The same features characteristic of PSCT, such as cytologic uniformity and nuclear regularity, as well as its tendency to contain vertically disposed melanocytes ("raining down") to the epidermal surface, help to distinguish PSCT from dysplastic nevus, in which the melanocytes are oriented more parallel to the epidermal surface and show more cytologic variability and atypia.[141] Dysplastic nevi are generally less cellular and often display a pronounced lentiginous melanocytic proliferation with elongation of the rete ridges and associated papillary dermal fibrosis, which are not typical features of PSCT. However, some atypical forms of PSCT show substantial overlap with conventional dysplastic nevi. Discrimination of the two lesions thus may not be reproducible. Such lesions may be designated as PSCT with architectural disorder and cytologic atypia or dysplastic nevus with features of PSCT.

DERMAL MELANOCYTOSES, BLUE NEVI, AND RELATED CONDITIONS

The classification of blue nevi and related lesions is based on assessing a number of features: clinical appearance; anatomic site of lesion; localization in the reticular dermis and subcutis; the extent to which the lesion is made up of dendritic versus spindle-shaped and other types of melanocytes; degree of cellularity of lesion; and degree of fibrosis (sclerosis) (Table 27-17).[150–161]

The bluish appearance of these various lesions is primarily related to depth of melanin in the dermis and the Tyndall phenomenon. The longer wavelengths of visible light penetrate the reticular dermis and are absorbed by the melanin. However, the shorter wavelengths representing the bluish part of the color spectrum do not penetrate so deeply and are reflected from the superficial dermis and epidermis.

The dermal melanocytoses and blue nevi are thought to result from the dermal arrest of cells migrating from the neural crest.[161,162] In contrast to ordinary nevi, it is believed that these migratory cells never reach the epidermis but instead give rise to melanocytic lesions with varying degrees of cellularity and melaninization.

Dermal Melanocytoses

Six entities—Mongolian spot, nevus of Ota, nevus fuscoceruleus zygomaticus (acquired nevus of Ota-like macules), acquired dermal melanocytosis of the face and extremities, nevus of Ito, and dermal melanocyte hamartoma—are related because they are all essentially bluish macular lesions that histologically demonstrate scattered dendritic melanocytes in the reticular dermis with little or no stromal alteration (Table 27-17).[1,23,150–161,163–171]

MONGOLIAN SPOT

Clinical and Histopathological Features   Mongolian spots are oval or round, often poorly defined, macules (about 1 to 10 cm) varying in color from slight gray to blue-black or dark brown, most often affecting the lumbosacral region but sometimes seen in other (ectopic, or aberrant) locations. These lesions are present at birth but usually spontaneously regress by age 3 to 4 years. Mongolian spots are observed primarily in persons of color. The mongolian spot is characterized by widely spaced dendritic melanocytes localized to the lower half or two-thirds of an unaltered reticular dermis (Fig. 27-35).[152]

TABLE 27-17

Dermal Melanocytoses

Feature	Mongolian spot	Nevus of Ota	Nevus of Ito	Blue nevus
Onset	Birth or soon after	Birth or soon after	Birth or soon after	Birth or later in life
Size	5 cm	5 cm	5 cm	1.5 cm
Color	Gray-tan, slate blue	Brown, slate blue	Brown, slate blue	Bluish black
Surface	Macular	Macular, rarely discrete papules	Macular, rarely discrete papules	Papular
Hair	Normal for site	Normal for site	Normal for site	Normal for site
Distribution	Midline	Unilateral	Unilateral	Unilateral
Number	Single, can be multiple	Single	Single	Single, rarely multiple
Site	Lumbosacral	First and second division trigeminal nerve	Shoulder and upper arm	Extensors of extremities: dorsa of hands and feet, buttocks, face
Racial incidence	Asians and dark-skinned races	Asians and dark-skinned races	Asians and dark-skinned races	More common in dark-skinned races
Familial incidence	Common	Rare	Rare	None
Sex	No difference	80% in females	80% in females	60% in females
Age of appearance	At birth	60% at birth	60% at birth	At or just after birth
Spontaneous fate	Usually disappears during first few years of life	Persist; rarely disappear	Persist; rarely disappear	Persist
Tendency to malignancy	Never reported	Rare	Rare	Rare
Histologic features	Scattered dermal melanocytes in lower half of dermis in low concentrations	Moderate number of dermal melanocytes in upper dermis	Moderate number of dermal melanocytes in upper dermis	Common form has high concentration of dermal melanocytes in middle and lower third of dermis; melanophages usually present; cellular form also contains bundles of spindle-shaped cells
Ultrastructure	Fully developed melanocytes with only mature melanosomes; virtually no premelanosomes	Fully developed melanocytes with only mature melanosomes; virtually no premelanosomes	Fully developed melanocytes with only mature melanosomes; virtually no premelanosomes	Fully developed melanocytes with only mature melanosomes; virtually no premelanosomes

NEVUS OF OTA

Synonym: *nevus fuscoceruleus ophthalmomaxillaris*

Clinical Features   This hamartomatous or nevoid condition usually presents at birth or in childhood as a unilateral speckled bluish macule involving the periorbital region, forehead, temple, cheek, or nose, corresponding to the distribution of the first two branches of the trigeminal nerve.[152,163,166] Examination may also disclose involvement of the sclera, conjunctiva, cornea, retina, or oral and nasal mucosae. Brownish lentigolike lesions and bluish papules or nodules are occasionally associated with nevus of Ota.

Histopathological Features   (See *dermal melanocyte hamartoma*.)

NEVUS FUSCOCERULEUS ZYGOMATICUS

Synonyms: *acquired nevus of Ota–like macules, Sun's nevus*

Clinical Features   The development of bilateral bluish macules in the zygomatic areas of the face has primarily been reported in Chinese and Japanese women.[168,169]

Histopathological Features   (See *dermal melanocyte hamartoma*.)

ACQUIRED DERMAL MELANOCYTOSIS OF THE FACE AND EXTREMITIES

Clinical Features   This particular disorder is associated with bilateral bluish or brownish discoloration of the face of adults somewhat similar to nevus of Ota but also associated with involvement of the extensor surfaces of the upper extremities and possibly the palms.[170]

Histopathological Features   (See *dermal melanocyte hamartoma*.)

NEVUS OF ITO

Synonym: *nevus fuscoceruleus acromiodeltoideus*

Clinical Features   The nevus of Ito is closely related to nevus of Ota but is distinguished by its unilateral distribution involving the supraclavicular, scapular, or deltoid regions.[163]

Histopathological Features   (See *dermal melanocyte hamartoma*.)

DERMAL MELANOCYTE HAMARTOMA

Clinical Features   The term *dermal melanocyte hamartoma* describes a small number of developmental abnormalities usually present at birth and exhibiting extensive involvement of the skin.[23,171]

Histopathological Features   Scattered dermal melanocytes with prominent dendritic processes are noted in the upper dermis without alteration of the dermal stroma. There may be aggregation of these cells about sebaceous glands, eccrine ducts, blood vessels, and cutaneous nerves. As in mongolian spot, the cells contain prominent deposits of fine melanin granules (Fig. 27-35). Melanophages, in general, are uncommon. The density of melanocytes is greater than in mongolian spot. A new histopathologic classification of nevus of Ota based on the location of melanocytes in the dermis has been reported: (1) superficial type, i.e., melanocytes present in the superficial dermis, (2) deep type, (3) diffuse type (melanocytes scattered throughout entire dermis), (4) superficial dominant type, and (5) deep dominant type.[166]

The brownish macules in any of these lesions demonstrate dermal melanocytes located very close to the epidermis or slight basilar melanocytic hyperplasia and basal layer hypermelanosis.[8] The slightly raised or papular lesions demonstrate an even greater concentration of dendritic melanocytes, resembling blue nevus.

Differential Diagnosis   The dermal melanocytoses as a group are distinguished from blue nevi by the lack of dermal fibrosis, sparse cellularity, and a single-cell disposition of dendritic melanocytes. Mongolian spots are distinguished from other dermal melanocytoses by location (sacral area), disappearance in infancy, and sparse number of dermal melanocytes without melanophages or fibrosis. Persistent ectopic "mongolian spots" may be difficult to discriminate from nevus of Ota or Ito. Some previously reported examples of ectopic mongolian spots are in fact nevus of Ota or Ito.

Blue Nevus

Historically, the classification of blue nevus has included two principal variants[150-161]; the more prevalent common blue nevus and the rela-

tively uncommon, larger variant, the cellular blue nevus. However, examination of sufficient numbers of blue nevi reveals that there is indeed a morphologic spectrum rather than necessarily two well-defined subtypes. The morphologic features that account for the spectrum of blue nevi include the relative number and density of dendritic and spindled melanocytes, melanophages, degree of fibrosis, the disposition and relationship of the latter components, and the overall size of the lesion. The spindle cells may be individually disposed, arranged in fascicles, or in compact nests. Finally, some blue nevi contain cellular elements from other nevi such as ordinary nevi or spindle and epithelioid cell tumors and have been designated combined nevi (see below).[156] The clinical characteristics of some blue nevi may also warrant attention such as a plaque-like or agminated appearance.[152,172-176] The following classification of blue nevi is based on the predominant histologic changes.

COMMON BLUE NEVUS

Clinical Features   The most common form of blue nevus usually presents as a well-demarcated, slightly raised, or dome-shaped bluish papule (Table 27-17).[150,152,153] The color is usually a uniform slate gray, blue-black, or black appearance. The borders are generally regular, and these nevi usually measure less than 1 cm in diameter. They are primarily located on the dorsal aspects of the hands and feet as well as involving the face and scalp. Onset is generally in childhood but may occur later in life. Melanoma has only rarely been reported to originate from this type of blue nevus.[177]

Histopathological Features   This form of blue nevus shows an aggregation of dendritic melanocytes that alters the normal configuration of the dermis (Figs. 27-36 and 27-37) (Table 27-17).[23,150,152,153] The lesion may occur anywhere in the reticular dermis and even in the papillary dermis, but most commonly involves the superficial dermis. In

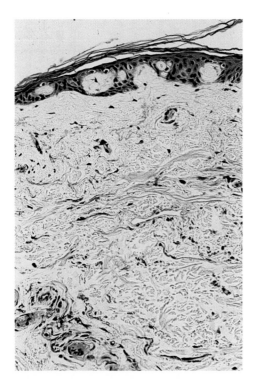

FIGURE 27-35   Mongolian spot. A punch biopsy shows a largely unaffected dermis. There are pigmented dendritic cells in the midreticular dermis scattered among collagen bundles. Neither fascicles of cells nor fibrosis are present as would be observed in blue nevus.

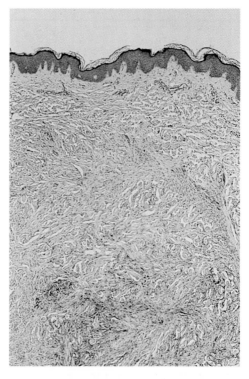

FIGURE 27-36   Blue nevus, ordinary type. The nevus is composed of numerous pigmented dendritic cells in a slightly fibrotic matrix.

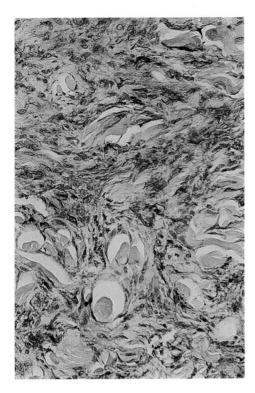

FIGURE 27-37 Blue nevus. The dendritic melanocytes are easily identified by their melanin content.

general, there are bundles of dendritic cells with frequent aggregation about appendages and neurovascular bundles. The cells are generally bipolar or stellate and characterized by lengthy dendritic processes (Fig. 27-37). Most cells contain a dense accumulation of relatively fine melanin granules. The nuclei are ovoid with uniform chromatin patterns. Melanophages are usually present and may be the principal cell type in some cases. Variable degrees of fibrosis are also present.

Differential Diagnosis This type of blue nevus shares the common dendritic cell type noted in the dermal melanocytoses already discussed. The blue nevus differs from the above entities by a greater concentration of dendritic melanocytes and is usually accompanied by varying degrees of fibrosis and melanophage accumulation. However, the papular and nodular lesions within nevus of Ota or Ito are indistinguishable from this variant of blue nevus. The differential diagnosis might also include primary or metastatic melanoma, possibly with some degree of regression. In general, blue nevi can be distinguished from melanoma by their small size, overall symmetry, lack of cytologic atypia, and absence of mitotic activity and necrosis.

SCLEROSING BLUE NEVUS

Clinical and Histopathological Features This variant is characterized by a symmetric and fairly well circumscribed fibrous nodule in the dermis. The fibrous component is conspicuous relative to a sparse number of dendritic and/or spindled melanocytes and melanophages.

Differential Diagnosis. Entities to be distinguished from sclerosing blue nevus include dermatofibroma, particularly the hemosiderotic variant, sclerosing Spitz tumor, and desmoplastic melanoma (Table 27-18). The type of dermatofibroma associated with prominent deposits of hemosiderin can closely mimic blue nevus. However, the typical epi-

---

TABLE 27-18

Sclerosing Blue Nevus and Desmoplastic-Neurotropic Melanoma

Sclerosing blue nevus	*Desmoplastic melanoma*
Clinical Features	
Common	Rare
Age mean 38.6 years	Age mean 60 years
Women affected more often than men	Men affected more often than women
Dorsal hands, feet, face	Head and neck, sun-exposed skin
Blue, blue-black	Flesh-colored papule or nodule, may have tan or brown component
Histopathological Features	
Usually no intraepidermal component	About 85% have intraepidermal component, often lentigo maligna
Symmetry	Asymmetry often
Well-demarcated fibrous nodule with rounded contours in dermis	Fibrous nodule often extending into deep reticular dermis or subcutis
Orderly arrangement of dendritic cells	Fascicles of cells oriented in all directions
Melanin often present	Melanin often absent
Little or no cytologic atypia	Often enlarged hyperchromatic spindle-shaped nuclei
Infiltration of cutaneous nerves (orderly)	Perineurial and endoneurial invasion
Usually no mitoses	Usually at least 1 or 2 mitoses/mm^2
Usually no mucin	Mucinous stroma on occasion
Immunohistochemistry	
S-100 protein +	S-100 protein +
HMB-45 +	HMB-45 − (in most cases)

---

dermal changes resembling seborrheic keratosis are usually found with dermatofibroma as well as the typical infiltrating pattern of cells in dermatofibroma. Close inspection of the pigment granules in dermatofibroma will usually reveal the golden refractile character of hemosiderin. If necessary, special stains for iron and melanin can be useful in distinguishing these two entities. The desmoplastic or sclerosing form of Spitz tumor is usually easily separated from blue nevus, since there is usually no pigment in the Spitz variant and the cell type is usually epithelioid. Desmoplastic melanoma is distinguished from sclerosing blue nevus by clinical features, the presence of an atypical lentiginous melanocytic proliferation, fascicles of atypical spindle cells, and inflammatory infiltrates in desmoplastic melanoma (Table 27-18). However, this distinction occasionally may be quite difficult. Diagnosis must be based on weighing the degree of cellularity, cytologic atypia, and mitotic activity.

"COMPOUND" BLUE NEVUS

These lesions exhibit basilar epidermal proliferation of heavily pigmented dendritic melanocytes.[178] Junctional nests are not present. The papillary and upper reticular dermis contain a fairly well circumscribed aggregate of spindle and dendritic melanocytes, usually heavily melanized with numerous melanophages.

Cellular Blue Nevus

Clinical Features

Onset birth, childhood, adolescence
Age mean 33 (range 6–85) years
Site—buttocks, sacrococcygeal area, forearm/wrist, leg/ankle/foot, scalp, face
Gray-blue to blue-black papule, nodule
Usually well-circumscribed
Regular borders
Size 0.3 to 3 cm

Histopathological Features

Symmetry
Localization to reticular dermis
Often deep extension with bulging, nodular configuration, rounded, well-demarcated inferior margin
Heterogeneity of patterns
    Biphasic pattern most common:
        Melanin-laden dendritic melanocytes and fibrosis and bundles of amelanotic fusiform cells
    Alveolar pattern:
        Fascicles or nests of fusiform cells compartmentalized by fibrous trabeculae
    Fascicular pattern
        Fascicles of spindle cells often with clear cytoplasm and prominent schwannian differentiation
    Atypical cellular blue nevus
        Marked cytologic atypia
        Enlarged bizarre cells
        Multinucleate cells
Lacunae containing melanophages
Cystic degeneration in central part of nevus with loose edematous stroma
Few or no mitotic figures
Necrosis absent or uncommon

Differential Diagnosis

Malignant blue nevus
Metastatic melanoma
Clear-cell sarcoma

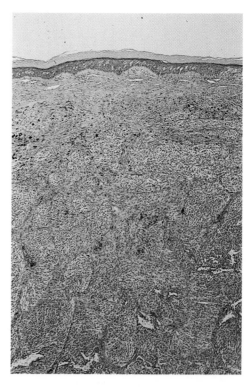

FIGURE 27-38   Blue nevus, cellular variant. This lesion occupies the entire dermis. Pale-staining areas correspond to nests and fascicles of fusiform cells.

Architecture of CBN[151,153–179]

CBN may show a single lobular mass with a well-defined horizontal inferior margin that parallels or bulges into the subcutaneous fat, or alternatively, there may be two or more lobules or digitate bulbous projections that extend into the deep reticular dermis or subcutaneous fat (Fig. 27-40).

Composition of CBN

CBN are heterogeneous, and their morphologic limits have not been clearly defined.[23] For example, the distinction from ordinary blue nevi, some pigmented peripheral nerve sheath tumors, and other unusual melanocytic nevi may be problematic (see below). Essential for the

CELLULAR BLUE NEVUS

Clinical Features   Cellular blue nevi (CBN) are generally 1 to 2 cm in diameter with a blue, blue-black, or black coloration and most commonly involve the buttocks, sacral area, or scalp (Table 27-19). They are generally diagnosed between the ages of 10 and 40 years and are usually asymptomatic. Rarely these lesions may undergo transformation to melanoma (malignant blue nevus). Incomplete excision of CBN is rarely associated with recurrence.

Histopathological Features   There is a continuum from ordinary blue nevi to "cellular" blue nevi, as discussed above (Figs. 27-38 to 27-41).[23] However, no criteria have been established as to what proportion of a blue nevus should consist of fusiform cells in order to qualify as a cellular blue nevus. The following criteria are proposed for diagnosis of CBN: The lesion should occupy the reticular dermis, at least a third to a half of the lesion should contain oval to fusiform cells, and the overall architecture should be multilobular or plexiform with deep involvement of the reticular dermis or subcutis (Table 27-19).

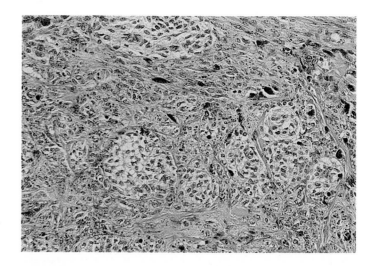

FIGURE 27-39   Cellular blue nevus. Discrete nests of round, oval, and slightly elongated cells with clear cytoplasm.

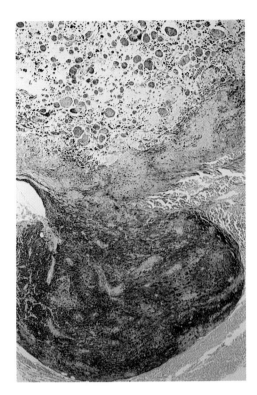

FIGURE 27-40 Cellular blue nevus. Characteristic bulbous configuration of cellular blue nevus extending into subcutis.

diagnosis are cellular foci of round, oval, elongate, or fusiform cells that constitute at least a third to a half if not most of the tumor (Fig. 27-39). These cells are arranged in a number of patterns and vary considerably as to melanin content. As opposed to the frequent diffuse distribution of melanin-laden dendritic melanocytes in the ordinary type of blue nevus, the fusiform cells of CBN are usually disposed in variably organized nests or bundles. These bundles may or may not be encapsulated by fibrous tissue. In some instances, fascicles of fusiform cells are oriented randomly in all directions without evidence of compartmentalization. However, a common pattern is that of compact highly cellular nests or fascicles separated by fibrous trabeculae. There may be linear or concentric arrangements of cells within these nests.

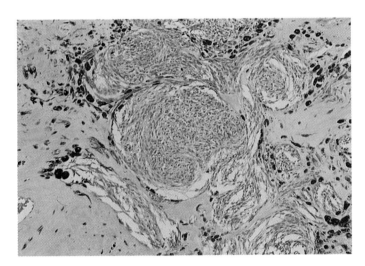

FIGURE 27-41 Cellular blue nevus with central cytic degeneration. Nests of cells are separated by edema.

Often pigmented dendritic melanocytes and melanophages are present in the peripheral fibrous tissue surrounding the cellular fascicles. The sizes of fascicles or nests may vary considerably. There may be large lobules of fusiform cells constituting much of the tumor without intervening fibrous tissue. Well-defined rounded nests of cells have been described as the *alveolar* pattern in CBN.[157,179] Fascicles of spindle cells may have Schwannian differentiation and may merge with and infiltrate cutaneous nerves.[159]

The cells comprising the "cellular" foci are most often fusiform or spindle-shaped but may also be round or oval.[23] These cells are usually somewhat enlarged but may be relatively small. The cells boundaries are often ill-defined, and the cytoplasm is usually either clear, vacuolated, slightly eosinophilic, or bluish. The fusiform cells do not contain readily apparent melanin by conventional microscopy. Because of the paucity or absence of melanin, these cellular foci appear pale or clear on scanning magnification, in contrast to the often heavily pigmented areas containing dendritic melanocytes, melanophages, and sclerosis. The latter pale areas are quite helpful in recognizing CBN. However, the degree of melaninization may vary from barely visible fine granular melanin to heavy pigmentation obscuring cytologic detail. Usually, the dendritic melanocytes and melanophages contain the heaviest deposition of melanin. However, the latter cells are usually located in peripheral fibrous trabeculae or in areas of sclerosis.

The nuclei of these cells are usually round, oval, or fusiform and commonly somewhat enlarged. The chromatin tends to be evenly dispersed, and one or more small nucleoli are often observed. Minimal or low-grade nuclear pleomorphism is noted in many CBN. However, this should not be pronounced. Similarly, occasional mitoses are noted in many CBN. As a general rule, if two or more mitoses are present per square millimeter, the lesion should be carefully evaluated for other corroborating evidence of malignancy.

Multinucleate giant cells are occasionally noted in the cellular areas and may be numerous. Such giant cells may also occur in areas of cystic degeneration (see below).[179]

Occasional CBN are composed of discrete nests of amelanotic round or oval cells analogous to the usual fusiform cells. Such nests are separated in the typical fashion by fibrous trabeculae that usually contain some dendritic melanocytes and melanophages. Recognition of other features of CBN such as the lobular well-demarcated configuration and clinical features are necessary for diagnosis as CBN.

Perhaps two-thirds or so of CBN have a so-called biphasic pattern, i.e., a component of common blue nevus, areas containing pigmented dendritic melanocytes, variable sclerosis, and melanophages, in addition to the cellular areas.[157,179] These areas are often in the superficial dermis overlying or at the periphery of cellular lobules.

A rather characteristic feature of CBN is cystic degeneration (*encystification*), which is often centrally located (Fig. 27-41)[155,181] and probably indistinguishable from similar changes in ancient schwannoma. The latter may have an ischemic or traumatic basis. These degenerative changes are typified by edema, myxoid stromal alteration, diminished cellularity, and scattered melanophages. Alterations of blood vessels also tend to be a prominent feature and include ectatic vessels with hyalinization of their walls and thrombosis.

ATYPICAL CELLULAR BLUE NEVUS

Atypical variants of CBN may be extremely difficult to distinguish from malignant blue nevus.[179,182] Morphologic criteria have not been clearly established for atypical CBN. However, atypical CBN are generally characterized by large size, deep extension, large expansile nests of spindle cells, prominent cellularity and cytologic atypia, and significant mitotic activity.[179,182]

TABLE 27-20

TABLE 27-20

Cellular Blue Nevus and Malignant Blue Nevus

Cellular blue nevus	*Malignant blue nevus*
Clinical Features	
Mean age 32.6 (7 to 60) years	Extremely rare 48.8 (30 to 75) years
Women affected more often than men	Men affected more often than women
Buttock, sacrococcygeal area, extremities	Scalp
Size 1.8 cm (1–2 cm)	Size 2.5 cm (1.3–4 cm)
Blue, blue-gray, blue-black nodule	Blue, blue-black nodule
Histopathological Features	
Component of ordinary blue nevus in 60%	Blue nevus component, cellular in 92%
Symmetry	Asymmetry
Lobular or multilobular	Lobular or multilobular
Cytologic atypia, low-grade or absent	Substantial cytologic atypia
Mitoses < 1 or 2/10 HPF	Mitoses 1–2/10 HPF
Usually no atypical mitoses	Atypical mitoses
Necrosis uncommon	Necrosis in 33%
	Pronounced heterogeneity in most tumors

Differential Diagnosis   The differential diagnosis of CBN (and atypical CBN) includes malignant blue nevus (MBN) (malignant melanoma arising in association with cellular blue nevus) (see below) (Table 27-20),[183,184] metastatic melanoma, and clear-cell sarcoma. The clinical history of a long-standing blue nevus with subsequent change or finding an associated benign blue nevus remnant (usually CBN) is extremely important for the diagnosis of MBN. Without the latter criterion, MBN cannot be distinguished from conventional melanoma, whether primary or metastatic. The MBN is discriminated from CBN by greater degrees of cytologic atypia, greater mitotic activity with atypical forms, and necrosis. There may be considerable heterogeneity within MBN, and the diagnosis has been missed because of this histologic variation.[183,184] The presence of a concomitant conventional blue nevus element favors a diagnosis of CBN. It cannot be overemphasized that although MBN is vanishingly rare, atypical CBN should be completely excised and the patients monitored very carefully for recurrence. Metastases from such lesions have been observed after the passage of several years. Thus, because of the unusual nature of these lesions, their rarity, and the lack of long-term follow-up, the biologic potential of atypical forms of CBN is largely unknown and requires further study.

LYMPH NODE INVOLVEMENT BY CELLULAR BLUE NEVUS

On occasion, foci of CBN may be detected in regional lymph nodes,[185,186] such as the axillary or inguinal lymph nodes proximal to a CBN on an extremity. These nodal foci of CBN have most commonly involved the subcapsular peripheral sinuses and parenchyma of the lymph nodes, which are sites involved by metastatic cancer, but also the lymph node capsule. Explanations for such nodal involvement have included benign metastases and aberrant histogenesis of CBN in lymph nodes.[185,186] The latter phenomenon should be recognized, carefully assessed, and not misdiagnosed as metastatic melanoma or MBN.

Similarly, a cutaneous lesion should not be misdiagnosed as MBN simply because of the lymph node involvement.

PATCHLIKE BLUE NEVUS

Clinical and Histopathological Features   A macular area of blue-gray pigmentation from 1 to several centimeters clinically resembles a mongolian spot.[187,188] In contrast to mongolian spot, the patchlike blue nevus contains a greater number of dendritic melanocytes in the dermis.

PLAQUE-TYPE BLUE NEVUS

Clinical and Histopathological Features   A palpable area of blue-gray pigmentation measures 1 to several cm or more in diameter.[152,173–176] The plaque is either a single lesion or composed of multiple but distinct papules. Eruptive or agminated blue nevi, patchlike blue nevus, pilar neurocristic hamartoma, and plaque-type blue nevus are probably closely related.[190] The histologic features are similar to ordinary blue nevi; there may be prominent periappendageal aggregation of dendritic melanocytes and compact bundles of spindle cells.

PILAR NEUROCRISTIC HAMARTOMA

Clinical and Histopathological Features   Multiple perifollicular papules occupy an area of skin measuring several centimeters in diameter.[190] Individual papules vary in color from tan to blue or black. There is some similarity to patch- and plaquelike blue nevi in humans and equine melanotic disease. There is prominent perifollicular accumulation of dendritic melanocytes that shows extension to nearby eccrine ducts. The intervening reticular dermis contains scattered pigmented dendritic cells resembling mongolian spot.

TARGET BLUE NEVUS

Clinical and Histopathological Features   A central dark-blue nodule is surrounded by a flesh-colored annulus and more peripheral blue-black macular annulus. The lesion measures about 1 cm in greatest diameter and has been reported to occur on the dorsal aspect of the foot.[191] The dark central nodule has the features of a typical blue nevus, i.e., a fibrotic tumor containing pigmented dendritic cells and fusiform cells. The flesh-colored annulus shows dermal sclerosis and significantly reduced numbers of pigment-containing cells. However, in contrast, the most peripheral zone has prominent numbers of the pigmented dendritic cells.

MELANOCYTIC NEVI WITH PHENOTYPIC HETEROGENEITY

Various nevi reported in the literature as *combined nevus, deep penetrating nevus, plexiform spindle cell nevus,* and *inverted type A nevus* are notable for unusual histologic features. These nevi also may show related clinical and histologic features.

The Combined Nevus

The term *combined nevus* was used initially to describe the combination of ordinary nevus and blue nevus elements[23] but was subsequently extended to include components of Spitz tumor and pigmented spindle cell tumor (deep-penetrating nevus and plexiform pigmented spindle

TABLE 27-21

The Combined Nevus

Clinical Features

Any age (3 to 74 years) but usually less than 40 years of age
Women more often affected than men
Head and neck (especially for blue nevus variants), upper trunk,
    proximal extremities
Often component of blue, blue-black
May have small (1–5 mm) blue, blue-black focus in ordinary nevus
Size less than 6 to 7 mm in most instances

Histopathological Features

Symmetric
Well-circumscribed
Orderly arrangements of cells
Two or more of the following
    Ordinary nevus component
    Pigmented dendritic melanocytes
    Pigmented spindle/epithelioid cells
    Amelanotic spindle cells
    Spitz tumor cells
Ordinary nevus component often overlies or is adjacent to other
    component
Deep involvement occurs
Plexiform configuration on occasion

Differential Diagnosis

Cellular blue nevus
Melanoma

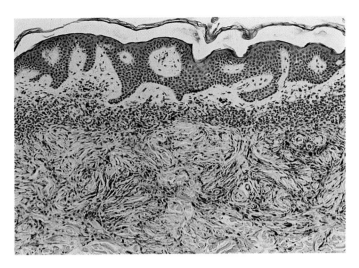

FIGURE 27-42 Combined nevus composed of ordinary compound nevus overlying blue nevus. Note well-defined zone of small nevus cells in superficial dermis overlying blue nevus.

Almost any combination of cell types is possible. Thus, one may encounter nevi containing various admixtures of ordinary nevus cells, dendritic melanocytes, Spitz tumor cells, and perhaps other transitional cell types. Atypical features may also be observed such as melanocytic dysplasia of the intraepidermal component.[192–194]

Inverted Type A Nevus and Melanocytic Nevus with Focal Atypical Epithelioid Cell Component

The morphologic pattern invoked by inverted type A nevus and melanocytic nevus with focal atypical epithelioid cell component, is one probably also encompassed by combined nevus.[195–196] The term describes discrete nests of epithelioid cells, usually pigmented, within the dermal component of an ordinary nevus. These nests are often deep and may be multifocal.

Differential Diagnosis   The histologic change of most concern is an aberrant focus of cytologically altered/atypical cells in an otherwise ordinary nevus, suggesting transformation to melanoma. However, the development of melanoma in the dermal component of a nevus is highly unusual. Although occasional aggregates of epithelioid cells are large, many are small and well-circumscribed. Cytologic atypia is usually low-grade or insignificant compared to melanoma. The surrounding nevus which commonly is of ordinary type is generally unremarkable with reference to atypicality. An occasional mitosis may be observed in such a focus without undue concern; however, the presence of two or more mitoses per high-power field should prompt careful inspection for melanoma. Although combined nevi are heterogenous, they tend to be present in fairly young individuals (younger than 40 years), measure less than 5 or 6 mm, and exhibit an overall symmetry and regular appearance.

cell nevus).[192–194] On morphologic grounds alone, the combined nevus also encompasses so-called inverted type A nevus and nevus with focal atypical epithelioid cell component.[195,196]

Clinical Features   The characteristics of the combined nevus are probably related to the predominant cellular population present, e.g., whether blue nevus or Spitz tumor (Table 27-21).[192–194] Most patients are young and female.[192,196] Combined nevi may demonstrate a small well-circumscribed blue or blue-black focus, e.g., often 1 to 3 mm in diameter, within an otherwise ordinary flesh-colored, tan, or brown nevus.

Histopathological Features   One of the most common patterns is that of an ordinary nevus and blue nevus (Table 27-21) (Fig. 27-42). The ordinary nevus component may be compound or dermal and often overlies or is adjacent to the blue nevus component. Another common pattern is an ordinary nevus in combination with discrete foci of pigmented spindle cells and/or pigmented epithelioid cells.[195,196] The latter cells are often enlarged, contain abundant granular melanin, and are disposed in nests or fascicles in the deep portions of or beneath the ordinary nevus, sometimes in a plexiform arrangement. The sizes of the nests or fascicles may vary from minuscule to large lobular or digitate aggregates. The nuclei are usually slightly enlarged round, oval, or elongate and uniform but on occasion show slight to moderate atypia. Melanophages are also frequently associated with these pigmented foci. This pattern may be morphologically identical to deep-penetrating nevus and plexiform pigmented spindle cell nevus.[197–199]

Spitz tumors uncommonly are observed in association with ordinary nevus elements.[193] The topographic relationships of these two components include the Spitz tumor component adjacent to, beneath, or admixed with the common nevus elements.

Deep-Penetrating Nevus

Deep-penetrating nevus (DPN) describes a group of unusual nevi with disturbing morphologic features[197] but that are nonetheless related to blue nevus, cellular blue nevus, and Spitz tumor.

Clinical and Histopathological Features   Most patients range in age from 10 to 30 years (Table 27-22). DPN most commonly involves the face, upper trunk, and proximal extremities, measures less than 1 cm in

TABLE 27-22

TABLE 27-22

Deep-Penetrating Nevus*

Clinical Features

Age range 10–30 years
Site—face, upper trunk, proximal extremities
Size less than 1 cm
Raised lesions with bluish color

Histopathological Features

Symmetric
Well-circumscribed
Wedge configuration
Extension of cellular fascicles into deep dermis or subcutis
Pigmented spindle cells in fascicles associated with neurovascular
    bundles
Occasional junctional nests
Diffuse involvement of superficial dermis
Occasional cytologic atypia

Differential Diagnosis

Spindle and epithelioid cell tumor
Cellular blue nevus
Melanoma

---

*Plexiform spindle-cell nevus is similar to deep-penetrating nevus but shows a striking plex-
iform configuration not always present in deep-penetrating nevus; neither does the plexiform
nevus always extend as deeply as deep-penetrating nevus.

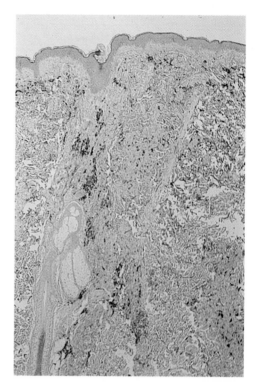

FIGURE 27-43 Plexiform pigmented spindle cell nevus. Characteristic
appearance on scanning magnification of fascicles of pigmented spindle cells in
plexiform arrangement. The fascicles are associated with appendages, blood vessels, and nerves. There is normal collagen separating these cellular aggregates.

greatest diameter, and is clinically diagnosed as blue nevus or cellular
blue nevus.

Scanning magnification discloses a symmetric, well-circumscribed
lesion with involvement of the deep reticular dermis and possibly subcutis (Table 27-22).[197] The overall architecture is usually that of a
wedge extending into the deep dermis (Fig. 27-43). The superficial dermal portion is characterized by a diffuse proliferation of pigmented
spindle cells that show progressive organization as discrete fascicles or
nests with descent into the deep dermis. Junctional nests are noted in
some lesions. The fascicles of spindle cells tend to be associated with
neurovascular and adnexal structures of the lower reticular dermis.
These cellular aggregates often exhibit bulbous contours and may bulge
into the subcutis, as do cellular blue nevi. Melanophages are usually
intimately associated with the spindle cells. Some nevi may show cytologic atypia.

Plexiform Spindle Cell Nevus

Clinical and Histopathological Features   Plexiform spindle cell nevus
is closely related to superficial pigmented spindle cell tumor, Spitz
tumor, blue nevus, and DPN.[198,199] The lesions thus far reported
occurred in young adults (mean age 22.5 years) and involved the shoulders and back.[198] Clinically, the lesions are raised, bluish or black, suggesting blue nevus, an atypical nevus, or melanoma.

Most lesions are slightly raised, symmetric, and exhibit a wedge-
shaped configuration in the reticular dermis.[198,190] The most striking
feature is the plexiform arrangement of fascicles of pigmented spindle
cells that track along adnexal structures and neurovascular bundles
(Fig. 27-43). Other common features include junctional nests, diffuse
involvement of the superficial dermis, and infiltration of cutaneous
nerves and arrector pili muscles. The spindle cells contain abundant
granular melanin and oval or elongate nuclei with delicate chromatin
patterns and inconspicuous nucleoli (Fig. 27-44). Occasional low-grade
cytologic and rare mitotic figures are observed.

Differential Diagnosis   Because of the presence of pigmented spindle
cells and frequent deep involvement, plexiform spindle cell nevi are
closely related to DPN. However, they are discriminated from DPN by
their striking plexiform configuration (often lacking in DPN) and frequent absence of bulbous cellular aggregates and deep involvement.

Because of the unusual nature of these nevi, the immediate concern
is melanoma, whether primary or metastatic (Table 27-22). Particular
features helping in this differential diagnosis include the usual size of
less than 6 or 7 mm (almost always less than 1 cm), overall symmetry,

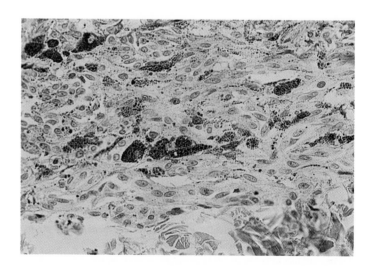

FIGURE 27-44 Plexiform pigmented spindle cell nevus. This field shows a
bundle of uniform-appearing fusiform cells. The cells contain fine granular
melanin and monotonous nuclei with dispersed chromatin.

nondisruptive growth patterns, lack of high-grade atypia, and lack of significant mitotic activity in such nevi. Nonetheless, some of these nevi are quite challenging because of large size, confluent masses of cells without evidence of maturation, and cytologic atypia. As a result, the biologic potential of a small minority of such lesions may be difficult to predict. Rare instances of lymph node metastases have been observed.[194] The most appropriate management is to communicate to the clinician the uncertain but possibly aggressive potential of such tumors.

Phenotypic Heterogeneity and Nomenclature

The nevi described above are related because of depth, architecture, and the presence of pigmented cells that may be oval, elongate, spindled, or perhaps dendritic. Discriminating features include, e.g., superficial or deep disposition; configuration, i.e., plexiform, bulbous; cell type, i.e., pigmented spindle cell, epithelioid cell, dendritic cell; and two or more populations of cells.

MELANOCYTIC PROLIFERATIONS WITH ARCHITECTURAL DISORDER AND CYTOLOGIC ATYPIA (MELANOCYTIC DYSPLASIA AND DYSPLASTIC NEVUS)

Melanocytic proliferations with disordered arrangements and cytologic atypia of melanocytes are an important but highly controversial subject.[200–255] Broadly defined, these lesions form a continuum extending from "typical," e.g., basilar melanocytes or ordinary nevi, to melanoma (Table 27-23).[233,243] The immediate significance of such lesions is

---

TABLE 27-23

Melanocytic Proliferations with Architectural Disorder and Cytologic Atypia (Melanocytic Dysplasia)

Intraepidermal
  Without dermal nevus remnant
    Intraepidermal melanocytic proliferation with architectural disorder and cytologic atypia (junctional dysplastic nevus)
    Lentiginous melanocytic proliferation with architectural disorder and cytologic atypia (melanocytic dysplasia) of acral skin
    Lentiginous melanocytic proliferation with architectural disorder and cytologic atypia (melanocytic dysplasia) of sun-damaged skin
      Lentigo maligna
    Other intraepidermal melanocytic proliferations with architectural disorder and cytologic atypia, not otherwise specified
  With dermal nevus remnant
    Intraepidermal melanocytic proliferation with architectural disorder and cytologic atypia (compound dysplastic nevus)
    Other intraepidermal melanocytic proliferations with architectural and cytologic atypia
    Spindle and epithelioid cell tumors
    Pigmented spindle cell tumors
    Congenital nevi
    Genital nevi
    Acral nevi
Dermal
  Dermal melanocytic proliferations with architectural disorder and cytologic atypia

whether they are markers of increased melanoma risk, whether they are precursors of melanoma, and in practical terms, their histologic distinction from outright melanoma.

Because of the controversy surrounding these nevi, an NIH Consensus Conference has recently recommended that the term *dysplastic nevus* be abandoned in favor of *nevus with architectural disorder and/or cytologic atypia*.[207,242]

The Significance of the Dysplastic Melanocytic Nevus

MARKERS OF INCREASED MELANOMA RISK

Based on studies of hereditary melanoma kindreds,[200,201,205,211,247,248] the presence of Dysplastic Melanocytic Nevus (DMN) on individuals in these kindreds confers a significantly increased risk for the development of melanoma. In fact, the presence of DMN in this setting confers a 48.9 percent cumulative risk for melanoma by age 50 years.[248] In prospective follow-up, only family members with DMN developed melanoma whereas those without DMN did not develop melanoma. Individuals in the general population have dysplastic nevi[203] which also serve as markers for increased melanoma risk, although not nearly so great as in familial melanoma.[205,211] Estimates of the relative risk for melanoma in persons with sporadic DMN may be in the range of 7 to 20 percent. The prevalence of individuals with sporadic DMN has been difficult to accurately gauge but may be in the range of 7 percent to 20 percent.[206,212,237] One particular reason for the difficulty in estimating prevalence of DMN has been the lack of standardized clinical and histopathologic criteria for DMN and for what constitutes the minimum essential criteria for the DMN phenotype, e.g., 50 or 100 or more clinically atypical nevi.[233,251] Classifications have been devised for individuals with DMN and the extent to which they have a personal or family history of melanoma and DMN.[205] Although much more information is needed on this subject, risk-stratification protocols have been formulated to facilitate assessment of melanoma risk and the management of patients.[205] Melanoma risk is probably a continuum with risk directly related to family history of melanoma, especially for individuals with at least two first-degree blood relatives with melanoma; total number of nevi on the skin surface; total number of clinically atypical nevi; and personal history of melanoma.

DYSPLASTIC NEVI AS PRECURSORS TO MELANOMA

DMN occasionally progress to melanoma and thus serve as precursors to melanoma. This progression has been observed through the use of serial photographs and the documentation histologically of focal melanoma developing in an otherwise stable DMN.[210] Various authors have also reported remnants of DMN associated with melanoma with an average frequency of about 33 percent.[204,220,222,224,251] A confounding problem in this situation is the inability in all instances to clearly distinguish the intraepidermal component of melanoma from DMN.

Clinical Features The numbers of clinically atypical nevi on the individual patient may vary from only one or two to in the hundreds or more.[22,200,201,210,211,215,220] Although the majority of DMN occur on the trunk, these nevi show a peculiar propensity for the scalp, female breasts, buttocks, and dorsal surfaces of the feet (Table 27-24). DMN tend to show considerable variation in size, shape, and coloration from nevus to nevus.

DMN (Table 27-24)[22,200,220,233,234] are usually larger than common nevi and smaller than melanoma (but not necessarily so) and generally measure 4 to 12 mm. They often show asymmetry, often irregular and ill-defined borders, and a relatively flat surface (at least part of the lesion is entirely flat). The surface may also be "pebbled" or have a cob-

Dysplastic Nevi

Clinical Features

General

Increased numbers of typical and atypical nevi

Variation in gross morphologic features among nevi

Increased numbers of nevi on scalp, female breasts, buttocks

Nevus characteristics

Increased size (4–12 mm, but not always)

Asymmetry

Macular component

Irregular border

Ill-defined border

Altered topography, pebbled or cobblestone surface

Haphazard, variegated, or greater complexity of coloration

Histopathological Features

Architectural features

Lentiginous melanocytic proliferation*

Variation in size, shape, location of junctional nests with bridging or confluence*

Lack of cellular cohesion of junctional nests

Lateral extension (the "shoulder" phenomenon) of junctional component

Cytologic features

Spindled-cell (with prominent retraction artifact of cytoplasm) pattern

Epithelioid cell pattern

Discontinuous nuclear atypia (not all nuclei atypical)*

Nuclear enlargement

Nuclear pleomorphism

Nuclear hyperchromatism

Prominent nucleoli

Prominent pale or "dusty" cytoplasm

Large melanin granules

Host response

Lymphocytic infiltrates

Fibroplasia

Concentric eosinophilic pattern

Lamellar pattern

Prominent vascularity

---

*Essential features needed for diagnosis. Either lentiginous melanocytic proliferation or variation in junctional nesting is acceptable.

blestone appearance. DMN in general have a more complex color than do ordinary nevi. There are often more than two colors present, i.e., tan, brown, dark brown, and the colors have an irregular or haphazard pattern.

Histopathological Features   The histologic criteria include parameters of architectural disorder, cytologic atypia, and host response (Figs. 27-45 to 27-49) (Table 27-24).[23,201–204,207,209,210,213,214,216,220–222,224,225,228–231,233,236]

Architecture.   The majority of DMN, perhaps 80 percent, are compound and the remainder junctional. Most are relatively flat with only slight expansion of the papillary dermis by limited dermal components. Many (but not all) DMN are lentiginous, i.e., the epidermal rete ridges are elongated, often club-shaped, accompanied by melanocytic hyperplasia and increased melanin content of the epidermis (Figs. 27-46 and 27-47).[230,233] Many heavily pigmented DMN also contain melanin

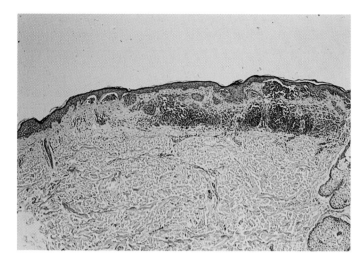

FIGURE 27-45   Compound dysplastic nevus. This field demonstrates the lateral extension of the intraepidermal component (to the left) beyond the dermal nevus component (right side of the field).

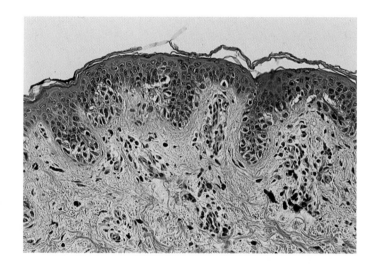

FIGURE 27-46   Junctional dysplastic nevus. Predominant lentiginous pattern of dysplastic nevus. The basilar melanocytes reach confluence along the rete ridges.

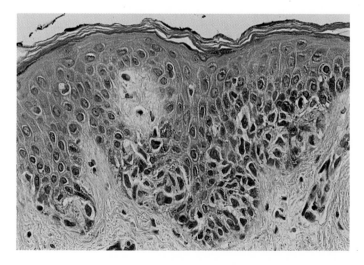

FIGURE 27-47   Junctional dysplastic nevus. Higher magnification discloses variation in size, shape, and staining of nuclei of basilar melanocytes. Some melanocytes have nuclei larger than those in spinous layer keratinocytes.

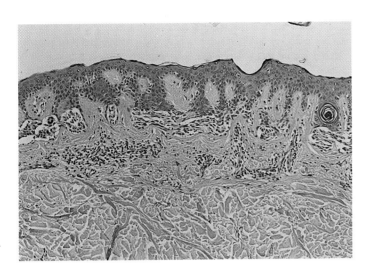

FIGURE 27-48   Compound dysplastic nevus. Mainly junctional nested pattern. There is some variation in the size, shape, and placement of junctional nests.

macroglobules in the basilar epidermis, an entirely nonspecific finding.[230] Many (perhaps the vast majority) compound DMN have lateral extension and poor circumscription of the intraepidermal components (Fig. 27-45). The latter features refer to the intraepidermal melanocytic component extending laterally or peripherally beyond the papillary dermal nevus elements (the *shoulder* phenomenon) and gradually diminishing in cellularity without clear demarcation. Although not a fundamental component of dysplasia as outlined above, lateral extension is a useful feature in recognizing most compound DMN particularly at scanning magnification and does correlate with the peripheral macular annulus observed clinically in many DMN. Junctional DMN by definition do not display lateral extension but tend to be poorly circumscribed.

The essential architectural feature is disordered intraepidermal melanocytic proliferation[230,233] which includes two patterns: (1) lentiginous melanocytic proliferation (Fig. 27-46) and (2) disordered or irregular junctional nesting (Fig. 27-48). Both patterns are often present to varying degree in many DMN, but either pattern may be present alone. The frequency of melanocytes in DMN is, as a rule, greater than in a lentigo, often reaching confluence and replacing basilar keratinocytes.

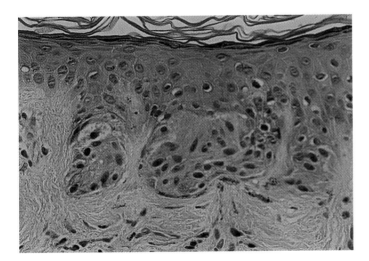

FIGURE 27-49   Compound dysplastic nevus, epithelioid cell variant. Junctional nests contain epithelioid melanocytes. Note abundant "dusty" cytoplasm of the epithelioid cells. The papillary dermis also shows fibrosis.

In its most extreme version, the proliferation of melanocytes may result in multilayered confluence of cells along the dermal-epidermal junction, often "bridging" between rete. The melanocytes present in this pattern commonly exhibit retraction of cytoplasm resulting in a vacuolated appearance of the basal layer, almost suggesting basal layer vacuolopathy. The nuclei within these vacuolated cells are commonly pleomorphic with angulated contours.[230,233]

Compared to typical nevi, junctional nests in DMN tend to vary significantly in size, shape (ovoid, elongate, or confluent along the dermal-epidermal junction), and spacing (nests are not present at equidistant intervals). Junctional nests instead of being located at the tips of rete are irregularly distributed on the sides and between rete, often with no regular pattern ("irregularly irregular"). Bridging of nests between rete is another feature of the abnormal nesting pattern. Often paralleling the variation in nesting is the loss of cellular cohesion in junctional nests. The individual nevus cells literally appear to fall apart with clear spaces forming between individual cells and aggregates of cells.

Although upward migration of melanocytes throughout the epidermis is not a common feature of DMN, it is seen on occasion but is often limited, focal, or orderly in appearance.

Cytology.   One of the fundamental criteria for DMN is variable (or discontinuous) cytologic atypia of intraepidermal melanocytes.[209,229,230,233] The latter refers to intraepidermal melanocytes that are not uniformly atypical but tend to vary from cell to cell as to the degree of nuclear atypia. In general, this nuclear atypia is a continuum and characterized by gradual nuclear enlargement, pleomorphism, variation in nuclear chromatin pattern, and the eventual development of prominent nucleoli. The beginnings of nuclear atypia may be almost imperceptible and may not be reproducible. Commonly with slight or low-grade cytologic atypia, the cells show retraction of cytoplasm, and the size of the melanocytic nuclei is increased and approximates that of or is slightly larger than the nuclei of spinous layer keratinocytes.[226] With greater (moderate) atypia, the nuclei are somewhat larger than the nuclei of spinous layer keratinocytes, and nucleoli are more commonly visible. With severe cytologic atypia, the melanocytes may contain abundant cytoplasm which often has a granular eosinophilic appearance or may contain finely divided ("dusty") melanin.[226] The nuclei may be enlarged to twice the size of spinous layer keratinocyte nuclei or larger (Fig. 27-47). Nucleoli are often enlarged and may be eosinophilic. The ultimate endpoint is a uniformly atypical population of cells which marks the development of melanoma.

The cell types that comprise DMN include basilar melanocytes with retracted cytoplasm, small rounded nevus cells, spindle cells, sometimes pigmented, and epithelioid cells (Fig. 27-49).[23,209,230,233] The basilar melanocytes with retraction of cytoplasm are often observed in predominantly lentiginous forms of DMN while the epithelioid cell type is often present in a much less prevalent, predominantly nested form of DMN (so-called epithelioid cell dysplasia).

Host Response.   Among mononuclear-cell infiltrates, fibroplasia, and prominent vascularity, the first two have received considerable attention as criteria for DMN.[23,209,210,214,230,233] Lymphocytic infiltrates are present in the overriding majority of DMN. These infiltrates vary from sparse perivascular lymphoid infiltrates (Fig. 27-48) to dense bandlike infiltrates filling the papillary dermis.

The more common form of fibroplasia is concentric eosinophilic fibrosis, which is hyalinized collagen that is compactly disposed about the epidermal rete ridges. Lamellar fibroplasia is less prevalent and notable for delicate stacking of horizontally disposed collagen, subjacent to the epidermal rete ridges (Fig. 27-49). Mesenchymal spindle cells typically line these filamentous strands of collagen. Both patterns of fibroplasia may be present in the same lesion or occur separately.

Histologic Variants of Dysplastic Nevus

EPITHELIOID CELL VARIANT

The *epithelioid* cells resemble the cell type in pagetoid melanoma except that they tend to be less cytologically atypical (Fig. 27-49).[209] The cells are round or polygonal and contain abundant pink or "dusty" (finely divided melanin) cytoplasm. Relatively small round nuclei are usually present in the center of the cell. The cells tend to have an almost exclusively nested distribution often without an associated lentiginous element.

HALO NEVUS VARIANT

These DMN display dense mononuclear cell infiltrates filling the papillary dermis and obscuring any nests of nevus cells present.[23] These nevi are distinguished from benign halo nevi by aberrant architectural features and cytologic atypia.

Specificity of Histologic Features of Dysplastic Nevus

Disordered arrangements of cells and cytologic atypia are encountered in a number of lesions thought to be distinct from conventional DMN.[23,243] The latter findings are often similar to those observed in DMN and provide evidence that almost any melanocytic proliferation may progress to an *intermediate* or dysplastic stage and possibly have some potential for giving rise to melanoma. Because these other "dysplastic" melanocytic lesions, such as congenital nevi, Spitz tumors, and vulvar nevi have received considerably less attention than conventional DMN, essentially no information is available concerning their melanoma risk.[23,243] As outlined in Table 27-25, it is proposed that these various lesions may be subjected to the same guidelines as have DMN (see below).

Differential Diagnosis   The DMN must be distinguished from in situ or invasive melanoma, atypical lentiginous melanocytic proliferations and melanoma in situ of sun-damaged skin (historically termed *lentigo maligna* and *Hutchinson's melanotic freckle*), lentiginous nevi, pigmented spindle cell tumor, Spitz tumor, halo nevus, congenital nevus, and recurrent nevus.

One of the most difficult problems is the discrimination of severely atypical DMN from in situ or microinvasive melanoma. This differential diagnosis is discussed below, and the most salient points are summarized in Table 27-26. In one sense, this distinction is somewhat arbitrary and subjective, since no consensus has been reached regarding criteria for separating the two entities. However, in another sense, the central issue is whether a particular lesion retains some degree of growth control, an orderly nevic appearance, and variable or discontinuous nuclear atypia versus loss of growth control, loss of an orderly nevic appearance, and continuous nuclear atypia.

DMN and lentiginous melanocytic proliferations and melanoma in situ (LMPS) of sun-damaged skin show histologic similarities on occasion and may be difficult to separate. LMPS is distinguished from DMN in most instances because LMPS is a dysplasia secondary to cumulative sun exposure and consequently develops on markedly sun-exposed skin of the elderly (average age 60 years). The most common locations are the cheek and nose, which are unusual sites for conventional DMN. LMPS is usually a de novo melanocytic dysplasia, since dermal nevus components are uncommon, whereas approximately 80 percent of DMN contain dermal nevus cells.[224]

LMPS developing on the central face most commonly shows a basilar proliferation of variably atypical melanocytes that often involve the appendageal epithelium. The epidermis is usually effaced, i.e., has no rete ridge pattern, and there is prominent solar elastosis in the dermis. In contrast, the DMN generally has elongated rete ridges with concentration of basilar melanocytes and many junctional nests along the rete ridges, and solar elastosis is usually minimal. LMPS may also have junctional nests, but they are often discohesive elongate nests composed of pigmented spindled cells. The latter nests on occasion show striking involvement of hair follicles and eccrine ducts, a finding not typically observed in DMN.

TABLE 27-25

Guidelines for Grading Architectural and Cytologic Atypia in Melanocytic Proliferations

	*Spectrum of Changes**		
	Low-grade		High-grade
Architectural features		Asymmetry[†]	
		Lateral extension	
	Lentiginous melanocytic hyperplasia[†]		Confluence of cells along basal layer
	Little or no upward migration[†]	Intradermal upward migration of cells	Fully developed pagetoid spread
	Little variation in nesting[†]	Variation in junctional nesting, bridging	Confluence of nests
	Cohesion of cells in nests[†]		Diminished cohesion of cells
	Elongated rete		Effacement (loss) of rete pattern
	Little disturbance in dermal maturation[†]	Failure of maturation of dermal cellular component	Rounded expansile nests of dermal cells
Cytologic features	Discontinuous atypia[†] (few cells atypical)		Continuous atypia (most cells atypical)
		Cellular enlargement[†]	
		Nuclear enlargement[†]	
		Nuclear pleomorphism[†]	
		Prominent nucleoli[†]	
		Hyperchromatism[†]	
	Uniform, nongranular cytoplasm	Abundant cytoplasm	Abundant granular eosinophilic or dusty cytoplasm

*Each variable or parameter is a continuous variable from low-grade to high-grade, e.g., the variable *asymmetry* would represent a spectrum from little or no asymmetry (low-grade) to prominent or marked asymmetry (high-grade). Thus, either the extremes for each parameter is specifically indicated or the parameter is simply stated without qualification of the extremes.

[†]A principal feature for grading architectural and cytologic atypia.

TABLE 27-26

Severely Atypical Dysplastic Nevus and Melanoma

Severely atypical dysplastic nevus*	In situ or microinvasive melanoma*
Some asymmetry	Prominent asymmetry
Poorly circumscribed	Poorly circumscribed
Rete ridges preserved	Tendency to loss or effacement of rete ridges
Some maintenance of nevus nesting pattern and order	Loss of orderly nesting pattern
Some diminished cohesion of nests	Diminished cohesion of nests may be prominent
Lentiginous melanocytic proliferation concentrated on rete ridges	Loss of rete-oriented melanocytic proliferation
Pagetoid spread absent, minimal, or not prominent	Pagetoid spread prominent
Discontinuous cytologic atypia	Fairly uniform (continuous) cytologic atypia
Often some maturation of dermal component	Often no maturation of dermal component
Usually no mitoses in dermal component	Uncommon mitoses in dermal component (microinvasive melanoma)
Usually perivascular lymphocytic infiltrates	Tendency to bandlike lymphocytic infiltrates

*The histologic guidelines listed in this table represent the most common presentation. However, there is considerable variation among these features.

LMPS arising on other sun-exposed sites may show a rete ridge pattern and thus present an even greater problem in differential diagnosis. Discriminating features favoring LMPS include a mainly lentiginous pattern of melanocytic proliferation, prominent involvement of appendages, presence of pigmented spindle cells, and solar elastosis. Overlap with DMN on occasion may be so great that separation may be difficult, often arbitrary, and not necessary. The various clinical and histologic features present must be assessed. If discrimination is not possible, a reasonable approach is a descriptive diagnosis, e.g., intraepidermal melanocytic proliferation with features of both LMPS and dysplastic nevus and severe cytologic atypia.

Another conundrum is the distinction of DMN from lentiginous nevi, particularly those from acral skin. Here, the main problem is one of threshold, i.e., is there sufficient disordered architecture and cytologic atypia for the diagnosis of DMN? Such lesions should be evaluated for poor circumscription, asymmetry, substantially increased frequency of basilar melanocytes, irregularity of junctional nesting with elongated confluent nests, bridging of nests between rete ridges, and finally cytologic atypia of intraepidermal melanocytes. Lesions having equivocal changes should not be diagnosed as DMN. It is reasonable to designate the latter lesions as showing some architectural disorder or, alternatively, as not having clear-cut melanocytic dysplasia.

As discussed below, a number of types of melanocytic nevi such as pigmented spindle cell tumor, Spitz tumor, and congenital nevus may on occasion demonstrate disordered architectural patterns and cytologic atypia, i.e., show evidence of melanocytic dysplasia. Yet, at the same time, these various nevi retain many of the histologic features that make them distinctive, e.g., fascicles of slender pigmented spindle cells in pigmented spindle cell nevus, large epithelioid cells in Spitz tumor, and extensive involvement of the reticular dermis in congenital nevus.

Recurrent melanocytic nevi may on occasion enter into the differential diagnosis of DMN (see above).

Grading of Dysplastic Nevi

The following guidelines for grading dysplastic nevi are suggested: (1) severely atypical or high-grade DMN should be recognized because of their overlap with melanoma in situ. Such lesions should be completely excised with margins of at least 5 mm. (2) DMN with moderate atypia (see earlier discussion) should be completely removed with clear margins. Because DNA aneuploidy has been documented in such lesions, there may possibly be a greater potential for progression to melanoma than less atypical lesions.[253] (3) DMN with slight or minimal atypia need not have reexcision if the bulk of the lesion has been removed, even if the margins are involved. Such lesions are common, and reproducible distinction from lentiginous nevi with architectural disorder and no cytologic atypia may not be possible. In general, slightly atypical DMN do not exhibit DNA aneuploidy.[253]

Histopathological Reporting of Dysplastic Nevi

The pathologist should communicate clearly to the clinician the nature of the lesion and its significance, regardless of terminology used. In one sense, the significance of the individual lesion is related to the degree of atypicality in that lesion. The immediate concern is to ensure proper management of the individual lesion, i.e., degree of atypicality is properly assessed and the need for additional therapy, i.e., surgery, if any, is communicated to the clinician (Table 27-27). In another sense, the significance of a DMN must be viewed from the perspective of global melanoma risk in the patient. Thus, the significance of the individual DMN can be viewed in quantitative terms and is directly related to family history of melanoma, family history of DMN, personal history of melanoma, the patient's nevus phenotype (total number of typical and atypical nevi on the skin surface), degree of atypia of previously removed nevi, and other risk factors for melanoma.

TABLE 27-27

Histopathologic Reporting of Dysplastic Nevi

Grade of lesion	Reexcision if margins involved
Low-grade lesions	
Junctional or compound nevus with architectural disorder (no cytologic atypia)	No
Junctional or compound dysplastic nevus with slight atypia* (or nevus with architectural disorder and slight cytologic atypia)	No, if bulk of lesion removed
High-grade lesions	
Junctional or compound dysplastic nevus with moderate atypia (or nevus with architectural disorder and moderate cytologic atypia)	Yes
Junctional or compound dysplastic nevus with severe cytologic atypia (or nevus with architectural disorder and severe cytologic atypia)	Yes, with at least 5-mm margins

*See text for criteria for grades of cytologic atypia.

MALIGNANT MELANOMA

Classification of Cutaneous Melanoma

The morphologic spectrum of cutaneous melanoma (Table 27-28) may be described according to (1) the location of melanoma cells in the skin, whether intraepidermal, dermal, subcutaneous, or soft tissue; (2) the disposition and frequency or density of melanocytes in these domains, e.g., *pagetoid* (dispersion of single and small groups of melanocytes throughout epidermis), *lentiginous* (a basilar epidermal single-cell proliferation of melanocytes), or *nested* arrangements of cells in the epidermis, single-cell infiltrating or aggregative (nodular) patterns in the

TABLE 27-28

Classification of Melanoma According to Tissue Localization, Organizational Attributes (Disposition) of Melanocytes, Other Morphologic Features, and Cytology

Location in the skin
  Intraepidermal
  Dermal
  Subcutaneous
  Soft tissue
Disposition and frequency
  Intraepidermal component
    Pagetoid
    Lentiginous
    Nested
    Two or more patterns
    Not melanoma
  Dermal component
    Single-cell infiltration
    Nests of cells
    Aggregative (nodule formation)
Specific morphologic features
  Epidermal surface configuration
    Verrucous
    Papillomatous
    Polypoid
  Stromal alterations
    Desmoplasia
    Myxoid alteration
  Other alterations
    Neurotropism
    Neural differentiation (neurogenic, neural transforming)
    Angiotropism
    Alveolar/glandular
Cell type
  Epithelioid
  Spindle
  Dendritic
  Nevuslike
  Small cell
  Balloon cell
  Clear cell
  Anaplastic giant cell
  Rhabdoid
  Signet ring
  Difficult to classify
Precursor lesion
  Nevus remnant of any kind
  Other precursor

TABLE 27-29

Historical Classification of Malignant Melanoma

Presence of radial growth phase
  Superficial spreading
  Lentigo maligna
  Acral lentiginous
  Unclassified
Absence of radial growth phase
  Nodular melanoma

dermis and subcutis; (3) unusual histologic features or stromal alterations, such as verrucous, papillomatous, or polypoid epidermal surface configurations; desmoplasia; myxoid stroma; neurotropism; neurogenic or neural differentiation; resemblance to melanomas developing in animals, experimentally or spontaneous; and (4) cytologic features such as epithelioid, spindled, dendritic, nevuslike, small, clear, balloon, "Spitz-tumor-"like, and other cell types.[256] Because most all melanomas are initiated in and localized to the epidermis (or epithelium) for some period of time, a classification of melanoma based on the presence or absence and patterns of intraepidermal involvement has been developed and utilized.[257–262] One idea behind such a classification was that particular intraepidermal patterns (also termed *radial* or *horizontal growth phases*) might correlate with differences in etiology and possibly prognosis. Four clinicopathologic subtypes of melanoma have been proposed (Table 27-29).[22,257–264] Melanoma with an adjacent lentiginous intraepidermal component of sun-exposed skin (so-called lentigo maligna melanoma) may be distinct from other forms of melanomas with intraepithelial components (the pagetoid and acral lentiginous forms of melanoma) because of its strong correlation with cumulative sunlight exposure, onset in older persons, and uncommon association with melanocytic nevi.[262] Melanomas with adjacent pagetoid intraepidermal component have been reported to correlate with intermittent sunlight exposure.[262] Acral melanomas develop in relatively sun-protected sites.[261,265,266] Nodular melanoma (NM) is described as having no adjacent intraepithelial component and is thought by some to be a final common pathway of rapid tumor progression irrespective of intraepithelial pattern or location.[23,260,267]

Although no correlation between intraepidermal pattern (so-called radial growth phase) and prognosis has been established,[268,269] some evidence indicates that etiologic factors might still explain some of the morphologic patterns of melanoma, as discussed above.[262] Nevertheless, an objective assessment of the classification of melanoma according to intraepidermal pattern or growth phase is that such a classification is a straw man and has not been clearly validated.[256,267,270] The reasons for this view are: (1) the tremendous morphologic heterogeneity of melanoma, (2) morphologic patterns may correlate with anatomic site, (3) the intraepithelial components of many melanomas are not easily classified (because of overlapping features) and classification is not reproducible,[271] (4) some intraepithelial components are difficult to recognize as either clearly benign, i.e., a potential precursor such as dysplastic nevus, or malignant, and (5) the idea that nodular melanomas develop as de novo invasive tumors without any initial intraepithelial melanocytic proliferation[261] is theoretically possible but has not been proved.

Despite the flaws in the current classification of melanoma outlined above, some form of classification is needed for both pathologic reporting and investigational purposes. The schema outlined in Table 27-28 provides the framework for such a classification. An (adjacent) intraepithelial component if present should be recorded and, if possible, described according to its pattern as predominantly pagetoid, lentigi-

TABLE 27-30

Clinical Features of Melanoma

In general onset after puberty but all ages

Most frequent ages 40–70 years

Caucasians more often affected than Africans, Asians

Women equally or more frequently affected than men

Most common sites—lower extremities and trunk of women
and trunk (back) of men

Pain, pruritus

Size often greater than 1 cm (range 2 mm to more than 15 cm)

Initially macular, later stages may be papular and nodular

Asymmetry

Irregular and often notched borders

Complexity and variation in color often with admixtures of tan,
brown, black, blue, gray, white, red

May be entirely skin-colored (amelanotic) or black

Ulceration and bleeding may be present

Longitudinal pigmented bands of nails, often larger than 9 mm in width

Periungual pigmentation (Hutchinson's sign)

to 27-54).[270] The latter proliferation may develop with or without a detectable melanocytic nevus. Estimates of the frequency of melanomas developing in continuity with a nevus of any kind vary widely; approximately a third of melanomas have nevus remnants. The duration of this intraepidermal phase ranges from months to many years, during which these proliferative lesions show progressive degrees of architectural and cytologic atypicality.

Increasing cytologic atypia of melanocytes accompanies the aberrant architectural appearance. The melanocytes vary in degree of atypia and the proportion of cells with nuclear atypia. However, atypical melanocytes usually have enlarged nuclei that exhibit variation in nuclear shapes and chromatin patterns, and may have large nucleoli. Thickening of nuclear membranes and irregular nuclear contours are also characteristic. The cytoplasm of such melanocytes may be abundant with a pink granular quality, may contain granular or finely divided (dusty) melanin (Figs. 27-50 and 27-51), or show retraction, resulting in a clear space around the nuclei. Melanocytes with scant cytoplasm typically have high nuclear-to-cytoplasmic ratios. Such proliferations have been variously labeled *atypical*

nous, nested, or any combination of these features, rather than necessarily applying a term such as *superficial spreading* or *lentigo maligna melanoma*. An invasive component should be recorded if present and measured in millimeters (see below), and certain features recorded such as stromal alterations, e.g., desmoplasia, invasion of nerves (neurotropism), cell type, and presence of a nevus remnant.

Clinical Features   In general, cutaneous melanoma is a disease of adult Caucasians and is rarely observed before puberty.[263] Men and women are equally affected, although some European studies have suggested a higher incidence in females.[262] Patients are most commonly diagnosed with melanoma in the fourth through seventh decades. The most common sites include the trunk (back) followed by the upper extremities and head and neck for men and the lower extremities followed by the back, upper extremities, and head and neck for women. Gross morphologic features of melanoma include size often greater than 1 cm (range 2 mm to greater than 15 cm); irregular or notched borders; asymmetry; complexity of color including a variable admixture of tan, brown, blue, black, red, pink, gray, and white; and ulceration and bleeding.[22,263,272] Early melanomas especially those involving sun-exposed and acral sites may be completely flat but with progression usually develop a papular or nodular component. Melanomas lacking pigment (amelanotic melanoma) and those resembling keratoses are particularly difficult to diagnose without a high index of suspicion. Acral melanoma, although accounting for 5 percent or less of melanomas among Caucasians, is the most frequent form of melanoma among Asians, blacks, and other ethnic groups of color (Table 27-30).[22,261,265,266] However, approximately the same incidence of acral melanoma occurs in all ethnic groups. Subungual melanoma (SM) is a distinctive variant of acral melanoma[273–276] that most often involves the nail bed of the great toe or thumb where it commonly presents as an ulcerated tumor.[22] However, the initial manifestations may include a longitudinal pigmented band of the nail plate (frequently 9 mm in width) or a mass under the nail plate.[277] A useful clinical sign is pigmentation extending from the nail onto the surrounding periungual skin (Hutchinson's sign).[22]

Histopathological Features

Intraepithelial component. Almost all melanomas begin as a proliferation of melanocytes initially confined to the epidermis (Figs. 27-50

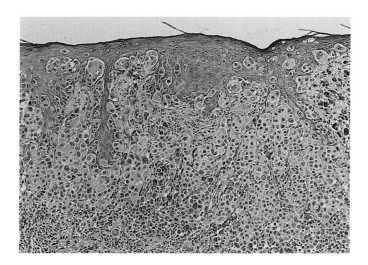

FIGURE 27-50   Pagetoid melanoma. Pagetoid spread of epithelioid cells throughout epidermis and confluent sheets of epithelioid cells in dermis.

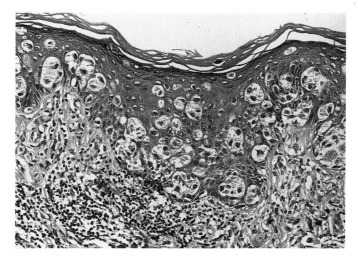

FIGURE 27-51   Pagetoid melanoma. Extensive pagetoid spread of epithelioid melanoma cells.

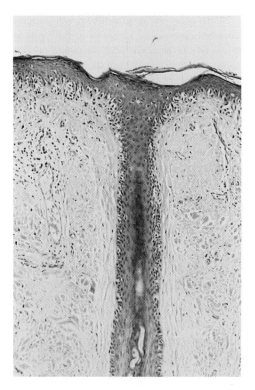

FIGURE 27-52 Lentiginous melanocytic proliferation of sun-exposed skin. There is a striking basilar proliferation of variably atypical melanocytes in both the epidermis and the follicular epithelium.

melanocytic hyperplasia, premalignant melanosis, melanocytic dysplasia, and, recently *pagetoid melanocytic proliferation,* as well as *melanoma in situ* (Table 27-31).[258,260,278,279]

Invasive melanoma. After the period of intraepidermal proliferation, there is often invasion of the papillary dermis,[14,258,261] primarily as single cells and small aggregates of cells.[280] Microinvasive melanoma is also remarkable for a striking host response in the papillary dermis, typically a dense cellular infiltrate of lymphocytes and monocyte/macrophages (Fig. 27-51). Presumably, in consequence of this host reaction, regression, often focal, is common in up to 50 percent of microinvasive melanomas (see below).[281]

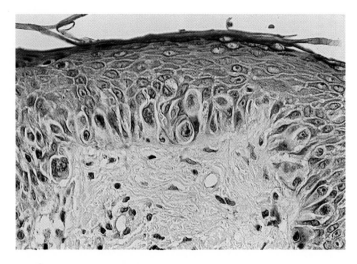

FIGURE 27-53 Lentiginous melanoma of sun-exposed skin. Higher magnification showing atypia of basilar melanocytes.

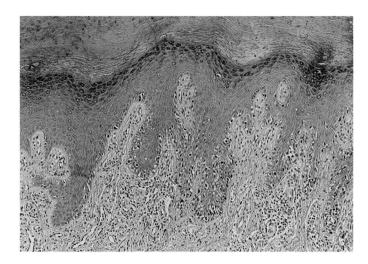

FIGURE 27-54 Lentiginous melanoma of acral skin. The epidermis is hyperplastic and exhibits characteristic lentiginous proliferation of pleomorphic melanoma cells.

The term *vertical growth phase* has been used by some to describe the proliferation of invasive melanoma cells as cohesive aggregates.[14,280] It has been postulated that the so-called vertical growth phase may signify the onset of the metastatic phenotype, since it may be indistinguishable from metastatic melanoma.[280,282] Melanomas with prominent invasive components may display polypoid morphologies such that more than half (sessile forms) or virtually all (pedunculated forms) of the tumor is above the epidermal surface. Amelanotic variants also may develop in any type of melanoma.[23]

Melanoma with adjacent predominately pagetoid intraepidermal component. *Pagetoid spread* (transepidermal migration of cells in a manner analogous to Paget's disease of the breast)[14,23,257–261,283] refers to single cells and small groups of cells randomly scattered throughout the epidermis reaching the granular layer and stratum corneum. The melanoma cells often have an epithelioid cell appearance, i.e., they resemble epithelial cells because of abundant cytoplasm that is usually granular and eosinophilic or contains finely divided (dusty) melanin (Figs. 27-50 and 27-51). The cells are usually larger than (sometimes two to three times) the surrounding keratinocytes. The epidermis may be hyperplastic, the epidermal rete pattern is often lost (effaced), and the surface of the epidermis abutting the intraepidermal tumor may exhibit a characteristically scalloped contour. Melanoma cells often proliferate as variably sized nests and horizontally disposed aggregates immediately underneath this scalloped epidermis. These aggregates are frequently large in size and have diminished cohesion of cells. In some instances, the latter proliferative pattern may predominate with little or no pagetoid spread.

TABLE 27-31

Anatomic Levels of Invasion

Level I—entirely intraepidermal; melanoma in situ
Level II—microinvasive into papillary dermis
Level III—expansion of papillary dermis by cohesive cellular nodule or plaque (but confined to papillary dermis)
Level IV—invasion of reticular dermis
Level V—invasion of subcutaneous fat

The most common cell in the invasive component is epithelioid (Fig. 27-50). Less frequently spindle cells, small cells, or large bizarre mononuclear or multinucleate cells may predominate or are admixed with the other cell types. Many melanomas show heterogeneity of cell type, such that the cells vary in nuclear size and shape and amount of cytoplasm from one focus to another.

Melanoma with adjacent predominately lentiginous intraepidermal component of sun-exposed skin (lentigo maligna melanoma; Hutchinson's melanotic freckle). *Lentigo maligna* is a confusing term, since it has been used to describe a histologic spectrum from slightly increased numbers of basilar melanocytes with variable low-grade cytologic atypia[23,257–261,284] that is not clearly melanoma in situ, to a contiguous and often nested intraepidermal proliferation of highly pleomorphic melanocytic cells that is melanoma in situ.[284] Furthermore, some pathologists consider all lentigo maligna to be melanoma in situ,[270] while others do not,[23,264] hence the confusion. Irrespective of terminology, the pathologist must clearly communicate to the clinician the meaning of the pathologic terms used to describe these lesions. For clarity, the author recommends the term *lentiginous melanocytic proliferation* with atypia (LMPS) (atypia may be graded as slight, moderate, or severe according to guidelines proposed for dysplastic nevi) for lesions judged to fall short of melanoma in situ; otherwise, *melanoma in situ* should be used for lesions showing sufficiently disordered melanocytic proliferation and cellular atypia, i.e., contiguous proliferation of uniformly markedly atypical melanocytes.

In addition to a mainly basilar proliferation of melanocytes (Figs. 27-52 and 27-53), this form of melanoma is also characterized by atrophy and effacement of the epidermis (Fig. 27-52), involvement of appendageal structures (Fig. 27-52), and marked solar elastosis.[23,257–261,284] However, the presence of the latter changes may simply be related to anatomic site, i.e., the skin of the cheek in older individuals usually exhibits a flattened epidermis and prominent solar elastosis. There may be prominent involvement of appendageal epithelium with large cellular nests. Recognition of prominent appendageal involvement by melanoma is of critical importance so that the lesion is not misdiagnosed as invasive rather than simply as intraepithelial or in situ. The most typical cell type has retracted cytoplasm and often an elongate, stellate, or spindled configuration[284] and a high nuclear-cytoplasmic ratio. The nuclei are commonly pleomorphic and hyperchromatic. With progression, the cells become more epithelioid in appearance and exhibit nuclear enlargement and prominent nucleoli (Fig. 27-53). Another characteristic feature is the presence of prominent spindle cell differentiation with formation of confluent fascicles of spindle cells along the dermal-epidermal junction and appendages.[23,284]

Extension of melanoma into the dermis may be difficult to recognize because of prominent cellularity of the stroma and activation of mesenchymal cells. The invasive dermal component is frequently composed of spindle cells either occurring singly or in bundles[260] with varying stromal desmoplasia and invasion of nerve twigs (see discussion of desmoplastic melanoma). However, the invasive component may contain any cell type. Invasion of the dermis may originate from appendageal-associated melanoma cells or nests. In the latter instances, depth of invasion (Breslow thickness) should not be measured from the granular layer of the epidermis, since this value would overestimate tumor depth. The measurement of tumor thickness instead should ideally be taken from the granular layer of the hair follicle or sweat gland.

Melanomas with adjacent predominately lentiginous intraepithelial component of acral skin, the nail apparatus, and mucosal surfaces. These tumors are usually advanced, often ulcerated, and characterized by a tumor nodule frequently extending deeply into the stroma.[23,260,261,265,266] Scanning magnification will usually reveal a hyperplastic epidermis and lentiginous proliferation of atypical melanocytic cells (Fig. 27-54). These cells are commonly contiguous with occasional clustering, appear to lie within lacunae, and display prominent dendrites that extend through the epidermis. Pagetoid patterns are also observed frequently, either alone or associated with lentiginous proliferation. The nuclei are enlarged, hyperchromatic, and often highly pleomorphic. With tumor progression, there is a tendency for upward migration and dermal invasion. Variable degrees of melanization are present.

The dermal component is most often composed of spindle cells, but epithelioid cells, small nevuslike cells, and highly pleomorphic cell types are occasionally noted.[266] A small proportion exhibit desmoplasia and neurotropism (see below).

Melanoma without adjacent intraepithelial component (nodular melanoma). Scanning magnification discloses a raised, dome-shaped, or polypoid tumor often but not always exhibiting some asymmetry (Fig. 27-55).[23,257–261] The epidermis over the tumor is usually thin and effaced, and may be ulcerated. Variable upward migration of melanoma cells in the epidermis may be present, but intraepidermal spread should not extend beyond the margins of the tumor. The dermal component is typified by a cohesive nodule or smaller nests of tumor cells that have a pushing or expansile pattern of growth.[14,261,280] The tumor cells most frequently are epithelioid, but other cell types including spindle cells and small epithelioid cells resembling nevus cells may predominate or be admixed with other cell types.[261]

Differential Diagnosis   The differential diagnosis includes various melanocytic proliferations (Table 27-32): markedly atypical dysplastic nevi, halo nevi, spindle and epithelioid cell (Spitz) tumors, pigmented spindle cell tumors, recurrent melanocytic nevi, and congenital nevi, particularly in the first year of life. Nevi associated with prominent pagetoid spread are commonly confused with melanoma.

Dysplastic nevi with pronounced atypia may be misdiagnosed as melanoma because of appearances suggestive of early pagetoid spread, confluence of cellular aggregates along the dermal-epidermal junction, prominent variation in nesting pattern, significant cytologic atypia, entrapment of nests of dermal nevus cells in the papillary dermis, and dense mononuclear cell infiltrates. On occasion, the distinction of dysplastic nevi from melanoma is exceedingly difficult. Nonetheless, discrimination of melanoma from dysplastic nevi is usually possible

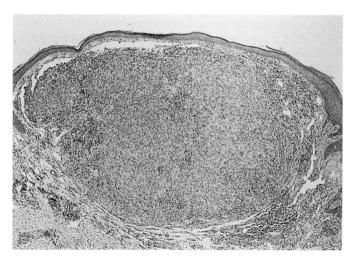

FIGURE 27-55   Nodular melanoma. The tumor has a dome-shaped configuration.

TABLE 27-32

Differential Diagnosis of Malignant Melanoma

Melanocytic tumors
    Dysplastic melanocytic nevus
    Halo nevus
    Spindle and epithelioid cell tumor
    Pigmented spindle cell tumor
    Recurrent melanocytic nevus
    Other melanocytic nevi with prominent pagetoid spread
    Metastatic melanoma
Nonmelanocytic tumors
    Squamous cell carcinoma
    Paget's disease, mammary or extramammary
    Sebaceous carcinoma
    Cutaneous T-cell lymphoma
    Epidermotropic eccrine carcinoma
    Metastatic carcinoma, other
    Angiosarcoma
    Kaposi's sarcoma
    Leiomyosarcoma
    Atypical fibroxanthoma
    Malignant fibrous histiocytoma

because of the greater asymmetry and disorder encountered in melanoma. Usually dysplastic nevi will maintain an overall symmetry, a nevic appearance as exemplified by fairly organized junctional nesting, a basilar proliferation of melanocytes that is still concentrated along the epidermal rete and with greater density toward the lower poles of the rete. Thus, the intervening epidermis between rete will contain a lesser density of melanocytes compared to that on the epidermal rete. If pagetoid spread is present, this architectural pattern is often more prominent about epidermal rete and confined to the lowermost epidermis. Occasional dysplastic nevi exhibit effacement of the epidermal rete pattern and confluence of melanocytic cells along the dermal-epidermal junction in this zone. The latter changes are commonly associated with dense mononuclear cell infiltrates. The latter changes may strongly suggest melanoma, and the findings must be carefully interpreted in the overall context of the lesion. Dysplastic nevi are generally characterized by variable or discontinuous cytologic atypia, i.e., the degree of nuclear enlargement, pleomorphism, and hyperchromatism varies from cell to cell.[23] This cytologic feature is very helpful in discriminating dysplastic nevi from the more uniform or contiguous cytologic atypia of melanoma.

A finding that raises the possibility of melanoma is entrapment of atypical nevus cells in a fibrotic papillary dermis of a dysplastic nevus. Such findings may even suggest partial regression of melanoma. A distinction from melanoma should be based on an assessment of all the cytologic and architectural characteristics of the lesion. Important, the dermal nevus cells in question usually lack the marked and uniform cytologic atypia, especially manifested as hyperchromasia, of melanoma cells.

In general, halo nevi have dense mononuclear cell infiltrates, histologic regression in some instances, and varying degrees of architectural and cytologic atypia that may suggest melanoma. The typical halo nevus of children and adolescents is characterized by overall symmetry, orderly appearance, and little or no cytologic atypia.[23] The lymphoid cells that permeate the dermal nevus have a uniform density and regular horizontal contour. The nevus cells of halo nevi may demonstrate cellular enlargement with prominent eosinophilic cytoplasm, but their

nuclear details are usually little altered. In contrast, there is a variant of halo nevus that has prominent pattern and cellular atypia and is perhaps best categorized as a dysplastic nevus. The discussion of dysplastic nevi (above) is relevant to this form of (atypical) halo nevus.

The misdiagnosis of other melanocytic nevi including spindle and epithelioid cell tumors, pigmented spindle cell tumors, congenital nevi, recurrent melanocytic nevi, and nevi in children as melanoma is primarily related to misinterpretation of patterns of minor pagetoid spread. Overall symmetry and a well-organized appearance, as well as little or no cytologic atypia, favor a benign melanocytic proliferation. Pagetoid spread in benign melanocytic nevi is generally characterized by an orderly pattern and is generally limited to the lower epidermis, and aggregates of cells predominate over single cells.

Spindle and epithelioid cell tumors pose particular diagnostic problems (see above). Lentiginous melanocytic proliferations with atypia (LMPS) and lentiginous melanomas from markedly sun-damaged skin (LM) must be distinguished from solar lentigo, dysplastic nevus, and pigmented spindle cell tumor (see previous discussions). The former lesions may in fact develop from some varieties of solar lentigo. Well-differentiated forms of LMPS and LM with spindle cells may cause confusion with pigmented spindle cell tumor (PSCT). Typical PSCT usually involves covered skin and commonly occurs in children and young adults[141]; whereas LMPS and LM invariably develop in sun-exposed skin and usually in older persons. An effaced epidermis, cellular nests with diminished cohesion, and a prominent basilar single-cell proliferation of markedly atypical spindle cells argue in favor of LMPS and LM. Pigmented spindle cell tumors are usually well-circumscribed with well-formed, orderly, and regular fascicles of pigmented spindle cells. Epidermal hyperplasia usually encountered in PSCT contrasts with the atrophy of LMPS and LM. Cytologically, PSCT is usually composed of monotonous fusiform cells with nuclei containing delicate chromatin.

The differential diagnosis for acral melanoma primarily includes lentigines and lentiginous melanocytic nevi of acral skin (Table 27-32). Lentigines of acral skin usually do not exhibit the frequency of melanocytic proliferation or cytologic atypia that is typical of acral melanoma.[266] Occasional acral nevi may have alarming features such as upward migration of cells throughout the epidermis, prominent lentiginous melanocytic proliferation, and some degree of cytologic atypia. Although upward migration may be noted in acral nevi, particularly in children, the constituent cells seldom reveal more than low-grade cytologic atypia, and the pattern of pagetoid spread is usually orderly and confined to the lowermost epidermis. Other characteristics of acral nevi include regular size, spacing, and cohesive qualities of the junctional nesting. One particular note of caution is that well-differentiated acral melanoma may exhibit dermal components with little or no inflammatory response. In such cases, careful evaluation for cytologic atypia, necrotic cells, and mitotic activity are helpful in recognizing melanoma.

NM may be confused with metastatic melanoma, spindle and epithelioid cell tumor, atypical cellular blue nevus, squamous cell carcinoma, atypical fibroxanthoma, fibrous histiocytoma, leiomyosarcoma, myoid fibroma, cellular capillary hemangioma, and Kaposi's sarcoma (Table 27-32). Epidermotropic metastatic melanoma involving the papillary dermis may prove difficult to distinguish from NM.[23,285] Metastatic melanoma is often fairly monomorphous with little stromal response while NM are often polymorphous and exhibit greater stromal response. However, distinction may be impossible in certain cases and discrimination must rely on clinical information and clinical course.

Spindle and epithelioid (Spitz's) cell tumors, particularly those with atypia, enter into the differential diagnosis of NM. Clinical information is pertinent to the diagnosis, since melanoma is uncommon in the young, whereas atypical lesions are more suspicious for melanoma in adults.

On occasion, nonmelanocytic lesions are considered in the differential diagnosis of melanoma. The principal conditions include Paget's disease, either mammary or extramammary, squamous cell carcinoma in situ, sebaceous carcinoma, epidermotropic eccrine carcinoma, cutaneous T-cell lymphoma, and other epidermotropic carcinomas. In most instances, the dilemma can be resolved simply by careful attention to histologic details in routinely stained sections.[286]

Unusual Variants of the Invasive Component of Melanoma

DESMOPLASTIC MELANOMA

Desmoplastic, neurotropic, and neurogenic melanoma are rare variants of melanoma that exhibit a continuum of histologic features corresponding to the neuroectodermal origin of the melanocyte.[287-300] The phenotype of the tumor may thus include any combination of the following: desmoplasia—fibroblastlike spindle cells usually in fascicles (predominant pattern), neurotropism (perineurial invasion)—invasion of nerve structures by tumor cells, neural differentiation (both schwannian and perineurial)—formation of nervelike structures recapitulating perineurium and endoneurium or delicate sheets of spindle cells reminiscent of neurofibroma, and less commonly neuroendocrine differentiation, as in Merkel cell carcinoma. Desmoplastic melanoma (DM) most frequently arises in association with lentiginous melanomas[23,261]; however, de novo variants of desmoplastic melanoma also occur.[296]

The pathogenesis of desmoplasia and the true nature of the spindle cells in desmoplastic melanoma remain a subject of controversy.[287-300] Some authors maintain that the fibroplasia results from the induction of collagen synthesis by benign fibroblasts whereas others believe that melanoma cells function as adaptive fibroblasts to promote collagenization in these tumors.[289,294,296] The latter conclusion is based on ultrastructural and immunohistochemical studies and because melanocytes are capable of collagen production as well as melanin synthesis and schwannian differentiation.[294-297]

Clinical Features The usual presentation is as a raised, firm nodule that is flesh-colored or associated with variable pigmentation (Table 27-33).[22,287-300] The irregular and variegated features of an associated intraepithelial component such as LMPS may be the most visible feature of desmoplastic melanoma. Difficulty in recognizing desmoplastic melanoma, clinically and histologically, usually causes a delay in recognition and appropriate surgery.

Histopathological Features Scanning magnification usually discloses a fibrous nodule displacing the normal dermal collagen or lamina propria, often extending into subcutaneous fat (Table 27-33) (Fig. 27-56).[294-296] An intraepidermal melanocytic proliferation is usually observed in the majority of cases.[296]

The most common histologic pattern of DM is a predominantly desmoplastic presentation.[294-296] Interspersed among dense collagenous fibers are individual spindle cells and variably sized fascicles of cells (Fig. 27-57). The nuclei may show considerable pleomorphism and wavy or serpiginous nuclear morphology, although most nuclei are enlarged and exhibit tapering contours. However, some nuclei are plump, and occasional bizarre multinucleate giant cell forms are noted. Most desmoplastic melanomas lack pigment, but occasional cells may contain fine melanin granules within cellular processes. The tumor stroma is usually fibrous, but myxoid alteration is occasionally encountered and uncommonly may be prominent.[296] A finding typical of desmoplastic melanoma and useful in its recognition is the presence of variably dense perivascular lymphocytic infiltrates which are usually scattered throughout the tumor.[296] The tumor cells in desmoplastic melanoma are also notable for infiltrating walls of blood vessels.

TABLE 27-33

Desmoplastic Neurotropic Melanoma

Clinical Features

Age 60–65 years
Men equally or more frequently affected than women
Sun-exposed skin, head and neck, but also acral, mucosal sites
Firm nodule
Flesh-colored or with pigmented lesion (29 to 43%)
1–3 cm
Occasional dysesthesias, nerve palsies

Histopathological Features

Intraepidermal melanocytic proliferation in > 75%; lentigo maligna, most common
Fibrous nodule in dermis and possibly subcutis
Often absence of pigment
Fascicles of atypical spindle cells
Schwannian, perineurial differentiation
Neurotropism common (perineurial and endoneurial invasion)
Patchy lymphoid infiltrates common
Variable myxoid stroma
Occasional mitoses in dermis

Differential Diagnosis

Sclerosing blue nevi including variants with hypercellularity
Desmoplastic (sclerosing) Spitz tumor
Neurothekeoma, particularly cellular variants
Malignant peripheral nerve sheath tumors
Myxoma
Dermatofibroma
Dermatofibrosarcoma protuberans
Atypical fibroxanthoma
Malignant fibrous histiocytoma
Scar
Fibromatosis
Spindle-cell squamous cell carcinoma
Leiomyosarcoma

Immunohistochemistry

S-100 protein +
Vimentin +
HMB-45 usually − (spindle cells)
Leu 7 −
Keratin −

Mitotic figures can usually be found even in the most paucicellular forms of this tumor.[294-296]

Desmoplastic melanomas are usually diagnosed at an advanced stage, since they are usually at least 4 or 5 mm in thickness and level IV or V (Table 27-33).[287-300] Because of misdiagnosis, they are commonly first recognized as recurrent or metastatic tumors. Desmoplastic melanomas frequently recur (range 25 to 82 percent).[287-293,296] Based on a series of 45 cases, local recurrence was associated with the following factors: failure to diagnose the tumor correctly, inadequate surgery (resection margins less than 1 cm), location on the head and neck, anatomic level V, and thickness greater than 4 mm.[293] Failure to completely extirpate desmoplastic melanoma is related to the difficulty of assessing margins, infiltration of nerves, and the fact that they are usually amelanotic.

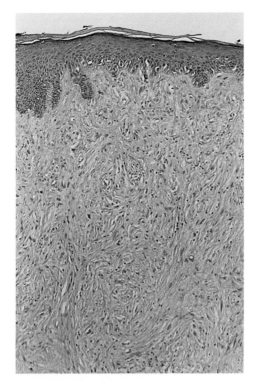

FIGURE 27-56 Desmoplastic melanoma. Fibrotic nodule occupies dermis.

Neurotropic and Neurogenic Melanoma

The term *neurotropism* refers to the involvement of perineurium and/or endoneurium of cutaneous nerves by melanoma cells (Fig. 27-58).[298] There may be considerable thickening of the perineurium and expansion of the endoneurial space by the tumor involvement.[292–295] Extension of tumor along the cutaneous nerves may, however, be extensive and subtle. Histologic clues to nerve involvement include the presence of hyperchromatic spindle cells in the perineurium or endoneurium and mucinous alteration of the nerve. Careful examination of cutaneous nerves at the surgical margins is mandatory to assess adequate excision. Melanoma spindle cells involving cutaneous nerves usually show nuclear enlargement, hyperchromatism, and pleomorphism.

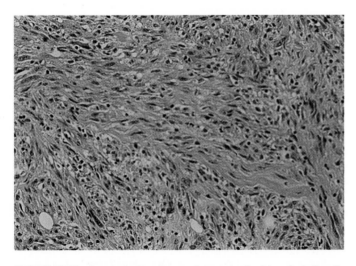

FIGURE 27-57 Desmoplastic melanoma. Intersecting fascicles of spindle cells with dense fibrous stroma.

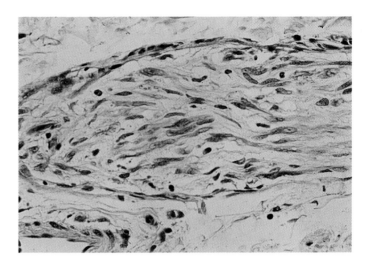

FIGURE 27-58 Desmoplastic-neurotropic melanoma. A cutaneous nerve shows prominent endoneurial infiltration by melanoma cells (neurotropism).

The term *neurogenic melanoma* describes neural or schwannian differentiation in a pattern resembling peripheral nerve sheath tumors such as neurofibromas or neuromas and the recapitulation of perineurium and endoneurium.[294–299] The tumor cells in such areas are characterized by serpiginous or wavy nuclear configurations and filamentous cytoplasmic processes. The cells are embedded in a variably mucinous and fibrous stroma. In some instances, the stroma may be so sufficiently myxoid as to suggest a myxoma. However, the tumor cells demonstrate loose fascicular arrangements, cytologic atypia, and occasional mitotic figures.

Differential Diagnosis The spectrum of tumors potentially confused with desmoplastic and neurotropic melanoma is varied and includes spindle cell proliferations and tumors with a fibrous appearance (Table 27-33).[287–300] The principal lesions to be considered include sclerosing blue nevus,[294] desmoplastic Spitz tumor,[144] neurothekeoma,[301] malignant peripheral nerve sheath tumor, dermatofibroma, atypical fibroxanthoma, malignant fibrous histiocytoma, scar, fibromatosis, myxoma, spindle cell squamous cell carcinoma, and leiomyosarcoma.[294] The epidermal lentiginous melanocytic proliferation commonly found in desmoplastic melanoma is usually absent in the other conditions.

Sclerosing blue nevus and desmoplastic Spitz tumor[144,294] both are characterized by an orderly infiltration of the fibrotic stroma and an overall benign cytologic appearance. Mitotic figures, usually encountered in desmoplastic melanoma, are exceedingly rare or absent in sclerosing blue nevus, but early forms of desmoplastic melanoma may be exceedingly difficult to distinguish from sclerosing blue nevus,[294,295] and it is vital to weigh all clinical and histologic features. For example, desmoplastic melanoma in a young individual on an anatomic site besides the head and neck or acral areas would be highly unusual, and such circumstances would argue against a diagnosis of desmoplastic melanoma.

The desmoplastic Spitz tumor is characterized by symmetry, a wedge-shaped configuration, and infiltration of the dermis by relatively monotonous epithelioid or spindle cells,[144] allowing its distinction from desmoplastic melanoma in most instances. Desmoplastic melanoma may also show a fascicular arrangement of cells that is generally lacking in desmoplastic Spitz tumor.

Relatively cellular variants of neurothekeoma (nerve sheath myxoma) may suggest desmoplastic melanoma.[301] Neurothekeoma commonly arises in the head and neck region, as does desmoplastic melanoma. Neurothekeoma generally occurs in young individuals (average age 20 years), does not demonstrate an intraepidermal melanocytic proliferation, and is typified by a lobular architecture in the dermis.[301] Concentric and fascicular arrangements of cells are often noted in neurothekeoma; the constituent cells may be epithelioid or bipolar and stellate, and multinucleate forms are seen. Low-grade nuclear pleomorphism and occasional mitotic figures are occasionally encountered. Distinction from desmoplastic melanoma is based on a regular, organized appearance, orderly infiltration of the dermis, and a lesser degree of cytologic atypia.[301]

Because of prominent schwannian differentiation, discrimination of desmoplastic-neurotropic melanoma from peripheral nerve sheath tumors may be difficult or impossible. All clinical and histologic characteristics must be considered. Tumors of the head and neck of elderly patients associated with lentiginous melanomas are usually not a diagnostic problem. Tumors in other anatomic sites without an intraepidermal component will cause difficulty, and immunohistochemistry may be of particular value in them (see below).[294,296,297,302]

Lesions demonstrating fibrous or fibrohistiocytic differentiation figure prominently in the differential diagnosis of desmoplastic melanoma and include dermatofibroma (fibrous histiocytoma), juvenile xanthogranuloma, dermatofibrosarcoma protuberans, atypical fibroxanthoma, superficial forms of malignant fibrous histiocytoma, scar, and fibromatosis. These lesions generally lack intraepidermal melanocytic proliferation, melanin pigment, and neurotropism.[294] Atypical fibroxanthoma and malignant fibrous histiocytoma enter the differential diagnosis and often require immunohistochemical evaluation, although they may contain xanthoma cells, not usually seen in desmoplastic melanoma. Fibrohistiocytic tumors as a general rule do not display neurotropism.

Desmoplastic melanomas with extensive mucin may raise problems of differential diagnosis, suggesting, e.g., a myxoma.[294] However, myxomas generally lack the cytologic atypia and neurotropism of desmoplastic-neurotropic melanoma, and the myxomatous variants of desmoplastic melanoma usually have zones of prominent cellularity.

Spindle cell squamous carcinoma and cutaneous leiomyosarcoma may be confused with desmoplastic melanoma, but each does not usually show intraepidermal melanocytic proliferation and melanin synthesis.[294] Squamous cell carcinoma may show keratinization, dyskeratosis, and intercellular bridges. Leiomyosarcoma may exhibit the cytologic characteristics of smooth-muscle cells, but immunohistochemistry may be essential to finalize the diagnosis.

Because of the serious consequences of this tumor, immunohistochemistry is needed in most desmoplastic melanomas to confirm the diagnosis. Almost 100 percent of desmoplastic-neurotropic melanomas demonstrate immunoreactivity with antibodies against vimentin and S-100 protein,[290–297,302] but uniquely almost all are negative for HMB-45. In recent studies, we have found that if there is positive immunostaining for HMB-45 in DM, it involves nondesmoplastic foci only, i.e., an intraepidermal component or superficial dermal focus of conventional melanoma cells.[296] A battery of markers must be utilized to evaluate such tumors. Other antibodies with variable reactivity with desmoplastic melanoma are neuron-specific enolase and NK1/C3. Antibodies against keratin, desmin, actin, and Leu-7 (specific for peripheral nerve sheath differentiation but negative in melanocytic tumors), in general, are negative in desmoplastic melanoma.[296,297,302]

Minimal Deviation Melanoma (MDM)

The term MDM was introduced to embrace the concept that a subset of melanomas is characterized by lesser cytologic atypia and a better prognosis than conventional melanomas of the same thickness.[41,303–306]

Thus, central to the concept of MDM is the presence of a cohesive nodule of dermal tumor cells. The growth pattern of such a nodule potentially indicates aggressive properties, such as recurrence or metastasis. Also implicit is the presence of a cell type lacking the characteristics of "fully-evolved" melanoma cells.[41,303–306] The cell types presumed to occur in MDM resemble ordinary nevus cells, spindled melanocytes, and epithelioid cells as from Spitz tumors.[303]

Because of the lack of specific histologic criteria and objective markers, data are not available that confirm or refute MDM as an entity. The diagnosis of MDM has probably been applied to a heterogenous collection of tumors of widely varying biologic potential from atypical nevi to conventional melanomas.

Nevoid Melanoma

The term *nevoid melanoma* was first used by Schmoeckel and colleagues[307] to describe a group of melanomas with histologic features suggesting a melanocytic nevus.[308,309] However, in their description of 33 patients with nevoid melanoma, Schmoeckel and colleagues noted that 15 patients developed metastases. They did not consider nevoid melanoma to have any better prognosis than conventional melanomas. The same caveats apply to nevoid melanoma as discussed above for minimal deviation melanoma.

Clinical and Histopathological Features   There were no distinctive clinical features compared to conventional melanomas (Table 27-34). Most tumors reported have been in adults. At scanning magnification, the most striking feature is a close resemblance to a nevus (Fig. 27-20).[307–309] Most of these lesions exhibit an overall symmetry, minimal or no intraepidermal pagetoid spread, and a monomorphous population of nevuslike cells in the dermis (Fig. 27-21). Although the base of the melanoma is often poorly defined, the lateral margins may be well-demarcated. In most instances, there is no host inflammatory response or surface ulceration. Histologic features favoring melanoma generally include the lack of maturation of dermal tumor cells, prominent cytologic atypia, mitoses in the dermal component, and infiltrative growth of cells into the deep dermis.[307–309]

TABLE 27-34

Nevoid Melanoma and Melanocytic Nevus

Nevoid melanoma	Melanocytic nevus
Clinical Features	
Older age	Younger age
Larger size, i.e., 1 to 2 cm	Smaller size, i.e., less than 6 mm
Some variation in color	More homogenous color
Greater asymmetry	Less asymmetry
Histopathological Features	
Greater asymmetry	Symmetry
Less well-circumscribed	Well-circumscribed
Greater likelihood of pagetoid spread	Little or no pagetoid spread
Intraepidermal basilar melanocytic proliferation common	Basilar proliferation less common
Infiltration of adnexae	No infiltration of adnexae
Reduced or no maturation	Maturation
Mitoses in dermis	Usually no dermal mitoses
Atypical mitoses	No atypical mitoses
Deep infiltration of dermis	No deep infiltration

Differential Diagnosis The principal dilemma is discrimination of such melanomas from melanocytic nevi, especially papillomatous dermal nevi. As outlined in Table 27-34, a constellation of factors must be considered in arriving at a final diagnosis. In some cases, it may be difficult to reach a final diagnosis. It is reasonable in such situations to communicate this uncertainty to the clinician and advise that the patient have appropriate treatment and periodic follow-up examinations, as for melanoma.

Verrucous Melanoma

Although *verrucous melanoma* was initially described in his classification of melanoma in 1967,[257] Clark subsequently discarded the term, since he believed that its features could be present in any type of melanoma.[258] Recent reports have emphasized the prominent clinical and histologic verrucous features of such melanomas and the difficulty in classifying many of these lesions.[310,311] Some of these melanomas might also be described as *nevoid melanoma*.

Clinical and Histopathological Features Most lesions are well-circumscribed, 1 to 2 cm in diameter, and characterized by a dark-brown, black, or grayish appearance and hyperkeratotic verrucous surface and diagnosed clinically as seborrheic keratosis or papillomatous nevi (Table 27-35).[310,311]

The most striking feature at scanning magnification is the prominent papillomatous or verrucoid epidermal hyperplasia suggesting a seborrheic keratosis, epidermal nevus, verruca, or papillomatous melanocytic nevus (Fig. 27-20).[257,310,311] Many such lesions also exhibit some degree of symmetry, although this feature should not be so common as in a benign process. Hyperkeratosis and parakeratosis may also be prominent.[310] The degree of epidermal hyperplasia may be marked and possibly pseudoepitheliomatous.[311] The intraepidermal melanocytic component may vary from minimal or absent or show prominent pagetoid spread. Also common is the frequent presence of a laterally extending intraepidermal component.[311] Some of these tumors may show a contiguous basilar and suprabasilar proliferation of atypical melanocytes, often involving adnexal epithelium.[310,311] In common with nevoid melanoma, the dermal component in some melanomas may show a startling resemblance to a dermal nevus.[23,310,311] The cell type in the latter tumors resembles a small nevus cell, but careful inspection should disclose prominent cellular pleomorphism, little or no maturation, and cells dispersed in confluent nests and sheets without orderly infiltration of stroma. The presence of mitotic figures (e.g., greater than 2 or 3 per section) and necrotic cells in the dermal component also argues against a benign process.

Differential Diagnosis Verrucous melanoma may suggest nonmelanocytic tumors such as seborrheic keratosis, verruca, and epidermal nevus. However, the melanocytic nature of the lesion should become clear with careful inspection. Of particular concern is the potential misdiagnosis of verrucous melanoma as a benign nevus, especially a papillomatous dermal nevus.[23]

Melanoma Arising in Association with Dermal Nevi

The development of melanoma in the dermal component of an acquired nevus is an uncommon or rare event.[312–314] Some of these melanomas may originate from adnexal-associated nevus elements.

Clinical and Histopathological Features Most patients are approximately 40 to 60 years of age, and the most common site is the head and neck area (Table 27-36).[312–314] The lesions are often larger than ordi-

---

TABLE 27-35

Verrucous Melanoma

Clinical Features

Age 50–60 years
Women more often affected than men
Location anywhere, but lower extremities more common
Well-circumscribed
1–2 cm
Dark-brown, black, grayish
Verrucous hyperkeratotic surface
Ulceration uncommon

Histopathological Features

Hyperkeratosis
Papillomatous epidermal hyperplasia
Occasional pseudoepitheliomatous hyperplasia
Symmetry on occasion
Epidermal involvement
   None
   Pagetoid spread
   Contiguous basilar melanocytic proliferation
   Involvement of adnexal structures
Dermal component
   Occasional striking nevuslike appearance
   Little or no maturation
   Confluent sheets or nests of cells
Mitoses in dermis
Necrotic cells
Little or no inflammation common
May resemble any other histological type of melanoma

Differential Diagnosis

Papillomatous dermal nevus

Prognosis

Same as other types of melanoma

---

nary dermal nevi, e.g., 1 to 2 cm, and there is usually a history of recent change or enlargement.

Usually within an otherwise ordinary dermal nevus, one encounters a distinct nodule of cytologically atypical melanocytes.[312–314] There is usually a transition from the ordinary dermal nevus component to the nodular aggregate of atypical cells. The latter cells are most commonly enlarged with abundant cytoplasm and pleomorphic nuclei. Mitotic figures are usually easily found within the cellular nodule.

Differential Diagnosis The most obvious dilemma is the differentiation of a focus of melanoma from dermal nevus, especially a nevus with cytologically bizarre nevus cells as in ancient schwannoma or a distinct focus of epithelioid or fusiform cells, i.e., so-called combined nevus, inverted type A nevus, or clonal nevus.[41,196] First of all, the nodular area in question should demonstrate a cohesive or expansile aggregate of cells with unequivocal cytologic atypia. Although these melanocytic cells will usually have a monomorphous or clonal appearance, inspection of individual cells should disclose substantial nuclear pleomorphism and often prominent nucleoli and hyperchromatism. Mitotic figures should also be present in this focus. A dermal nevus with bizarre or ancient cytologic features usually will not show mitoses. One should also consider clinical factors such as age of the patient (melanoma usually develops in persons greater than 30 to 40 years of age), size (such

TABLE 27-36

Melanoma Arising in Association with Dermal Nevus

Clinical Features

Age 40–60 years
Head and neck most common site
Often 1 to 2 cm
Resembles dermal nevus
Often uniform pink, tan, or brown
Often history of recent enlargement

Histopathological Features

Focal cohesive nodules of atypical melanocytes
Background of ordinary dermal nevus
Monomorphous cells in nodules
Cellular and nuclear enlargement
Nuclear pleomorphism
Melanin content variable
Mitotic figures usually present

Differential Diagnosis

Dermal nevus
Combined nevus

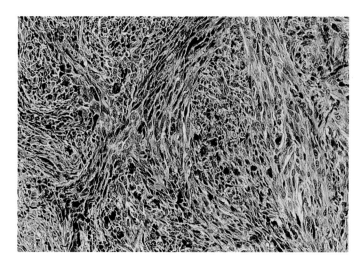

FIGURE 27-59 Malignant blue nevus (melanoma arising in association with blue nevus). Fascicular arrangements of spindle cells, many of which contain melanin, can be observed in this field.

lesions are often greater than 1 cm in diameter), and history of recent change or enlargement. However, so-called combined nevi are often present in younger individuals, are characterized by a small dark nodule or papule in a relatively small symmetric nevus, and usually show low-grade or no cytologic atypia of the epithelioid/fusiform cells. Often the latter cells display prominent melaninization of melanocytes and are accompanied by melanophages.

Malignant Blue Nevus (MBN)

MBN is an extremely rare form of melanoma originating from or associated with a preexisting blue nevus and characterized by a dense proliferation of variably pigmented spindle cells without involvement of the epidermis.[180,183,184] If strict criteria are applied, as outlined above, only 33 cases of MBN have been reported.[183,184]

Clinical Features The average age at diagnosis is 45 years, two-thirds of the patients are men, and the commonest site is the scalp (Table 27-20). Malignant blue nevi most frequently present as blue or blue-black plaques or nodules ranging from 1 to 4 cm (most larger than 3 cm)[184] that are often multinodular. There is usually a history of recent enlargement or change in a previously stable blue nevus. MBN are highly aggressive with metastasis to lymph nodes and a variety of visceral sites in 82 percent of the 33 cases reported.[184]

Histopathological Features Malignant blue nevi are characterized by nodular or multinodular aggregations of spindle cells in tightly packed fascicles in the dermis and often the subcutis (Table 27-20) (Fig. 27-59).[180,183,184] By definition, there is sparing of the epidermis. Occasional epithelioid cells and multinucleate giant cells are encountered. Melanin pigment and cytoplasmic vacuolization are noted in approximately two-thirds of cases. However, in the M.D. Anderson series, only about a third were heavily melaninized.[184] Necrosis, a feature previously thought characteristic of MBN, was observed in only 4 of 12 cases reported by Connelly and Smith.[184] In general, there is striking cytologic atypia, prominent nuclear pleomorphism, infrequent mitotic fig-

ures (approximately 1 mitosis per 10 high power fields, but some have more), and uncommonly atypical mitoses. Most MBN have a component of cellular blue nevus (CBN), but elements of common blue nevus (pigmented dendritic melanocytes, fibrosis, and melanophages) and rarely nevus of Ota may be observed.

Differential Diagnosis Malignant blue nevus must be distinguished from CBN (see *differential diagnosis for CBN*)[23,157,182] and metastatic melanoma.[183,184]

Because there are no histologic features specific for MBN, a contiguous remnant of blue nevus should be identified or a history of an antecedent blue nevus documented to distinguish MBN from either NM or metastatic melanoma.[184]

Clear-Cell Sarcoma (Malignant Melanoma of Soft Parts) (CCS)

CCS has been a perplexing tumor because of its origin in soft tissue, classification in the past as synovial sarcoma or fibrosarcoma,[315–318] and a pattern of biologic behavior that is consistent with a sarcoma.[318] However, at present, CCS is best considered an unusual variant of melanoma. It develops in young adults between the ages of 20 and 40 and most commonly involves the distal extremities (the foot being the most common site) (Table 27-37). The tumor typically presents as a slowly enlarging deep-seated mass because of its association with tendons and aponeuroses, and there may be occasional tenderness or pain. Clear-cell sarcoma is slightly more prevalent in women.

Clinical and Histopathological Features The tumor is characterized by a well-circumscribed, multilobulated appearance.[315–318] Oval or fusiform cells with clear or eosinophilic granular cytoplasm are arranged in well-defined nests and fascicles (Fig. 27-60). Tumor aggregates are generally compartmentalized by fibrous tissue of variable thickness that merges with aponeurotic or tendinous structures. There is variation in nuclear size and shape, and the nuclei are notable for vesicular qualities and prominent nucleoli. Distinctive multinucleate giant cells occur in about two-thirds of cases.[315,316] Melanin may be detected in approximately half of these tumors. Special stains will yield more tumors containing melanin. Most tumors react with antibodies to vimentin, S-100 protein, HMB-45, and neuron-specific enolase.[317]

Clinical Features

Age 20–40 years
Women equally or more frequently affected than men
Distal extremities, the foot most commonly involved
Deep location—tendons and aponeuroses
Slowly enlarging mass
Tenderness, pain

Histopathological Features

Multilobulated tumor
Oval or fusiform cells in nests and fascicles
Fibrous trabeculae separate cellular aggregates
Clear or eosinophilic cytoplasm
Multinucleate giant cells
Melanin in over half of cases

Immunohistochemistry

S-100 protein +
HMB-45 +

Electron Microscopy

Premelanosomes
Melanosomes

Differential Diagnosis

Metastatic melanoma
Cellular blue nevus
Malignant blue nevus
Malignant peripheral nerve sheath tumor
Epithelioid sarcoma
Synovial sarcoma
Fibrosarcoma

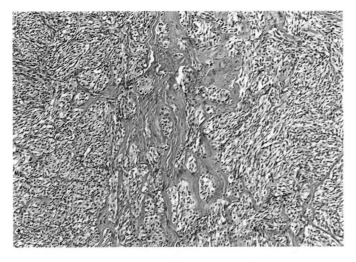

FIGURE 27-60   Clear-cell sarcoma. The tumor is remarkable for intersecting fascicles of spindle cells, compartmentalized by fibrous tissue.

There is no staining with antibodies against cytokeratin, epithelial membrane antigen, or leukocyte common antigen.[317] Melanosomes and premelanosomes are noted on electron microscopy.[317]

Local recurrences are frequent, 70 percent of patients in one series experiencing at least one recurrence during a mean period of 4.2 years.[316] The recurrences are often multiple and followed by less frequent regional node and lung metastases. In the series above, 43 percent of the individuals died of metastases.[316]

Differential Diagnosis   CCS may be confused with CBN, MBN, metastatic melanoma, malignant peripheral nerve sheath tumors, epithelioid sarcoma, synovial sarcoma, and fibrosarcoma.[315–318] The tumor probably most closely resembles CBN with atypia and MBN, but the latter do not usually occur in soft tissue. CCS is distinguished by the typical clinical presentation in young adults, involvement of distal extremities, typical histology, and immunohistochemistry. Epithelioid sarcoma and synovial sarcoma immunostain with cytokeratin and epithelial membrane antigen but not with S-100 protein and HMB-45.

Balloon Cell Melanoma

Balloon cell melanoma (BCM) exhibits ballooning in at least 50 percent of the melanoma cells.[319,320] The individual "balloon cells" have abundant vacuolated cytoplasms that impart a clear-cell appearance. Although BCM is extremely rare, knowledge of BCM is important for its distinction from the much more common balloon cell nevus and from other clear-cell tumors of the skin. BCM is reported to have a particular propensity for multiple skin and subcutaneous metastases.[319]

The balloon cell change has been attributed to (1) degeneration and coalescence of melanosomes, (2) defective melanosome formation and subsequent generation of large membrane-bound vesicles, (3) blocked melanin synthesis and subsequent accumulation of protyrosinase vesicles, and (4) lipoidal degeneration of melanocytes.[320] Recent ultrastructural studies have provided evidence supporting the first three explanations mentioned above. In addition, the presence of abundant RNA in the balloon cells and immunostaining with HMB-45 suggest that the cells are metabolically active rather than degenerative.[320]

Clinical and Histopathological Features   There were no distinctive clinical features of BCM. The balloon cells are large, round, or polygonal cells with clear or eosinophilic, slightly granular, cytoplasm.[319,320] The nuclei are irregularly placed and exhibit only slight to moderate atypia. Mitotic activity is also generally low. Melanin has been noted in about a quarter of cases.[320] Metastases from BCM often show balloon cell change but may be difficult to diagnose because they are amelanotic and fail to exhibit nesting. Virtually all BCM studied thus far show positive immunostaining with S-100 protein and HMB-45.[320] A small number may be positive for carcinoembryonic antigen.

Differential Diagnosis   BCM may be confused with balloon cell nevus, xanthoma, hibernoma, granular cell tumor, metastatic clear-cell carcinomas such as renal cell or adenocarcinoma, liposarcoma, and clear-cell appendage tumors.[319,320] Perhaps, the greatest problem is distinction of BCM from balloon cell nevus. In general, balloon cell nevi occur in young individuals (under age 30 years), show "maturation" of nevus cells (decreased size of cells and nuclei with depth), the presence of multinucleate giant cells; in contrast, BCM tends to develop in older patients, to lack "maturation" of melanoma cells, and to have cellular atypia and mitotic activity.[320]

TABLE 27-38

Unusual or Rare Presentations of Primary Melanoma

Spitzoid melanoma[121]	Cellular composition resembles enlarged epithelioid/fusiform cells of Spitz tumor.
Myxoid melanoma[122–124]	Prominent myxoid stroma suggesting mucinous carcinoma or peripheral nerve sheath tumors.
Melanoma resembling experimentally induced and spontaneous melanomas in animals[125]	Raised dermal tumor composed of heavily melanized epithelioid cells, fusiform cells often with dendrites, and histiocytes. The striking melanin content tends to obscure cytologic detail and bleaching is often needed.
Small-cell melanoma[122, 125]	Melanoma composed of uniform small cells, sometimes in organoid arrangements (Figs. 27-20 and 27-21), developing in congenital nevi and mucosal sites such as vulva, vagina.

Other Rare or Unusual Variants of Melanoma[321–324] (Table 27-38)

REGRESSION

Melanoma is notable for its frequency of spontaneous regression.[23,281] The prevalence of histologic regression varies according to the definition of regression used and the thickness range of the melanomas reported.[281,325,326] In a study of 563 cases of primary melanoma, histologic regression was noted in 46 percent of thin (less than 1.5 mm), 32 percent of intermediate (1.5 to 3.0 mm), and 9 percent of thick (greater than 3.0 mm) melanomas.[326] McGovern has also recorded regression in 58 percent of melanomas less than 0.70 mm in thickness.[325,327] Complete regression of melanoma is uncommon and has been reported to occur with a frequency of 2.4 to 8.7 percent (Fig. 27-61).[328,329] Many cases of metastatic melanoma with unknown primary

TABLE 27-39

Stages of Histologic Regression of Malignant Melanoma

Early (or active):   Zone of papillary dermis and epidermis within a recognizable melanoma, characterized by dense infiltrates of lymphocytes disrupting/replacing nests of melanoma cells within the papillary dermis and possibly the epidermis, as compared to adjoining zones of tumor; degenerating melanoma cells should be recognizable. There is no obvious fibrosis.

Intermediate: Zone of papillary dermis and epidermis within a recognizable melanoma, characterized by reduction (loss) in the amount of tumor (a disruption in the continuity of the tumor) or absence of tumor in papillary dermis and possibly within the epidermis, compared to adjacent zones of tumor, and replaced by varying admixtures of lymphoid cells and increased fibrous tissue (as compared to normal papillary dermis) in this zone. Variable telangiectasia (and new blood vessel formation) and melanophages may also be present.

Late: Zone of papillary dermis and epidermis within a recognizable melanoma, characterized by marked reduction in the amount of tumor compared to adjacent areas of tumor, or absence of tumor in this zone, and replacement and expansion of the papillary dermis in this zone by extensive fibrosis (usually dense fibrous tissue, horizontally disposed) and variable telangiectasia (and new blood vessel formation), melanophages, sparse or no lymphoid infiltrates, and effacement of the epidermis. (Other than fibrosis, the latter features are frequently present but not essential for recognizing regression.)

are thought to be explained by spontaneous regression of the primary melanoma.

Spontaneous regression is thought to be immunologically mediated because of mononuclear cell infiltrates containing T lymphocytes, and monocyte/macrophages at the site of regression.[330] Regression is seen most often in microinvasive or thin melanoma and is present as focal, partial, and rarely complete regression of the tumor.[281,331] The changes of regression form a continuum, but may be arbitrarily categorized into three stages (Table 27-39).[331]

METASTATIC MELANOMA

Melanoma can spread hematogenously, through lymphatic channels, or by direct local invasion and thus may occur in any site of the body. Metastases are more frequent to lymph nodes, skin, and subcutaneous tissue (nonvisceral sites) than to visceral organs.[285,332–334] Lymph nodes are the most common site of metastases and 60 to 80 percent of patients with metastatic melanoma develop lymph node metastases.[263,334] The lymph node groups most commonly involved are ilioinguinal, axillary, intraparotid, and cervical lymph nodes.[335] The metastatic tumor may be clinically apparent (macroscopic metastasis) or detected only by histologic examination (microscopic metastasis).

Nearly half of the patients with metastatic melanoma develop skin metastases,[333,334] which may occur in the area of loco-regional lymphatic drainage or at a remote location. Two subtypes of regional cutaneous metastases are arbitrarily distinguished by their distance from the primary melanoma.[336]

Cutaneous satellites are discontinuous tumor cell aggregates that are located in the dermis and/or subcutis within 5 cm of the primary tumor, whereas *in-transit metastases* are located more than 5 cm away from the primary melanoma. The finding of the latter metastases has poor prog-

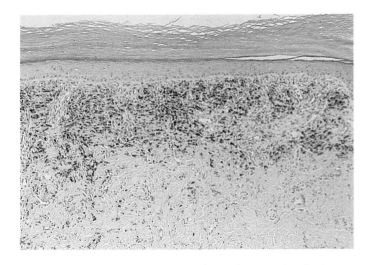

FIGURE 27-61   Tumoral melanosis. There is complete regression of melanoma with residual aggregates of melanophages.

nostic implications, since the majority of patients with such lesions develop disseminated metastatic disease.[336] Although virtually any organ may be involved, the most common first sites of visceral metastases reported in clinical studies are lung (14 to 20 percent), liver (14 to 20 percent), brain (12 to 20 percent), bone (11 to 17 percent), and intestine (1 to 7 percent), and first metastases at other sites are very rare (<1 percent).[332]

Metastatic melanoma has a tendency to grow in nests, sheets, or fascicles, often with an infiltrative border, pleomorphism, mitoses, and necrosis.[285] Cytologically, epithelioid and/or spindle cells are commonly found in metastatic melanoma.[285] Melanin, which greatly facilitates the recognition of metastatic melanoma, may be apparent, subtle, or absent (amelanotic melanoma).

Several situations may arise in which the diagnosis of metastatic melanoma is not straightforward. The problem may lie in the identification of a metastatic-appearing lesion as melanocytic or in the distinction between a primary and secondary melanoma.[23,285]

MELANOMA SIMULATING OTHER NEOPLASMS

Metastatic melanoma may assume a great variety of morphologic appearances and may mimic a number of nonmelanocytic tumors, such as lymphoma, undifferentiated carcinoma, adenocarcinoma, a variety of sarcomas, and many others.[322] The differential diagnosis is particularly difficult in amelanotic melanoma. Often, additional studies are needed, such as melanin stains, immunohistochemistry using a panel of antibodies, and electron microscopy, to identify conclusively a metastatic tumor as melanocytic.

PRIMARY CUTANEOUS VERSUS CUTANEOUS METASTATIC MELANOMA

A common problem is distinguishing an epidermotropic metastasis from a primary melanoma (or possibly a nevus in some instances) (Table 27-40). Cutaneous metastases usually lie within the reticular dermis or subcutis and only rarely involve the overlying epidermis, whereas primary cutaneous melanomas typically have an intraepidermal component.[23,336] Also metastases tend to be smaller (often less than 4 mm) than primary tumors (usually larger than 4 or 5 mm). In cases of metastatic melanoma showing epidermotropism,[337] the epidermal component is usually relatively limited compared to the dermal component (Fig. 27-62). If the dermal metastasis is superficial, the overlying epi-

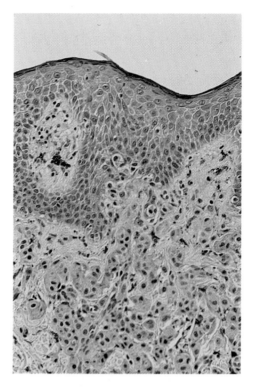

FIGURE 27-62 Epidermotropic metastatic melanoma. There is focal involvement of epidermis. The metastasis resembles a compound nevus.

dermis may be thinned, and the lateral borders may show hyperplastic elongated rete ridges turned inward forming a *collarette*. Tumor cells within vascular lumina are more likely to be found in and around a metastatic lesion than near a primary tumor.[337]

Primary tumors generally display more pleomorphism than metastatic lesions, which often appear as an atypical, but rather monomorphous, population of cells.[338] Primary tumors tend to show more variation in the overall composition of the lesion. There is often more fibrosis and more of an inflammatory host response.[339,340] When deciding whether a melanocytic tumor is a metastasis or a primary lesion, one must weigh the histologic appearance against a detailed clinical history to arrive at the correct diagnosis.

TABLE 27-40

Primary Cutaneous Melanoma versus Cutaneous Metastasis

	Primary melanoma	*Cutaneous metastasis*
Location of tumor	Usually both dermis and epidermis	Dermis and/or subcutis
If epidermal involvement	Usually prominent; pagetoid horizontal and vertical spread commonly present; usually epidermal component extends laterally beyond dermal component	Usually dermal component extends laterally beyond epidermal component; pagetoid spread less common
Size	Usually larger than 0.4 cm and usually larger than 1.0 cm	Often small; may be smaller than 1.0 cm and occasionally smaller than 0.4 cm
Epidermal collarette	Usually less common	More likely present
Cytology	Usually pleomorphic	Usually monotonous
Reactive fibrosis	May be marked	Usually mild
Vascular invasion	Rarely seen	More likely present

MELANOCYTIC AGGREGATES VERSUS MICROMETASTASES

Collections of small melanocytes are occasionally seen within lymph nodes draining the skin.[341–344] These aggregates are usually small and inconspicuous but may occupy as much as a third of a lymph node.[341–344] They are usually located in the fibrous capsule of the node rather than the marginal sinus[342] but rarely can be found in the lymphatic tissue proper.[341] Their bland appearance, frequent resemblance to nevus cells, and their location in the fibrous capsule of the lymph node help to distinguish them from micrometastases. However, especially in frozen sections or in the rare situation of intranodal location, such aggregates in lymph nodes may lead to diagnostic confusion. There has been considerable debate as to whether these nodal melanocytic lesions derive from aberrant migration of melanoblasts from the neural crest during embryogenesis or represent lymphatic spread from a benign cutaneous nevus.

METASTATIC MELANOMA WITH UNKNOWN PRIMARY SITE

Approximately 4 percent to 12 percent of patients with melanoma develop metastases without a clinically detectable primary tumor.[345,346] Although it is possible that some melanomas may arise *de novo* within a lymph node or visceral site, it is generally believed that many of these cases are related to complete regression of a primary cutaneous melanoma.[329,347] Metastatic melanomas with unknown primary site are twice as common in men as in women, which is in agreement with the observation that tumor regression is more commonly observed in men than in women.[348] The most common site of presentation[349] is in lymph nodes (64 percent), whereas 21 percent of the cases present with visceral metastases.[332,346,349]

MELANOSIS IN METASTATIC MELANOMA

Cutaneous or generalized melanosis is a rare complication of metastatic melanoma.[332,350–352] Hyperpigmentation may be focal or diffuse, limited to the skin or generalized, involving internal organs.

THE HISTOLOGICAL DIAGNOSIS OF MALIGNANT MELANOMA

The histological diagnosis of malignant melanoma remains rather imprecise and depends on the recognition of a constellation of histologic features, no single feature in and of itself being diagnostic of melanoma (Table 27-41).[23] However, a large percentage of melanomas are diagnosed correctly by a majority of knowledgeable histopathologists. It is also true that a small percentage of melanocytic tumors are histologically challenging and will produce no consensus even among expert histopathologists.

In general, melanomas are characterized by overall asymmetry, whereas benign melanocytic lesions tend to have symmetry and orderliness. Although there is no absolute size criterion, the larger the lesion in breadth (generally over 4 to 5 mm and especially over 10 mm), the greater the likelihood that the lesion is melanoma. Melanomas are also characterized by poor circumscription of the peripherally extending intraepidermal component. Other architectural attributes suggesting melanoma include considerable variation in the sizes and shapes of intraepidermal cellular nests and diminished cohesiveness of the nests of cells. The elongated epidermal rete pattern that typifies melanocytic nevi is frequently lost in melanoma, and there may be an accompanying confluence of melanoma cells along the dermal-epidermal junction.

TABLE 27-41

Criteria for the Histologic Diagnosis of Melanoma

Architecture
  Asymmetry
  Large size (usually larger than 4 to 5 mm) but many exceptions
  Poor circumscription
  Variation in size, shape, placement of nests
  Diminished cohesiveness of cells in nests
  Confluence of nests
  Loss of epidermal rete pattern (effacement)
  Upward migration of melanocytes (pagetoid spread) in random pattern, single cells predominate over nests, cells reach granular and cornified layers
  Rich mononuclear cell infiltrates, usually bandlike
  Confluent cellular aggregates
  Pushing, expanding pattern without regard for stroma
  Fibroplasia of papillary dermis
  Regression frequently present
Cytology
  Nuclear changes
    Majority of melanocytes uniformly atypical
    Nuclear enlargement
    Nuclear pleomorphism (variation in sizes and shapes)
    Nuclear hyperchromasia with coarse chromatin
    One or more prominent nucleoli
  Cytoplasmic changes
    Abundant granular eosinophilic cytoplasm in epithelioid cells
    Finely divided ("dusty") melanin
    Variation in size of melanin granules
    High nuclear-to-cytoplasmic ratios in spindle cells
    Retraction of cytoplasm
    Mitoses (unusual in dermal component)
  Atypical mitoses
  Necrotic cells

One of the features most characteristic of melanoma, yet one that is not specific to melanoma, is upward migration or pagetoid spread of melanocytes in a random pattern. A predominance of single cells over small aggregates or nests typifies this pattern in melanoma. Melanoma cells are usually present at all levels of the epidermis including the granular and cornified layers.

Cytologic atypia is mandatory for a diagnosis of melanoma (Table 27-41). There is a uniformity or monomorphous quality of the atypia in melanoma rather than the discontinuous pattern of atypia found in dysplastic nevi. Melanoma is also notable for hypercellularity and high nuclear-to-cytoplasmic ratios of melanoma cells.

PROGNOSTIC FACTORS IN MELANOMA

Over the past 20 years there has been extensive investigation of prognostic factors in melanoma using large databases and multivariate techniques.[23,268,269,280,353] The most powerful predictors of survival from many such studies have been thickness of the primary melanoma (measured in millimeters from the granular layer of the epidermis vertically to the greatest depth of tumor invasion) and stage or extent of disease, i.e., localized tumor, nodal metastases, distant metastases.

Although a number of studies have described "breakpoints" for tumor thickness and prognosis, e.g., patients with melanomas smaller

TABLE 27-42

Prognostic Factors for Localized Melanoma

Prognostic factor	Effect on prognosis
Tumor thickness (mm)*	Worse with increasing thickness
Levels of invasion	Worse with deeper levels
Ulceration	Worse with ulceration
Mitotic rate	Worse with increasing mitotic rate
Tumor-infiltrating lymphocytes (TILs)	Better with TILs
Regression	Unsettled; some studies have shown an adverse outcome while others no effect or a favorable outcome
Growth phase	Risk of metastasis associated with vertical growth phase
Microscopic satellites	Worse prognosis
Vascular/lymphatic invasion	Worse prognosis but rare
Tumor cell type	Better prognosis with spindle cells versus other cell types
Age	Worse prognosis with increasing age
Sex	Women have better prognosis than men
Anatomic site	Extremity lesions have better prognosis than axial lesions (trunk, head and neck, palms and soles)

*Most important prognostic factor

TABLE 27-43

Histopathologic Reporting of Melanoma

Essential information
    Diagnosis: Malignant melanoma, in situ or invasive
    Measured depth (mm)
    Adequacy of surgical margins
Other prognostic information reported to be significant in
    some databases
    Histologic ulceration
    Mitotic rate (per mm^2)
    Anatomic level, i.e, I, II, III, IV, V
    Presence of desmoplasia, neurotropism, or both
    Presence of marked or virtually complete regression
    Presence of vascular/lymphatic invasion
    Presence of microscopic satellites
    Radial or vertical growth phase
    Histologic subtype, e.g., lentigo maligna
    Tumor-infiltrating lymphocytes

prognostic factors such as ulceration, mitotic rate per square millimeter, anatomic level, histologic type of melanoma, radial or vertical growth phase, and tumor-infiltrating lymphocytes might be reported as well. However, many of the latter factors are highly correlated with tumor thickness and thus may not add significant information beyond thickness alone.

REFERENCES

1. Hodgson C: Senile lentigo. *Arch Dermatol* 87:197–207, 1963.
2. Braun-Falco O, Schoefinius H-H: Lentigo senilis. Übersicht und eigene Unter-suchungen. *Hautarzt* 7:277–283, 1971.
3. Bean WB: Senile freckles. *JAMA* 234(10):1059, 1975.
4. Montagna W, Hu F, Carlisle K: A reinvestigation of solar lentigines. *Arch Dermatol* 116:1151–1154, 1980.
5. Rhodes AR, Harrist TJ, Momtaz KT: The PUVA-induced pigmented macule: A lentig-inous proliferation of large, sometimes cytologically atypical, melanocytes. *J Am Acad Dermatol* 9:47–58, 1983.
6. Rhodes AR, Stern RS, Melski JW: The PUVA lentigo: An analysis of predisposing factors. *J Invest Dermatol* 81:459–463, 1983.
7. Kanerva L, Niemi K-M, Lauharanta J: A semiquantitative light and electron micro-scopic analysis of histopathologic changes in photochemotherapy-induced freckles. *Arch Dermatol Res* 276:2–11, 1984.
8. Bolognia JL: Reticulated black solar lentigo ("ink spot" lentigo). *Arch Dermatol* 128:934–940, 1992.
9. Rhodes AR, Albert L, Barnhill RL, Weinstock MA: Sun-induced freckles in children and young adults: A correlation of clinical and histopathologic features. *Cancer* 67: 1990–2001, 1991.
10. Roewert HJ, Ackerman AB: Large-cell acanthoma is a solar lentigo. *Am J Der-matopathol* 14:122–132, 1992.
11. Mehregan AH: Lentigo senilis and its evolutions. *J Invest Dermatol* 65:429–433, 1975.
12. Stegmaier OC, Montgomery H: Histopathologic studies of pigmented nevi in children. *J Invest Dermatol* 20:51–62, 1953.
13. Stegmaier OC, Becker SW Jr: Incidence of melanocytic nevi in young adults. *J Invest Dermatol* 34:125–129, 1960.
14. Clark WH Jr, Elder DE, Guerry D IV, et al: A study of tumor progression: The pre-cursor lesions of superficial spreading and nodular melanoma. *Human Pathol* 15:1147–1165, 1984.
15. LeDouarin N: Migration and differentiation of neural crest cells. *Curr Top Dev Bio* 16:31–85, 1980.
16. Quevedo WC, Fleischman RD: Developmental biology of mammalian melanocytes. *J Invest Dermatol* 75:116–120, 1980.
17. Lund HZ, Stobbe GD: The natural history of the pigmented nevus; factors of age and anatomic location. *Am J Pathol* 1949;25:1117–1155.
18. Maize JC, Foster G: Age-related changes in melanocytic naevi. *Clin Exp Dermatol* 4:49-58, 1979.
19. Hu F: Melanocyte cytology in normal skin, melanocytic nevi, and malignant

than 0.76 mm have almost 100 percent 5-year survival,[354] there is now good evidence that this inverse relationship between thickness and sur-vival is essentially linear.[353,355] Whereas thickness is the best prog-nostic factor available for localized melanoma, there are occasional melanomas that defy this relationship, i.e., thin melanomas that metas-tasize and thick ones that do not.[268] A number of other factors also have been reported to influence outcome in patients with localized melanoma (Table 27-42). However, these various factors largely derive their effect from a correlation with melanoma thickness and generally fail to remain significant after multivariate analysis.[268,269] Once regional lymph node metastases have developed, 5-year survival drops to the range of about 10 to 50 percent and is largely related to the number and extent of lymph nodes involved.[356] The median survival for patients with distant metas-tases is approximately 6 months.[353] The only factors influencing the time to death include number of metastatic sites, surgical resectability of the metastases, duration of remission, and location of metastases, i.e., nonvisceral (skin, subcutaneous tissue, distant lymph nodes) versus vis-ceral sites (lung, liver, brain, bone).[353]

HISTOPATHOLOGICAL REPORTING OF MELANOMA

The pathology report should include the following minimum informa-tion: diagnosis, i.e., malignant melanoma, in situ or invasive; depth of tumor invasion in millimeters measured vertically from the granular layer of the epidermis or from the surface of an ulcer with an ocular micrometer; and the adequacy of surgical margins (Table 27-43).[23] The following histologic changes should also be mentioned if present: des-moplasia or neurotropism; marked or virtually complete regression; true vascular lymphatic invasion; and true microscopic satellites. Other

melanomas, in Ackerman AB (ed): *Pathology of Malignant Melanoma*. New York, Masson Publishing USA, 1981, pp 1–21.

20. Mishima Y: Macromolecular changes in pigmentary disorders. *Arch Dermatol* 519–557, 1965.

21. Stegmaier OC: Natural regression of the melanocytic nevus. *J Invest Dermatol* 32:413–419, 1959.

22. Barnhill RL, Fitzpatrick TB, Fandrey K, et al: *The Pigmented Lesion Clinic: A Color Atlas and Synopsis of Benign and Pigmented Lesions*. New York, McGraw-Hill, 1995.

23. Barnhill RL: *The Pathology of Melanocytic Nevi and Malignant Melanoma*. Boston, Butterworth-Heineman, 1995.

24. Barnhill RL, Albert LS, Shama SK, et al: Genital lentiginosis: A clinical and histopathologic study. *J Am Acad Dermatol* 22:453–460, 1990.

25. Folberg R, McLean IW: Primary acquired melanosis and melanoma of the conjunctiva: Terminology, classification and biologic behavior. *Hum Pathol* 16:129–135, 1985.

26. Jeghers H, McKusick BA, Katz KH: Generalized intestinal polyposis and melanin spots of the oral mucosa, lips and digits. *N Engl J Med* 241:993–1005, 1031–1036, 1949.

27. Utsunomiya J, Gocho H, Miyanaga T, et al: Peutz-Jeghers syndrome: Its natural course and management. *Johns Hopkins Med J* 1975;136:71-82.

28. Easton DF, Cox GM, MacDonald AM, Ponder BA: Genetic susceptibility to naevi—a twin study. *Br J Cancer* 64:1164–1167, 1991.

29. Goldgar DE, Cannon-Albright LA, Meyer LJ, et al: Inheritance of nevus number and size in melanoma and dysplastic nevus syndrome kindreds. *JNCI* 83:1726–1733, 1991.

30. Armstrong BK, de Klerk NH, Holman CDJ: The aetiology of common acquired melanocytic moles: Constitutional variables, sun exposure, and diet. *JNCI* 77:329–335, 1986.

31. Green A, Bain C, MacLennan R, et al: Risk factors for cutaneous melanoma in Queensland, in Gallagher RP (ed): *Recent Results in Cancer Research: Epidemiology of Malignant Melanoma*. Berlin, Springer-Verlag, 1986.

32. Armstrong BK, English DR: The epidemiology of acquired melanocytic naevi and their relationship to malignant melanoma, in Elwood JM (ed): *Melanoma and Naevi*. Basel, Karger, 1988, pp 27–47.

33. Hughes BR, Cunliffe WJ, Bailey CC: Excess benign melanocytic naevi after chemotherapy for malignancy in childhood. *Br Med J* 299:88–91, 1989.

34. de Wit PEJ, de Vaan GAM, de Booth M, et al: Prevalence of naevocytic naevi after chemotherapy for childhood cancer. *Med Pediatr Oncol* 18:336–338, 1990.

35. MacKie RM, English J, Aitchison TC, et al: The number and distribution of benign pigmented moles (melanocytic naevi) in a healthy British population. *Br J Dermatol* 113:167–174, 1985.

36. Rampen FHJ, de Wit PEJ: Racial differences in mole proneness. *Acta Derm Venereol (Stock)* 69:234–236, 1989.

37. Sigg C, Pelloni F: Frequency of acquired melanocytic nevi and their relationship to skin complexion in 939 schoolchildren. *Dermatologica* 179:123–128, 1989.

38. Coleman WP III, Gately LE III, Krementz AB, et al: Nevi, lentigines, and melanomas in blacks. *Arch Dermatol* 116:548–551, 1980.

39. Kopf AW, Andrade R: A histologic study of the dermoepidermal junction in clinically "intraepidermal" nevi, employing serial sections: I. Junctional theques. *Ann NY Acad Sci*, 100:200–222, 1960.

40. Masson P: My conception of cellular nevi. *Cancer* 4:9–38, 1951.

41. Reed RJ, Ichinose H, Clark WH Jr, Mihm MC Jr: Common and uncommon melanocytic nevi and borderline melanomas. *Semin Oncol* 2:119–147, 1975.

42. Masson P: Melanogenic system: nevi and melanomas. *Pathol Ann* 2:351–397, 1967.

43. Barr RJ, King DF: The significance of pseudoinclusions within the nuclei of melanocytes of certain neoplasms, in Ackerman AB (ed): *Pathology of Malignant Melanoma*. New York, Masson, 269–272, 1981.

44. Boyd AS, Rapini RP: Acral melanocytic neoplasms: A histologic analysis of 158 lesions. *J Am Acad Dermatol* 31:740–745, 1994.

45. McCalmont TH, Brinsko R, LeBoit PE: Melanocytic acral nevi with intraepidermal ascent of cells (MANIACs): A reappraisal of melanocytic lesions from acral sites. *J Cutan Pathol* 18:378[abstract], 1991.

46. Fallowfield ME, Collina G, Cook MG: Melanocytic lesions of the palm and sole. *Histopathol* 24:463–467, 1994.

47. Clemente C, Zurrida S, Bartoli C, et al: Acral-lentiginous naevus of plantar skin. *Histopathol* 27:549–555, 1995.

48. Schrader WA, Helwig EB: Balloon cell nevi. *Cancer* 20:1502–1514, 1967.

49. Goette DK, Doty RD: Balloon cell nevus: Summary of the clinical and histologic characteristics. *Arch Dermatol* 109–111, 1978.

50. Hashimoto K, Bale GF: An electron microscopic study of balloon cell nevus. *Cancer* 30:530–540, 1972.

51. Okun MR, Donnellan B, Edelstein L: An ultrastructural study of balloon cell nevus: Relationship of mast cells to nevus cells. *Cancer* 34:615–625, 1974.

52. Weedon D: Unusual features of nevocellular nevi. *J Cutan Pathol* 9:284–292, 1982.

53. Sutton RL: An unusual variety of vitiligo (leucodermal acquisitum centrifugum). *J Cutan Dis* 34:797–800, 1916.

54. Frank SB, Cohen HJ: The halo nevus. *Arch Dermatol* 89:367–373, 1964.

55. Kopf AW, Morrill SD, Silberberg I: Broad spectrum of leukoderma acquisitum centrifugum. *Arch Dermatol* 92:14–35, 1965.

56. Wayte DM, Helwig EB: Halo nevi. *Cancer* 22:69–90, 1968.

57. Brownstein MH, Kazam BB, Hashimoto K: Halo congenital nevus. *Arch Dermatol* 113:1572–1575, 1977.

58. Larsson PA, Liden S: Prevalence of skin diseases among adolescents 12-16 years of age. *Acta Derm Venereol (Stockh)* 60:415–423, 1980.

59. Bergman W, Willemze R, de Graaff-Reitsma C, Ruiter DJ: Analysis of major histocompatibility antigens and the mononuclear cell infiltrate in halo nevi. *J Invest Dermatol* 85:25–29, 1985.

60. Copeman PWM, Lewis MG, Phillips TM, Elliott PG: Immunological associations of the halo nevus with cutaneous malignant melanoma. *Br J Dermatol* 88:127–137, 1973.

61. Bennett C, Copeman PWM: Melanocyte mutation in halo naevus and malignant melanoma? *Br J Dermatol* 100:423–436, 1979.

62. Whimster I: The halo naevus and cutaneous malignant melanoma. *Br J Dermatol* 90:111–113, 1974.

63. Gauthier Y, Surlève J-E, Texier L: Halo nevi without dermal infiltrate. *Arch Dermatol* 114:1718 (Letter), 1978.

64. Mitchell MS, Nordlund JJ, Lerner AB: Comparison of cell-mediated immunity to melanoma cells in patients with vitiligo, halo nevi or melanoma. *J Invest Dermatol* 75:144–147, 1980.

65. Cohen HJ, Minkin W, Frank SB: Nevus spilus. *Arch Dermatol* 102:433–437, 1970.

66. Matsudo H, Reed WB, Homme D, et al: Zosteriform lentiginous nevus. *Arch Dermatol* 107:902–905, 1973.

67. Stewart DM, Altman J, Mehregan AH: Speckled lentiginous nevus. *Arch Dermatol* 114:895–896, 1978.

68. Port M, Courniotes J, Podwal M: Zosteriform lentiginous naevus with ipsilateral rigid cavus foot. *Br J Dermatol* 98:693–698, 1978.

69. Falo LD Jr, Sober AJ, Barnhill RL: Evolution of nevus spilus. *Dermatology* 189: 382–383, 1994.

70. Rhodes AR, Mihm MC Jr: Origin of cutaneous melanoma in a congenital dysplastic nevus spilus. *Arch Dermatol* 126:500–505, 1990.

71. Stern JB, Haupt HM, Aaronson CM: Malignant melanoma in a speckled zosteriform lentiginous nevus. *Int J Dermatol* 29:583–584, 1990.

72. Kurban RS, Preffer FI, Sober AJ, et al: Occurrence of melanoma in "dysplastic" nevus spilus: Report of case and analysis by flow cytometry. *J Cutan Pathol* 19:423–428, 1992.

73. Kornberg R, Ackerman AB: Pseudomelanoma. *Arch Dermatol* 111:1588–1590, 1975.

74. Park HK, Leonard DD, Arrington JH, Lund HZ: Recurrent melanocytic nevi: Clinical and histologic review of 175 cases. *J Am Acad Dermatol* 17:285–292, 1987.

75. Friedman RJ, Ackerman AB: Difficulties in the histologic diagnosis of melanocytic nevi on the vulvae of premenopausal women, in Ackerman AB (ed): *Pathology of Malignant Melanoma*. New York, Masson, 1981, pp 119–127.

76. Christensen WN, Friedman KJ, Woodruff JD, Hood AF: Histologic characteristics of vulvar nevocellular nevi. *J Cutan Pathol* 14:87–91, 1986.

77. Thompson GW, Diehl AK: Partial unilateral lentiginosis. *Arch Dermatol* 116:356, 1980.

78. MacDonald DM, Black MM: Secondary localized cutaneous amyloidosis in melanocytic nevi. *Br J Dermatol* 103:553–556, 1980.

79. Söderström K-O: Angiomatous type of intradermal nevi. *Am J Dermatopathol* 9: 549–551, (Letter), 1987.

80. Collina G, Eusebi V: Naevocytic naevi with vascular-like spaces. *Br J Dermatol* 124:591–595, 1991.

81. James MP, Wells RS: Cockade naevus: An unusual variant of the benign cellular naevus. *Acta Derm Venereol* 60:360–363, 1980.

82. Freeman RG, Knox JM: Epidermal cysts associated with pigmented nevi. *Arch Dermatol* 85:590–594, 1962.

83. Canizares O: Subnevic folliculitis resembling melanoma. *Arch Dermatol* 97:363, 1968.

84. Meyerson LB: A peculiar papulosquamous eruption involving pigmented nevi. *Arch Dermatol* 103:510–512, 1971.

85. Weedon D, Farnsworth J: Spongiotic changes in melanocytic nevi. *Am J Dermatopathol* 6(Suppl):257–259, 1984.

86. Burgdorf W, Nasemann T: Cutaneous osteomas: A clinical and histopathologic review. *Arch Dermatol Res* 260:121–135, 1977.

87. Yesudian P, Thambiah AS: Perinevoid alopecia: An unusual variant of alopecia areata. *Arch Dermatol* 112:1432—1434, 1976.

88. Weitzner S: Intradermal nevus with psammoma body formation. *Arch Dermatol* 98: 287–289, 1968.

89. Mark GJ, Mihm MC, Liteplo MG, et al: Congenital melanocytic nevi of the small and garment type. *Hum Pathol* 4:395–418, 1973.

90. Walton RG, Jacobs AH, Cox AJ: Pigmented lesions in newborn infants. *Br J Dermatol* 95:389–396, 1976.

91. Cramer SF: The melanocytic differentiation pathway in congenital melanocytic nevi: Theoretical considerations. *Pediatr Pathol* 8:253–265, 1988.

92. Stenn KS, Arons M, Hurwitz S: Patterns of congenital nevocellular nevi. *J Am Acad Dermatol* 9:388–393, 1983.

93. Rhodes AR, Silberman RA, Harrist TJ, Melski JW: A histologic comparison of congenital and acquired nevomelanocytic nevi. *Arch Dermatol* 121:1266–1273, 1985.

94. Everett MA: Histopathology of congenital pigmented nevi. *Am J Dermatopathol* 11:11–12, 1989.

95. Reed WB, Becker SW Sr, Becker SW Jr, Nickel WR: Giant pigmented nevi, melanoma, and leptomeningeal melanocytosis. *Arch Dermatol* 91:100–118, 1965.

96. Rhodes AR: Neoplasms; benign neoplasias, hyperplasias, and dysplasia of melanocytes, in Fitzpatrick TB, Eisen AZ, Wolff K, et al (eds): *Dermatology in General Medicine*, 4th ed. New York, McGraw-Hill, 1026–1037, 1993.

97. Kopf AW, Bart RS, Hennessey P: Congenital nevocytic nevi and malignant melanoma. *J Am Acad Dermatol* 1:123–130, 1979.

98. Rhodes AR, Sober AJ, Day CL, et al: The malignant potential of small congenital nevocellular nevi: An estimate of association based on a histologic study of 234 primary cutaneous melanomas. *J Am Acad Dermatol* 6:230–241, 1982.

99. Rhodes AR, Melski JW: Small congenital nevocellular nevi and the risk of cutaneous melanoma. *J Pediatr* 100:219–224, 1982.

100. Illig L, Weidner F, Hundeiker M, et al: Congenital nevi less than or equal to 10 cm as precursors to melanoma: 52 cases, a review, and a new conception. *Arch Dermatol* 121:1274–1281, 1985.

101. Castilla EE, da Graca Dutra M, Orioli-Parreiras IM: Epidemiology of congenital pigmented naevi: I. Incidence rates and relative frequencies. *Br J Dermatol* 104:307–315, 1981.

102. Lorentzen M, Pers M, Bretteville-Jensen G: The incidence of malignant transformation in giant pigmented nevi. *Scand J Plast Reconstr Surg* 71:163–167, 1977.

103. Rhodes AR, Wood WC, Sober AJ, Mihm MC Jr: Nonepidermal origin of malignant melanoma associated with a giant congenital nevocellular nevus. *Plast Reconstr Surg* 67:782–790, 1981.

104. Reed RJ: Giant congenital nevi: A conceptualization of patterns. *J Invest Dermatol* 100:(Suppl):300S–312S, 1993.

105. Barnhill RL, Fleischli M: Histologic features of congenital melanocytic nevi in infants less than a year of age. *J Am Acad Dermatol* 33:780–785, 1995.

106. Silvers DN, Helwig EB: Melanocytic nevi in neonates. *J Am Acad Dermatol* 4:166–175, 1981.

107. Clemmensen OJ, Kroon S: The histology of "congenital features" in early acquired melanocytic nevi. *J Am Acad Dermatol* 19:742–746, 1988.

108. Walsh MY, MacKie RM: Histologic features of value in differentiating small congenital melanocytic nevi from acquired naevi. *Histopathology* 12:145–154, 1988.

109. Solomon L, Eng AM, Bené M, Loeffel D: Giant congenital neuroid melanocytic nevus. *Arch Dermatol* 116:318–320, 1980.

110. Hendrickson MR, Ross JC: Neoplasms arising in congenital giant nevi: Morphologic study of seven cases and a review of the literature. *Am J Surg Pathol* 5:109–135, 1981.

111. Mancianti ML, Clark WH, Hayes FA, Herlyn M: Malignant melanoma simulants arising in congenital melanocytic nevi do not show experimental evidence for a malignant phenotype. *Am J Pathol* 136:817–829, 1990.

112. Clark WH Jr, Elder DE, Guerry D IV: Dysplastic nevi and malignant melanoma, in Farmer ER, Hood AF (eds): *Pathology of the Skin*. Norwalk, CT, Appleton and Lange, 1990, pp 684–756.

113. Weidner N, Flanders DJ, Jochimsen PR, Stamler FW: Neurosarcomatous malignant melanoma arising in a neuroid giant congenital melanocytic nevus. *Arch Dermatol* 121:1302–1306, 1985.

114. Jauniaux E, de Meeus M-C, Verellen G: Giant congenital melanocytic nevus with placental involvement: Long-term follow-up of a case and review of the literature. *Pediatr Pathol* 13:717–721, 1993.

115. Hara K: Melanocytic lesions in lymph nodes associated with congenital naevus. *Histopathol* 23:445–451, 1993.

116. Skov-Jensen T, Hastrup J, Lambrethsen E: Malignant melanoma in children. *Cancer* 19:620–626, 1966.

117. Trozak DJ, Rowland WD, Hu F: Metastatic malignant melanoma in prepubertal children. *Pediatr* 55:191–204, 1975.

118. Roth ME, Grant-Kels JM, Kuhn K, et al: Melanoma in children. *J Am Acad Dermatol* 22:265–274, 1990.

119. Ceballos PI, Ruiz-Maldonado R, Mihm MC Jr: Melanoma in childhood. *N Engl J Med* 332:656–662, 1995.

120. Reintgen DS, Vollmer R, Seigler HF: Juvenile malignant melanoma. *Surg Gyn Obstet* 168:249–253, 1989.

121. Barnhill RL, Flotte T, Fleischli M, Perez-Atayde AR: Childhood melanoma and atypical Spitz-tumors *Cancer* 76:1833–1845, 1995.

122. Handfield-Jones SE, Smith NP: Malignant melanoma in childhood. *Br J Dermatol* 134:607–613, 1996.

123. Spitz S: Melanomas of childhood. *Am J Pathol* 24:591–609, 1948.

124. Allen A, Spitz S: Malignant melanoma: A clinico-pathological analysis of the criteria for diagnosis and prognosis. *Cancer* 6:1–45, 1953.

125. Kernen J, Ackerman L: Spindle cell nevi and epithelioid cell nevi (so-called juvenile melanomas) in children and adults: A clinicopathological study of 27 cases. *Cancer* 13:612–625, 1960.

126. Kopf A, Andrade R: Benign juvenile melanoma, in Kopf A, Andrade R (eds): *Yearbook of Dermatology 1965-1966*. Chicago, Year Book Medical Publishers pp 7–52.

127. Echevarria R, Ackerman L: Spindle and epithelioid nevi in the adult: Clinicopathologic report of 26 cases. *Cancer* 20:175–189, 1967.

128. Paniago-Pereira C, Maize J, Ackerman A: Nevus of large spindle and/or epithelioid cells (Spitz's nevus). *Arch Dermatol* 114:1811–1823, 1978.

129. Weedon D, Little J: Spindle and epithelioid cell nevi in children and adults: A review of 211 cases of the Spitz nevus. *Cancer* 40:217–225, 1977.

130. Allen A: Juvenile melanomas of children and adults and melanocarcinomas of children. *Arch Dermatol* 82:325–335, 1960.

131. Coskey R, Mehregan A: Spindle cell nevi in adults and children. *Arch Dermatol* 108:535–536, 1973.

132. Weedon D: The Spitz nevus. *Clin Oncol* 3:493–507, 1984.

133. Binder S, Asnog C, Paul E, Cochran A: The histology and differential diagnosis of Spitz nevus. *Semin Diagn Pathol* 10:36–46, 1993.

134. Busam KJ, Barnhill RL: The spectrum of spitz tumors, in Kirkham N, Lemoine NR (eds): *Progress in Pathology*, vol 2. Edinburgh, Churchill Livingstone, 1995, pp 31–46.

135. Hamm H, Happle R, Broecker E: Multiple agminate Spitz nevi: Review of the literature and report of a case with distinctive immunohistologic features. *Br J Dermatol* 117:511–522, 1987.

136. Smith K, Skelton H, Lupton G, Graham J: Spindle cell and epithelioid cell nevi with atypia and metastasis (malignant Spitz nevus). *Am J Surg Pathol* 13:931–939, 1989.

137. Merot Y, Frenk E: Spitz nevus (large spindle and/or epithelioid cell nevus): Age-related involvement of the suprabasal epidermis. *Virchows Arch A (Pathol Anat)* 415:97–101, 1989.

138. Kamino H, Misheloff E, Ackerman A, et al: Eosinophilic globules in Spitz's nevi: New findings and a diagnostic sign. *Am J Surg Pathol* 1:319–324, 1979.

139. Arbuckle S, Weedon D: Eosinophilic globules in the Spitz nevus. *J Am Acad Dermatol* 7:324–327, 1982.

140. Havenith M, van Zandvoort E, Cleutjens J, Bosman F: Basement membrane deposition in benign and malignant nevomelanocytic lesions: An immunohistochemical study with antibodies to type IV collagen and laminin. *Histopathology* 15:137–146, 1989.

141. Barnhill RL, Barnhill MA, Berwick M, Mihm MC Jr: The histologic spectrum of pigmented spindle cell nevus: A review of 120 cases with emphasis on atypical variants. *Hum Pathol* 22:52–58, 1991.

142. Busam KJ, Barnhill RL: Pagetoid Spitz nevus. *Am J Surg Pathol* 19:1061–1067, 1995.

143. Mooi W, Krausz T: Spitz naevus, desmoplastic Spitz naevus and pigmented spindle cell naevus, in Mooi W, Krausz T (eds): *Biopsy: Pathology of Melanocytic Disorders*. London, Chapman and Hall, 1992, pp 156–185.

144. Barr R, Morales R, Graham J: Desmoplastic nevus: A distinct histologic variant of mixed spindle and epithelioid cell nevus. *Cancer* 46:557–564, 1980.

145. MacKie RM, Doherty VR: The desmoplastic melanocytic naevus: A distinct histologic entity. *Histopathology* 20:207–211, 1992.

146. Gartmann H: Der pigmentierte Spindelzellentumor. *Z Hautkrankh* 56:862–876, 1981.

147. Sagebiel R, Chinn E, Egbert B: Pigmented spindle cell nevus: Clinical and histologic review of 90 cases. *Am J Surg Pathol* 8:645–653, 1984.

148. Smith N: The pigmented spindle cell tumor of Reed: An underdiagnosed lesion. *Sem Diagn Pathol* 4:75–87, 1987.

149. Barnhill RL, Mihm MC: Pigmented spindle cell nevus and its variants: Distinction from melanoma. *Br J Dermatol* 121:717–726, 1989.

150. Montgomery H: The blue nevus (Jadassohn-Tieche): Its distinction from ordinary moles and malignant melanomas. *Am J Cancer* 36:527–539, 1939.

151. Allen AC: A reorientation on the histogenesis and clinical significance of cutaneous nevi and melanomas. *Cancer* 2:28–56, 1949.

152. Dorsey CS, Montgomery H: Blue nevus and its distinction from Mongolian spot and the nevus of Ota. *J Invest Dermatol* 22:225–236, 1954.

153. Lund HZ, Kraus JM: *Melanotic Tumors of the Skin. Atlas of Tumor Pathology*. Washington, DC, Armed Forces Institute of Pathology, 1962, pp 104–106.

154. Gartmann VH: Neuronaevus blue Masson—cellular blue nevus Allen. *Archiv für klinische u. experimentelle Dermatologie* 221:109–121, 1965.

155. Leopold JG, Richards DB: Cellular blue nevi. *J Path Bact* 94:247–255, 1967.

156. Leopold JG, Richards DB: The interrelationship of blue and common naevi. *J Path Bact* 95:37–46, 1968.

157. Rodriguez HA, Ackerman LV: Cellular blue nevus: Clinicopathologic study of forty-five cases. *Cancer* 21:393–405, 1968.

158. Merkow LP, Burt RC, Hayeslip DW, et al: A cellular and malignant blue nevus: A light and electron microscopic study. *Cancer* 24:888–896, 1969.

159. Bird CC, Willis RA: The histogenesis of pigmented neurofibromas. *J Path* 97:631–637, 1969.

160. Mishima Y: Cellular blue nevus: Melanogenic activity and malignant transformation. *Arch Dermatol* 101:104–110, 1970.

161. Levene A: On the natural history and comparative pathology of the blue naevus. *Annu Rep Coll Surg Engl* 62:327–334, 1980.

162. Sun J, Morton TH, Gown AM: Antibody HMB-45 identifies the cells of blue nevi. *Am J Surg Pathol* 14:748–751, 1990.

163. Mishima Y, Mevorah B: Nevus Ota and nevus of Ito in American Negroes. *J Invest Dermatol* 36:133–154, 1961.

164. Kopf AW, Weidman AI: Nevus of Ota. *Arch Dermatol* 85:195–208, 1962.

165. Hidano A, Kajima H, Ikeda S, et al: Natural history of nevus of Ota. *Arch Dermatol* 95:187–195, 1967.

166. Hirayama T, Suzuki T: A new classification of Ota's nevus based on histopathologic features. *Dermatologica* 183:169–172, 1991.

167. Kopf AW, Bart RS: Malignant blue (Ota's?) nevus. *J Dermatol Surg Oncol* 8:442–445, 1982.

168. Hori Y, Kawashima M, Oohara K, Kukita A: Acquired, bilateral nevus of Ota-like macules. *J Am Acad Dermatol* 10:961–964, 1984.

169. Sun C-C, Lu Y-C, Lee EF, Nakagawa H: Naevus fusco-caeruleus zygomaticus. *Br J Dermatol* 117:545–553, 1986.

170. Hidano A, Kaneko K: Acquired dermal melanocytosis of the face and extremities. *Br J Dermatol* 124:96–99, 1991.

171. Burkhart CG, Gohara A: Dermal melanocytic hamartoma. *Arch Dermatol* 117:102–104, 1981.

172. Shenfield HT, Maize JC: Multiple and agminated blue nevi. *J Dermatol Surg Oncol* 6:725–728, 1980.

173. Upshaw BY, Ghormley RK, Montgomery H: Extensive blue nevus of Jadassohn-Tièche: Report of case. *Surgery* 22:761–765, 1947.

174. Pittman JL, Fisher BK: Plaque-type blue nevus. *Arch Dermatol* 112:1127–1128, 1976.

175. Hendricks WM: Eruptive blue nevi. *J Am Acad Dermatol* 4:50–53, 1981.

176. Heymann WR, Yablonsky TM: Congenital plaque-type blue nevus. *Arch Dermatol* 127:587, 1991.

177. Modly C, Wood C, Horn T: Metastatic malignant melanoma arising from a common blue nevus in a patient with subacute cutaneous lupus erythematosus. *Dermatologica* 178:171–175, 1989.

178. Kamino H, Tam ST: Compound blue nevus: A variant of blue nevus with an additional junctional dendritic component. A clinical, histopathologic, and immunohistochemical study of six cases. *Arch Dermatol* 126:1330–1333, 1990.

179. Sterchi JM, Muss HB, Weidner N: Cellular blue nevus simulating metastatic melanoma: Report of an unusually large lesion associated with nevus-cell aggregates in regional lymph nodes. *J Surg Oncol* 36:71–75, 1987.

180. Temple-Camp CRE, Saxe N, King H: Benign and malignant cellular blue nevus: A clinicopathological study of 30 cases. *Am J Dermatopathol* 10:289–296, 1988.

181. Michal M, Baumruk K, Skalova A: Myxoid change within cellular blue naevi: A diagnostic pitfall. *Histopathology* 20:527–530, 1992.

182. Avidor I, Kessler E: "Atypical" blue nevus—a benign variant of cellular blue nevus. *Dermatologica* 154:39–44, 1977.

183. Goldenhersh MA, Savin RC, Barnhill RL, Stenn KS: Malignant blue nevus. *J Am Acad Dermatol* 19:712–722, 1988.

184. Connelly J, Smith JL Jr: Malignant blue nevus. *Cancer* 67:2653–2657, 1991.

185. Lambert WC, Brodkin RH: Nodal and subcutaneous cellular blue nevi: A pseudometastasizing pseudomelanoma. *Arch Dermatol* 120:367–370, 1984.

186. Lamovec J: Blue nevus of the lymph node capsule: Report of a new case with review of the literature. *Am J Clin Pathol* 81:367–372, 1984.

187. Pariser H, Beerman H: Extensive blue patchlike pigmentation. A morphologic variant of blue nevus? Persistent extrasacral Mongolian blue spot? Diffuse mesodermal pigmentation? *Arch Dermatol Syphil* 59:396–404, 1949.

188. Radentz WA, Vogel P: Congenital common blue nevus. *Arch Dermatol* 126:124–125, 1990.

189. Pfaltz M, Schnyder UW: Verlauf und ultrastruktur beim plaqueartigen naevus bleu. *Hautarzt* 40:355–357, 1989.

190. Tuthill RJ, Clark WH Jr, Levene A: Pilar neurocristic hamartoma: Its relationship to blue nevus and equine melanotic disease. *Arch Dermatol* 118:592–596, 1982.

191. Bondi EE, Elder D, Guerry D IV, Clark WH Jr: Target blue nevus. *Arch Dermatol* 119:919–920, 1983.

192. Fletcher V, Sagebiel RW: The combined nevus: Mixed patterns of benign melanocytic lesions must be differentiated from malignant melanomas, in Ackerman AB (ed): *Pathology of Malignant Melanoma.* New York, Masson, 1981, pp 273–283.

193. Rogers GS, Advani H, Ackerman AB: A combined variant of Spitz's nevi. *Am J Dermatopathol* 7:61–78, 1985.

194. Pulitzer DR, Martin PC, Cohen AP, Reed, RJ: Histologic classification of the combined nevus: Analysis of the variable expression of melanocytic nevi. *Am J Surg Pathol* 15:1111–1122, 1991.

195. Mihm MC Jr, Googe PB: *Problematic Pigmented Lesions.* Philadelphia, Lea & Febiger, 1990, pp 76–77.

196. Ball NJ, Golitz LE: Melanocytic nevi (with focal atypical epithelioid cell components): A review of 73 cases. *J Am Acad Dermatol* 30:724–729, 1994.

197. Seab JA Jr, Graham JH, Helwig EB: Deep penetrating nevus. *Am J Surg Pathol* 13:39–44, 1989.

198. Barnhill RL, Mihm MC Jr, Magro CM: Plexiform spindle cell naevus: A distinctive variant of plexiform melanocytic naevus. *Histopathology* 18:243–247, 1991.

199. Cooper PH: Deep penetrating (plexiform spindle cell) nevus: A frequent participant in combined nevus. *J Cutan Pathol* 19:172–180, 1992.

200. Lynch HT, Frichot BC III, Lynch JF: Familial atypical multiple mole-melanoma syndrome. *J Med Genet* 15:352–356, 1978.

201. Clark WH Jr, Reimer RR, Greene M, et al: Origin of familial malignant melanomas from heritable melanocytic lesions: The B-K mole syndrome. *Arch Dermatol* 114:732–738, 1978.

202. Sagebiel RW: Histopathology of borderline and early malignant melanomas. *Am J Surg Pathol* 3:543–552, 1979.

203. Elder DE, Goldman LI, Goldman SC, et al: Dysplastic nevus syndrome: A phenotypic association of sporadic cutaneous melanoma. *Cancer* 46:1787–1794, 1980.

204. Elder DE, Greene MH, Bondi EE, Clark WH Jr: Acquired melanocytic nevi and melanoma: The dysplastic nevus syndrome, in Ackerman AB (ed): *Pathology of Malignant Melanoma.* New York, Masson 1981, pp 185–215.

205. Kraemer KH, Greene MH, Tarone R, et al: Dysplastic naevi and cutaneous melanoma risk [letter]. *Lancet* 2:1076–1077, 1983.

206. Crutcher WA, Sagebiel RW: Prevalence of dysplastic nevi in a community practice (letter). *Lancet* 1:729, 1984.

207. NIH Consensus Conference: Precursors to malignant melanoma. *JAMA* 251:1864–1866, 1984.

208. Ackerman AB, Mihara I: Dysplasia, dysplastic melanocytes, the dysplastic nevus syndrome, and the relation between dysplastic nevi and malignant melanoma. *Hum Pathol* 16:87–91, 1985.

209. Elder DE: The dysplastic nevus. *Pathology* 17:291–297, 1985.

210. Greene MH, Clark WH Jr, Tucker MA, et al: Acquired precursors of cutaneous malignant melanoma: The familial dysplastic nevus syndrome. *N Engl J Med* 312:91–97, 1985.

211. Greene MH, Clark WH Jr, Tucker MA, et al: High risk of malignant melanoma in melanoma-prone families with dysplastic nevi. *Ann Intern Med* 102:458–465, 1985.

212. Nordlund JJ, Kirkwood J, Forget BM, et al: Demographic study of clinically atypical (dysplastic) nevi in patients with melanoma and comparison subjects. *Cancer Res* 45:1855–1861, 1985.

213. Sagebiel RW: Histopathology of precursor melanocytic lesions. *Am J Surg Pathol* 9:41–52, 1985.

214. Sagebiel RW: Diagnosis and management of premalignant melanocytic proliferations. *Pathology* 17:285–290, 1985.

215. Kelly JW, Crutcher WA, Sagebiel RW: Clinical diagnosis of dysplastic melanocytic nevi: A clinicopathological correlation. *J Am Acad Dermatol* 14:1044–1052, 1986.

216. Roush GC, Barnhill RL, Duray PH, et al: Diagnosis of the dysplastic nevus in different population. *J Am Acad Dermatol* 14:419–425, 1986.

217. Seywright MM, Doherty VR, MacKie RM: Proposed alternative terminology and subclassification of so-called "dysplastic naevi." *J Clin Pathol* 39:189–194, 1986.

218. Rhodes AR, Weinstock MA, Fitzpatrick TB, et al: Risk factors for cutaneous melanoma: A practical method of recognizing predisposed individuals. *JAMA* 258:3146–3154, 1987.

219. Ackerman AB: What naevus is dysplastic, a syndrome and the commonest precursor of malignant melanoma? A riddle and an answer. *Histopathology* 13:241–256, 1988.

220. Barnhill RL, Hurwitz S, Duray PH, Arons MS: The dysplastic nevus: Recognition and management. *Plast Reconstr Surg* 81(2):280–289, 1988.

221. Bergman W, Ruiter DJ, Scheffer E, van Vloten WA: Melanocytic atypia in dysplastic nevi: Immunohistochemical and cytophotometrical analysis. *Cancer* 61:1660–1666, 1988.

222. Black WC: Residual dysplastic and other nevi in superficial spreading melanoma: Clinical correlations and association with sun damage. *Cancer* 62:163–173, 1988.

223. Steijlen PM, Bergman W, Hermans J, et al: The efficacy of histopathological criteria required for diagnosing dysplastic naevi. *Histopathology* 12:289–300, 1988.

224. Gruber SB, Barnhill RL, Stenn KS, Roush GC: Nevomelanocytic proliferations in association with cutaneous malignant melanoma: A multivariate analysis. *J Am Acad Dermatol* 21(4 Pt 1):773–780, 1989.

225. Piepkorn M, Meyer LJ, Goldgar D: The dysplastic melanocytic nevus—a prevalent lesion that correlates poorly with clinical phenotype. *J Am Acad Dermatol* 20:407–415, 1989.

226. Rhodes AR, Mihm MC Jr, Weinstock MA: Dysplastic melanocytic nevi: A reproducible histologic definition emphasizing cellular morphology. *Mod Pathol* 2:306–319, 1989.

227. Rigel DS, Rivers JK, Kopf AW, et al: Dysplastic nevi markers for increased risk of melanoma. *Cancer* 63:386–389, 1989.

228. Ahmed I, Piepkorn MW, Rabkin MS, et al: Histopathologic characteristics of dysplastic nevi: Limited association of conventional histologic criteria with melanoma risk group. *J Am Acad Dermatol* 22:727–733, 1990.

229. Barnhill RL, Roush GC: Histopathologic spectrum of clinically atypical melanocytic nevi: II. Studies of nonfamilial melanoma. *Arch Dermatol* 126(10):1315–1318, 1990.

230. Barnhill RL, Roush GC, Duray PH: Correlation of histologic and cytoplasmic features with nuclear atypia in atypical (dysplastic) nevomelanocytic nevi. *Hum Pathol* 21:51–58, 1990.

231. Black WC, Hunt WC: Histologic correlations with the clinical diagnosis of dysplastic nevus. *Am J Surg Pathol* 14:44–52, 1990.

232. Klein LJ, Barr RJ: Histologic atypia in clinically benign nevi: A prospective study. *J Am Acad Dermatol* 22:275–282, 1990.

233. Barnhill RL: Current status of the dysplastic melanocytic nevus. *J Cutan Pathol* 18:147–159, 1991.

234. Barnhill RL, Roush GC: Correlation of clinical and histopathological features in clinically atypical melanocytic nevi. *Cancer* 67:3157–3164, 1991.

235. Clark WH Jr: Tumour progression and the nature of cancer. *Br J Cancer* 64:631–644, 1991.

236. Clemente C, Cochran AJ, Elder DE, et al: Histopathologic diagnosis of dysplastic nevi: Concordance among pathologists convened by the World Health Organization Melanoma Programme. *Hum Pathol* 22:313–319, 1991.

237. Halpern AC, Guerry D, Elder DE, et al: Dysplastic nevi as risk markers of sporadic (nonfamilial) melanoma. *Arch Dermatol* 127:995–999, 1991.

238. Roush GC, Barnhill RL: Correlation of clinical pigmentary characteristics with histopathologically-confirmed dysplastic nevi in nonfamilial melanoma patients. Studies of melanocytic nevi IX. *Br J Cancer* 64(5):943–947, 1991.

239. Titus-Ernstoff L, Ernstoff MS, Duray PH, et al: A relation between childhood sun exposure and dysplastic nevus syndrome among patients with nonfamilial melanoma. *Epidemiology* 2(3):210–214, 1991.

240. Barnhill RL, Roush GC, Titus-Ernstoff L, et al: Comparison of nonfamilial and familial melanoma. *Dermatology* 184(1):2–7, 1992.

241. Duray PH, DerSimonian R, Barnhill RL, et al: An analysis of inter-observer recognition of the histopathologic features of dysplastic nevi from a mixed group of nevomelanocytic lesions. *J Am Acad Dermatol* 27(5 Pt 1):741–749, 1992.

242. NIH Consensus Development Panel on Early Melanoma: Diagnosis and treatment of early melanoma. *JAMA* 268:1314–1319, 1992.

243. Barnhill RL: Melanocytic nevi and tumor progression: Perspectives concerning histomorphology, melanoma risk, and molecular genetics. *Dermatology* 187:86–90, 1993.

244. Bruijn JA, Berwick M, Mihm MC Jr, Barnhill RL: Common acquired melanocytic nevi, dysplastic melanocytic nevi and malignant melanomas: An image analysis cytometric study. *J Cutan Pathol* 20(2):121–125, 1993.

245. Duncan LM, Berwick MA, Bruijn JA, et al: Histopathologic recognition and grading of dysplastic melanocytic nevi: an inter-observer agreement study. *J Invest Dermatol* 100(3)Suppl:318S–321S, 1993.

246. Titus-Ernstoff L, Barnhill RL, Duray PH, et al: Dysplastic nevi in relation to superficial spreading melanoma. *Cancer Epidemiol Biomarkers Prev* 2(2):99–101, 1993.

247. MacKie RM, McHenry P, Hole D: Accelerated detection with prosepective surveillance for cutaneous malignant melanoma in high-risk groups. *Lancet* 341:1618–1620, 1993.

248. Tucker MA, Fraser MC, Goldstein AM, et al: Risk of melanoma and other cancers in melanoma-prone families. *J Invest Dermatol* 100:350S–355S, 1993.

249. Halpern AC, Guerry DP IV, Elder DE, et al: A cohort study of melanoma in patients with dysplastic nevi. *J Invest Dermatol* 100:346S–349S, 1993.

250. Barnhill RL: Moles and melanoma—New method in the madness. *West J Med* 160:381–383, 1994.

251. Williams ML, Sagebiel RW: Melanoma risk factors and the atypical mole: Controversies and consensus. *Western J Med* 160:343–350, 1994.

252. Piepkorn MW, Barnhill RL, Rabkin MS, et al: Histologic diagnosis of the dysplastic nevus: An analysis of inter- and intra-observer concordance, correlation with clinical phenotype, and prevalence in population controls. *J Am Acad Dermatol* 30:707–714, 1994.

253. Schmidt B, Hollister K, Weinberg D, Barnhill RL: Analysis of dysplastic nevi by DNA image cytometry. *Cancer* 73:2971–2977, 1994.

254. Kang S, Barnhill RL, Mihm MC Jr, et al: Melanoma risk in individuals with clinically atypical nevi. *Arch Dermatol* 130:999–1001, 1994.

255. Hastrup N, Clemmensen OJ, Spaun E, Sondergarrd K: Dysplastic naevus; histological criteria and their inter-observer reproducibility. *Histopathology* 24:503–509, 1994.

256. Barnhill RL: Malignant melanoma: Histology, in Miller SJ, Maloney ME (eds): *Cutaneous Oncology: Pathophysiology, Diagnosis and Treatment*. Cambridge, MA, Blackwell Science. In press, 1997.

257. Clark WH Jr: A classification of malignant melanoma in man correlated with histogenesis and biologic behavior, in Montagna W, Hu F (eds): *Advances in the Biology of the Skin*, vol. 8. New York, Pergamon Press, 1967, pp 621–647.

258. Clark WH Jr, From L, Bernardino EA, Mihm MC: The histogenesis and biologic behavior of primary human malignant melanomas of the skin. *Cancer Res* 29:705–727, 1969.

259. McGovern VJ, Mihm MC Jr, Bailly C, et al: The classification of malignant melanoma and its histologic reporting. *Cancer* 32:1446–1457, 1973.

260. Reed RJ: The pathology of human cutaneous melanoma, in Costanzi JJ (ed): *Malignant Melanoma I*. The Hague, Martinus Nijhoff, 1983, pp 85–116.

261. Clark WH Jr, Elder DE, Van Horn M: The biologic forms of malignant melanoma. *Human Pathol* 17:443–450, 1984.

262. Heenan PJ, Armstrong BK, English DE, et al: Pathological and epidemiological variants of cutaneous malignant melanoma, in Elder DE (ed): *Pathobiology of Malignant Melanoma*. Basel, Karger, 107–146, 1987.

263. Barnhill RL, Mihm MC, Fitzpatrick TB, Sober AJ: Neoplasms: Malignant melanoma, in Fitzpatrick TB, Eisen AZ, Wolff K, et al (eds): *Dermatology in General Medicine*, vol 1. New York, McGraw-Hill, 1993, pp 1078–1115.

264. Barnhill RL, Mihm MC Jr: The histopathology of cutaneous malignant melanoma. *Semin Diagn Pathol* 10:47–75, 1993.

265. Reed RJ: Acral lentiginous melanoma, in *New Concepts in Surgical Pathology of Skin*. New York, John Wiley & Sons, 1976, pp 89–90.

266. Arrington JH III, Reed RJ, Ichinose H, Krementz ET: Plantar lentiginous melanoma: A distinctive variant of human cutaneous malignant melanoma. *Am J Surg Pathol* 1:131–143, 1977.

267. Heenan PJ, Holman CDJ: Nodular malignant melanoma: A distinct entity or a common end stage? *Am J Dermatopathol* 4:477–478, 1982.

268. Vollmer RT: Malignant melanoma: A multivariate analysis of prognostic factors. *Pathol Ann* 24:383, 1989.

269. Barnhill RL, Fine J, Roush GC, Berwick M: Predicting five-year outcome from cutaneous melanoma in a population-based study. *Cancer.* 78:427–432, 1996.

270. Ackerman AB: Malignant melanoma: A unifying concept. *Human Pathol* 11:591–595, 1980.

271. Heenan PJ, Matz LR, Blackwell JB, et al: Inter-observer variation between pathologists in the classification of cutaneous malignant melanoma in western Australia. *Histopathology* 8:717–729, 1984.

272. Mihm MC Jr, Fitzpatrick TB, Brown MM, et al: Early detection of primary cutaneous malignant melanoma: A color atlas. *N Engl J Med* 289:989–996, 1973.

273. Patterson RH, Helwig EB: Subungual malignant melanoma: A clinical-pathologic study. *Cancer* 46:2074–2087, 1980.

274. Saida T, Yoshida N, Ikegawa S, et al: Clinical guidelines for the early detection of plantar malignant melanoma. *J Am Acad Dermatol* 23:37–40, 1990.

275. Blessing K, Kernohan NM, Park KGM: Subungual malignant melanoma: Clinicopathological features of 100 cases. *Histopathology* 19:425–429, 1992.

276. Rigby HS, Briggs JC: Subungual melanoma: A clinicopathological study of 24 cases. *Br J Plast Surg* 45:275–278, 1992.

277. Saida T, Ohshima Y: Clinical and histopathologic characteristics of early lesions of subungual malignant melanoma. *Cancer* 63:556–560, 1989.

278. Ten Seldam R, Helwig E, Sobin L, et al: Histological typing of skin tumours, in *Histological Typing of Skin Tumours. International Histological Classification of Tumors*, No. 12. Geneva, WHO, 1974.

279. Clark WH Jr, Evans HL, Everett MA, et al: Early melanoma: Histologic terms. *Am J Dermatopathol* 13:579–582, 1991.

280. Clark WH Jr, Elder DE, Guerry D IV, et al: Model predicting survival in Stage I melanoma based on tumor progression. *JNCI* 81:1893–1904, 1989.

281. McGovern VJ: Spontaneous regression of melanoma. *Pathology* 7:91–99, 1975.

282. Herlyn M, Clark WH, Rodeck U, et al: Biology of tumor progression in human melanocytes. *Lab Invest* 56:461–474, 1987.

283. Price NM, Rywlin AM, Ackerman AB: Histologic criteria for the diagnosis of superficial spreading malignant melanoma: Formulated on the basis of proven metastatic lesions. *Cancer* 38:2434–2441, 1976.

284. Clark WH Jr, Mihm MC Jr: Lentigo maligna and lentigo maligna melanoma. *Am J Pathol* 55:39–67, 1969.

285. Elder DE: Metastatic melanoma, in Elder DE (ed): *Pigment Cell*, vol. 8. Basel, Karger, 1987, pp 182–204.

286. Fitzpatrick JE: The histologic diagnosis of intraepithelial pagetoid neoplasms. *Clin Dermatol* 9:255–259, 1991.

287. Connelly J, Lattes R, Orr W: Desmoplastic malignant melanoma (a rare variant of spindle cell melanoma). *Cancer* 28:914–936, 1971.

288. Valensi QJ: Desmoplastic malignant melanoma: A light and electron microscopic study of two cases. *Cancer* 43:1148–1155, 1979.

289. From L, Hanna W, Kahn HJ, et al: Origin of the desmoplasia in desmoplastic malignant melanoma. *Hum Pathol* 14:1072–1080, 1983.

290. Egbert B, Kempson R, Sagebiel R: Desmoplastic malignant melanoma: A clinicohistopathologic study of 25 cases. *Cancer* 62:2033–2041, 1988.

291. Walsh NM, Roberts JT, Orr W, Simon GT: Desmoplastic malignant melanoma: A clinico-pathologic study of 14 cases. *Arch Pathol Lab Med* 112:922–927, 1988.

292. Jain S, Allen PW: Desmoplastic malignant melanoma and its variants: A study of 45 cases. *Am J Surg Pathol* 13:358–373, 1989.

293. Smithers BM, McLeod GR, Little JH: Desmoplastic, neural transforming and neurotropic melanoma: A review of 45 cases. *Aust N Z J Surg* 60:967–972, 1990.

294. Bruijn JA, Mihm MC Jr, Barnhill RL: Desmoplastic melanoma. *Histopathology* 20:197–205, 1992.

295. Bruijn JA, Salasche SJ, Sober AJ, et al: Desmoplastic melanoma: Clinicopathologic aspects of six cases. *Dermatology* 185:3–8, 1992.

296. Carlson JA, Dickersin GR, Sober AJ, Barnhill RL: Desmoplastic neurotropic malignant melanoma: A clinicopathologic analysis of 28 cases. *Cancer* 75:478–494, 1994.

297. Skelton HG, Smith KJ, Laskin WB, McCarthy WF, et al: Desmoplastic malignant melanoma. *J Am Acad Dermatol* 32:717–725, 1995.

298. Reed RJ, Leonard DD: Neurotropic melanoma: A variant of desmoplastic melanoma. *Am J Surg Pathol* 3:301–311, 1979.

299. Kossard S, Doherty E, Murray E: Neurotropic melanoma. A variant of desmoplastic melanoma. *Arch Dermatol* 123:907–912, 1987.

300. Barnhill RL, Bolognia JL: Neurotropic melanoma with prominent melaninization. *J Cutan Pathol* 22:450–459, 1995.

301. Barnhill RL, Mihm MC: Cellular neurothekeoma: A distinctive variant of neurothekeoma mimicking nevomelanocytic tumors. *Am J Surg Pathol* 14:113–120, 1990.

302. Anstey A, Cerio R, Ramnarain N, et al: Desmoplastic malignant melanoma: An immunocytochemical study of 25 cases. *Am J Dermatopathol* 16:14–22, 1994.

303. Muhlbauer JE, Margolis RJ, Mihm MC Jr, Reed RJ: Minimal deviation melanoma: A histologic variant of cutaneous malignant melanoma in its vertical growth phase. *J Invest Dermatol* 80(Suppl):63S–65S, 1983.

304. Phillips ME, Margolis RJ, Merot Y, et al: The spectrum of minimal deviation melanoma: A clinicopathologic study of 21 cases. *Hum Pathol* 17:796–806, 1986.

305. Reed RJ: Minimal deviation melanoma, in Mihm MC Jr, Murphy GF, Kaufman N, (eds): *Pathobiology and Recognition of Malignant Melanoma*. Baltimore, Williams and Wilkins, 1988, pp 110–152.

306. Reed RJ, Webb S, Clark WH Jr: Minimal deviation melanoma (Halo nevus variant). *Am J Surg Pathol* 14:53–68, 1990.

307. Schmoeckel C, Castro CE, Braun-Falco O: Nevoid malignant melanoma. *Arch Dermatol Res* 277:362–369, 1985.

308. Wong TY, Suster S, Duncan LM, Mihm M Jr: Nevoid melanoma: A clinicopathological study of seven cases of malignant melanoma mimicking spindle and epithelioid cell nevus and verrucous dermal nevus. *Human Pathol* 26:171–179, 1995.

309. McNutt NS, Urmacher C, Hakimian, et al: Nevoid malignant melanoma: Morphologic patterns and immunohistochemical reactivity. *J Cutan Pathol* 22:502–517, 1995.

310. Steiner A, Konrad K, Pehamberger H, Wolff K: Verrucous malignant melanoma. *Arch Dermatol* 124:1534–1537, 1988.

311. Blessing K, Evans AT, Al-Nafussi A: Verrucous naevoid and keratotic malignant melanoma: A clinico-pathological study of 20 cases. *Histopathology* 23:453–458, 1993.

312. Okun M, Bauman L: Malignant melanoma arising from an intradermal nevus. *Arch Dermatol* 92:69–72, 1965.

313. Okun MR, Di Mattia A, Thompson J, Pearson SH: Malignant melanoma developing from intradermal nevi. *Arch Dermatol* 110:599–601, 1974.

314. Benisch B, Peison B, Kannerstein M, Spivack J: Malignant melanoma originating from intradermal nevi: A clinicopathologic entity. *Arch Dermatol* 116:696–698, 1980.

315. Enzinger FM: Clear-cell sarcoma of tendons and aponeuroses: An analysis of 21 cases. *Cancer* 18:1163–1174, 1965.

316. Chung EB, Enzinger FM: Malignant melanoma of soft parts: A reassessment of clear-cell sarcoma. *Am J Surg Pathol* 7:405–413, 1983.

317. Swanson PE, Wick MR: Clear cell sarcoma: An immunohistochemical analysis of six cases and comparison with other epithelioid neoplasms of soft tissue. *Arch Pathol Lab Med* 113:55–60, 1989.

318. Sara AS, Evans HL, Benjamin RS: Malignant melanoma of soft parts (clear cell sarcoma): A study of 17 cases, with emphasis on prognostic factors. *Cancer* 65:367–374, 1990.

319. Peters MS, Su WPD: Balloon cell malignant melanoma. *J Am Acad Dermatol* 13:351–354, 1985.

320. Kao GF, Helwig EB, Graham JH: Balloon cell malignant melanoma of the skin: A clinicopathologic study of 34 cases with histochemical, immunohistochemical, and ultrastructural observations. *Cancer* 69:2942–2952, 1992.

321. Okun MR: Melanoma resembling spindle and epithelioid cell nevus. *Arch Dermatol* 115:1416–1420, 1979.

322. Nakhleh RE, Wick MR, Rocamora A, et al: Morphologic diversity in malignant melanomas. *Am J Clin Pathol* 93:731–740, 1990.

323. Prieto VG, Kanik A, Salob S, McNutt NS: Primary cutaneous myxoid melanoma: Immunohistologic clues to a difficult diagnosis. *J Am Acad Dermatol* 30:335–339, 1994.

324. Clark WH Jr, Elder DE, Guerry D IV: Dysplastic nevi and malignant melanoma, in Farmer ER, Hood AF (eds): *Pathology of the Skin*. Norwalk, CT, Appleton and Lange, 1990, pp 684–756.

325. McGovern VJ: Melanoma—growth patterns, multiplicity and regression, in *Melanoma and Skin Cancer. Proceedings of the International Cancer Conference*, Sydney. VCN Blight, Government Printer, 1972, pp 95–106.

326. Blessing K, McLaren KM: Histological regression in primary cutaneous melanoma: Recognition, prevalence and significance. *Histopathology* 20:315–322, 1992.

327. McGovern VJ, Shaw HM, Milton GW: Prognosis in patients with thin malignant melanoma: Influence of regression. *Histopathology* 7:673–680, 1983.

328. Pack GT, Miller TR: Metastatic melanomas with indeterminate primary site. *JAMA* 176:55–56, 1961.

329. Smith JL Jr, Stehlin JS Jr: Spontaneous regression of primary malignant melanomas with regional metastases. *Cancer* 18:1399–1415, 1965.

330. Tefany FJ, Barnetson RS, Halliday GM, et al: Immunocytochemical analysis of the cellular infiltrate in primary regressing and non-regressing malignant melanoma. *J Invest Dermatol* 97:197–202, 1991.

331. Kang S, Barnhill RL, Mihm MC, Sober AJ: Regression in malignant melanoma: An interobserver concordance study. *J Cutan Pathol* 20:126–129, 1993.

332. Balch C, Milton G: Diagnosis of metastatic melanoma at distant sites, in Balch C, Milton G, Shaw HM, Soong S-J (eds): *Cutaneous Melanoma. Clinical Management and Treatment Results Worldwide*. Philadelphia, J.B. Lippincott, 221–250, 1985.

333. McNeer G, Das Gupta T: Life history of melanoma. *AJR* 93:686–694, 1956.

334. Peterson N, Bodenham D, Lloyd O: Malignant melanoma of the skin: A study of the origin, development, etiology, spread, treatment and prognosis. *Br J Plast Surg* 15:49–116, 1962.

335. Balch CM, Urist MM, Maddox WA, et al: Management of regional metastatic melanoma, in Balch CM, Milton GW, Shaw HM, Soong S-J (eds): *Cutaneous Melanoma. Clinical Management and Treatment Results Worldwide*. Philadelphia, JB Lippincott, 1985, pp 93–130.

336. Elder DE, Murphy G: Metastatic malignant melanoma, in Elder DE, Murphy G (eds): *Melanocytic Tumors of the Skin*. Washington, DC, American Registry of Pathology, Armed Forces Institute of Pathology, 1991, pp 191–205.

337. Kornberg R, Harris M, Ackerman A: Epidermotropically metastatic malignant melanoma. *Arch Dermatol* 114:67–69, 1978.

338. Elder DE, Ainsworth A, Clark W: The surgical pathology of cutaneous malignant melanoma, in Clark W (ed): *Human Malignant Melanoma*. New York, Grune and Stratton, 1979, pp 55–108.

339. Bengoechea-Beeby M, Velasco-Oses A, Fernandez F, et al: Epidermotropic metastatic melanoma. *Cancer* 72:1909–1913, 1993.

340. Abernethy JL, Soyer HP, Kerl H, et al: Epidermotropic metastatic malignant melanoma simulating melanoma in situ: A report of 10 examples from two patients. *Am J Surg Pathol* 18:1140–1149, 1994.

341. McCarthy S, Palmer A, Bale P, Hist E: Nevus cells in lymph nodes. *Pathology* 6:351–358, 1974.

342. Johnson W, Helwig E: Benign nevus cells in the capsule of lymph nodes. *Cancer* 23:747–753, 1969.

343. Ridolfi R, Rosen P, Thaler H: Nevus cell aggregates associated with lymph nodes: Estimated frequency and clinical significance. *Cancer* 39:164–171, 1977.

344. Andreola S, Clemente C: Nevus cells in axillary lymph nodes from radical mastectomy specimens. *Pathol Res Pract* 179:616–618, 1985.

345. Das Gupta T, Bowden L, Berg J: Malignant melanoma of unknown primary origin. *Surg Gynecol Obstetr* 117:341–345, 1963.

346. Giuliano A, Cochran AJ, Morton D: Melanoma from unknown primary site and amelanotic melanoma. *Semin Oncol* 9:442–447, 1982.

347. Pellegrini A: Regressed primary malignant melanoma with regional metastases. *Arch Dermatol* 116:585–586, 1980.

348. Chang P, Knapper W: Metastatic melanoma of unknown primary. *Cancer* 49:1106–1111, 1982.

349. Reintgen D, McCarty K, Woodard B, et al: Metastatic malignant melanoma with an unknown primary. *Surg Gynecol Obstet* 156:335–340, 1983.

350. Silberberg I, Kopf A, Gumport S: Diffuse melanosis in malignant melanoma. *Arch Dermatol* 97:671–677, 1968.

351. Eide J: Pathogenesis of generalized melanosis with melanuria and melanoptysis secondary to malignant melanoma. *Histopathology* 5:285–294, 1981.

352. Rowden G, Sulicca V, Butler T, Manz H: Malignant melanoma with melanosis: Ultrastructural and histologic studies. *J Cutan Pathol* 7:125–139, 1980.

353. Balch CM, Soong S-J, Shaw HM, et al: An analysis of prognostic factors in 8500 patients with cutaneous melanoma, in Balch CM, Houghton AN, Milton GW, et al (eds): *Cutaneous Melanoma*, 2nd ed. Philadelphia, JB Lippincott, 1992, pp 165–187.

354. Day CL Jr, Lew RA, Mihm MC Jr, et al: The natural break points for primary tumor thickness in clinical stage I melanoma [letter]. *N Engl J Med* 305:1155, 1981.

355. Keefe M, MacKie RM: The relationship risk of death from clinical stage I cutaneous melanoma and thickness of primary tumour: No evidence for steps in risk. *Brit J Cancer* 64: 598–602, 1991.

356. Balch CM, Soong S-J, Murad TM, et al: A multifactorial analysis of melanoma: III. Prognostic factors in melanoma patients with lymph node metastases (stage II). *Ann Surg* 193:377, 1981.

CHAPTER 28

SEBACEOUS AND PILAR TUMORS

Mark R. Wick / Paul E. Swanson / Raymond L. Barnhill

As stated in the introduction to the previous chapter, the pathology of adnexal tumors of the skin—including sudoriferous, sebaceous, and pilar neoplasms—is a complex and voluminous subject. In keeping with the aims of the antecedent section on sweat gland lesions, the following discussion of pilosebaceous tumors is meant to be practical and diagnostically oriented in its focus. Those readers wishing to supplement the information presented here are referred to several comprehensive texts covering appendageal cutaneous neoplasms.[1–3]

SEBACEOUS TUMORS AND TUMOR-LIKE CONDITIONS

Sebaceous proliferations are seemingly less common than those showing differentiation toward the sweat glands. Moreover, sebocytic neoplasms manifest less morphological diversity than sudoriferous tumors and therefore are not as complicated nosologically.

Benign Sebaceous Proliferations

SEBACEOUS HYPERPLASIA

Clinical Features The most common proliferative abnormality of the sebaceous glands is that of hyperplasia, which most often is seen in elderly individuals (Table 28-1).[4–11] Clinically, this condition most commonly presents itself in the form of a localized eruption of yellowish-tan umbilicated papules—usually on the face or eyelids, but occasionally affecting the mammary areola or genital skin—with the potential for confluence.[12–14] The lesion also may resemble the papulonodular profile of basal cell carcinoma macroscopically, and rare forms have been termed "linear" (zosteriform) or "giant solitary" sebaceous hyperplasia (SH).[4,7,8] In "premature" SH, an autosomal dominant pattern of inheritance may be noted, and the clinical onset of the process occurs early in life.[8,9] Farina et al. have suggested that SH is the sebaceous analogue of trichofolliculoma (see the following), and because the former of these lesions does not involute clinically, they conclude that it is probably a benign neoplasm rather than a form of hyperplasia.[13]

Histopathological Features One may define SH by the presence of four or more sebaceous lobules attached to the infundibulum of each pilosebaceous unit seen in the biopsy specimen (Table 28-1; Fig. 28-1). The cells comprising the lobules are predominantly fully mature sebocytes, showing compact nuclei and abundant multivacuolated lucent cytoplasm. However, a thin rim of basaloid cells often is present at the periphery of the sebocytic aggregates. The overlying epidermis may be atrophic in unusually expansive examples of SH.

Differential Diagnosis The primary entities to be considered are nevus sebaceus and sebaceous adenoma. Nevus sebaceus differs from SH by its general breadth, the presence of hamartomatous (rudimentary) folliculo-sebaceous units, papillomatous epidermal hyperplasia, and frequent apocrine elements. Sebaceous adenoma is distinguished from SH by showing a larger basaloid germinative component (up to half of the sebaceous lobules) than is observed in SH.

SEBACEOUS ADENOMA

Clinical Features Sebaceous adenoma (SA) presents itself as a pale yellow nodular facial lesion that slowly enlarges and makes its appearance after the age of 50 years (Table 28-2). This tumor ranges in size from less than 1 cm (the usual size) to greater than 5 cm in maximum dimension.[15–20] Clinical misdiagnosis of SA as basal cell carcinoma is again a common problem. There may be an association with the Muir-Torre syndrome, wherein the patient has metachronous or synchronous visceral malignancies and cutaneous sebaceous adenomas, sebaceous carcinomas, basal cell carcinomas with sebaceous differentiation, or squamous carcinomas of the "keratoacanthoma" type.[21–28] Malignant tumors of internal organs in the Muir-Torre syndrome are most often carcinomas of the larynx and gastrointestinal tract, but virtually any visceral site may be affected; rarely, nodal or extranodal malignant lymphomas may be encountered as well.[24,26,28] The SAs seen in this context may either be "classical" microscopic lesions, or they may demonstrate histological peculiarities and thus be labeled as "variant" adenomas (see the following).[27]

Histopathological Features The microscopic characteristics of "classical" SA are probably the most clear-cut of any sebaceous proliferation, except for SH (Table 28-2).[17,19,20] They are represented by the sharply circumscribed proliferation of enlarged sebaceous lobules, comprised by fully mature sebocytes, frequently attenuating the overlying epidermis and sometimes attaching to its basal aspect (Fig. 28-2). A fibrous pseudocapsule commonly surrounds the lesion and attests to its slow growth, as do appendageal "collarettes" that may form at the periphery of the tumors. The cellular lobules of SA may contain duct-like structures into which holocrine secretion occurs, and this phenomenon can result in the formation of intralesional cysts. Modest nucleolar prominence may be appreciated in the constituent cells of SA, but nuclear hyperchromasia or pleomorphism and mitotic activity are only rarely observed.

"Variant" sebaceous adenomas of the Muir-Torre type differ from the preceding description in several regards. First, they may lack the exquisite demarcation from the adjacent dermis that is shown by classical SA. Second, the component cellular lobules are composed of an

TABLE 28-1

Sebaceous Hyperplasia

Clinical Features

Older individuals
Face, mammary areola, genital skin
Yellowish to tan papules, often umbilicated
Rare linear or giant forms

Histopathological Features

Single follicular canal opens to umbilicated epidermal surface
Four or more sebaceous lobules attached to central infundibulum of sebaceous follicle
Fully mature sebaceous lobules composed of sebocytes with compact nuclei and abundant multivacuolated clear cytoplasm

Differential Diagnosis

Sebaceus adenoma
Nevus sebaceus

TABLE 28-2

Sebaceous Adenoma

Clinical Features

Often more than 50 years of age
Head and neck, especially face
Yellowish nodule
Usually <1 cm but up to 5 cm or more
Association with Muir-Torre syndrome (sebaceous neoplasms, squamous cell carcinomas, and visceral carcinomas [laryngeal and gastrointestinal])

Histopathological Features

Classical type
    Well-defined enlarged sebaceous lobules
    Frequent attachment to epidermis with epidermal thinning
    Fully mature sebocytes
    Lobules may contain duct-like structures
Variant type (Muir-Torre)
    Sharp demarcation of lobules may be lacking
    Lobules show admixture of peripherally located basaloid epithelium (up to 50%) centrally mature sebocytes
    Basaloid epithelium may show slight nuclear pleomorphism, distinct nucleoli, and occasional mitoses

Differential Diagnosis

Sebaceous hyperplasia
Basal cell carcinoma with sebaceous differentiation

admixture of peripherally-disposed basaloid, germinative-type epithelial cells—often with mild nuclear pleomorphism, distinct nucleoli, and modest mitotic activity—and centrally mature sebocytes (Figs. 28-3 and 28-4).[27]

It must be emphasized that even though the term "Muir-Torre-type" has just been used in reference to variant SAs, only a distinct minority of patients with such lesions ultimately will be proven to have the syndrome; most adenomatous sebaceous tumors containing a significant number of basaloid cells occur as solitary sporadic neoplasms. In fact, although it is the authors' opinion that patients with the Muir-Torre complex more often have variant-form than classical sebaceous adenomas, it is forthrightly stipulated that there has been no systematic analysis of this contention to date.

In recognition of the confusion that often surrounds sebaceous tumors which contain a proportion of basaloid cells, Sanchez-Yus et al. have proposed that yet another term, "sebomatricoma," be added to the lexicon of sebaceous neoplasia to encompass *all* such lesions.[33]

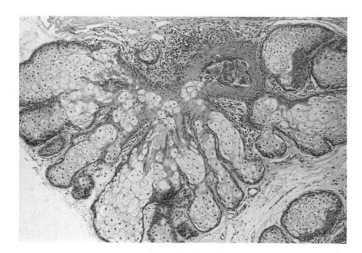

FIGURE 28-1 Sebaceous Hyperplasia. Numerous sebaceous lobules are attached to the infundibulum of a single pilosebaceous unit.

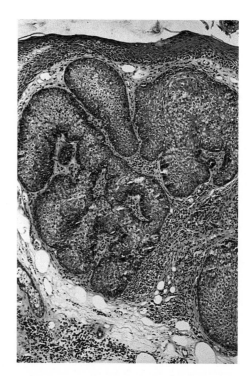

FIGURE 28-2 Sebaceous Adenoma. Sharply circumscribed lobules of sebaceous glands are separated from adjacent dermis by an induced cellular fibrous stroma.

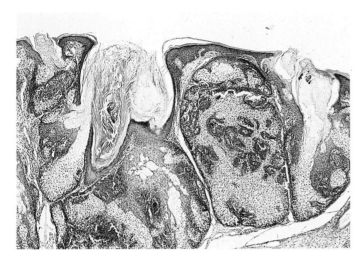

FIGURE 28-3 Sebaceous Adenoma, Muir-Torre Variant. The architectural features of lesions in Muir-Torre syndrome have been likened to keratoacanthoma. Tumor lobules are less distinct than in typical forms of sebaceous adenoma.

According to that nosological construction, one would recognize SH, "sebomatricoma," and sebaceous carcinoma as the only "true" sebocytic proliferations, eschewing all prior pertinent terminology. The authors have no particular conceptual or practical objections to this suggestion, except for the fact that it would undoubtedly result in the erroneous inclusion of some examples of basal cell carcinoma in the "sebomatricoma" group. Whether or not this would have adverse clinical effects is a debatable point.

Differential Diagnosis   Muir-Torre-type SAs may be difficult to distinguish diagnostically from basal cell carcinoma with sebaceous differentiation (BCCSD) (also known as "basosebaceous epithelioma" or "sebaceous epithelioma").[29–32] The salient points of difference between these tumors are subtle but reproducible; BCCSD manifests an at-least-

focally fibromyxoid stroma and epithelial-stromal "clefts," in similarity to ordinary basal cell carcinoma, whereas Muir-Torre adenomas does not. Moreover, BCCSD is *dominated* by its basaloid cell constituents, with only a minor proportion of sebocytic elements; SAs of the Muir-Torre type contain no more than 50 percent germinative-type cells.

SUPERFICIAL EPITHELIOMA WITH SEBACEOUS DIFFERENTIATION

Clinical Features   A rare form of sebaceous neoplasia is that represented by the "superficial epithelioma with sebaceous differentiation" (SESD).[34,35] Based on observation of a limited number of examples, SESD appears to present itself as a slowly evolving, smooth-surfaced papule or an erythematous hyperkeratotic nodule; lesions have been observed in the skin of the face, trunk, and thigh, and multiplicity in the same patient is potentially observed. A possible association with the Muir-Torre syndrome is as yet unproven.

Histopathological Features   There are certain similarities between SESD and tumor of the follicular infundibulum, inverting follicular keratosis, and superficial basal cell carcinoma. The first of these lesions is composed of an interanastomosing, "fenestrated" constellation of compact polyhedral cells that connects broadly to the basal epidermis over a limited span and is sharply circumscribed (Fig. 28-5). As such, SESD forms a plate-like growth in the superficial corium. Peripheral palisading of nuclei—as seen in superficial basal cell carcinoma—may be observed in the cellular cords of SESD, but this finding is inconstant.[35] Squamoid elements (as seen in inverting keratoses) also may be seen focally, with formation of cellular "eddies," and duct-like lumina are also appreciated in most cases. The latter have an eosinophilic cuticle like that seen in eccrine ducts. Mature sebocytes are dispersed to the periphery and the deep aspects of SESD, and they are usually observed in small aggregates.

Differential Diagnosis   Fibromyxoid stroma, matrical-epithelial clefting, apoptosis, mitotic activity, continuity with the skin surface, and stromal hypercellularity are all absent in SESD, unlike the anticipated attributes of basal cell carcinomas, keratoses, or tumors of the follicular infundibulum.

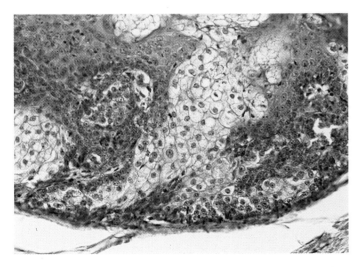

FIGURE 28-4 Sebaceous Adenoma, Muir-Torre Variant. At higher magnification, an admixture of basaloid cells and sebocytes replaced the more orderly transition seen in typical sebaceous adenoma. The cells nonetheless are benign, and most sebocytes assume a mature phenotype.

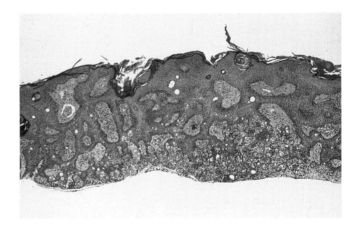

FIGURE 28-5 Superficial Epithelioma with Sebaceous Differentiation. The plate-like growth of this lesion resembles the so-called tumor of follicular infundibulum (see Fig. 28-14). Clusters of sebaceous cells, some with sebaceous ducts, are admixed with squamous elements. In this example, the sebaceous cells are clustered at the base of the lesion.

Sebaceoma

The tumor called "sebaceoma" by Troy and Ackerman also has been addressed in the previous chapter.[36] To recapitulate briefly, this circumscribed nodular dermal lesion is basically a histological amalgam of SESD, classical trichoepithelioma, "dermal duct tumor," and cylindroma. As such, it has also been dubbed "sebocrine adenoma" and "infundibular adenoma" by other authors.[37,38] A more general—and, it is felt, more appropriate—term for neoplasms such as "sebaceoma" would be that of "benign adnexal neoplasm with divergent differentiation."

Sebaceous Neoplasms of "Borderline" Malignancy

There is only one cutaneous tumor with sebaceous differentiation that is properly classified as a "borderline" malignancy; that is, a neoplasm that may recur locally but is extremely unlikely to metastasize distantly. This is the basal cell carcinoma with sebaceous differentiation, as briefly discussed previously.[29–32]

BCCSD differs from ordinary basal cell carcinomas (BCCs) in that its constituent cells are generally somewhat larger, with more eosinophilic cytoplasm (Fig. 28-6). Furthermore, the expected stromal change of conventional BCCs—with fibromyxoid alteration and cleavage away from epithelial cell nests—is only focally seen and therefore feebly represented in BCCSD. Points of synonymity include a potential for peripherolobular nuclear palisading, zones of typical basaloid cell differentiation with internal apoptosis, the potential for multilineage differentiation (including formation of melanin and eccrine ductal structures), and connection to the stratum basalis or to dermal epithelial appendages, as well as possible recurrence of the BCCSD after electrodessication or curettage.[18] The sebaceous elements of the latter lesion are fully mature, and are usually disposed toward the centers of cellular lobules.

In the authors' experience, BCCSD is an important entity with which pathologists should be familiar. It is often confused with sebaceous adenoma on one hand and sebaceous carcinoma on the other, and is certainly more common than either of those neoplasms.

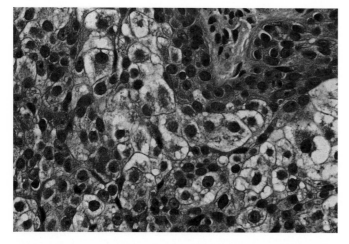

FIGURE 28-6 Basal Cell Carcinoma with Sebaceous Differentiation. Immature and mature sebocytes are admixed with a basaloid population that contains more abundant eosinophilic cytoplasm than normally encountered in typical variants of basal cell carcinoma.

Sebaceous Carcinomas

Traditionally, sebaceous carcinomas (SCs) have been considered in two categories, ocular and extraocular.[17–19,39–50] The proposed justification for this paradigm was based on a putative difference in the behavior of these two groups of tumors; it was contended that ocular SC had a more aggressive nature than that of extraocular lesions. However, a redactive examination of the pertinent literature fails to support that premise. *Both ocular and extraocular sebaceous malignancies are attended by an approximate risk of 30 to 40 percent for local tumor recurrence, 25 to 25 percent for distant metastases, and 10 to 20 percent for tumor-related death.*[40] Hence, there is, in fact, no inherent biological difference between them, with the exception that an ocular *location* is, by far, more common than an origin in the skin outside of the eyelids.

Clinical Features Sebaceous carcinoma typically is seen in middle-aged or elderly patients, with a mean age of 62 years (Table 28-3). For unexplained reasons, ocular neoplasms show a marked predilection for Asian individuals. These patients present with non-tender masses at the lid margin or in the conjunctiva, and, as such, they are commonly misdiagnosed as chalazions, blepharitis, or conjunctivitis. Multicentricity is

---

TABLE 28-3

Sebaceous Carcinoma

Clinical Features

Middle-aged and elderly patients (mean age 62 years)
Predilection for Asians
Ocular (eyelids) more often than extraocular sites (head and neck more often than trunk, genitalia, extremities)
Nontender mass

Histopathological Features

Pagetoid spread of atypical epithelial cells within epidermis or conjunctival epithelium
Lobular dermal aggregates of variably atypical polyhedral cells
Central necrosis ("comedo" pattern) common
Well-differentiated tumors
  Cells with abundant multivacuolated cytoplasm, vesicular nuclei, and discernible nucleoli
Poorly differentiated tumors
  Nondescript cells with high nucleocytoplasmic ratios, prominent nuclear pleomorphism, prominent nucleoli, prominent mitotic activity
Basaloid SC
  Small cells with scanty cytoplasm, peripheral palisading, nuclear anaplasia
Squamoid SC
  Prominent squamous metaplasia with keratin pearls
Sarcomatoid SC
  Spindle cell features

Differential Diagnosis

Balloon cell melanoma
Clear cell squamous cell carcinoma
Clear cell basal cell carcinoma
Clear cell eccrine carcinoma
Trichilemmal carcinoma
Metastatic clear cell carcinomas of visceral origin

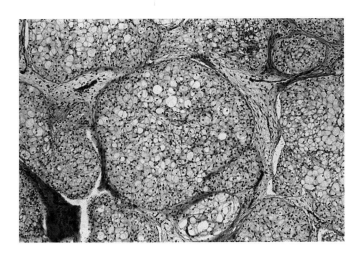

FIGURE 28-7   Sebaceous Carcinoma. Typical examples of sebaceous carcinoma consist of discrete tumor lobules separated by a nondesmoplastic fibrous stroma.

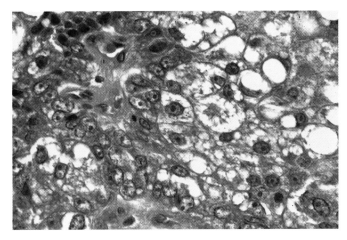

FIGURE 28-9   Sebaceous Carcinoma. In well-differentiated sebaceous carcinoma, abundant multivacuolated cytoplasm is identified readily. Nuclei are large, with variably prominent nucleoli, but mitoses are few.

observed in 5 to 10 percent of cases, and other ophthalmological conditions confused with SC include cicatricial ocular pemphigoid, basal cell or squamous cell carcinoma, or cutaneous horn.[41]

In reference to extraocular tumors, most SCs are seen on the head and neck, followed in relative order by the trunk, genitalia, and extremities.[39,40,44–46,48,51] They present themselves as relatively nondescript nodular masses that are occasionally painful or rapidly growing; a proportion are ulcerated as well. As cited previously, a subpopulation of patients has the Muir-Torre syndrome.[27]

Histopathological Features   The microscopic characteristics of SC feature the presence of lobular dermal aggregates of variably atypical polyhedral cells, separated from one another by fibrovascular stroma that lacks obvious desmoplasia (Table 28-3; Fig. 28-7). The resulting image is that of an organoid neoplasm. Central portions of the tumor cell nests may become necrotic, yielding a "comedo" pattern on scanning microscopy (Fig. 28-8). Cytologically, the constituent elements of well-differentiated SCs show abundant multivacuolated lucent cytoplasm and oval vesicular nuclei with discernible nucleoli, but sparse mitoses (Fig. 28-9). At the other end of this spectrum, poorly differ-

entiated tumors are composed of more nondescript cells with high nucleocytoplasmic ratios, more prominent nuclear pleomorphism, prominent nucleoli, brisk mitotic activity with possibly atypical division figures, and amphophilic to basophilic cytoplasm (Fig. 28-10).[17–19,39–41] Intracellular compartmentalized vacuoles are not nearly as prominent in the latter lesions, and may require the use of special techniques—such as oil-red-O or Sudan IV stains on fresh tissue or epithelial membrane antigen (EMA) immunostains in paraffin sections—to highlight their presence.

Grading of SCs is accomplished most reproducibly using tumor *growth patterns* rather than nuclear features.[40] Neoplasms that are composed of generally rounded, demarcated, roughly equally sized lobules of cells are graded as I/III, whereas those that show an admixture of rounded and distinct with infiltrative and confluent cell nests are grade II/III. Grade III SCs feature the presence of highly permeative cellular aggregates with jagged profiles, or demonstrate medullary sheet-like growth.

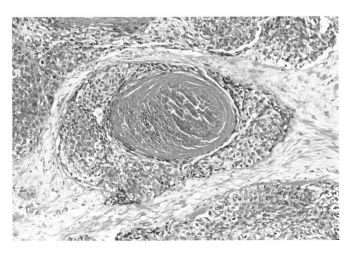

FIGURE 28-8   Sebaceous Carcinoma. Comedonecrosis may be conspicuous in high-grade lesions.

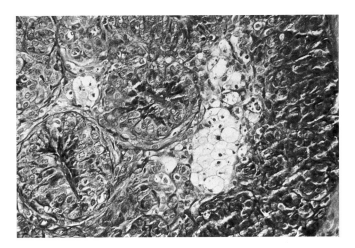

FIGURE 28-10   Sebaceous Carcinoma. Poorly differentiated lesions consist predominantly of cells with less well-defined intracytoplasmic compartments, although lower grade elements may be admixed. Nuclei are pleomorphic, with striking atypia.

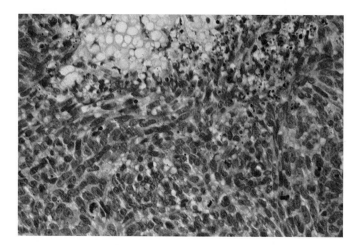

FIGURE 28-11   Sebaceous Carcinoma. Basaloid variants of sebaceous carcinoma contain cells with less abundant cytoplasm, and inconspicuous compartmentalization. Mitotic activity is brisk in basaloid lesions.

Regardless of grade, all examples of SC share a possible association with in situ carcinoma, or extramammary Paget's disease (EPD) of the sebaceous type, or both, in the surface epithelium overlying the dermal tumor mass.[40,41,47,52] The mechanisms linking these abnormalities are similar to those attending sudoriferous Paget's disease, as considered in the previous chapter. From a practical perspective, the pathologist should especially think of an underlying invasive oculocutaneous SC whenever a conjunctival or eyelid biopsy demonstrates such pathologic changes, because it is in those sites that its relationship with intraepithelial neoplasia is strongest. Outside of the ocular region, however, EPD that does not label for epithelial mucin content or apocrine-selective immunohistologic markers also may have this association.

Particular histologic variants of SC are worthy of special attention because they are capable of causing diagnostic confusion with other cutaneous lesions.[17–19,39–41,53] Basaloid SC is a form that is composed of small cells with scant cytoplasm and the common presence of nuclear palisading at the periphery of cell nests (Fig. 28-11). It most often has a high-grade growth pattern—with nuclear anaplasia—and demonstrates only a small minority of dispersed, vacuolated, obviously sebocytic elements. Squamoid SC is dominated by foci of prominent squamous metaplasia, complete with keratin pearls; spindle-cell change, with assumption of a "sarcomatoid" morphotype, is yet another potentiality of this tumor variant.[6,7]

Differential Diagnosis   As one might expect, the pathologic differential diagnosis of SC is broad, encompassing virtually all of the malignant clear-cell tumors of the skin. These have been well-summarized by Suster, and include such entities as "balloon cell" melanoma, hydropic squamous carcinoma and basal cell carcinoma, clear cell eccrine carcinoma, trichilemmal carcinoma, and metastatic clear cell carcinomas of visceral origin.[54] With the possible exception of selected balloon cell melanomas, however, none of these neoplasms exhibits the particular vacuolization pattern that is seen in sebocytes, which is a multivesicular "bubbly" compartmentalization of the cytoplasm of each cell, rather than a unilocular vacuole.[40,54] As discussed, immunostains for EMA or histochemical analyses for neutral lipid may be necessary to confirm the presence of the former of these two patterns. Furthermore, SC lacks several specialized protein products that may be seen in sweat gland tumors or metastatic visceral carcinomas; included among these are carcinoembryonic antigen, S100 protein, gross cystic disease fluid protein-15, CA-125, and CA19.9.[55]

Basaloid SC is distinguishable from basal cell carcinoma on a cytological basis, because the nuclei of poorly differentiated sebaceous tumors are much more vesicular than those of BCC. In addition, the stroma of basaloid SC is not fibromyxoid in nature, and the number of obviously identifiable sebocytes is extremely small in that variant. In contrast, BCCSD regularly demonstrates easily observable clusters of mature sebaceous elements. Both basaloid SC and BCCSD appear to be capable of expressing the glycoprotein target for the BER-EP4 antibody in immunohistochemical studies, but they do differ in their expression of EMA. SC is diffusely EMA-reactive, whereas BCCSD is either completely EMA-negative or it shows discrete positivity only in foci of obvious sebocytic differentiation.[55] Squamoid SC can be separated diagnostically from ordinary squamous cell carcinoma by attention to the presence of multivesiculated sebocytes in the first of these lesions, as well as a usual lack of continuity of the dermal tumor with the epidermis and a dissimilarity in BER-EP4-immunoreactivity. (SC is positive; squamous carcinoma is negative.)[56] Sarcomatoid forms of SC are recognizable generically as epithelial malignancies if small foci of ordinary carcinoma are interspersed throughout them; otherwise, immunoreactivity for keratin is necessary to exclude a true mesenchymal tumor.[57] Unfortunately, a specific diagnosis of sarcomatoid SC may not be possible even with special techniques if vesiculated clear cell elements are altogether lacking, because the neoplastic cells appear to abjure their ability to display sebocytic features with a progressive loss of differentiation.

Pseudoneoplastic Sebaceous Proliferations: Nevus Sebaceus (of Jadassohn)

Clinical Features   Nevus sebaceus (also known as organoid nevus or pilosyringosebaceous nevus) typically is present at birth, and gradually enlarges thereafter (Table 28-4). It produces a localized area of alopecia, or is a tan-brown, roughly surfaced plaque in the skin of the face or neck that becomes overtly verrucoid during puberty. A minor proportion of these lesions also is associated with multisystem abnormalities, including structural oculocerebrocranial defects that may cause seizures, mental retardation, and visual field cuts.[58–63]

Histopathological Features   Nevus sebaceus (NS) is characterized by slight epidermal papillomatosis in its earliest form, often with an accompanying proliferation of basaloid cells that take on an appearance resembling that of germinative or rudimentary hair follicles (Table 28-4). Sebaceous and apocrine glands are not conspicuous in NS during childhood, but they become so in adolescence and are associated with more striking surface papillomatosis of the lesion (Figs. 28-12 and 28-13).

A variety of cutaneous tumors have been reported to arise potentially in NS, including basal cell carcinoma, trichilemmoma, proliferating pilar tumor, syringocystadenoma papilliferum, apocrine adenoma, sebaceous adenoma, and pilar leiomyoma.[64] Ng has offered the opinion that these contextual proliferations are not truly neoplastic in nature, but rather are hamartomatous in keeping with the general character of NS.[65] This is an attractive hypothesis, but it is one which the author believes to be oversimplified. Several examples have been documented wherein NS gave rise to undisputed neoplasms that demonstrated aggressive behavior, including squamous cell carcinoma and ductal apocrine adenocarcinoma.[66,67]

Differential Diagnosis   The papillomatous epidermal hyperplasia in NS may suggest verruca and epidermal nevus. NS is distinguished from the latter conditions by the presence of rudimentary hair follicles, usually but not always prominent sebaceous elements, and apocrine glandular elements. NS is discriminated from SH by greater breadth, the latter morphological features, and clinical presentation.

Clinical Features

Congenital onset
Head and neck, usually scalp; upper trunk
Oval or elongate yellowish or tan-brown alopecic plaque
Rough to verrucous surface
An association with other developmental abnormalities, including
    oculocerebrocranial defects that may result in seizures, mental
    retardation, visual field loss

Histopathological Features

All ages
    Rudimentary hair follicle structures with basaloid epithelium
        resulting in clinical alopecia
    Variable papillomatosis of epidermis and sebaceous gland under-
        development or prominence
After puberty
    Prominent papillomatosis of epidermis
    Prominence of sebaceous glands
    Prominent apocrine glands in a subset
Development of various hamartomas and tumors
    Basaloid (basal cell) hamartomas
    Trichilemmoma
    Proliferating pilar tumor
    Syringocystadenoma papilliferum
    Apocrine hamartomas or adenomas
    Sebaceous hamartomas or adenomas
    Basal cell carcinoma
    Ductal apocrine adenocarcinoma

Differential Diagnosis

Epidermal nevus
Verruca
Sebaceous hyperplasia
Sebaceous adenoma

PILAR NEOPLASMS AND PSEUDONEOPLASTIC LESIONS

Because the hair follicles are more complicated than the sebaceous glands at a microanatomic level, the nosological scheme pertaining to pilar neoplasms is also more extensive. One can approach this topic by dividing hair follicle tumors into those that differentiate toward the outer hair sheath epithelium; others whose target is the germinative epithelium; and lesions with mixed epithelial-mesenchymal features or lineages resembling those of the follicle-related mesenchymal tissues. It must be admitted before embarking on this nosological enterprise that it is perhaps the most contentious area of cutaneous adnexal pathology at the present time. Several competing classification schemes for pilar tumors have been advocated in the past and new variations continue to appear, often with little more to recommend them than rather ethereal theoretical considerations.[1]

Benign Hair Follicle Tumors

For reasons that are unknown (at least to the authors), there are many more benign pilar tumors than malignant ones. These will be covered as

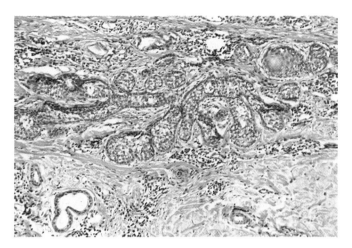

FIGURE 28-12   Nevus Sebaceus. In early stages of this lesion, irregular lobular proliferations of basaloid (immature sebaceous) cells proliferate in superficial dermis.

a group in respect to their presumed targets of differentiation, followed by a general discussion of pilar carcinomas and tumor-like conditions of the follicular apparatus.

TUMORS OF THE OUTER HAIR SHEATH AND INFUNDIBULUM

Despite the fact that it shows many morphological similarities to the epidermis, the follicular infundibulum (the hair pore and the follicular segment above the insertion of the sebaceous duct) is a specialized modification of the outer hair sheath. Cells in that structure mature with an outward polarity, whereas maturation in the isthmic portion of the follicle—between the sebaceous duct and the insertion of the arrector pili muscles—shows the converse of that orientation. Moreover, infundibular keratinization features an intermediary granular cell layer, whereas isthmic keratin formation is "abrupt," and lacks keratohyaline granules. These keratinization patterns are used, in part, to classify the differentiation of pilar neoplasms and provide a nosological structure for them. However, follicular tumors that lack overt keratin formation must be categorized in a more indirect fashion.

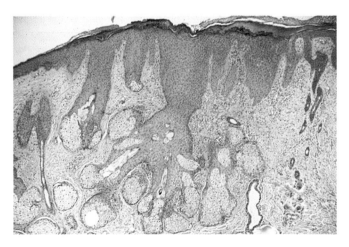

FIGURE 28-13   Nevus Sebaceus. In older lesions, mature sebaceus lobules become prominent. Epidermal hyperplasia also is evident.

TABLE 28-5
Tumor of the Follicular Infundibulum

Clinical Features

Middle-aged or elderly patients
Women more often than men
Head and neck
Solitary papule or nodule
Usually <1 cm

Histopathological Features

Well-demarcated
Subepidermal plate of compact polyhedral cells
Multifocal connection to overlying epidermis by strands of
    epithelium
Peripheral palisading of nuclei
Variable clear cell change (glycogen)
Cytological atypia usually absent

Differential Diagnosis

Trichilemmoma
Basal cell carcinoma

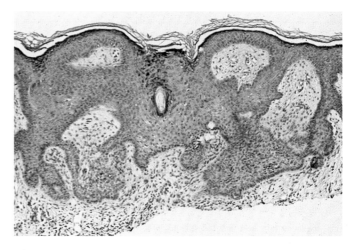

FIGURE 28-14   Tumor of Follicular Infundibulum. A peripheral palisade of basaloid cells is evident in this lesion.

Tumor of the Follicular Infundibulum

Clinical Features   Tumor of the follicular infundibulum (TFI) is also known as "basal cell hamartoma with follicular differentiation" or "infundibuloma" (Table 28-5).[68–73] It is a relatively uncommon lesion that shows a marked predilection for middle-aged or elderly women and presents as a solitary papulonodular tumor measuring less than 1 cm in greatest dimension. Multiplicity is rarely seen but has indeed been reported, and there may be an association with concomitant nevus sebaceus or Cowden's syndrome (see section on trichilemmoma that follows).[73]

Histopathological Features   Tumor of the follicular infundibulum is typified microscopically by a subepidermal plate of compact polyhedral cells that forms a lattice-work structure and connects to the stratum basalis multifocally (Table 28-5). The lesion is sharply demarcated laterally, and its internal image has been described as "fenestrated." Peripherally disposed tumor cells in the constituent cellular cords may demonstrate nuclear palisading and contain glycogen, in likeness to the trichilemmal sheath. A prominent layer of eosinophilic basement membrane material often is seen surrounding the cords as well. Nuclei are bland, and mitotic activity and apoptosis are consistently absent (Fig. 28-14). Hair is not formed in TFI, but "bystander" follicles may be entrapped in the tumor and intralesional acrosyringia are seen in some examples.[74] Cribier and Grosshans have found that there is an accentuated deposition of dermal elastic tissue immediately beneath TFIs.[73] An infundibular nature for the lesion is more inferential than proven, and it is predicated largely on the microanatomic relationship of TFI to the acrotrichium.

Differential Diagnosis   The distinction of TFI and superficial BCC may be challenging in selected cases. However, the former of these neoplasms is more highly differentiated—with regular formation of basement membrane and more voluminous cytoplasm—and TFI also differs from BCC in being negative with the BER-EP4 antibody immunohistochemically.[56]

Pilar Sheath Acanthoma

Clinical Features   Middle-aged or elderly patients, with no gender predilection, are typically affected by pilar sheath acanthoma (PSA),

which manifests itself as a single tan-pink papule or plaque, usually on the upper lip or in the central facial skin (Table 28-6). A small central keratotic plug is often appreciated clinically.[75–77]

Histopathological Features   This tumor has a central infundibular microcyst that contains keratinous material and opens focally to the epidermal surface (Table 28-6). The wall of the cyst is acanthotic and proliferative, sending many lobular cellular buds out radially into the adjacent dermis (Fig. 28-15). Constituent cells are variably polygonal, with pale eosinophilic or clear cytoplasm (which is glycogenated as shown by the periodic acid-Schiff [PAS] stain), or basaloid. The proliferating cellular projections may themselves contain small keratinous accumulations ("horn cysts"). Nuclei are bland, mitoses are absent, and hair is not formed in PSA. The histologic features of this tumor are so singular that differential diagnosis is academic.

In view of the probable incorporation of cellular elements in PSA that show infundibular as well as follicular-isthmic differentiation, Hurt has proposed that the term "lobular infundibuloisthmicoma" as a replacement for "pilar sheath acanthoma."[78] However, the latter of these two names has the benefits of greater familiarity and brevity, and it is likely to persist in common usage for the foreseeable future.

Dilated Pore of Winer

Clinical and Histopathological Features   Although "Winer's pore" (DPW) is a rather common clinical entity—occurring as a solitary or multifocal nodular lesion in the skin of the head and neck in adults—the microscopic distinction between PSA and DPW is, perhaps, more imagined than real (Table 28-6).[79,80] The only morphological differences between these lesions are that DPW shows a larger, more obvious cystic opening to the skin surface, often has small sebaceous glands or vellus hairs incorporated into its base, and demonstrates a lesser degree of peripheral epithelial proliferation that assumes the appearance of accentuated rete ridges (Fig. 28-16). Occasional examples of DPW may exhibit a superficial dish-like invagination.

Differential Diagnosis   As discussed previously for PSA, DPW is distinctive. On occasion the differential diagnosis might include an epidermoid cyst, trichofolliculoma, fibrofolliculoma, and perifollicular fibroma.

Trichoadenoma

Clinical Features   Trichoadenoma (of Nikolowski) (TA) is an infrequently encountered neoplasm that is represented clinically by a nonde-

TABLE 28-6

Comparison of Pilar Sheath Acanthoma and Dilated Pore of Winer

Pilar Sheath Acanthoma	Dilated Pore of Winer
Clinical Features	
Middle-aged or elderly patients	
Women equal to men	
Face, especially upper lip	
Solitary tan-ink papule or plaque	
Central keratotic plug or comedone	
Histopathological Features	
Central infundibular microcyst	
Cystic opening to epidermal surface	
Keratinous material in cyst	
Polygonal cells in epithelial lining with variably pale or clear cytoplasm (containing glycogen) or basaloid appearance	
Bland cytological characteristics	
No hair formation	
Epithelial wall proliferative with lobular cellular buds	Greater cystic opening to surface
Proliferative buds may contain keratinous accumulations	Cystic wall less proliferative than PSA
Differential Diagnosis	
Epidermoid cyst	
Trichofolliculoma	
Perifollicular fibroma	
Fibrofolliculoma	

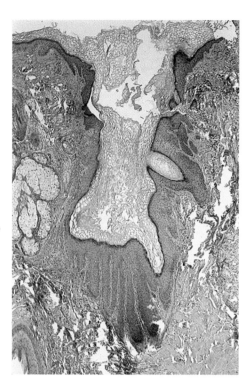

FIGURE 28-16   Dilated Pore of Winer. Although dilated pore characteristically opens at the epidermal surface through a cystic infundibulum, cross sections of the intradermal component may be difficult to distinguish form pilar sheath acanthoma.

bland, without nucleoli or mitotic figures (Fig. 28-17). There are no basaloid elements, and only a minor component of non–cyst-forming epithelial cells, in the form of solid "buds" from microcysts, is apparent.

Differential Diagnosis   The lack of both basaloid epithelium and non–cyst-forming epithelium distinguishes TA from syringoma, desmoplastic trichoepithelioma (see the following), and microcystic adnexal carcinoma, all of which feature prominent non-cystic cellular proliferations.

TABLE 28-7

Trichoadenoma

Clinical Features

Adults usually
Head, neck, and trunk
Nondescript papule
<1 cm

Histopathological Features

Dome-shaped
Symmetrical
Keratinous cysts lined by uniform cuboidal cells
Eosinophilic or clear cytoplasm
Granular layer
No basaloid epithelium

Differential Diagnosis

Syringoma
Trichoepithelioma, especially desmoplastic type
Microcystic adnexal carcinoma
Tumor of the follicular infundibulum
Basal cell carcinoma

script solitary nodule in the skin of the head, neck, or trunk (Table 28-7).[81–85] It generally measures less than 1 cm in greatest dimension.

Histopathological Features   The histologic image of TA is one featuring a proliferation of microcystic arrays of pilar-type keratinizing epithelium, separated from one another by fibroblastic stroma in the dermis, without any attachment to the epidermis (Table 28-7). The keratin-filled cysts are comprised by polyhedral cells that often contain keratohyaline granules and eosinophilic or clear cytoplasm. Nuclei are

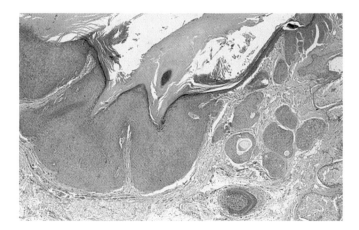

FIGURE 28-15   Pilar Sheath Acanthoma. A central microcyst derived from the infundibulum (complete with epidermal-type keratinization) has areas of acanthosis with small lobules of keratinocytes budding into adjacent dermis.

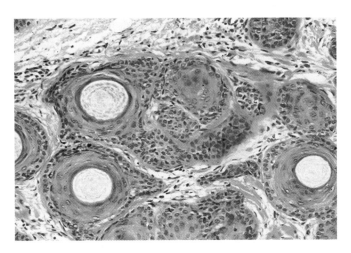

FIGURE 28-17 Trichoadenoma (of Nikolowski). A nodular growth of keratinizing epithelium, trichoadenoma is distinguished from dilated pore and pilar sheath acanthoma by the presence of trichilemmal type keratin within small horn cysts and the absence of an obvious connection to the epidermis.

Trichilemmoma

Clinical Features   Trichilemmoma (TL) is a relatively frequently encountered lesion of the face or neck that may be seen throughout life, but with a predominance in adults (Table 28-8).[86–88] There is also a potential association between *multiple* TLs and Cowden's syndrome.[89–91] This disorder features the autosomally determined presence of multifocal hamartomatous polyposis of the intestines, an increased risk of mammary carcinoma or other internal malignancies, and various other cutaneous tumors such as sclerotic fibromas ("collagenomas") and adnexal hamartomas or nevi. These associated lesions may be synchronously or metachronously in reference to the TLs.

TABLE 28-8

Trichilemmoma

Clinical Features

    Adults
    Head and neck, especially upper lip and nose
    Keratotic pink papules
    Solitary or multiple
    Association with Cowden's syndrome
        Multifocal hamartomatous polyposis of the intestines
        Increased risk of breast carcinoma and other internal
            malignancies
        Autosomal dominant

Histopathological Features

    Verrucous surface configuration often
    Lobular proliferation of polygonal cells with variably clear cyto-
        plasm (containing glycogen)
    Peripheral palisading of nuclei
    Occasional apoptotic bodies
    Lobules bounded by eosinophilic basement membranes

Differential Diagnosis

    Tumor of the follicular infundibulum
    Inverted follicular keratosis
    Verruca
    Eccrine acrospiroma
    Basal cell carcinoma

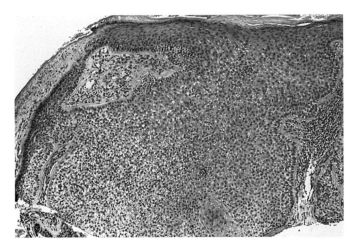

FIGURE 28-18 Trichilemmoma. A lobular proliferation of bland cells with clear or pale eosinophilic cytoplasm is surrounded by a distinct basal lamina.

Histopathological Features   Regardless of whether TL is sporadic and solitary or syndromic and multicentric, its histological attributes are the same (Table 28-8). One sees a prototypically lobular, folliculocentric proliferation of bland, amitotic, relatively uniform polygonal cells with variably clear PAS-positive cytoplasm, surrounded by a distinct cuff of eosinophilic basement membrane material (Fig. 28-18). The tumor commonly shows peripheral nuclear palisading within the cellular lobules, and may encroach upon the overlying basilar epidermis (Fig. 28-19). However, the interfollicular surface epithelium is normal. Sometimes, adjacent lobular profiles in TL may coalesce, yielding a nodular dermal mass. Circular profiles ("eddies") of squamoid cells are lacking in this neoplasm, as are foci of overt keratinization.[92,93]

    Hunt et al. and Tellechea and coworkers have described a peculiar variant of TL in which there is a pseudoinvasive interface between tumor cell clusters and the subjacent dermal stroma, instead of a "pushing" lobular configuration (Fig. 28-20).[94,95] The corium underneath such lesions manifests a fibromyxoid proliferative response, accounting for the proposed name of "desmoplastic trichoepithelioma." Limited mitotic activity may be observed in the neoplastic cell population, and this observation, together with the overall growth pattern, may result in a mistaken diagnosis of basal cell carcinoma or infiltrative squamous cell carcinoma. A helpful clue to the correct interpretation in these cases

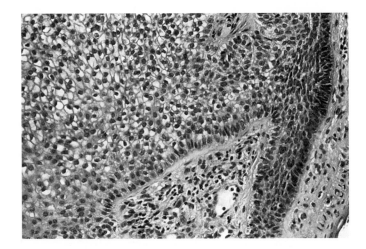

FIGURE 28-19 Trichilemmoma. Nuclear palisades are evident at the periphery of the lesion. Basement membrane material is conspicuous at this magnification.

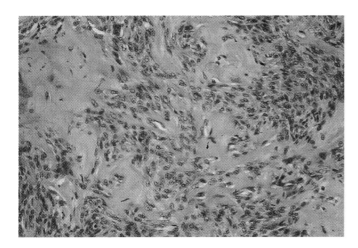

FIGURE 28-20 Trichilemmoma. Within the lesion or at the dermal interface, nests of cells may divide a fibromyxoid stroma in a pattern suggestive of invasion.

is the previously cited peritumoral basement membrane in desmoplastic TLs, which is retained in spite of the other disturbing histologic findings and is potentially highlighted with the PAS method or immunostains for collagen type IV or laminin.

Differential Diagnosis   TL shows significant overlap with tumor of the follicular infundibulum. TL is notable for a lobular configuration, whereas TFI has a plate-like pattern with inter-connecting epithelial cords. Two histologically similar pilar proliferations, namely, follicular verruca vulgaris and inverted follicular keratosis (which may, in fact, be one and the same lesion), must be considered. In general, TL differs from the latter entities by the lack of squamous eddies and overt keratinization.

Benign Proliferating Pilar Tumor

Clinical Features   Benign proliferating pilar tumor (BPPT) (also known as "proliferating trichilemmal tumor," "proliferating trichilemmal cyst," and "pilar tumor") shows a marked predilection to occur during middle or old age, with striking preference for women (Table 28-9).[96–101] Its usual location is in the scalp, but isolated examples of this nodular lesion also have been reported in other topographic sites.[98] The neoplasm arises in the deep dermis and grows slowly over the span of years, typically to a size of several centimeters before the patient seeks medical attention. Erosion through the skin surface may occur.

Histopathological Features   Benign proliferating pilar tumor is characterized by sharp peripheral circumscription on scanning microscopy (Table 28-9). This is an important observation, because the *architecture* of proliferating pilar tumors is crucial to determining their biologic potential, as discussed in the following. Accordingly, piecemeal excisions or curettage should be strongly discouraged if BPPT is in the clinical differential diagnosis. Cords of large polyhedral tumor cells with obviously squamoid characteristics comprise this neoplasm; these interanastomose with one another, often encompassing a central cystic area that is filled with trichilemmal-type keratinous debris (Fig. 28-21). Clear cells are often present in the tumor cell population, and a cuff of basement membrane material may enclose the advancing edge of the tumor. These features link BPPT to other tumors of the outer hair sheath.

The cytologic features of BPPT differ substantially from those of other benign pilar neoplasms, in that they often include nuclear pleomorphism, vesicular nuclear chromatin, prominent nucleoli, and brisk mitotic activity (up to 10 per 10 high-power [X400] fields) (Fig. 28-22).

Benign Proliferating Pilar Tumor

Clinical Features

Usually older individuals
Women more often than men
Scalp, most common site
Often large exophytic tumors, measuring up to 10 cm in diameter
Recurrence after removal is infrequent
Metastases to regional lymph nodes occur rarely

Histopathological Features

Lobular proliferation of squamous epithelium with tricholemmal differentiation
Usually well demarcated at periphery
A trichilemmal cyst remnant usually present
The epithelium often shows
    Variable clear cell change
    Disordered proliferation
    Nuclear pleomorphism
    Prominent nucleoli
    Mitoses

Differential Diagnosis

Squamous cell carcinoma

Because of this constellation of findings, it is easy to understand why a number of such tumors have been confused with squamous cell carcinomas (SCCs) in the past.[102] Nevertheless, it must be reiterated that the architecture of BPPT, rather than its cytomorphology, is of paramount behavioral importance. If the lesion shows a well-demarcated, generally rounded interface with the surrounding connective tissue, it will behave in a benign fashion. Alternatively, infiltrative margins should be viewed with concern (see the following). Foci of dystropic calcification are common in the stroma and within the cell nests of BPPT, and areas of "abrupt" trichilemmal keratinization are regularly interspersed throughout the lesion.

Differential Diagnosis   The principal distinction is between BPPT and SCC. The overall growth pattern of squamous cancers typically is

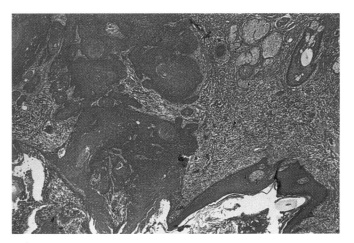

FIGURE 28-21 Proliferating Pilar Tumor. A central cystic area is encompassed by nests and cords of keratinizing epithelial cells. Communication with the epidermis is present.

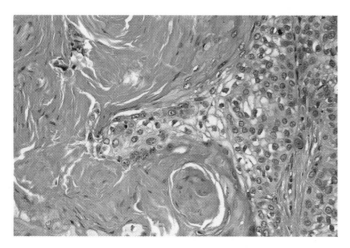

FIGURE 28-22   Proliferating Pilar Tumor. Abrupt (trichilemmal) keratinization typifies this lesion. Cells relatively uniform in size, cytoplasm is clear or weakly eosinophilic, and mild cytologic atypia and mitotic activity may be seen.

infiltrative, unlike that just described, and SCC does not feature the presence of pilar-type keratinization. Last, the clinical history has an important role in this contextual diagnosis, because BPPT typically evolves over a much longer period of time than SCC does.

TUMORS OF THE GERMINATIVE FOLLICULAR EPITHELIUM

The germinative components of the hair follicle include matrical cells, cortical cells, and cells of the inner hair sheath. Neoplasms differentiating toward these elements are capable of reproducing the entire gamut of hair formation in embryonic and mature skin. A pathognomonic pattern of cellular maturation typifies a subset of such tumors, in which immature matrical cells lose their cytoplasmic organelles and, at the same time, accumulate intracellular keratin. The resulting elements are called "ghost" cells or "shadow" cells, in that they have been transformed into homogeneously eosinophilic cells with ghost-like, karyolytic nuclear profiles. Accordingly, "shadow" cells are synonymous with matrical follicular differentiation, in either monolinear or multilinear neoplasms of the cutaneous adnexa.[103] Four appendageal neoplasms are commonly classified as showing germinative pilar features: trichofolliculoma, trichoepithelioma, pilomatricoma, and trichogerminoma.

Trichofolliculoma

Clinical Features   Trichofolliculoma (TF) is an infrequently seen lesions that is restricted in topographic distribution to the head and neck (Table 28-10). Generally it affects adults and presents as a small flesh-colored nodule with a central keratinous plug from which vellus hairs emanate.[104,105]

Histopathological Features   Trichofolliculoma is a pilar proliferation that is centered on a dilated primary follicle that is lined by infundibular or isthmic-type epithelium and opens to the epidermal surface (Table 28-10; Fig. 28-23). From that central structure, several secondary follicles bud in a radial fashion, and these either differentiate toward germinative epithelium or form mature hairs (Fig. 28-24). The dermal stroma within and around TFs are densely collagenized, and is arranged in parallel layers. This process clearly demarcates the tumor from the adjacent corium. Constituent cells of TF show a range of cytologic features, with some representing isthmic, keratinizing elements; others showing outer hair sheath features with clear cytoplasm and peripheral nuclear palisading in cell groups; and still others having a compact polyhedral or

---

TABLE 28-10

Trichofolliculoma

Clinical Features

Usually adults
Head and neck, especially the nose
Small skin-colored papule or nodule, usually solitary
Central keratinous plug with vellus hairs

Histopathological Features

Dilated hair follicle structure opening to surface
Infundibulum or isthmic-type epithelium
Secondary follicular structures radiate (or "bud") from the central structure
The secondary follicles show varying degrees of differentiation from germinative to formation of mature hair
An organoid fibrous stroma surrounding the follicle structure, well-demarcated from adjacent dermis
Considerable heterogeneity of epithelial cells
  Isthmic, clear cells with peripheral nuclear palisading, basaloid matrical cells

Differential Diagnosis

Trichoepithelioma
Basal cell carcinoma
Fibrofolliculoma

---

basaloid matrical appearance. Rare examples of TF may exhibit partial sebocytic differentiation in the secondary follicles, spurring some authors to modify the name of the lesion to *sebaceous* trichofolliculoma."[106,107]

Differential Diagnosis   Trichofolliculoma must be distinguished from another follicular tumor, trichoepithelioma, as well as "keratotic" (pilar-type) BCC.[108] Trichoepithelioma does not have a dilated primary follicle at its center, and, in addition, is typically dominated by basaloid cells rather than showing the mixture that is characteristic of TF. The stromal collagen pattern in TF is altogether different from the loose, fibromyxoid matrix of BCC, and the former of these tumors demonstrates a much higher degree of cytologic differentiation than the latter.

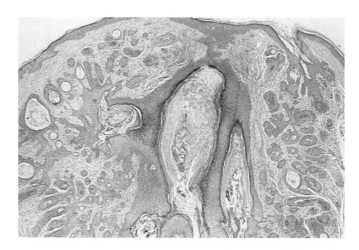

FIGURE 28-23   Trichofolliculoma. A dilated infundibulum supports a complex proliferation of small germinative hair elements and small follicles.

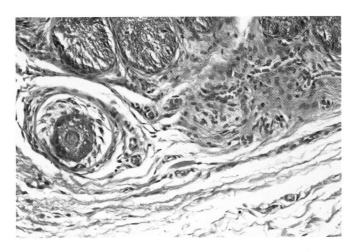

FIGURE 28-24   Trichofolliculoma. Both basaloid clusters and small immature hair follicles are evident at higher magnification.

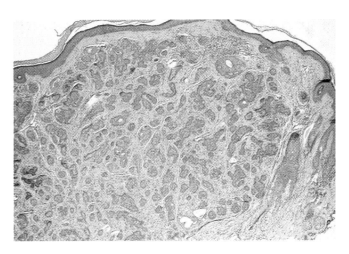

FIGURE 28-25   Trichoepithelioma. This lobular proliferation of basaloid cells induces its own tumoral stroma that sharply demarcates the lesion from corium. The epidermis is not involved.

Trichoepithelioma

Clinical Features   Trichoepithelioma of the "classical" type (TE) usually is seen as a solitary, slowly growing, flesh-colored nodule in the skin of the face, which typically arises during childhood (Table 28-11).[109–111] The clinical distinction between TE and BCC is nearly impossible in some cases, and, as discussed subsequently, this dilemma may extend to a microscopic level as well. *Multiple* TEs are seen in the "epithelioma adenoides cysticum" (Brooke-Fordyce) syndrome, which is transmitted in an autosomal dominant fashion.[112–115] In that disease complex, TEs may literally cover the face, with each lesion being less than 1 cm; extracranial skin fields may be involved as well. It is interesting that multiple TEs may coexist with multifocal cylindromas, spiradenomas, salivary glandular "dermal analogue tumors" (which

resemble cylindromas), trichilemmomas, or BCCs, in the context of the Brooke-Fordyce or Cowden syndromes or in related, "derivative" genodermatoses.[112–116] Systemic conditions that may potentially coexist with multifocal trichoepitheliomatosis include the Rombo syndrome (milia, hypotrichosis, atrophoderma, TEs, BCCs, and vasodilatation with cyanosis), systemic lupus erythematosus, and myasthenia gravis.[117,118]

Histopathological Features   Regardless of whether they are sporadic or syndromic tumors, TEs have the same histologic image (Table 28-11). They are composed of lobular arrays of relatively uniform basaloid cells in the dermis, separated from one another by mature, collagenous, hypocellular stroma (Fig. 28-25). The lobular constituents often connect to one another focally, and contain variably sized keratinous microcysts mantled by cells showing infundibular or isthmic differentiation (Fig. 28-26). The remaining (predominant) cell population is embryonic and germinative in appearance, and, as such, is very similar to that encountered in nodulocystic or pilar-type BCCs. The likeness between those tumors is even more problematic in examples of TE that exhibit retiform or adenoid foci, as commonly seen in BCC. The cited distinction also is particularly difficult in those TEs that lack obvious keratinous microcyst formation and are composed of solidly cellular basaloid clusters; such variants have been termed "immature trichoepitheliomas" (Fig. 28-27).[119]

Differential Diagnosis   Traditionally, several points of difference between TE and BCC have been cited. Those include the lack of a loose, fibromyxoid BCC-like stroma in TE; the presence of abortive hair papilla formation in TE but not BCC; an absence of apoptotic foci in TE and their existence in BCC; and melanin pigmentation in the latter but not the former of the two neoplasms.[120] Although these dissimilarities do indeed exist in most instances, the authors have been increasingly struck over the years that TE and BCC may have such similar images *because they may, in fact, be points in a single continuum of tumors.* This somewhat iconoclastic view is not novel, and it is supported by the previously cited clinical observation that multiple "trichoepitheliomas" can co-mingle with BCCs in selected patients and kindreds, as well as histopathologic cases-in-point where the microscopic "discriminants" mentioned are *shared* by the two neoplasms under discussion here.[114,121,122]

Other investigators have attempted to utilize immunostains for *bcl-2* protein and CD34 to separate TE from BCC; reported observations in those studies have included a lack of *bcl-2* protein in TE and the

---

TABLE 28-11

Trichoepithelioma

Clinical Features

Children and adults
Solitary or multiple ("epithelioma adenoides cysticum"—Brooke-Fordyce syndrome)
Head and neck, especially face
Skin-colored papule or nodule, pearly appearance
Usually <1 cm
Multiple TE associated with multiple cylindromas, spiradenomas, salivary glandular tumors, trichilemmomas, or basal cell carcinomas

Histopathological Features

Organoid arrangement of mature collagenous hypocellular stroma about lobules of uniform basaloid cells, well-demarcated from surrounding dermis
Basaloid cells tend to show peripheral palisading of nuclei, lace-like or cribiform in patterns, and hair matrix-like differentiation
Keratinous microcysts frequent
Often hair papilla-like structures ("mesenchymal papillary bodies") in stroma adjacent to hair matrical-like epithelium
Minimal or no mitotic figures and necrotic cells

Differential Diagnosis

Trichofolliculoma
Basal cell carcinoma

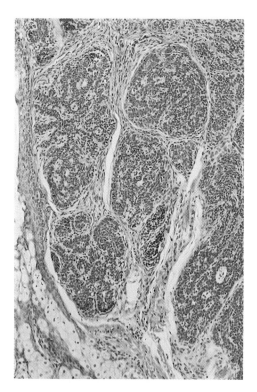

FIGURE 28-26 Trichoepithelioma. Note organoid basaloid epithelial aggregates with fibrous stroma resembling hair papillae.

regular presence of that marker in BCC, and the presence of CD34 in the stroma immediately adjacent to cellular clusters in TE but not in BCC.[123–126] Our laboratories, however, have been unable to reproduce those findings, and therefore we must conclude that there are no reproducible adjunctive-morphologic methods to separate the two neoplasms in question at the present time.[127]

Whether one espouses the view that TE and pilar-type BCC are truly distinct from one another, or, alternatively, that TE represents a differentiated form of BCC, the clinical impact of that opinion probably is negligible. Dermatologists aim to conservatively but completely excise both tumor types, and should do so.

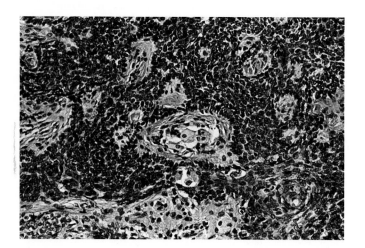

FIGURE 28-27 Trichoepithelioma. Solid basaloid proliferations devoid of keratocyst formation comprise a pattern referred to as immature trichoepithelioma.

Desmoplastic Trichoepithelioma

Another contentious point surrounds the question of whether "desmoplastic" trichoepithelioma (DTE), also known as "sclerosing epithelial hamartoma," does indeed have a nosological relatedness to TE (Table 28-12).[128,129]

Clinical Features The former of those neoplasms is virtually always solitary; is not seen in the epithelioma adenoides cysticum syndrome or in association with systemic diseases; and typically presents as a slightly umbilicated nodule or plaque in the central facial skin of young or middle-aged women.[130,131]

Histopathological Features More histological than clinical dissimilarities can be seen between TE and DTE. The second of those tumors is usually represented by a discoid lesion in the dermis that is wider than it is deep, and whose lateral margins are sharply circumscribed (Table 28-12). Narrow linear or slightly branching cords of compact polygonal cells comprise DTE, without a truly basaloid component. There is also an admixture of keratinous microcysts that are very often filled with calcified material and are connected directly to the linear polyhedral-cell configurations (Fig. 28-28). The intervening stroma is densely collagenized and hypocellular, without fibromyxoid foci or retraction from the epithelial cell groups.[132] Unlike both TE and BCC, DTE is immunoreactive for EMA as well.[133]

Differential Diagnosis The last of these points is helpful in making the distinction between DTE and its principal differential diagnostic alternative, morpheaform BCC (MBCC). The latter tumor likewise shows a composition by narrow, slightly branching cords of epithelial cells—often with areas of dystrophic calcification as well—embedded in a hypocellular stroma. In addition to noting the EMA-reactivity of DTE and EMA-negativity of MBCC, it is useful to remember that basal cell carcinomas of all types lack sharp circumscription and are composed of

TABLE 28-12

Desmoplastic Trichoepithelioma

Clinical Features

   Young to middle-age adults
   Women more than men
   Central face, especially cheek
   Solitary, often skin-colored or slightly yellowish plaque
   Raised borders and slightly depressed central area
   Firm or scar-like

Histopathological Features

   Discoid lesion in upper dermis with well-defined margins
   Narrow linear or slightly branching cords of compact polygonal cells
   Keratinous microcysts often filled with calcified material
   Densely collagenized stroma surrounds epithelial elements
   Dystrophic calcification
   Foreign body giant cell reaction to keratin
   No appreciable cytological atypia or mitotic activity

Differential Diagnosis

   Morphea form basal cell carcinoma
   Syringoma

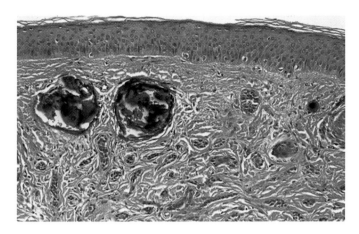

FIGURE 28-28 Desmoplastic Trichoepithelioma. Keratocysts commonly contain calcified material.

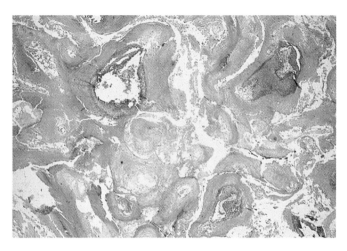

FIGURE 28-29 Pilomatrixoma. Islands of basaloid cells that resemble hair matrix are associated with abundant keratinous debris.

truly basaloid elements. Moreover, MBCC, in fact, does exhibit small zones in which the stroma is fibromyxoid and retracted—in likeness to other BCCs—and it also focally manifests larger cellular aggregates than those seen in DTE.[132]

Pilomatricoma

Clinical Features Pilomatricoma (PM)—also known as "calcifying epithelioma of Malherbe," "pilomatrixoma," and "trichomatricoma"—is a distinctive neoplasm that represents the prototype of matrical follicular differentiation (Table 28-13). It is most often seen in children and adolescents as a slowly growing, deeply seated, cystic nodule in the skin of the head and neck, but this neoplasm may certainly be observed in adults as well as in extracranial locations.[134–139]

Histopathological Features Several stages of development have been observed for PM, and distinctive clinicopathologic variants of the tumor also exist (Table 28-13). Ackerman has suggested that PM begins as a subepidermal cyst that is lined in part by infundibular-type epithelium and, in its inferior-peripheral aspects, by germinative-matrical cells.[1] The latter elements are the most distinctive component of this neoplasm; they are represented by compact basaloid polygonal cells with monotous round nuclei, dark chromatin, small nucleoli, consistently observable and often-brisk mitotic activity, and amphophilic cytoplasm (Figs. 28-29 and 28-30). The peripherally disposed germinative cells blend into an intermediate zone nearer the cyst lumen, where nuclei variably assume a washed-out, "ghost"-like appearance and the cytoplasm becomes more uniformly cornified and eosinophilic. In the center of the lesion, ghost cells are seen exclusively (Fig. 28-31), and these often undergo regional dystrophic calcification.

With the passage of time, the number of basaloid cells in PM decreases progressively, eventually to be replaced entirely by aggregates of ghost cells, calcium deposits, and even foci of metaplastic bone. Extravasated keratin often elicits a foreign body-type giant cell reaction in the surrounding dermis; in fact, these changes may dominate "ancient" PMs.[138,139] Moreover, extensive secondary heterotopic

TABLE 28-13

Pilomatricoma

Clinical Features

Children and adolescents, but any age
Head and neck most common
Solitary slowly developing hard nodule, usually deeply seated

Histopathological Features

Well-defined lobular tumor in dermis or subcutis
Initially the tumor may be cystic with infundibular and germinative-matrical cellular components
Germinative-matrical cells are uniform basaloid cells with monotonous round nuclei, dark chromatin, and small nucleoli
Prominent mitotic activity
Transition of matrical epithelium to "ghost" or "shallow" cells that exhibit an imprint of a nucleus that has been lost
Formation of hard nail-like keratin
Progressive loss of basaloid epithelium
Foreign body giant cell reaction to keratin
Calcification, ossification

Differential Diagnosis

Basal cell carcinoma
Pilomatrical carcinoma

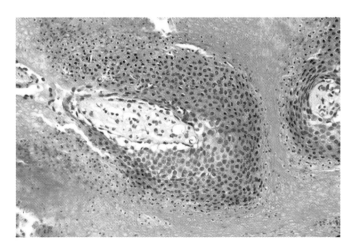

FIGURE 28-30 Pilomatrixoma. At higher magnification, the morphologic analogy of this neoplastic lesion to hair matrix is obvious.

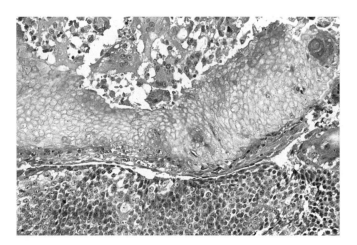

FIGURE 28-31   Pilomatrixoma. Matrical keratinization results in preservation of cell borders, but loss of nuclei (ghost cells).

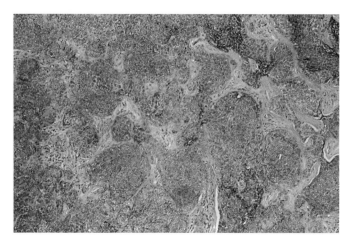

FIGURE 28-32   Trichogerminoma. Interconnected lobules of basaloid epithelial cells with pale eosinophilic cytoplasm for a nodular mass in the dermis.

ossification may simulate the appearance of a cutaneous osteoma, if attention is not paid to residual basaloid or ghost cell elements.

Histological variants of PM include a "perforating" form of the tumor in which it is seemingly eliminated through the overlying epidermis; it may be posited that PMs associated with clinical anetoderma illustrate an earlier stage of this phenomenon.[138,140–145] Transepidermal extrusion therefore would appear to be one way in which PMs "resolve" or mature; conversely, transformation of the lesion into an osteocalcific mass is the apparent outcome for those neoplasms that are "retained" in the dermis. Another unusual form of PM is that in which peripheral "buds" of tumor cells are seen to infiltrate from the main mass into the surrounding corium and incite a desmoplastic response, in analogy to the image of low-grade malignant acrospiromas (see previous chapter). These lesions are otherwise typical morphologically, and may therefore be labeled appropriately as "invasive" (or, alternatively, low-grade malignant) pilomatricomas.[138,139,146] The biological correlate of such findings is a potential for local recurrence that is virtually unknown in banal PM.

Differential Diagnosis   The differential diagnosis of PM principally concerns the subtype of "pilar" BCC in which follicular matrical differentiation—complete with aggregates of ghost cells—may be seen.[147] Overall, however, there are many points of cytological and architectural dissimilarity between these neoplasms, as enumerated previously.

Trichogerminoma

In 1992, Sau et al. seminally reported 14 cases of a rare cutaneous adnexal neoplasm that they elected to designate as "trichogerminoma," because of the conclusion that it demonstrated differentiation toward the hair germ epithelium.[148]

Clinical Features   Patients with this lesion ranged in age from 16 to 73 years, and males predominated by a factor of two. They presented with slowly growing, dermal or subcutaneous masses on the head and neck, trunk, or extremities, ranging up to 4 cm in maximum dimension. Followup showed that the patients all had an uneventful course after excision of their masses, except for one who suffered a transformation of his tumor into a high-grade carcinoma and died from distant metastasis of that component.

Histopathological Features   Trichogerminoma (TG) is a well-demarcated, highly cellular lesion that has its epicenter in the deep dermis (Fig. 28-32). The neoplastic cells are basaloid and monotonous, with round nuclei, dispersed chromatin, distinct nucleoli, and often-numer-

ous mitoses. They are arranged in lobules that are separated from one another by variably cellular fibrovascular stroma, which may contain matrical mucin. The most characteristic feature of this tumor is the formation of "cell balls" throughout the mass, represented by micronodular aggregates of neoplastic cells with internal concentricity and peripheral condensation, or nuclear palisading, or both. Many cell groups are surrounded by PAS-positive eosinophilic membranes, resembling the vitreous layer of the outer root sheath. Small keratin microcysts may be appreciated within the cellular balls, as may foci of apoptosis, clear cell change (Fig. 28-33), structures resembling abortive hair bulbs, and divergent sebaceous differentiation.

Differential Diagnosis   Because of its diverse microscopic attributes, TG has a lengthy differential diagnosis, which includes BCC, TE, and trichoblastoma (see the following). Indeed, skeptics may choose to regard this neoplasm as a variant of pilar-type BCC, because of several points of microscopic similarity with TG as outlined previously. However, in light of the *aggregate* clinicopathologic characteristics of TG, I believe that it does withstand scrutiny as a distinctive entity. More complete delineation of its biological nature and morphologic spectrum will require study of additional cases.

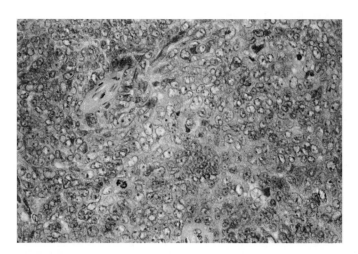

FIGURE 28-33   Trichogerminoma. At higher magnification, nuclei with vesicular chromatin and prominent nucleoli are seen. Mitotic activity is readily identified, as are apoptotic cells.

TABLE 28-14

Basaloid Follicular Hamartoma

Clinical Features

Children or adults
Any location
Solitary or multiple forms
   Localized, linear, or generalized
Papules, plaques
Comedones, keratotic plugs
Alopecia may occur

Histopathological Features

Folliculocentric
Proliferation of bland uniform basaloid cells
   in cords and aggregates
Organized fibrous stroma
Adenoid or reticulated patterns
Small keratinous cysts
Calcification may occur

Differential Diagnosis

Fibroepithelioma of Pinkus
Superficial basal cell carcinoma
Trichoepithelioma
Reticulated seborrheic keratosis

MIXED EPITHELIAL AND MESENCHYMAL FOLLICULAR PROLIFERATIONS

Two adnexal neoplasms are typified by conjoint differentiation toward the follicular epithelium and follicle-related mesenchyme. These representatives are basaloid follicular hamartoma—arguably included in this section as a tumor in the generic sense of that term—and trichoblastoma.

Basaloid Follicular Hamartoma

Clinical Features Basaloid follicular hamartoma (BFH)—also known as "generalized hair follicle hamartoma" and "linear unilateral basal cell nevus"—is generally regarded today as a malformative developmental lesion rather than a true neoplasm (Table 28-14).[149–154] However, it should be noted in that regard that this condition may develop for the first time during adulthood. It likewise may be linear or regionalized, pale or erythematous, plaquelike or papular, and solitary or generalized. Some examples of BFH have caused alopecia or arisen in patients with myasthenia gravis.[151,152] In the author's opinion, the lesion described by Alessi and Azzolini as "localized hair follicle hamartoma" is a "hybrid" variant of BFH that also incorporates some of the elements of nevus sebaceus.[155]

Histopathological Features The microscopic image of this lesion features a folliculocentric proliferation of bland, uniform basaloid cells, which are arranged in cords and clusters and separated from one another by an organized fibrous stroma (Table 28-14). Adenoid or reticulated patterns can often be appreciated in the epithelial component, and small keratinous cysts may be evident as well (Figs. 28-34, 28-35, and 28-36). These can become calcified; vellus hairs or sebaceous glands also may be included in BFH.

Differential Diagnosis Because of the particular nature of the interface between the epithelium and stroma in individual lesions of BFH, differential diagnosis with the "fibroepitheliomatous" variant of BCC may be difficult, as may the distinction between BFH and multifocal-

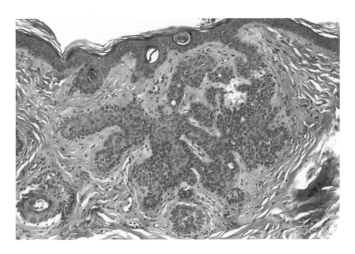

FIGURE 28-34 Basaloid Follicular Hamartoma. A small folliculocentric proliferation of basaloid cells is present.

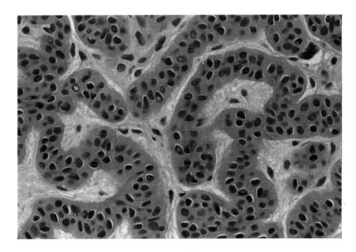

FIGURE 28-35 Basaloid Follicular Hamartoma. A reticular pattern of growth may be seen.

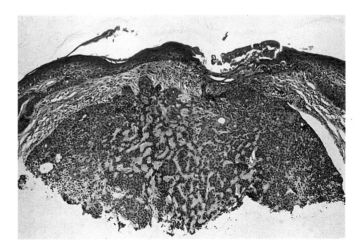

FIGURE 28-36 Trichoblastoma. Cords and clusters of basaloid cells form a discrete mass in the dermis.

superficial BCC in other instances. Follicular hamartomas lack the foci of apoptosis, myxoid alterations in tumoral stroma, and epithelial-stromal retraction seen in BCC. Also, clinical information obviously is extremely useful in making the interpretative separation under discussion.

Trichoblastoma

Following publication of a textbook by Ackerman et al. on follicular neoplasms in 1993, it has become fashionable to follow the recommendation of those authors to utilize the term "trichoblastoma" in a nosologically egalitarian fashion, as an umbrella over not only the bulk of benign pilar tumors, but also many lesions that classically would be considered as BCC variants.[1,156,157] This practice is defended by some on conceptual grounds, and certainly by many others who are interested in a condensed and "user-friendly" nomenclatural scheme as applied to adnexal neoplasms.[158]

However, the authors believe that a negative impact would accrue from such an approach. Headington's original intent in creating the term "trichoblastoma" (with the synonym "trichogenic adnexal tumor") was to bring two salient elements of this lesion into focus. These are its relatively primitive histologic appearance, resembling that of the embryonic hair, and other morphologic attributes that suggest an epithelial–stromal interaction as the underlying mechanism for the peculiar image of this tumor.[159] Depending on whether the epithelium or stroma is predominant in neoplasms in this category, additional diagnostic modifications, such as "trichoblastic trichoblastoma" or "trichoblastic fibroma" may be used as desired.[160] However, we would stress that regardless of such nuance, the basic designation of "trichoblastoma" (TBL) is associated with a distinctive, well-recognized, visual and clinicopathologic profile, and the correspondingly narrow meaning of the term therefore should be retained. To do otherwise would, in our opinion, be tantamount philosophically to describing all malignant epithelial tumors of the viscera as "carcinoma, not further specified." Experience has taught us the inadvisability of that particular contextual approach.

Clinical Features   In this narrow sense, TBL may arise in almost any skin field, except possibly for the distal extremities (Table 28-15). It is generally a solitary, nondescript, nodular lesion that is situated at any level of the dermis; the size is usually less than 2 cm, but "giant" tumors of this type have been documented. No syndromic associations pertain.[159,161]

Histopathological Features   Trichoblastoma is a basaloid proliferation in which the neoplastic cells are arranged in cords, sheets, or discrete clusters (Table 28-15). The most common of these patterns is the first, in which strands of two to three cells in thickness anastomose with one another and are separated by cellular stroma (Figs. 28-37 and 28-38). A hyaline membrane may invest the cellular cords as well, and globular deposits of eosinophilic matrix may be seen between them or in the adjacent stroma. Hair differentiation is evident either as immature cellular clusters that bud from the mass and are indented by stroma in the manner of a primitive hair papilla and hair bulb, or as more mature proliferative foci that resemble hair root structures.[159–162] Occasional examples of TBL may exhibit the formation of melanin pigment, as described by Aloi and coworkers.[163] A multinodular variant of TBL showing desmoplastic stroma has been reported by Chan et al; this lesion also differed from classical forms of the tumor in showing small foci of keratinization, mucomyxoid stromal alteration, and focal spindle-cell differentiation with infiltration of perineural spaces and arrector muscles.[164] Despite these worrisome findings, the clinical evolution was innocuous.

TABLE 28-15
Trichoblastoma and Related Tumors

Clinical Features

   Adults
   Women as often as men
   Almost any location, especially face and scalp
   Usually does not involve distal extremities
   Solitary nondescript papule or nodule
   <2 cm usually, but may be giant

Histopathological Features

   Well-demarcated from surrounding tissue
   Symmetrical
   Basaloid epithelial proliferation in cords, sheets, or discrete clusters
   Fibrotic investment of epithelium
   Follicular germinative epithelium
   Peripheral palisading of nuclei
   Follicular differentiation resembling hair bulbs and papillae
   Keratinous cysts on occasion
   Fibrotic stroma
   Occasional necrosis
   Limited numbers of mitoses

Differential Diagnosis

   Basal cell carcinoma

Differential Diagnosis   Depending on its particular histologic constituency, the differential diagnosis of TBL encompasses BCC of the nodulocystic and morpheaform types, trichogerminoma, and BFH. Of these, the most difficult distinction is between TBL and BFH, because of their shared potential for cellular growth in single-file strands and an "interactive" interface between epithelial and stromal cells in those lesions. However, structures resembling embryonic hairs are not a part of the histopathological repertoire of BFH, as they are in TBL.[152]

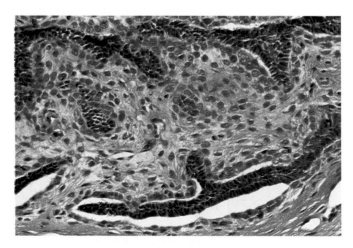

FIGURE 28-37 Trichoblastoma. Basaloid cells are often arranged in cords that are two or three cells thick. The cellular fibrous matrix induced by the tumor is analogous to normal perifollicular mesenchyme.

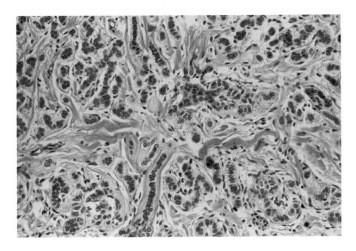

FIGURE 28-38   Trichoblastoma. A more sclerotic stroma typifies a variant that has been referred to as trichoblastic fibroma.

NEOPLASMS SHOWING DIFFERENTIATION TOWARD FOLLICLE-RELATED MESENCHYME

Tumors demonstrating differentiation toward the stromal elements that are associated with developing hair follicles are extremely rare. Moreover, their clinical presentations and histologic images are quite similar. All of these factors taken together make it easy to understand why this small area of adnexal tumor pathology is unfamiliar to most pathologists. Those lesions that are grouped in this category include trichodiscoma, perifollicular fibroma, fibrofolliculoma, follicular myxoma, and pilar leiomyoma.

Trichodiscoma

Trichodiscoma was so named because this tumor was presumed to show differentiation toward the hair discs, or *Haarscheibe*.[165] In normal skin, the latter structures are receptor complexes composed of nerve ends and supporting fibrovascular stroma, which are associated with intraepidermal Merkel cells. In reality, there has been no objective evidence to support the presence of morphological or functional attributes of the hair disc in trichodiscoma.

Clinical Features   This neoplasm becomes manifest as a grouping of otherwise banal small nodules in the skin, most often in the head and neck region but also possibly in other locations, in patients of virtually any age (Table 28-16).[165–168] These nodules may be grouped in a regional fashion, or the patient may have a generalized "trichodiscomatosis."[166,169] Contrary to what may be expected intuitively because of its putative relationship with the Haarscheibe, trichodiscoma is not a painful lesion. There may be an association between this lesion and other follicular malformations or neoplasms in the same individual.[170]

Histopathological Features   The histologic diagnosis of trichodiscoma is predicated on the presence of a superficial dermal "plate" of paucicellular fibrovascular tissue containing nerve twigs (seen only by silver impregnation stains), stromal mucin, and elastin (Table 28-16).[165,169] The overlying epidermis is attenuated and hair follicles usually are present at the periphery of the dermal abnormality (Fig. 28-39). Interestingly, immunostains have shown an absence of Merkel cells in the overlying epithelium, contrary to theoretical predictions.

Differential Diagnosis   The microscopic image of trichodiscoma is so distinctive that there is virtually no tenable differential diagnosis. In fact, this same truism also applies to most of the remaining lesions presented in this section.

Perifollicular Fibroma

Perifollicular fibroma (PF) is also primarily a fibroblastic proliferation, with clinical features that are similar, if not identical, to those of trichodiscoma (Table 28-16).[171–175] Much literature was devoted in the past to a consideration of whether PF was kin to fibrous papule of the face and adenoma sebaceum.[176,177] Inasmuch as those proliferations are basically angiofibromatous, we do not recognize any relatedness between them and PF.[178] The latter lesion differs from them histologically in showing a vaguely nodular proliferation of bland, paucicellular fibrous stroma—with or without mucin deposition—around hair follicles. This process assumes a lamellar image and may or may not be associated with fibrosis of the adjacent interfollicular dermis as well (Fig. 28-40).

Junkins-Hopkins and Cooper have considered the significance of a multiplicity of PFs, revisiting traditional teaching that this finding was

TABLE 28-16

Comparison of Trichodiscoma, Perifollicular Fibroma, and Fibrofolliculoma

Trichodiscoma	Perifollicular fibroma	Fibrofolliculoma
	Clinical Features	
	Adults usually Head and neck, trunk, extremities Often multiple May be generalized Small skin-colored papules, flat or dome-shaped	
	Histopathological Features	

Stromal component expands dermis,
    forming nodule
	Stromal component: Stroma composed of
	    delicate collagen bundles, scattered
	    fibroblasts, mucin deposition, and
	    numerous microvessels
		Well-demarcated stromal component
		    oriented about central hair follicular
		    infundibular structure. Thin epithelial
		    cords extend from infundibular structure
		    into surrounding stroma. The cords
		    have an anastomosing pattern.

	Stromal component oriented about central hair follicle	

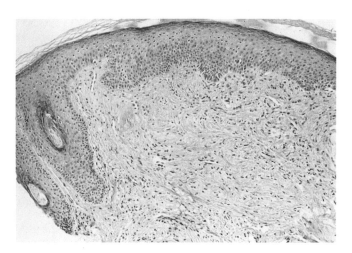

FIGURE 28-39   Trichodiscoma. A superficial plate of paucicellular fibrous stroma expands the corium. The lesion is bordered by a hair follicle.

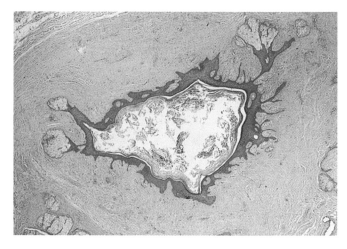

FIGURE 28-41   Fibrofolliculoma. Perifollicular fibrous proliferation is identical to that seen in perifollicular fibroma, but the central follicle is dilated, and septa of proliferating epithelium and sebaceous lobules divide the fibrous mantle.

sometimes associated with familial colonic polyposis and an increased risk of colorectal carcinoma.[179,180] Those authors concluded that the latter paradigm was erroneous, and that multiple fibrofolliculomas (vide infra)—as seen with multiple trichodiscomas and acrochordons in the autosomal dominant Birt-Hogg-Dube' syndrome—were the real culprits in regard to related colonic pathology.[181,182]

Fibrofolliculoma

Fibrofolliculoma is closely similar to PF clinicopathologically, but differs from that tumor in being associated with central follicular dilatation or distortion, and showing interanastomosing septa of follicular epithelium that traverse the lamellated fibrous mantle around the affected pilosebaceous unit or units (Table 28-16; Fig. 28-41).[183,184] Weintraub

and Pinkus have referred to this as an "epithelial net."[185] Besides the previously mentioned role played in the Birt-Hogg-Dube' syndrome, fibrofolliculoma also may be linked in selected patients to the concurrent presence of connective tissue nevi.[185]

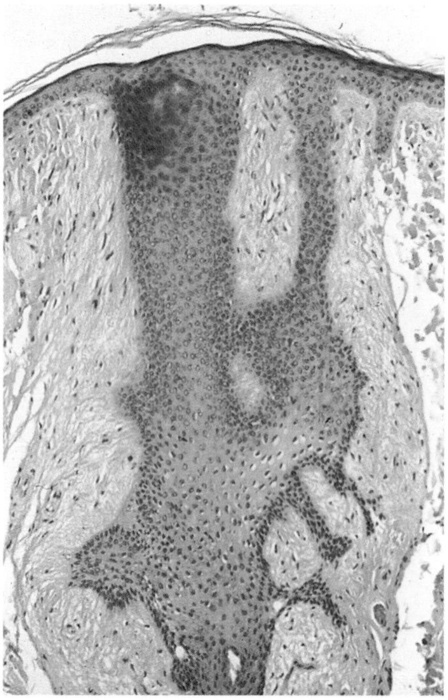

Steffen has described several examples of neoplasms that were called "mantleomas," wherein cords of nondescript bland polygonal cells were attached to the follicular infundibulum and proliferated in parallel to the hair follicle as a "mantle."[186] Because small nests of sebocytes were seen at the termini of the cellular cords in such lesions, they were classified as sebaceous in nature. However, we believe it is just as likely that the cited neoplasms may have been benign pilar sheath tumors, akin but not identical to fibrofolliculomas, with divergent sebaceous differentiation.

Follicular Myxoma

Clinical and Histopathological Features   Follicular myxoma is an extraordinarily rare tumor that is seen in patients under the age of 25, and it may coexist with other follicular tumors showing germinative epithelial differentiation. This neoplasm is typified by the localized deposition of myxoid stroma surrounding a confined group of pilosebaceous units; the latter structures are often distorted and may interconnect with one another, yielding a lobular configuration (Fig. 28-42).[159,187,188] Arborizing capillaries are present within the myxoid matrix, as well as small aggregates of presumably follicular epithelial cells—sometimes showing matrical differentiation—and rare foci in which diminuitive hair follicles or follicular cysts are formed. The overlying epidermis often exhibits papillomatous change that is probably reactive in nature. Lesions that are similar to follicular myxomas have been described in patients with the NAME (nevi-atrial myxomas-myxoid neurofibromas [or cutaneous myxomas]-ephelides) syndrome.[189]

Pilar Leiomyoma (see Chapter 32)

Leiomyomas of the skin that are confined to the superficial half of the corium are presumed to be of pilar origin, although direct continuity between the tumor and the arrector pili muscles is extremely rare.

Clinical Features   As such, "pilar" leiomyomas (PL) are usually solitary, sometimes tender, nodular lesions that generally measure less than 1 cm in greatest dimension.[190,191] However, a regionally "eruptive" multifocal version of this neoplasm also is recognized.[192] Patients of all ages and both genders may be affected without preference.

FIGURE 28-40   Perifollicular Fibroma. The perifollicular mesenchyme is expanded by a paucicellular fibrous stroma not unlike that seen in trichodiscoma.

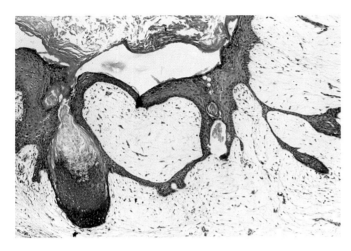

FIGURE 28-42   Follicular Myxoma. A prominent myxoid stroma distorts a follicle-based epithelial proliferation which, in this example, includes diminutive hair follicles.

Histopathological Features   The microscopic profile of PL features skeins of spindle cells with blunt-ended, fusiform nuclear profiles and fibrillar eosinophilic cytoplasm, which are intertwined in a "whorling" fashion. Fascicles of tumor cells cut in cross section often exhibit zones of perinuclear clarity; areas demonstrating nuclear palisading—in likeness to those of neural tumors—may sometimes be seen. PLs are sharply demarcated and amitotic, and similarly they lack nuclear pleomorphism and necrosis.

Differential Diagnosis   One must primarily consider solitary myofibroma of the skin, cutaneous neurilemmoma, or palisaded neuroma.[193] The first of these three alternatives does not show the tightly whorled microscopic pattern of "pure" smooth muscle tumors. Instead, myofibromas are composed of loosely aggregated micronodular arrays of bland spindle cells in a variably myxoid stroma, often with a biphasic pattern of cellular density and prominently branching ("staghorn"-shaped) stromal blood vessels. Neural tumors such as neuromas and neurilemmomas may be perplexingly similar to smooth muscle neoplasms in selected cases, and immunohistology may be necessary to distinguish between these classes of tumors. PLs are reactive for actin or desmin or both, whereas benign neurogenic lesions lack those determinants.[55]

Malignant Pilar Neoplasms

Malignant tumors of the follicular apparatus are rare, even more so than adnexal malignancies that demonstrate sweat glandular differentiation. This factor probably explains why, in the experience of the authors, most pilar carcinomas are mistaken for other lesions or otherwise misdiagnosed. Also, it is a truism of this group of tumors that they commonly demonstrate a mixture of features that defy facile classification into neoplasms of the outer hair sheath, germinative follicular cells, and so on. Hence, diagnostic categorization in this context is a "best fit" enterprise.

TRICHILEMMAL CARCINOMA

Trichilemmal carcinoma (TLC) was introduced as an entity by Headington in 1976, but that diagnosis was not embraced by pathologists for several years thereafter.[159,196–199] Recently, publication of a number of series has made it clear that TLC does exist as a distinctive lesion in the follicular tumor group.[200–203]

Trichilemmal Carcinoma

Clinical Features

Often more than 50 years of age
Head and neck
Nodular or plaque-like lesion, whitish and hyperkeratotic, reddish with smooth surface, or ulcerated
Usually <3 cm

Histopathological Features

Lobulated, folliculocentric tumor
Atypical epithelium replaces epithelial sheath of one or more hair follicles
There may be intervening unaffected epidermis between the hair follicles affected
Invasion of dermis may occur from the involved hair follicles
Some tumor cells have PAS-positive, diastase labile clear cytoplasm
Peripheral palisading of tumor lobules
Trichilemmal keratinization
The tumor otherwise shows cytological atypia and mitotic activity as in squamous cell carcinoma
Pagetoid spread in epidermis on occasion

Differential Diagnosis

Clear cell tumors as listed for sebaceous carcinoma

Clinical Features   This lesion arises in hair-bearing skin that also are actinically-damaged, and therefore usually affects the face, scalp, or ears (Table 28-17). Patients over the age of 50 are favored, with no gender predilection. Clinically, TLC may be nodular or plaque-like, whitish and hyperkeratotic or reddish and smooth-surfaced, or ulcerated, and it typically is less than 3 cm in diameter. It is commonly mistaken for proliferative actinic keratoses, BCC, or squamous carcinoma by dermatologists; more uncommonly "keratoacanthoma" is favored because of relatively rapid tumor growth. There is no known association between TLC and Cowden's syndrome, unlike the case with trichilemmomas (see the preceding), and "remnants" of the latter of these two neoplasms are never seen in conjunction with TLC. Therefore, it would appear that they both arise as de novo proliferations and do not share a common pathogenesis.

Histopathological Features   Trichilemmal carcinoma is a lobulated, folliculocentric tumor that may replace the epithelial sheath of one, or more commonly, several hair follicles, yielding a pattern wherein groups of neoplastic cells replace the perifollicular epidermis but are separated by normal surface epithelium (Table 28-17). The general image may thus be one of multifollicular and perifollicular-epidermal carcinoma in situ. Alternatively, invasive foci may emanate from either of these two sites and involve the adjacent dermal connective tissue in an irregular fashion, with surrounding lymphoplasmacytic inflammation and stromal desmoplasia (Fig. 28-43). At least a portion of the tumor cells have PAS-positive, diastase-labile lucent cytoplasm, and many lobules in TLC show peripheral nuclear palisading (Fig. 28-44). Foci of trichilemmal-type keratinization are scattered randomly throughout the lesion, which otherwise resembles squamous carcinoma in regard to the degree of nuclear atypia, mitotic activity, and cytoplasmic eosinophilia that is apparent. Some examples of TLC are singular in that they include pagetoid spread of the tumor cells into the overlying epidermis. Perineural or vascular infiltration in the dermis is unusual but may be observed.

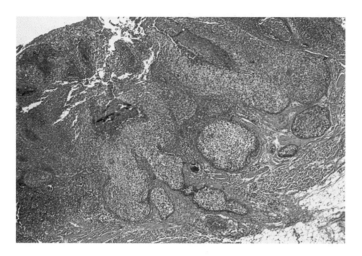

FIGURE 28-43   Trichilemmal Carcinoma. Infiltrating lobules of tumor cells incite a focally prominent inflammatory infiltrate in a desmoplastic stroma. The clear cell appearance of proliferating epithelial cells is striking.

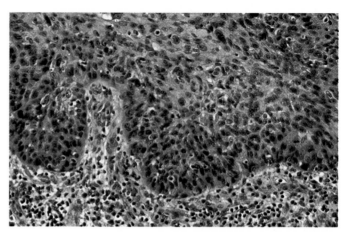

FIGURE 28-44   Trichilemmal Carcinoma. At the periphery of tumor lobules, nuclear palisades may be seen.

Differential Diagnosis   One must consider virtually all other cutaneous malignancies that may show an epithelioid clear-cell constituency. These include hydropic BCC or squamous carcinoma, clear cell eccrine carcinoma, sebaceous carcinoma, balloon cell melanoma, and metastatic clear-cell adenocarcinomas of the viscera. Attention to the constellation of histologic findings presented in concert with procurement of clinical information (regarding duration of growth and macroscopic appearance of the lesion) usually allows for satisfactory recognition of TLC. Nonetheless, application of PAS stains and selected immunostains may be necessary in some instances for definitive interpretation (Table 28-18). In particular, the application of antibodies to pilar-selective keratins (e.g., AE13/AE14) may be helpful in this context.

MALIGNANT PROLIFERATING PILAR TUMOR

Clinical and Histopathological Features   The basic clinicopathologic profile attending "malignant proliferating pilar tumor" (MPPT) (also known as "malignant trichilemmal cyst," "malignant pilar tumor," "giant hair matrix tumor," and "trichochlamydocarcinoma") is basically identical to that which was delineated previously in reference to benign proliferating pilar tumor (Table 28-19).[204–215] That is true, at least in part, because it appears that some MPPTs arise in transition from BPPT, in a manner like that attending sweat gland carcinoma ex dermal cylindroma or eccrine spiradenoma.

The first pathologic issue that must be addressed in connection with this neoplasm is the caution with which it should be diagnosed. Brownstein and Arluk properly drew attention to the fact that benign proliferating pilar tumors have cytologic features that, at first glance, suggest an interpretation of carcinoma.[102] However, as stated previously in this chapter, the pattern of growth is of greater importance in determining the biological potential of pilar neoplasms of this type.

With that caveat in mind, there are two forms of MPPT with dissimilar behavioral attributes (Table 28-19). The first is a close mimic of benign proliferating pilar tumor, except for the fact that low-grade malignant proliferating pilar tumor demonstrates irregular invasion of the surrounding and intervening connective tissue by irregularly shaped and -sized cords and nests of neoplastic cells (Figs. 28-45 and 28-46). The cytologic attributes and the remaining architectural features of low-grade MPPT are synonymous with those of BPPT. In contrast, high-grade malignant proliferating pilar tumor lacks the lobular growth pattern of BPPT and demonstrates foci of obvious geographic necrosis.[211]

TABLE 28-18

Special Stains in the Differential Diagnosis of Clear-cell Cutaneous Tumors

Tumor	PAS-w	PAS-s	AE13/14	S100	EMA*	CEA	CA-125	CA19-9
TLC	0	+	+	0	+	0	0	0
HBCC	0	+/−	0	0	0	0	0	0
HSCC	0	+/−	0	0	+/−	0	0	0
CCEC	0	+	0	+/−	+	+/−	0	0
SC	0	+/−	0	0	+*	0	0	0
BCM	0	+/−	0	+	0	0	0	0
MCCA	+/−	+/−	0	+/−	+	+/−	+/−	+/−

Key:
PAS-w = Periodic acid-Schiff (PAS) stain with diastase digestion
PAS-s = PAS stain without diastase digestion
AE13/14 = Pilar-selective keratin immunostains
S100 = S100 protein
EMA = Epithelial membrane antigen
CEA = Carcinoembryonic antigen
TLC = Trichilemmal carcinoma
HBCC = Hydropic basal cell carcinoma
HSCC = Hydropic squamous cell carcinoma
CCEC = Clear cell eccrine carcinoma
SC = Sebaceous carcinoma
BCM = Balloon cell melanoma
MCCA = Metastatic visceral clear-cell adenocarcinomas
*EMA-reactivity in sebaceous carcinomas is uniquely multivacuolated within the cytoplasm of the tumor cells.

TABLE 28-19

Malignant Proliferating Pilar Tumor (MPPT)

Clinical Features

  Similar to benign proliferation pilar tumor (BPPT)
  Middle-aged to elderly females
  Scalp
  Nodules, often ulcerated

Histopathological Features

  Low-grade MPPT
    Features similar to BPPT except
      Irregular invasion of surrounding connective tissue by irregu-
        larly shaped and sized cords of epithelium
  High-grade MPPT
  Lack of lobular growth pattern of BPPT
  Foci of geographic necrosis
  Cellular anaplasia
  Abnormal mitotic figures
  Spindle-cell transformation

Differential Diagnosis

  Low-grade MPPT
    Squamous cell carcinoma
  High-grade MPPT
    Poorly-differentiated eccrine ductal carcinoma
    Metastatic carcinoma with squamous metaplasia

Moreover, it shows a much more anaplastic cytologic image with strik-ing nuclear pleomorphism, abnormally shaped mitotic figures, and potential spindle-cell transformation.[213,214]

Separation of MPPT into the mentioned subtypes facilitates the prog-nostication of these lesions. Low-grade tumors are expected to show the potential for local recurrence only (which may, nevertheless, be muti-lating and difficult to control), whereas high-grade neoplasms also pos-sess the capability for distant metastasis.[204,205]

Differential Diagnosis One principally focuses attention on squamous cell carcinoma, but high-grade MPPT also may be confused with poorly differentiated ductal eccrine adenocarcinomas or metastatic carcinomas showing extensive squamous metaplasia. Unlike primary cutaneous squamous carcinomas, MPPTs do not communicate with the overlying epidermis, and they manifest the presence of trichilemmal keratiniza-tion. Ductal eccrine carcinomas lack the last of these findings and also exhibit at least limited foci of glandular differentiation that is absent in MPPTs. The distinction between metastatic carcinoma and MPPT is best made on the basis of clinical information, typically revealing the solitary nature and relatively long duration of growth attending follicu-lar neoplasms in general, but application of pilar keratin-selective immunostains may again may be helpful in this setting.[55]

INVASIVE PILOMATRICOMA AND PILOMATRIX CARCINOMA

Clinical and Histopathological Features Many similarities can be drawn between the foregoing discussion of proliferating pilar tumors and pilomatrical neoplasms, in regard to features that can be used in a determination of their biological potentials. Invasive pilomatricoma dif-fers from type ordinaire PM only in demonstrating irregular "budding" cellular growth into the surrounding stroma at the periphery of the lesion, much in the same way that low-grade MPPT infiltrates the der-mis or subcutis (Table 28-20).[138,139,146,216–227] On the other hand, overt pilomatrix carcinoma (PMC) is typified by broad zones of geographic necrosis, infiltrative growth, and, most important, an alteration in the cytologic features of the tumor cells.[216–227] They acquire high nucleo-cytoplasmic ratios, obviously vesicular nuclear chromatin, and large nucleoli, and as such resemble the neoplastic elements of lymphoep-ithelioma-like carcinomas of the skin (Figs. 28-47 and 28-48). How-ever, the retention of focal ghost- or "shadow-"cell keratinization be-trays the matrical differentiation of PMC.

Behaviorally, invasive PM has the potential for local recurrence but not for distant metastasis.[138] In contrast, PMC may spread secondarily to the regional lymph nodes or the viscera, and tumor-related fatality obviously is a possibility under those circumstances.[219,227]

Differential Diagnosis Because of the unique histologic image of pilomatrical tumors, with ghost-cell keratinization, recognition of PMC

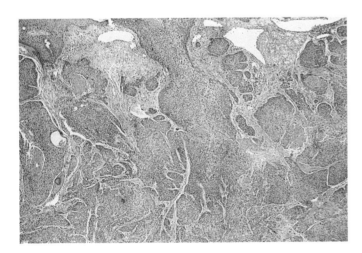

FIGURE 28-45 Malignant Proliferating Pilar Tumor. Irregular shaped nests of cells infiltrate dermis. Communication with epidermis is evident in this example.

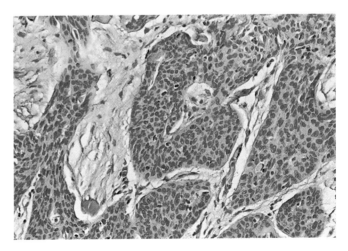

FIGURE 28-46 Malignant Proliferating Pilar Tumor. Basaloid and polygonal cells populate these invasive tumor lobules.

TABLE 28-20

Invasive Pilomatricoma and Pilomatrix (Matrical) Carcinoma

Invasive Pilomatricoma	Pilomatrix Carcinoma
Clinical Features	
Features similar to pilomatricoma	Adults Face, trunk, and extremities Nodules, possibly ulcerated
Histopathological Features	
Features similar to pilomatricoma except Invasion of surrounding tissue at periphery of tumor by irregular cords of cells	Large tumors with atypical matrical epithelium and shadow cells Zones of geographic necrosis Infiltrative growth Sheets of atypical epithelium High nucleocytoplasmic ratios Vesicular nuclear chromatin Large nucleoli Prominent mitoses
Differential Diagnosis	
Pilomatricoma	Lymphoepithelioma-like carcinoma of the skin Metastatic undifferentiated carcinoma

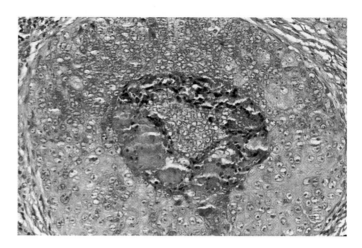

FIGURE 28-48 Pilomatrix Carcinoma. Large polygonal cells with abundant cytoplasm, large vesicular nuclei and prominent nucleoli impart a resemblance to lymphoepithelioma. Central zones of matrical (ghost cell) keratinization are seen.

generally is not a problem. However, small biopsies might yield specimens that could be confused with lymphoepithelioma-like carcinoma of the skin (LELCS) or metastatic undifferentiated carcinoma. Once again, clinical information would allow for exclusion of the latter possibility, but there are no adjunctive methods capable of separating the carcinomatous epithelium of PMC from that of LELCS in limited tissue samples.

MALIGNANT TRICHOEPITHELIOMA

Scattered reports may be found in the pertinent literature on "malignant trichoepitheliomas" (or "trichoepitheliocarcinomas").[215,228–230] These appear to be defined as tumors with the general structure of banal trichoepithelioma, but with either infiltrative growth, or cytologic atypia, or both. In any event, the clinical evolution of such tumors has been uneventful after simple excision.

As elucidated in an earlier section of this chapter, the authors have a bias toward the interpretation that even ordinary TE is, in fact, a highly differentiated variant of "pilar" BCC.[216,231] Acceptance of this view as correct (a debatable decision) would make the term "malignant trichoepithelioma" nosologically redundant. In any event, there are no accepted pathologic criteria to define the latter entity, and therefore it is not a diagnosis that we would care to make or encourage others to render.

ADNEXAL CARCINOMAS WITH MIXED DIFFERENTIATION

As introduced in the preceding chapter, pathologists who evaluate a substantial number of adnexal skin tumors not infrequently encounter some that are not easily classified, according to accepted diagnostic schemes. Often, these manifest multi-lineage differentiation along more than one appendageal route, and therefore include elements showing a combination of sudoriferous, sebaceous, and pilar characteristics.[232] General categorization as carcinomas of lesions in this group that are infiltrative, or cytologically anaplastic, or both, is not difficult, and the best approach to labeling them more precisely is to use the designation of "adnexal carcinoma with mixed (or divergent) differentiation." A similar tactic can be used in dealing with benign mixed-lineage appendage neoplasms as well. In the authors' view, this is preferable to the application of such alternative but complicated diagnostic terms as "pilary complex carcinoma" or "complex adnexal tumor of the primary epithelial germ with distinct patterns of superficial epithelioma with sebaceous differentiation, immature trichoepithelioma, and apocrine adenocarcinoma."[233,234]

As discussed, LELCS may be a primitive member of this group of tumors. Two reports have now documented the presence of focal sweat glandular, follicular, or sebaceous differentiation in this otherwise cytologically anaplastic neoplasm.[235,236]

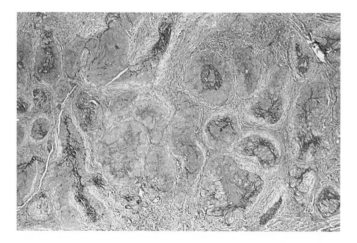

FIGURE 28-47 Pilomatrix Carcinoma. Irregular nests and lobules of large polygonal cells infiltrate dermis. Cytoplasm is pale eosinophilic or amphophilic, and central zones of keratinization and necrosis are evident.

PILAR LEIOMYOSARCOMA
(SEE CHAPTER 32)

The classification of superficial (dermal) leiomyosarcomas as "pilar" in nature has more inferential than objective support. In general, these lesions differ from cutaneous leiomyomas in showing infiltrative rather than circumscribed growth; more striking nuclear atypia; and the presence of mitotic activity.[237–239] An arrector pili-like lineage for "pilar leiomyosarcoma" (PLMS) is implied by its occurrence in a compartment of the dermis that harbors the former normal structures, as well as shared immunoreactivity in both the normal hair-related musculature and in PLMS for such determinants as S100 protein.[239] The typical biology of this usually well-differentiated neoplasm is that of a "borderline" mesenchymal malignancy, with limited potential for local recurrence but only rare examples of metastasis.[239,240]

Differential diagnosis is not commonly a problem in cases of PLMS, but it theoretically involves several other spindle-cell malignancies of the skin. These principally include spindle-cell squamous carcinoma, sarcomatoid melanoma, and atypical fibroxanthoma. Immunohistochemistry is a cost-effective and timely technique that can be used for the separation of these tumor entities, as summarized in Table 28-21.[239]

TABLE 28-21

Immunohistochemical Differential Diagnosis of Pilar Leiomyosarcoma

Tumor	KER	VIM	S100	CD57	DES	CD31/UEA
Leiomyosarcoma	0	+	+/−	0	+	0
MPNST	0	+	+/−	+/−	0	0
Spindle-cell angiosarcoma	0	+	0	0	0	+
Spindle-cell squamous cell carcinoma	+	+/−	0	0	0	0
Spindle-cell malignant melanoma	0	+	+	+/−	0	0
Kaposi's sarcoma	0	+	0	0	0	+/−

Key:
KER = Keratin
VIM = Vimentin
S100 = S100 protein
DES = Desmin
UEA = Ulex europaeus I lectin binding
MNPST = Malignant peripheral nerve sheath tumor

Pseudoneoplastic Proliferations of Hair Follicles and Follicle-Related Mesenchyme

Several other tumefactive lesions of the skin demonstrate pilar features, and may be mistaken for true neoplasms. In fact, some of these—such as basaloid follicular hamartoma—have already been discussed somewhat arbitrarily as neoplastic in the preceding material. Others are considered in the following.

HAIR FOLLICLE HAMARTOMA

A form of "follicular hamartoma" has been described that is probably related to BFH (see the preceding). It resembles a multifocal-superficial of trichoepithelioma (TE), replacing each hair follicle in a confined segment of skin and also featuring an association with hyperplastic sebaceous glands.[155]

Differential Diagnosis   Points of distinction from true TE include the presence of mature hair and proliferating outer root sheath elements in this form of follicular hamartoma.

HAIR FOLLICLE NEVUS

Clinical and Histopathological Features   Hair follicle nevi are seen in patients of all ages, as nondescript, 1- to 5-mm, flesh-colored, smooth-surfaced papules in hair-bearing skin. Histologically, they are constituted by a localized proliferation of miniature hair follicles, the contents of which approximate the size of vellus hairs.[241–243] The interfollicular stroma is composed of variably dense fibrovascular tissue.

Differential Diagnosis   Misdiagnosis as a form of trichoepithelioma may be avoided by attention to the fact that TE does not demonstrate the advanced degree of hair formation seen in follicular nevi. Constituent cell populations are also different in these lesions, with TE featuring much more basaloid elements.

SMOOTH MUSCLE HAMARTOMA AND BECKER'S NEVUS

Clinical Features   Cutaneous smooth muscle hamartomas (SMHs), which may be confused with either pilar leiomyoma or pilar leiomyosarcoma, may be either congenital or acquired in childhood. In addition, they probably comprise part of the spectrum of "Becker's nevus."[244–253] These proliferations are solitary and usually are seen on the trunk or the extremities; they are manifest as lightly pigmented patches or plaques and measure up to 10 cm in diameter. Hypertrichosis also is commonly associated with SMH. Slight manual irritation of the lesion produces "pseudo-Darier's sign," in which a short-lived elevation ("pseudo-urtication") of the lesion eventuates; however, SMHs are painless.

Histopathological Features   There are abnormal bundles of smooth muscle in the reticular dermis and subcutis, arranged in haphazard or widely separated skeins. These often have an attachment to arrector pili muscles. "Pure" myogenous hamartomas are not associated with abnormalities in the epidermis. Nevertheless, Slifman and colleagues reported that some examples of Becker's nevus—in which surface acanthosis, papillomatosis, hypertrichosis, and hyperpigmentation are observed—also exhibit the presence of dermal myogenic proliferations that are indistinguishable from those of SMH.[256]

Differential Diagnosis   The distinction between SMH and true cutaneous smooth muscle tumors necessitates correlation between clinical data and histologic findings. Myogenous neoplasms of the skin are rare in children, whereas it is typical for SMH to be found in early life. Moreover, leiomyomas usually have a sharp microscopic interface with the adjacent stroma, whereas SMH exhibits a "ragged" peripheral margin and disorganized fascicular growth like that of muscular sarcomas. In specific counterpoint to the latter tumors, it is important to note that mitoses, nuclear atypia, and necrosis are not apparent in SMH.

NEUROFOLLICULAR AND PILAR-NEUROCRISTIC HAMARTOMAS

Two other peculiar dermal mesenchymal proliferations that are putatively related to the hair follicles have been described within the last 15 years. These have been dubbed "neurofollicular hamartoma" (NH) and "pilar neurocristic hamartoma" (PNH), although a true relationship of such lesions to the hair follicles is inferred at best, and their hamartomatous nature is also questionable.[254–257]

Clinical and Histopathological Features　Neurofollicular hamartoma is said to present as a solitary papule in the skin of the face, in children as well as adults. Histologically, it bears a resemblance to both angiofibroma and neurofibroma, consisting of a tangle of bland spindle cell fascicles that are laterally bounded by hyperplastic pilosebaceous units. S100 protein and silver-positive material is seen in NH by special staining methods, and it is therefore thought to represent a malformation of nerve endings serving the hair follicles. However, it should be noted that Sangueza and Requena found no reproducible differences between NH and trichodiscoma in a formal comparative analysis, making it more than possible that these tumefactions are synonymous.[265]

Clinical and Histopathological Features　Pilar-neurocristic hamartoma differs from the description just given, both clinically and pathologically. It is a pigmented papule or plaque in the skin of the head and neck, potentially affecting patients of all ages. Microscopically, one sees an interdigitating proliferation of bland, spindle cells—with some containing melanin pigment—in a tight perifollicular configuration in the dermis. Ultrastructural studies have demonstrated a mixture of melanocytic and Schwann cell features in this lesion, likening it to the blue nevus.[257] Moreover, Pathy et al. and Pearson and coworkers have described several cases in which malignant melanomas have arisen secondarily in PNH.[258,259] Based on those findings, the authors prefer to view the latter lesion as a melanocytic nevus variant rather than a pilar-related hamartoma.

REFERENCES

1. Ackerman AB, DeViragh PA, Chongchitnant N: *Neoplasms with Follicular Differentiation*, Lea & Febiger, Philadelphia, 1993.
2. Hashimoto K, Mehregan AH, Kumakiri M: *Tumors of Skin Appendages*, Butterworths, Boston, 1987.
3. Wick MR, Swanson PE: *Cutaneous Adnexal Tumors: A Guide to Pathologic Diagnosis*, ASCP Press, Chicago, 1991.
4. Czarnecki UB, Dorevitch AP: Giant senile sebaceous hyperplasia. *Arch Dermatol* 122:1101–1102, 1986.
5. Kumar P, Marks R: Sebaceous gland hyperplasia and senile comedones: A prevalence study in elderly hospitalized patients. *Br J Dermatol* 117:231–236, 1987.
6. Luderschmidt C, Plewig G: Circumscribed sebaceous gland hyperplasia: autoradiographic and histoplanometric studies. *J Invest Dermatol* 70:207–209, 1978.
7. Kudoh K, Hosokawa M, Miyazawa T, Tagami H: Giant solitary sebaceous gland hyperplasia clinically simulating epidermoid cyst. *J Cutan Pathol* 15:396–398, 1988.
8. Bhawan J, Calhoun J: Premature sebaceous gland hyperplasia. *J Am Acad Dermatol* 8:136, 1983.
9. De Villez RL, Roberts JC: Premature sebaceous gland hyperplasia. *J Am Acad Dermatol* 6:933–935, 1982.
10. Dupre A, Bonafe J, Lamon R: Functional familial sebaceous hyperplasia of the face: reverse of the Cunliffe acne-free nevus? Its inclusion among naevoid sebaceous receptor disease. *Clin Exp Dermatol* 5:202–207, 1980.
11. Graham-Brown RAC, McGibbon DH, Sarkany I: A papular placque-like eruption of the face due to naevoid sebaceous gland hyperplasia. *Clin Exp Dermatol* 8:379–382, 1983.
12. Catalano PM, Ioannides A: Areolar sebaceous hyperplasia. *J Am Acad Dermatol* 13:867–868, 1985.
13. Farina MC, Soriano ML, Escalonilla P, Pique E, Martin L, Barat A, Requena L: Unilateral areolar sebaceous hyperplasia in a male. *Am J Dermatopathol* 18:417–419, 1996.
14. Rocamora A, Santonja C, Vives R, Varona C: Sebaceous gland hyperplasia of the vulva: a case report. *Obstet Gynecol* 68:63s–65s, 1986.
15. Lever WF: Sebaceous adenoma: Review of the literature and report of a case. *Arch Dermatol* 57:102–111, 1948.
16. Warren S, Warvi WN: Tumors of sebaceous glands. *Am J Pathol* 19:441–460, 1943.
17. Prioleau PG, Santa Cruz DJ: Sebaceous gland neoplasia. *J Cutan Pathol* 11:396–414, 1984.
18. Rulon DB, Helwig EB: Cutaneous sebaceous neoplasms. *Cancer* 33:82–102, 1974.
19. Brownstein MH, Shapiro L: The pilosebaceous tumors. *Int J Dermatol* 16:340–352, 1977.
20. Mehregan AH, Rahbari H: Benign epithelial tumors of the skin. II. Benign sebaceous tumors. *Cutis* 19:317–320, 1977.
21. Reiffers J, Laugier P, Hunziker N: Sebaceous hyperplasias, keratoacanthomas, epitheliomas of the face, and cancer of the colon: A new entity? *Dermatologica* 153:23–33, 1976.
22. Rulon DB, Helwig EB: Multiple sebaceous neoplasms of the skin: An association wtih multiple visceral carcinomas, especially of the colon. *Am J Clin Pathol* 60:745–753, 1973.
23. Sciallis GF, Winkelmann RK: Multiple sebaceous adenomas and gastrointestinal carcinoma. *Arch Dermatol* 110:913–916, 1974.
24. Housholder MS, Zeligman I: Sebaceous neoplasms associated with visceral carcinomas. *Arch Dermatol* 116:61–64, 1980.
25. Tschang TP, Poulos E, Ho CK: Multiple sebaceouss adenomas and internal malignant disease: a case report with chromosomal analysis. *Hum Pathol* 7:589–594, 1976.
26. Fahmy A, Burgdorf WHC, Schosser RH, Pitha J: Muir-Torre syndrome: Reevaluation of the dermatological features and consideration of its relationship to the family cancer syndrome. *Cancer* 49:1898–1903, 1973.
27. Burgdorf WHC, Pitha J, Fahmy A: Muir–Torre syndrome: Histologic spectrum of sebaceous proliferations. *Am J Dermatopathol* 8:202–208, 1986.
28. Davis DA, Cohen PR: Genitourinary tumors in men with the Muir-Torre syndrome. *J Am Acad Dermatol* 33:909–912, 1995.
29. Lasser A, Carter DM: Multiple basal cell epitheliomas with sebaceous differentiation. *Arch Dermatol* 107:91–93, 1973.
30. McMullan FH: Sebaceous epithelioma. *Arch Dermatol* 71:725–727, 1955.
31. Zackheim HS: The sebaceous epithelioma. *Arch Dermatol* 89:711–724, 1964.
32. Okuda C, Ito M, Fujiwara H, Takenouchi T: Sebaceous epithelioma with sweat gland differentiation. *Am J Dermatopathol* 17:523–528, 1995.
33. Sanchez-Yus E, Requena L, Simon P, del Rio E: Sebomatricoma: A unifying term that encompasses all benign neoplasms with sebaceous differentiation. *Am J Dermatopathol* 17:213–221, 1995.
34. Rothko F, Farmer ER, Zeligman I: Superficial epithelioma with sebaceous differentiation. *Arch Dermatol* 116:329–331, 1980.
35. Friedman KJ, Boudreau S, Farmer ER: Superficial epithelioma with sebaceous differentiation. *J Cutan Pathol* 14:193–197, 1987.
36. Troy JL, Ackerman AB: Sebaceoma: A distinctive benign neoplasm of adnexal epithelium differentiating toward sebaceous cells. *Am J Dermatopathol* 6:7–13, 1984.
37. Zaim MT: Sebocrine adenoma: An adnexal adenoma with sebaceous and apocrine poroma-like differentiation. *Am J Dermatopathol* 10:311–318, 1988.
38. Grosshans E, Hanau D: L'adenome infundibulaire: un porome folliculaire a' differenciation sebacee et apocrine. *Ann Dermatol Venereol* 108:59–66, 1981.
39. Wick MR, Goellner JR, Wolfe JT III, Su WPD: Adnexal carcinomas of the skin. II. Extraocular sebaceous carcinomas. *Cancer* 56:1163–1172, 1985.
40. Wolfe JT III, Wick MR, Campbell RJ: Sebaceous carcinomas of the oculocutaneous adnexa and extraocular skin, in Wick MR (ed): *Pathology of Unusual Malignant Cutaneous Tumors*. New York: Marcel Dekker, 1985, pp. 77–106.
41. Wolfe JT III, Campbell RJ, Yeatts RP, Waller RR, Wick MR: Sebaceous carcinoma of the eyelid: Errors in clinical and pathologic diagnosis. *Am J Surg Pathol* 8:597–606, 1984.
42. Rao NA, Hidayat AA, McLean IW, Zimmerman LE: Sebaceous carcinoma of the ocular adnexa: A clinicopathologic study of 104 cases, with five-year followup data. *Hum Pathol* 13:113–122, 1982.
43. Ni C, Kuo PK: Meibomian gland carcinoma: A clinicopathological study of 156 cases with long-period followup of 100 cases. *Jpn J Ophthalmol* 23:388–401, 1979.
44. Graham RM, McKee PH, McGibbon D: Sebaceous carcinoma. *Clin Exp Dermatol* 9:466–471, 1984.
45. Doxanas MT, Green WR: Sebaceous gland carcinoma: Review of 40 cases. *Arch Ophthalmol* 102:245–249, 1984.
46. Ausidio RA, Lodeville O, Quaglivolo V, Clemente C: Sebaceous carcinoma arising from the eyelid and from extraocular sites. *Tumori* 73:531–535, 1987.

47. Nguyen GK, Mielke BW: Extraocular sebaceous carcinoma with intraepidermal (pagetoid) spread. *Am J Dermatopathol* 9:304–305, 1987.

48. Nelson BR, Hamlet KR, Gillard M, Railan D, Johnson TM: Sebaceous carcinoma. *J Am Acad Dermatol* 33:1–15, 1995.

49. Harvey PA, Parsons MA, Rennie IG: Primary sebaceous carcinoma of lacrimal gland: A previously unreported primary neoplasm. *Eye* 8:592–595, 1994.

50. Ansai S, Hashimoto H, Aoki T, Hozumi Y, Aso K: A histochemical and immunohistochemical study of extraocular sebaceous carcinoma. *Histopathology* 22:127–133, 1993.

51. Oppenheim AR: Sebaceous carcinoma of the penis. *Arch Dermatol* 117:306–307, 1981.

52. Russell WB, Page DL, Hough AJ, Lodgers LW: Sebaceous carcinoma of meibomian gland origin: Tthe diagnostic importance of pagetoid spread of neoplastic cells. *Am J Clin Pathol* 73:504–511, 1980.

53. Nakamura SI, Nakayama K, Nishihara K, Imai T: Sebaceous carcinoma, with special reference to the histopathologic differential diagnosis. *J Dermatol* 15:55–59, 1988.

54. Suster S: Clear cell tumors of the skin. *Semin Diagn Pathol* 13:40–59, 1996.

55. Swanson PE, Wick MR: Immunohistochemistry of cutaneous tumors, in Leong ASY (ed): *Applied Immunohistochemistry for the Surgical Pathologist*. London: Edward Arnold, pp. 269–308.

56. Jimenez FJ, Burchette JL Jr, Grichnik JM, Hitchcock MG: BER–EP4 immunoreactivity in normal skin and cutaneous neoplasms. *Mod Pathol* 8:854–858, 1995.

57. Wick MR, Fitzgibbon JF, Swanson PE: Cutaneous sarcomas and sarcomatoid neoplasms of the skin. *Semin Diagn Pathol* 10:148–158, 1993.

58. Mehregan AH, Pinkus H: Life history of organoid nevi: Special reference to nevus sebaceus of Jadassohn. *Arch Dermatol* 91:574–587, 1965.

59. Morioka S: The natural history of nevus sebaceus. *J Cutan Pathol* 12:200–213, 1985.

60. Lentz CL, Altman J, Mopper C: Nevus sebaceus of Jadassohn. *Arch Dermatol* 97:294–296, 1968.

61. Wilson–Jones E, Heyl T: Nevus sebaceus: A report of 140 cases with special regard to the development of secondary malignant tumors. *Br J Dermatol* 82:99–105, 1970.

62. Clancy RR, Kurtz MB, Baker D, Sladky JT, Honig PJ, Younkin DP: Neurologic manifestations of the organoid nevus syndrome. *Arch Neurol* 42:236–240, 1985.

63. Zaremba J: Jadassohn's nevus phakomatosis: A study based on a review of 37 cases. *J Ment Defic Res* 22:103–122, 1977.

64. Alessi E, Wong SN, Advani HH, Ackerman AB: Nevus sebaceus is associated with unusual neoplasms: An atlas. *Am J Dermatopathol* 10:116–127, 1988.

65. Ng WK: Nevus sebaceus with apocrine and sebaceous differentiation. *Am J Dermatopathol* 18:420–423, 1996.

66. Domingo J, Helwig EB: Malignant neoplasms associated with nevus sebaceus of Jadassohn. *J Am Acad Dermatol* 1:545–556, 1979.

67. Tarkhan H, Domingo J: Metastasizing eccrine porocarcinoma developing in a nevus sebaceus of Jadassohn: Report of a case. *Arch Dermatol* 121:413–415, 1985.

68. Mehregan AH, Butler JD: A tumor of the follicular infundibulum: Report of a case. *Arch Dermatol* 1961; 83:924–927, 1961.

69. Mehregan AH: Tumor of follicular infundibulum. *Dermatologica* 142:177–183, 1971.

70. Trunell TN, Waisman M: Tumor of the follicular infundibulum. *Cutis* 23:317–318, 1979.

71. Mehregan AH: Infundibular tumors of the skin. *J Cutan Pathol* 11:387–395, 1984.

72. Kossard S, Finley AG, Poyzer K, Kocsard E: Eruptive infundibulomas: A distinctive presentation of the tumor of follicular infundibulum. *J Am Acad Dermatol* 21:361–366, 1989.

73. Cribier B, Grosshans E: Tumor of the follicular infundibulum: A clinicopathologic study. *J Am Acad Dermatol* 33:979–984, 1995.

74. Horn TD, Vennos EM, Bernstein BD, Cooper PH: Multiple tumors of follicular infundibulum with sweat duct differentiation. *J Cutan Pathol* 22:281–287, 1995.

75. Bhawan J: Pilar sheath acanthoma: A new benign follicular tumor. *J Cutan Pathol* 6:438–440, 1979.

76. Mehregan AH, Brownstein MH: Pilar sheath acanthoma. *Arch Dermatol* 114:1495–1497, 1978.

77. Lee JYY, Hiesch G: Pilar sheath acanthoma. *Arch Dermatol* 123:569–570, 1987.

78. Hurt MA: Pilar sheath acanthoma (lobular infundibuloisthmicoma). *Am J Dermatopathol* 18:435, 1996.

79. Winer LH: The dilated pore, a trichoepithelioma. *J Invest Dermatol* 23:181–188, 1954.

80. Klovekorn G, Klovekorn W, Plewig G, Pinkus H: Riesenpore und haarseidenakanthom: Klinische und histologische diagnose. *Hautarzt* 34:209–216, 1983.

81. Rahbari H, Mehregan AH, Pinkus H: Trichoadenoma of Nikolowski. *J Cutan Pathol* 4:90–98, 1977.

82. Yamaguchi J, Takino C: A case of trichoadenoma arising in the buttock. *J Dermatol* 19:503–506, 1992.

83. Nikolowski W: Trichoadenom. *Z Hautkr* 53:87–90, 1978.

84. Undeutsch W, Rassner G: Das Trichoadenom (Nikolowski): Ein klinischer und histologischer Fallbericht. *Hautarzt* 35:650–652, 1984.

85. Sieron J, Thein T, Pirsig W, Hemmer J: The Nikolowski trichoadenoma: A rare tumor of the ENT area. *Laryngo Rhino Otologie* 72:140–142, 1993.

86. Brownstein MH, Shapiro L: Trichilemmoma: Analysis of 40 new cases. *Arch Dermatol* 107:866–869, 1973.

87. Hidayat AA, Font RL: Trichilemmoma of the eyelid and eyebrow: A clinicopathologic study of 31 cases. *Arch Ophthalmol* 98:844–847, 1980.

88. Reifler DM, Ballitch HA II, Kessler DL, Stawiski MA, O'Gawa GM: Tricholemmoma of the eyelid. *Opthalmology* 94:1272–1275, 1987.

89. Brownstein MH, Wolf H, Bikowski JB: Cowden's disease: A cutaneous marker of breast cancer. *Cancer* 41:2393–2398, 1978.

90. Brownstein MH, Mehregan AH, Bikowski JB, Lupulescu A, Patterson JC: The dermatopathology of Cowden's syndrome. *Br J Dermatol* 100:667–673, 1979.

91. Starink TM, Meijer CJLM, Brownstein MH: The cutaneous pathology of Cowden's disease: Nnew findings. *J Cutan Pathol* 12:83–93, 1985.

92. Reed RJ, Pulitzer DR: Inverted follicular keratosis and human papillomaviruses. *Am J Dermatopathol* 5:453–465, 1983.

93. Spielvogel RL, Austin C, Ackerman AB: Inverted follicular keratosis is not a specific keratosis but a verruca vulgaris (or seborrheic keratosis) with squamous eddies. *Am J Dermatopathol* 5:427–442, 1983.

94. Hunt SJ, Kilzer PB, Santa Cruz DJ: Desmoplastic trichilemmoma: Histologic variant resembling invasive carcinoma. *J Cutan Pathol* 17:45–52, 1990.

95. Tellechea O, Reis JP, Baptista AP: Desmoplastic trichilemmoma. *Am J Dermatopathol* 14:107–114, 1992.

96. Leppard BJ, Sanderson KV: The natural history of trichilemmal cysts. *Br J Dermatol* 95:379–390, 1976.

97. Laing V, Knipe RC, Flowers FP, Stoer CB, Ramcos-Caro FA: Proliferating trichilemmal tumor: Report of a case and review of the literature. *J Dermatol Surg Oncol* 17:295–298, 1991.

98. Yamaguchi J, Irimajiri T, Ohara K: Proliferating trichilemmal cyst arising in the arm of a young woman. *Dermatology* 189:90–92, 1994.

99. Mann B, Salm R, Azzopardi JG: Pilar tumor: A distinctive type of trichilemmoma. *Diagn Histopathol* 5:157–167, 1982.

100. Baptista AP, Silva LGE, Born MC: Proliferating trichilemmal cyst. *J Cutan Pathol* 10:178–187, 1983.

101. Janitz J, Wiedersberg H: Trichilemmal pilar tumors. *Cancer* 45:1594–1597, 1980.

102. Brownstein MH, Arluk DJ: Proliferating trichilemmal cyst: A simulant of squamous cell carcinoma. *Cancer* 48:1207–1214, 1981.

103. Jacobson M, Ackerman AB: "Shadow" cells as clues to follicular differentiation. *Am J Dermatopathol* 9:51–57, 1987.

104. Pinkus H, Sutton RL: Trichofolliculoma. *Arch Dermatol* 91:46–49, 1965.

105. Gray HR, Helwig EB: Trichofolliculoma. *Arch Dermatol* 86:619–625, 1962.

106. Plewig G: Sebaceous trichofolliculoma. *J Cutan Pathol* 7:394–403, 1980.

107. Shuttleworth D, Graham-Brown RAC, Barton RPE: Median nasal dermoid fistula. *Clin Exp Dermatol* 10:262–273, 1985.

108. Foot NC: Adnexal carcinoma of the skin. *Am J Pathol* 23:1–21, 1947.

109. Gray HR, Helwig EB: Epithelioma adenoides cysticum and solitary trichoepithelioma. *Arch Dermatol* 87:102–114, 1963.

110. Zeligman I: Solitary trichoepithelioma. *Arch Dermatol* 82:35–41, 1960.

111. Lever WF: Pathogenesis of benign tumors of cutaneous appendages and of basal cell epithelioma. *Arch Dermatol Syphilol* 57:679–689, 1948.

112. Gaul LE: Heredity of multiple benign cystic epithelioma: "Tthe Indiana family." *Arch Dermatol* 68:517–524, 1953.

113. Guillot B, Buffiere I, Barneon G, Bensadoun D, Guilhou JJ, Meynadier J: Trichoepithelioma multiples, cylindromes, grains de milium: Une entite. *Ann Dermatol Venereol* 114:175–182, 1987.

114. Pariser RJ: Multiple hereditary trichoepitheliomas and basal cell carcinomas. *J Cutan Pathol* 13:111–117, 1986.

115. Rasmussen JE: A syndrome of trichoepitheliomas, milia, and cylindroma. *Arch Dermatol* 111:610–614, 1975.

116. Rockerbie N, Solomon AR, Woo TY, Beals TF, Ellis LN: Malignant dermal cylindroma in a patient with multiple dermal cylindromas, trichoepitheliomas, and bilateral dermal analogue tumors of the parotid gland. *Am J Dermatopathol* 11:353–359, 1989.

117. Michaelsson G, Olsson E, Westermark P: The Rombo Syndrome: A familial disorder with vermiculate atrophoderma, milia, hypotrichosis, trichoepitheliomas, basal cell carcinoma, and peripheral vasodilatation with cyanosis. *Acta Dermatol Venereol* 61:497–503, 1981.

118. Starink TM, Lane EB, Meijer CJ: Generalized trichoepitheliomas with alopecia and myasthenia gravis: Clinicopathologic and immunohistochemical study and comparison with classic and desmoplastic trichoepithelioma. *J Am Acad Dermatol* 15:1104–1112, 1986.

119. Long SA, Hurt MA, Santa Cruz DJ: Immature trichoepithelioma: Report of six cases. *J Cutan Pathol* 15:353–358, 1988.

120. Brook JD, Fitzpatrick JE, Golitz LE: Papillary mesenchymal bodies: A histological finding useful in differentiating trichoepitheliomas from basal cell carcinomas. *J Am Acad Dermatol* 21:523–528, 1989.

121. Chen S: Trichoepitheliocarcinoma: Report of five cases. *Zhonghua Binglixue Zazhi* 11:143–145, 1982.

122. Howell JB, Anderson DE: Transformation of epithelioma adenoides cysticum into multiple rodent ulcers: Fact or fallacy?. *Br J Dermatol* 95:233–242, 1976.

123. Kirchmann TT, Prieto VG, Smoller BR: CD34 staining pattern distinguishes basal cell carcinoma from trichoepithelioma. *Arch Dermatol* 130:589–592, 1994.

124. Bryant D, Penneys NS: Immunostaining for CD34 to determine trichoepithelioma. *Arch Dermatol* 131:616–617, 1995.

125. Morales–Ducret CR, van de Rijn M, LeBrun DP, Smoller BR: *bcl–2* expression in primary malignancies of the skin. *Arch Dermatol* 131:909–912, 1995.

126. Nakagawa K, Yamamura K, Maeda S, Ichihashi M: *bcl–2* expression in epidermal keratinocytic diseases. *Cancer* 74:1720–1724, 1994.

127. Fitzpatrick M, Adesokan PN, Ritter JH, et al: Immunohistologic differential diagnosis of basal cell carcinoma, squamous cell carcinoma, and trichoepithelioma in small cutaneous biopsy specimens. *Am J Clin Pathol* 103:508, 1995.

128. Brownstein MH, Shapiro L: Desmoplastic trichoepithelioma. *Cancer* 40:2979–2986, 1977.

129. Bernstein G, Roth GJ: Sclerosing epithelial hamartoma. *J Dermatol Surg Oncol* 4: 87–90, 1978.

130. Dammert K, Kallionen M: Das desmoplastiche Trichoepitheliom: Klinik, Histologie, und Differentialdiagnose. *Hautarzt* 38:606, 1987.

131. MacDonald DM, Wilson-Jones E, Marks R: Sclerosing epithelial hamartoma. *Clin Exp Dermatol* 2:153–160, 1977.

132. Takei Y, Fukushiro S, Ackerman AB: Criteria for histologic differentiation of desmoplastic trichoepithelioma (sclerosing epithelial hamartoma) from morphea-like basal cell carcinoma. *Am J Dermatopathol* 7:207–211, 1985.

133. Wick MR, Cooper PH, Swanson PE, Kaye VN, Sun TT: Microcystic adnexal carcinoma: An immunohistochemical comparison with other cutaneous appendage tumors. *Arch Dermatol* 126:189–194, 1990.

134. Forbis R, Helwig EB: Pilomatrixoma (calcifying epithelioma). *Arch Dermatol* 83: 606–618, 1961.

135. Moehlenbeck FW: Pilomatrixoma (calcifying epithelioma). *Arch Dermatol* 108: 532–534, 1973.

136. Taaffe A, Wyatt EH, Bury HPR: Pilomatrixoma (Malherbe). A clinical and histological survey of 78 cases. *Int J Dermatol* 27:477–480, 1988.

137. Kaddu S, Soyer HP, Cerroni L, Salmhofer W, Hodl S: Clinical and histopathological spectrum of pilomatricoma in adults. *Int J Dermatol* 33:705–708, 1994.

138. Marrogi AJ, Wick MR, Dehner LP: Pilomatrical neoplasms in children and young adults. *Am J Dermatopathol* 14:87–94, 1992.

139. Kaddu S, Soyer HP, Hodl S, Kerl H: Morphological stages of pilomatricoma. *Am J Dermatopathol* 18:333–338, 1996.

140. Ter Poorten HJ, Sharbaugh AH: Extruding pilomatricoma: Report of a case. *Cutis* 22:47–49, 1978.

141. Tsoitis G, Mandinaos C, Kanitakis JC: Perforating calcifying epithelioma of Malherbe with a rapid evolution. *Dermatologica* 168:233–237, 1984.

142. Zulaica A, Peteiro C, Quintas C, Pereiro M Jr, Toribio J: Perforating pilomatricoma. *J Cutan Pathol* 15:409–411, 1988.

143. Alli N, Gungor E, Artuz F: Perforating pilomatricoma. *J Am Acad Dermatol* 35: 116–118, 1996.

144. Lee WS, Yoo MS, Ahn SK: Anetodermic cutaneous changes overlying pilomatricoma. *Int J Dermatol* 34:144–145, 1995.

145. Shames BS, Nassif A, Bailey CS, Saltzstein SL: Secondary anetoderma involving a pilomatricoma. *Am J Dermatopathol* 16:557–560, 1994.

146. Inglefield CJ, Muir IF, Gray ES: Aggressive pilomatricoma in childhood. *Ann Plast Surg* 33:656–658, 1994.

147. Aloi FG, Molinero A, Pippione M: Basal cell carcinoma with matrical differentiation. *Am J Dermatopathol* 10:509–513, 1988.

148. Sau P, Lupton GP, Graham JH: Trichogerminoma: Report of 14 cases. *J Cutan Pathol* 19:357–365, 1992.

149. Mehregan AH, Baker S: Basaloid follicular hamartoma: Report of three cases with localized and systematized unilateral lesions. *J Cutan Pathol* 12:55–65, 1985.

150. Anderson TE, Best PV: Linear basal cell nevus. *Br J Dermatol* 74:20–23, 1962.

151. Brown AC, Crounse RG, Winkelmann RK: Generalized hair follicle hamartoma: Associated with alopecia, aminoaciduria, and myasthenia gravis. *Arch Dermatol* 99: 478–493, 1969.

152. Brownstein MH: Basaloid follicular hamartoma: Solitary and multiple types. *J Am Acad Dermatol* 27:237–240, 1992.

153. Bleiberg J, Brodkin RH: Linear unilateral basal cell nevus with comedones. *Arch Dermatol* 100:187–190, 1969.

154. Delacretaz J, Balsiger F: Hamartoma folliculaire multiple familial. *Dermatologica* 159:316–324, 1979.

155. Alessi E, Azzolini A: Localized hair follicle hamartoma. *J Cutan Pathol* 20:364–367, 1993.

156. Requena L, Barat A: Giant trichoblastoma on the scalp. *Am J Dermatopathol* 15: 497–502, 1993.

157. Schirren CG, Rutten A, Sander C, McClain S, Diaz C, Kind P: Trichoblastoma: a tumor with follicular differentiation. *Hautarzt* 46:81–86, 1995.

158. Rosen LB: A review and proposed new classification of benign acquired neoplasms with hair follicle differentiation. *Am J Dermatopathol* 12:496–516, 1990.

159. Headington JT: Tumors of the hair follicle: A review. *Am J Pathol* 85:480–505, 1976.

160. Altman DA, Mikhail GR, Johnson TM, Lowe L: Trichoblastic fibroma: A series of 10 cases with a report of a new plaque variant. *Arch Dermatol* 131:198–201, 1995.

161. Imai S, Nitto H: Trichogenic trichoblastoma. *Hautarzt* 33:609–611, 1982.

162. Wong TY, Reed JA, Suster S, Flynn SD, Mihm MC Jr: Benign trichogenic tumors: A report of two cases supporting a simplified nomenclature. *Histopathology* 22:575–580, 1993.

163. Aloi F, Tomasini C, Pippione M: Pigmented trichoblastoma. *Am J Dermatopathol* 14:345–349, 1992.

164. Chan JK, Ng CS, Tsang WY: Nodular desmoplastic variant of trichoblastoma. *Am J Surg Pathol* 18:495–500, 1994.

165. Pinkus H, Coskey R, Burgess GH: Trichodiscoma: A benign tumor related to *Haarscheibe* (hair disc). *J Invest Dermatol* 63:212–218, 1974.

166. Camarasa JG, Calderon P, Moreno A: Familial multiple trichodiscomas. *Acta Dermatol Venereol* 68:163–165, 1988.

167. Coskey RJ, Pinkus H: Trichodiscoma. *Int J Dermatol* 15:600–601, 1976.

168. Grosshans E, Dungler T, Hanau D: Le trichodiscome de Pinkus. *Ann Dermatol Venereol* 108:837–846, 1981.

169. Starink TM, Kisch LS, Meijer CJLM: Familial multiple trichodiscomas: A clinicopathologic study. *Arch Dermatol* 121:888–891, 1985.

170. Moreno A, Puig LL, deMoragas JM: Multiple fibrofolliculomas and trichodiscomas. *Dermatologica* 171:338–342, 1985.

171. Duperrat B, Menanteau Y: Le fibrome perifolliculaire. *Ann Dermatol Syphilol* 96: 121–128, 1969.

172. Pinkus H: Perifollicular fibromas: Pure periadnexal adventitial tumors. *Am J Dermatopathol* 1:341–342, 1979.

173. Freeman RG, Chernosky ME: Perifollicular fibroma. *Arch Dermatol* 100:66–69, 1969.

174. Zackheim MS, Pinkus H: Perifollicular fibromas. *Arch Dermatol* 82:913–917, 1960.

175. Steigleder GK: Perifollikulaeres Fibrom (Zackheim und Pinkus). *Hautarzt* 13:370–371, 1962.

176. Miegel WN, Ackerman AB: Fibrous papules of the face. *Am J Dermatopathol* 1:329–340, 1979.

177. Reed RJ, Hairston MA, Palomeque RE: The histologic identity of adenoma sebaceum and solitary melanocytic angiofibroma. *Dermatologica Int* 5:3–7, 1966.

178. Sanchez NP, Wick MR, Perry HO: Adenoma sebaceum of Pringle: A clinicopathologic review, with a discussion of related pathologic entities. *J Cutan Pathol* 8:395–403, 1981.

179. Junkins-Hopkins JM, Cooper PH: Multiple perifollicular fibromas: Review of a case and analysis of the literature. *J Cutan Pathol* 21:467–471, 1994.

180. Schachtschabel AA, Kuster W, Happle R: Perifollicular fibroma of the skin and colonic polyps: Hornstein-Knickenberg syndrome. *Hautarzt* 47:304–306, 1996.

181. Balus L, Fazio M, Sacerdoti G, Morrone A, Marmo W: Fibrofolliculomes, trichodiscomes, et acrochordons: syndrome de Birt-Hogg-Dube. *Ann Dermatol Venereol* 110: 601–609, 1983.

182. Birt AR, Hogg GR, Dube WJ: Hereditary multiple fibrofolliculomas with trichodiscomas and acrochordons. *Arch Dermatol* 113:1674–1677, 1977.

183. Foucar K, Rosen T, Foucar E, Cochran R: Fibrofolliculoma: A clinicopathologic study. *Cutis* 28:429–432, 1981.

184. Scully K, Bargmann H, Assaad D: Solitary fibrofolliculoma. *J Am Acad Dermatol* 11:361–363, 1984.

185. Weintraub R, Pinkus H: Multiple fibrofolliculomas (Birt-Hogg-Dube) associated with a large connective tissue nevus. *J Cutan Pathol* 4:289–299, 1977.

186. Steffen C, Mantleoma: A benign neoplasm with mantle differentiation. *Am J Dermatopathol* 15:306–310, 1993.

187. Headington JT: Differentiating neoplasms of hair germ. *J Clin Pathol* 23:464–471, 1970.

188. Carney JA, Headington JT, Su WPD: Cutaneous myxomas: A major component of the complex of myxomas, spotty pigmentation, and endocrine overactivity. *Arch Dermatol* 122:790–798, 1986.

189. Aterhton DJ, Pitcher DW, Wells RS, MacDonald DM: A syndrome of various cutaneous pigmented lesions, mxyoid neurofibromata, and atrial myxoma: The NAME syndrome. *Br J Dermatol* 103:421–429, 1980.

190. Montgomery H, Winkelmann RK: Smooth muscle tumors of the skin. *Arch Dermatol* 79:32–40, 1959.

191. Fisher WC, Helwig EB: Leiomyomas of the skin. *Arch Dermatol* 88:510–521, 1963.

192. Sangueza P, Sangueza O, Sangueza L, Martin-Sangueza J: Eruptive and progressive cutaneous leiomyomatosis associated with cerebrovascular abnormalities and osteoma of the petrous bone. *Med Cutan Ibero Latino Am* 17:169–173, 1989.

193. Beham A, Badve S, Suster, Fletcher CDM: Solitary myofibroma in adults: Clinicopathological analysis of a series. *Histopathology* 22:335–341, 1993.

194. Argenyi ZB: Recent developments in cutaneous neural neoplasms. *J Cutan Pathol* 20:97–108, 1993.

195. Megahed M: Palisaded encapsulated neuroma (solitary circumscribed neuroma): A clinicopathologic and immunohistochemical study. *Am J Dermatopathol* 16:120–125, 1994.

196. Ten Seldam REJ: Tricholemmocarcinoma. *Australas J Dermatol* 18:62–72, 1977.

197. Krumrey KW: The tricholemmal carcinoma: Report of a case with review of the literature. *Aktuel Dermatol* 10:70–72, 1984.

198. Schell H, Haneke E: Tricholemmal carcinoma: Report of 11 cases. *Hautarzt* 37: 384–387, 1986.

199. Grouls V: Tricholemmale Keratose und tricholemmales Karzinom. *Hautarzt* 38: 335–341, 1987.

200. Boscaino A, Terracciano LM, Donofrio V, Ferrara G, DeRosa G: Trichilemmal carcinoma: A study of seven cases. *J Cutan Pathol* 19:94–99, 1992.

201. Swanson PE, Marrogi AJ, Williams DJ, Cherwitz DL, Wick MR: Trichilemmal carcinoma. *J Cutan Pathol* 19:100–109, 1992.

202. Reis JP, Tellechea O, Cunha MF, Baptista AP: Trichilemmal carcinoma: Review of eight cases. *J Cutan Pathol* 20:44–49, 1993.

203. Wong TY, Suster S: Trichilemmal carcinoma: A clinicopathologic study of 13 cases. *Am J Dermatopathol* 16:463–473, 1994.

204. Amaral A, Nascimento A, Goellner JR: Proliferating pilar (trichilemmal) cyst: report of 2 cases, one with carcinomatous transformation and one with distant metastases. *Arch Pathol Lab Med* 108:808–810, 1984.

205. Batman PA, Evans HJR: Metastasizing pilar tumor of the scalp. *J Clin Pathol* 39: 757–760, 1986.

206. Dabska M: Giant hair matrix tumor. *Cancer* 28:701–706, 1971.

207. Dominguez-Arranz M, Morandeira-Garcia MJ, Arraiza-Goicoechea A, Morandeira-Garcia JR, Grasa-Jordan MP: Malignant proliferative tricholemmal tumor: A clinical, morphologic, and ultrastructural study. *Rev Esp Oncol* 31:611–621, 1984.

208. Jaworski R: Malignant trichilemmal cyst. *Am J Dermatopathol* 10:276–277, 1988.

209. Kishimoto S, Miyashi A, Araki K, Uyeda K, Saito H: Malignant proliferating trichilemmal cyst with metastasis. *Acta Dermatol* 77:125–129, 1982.

210. Mehregan AH, Lee KC: Malignant proliferating trichilemmal tumors: Report of three cases. *J Dermatol Surg Oncol* 13:1339–1342, 1987.

211. Saida T, Oohara K, Hori Y, Tsuchiya S: Development of a malignant proliferating trichilemmal cyst in a patient with multiple trichilemmal cysts. *Dermatologica* 166: 203–208, 1983.

212. Weiss J, Heine M, Grimmel M, Jung EG: Malignant proliferating trichilemmal cyst. *J Am Acad Dermatol* 32:870–873, 1995.

213. Mori O, Hachisuka H, Sasai Y: Proliferating trichilemmal cyst with spindle cell carcinoma. *Am J Dermatopathol* 12:479–484, 1990.

214. Alvarez-Quinones M, Garijo MF, Fernandez F, Val-Bernal JF: Malignant aneuploid spindle cell transformation in a proliferatiing trichilemmal tumor. *Acta Dermatol Venereol* 73:444–446, 1993.

215. Waligora MJ, Chor PJ, Schneider TA, et al: Malignant proliferating trichilemmal tumor. *Eur J Dermatol* 3:279–281, 1993.

216. Lopansri S, Mihm MC: Pilomatrix carcinoma or calcifying epitheliocarcinoma of Malherbe: A case report and review of the literature. *Cancer* 45:2368–2373, 1980.

217. Gray M, Parhizgar B, Beerman H: Malignant pilomatrixoma. *Arch Dermatol* 120: 770–773, 1984.

218. Manivel JC, Wick MR, Mukai K: Pilomatrix carcinoma: An immunohistochemical comparison with benign pilomatrixoma and other benign lesions of pilar origin. *J Cutan Pathol* 13:22–29, 1986.

219. Gould E, Kurzon R, Kowalczyk AP, Saldana M: Pilomatrix carcinoma with pulmonary metastases: A report of a case. *Cancer* 54:370–372, 1984.

220. Van der Walt JD, Rohlova B: Carcinomatous transformation in a pilomatrixoma. *Am J Dermatopathol* 6:63–69, 1984.

221. Weedon D, Bell J, Maize J: Matrical carcinoma of the skin. *J Cutan Pathol* 7:39–42, 1980.

222. Reed RJ, Lamar LM: Invasive hair matrix tumors of the scalp: Invasive pilomatrixoma. *Arch Dermatol* 94:310–316, 1966.

223. Martelli G, Giardini R: Pilomatrix carcinoma: A case report and review of the literature. *Eur J Surg Oncol* 20:703–704, 1994.

224. Panico L, Manivel JC, Pettinato G, et al.: Pilomatrix carcinoma. *Tumori* 80:309–314, 1994.

225. Sau P, Lupton GP, Graham JH: Pilomatrix carcinoma. *Cancer* 71:2491–2498, 1993.

226. Zagarella SS, Kneale KL, Stern HS: Pilomatrix carcinoma of the scalp. *Aust J Dermatol* 33:39–42, 1992.

227. Niedermeyer HP, Peris K, Hofler H: Pilomatrix carcinoma with multiple visceral metastases: Report of a case. *Cancer* 77:1311–1314, 1996.

228. Liubskaia OG, Papadiuk VI: A rare case of malignant trichoepithelioma of the external acoustic meatus. *Vestnik Otorinolaringologii* 2:50–51, 1995.

229. Aygun C, Blum JE: Trichoepithelioma 100 years later: A case report supporting the use of radiotherapy. *Dermatology* 187:209–212, 1993.

230. D'Souza M, Garg BR, Ratnakar C, Agrawal K: Multiple trichoepitheliomas with rare features. *J Dermatol* 21:582–585, 1994.

231. San Juan EB, Guana AL, Goldberg LH, Kolbusz RV, Orengo IF, Alford E: Aggressive trichoepithelioma versus keratotic basal cell carcinoma. *Int J Dermatol* 32:728–730, 1993.

232. Nakhleh RE, Swanson PE, Wick MR: Cutaneous adnexal carcinomas with mixed differentiation. *Am J Dermatopathol* 12:325–334, 1990.

233. Rahbari H, Mehregan AH: Pilary complex carcinoma: An adnexal carcinoma of the skin with differentiation towards the components of the pilary complex. *J Dermatol* 20:630–637, 1993.

234. Sanchez-Yus E, Requena L, Simon P, Sanchez M: Complex adnexal tumor of the primary epithelial germ with distinct patterns of superficial epithelioma with sebaceous differentiation, immature trichoepithelioma, and apocrine adenocarcinoma. *Am J Dermatopathol* 14:245–252, 1992.

235. Wick MR, Swanson PE, LeBoit PE, Cooper PH: Lymphoepithelioma-like carcinomas of the skin with adnexal differentiation. *J Cutan Pathol* 18:93–102, 1991.

236. Requena L, Sanchez-Yus E, Jimenez E, Roo E: Lymphoepithelioma-like carcinoma of the skin: A light microscopic and immunohistochemical study. *J Cutan Pathol* 21: 541–548, 1994.

237. Dahl I, Angervall L: Cutaneous and subcutaneous leiomyosarcoma: A clinicopathologic study of 47 patients. *Pathol Eur* 9:307–314, 1974.

238. Fields JP, Helwig EB: Leiomyosarcoma of the skin and subcutaneous tissue. *Cancer* 47:156–169, 1981.

239. Swanson PE, Stanley MW, Scheithauer BW, Wick MR: Primary cutaneous leiomyosarcoma: A histologic and immunohistochemical study of 9 cases, with ultrastructural correlation. *J Cutan Pathol* 15:129–141, 1988.

240. Wolff M, Rothenberg A: Dermal leiomyosarcoma: A misnomer? *Prog Surg Pathol* 7:147–162, 1986.

241. Choi EH, Ahn SK, Lee SH, Barg D: Hair follicle nevus. *Int J Dermatol* 31:578–581, 1992.

242. Komura A, Tani M: Hair follicle nevus. *Dermatology* 185:154–155, 1992.

243. Happle R: Epidermal nevus syndromes. *Semin Dermatol* 14:111–121, 1995.

244. Johnson MD, Jacobs AH: Congenital smooth muscle hamartoma. *Arch Dermatol* 125:820–822, 1989.

245. Tsambaos D, Orfanos CE: Cutaneous smooth muscle hamartoma. *J Cutan Pathol* 9:33–42, 1982.

246. Bronson DM, Fretzin DF, Farrell LN: Congenital pilar and smooth muscle nevus. *J Am Acad Dermatol* 8:111–114, 1983.

247. Slifman NR, Harrist TJ, Rhodes AR: Congenital arrector pili hamartoma. *Arch Dermatol* 121:1034–1037, 1985.

248. Goldman MP, Kaplan RP, Heng MCY: Congenital smooth muscle hamartoma. *Int J Dermatol* 26:448–452, 1987.

249. Darling TN, Kamino H, Murray JC: Acquired cutaneous smooth muscle hamartoma. *J Am Acad Dermatol* 28:844–845, 1993.

250. Wong RC, Solomon AR: Acquired dermal smooth muscle hamartoma. *Cutis* 35: 369–370, 1985.

251. Chapel TA, Tavafoghi V, Mehregan AH, et al.: Becker's melanosis: An organoid hamartoma. *Cutis* 27:405–415, 1981.

252. Karo KR, Gange RW: Smooth muscle hamartoma: possible congenital Becker's nevus. *Arch Dermatol* 117:678–679, 1981.

253. Urbanek RW, Johnson WC: Smooth muscle hamartoma associated with Becker's nevus. *Arch Dermatol* 114:104–106, 1978.

254. Barr RJ, Goodman MM: Neurofollicular hamartoma: A light microscopic and immunohistochemical study. *J Cutan Pathol* 16:336–341, 1989.

255. Nova MP, Zung M, Halperin A: Neurofollicular hamartoma: A clinicopathological study. *Am J Dermatopathol* 13:459–462, 1991.

256. Sangueza OP, Requena L: Neurofollicular hamartoma: A new histogenetic interpretation. *Am J Dermatopathol* 16:150–154, 1994.

257. Tuthill RJ, Clark WH Jr, Levene A: Pilar neurocristic hamartoma: Its relationship to blue nevus and equine melanotic disease. *Arch Dermatol* 118:592–596, 1982.

258. Pathy AL, Helm TN, Elston D, Bergfeld WF, Tuthill RJ: Malignant melanoma arising in a blue nevus with features of pilar neurocristic hamartoma. *J Cutan Pathol* 20: 459–464, 1993.

259. Pearson JP, Weiss SW, Headington JT: Cutaneous malignant melanotic neurocristic tumors arising in neurocristic hamartomas: A melanocytic tumor morphologically and biologically distinct from common melanoma. *Am J Surg Pathol* 20:665–677, 1996.

C H A P T E R   2 9

SWEAT GLAND TUMORS

Mark R. Wick / Paul E. Swanson / Raymond L. Barnhill

Cutaneous neoplasms showing differentiation toward the sweat gland units are relatively uncommon specimens in general pathology but are not so uncommon in dermatopathology. Despite that fact, their histologic diversity—and the plethora of nosologic schemes that have been applied to them in the past—can be daunting at first glance. In this specific context, one is faced with a decision to adopt a stance of terminologic minimalism, using such diagnostic terms as *benign sweat gland neoplasm*, or to embrace more eclectic nomenclature as applied to adnexal tumors. This chapter (and Chap. 30) will present a moderate stance in reference to the latter issue, using a classification system that is attuned as much as possible to concepts and terms that are commonly embraced in surgical pathology. Because of the relatively nondescript clinical features attending many sweat gland tumors, these will not be covered in any detail except for those lesions where they are distinctive and contribute meaningfully to pathologic diagnosis.

The topic of cutaneous adnexal neoplasia is a broad and complicated one; indeed, several entire textbooks have been devoted to it.[1–3] Hence, the following material is intended to present a practical, diagnostically directed synopsis rather than an encyclopedic treatment of the subject, and the interested reader is referred to the reference sources cited above for additional information.

BENIGN SWEAT GLAND NEOPLASMS

Eccrine Tumors

Benign neoplasms showing differentiation toward the eccrine unit are generally the most commonly encountered adnexal cutaneous lesions. They may be found in virtually all topographic sites and are seen in children and adults alike.

ECCRINE CYLINDROMA

Clinical Features   Several adnexal tumors with sweat glandular differentiation are observed with regularity in the skin of the face, neck, and scalp (Table 29-1). One such tumor, dermal cylindroma, may be encountered as a solitary sporadic nodular lesion or as a multifocal process in the context of the autosomal dominant "turban tumor" (Ancell-Spiegler) syndrome.[4–9] In the latter condition, multiple raised reddish tumors may cover the entire scalp but also may involve the face and upper body. Cylindromas may develop at any age but most commonly are noted in young adults aged 20 to 40 years and are more common in women. Although in most instances this tumor is asymptomatic, a certain proportion are reported to be painful. Cylindromas show an association with both eccrine spiradenoma (see below) and trichoepitheliomas involving the central face (Brook's syndrome).

Histopathological Features   In either of these contexts, the neoplasm demonstrates two cell populations, one compact and basaloid and the other having a polygonal shape with more abundant amphophilic cyto-

plasm (Table 29-1). Nuclear chromatin is dispersed, nucleoli are inconspicuous, and mitotic activity is typically limited in scope. Two salient aspects of this neoplasm facilitate its recognition on low-power microscopy; these are represented by a "jigsaw puzzle" growth pattern—with angular cell nests that are molded to one another in a fibrous matrix (Fig. 29-1)—and the regular deposition of eosinophilic hyaline basement membrane material throughout the cellular clusters and immediately around them in the interstitium (Fig. 29-2). Cylindroma often displays an irregular pattern of peripheral growth, with "buds" of tumor being seen in the dermis or subcutis, seemingly detached from the main mass. This finding has no untoward prognostic significance and should not be used to label such lesions as *malignant*. Similarly, rare examples of cylindroma that exhibit easily appreciable mitotic activity show no adverse behavior if the nuclear characteristics and overall microscopic structure are characteristic of that tumor entity.[10] As discussed subsequently, truly malignant tumors arising from eccrine cylindroma have a distinctive histologic configuration; they are comprised of obviously anaplastic cells and lack the organoid qualities seen in banal sweat gland adenomas.

Differential Diagnosis   Cylindroma must be distinguished from eccrine spiradenoma and basal cell carcinoma. As mentioned, there may be considerable overlap between cylindroma and spiradenoma, and some tumors may be hybrid lesions. The essential discriminating feature is the mosaic pattern of many small epithelial aggregates in cylindroma versus the isolated rounded tumor lobules that are often few in number in spiradenoma. Basal cell carcinoma differs from cylindroma by showing frequent origin from the epidermis, peripheral palisading of nuclei, separation artifact (from the surrounding stroma), a mucinous stroma, and necrosis and mitoses.

ECCRINE SPIRADENOMA

Clinical Features   This tumor most commonly develops in young adults as a solitary skin-colored or bluish nodule usually less than 1 cm but occasionally up to 5 cm in diameter with a cystic or spongelike consistency on the ventral surfaces of the upper body (Table 29-2). Multiple forms of spiradenoma have been reported, and they may be grouped or linear in configuration. Approximately half of spiradenomas have been described as painful and another third as tender.

Histopathological Features   Eccrine spiradenoma differs in appearance only slightly from the histologic description just given for cylindromas. However, the first of these two neoplasms generally is devoid of a jigsaw puzzle profile and instead demonstrates the presence of intratumoral vascular spaces that are often dilated and are most numerous at the periphery of tumor cell clusters (Table 29-2) (Fig. 29-3). These channels may contain lymphatic fluid, erythrocytes, or both and occasionally may be so prominent that they impart a vasogenic appearance to cylindroma at both the clinical and microscopic levels.[11–14]

TABLE 29-1

Eccrine Cylindroma

Clinical Features

Head, neck, especially scalp
Multiple tumors (turban tumors)
  Autosomal dominant
Association with eccrine spiradenomas and trichoepitheliomas
  (Brook's syndrome)

Histopathological Features

Mosaic or jigsaw puzzle pattern of tumor islands
Tumor aggregates delimited by basement membrane material that also
  results in "hyaline" droplets within aggregates.
Basaloid tumor aggregates with two cellular populations
  Outer layer composed of small round cells with scant cytoplasm
  Inner layer comprised of larger polygonal cells with more abundant
  cytoplasm
Irregular pattern at periphery of tumor (budding)
Occasional mitotic figures

Differential Diagnosis

Basal cell carcinoma
Eccrine spiradenoma

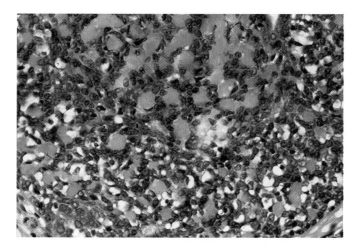

FIGURE 29-2   Cylindroma. Hyalin matrical material is regularly dispersed in a basaloid cell proliferation.

to spiradenoma and cylindroma. In occasional instances, it may be a challenge to distinguish between these two pathologic entities microscopically; indeed, some patients have been described who have the Ancell-Spiegler syndrome as well as multifocal spiradenomatosis.[8,9,12]

Differential Diagnosis   The principal entities to be considered in the differential diagnosis include cylindroma, glomus tumor, and basal cell carcinoma. As discussed above, spiradenoma and cylindroma may overlap considerably. The various points in differential diagnosis are discussed above in the section on differential diagnosis for cylindroma. Both spiradenoma and glomus tumors may be vascular. Spiradenoma, in general, is distinguished from glomus tumor by the presence of a peripheral hyalinized basement membrane, hyaline globules within the tumor, the two-cell populations, and the presence of occasional tubular structures. Spiradenoma differs from basal cell carcinoma by the usual

Such lesions have been described as *giant vascular spiradenomas*.[15] Other singular characteristics of spiradenoma include the regular distribution of mature lymphocytes throughout the neoplasm much as one would see in tumors of the thymic epithelium (Fig. 29-4), and the capacity to present as a deeply seated tumor of the lower corium and subcutis.[16] Otherwise, the potentials for deposition of basement membrane and irregular, permeative, peripheral growth of the lesion are common

TABLE 29-2

Eccrine Spiradenoma

Clinical Features

Trunk
Ventral surfaces
Skin-colored or bluish with cystic or spongelike consistency
Painful or tender

Histopathological Features

Rounded tumor lobules, often large and few in number
No epidermal connection or jigsaw puzzle pattern
Tumor lobules delimited by basement membrane material and contain
  hyaline droplets
    Smaller outer cell
    Larger inner polygonal cells
Often highly vascular and infiltrated by lymphocytes
Overlap with eccrine cylindroma

Differential Diagnosis

Basal cell carcinoma
Eccrine cylindroma
Vascular and glomus tumors

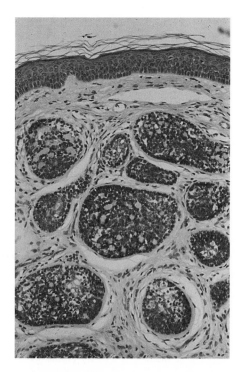

FIGURE 29-1   Cylindroma. Angular and ovoid nests of basaloid cells are molded to one another in a fibrous matrix. Hyalin matrical cylinders are conspicuous.

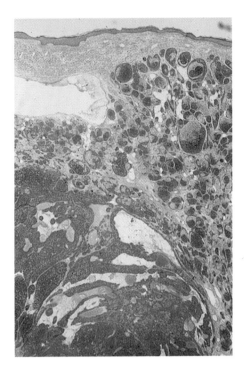

FIGURE 29-3   Spiradenoma. An organoid pattern of epithelial cells is interrupted by dilated intratumoral vascular channels.

lack of connection to the overlying epidermis, the well-demarcated round, lobular character of spiradenoma, the presence of peripheral basement membrane material and hyaline globules within the tumor, the uniformity of cells versus that in basal cell carcinoma, and the lack of significant necrosis and mitotic figures in spiradenoma as compared to basal cell carcinoma.

SYRINGOMA

Clinical Features   Syringoma represents another benign eccrine proliferation that is likely malformative in nature rather than neoplastic in most instances. This tumor commonly is multifocal and is largely restricted to the skin of the upper face (particularly the lower eyelids) and the genital region (Table 29-3).[17–25] However, solitary lesions do exist; in general, syringomas have a nondescript papular configuration,

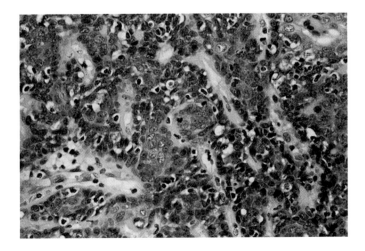

FIGURE 29-4   Spiradenoma. Lymphocytes are scattered throughout the lesion.

TABLE 29-3
Syringoma

Clinical Features

Usually multiple
Plaquelike, milialike, linear, and eruptive variants
Upper cheeks, below eyelids, genitalia, thighs
Small, discrete, whitish or yellowish papules, 1–4 mm in diameter

Histopathological Features

Superficial dermal well-defined tumor
Small tubule or epithelial aggregates, often comma-shaped
Central lumina with luminal cuticle
Polygonal or flattened tumor cells with eosinophilic or clear cytoplasm
Absence of cytologic atypia, mitoses, and infiltrative growth

Differential Diagnosis

Basal cell carcinoma
Desmoplastic trichoepithelioma
Microcystic adnexal carcinoma

are usually white or yellowish, and measure 1 to 4 mm in diameter.[19] A number of variants of syringoma have been described: plaquelike lesions; linear forms; variants localized to the penis, vulva, scalp, and acral surfaces; milialike forms; and eruptive and disseminated variants.

Histopathological Features   Microscopically, small, comma-shaped tubules of cells—many of which manifest central lumina and have luminal cuticles—are dispersed throughout a collagenous stroma in the dermis (Table 29-3). The tumor cells are polygonal or flattened and have either eosinophilic or clear cytoplasm.[17,19,24,25] Nuclei are compact, with no nucleoli or mitoses. Syringomas demonstrate sharp circumscription on low-power histologic examination, and they lack mitotic activity, nuclear atypia, and infiltrative growth (Figs. 29-5, 29-6). Nevertheless, a small superficial biopsy through the center of such a tumor can provide an image which recapitulates a form of appendageal *carcinoma*[19] (see below), making excision the recommended initial approach to the management of syringoma, if at all feasible clinically. A clear-cell variant shows the epithelial tubular structures to be composed of somewhat large cuboidal cells with pale or clear cytoplasm. This clear-cell change results from glycogen accumulation. The clear-cell alteration may involve the entire tumor, a portion of the tumor, or only the cells lining the ductal lumina.

Differential Diagnosis   Syringoma must be distinguished from desmoplastic trichoepithelioma, morpheaform basal cell carcinoma, and microcystic adnexal carcinoma (MAC) (sclerosing sweat duct carcinoma). Syringoma may be distinguished from desmoplastic trichoepithelioma by the presence of basophilic material within tubular lumina rather than keratinous material in general (occasional tubular structures near the epidermis in syringoma may contain keratinous material), the presence of eosinophilic cuticles lining the lumina in syringoma, the common presence of clear-cell change in cells lining the lumina in syringoma, and the much less frequent foreign-body giant cell reactions to extruded keratin and dystrophic calcification that are typically seen in trichoepithelioma. Syringoma also tends to show tubular structures with a tadpolelike configuration much more frequently than trichoepithelioma. In general, morpheaform basal cell carcinoma differs from syringoma by showing a less well defined tumor, the presence of epidermal connection, the predominance of basaloid epithelial strands

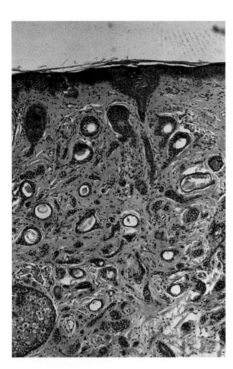

FIGURE 29-5 Syringoma. Small ductules, some with inspissated secretory material, populate a densely fibrous stroma.

without ductal lumina or keratinous cysts, the frequent presence of perineurial infiltration, and much greater frequency of mitotic figures and necrotic cells as compared to syringoma. Syringoma may be distinguished from MAC by the superficial and well-demarcated configuration of syringoma versus the deep infiltration of reticular dermis, subcutaneous fat, skeletal muscle, and cutaneous nerves by MAC. In addition, MAC may show follicular differentiation with prominent formation of keratinous cysts, more prominent epithelial lobules, and some degree of cytologic atypia with occasional mitoses.

ECCRINE POROMA GROUP

Poroma is a lesion which is so named because of a microscopic resemblance between epidermal and dermal components of this neoplasm and elements of the acrosyringeal-eccrine coil unit.[26–32]

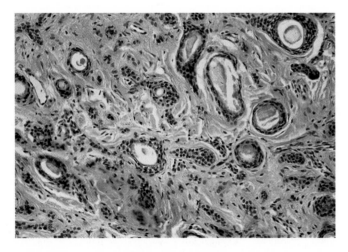

FIGURE 29-6 Syringoma. These characteristically shaped ductular elements are lined by cytologically bland cells. Mitotic figures are not present.

TABLE 29-4

Eccrine Poroma

Clinical Features

Hidroacanthoma simplex
  Lower extremities common
  Slightly raised verrucous plaques
  Skin-colored or brownish
Poroma and dermal duct tumor
  Palms, soles, other sites
  Papules or nodules
  May have verrucous or moist eroded surface

Histopathological Features

Hidroacanthoma simplex
  Discrete intraepidermal nests of basaloid cuboidal cells
  Association with sweat ducts
Poroma
  Anastomosing ribbons of cuboidal epithelium, sharply demarcated
    from epidermis
  Ductal structures
  Vascular stroma
  Uniformity of cuboidal epithelial cells
  Occasional focal atypia and mitoses
Dermal duct tumor
  Rounded lobules of epithelium in dermis with little or no epidermal
    connection

Differential Diagnosis

Hidroacanthoma simplex
  Clonal seborrheic keratosis
  Squamous cell carcinoma in situ
  Basal cell carcinoma
  Paget's disease
  Melanoma
Poroma
  Acrospiroma
  Basal cell carcinoma
  Porocarcinoma

Clinical Features Intraepidermal forms of poroma (hidroacanthoma simplex) are generally flat or slightly raised brownish lesions often involving the lower extremities of older women (Table 29-4). There may be a slightly verrucous surface suggesting seborrheic keratosis. Other variants of poroma usually present as papules or nodules on the distal extremities, including the palms and soles, but they may be seen in any location. The surface may be keratotic or eroded and often suggests a verruca, pyogenic granuloma, or amelanotic melanoma. Children are potentially affected, as well as adults of all ages. Entirely dermal variants (dermal duct tumor) of poroma are usually nondescript papules or nodules.

Histopathological Features The hallmark of eccrine poroma is the presence of intraepidermal "lakes" of compact, monotonous polyhedral cells, which are sharply marginated from adjacent keratinocytes of the epidermis (Table 29-4). Nuclei are bland, without nucleoli or significant mitotic activity, and cytoplasm is moderate in amount and amphophilic.[26–28,32]

  The form of poroma in which *only* an intraepidermal component is seen has been called *hidroacanthoma simplex*[33] (Fig. 29-7); conversely,

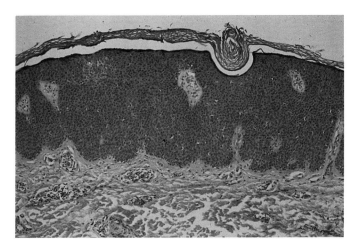

FIGURE 29-7   Intraepidermal poroma (hidroacanthoma simplex). The epidermis is expanded by a monotonous population of small basaloid cells.

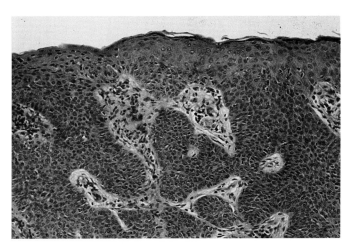

FIGURE 29-9   Poroma. As evident in most examples of poroma, both intraepidermal and dermal elements are in continuity.

the form in which a *dermal* component predominates—with the formation of ductlike spaces within tumor cell nests—is commonly known as *dermal duct tumor*[34,35] (Fig. 29-8). Nonetheless, these represent the poles in a continuum, most members of which manifest cellular growth in both compartments of the skin (Fig. 29-9). Variations in the dermal portion of poromas include the presence of focal squamous metaplasia, limited areas of clear-cell changes, and sometimes extensive formation of glandular lumina.[32]

The usual features in each variant of this tumor are those of cytologic blandness and relative monotony. Nevertheless, occasional examples do demonstrate focal nuclear enlargement or nucleolation, with or without limited mitotic activity.[32] If the overall pattern of the lesion is still that of a banal poroma, one should not succumb to the temptation to label

such tumors as malignant; true porocarcinomas (as described below) show the mandatory presence of infiltrative growth, and foci of spontaneous necrosis are also common therein. Lastly, one sometimes encounters poromatous tumors that differ from usual lesions in this category by their possession of an acanthotic or papillomatous surface. Rahbari has suggested that the term *syringoacanthoma* be applied to such neoplasms,[36] but they probably are variations on the basic structure of poroma.

Differential Diagnosis   Intraepidermal forms of poroma (hidroacanthoma simplex) raise the differential diagnosis of so-called intraepidermal epithelioma or the Borst-Jadassohn phenomenon. The major entities to be considered include clonal forms of seborrheic keratosis, squamous cell carcinoma in situ, mammary and extramammary Paget's disease, basal cell carcinoma, and melanoma in situ. In general, seborrheic keratoses of the clonal type do not exhibit epithelial cells as small as those observed in poroma or the association with intraepidermal sweat ducts. The other entities can be discriminated from poroma by characteristic histopathologic features; rarely one might have to resort to immunohistochemistry to resolve the issue.

Deeper variants of poroma must be distinguished from eccrine acrospiroma, basal cell carcinoma, and trichilemmoma and tumor of the follicular infundibulum. There may be considerable overlap between poroma and acrospiroma, and some authors believe them to be variations of a single entity. In general, poroma is characterized by a monomorphous population of basaloid cuboidal cells and tends not to show the squamous differentiation, large cystic spaces, and prominent clear-cell change that typifies acrospiroma. Poroma differs from BCC by displaying a more organoid appearance, i.e., fairly uniform anastomosing cords of epithelium, the general lack of peripheral palisading of nuclei and separation artifact, the uniformity of the cuboidal cells, and the lack of consistent mitoses and necrotic cells throughout the tumor. Poroma differs from trichilemmoma and tumor of the follicular infundibulum by the lack of a hyalinized basement membrane at the periphery of the tumor, the degree of dyskeratosis noted in trichilemmoma, and often greater depth of involvement than typically observed in trichilemmoma and tumor of the follicular infundibulum.

ECCRINE SYRINGOFIBROADENOMA

Clinical and Histopathological Features   In the few cases reported, this exceedingly rare neoplasm (also known as *acrosyringeal nevus*) usually presents as a nondescript solitary hyerkeratotic nodule on the

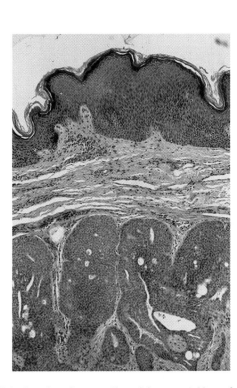

FIGURE 29-8   Intradermal poroma (dermal duct tumor). Nests of cytologically uniform cells do not communicate with overlying epidermis. Small, irregular ductlike spaces are evident.

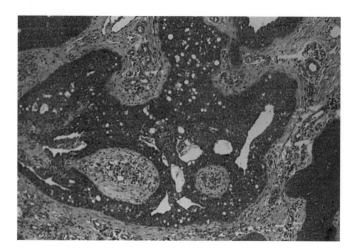

FIGURE 29-10 Eccrine syringofibroadenoma. Irregular nests of squamoid cells with distinct ductular lumens rest in a cellular fibrous stroma.

extremities. Contrary to the implications of its name, eccrine syringofibroadenoma bears more of a visual resemblance to poroma than to syringoma. This rare neoplasm demonstrates a complex interconnection of regularly spaced cellular cords in the corium with others in the epidermis. The surface epithelium is generally hyperplastic and may be overtly pseudocarcinomatous; the dermal element features the presence of a variably cellular fibroblastic and vascular stroma between the epithelial cellular columns, which are definitely squamoid in character and may demonstrate small intercellular ductal lumina[37,38] (Fig. 29-10). Hence, the overall appearance simulates that of mammary fibroadenoma and has a vague likeness to fibroepithelioma of Pinkus (fibroepitheliomatous basal cell carcinoma). Weedon and Lewis have used the alternate designation of *acrosyringeal nevus* to describe syringofibroadenoma, preferring the interpretation that it represents a malformative proliferation of the terminal eccrine duct.[39] In any event, this lesion is typically sharply circumscribed and lacks nuclear atypia and mitotic activity in either component. It is likely that the stroma is "induced" by the epithelial proliferation in syringofibroadenoma, as is thought to be true of its counterpart in the breast.

Differential Diagnosis   The major lesions to be considered are fibroepithelioma of Pinkus and a reticulated form of seborrheic keratosis. The syringofibroadenoma differs from the latter two entities by demonstrating a uniform population of cuboidal basaloid cells and the presence of ducts in the anastomosing bands of epithelium.

PAPILLARY ECCRINE ADENOMA

Clinical and Histopathological Features   This lesion, also known as *tubulopapillary eccrine hidradenoma*, develops as a dome-shaped nodule or plaque often measuring approximately 1 cm on the extremities and is more common in black women (Table 29-5). Papillary eccrine adenoma shows a basic composition by uniform polygonal cells that are aggregated into discrete multilayered ductal profiles in the corium, subdivided from one another by fibrovascular stroma of variable density. In addition, the tumor cells line the peripheral aspects of dermal microcysts and form intradermal tubulopapillary complexes[40–45] (Fig. 29-11). The latter feature accounts for the designation of *tubulopapillary hidradenoma* that was applied to this tumor by Falck and Jordaan.[46] Both eccrine and apocrine cytologic features may be observed in such lesions (hence, the synonym of *tubular apocrine adenoma*),[47] but eccrine differentiation is more common by far. Communication between

TABLE 29-5

Papillary Eccrine Adenoma

Clinical Features

Women >> men
Blacks >> whites
Extremities
Solitary dome-shaped nodule, about 1 cm in diameter

Histopathological Features

Well-defined dermal tumor
Epithelial aggregates containing cystic or ductal structures
Multilayered and papillary appearance of the cystic/ductal structures
The epithelium composed of polygonal cells
Variable clear-cell change and squamous differentiation
No significant cytologic atypia or mitotic activity
Fibrovascular stroma of variable density
Eccrine >> apocrine features

Differential Diagnosis

Microcystic adnexal carcinoma
Syringocystadenoma papilliferum
Hidradenoma papilliferum
Nipple adenoma
Papillary eccrine carcinoma

cellular nests in the corium and similar aggregates in the epidermis may focally occur via columns of cells which superficially resemble the normal acrosyringia, as seen prototypically in poromas (see above). Ductal spaces in these structures may contain luminal "cuticles," as mentioned in reference to syringoma. Cytologic attributes of papillary eccrine adenoma are again banal, without nucleoli, nuclear anaplasia, or appreciable mitotic activity (Fig. 29-12). The overall image is nearly identical to

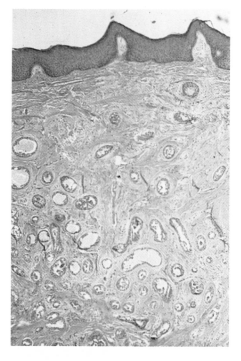

FIGURE 29-11 Papillary eccrine adenoma. Discrete ductular profiles, some with papillary intraluminal excrescences, loosely infiltrate the corium.

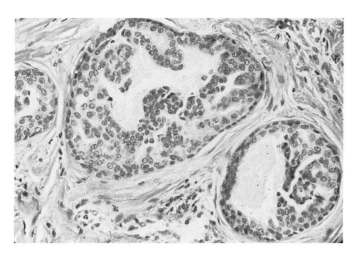

FIGURE 29-12   Papillary eccrine adenoma. A peripheral cell layer of uniform basaloid cells is overgrown by a cytologically bland micropapillary proliferation.

that of localized, florid intraductal hyperplasia of the female breast; however, the potential for recurrence of this skin tumor attests to its neoplastic nature.

Differential Diagnosis   The major entities to be considered include microcystic adnexal carcinoma, syringocystadenoma papilliferum, hidradenoma papilliferum, nipple adenoma, and papillary eccrine carcinoma. Although there may be some confusion between papillary eccrine adenoma and MAC, MAC differs from eccrine papillary adenoma by prominence of keratinous cysts and often some degree of follicular differentiation, the lack of papillary differentiation as the predominant feature, deep infiltration, perineurial invasion, and frequent localization to the head and neck. Eccrine papillary adenoma and apocrine tubular adenoma, as discussed above, show considerable overlap and may be part of the same spectrum. Such apocrine tumors may differ only by showing greater or exclusive decapitation secretion. Syringocystadenoma papilliferum may be distinguished from eccrine papillary adenoma by a prominent cystic invagination lined by squamoid epithelium, prominent plasmacellular infiltrates in the stroma, localization to the head and neck area, and frequent association with nevus sebaceus. Hidradenoma papilliferum differs from eccrine papillary adenoma by its well-defined dermal nodular configuration, an almost exclusive localization to the vulvar and perineal area, and predominance in women. The nipple adenoma may show significant overlap with eccrine papillary adenoma but is distinguished by its localization to the breast. In general, eccrine papillary carcinomas are characterized by larger size, infiltrating features, greater cellularity, more frequent necrosis, and greater numbers of mitoses than in eccrine papillary adenoma. However, in many instances the latter distinction is quite difficult, and one must assess all features in arriving at a final interpretation.

ECCRINE ACROSPIROMA

Clinical Features   These tumors, also known as *solid-cystic hidradenoma*, *clear-cell hidradenoma*, *clear-cell myoepithelioma*, or *nodular eccrine hidradenoma*, often present as solitary nodules or sometimes cystic lesions usually 1 to 2 cm (but occasionally up to 6 cm) in diameter (Table 29-6). They may occur in any location and affect women slightly more often than men.

Histopathological Features   This form of eccrine adenoma has a micronodular growth pattern in the dermis, with each of the nodules being comprised of a monomorphous population of polygonal cells

TABLE 29-6
Eccrine Acrospiroma

Clinical Features

Wide age range
Women > men
Almost any location
Papule or nodule, 1–2 cm
Often skin-colored

Histopathological Features

Frequent origin from epidermis
Large lobular epithelial aggregates, well demarcated
Often solid nodules of cuboidal cells with varying degrees of squamous differentiation and clear-cell change
Occasional focal spindled epithelial cells
Ductal structures
Cystic spaces
Focal decapitation secretion
Variable focal cytologic atypia and occasional mitoses
Variable hyalinized stroma

Differential Diagnosis

Eccrine poroma
Mixed tumor
Squamous cell carcinoma

(Table 29-6). These aggregates variably demonstrate internal microcystic change, with or without foci of ductal differentiation and the formation of lumina[48,49] (Figs. 29-13 and 29-14). The latter characteristics led Winkelmann and Wolff to coin the term *solid and cystic hidradenoma* in reference to this neoplasm.[50] The peripheral aspects of eccrine

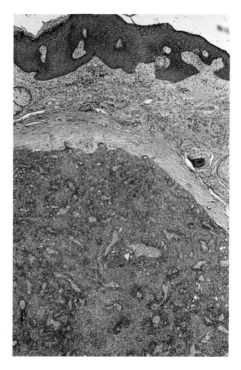

FIGURE 29-13   Eccrine acrospiroma (hidradenoma). A solid nest of cells with focal ductal differentiation is sharply demarcated from dermis.

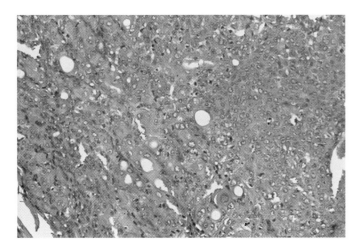

FIGURE 29-14 Eccrine acrospiroma (hidradenoma). Small ductal lumens are evident at higher magnification.

acrospiromas have a "pushing" interface with the surrounding dermal stroma, and the lesion is accordingly well circumscribed on scanning microscopy. This is the most important aspect of the tumor in assessing its biologic potential, because even those acrospiromas that show extremely bland cytologic features may recur if they exhibit budding or irregular peripheral permeation of the corium by cords of neoplastic cells (Fig. 29-15). Indeed, the latter lesions should be considered low-grade hidradenocarcinomas. Other features thought to predict aggressiveness in eccrine acrospiromas include broad zones of clear-cell change, global nuclear anaplasia, areas of spontaneous tumor necrosis, and the presence of tumor giant cells.[51] However, squamous metaplasia is a common finding in eccrine acrospiroma and has no untoward biologic significance. In fact, it is the underlying characteristic used by Stanley and coworkers to define the variant of this tumor known as *epidermoid hidradenoma*.[52] Mitoses may sometimes be disturbingly obvious in acrospiromas, but, as documented by Cooper, these do not imply adverse behavior.[10] Focal connections between neoplastic dermal cellular aggregates and the basal epidermis also are appreciated in roughly

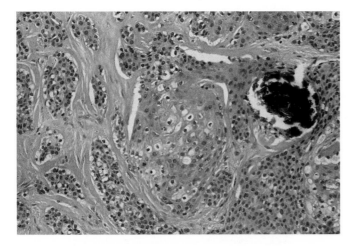

FIGURE 29-15 Eccrine acrospiroma (hidradenoma). Permeative growth may be seen at the periphery of some examples of acrospiroma and should lead one to consider a low-grade malignancy in such cases. Squamoid nests are commonly seen.

50 percent of cases; this observation has, in part, prompted rather egalitarian authors to use the term *acrospiroma* as a broad designation that encompasses tubulopapillary hidradenomas, nodular hidradenomas, and poromas.[53]

Differential Diagnosis   As discussed above, there is considerable overlap between eccrine acrospiroma and the eccrine poroma group. In some instances, a tumor may present with an intraepidermal portion resembling poroma (hidroacanthoma simplex) and with a deeper dermal component typical of acrospiroma. Final diagnosis may be based on the predominant features present. Other entities to be considered in the differential diagnosis of acrospiroma include mixed tumor (chondroid syringoma), squamous cell carcinoma, basal cell carcinoma, and a malignant form of acrospiroma. On occasion there may be overlap between acrospiroma and mixed tumor with some lesions showing prominent cystic spaces, hyalinized stroma, and anastomosing cords of epithelium. Final categorization must be based on the prominence of the stromal component in relationship to the other features present. Thus for a diagnosis of mixed tumor, a lesion should exhibit a rounded configuration with a significant component of stroma, whether it be chondroid, myxoid, or hyalinized. In contrast, acrospiroma primarily exhibits nodular aggregates of epithelium. A proportion of acrospiromas may show prominence of squamous differentiation raising the possibility of squamous cell carcinoma. However, careful examination should disclose the lack of significant atypicality and the presence of other features typical of acrospiroma, including ductal structures, cystic spaces, variable degrees of clear-cell change, and a hyalinized stroma. Eccrine acrospiroma differs from basal cell carcinoma by the lack of peripheral palisading of nuclei, separation artifact, a mucinous stroma, and the overall basaloid appearance of the tumor that typifies basal cell carcinoma. Eccrine acrospiromas may show slight cytologic atypia and mitotic figures, raising the possibility of malignancy. In general, benign tumors are characterized by a well-circumscribed appearance without evidence of infiltration of the adjacent tissue, only modest nuclear atypia, and a mitotic rate that is usually less than 5 mitoses per 10 hpf. Nonetheless, the presence of mitotic activity and cytologic atypia in acrospiroma has been correlated with an increased rate of local recurrence and indeed may be equated to low-grade malignancy.

Apocrine Neoplasms

Benign apocrine tumors are, in general, much less common than eccrine adenomas. Their topographic distribution is also more restricted; it largely centers on the head and neck, axillae, groin, and perineum, where normal apocrine glands are relatively prominent.

SYRINGOCYSTADENOMA PAPILLIFERUM

Clinical Features   Syringocystadenoma papilliferum (SP) is a distinctive lesion that is largely restricted to the skin of the head and neck and particularly affects the scalp (Table 29-7). It is one of several neoplasms that may be associated with nevus sebaceus of Jadassohn, but it most often occurs as a sporadic tumor.[54–57]

Histopathological Features   The histologic attributes of SP are distinctive. As its name implies, the tumor has a papillary configuration, but it sits in a semicystic "dell" in the integument that is in continuity with the surface epithelium (Table 29-7) (Fig. 29-16). At the interface between the epidermis and the neoplasm, keratinocytes give way to aggregates of cuboidal or low columnar glandular cells that often exhibit decapitation "snouts" at their apices. These elements line micropapillary structures with easily discernible fibrovascular cores, which are filled with plasma cells and other chronic inflammatory elements

Syringocystadenoma Papilliferum

Clinical Features

Head and neck, especially scalp
Solitary verrucouslike plaque or nodule
Often moist or oozing surface
Often 2–3 cm
Frequently congenital and associated with nevus sebaceus

Histopathological Features

Epidermal cystic invagination lined by squamous epithelium with transition to epithelial lining with two cell layers
Often verrucous epidermal surface
Cystic invagination contains papillary projections lined by luminal columnar cells and inner cuboidal cells
Decapitation secretion
The stroma of the papillary epithelial structures contains numerous plasma cells
Background nevus sebaceus common

Differential Diagnosis

Nevus sebaceus
Hidradenoma papilliferum

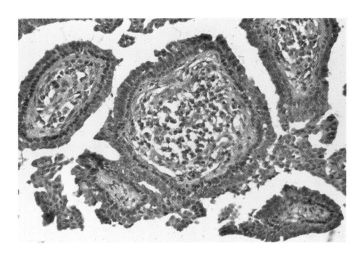

FIGURE 29-17 Syringocystadenoma papilliferum. Low columnar cells with apocrine-type decapitation secretion line inflamed fibrovascular cores. The cores are populated by a plasma-cell-rich mononuclear infiltrate.

Differential Diagnosis Uncommonly, SP must be distinguished from hidradenoma papilliferum (HP). SP can be distinguished from HP in almost all cases by epidermal invagination and verrucous surface alteration and a location on the head or neck.

HIDRADENOMA PAPILLIFERUM

Clinical and Histopathological Features Hidradenoma papilliferum (HP) is a dermal neoplasm having a central cystic space into which cellular proliferations project (Table 29-8). It occurs almost exclusively in the genitoperineal skin in women,[58–61] although rare examples have been described elsewhere in the body[62] and in males. As implied by its name, the basic configuration of the intracystic component of HP is micropapillary; cells mantling the fibrovascular cores of the papillae are very similar in appearance to those in SP, as described above (Figs. 29-18 and 29-19). However, there are more solid zones of cellular proliferation in HP, with more elaborately branching and interconnecting papillae than those seen in SP; limited extracystic dermal growth of tubular cell profiles may also be observed at the periphery of HP (Fig. 29-19).

(Fig. 29-17). Tubular structures, lined by tumor cells, are seen to take origin from the base of the indentation ("cyst") in which the tumor resides; these grow randomly into the subjacent and intervening dermis in a limited fashion, such that the tumor has a circumscribed image on scanning microscopy. The neoplastic cells have compact oval nuclei and amphophilic to eosinophilic cytoplasm, and overt mucinous metaplasia may sometimes be seen. Cytologic atypia is variable but generally is unremarkable; however, those tumors that have been subjected to mechanical trauma or other insults may show a frightening degree of nuclear pleomorphism and mitotic activity. Despite such findings, a well-documented case of malignant transformation in SP has yet to be described. Accordingly, simple excision represents adequate therapy for this lesion.

Hidradenoma Papilliferum

Clinical Features

Women, almost exclusively
Vulva, rarely other sites such as breast, eyelid, ear canal
Dome-shaped nodule with occasional bleeding pain, usually solitary

Histopathological Features

Well-circumscribed dermal nodule, solid or cystic
Usually no epidermal connection
Complex pattern of anastomosing papillary structures, tubules
Epithelial lining with myoepithelial cells and luminal columnar or cuboidal cells
Decapitation secretion
Occasional slight nuclear pleomorphism, mitoses

Differential Diagnosis

Syringocystadenoma papilliferum
Tubular apocrine adenoma

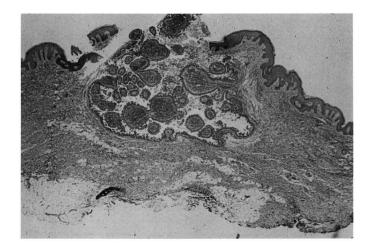

FIGURE 29-16 Syringocystadenoma papilliferum. A papillary proliferation lines a semicystic depression in the dermis that is in continuity with the epidermis.

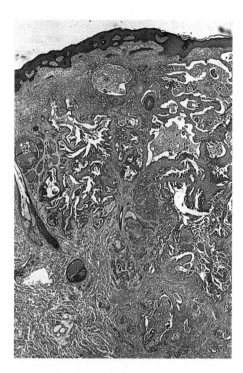

FIGURE 29-18 Hidradenoma papilliferum. This intradermal lesion is composed of variably sized cystic spaces into which papillary cellular proliferations project.

As is true of SP, the cytologic attributes of HP may occasionally be worrisome, and that feature has accounted for past misdiagnosis of the lesion as a malignancy.[63] This problem may be avoided by attention to the characteristically circumscribed low-power image of HP, as well as the regular presence of decapitation "snouts" on many individual tumor cells.

Differential Diagnosis   The major entities to be considered include syringocystadenoma papilliferum and other apocrine adenomas, e.g., tubulopapillary adenoma. In general, hidradenoma papilliferum is distinguished from other entities by its well-demarcated nodular appearance in the dermis, usually without epidermal connection, localization

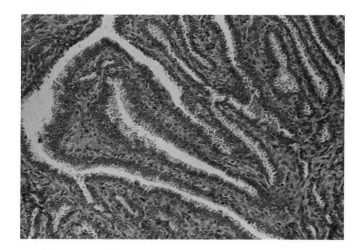

FIGURE 29-19 Hidradenoma papilliferum. Frondlike growth and decapitation secretion are apparent.

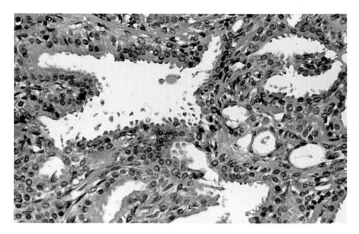

FIGURE 29-20 Tubular apocrine adenoma. Unlike hidradenoma papilliferum, this lesion is composed predominantly of tubuloductal profiles, although a distinct pattern of apocrine secretion is retained.

to the vulvar and perineal area, and almost exclusive occurrence in women.

TUBULAR APOCRINE ADENOMA

Clinical and Histopathological Features   Tubular apocrine adenoma is, for all intents and purposes, largely synonymous with the apocrine counterpart of papillary eccrine adenoma (tubulopapillary hidradenoma, see above), in regard not only to its clinical features but also to its basic histologic structure.[46,47,64–66] However, occasional tumors have been described under this term that assumed more of the configuration of an acrospiroma but were composed of cells which had unequivocally apocrine cytologic characteristics (Fig. 29-20). One can decide on an individual basis whether to label such lesions as apocrine hidradenomas.

Differential Diagnosis   See above discussion for differential diagnosis of eccrine papillary adenoma.

Sweat Gland Adenomas Showing Mixed Differentiation

BENIGN MIXED TUMORS OF THE SKIN ("CHONDROID SYRINGOMAS")

Clinical and Histopathological Features   Mixed tumor of the skin (MTS) arises most often on the head and neck as a nondescript dermal or subcutaneous nodule (Table 29-9).[67–69] However, this tumor occasionally may be sufficiently chondroid at a histologic level that it assumes a hard consistency macroscopically. The latter potential—that is, for formation of cartilagelike matrix—accounts in part for the historic synonym that was applied to MTS; namely, *chondroid syringoma*. That designation is not recommended because MTS is not universally chondroid and has little or no clinicopathologic resemblance to syringoma.

MTS represents a biologic paradigm for a nearly universal potentiality among human tumors. This is the ability for a primordial "stem cell" population (from which virtually all neoplasms emanate) to pursue divergent differentiation at a morphologic level into dissimilar target tissues.[70] Electron microscopic and immunohistologic studies support the concept that *all* tumor cells in MTS are basically epithelial,[70–73] but some of them acquire the capacity to assume cartilagelike, fibroblastoid,

Mixed Tumor (Chondroid Syringoma)

Clinical Features

Head and neck, especially face
Men > women
Firm dermal or subcutaneous nodule

Histopathological Features

Well-circumscribed dermal or subcutaneous lobular tumor
Only rare epidermal connection
Stromal component
   Variable chondroid, mucinous, hyalinized, or osteoid matrix
Epithelial component heterogenous
   Eccrine, apocrine, sebaceous, pilar, simple glandular, or squamous
     differentiation
Often small tubular lumina lined by cuboidal epithelium or complex
   pattern of anastomosing tubular lumina lined by one or two cell lay-
   ers that are cuboidal or columnar
Occasional prominent cystic spaces

Differential Diagnosis

Cutaneous chondroma
Eccrine acrospiroma

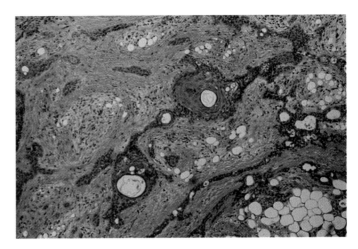

FIGURE 29-22   Benign mixed tumor (chondroid syringoma). Ductular and squamous epithelial elements permeate a chondroid-myxoid stroma that also contains mature adipose tissue.

myoid, myoepithelioid, lipoid, or even osteogenic microscopic appearances. Hence, one is faced with a structural phenotype in which slightly branching tubules and clusters of epithelial cells with variable cytologic appearances (e.g., eccrine, apocrine, sebaceous, pilar, mucinous, simple glandular, or squamoid) are admixed intimately but randomly with zones of matrical tissue that look like cartilage, bone, muscle, myxoid mesenchyme, and fat, sometimes all in the same mass[74,75] (Figs. 29-21 and 29-22). Thus, the name *mixed* tumor is particularly apropos, because not only are epithelial and mesenchymal tissues interspersed, but the *subtypes* of those tissues *also* are heterogeneous, and their relative proportions are greatly variable.

   The cytologic characteristics of the individual cellular elements of MTS are generally bland, but occasionally prominent nucleoli and mitotic activity can be observed regionally or diffusely in the obviously

epithelial component. Providing that the global image of the tumor is that of a well-circumscribed (but potentially multinodular) lesion, these findings have no biologic consequence. Similar comments apply to tumors showing focally dense spindle-cell growth or clear-cell change.[76]

Differential Diagnosis   In general the features of cutaneous mixed tumor are distinctive. Nonetheless, the differential diagnosis, on occasion, may include cutaneous cartilaginous tumors, such as chondroma and other appendageal tumors, particularly eccrine acrospiroma. On occasion some mixed tumors may show a limited epithelial component consisting of single epithelial cells and minimal tubular structures. Such tumors must be distinguished from cutaneous chondromas. Careful examination of the tumor should reveal tubular structures. However rarely these may not be present. It may be necessary to resort to immunohistochemistry to distinguish these two processes. In addition, mixed tumors are more common in the head and neck area, whereas cartilaginous tumors are more commonly localized to the distal extremities and frequently show prominent calcification. In some cases, mixed tumor must be distinguished from eccrine acrospiroma. As previously discussed, a prominent stromal component is characteristic of mixed tumor versus the predominance of a lobular epithelial proliferation in acrospiroma.

OTHER MIXED-LINEAGE ADNEXAL ADENOMAS

Those who are experienced in examining appendageal tumors of the skin are accustomed to the fact that one regularly encounters lesions which are undoubtedly benign but that show more than one route of epithelial adnexal differentiation. In that vein, admixtures of eccrine and apocrine, sudoriferous and pilar, pilar and sebaceous, or sweat glandular and sebaceous tissues may be observed in those neoplasms (Fig. 29-23). Rather than invoking the use of such nebulous terms as *sebocrine adenoma*, *infundibular adenoma*, or *sebaceoma*—as proposed by other authors[77–79]—or forcing the diagnosis into another ill-fitting nomenclatural compartment in describing lesions with the just-cited characteristics, the generic labels of *adnexal adenoma with divergent differentiation* or *mixed sweat gland adenoma*[80] are preferable. One can then provide the details of microscopic structure in a commentary in the diagnostic report and offer an opinion on which "standard" appendageal neoplasm is most related in a nosologic sense.

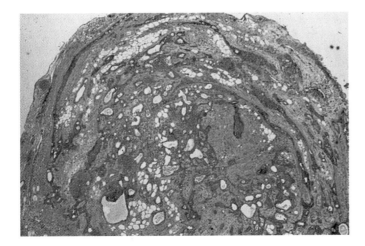

FIGURE 29-21   Benign mixed tumor (chondroid syringoma). An admixture of epithelial and stromal elements is conspicuous at low magnification.

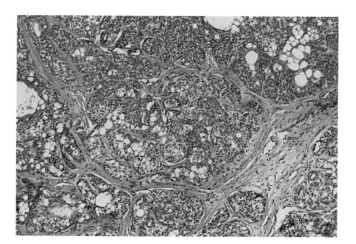

FIGURE 29-23   Adnexal adenoma with divergent differentiation. Small basaloid nests with focal sebaceous differentiation are seen.

MALIGNANT SWEAT GLAND TUMORS

Over the past 30 years, substantial revisionism has occurred in reference to definitions of sweat gland carcinomas. One must no longer rely on metastasis as the only "reliable" determinant of aggressiveness in that context, because several histologic factors have been delineated which can be used as prospective predictors of potentially malignant behavior.

The categorization of carcinomas of the sweat glands obviously represents a microcosm of the nosology of cutaneous adnexal neoplasms in general. One can either pursue a broadly based approach to classification, utilizing the term *sweat gland carcinoma* to describe most lesions, or one can adopt a more individualized approach. Because *differential diagnostic* considerations vary considerably in reference to various specific malignant sudoriferous tumors (and, selectively, biologic characteristics as well), a relatively detailed nomenclatural scheme for such neoplasms is again appropriate.

Eccrine Carcinomas

In general, the best model for understanding the range of microscopic patterns expressed by cutaneous eccrine malignancies is the spectrum of carcinoma morphotypes seen in the female breast.[81] This similarity is not difficult to understand theoretically, because it is widely acknowledged that the mammary glands represent large and somewhat specialized versions of the sudoriferous apparatus. In accord with this information, it is a logical extension for dermatopathologists to apply to sweat gland carcinomas a terminologic system which is similar to that used for breast cancer. One might also expect that some malignant adnexal tumors will have clinicopathologic characteristics which are sufficiently singular as to ensure their primary nature, whereas others are, for all intents and purposes, indistinguishable from metastases *to* the skin. These two major subgroups will be presented below.

ECCRINE CARCINOMAS THAT ARE DEFINABLE AS PRIMARY TUMORS

Eccrine Porocarcinoma

Clinical Features   This tumor most commonly presents as a verrucous plaque or nodule with frequent ulceration, commonly measuring up to 5 cm in diameter and localized to the lower extremities, followed by the head and neck, upper extremities, and trunk (Table 29-10). In general, these tumors tend to present in older individuals, most frequently in the seventh decade. In many cases there is a history of a relatively long-standing lesion.

TABLE 29-10

Eccrine Porocarcinoma

Clinical Features

Older individuals, often > 60 years
Lower extremities, head and neck, upper extremities, trunk
Verrucous papule or nodule up to 5 cm in diameter
High rate of local recurrence
Regional lymph node metastases
Tendency to multiple epidermotropic metastases

Histopathological Features

Many features in common with poroma
Infiltrative features
Desmoplastic stroma often
Tumor necrosis
Cytologic atypia
Mitoses
Extensive clear-cell change frequent

Differential Diagnosis

Eccrine poroma
Squamous cell carcinoma
Malignant acrospiroma
Malignant trichilemoma
Amelanotic melanoma

Histopathological Features   Eccrine porocarcinomas are notable for the high frequency of local recurrence, regional lymph node metastases, and a peculiar tendency to multiple epidermotropic metastases.

Eccrine porocarcinoma is closely related clinically and structurally to ordinary eccrine poroma, as described below. The points of histologic dissimilarity between the benign and malignant lesions in this category include the presence in porocarcinomas of infiltrative growth (with desmoplastic stromal response); spontaneous tumor necrosis; obvious global cytologic anaplasia, with high nucleocytoplasmic ratios and nucleolation; extensive clear-cell change; or perineural or vascular invasion[82–90] (Table 29-10) (Fig. 29-24). Not all those features need be present in order to assign a diagnosis of malignancy; in fact, infiltrative growth is sufficient unto itself in this regard.

As expected, invasive porocarcinoma has both acrosyringiumlike and dermal components, by definition. However, a solely *intraepidermal* form of the tumor has been recognized (and formally termed *malignant hidroacanthoma simplex*[91–94]) that falls into the category of Borst-Jadassohn lesions. As such, it shows the clonal, micronodular growth of atypical polygonal cells within the surface epithelium, yielding nests of tumor cells that are sharply marginated from adjacent keratinocytes (Fig. 29-25). It may be necessary to perform immunostains, for such markers as carcinoembryonic antigen (CEA) or S-100 protein, to distinguish intraepidermal porocarcinoma (which is potentially CEA-positive and S-100 protein–positive)[95] from other histologic look-alikes such as clonal Bowen's disease or seborrheic keratosis (both CEA-negative and S-100-negative) or melanoma in situ (CEA-negative and S-100-positive).[96] In addition, the scattering of single malignant cells throughout the epidermis—as typically seen in Paget's disease of the skin or amelanotic superficial spreading malignant melanoma—is not a feature of porocarcinoma. The last of these considerations is particularly important in cases of porocarcinoma where the neoplastic cells divergently synthesize melanin (often causing clinicians to make a diagnosis of melanoma)—a well-recognized but rare potentiality of that tumor.[97]

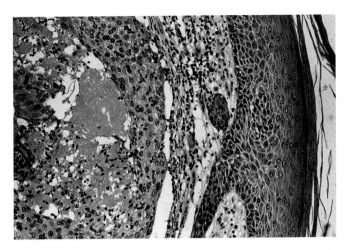

FIGURE 29-24 Eccrine porocarcinoma. The presence of necrosis helps to distinguish this cytologically atypical proliferation from architecturally similar examples of poroma.

Together with the extreme rarity with which secondary cutaneous carcinomas involve the epidermis, the particular microscopic attributes of eccrine porocarcinoma make the diagnostic consideration of metastasis *to* the skin from another organ site a largely academic matter. Isolated cases with intraepidermal growth have been documented in reference to metastatic carcinomas in the skin,[98] but this eventuality is so uncommon that the author has seen only two examples of it.

Differential Diagnosis   Mainly intraepidermal forms of porocarcinoma must be distinguished from hidroacanthoma simplex, squamous cell carcinoma in situ, mammary and extramammary Paget's disease, and melanoma (see previous discussion). Deeper forms of the tumor must be distinguished from invasive squamous cell carcinoma and malignant acrospiroma. In general, eccrine porocarcinoma is characterized by a small cuboidal cell population as opposed to somewhat larger cells in conventional squamous cell carcinoma. Porocarcinoma also shows prominent epidermal involvement and ductal or tubular structures. Porocarcinomas also have more frequent epidermal involvement as opposed to a more prevalent dermal location of malignant acrospiroma.

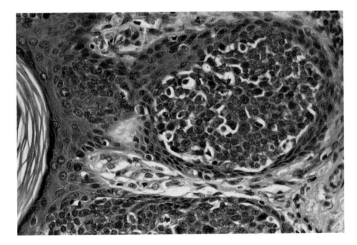

FIGURE 29-25 Intraepidermal porocarcinoma (malignant hidroacanthoma simplex). This classic pattern of a clonal intraepidermal proliferation of atypical cells has been referred to as the "Borst-Jadassohn" effect. It is typical of examples of porocarcinoma limited to the epidermis but may also be present in lesions that infiltrate the corium.

Finally, in rare instances, cutaneous metastases must be differentiated from porocarcinoma. Careful clinicopathologic correlation may be needed to arrive at a final diagnosis.

Malignant Acrospiroma

This category of carcinoma, also called *hidradenocarcinoma*, probably encompasses a heterogenous group of tumors including porocarcinoma and clear-cell eccrine carcinoma (see below).

Clinical Features   The cases previously reported have presented as ulcerated nodules involving the head and neck area and extremities of older individuals (Table 29-11).[1,2,12,90,137] In general these tumors have been associated with frequent metastases.

Histopathological Features   In general these are dermal-based tumors that are composed of lobules of polygonal clear cells with greater atypicality than that associated with benign acrospiromas (Table 29-11).[1,2,12,90,137] Three morphologic variants have been described: (1) tumors with a polypoid configuration, (2) tumors characterized by marked desmoplasia, and (3) comedo variants showing central necrosis within lobular epithelial aggregates. Both basaloid and squamous foci may occur to varying extents in a given tumor and may predominate over clear-cell alteration. Ductal structures can be detected in the majority of cases. Particular features suggesting malignancy include cytologic atypia, infiltrative pattern at the periphery of the tumor, necrosis, and mitoses in significant number. It should be pointed out that cytologic features may vary from being well-differentiated to anaplastic.

Differential Diagnosis   The major entities to be considered include other clear-cell epithelial malignancies such as porocarcinoma, clear-cell eccrine carcinoma, sebaceous carcinoma, tricholemmal carcinoma,

TABLE 29-11

Malignant Acrospiroma

Clinical Features

Older individuals
Face and extremities
Ulcerated nodules frequent
Metastases frequent

Histopathological Features

Three morphologic variants:
   Polypoid configuration of tumor
   Sclerosing variant with marked desmoplasia
   Comedo variant showing central necrosis within lobular epithelial
     aggregates
Dermal-based tumor composed of lobules of polygonal clear cells
Occasional basaloid and squamous foci
Ductal structures
Degree of cytologic atypia varies from well differentiated to anaplastic
Infiltrative growth pattern
Mitoses usually significant in number
Necrosis

Differential Diagnosis

Eccrine porocarcinoma
Squamous cell carcinoma
Sebaceous carcinoma
Clear-cell eccrine carcinoma

TABLE 29-12

TABLE 29-12

Mucinous Eccrine Carcinoma

Clinical Features

Older individuals (50–70 years)
Head and neck, especially eyelids, scalp
Skin-colored or discolored nodule up to 3 cm in diameter
Recurrences common
Low rate of metastasis

Histopathological Features

Aggregates of epithelial cells in lakes of mucin
Epithelial nests may be solid, contain lumina, or show cribriform
   patterns
Minimal cytologic atypia
Mitoses uncommon

Differential Diagnosis

Metastases from the breast, gastrointestinal tract, and ovary (unlikely)
Myxoid melanoma

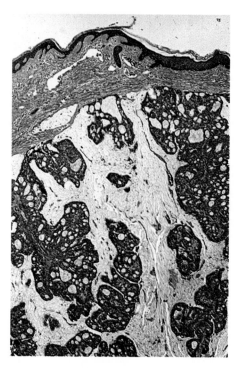

FIGURE 29-26 Mucinous eccrine carcinoma. Rounded or irregular ducto-glandular nests rest in a mucinous matrix.

squamous cell carcinoma, clear-cell basal cell carcinoma, and occasional metastases to the skin. There is substantial overlap of malignant acrospiroma with porocarcinoma and clear-cell eccrine carcinoma, and such a distinction in some cases may be more artificial than a viable exercise. Separation of the former tumor from the other entities is based on predominant morphologic pattern, particular features such as sebaceous differentiation (vacuolated cells), and on occasion the use of other techniques such as special stains (for glycogen and lipid), immunohistochemistry, or electron microscopy.

Mucinous Eccrine Carcinoma

Clinical Features   Mucinous carcinoma is a distinctive tumor often presenting on the face and especially the eyelids as a skin-colored or occasionally slightly discolored nodule, measuring up to 3 cm in diameter (Table 29-12). In many cases the tumor has a soft or spongelike consistency. The vast majority of tumors develop in older individuals in their sixth and seventh decades. It is possible that these tumors may be more common in men and African-Americans. In general, mucinous carcinoma is prone to local recurrence but has a relatively low rate of regional lymph node metastasis.

Histopathological Features   Mucinous eccrine carcinoma (MEC) represents a form of sweat gland carcinoma which lacks a benign counterpart (Table 29-12). It is extremely similar—if not identical—histologically to mucinous (*colloid*) carcinoma of the breast or gastrointestinal tract. Thus, when this tumor is encountered in the skin, it often causes concern over the diagnostic possibility of metastasis from an occult visceral lesion. Nevertheless, on empirical grounds, this is not a known potentiality of mammary or alimentary tract mucinous carcinomas and may be dismissed for that reason. In other words, "colloid" carcinomas of the breasts, stomach, and intestines do not ever involve the skin unless the patient has a long-standing and disseminated tumor[99]; these neoplasms appear to lack the ability to selectively affect the dermis early in the course of disease. Thus, as true of porocarcinomas, one can again use the histologic details attending MEC to render a certain interpretation that this cutaneous lesion is primary in nature.

Mucinous carcinoma is characterized by the presence of large extracellular pools of epithelial mucin in the dermis and possibly the subcutis, in which rounded or irregular nests and slightly branching cords of polyhedral tumor cells are suspended (Figs. 29-26 and 29-27). The

overall growth of the lesion is infiltrative, and fibrovascular septa of variable width and prominence subdivide the epithelial elements and mucinous matrix in MEC.[100–108] Nuclei are generally oval with dispersed chromatin and small nucleoli; cytoplasm is amphophilic or slightly eosinophilic and may be vacuolated. Mitotic figures are usually limited in number, and vascular or neural permeation is relatively

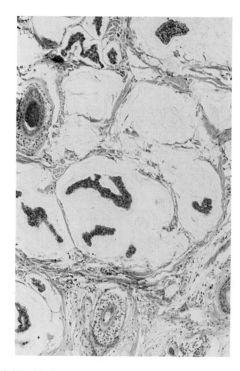

FIGURE 29-27 Mucinous eccrine carcinoma. Mucin pools dissect through dermis. As in mucinous carcinomas in other sites, cords of malignant epithelial cells may only sparsely populate areas of the lesion.

uncommon. The mucin produced in this tumor is strongly labeled by the mucicarmine or diastase-digested periodic acid–Schiff (PAS-D) methods; it will also stain with the colloidal iron or alcian blue techniques.[103]

Differential Diagnosis Virtually the only tenable differential diagnosis in cases of MEC is that of "hyper-myxoid" mixed tumor of the skin. The distinction between those lesions is usually easily made by conventional microscopy, in that the mesenchymoid zones of such mixed tumors do contain fusiform stromal cells, albeit widely scattered. In contrast, the mucinous pools of MEC are strictly acellular except for the neoplastic polyhedral cell clusters themselves. Results of histochemical investigations also differ in this context, because the mucomyxoid stromal zones of mixed tumors are negative with the mucicarmine and PAS-D procedures.[68]

As discussed above, one must consider the possibility of metastatic mucinous carcinoma from the breast, gastrointestinal tract, or ovary. However, as mentioned above, the probability of an occult metastasis in the skin with features of mucinous carcinoma is almost nonexistent. If this does occur it is usually a manifestation of very late-stage disease. Note that metastatic breast carcinoma almost always follows obvious disease in the breast.

Adenoid Cystic Carcinoma of the Skin

Clinical Features Adenoid cystic carcinoma (ACC) represents a morphotype common to a number of organs and tissues, including the salivary glands, respiratory tract, breast, skin, uterine cervix, thymus, and prostate gland. In each of these sites, the usual evolution of the tumor is one of relatively slow growth with aggressive local behavior; secondary spread to other locations occurs only late in the clinical course. The most common sites of cutaneous involvement are the scalp and chest. Thus, for most of the same reasons cited in connection with MEC, cutaneous ACC can reasonably be considered to represent a primary tumor whenever it is encountered.

Histopathological Features This neoplasm is felt to demonstrate eccrine differentiation; it is composed of a "pure" population of monomorphic basaloid cells that are arranged in tubules, elongated nests, and cords. Ductal lumina may be formed by the neoplastic elements, or they may enclose "cylinders" of mucoid matrix with a lightly basophilic hue. Another common feature is the deposition of linear profiles or globules of brightly eosinophilic basement membrane material in the intercellular spaces[109–120] (Figs. 29-28 and 29-29). Nuclei are compact, with dispersed chromatin and indistinct nucleoli; mitoses are sparse. Cytoplasm is scant and amphophilic.

Differential Diagnosis Importantly, the dermal stroma adjacent to clusters of tumor cells in ACC does not show retraction artifact or fibromyxoid alteration, as seen in basal cell carcinomas. This is a crucial distinction, because most tumors thought to be cutaneous ACCs are actually adenoid basal cell carcinomas (ABCCs).[113] The overall growth pattern of both of those tumor types is infiltrative, and permeation of vascular adventitia and perineural spaces is potentially common to each of them as well. Additional minor points of difference between ACCs and ABCCs is that the latter neoplasm manifests the regular presence of apoptotic cells in the center of tumor cell nests and may even show cohesive foci of geographic necrosis, whereas those observations are rare in ACCs. Moreover, basal cell carcinomas of *all* types commonly display evidence of multilinear differentiation (e.g., a mixture of adenoid and pilar-keratotic foci) and may contain true melanin pigment. Such attributes are again not part of the morphologic spectrum of ACC. Whenever it is needed, immunostaining is again capable of distinguishing between these tumors; ABCC is EMA-negative, whereas ACC regularly expresses that marker.[95,113]

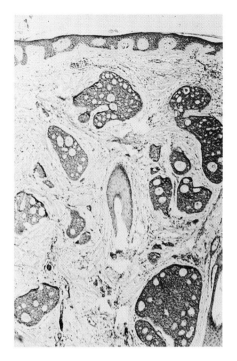

FIGURE 29-28 Adenoid cystic carcinoma. Large angular clusters of basaloid cells are dispersed in the dermis. Uniform, rounded matrical cylinders interrupt these monomorphic basaloid nests.

Papillary Digital Eccrine Adenocarcinoma

In 1987, Kao and coworkers published the seminal description of a distinctive group of eccrine neoplasms that are unique to the distal extremities, particularly the digits.[121] Although these tumors were originally segregated into two groups by those authors—as "aggressive digital papillary adenomas" and "aggressive digital papillary adenocarcinomas"—it is considered that they represent points in the same continuum of what is basically a family of universally malignant neoplasms. Thus, the more unifying term of *papillary digital eccrine adenocarcinoma* (PDEA) in reference to such lesions is preferable. The most helpful image to bear in mind in reference to PDEA is that of invasive papillary large-duct carcinoma of the female breast,[81] because they are identical for practical purposes. Nevertheless, because metastasis to the skin of

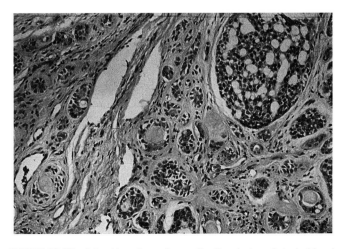

FIGURE 29-29 Adenoid cystic carcinoma. Smaller clusters of atypical basaloid cells (with or without cylinders of basement-membrane-like material) may loosely infiltrate the dermis.

TABLE 29-13

Papillary Digital Eccrine Adenocarcinoma

Clinical Features

Older individuals
Digits, palms, soles
Firm nodules

Histopathological Features

Micropapillae projecting into cystic spaces
Solid nests and tubules composed of polygonal cells
Infiltration of surrounding tissue
Nuclear features varying from dispersed chromatin and small nucleoli
to vesicular nuclei with prominent nucleoli

Differential Diagnosis

Hidradenoma papilliferum

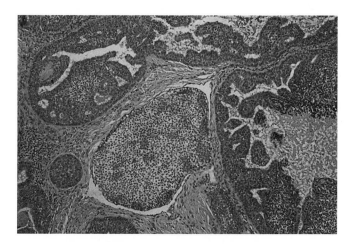

FIGURE 29-30 Papillary digital eccrine adenocarcinoma. Solid nests and papillary structures are evident in this intradermal neoplasm.

occult forms of the latter mammary tumor is empirically unknown, differential diagnosis centering on that point is hypothetical rather than real. Thus, one may once more rightly conclude that a cutaneous lesion with the configuration of papillary adenocarcinoma is a primary neoplasm.

Clinical Features   These tumors most commonly present in older individuals as solitary nodules up to 2 cm in diameter localized to the fingers, toes, palms, and soles (Table 29-13). There is a high rate of local recurrence, and about 50 percent of tumors eventuate in distant metastases with a predilection for the lungs.

Histopathological Features   On scanning microscopy, PDEAs feature the formation of *macro*papillae that project into large cystic spaces and, in addition, contain solid nests and tubules comprised of polygonal cells that irregularly infiltrate the surrounding dermis and subcutis (Table 29-13) (Figs. 29-30 and 29-31); involvement of the underlying bone may sometimes be present as well. Nuclear characteristics are bimorphic; one subgroup of PDEAs (so-called aggressive papillary digital adenomas) shows dispersed chromatin, small or indistinct nucleoli, and limited mitotic activity[121,122] and may accordingly be considered as the low-grade member of the spectrum under consideration here. However, the second variant (i.e., aggressive digital papillary adenocarcinoma) manifests vesicular nuclei; prominent nucleoli; numerous, often pathologically shaped mitotic figures; and foci of spontaneous geographic necrosis[121] (Fig. 29-31). The latter tumor is a more poorly differentiated form of PDEA. Perineural and lymphatic invasion may be observed regardless of tumor grade, but *only* poorly differentiated tumors in this category will produce distant metastases. Squamous metaplasia, and clear, ovoid, possibly myoepithelial cells are seen more often in low-grade than high-grade PDEA.

Differential Diagnosis   On morphologic grounds, the only vaguely plausible differential diagnostic alternative to PDEA is that of hidradenoma papilliferum, as described above, but that lesion is never observed on the digits and has never been documented convincingly in malignant form. Despite an overlap with PDEA in nomenclature, *papillary eccrine adenoma* forms *micro*papillae that project into tubular lumina[122] (see above), unlike the features of the former lesion. Therefore, the comparative but dissimilar images of these two skin tumors correspond to papillary carcinoma *versus* intraductal hyperplasia of the breast.

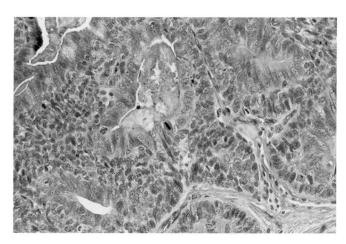

FIGURE 29-31 Papillary digital eccrine adenocarcinoma. At higher magnification, areas of mitotic activity are associated with atypical cells with vesicular nuclei and prominent nucleoli.

Microcystic Adnexal Carcinoma

In 1982, a peculiar tumor of the skin was recognized in which syringomalike profiles of bland cuboidal epithelial cells—largely lacking nucleoli and mitotic activity—were seen to infiltrate the dermis and subcutis in a random and permeative fashion[123] (Fig. 29-32). These cellular aggregates were occasionally punctuated by microcystic arrays containing pilar-type (trichilemmal) keratin. The name "microcystic adnexal carcinoma" (MAC) was chosen to describe the lesion, which has, in the interim, been shown to demonstrate mixed eccrine and pilar differentiation.[124,125] Cooper and colleagues assigned the synonym of *sclerosing sweat duct carcinoma* in reference to the densely collagenized stroma that separates the tumor cell aggregates from one another in a variant of MAC that *lacks* pilar microcysts[126,127]; this neoplastic subtype had been referred to as *anaplastic syringoma* or *syringoid carcinoma* in the prior literature[128,129] (Fig. 29-33). It is for those reasons that the tumor has been discussed in this section rather than in the one which considers mixed-lineage neoplasms (see below).

Clinical Features   MAC usually presents as an indurated lesion involving the face, particularly the upper lip, but also in other locations

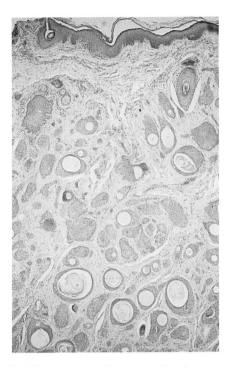

FIGURE 29-32 Microcystic adnexal carcinoma. Small rounded or syringoid profiles consisting of basaloid and squamoid cells—some with keratinization—loosely infiltrate the dermis.

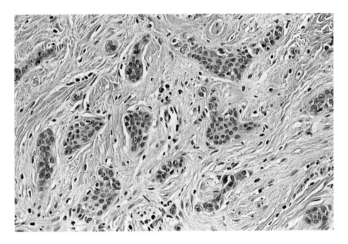

FIGURE 29-33 Microcystic adnexal carcinoma. The absence of microcysts typifies a subset of microcystic adnexal carcinomas. Small angular clusters in these lesions are associated with a desmoplastic stromal response. The term *sclerosing sweat duct carcinoma* has been applied to such tumors.

such as the axilla (Table 29-14). These tumors are generally perceived as slow-growing indolent tumors and may develop in individuals of any age, but especially young women. The rate of local recurrence approaches 50 percent, but true metastasis is unknown.

Histopathological Features   The features of MAC are basically those that have just been described above (Table 29-14). Infiltration of perineural sheaths, vascular adventitia, and even subjacent muscle is a common finding in this lesion.[130-137] The neoplastic cells may focally aggregate themselves into whorled, concentric profiles in the dermis, and clear-cell change also has been described.[138] The latter feature links

---

TABLE 29-14

Microcystic Adnexal Carcinoma

Clinical Features

Adults, 20–76 years
Women = men
Face, especially upper lip, axilla
Slowly developing indurated plaque or nodule
Skin-colored, yellowish
Local recurrence common
Metastasis rare

Histopathological Features

Small epithelial aggregates with keratinous cysts, especially superficially
Solid epithelial islands and cords, some with lumina
Fibrotic to densely sclerotic stroma
Deeply invasive with frequent infiltration of subcutis, skeletal muscle, and nerves
Minimal or low-grade atypia
Mitotic figures generally uncommon

Differential Diagnosis

Syringoma
Desmoplastic trichoepithelioma
Morpheaform basal cell carcinoma
Papillary eccrine adenoma

MAC to "low-grade clear-cell carcinoma," as described by Cooper and colleagues.[139] Secretory material can be observed in the lumina of the syringomalike profiles of cells as well.[126] Another variant of MAC shows a *predominance* of keratinous microcysts, simulating the *trichoadenoma of Nikolowsky*.[137] Nonetheless, this variant differs from the latter tumor in exhibiting syringoid cell profiles and deeply infiltrative growth as well. In accord with the general capacity for divergent differentiation in MAC, it should come as no surprise that occasional examples demonstrate sebaceous foci as well as eccrine and pilar elements.[133]

Differential Diagnosis   The differential diagnosis of MAC does *not* include metastatic carcinomas of visceral origin, all of which would be expected to show a more confined growth pattern and a higher degree of cytologic anaplasia. Instead, other lesions that must be considered include conventional syringoma, desmoplastic trichoepithelioma, morpheaform basal cell carcinoma, trichoadenoma, and primary adenosquamous carcinoma of the skin. The last two of these entities will be discussed in later sections of this chapter.

Conventional syringoma and desmoplastic trichoepithelioma (DTE) both are separable from MAC simply by attention to adequate clinical information. All are predominantly facial lesions, but the first two tumors are small, exquisitely circumscribed papulonodular lesions, whereas MAC is an ill-defined, fixed plaque.[17,126,140] Microscopically, an analogy to this information can also be observed; syringoma and DTE show a profile in which the dermal tumor is broader than it is deep, with sharply defined peripheral borders. In contrast, MAC extends to the base of even generous biopsy specimens and "shades off" into the surrounding tissue.[19,140] Given these observations, one can readily appreciate the wisdom of diagnostic equivocation if faced with a shave biopsy containing a tumor that *may* represent MAC in the absence of clinical data. Lastly, morphealike BCC shows more branched cellular nests than those seen in MAC, and luminal differentiation is not apparent therein; the stroma of the former of these lesions also shows a characteristic "cleavage" away from tumor cell clusters,[141] but this feature is not evident in MAC.

Primary Cutaneous Adenosquamous Carcinoma

Clinical Features   A primary neoplasm of the skin has been described that occurs more commonly on the head and neck, without regard to gender or age. This neoplasm demonstrates continuity with the epidermis and conjoint glandular and squamous differentiation microscopically and has been called *adenosquamous carcinoma* (ASC) in order to distinguish it from MAC and other malignant adnexal neoplasms.[142–144] The behavior of ASC has been aggressive, with 7 of 10 patients in the largest series succumbing to their tumors or being likely to do so.[142] Regional lymph node metastases were observed in some cases.

Histopathological Features   One sees in ASC a growth pattern which closely simulates that of MAC, except that the lesion is multifocally connected to the epidermis in the former neoplasm, and the tumor cells show obvious nuclear anaplasia. As its name suggests, squamous carcinomalike and glandular foci are interspersed in ASC, with the adenocarcinomatous areas having a potential for mucinous differentiation as well. Mitoses are numerous, and zones of geographic necrosis may be evident. The same propensity for neural and vascular invasion that is manifested in MAC is also seen in ASC.[142–144]

Differential Diagnosis   One must principally consider other primary tumors of the skin, rather than metastases, because of the prominent epidermal continuity that is appreciable in ASC cases. Obviously, one may have difficulty in excluding ordinary squamous carcinoma if only a small biopsy specimen is obtained; however, if foci of epidermal connection are not seen because of sampling limitations, metastases may indeed be considered diagnostically. Procurement of historical details—providing the information that ASC is a solitary, relatively slowly evolving lesion—is the best method for distinguishing between primary and secondary (multifocal and rapidly growing) adenosquamous tumors in this context. Last, one might consider ductal eccrine adenocarcinoma with prominent squamous metaplasia (see below) as an alternative interpretation to one of ASC, but, as Banks and Cooper[142] have indicated, the distinction between these two tumors may be somewhat arbitrary.

Primary Mucoepidermoid Carcinoma of the Skin

Mucoepidermoid carcinomas (MEDC) usually arise in the salivary glands or respiratory tree and assume a well-differentiated appearance histologically.[145–147] In accord with the latter point, these tumors are slowly growing in most instances and only uncommonly metastasize to distant sites. When the latter eventuality occurs, it is virtually always after the primary neoplasm has been recognized and treated in some manner. These same precepts apply to involvement of the skin by metastatic MEDCs[148–151]; in other words, when this rare event is observed, it is in a patient who is well-known to have carcinoma historically, rather than in the face of an occult visceral neoplasm. Hence, we would take some issue with other authors over the contention that metastatic MEDC is a "mimic of sweat gland carcinoma."[148]

Histopathological Features   There are points of difference between primary and metastatic MEDCs; the latter tumors are usually multinodular and show a sharp interface with the surrounding dermis or subcutis, whereas primary neoplasms of this type have indistinct peripheries and grow as single nodules or with a uninodular predominance.

There is also commonly an admixture of chronic inflammatory cells with the neoplastic elements in *primary* cutaneous MEDC but not in metastases. Otherwise, MEDCs in general are comprised of polygonal squamous cells that are admixed with nondescript cuboidal tumor cells and obviously mucin-forming cuboidal or low columnar elements.[145–147] Mucin-filled microcysts also may be appreciated, as may areas of clear-cell change.[151] The nuclear features of all cell types in this tumor are bland, with only small inconspicuous nucleoli and dispersed chromatin; mitoses are sparse. Irregular peripheral infiltration of the dermis is evident, and perineural or (rarely) lymphatic invasion also may be present.

Differential Diagnosis   The microscopic attributes of MEDC are so typical that differential diagnosis is largely academic. It is conceivable that one might confuse that tumor with the pseudoneoplastic-metaplastic proliferative lesions of sweat glands that are sometimes seen in response to chronic mechanical or pharmacologic insults (see below). Nevertheless, the latter processes rarely produce a mass lesion and should be separable from MEDC on that basis.

Carcinoma ex Dermal Cylindroma and Eccrine Spiradenoma

Despite the knowledge that they are usually slowly growing tumors that may have been present for years before coming to clinical attention, sweat gland carcinomas in general do *not* derive from preexisting adenomas. The only exceptions to that general rule which have any frequency are carcinomas that evolve from "parent" cylindromas or spiradenomas.[152] A good number of these neoplasms have been documented in the literature[152–167]; it appears that their presence is most often signaled by the rapid expansion of a previously indolent cutaneous nodule of long standing, with or without ulceration or pain (Table 29-15). In order for this diagnosis to be accepted pathologically, there must be remnants of the "parent" lesion along with a carcinomatous component in the excised tissue (Fig. 29-34), *or* one must be able to confirm that a banal cylindroma or spiradenoma was removed previously from the *exact* site at which a sweat gland carcinoma is now present. Because of such restrictive requirements, it is beyond reason that one would diagnostically consider metastasis to the skin from a visceral carcinoma in this context.

TABLE 29-15

Carcinoma ex Dermal Cylindroma and Eccrine Spiradenoma

Clinical Features

Long-standing lesion with recent enlargement, ulceration, pain
Common disparity between high-grade appearance of tumor and lack of aggressive behavior

Histopathological Features

Remnant of benign cylindroma or spiradenoma
Anaplastic epithelium in sheets or nests
Epithelioid, stellate, or fusiform tumor cells with pronounced cytologic atypia
Resemblance to squamous cell carcinoma, adenosquamous carcinoma, adenocarcinoma, clear-cell adenocarcinoma, sarcomatoid carcinoma
Prominent mitotic rate

Differential Diagnosis

Any anaplastic tumor

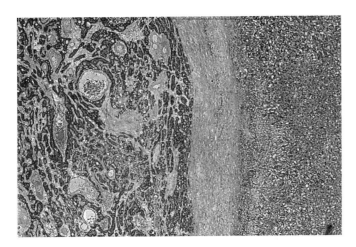

FIGURE 29-34   Carcinoma ex eccrine spiradenoma. Invasive carcinoma is juxtaposed with residual benign spiradenoma.

Histopathological Features   Remnants of the parent neoplasm have the typical appearance of cylindroma or spiradenoma, as detailed above (Table 29-15). The malignant elements most often assume the character of an undifferentiated carcinoma, showing sheets or clusters of nondescript but highly anaplastic epithelioid, stellate, or fusiform tumor cells with marked anisonucleosis, nucleolar prominence, cellular pleomorphism, and brisk mitotic activity.[154,157,162] As such, the image of a "sarcomatoid" carcinoma may be encountered.[167] Less commonly, more definable carcinoma morphotypes are reflected in the malignant components of carcinoma ex cylindroma or spiradenoma (CECS)[152]; these may include squamous carcinoma, adenosquamous carcinoma, or pure adenocarcinoma, and various subtypes of the last of these three possibilities may be evident (e.g., clear-cell adenocarcinoma) (Fig. 29-35). Under those circumstances, the *only* factor distinguishing such lesions from "ordinary" malignancies of the skin is the presence of the remnant adenoma.

One behavioral peculiarity of CECS merits some attention; that is, there may be an inexplicable disparity between the grade of the carcinomatous elements and the biologic evolution of the neoplasm. Several examples have been reported in which highly undifferentiated forms of CECS were attended by a lack of metastasis and long-term disease-free survival.[159,162,163]

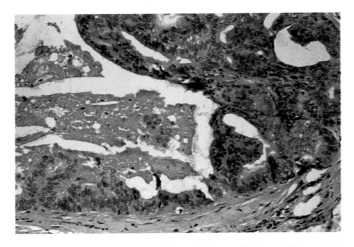

FIGURE 29-35   Carcinoma ex eccrine spiradenoma. Without evidence of origin in or from a preexisting spiradenoma, this high-grade adenocarcinoma is indistinguishable from other primary adnexal carcinomas.

ECCRINE CARCINOMAS THAT HISTOLOGICALLY SIMULATE METASTATIC TUMORS

As implied in the foregoing discussion, there are indeed some forms of eccrine carcinoma where uncertainties of the clinical picture or the histologic appearance of the mass make it virtually impossible to exclude metastasis *to* the skin on routine microscopic evaluation. The following sections address such lesions.

Ductal Eccrine Adenocarcinoma

Ductal eccrine adenocarcinoma (DEA) is, perhaps, the most common of the eccrine carcinomas. Its histologic features are virtually identical to those seen in "conventional" invasive ductal carcinoma of the *breast*,[81] metastases of which, for obvious reasons, represent the principal differential diagnostic consideration.[128,168] Obtaining a detailed clinical history of the skin lesion in question is therefore most important.

Clinical Features   DEA is virtually always a solitary, slowly growing mass measuring up to 5 cm in diameter that has been present for many months or even years before the patient seeks medical attention (Table 29-16). In contrast, metastases of mammary carcinoma are typically multiple and occur in "crops" that manifest a rapid clinical evolution.[168] The reason for emphasis on historical data is that, as one might expect, the detailed pathologic (ultrastructural and immunohistologic) features of ductal breast and eccrine carcinomas are identical; this synonymity even extends to the expression of estrogen and progesterone receptors by both tumors.[169] DEA is notable for a relatively high rate of metastasis, i.e., approximately half of the cases metastasize.

Histopathological Features   The salient histologic characteristics of DEA include the proliferation of solid cords or tubules of obviously atypical polygonal cells that randomly infiltrate the dermal connective tissue[170–174] (Table 29-16) (Fig. 29-36). Focal formation of ductal lumina is often apparent, and entrapped eccrine ducts sometimes may demonstrate the changes of carcinoma in situ.[170] The intratumoral stroma is variably desmoplastic and may contain chronic inflammatory cells (Fig. 29-37). When such features are prominent (as they are in only a minority of cases), one can be somewhat confident of the primary nature of the neoplasm; however, their absence does not conversely

TABLE 29-16

Ductal Eccrine Adenocarcinoma

Clinical Features

Solitary, slow-growing tumor
Up to 5 cm in diameter
Approximately 50% metastatic

Histopathological Features

Solid cords and tubules of polygonal cells
Ductal structures
Variable squamous differentiation
Infiltrating features
Variably desmoplastic stroma
Cytologic atypia
Mitotic figures usually readily apparent

Differential Diagnosis

Metastatic adenocarcinoma, particularly breast carcinoma
Basal cell carcinoma
Squamous cell carcinoma

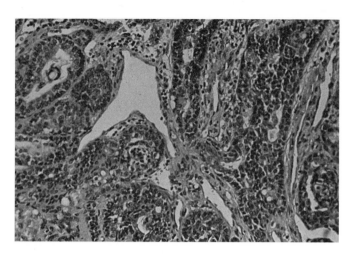

FIGURE 29-36   Ductal eccrine carcinoma. This solid and ductular proliferation is composed of pleomorphic cellular elements. Mononuclear inflammatory cells are evident within tumoral stroma.

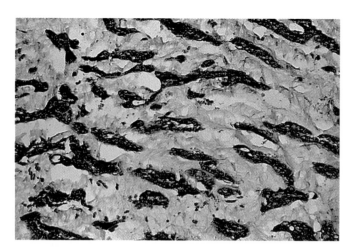

FIGURE 29-38   Ductal eccrine carcinoma with fibromyxoid stroma. In a small percentage of ductal eccrine carcinomas, cells appear more basaloid and form cords and nests that infiltrate a fibromyxoid matrix.

equate with a diagnosis of metastatic disease. Nuclear chromatin is either dense or vesicular, and prominent nucleoli are commonly present; mitotic activity is almost always appreciable but may be limited in scope. Cytoplasm is usually amphophilic, and small intracytoplasmic vacuoles may be evident; sometimes, well-defined areas of overtly squamoid differentiation are seen in DEA as well, such that differential diagnosis with a form of squamous cell carcinoma may be considered.

One variant of DEA that is site-related has been termed *ductal eccrine adenocarcinoma with fibromyxoid stroma* (DEAFS).[95,170] This lesion was probably included under the rubrics of *malignant chondroid syringoma* or *syringoid carcinoma* in the past, and the lesion occurs more commonly on the distal extremities (particularly the sole of the foot). As its name implies, DEAFS differs from "usual" DEA by its possession of a uniformly fibromyxoid stroma that recalls one of the attributes of cutaneous mixed tumor (Fig. 29-38). Other peculiarities of this tumoral subtype are its ability to communicate with the surface epithelium in a similar manner to that of poroma and to be comprised of compact, almost basaloid cells. Because of the concatenation of these features (i.e., a fibromyxoid matrix and an epidermal connection to cords of relatively small polyhedral cells), a mistaken diagnosis of basal cell carcinoma also may be rendered in such cases. When selected circumstances (such as limited, artifactually distorted biopsy material) make it

necessary, the latter problem can be addressed by performing immunostains for epithelial membrane antigen (EMA). Virtually all forms of sweat gland carcinoma are EMA-positive, whereas basal cell carcinomas are consistently nonreactive for that determinant.[95,175]

Another variant of DEA is a form in which the neoplastic cells partially or globally assume a fusiform configuration.[170] This feature may reflect the presence of myoepithelial differentiation, although that point has not been addressed systematically to date. The spindle cells are capable of focal concentric growth—yielding "tactoid"-like structures, and they often blend imperceptibly with conventional epithelioid areas. Lastly, uncommon examples of DEA have been described in which there was a histologic admixture of MEC-like foci, as described above; this pattern is mirrored in primary breast tumors as well.[176] In such instances, the ductal adenocarcinomatous component confers a significant metastatic risk to the lesions (which approximates 40 percent overall for DEA).

Differential Diagnosis   Metastatic adenocarcinoma from the breast or a visceral site must be considered in the differential diagnosis of DEA. However, for practical purposes only metastatic breast carcinoma closely resembles DEA and, as discussed above, may be indistinguishable from DEA without clinical information. Carcinomas with the appearance of DEA may occasionally be seen in the skin of the breast or the mammary tails in the axillae. The question arises under these circumstances as to whether the tumor is a primary cutaneous malignancy or a carcinoma of the breast proper. By convention, the diagnosis of sweat gland carcinoma *of any type* is not made in the skin of the breast, and the clinician should be told to manage such cases as *mammary parenchymal* neoplasms. As mentioned above, other considerations in particular tumors include basal cell carcinoma and squamous cell carcinoma.

Clear-Cell Eccrine Carcinoma

As suggested at intervals in the foregoing descriptions, several eccrine neoplasms feature the potential presence of clear-cell change; these tumors include acrospiromas, MACs, poromas, and mixed tumors of the skin. However, one particular type of eccrine malignancy is so dominated by clear cells that it derives its name from them, namely, *clear-cell eccrine carcinoma* (CCEC).[177,178] Nosologically, the latter lesion is most closely related to low-grade *malignant acrospiroma* (hidradenocarcinoma),[179–186] but its major significance derives from a potential pathologic confusion with metastases of renal cell carcinoma and other adenocarcinomas of urogenital or pulmonary origin.[187]

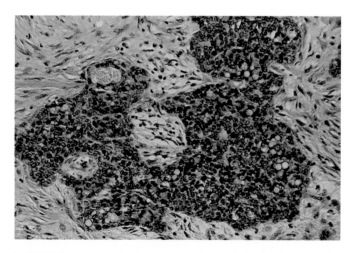

FIGURE 29-37   Ductal eccrine carcinoma. Stromal desmoplasia may be prominent in some examples of ductal carcinoma.

Clinical Features The surest approach to excluding the possibilities discussed above is to obtain detailed clinical information on the solitary or multifocal nature of the lesion and its duration of antecedent growth. In the same line of thought, it should also be remembered that CCEC is most often seen in the skin of the head and neck, whereas the metastatic tumors that may simulate it histologically show a predilection for the truncal surface.[168]

Histopathological Features CCEC is a multilobulated dermal neoplasm that lacks connections to the epidermis and shows a vague peripheral interface with the surrounding dermis and subcutis. Broad sheets or large clusters of polyhedral tumor cells with lucent cytoplasm are separated from one another by fibrovascular stroma of variable density. Nuclei may either be compact with evenly distributed chromatin and small nucleoli, or vesicular with prominent nucleoli (Fig. 29-39). Mitotic activity is likewise heterogeneous from lesion to lesion. Spontaneous tumor necrosis and infiltration of perineural or perivascular spaces are other potential observations in CCEC cases.[177,178]

Differential Diagnosis As discussed above, the major concerns are metastases of renal cell carcinoma and other adenocarcinomas of urogenital or pulmonary origin. Important, one does *not* see "hobnail" cell profiles or intercellular blood lakes in CCEC, such as those that have been described in a proportion of clear-cell carcinomas of urogenital or renal origins, respectively.[187–189] Immunostains for carcinoembryonic antigen and the CA-125 glycoprotein are potentially discriminatory in this context as well. If the CEA stain is positive, such results would tend to militate in favor of CCEC, because renal cell carcinomas are quite uniformly negative, and clear-cell urogenital carcinomas usually lack CEA also.[175] Similarly, carcinomas of the female genital tract are expected to express CA-125 (and renal carcinomas may sometimes do so as well), whereas that determinant has not been seen in CCEC.

Primary Malignant Mixed Tumor of the Skin (So-Called Carcinosarcoma)

Contrary to intuitive expectations, the exceedingly rare neoplasms called *malignant mixed tumors* of the skin are *not* synonymous with carcinomas ex mixed tumors, as true in the salivary glands. Instead, almost all reports of these cutaneous lesions have shown neoplasms that lack any type of "parent" adenoma and appear to represent de novo sweat gland carcinomas manifesting divergent mesenchymallike differentia-

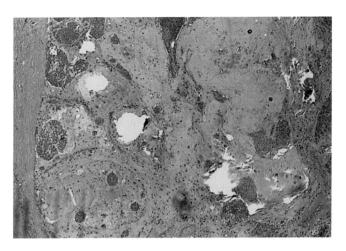

FIGURE 29-40 Malignant mixed tumor of skin. Chondroid nests harbor nests of atypical epithelial cells in this example of malignant mixed tumor.

tion.[190–200] An exception is the case reported by Sharvill,[201] which is more aptly considered a *carcinoma ex cutaneous mixed tumor*. In the usual malignant mixed tumor, recognizable eccrine carcinoma morphotypes are admixed histologically with tissue foci resembling chondrosarcoma, osteosarcoma, rhabdomyosarcoma, fibrosarcoma, leiomyosarcoma, or undifferentiated sarcoma, all in the same mass[190–200] (Fig. 29-40). The biologic evolution of such tumors is again paradoxical, in that relatively few of them have demonstrated aggressive behavior despite their alarming pathologic characteristics.

Differential Diagnosis Metastases to the skin from carcinosarcomas (more properly termed sarcomatoid carcinomas) of the kidney, lung, genital tract, and other sites[202] must be excluded through clinical investigations before a diagnosis of primary cutaneous malignancy can be assigned confidently in these circumstances.

Basaloid (Small-Cell) Eccrine Carcinoma

Past treatises on sweat gland tumors have anecdotally mentioned the existence of a small-cell variant of eccrine carcinoma, with "basaloid" features.[1,128,203] In fact, Berg and McDivitt mentioned 14 such neoplasms in their report on the subject in 1968,[128] but it is likely that many of those cases ultimately proved to be examples of Merkel cell carcinoma as introduced by Toker in 1972.[204] Matsuo and coworkers[205] documented a similar case which was classified as "small-cell carcinoma of the skin, non-Merkel cell type."

Clinical Features The authors have seen four cases of basaloid eccrine carcinoma (BEC); one arose in a male child, whereas the others were observed in two men and one woman. All the lesions arose in the skin of the arms or legs and were solitary, nodular, tan-pink, nonulcerated tumors that had been present for at least 1 year before diagnosis. Two of the lesions metastasized to regional lymph nodes, and one proved fatal with distant spread to visceral organs.

Histopathological Features BEC is typified by nests and cords of small, uniform tumor cells with hyperchromatic or vesicular chromatin, distinct nucleoli, and obvious mitotic activity. Cytoplasm is scant and amphophilic, and single-cell necrosis or small foci of geographic necrosis are commonly present. The latter feature may produce zones of apparent microcystification (Fig. 29-41). Lesional stroma in BEC cases is desmoplastic and moderately cellular, but the density of matrical blood vessels is low.

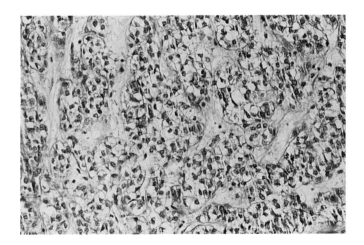

FIGURE 29-39 Clear-cell eccrine carcinoma. At higher magnification, the cytoplasm is lucent, and nuclei are variably pleomorphic.

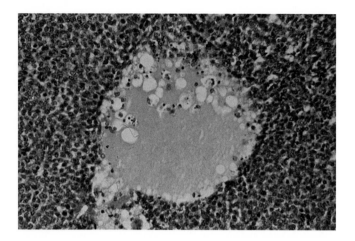

FIGURE 29-41　Basaloid (small-cell) eccrine carcinoma. Solid nests of cyto-logically uniform basaloid cells dominate this lesion. Necrosis, mitotic activity, and prominent nucleoli are evident even at intermediate magnification.

Differential Diagnosis　All the other small-cell tumors of the skin, including not only Merkel cell carcinoma but also metastatic visceral neuroendocrine carcinoma, small-cell melanoma, primitive neuroecto-dermal tumor or Ewing's sarcoma, malignant lymphoma, and small-cell (basaloid) squamous carcinoma, must be considered. Either electron microscopy or immunohistology are effective in recognizing BEC among the stated possibilities.[1] Results of such studies are outlined in Tables 29-17 and 29-18.

Apocrine Carcinomas

In likeness to eccrine malignancies, apocrine carcinomas may be divided into those that are histologically distinctive as primary lesions and others that may simulate metastases from visceral tumors to the skin. These are considered as such, below.

APOCRINE CARCINOMAS HISTOLOGICALLY DEFINABLE AS PRIMARY TUMORS

Two forms of apocrine carcinoma have sufficiently singular attributes that they may reliably be diagnosed as primary cutaneous disorders. These are ductopapillary apocrine carcinoma and the apocrine type of mammary or extramammary Paget's disease of the skin.

Ductopapillary Apocrine Carcinoma

Clinical Features　Ductopapillary apocrine carcinoma (DPAC) is vir-tually identical to papillary digital eccrine carcinoma (see above) on architectural grounds (Table 29-19) (Fig. 29-42), but the first of these two tumor types is most often encountered in the eyelids, axillae, and genitoperineal skin instead of the distal extremities.[128,206–214] There may be an association with nevus sebaceus on the scalp or extramam-mary Paget's disease in the groin. DPAC most commonly presents as a solitary often multinodular nondescript lesion measuring a few cen-timeters in diameter. DPAC often results in regional lymph node metas-tases followed by visceral spread in about 40 percent of cases.

Histopathological Features　DPAC is definable as apocrine because the tumor cells possess a generous amount of finely granular eosinophilic cytoplasm, with or without decapitation "snouts" at the

---

TABLE 29-17

Ultrastructural Differential Diagnosis of Cutaneous Small-Cell Tumors

TUMOR	ICJ	Type 1MF	NSG	MEL	MCL	PNFW
BEC	+	±	0	0	+	0
MCC	+	Usually 0	+	0	Usually 0	+
MSCC	+	0	+	0	0	±
PNET/ES	+	0	±	0	0	0
SCMM	±	0	±	+	0	0
SCSCC	+	+	0	0	0	0
ML	0	0	0	0	0	0

KEY: ICJ = intercellular junctional complexes; NSG = neurosecretory granules; MCL = intercellular microlumina; BEC = basaloid eccrine carcinoma; MSCC = metastatic visceral small-cell carcinoma; PNET/ES = primitive neuroectodermal tumor/Ewing's sarcoma; SCMM = small-cell malignant melanoma; SCSCC = small-cell squamous cell carcinoma; ML = malignant lymphoma; MF = microfilaments; MEL = premelanosomes; PNFW = perinuclear filament whorls; MCC = Merkel cell carcinoma.

TABLE 29-18

Immunohistochemical Differential Diagnosis of Cutaneous Small-Cell Tumors

TUMOR	CK	CGA	CEA	S-100	LCA	MIC2
BEC	+	0	+	±	0	0
MCC	+*	+ (33%)	0	0	0	±
MSCC	+	+ (30–50%)	±	0	0	±
PNET/ES	0	0	0	0	0	+
SCMM	0	0	0	+	0	0
SCSCC	+	0	0	0	0	0
ML	0	0	0	0	+	0†

KEY: CK = cytokeratin; CEA = carcinoembryonic antigen; LCA = leukocyte common antigen (CD45); CGA = chromogranin-A; S-100 = S-100 protein; MIC2 = p30/32^MIC2 protein.
*Keratin reactivity in Merkel cell carcinoma typically shows a characteristic perinuclear globular pattern.
†Lymphoblastic non-Hodgkin's lymphoma may be MIC2-positive.

TABLE 29-19

Ductopapillary Apocrine Carcinoma

Clinical Features

Older individuals
Eyelids, axillae, genitoperineal skin
Solitary multinodular lesion, usually a few cm in diameter
Association with nevus sebaceus and extramammary Paget's disease
Frequent lymph node metastases and visceral metastases in 40% of
 cases

Histopathological Features

Similar to digital papillary eccrine carcinoma
Polygonal cells with finely granular eosinophilic cytoplasm
Often decapitation secretion
Infiltration of surrounding tissue
Cytologic atypia and mitoses
Prussian blue iron stain–positive in 40–50%
Gross cystic disease fluid protein-15–positive

Differential Diagnosis

Digital papillary eccrine carcinoma
Hidradenoma papilliferum

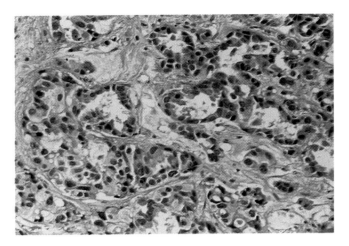

FIGURE 29-43   Ductal growth in ductopapillary apocrine carcinoma. Finely granular eosinophilic cytoplasm and decapitation secretion are evident in this glandular neoplasm.

luminal aspects of tubular or microcystic profiles within the tumor (Fig. 29-43). Nuclear atypia is obvious—well beyond that which may be present in hidradenoma papilliferum—and mitotic activity is easily appreciated.[209] Like papillary eccrine carcinomas, DPAC manifests irregular infiltration of the surrounding skin and may invade perineural sheaths or vascular adventitia.

Histochemical and immunohistochemical studies of this tumor may be useful in helping to define its apocrine lineage when morphologic markers of it are less than definitive. The Prussian blue stain for iron is positive in the cytoplasm of tumor cells in DPAC (and apocrine tumors in general) in approximately 40 to 50 percent of cases,[206] and immunostains for gross cystic disease fluid protein-15 (GCDFP-15; an apocrine-selective protein derived from fibrocystic mammary epithelium) are intensely and uniformly positive.[175]

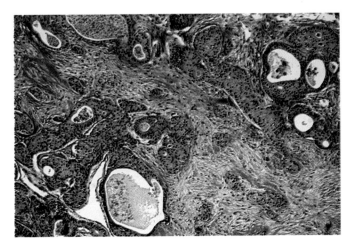

FIGURE 29-42   Ductopapillary apocrine carcinoma. Architectural similarities between ductal apocrine and ductal eccrine carcinomas are obvious at low magnification, although the abundance of eosinophilic cytoplasm in the malignant epithelial cells may suggest apocrine differentiation.

Differential Diagnosis   For the same reasons cited in connection with PDEA in the foregoing discussion of that tumor, the differential diagnosis is limited. Papillary carcinoma of the breast may have apocrine features in selected cases, but it lacks the capacity to metastasize to the skin in the absence of systemic dissemination. Thus, it would never present a worry with regard to its possibly occult existence as a cause of secondary skin disease. As mentioned, hidradenoma papilliferum bears a superficial resemblance to DPAC, but it lacks the degree of nuclear atypia, architectural complexity, and infiltrative growth seen in the latter of these two lesions. Spontaneous necrosis and dystrophic calcification are also potential attributes of DPAC[206–214] but are not observed in hidradenoma papilliferum.

Paget's Disease of the Skin, Apocrine Type
Conventional dogma of today still teaches that mammary and extramammary Paget's disease of the skin represents two separate diseases. Mammary Paget's disease (MPD) is said to emanate from the "migration" of neoplastic cells into the epidermis from an underlying carcinoma of the breast,[215] whereas extramammary Paget's disease (EPD) is thought to originate *within* the epidermis by the proliferation of primitive native stem (basal) cells with the potential for glandular differentiation.[216] A somewhat iconoclastic view of this topic holds that *both* forms of pagetoid proliferation derive from the latter pathogenetic mechanism, as cited traditionally only in connection with EPD. Perhaps the strongest support for this opinion comes from the observation that approximately 3 to 5 percent of MPD cases are *not* found to be associated with an underlying carcinoma, despite extensive sampling of the breast.[217,218] Thus, we believe that MPD and EPD can be considered together as a unified disorder. Moreover, the classification of that condition as a principally apocrine tumor is justified by the results of GCDFP-15 immunostains, demonstrating positivity in the overwhelming majority of both MPD and EPD lesions.[219] (Parenthetically, it must be acknowledged that other cellular lineages are occasionally manifest in Paget's disease, including sebaceous, eccrine, and visceral-enteric pathways. However, these account for a small minority of cases.)

Clinical Features   Both mammary and extramammary Paget's disease present as erythematous scaling or weeping lesions involving the nipple and areolae on the one hand and extramammary sites such as the vulva, penis and scrotum, perineum, umbilicus, axillae, eyelids, and ear canal (Table 29-20) on the other. Mammary Paget's disease is almost always unilateral, affecting mainly women aged 40 to 60 years. The clinical

TABLE 29-20

Mammary and Extramammary Paget's Disease

Mammary	*Extramammary*
Clinical Features	
40–60 years	Often > 50 years
Women >> men	Women ≥ men
Nipple and areolae	Vulva, penis and scrotum, perineum, umbilicus, axillae, eyelid, ear canal
Erythematous oozing or scaling plaque	Erythematous oozing or scaling plaque

Histopathological Features

Hyperkeratosis, parakeratosis
Epidermal hyperplasia
Epidermis permeated by aggregates of polygonal cells and single cells with abundant pale-staining or eosinophilic cytoplasm
Lumen formation may occur
Vesicular nuclei with prominent nucleoli
Intracellular mucin stained by PAS+D, mucicarmine, alcian blue in 50–60% of cases
Immunoreactivity for CEA, GCDFP-15, and keratin-7

Differential Diagnosis

Squamous cell carcinoma in situ
Pagetoid melanoma

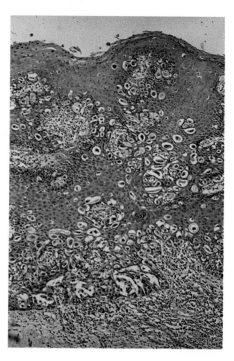

FIGURE 29-44   Paget's disease of the skin, apocrine type. Large epithelioid cells with clear cytoplasm infiltrate appear singly or in clusters in the epidermis.

findings usually suggest eczema or a related process. In contrast, EPD is much less common than MPD, develops in patients often over 50 years of age, and affects men almost as frequently as women.

Histopathological Features   Paget's disease shows the presence of "foreign" epithelioid tumor cells within the epidermis (Table 29-20) (Fig. 29-44). The adjacent skin commonly exhibits hyperkeratosis and acanthosis. The cells are dispersed singly or as small clusters throughout the surface epithelium. Typically, tumor cells in both MPD and EPD are round to ovoid and have pale, amphophilic cytoplasm, which is sometimes vacuolated (Fig. 29-45). The nuclei generally contain evenly distributed or vesicular chromatin, often with a discernible but small nucleolus; mitotic figures are infrequent.[220–225] An "anaplastic" form of Paget's disease has also been documented.[226] This subtype manifests marked variation in the size, shape, and density of tumor cell nuclei, as well as anisocytosis. Another histologic idiosyncrasy of Paget's disease is caused by its potentially confluent growth in the basal epidermis. Because the tumor cells have relatively poor intercellular cohesion, they often undergo detachment from one another. This phenomenon results in the formation of "pseudobullae" which can imitate the acantholysis that typifies forms of pemphigus.[203] Tumor cells in MPD and EPD contain mucopolysaccharides that are positive with PAS-D, mucicarmine, and alcian blue methods in 50 to 60 percent of cases.

Differential Diagnosis   One must consider pagetoid forms of amelanotic melanoma and bowenoid intraepidermal squamous carcinoma. Paget's cells may contain granules of melanin, which are produced by neighboring melanocytes and secondarily engulfed by the tumor cells. Hence, this may lead to diagnostic confusion with melanoma.

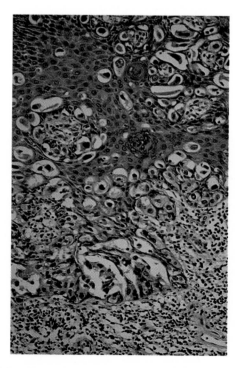

FIGURE 29-45   Paget's disease of the skin, apocrine type. Nuclei are large and pleomorphic. Cytoplasm is clear or amphophilic.

Conventional histochemistry can be helpful in confirming the diagnosis of Paget's disease, because neither melanoma nor squamous carcinoma produces mucin. Immunostains also can be beneficial diagnostically.[95,96,219,227–229] Reactivity for CEA, GCDFP-15, or keratin type 7 confirms the diagnosis of Paget's disease in the narrow context under discussion here. Additional positivity for CA19.9 or keratin type 20 in genitoperineal disease should direct attention to the possibility of an associated adenocarcinoma in the rectum, urinary bladder, or endocervix,[230–233] because those markers reflect the presence of an "enteric" immunophenotype in EPD.

APOCRINE CARCINOMAS THAT MAY SIMULATE METASTASES

There are basically two forms of apocrine carcinoma whose histologic images simulate those of metastatic tumors: ductal apocrine adenocarcinoma and primary signet-ring cell carcinoma of the skin. Their features are considered below.

Ductal Apocrine Carcinoma

Clinical and Histopathological Features   As mentioned earlier in this chapter, the anatomic distribution of apocrine tumors in general is relatively restricted. In addition to this topographic relatedness, there are many similarities between the *histologic* attributes of ductal apocrine adenocarcinoma (DAA) and ductal eccrine adenocarcinoma. Both are composed of irregular, randomly oriented, proliferations of neoplastic ductal profiles in the dermis, with or without changes in entrapped sweat ducts that simulate those of carcinoma in situ of the breast. Obvious cytologic atypia, mitotic activity, spontaneous necrosis, and infiltration of nerves and blood vessels are features which are common to both of these two classes of apocrine gland carcinoma[207–214] (Figs. 29-46 and 29-47). The distinguishing features of DAA are much the same as those of DPAC; namely, the presence of decapitation secretion snouts and abundant, finely granular, eosinophilic cytoplasm. Histochemical and immunohistologic findings also mirror those of DPAC, as described above. Thus, the only real (but nonetheless important) difference between these tumor variants is the potential for papillary differentiation in DPAC.

Differential Diagnosis   One must consider cutaneous metastases of those visceral adenocarcinomas that potentially feature a constitution by

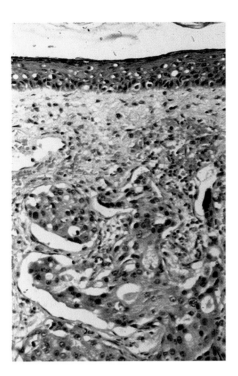

FIGURE 29-47   Ductal apocrine carcinoma. Vascular infiltration is a common feature in apocrine carcinomas.

large "pink" cells; these metastases include apocrine tumors of the breast and selected carcinomas of the lung, kidney, adrenal, and liver.[234] Immunohistologic evaluation for GCDFP-15 reactivity is capable of narrowing considerations to two tumor entities, DAA and apocrine carcinoma of the breast.[95] Nevertheless, as is true of DEA, no reliable discriminators can be applied by the pathologist to refine the diagnosis further. Hence, any patient with a carcinoma of the skin showing an apocrine immunophenotype should have a thorough examination of the breasts—including mammography—before a diagnosis of DAA is made. Historical data concerning duration of lesional growth and potential multifocality are also essential in this process, as outlined above in reference to DEA.

Primary Signet-Ring Cell Adenocarcinoma of the Skin

Clinical and Histopathological Features   Among all the favored skin fields for apocrine neoplasia, one of them—the eyelids—is virtually the *only* location in which primary signet-ring cell adenocarcinoma (PSRCA) is seen, as a nodular or plaquelike lesion.[235] This information is useful in narrowing differential diagnostic considerations (see below), but the possibility of metastasis still remains as a possibility in such cases.

PSRCA exhibits the random growth of small epithelioid cells in the dermis or subcutis or both, and they are often arranged in single file or cords (Fig. 29-48). Small clusters of tumor cells also may be evident. Perineural invasion is apparent in only a small minority of cases, but this finding is particularly important because it tends to support a primary origin in the skin. Vascular invasion may be seen as well. The individual neoplastic cells have round nuclei with dispersed chromatin and small nucleoli, and they are displaced to the periphery of the cell by single cytoplasmic vacuoles that actually represent primitive lumina. Secretory material may be observed focally within such spaces. Necrosis is rare, and mitotic activity is usually surprisingly scant in PSRCA.

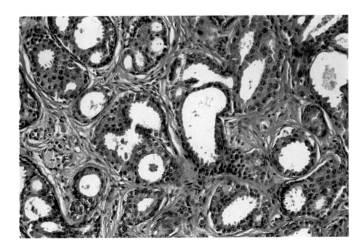

FIGURE 29-46   Ductal apocrine carcinoma. Randomly oriented ductal profiles are lined by cells with eosinophilic cytoplasm and apocrine snouts.

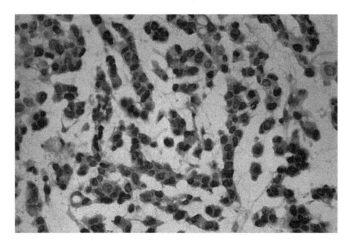

FIGURE 29-48 Primary signet-ring cell carcinoma of the skin. Intracytoplasmic mucin droplets displace the nucleus, yielding the characteristic signet-ring cell appearance.

Differential Diagnosis A metastasis should be favored when one is confronted with the miscroscopic image just cited, because of the rarity of PSRCA. (The authors have seen only two cases in the past 10 years.) Several visceral organs have a capacity to harbor signet-ring cell carcinomas, including the breasts, stomach, intestines, biliary tree, urinary tract, and female genitalia.[236–239] Knowledge of the distribution of disease is helpful in diagnosis, because, as mentioned earlier, PSRCA is seemingly limited to the eyelids. In contrast, signet-ring cell carcinomas of the abdominal and pelvic organs tend to metastasize to the skin of the trunk. Once more, however, metastatic lobular carcinoma of the breast is capable of perfectly simulating the clinicopathologic attributes of PSRCA, including its immunophenotype.[237] Thus, historical, physical, and mammographic information is paramount in securing a final interpretation.

Sweat Gland Carcinomas of Uncertain or Mixed Lineage

Selected malignant adnexal tumors remain that are capable of exhibiting sudoriferous differentiation but exhibit this feature as histologically occult or simultaneous with obviously divergent appendageal elements. The two neoplasms in this group are *lymphoepitheliomalike carcinoma of the skin* and *adnexal carcinoma with mixed differentiation*.

LYMPHOEPITHELIOMALIKE CARCINOMA OF THE SKIN

In 1988, Swanson and coworkers[240] described several cutaneous tumors that apparently arose in the skin primarily but which were seemingly identical microscopically to lymphoepitheliomalike carcinomas (LELCs) of the nasopharynx and other organ sites.

Clinical and Histopathological Features These lesions were nondescript, slowly growing nodules, most often seen in the skin of the head and neck in adults (Table 29-21).[240] Microscopically, they were composed of syncytial or vague clusters of large epithelioid cells in the dermis, with vesicular nuclear chromatin, prominent nucleoli, and obvious mitoses (Fig. 29-49). Mature lymphocytes permeated the lesions diffusely and surrounded them as well. Subsequent studies have shown

TABLE 29-21
Lymphoepitheliomalike Carcinoma

Clinical Features

Older individuals
Head and neck, especially face and scalp
Papules and nodules

Histopathological Features

Sheets or nodular aggregates of polygonal cells with vesicular nuclei
Monotonous appearance
Occasional intracellular vacuoles and mucin
Adnexal differentiation may be present
    Keratinization as in a pilar cyst
    Sweat gland differentiation
Cytologic atypia
Mitoses
Dense mononuclear cell infiltrate
Immunostaining:
    Cytokeratin +
    Epithelial membrane antigen +

Differential Diagnosis

Adnexal tumor, benign or malignant
Squamous cell carcinoma
Neuroendocrine carcinoma
Lymphoma
Melanoma

that eccrine or pilar differentiation may be evident in LELC of the skin, with the focal formation of intercellular ductal spaces or areas of trichilemmal-type keratinization.[241] That information, together with the exclusive localization of the tumors to the corium—with no epidermal connection—makes it likely that cutaneous LELC is a primitive appendageal neoplasm.

Interestingly, although the histologic features of this tumor are those of a largely undifferentiated epithelial proliferation, its biologic behav-

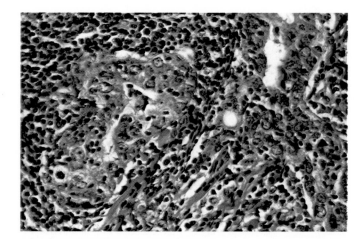

FIGURE 29-49 Primary lymphoepitheliomalike carcinoma of the skin. Syncytial clusters of large pleomorphic epithelial cells occasionally form ductal profiles, bespeaking their apparent adnexal attributes. The admixture of mature lymphocytes and plasma cells typifies this entity.

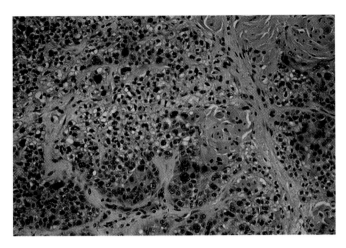

FIGURE 29-50 Adnexal carcinoma with mixed differentiation. Areas of pilar keratinization are present in a clear-cell and basaloid population that exhibits features of sebaceous differentiation.

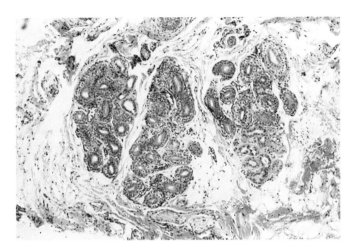

FIGURE 29-51 Eccrine nevus. An increased number of slightly disordered sweat glands form small lobules in association with a small peripheral nerve.

ior is indolent, and few patients with LELC have had metastases of their lesions.[240–247] Another intriguing fact is that, unlike LELCs of the nasopharynx, pharyngeal tonsils, salivary glands, and lungs, similar tumors of the skin do *not* exhibit integration of genomic nucleic acid from the Epstein-Barr virus upon in situ hybridization or polymerase chain reaction studies.[241]

Differential Diagnosis LELC must be distinguished from conventional adnexal carcinomas, squamous cell carcinoma, neuroendocrine carcinoma, primary or metastatic melanoma, and lymphoma.

ADNEXAL CARCINOMA WITH MIXED DIFFERENTIATION

The examination of a meaningful number of cutaneous adnexal tumors cannot be done without realizing that some of them defy predefined nosologic schemes. These most often exhibit bilinear or even multilinear differentiation, showing mixtures of eccrine, apocrine, sebaceous, and pilar elements. This phenomenon has been cited above in reference to adenomas, and it applies to appendageal carcinomas as well. Several tumors have been documented that amalgamate the features of DEA, porocarcinoma, DAA, sebaceous carcinoma, pilomatrix carcinoma, and malignant proliferating pilar tumors (see Chap. 30), all intimately admixed within the same mass[248] (Fig. 29-50). The most appropriate diagnostic label for such lesions is simply the descriptive one of *adnexal carcinoma with mixed differentiation* (ACMD). Basic recognition of these tumors as malignant is accomplished by attention to the features that have been stressed repeatedly throughout this chapter, namely, infiltrative growth, obvious cytologic anaplasia, spontaneous necrosis, and invasion of nerves or blood vessels. The behavior of ACMDs has been indolent, and no fatalities have been ascribed to them as of this writing.

PSEUDONEOPLASTIC LESIONS OF SWEAT GLANDS

Occasionally, the pathologist may be faced with biopsy specimens in which reactive proliferations of the sweat glands invoke a consideration of neoplastic disease. This is most often true when clinical information on the case is inadequate, but exceptions to that caveat do occur. Such "pseudoneoplastic" adnexal lesions are considered below.

Eccrine and Apocrine Nevi

Nevi (malformations) of the eccrine and apocrine apparatus are composed of cellular arrays that recall the images of embryonic sweat glands. Hence, they exhibit well-formed sudoriferous coils that are comprised of compact polygonal cells, sometimes with a luminal cuticle. Each of these tubular aggregates is invested by a basement membrane, and small nerves also may be seen at the lesional periphery. The sweat gland units are slightly disordered structurally, and they are more numerous than those found in mature skin appendages[249–257] (Fig. 29-51). This explains the fact that such lesions are commonly felt to represent such neoplasms as hidradenomas (acrospiromas) or syringomas. However, sweat gland nevi do not show the confluent cellular growth of the former of these two tumors or the "comma-tail" glandular configurations of the latter.

The lesion known as *eccrine angiomatous hamartoma* (EAH) is, in all likelihood, also a nevocytic malformation that incorporates sweat glands and mesenchymal elements.[258] The lesion commonly is seen in early childhood as a red, yellow, brownish, or tan papule or plaque on the distal extremities and may be associated with localized sweating and pain on palpation. Histologically, EAH differs slightly from uncomplicated adnexal nevi, because it incorporates venular blood vessels and small nerve twigs between the nevoid sweat gland coils. These "extra" components probably explain the aforementioned pressure sensitivity of EAH.

Syringometaplasias

Other lesions that resemble sweat gland nevi have been documented by Mehregan in patients with scarring alopecia or near keratoacanthomas or squamous cell carcinomas.[259] Similar lesions may be observed in fibrosing dermatitides and adjacent to basal cell carcinomas and malignant melanomas. Other authors have likewise documented the appearance of cutaneous syringomalike proliferations—with the additional elements of squamous or mucin-forming glandular cells—after the use of oral nonsteroidal anti-inflammatory and antineoplastic drugs[260,261] (Fig. 29-52). It is probable that these lesions are reactive or metaplastic in nature (*syringometaplasias*) and arise after appendageal injuries. Several of them have regressed after removal of the offending agent.

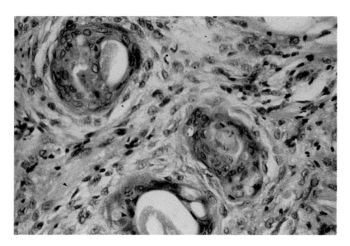

FIGURE 29-52 Syringometaplasia. Dermal appendageal injury often results in squamous metaplasia in the eccrine duct.

Eccrine and Apocrine Hidrocystomas

Selected cystic lesions of the eccrine and apocrine sweat gland units—usually seen on the face in patients living in warm climates—have variously been described as neoplasms or reaction patterns. Most often, these are termed *eccrine and apocrine hidrocystomas*, and they are characterized by dilation of the sweat ducts and secondary proliferation—which is architecturally bland—of the ductal epithelium.[262–264]

The latter phenomenon may produce micropapillary intraluminal cell profiles (as in so-called cystadenomas).[265,266] Apocrine hidrocystomas have also been described as *Moll's gland cysts* in the ophthalmologic literature.[267] Tumefactions in this general category probably are pseudoneoplastic in nature and represent reactions to terminal sweat duct obstruction and inspissation of sweat glandular secretions.

Some authors maintain that the eccrine variant is more likely to be a retention cyst, whereas the apocrine counterpart is a true organoid proliferation, hence the term *cystadenoma*. It must be emphasized that in many instances one cannot easily categorize a lesion as clearly eccrine or apocrine. Such a discrimination in reality is probably not important, and describing the lesion simply as *hidrocystoma* should suffice. Also, apocrine hidrocystoma and cystadenoma are probably variants of a single pathologic entity based on the degree to which the cyst lining is proliferative.

Clinical Features   Both eccrine and apocrine variants tend to present as skin-colored, bluish, or even blue-brown papules or nodules with a translucent quality (Table 29-22). The lesions generally measure less than 1 cm but on occasion may be larger or, rarely, giant (up to 7 cm). The periorbital areas of the face are most commonly affected. Other sites may be involved such as the head, neck, and upper trunk, genital, and perineal areas, particularly for apocrine variants. Such lesions occurring on the penis are best classified as a *median raphe cyst*. Most such lesions are solitary, especially the apocrine variant. Eccrine hidrocystomas may be numerous and exacerbated by heat exposure.

Histopathological Features   The hidrocystomas, notably the eccrine forms, usually show a dilated cyst with edematous or compacted fibrous stroma that is occasionally hyalinized (Table 29-22) (Fig. 29-53). The epithelial lining consists of two layers of cuboidal epithelium, sometimes flattened and in some instances a single-cellular layer. The epithelial lining also may show both hyperplasia and squamous metaplasia. In many cases the cyst is connected to an eccrine duct.

TABLE 29-22

Eccrine and Apocrine Hidrocystoma/Cystadenoma

Eccrine	Apocrine
Clinical Features	
	Usually adults
	Men = Women
	Periorbital sites but also head and neck, upper trunk
Solitary > multiple	Solitary almost exclusively
	Skin-color or bluish papules, nodules
	Commonly translucent
	Often < 1 cm but rarely up to 7 cm
Precipitated or exacerbated by heat	
Histopathological Features	
	Often dilated cystic structure in dermis
Epithelial lining:	Epithelial lining:
One or two cell layers	Two cell layers
Cuboidal or flattened	Luminal cell is columnar or cuboidal with decapitation secretion
Squamous metaplasia	Outer layer composed of myoepithelial cells (cuboidal or flattened)
Hyperplasia of lining	Hyperplasia of lining with papillary projections, folding
	Occasional mitoses, slight pleomorphism
Differential Diagnosis	
Other cysts, e.g., epidermoid cyst	Other cysts
	Papillary adenoma
	Papillary carcinoma

Apocrine variants exhibit an epithelial lining composed of a two-cell layer. The inner (luminal) layer consists of cuboidal or columnar cells with decapitation secretion (snouts). The outer layer usually is composed of cuboidal or elongated myoepithelial cells. The epithelial lining may be proliferative and show papillary projections. On occasion the

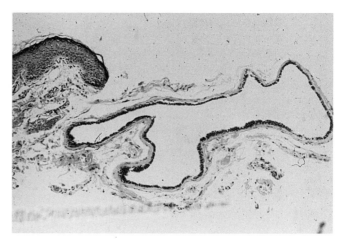

FIGURE 29-53 Apocrine hidrocystoma. Hidrocystomas are simple cysts of the sweat gland apparatus formed by dilation of sweat ducts with secondary epithelial proliferation. The presence of cuboidal eccrine or low columnar epithelium further defines these cystic lesions.

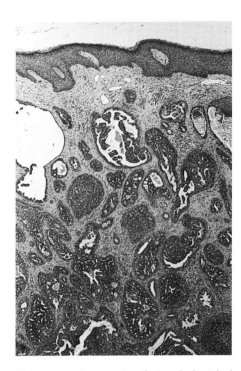

FIGURE 29-54 Erosive adenomatosis of the nipple (nipple adenoma). Ductopapillary proliferations are centered on large ducts and lactiferous sinuses beneath the skin of the nipple.

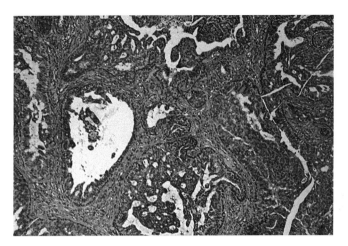

FIGURE 29-55 Erosive adenomatosis of the nipple (nipple adenoma). Complex glandular and papillary proliferations are arranged in a nodular array.

latter proliferative foci may be somewhat cellular and exhibit mitoses and slight cellular pleomorphism.

Differential Diagnosis   These lesions are usually distinctive. On occasion one might consider other entities in the differential diagnosis because of squamous metaplasia or proliferation of the cyst lining. A papillary adenoma or even a malignant tumor might be considered in the latter instance.

EROSIVE ADENOMATOSIS OF THE NIPPLE (NIPPLE ADENOMA)

By tradition, the lesion known as *erosive adenomatosis of the nipple* (EAN) or *nipple adenoma*[268–275] has been included in discussions of cutaneous adnexal tumors. We believe that this decision has more historic than pathologic justification, inasmuch as the proliferation in question probably originates in the terminal subareolar mammary ducts rather than the skin of the nipple itself.[268,274] However, for the sake of completeness, a brief discussion of EAN is included here.

Clinical Features   Erosive adenomatosis can present as a nondescript mass that is centered under the areolar complex, or it may also distort the nipple and cause eczematoid changes in the overlying skin. As such, EAN is in the macroscopic differential diagnosis of mammary Paget's disease, especially because women between the ages of 40 and 90 years are principally affected.[271,272] In light of these facts, and the particular microscopic attributes of nipple adenoma—as described below—the latter condition has been misdiagnosed as a carcinoma. However, EAN is a uniformly benign lesion which may, in fact, have more in common with mammary fibrocystic change than with true neoplasms of the breast or skin.

Histopathological Features   The usual lesions of EAN consist of proliferations of small glands that are centered on large lactiferous ducts

beneath the nipple (Figs. 29-54 and 29-55). The skin surface may be ulcerated or spongiotic and inflamed. The constituent glandular arrays of EAN are configured in a vaguely nodular fashion, but they lack the specialized stroma of true mammary lobules. "Pseudoinvasion" of lesional glands may be observed within bundles of the subareolar musculature. Two cell layers are evident in each gland, with basal elements being bluntly fusiform and occasionally possessing optically lucent cytoplasm, whereas the luminal cells have bland oval nuclei, relatively abundant eosinophilic cytoplasm, and frequent apocrine snouts. Glandular profiles are irregular, and many assume pointed images resembling the prows of ships. Entrapped lactiferous ducts demonstrate intraluminal papillary hyperplasia of ductal epithelial cells, but the rigid bridging patterns of ductal carcinoma in situ are usually absent. In reference to the latter point, however, occasional examples of EAN have featured an admixture of overt ductal breast carcinoma.[271] Thus, it is notable that mitoses and foci of single-cellular or geographic necrosis are lacking or extremely scarce in uncomplicated EAN. However, squamous metaplasia—sometimes with formation of squamous microcysts—is a relatively common observation in the lactiferous ducts immediately beneath the skin surface in this condition.

Differential Diagnosis   MAC, as well as tubular carcinoma of the breast, must be considered in the differential diagnosis. The demonstration of muscle-specific actin-positive basal cells in each of the proliferating glands in EAN distinguishes it from those pathologic alternatives.[275]

IMMUNOHISTOCHEMISTRY OF SWEAT GLAND TUMORS

Immunohistology does have some application in the differential diagnosis of sweat gland neoplasms, as referenced at several points in this chapter. However, this technique *must* be applied very specifically to tightly confined questions of interpretation, because the immunophenotypes of sudoriferous tumors overlap with one another and—in the case of sweat gland carcinomas—also with the antigenic profiles of visceral malignancies.[1,95,169,175] Hence, the greatest utility of immunostains in this context is in the separation of sweat gland tumors from *other primary skin lesions*, such as variants of squamous cell carcinoma, basal cell carcinoma, malignant melanoma, or mesenchymal neoplasms with epithelioid cytologic features. Determinants of interest and expected reactivity patterns are outlined in Table 29-23.

TABLE 29-23

Immunohistochemical Findings in Sweat Gland Tumors and Differential Diagnositc Alternatives

TUMOR	CK	EMA	CK7	CEA	S-100	GCDFP	CA19.9	CA125	CD31	VIM
Benign and malignant eccrine neoplasms	+	+	7	±	±	±	0	0	0	±
Benign and malignant apocrine neoplasms	+	+	+	±	0	+	0	0	0	0
EPD and MPD	+	+	+	+	0	±	±	±	0	0
Metastatic visceral carcinoma	+	±	±	±	±	±	±	±	0	±
Melanoma	0	0	0	0	+	0	0	0	0	+
Adenoid basal cell carcinoma	+	0	0	0*	0*	0*	0	0	0	0
Adenoid squamous carcinoma	+	±	±	0	0	0	0	0	0	±
Epithelioid sarcoma	+	±	±	±	±	0	0	0	0	±
Epithelioid angiosarcoma	±	0	0	0	0	0	0	0	+	+

KEY: CK = broad-spectrum cytokeratin proteins; CK7 = keratin type 7; S-100 = S-100 protein; VIM = vimentin; MPD = mammary Paget's disease; EMA = epithelial membrane antigen; CEA = carcinoembryonic antigen; GCDFP = gross cystic disease fluid protein-15; EPD = extramammary Paget's disease.
*Foci of divergent sudoriferous differentiation in basal cell carcinoma may show limited reactivity for these determinants.

REFERENCES

1. Wick MR, Swanson PE: *Cutaneous Adnexal Tumors: A Guide to Pathologic Diagnosis.* Chicago, ASCP Press, 1991.
2. Hashimoto K, Mehregan AH, Kumakiri M: *Tumors of the Skin Appendages.* Boston, Butterworth, 1987.
3. Abenoza P, Ackerman AB: *Neoplasms with Eccrine Differentiation.* Philadelphia, Lea & Febiger, 1990.
4. Sharma HS, Meorkamal MZ, Zainol H, Dharap AS: Eccrine cylindroma of the ear canal—report of a case. *J Laryngol Otol* 108:706–709 1994.
5. Wollina U, Rulke D, Schaarschmidt H: Dermal cylindroma: Expression of intermediate filaments, epithelial and neuroectodermal antigens. *Histol Histopathol* 7:575–582, 1992.
6. Crain RC, Helwig EB: Dermal cylindroma (dermal eccrine cylindroma). *Am J Clin Pathol* 35:504–515, 1961.
7. Goette DK, McConnell MA, Fowler VR: Cylindroma and eccrine spiradenoma coexistent in the same lesion. *Arch Dematol* 118:273–274, 1982.
8. Welch JP, Wells RS, Kerr CB: Ancell-Spiegler cylindromas (turban tumors) and Brooke-Fordyce trichoepitheliomas: Evidence for a single genetic entity. *J Med Genet* 5:29–35, 1968.
9. Cecchi R, Crudeli F, Fedi E, Giomi A: Multiple trichoepitheliomas, cylindromas, and eccrine spiradenomas observed in the same family. *G Ital Dermatol* 120:149–152, 1985.
10. Cooper PH: Mitotic figures in sweat gland adenomas. *J Cutan Pathol* 14:10–14, 1987.
11. Mambo NC: Eccrine spiradenomas: Clinical and pathologic study of 49 tumors. *J Cutan Pathol* 10:312–320, 1983.
12. Van der Putte SC: The pathogenesis of familial multiple cylindromas, trichoepitheliomas, milia, and spiradenomas. *Am J Dermatopathol* 17:271–280, 1995.
13. Kersting DW, Helwig EB: Eccrine spiradenoma. *Arch Dermatol* 73:199–227, 1956.
14. Shelley WB, Wood MG: A zosteriform network of spiradenomas. *J Am Acad Dermatol* 2:59–61, 1980.
15. Cotton DW, Slater DN, Rooney N, et al: Giant vascular eccrine spiradenomas: A report of two cases with histology, immunohistology, and electron microscopy. *Histopathology* 10:1093–1099, 1986.
16. Kao GF, Laskin WB, Weiss SW: Eccrine spiradenoma occurring in infancy, mimicking a mesenchymal tumor. *J Cutan Pathol* 17:214–219, 1990.
17. Pruzam DL, Esterly NB, Prose NS: Eruptive syringoma. *Arch Dermatol* 125:1119–1120, 1989.
18. Isaacson D, Turner ML: Localized vulvar syringomas. *J Am Acad Dermatol* 1:352–356, 1979.
19. Henner MS, Shapiro PE, Ritter JH, et al: Solitary syringoma: A report of five cases and comparison with microcystic adnexal carcinoma. *Am J Dermatopathol* 17:465–470, 1995.
20. Karam P, Benedetto AN: Syringomas: New approach to an old technique. *Int J Dermatol* 35:219–220, 1996.
21. Hashimoto K, DiBella D, Borsuk GM: Eruptive hidradenoma and syringoma. *Arch Dermatol* 96:500–519, 1967.
22. Brown SM, Freeman RG: Syringoma limited to the vulva. *Arch Dermatol* 114:331–333, 1971.
23. Yesudian P, Thambiah A: Familial syringoma. *Dermatologica* 151:32–35, 1975.
24. Feibelman CE, Maize JC: Clear cell syringoma: A study by conventional and electron microscopy. *Am J Dermatopathol* 6:139–150, 1984.
25. Ambrojo P, Caballero-Martinez AA, Sanchez-Yus E, Furio V: Clear cell syringoma. *Dermatologica* 178:164–166, 1989.
26. Pinkus H, Rogin JR, Goldman P: Eccrine poroma. *Arch Dermatol* 74:511–521, 1956.
27. Freeman RG, Knox JM, Spiller WF: Eccrine poroma. *Am J Clin Pathol* 36:444–450, 1961.
28. Hyman AB, Brownstein MH: Eccrine poroma: An analysis of 45 new cases. *Dermatologica* 138:29–38, 1969.
29. Goldner R: Eccrine poromatosis. *Arch Dermatol* 101:606–608, 1970.
30. Wilkinson RD, Schopflocher P, Rozenfeld M: Hidrotic ectodermal dysplasia with diffuse eccrine poromatosis. *Arch Dermatol* 113:472–476, 1977.
31. Palazzo J, Stenn KS, Wolf ER: Eccrine tubular poroma. *J Cutan Pathol* 14:365, 1987.
32. Pylyser K, DeWolf-Peeters C, Marien K: The histology of eccrine poroma: A study of 14 cases. *Dermatologica* 167:243–249, 1983.
33. Mehregan AH, Levson DN: Hidroacanthoma simplex. *Arch Dermatol* 100:303–305, 1969.
34. Hu CH, Marques AS, Winkelmann RK: Dermal duct tumor. *Arch Dermatol* 114:1659–1664, 1978.

35. Aloi FG, Pippione M: Dermal duct tumor. *Appl Pathol* 4:175–178, 1986.

36. Rahbari H: Syringoacanthoma: Acanthotic lesion of the acrosyringium. *Arch Dermatol* 120:751–756, 1984.

37. Kanitakis J, Zambruno G, Euvrard S, et al: Eccrine syringofibroadenoma. *Am J Dermatopathol* 9:37–40, 1987.

38. Civatte J, Jeanmougin M, Barrandon Y, Simenez-DeFranch A: Syringofibroadenoma eccrino de Mascaro. *Med Cutan Ibero Lat Am* 9:193–196, 1981.

39. Weedon D, Lewis J: Acrosyringeal nevus. *J Cutan Pathol* 4:166–168, 1977.

40. Rulon DB, Helwig EB: Papillary eccrine adenoma. *Arch Dermatol* 113:596–598, 1977.

41. Cooper PH, Frierson HF Jr: Papillary eccrine adenoma. *Arch Pathol Lab Med* 108:55–57, 1984.

42. Urmacher C, Lieberman PH: Papillary eccrine adenoma: A light microscopic and immunohistochemical study. *Am J Dermatopathol* 9:243–249, 1987.

43. Sexton M, Maize JC: Papillary eccrine adenoma: A light microscopic and immunohistochemical study. *J Am Acad Dermatol* 18:1114–1120, 1988.

44. Biernat W, Kordek R, Wozniak L: Papillary eccrine adenoma: A case of cutaneous sweat gland tumor with secretory and ductular differentiation. *Pol J Pathol* 45:319–322, 1994.

45. Aloi F, Pich A: Papillary eccrine adenoma: A histopathological and immunohistochemical study. *Dermatologica* 182:47–51, 1991.

46. Falck VG, Jordaan JH: Papillary eccrine adenoma: A tubulopapillary hidradenoma with eccrine differentiation. *Am J Dermatopathol* 8:64–72, 1986.

47. Tellechea O, Reis JP, Marques C, Baptista AP: Tubular apocrine adenoma with eccrine and apocrine immunophenotypes or papillary tubular adenoma? *Am J Dermatopathol* 17:499–505, 1995.

48. Johnson BL Jr, Helwig EB: Eccrine acrospiroma. *Cancer* 23:641–657, 1969.

49. Hashimoto K, DiBella RJ, Lever WF: Clear cell hidradenoma. *Arch Dermatol* 96:18–38, 1967.

50. Winkelmann RK, Wolff K: Solid-cystic hidradenoma of the skin. *Arch Dermatol* 97:651–661, 1968.

51. Mambo NC: The significance of atypical nuclear changes in benign eccrine acrospiromas: A clinical and pathological study of 18 cases. *J Cutan Pathol* 11:35–44, 1984.

52. Stanley RJ, Sanchez NP, Massa MC, et al: Epidermoid hidradenoma: A clinicopathologic study. *J Cutan Pathol* 9:293–302, 1982.

53. Santa Cruz DJ: Sweat gland carcinoma: A comprehensive review. *Semin Diagn Pathol* 4:38–74, 1987.

54. Helwig EB, Hackney VC: Syringocystadenoma papilliferum. *Arch Dermatol* 71:361–372, 1955.

55. Pinkus H: Life history of naevus syringocystadenomatosus papilliferus. *Arch Dermatol* 69:305–322, 1954.

56. Niizuma K: Syringocystadenoma papilliferum: Light and electron microscopic studies. *Acta Dermatol Venereol* 56:327–336, 1976.

57. Grund JL: Syringocystadenoma papilliferum and nevus sebaceus (Jadassohn) occurring as a single tumor. *Arch Dermatol* 65:340–347, 1952.

58. Woolworth H Jr, Dockerty MB, Wilson RB, Pratt JH: Papillary hidradenoma of the vulva. *Am J Obstet Gynecol* 110:501–508, 1971.

59. Meeker JH, Neubechker RD, Helwig EB: Hidradenoma papilliferum. *Am J Clin Pathol* 37:182–195, 1962.

60. Hashimoto K: Hidradenoma papilliferum: An electron microscopic study. *Acta Dermatol Venereol* 53:22–30, 1973.

61. Novak E, Stevenson RR: Sweat gland tumors of the vulva: Benign (hidradenoma) and malignant (hidradenocarcinoma). *Am J Obstet Gynecol* 50:641–654, 1945.

62. Santa Cruz DJ, Prioleau PG, Smith ME: Hidradenoma papilliferum of the eyelid. *Arch Dermatol* 117:55–56, 1981.

63. Shenoy YMV: Malignant perianal papillary hidradenoma. *Arch Dermatol* 83:965–967, 1961.

64. Umbert P, Winkelmann RK: Tubular apocrine adenoma. *J Cutan Pathol* 3:75–87, 1976.

65. Toribio J, Zulaica A, Peteiro C: Tubular apocrine adenoma. *J Cutan Pathol* 14:114–117, 1987.

66. Ansai S, Watanabe S, Aso K: A case of tubular apocrine adenoma with syringocystadenoma papilliferum. *J Cutan Pathol* 16:230–236, 1989.

67. Headington JT: Mixed tumors of the skin. *Arch Dermatol* 84:989–996, 1961.

68. Fernandez RJ: Mixed tumors of the skin of the salivary gland type. *J Invest Dermatol* 60:49–58, 1976.

69. Hassab-El-Naby HM, Tam S, White WL, Ackerman AB: Mixed tumors of the skin: A histological and immunohistochemical study. *Am J Dermatopathol* 11:413–428, 1989.

70. Mills SE: Mixed tumor of the skin: A model of divergent differentiation. *J Cutan Pathol* 11:382–386, 1984.

71. Mohri S, Andoh S: An immunohistochemical study of mixed tumor of the skin. *J Dermatol* 18:414–419, 1991.

72. Hara K: Mixed tumors of the skin: A histopathological, enzyme-histochemical, and immunohistochemical study. *Histopathology* 26:145–152, 1995.

73. Jaworski RC: The ultrastructure of chondroid syringoma (mixed tumor of the skin). *Ultrastruct Pathol* 6:153–159, 1984.

74. Kunikane H, Ishikura H, Yamaguchi J, et al: Chondroid syringoma (mixed tumor of the skin): A clinicopathologic study of 13 cases. *Acta Pathol Jpn* 37:615–625, 1987.

75. Requena L, Sanchez-Yus E, Santa Cruz DJ: Apocrine type of cutaneous mixed tumor with follicular and sebaceous differentiation. *Am J Dermatopathol* 14:186–194, 1992.

76. Efskind J, Eker R: Myoepitheliomas of the skin. *Acta Dermatol Venereol* 34:279–283, 1954.

77. Zaim MT: Sebocrine adenoma. *Am J Dermatopathol* 10:311–318, 1988.

78. Troy JL, Ackerman AB: Sebaceoma: A distinctive benign neoplasm of adnexal epithelium, differentiating towards sebaceous cells. *Am J Dermatopathol* 6:7–14, 1984.

79. Hanau D, Grosshans E, Laplanche G: A complex poroma-like adnexal adenoma. *Am J Dermatopathol* 6:567–572, 1984.

80. Letizia C, Marcheggiano A, DeToma G, et al: Mixed type sweat gland adenoma: A case report. *Ann Ital Med Intern* 8:248–249, 1993.

81. Page DL, Anderson TJ, Sakamoto G: Infiltrating carcinoma: Major histological types, in Page DL, Anderson TJ (eds): *Diagnostic Histopathology of the Breast.* New York, Churchill-Livingstone, 1987, pp 193–295.

82. Goedde TA, Bumpers H, Fiscella J, et al: Eccrine porocarcinoma. *J Surg Oncol* 55:261–264, 1994.

83. Poiares-Baptista A, Tellechea O, Reis JP, et al: Eccrine porocarcinoma: A review of 24 cases. *Ann Dermatol Venereol* 120:107–115, 1993.

84. Snow SN, Reizner GT: Eccrine porocarcinoma of the face. *J Am Acad Dermatol* 27:306–311, 1992.

85. Yamamoto O, Haratake J, Yokoyama S, et al: A histopathological and ultrastructural study of eccrine porocarcinoma with special reference to its subtypes. *Virchows Arch A Pathol Anat Histopathol* 420:395–401, 1992.

86. Turner JJ, Maxwell L, Bursle CA: Eccrine porocarcinoma, *Pathology* 14:469–475, 1982.

87. Shaw M, McKee PH, Lowe D, Black MM: Malignant eccrine poroma: A study of twenty-seven cases. *Br J Dermatol* 107:675–680, 1982.

88. Bottles K, Sagebiel RW, McNutt NS, et al: Malignant eccrine poroma. *Cancer* 53:1579–1585, 1984.

89. Ryan JF, Darley CR, Pollock DJ: Malignant eccrine poroma: Report of three cases. *J Clin Pathol* 39:1099–1104, 1986.

90. Mehregan AH, Hashimoto K, Rahbari H: Eccrine adenocarcinoma: A clinicopathologic study of 35 cases. *Arch Dermatol* 119:104–114, 1983.

91. Miyashita M, Suzuki H: In situ porocarcinoma: A case with malignant expression in clear tumor cells. *Int J Dermatol* 32:749–750, 1993.

92. Bardach H: Hidroacanthoma simplex with in situ porocarcinoma. *J Cutan Pathol* 5:236–248, 1978.

93. Isikawa K: Malignant hidroacanthoma simplex. *Arch Dermatol* 104:529–532, 1972.

94. Moreno R, Salvatella N, Guix M, et al: Malignant hidroacanthoma simplex. *Dermatologica* 169:318–322, 1984.

95. Swanson PE, Cherwitz DL, Neumann MP, Wick MR: Eccrine sweat gland carcinoma: An histologic and immunohistochemical study of 32 cases. *J Cutan Pathol* 14:65–86, 1987.

96. Guldhammer B, Norgaard T: The differential diagnosis of intraepidermal malignant lesions using immunohistochemistry. *Am J Dermatopathol* 8:295–301, 1986.

97. Hara K, Kamiya S: Pigmented eccrine porocarcinoma: A mimic of malignant melanoma. *Histopathology* 27:86–88, 1995.

98. Manteaux A, Cohen PR, Rapini RP: Zosteriform and epidermotropic metastasis: Report of two cases. *J Dermatol Surg Oncol* 18:97–100, 1992.

99. Rosen T: Cutaneous metastases. *Med Clin North Am* 64:885–900, 1980.

100. Fukamizu H, Tomita K, Inoue K, Takigawa M: Primary mucinous carcinoma of the skin. *J Dermatol Surg Oncol* 19:625–628, 1993.

101. Ghamande SA, Kasznick J, Griffiths CT, et al: Mucinous adenocarcinomas of the vulva. *Gynecol Oncol* 57:117–120, 1995.

102. Katoh N, Hirano S, Hosokawa Y, et al: Mucinous carcinoma of the skin: Report of a case with DNA cytofluorometric study. *J Dermatol* 21:117–121, 1994.

103. Mendoza S, Helwig EB: Mucinous (adenocystic) carcinoma of the skin. *Arch Dermatol* 103:68–78, 1971.

104. Rodriguez MM, Lubowitz RM, Shannon GM: Mucinous (adenocystic) carcinoma of the eyelid. *Arch Ophthalmol* 89:493–494, 1973.

105. Grossman JR, Izuno GT: Primary mucinous (adenocystic) carcinoma of the skin. *Arch Dermatol* 110:274–276, 1974.

106. Santz Cruz DJ, Meyers JH, Gnepp DR, Perez BM: Primary mucinous carcinoma of the skin. *Br J Dermatol* 68:645–653, 1978.

107. Yeung KY, Stinson JC: Mucinous (adenocystic) carcinoma of sweat glands with widespread metastases. *Cancer* 39:2556–2562, 1977.

108. Pilgram JP, Kloss SG, Wolfish PS, Heng MCY: Primary mucinous carcinoma of the skin with metastases to the lymph nodes. *Am J Dermatopathol* 7:461–469, 1985.

109. Wassef M, Thomas V, Deffrennes D, Saint-Guily JL: Primary adenoid cystic carcinoma of the skin: Histologic and ultrastructural study of two cases localized in the external auditory canal. *Ann Pathol* 15:150–155, 1995.

110. Eckert F, Pfau A, Landthaler M: Adenoid cystic sweat gland carcinoma: A clinicopathologic and immunohistochemical study. *Hautarzt* 45:318–323, 1994.

111. Matsumura T, Kumakiri M, Ohkaware A, Yoshida T: Adenoid cystic carcinoma of the skin: An immunohistochemical and ultrastructural study. *J Dermatol* 20:164–170, 1993.

112. Cooper PH, Adelson GL, Holthaus WH: Primary cutaneous adenoid cystic carcinoma. *Arch Dermatol* 120:774–777, 1984.

113. Wick MR, Swanson PE: Primary adenoid cystic carcinoma of the skin. *Am J Dermatopathol* 8:2–13, 1986.

114. Seab JA, Graham JH: Primary cutaneous adenoid cystic carcinoma. *J Am Acad Dermatol* 17:113–118, 1987.

115. Van der Kwast TH, Vuzevski VD, Ramaekers F: Primary cutaneous adenoid cystic carcinoma. *Br J Dermatol* 118:567–576, 1988.

116. Kuramoto Y, Tagami H: Primary adenoid cystic carcinoma masquerading as syringoma of the scalp. *Am J Dermatopathol* 12:169–174, 1990.

117. Sanderson KV, Batten JC: Adenoid cystic carcinoma of the scalp with pulmonary metastases. *Proc R Soc Med* 68:649–650, 1975.

118. Headington JT, Teears R, Niederhuber JE: Primary adenoid cystic carcinoma of the skin. *Arch Dermatol* 114:421–424, 1978.

119. Boggio R: Adenoid cystic carcinoma of the scalp. *Arch Dermatol* 111:793–794, 1975.

120. Beck HG, Lechner W, Wunsch PH: Adenoid-zystisches Schwiessdrusenkarzinom. *Hautarzt* 37:405–409, 1986.

121. Kao GF, Helwig EB, Graham JH: Aggressive digital papillary adenoma and adenocarcinoma. *J Cutan Pathol* 14:129–146, 1987.

122. Smith KJ, Skelton HG, Holland TT: Recent advances and controversies concerning adnexal neoplasms. *Dermatol Clin* 10:117–160, 1992.

123. Goldstein DJ, Barr RJ, Santa Cruz DJ: Microcystic adnexal carcinoma: A distinct clinicopathologic entity. *Cancer* 50:566–572, 1982.

124. Wick MR, Cooper PH, Swanson PE, et al: Microcystic adnexal carcinoma: An immunohistochemical comparison with other cutaneous appendage tumors. *Arch Dermatol* 126:189–194, 1990.

125. Nickoloff BJ, Fleischmann HE, Carmel J: Microcystic adnexal carcinoma: Immunohistologic observations suggesting dual (pilar and eccrine) differentiation. *Arch Dermatol* 122:290–294, 1986.

126. Cooper PH, Mills SE, Leonard DD, et al: Sclerosing sweat duct (syringomatous) carcinoma. *Am J Surg Pathol* 9:422–433, 1985.

127. Cooper PH: Sclerosing carcinomas of sweat ducts (microcystic adnexal carcinoma). *Arch Dermatol* 122:261–264, 1986.

128. Berg JW, McDivitt RW: Pathology of sweat gland carcinomas. *Pathol Annu* 3: 123–144, 1968.

129. Lipper S, Peiper SC: Sweat gland carcinoma with syringomatous features. *Cancer* 44:157–163, 1979.

130. Cooper PH, Mills SE: Microcystic adnexal carcinoma. *J Am Acad Dermatol* 10:908–914, 1984.

131. McAlvany JP, Stonecipher MR, Leshin B, et al: Sclerosing sweat duct carcinoma in an 11 year old boy. *J Dermatol Surg Oncol* 20:767–768, 1994.

132. Batsakis JG, El-Naggar AK, Weber RS: Two perplexing skin tumors: Microcystic adnexal carcinoma and keratoacanthoma. *Ann Otol Rhinol Laryngol* 103:829–832, 1994.

133. LeBoit PE, Sexton M: Microcystic adnexal carcinoma of the skin. A reappraisal of the differentiation and differential diagnosis of an underrecognized neoplasm. *J Am Acad Dermatol* 29:609–618, 1993.

134. Hesse RJ, Scharfenberg JC, Ratz JL, Griener E: Eyelid microcystic adnexal carcinoma. *Arch Ophthalmol* 113:494–496, 1995.

135. Verdier-Sevrain S, Thomine E, Lauret P, Hemet J: Syringomatous carcinoma: Apropos of three cases with a review of the literature. *Ann Pathol* 15:280–284, 1995.

136. Schlipper JH, Holecek BU, Sievers KW: A tumor derived from Ebner's glands: Microcystic adnexal carcinoma of the tongue. *J Laryngol Otol* 109:1211–1214, 1995.

137. Cooper PH: Carcinomas of sweat glands. *Pathol Annu* 22(Part 1):83–124, 1987.

138. Yus ES, Caballero LR, Salazar IG, Menchero SC: Clear cell syringoid eccrine carcinoma. *Am J Dermatopathol* 9:225–231, 1987.

139. Cooper PH, Robinson CR, Greer KE: Low grade clear cell eccrine carcinoma. *Arch Dermatol* 120:1076–1078, 1984.

140. Brownstein MH, Shapiro L: Desmoplastic trichoepithelioma. *Cancer* 40:2979–2986, 1977.

141. Salasche SJ, Amonette RA: Morpheaform basal cell epitheliomas. *J Dermatol Surg Oncol* 7:387–394, 1981.

142. Banks ER, Cooper PH: Adenosquamous carcinoma of the skin: A report of 10 cases. *J Cutan Pathol* 18:227–234, 1991.

143. Weidner N, Foucar E: Adenosquamous carcinoma of the skin: An aggressive mucin- and gland-forming squamous carcinoma. *Arch Dermatol* 121:775–779, 1985.

144. Sakamoto F, Ito M, Oguro K, et al: Adenosquamous carcinoma of the skin: Ultrastructural and immunohistochemical studies. *Jpn J Dermatol* 100:1183–1190, 1990.

145. Landman G, Farmer ER: Primary cutaneous mucoepidermoid carcinoma: Report of a case. *J Cutan Pathol* 18:56–59, 1991.

146. Wenig BL, Sciubba JJ, Goodman RS, Platt N: Primary cutaneous mucoepidermoid carcinoma of the anterior neck. *Laryngoscope* 93:464–467, 1983.

147. Friedman KJ: Low-grade primary cutaneous adenosquamous (mucoepidermoid) carcinoma. *Am J Dermatopathol* 11:43–50, 1989.

148. Smoller BR, Narurkar V: Mucoepidermoid carcinoma metastatic to the skin: An histologic mimic of a primary sweat gland carcinoma. *J Dermatol Surg Oncol* 18:365–368, 1992.

149. Metcalf JS, Maize JC, Shaw EB: Bronchial mucoepidermoid carcinoma metastatic to skin: Report of a case and review of the literature. *Cancer* 58:2556–2559, 1986.

150. Barsky SH, Martin SE, Matthews M, et al: "Low grade" mucoepidermoid carcinoma of the bronchus with "high grade" biological behavior. *Cancer* 51:1505–1509, 1983.

151. Revercomb CH, Reitmeyer WJ, Pulitzer DR: Clear cell variant of mucoepidermoid carcinoma of the skin. *J Am Acad Dermatol* 29:642–644, 1993.

152. Galadari E, Mehregan AH, Lee KC: Malignant transformation of eccrine tumors. *J Cutan Pathol* 14:15–22, 1987.

153. Bondeson L: Malignant dermal eccrine cylindroma. *Acta Dermatol Venereol* 59: 92–94, 1979.

154. Boulond A, Clerens A, Signard H: Cylindrome malin. *Dermatologica* 158:203–207, 1979.

155. Urbanski SJ, From L, Abramowicz A: Metamorphosis of dermal cylindroma: Possible relation to malignant transformation. *J Am Acad Dermatol* 12:188–195, 1985.

156. Rockerbie N, Solomon AR, Woo TY, et al: Malignant dermal cylindroma in a patient with multiple dermal cylindromas, trichoepitheliomas, and bilateral dermal analogue tumors of the parotid gland. *Am J Dermatopathol* 11:353–359, 1989.

157. Lyon JB, Rouillard LM: Malignant degeneration of turban tumor of the scalp. *Trans St John's Hosp Dermatol Soc* 46:74–77, 1961.

158. Grouls V, Iwaszkiewicz J, Berndt R: Malignant dermal cylindroma. *Pathologe* 12: 157–160, 1991.

159. Dabska M: Malignant transformation of eccrine spiradenoma. *Pol Med J* 11:388–396, 1972.

160. Evans HL, Su WPD, Smith JL, Winkelmann RK: Carcinoma arising in eccrine spiradenoma. *Cancer* 43:1881–1884, 1979.

161. Cooper PH, Frierson HF Jr, Morrison AG: Malignant transformation of eccrine spiradenoma. *Arch Dermatol* 121:1445–1448, 1985.

162. Wick MR, Kaye VN, Swanson PE, Pittelkow MR: Sweat gland carcinoma *ex* eccrine spiradenoma. *Am J Dermatopathol* 9:90–98, 1987.

163. Argenyi AZ, Nguyen AV, Balogh K, et al: Malignant eccrine spiradenoma: A clinicopathologic study. *Am J Dermatopathol* 12:335–343, 1990.

164. Varsa EW, Jordan SW: Fine needle aspiration cytology of malignant spiradenoma arising in congenital eccrine spiradenoma. *Acta Cytol* 34:275–277, 1990.

165. Zamboni AC, Zamboni WA, Ross DS: Malignant eccrine spiradenoma of the hand. *J Surg Oncol* 43:131–133, 1990.

166. Yaremchuk MJ, Elias LS, Graham RR, Wilgis EF: Sweat gland carcinoma of the hand: Two cases of malignant eccrine spiradenoma. *J Hand Surg* 9:910–914, 1984.

167. McKee PH, Fletcher CDM, Stavrinos P, Pambakian H: Carcinosarcoma arising in eccrine spiradenoma: A clinicopathologic and immunohistochemical study of two cases. *Am J Dermatopathol* 12:335–343, 1990.

168. Brownstein MH, Helwig EB: Patterns of cutaneous metastasis. *Arch Dermatol* 105:862–868, 1972.

169. Swanson PE, Mazoujian G, Mills SE, et al: Immunoreactivity for estrogen receptor protein in sweat gland tumors. *Am J Surg Pathol* 15:835–841, 1991.

170. Wick MR, Goellner JR, Wolfe JT III, Su WPD: Adnexal carcinomas of the skin: I. Eccrine carcinomas. *Cancer* 56:1147–1162, 1985.

171. El-Domeiri AA, Brasfield RD, Huvos AG, Strong EW: Sweat gland carcinoma: A clinicopathologic study of 83 patients. *Ann Surg* 173:270–274, 1971.

172. Kay S, Hall WEB: Sweat gland carcinoma with proved metastases. *Cancer* 7:373–376, 1954.

173. Okada N, Ota J, Sato K, Kitano Y: Metastasizing sweat gland carcinoma. *Arch Dermatol* 120:768–769, 1984.

174. Miller WL: Sweat gland carcinoma: A clinicopathologic problem. *Am J Clin Pathol* 47:767–780, 1967.

175. Swanson PE, Wick MR: Immunohistochemistry of cutaneous tumors, in Leong ASY (ed): *Applied Immunohistochemistry for the Surgical Pathologist.* London, Edward Arnold, 1993, pp 269–308.

176. Yamamoto O, Nakayama K, Asahi M: Sweat gland carcinoma with mucinous and infiltrating duct-like patterns. *J Cutan Pathol* 19:334–339, 1992.

177. Wong TY, Suster S, Nogita T, et al: Clear cell eccrine carcinomas of the skin: A clinicopathologic study of nine patients. *Cancer* 73:1631–1643, 1994.

178. Suster S: Clear cell tumors of the skin. *Semin Diagn Pathol* 13:40–59, 1996.

179. Headington JT, Niederhuber JE, Beals TF: Malignant clear cell acrospiroma. *Cancer* 41:641–647, 1978.

180. Kersting DW: Clear cell hidradenoma and hidradenocarcinoma. *Arch Dermatol* 87:323–333, 1963.

181. Keasbey LE, Hadley GG: Clear cell hidradenoma: Report of three cases with widespread metastases. *Cancer* 7:934–952, 1954.

182. McKenzie DH: A clear-cell hidradenocarcinoma with metastases. *Cancer* 10:1021–1023, 1957.

183. Chung CK, Hefferman AH: Clear cell hidradenoma with metastasis. *Plast Reconstr Surg* 48:177–179, 1971.

184. Czarnecki DB, Aarous I, Dowling JP: Malignant clear cell hidradenoma: A case report. *Acata Dermatol Venereol* 62:173–176, 1982.

185. Hernandez-Perez E, Cestoni-Parducci R: Nodular hidradenoma and hidradenocarcinoma: A 10 year review. *J Am Acad Dermatol* 12:15–20, 1985.

186. Wick MR, Goellner JR, Wolfe JT III, Su WPD: Vulvar sweat gland carcinomas. *Arch Pathol Lab Med* 109:43–47, 1985.

187. Brownstein MH, Helwig EB: Metastatic tumors of the skin. *Cancer* 29:1298–1307, 1972.

188. Tolia BM, Whitmore WF: Solitary metastasis from renal cell carcinoma. *J Urol* 114:836–838, 1975.

189. Connor DH, Taylor HB, Helwig EB: Cutaneous metastases of renal cell carcinoma. *Arch Pathol* 76:339–346, 1963.

190. Rosborough D: Malignant mixed tumors of the skin. *Br J Surg* 50:697–699, 1963.

191. Matz LR, McCully DJ, Stokes BAR: Metastasizing chondroid syringoma: A case report. *Pathology* 1:77–81, 1961.

192. Hilton JMN, Blackwell JB: Metastasizing chondroid syringoma. *J Pathol* 167–170, 1972.

193. Webb JN, Stott WG: Malignant chondroid syringoma of the thigh. *J Pathol* 116:43–46, 1975.

194. Botha JBC, Kahn LB: Aggressive chondroid syringoma. *Arch Dermatol* 114:954–955, 1978.

195. Ishimura E, Iwamoto H, Kobashi Y, et al: Malignant chondroid syringoma. *Cancer* 52:1966–1973, 1983.

196. Scott A, Metcalf S: Cutaneous malignant mixed tumor. *Am J Dermatopathol* 10:335–342, 1988.

197. Shvili D, Rothem A: Fulminant metastasizing chondroid syringoma of the skin. *Am J Dermatopathol* 8:321–325, 1986.

198. Harrist TJ, Aretz TH, Mihm MC Jr, et al: Cutaneous malignant mixed tumor. *Arch Dermatol* 117:719–724, 1981.

199. Pinto de Moraes H, Herrera GA, Mendonca AM, Estrela RR: Metastatic malignant mixed tumor of the skin: Ultrastructural and immunohistochemical characterization, histogenetic considerations, and comparison with benign mixed tumors of skin and salivary glands. *Appl Pathol* 4:199–208, 1986.

200. Redono C, Rocamora A, Villoria F, Garcia M: Malignant mixed tumor of the skin: Malignant chondroid syringoma. *Cancer* 49:1690–1696, 1982.

201. Sharvill DE: Mixed salivary-type tumor of the skin with malignant recurrence. *Br J Dermatol* 74:103–104, 1962.

202. Wick MR, Swanson PE: "Carcinosarcomas"—current perspectives and a historical review of nosological concepts. *Semin Diagn Pathol* 10:118–127, 1993.

203. Wick MR, Coffin CM: Sweat glands and pilar carcinomas, in Wick MR (ed): *Pathology of Unusual Malignant Cutaneous Tumors.* New York, Marcel Dekker, 1985, pp 1–76.

204. Toker C: Trabecular carcinoma of the skin. *Arch Dermatol* 105:107–110, 1972.

205. Matsuo K, Sakamoto A, Kawai K, et al: Small-cell carcinoma of the skin, "non-Merkel cell type." *Acta Pathol Jpn* 35:1029–1036, 1985.

206. Horn RC Jr: Malignant papillary cystadenoma of sweat glands with metastases to the regional lymph nodes. *Surgery* 16:348–355, 1944.

207. McDonald JR: Apocrine sweat gland carcinoma of the vulva. *Am J Clin Pathol* 11:890–897, 1941.

208. Kipke GF, Haust MD: Carcinoma of apocrine glands. *Arch Dermatol* 78:440–445, 1958.

209. Warkel RL, Helwig EB: Apocrine gland adenoma and adenocarcinoma of the axilla. *Arch Dermatol* 114:198–203, 1978.

210. Saigal RK, Khanna SD, Chandler J: Apocrine gland carcinoma in axilla. *Indian J Dermatol* 37:177–180, 1971.

211. Aurora AL, Luxenberg MN: Case report of adenocarcinoma of glands of Moll. *Am J Ophthalmol* 70:984–990, 1970.

212. Paties C, Taccagni GL, Papotti M, et al: Apocrine carcinoma of the skin: A clinico-pathologic, immunocytochemical, and ultrastructural study. *Cancer* 71:375–381, 1993.

213. Van der Putte SCJ, Van Gorp LHM: Adenocarcinoma of the mammary-like glands of the vulva. *J Cutan Pathol* 21:157–163, 1994.

214. Yamamoto O, Haratake J, Hisaoka M, et al: A unique case of apocrine carcinoma on the male pubic skin: Histopathologic and ultrastructural observations. *J Cutan Pathol* 20:378–383, 1993.

215. Chaundary MA, Millis RR, Lane B, Miller NA: Paget's disease of the nipple: A ten-year review including clinical, pathological, and immunohistochemical findings. *Breast Cancer Res Treat* 8:139–146, 1986.

216. Jones RE, Ackerman AB: Extramammary Paget's disease: A critical reappraisal. *Am J Dermatopathol* 1:101–132, 1979.

217. Jones RE: Mammary Paget's disease without underlying carcinoma. *Am J Dermatopathol* 7:361–365, 1985.

218. Mori O, Hachisuka H, Nakano S, et al: A case of mammary Paget's disease without an underlying carcinoma: Microscopic analysis of the DNA content in Paget cells. *J Dermatol* 21:160–165, 1994.

219. Mazoujian G, Pinkus GS, Haagensen DE: Extramammary Paget's disease: Evidence for an apocrine origin. *Am J Surg Pathol* 8:43–50, 1984.

220. Lee SC, Roth LM, Ehrlich C, Hall JA: Extramammary Paget's disease of the vulva: A clinicopathologic study of 13 cases. *Cancer* 39:2540–2549, 1977.

221. Boehm F, Morris JML: Paget's disease and apocrine gland carcinoma of the vulva. *Obstet Gynecol* 38:185–192, 1971.

222. Hart WR, Millman JB: Progression of intraepithelial Paget's disease of the vulva to invasive carcinoma. *Cancer* 40:2333–2337, 1977.

223. Mitsudo S, Nakanishi I, Koss LG: Paget's disease of the penis and adjacent skin: Its association with fatal sweat gland carcinoma. *Arch Pathol Lab Med* 105:518–520, 1981.

224. Knauer WJ Jr, Whorton CM: Extramammary Paget's disease originating in Moll's glands of the eyelid. *Trans Am Acad Ophthalmol Otolaryngol* 67:829–833, 1963.

225. Nadji M, Morales AR, Girtanner RE, et al: Paget's disease of the skin: A unifying concept of histogenesis. *Cancer* 50:2203–2206, 1982.

226. Rayne SC, Santa Cruz DJ: Anaplastic Paget's disease. *Am J Surg Pathol* 16:1085–1091, 1992.

227. Helm KF, Goellner JR, Peters MS: Immunohistochemical stains in extramammary Paget's disease. *Am J Dermatopathol* 14:402–407, 1992.

228. Hitchcock A, Topham S, Bell J, et al: Routine diagnosis of mammary Paget's disease. *Am J Surg Pathol* 16:58–61, 1992.

229. Kariniemi AL, Ramaekers F, Lehto VP, Virtanen I: Paget cells express cytokeratins typical of glandular epithelia. *Br J Dermatol* 112:179–183, 1985.

230. Takeshita K, Kzumoi S, Ebuchi M, et al: A case of rectal carcinoma concomitant with pagetoid lesion in the perianal region. *Gastroenterol Jpn* 13:85–95, 1978.

231. McKee PH, Hertogs KT: Endocervical adenocarcinoma and vulvar Paget's disease: A significant association. *Br J Dermatol* 103:443–448, 1980.

232. Degefu S, O'Quinn AG, Dhurandhar HN: Paget's disease of the vulva and urogenital malignancies. *Gynecol Oncol* 25:347–354, 1986.

233. Ojeda VJ, Heenen PJ, Watson SH: Paget's disease of the groin associated with adeno-carcinoma of the urinary bladder. *J Cutan Pathol* 14:227–231, 1987.

234. Gaffey MJ, Traweek ST, Mills SE, et al: Cytokeratin expression in adrenocortical neo-plasia: An immunohistochemical and biochemical study with implications for the differential diagnosis of adrenocortical, hepatocellular, and renal cell carcinoma. *Hum Pathol* 23:144–153, 1992.

235. Jakobiec FA, Austin P, Iwamoto T, et al: Primary infiltrating signet ring carcinoma of the eyelids. *Ophthalmology* 90:291–299, 1983.

236. Vidmar D, Baxter DL Jr, Devaney K: Extensive dermal metastases from primary signet ring carcinoma of the urinary bladder. *Cutis* 49:324–328, 1992.

237. Hood CI, Font RL, Zimmerman LE: Metastatic mammary carcinoma in the eyelid with histiocytoid appearance. *Cancer* 31:793–800, 1973.

238. Almagro UA: Primary signet ring carcinoma of the colon. *Cancer* 52:1453–1457, 1983.

239. Lauren P: The two histological main types of gastric carcinoma: Diffuse and so-called intestinal type carcinoma. *Acta Pathol Microbiol Scand* 64:31–49, 1965.

240. Swanson SA, Cooper PH, Mills SE, Wick MR: Lymphoepithelioma-like carcinoma of the skin. *Mod Pathol* 1:359–365, 1988.

241. Wick MR, Swanson PE, LeBoit PE, et al: Lymphoepithelioma-like carcinoma of the skin with adnexal differentiation. *J Cutan Pathol* 18:93–102, 1991.

242. Axelsen SM, Stamp IM: Lymphoepithelioma-like carcinoma of the vulvar region. *Histopathology* 27:281–283, 1995.

243. Jimenez F, Clark RE, Buchanan MD, Kamino H: Lymphoepithelioma-like carcinoma of the skin treated with Mohs micrographic surgery in combination with immune staining for cytokeratins. *J Am Acad Dermatol* 32:878–881, 1995.

244. Robins P, Perez MI: Lymphoepithelioma-like carcinoma of the skin treated by Mohs micrographic surgery. *J Am Acad Dermatol* 32:814–816, 1995.

245. Dozier SE, Jones TR, Nelson-Adesokan P, Hruza GJ: Lymphoepithelioma-like carcinoma of the skin treated by Mohs micrographic surgery. *Dermatol Surg* 21:690–694, 1995.

246. Requena L, Sanchez-Yus E, Jimenez E, Roo E: Lymphoepithelioma-like carcinoma of the skin: A light microscopic and immunohistochemical study. *J Cutan Pathol* 21:541–548, 1994.

247. Ortiz-Frutos FJ, Zarco C, Gil R, et al: Lymphoepithelioma-like carcinoma of the skin. *Clin Exp Dermatol* 18:83–86, 1993.

248. Nekhleh RE, Swanson PE, Wick MR: Cutaneous adnexal carcinomas with mixed differentiation. *Am J Dermatopathol* 12:325–334, 1990.

249. Goldstein N: Ephidrosis (local hyperhidrosis): Nevus sudoriferus. *Arch Dermatol* 96:67–71, 1967.

250. Kin JH, Hur H, Lee CW, Kim YT: Apocrine nevus. *J Am Acad Dermatol* 18:579–581, 1988.

251. Romer JC, Taira JW: Mucinous eccrine nevus. *Cutis* 53:259–261, 1994.

252. Ruiz-de Erenchun F, Vazquez-Doval FJ, Contreras-Mejuto F, Quintanilla E: Localized unilateral hyperhidrosis: Eccrine nevus. *J Am Acad Dermatol* 27:115–116, 1992.

253. Imai S, Nitto H: Eccrine nevus with epidermal changes. *Dermatologica* 166:84–88, 1983.

254. Mori O, Hachisuka H, Sasai Y: Apocrine nevus. *Int J Dermatol* 32:448–449, 1993.

255. Neill JS, Park HK: Apocrine nevus: Light microscopic, immunohistochemical, and ultrastructural studies of a case. *J Cutan Pathol* 20:79–83, 1993.

256. Ando K, Hashikawa Y, Nakashima M, et al: Pure apocrine nevus: A study of light microscopic and immunohistochemical features of a rare tumor. *Am J Dermatopathol* 13:71–76, 1991.

257. Schwartz RA, Rojas-Corona R, Lambert WC: The polymorphic apocrine nevus: A study of a unique tumor including carcinoembryonic antigen staining. *J Surg Oncol* 26:183–186, 1984.

258. Challa VE, Jona J: Eccrine angiomatous hamartoma: A rare skin lesion with diverse histological features. *Dermatologica* 155:216–219, 1977.

259. Mehregan AH: Proliferation of sweat ducts in certain diseases of the skin. *Am J Dermatopathol* 3:27–31, 1981.

260. Bhawan J, Malhotra R: Syringosquamous hyperplasia and eccrine squamous syringometaplasia associated with benoxaprofen therapy. *Arch Dermatol* 123:1202–1204, 1987.

261. King DT, Barr RJ: Syringometaplasia: Mucinous and squamous variants. *J Cutan Pathol* 6:284–291, 1979.

262. Farina MC, Pique E, Olivares M, et al: Multiple hidrocystoma of the face: Three cases. *Clin Exp Dermatol* 20:323–327, 1995.

263. Yasaka N, Iozumi K, Nashiro K, et al: Bilateral periorbital eccrine hidrocystoma. *J Dermatol* 21:490–493, 1994.

264. Shields JA, Eagle RC Jr, Shields CL, et al: Apocrine hidrocystoma of the eyelid. *Arch Ophthalmol* 111:866–867, 1993.

265. Hassan MO, Khan MA, Kruse TV: Apocrine cystadenoma. *Arch Dermatol* 115:194–200, 1979.

266. Kruse TV, Khan MA, Hassan MO: Multiple apocrine cystadenomas. *Br J Dermatol* 100:675–681, 1979.

267. Hashimoto K, Zagula-Mally ZW, Youngberg G, Leicht S: Electron microscopic studies of Moll's gland cyst. *J Cutan Pathol* 14:23–26, 1987.

268. Jones DB: Florid papillomatosis of the nipple ducts. *Cancer* 8:315–319, 1955.

269. Myers JL, Mazur MT, Urist MM, Peiper SC: Florid papillomatosis of the nipple: Immunohistochemical and flow cytometric analysis of two cases. *Mod Pathol* 3:288–293, 1990.

270. Smith NP, Jones EW: Erosive adenomatosis of the nipple. *Clin Exp Dermatol* 2:79–83, 1977.

271. Rosen PP, Caicco JA: Florid papillomatosis of the nipple: A study of 51 patients, including nine with mammary carcinoma. *Am J Surg Pathol* 10:87–101, 1986.

272. Goldman RL, Cooperman H: Adenoma of the nipple: A benign lesion simulating carcinoma clinically and pathologically. *Am J Surg* 119:322–325, 1970.

273. Brownstein MH, Phelps RG, Magnin PH: Papillary adenoma of the nipple: Analysis of fifteen new cases. *J Am Acad Dermatol* 12:707–715, 1985.

274. Perzin KH, Lattes R: Papillary adenoma of the nipple (florid papillomatosis, adenoma, adenomatosis): A clinicopathologic study. *Cancer* 29:996–1009, 1972.

275. Diaz NM, Palmer JO, Wick MR: Erosive adenomatosis of the nipple: Histology, immunohistology, and differential diagnosis. *Mod Pathol* 5:179–184, 1992.

CHAPTER 30

FIBROUS AND FIBROHISTIOCYTIC TUMORS

Scott R. Granter / Christopher D. M. Fletcher

Tumors of fibrous tissue are common and histologically diverse. In addition, new entities continue to be described. The behavior and overall prognosis of these lesions is highly varied and thus precise classification is required. It cannot be emphasized enough that behavior of fibrous tumors may be difficult to predict based on traditional histologic concepts. For example, the morphologic features of some tumors, such as low-grade fibromyxoid sarcoma and atypical fibroxanthoma, do not reflect their biologic behavior. For this reason, the pathologist should not attempt to predict the clinical behavior of mesenchymal tumors without a firm histologic diagnosis.

BENIGN FIBROUS PROLIFERATIONS AND TUMORS

Hypertrophic Scar and Keloid

Clinical Features   Wound healing may be associated with an abnormal connective tissue response and result in exuberant scar formation. Hypertrophic scars and keloids occur most commonly in children and young adults (Table 30-1). Keloids show a strong predilection for darkly pigmented races, particularly African Americans. Keloids occur most commonly in the head and neck, upper chest, and shoulder region. Most hypertrophic scars and keloids develop soon after surgical or other traumatic injury. Keloids are raised, shiny, smooth, and well-circumscribed plaques. They tend to extend beyond the original site of injury and may attain very large size through progressive growth and thereby become unsightly. Hypertrophic scars, in contrast to keloids, do not usually extend beyond the site of original injury and tend to regress with time.

Histopathological Features   Early scars may be fairly cellular and are composed of plump myofibroblasts and fibroblasts arranged in parallel array (Table 30-1). Sparse chronic inflammatory cells may be present, particularly in early scars. As the scar ages, cellularity decreases and collagenization increases. A characteristic feature of hypertrophic scars, which often tend to be nodular, is the presence of long, slender, blood vessels oriented perpendicular to the epidermis. Keloids are similar histologically to hypertrophic scars but with the addition of characteristic thick bands of "glassy" hyalinized collagen (Fig. 30-1).

Differential Diagnosis   The hyalinized bands of collagen seen in keloids are distinctive and therefore these lesions rarely pose a diagnostic problem. Dermatofibroma is distinguished from hypertrophic scar by its storiform pattern and characteristic entrapment of hyaline collagen bundles. The epidermis usually is hyperplastic in dermatofibroma and atrophic in hypertrophic scars. Fibromatosis is distinguished from scars

by increased cellularity and a more infiltrative growth pattern; furthermore, a superficial location would be exceptional. Blood vessels oriented perpendicularly to the epidermis are not seen in fibromatosis.

Fibroepithelial Polyp (Acrochordon, Skin Tag) and Soft Fibroma

Clinical Features   The fibroepithelial polyp, also know as skin tag or acrochordon, is one of the most common skin lesions. They are polypoid, soft, often slightly hyperpigmented, and attached by a thin fibrovascular stalk. Fibroepithelial polyps are most common in middle-aged and elderly adults, are frequently multiple, and range in size from a millimeter to larger than a centimeter (Table 30-2). They are particularly common in the neck and axillary area and usually are removed for cosmetic reasons only. Not uncommonly, fibroepithelial polyps twist about their stalk and infarct, causing a change in color from tan to black. This change in color often alarms the patient and a clinical opinion is sought. Fibroepithelial polyps with dense collagenous stroma are often designated fibroma. Patients with Cowden's syndrome may have multiple fibromas.[1]

Histopathological Features   These lesions are digitate or polypoid with a collagenous core that varies from loosely textured to densely sclerotic collagen (Table 30-2) (Fig. 30-2). Ectatic thin-walled vessels are common. Those polyps with a core of dense sclerotic collagen often are diagnosed as fibromas. Polyps containing significant amounts of adipose tissue are often designated soft fibromas or even, mistakenly, nevus lipomatosus superficialis. The epidermis may be unremarkable or show features of lichen simplex chronicus; the result of rubbing by the patient or friction from clothing. Many fibroepithelial polyps show epithelial changes similar to seborrheic keratosis, including acanthosis with horn cysts.

Differential Diagnosis   Distinction between some fibroepithelial polyps and seborrheic keratosis can be difficult. We designate clinically polypoid lesions as fibroepithelial polyps, but this is admittedly an arbitrary decision. Alternatively, lesions with prominent epidermal changes may be designated pedunculated seborrheic keratosis. Soft fibromas with large amounts of fat may mimic nevus lipomatosus superficialis. Broad-based, plaque-like lesions with fat extending into the dermis are more characteristic of nevus lipomatosus superficialis. In contrast to fibroepithelial polyps and soft fibroma, nevus lipomatosus superficialis most often is located on the posterior upper thigh and buttocks. Angiofibromas are distinguished by a prominent vascular component; however, a spectrum between fibroepithelial polyp and angiofibroma exists.

TABLE 30-1
Hypertrophic Scar and Keloid

Clinical Features

Most common in children and young adults
Keloids
    Predilection for African Americans
    Head and neck, upper chest, and shoulder region
    Raised, shiny, smooth, and well-circumscribed plaques
    Extend beyond the original site of injury
    Tend to grow progressively
Hypertrophic scar
    Does not extend beyond the original site of injury and tends to regress

Histopathological Features

Early scars—fairly cellular, fibroblasts arranged in parallel array
Sparse chronic inflammatory cells may be present
Cellularity decreases and collagenization increases with age
Long, slender, blood vessels oriented perpendicularly to the epidermis
Keloids have thick bands of "glassy" hyalinized collagen

Differential Diagnosis

Dermatofibroma
Fibromatosis

TABLE 30-2
Fibroepithelial Polyp

Clinical Features

Commonly involving the skin of the neck and axillary area of middle-aged and elderly
Frequently multiple
1–15 mm in size
Polypoid, soft, and attached by a thin fibrovascular stalk
Often slightly hyperpigmented

Histopathological Features

Polypoid with a collagenous core of loosely textured to dense sclerotic collagen
Soft fibromas are larger with adipose tissue
Epidermis may show features of lichen simplex chronicus or seborrheic keratosis

Differential Diagnosis

Seborrheic keratosis
Nevus lipomatosus superficialis
Angiofibroma
Pedunculated nevus

Commonly, pedunculated melanocytic nevi are mistaken for fibroepithelial polyps by clinicians. Indeed, some fibroepithelial polyps may represent involuted nevi. Not uncommonly, a small nest of nevomelanocytes are noted within an otherwise typical fibroepithelial polyp.

Angiofibroma

Angiofibromas comprise a clinically heterogenous group of lesions with similar histopathology (Table 30-3). Three distinct clinical variants of angiofibroma include adenoma sebaceum, fibrous papule, and pearly penile papule.

ADENOMA SEBACEUM

Clinical Features   Adenoma sebaceum is one manifestation of tuberous sclerosis, an autosomal dominantly inherited disorder with protean

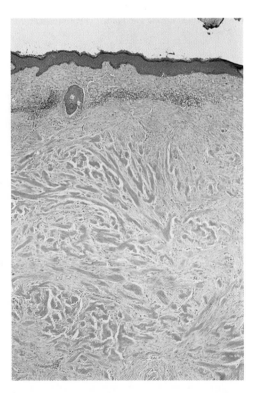

FIGURE 30-1   Keloid. The reticular dermis is expanded by a nodular aggregate of hyalinized eosinophilic bundles of collagen.

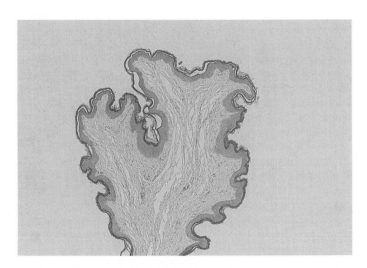

FIGURE 30-2   Acrochordon. Fibroepithelial polyp with squamous epithelium surrounding loose collagenous stroma.

clinical manifestations. Central nervous system manifestations include mental retardation, epilepsy, glial hamartomas, and subependymal giant cell astrocytomas. Systemic manifestations include cardiac rhabdomyomas, angiomyolipomas of the kidney, renal cysts, and carcinomas, pulmonary lymphangioleiomyomatosis, and fibrous dysplasia of bone. Mucocutaneous lesions commonly seen in tuberous sclerosis include adenoma sebaceum, subungual fibromas, cafe-au-lait spots, patches of cutaneous hypopigmentation (ash-leaf spots), fibromas, and connective tissue nevi (shagreen patch).[2]

The term adenoma sebaceum is a misnomer: It is distributed in the "sebaceous" area of the face where the greatest concentration of sebaceous glands reside; however, the lesion is not derived from sebaceous glands. These lesions present as multiple skin colored to pink-red papules and nodules on the cheeks, forehead, chin, and often are most dense in the nasolabial folds. They range from minute papules to large coalescent nodules. They develop at birth or in early childhood and may be the first sign of disease. Clinical recognition of these lesions as a manifestation of tuberous sclerosis is important, as new mutations are believed to account for approximately two-thirds of patients.

FIBROUS PAPULE

Clinical Features   Fibrous papule, a variant of angiofibroma, is a small shiny cutaneous papule that is located on the face, most commonly on the nose of adults. It is usually only a few millimeters in diameter. Dermatologists often biopsy these lesions to exclude basal cell carcinoma. They also may be indistinguishable from small nevi.

PEARLY PENILE PAPULES

Clinical Features   Pearly penile papules present as tiny papules, usually no more than a few millimeters in diameter, on the glans penis. They often are oriented circumferentially about the coronal sulcus of the glans.[3] Most patients are under 40 years of age and these lesions are more common in African Americans and uncircumcised men.[4]

Histopathological Features   Histologically, these three types of lesion are dermal fibroblastic proliferations associated with variable numbers of thin-walled slightly ectatic vessels (Table 30-3) (Fig. 30-3). The composite fibroblasts often are multinucleated and stellate shaped, resembling ganglion cells or radiation fibroblasts. Concentric fibrosis surrounding adnexal structures is a characteristic feature.

Differential Diagnosis   Pleomorphic fibroma differs by its typical location on the extremities and the presence of large pleomorphic and hyperchromatic nuclei, in comparison with the more reactive-appearing fibroblasts seen in adenoma sebaceum. In addition, pleomorphic fibroma lacks the rich vascular pattern seen in angiofibromas. Fibrous papules, predominantly composed of plump, rounded fibroblasts, may be mistaken for dermal nevi. Dermal nevi are distinguished from fibrous papules by nests of nevus cells. The fibroblasts in fibrous papule are not reactive for S-100 protein allowing immunohistochemical distinction from nevomelanocytes. Pearly penile papules are clinicopathologically distinctive and rarely pose a diagnostic problem.

Acral Fibrokeratoma (Acquired Digital Fibrokeratoma) and Periungual Fibroma

Clinical Features   Acral fibrokeratoma occurs most frequently on the fingers; however, it is also seen on the toes, palms and soles, feet, and legs of adults (Table 30-4).[5–8] Fibrokeratomas are small (less than

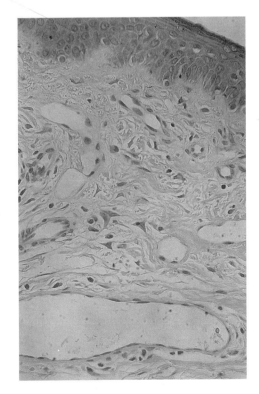

FIGURE 30-3   Fibrous papule. Ectatic vessels are surrounded by spindled and stellate fibroblasts.

TABLE 30-4

Acral Fibrokeratoma and Periungual Fibroma

Clinical Features

Fibrokeratoma

Fingers, toes, palms and soles, feet, and legs of adults

Small (<1.5 cm) nodules

Slightly elevated to dome-shaped or tall protrusions

Periungual fibroma

Arise in the peripubertal period in patients with tuberous sclerosis

Flesh-colored nodules that arise from the nail folds

Few millimeters to over 1 cm

Histopathological Features

Fibrokeratoma

Dense irregular collagen bundles

Variable numbers of fibroblasts

Sparse to numerous thin-walled vessels

Vessels and collagen bundles often arranged perpendicular to the epidermis

Epidermis usually shows some degree of hyperkeratosis and acanthosis

Periungual fibroma

May be indistinguishable from fibrokeratoma, except some cases may have multinucleated giant cells and stellate cells resembling ganglion cells

Differential Diagnosis

Supernumerary digit

Dermatofibroma

Angiofibroma

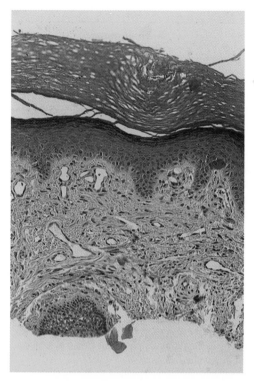

FIGURE 30-4   Periungual fibroma. The epidermis shows acanthosis and hyperkeratosis. The underlying dermis is expanded by dense collagen associated with a few ectatic vessels.

1.5 cm) nodules that range from slightly elevated to protuberant lesions that often are exophytic with a narrow base. The overlying epidermis usually is hyperkeratotic. Trauma does not appear to play a role in the pathogenesis.[8]

Periungual fibromas are smooth, shiny, flesh-colored nodules that arise from the nail folds (Table 30-4). They range in size from a few millimeters to over 1 cm. They usually present as multiple lesions in the peripubertal period. As with adenoma sebaceum, the presence of periungual fibromas should prompt a careful family history and clinical examination for evidence of tuberous sclerosis. Periungual fibromas are seen in approximately half of patients with this disorder.

Histopathological Features   Fibrokeratoma is composed of dense hyalinized and irregularly arranged collagen bundles with variable numbers of fibroblasts. Sparse to numerous thin-walled vessels may be present (Table 30-4) (Fig. 30-4). Vessels and collagen bundles often are arranged perpendicular to the overlying epidermis. The overlying epidermis usually shows some degree of hyperkeratosis and acanthosis. Elastic tissue stains usually fail to show elastic fibers.

Periungual fibromas also are composed of dense collagen bundles arranged in parallel array and may be associated with a variable number of blood vessels. They may be indistinguishable from acral fibrokeratoma.[9] Some cases have multinucleated giant cells and stellate cells resembling ganglion cells. Similar cells are seen in some variants of angiofibroma.

Differential Diagnosis   Clinically, supernumerary digit may resemble fibrokeratoma, but true supernumerary digit contains a proliferation of nerve bundles as well as fibrous tissue. Periungual fibromas of tuberous

sclerosis demonstrate concentric perivascular fibrosis and contain stellate and multinucleated fibroblasts, features generally not seen in fibrokeratoma. Others have not found these features helpful in distinguishing periungual fibroma from fibrokeratoma. These features are, however, seen in angiofibromas, a group of tumors within which periungual fibroma may be classified. In contrast to dermatofibroma, a well-developed storiform pattern and encapsulation of collagen is not seen in periungual fibroma and angiokeratoma.

Circumscribed Storiform Collagenoma (Sclerotic Fibroma)

Clinical Features   Storiform collagenoma is seen most commonly in young and middle-aged adults (Table 30-5). These lesions usually measure less than a centimeter and present as slow-growing solitary nodules on the head and neck region, or upper extremities.[10,11] Recurrence is not a feature.

Histopathological Features   These tumors are symmetric and well-circumscribed but unencapsulated (Table 30-5). The tumor is composed of paucicellular hyaline collagen containing numerous cleft-like spaces (Fig. 30-5). Cellularity varies; however, most tumors contain only rare scattered fibroblasts interposed between collagen bands. The clefts are randomly oriented and impart a storiform pattern at low magnification. Multiple fibromas with identical histologic appearance may be seen in Cowden's disease.

Differential Diagnosis   Epidermal acanthosis and the presence of inflammatory cells, including multinucleated giant cells, help to distinguish sclerotic dermatofibroma and circumscribed storiform collagenoma. Circumscribed storiform collagenoma tends to expand and efface the overlying epidermis, in contrast to the thickened epithelium

TABLE 30-5

Circumscribed Storiform Collagenoma

Clinical Features

Young and middle-aged adults
Usually <1 cm
Slow-growing solitary nodules on the head and neck region and
    upper extremities

Histopathological Features

Symmetric, well-circumscribed but unencapsulated
Paucicellular hyaline collagen with numerous cleft-like spaces
Rare scattered fibroblasts between collagen bands
Clefts impart a storiform pattern to the tumor

Differential Diagnosis

Sclerotic dermatofibroma/myofibroma
Keloids

TABLE 30-6

Fibroma of Tendon Sheath

Clinical Features

Young to middle-aged men
Slow-growing painless nodule of hands and feet
25% recur following excision

Histopathological Features

Well-circumscribed
Variably cellular, composed of fibroblasts and myofibroblasts in
    short fascicles
Slit-like vascular spaces

Differential Diagnosis

Giant cell tumor of tendon sheath
Angioleiomyoma
Fibromatosis

---

over dermatofibroma. However, it seems that occasional examples of this entity may represent an end-stage dermatofibroma or solitary myofibroma. This perspective is supported by occasional examples resembling collagenoma with small foci recognizable as dermatofibroma or solitary myofibroma. Keloids can be distinguished by the association of typical hypertrophic scar and poor circumscription. Storiform collagenoma shows more uniform hyalinization compared to keloid.

Fibroma of Tendon Sheath

Clinical Features   Fibroma of tendon sheath is a tumor of unclear pathogenesis. It is seen most frequently on the hands and feet of young adults, particularly men (Table 30-6).[12] Most tumors are painless, slowly growing nodules or masses on a finger, measuring under 3 cm in diameter. Attachment to the tendon or tendon sheath usually can be demonstrated at the time of surgery.[13] Up to 25 percent of tumors may

recur following surgical excision.[14] Serious functional impairment is almost never seen.

Histopathological Features   These tumors are well-circumscribed and show variable cellularity (Table 30-6). They are composed of uniform spindled fibroblasts and myofibroblasts with slender tapered nuclei arranged in short fascicles. Paucicellular tumors may be markedly hyalinized and demonstrate concentric whorls of dense eosinophilic collagen. A characteristic feature is the presence of slit-like vascular channels that appear compressed by surrounding stroma (Fig. 30-6). The presence of multinucleated giant cells in occasional tumors suggests the existence of a morphologic spectrum with giant cell tumor of tendon sheath.[15]

Differential Diagnosis   Cellular tumors with giant cells may be difficult, if not impossible, to distinguish from giant cell tumor of tendon sheath.[15] The presence of slit-like vessels and tumor cells arranged in short fascicles favors fibroma of tendon sheath. These features, together

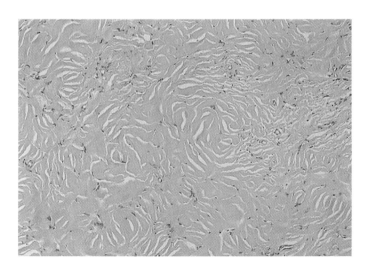

FIGURE 30-5 Circumscribed storiform collagenoma. The tumor is composed of paucicellular hyaline collagen containing numerous cleft-like spaces and only rare scattered fibroblasts. The pattern of randomly oriented bands of collagen often creates a storiform pattern at low magnification.

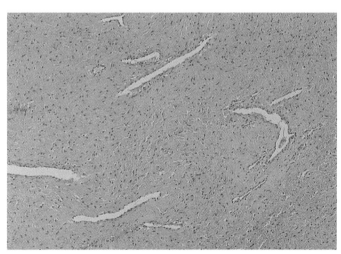

FIGURE 30-6 Fibroma of tendon sheath. This tumor is composed of uniform spindled fibroblasts and myofibroblasts with slender tapered nuclei in a densely collagenous stroma. The presence of slit-like vascular channels that appear compressed by surrounding stroma is characteristic.

TABLE 30-7

Dermatomyofibroma

Clinical Features

Pale pink or hypopigmented plaque
Upper trunk
Adolescents and young adults, usually females

Histopathological Features

Fascicles oriented parallel to the skin surface
Grenz zone
Composite cells are myofibroblasts with eosinophilic cytoplasm
Significant extension into fat and subcutaneous tissue is not seen

Differential Diagnosis

Dermatofibroma
Dermatofibrosarcoma protuberans (plaque-stage)

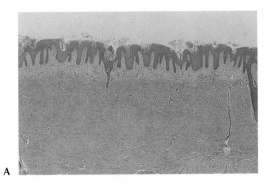

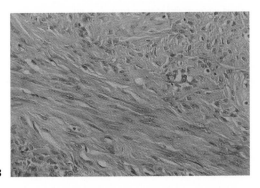

FIGURE 30-7   Dermatomyofibroma. *A.* The tumor exhibits a plaque-like growth pattern in the reticular dermis with a grenz zone sparing the superficial dermis. *B.* The tumor is composed of fascicles of spindled cells with a myoid appearance.

with overall circumscription of the tumor, allows distinction from fibromatosis. Angioleiomyoma may resemble fibroma of tendon sheath at low-power magnification; however, the vessels of angioleiomyoma have thick walls with smooth muscle cells radiating from them. The absence of myxoid "feathery" areas alternating with more cellular areas distinguishes fibroma of tendon sheath from nodular fasciitis.

Dermatomyofibroma

Clinical Features   Dermatomyofibroma usually presents as a pale pink or hypopigmented plaque on the upper trunk or neck of adolescents and young adults, particularly females (Table 30-7). Lesions may resemble keloid or plaque-like dermatofibrosarcoma protuberans (DFSP), grow slowly over many years, and attain a size of up to 5 cm.[16–18] Surgical excision appears curative in the small number of cases reported.

Histopathological Features   The tumor exhibits a band-like configuration in the reticular dermis with a grenz zone sparing the superficial dermis (Table 30-7) (Fig. 30-7). The latter band-like structure is composed of fascicles of spindle cells oriented parallel to the surface. Adnexal structures tend to be spared. Prominent extension into subcutaneous tissue usually is not seen although focal involvement of subcutaneous fat is present in some cases. The composite cells are uniformly actin-positive myofibroblasts with eosinophilic cytoplasm.

Differential Diagnosis   Dermatofibroma usually does not appear as a plaque clinically and displays a prominent storiform pattern of growth with "encapsulation" of individual collagen bundles. Dermatomyofibroma is distinguished from dermatofibrosarcoma protuberans by the lack of a uniform storiform pattern and absence of extensive infiltration into fat and subcutaneous tissue. In difficult cases, CD34 negativity and smooth muscle actin positivity help to rule out dermatofibrosarcoma protuberans.[18]

Nodular Fasciitis

Nodular fasciitis is a reactive myofibroblastic proliferation notorious for being misinterpreted as a sarcoma. In addition, sarcomas also may be misinterpreted as nodular fasciitis, resulting in patients not receiving appropriate therapy promptly. To complicate matters, this reactive proliferation shows a variety of distinct histological patterns. Nodular fasciitis is also discussed in Chapter 32.

Clinical Features   Most lesions are rapidly growing, often painful, subcutaneous or deep soft tissue masses, usually several centimeters in greatest dimension (Table 30-8). Comparable lesions may arise primarily in the dermis.[19] Alarmed patients often present with the history of a mass growing rapidly over the course of a week to several weeks, and some patients even testify to lesions growing "overnight." Most patients are young adults; however, the overall age range is wide. The upper limb, particularly the forearm, is the most common site of involvement. In children, most lesions are seen in the head and neck region.[20] Cranial fasciitis, a distinctive form of nodular fasciitis seen in infants, involves the soft tissue of the scalp and may erode into underlying bone.[21] Recurrence is observed in 1 to 2 percent of cases and is most likely due to inadequate surgical excision of growing lesions.[22] Biopsy material from recurrent tumors must be reevaluated carefully to ensure that the original lesion was diagnosed correctly.

Histopathological Features   This process most commonly involves the fascia and subcutaneous fat but a rare dermal variant has been described (Table 30-8). Most lesions are well-circumscribed; however, nodular fasciitis may also show infiltrative borders and extend along the fibrous septa of subcutaneous fat. At low power the cellularity varies from one area to another. Areas of low cellularity have a distinctive microcystic or myxoid background creating a loosely textured "feathery" appearance (Fig. 30-8). Cells in both the cellular and paucicellular zones tend to be arranged in broad sweeping and interlacing fascicles associated with thin-walled blood vessels. A storiform pattern may be seen focally. The dominant cell types are fibroblasts and myofibroblasts

TABLE 30-8

Nodular Fasciitis

Clinical Features

Rapidly growing and often tender
Subcutaneous or deep soft tissue masses, usually several centimeter in greatest dimension
Young adults
Upper limb, particularly the forearm
In children, most lesions in the head and neck region
Recurrence is rare

Histopathological Features

Usually well circumscribed, but may also show infiltrative borders
Cellularity varies within the tumor
Areas of low cellularity have a distinctive myxoid, feathery background
Short to broad sweeping fascicles, focal storiform pattern
"Tissue-culture" myofibroblasts with vesicular nucleus with occasional prominent nucleoli
Essentially no cytological atypia
Mitoses may be abundant
Inflammatory cells and multinucleated osteoclast-like giant cells may be seen
Ganglion-like cells in proliferative fasciitis

Differential Diagnosis

Fibromatosis
Sarcoma, particularly low-grade myxofibrosarcoma and fibrosarcoma
Fibrous histiocytoma

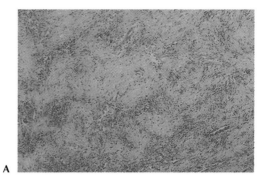

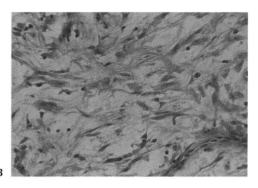

FIGURE 30-8 Nodular fasciitis. *A.* The low-power appearance of nodular fasciitis is characteristic: The cellularity varies from one area to another with areas of low cellularity having a distinctive "feathery" appearance. *B.* At high power, the composite cells show abundant tapering eosinophilic cytoplasm with frequent stellate forms. They resemble fibroblasts grown in tissue culture.

with spindled shape and vesicular nuclei and occasional prominent nucleoli. Many of these cells show abundant tapering eosinophilic cytoplasm with frequent stellate forms. Their morphology has been likened to fibroblasts grown in tissue culture. Mitoses may be abundant, but are never atypical. Pleomorphism and nuclear hyperchromasia are absent. Variable numbers of acute and chronic inflammatory cells usually are seen. Multinucleated osteoclast-like giant cells are present quite often.

Proliferative fasciitis is a variant of nodular fasciitis that is distinguished by the presence of larger polygonal cells with abundant amphophilic or basophilic cytoplasm that imparts a resemblance to ganglion cells or even rhabdomyoblasts (Fig. 30-9). These distinctive cells, which may be abundant or rare, are superimposed on a background of typical nodular fasciitis. Intramuscular tumors with the same histology have been designated proliferative myositis.[23] Ischemic fasciitis, also termed "atypical decubital fibroplasia," is a nodular fasciitis-like reaction thought to be secondary to ischemia. This lesion is characterized by fibrinoid necrosis associated with a nodular fasciitis-like fibroblastic reaction in the dermis and subcutis near bony protuberances of elderly and debilitated patients.[24,25] Cranial fasciitis is histologically similar to nodular fasciitis, and has a propensity to erode underlying bone and may even extend to the dura and meninges. This lesion usually occurs in infants and may be related to trauma during delivery.[26] Comparable lesions may occur at other parosteal locations. Intravascular fasciitis is an uncommon variant that involves veins, usually in the upper extremities and the head and neck region. This subtype is characterized by multinodular growth of nodular fasciitis within vessels.[27]

The majority of cases of nodular fasciitis show immunoreactivity for smooth muscle actin and muscle specific actin; however, reactivity for desmin usually is not seen, although sometimes this may be affected by the antibody used. The immunohistochemical profile and ultrastructural characteristics support a myofibroblastic origin for nodular fasciitis.

Differential Diagnosis Because of rapid growth, high mitotic activity, and infiltrative pattern, nodular fasciitis often is mistaken for a malig-

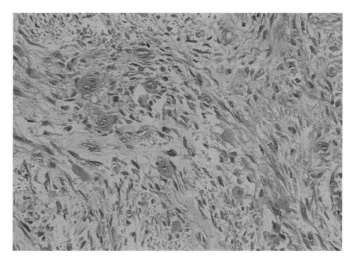

FIGURE 30-9 Proliferative fasciitis. The lesion resembles nodular fasciitis in all aspects with the additional finding of plump cells resembling ganglion cells.

nant neoplasm. The low-power pattern of nodular fasciitis, with distinctive alternating cellular and paucicellular "feathery" myxoid zones, taken with the bland cytologic features, establishes the correct diagnosis. At higher power, "tissue culture" fibroblast-like cells with vesicular nuclei, absence of nuclear hyperchromasia, together with absence of atypical mitoses, help to exclude a diagnosis of sarcoma. Areas of nodular fasciitis showing storiform patterns may be indistinguishable from fibrous histiocytoma. Nodular fasciitis is discriminated from fibrous histiocytoma-based on the other characteristic of "feathery" arrangements of uniform fibroblasts in broad sweeping fascicles, myxoid alteration, and depth typical of nodular fasciitis. In addition, nodular fasciitis does not show encapsulation of collagen that is characteristic of fibrous histiocytoma. Fibromatosis is more uniformly cellular and fascicular, is associated with more abundant dense collagen, and lacks the myxoid areas seen in nodular fasciitis. The fibroblasts in fibromatosis are more uniform and tend to have wavy nuclei. Fibrosarcoma, which is rare, is much more cellular, lacks the loose "feathery" pattern seen in nodular fasciitis, and is characterized by a herringbone fascicular pattern. Low-grade myxofibrosarcoma (myxoid malignant fibrous histiocytoma) occasionally is misdiagnosed as nodular fasciitis. This tumor is distinguished from nodular fasciitis by characteristic curvilinear vessels and the presence of cells with atypical hyperchromatic nuclei and vacuolated cytoplasm that may resemble lipoblasts.

Recurrent nodular fasciitis is rare and pathological material from patients with recurrent lesions must be *examined* critically and the original diagnosis carefully reassessed. It is the authors' experience that a significant proportion of cases diagnosed as recurrent nodular fasciitis are sarcomas.

Knuckle Pad

Clinical Features   Knuckle pads are considered by some to be a form of fibromatosis. They are hyperkeratotic papules on the dorsum of the interphalangeal or metacarpophalangeal joints.[28] They usually are seen in adults and rarely cause symptoms or functional impairment. Some cases may be familial or associated with superficial fibromatosis such as Dupuytren's disease. They show no apparent tendency to recur.

Histopathological Features   Microscopically, knuckle pads are composed of a bland fibrous proliferation, usually less cellular than fibromatosis. They usually are associated with overlying epidermal acanthosis and hyperkeratosis.

Differential Diagnosis   Knuckle pad may resemble scarring fibrosis secondary to trauma but is distinguished by clinical history.

Palmar and Plantar Fibromatosis

The fibromatoses are a family of fibroblastic proliferations sharing similar histology, an infiltrative pattern of growth, and a tendency to recur following excision. Tumors located at some sites show the capacity for locally aggressive and destructive growth; however, these tumors never metastasize.[29,30] The clinical behavior of fibromatoses is very site-dependent; however, in general the superficially located tumors are less aggressive. There is some evidence for an association with alcoholism and epilepsy in patients with superficial lesions.

Clinical Features   Palmar fibromatosis (syn. Dupuytren's contracture) is an extremely common tumor affecting mostly older individuals, with a male predominance (Table 30-9). Frequently both hands are involved. Uncommonly, both palmar and plantar fibromatosis occur in the same

TABLE 30-9
Palmar and Plantar Fibromatosis

Clinical Features

Palmar fibromatosis
   Both hands are commonly involved
   Small nodule that progressively enlarges to form a cord-like band that causes puckering of overlying skin
   Flexion contracture and functional impairment of the hand
Plantar fibromatosis
   Occurs in younger age groups
   May cause minor discomfort when walking
   Rarely associated with functional impairment

Histopathological Features

Interlacing fascicles with wavy collagenous stroma
Tumor cells are spindle-shaped; tapering or vesicular nuclei
Early lesions are fairly cellular, mitotically active, and composed of plumper myofibroblasts
Later stage lesions are less cellular, less mitotically active, with more abundant hyalinized collagen
Plantar form tends to be more cellular

Differential Diagnosis

Fibrosarcoma
Desmoid fibromatosis

patient. This tumor generally begins as small nodules that progressively enlarge to form a cord-like band. Many patients eventually develop flexion contracture with significant functional impairment. Flexion causes characteristic puckering of skin overlying the tumor. Fasciectomy with surgical division of the fibrous bands or complete removal of the lesion often are performed to give functional improvement.

Plantar fibromatosis (syn. Ledderhose's disease) differs from its palmar counterpart by its tendency to occur in younger age groups and is less commonly associated with functional impairment. Plantar fibromatosis may cause minor discomfort when walking, but rarely causes contractures. However, there is a significant tendency for local recurrence.

Histopathological Features   Superficial fibromatoses involve mainly fibrotendinous and subcutaneous tissue and appear to proceed through several histologic stages as the lesion ages (Table 30-9). Early lesions tend to be more cellular, more mitotically active, and composed of plumper myofibroblasts. Later stage lesions are much less cellular, less mitotically active, and tend to have more abundant hyalinized stromal collagen. Intermediate stage lesions (when biopsy is commonest) contain features of both phases in alternating areas. Tumor cells are spindle-shaped, often with wavy nuclei, and are arranged in interlacing fascicles within a wavy collagenous stroma (Fig. 30-10). Histologically, the plantar form of the disease tends to be more uniformly hypercellular at all stages in the disease process.

Differential Diagnosis   The main differential diagnosis is with fibrosarcoma; however, this distinction is rarely difficult. Fibrosarcoma is more cellular, shows significant nuclear atypia and hyperchromasia, and has a higher mitotic rate. Desmoid-type fibromatosis is almost invariably more deep-seated.

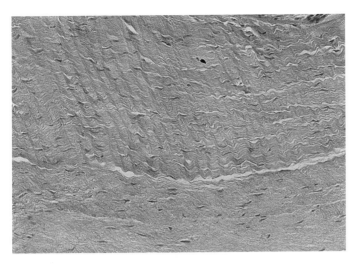

FIGURE 30-10   Palmar fibromatosis. The composite cells are spindle-shaped, often with wavy nuclei and are arranged in interlacing fascicles within dense wavy collagenous stroma.

Penile Fibromatosis

Clinical Features   Penile fibromatosis (Peyronie's disease) is considered by some a form of fibromatosis. Middle-aged and older males develop a slowly enlarging fibrous thickening of the penis, usually on the dorsum (Table 30-10).[31] With time, pain and curvature of the penis develops, which are exacerbated by erection. The pathogenesis and relationship to other forms of fibromatosis are poorly understood; however, it seems probable that Peyronie's disease has an inflammatory basis, possibly vasculitic in nature.[32]

Histopathological Features   The histological pattern depends on the age of the lesion.[33] Early lesions are associated with chronic inflammation, often perivascular in location (Table 30-10).[32] Older lesions tend to show less inflammation and more scar-like fibrous proliferation (hence the resemblance to fibromatosis) involving the corpus cavernosum. Calcification and metaplastic ossification are prominent features in some cases.

Differential Diagnosis   The absence of a history of trauma and progressive slow growth over years help to distinguish penile fibromatosis from a simple cicatrix. In the appropriate clinical setting there is no real differential diagnosis.

TABLE 30-10

Penile Fibromatosis

Clinical Features

  Middle-aged and older adults
  Slowly enlarging fibrous thickening of the penis, usually
    on the dorsum
  Pain and curvature of the penis, exacerbated by erection

Histopathological Features

  Chronic inflammation in early lesions
  Scar-like fibrous proliferation as lesion ages
  Calcification and metaplastic ossification in some cases

Differential Diagnosis

  Cicatrix

TABLE 30-11

Calcifying Aponeurotic Fibroma

Clinical Features

  Usually adolescents and young children
  Slowly growing mass in the palm or sole
  Not associated with pain or functional impairment
  Approximately half of cases recur

Histopathological Features

  Fibrous proliferation of spindled to rounded fibroblasts within a
    densely collagenous background
  Plump fibroblasts palisade around foci of calcification
  Cartilage formation in some cases

Differential Diagnosis

  Fibromatosis
  Fibro-osseous pseudotumor
  Calcium pyrophosphate deposition disease (pseudogout)

Calcifying Aponeurotic Fibroma

Clinical Features   Calcifying aponeurotic fibroma is an extremely rare tumor that classically presents as a slowly growing mass in the hands or, less commonly, the feet of adolescents and young children, although older patients may be affected (Table 30-11).[34] This tumor usually is not associated with pain or functional impairment. The mass often is attached to tendons or fascia. Approximately half of the cases recur. The pathogenesis and relationship with fibromatosis are unclear.

Histopathological Features   The histologic findings are distinctive; a fibrous proliferation of spindled to epithelioid cells is present within a densely collagenous background (Table 30-11). The more plump fibroblasts often line up in single-file array and palisade around foci of calcification (Fig. 30-11). Areas of calcification may be associated with cartilage formation, particularly in long standing lesions.

Differential Diagnosis   Calcifying aponeurotic fibroma is distinguished from fibromatosis by the presence of rounded epithelioid

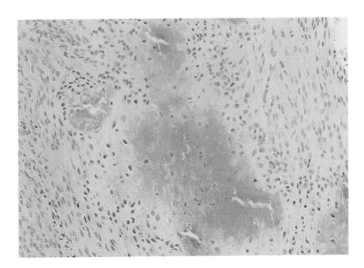

FIGURE 30-11   Calcifying aponeurotic fibroma. Plump epithelioid cells present within cellular fibrous stroma are arranged in single-file array palisading around a focus of calcification.

fibroblasts and calcification surrounded by palisaded fibroblasts. The presence of metaplastic cartilage in some cases is also helpful in this distinction. Fibro-osseous pseudotumor may also contain cartilage, however, fasciitis-like proliferation associated with osteoid is distinctive. The palisade of fibroblasts helps distinguish calcifying aponeurotic fibroma from calcium pyrophosphate deposition disease (pseudogout).

BENIGN AND INTERMEDIATE FIBROHISTIOCYTIC TUMORS

Dermatofibroma (Benign Fibrous Histiocytoma)

Dermatofibroma is one of the most common dermal tumors encountered in dermatopathology practice. Recognition of some variants of dermatofibroma is critical because they may mimic malignant neoplasms (Table 30-12). The pathogenesis is unknown. Many authors believe these tumors (at least in their commonest form) to be a reactive process; however, this has not been proven.

Clinical Features   Dermatofibroma may be seen in any age group, but is especially common in young to middle-aged adults (Table 30-13). Females seem to be affected more than males. Most tumors are less than 1.5 cm. The overlying skin may be erythematous or hyperpigmented with the borders gradually fading to normal skin color. Tumors characteristically exhibit the "dimple sign"—compression of the lateral borders of the tumor causes central depression or dimpling. Dermatofibromas are most commonly seen on the legs, arms, and trunk. Clinically, tumors with extensive hyperpigmentation may be mistaken for a melanocytic lesion. Lesions may persist for many years and some may regress spontaneously. Recurrence is infrequent following excision of the classical type, but the aneurysmal and cellular variants (see the following) recur in 20 to 25 percent of cases, especially if marginally or incompletely excised. The aneurysmal benign fibrous histiocytoma variant often shows rapid growth and can attain large size, causing clinical concern. Clinically, aneurysmal fibrous histiocytoma is often is mistaken for a melanocytic or vascular neoplasm owing to its red-brown color secondary to hemorrhage and hemosiderin deposition. The epithelioid variant is noted for often being polypoid (see the following).

Histopathological Features   Dermatofibroma is a remarkably heterogenous tumor with many variants described (Table 30-12). This tumor varies tremendously with regard to cellularity, vascularity, hemmorhage/hemosiderin deposition, degree of sclerosis (a feature of later stage lesions), and types of composite cells (giant cells, atypical cells, lipid-laden histocytes, etc.). Attention to the characteristic growth pattern at scanning magnification is critical to recognizing variants of dermatofibroma. At low-power, dermatofibromas are symmetrical and

---

TABLE 30-12

Variants of Dermatofibroma

Sclerosing hemangioma
Hemosiderotic histiocytoma
Aneurysmal benign histiocytoma
Dermatofibroma with monster cells (atypical benign fibrous histiocytoma)
Epithelioid cell benign fibrous histiocytoma
Cellular variant
Palisading variant
Clear cell variant

TABLE 30-13

Benign Fibrous Histiocytoma

Clinical Features

Young to middle-aged adults
Papule or nodule, most tumors <1.5 cm
Overlying skin may be erythematous or hyperpigmented, with borders gradually fading to normal skin color
"Dimple sign"
May persist for many years, some may regress spontaneously
Recurrence is infrequent following excision, except in the cellular and aneurysmal variants

Histopathological Features

Symmetric
Well-circumscribed but not encapsulated
Most tumors confined to dermis or minimal extension into subcutaneous tissue
Tightly whorled fascicles in a storiform pattern
Fibrohistiocytic cells entrap preexisting collagen bundles
Lymphocytes, xanthoma cells, histiocytes, multinucleated giant cells
Touton type giant cells may be seen in variable numbers
Overlying epidermis is often acanthotic with basilar hyperpigmentation

Differential Diagnosis

Dermatofibrosarcoma protuberans
Kaposi's sarcoma
Spindle cell hemangioendothelioma
Melanocytic lesions

---

fairly well circumscribed, but not encapsulated, round to lens-shaped nodules centered in the reticular dermis (Fig. 30-12). The common denominator for this family of tumors is the presence of tightly whorled fascicles of fibroblasts arranged in a storiform or pinwheel pattern (Fig. 30-13). In addition, some lesions show prominent fascicular arrangements of spindle cells. The composite cells are spindled to oval with vesicular nuclei and variable amounts of amphophilic cytoplasm. Dermatofibromas infiltrate the dermis in a very characteristic manner—the cells wrap themselves around preexisting collagen bundles to encapsulate them. Often the entrapped collagen bundles appear hyaline or keloidal. This entrapment of collagen is observed in its most characteristic pattern at the periphery of the tumor. Polarization microscopy may be used to demonstrate these residual collagen bundles. In addition to the fibrohistiocytic cells, lymphocytes, xanthoma cells, histiocytes, osteoclast-like giant cells, and Touton-type giant cells may be seen in variable numbers. Typically the overlying epidermis is acanthotic with basilar hyperpigmentation, often suggesting a lentigo or seborrheic keratosis (Fig. 30-14). In contrast, epidermal effacement may be seen over some lesions. In some cases a striking basaloid hyperplasia occurs that may mimic basal cell carcinoma. Occasional mitoses may be seen.

Occasional dermatofibromas extend into the superficial subcutaneous fat along with the fibrous trabecula separating fat lobules, resulting in a starburst or spokewheel pattern. Some of these tumors may infiltrate the most superficial and peripheral rims of fat lobules, entrapping fat in a pattern similar to that of dermatofibrosarcoma protuberans (see the following). However, these lesions otherwise exhibit typical features of dermatofibromas.

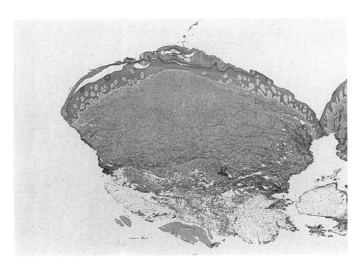

FIGURE 30-12   Dermatofibroma. At low-power, dermatofibromas are symmetrical, fairly well-circumscribed, but not encapsulated, round to lens-shaped nodules centered in the reticular dermis. Note the overlying epidermal hyperplasia.

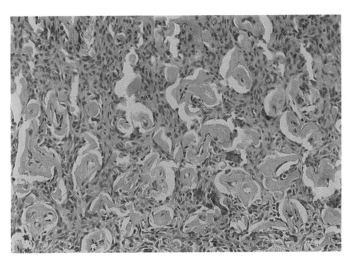

FIGURE 30-14   Dermatofibroma is characterized by tightly whorled fascicles of bland fibroblasts arranged in a storiform or pinwheel pattern. These cells wrap themselves around preexisting collagen bundles to encapsulate them. Note also hemosiderin deposition and scattered giant cells.

Some dermatofibromas are highly vascular and have been designated sclerosing hemangioma. Examples with extensive hemosiderin deposition are designated hemosiderotic histiocytoma. Aneurysmal benign fibrous histiocytoma is an important variant to recognize because it is frequently misdiagnosed.[35–37] Histologically, the tumor tends to be very cellular with characteristic cleft-like or gaping pseudovascular spaces but these spaces have no endothelial lining (Fig. 30-15). Hemorrhage into these spaces causes confusion with vascular neoplasms, particularly Kaposi's sarcoma. The cleft-like spaces have an artifactual appearance, giving the impression that the histotechnician cut the section using a dull blade. Examination of the periphery of the tumor shows features characteristic of dermatofibroma, with characteristic encapsulation of collagen by fibroblasts. "Dermatofibroma with monster cells" (or atypical benign fibrous histiocytoma) denotes a variant with scattered bizarre giant cells superimposed on an otherwise typical dermatofibroma (Fig. 30-16).[38] Epithelioid benign fibrous histiocytoma is an underrecognizsed variant of dermatofibroma comprised largely of polygonal or rounded, often binucleate cells with abundant eosinophilic cytoplasm (Fig. 30-17).[39–41] This variant often is exophytic with a collarette. The nuclei often are vesicular with small nucleoli. As with many variants of dermatofibroma, the periphery of the lesion often shows typical features of fibrous histiocytoma. Perhaps the most problematic variant of dermatofibroma is the cellular variant (Fig. 30-18).[42] This variant shows a more densely cellular fascicular growth pattern and may infiltrate fat, causing confusion with dermatofibrosarcoma protuberans or leiomyosarcoma. An admixture of inflammatory, foam cells, and giant cells often is present but sparse. Necrosis may be present.[42] The palisading variant of fibrous histiocytoma is characterized by focally prominent nuclear palisading.[43] Tumors composed predominantly of clear cells are designated clear cell dermatofibroma (Fig. 30-19).[44]

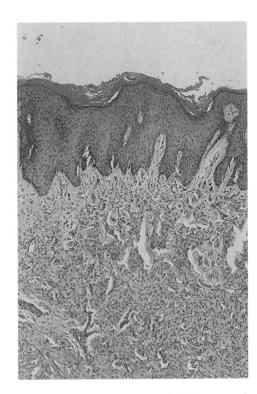

FIGURE 30-13   Dermatofibroma. A characteristic feature seen in many dermatofibromas is acanthosis with basilar hyperpigmentation of the overlying epidermis. Note the entrapment of collagen.

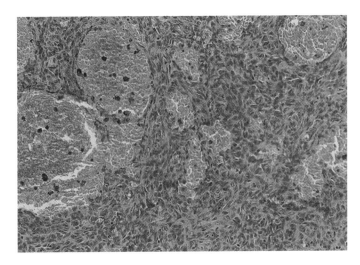

FIGURE 30-15   Aneurysmal benign fibrous histiocytoma usually is cellular with characteristic cleft-like hemorrhagic pseudovascular spaces.

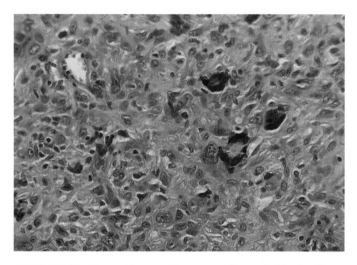

FIGURE 30-16 Dermatofibroma with monster cells (atypical benign fibrous histiocytoma). This variant shows scattered bizarre giant cells and cells with unusually plump nuclei superimposed on an otherwise typical dermatofibroma.

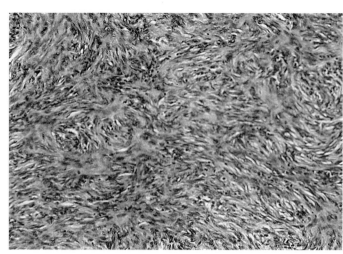

FIGURE 30-18 Cellular dermatofibroma. This variant is hypercellular with a fascicular growth pattern.

Differential Diagnosis The cellular variant must be distinguished from dermatofibrosarcoma protuberans and leiomyosarcoma. Fascicular growth of eosinophilic spindled cells with ovoid to cigar-shaped nuclei and perinuclear vacuoles are characteristic of leiomyosarcoma. Extensive infiltration into fat in a sieve-like pattern and CD34 immunoreactivity also favor a diagnosis of dermatofibrosarcoma. DFSP also is characterized by a more monomorphic population of slightly smaller cells compared to dermatofibroma. The presence of inflammatory cells, multinucleated giant cells, Touton-type giant cells, and xanthoma cells are supportive of dermatofibroma. The aneurysmal variant of fibrous histiocytoma may be confused with vascular tumors such as spindle-cell hemangioendothelioma and Kaposi's sarcoma. The presence of slit-like vessels and immunoreactivity for vascular tumor markers favors a vascular origin. The artifact-like pseudovascular spaces are characteristic of aneurysmal fibrous histiocytoma and are not found in true vascular tumors. The presence of thick-walled muscular vessels and/or organizing thrombi favor spindle-cell hemangioendothelioma.

Examining the periphery of aneurysmal fibrous histiocytoma shows characteristic encapsulation of collagen fibers. This feature is particularly helpful in the distinction from Kaposi's sarcoma. Epithelioid fibrous histiocytoma may be confused with melanocytic lesions including epithelioid nevi, and Spitz nevus in particular. A junctional component and immunoreactivity for S-100 protein establish the diagnosis of a melanocytic tumor.

Atypical Fibroxanthoma

Atypical fibroxanthoma is characterized by a highly pleomorphic histologic phenotype usually associated with malignant neoplasms. Despite its seemingly malignant histologic features, atypical fibroxanthoma has little, if any, potential for metastasis and essentially is a benign tumor when strict diagnostic criteria are applied. Given the differences in

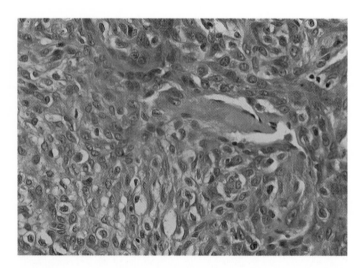

FIGURE 30-17 Epithelioid benign fibrous histiocytoma. This variant of dermatofibroma is comprised of polygonal or rounded cells with abundant eosinophilic cytoplasm.

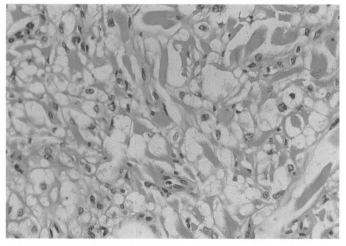

FIGURE 30-19 Clear cell dermatofibroma. This variant is composed predominantly of clear cells. The growth pattern is typical of dermatofibroma.

TABLE 30-14

Atypical Fibroxanthoma

Clinical Features

    Sun-damaged skin of adults
    Head and neck
    Frequently rapidly enlarging, usually <2 cm
    Mistaken for squamous cell carcinoma, basal cell carcinoma
      clinically

Histopathological Features

    Well-circumscribed, symmetric at scanning magnification
    Located in the dermis with minimal extension in to subcutaneous
      tissue
    Marked nuclear pleomorphism, prominent nucleoli, hyperchroma-
      sia, and frequent multinucleated giant cells
    Mitoses are numerous and frequently atypical
    No necrosis or vascular invasion

Differential Diagnosis

    Squamous cell carcinoma
    Melanoma
    Pleomorphic sarcomas
    Metastasis

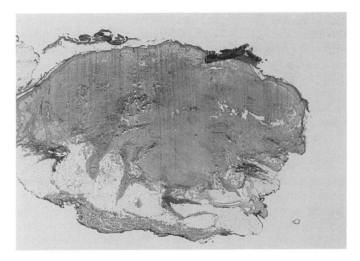

FIGURE 30-20 Atypical fibroxanthoma. Atypical fibroxanthomas are relatively symmetrical, well-circumscribed tumors at scanning magnification. Some tumors like this one show superficial extension into subcutaneous fat.

lymphocytes and histiocytes, including lipidized cells, are frequently seen within the tumor. Multinucleated giant histiocytes, including Touton-type giant cells, are also commonly noted. Importantly, however, necrosis and vascular or perineural invasion are not seen.

Differential Diagnosis   The diagnosis of atypical fibroxanthoma must be carefully approached as a diagnosis of exclusion since all other tumors considered in the differential diagnosis are metastasizing malig-

behavior of atypical fibroxanthoma compared to other pleomorphic tumors, particularly melanoma, the pathologist must always approach atypical fibroxanthoma as a diagnosis of exclusion.

Clinical Features   Atypical fibroxanthoma occurs almost exclusively in the sun-damaged skin of older adults (Table 30-14). Most tumors occur in the head and neck region, frequently are rapidly enlarging, and usually are less than 2 cm in greatest dimension. Because they are not clinically distinctive, the diagnosis is rarely made clinically. Atypical fibroxanthoma may be mistaken for squamous cell carcinoma, basal cell carcinoma, and even melanoma.[45] Complete excision is adequate therapy. Lesions with atypical features require a more generous excision and careful follow-up.

Histopathological Features   Atypical fibroxanthomas are relatively symmetrical, well-circumscribed, exophytic tumors at scanning magnification (Table 30-14) (Fig. 30-20). The bulk of the tumor is located in the dermis; however, some tumors show very superficial extension into subcutaneous fat. Tumors involving the superficial dermis may exhibit a grenz zone between the epidermis and the neoplasm or extend to the dermal–epidermal interface, often with ulceration. Intraepidermal pagetoid spread is not seen and the presence of intraepidermal malignant cells should raise the possibility of melanoma or pleomorphic squamous cell carcinoma with pagetoid spread. An epidermal collarette is quite common.

   The compostite cells range from highly pleomorphic bizzare forms with marked hyperchromasia and irregular nuclear outlines to more uniform spindled cells (Fig. 30-21). Although the degree of pleomorphism varies from case to case, the degree of cytologic atypia generally is uniform throughout a given tumor. Most cases show marked nuclear pleomorphism, prominent nucleoli, hyperchromasia, and frequent bizarre multinucleated tumor giant cells.[46,47] Mitoses often are numerous and frequently atypical. Tumors cells often are arranged in a focally storiform pattern. Some tumors show a relatively monomorphic fascicular pattern that mimics leiomyosarcoma.[48] Inflammatory cells, especially

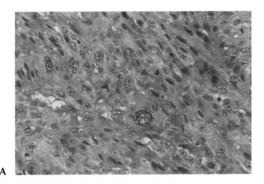

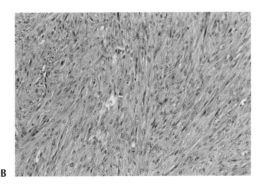

FIGURE 30-21 Atypical fibroxanthoma. *A.* The composite cells range from highly pleomorphic bizarre forms with marked hyperchromasia and irregular nuclear outlines. *B.* Occasional cases are composed of more uniform spindled cells. Mitoses often are numerous and frequently atypical. The tumor cells often are arranged in a storiform or fascicular pattern.

nant neoplasms. If strict criteria are followed, atypical fibroxanthoma may be regarded as benign neoplasms cured by simple excision. Tumors with atypical features are best regarded as potentially malignant and the clinician should be alerted to this possibility. An unequivocal diagnosis of atypical fibroxanthoma should not be rendered in cases with atypical features. Atypical features that raise the possibility of aggressive behavior include significant extension into adipose tissue, necrosis, and vascular invasion. Cases reported as metastatic atypical fibroxanthoma have demonstrated some of these features and form the rationale for requiring strict criteria to establish a diagnosis of atypical fibroxanthoma.[49] Tumors frequently show some infiltration into superficial fat near the cutaneous–subcutaneous junction; however, tumors with significant extension into fat should be regarded as potentially malignant. Because the entire base of the lesion must be examined to make this determination, a diagnosis based on a poorly sampled specimen, shave biopsy, or punch biopsy is not advised. Final diagnosis can only be made after the entire base of the lesion has been examined. Even if strict criteria are followed, perhaps some atypical fibroxanthomas may have the potential to metastasize; however, this has not been our experience. In a series of 140 atypical fibroxanthomas, nine patients developed recurrence; however, none developed metastatic disease.[45]

Deeply invasive tumors raise the possibility of pleomorphic sarcomas including leiomyosarcoma, malignant fibrous histiocytoma, pleomorphic liposarcoma, malignant peripheral nerve sheath tumor, extraosseous osteosarcoma, and pleomorphic rhabdomyosarcoma. Immunohistochemical studies may be helpful in the differential diagnosis. These studies should never be used to "rule-in" a diagnosis of atypical fibroxanthoma, but rather are used to rule out other tumors.[47] This approach is based on the fact that atypical fibroxanthoma is variably immunoreactive for vimentin, alpha-1-antitrypsin, and alpha-1-antitrypsin; all markers that are very non-specific. More specific immunohistochemical markers such as desmin, S-100, HMB-45, and keratins should be used to exclude other pleomorphic tumors. Reactivity with keratins suggest spindle cell squamous cell carcinoma, perhaps the commonest simulant of atypical fibroxanthoma. Because atypical fibroxanthoma arises in severely sun-damaged skin, the presence of actinic keratosis or squamous cell carcinoma in situ in the same biopsy should not reflexively lead to a diagnosis of pleomorphic squamous cell carcinoma, but nevertheless should be sought carefully. Keratin immunoreactivity is helpful in this situation. It is not surprising that atypical fibroxanthoma may coexist with other tumors related to sun exposure, especially basal cell carcinoma and squamous cell carcinoma.

Pleomorphic or spindle cell melanoma also must be considered in the differential diagnosis of atypical fibroxanthoma. The epidermis should be examined for atypical intraepidermal malignant melanocytes and precursor lesions. Immunoreactivity for S-100 protein and HMB-45 suggest melanoma, although HMB-45 often is negative in spindle-cell or pleomorphic melanomas. It should be noted that scattered Langerhans cells and histiocytes immunoreactive for S-100 protein commonly are present within atypical fibroxanthoma and must be distinguished from immunoreactivity in tumor cells.[50,51]

Giant Cell Tumor of Tendon Sheath

Clinical Features   Giant cell tumor of tendon sheath (GCTTS) is usually located on the fingers, and much less commonly on the toes of young adults (Table 30-15).[52] There is a female predominance. GCTTS presents as a slowly growing painless mass, usually less than 3 cm. Tumors may erode adjacent bone. Approximately 10 percent of cases recur following excision.[53] Extremely rare examples of malignant GCTTS have been documented.[54] Pigmented villonodular tenosynovitis is a diffuse form of giant cell tumor and tends to be more aggressive.

TABLE 30-15

Giant Cell Tumor of Tendon Sheath

Clinical Features

Predilection for young female adults
Fingers, much less commonly in the toes
Slowly growing painless mass, <3 cm
May recur following excision

Histopathological Features

Multilobulated
Varying proportions of histicytoid mononuclear cells, osteoclast-like multinucleated giant cells, xanthoma cells, chronic inflammatory cells, hemosiderin-laden macrophages, collagenized stroma
Multinucleated cells may be difficult to find
Mitotic figures may be present

Differential Diagnosis

Fibroma of tendon sheath
Fibrous histiocytoma
Epithelioid sarcoma

Because of its deeper location involving the synovium of large joints, this form is usually not encountered by dermatopathologists.

Histopathological Features   GCTTS is usually multilobulated. Lobules are sometimes separated by synovial-lined spaces (Table 30-15). The tumor is composed, in variable proportion, of sheets of histicytoid mononuclear cells, osteoclast-like multinucleate giant cells, xanthoma cells, chronic inflammatory cells, hemosiderin-laden macrophages, and collagenized stroma (Fig. 30-22). The degree of cellularity and collagenization varies and is probably related to age of the lesion. As lesions age they tend to become less cellular and the stroma becomes more hyalinized. Multinucleated cells may be difficult to find and are entirely absent in some tumors. Mitotic figures frequently are present and on occasion may be numerous.

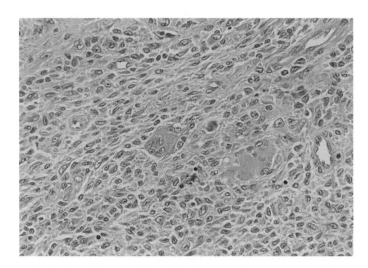

FIGURE 30-22   Giant cell tumor of tendon sheath. GCTTS is composed predominantly of sheets of histicytoid mononuclear cells and osteoclast-like multinucleate giant cells within variable amounts of collagenous stroma. In addition, xanthoma cells, chronic inflammatory cells and hemosiderin-laden macrophages may be present.

Differential Diagnosis   Hyalinized examples of GCTTS may resemble fibroma of tendon sheath, and distinction may be difficult.[55] The presence of cleft like vascular spaces and absence of giant cells favors fibroma of tendon sheath. GCTTS with prominent fascicular arrangements of spindle cells may closely resemble fibrous histiocytoma. However, the other features typical of GCTTS and the location facilitate the distiction of GCTTS from fibrous histiocytoma. Occasional epithelioid sarcomas may contain multinucleated giant cells. The presence of a monomorphic population of epithelioid cells with characteristic necrosis surrounded by a palisade of tumor cells and cytologic atypia helps distinguish epithelioid sarcoma from GCTTS. In difficult cases keratin immunoreactivity helps confirm a diagnosis of epithelioid sarcoma.

FIBROUS AND FIBROHISTIOCYTIC TUMORS OF CHILDHOOD

Infantile Digital Fibromatosis

Infantile digital fibromatosis of childhood, also called inclusion body fibromatosis and recurring digital fibrous tumor of childhood, is a distinctive myofibroblastic proliferation occurring mainly in the fingers and toes of infants and young children. A perplexing feature of this tumor is sparing of the thumb and great toe in all cases. The pathognomonic histological finding is the presence of cytoplasmic eosinophilic inclusion bodies.

Clinical Features   Infantile digital fibromatosis occurs nearly exclusively in young children and infants (Table 30-16). Most occur in children under 1 year of age and one-third are present at birth. Approximately one-third of patients have multiple tumors that may affect both hands and feet and these may be asynchronous. Most tumors are under 2 cm, asymptomatic, and tend to be located on the lateral aspect of the digit.[56,57] Rare tumors with identical pathological features have been observed in adults. In this population, the lesion tends to occur in non-digital locations.[58,59] Because recurrence is common following excision, and most of these lesions regress eventually without therapy, only clinical follow-up of these lesions is warranted unless functional compromise or symptoms dictate otherwise.[60]

Histopathological Features   The tumor is poorly circumscribed and composed of interlacing bundles of fibroblasts and myofibroblasts in variably collagenous stroma (Table 30-16). Lesions may be located primarily in the dermis or extend deeply into the subcutaneous tissue, even to periosteum. Nuclei are uniform, spindled, and somewhat wavy. The pathognomonic intracytoplasmic eosinophilic (often orange-red) inclusions vary from a fraction of the size of a red blood cell to several times larger, and are frequently located next to the nucleus (Fig. 30-23). The inclusions may be rare or numerous. Staining with trichrome or PTAH stain is helpful to identify inclusions in cases in which they are difficult to locate on routine HE staining. The inclusions have been shown to be composed of actin filaments by immunoelectron microscopy.[61]

Differential Diagnosis   Because of the unique clinical setting and pathognomonic inclusions, the diagnosis of infantile digital fibromatosis rarely is a challenge. As mentioned, PTAH and trichrome stains will help highlight the inclusions in cases in which they are difficult to find. It is interesting to note that comparable inclusions are now being recognized in other types of myofibroblastic or myoid lesions.[62]

Infantile Myofibromatosis and Solitary Myofibroma

Infantile myofibromatosis is a disease of infants and young children with a predilection for males. Some cases appear to be inherited; however, the pattern of inheritance is unclear.[63] The disease may be limited to a single lesion, or multifocal lesions involving bones and viscera, particularly the lungs and gastrointestinal tract, may be present. Early liter-

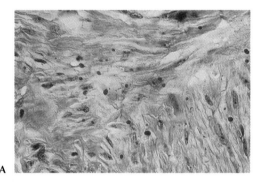

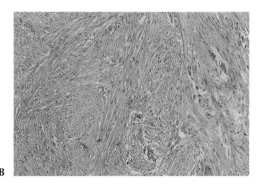

FIGURE 30-23   Infantile digital fibromatosis. Note the interlacing bundles of fibroblasts and myofibroblasts within collagenous stroma. *A.* The nuclei are uniform, spindled and somewhat wavy. The pathognomonic intracytoplasmic eosinophilic inclusions are usually appreciated in standard H+E stained sections. *B.* However, a trichrome (illustrated) or PTAH stain is helpful to identify inclusions in cases in which they are difficult to locate.

TABLE 30-16

Infantile Digital Fibromatosis

Clinical Features

- Asymptomatic dermal or subcutaneous nodule, <2 cm
- Involvement of fingers and toes, especially lateral aspect
- Sparing of the great toe and thumb
- Over half recur following excision
- Spontaneous regression in most cases
- Rare cases in adults and at extradigital sites

Histopathological Features

- Poorly circumscribed
- Sweeping fascicles of (myo)fibroblasts
- Pathognomonic eosinophilic inclusions, stain with trichrome and PTAH

Differential Diagnosis

- Dermal scar
- Dermatofibroma

Infantile Myofibromatosis and Solitary Myofibroma

Clinical Features

Mainly infants and young children
Predilection for males
Subcutaneous or soft tissue nodule, <3–4 cm
Head and neck and trunk are the most common sites
Lesions may recur following surgical excision
Many lesions show spontaneous regression
Minority of patients have bone or visceral involvement

Histopathological Features

Circumscribed, but unencapsulated
Sweeping fascicles or whorls of spindle cells with bland nuclei and
   abundant eosinophilic cytoplasm
More cellular zones of smaller round to spindled cells with scant
   cytoplasm associated with hemangiopericytoma-like vascular
   pattern
Necrosis, vascular invasion, and mitoses may be present

Differential Diagnosis

"Infantile hemangiopericytoma"
Fibromatosis
Fibrous hamartoma of infancy

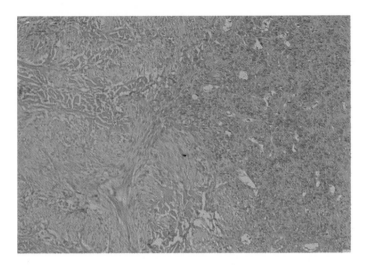

FIGURE 30-24   Myofibroma(tosis). Infantile myofibromatosis and adult myofibroma are histologically similar. These tumors are composed of broad sweeping fascicles or whorled nodules of spindle cells with bland nuclei and abundant eosinophilic cytoplasm (left) in addition to more cellular areas of primitive small round to spindled cells with scant cytoplasm and notable vascular pattern (right).

ature emphasized cases with systemic involvement, giving the false impression that this was the most common form of the disease. Larger series have concluded that the solitary tumors predominate.[64,65] Immunohistochemical and ultrastructural evidence suggest that these tumors are myofibroblastic in origin.[64,66]

Adults may be affected by tumors that are histologically identical to infantile myofibromatosis; however, multiple lesions are rare in this population.[65,66] For this reason, the tumors are termed solitary myofibromas in adults.

Clinical Features   Skin and soft tissue lesions tend to be less than 3 to 4 cm and often present in the perinatal period as small subcutaneous or soft tissue nodules, or a poorly defined swelling (Table 30-17). The head and neck, and trunk are the most common sites of skin and soft tissue involvement. Because lesions may recur following surgical excision, and most lesions eventually show spontaneous regression if left untreated, close clinical follow-up after diagnosis is a reasonable clinical approach. Children with multiple lesions often show involvement of bones. Patients with visceral involvement, particularly lung and gastrointestinal tract, have a worse prognosis with potentially fatal outcome.[67]

The adult solitary myofibroma usually presents as a solitary subcutaneous nodule or mass in a wide variety of sites, but a head and neck location is most common. Visceral involvement is not seen in adults. Recurrence is rare.[68]

Histopathological Features   The tumors are well-circumscribed but unencapsulated, and are composed of two distinct elements that are present in varying proportions (Table 30-17) (Fig. 30-24). First, broad sweeping fascicles or whorled nodules of spindle cells with bland nuclei and abundant eosinophilic cytoplasm resembling myofibroblasts are present. The second component is characterized by more cellular areas of primitive small round to spindled cells with scant cytoplasm. This

primitive cellular component is often associated with a hemangiopericytoma-like pattern of branching vessels (Fig. 30-25). Several features may lead to a mistaken diagnosis of malignancy: necrosis, vascular invasion, and mitoses may be present. The spindled cells usually stain with actin.

Solitary myofibroma of adults is histologically similar to the infantile form, except that there is often only a small component of primitive cells with a hemangiopericytoma-like vascular pattern.[69] Stromal hyalinization, sometimes with a pseudochondroid appearance, is quite common.

Differential Diagnosis   Careful search for the more differentiated spindle-cell fascicles will prevent confusion with hemangiopericytoma in cases where the slit-like vascular pattern is prominent. Probably most, if not all, cases of "infantile hemangiopericytoma" represent cellular variants of infantile myofibromatosis in which the hemangiopericytoma pattern predominates.[68] The biphasic pattern also allows differentiation

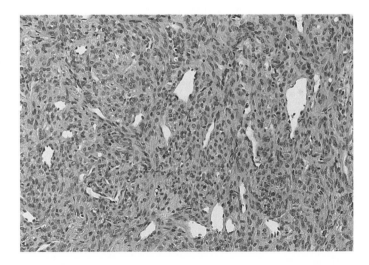

FIGURE 30-25   Myofibroma(tosis). The primitive cellular component often is associated with a hemangiopericytoma-like pattern of branching vessels.

from fibromatosis. Fibrous hamartoma of infancy contains fascicles of myofibroblasts that are similar to those seen in infantile myofibromatosis. The former is distinguished by the presence of distinctive whorled organoid nests of primitive spindled cells in myxoid stroma as well as areas of disorderly fibrosis and mature adipose tissue.

Most important is the recognition that mitoses, necrosis, and vascular invasion may be observed in infantile myofibromatosis, and are not indicative of a malignant neoplasm. Vascular invasion is also a feature in up to one-third of adult lesions.

Juvenile Hyaline Fibromatosis

Juvenile hyaline fibromatosis is an extremely rare disease of uncertain pathogenesis that affects young children. Siblings often are affected and the disease shows an autosomal recessive pattern of inheritance. This disorder may also be associated with impaired intellect, gingival hypertrophy, flexural contractures, and bone lesions.[70] In fact, it may represent an inherited abnormality of collagen metabolism rather than a neoplastic process.

Clinical Features   The onset of this disease is usually before 5 years of age; however, new lesions may continue to develop during adulthood (Table 30-18). Patients develop multiple exophytic lesions ranging from small papules measuring several millimeters to large masses many centimeters in diameter. The lesions have a predilection for the head and neck, and upper trunk. They are slow-growing and usually asymptomatic. However, some patients develop multiple disfiguring nodules that require multiple surgical procedures over many years.[72]

Histopathological Features   The tumors are poorly circumscribed and show variable but usually low cellularity. Separating strands of bland appearing fibroblasts are ribbons of glassy hyaline eosinophilic material (Fig. 30-26). Early lesions appear more cellular (Table 30-18).[62] Fibroblasts are sometimes surrounded by prominent clear halos caused by retraction artifact. The bands of homogeneous eosinophilic material, the defining feature of this disorder, stain with PAS, and alcian blue stains.[70]

Differential Diagnosis   The diagnosis is not difficult if the pathologist is cognizant of this entity. The presence of affected siblings is sugges-

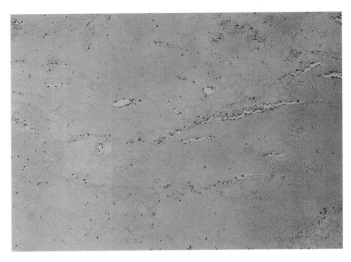

FIGURE 30-26   Juvenile hyaline fibromatosis. This unusual and rare lesion is characterized by paucicellular ribbons of glassy hyaline eosinophilic material.

tive of this diagnosis. The broad bands of hyaline eosinophilic material are distinctive but could be confused with the bands of collagen seen in keloidal scars. The bands of amorphous hyaline material lack the fibrillar appearance of keloidal collagen. Infantile myofibromatosis could be confused clinically; however, the latter is usually more cellular, often has a hemangiopericytoma-like vascular pattern, and most importantly, lacks hyaline material. Nodular fasciitis also may show keloidal hyalinization as a pattern of regression but the typical "feathery" appearance of the cellular component allows ready distinction.

Fibrous Hamartoma of Infancy

Clinical Features   Fibrous hamartoma of infancy is a distinctive fibrous proliferation that occurs most often in children less than two years of age and shows a predilection for males (Table 30-19).[73,74] Approximately 15 percent of tumors are present at birth. The patient

TABLE 30-18

Juvenile Hyaline Fibromatosis

Clinical Features

Onset in first 5 years of life
Siblings may be affected
Lesions often are multiple
Size ranges from small papules to large masses
May be associated with gingival hypertrophy, flexion contractures, and bone lesions, impaired intellect

Histopathological Features

Bands of homogeneous "glassy" hyaline material
Bland fibroblasts, cellularity varies

Differential Diagnosis

Keloid
Infantile myofibromatosis

TABLE 30-19

Fibrous Hamartoma of Infancy

Clinical Features

Children <2 years of age and predilection for males
15% of tumors are present at birth
Slowly or rapidly growing ill-defined subcutaneous mass
Shoulder, upper arm, or axillary region
Usually no spontaneous regression
No recurrence following surgical excision

Histopathological Features

Fascicles of eosinophilic spindle cells
Organoid nests of primitive appearing round to spindle cells within a myxoid matrix. Mature fat dispersed in varying amounts
Scar-like fibrous tissue

Differential Diagnosis

Infantile myofibromatosis
Connective tissue nevus

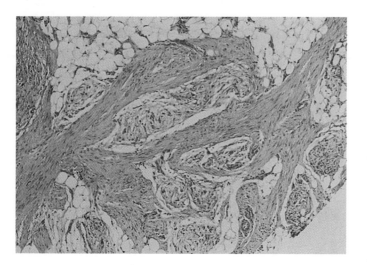

FIGURE 30-27   Fibrous hamartoma of infancy. Note the fascicles of palely eosinophilic spindle cells, organoid nests of primitive cells within a myxoid background, and fat.

TABLE 30-20

Giant Cell Fibroblastoma

Clinical Features

> Young children, particularly boys
> Asymptomatic subcutaneous lesions of the trunk, groin, and lower
>   extremities
> 30–50% of cases recur following surgical excision

Histopathological Features

> Irregular pseudovascular spaces lined by multinucleated giant cells
> Hypocellular hyalinized ribbons of collagenous tissue
> Diffuse spindle cells
> Storiform pattern resembling dermatofibrosarcoma protuberans in
>   some cases

Differential Diagnosis

> Vascular tumor/hemangioma
> Dermatofibrosarcoma protuberans
> Giant cell angiofibroma

presents with an ill-defined subcutaneous mass usually in the shoulder, upper arm, or axillary region. Less common sites include extremities, pubic area, and scrotum.[75] Most tumors are less than 5 cm, they may develop slowly or rapidly, and may be mobile or adherent to muscle or fascia.[73] These tumors are not prone to spontaneous regression if followed clinically or recurrence following surgical excision.[76,77]

Histopathological Features   Tumors are situated in the deep dermis, are unencapsulated but relatively circumscribed and are composed of four distinctive elements (Table 30-19) (Fig. 30-27).

1. Fascicles of palely eosinophilic spindle cells of varying width.
2. Organoid nests of primitive appearing, round to spindled cells within a myxoid background. The myxoid matrix is alcian blue positive and staining is abolished with hyaluronidase pretreatment.
3. Mature fat dispersed in varying amounts.
4. Scar-like fibrous tissue.

These four elements may be present in varying proportions. The spindle cells appear to be composed of actin-positive myofibroblasts and fibroblasts.[77]

Differential Diagnosis   In most cases the findings are so distinctive that differentiation from other tumors is not difficult. However, in cases with only a minor component of the primitive myxoid foci, diagnosis may be difficult. Careful search for and identification of this element allow distinction from infantile myofibromatosis and connective tissue nevus. In addition, the hemangiopercytoma-like vascular pattern seen in myofibromatosis is not seen in fibrous hamartoma.

Giant Cell Fibroblastoma

Giant cell fibroblastoma is a rare tumor of children that shares some pathological features with dermatofibrosarcoma protuberans. Tumors showing elements resembling both giant cell fibroblastoma and dermatofibrosarcoma protuberans have been documented.[78] Giant cell fibroblastoma may recur with histologic features of dermatofibrosarcoma protuberans.[79] In addition, dermatofibrosarcoma protuberans may recur with a histologic phenotype similar to giant cell fibroblastoma.[80] Both tumors are reactive for CD34. Finally, abnormalities involving

chromosome 17 and 22 have been documented in both of these tumors.[81] Evidence points to a fibroblastic origin for this tumor.[82]

Clinical Features   This tumor occurs mainly, but not exclusively, in young children, particularly boys (Table 30-20).[83] Cases in adulthood are distinctly rare. There is a predilection for the trunk, groin, and lower extremities. Most lesions are a few centimeters in size and asymptomatic. These tumors are situated in the dermis or superficial subcutaneous tissue. The overlying skin is usually unremarkable. Between 30 to 50 percent of cases recur following surgical excision. For this reason, wide local excision is advocated, if clinically feasible. Metastases have not been recorded.

Histopathological Features   The principal histologic hallmark of this tumor is the presence of irregular pseudovascular spaces lined by multinucleated, often floret-like giant cells (Table 30-20) (Fig. 30-28). The cells lining the pseudovascular spaces are not immunoreactive for endothelial markers.[84] The pseudovascular spaces are frequently separated by hypocellular hyalinized ribbons of collagenous tissue arranged in a parallel array. The bulk of the tumor is composed of diffusely infiltrative sheets of fibroblastic spindle cells in a matrix that is often myxoid. Such cellular areas usually involve the subcutaneous adipose tissue. Some cases show hypercellular areas with a storiform pattern resembling dermatofibrosarcoma protuberans. Transition between cellular and myxoid areas may be gradual or abrupt. Giant cells, similar to those lining the pseudovascular spaces, are seen in variable numbers in both myxoid and cellular areas of the tumor.

Differential Diagnosis   The differential diagnosis is not difficult if the angiectoid spaces are recognized as pseudovascular; otherwise, confusion with vascular neoplasms is possible. Because the tumor cells are immunoreactive for CD34, a marker for endothelial cells, there is further potential for confusion with vascular tumors. As already noted, cellular tumors with a storiform architectural pattern share more than a superficial resemblance to dermatofibrosarcoma protuberans. Giant cells, pseudovascular spaces, and the young age of the patient should allow distinction. Another morphologically similar but rare lesion is giant cell angiofibroma that, in contrast, occurs mainly around the orbit, is well-circumscribed, and is much more vascular.[85]

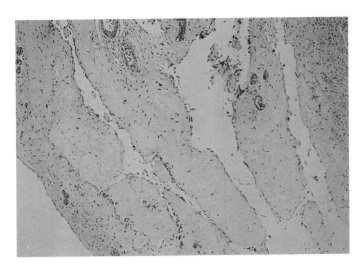

FIGURE 30-28 Giant cell fibroblastoma. Scanning magnification shows pseudovascular spaces separated by ribbons of fibrous tissue.

FIBROUS AND FIBROHISTIOCYTIC TUMORS OF LOW-GRADE MALIGNANCY

Dermatofibrosarcoma Protuberans

Dermatofibrosarcoma protuberans (DFSP) has long been considered a tumor of fibrohistiocytic lineage, possibly because of its resemblance to fibrous histiocytoma. More recently, the cell of origin for DFSP has

---

TABLE 30-21

Dermatofibrosarcoma Protuberans

Clinical Features

Most common in young and middle-aged adults
Slowly enlarging nodule or plaque
Trunk and proximal extremities
Tumors may enlarge rapidly
Recurrence rate (20%) dependent on wide local excision with generous free clear margins
Occasional tumors metastasize

Histopathological Features

Diffuse infiltration of subcutaneous tissue with entrapment of fat creating a sieve-like pattern
Uniform population of cells with spindled nuclei, scant cytoplasm
Whorled or storiform pattern
Inflammatory cells and xanthoma cells are absent or sparse
Mitotic rate is usually <5 mitoses per 10 high powered fields
Variants: myxoid change, fibrosarcoma-like areas, giant cell fibroblastoma-like foci, dendritic melanin-containing cells, myoid nodules

Differential Diagnosis

Cellular dermatofibroma
Neurofibroma
Malignant fibrous histiocytoma
Myxoid liposarcoma
Myxofibrosarcoma (myxoid malignant fibrous histiocytoma)

---

been questioned. Ultrastructural examination has pointed to fibroblastic or fibrohistiocytic lineage.[86] A discontinuous basal lamina has also suggested perineurial differentiation.[87,88] Immunoreactivity with CD34 has also been interpreted as evidence of an unusual nerve sheath tumor.[89] However, the bulk of evidence supports the view that DFSP is a low-grade fibroblastic sarcoma. Cytogenetic analysis of some cases has identified a ring chromosome involving chromosomes 17 and 22.[90,91]

Clinical Features   Dermatofibrosarcoma protuberans affects individuals over a wide age range, from children to the elderly, but occurs most commonly in young and middle-aged adults (Table 30-21). The tumor presents as a slowly enlarging plaque and subsequent nodule that is frequently present for many years prior to diagnosis. After long periods of stable size or slow growth, tumors may enlarge rapidly. The most commonly affected sites are the trunk and proximal extremities. The extent of tumor is frequently underestimated. Tumors with uninvolved surgical margins of 3 cm or greater have a lower recurrence rate (20%) than tumors with narrower margins.[92] Although it has been difficult to estimate the incidence of metastatic disease, occasional tumors metastasize.[93] Metastases seem to follow recurrent lesions that have undergone high grade transformation. The overall incidence appears to be less than 0.5 percent.

Histopathological Features   The histopathology of DFSP is remarkably similar from case to case (Table 30-21). Tumors tend to be localized to the reticular dermis and subcutis, usually sparing the papillary dermis. The epidermis frequently is unremarkable, but ulceration may occur. Epidermal hyperplasia with basilar hyperpigmentation, as one observes in dermatofibroma, may be seen occasionally, particularly with tumors involving the superficial dermis.

At scanning magnification there is diffuse infiltration of subcutaneous tissue with entrapment of fat by tumor cells, resulting in a sieve-like or honeycomb pattern (Fig. 30-29). The tumor is composed of a remarkably uniform population of cells with relatively small oval or spindled nuclei and scant pale cytoplasm, arranged in a whorled or storiform pattern. In general this storiform pattern is maintained throughout the tumor. DFSP usually have prominent cellularity, and this cellularity usually is greatest near the center of the lesion. Despite the monomorphic appreareance, mild cytological atypia is present in DFSP. Multinucleate cells, xanthoma cells, and inflammatory cells are generally sparse or absent. The mitotic rate is usually less than five mitoses per 10 high-powered fields.[94] Although most DFSPs are remarkably similar histologically, some tumors display heterogeneity including extensive myxoid change, hyalinization, fibrosarcoma-like areas (Fig. 30-30), and giant cell fibroblastoma-like foci.[95,96] Tumors with a significant degree of fibrosarcoma-like areas may have a worse prognosis.[97] In our experience, the metastatic rate approximates 20 percent, which is substantially more than previously published data would suggest. DFSP containing dendritic melanin-containing cells have been termed pigmented DFSP or Bednar tumor (Fig. 30-31).[98,99] Nodular myoid differentiation, most notably in the fibrosarcomatous variant has been documented recently.[100]

Differential Diagnosis   For small biopsy specimens the main differential diagnosis is cellular dermatofibroma. Hyperplastic pigmented epidermal rete, inflammatory cell infiltrates, foam cells, and entrapment of collagen all favor dermatofibroma. Less cellular DFSPs can be very difficult to distinguish from superficially biopsied dermatofibromas in which the characteristic infiltration of fat is not appreciated. Fortunately, the clinical appearance of dermatofibroma, that is, a small firm hyperpigmented nodule, is quite different from the gross appearance of DFSP. Thus, clinical information may be helpful in difficult

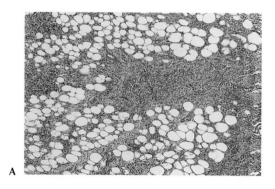

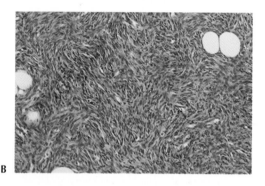

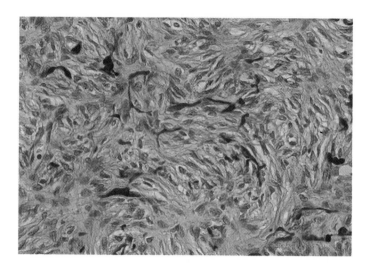

FIGURE 30-31   Pigmented dermatofibrosarcoma protuberans (Bednar tumor). This tumor has dendritic melanin-containing cells. Otherwise, the tumor has typical features of DFSP.

FIGURE 30-29   Dermatofibrosarcoma protuberans. *A*. At scanning magnification diffuse infiltration of subcutaneous tissue with entrapment of fat by tumor cells results in a sieve-like or "Swiss cheese" pattern. *B*. The tumor is composed of a uniform population of small oval or spindled cells arranged in a whorled or storiform pattern (b).

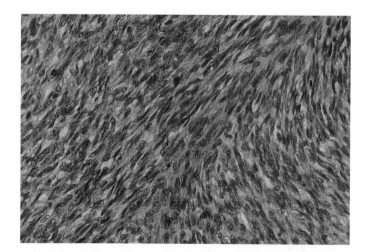

FIGURE 30-30   Dermatofibrosarcoma protuberans. This DFSP shows areas identical to fibrosarcoma. Tumors with a significant degree of fibrosarcoma-like areas have a worse prognosis.

cases. For equivocal tumors in which the base of the lesion is not visualized, it is prudent to request re-excision so that the entire lesion may be examined. Nearly all cases of DFSP are immunoreactive for CD34, an attribute helpful in distinguishing DFSP from dermatofibroma.[89] DFSP may mimic neurofibroma, particularly in small biopsies. Careful search for more cellular areas with a storiform pattern usually will lead to the correct diagnosis. Immunostaining for S-100 protein is very helpful since DFSP is not immunoreactive with this marker. In contrast, vir-

tually all neurofibromas are immunoreactive for S-100. Pleomorphic sarcomas, particularly so-called malignant fibrous histiocytoma, may also have a prominent storiform pattern. Although focal pleomorphism may occur in DFSP, marked pleomorphism favors pleomorphic sarcoma. DFSP with extensive myxoid change may mimic myxoid liposarcoma; however, "chicken wire" vasculature and the lipoblasts are diagnostic of liposarcoma. Extensive sampling of DFSP with myxoid change almost always reveals areas with more typical histological features. Scattered cells with marked pleomorphism and characteristic arcuate vessels distinguish myxofibrosarcoma (myxoid malignant fibrous histiocytoma) from myxoid DFSP.

Plexiform Fibrohistiocytic Tumor

Plexiform fibrohistiocytic tumor is a distinctive tumor that is easily mistaken for a primary granulomatous process. This tumor is considered to be a low-grade neoplasm based on frequent and, in some cases, persistent recurrence as well as the potential for metastasis. Ultrastructural and immunohistochemical studies favor a myofibroblastic origin for this tumor.[101]

Clinical Features   This tumor occurs primarily in children and young adults, and is more common in males (Table 30-22). In the largest series reported, the median age was 14.5 years.[102] The tumor is an ill-defined, slow-growing nodule or mass, usually between 1 and 3 cm., but ranges up to 6 cm in diameter.[102] The tumor is located in the upper extremity in nearly two-thirds of patients, with a predilection for the shoulder and forearm. Nearly 40 percent recur following excision. In addition, two patients with metastasis to local lymph nodes have been reported, as has one very recent case with lung metastasis.[102,102a] Occasionally, tumors regress spontaneously.[101]

Histopathological Features   The tumor is composed of two elements in varying proportions-fascicles of fibroblastic cells and well-delineated, often nodular aggregates of histiocyte-like cells (Table 30-22) (Fig. 30-32). The fascicles of fibroblastic cells are arranged in a complex plexiform pattern, may form thin or broad bands, and tend to trap adipose tissue between them. Dispersed throughout this background are nodular aggregates of histiocyte-like cells, frequently associated with

TABLE 30-22

Plexiform Fibrohistiocytic Tumor

Clinical Features

Mainly children and young adults, more common in males

Ill-defined, slow-growing nodule or mass, usually between 1–3 cm

Upper extremity in nearly two-thirds of patients, particularly the shoulder and forearm

38% recur following excision; rare nodal or lung metastasis

Histopathological Features

Fascicles of fibroblastic cells arranged in complex plexiform pattern

Aggregates of histiocyte-like cells, often with osteoclast-like multi-nucleated cells and associated lymphocytes

Hemorrhage common in histiocytic nodules

Pleomorphism is usually not present and mitoses are rare

Differential Diagnosis

Infectious process

Primary granulomatous disease

Fibromatosis

Fibrous hamartoma of infancy

Giant cell tumor tendon sheath

"Giant cell malignant fibrous histiocytoma"

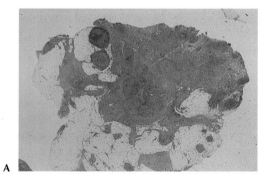

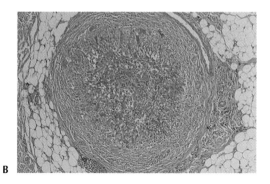

FIGURE 30-32 Plexiform fibrohistiocytic tumor. *A.* Scanning magnification shows fascicles of fibroblastic cells are arranged in a complex plexiform pattern. *B.* High-power shows aggregates of histiocyte-like cells associated with osteo-clast-like multinucleated forms surrounded by fibrous tissue.

osteoclast-like multinucleated forms. A lymphocytic infiltrate is often seen, usually associated with the histiocytic foci. The transition between the fibroblastic fascicles and aggregates of histiocyte-like cells may be abrupt in some foci and gradual in others. Extravasation of red blood cells and hemosiderin deposition is common in the nodular histiocytic areas. Although all tumors have a mixture of both elements, some tumors are composed almost exclusively of the fibroblastic pattern. Rare tumors may be predominantly composed of the histiocytic component.[101] Significant pleomorphism usually is not present and mitoses are infrequent. However, vascular invasion is evident in some cases. The spindled and mononuclear cells usually express actin, and the osteo-clast-like giant cells are immunoreactive for CD68.[102] Reactivity for actin and ultrastructural demonstration of contractile filaments with focal densities suggests a myofibroblastic origin for this tumor.

Differential Diagnosis   Plexiform fibrohistiocytic tumor must be distinguished from an infectious process and primary granulomatous disease such as sarcoidosis. Confusion is most likely to occur in the rare tumors with a predominantly histiocytic pattern. The presence of central necrosis within histiocytic nodules is strongly suggestive of a infectious etiology. A conspicuous fibroblastic component with a plexiform growth pattern is present in most tumors and allows easy distinction from an infectious process. Whenever there is any doubt regarding the diagnosis, special stains for organisms should be examined and tissue submitted for culture. Predominantly fibroblastic tumors could be confused with fibromatosis; however, close inspection will show at least a few histiocytic nodules. This tumor must be distinguished from fibrous hamartoma of infancy, another tumor with a predilection for the shoulder area. The distinctive myxoid areas with an organoid arrangement that characterize fibrous hamartoma of infancy are not seen in plexiform fibrohistiocytic tumor. Location in fingers and the relative lack of inflammatory and spindle cell components, help to distinguish giant cell tumor of tendon sheath from plexiform fibrohistiocytic tumor. In addition to osteoclast-like giant cells, the presence of markedly pleomorphic tumor cells easily distinguishes so-called "giant cell malignant fibrous histiocytoma" from the bland population of cells in plexiform fibrohistiocytic tumor.

MALIGNANT FIBROUS AND FIBROHISTIOCYTIC TUMORS

Malignant Fibrous Histiocytoma

Once the most commonly diagnosed malignant soft tissue tumor, the pleomorphic variant of malignant fibrous histiocytoma (MFH), recently has been critically re-evaluated.[103] Using ultrastructural and immuno-histochemical techniques, it has now been shown that tumors once designated as the pleomorphic variant of MFH are not histiocytic in nature and actually represent a diverse group of tumors that have in common marked cytologic pleomorphism, rather than a distinct entity. The criteria used to diagnose MFH, including cytologic pleomorphism, multinu-cleated giant cells, and storiform cellular pattern, are not reproducible and this diagnosis became a "wastebasket" for pleomorphic tumors. If pleomorphic tumors are thoroughly sampled, and examined ultrastruc-turally and immunohistochemically, most can be precisely diagnosed (Fig. 30-33). Admittedly, there are pleomorphic tumors that defy such precise categorization. We diagnose such tumors as "high-grade pleo-morphic sarcoma, not otherwise specified" rather than apply a specific name to these tumors. Only if the pathologist strives for precise cate-gorization of pleomorphic tumors will relevant clinical correlation be possible. The classification of giant cell variant of malignant fibrous histiocytoma is fraught with similar problems. This variant is similar to

TABLE 30-23

Malignant Fibrous Histiocytoma

Clinical Features

Myxofibrosarcoma

Usually located in the extremities of elderly adults

Often located in subcutaneous tissue or deep dermis

Better prognosis than the pleomorphic variant of MFH

Correlation between histologic grade and prognosis; low-grade tumors have little metastatic potential

Overall survival is 60–70%

Angiomatoid MFH

Affects children and young adults

Superficial soft tissues of the extremities and less commonly the trunk

May be associated with pyrexia, anemia, paraproteinemia, and weight loss

20% develop local recurrence following excision

Histopathological Features

Myxofibrosarcoma

Myxoid hypocellular areas composed of acid mucopolysaccharide

Arcuate vessels in myxoid areas

Cells within the myxoid areas are spindled and stellate with atypical nuclei

Mucin-containing "pseudolipoblasts"

Abrupt transition to more cellular or high-grade pleomorphic areas

Angiomatoid "MFH"

Well-circumscribed

Multiple nodules and sheets of uniform epithelioid to spindled cells with abundant eosinophilic cytoplasm and uniform vesicular nuclei

Highly vascular with frequent hemorrhage; spaces lined by neoplastic cells

Frequently surrounded by a pseudocapsule and cuff of chronic inflammatory cells

Immunoreactive for desmin and muscle actin in 50% of cases, but not smooth muscle actin

Differential Diagnosis

Myxofibrosarcoma

Nodular fasciitis

Benign myxomas

Superficial angiomyxoma

Myxoid liposarcoma

Low-grade fibromyxoid sarcoma

Angiomatoid "MFH"

Epithelioid vascular neoplasms

Epithelioid sarcoma

Aneurysmal benign fibrous histiocytoma

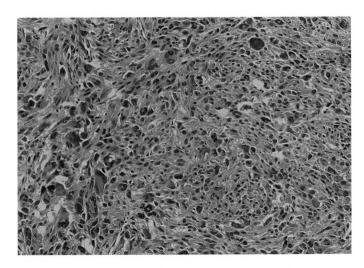

FIGURE 30-33 Pleomorphic malignant fibrous histiocytoma. This markedly pleomorphic tumor originally was diagnosed as malignant fibrous histiocytoma. On review, focal areas of fascicular growth suggesting leiomyosarcoma was noted and the tumor proved to be immunoreactive for desmin. Based on this data, a revised diagnosis of pleomorphic leiomyosarcoma was issued.

ogists. The clinical and pathological features of these definable entities are discussed in the following text, albeit it is now understood that neither of these lesions is truly histiocytic.

Clinical Features　Myxofibrosarcoma usually is located in the extremities of elderly adults, but may be seen in younger patients as well (Table 30-23).[105] This form of MFH is distinguished by its propensity for location in subcutaneous tissue, distinctive histology, and significantly better prognosis than the pleomorphic variant of MFH. There is good correlation between histologic grade and prognosis; low-grade tumors have little metastatic potential.[106,107] Overall survival is 60 to 70 percent for all grades.

Angiomatoid MFH is another clinically and histologically distinct entity that has been placed under the rubric of MFH.[108,109] More recent clinicopathologic evaluation of a large number of patients indicates that this tumor can be considered a low-grade malignant neoplasm.[109] These tumors are clinically distinguished from other forms of MFH by their proclivity for children and young adults and a superficial location. Interestingly, a small number of cases are associated with systemic features, including pyrexia, anemia, paraproteinemia, and weight loss. These tumors usually are located in the superficial soft tissues of the extremities, and less commonly the trunk. Approximately 20 percent develop local recurrence following excision. Metastasis occurs in no more than 5 percent of cases and a fatal outcome is extremely rare.[109]

Histopathological Features　Myxofibrosarcoma demonstrates a broad histological spectrum, from low-grade tumors that must be distinguished from a benign myxoma to high-grade sarcomas (Table 30-23). Myxofibrosarcoma is characterized by myxoid hypocellular areas composed of acid mucopolysaccharide (mainly hyaluronic acid), often with a multinodular growth pattern (Fig. 30-34). Characteristic arcuate or curvilinear vessels are seen in these myxoid areas. The cells within myxoid areas are spindled and stellate and have atypical hyperchromatic nuclei. "Pseudolipoblasts" frequently are seen in the myxoid areas. These hyperchromatic cells with bubbly cytoplasm that indent the nucleus share more than a passing resemblance to true lipoblasts; however, they contain acid mucin rather than lipid. Furthermore, they are generally smaller than lipoblasts and tend to have non-indented, often central nuclei. The myxoid zones often show transition to more cellular

pleomorphic MFH with numerous osteoclast-like giant cells. Approximately half of the cases are associated with osteoid production.[104] Such tumors might be more logically designated soft tissue osteosarcomas. Critical reappraisal of these tumors is needed to better understand their pathogenesis. Two tumors that have been categorized in the MFH family of tumors, myxofibrosarcoma (myxoid MFH) and angiomatoid MFH, appear to be distinct clinicopathologic entities and often are superficially located, thereby coming to the attention of dermatopathol-

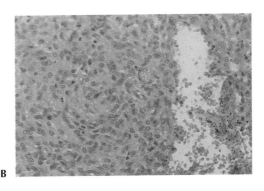

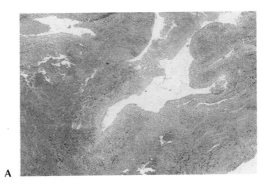

FIGURE 30-34 Myxofibrosarcoma (Myxoid Malignant Fibrous Histiocytoma). At low-power this low to intermediate grade myxofibrosarcoma is shows myxoid hypocellular areas and characteristic arcuate or curvilinear vessels.

FIGURE 30-35 Angiomatoid "MFH." *A.* At low magnifications this tumors shows large hemorrhagic spaces that may suggest a vascular neoplasm. *B.* Higher magnification shows this tumor is composed of sheets of uniform epithelioid to spindled cells with abundant eosinophilic cytoplasm and uniform ovoid vesicular nuclei. These cells are not immunoreactive for endothelial cell makers.

areas and even to high-grade pleomorphic sarcoma. Diagnosis based on pleomorphic areas alone is not possible.

Angiomatoid "MFH" usually is well-circumscribed, and composed of multiple nodules and sheets of uniform epithelioid to spindled cells with abundant eosinophilic cytoplasm and uniform ovoid vesicular nuclei.[108–110] These nodules tend to be distributed in a densely collagenous stroma often containing hemosiderin pigment. Significant pleomorphism is only rarely seen and mitoses usually are infrequent. These tumors tend to contain frequent hemorrhagic spaces lined by neoplastic cells suggestive of a vascular neoplasm (Fig. 30-35). The tumor frequently is surrounded by a pseudocapsule. Frequently a cuff of chronic inflammatory cells, that may be dense and associated with germinal center formation, is present at the periphery of the tumor. Tumor cells are not immunoreactive for vascular markers. Approximately 50 percent of tumors are immunoreactive for desmin and/or muscle actin, but not smooth muscle actin. These observations suggest myoid differentiation, but this remains controversial.[111]

Differential Diagnosis   At the low-grade end of the spectrum, myxofibrosarcoma must be distinguished from myxomas and reactive proliferations, including nodular fasciitis. At the other end of the spectrum, pleomorphic malignant tumors must be considered. Nodular fasciitis and benign myxomas lack significant nuclear atypia and a curvilinear vascular pattern. Superficial angiomyxoma also lacks pleomorphism and arcuate vessels, and approximately one-third of cases are associated with an epithelial cyst. If myxofibrosarcoma is not properly sampled and myxoid areas are not observed, confusion with pleomorphic sarcomas is possible. Pseudolipoblasts may suggest myxoid liposarcoma; however, myxoid liposarcoma lacks significant nuclear atypia and has a characteristic "chicken-wire" vascular pattern. Low-grade fibromyxoid sarcoma is composed of uniform fibroblasts without significant atypia, arranged in a whorled fashion, and lacks arcuate vessels.

Absence of immunoreactivity for endothelial markers distinguishes angiomatoid "MFH" from epithelioid vascular neoplasms. Epithelioid sarcoma is distinguished by keratin immunoreactivity and its characteristic pattern of necrosis. Aneurysmal benign fibrous histiocytoma also often is highly vascular, shows hemorrhagic cleft-like spaces, and at scanning magnification may mimic angiomatoid "MFH." Closer inspection, however, reveals the typical polymorphic cytology and

growth pattern of benign fibrous histiocytoma; furthermore, the latter lesions almost always are based in the dermis.

Fibrosarcoma

A report from the Mayo clinic published in 1936 designated 65 percent of soft tissue sarcomas as fibrosarcoma.[112] Using current routine diagnostic techniques, including electron microscopy and immunohistochemical studies, it is now clear that many tumors formerly designated fibrosarcoma were actually malignant peripheral nerve sheath tumors, monophasic synovial sarcomas, fibromatosis, and nodular fasciitis, among others. It is now realized that this once frequently diagnosed tumor is very uncommon.

Clinical Features   Two clinically distinct forms of fibrosarcoma are recognized, an adult form and a juvenile form (Table 30-24). Fibrosarcoma in adults usually presents in young and middle-aged adults as a deep-seated, slow growing, and sometimes painful mass, in the thigh or trunk.[113] In contrast, the infantile fibrosarcoma affects children under 2 years of age, is often congenital, tends to be more superficially located and smaller than the adult form, and usually arises in the extremities.[114] The prognosis of infantile fibrosarcoma is much better compared to the adult form. A 35 percent 5-year survival has been reported in high-grade adult fibrosarcomas.[115] The outcome of patients treated with radical surgery appears superior to local excision.[116] The infantile form has a much more optimistic outlook, with a 5-year survival of at least 85 percent.[117]

TABLE 30-24

Fibrosarcoma

Clinical Features

Adult form—deep-seated slow growing mass in the thigh or trunk
Infantile form—children under 2 years of age, often congenital, superficially located
Prognosis of infantile fibrosarcoma is much better than the adult form

Histopathological Features

Uniform spindled cells arranged in herringbone fascicles
Nuclei are slender with uniform chromatin and small inconspicuous nucleoli
Cytoplasmic borders not distinct
High-grade tumors may have marked nuclear pleomorphism
Hemangiopericytoma-like vascular spaces common in infantile tumors

Differential Diagnosis

Fibromatosis
Nodular fasciitis
Malignant peripheral nerve sheath tumor
Monophasic synovial sarcoma

Histopathological Features   Adult fibrosarcoma tends to be larger and more deeply located than the infantile form (Table 30-24). The histopathological characteristics of the adult and infantile forms of fibrosarcoma are similar. The tumor is composed of strikingly uniform, spindled cells, arranged in herringbone fascicles (Fig. 30-36). The nuclei are slender, with uniform chromatin and small inconspicuous nucleoli. Cytoplasmic borders are indistinct. Some tumors have variable amounts of dense wire-like collagen. Marked nuclear pleomorphism with clumped chromatin and prominent nucleoli may be seen in some high-grade tumors, making distinction from other high grade sarcomas difficult. Some tumors are composed or more rounded cells, a feature not uncommon in the infantile form. Hemangiopericytoma-like branching vascular spaces are seen in many infantile fibrosarcomas. Immunoreactivity for actin is common in the infantile (but not adult) type.

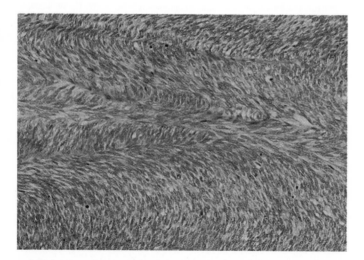

FIGURE 30-36   Fibrosarcoma. This tumor is composed of strikingly uniform, spindled cells, arranged in herringbone fascicles.

Differential Diagnosis   Fibrosarcoma should be approached as a diagnosis of exclusion. Fibrosarcoma should not be immunoreactive for keratins, desmin, S-100 protein, and epithelial membrane antigen. Distinction between low-grade fibrosarcoma and fibromatosis may be difficult. Fibromatosis is less cellular and shows more regular nuclei and less frequent mitotic figures. Nodular fasciitis is distinguished by its distinctive low-power pattern—a mixture of cellular areas alternating with myxoid paucicellular zones. Prior to sophisticated diagnostic techniques, some cases of malignant peripheral nerve sheath tumor were interpreted as fibrosarcoma. Tumors arising from neurofibromas and large nerves are most likely neural. Although a herringbone pattern may be seen focally in malignant peripheral nerve sheath tumors, other histologic patterns usually are present, such as myxoid zones and perivascular whorling. Immunoreactivity for S-100 protein is observed in approximately half of malignant peripheral nerve sheath tumors. Ultrastructural examination may be helpful in malignant peripheral nerve sheath tumors that are not immunoreactive for S-100 protein. A hemangiopericytoma-like vascular pattern may occur in fibrosarcoma, particularly in the infantile form, and cause confusion with monophasic synovial sarcoma. Immunoreactivity for epithelial membrane antigen and keratin distinguish monophasic synovial sarcoma from fibrosarcoma. Cytogenetic analysis also may be helpful in this distinction since synovial sarcoma is associated with an X;18 translocation and infantile fibrosarcoma with trisomies of chromosomes 8, 11, 17, and 20.[118,119]

Low-grade Fibromyxoid Sarcoma

Low-grade fibromyxoid sarcoma is a recently described sarcoma notable for its deceptively bland appearance. At the time of this writing, there is relatively little experience with this entity and, undoubtedly, more cases need to be examined to further define the clinicopathologic spectrum of this tumor.

Clinical Features   Most affected patients are in their second to fourth decades of life (Table 30-25). Experience with the few tumors reported indicate that low-grade fibromyxoid sarcoma may be seen in a variety

TABLE 30-25

Low-grade Fibromyxoid Sarcoma

Clinical Features

Most common in young adults
Wide variety of locations, mainly axial
Size—few centimeters to 15cm
Recurrence following excision is common
At least 30% metastasize
Mortality at least 30%, often many years after presentation

Histopathological Features

Remarkably bland and uniform fibroblasts
Paucicellular
Whorled growth pattern
Background varies from collagenous to myxoid
Mitotic rate usually is low and pleomorphism is only slight

Differential Diagnosis

Easily mistaken for a benign tumor or reactive process
Fibromatosis
Low-grade myxofibrosarcoma

of locations, including thigh, inguinal region, axilla, shoulder, chest wall, neck, buttock, and retroperitoneum.[120–122] Most tumors are deeply located, but we have encountered rare cases involving dermis and subcutis. The tumor has a propensity for recurrences that often are multiple. Metastatic disease develops in at least a third of cases but may be delayed for 10 to 20 years following initial diagnosis. Long-term follow-up studies are needed to clearly define the prognosis of this tumor.

Histopathological Features   This tumor ranges from a few centimeters to 15 cm in diameter and arises in the fascia and soft tissue deep to fascia (Table 30-25).[121] The tumor is composed of remarkably bland and uniform fibroblasts. Cellularity often is low. At low power, the neoplasm typically shows a swirling growth pattern. The background varies from myxoid to collagenous (Fig. 30-37). Mitotic rate is usually low and pleomorphism is only slight. Cellularity may increase within recurrent tumors. Tumors are variably immunoreactive for smooth muscle actin, desmin, and a few cases have shown rare cells immunoreactive for keratins.[122] Tumors are not immunoreactive for antibodies against S-100 protein, epithelial membrane antigen, and CD34.[122]

Differential Diagnosis   Low-grade fibromyxoid sarcoma emphasizes that morphologic features of some malignant tumors do not reflect the customary cytological concepts of malignancy. Without prior knowledge of this entity, it is highly likely to be mistaken for a benign tumor or reactive process. Low-grade fibromyxoid sarcoma might be confused with fibromatosis. The alternating myxoid and collagenous areas with a whorled low-power pattern favor low-grade fibromyxoid sarcoma. Low-grade myxofibrosarcoma, despite its similar name, is easily distinguished by characteristic curvilinear vessels, pseudolipoblasts, and greater nuclear atypia and pleomorphism.

MISCELLANEOUS TUMORS

Epithelioid Sarcoma

Epithelioid sarcoma is a distinctive neoplasm of uncertain pathogenesis. Recognition of this tumor is critical because it may be mistaken for a benign granulomatous process or infection. Even when this tumor appears localized clinically, early multifocal locoregional spread often is present, making surgical control a challenge. Patients often suffer multiple recurrences and 5-year survival is approximately 50 percent.[123] In our experience at least 70 percent of patients eventually die of their tumor with long-term follow-up. Prognosis correlates with tumor size and degree of tumor necrosis.[123,124] Males tend to fare worse than females, and tumors in the distal extremities tend to do better than proximal and more centrally located tumors.[123]

Clinical Features   Tumors are most commonly located in the distal extremities, particularly the hand and fingers, of young adult men (Table 30-26).[123] Despite a striking predilection for the hand, the tumor is seen in wide variety of sites and age groups. Ulceration of the skin overlying superficial tumors is common. Deep-seated tumors tend to be slow-growing and show a multifocal growth pattern of local spread. Most tumors are a few centimeters in size at the time of presentation. Despite the initial clinical appearance of a single localized mass, patho-

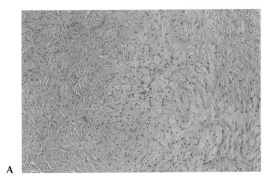
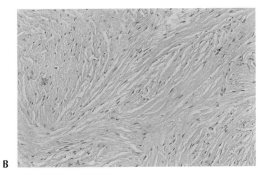

FIGURE 30-37   Low-grade fibromyxoid sarcoma. *A.* This tumor shows transition from myxoid areas to more dense fibrous areas. *B.* At low power, another example shows the characteristic swirling growth pattern. Cellularity is often low and the tumor is composed of remarkably bland and uniform fibroblasts. It is not surprising that this tumor often is mistaken for a benign neoplasm or reactive process.

TABLE 30-26

Epithelioid Sarcoma

Clinical Features

Most commonly located in the extremities, particularly in the hand and fingers
Young adults, males more often than females
Tend to be slow growing and multifocal
Propensity for multiple recurrences
Metastases develop in 50%, usually to lymph nodes and lung
Poor long-term prognosis

Histopathological Features

Spindled to round cells with abundant eosinophilic cytoplasm
Palisade around areas of necrosis
Some tumors show a marked chronic inflammatory infiltrate
Immunoreactivity for keratins, vimentin, and epithelial membrane antigen

Differential Diagnosis

Primary necrobiotic granulomatous processes (granuloma annulare, necrobiosis lipoidica, rheumatoid nodule)
Granulomatous infection
Giant cell tumor of tendon sheath
Epithelioid angiosarcoma and epithelioid hemangioendothelioma
Squamous cell carcinoma
Melanoma
Synovial sarcoma

logical examination often documents multifocal spread along tendons, nerves, and fascial structures in a serpiginous fashion. The characteristic early multifocal spread of this tumor and propensity for multiple recurrences demands early radical surgery. Metastases, usually to lymph nodes and lung, develop in at least one-half of patients.

Histopathological Features   Tumors frequently are multifocal with a plexiform and diffusely infiltrative pattern (Table 30-26). Tumors are composed of spindled to round cells with abundant eosinophilic cytoplasm and relatively uniform medium-sized nuclei. The spindled and epithelioid areas tend to gradually merge and have similar nuclear and cytoplasmic characteristics. A characteristic finding in approximately 40 to 50 percent of cases are tumor cells arranged in a palisade around areas of necrosis (Fig. 30-38). This feature frequently leads to confusion with granulomatous processes. Cellular discohesion, producing a pseudovascular pattern, also is a common finding. Some tumors show a marked chronic inflammatory infiltrate, further contributing to this confusion. Epithelioid sarcoma has a propensity for neural and tendon sheath invasion. The tumor is immunoreactive for keratins, vimentin, and epithelial membrane antigen. Approximately 50 percent of cases are CD34-positive. Immunoreactivity for keratins varies from focal to diffuse, but invariably is present. Electron microscopic examination, although usually not helpful in establishing the diagnosis, demonstrates poorly differentiated cells with features of myofibroblasts, and some cells with features of primitive epithelial cells.

Differential Diagnosis   Distinction from necrobiotic granulomatous processes, such as granuloma annulare, necrobiosis lipoidica, and rheumatoid nodule, and infection may be difficult, particularly in small biopsies. Keratin immunoreactivity distinguishes epithelioid sarcoma from any of these granulomatous diseases. Tumors that are discohesive, form cleft-like pseudovascular spaces, and show intracytoplasmic vacuole formation, may be mistaken for an epithelioid vascular neoplasm. Expression of vascular immunomarkers, such as CD31, establish the diagnosis of a vascular neoplasm. It should be noted that epithelioid angiosarcoma and epithelioid hemangioendothelioma also are quite frequently immunoreactive for keratin. Therefore, keratin stains may not allow distinction from some vascular neoplasms. The presence of overlying squamous cell carcinoma in situ, dyskeratosis, intercellular bridges, and squamous pearls, all help distinguish squamous cell carcinoma from epithelioid sarcoma. Melanoma is distinguished by the presence of melanin, associated melanoma-in-situ, or other precursor melanocytic lesions. In problematic cases, the immunohistochemical profile of melanoma allows distinction from epithelioid sarcoma-melanomas are in general non-reactive for keratins, immunoreactive for S-100 protein, and, at least when epithelioid, frequently express HMB-45. Epithelioid sarcoma has many immunophenotypic features in common with synovial sarcoma, and distinction between these two neoplasms may be problematic. However, abrupt transition from spindled to epithelioid cells and gland-like spaces are typical of synovial sarcoma and the latter tumor generally has a much more basophilic hue. In contrast, the spindled cells gradually merge with more epithelioid areas and pseudoglandular structures are not seen in epithelioid sarcoma. The characteristic hemangiopericytoma-like vessels present in synovial sarcoma usually are not seen in epithelioid sarcoma.

Superficial Angiomyxoma and Cutaneous Myxoma

Clinical Features   Superficial angiomyxoma is a slow-growing dermal or subcutaneous nodule occurring most commonly in the head and neck region of adults (Table 30-27).[125] Most tumors are under 3 to 4 cm and

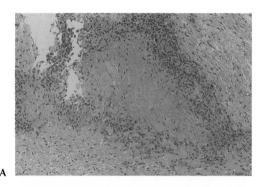

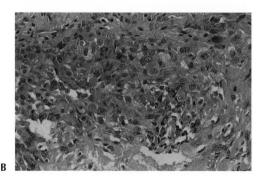

FIGURE 30-38   Epithelioid sarcoma. *A.* This tumor shows tumor cells arranged in a palisade around areas of necrosis. This feature frequently leads to confusion with granulomatous processes. *B.* High magnification shows the composite cells are round to spindled with abundant eosinophilic cytoplasm and relatively uniform nuclei.

TABLE 30-27
Superficial Angiomyxoma and Cutaneous Myxoma

Clinical Features

   May be associated with the Carney Complex
   Head and neck region of adults
   Slow growing dermal or subcutaneous nodule, <3–4 cm
   May recur following surgical resection

Histopathological Features

   Poorly circumscribed, paucicellular
   Myxoid matrix with widely scattered bland stellate and spindle
     fibroblasts
   Thin-walled blood vessels, lymphocytes, and neutrophils in varying
     numbers
   Mitoses may be seen
   Frequent association with epithelial proliferation, particularly cysts

Differential Diagnosis

   Low-grade myxofibrosarcoma (myxoid "malignant fibrous histio-
     cytoma")
   Myxoid liposarcoma
   Aggressive angiomyxoma

may recur following surgical resection.[126] Cutaneous myxomas identical to superficial angiomyxoma may be associated with the Carney complex, an autosomal dominant disorder with multiple manifestations.[127] The complex has three major components: myxomatous masses (cardiac myxomas, cutaneous myxomas, myxoid fibroadenomas of the breast), spotty pigmentation of the skin (lentigines, blue nevi), and endocrine disorders (primary pigmented nodular adrenocortical disease, large cell calcifying Sertoli cell tumor of the testes, and pituitary adenomas).[127–129] Recently, psammomatous melanotic schwannomas have been described in patients with Carney complex.[130] The presence of angiomyxoma in the external ear seems pathognomonic of Carney complex.[131]

Histopathological Features   These tumors are poorly circumscribed, sometimes multinodular, paucicellular lesions involving the dermis and superficial subcutaneous tissue (Table 30-27). Embedded in the myxoid matrix are scattered stellate and spindled fibroblasts with bland nuclei (Fig. 30-39). Thin-walled blood vessels, lymphocytes, and neutrophils often are present in varying numbers. Lesions frequently are associated with epithelial proliferation (particularly follicular), most often in the form of cysts, basaloid buds, and pseudoepitheliomatous hyperplasia. Occasional mitoses may be seen; however, significant nuclear atypia is not present.

Differential Diagnosis   Distinction between angiomyxomas and cutaneous myxomas associated with the Carney complex may not be possible. Cutaneous myxomas may be the first presentation of this syndrome, and the clinician should be alerted to this possibility. The bland fibroblasts and lack of curvilinear vascular pattern allows myxoma to be distinguished from low-grade myxofibrosarcoma (myxoid malignant fibrous histiocytoma). Although myxoid liposarcoma is composed of very bland cells, the characteristic "chicken wire" vascular pattern and presence of occasional lipoblasts establishes this diagnosis. Aggressive angiomyxoma is distinguished by a more infiltrative and less nodular growth pattern associated with thickened vessels and a generally deeper location. The typical sites for aggressive angiomyxoma in the vulva, perineum, and scrotum would be somewhat more unusual for angiomyxoma and myxoma. Because of its capacity for local destructive growth, distinguishing aggressive angiomyxoma from superficial angiomyxoma is critical.

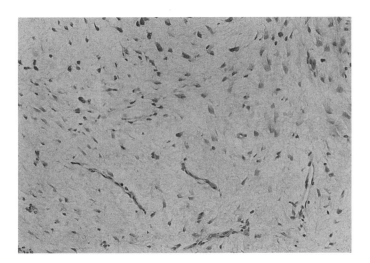

FIGURE 30-39   Superficial angiomyxoma. Typical cytologically bland tumor with thin-walled vessels.

QUICK REFERENCE GUIDE TO FIBROUS AND FIBROHISTIOCYTIC TUMORS

Tumors with Storiform Pattern

Confined to dermis with overlying epithelial hyperplasia = dermatofibroma

Less uniform storiform pattern mixed with fascicles parallel to epidermis = dermatomyofibroma

Extensive infiltration of fat and CD34+ = dermatofibrosarcoma protuberans

Marked atypia, sun-damaged skin, minimal infiltration of fat = atypical fibroxanthoma

Marked atypia, significant infiltration subcutaneous fat = pleomorphic sarcoma, sarcomatoid carcinoma, melanoma

Storiform pattern produced by cleft-like spaces in paucicellular hyaline nodule = storiform collagenoma

Tumors with a Prominent Myxoid Component

Curvilinear vessels, atypical cells, pseudolipoblasts = myxofibrosarcoma (myxoid "malignant fibrous histiocytoma")

Tissue culture fibroblasts within tumor with myxoid feathery zones alternating with hypercellular zones = nodular fasciitis

Myxoid tumor in child with giant cells lining pseudovascular spaces, CD34+ = giant cell fibroblastoma

Paucicellular nodule with very bland stellate and spindled cells, inflammatory cells and thin-walled blood vessels = myxoma, angiomyxoma

Paucicellular tumor with myxoid areas admixed with whorled collagenous component, very bland cells = low-grade fibromyxoid sarcoma

Fibrous and Fibrohistiocytic Tumors in Children

Tumor of finger or toes composed of myofibroblasts in fascicles, characteristic eosinophilic inclusions = infantile digital fibromatosis

Biphasic tumor composed of sweeping or whorled fascicles of myofibroblasts alternating with hemangiopericytoma-like areas = infantile myofibromatosis

Paucicellular nodules composed of ribbons of PAS+ glassy hyaline eosinophilic material = juvenile hyaline fibromatosis

Biphasic tumor composed of anastomosing bands of fibrous tissue and nodular aggregates of histiocyte-like cells resembling granulomas, creating a plexiform pattern = plexiform fibrohistiocytic tumor

Myxoid tumor with giant cells lining pseudovascular spaces, CD34+ = giant cell fibroblastoma

Tumor of hand or feet composed of spindled to epithelioid cells, with palisading around foci of calcification cells = calcifying aponeurotic fibroma

Tumor composed of fascicles of eosinophilic spindle cells, distinctive organoid nests within a myxoid background, mature fat dispersed and fibrous tissue = fibrous hamartoma of infancy

Tumors Composed of Fibrous Tissue

Tumor composed of cellular "herringbone" fascicles with atypia, necrosis, high cellularity, necrosis and mitoses = fibrosarcoma

Paucicellular tumor with dense hyalinized collagen and spindled or wavy nuclei = fibromatosis, knuckle pad, Peyronie's disease

Dense fibrous tissue with lobules of orderly bands of collagen parallel to the epidermis separated by blood vessels = hypertrophic scar

Features of hypertrophic scar with thick bands of glassy collagen = keloid

Tumor of hand or feet in young patient composed of spindled to epithelioid cells, with palisading around foci of calcification = calcifying aponeurotic fibroma

Exophytic lesion on hand with irregular thick bundles of collagen and variable numbers of blood vessels = acral fibrokeratoma and periungual fibroma

Angiofibromas

Central face in child with stigmata of tuberous sclerosis = adenoma sebaceum

Shiny papule on face, especially nose with clinical appearance often mistaken for basal cell carcinoma = fibrous papule

Tiny papules on the glans penis = pearly penile papules

Tumors of Digits

Tumor in young child composed of myofibroblasts in fascicles, characteristic eosinophilic inclusions = infantile digital fibromatosis

Exophytic lesion on hand with irregular thick bundles of collagen and variable numbers of blood vessels = acral fibrokeratoma and periungual fibroma

Nodule over knuckles composed of bland fibrous tissue often with overlying epithelial hyperplasia = knuckle pad

Lobulated tumor with giant cells, mononuclear cells, xanthoma cells, hemosiderin-laden macrophages, and collagenized stroma = giant cell tumor of tendon sheath

Paucicellular tumor with slit-like vascular spaces and rare, if any, giant cells = fibroma of tendon sheath

Tumor composed of keratin positive spindled and epithelioid cells with palisading around areas of necrosis = epithelioid sarcoma

REFERENCES

1. Starink TM, Meijer CJ, Braunstein MH: The cutaneous pathology of Cowden's disease: new findings. *J Cutan Pathol* 12:83–93, 1985.
2. Nickel WRY, Reed WB: Tuberous sclerosis (review of cutaneous lesions). *Arch Dermatol* 85:209–226, 1962.
3. Ackerman AB, Kornberg R: Pearly penile papules. Acral angiofibromas. *Arch Dermatol* 108:673–675, 1973.
4. Rehbein HM. Pearly penile papules: incidence. *Cutis* 19(1):54–57, 1977.
5. Bart RS, Andrade R, Kopf AW, et al: Acquired digital fibrokeratoma. *Arch Dermatol* 97:120–128, 1968.
6. Kint A, Baran R, DeKeyser H: Acquired (digital) fibrokeratomas. *J Am Acad Dermatol* 12:816–821, 1985.
7. Verallo WM: Acquired digital fibrokeratomas. *Br J Dermatol* 80:730–736, 1968.
8. Cooper PH, Mackel SE: Acquired fibrokeratoma of the heel. *Arch Dermatol* 121:386–388, 1985.
9. Kint A, Baran R: Histopathologic study of koenen tumors. Are they different from acquired digital fibrokeratoma? *J Am Acad Dermatol* 18:369–372, 1988.
10. Metcalf JS, Maize JC, LeBoit PE: Circumscribed storiform collagenoma (sclerosing fibroma). *Am J Dermatopathol* 13:122–129, 1991.
11. Maize J, Leidel G, Mullens S, et al: Circumscribed storiform collagenoma *Am J Dermatopathol* 11:287 (abs), 1989.
12. Pulitzer DR, Martin PC, Reed RJ: Fibroma of tendon sheath. A clinicopathologic study of 32 cases. *Am J Surg Pathol* 13(6):472–479, 1989.
13. Chung EB, Enzinger FM: Fibroma of tendon sheath. *Cancer* 44:1945–1954, 1979.
14. Humphreys S, McKee PH, Fletcher CDM: Fibroma of tendon sheath: A clinicopathologic study. *J Cutan Pathol* 13:331–338, 1986.
15. Satti MB: Tendon sheath tumours: A pathological study of the relationship between giant cell tumour and fibroma of tendon sheath. *Histopathology* 20:213–220, 1992.
16. Hugel H: Die plaqueformige dermale Fibromatose. *Hautarzt* 42:223–226, 1991.
17. Kamino H, Reddy VB, Gero M, et al: Dermatomyofibroma. A benign cutaneous plaque-like proliferation of fibroblasts and myofibroblasts in young adults. *J Cutan Pathol* 19:85–93, 1992.
18. Mentzel T, Calonje E, Fletcher CDM: Dermatomyofibroma: Additional observations of a distinctive cutaneous myofibroblastic tumour with emphasis on differential diagnosis. *Br J Dermatol* 129:60–73, 1993.
19. Goodlad JL, Fletcher CDM:. Intradermal variant of nodular fasciitis. *Histopathology* 17:569–571, 1991.
20. Allen PW: Nodular fasciitis. *Pathology* 4:9–26, 1972.
21. Lauer DH, Enzinger FM: Cranial fasciitis of childhood. *Cancer* 45:401–406, 1980.
22. Meister P, Buckmann FW, Konrad EA: Nodular fasciitis: Analysis of 100 cases and review of the literature. *Pathol Res Pract* 162:133–165, 1978.
23. Meis JM, Enzinger FM: Proliferative fasciitis and myositis of childhood. *Am J Surg Pathol* 16:364, 1992.
24. Perosio PM, Weiss SW: Ischemic fasciitis: A juxta-skeletal fibroblastic proliferation with a predilection for elderly patients. *Mod Pathol* 6:69–72, 1993.
25. Montgomery EA, Meis JM, Mitchell MS, et al: Atypical decubital fibroplasia. A distinctive fibroblastic pseudotumor occurring in debilitated patients. *Am J Surg Pathol* 16:708–715, 1992.
26. Lauer DH, Enzinger FM: Cranial fasciitis of childhood. *Cancer* 1980;45:401–406, 1980.
27. Patchefsky AS, Enzinger FM. Intravascular fasciitis: A report of 17 cases. *Am J Surg Pathol* 5:29–36, 1981.
28. Allison JR Jr, Allison JR Sr: Knuckle pads. *Arch Dermatol* 93:311–316, 1966.
29. Allen PW: The fibromatoses: A clinicopathologic classification based on 140 cases. Part I. *Am J Surg Pathol* 1:255–270, 1977.
30. Ushiima M, Tsuneyoshi M, Enjoji M: Dupuytren's type fibromatosis. A clinicopathologic study of 62 cases. *Acta Pathol Jpn* 34:991–1001, 1984.
31. Billig R, Baker R, Immergut M, Maxrud W: Peyronie's disease. *Urology* 6:409–418, 1975.
32. Smith BH: Peyronie's disease. *Am J Clin Pathol* 45:670– 678, 1966.
33. Smith BH:. Subclinical Peyronies disease. *Am J Clin Pathol* 52(4):385, 1969.
34. Allen PW, Enzinger FM: Juvenile aponeurotic fibroma. *Cancer* 26:857, 1970.
35. Santa Cruz DJ, Kyriakos M: Aneurysmal ("angiomatoid") fibrous histiocytoma of the skin. *Cancer* 8:467–471, 1981.
36. Caljone E, Fletcher CDM: Aneurysmal benign fibrous histiocytoma: Clinicopathologic analysis of 40 cases of a tumor frequently misdiagnosed as a vascular neoplasm. *Histopathology* 26:323–331, 1995.
37. Calonje E, Fletcher CDM. Cutaneous fibrohistiocytic tumors: An update. *Adv Pathol* 1:2–15, 1994.
38. Tamada S, Ackerman AB: Dermatofibroma with monster cells. *Am J Dermatopathol* 9:380–387, 1987.
39. Singh Gomez C, Calonje E, Fletcher CDM: Epithelioid benign fibrous histiocytoma of skin: Clinicopathological analysis of 20 cases of a poorly known variant. *Histopathology* 24:123–129, 1994.
40. Wilson Jones E, Cerio R, Smith NP. Epithelioid benign fibrous histiocytoma: A new entity. *Br J Dermatol* 120:185–195, 1989.
41. Glusac EJ, Barr RJ, Everett MA, Pitha J, Santa Cruz DJ: Epithelioid cell histiocytoma. A report of 10 cases including a new cellular variant. *Am J Surg Pathol* 18(6):583–590, 1994.
42. Calonje E, Mentzel T, Fletcher CDM: Cellular benign fibrous histiocytoma: Clinicopathologic analysis of 74 cases with a distinctive variant of cutaneous fibrous histiocytoma with frequent recurrence. *Am J Surg Pathol* 18:668–676, 1994.
43. Schwob VS, Santa Cruz DJ: Palisading cutaneous fibrous histiocytoma. *J Cutan Pathol.* 13:403–407, 1986.
44. Zelger BW, Steiner H, Kutzner H: Clear cell dermatofibroma. Case report of an unusual fibrohistiocytic lesion. *Am J Surg Pathol* 20(4):483–491, 1996.
45. Fretzin DF, Helwig EB: Atypical fibroxanthoma of the skin. A clinicopathologic study of 140 cases. *Cancer* 31:1541–1552, 1973.
46. Leong A S-Y, Milios J: Atypical fibroxanthoma of the skin: A clinicopathological and immunohistochemical study of 30 cases. *Histopathology* 11:463–475, 1987.
47. Longacre TA, Smoller BR, Rouse RV: Atypical fibroxanthoma. Multiple immunohistologic profiles. *Am J Surg Pathol* 17(12):1199–1209, 1993.
48. Calonje E, Wadden C, Jones EW, et al: Spindle cell non-pleomorphic atypical fibroxanthoma: Analysis of a series and delineation of a distinctive variant. *Histopathology* 22:247–254, 1993.
49. Helwig EB, May D: Atypical fibroxanthoma of the skin with metastasis. *Cancer* 57:368–376, 1986.
50. Winkelmann RK, Peters MS: Atypical fibroxanthoma. a study with antibody to S-100 protein. *Arch Dermatol* 121:753–755, 1985.
51. Ricci AR Jr, Cartun RW, Zakowski MF: Atypical fibroxanthoma. A study of 14 cases emphasizing the presence of Langerhans histiocytes with implications for differential diagnosis by antibody panels. *Am J Surg Pathol* 12:591–598, 1988.
52. Ushijima M, Hashimoto H, Tsuneyoshi M, et al: Giant cell tumor of tendon sheath (nodular tenosynovitis). A study of 207 cases to compare the large joint group with the common digit group. *Cancer* 57:875–884, 1986.
53. King DT, Millman AJ, Gurevitch AW, et al: Giant cell tumor of the tendon sheath involving skin. *Arch Dermatol* 114:944–946, 1978.
54. Churg AM, Kahn LB: Myofibroblasts and related cells in malignant fibrous and fibrohistiocytic tumors. *Hum Pathol* 8:205–218, 1977.

55. Satti MB:. Tendon sheath tumors: A pathological study of the relationship between giant cell tumor and fibroma of tendon sheath. *Histopathology* 20:213–220, 1992.

56. Reye RDK: Recurring digital fibrous tumors of childhood. *Arch Pathol* 80:228, 1965.

57. Enzinger FM: Dermal fibromatosis, in: *Tumors of Bone and Soft Tissue*. Chicago: Year Book, 1965, pp. 375–396.

58. Purdy LJ, Colby TV: Infantile digital fibromatosis occurring outside the digit. *Am J Surg Pathol* 8:787–790, 1984.

59. Canioni D, Rickard S, Rambaud C, et al: Lingual localization of an inclusion body fibromatosis (Reye's tumor). *Pathol Res Pract* 187:886–889, 1991.

60. Allen PW: Recurring digital fibrous tumors of childhood. *Pathology* 4:215–233, 1972.

61. Iwasaki H, Kikuchi M, Ohtsuki I, et al: Infantile digital fibromatosis. Identification of actin filaments in cytoplasmic inclusions by heavy meromyosin binding. *Cancer* 52:1653–1661, 1983.

62. Bittesini L, Dei Tos AP, Doglioni C, Della Libera D, Laurino L, Fletcher CD: Fibroepithelial lesion of the breast with digital fibroma-like inclusions in the stromal component. Case report and immunohistochemical and ultrastructural analysis. *Am J Surg Pathol* 18(3):296–301, 1994.

63. Bracko M, Cindro L, Golouh R: Familial occurrence of infantile myofibromatosis. *Cancer* 69:1294–1299, 1992.

64. Chung EB, Enzinger FM: Infantile myofibromatosis. *Cancer* 48:1807, 1981.

65. Smith KJ, Skelton HG, Barrett TL, et al: Cutaneous myofibroma. *Mod Pathol* 2:603, 1989.

66. Fletcher CD, Achu P, Van Noorden S, et al: Infantile myofibromatosis: A light microscopic, histochemical and immunohistochemical study suggesting true smooth muscle differentiation. *Histopathology* 11:245, 1987.

67. Spraker MK, Stack C, Esterly N: Congenital generalized fibromatosis: A review of the literature and report of a case associated with porencephaly, hemiatrophy and cutis marmorata telangiectatica congenita. *J Am Acad Dermatol* 10:365–371, 1984.

68. Daimaru Y, Hashimoto H, Enjoji M. Myofibromatosis in adults (adult counterpart of infantile myofibromatosis). *Am J Surg Pathol* 13(10):859–865, 1989.

69. Beham A, Badve S, Suster S, et al: Solitary myofibroma in adults: Clinicopathological analysis of a series. *Histopathology* 22:335–341, 1993.

70. Fayad MN, Tacoub A, Salman S, et al: Juvenile hyaline fibromatosis. Two new patients and review of the literature. *Am J Med Genet* 26:123–131, 1987.

71. Woyke S, Domagala W, Markiewicz D: A 19 year follow-up of multiple juvenile fibromatosis. *J Pediatr Surg* 19:302, 1984.

72. Mayer-da-Silva A, Poiares-Baptista A, Rodrigo FG, et al: Juvenile hyaline fibromatosis. A histologic and histochemical study. *Arch Pathol Lab Med* 112:928–931, 1988.

73. Enzinger FM: Fibrous hamartoma of infancy. *Cancer* 18:241–248, 1965.

74. Paller AS, Gonzalez-Crussi F, Sherman JO: Fibrous hamartoma of infancy. Eight additional cases and a review of the literature. *Arch Dermatol* 125:88–91, 1989.

75. Groisman G, Kerner H: A case of fibrous hamartoma of infancy in the scrotum, including immunohistochemical findings. *J Urol* 144:340, 1990.

76. Efem SEE, Ekpo MD: Clinicopathologic features of untreated fibrous hamartoma of infancy. *J Clin Pathol* 46:522–524, 1993.

77. Fletcher CDM, Powell G, van Noorden S, et al: Fibrous hamartoma of infancy: a histochemical and immunohistochemical study. *Histopathology* 12:65–74, 1988.

78. Beham A, Fletcher CDM: Dermatofibrosarcoma protuberans with areas resembling giant cell fibroblastoma: report of two cases. *Histopathology* 17:165–167, 1990.

79. Alguacil-Garcia A: Giant cell fibroblastoma recurring as dermatofibrosarcoma protuberans. *Am J Surg Pathol* 15:798–801, 1991.

80. Coyne J, Kafton SM, Craig RDP: Dermatofibrosarcoma protuberans recurring as a giant cell fibroblastoma. *Histopathology* 21:184–187, 1992.

81. Craver RD, Correa H, Kao YS, Van Brunt T, Golladay ES: Aggressive giant cell fibroblastoma with a balanced 17;22 translocation. *Cancer Genet Cytognet* 80(1):20–22, 1995.

82. Abdul-Karim FW, Evans HL, Silva EG: Giant cell fibroblastoma: A report of 3 cases. *Am J Clin Pathol* 83:165–170, 1985.

83. Shmookler BM, Enzinger FM, Weiss SW: Giant cell fibroblastoma. A juvenile form of dermatofibrosarcoma protuberans. *Cancer* 64:2154–2161, 1989.

84. Fletcher CDM: Giant cell fibroblastoma of soft tissue: A clinicopathological and immunohistochemical study. *Histopathology* 13:499–508, 1988.

85. Dei Tos AP, Seregard S, Calonje E, Chan JK, Fletcher CD: Giant cell angiofibroma. A distinctive orbital tumor in adults. *Am J Surg Pathol* 19(11):1286–1293, 1995.

86. Schmoeckel C, Albini A, Krieg T, et al: The fibroblastic nature of dermatofibrosarcoma protuberans: Morphological investigations in vivo and in vitro. *Arch Dermatol Res* 278:138–147, 1985.

87. Hashimoto K, Brownstein MH, Jakobiec FA: Dermatofibrosarcoma protuberans. A tumor with perineural and endoneural cell features. *Arch Dermatol* 110:874–885, 1974.

88. Alguacil-Garcia A, Unni KK, Goellner JR: Histogenesis of dermatofibrosarcoma protuberans. An ultrastructural study. *Am J Clin Pathol* 69:427–434, 1978.

89. Weiss SW, Nickoloff BJ: CD34 is expressed by a distinctive cell population in peripheral nerve, nerve sheath tumors, and related lesions. *Am J Surg Pathol* 17:1039, 1993.

90. Bridge JA, Neff JR, Sandberg AA: Cytogenetic analysis of dermatofibrosarcoma protuberans. *Cancer Genet Cytogenet* 49:199–202, 1990.

91. Stephenson CF, Berger CS, Leong SP. Ring chromosome in a dermatofibrosarcoma protuberans. *Cancer Genet Cytogenet* 58:52–54, 1992.

92. Roses DF, Valensi Q, Latrenta G, et al: Surgical treatment of dermatofibrosarcoma protuberans. *Surg Gynecol Obstet* 162:449, 1986.

93. Volpe R, Carbone A: Dermatofibrosarcoma protuberans metastatic to lymph nodes and showing a dominant histiocytic component. *Am J Dermatopathol* 5:327–334, 1983.

94. Fletcher CDM, Evans BJ, Macartney JC, et al: Dermatofibrosarcoma protuberans: A clinicopathological and immunohistochemical study with a review of the literature. *Histopathology* 9:921–938, 1985.

95. Frierson HF, Cooper PH: Myxoid variant of dermatofibrosarcoma protuberans. *Am J Surg Pathol* 1(5):445–450, 1983.

96. Beham A, Fletcher CDM: Dermatofibrosarcoma protuberans with areas resembling giant cell fibroblastoma: Report of two cases. *Histopathology* 17:165–167, 1990.

97. Connelly JH, Evans HL: Dermatofibrosarcoma protuberans: A clinicopathologic review with emphasis on fibrosarcomatous areas. *Am J Surg Pathol* 16:921–925, 1992.

98. Dupree WB, Langloss JM, Weiss SW: Pigmented dermatofibrosarcoma protuberans (Bednar tumor). *Am J Surg Pathol* 9:630–639, 1985.

99. Fletcher CDM, Theaker JM, Flanagan A, et al: Pigmented dermatofibrosarcoma protuberans (Bednar tumor): Melanocytic colonization or neuroectodermal differentiation? A clinicopathologic and immunohistochemical study. *Histopathology* 13:631–643, 1988.

100. Calonje E, Fletcher CDM: Myoid differentiation in dermatofibrosarcoma protuberans and its fibrosarcomatous variant: Clinicopathologic analysis of 5 cases. *J Cutan Pathol* 23:30–36, 1996.

101. Hollowood K, Holley MP, Fletcher CD: Plexiform fibrohistiocytic tumour: Clinicopathological, immunohistochemical and ultrastructural analysis in favour of a myofibroblastic lesion. *Histopathology* 1992;19:503, 1992.

102. Enzinger FM, Zhang RY: Plexiform fibrohistiocytic tumor presenting in children and young adults: An analysis of 65 cases. *Am J Surg Pathol* 12:818, 1988.

102a. Salomao DR, Nascimento AG: Plexiform fibrohistiocytic tumor with lung metastasis. *Am J Surg Pathol* 21:469–476, 1997.

103. Fletcher CDM: Pleomorphic malignant fibrous histiocytoma: Fact or fiction? A critical reappraisal based on 152 cases. *Am J Surg Pathol* 16:213–228, 1992.

104. Guccion JG, Enzinger FM: Malignant giant cell tumor of soft parts. An analysis of 32 cases. *Cancer* 29:1518–1529, 1979.

105. Mentzel T, Calonje E, Wadden C, Camplejohn RS, Beham A, Smith MA, et al: Myxofibrosarcoma: Clinicopathologic analysis of 75 cases with emphasis on low-grade variant. *Am J Surg Pathol* 20(4):391–405, 1996.

106. Merck C, Angervall L, Kindblom L-G, et al: Myxofibrosarcoma. A malignant soft tissue tumour of fibroblastic-histiocytic origin. A clinicopathologic and prognostic study of 110 cases using multivariate analysis. *Acta Pathol Microbiol Immunol Scan Sect A*91(suppl 282):1–40, 1983.

107. Weiss SW, Enzinger FM: Myxoid variant of malignant fibrous histiocytoma. *Cancer* 39:1672–1685, 1977.

108. Enzinger FM. Angiomatoid malignant fibrous histiocytoma: A distinctive fibrohistiocytic tumor of children and young adults simulating a vascular neoplasm. *Cancer* 44:2147, 1979.

109. Costa MJ, Weiss SW: Angiomatoid malignant fibrous histiocytoma: A follow-up study of 108 cases with evaluation of possible histologic predictors of outcome. *Am J Surg Pathol* 14:1126–1132, 1990.

110. Pettinato G, Manivel JC, DeRosa G, et al: Angiomatoid malignant fibrous histiocytoma: Cytologic, immunohistochemical, ultrastructural and flow cytometric study of 20 cases. *Mod Pathol* 3:479–487, 1990.

111. Fletcher CDM: Angiomatoid "malignant fibrous histiocytoma": An immunohistochemical study indicative of myoid differentiation. *Hum Pathol* 22:563-568, 1991.

112. Meyerding HW, Broders AC, Hargrave RL: Clinical aspects of fibrosarcoma of the soft tissues of the extremities. *Surg Gynecol Obstet* 62:1010, 1936.

113. Scott SM, Reiman HM, Pritchard DJ, et al: Soft tissue fibrosarcoma. A clinicopathologic study of 132 cases. *Cancer* 24:925–931, 1989.

114. Chung EB, Enzinger FM: Infantile fibrosarcoma. *Cancer* 38:729–739, 1976.

115. MacKenzie DH: Fibrosarcoma: A dangerous diagnosis. A review of 2056 cases of fibrosarcoma of soft tissues. *Br J Surg* 51:607–613, 1964.

116. Bizer LJ: Fibrosarcoma: Report of 64 cases. *Am J Surg* 121:586–687, 1971.

117. Pritchard DJ, Soule EH, Taylor WF, et al: Fibrosarcoma, a clinicopathologic and statistical study of 199 tumors of the soft tissues of the extremities and trunk. *Cancer* 33:888–897, 1974.

118. Dal Cin P, Brock P, Casteels-Van Daele M, et al: Cytogenetic characterization of congenital or infantile fibrosarcoma. *Eur J Pediatr* 150:579, 1991.

119. Schofield DE, Fletcher JA, Grier HE, et al: Fibrosarcoma in infants and children: Application of new techniques. *Am J Surg Pathol* 18:14, 1994.

120. Evans HL: Low-grade fibromyxoid sarcoma. A report of two metastasizing neoplasms having a deceptively benign appearance. *Am J Clin Pathol* 88:616–619, 1987.

121. Evans HL: Low-grade fibromyxoid sarcoma. A report of 12 cases. *Am J Surg Pathol* 17:595–600, 1993.

122. Goodlad JR, Mentzel T, Fletcher CDM: Low-grade fibromyxoid sarcoma: Clinico-

pathologic analysis of eleven new cases in support of a distinct entity. *Histopathology* 26:229–237, 1995.

123. Chase DR, Enzinger FM: Epithelioid sarcoma. Diagnosis, prognostic indicators and treatment. *Am J Surg Pathol* 9:241–263, 1985.

124. Evans HL, Baer SC: Epithelioid sarcoma: A clinicopathologic and prognostic study of 26 cases. *Semin Diagn Pathol* 10:286–291, 1993.

125. Allen PW, Dymock RB, MacCormack WB: Superficial angiomyxomas with and without epithelial components. Report of 30 tumors in 28 patients. *Am J Surg Pathol* 12:519–350, 1988.

126. Guerin D, Calonje E, McCormick D: Superficial angiomyxoma: Clinicopathological analysis of 26 cases of a distinctive cutaneous tumour with a tendency for recurrence. *J Pathol* 176(Suppl):51A (Abstract), 1995.

127. Carney JA, Hruska LS, Beauchamp GD, et al: Dominant inheritance of the complex of myxomas, spotty pigmentation, and endocrine overactivity. *Mayo Clin Proc* 61:165, 1986.

128. Carney JA: Differences between nonfamilial and familial cardiac myxoma. *Am J Surg Pathol* 9:53, 1985.

129. Carney JA, Toorkey BC: Myxoid fibroadenoma and allied conditions (myxomatosis) of the breast: a heritable disorder with special associations including cardiac and cutaneous myxomas. *Am J Surg Pathol* 15:713, 1992.

130. Carney JA: Psammomatous melanotic schwannoma: A distinctive heritable tumor with special associations including cardiac myxoma and the Cushing syndrome. *Am J Surg Pathol* 14:206, 1990.

131. Ferreiro JA, Carney JA: Myxomas of the external ear and their significance. *Am J Surg Pathol* 18(3):274–280, 1994.

CHAPTER 31

VASCULAR TUMORS

Steven J. Hunt / Daniel J. Santa Cruz / Raymond L. Barnhill

The nomenclature of vascular lesions is at best confusing and often incoherent, since the pathogenesis of many lesions is understood poorly or not at all. Thus, many classification schemes have been proposed but none are entirely satisfactory at present.[1-4] For example, vascular lesions may be classified as to the type and/or caliber of vascular channel present, e.g., capillary, venule, vein, arteriole, artery, lymphatic, and glomus vessel; proliferative versus nonproliferative lesions; congenital versus acquired lesions; malformations versus reactive, proliferative, or neoplastic lesions; and other features such as distribution and multicentricity. This chapter discusses the various entities in general terms as (1) benign vascular lesions which will include: ectasias/telangiectasias, proliferative lesions such as capillary hemangioma, and various malformations; (2) lesions with indeterminate or borderline status, e.g., the so-called hemangioendotheliomas; and (3) malignant vascular lesions such as angiosarcoma. We will attempt to maintain a balanced perspective in discussing each entity without trying to resolve the often controversial issues of nomenclature and pathogenesis.

Although the capillary differentiation of hemangiomas is frequently mentioned in the literature, the vast majority of vascular neoplasms have in addition to the inner endothelial lining a peripheral coat of smooth-muscle cells. Therefore, most of the so-called capillary hemangiomas are, in fact, venular lesions. This bias is reflected in the literature by the almost universal reference to endothelial cell markers as *vascular markers*. Strictly speaking, only telangiectasias and perhaps lymphatics are characterized by an endothelial lining alone. Paradoxically, the so-called venous lakes do not seem to have a substantial smooth-muscle component, thus better qualifying as a telangiectatic condition.

There is undoubtedly considerable heterogeneity of endothelial and smooth-muscle-cell phenotypes and functions in normal blood vessels which are today poorly understood. It is likely that there are specialized capacities in endothelial cells, including antigen presentation, secretion of cytokines, and so on, beyond the simple and obvious blood-containing function.

Finally, although well-defined clinicopathologic entities can be recognized, there is frequent morphologic overlap of some lesions.

BENIGN VASCULAR LESIONS

Hereditary Benign Telangiectasia

Affected individuals exhibit widespread telangiectases without evidence of visceral organ involvement or systemic disease.[5] The inheritance is thought to be autosomal dominant.

Clinical Features The lesions may involve the face, trunk, and extremities and may have a polymorphic appearance as discrete reddish papules resembling cherry angiomas, plaquelike lesions, lesions with an erythematous flush, or arborizing lesions.[5]

Histopathological Features The principal findings are widely dilated capillaries in the superficial dermis.[5]

Differential Diagnosis This condition must be distinguished from other telangiectases.

Hereditary Hemorrhagic Telangiectasia

Also known as *Osler's disease* or *Osler-Weber-Rendu disease*, hereditary hemorrhagic telangiectasia is a rare autosomal dominant disorder that typically presents with recurrent epistaxis in childhood and mucocutaneous telangiectases by the third and fourth decades of life.[6] Visceral involvement by telangiectases and arteriovenous malformations can result in variable hemorrhage and even death.

Clinical Features Telangiectases occur as nonpulsatile, punctate, or linear lesions that may involve any cutaneous site; commonly involved are the face, ears, lips, fingers, nail beds, palms, and soles (Table 31-1). Mucous membrane involvement is also diverse and ranges from the nasopharynx and oral mucosa to throughout the gastrointestinal tract.[6] Vascular aneurysms and arteriovenous malformations of organs such as the brain and lungs may occur. Recurrent nosebleeds beginning in childhood may herald the presence of the disorder, but the characteristic mucocutaneous telangiectases are usually not seen before puberty. Gastrointestinal hemorrhages may produce recurrent episodes of melena. The clinical severity of hemorrhagic hereditary telangiectasia depends on the location and frequency of hemorrhage.

Histopathological Features Dilated, thin-walled, irregular capillaries and venules occur directly beneath the surface of mucocutaneous epithelia (Fig. 31-1). Anomalies of endothelial cells, endothelial cell junctions, and perivascular connective tissue have been described.[6]

Differential Diagnosis Telangiectases may be seen as primary cutaneous lesions in other disorders such as ataxia telangiectasia, generalized essential telangiectasia, hereditary benign telangiectasia, and unilateral nevoid telangiectasia syndrome, as well as secondary to many other conditions or insults (see below). In particular, the extensive mucocutaneous telangiectases with recurrent mucosal hemorrhages and the presence of systemic visceral involvement serve to distinguish hereditary hemorrhagic telangiectasia from other telangiectases.

Ataxia-Telangiectasia (Louis-Bar Syndrome)

Clinical Features Patients present with telangiectases, cutaneous atrophy, and mottled hyper- and hypopigmentation involving the head and neck and commencing in childhood.[7] There may also be ectasia of bulbar conjunctival vessels and premature graying of hair. Other important

Hereditary Hemorrhagic Telangiectasia

Clinical Features

Autosomal dominant
Telangiectases involving mucocutaneous sites, developing at puberty
Face, lips, ears, fingers, nail beds, palms, soles, nasopharynx, oral mucosa involved
Nonpulsatile, punctate or linear vascular lesions
Recurrent epistaxis
Vascular anomalies and arteriovenous malformations sometimes involving viscera, especially the brain and lungs
Melena from GI hemorrhage
Anemia

Histopathological Features

Dilated, thin-walled irregular capillaries and venules beneath epithelial layers

Differential Diagnosis

Telangiectases in many other conditions
Hereditary benign telangiectasia
Ataxia-telangiectasia
Generalized essential telangiectasia
Unilateral nevoid telangiectasia.

components of this autosomal recessive syndrome include progressive cerebellar ataxia from cerebellar cortical atrophy, a combined immunodeficiency involving both cellular and humoral immunity, recurrent infections, chromosomal instability from a striking sensitivity to ionizing radiation, and a markedly increased incidence of neoplasia, particularly lymphoma and leukemia.

Histopathological Features   There is ectasia of venules in the superficial vascular plexus.[7]

Differential Diagnosis   One must distinguish ataxia-telangiectasia from other genodermatoses associated with chromosomal instability and telangiectasia such as Bloom's syndrome, Rothmund-Thomson syndrome, and xeroderma pigmentosum.

Generalized Essential Telangiectasia

Clinical Features   This condition most commonly affects adult women and is typified by onset on the lower extremeties with subsequent involvement of the trunk, upper extremities, head, and neck.[8] There is no evidence of systemic disease or visceral organ involvement.

Histopathological Features   The major finding is a dilated capillary vessel in the papillary dermis without inflammation[8] (Fig. 31-2).

Unilateral Nevoid Telangiectasia

Clinical Features   In this condition delicate telangiectases with a unilateral and often dermatomal distribution are noted at birth or later in life.[9] The process most frequently involves the face followed by the neck, chest, and arms.

Histopathological Features   One observes dilated capillaries in the superficial and middle dermis.[9]

Cutis Marmorata Telangiectatica Congenita (Congenital Generalized Phlebectasia)

Clinical Features   Neonates present with a localized or generalized reticular or netlike vascular mottling of the skin that suggests livedo reticularis but is persistent rather than transient.[10] The mottling is explained by ectasia of a range of vessel types including capillaries and venous channels. There may be atrophy of the overlying skin and ulceration. There is a tendency of the vascular abnormalities to improve with age. Other abnormalities reported include enlargement or hypoplasia of an affected limb, skeletal anomalies, glaucoma, and mental retardation. The disorder may be inherited as autosomal dominant.

Histopathological Features   One observes dilated capillaries, venules, and venous vessels throughout the dermis and possibly the subcutis.[10]

Differential Diagnosis   The clinical findings are usually distinctive. Livedo reticularis is a transient mottling that is related to sluggish blood flow (from many causes) rather than a vascular structural abnormality.

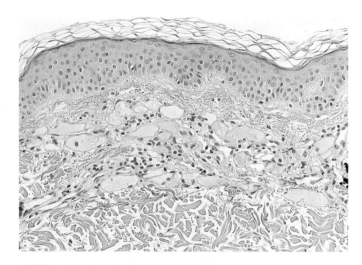

FIGURE 31-1   Hereditary hemorrhagic telangiectasia. Dilated venules are present in the papillary dermis.

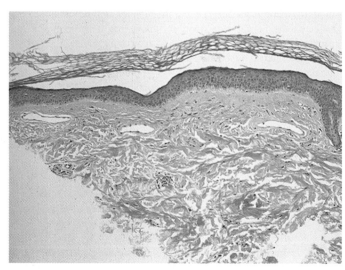

FIGURE 31-2   Essential telangiectasia. There are telangiectases in the superficial dermis.

Secondary Telangiectases

Secondary causes of telangiectasia are manifold and include conditions such as acne rosacea, varicose veins, trauma, lupus erythematosus, dermatomyositis, scleroderma and sclerodactyly (CREST syndrome), radiation dermatitis, poikiloderma, xeroderma pigmentosum, chronic sun exposure, and mastocytosis.

Venous Lake

The venous lake is an acquired venular ectasia developing on exposed skin of the head and neck in elderly patients probably from lack of support from the surrounding tissue.[11]

Clinical Features The lesions are often solitary dark-bluish papules 3 to 10 mm in diameter and commonly involve the ears, lips, face, and neck[11] (Table 31-2).

Histopathological Features The lesion is an ectatic vascular space localized to the superficial to middle dermis and is usually lined by a single layer of endothelium (Fig. 31-3); however, smooth muscular elements may occasionally be associated with the wall of the vessel.[11,12] The surrounding dermis usually shows solar elastosis and diminished collagen.

Differential Diagnosis The lesion is distinctive; however, other vascular ectasias might be considered in the differential diagnosis.

Capillary Aneurysm (or Thrombosed Capillary Aneurysm)

Clinical Features The lesion usually presents as a solitary bluish papule on the face or trunk occasionally with itching or tenderness.[13] The lesion may have developed slowly or abruptly. The sudden development of such a lesion is attributed to occlusion of the vessel by a thrombus. The primary clinical concern in many instances is to rule out melanoma.

Histopathological Features The principal finding is a single ectatic vascular structure (usually a venule) often containing a thrombus.[13] The vascular channel is characterized by an unremarkable endothelial lining

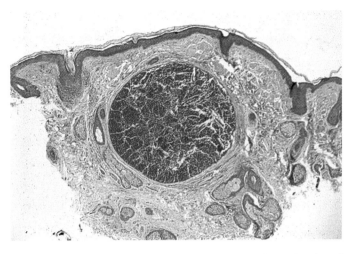

FIGURE 31-3 Venous lake. A widely dilated, thin-walled vascular channel filled with red blood cells is present in the dermis.

that is surrounded by a concentric layering of fibrous tissue without smooth muscle or elastic lamina.

Differential Diagnosis The differential diagnosis includes other ectatic vascular channels with or without thrombosis such as venous lake, enlarged and torturous arterial and lymphatic channels, and angiokeratoma.

Spider Angioma

Also known as *nevus araneus*, *spider nevus*, *arterial spider*, or *spider telangiectasis*, the spider angioma is a common cutaneous vascular lesion that is often seen as an incidental finding in healthy children.[14,15] Some of the these lesions persist into adulthood, and other spider angiomas occur as acquired manifestations of pregnancy, hepatic cirrhosis, and thyrotoxicosis.

Clinical Features The most common sites of involvement are the face, particularly the upper infraorbital cheeks, the neck, trunk, and hands (Table 31-3). An erythematous central punctum, which may be slightly elevated and may be seen to be pulsatile on diascopy, gives forth an

---

TABLE 31-2
Venous Lake

Clinical Features

Predilection for exposed ("weathered") skin of older individuals—
    face, ears, lips
Dark-blue papule, 3–10 mm, suspicious for melanoma

Histopathological Features

Dilated thin-walled vascular channel in dermis
Uncommon smooth muscle in wall
Occasional intraluminal thrombosis
Solar elastosis and lack of supporting dermal collagen

Differential Diagnosis

Telangiectasis

TABLE 31-3
Spider Angioma

Clinical Features

Common in adolescents, young adults, women more than men,
    individuals with liver disease and thyrotoxicosis
Involves face, neck, trunk, and hands
Pulsatile red punctum with arborizing channels
Blanches with pressure

Histopathological Features

Vertically oriented arterial vascular channel in dermis
Branching into smaller vessels

Differential Diagnosis

Telangiectases

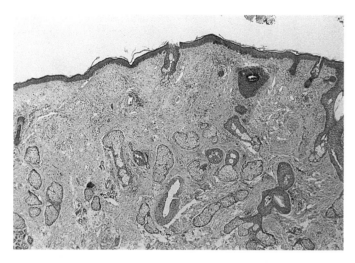

FIGURE 31-4 Spider angioma. There is a small arterial vessel in the lower dermis.

array of peripherally radiating fine vessels. A spider angioma typically blanches with pressure, and upon release refills rapidly by blood flow originating from its center. Often solitary, multiple spider angiomas may occasionally occur, and particularly in the setting of chronic liver disease they may be numerous.

Histopathological Features A central artery rises in the dermis (Fig. 31-4) and branches into smaller vessels that supply blood to the radiating array of fine capillaries.[14] Rarely, the wall of the artery may contain glomus cells.[14]

Differential Diagnosis The clinical appearance of the spider angioma with its pulsatile nature is distinct and allows distinction from simple telangiectases. In contrast to spider angiomas, the lesions of hereditary hemorrhagic telangiectasia, an inherited mucocutaneous disorder that is described further in this chapter, are numerous and consist of nonpulsatile, punctate, or linear telangiectases.

Angioma Serpiginosum

Angioma serpiginosum is an unusual benign vascular lesion that was first described by Hutchinson in 1889 as a peculiar form of serpiginous and infective nevoid disease. It was named by Crocker in 1894, and additional reports over time have clarified its clinicopathologic features.

Clinical Features Angioma serpiginosum typically occurs during the first two decades of life, is more common in women, and occurs at any site.[16,17] Although the lower extremities are the most common site, the palms and soles are typically spared. Minute violaceous-red puncta, at times requiring magnification for adequate visualization, occur in gyrate or serpiginous configurations. Groups of puncta may coalesce into patches. Peripheral extension occurs through the formation of satellite puncta. Angioma serpiginosum usually occurs sporadically in individuals, but familial transmission has been reported. Autosomal dominant inheritance with variable penetrance favoring women was suggested, but the possibility of recessive inheritance could not be excluded.[17] Angioma serpiginosum may spontaneously regress but is usually slowly progressive. There may, however, be periods of relative quiescence or prolonged stability.

Histopathological Features Angioma serpiginosum is characterized by increased numbers of dilated capillaries in the upper dermis.[16] The

overlying epidermis is normal, and there is no significant inflammation. Red cell extravasation and hemosiderin are absent. The dilated capillaries are relatively thick-walled.

Differential Diagnosis The absence of red cell extravasation and hemosiderin differentiates angioma serpiginosum from the pigmented purpuric dermatoses. Clinical similarities to angiokeratoma circumscriptum exist, but the latter condition differs from angioma serpiginosum by developing a verrucous, hyperkeratotic surface.

Angiokeratoma

Angiokeratomas traditionally occur as five clinical types[18–21] (Table 31-4):

1. Mibelli type, with hyperkeratotic lesions on the dorsal fingers and toes
2. Fordyce type, with involvement of the scrotum and vulva
3. Angiokeratoma corporis diffusum (ACD), a lysosomal storage disease inherited as an X-linked recessive disorder in Fabry's disease (alpha-galactosidase A deficiency) but also seen with the autosomal recessive disorder, fucosidosis (alpha-L-fucosidase deficiency), and rarely with beta-galactosidase deficiency, alone or in combination with neuraminidase deficiency
4. The solitary or multiple type which may occur anywhere but favors the lower extremities
5. Angiokeratoma circumscriptum, with lesions in groups or bands usually on an extremity

---

TABLE 31-4

Angiokeratoma

Clinical Features

Onset in first two decades common, but also older individuals
Solitary or multiple
Sites vary (see below)
Hyperkeratotic lesions that may be pink-red, purple, brown, blue, or black
Melanoma often a clinical concern
Five clinical types:
    Mibelli type: lesions on dorsal fingers and toes
    Fordyce type: lesions on scrotum and vulva
    Angiokeratoma corporis diffusum:
        Fabry's disease (alpha-galactosidase A deficiency)
        Fucosidosis (alpha-L-fucosidase deficiency)
        Beta-galactosidase deficiency
    Solitary or multiple type: common on lower extremities but may occur anywhere
    Angiokeratoma circumscriptum: usually on the extremities

Histopathological Features

Ectatic thin-walled vascular channels in papillary dermis
Vascular spaces intimately associated with or encased by epidermis
Epidermal hyperplasia and hyperkeratosis often present
Intraluminal thrombosis and organization common

Differential Diagnosis

Verrucous hemangioma (malformation)
Telangiectases

However, this last type of angiokeratoma has deep angiomatous involvement in contrast to the telangiectatic nature of angiokeratomas, in general, and may be better classified with verrucous hemangiomas. The existence of a sixth type of angiokeratoma, angiokeratoma serpiginosum, clinically simulating angioma serpiginosum, has been suggested.

Clinical Features   Most forms of angiokeratoma present during the first two decades of life (Table 31-4). Angiokeratoma circumscriptum may be visible at birth. In contrast, angiokeratomas of ACD typically present in late childhood; and angiokeratoma scroti and the solitary or multiple types of angiokeratoma generally arise during the second to fourth decades. Vulvar angiokeratomas usually occur in the third and fourth decades and have been regarded as analogous to angiokeratoma scroti, particularly in regards to their anatomic location and a pathogenesis related to conditions of increased venous pressure. ACD is a manifestation of a systemic disorder, the clinicopathologic features of which are beyond the scope of this discussion.

Angiokeratomas occur as variably hyperkeratotic lesions that may be pink-red to purple, brown, or occasionally blue to black. Clinically, the differential diagnosis includes hemangioma, verruca, nevus, and, when thrombosed and deeply pigmented, malignant melanoma. The latter occurrence has been emphasized in individual case reports. Angiokeratomas usually offer no symptoms, but with local trauma they may become irritated and can bleed, given their highly vascular nature.

Histopathological Features   Angiokeratomas are telangiectasias, and all angiokeratomas are histologically similar but for the addition of certain features for angiokeratoma corporis diffusum[20,21] (Table 31-4). Ectatic, thin-walled vascular spaces occur in the papillary dermis intimately associated with, and variably encased by, acanthotic epidermis with elongated rete ridges and hyperkeratosis that is often slight but accentuated on acral sites (Fig. 31-5). Partial or virtually complete occlusion of these dilated vessels by intravascular fibrin thrombi, in various degrees of organization, may be present. Dilated veins often drain the vascular lacunae of angiokeratoma scroti and vulvar angiokeratoma.

Careful examination of angiokeratomas of ACD may show subtle vacuolization of the endothelium, arrector pili muscle, and vascular smooth-muscle cells, but these vacuoles are better seen by lipid stains, such as Sudan black B, or by periodic acid–Schiff stain (PAS) of the

glycolipid. The lipid is doubly refractile and can be visualized in frozen tissue sections examined by polarized light. Ultrastructural examination will reveal characteristic electron-dense, lamellar inclusion bodies.

Differential Diagnosis   The diagnosis of angiokeratoma is seldom difficult, and the clinical setting allows appropriate subclassification. Verrucous hemangiomas because of their superficial component may mimic angiokeratomas and when small may enter into the differential diagnosis. However, because angiokeratomas are telangiectasias, they lack the deep hemangiomatous component so characteristic of verrucous hemangioma. It is important of course to distinguish those with enzyme deficiencies, due to the obvious systemic implications.

Nevus Flammeus

Also known as *Salmon patch* or *port-wine stain*, this congenital vascular anomaly often involves the head and neck with a unilateral distribution but may occur anywhere.[2,3,4,14,22] Some variants, e.g., the so-called salmon patch, may regress in the postnatal period, whereas other variants are persistent, e.g., the port-wine stain. There may be an association with syndromes involving other organs.

Clinical Features   The initial lesions present at birth are pink to reddish macules that are often irregular in configuration and involve the nape of the neck (so-called stork bite), the eyelids and glabella (the salmon patch), other areas of the face, or any anatomic site (Table 31-5). The persistent lesions may become papular and keratotic.

TABLE 31-5
Nevus Flammeus

Clinical Features

Onset at birth
Often involves head and neck but may occur anywhere
Pink macular lesions but may become papular and keratotic
Some lesions regress:
 "Stork bite" on nape of neck
 "Salmon patch" on eyelids
Some persistent lesions, e.g., the port-wine stain, associated with
    particular sydromes:
 Cobb's syndrome: vascular malformation in spinal cord and
    port-wine stain in corresponding dermatome
 Sturge-Weber syndrome: unilateral port-wine stain involving the
    ophthalmic branch of trigeminal cranial nerve; seizures,
    hemiparesis, hemiplegia from vascular malformation of
    contralateral leptomeninges; occasional vascular malformations
    in other sites such as the choroid; mental retardation; glaucoma
 Klippel-Trenaunay-Weber syndrome: unilateral hypertrophy of a
    limb (bone and soft tissue overgrowth); varicosities; arteriovenous malformation often present; other vascular malformations
    on occasion

Histopathological Features

Widely dilated thin-walled venules in upper dermis or throughout
    reticular dermis

Differential Diagnosis

Telangiectases
Spider angioma

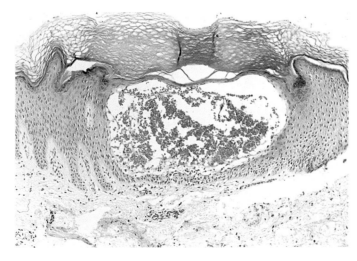

FIGURE 31-5   Angiokeratoma. A thin-walled ectatic vascular channel is surrounded by epidermis.

Persistent lesions may be associated with particular syndromes, termed *congenital dysplastic angiopathies* by Bean, that are highly variable in their clinical findings.[14] The following syndromes are commonly associated with port-wine stains:

- *Cobb's syndrome*: Individuals with this syndrome have a vascular malformation involving the spinal cord and usually a port-wine stain in the distribution of the corresponding dermatome of the skin.[23]
- *Sturge-Weber syndrome (encephalotrigeminal angiomatosis)*: This syndrome is characterized by a unilateral port-wine stain often in the distribution of the ophthalmic branch of the fifth (trigeminal) cranial nerve; seizures and hemiplegia or hemiparesis related to a vascular malformation involving the contralateral leptomeninges; possible choroidal vascular malformations; mental retardation; and glaucoma.[14,24]
- *Klippel-Trenaunay-Weber syndrome (hemihemangiectatic hypertrophy; congenital dysplastic angiopathies; angioosteohypertrophy)*: In addition to a port-wine stain (usually involving the affected limb) the primary defining feature is the unilateral hypertrophy of a limb, most commonly the lower extremity, often with associated varicosities.[14,25,26] There is overgrowth of both bone and soft tissue in most instances. Commonly there is an underlying arteriovenous malformation, but other vascular anomalies may be present including angiokeratomas and venous (cavernous) and lymphatic malformations.

Histopathological Features   The essential findings are widely dilated, thin-walled venules scattered throughout the upper dermis or throughout the entire reticular dermis[2,3,14] (Fig. 31-6). Papular lesions developing in nevus flammeus are composed of a proliferation of thin-walled vascular channels with lumina that vary in size.

Differential Diagnosis   Other vascular ectasias such as generalized essential telangiectasia, hereditary benign telangiectasia, hereditary hemorrhagic telangiectasia, unilateral nevoid telangiectasia, and spider angioma enter into the differential diagnosis. Nevus flammeus differs from the other conditions because of the onset of lesions at birth, rather distinctive macular to papular clinical lesions, and fairly discrete dilated venules in the upper reticular dermis.

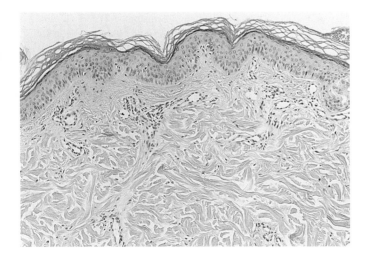

FIGURE 31-6   Nevus flammeus. There are dilated thin-walled microvessels in the superficial dermis.

Cavernous Malformation

Also known as *cavernous hemangioma* or *venous malformation*, this rather characteristic type of vascular proliferation usually presents at birth or in childhood but may develop in older individuals and may be associated with a number of syndromes such as blue rubber bleb nevus syndrome and Maffucci's syndrome.[2,3,14,27–29] The term *cavernous* refers to widely dilated vascular channels that resemble those in corpus cavernosum.

Clinical Features   The individual vascular lesion usually presents as soft, red to purple nodules or plaques that have a compressible quality (Table 31-6). The most common sites include the head and neck, but lesions may occur anywhere. Onset may be at birth, in the first few weeks of life, or later.

Individuals with blue rubber bleb nevus syndrome, an autosomal dominant condition, present at birth with numerous cavernous vascular malformations involving the skin, gastrointestinal tract, central nervous system, liver, and spleen.[14,27,28] Patients may exhibit pain and hyperhidrosis from the cutaneous lesions and melena and anemia from those situated in the GI tract.

TABLE 31-6

Cavernous Malformation

Clinical Features

Onset commonly at birth or in childhood
Involve head and neck most commonly but may occur anywhere
Soft, red to purple nodules or plaques
Compressible and rubbery
Associated with particular syndromes:
  Blue rubber bleb nevus syndrome: autosomal dominant; cavernous malformations involving the skin, GI tract, liver, spleen, and CNS; pain and hyperhidrosis; melena and anemia.
  Maffucci's syndrome: cavernous malformations, lymphatic malformations, and phlebectasias; multiple enchondromas and bony deformities from nonossifying cartilage; high risk of chondrosarcoma and angiosarcoma

Histopathological Features

Location usually in deep dermis or subcutis
Often well-circumscribed but may be diffuse
Vascular channels are dilated and often encased in fibrous tissue with lobular configuration
Vessels contain single layer of endothelium surrounded by fibrous tissue in vessel wall
Smooth muscle may be observed in the vessel wall but is often inconspicuous
Commonly part of combined or complex vascular malformations, e.g.:
  Capillary-cavernous (venous) malformation
  Lymphaticocavernous malformation
  Arteriocavernous malformation

Differential Diagnosis

Cavernous lymphatic malformation
Glomangioma
Port-wine stain
Arteriovenous and other malformations
Involuting juvenile capillary hemangioma

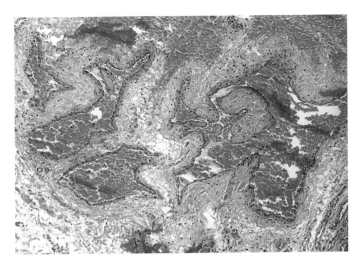

FIGURE 31-7 Cavernous (venous) malformation. A circumscribed aggregate of large vascular channels with walls thickened by smooth muscle and fibrous tissue.

TABLE 31-7

Angiomatosis

Clinical Features

Usually presents in childhood
Swelling of a large contiguous area of soft tissue and dermis
High recurrence rate

Histopathological Features

Infiltration of dermis and soft tissue by a mixture of veins, cavernous
     vascular spaces, and capillary-sized vessels

Differential Diagnosis

Intramuscular hemangioma
Lymphatic malformations
Angiolipoma

The principal findings with Maffucci's syndrome include three varieties of vascular lesions: cavernous malformations, lymphatic malformations, and phlebectasias; multiple enchondromas and bony deformities resulting from nonossifying cartilage in the metaphyses of growing bones; frequent fractures of bone from the latter defects; and the frequent development of chondrosarcoma and angiosarcoma in up to 50% of affected individuals.[14,29]

Histopathological Features The lesions are usually situated in the deep dermis or subcutis and are often well-circumscribed but may be diffuse[2,13,14] (Fig. 31-7). The vascular channels are often encased in fairly dense fibrous tissue that has a lobular configuration. The vessels exhibit a single layer of endothelium surrounded by fibrous tissue. Smooth-muscle elements may be observed in the fibrous lining of the vessels. It must be emphasized that cavernous malformations may occur as a component of almost any complex or combined vascular malformation or as part of any of the syndromes described above. Thus, for example, one may have capillary-lymphatic, capillary-cavernous (venous), lymphaticocavernous (venous), and arteriocavernous (venous) malformations, or even more complex combinations of channels.

Differential Diagnosis Cavernous (venous) malformation must be distinguished from cavernous lymphatic malformation, glomangioma, port-wine stain, arteriovenous and other malformations, and juvenile capillary hemangioma (involuting stage). A cavernous lymphatic malformation differs from a cavernous (venous) malformation only by the lumina containing eosinophilic proteinaceous fluid and numerous lymphocytes. Glomangiomas are structurally similar to cavernous (venous) malformations but have glomus cells in their walls. Arteriovenous malformations differ by having arterial-type channels usually with a well-developed internal elastic lamina. Lobular capillary hemangiomas usually exhibit striking lobules of vascular channels with variable cellularity separated by fibrous septa.

Angiomatosis

Clinical Features Angiomatosis is a rare condition that usually presents in childhood as symptoms of persistent swelling of a large contiguous area of soft tissue and dermis.[30] Occasional lesions extend into bone (Table 31-7). This condition is sometimes painful. Cases associated with visceral and central nervous system hemangiomas have been

described. Angiomatosis has a very high recurrence rate, up to 90% in one series.

Histopathological Features Angiomatosis is characterized by infiltration of dermis and soft tissue by a mixture of veins, cavernous vascular spaces, and capillary-sized vessels (Fig. 31-8).[30] A characteristic feature is the presence of large amounts of adipose tissue. This feature may cause confusion with adipose tumors. A distinctive subtype of angiomatosis is composed of capillary-size vessels with occasional larger "feeder" vessels.

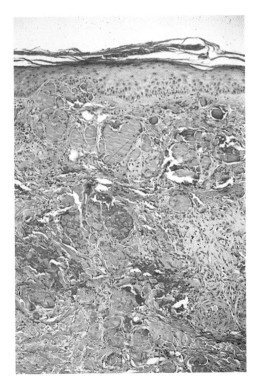

FIGURE 31-8 Angiomatosis. Dilated vascular channels are diffusely scattered throughout the dermis.

Differential Diagnosis Distinction between intramuscular hemangioma and angiomatosis essentially depends on the extent of the lesion. Intramuscular hemangioma tends to be limited to a group of muscles compared to the more extensive involvement by angiomatosis. The small size and discrete nature of angiolipoma preclude confusion with angiomatosis.

Verrucous Hemangioma

Also known as *keratotic hemangioma, unilateral verrucous hemangioma, angiokeratoma circumscriptum naeviforme, nevus keratoangiomatosus*, and *naevus vascularis unius lateralis*, verrucous hemangioma (VH) is an uncommon vascular malformation that tends to arise near birth or in childhood.[31,32] In 1967, Imperial and Helwig at the Armed Forces Institute of Pathology defined the clinicopathologic features of 21 verrucous hemangiomas identified during a retrospective review of 1175 cases that previously had been classified as angiokeratoma or various types of hemangioma.[31]

Clinical Features In Imperial and Helwig's series, approximately half of VH developed in the perinatal period whereas six others presented by the age of 17 years[31] (Table 31-8). The most common site is the lower extremity, particularly distally. VH typically occurs as unilateral, grouped, sometimes linear or serpiginous, discrete to confluent, hyperkeratotic angiomatous papules. Early lesions are bluish-red, well demarcated, soft, and compressible. Over time, VH gradually enlarge, satellite nodules may arise, and ultimately a verrucous hyperkeratotic appearance develops. An unusual case of a young girl with multiple eruptive VH papules developing and progressing since birth, and suggesting multiple hemangiomatosis, has been reported.

VH papules enlarge with body growth and tend to recur after surgical excision. Accordingly, they are best removed earlier in life when still small. In contrast to angiokeratomas, which respond to various superficial means of therapy, removal of VH requires a deep and relatively wide surgical excision. Otherwise, the lesions are apt to recur.

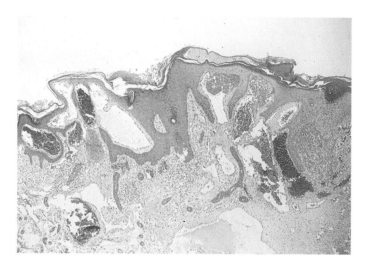

FIGURE 31-9 Verrucous hemangioma. The epidermis shows papillomatous hyperplasia and is intimately associated with ectatic vascular channels containing erythrocytes. The features are indistinguishable from angiokeratoma. However, a deep vascular component is present.

Histopathological Features Verrucous hemangioma is a variant of capillary or cavernous malformation (venous malformation, cavernous hemangioma) that may have mixed features of both and is associated with secondary, reactive epidermal changes, such as acanthosis, papillomatosis, and hyperkeratosis[31,32] (Fig. 31-9). Although the superficial portion of VH may bear resemblance to an angiokeratoma, the VH is distinct in that an angiomatous component extends deeply into the reticular dermis and underlying subcutaneous tissue. Often, the vascularity extends laterally into adjacent skin that clinically appears normal. The upper dermis can show fibrosis, hemosiderin, and inflammation. The surface may hold inflammatory and hemorrhagic crusts and may show occasional ulceration.

Differential Diagnosis Clinically, the differential diagnosis includes angiokeratoma, Cobb's syndrome, angioma serpiginosum, lymphangioma circumscriptum, verrucae, and, perhaps, pigmented tumors. Angiokeratoma corporis diffusum, scrotal angiokeratomas, and angiokeratoma of Mibelli on the fingers and toes are clinically distinct. Except for angiokeratoma circumscriptum, which may actually represent a verrucous hemangioma, angiokeratomas are telangiectasias and can be differentiated from VH by the absence of a deep angiomatous component. Angioma serpiginosa, occurring often on the legs, does not have a verrucous, hyperkeratotic surface and typically presents as minute violaceous-red puncta in gyrate or serpiginous configurations. Cobb's syndrome is a rare congenital vascular nevus in a dermatomal distribution on the trunk, with the appearance of angiokeratoma circumscriptum or nevus flammeus and an associated meningospinal angioma. Finally, cutaneous keratotic hemangioma is histologically similar to verrucous hemangioma but is clinically distinct, occurring as an acquired vascular tumor on the volar side of the fingers.

Spindle Cell Hemangioendothelioma

In 1986, Weiss and Enzinger delineated the features of this unique vascular lesion and coined its name, spindle cell hemangioendothelioma (SCH).[33] It was considered to be a low-grade angiosarcoma, with features of both a cavernous malformation and Kaposi's sarcoma. Because of its favorable prognosis and limited capability for metastasis, it was considered that biologically the spindle cell hemangioendothelioma

---

TABLE 31-8

Verrucous Hemangioma

Clinical Features

Origin in infancy and childhood
Distal lower extremity
Hyperkeratotic angiomatous papules
Grouped, discrete to confluent, sometimes linear or serpiginous
Verrucous appearance developing over time

Histopathological Features

Capillary to cavernous angiomatous proliferation
Pandermal involvement with extension into the subcutis
Lateral extension into clinically normal-appearing skin
Reactive acanthosis, papillomatosis, and hyperkeratosis
Occasional inflammatory crusting or ulceration

Differential Diagnosis

Angiokeratomas
"Angiokeratoma circumscriptum"
Angioma serpiginosa
Cutaneous keratotic hemangioma

TABLE 31-9

Spindle Cell Hemangioendothelioma

Clinical Features

Men more than women
Any age, often in the young
Favors the extremities, particularly distal
Solitary or multiple, circumscribed, reddish nodules
Gradually increase in size/number
Cystic hemorrhagic cavities, occasionally with a phlebolith
Associations with Maffucci's disease, varicose veins, congenital
   lymphedema

Histopathological Features

Cavernous, thin-walled blood vessels
Organizing thrombi and phleboliths
Solid, cellular areas of spindled cells
Network of slitlike spaces
Short fascicles
Plumper, more epithelioid cells, occasionally vacuolated
Relative lack of cytologic atypia and mitotic activity

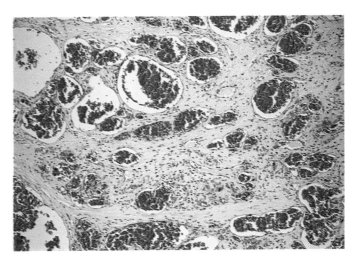

FIGURE 31-10   Spindle cell hemangioendothelioma. The lesion contains cavernous vascular channels.

might be categorized with the epithelioid hemangioendothelioma and the endovascular papillary angioendothelioma (Dabska tumor).

Additional cases of SCH were reported by Scott and Rosai in 1988, and despite the tendency toward slow progression and local recurrence, it was believed that there was insufficient evidence to view SCH as a low-grade angiosarcoma.[34] With further study, it now appears that SCH is a nonneoplastic, reactive vascular proliferation, associated with malformed blood vessels and repeated cycles of recanalization after thrombosis.[35,36]

Clinical Features   SCH occurs in individuals at any age and in both sexes but is more common in men (Table 31-9).[33] Lesions have arisen as early as the perinatal period, and nearly half of cases have presented during the first two and a half decades of life. SCH has a predilection for the extremities, particularly distally, with the hand being more common than the foot. Typically arising in the dermis or subcutaneous tissue, SCH presents as either solitary or multiple asymptomatic nodules that over a period of months or years gradually increase in size or number and often eventuate in extensive disease. When lesions are multiple, they usually occur in the same general area; however, bilateral lesions of the hands have been described and rare patients may have multiple lesions on diverse sites.[34]

SCH has occurred in Maffucci's syndrome and rarely in the Klippel-Trenaunay syndrome, early-onset varicose veins, and congenital lymphedema of Milroy's disease.[33–36] One case of SCH arose as multiple lesions adjacent to an epithelioid hemangioendothelioma, and another case presented as multiple lesions of SCH on the arm and chest in a patient with Maffucci's syndrome and a high-grade angiosarcoma of the abdominal wall.

Grossly, the tumors may be several centimeters in diameter and generally appear as small, circumscribed reddish nodules that on sectioning show variably sized, cystic, hemorrhagic spaces. On occasion, a phlebolith may be present and "pop out" from these cavities.

Local recurrence frequently occurs after simple excision, and multiple recurrences may occur in individual patients. Although several patients have developed extensive local disease, none have developed visceral metastasis and none have died, despite having received only conservative surgical therapy.

Histopathological Features   SCH is characterized histologically by two distinctive components: (1) thin-walled, cavernous blood vessels that sometimes are filled with organizing thrombi and phleboliths (Fig. 31-10) and (2) more solid, cellular areas composed predominantly of spindled cells (Fig. 31-11) (Table 31-9). The proportion of cavernous spaces to areas of spindled cells is variable.[33–36] The spindled cells may form a network of slitlike spaces and may form short fascicles. Small aggregates of plump, epithelioid cells are commonly interspersed among the spindled cells. Intracytoplasmic lumen formation is often present, usually in association with these epithelioid or "histiocytoid" areas. On occasion, these vacuolated cells may line vascular spaces. Cytologic atypia and mitotic activity are inconspicuous.

Factor VIII–related antigen is expressed by most of the endothelial lining cells and by the occasional plump cells but rarely, if ever, by the spindled cells. One case stained for Ulex europaeus lectin showed a similar pattern. The spindled-cell component was negative. Because of the histologic similarities to Kaposi's sarcoma, two cases were examined for HIV-1 antibody titers; both individuals were found to be negative.

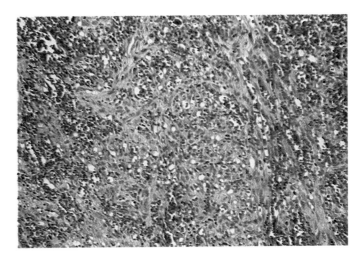

FIGURE 31-11   Spindle cell hemangioendothelioma. Cellular areas containing epithelioid cells with intracellular lumina.

Differential Diagnosis The most problematic entity in differential diagnosis is Kaposi's sarcoma (KS). In particular, the solid, cellular areas of spindled cells in SCH bear a resemblance to Kaposi's sarcoma but differ by containing an admixture of plump endothelial cells with clear to vacuolated cytoplasm. Ectatic, irregular vascular spaces are a component of plaque-stage KS, but frankly cavernous spaces containing thrombi and phleboliths are not.

Arteriovenous Hemangioma

Synonyms for arteriovenous hemangioma and related terms include *venous hemangioma, acral arteriovenous tumor, arteriovenous shunt, cirsoid aneurysm,* and *arteriovenous malformation.* Biberstein and Jessner reported the first case of arteriovenous hemangioma (AH) in 1956 as "cirsoid aneurysm."[37] The entity then lay relatively dormant in the literature until 1974 when Girard and coworkers characterized the salient clinical and histologic features of this benign entity in a report of 69 patients with histologically similar lesions that they termed *arteriovenous hemangioma.*[38] Subsequent reports have confirmed the benign nature of these vascular tumors and have emphasized the acral pattern of distribution by the assignment of the name *acral arteriovenous tumor.*[39,40]

The origin of these benign tumors is uncertain. Biberstein and Jessner considered their tumors to be true "cirsoid" aneurysmal dilatations of cutaneous arterial structures.[37] Other authors point out the resemblance of the fibromuscular vessels in AH to the Sucquet-Hoyer canal of the glomus and suggest that AH might be a hamartomatous proliferation of that structure. The issue remains unsettled.

Clinical Features The exact incidence of AH is unknown. The large number of cases included in most reports suggests that AH is a relatively common lesion. Our personal case files support this observation. AH primarily is a tumor of middle-aged to elderly adults with a peak incidence in the fourth and fifth decades of life (Table 31-10).[37–40] Rare

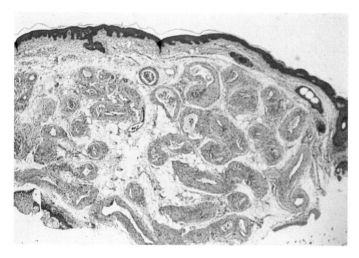

FIGURE 31-12 Arteriovenous hemangioma. Note thick-walled vessels in the dermis.

cases have occurred in childhood, the youngest patient being 6 weeks of age.

In most series, except that of Girard and coworkers,[38] males predominate. The lesions most commonly present as single, red or violaceous papules on the head or neck. They may be cutaneous or mucosal. Tumors have ranged in size from 1 mm to 3 cm, with an average of 4 to 6 mm. All are contained within the dermis in cutaneous sites and the submucosa in mucosal sites. Most are asymptomatic, but a minority of patients complain of enlargement, pain, or pruritus. Local excision is curative.

Histopathological Features AH lesions are well-circumscribed but unencapsulated (Table 31-10) [37–40] (Fig. 31-12). They are composed of an intimate admixture of thick-walled and thin-walled blood vessels distributed within the superficial and middle dermis. The proportion of thick-walled to thin-walled vessels is variable, although the former typically predominates (Fig. 31-13). The vessels may be closely approximated to and dispersed between the cutaneous and mucosal adnexae. The lining endothelium is a single layer in thickness and typically bland.

TABLE 31-10

Arteriovenous Hemangioma

Clinical Features

Most common in individuals 30 to 50 years of age
Men more than women
Head and neck, acral sites
Red or purple papules
Usually solitary, 4 to 6 mm (up to 3 cm)
Cutaneous or mucosal

Histopathological Features

Well-circumscribed, not encapsulated
Aggregates of thick-walled and thin-walled vessels
Variation in vessel caliber
Single layer of bland endothelium in vessels but occasional hobnail
    features present
Vessel walls contain fibrous tissue with occasional small smooth-
    muscle component
A true arterial component usually present

Differential Diagnosis

Cherry angioma
Lobular capillary hemangioma
Venous lake
Angioleiomyoma

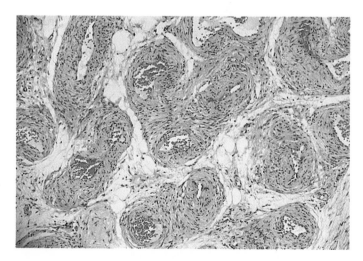

FIGURE 31-13 Arteriovenous hemangioma. Some of the vessels resemble arteries.

Occasionally the endothelial cells are prominent and protrude into the vessel lumen in a "hobnail" fashion. Thrombi, often showing organization and recanalization, are an occasional finding. The tumor stroma is characteristically collagenous. Girard and colleagues described direct communication between arteries and veins in a subset of their cases, whereas other authors have emphasized apparent "hybrid" fibromuscular channels reminiscent of the Sucquet-Hoyer canal of the glomus. Inflammation is an infrequent feature; when present it is described as a mixed, chronic inflammatory cell infiltrate associated with accentuation of fibrous changes within vessel walls.

Trichrome stains show the walls of thick-walled vessels to be predominantly fibrous with an inconspicuous smooth-muscle component. Elastin stains typically show finely fibrillar elastinophilic fibers scattered throughout the vessel wall. In most tumors, a true arterial component with an internal elastic lamina can be demonstrated.

Differential Diagnosis   The morphology of AH is characteristic, and a limited number of entities enter into the differential diagnosis. Clinically, venous lakes and cherry angiomas are a consideration due to their occurrence in a distribution and age group similar to AH's. The histology of each is distinct and easily distinguished from AH. Histologically, vascular leiomyomas are a consideration. The abundance of smooth muscle associated with these lesions is distinct from AH, as is the clinical setting.

Capillary Hemangioma

Also known as *juvenile capillary hemangioma* and *strawberry hemangioma*, capillary hemangiomas (CHs) are the most common tumors of infancy[2,3,4,22,41] (Table 31-11). The majority of such lesions present in the first few weeks of life as a solitary localized tumor in the skin. However, lesions involving multiple sites may occur. The incidence at birth is 1 to 2% and rises to 12% by age 1 year. Caucasians are most commonly affected relative to other racial groups, and females outnumber males by a ratio of 3 to 1. CHs are typified by a fairly predictable natural history in the great majority of cases: (1) rapid proliferation and enlargement in the first 8 to 12 months of life (the proliferating phase) and (2) regression of the lesion over a period of 1 to 5 years (the involuting phase). Over 50% of patients have complete regression of the CH by age 5 years, 70 to 90% by age 7 years, and there is continued involution in the remainder of patients to an age of 10 to 12 years. About 90% of CHs are associated with no adverse effects in children and do not necessitate any treatment. The remaining 10% require intervention, often because of local destructive effects or impingement on a vital structure such as an airway or the eye. In addition, large CH may result in shunting of blood and high-output cardiac failure or entrapment of platelets and a thrombocytopenic coagulopathy and a potentially life-threatening hemorrhage (the Kasabach-Merritt syndrome or phenomenon).[42] The pathogenesis of CH is poorly understood. There is an association with prematurity.

Clinical Features   CHs often present in the first month to first year of life as a pink macule often involving the head and neck and varying greatly in size. With growth these lesions become red to purplish papules or nodules that often have a rubbery texture. Some may occupy large areas, greatly distorting the normal anatomy and threatening vital structures. Some may exhibit ulceration usually from rapid growth. Involuting lesions develop whitish streaks which correspond to fibrosis.

Histopathological Features   In the initial proliferative phase, CHs are usually characterized by lobules of uniform endothelial cells with an admixture of pericytes and mast cells occupying the dermis and frequently the subcutaneous fat[2,3,4,22,41] (Fig. 31-14) (Table 31-11).

TABLE 31-11

Capillary Hemangioma

Clinical Features

Incidence at birth 1–2%, and 12% by 1 year
Most develop in the first month of life or in the first year
Females outnumber males by a ratio of 3:1
Caucasians most commonly affected racial group
Head and neck most common sites but may occur anywhere
Present initially as pink macular lesions that usually become red to purple nodules
Involution occurs with the development of whitish streaks
Natural history:
   Rapid proliferation and enlargement in the first 8 to 12 months of life
   Regression of the lesion over 1 to 5 years or longer
Occasional lesions may be life-threatening:
   Impingement on vital structures such as an airway
   The Kasabach-Merritt phenomenon, i.e., hemorrhage from entrapment of platelets in the hemangioma and development of a thrombocytopenic coagulopathy
   Shunting of blood and high-output cardiac failure

Histopathological Features

Proliferative phase:
   Highly cellular lobules separated by fibrous septa
   Lobules contain uniform endothelial cells with an admixture of pericytes and mast cells
   Mitoses are common
   Inconspicuous vascular lumina
   With time, the lobules become less cellular and vascular lumina become more prominent
Involuting phase:
   Vascular lobules composed almost entirely of microvessels
   Gradual replacement of lobules by myxoid fibrous tissue

Differential Diagnosis

Vascular malformations
Kaposiform hemangioendothelioma
Tufted angioma
Nonvascular tumors

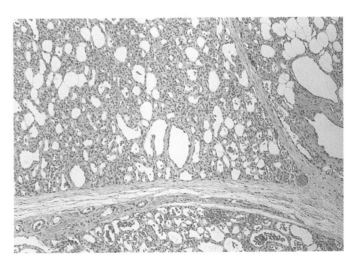

FIGURE 31-14   Juvenile capillary hemangioma, proliferative stage. The lesion contains lobules separated by fibrous septa. The lobules are composed of endothelial cells and small vascular channels.

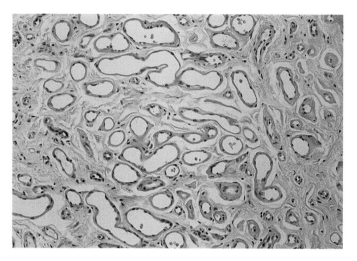

FIGURE 31-15 Juvenile capillary hemangioma, involutional stage. The vascular lobules at this stage are comprised of microvessels only, some of which have slightly hyalinized walls.

Vascular lumina may be difficult to discern but are usually present within the cellular lobules. The mitotic rate is usually significant at this stage. With time, the lobular character of the tumor becomes more evident, the degree of cellularity diminishes, and the vascular lumina are more readily identified (Fig. 31-15). With involution the vascular lobules are gradually replaced by fibrous tissue.

Differential Diagnosis   The clinical presentation of CH in children is usually distinctive. However, the differential diagnosis includes vascular malformations, kaposiform hemangioendothelioma, tufted angioma, and cellular nonvascular tumors of infancy. In the great majority of cases the lobular architecture of the tumor composed of aggregates of endothelial cells and pericytes and small well-formed vascular lumina is diagnostic. Vascular malformations often lack the well-defined lobular architecture and cellularity of CH. Vascular malformations also are often large, poorly delineated, and dominated by ectatic vascular channels with thin or thick walls or both or an admixture of various types of vascular channels such as capillary, venous, arterial, and even malformed vessels. Kaposiform hemangioendothelioma differs from conventional CH by showing spindle cell foci that contain irregular vascular channels and have resemblance to Kaposi's sarcoma. Tufted angioma is closely related to CH and differs only in degree by the discrete cellular nodules with cannonball-like appearance in the dermis.

Lobular Capillary Hemangioma (Pyogenic Granuloma)

Also known as *granuloma pyogenicum*, *granuloma gravidarum*, *botryomycosis humaine*, and *botryomycoma*, this common vascular lesion was once considered to be secondary to pyogenic infection or arising as exuberant granulation tissue in response to trauma. At present, it is best understood as a specific form of hemangioma, designated *lobular capillary hemangioma* because of its lobular architecture on low-power magnification.[43–48]

Clinical Features   Lobular capillary hemangioma (LCH) typically appears as a solitary, rapidly growing, dark red, exophytic, raised to polypoid, vascular lesion that frequently has superficial ulceration (Table 31-12). Many LCHs arise spontaneously without a known cause, and others are associated with trauma, pregnancy, or retinoid therapy. The most common sites for LCHs are the fingers, face, and oral cavity.

TABLE 31-12

Lobular Capillary Hemangioma

Clinical Features

Etiology: idiopathic, posttraumatic, pregnancy-, or retinoid-related
Many sites but most common: fingers, face, mouth
Rapidly growing, red, papule or polyp, frequently ulcerated
Satellite lesions, occasionally arise after trauma or removal
Rare eruptive, disseminated form
Rare wholly intradermal, subcutaneous, or intravenous forms

Histopathological Features

Lobular proliferations of capillaries
Cytologically bland endothelial cells
Epidermal flattening and peripheral collarette
Frequent superficial ulceration with secondary edema, hemorrhage, fibrin, necrosis, and acute inflammation

Differential Diagnosis

Capillary hemangioma
Bacillary angiomatosis
Acquired tufted angioma

In the latter location, lesions may be seen on the gingiva, lips, and tongue. The name, *granuloma gravidarum*, applies to a pyogenic granuloma arising on the gingival surface during pregnancy.

Pyogenic granuloma–like lesions consisting of granulation tissue have been described in cystic acne, treated with oral isotretinoin or secondarily infected with *Escherichia coli*. Etretinate, a retinoid akin to isotretinoin, has similarly been linked with the development of pyogenic granuloma–like lesions in patients with psoriasis. LCHs have been reported to occur intravenously and in subcutaneous tissue.

The phenomenon of satellite lesions arising after surgical removal, laser excision, or trauma to a pyogenic granuloma is well known. Satellite lesions usually occur on the trunk, particularly on the upper back of individuals less than 25 years of age. A rare, eruptive, disseminated, self-limited form with lesions that may number in the hundreds has been described. In most cases they have appeared spontaneously, although they have also arisen after a second-degree burn and after the removal of an ocular neoplasm. Underlying malignancy has been documented in some patients with disseminated pyogenic granulomas, but causation has not been established. The notion of a circulating angiogenic factor being involved in the pathogenesis is certainly intriguing but is still entirely speculative.

In one study, pyogenic granulomas from pregnant women showed no immunoreactivity for estrogen and progesterone receptor proteins. The negative results led to the conclusion that these steroid hormones are not directly involved in the formation of these vascular lesions.

Histopathological Features   Lobular capillary hemangiomas evolve through three, more or less, distinct phases (Table 31-12). In the early phase there is a compact vascular proliferation of solid, largely unopened vascular structures (Figs. 31-16 to 31-19). The histology is atypical with endothelial cells arranged seemingly in solid sheets with prominent nuclei and numerous mitotic figures. Later, there is a frank evolution into vascular structures with a multilobular arrangement and regular appearing lumina. In the final stage, there is a progressive development of pericytic cells, transformation into spindled smooth muscle, and evolution into veins. At the beginning, one or two veins dominate each lobule, but later there is extensive venulization of the whole lesion.

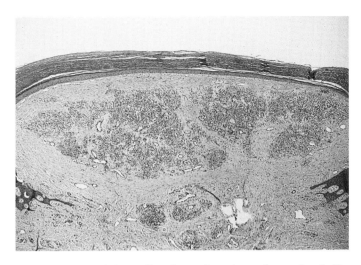

FIGURE 31-16   Lobular capillary hemangioma (pyogenic granuloma). The lesion is dome-shaped, has epidermal collarettes at the base, and exhibits a well-developed lobular architecture.

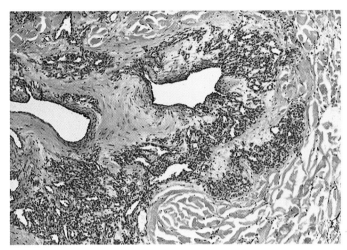

FIGURE 31-19   Lobular capillary hemangioma. There is "venulization" of the vascular lobules.

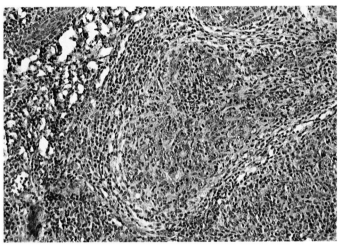

FIGURE 31-17   Lobular capillary hemangioma. Cellular phase with open vascular lumina.

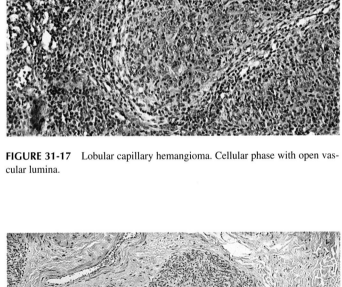

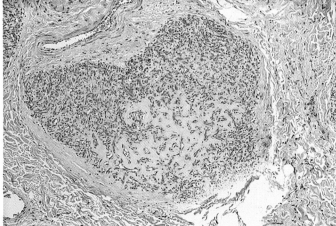

FIGURE 31-18   Lobular capillary hemangioma. Typical lobulated vascular phase with focal sclerosis.

Intra- and interlobular fibrosis ensues, and the lesion becomes progressively avascular and fibrotic. Rare examples may show a cavernous hemangioma appearance, but the typical lobular arrangement can be seen.

The typical LCH contains variably cellular but cytologically bland, lobular capillary proliferations with variable mitotic activity. The overlying epidermis is flattened, forms a peripheral collarette, and frequently shows erosion. As a result, LCHs often show secondary changes such as edema, hemorrhage, fibrin, necrosis, and acute inflammation. Intravenous LCHs extend into vascular lumina as polypoid lesions that connect with the wall of the vein by a fibrovascular stalk.

Immunohistochemically, the endothelial cells of the well-formed capillaries are positive for both factor VIII–related antigen and Ulex europaeus lectin. The endothelial cells of the more compact, cellular areas have shown similar results, although in one study the staining for factor VIII was equivocal. Vimentin stains all the endothelial cells as well as a concentrically arranged, perivascular spindled-cell proliferation that marks for muscle-specific actin and collagen type IV, and are likely to be pericytic. The immunopathologic and ultrastructural features of localized and disseminated pyogenic granulomas have been reported to be virtually identical.

Differential Diagnosis   The differential diagnosis of LCH is as varied as its clinical presentations and evolutionary stages. It may be confused clinically with amelanotic melanoma and eccrine poroma. Histologically, LCH has features that link it with tufted hemangioma. On occasion, the endothelial cells can be prominent and epithelioid, and a differential diagnosis with ALHE (epithelioid hemangioma) is required. The dermal form is sometimes confused with a glomus tumor.

Acquired Tufted Angioma

Also known as *angioblastoma (Nakagawa), progressive capillary hemangioma,* or *tufted hemangioma,* this entity was described by Wilson Jones and Orkin in 1976, and additional cases have better defined its clinicopathologic features.[49–51] Progressive capillary hemangioma (MacMillan) and angioblastoma (Nakagawa), an entity better known in the Japanese literature, have been regarded by many as similar or identical.[51] Acquired tufted angioma is considered to be a distinct clinicopathologic entity, related to the pyogenic granuloma (lobular capillary hemangioma), and peripheral satellite nodules resembling pyogenic granulomas have been observed. Furthermore, lesions reported as dermal pyogenic granulomas have been purported to be acquired tufted angioma.

Clinical Features   Classically, acquired tufted angioma (ATA) arises as slowly enlarging erythematous macules and plaques that often have a deep component and typically occur on the neck and upper trunk of children and young adults.[49,50] More than half of the cases have occurred during the first 5 years of life, and a few cases have presented at birth. ATA may present in adults; however, some of these cases have arisen within a preexisting, fixed vascular blemish or port-wine stain. ATAs are usually dull red in color, but occasionally the superficial component may appear more brightly red. ATAs are benign lesions that slowly enlarge over years and may attain considerable size.

ATA generally occurs sporadically. However, there has been one report of familial lesions with an autosomal dominant inheritance. One case of eruptive ATA of the right axilla and arm appearing in an older man soon after liver transplantation is documented. Surprisingly, the lesions were self-limited, involuting spontaneously over several months.

Histopathological Features   The hallmark of this hemangioma is the presence of small cellular, capillary tufts dispersed as "cannonballs" throughout the dermis[49–51] (Fig. 31-20). The tufts tend to be larger in the middle and lower dermis. The subcutaneous tissue is spared. Dilated lymphaticlike vessels may be present in the dermis and often appear as cleftlike lumina at the periphery of capillary tufts (Fig. 31-21). Protrusion of the tuft into the lumen may impart a glomerularlike appearance. The degree of cellularity within tufts may be so dense that capillary lumina may not be readily evident. Reticulin stains will reveal a rich network of reticulin that ensheathes individual endothelial cells. Mitotic figures may be seen, but cellular atypia is absent.

Immunoreactivity for factor VIII–related antigen and Ulex europaeus lectin is best seen in endothelial cells of larger, well-formed vascular channels. Ulex europaeus lectin also outlines the capillaries of the vascular tufts, but, except for occasional dilated lumina within these tufts, there is little to no staining for factor VIII–related antigen. Crystalline lamellae in endothelial cells have been identified in some but not all cases of ATA. They are not specific for ATA, since they have also been seen in strawberry hemangiomas and in fetal skin, apparently as an aspect of immature endothelial cells.

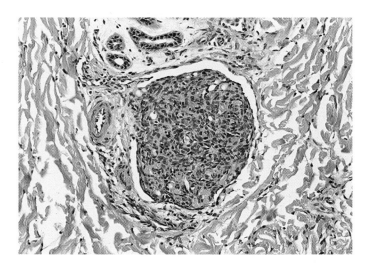

FIGURE 31-21   Acquired tufted angioma. There are typical crescent-shaped vessels at the periphery of the lobules (courtesy of Dr. C.D.M. Fletcher).

A more recent report of children with angioblastoma (Nakagawa) identified light microscopic features not previously reported with ATA, namely proliferation of eccrine glands near capillary tufts in all four patients and mucinous replacement of some capillary tufts in a single patient. Further review of cases of ATA might serve to clarify whether these are true differential features. For now, the literature seems to favor the view that ATA and angioblastoma are synonymous.

Differential Diagnosis   Although the progressive nature of ATA may invoke consideration of a low-grade angiosarcoma or Kaposi's sarcoma, the clinicopathologic features and particularly the early onset of most cases allow distinction. The most likely differential diagnosis is with lobular capillary hemangioma, a condition with which ATA may be related. Although the vascular lobules are very similar, the scattered nature of ATA is fairly characteristic. Glomeruloid hemangioma also can be very similar, but the systemic manifestations and the characteristic intralobular PAS-positive eosinophilic bodies are sufficient to allow the distinction. Similar thoughts are true for reactive angioendotheliomatosis. The heterogeneous appearance of the vascular lobules and different clinical presentations allow for a precise diagnosis. Dabska's tumor also may have a superficial resemblance to ATA. The endotheliotropic lymphocytes are, however, characteristic.

Glomeruloid Hemangioma

This rare hemangioma derives its name from its distinctive histologic resemblance to renal glomeruli and occurs in the setting of POEMS syndrome, a multisystem disorder consisting of polyneuropathy, organomegaly, endocrinopathy, M-protein, and skin changes.[52,53] The cutaneous manifestations include hyperpigmentation, hypertrichosis, hyperhidrosis, sclerodermalike skin thickening, and hemangiomas. Many patients with POEMS syndrome show overlapping features with multicentric Castleman's disease and its characteristic angiofollicular lymphoid hyperplasia of lymph nodes.

The glomeruloid hemangioma is considered to be a reactive endothelial proliferation, perhaps akin to reactive angioendotheliomatosis and the result of circulating angiogenic factors from activated lymphocytes. A very similar etiopathogenic situation, but with very different clinical and histologic presentation, is seen in patients with angiomatosis with luminal cryoprecipitates. These patients have circulating cryoproteins that when captured by endothelial cells of peripheral vessels produce

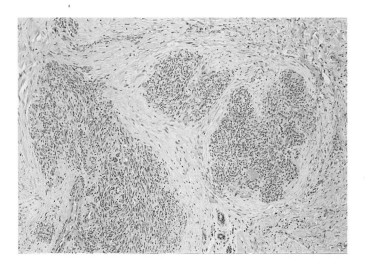

FIGURE 31-20   Acquired tufted angioma. Note discrete cellular lobules in dermis (courtesy of Dr. C.D.M. Fletcher).

TABLE 31-13

Glomeruloid Hemangioma

Clinical Features

Japanese > other populations
Fifth to sixth decades of life
Multiple, punctate to a few millimeters, erythematous or violaceous
  papules
Most common sites: trunk and proximal limbs

Histopathological Features

Conglomerates of capillaries within ectatic spaces, giving a
  glomeruluslike appearance
Generally bland endothelial cells
Occasional plump endothelial and stromal cells with pale cytoplasm,
  clear vacuoles, or eosinophilic globules
Little to absent inflammation

Differential Diagnosis

Acquired tufted angioma
Intravascular pyogenic granuloma
Intravascular papillary endothelial hyperplasia
Reactive angioendotheliomatosis
Endovascular papillary angioendothelioma (Dabska tumor)

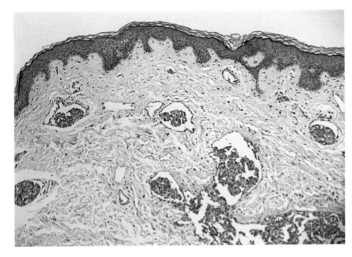

FIGURE 31-22   Glomeruloid hemangioma. Vascular channels throughout the dermis show the typical intravascular proliferation of endothelium reminiscent of renal glomeruli.

their proliferation with widespread inspissated cryoproteins in vascular lumina.

Clinical Features   Glomeruloid hemangiomas appear to be more common in the Japanese than other ethnic groups (Table 31-13). Only a few cases have been reported in the Caucasian population, affecting the fifth to sixth decades of life with no preponderance of sex. Patients with POEMS syndrome and hemangiomas have multiple, punctate-to-several-millimeter-sized, red or violaceous papules favoring the trunk and proximal limbs. Most of the hemangiomas are actually cherrylike capillary hemangiomas, with the glomeruloid hemangiomas being fairly rare. We have seen a case associated with multiple myeloma.

Histopathological Features   Ectatic vascular spaces are present in the dermis, and these contain glomeruluslike structures formed by conglomerates of blood-filled capillaries lined generally by flat endothelial cells[52,53] (Table 31-13) (Figs. 31-22 and 31-23). An occasional endothelial cell may be plump with pale cytoplasm, clear vacuoles, or eosinophilic globules. Similar cells that may be immature endothelial cells are interspersed as stromal cells between the capillary loops. The eosinophilic globules, PAS-positive and diastase-resistant, show polytypic immunoglobulin staining and presumably represent circulatory-derived immunoglobulin and other proteinaceous material. Mitoses are inconspicuous, numbering fewer than 1 per 10 high-power fields. There is little if any inflammation.

The cherry-type capillary hemangiomas may demonstrate rare, miniature glomeruloid tufts. The endothelial cells are positive for both factor VIII–related antigen and Ulex europaeus lectin 1. Many of the plump "stromal" cells are also positive for factor VIII–related antigen. Glomeruloid hemangiomas may have a striking degree of eosinophilic droplets.

Differential Diagnosis   Acquired tufted hemangioma is frequently associated with peripheral vascular clefts, but there is no actual intravascular angiomatous growth and they are devoid of eosinophilic globules.

The lesions occur in children and young adults as slowly growing macules and plaques that are larger than the small papules of glomeruloid hemangioma. Lobular capillary hemangioma (pyogenic granuloma) may rarely occur intravascularly but do not show the glomeruloid appearance of glomeruloid hemangioma. Intravascular papillary endothelial hyperplasia differs from glomeruloid hemangioma by having fibrous cores lined by plump endothelial cells and largely represents the organization of thrombotic matrix. Reactive angioendotheliomatosis shows dilated vessels that contain proliferations of endothelial cells that often fill lumina, have associated fibrin thrombi, and appear swollen or, at times, display mild cytologic atypia. In contrast to glomeruloid hemangioma, endovascular papillary angioendothelioma (Dabska tumor) shows intraluminal papillations lined by endothelium displaying some degree of pleomorphism. The vascular channels of endovascular papillary angioendothelioma are more primitive, and endothelial cells may appear to float free as single cells or clumps within vascular lumina. The hemorrhage and necrosis of more cellular lesions are not features of glomeruloid hemangioma.

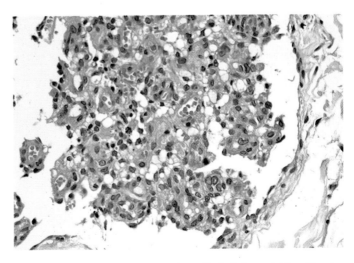

FIGURE 31-23   Glomeruloid hemangioma. Typical glomeruloid proliferation of blood vessels.

TABLE 31-14

Cherry Angioma

Clinical Features

Prevalent lesion that increases in frequency with age
Often multiple involving trunk and extremities
Well-defined papules 2–10 mm
Bright red to dusky purple

Histopathological Features

Dome-shaped
Epidermal collarettes
Lobular vascular proliferation
   Lobules containing thin-walled vascular channels, variable
     cellularity
   Lobules often separated by fibrous septa

Differential Diagnosis

Pyogenic granuloma
Arteriovenous hemangioma (malformation)
Venous malformation

Cherry Angioma

Also known as *senile angioma* or *Campbell de Morgan spot*, the cherry angioma is the most common vascular tumor encountered in the skin. The lesions develop in adults and increase in number with age.[14]

Clinical Features Cherry angiomas often develop in adults beginning in adolescence and are especially common in older adults[14] (Table 31-14). These angiomas occur at all sites but especially involve the trunk. They present as uniform bright to dull red papules ranging in size from 2 or 3 to 10 mm or so.

Histopathological Features Cherry angiomas are usually raised dome-shaped lesions that exhibit an epidermal collarette at the base of the tumor (Table 31-14). They are composed of fairly well-defined lobules composed of thin-walled dilated vascular channels that are largely confined to the papillary dermis (Fig. 31-24). In one sense they are a variant of lobular capillary hemangioma. The vascular lobules are

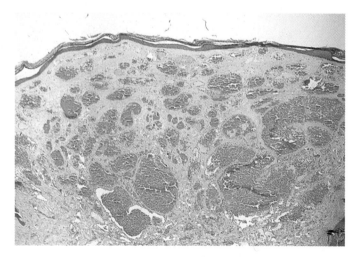

FIGURE 31-24   Cherry angioma. A dome-shaped lesion contains dilated vascular channels in a vaguely lobular configuration.

separated by fibrous septa that vary in thickness depending on the age of the lesion. The vascular channels comprising the proliferation are venular.

Differential Diagnosis The entities to be considered include pyogenic granuloma and bacillary angiomatosis because of the lobular architecture and epidermal collarettes. Cherry angioma does not show the endothelial proliferation noted in pyogenic granuloma or the inflammation, granular debris, and epithelioid endothelium observed in bacillary angiomatosis.

Bacillary Angiomatosis

This characteristic disorder, also known as *epithelioid angiomatosis*, typically occurs in patients with the acquired immunodeficiency syndrome.[54–56] In this setting, the clinical appearance may be mistaken for Kaposi's sarcoma, and this suspicion is raised by the highly vascular features of bacillary angiomatosis (BA).

Clinical Features BA most commonly presents as multiple angiomatous papules and nodules[54] (Table 31-15). However, clinical lesions vary in appearance and range greatly in number, from being solitary to numbering in the thousands. Minute papules; several-centimeter-sized nodules; flesh-colored, deep-seated subcutaneous lesions; an ulcerated, fungating mass; and involvement of underlying bone have all been described. The anatomic sites are diverse, and lesions may be widespread, with ocular, oral, and gastrointestinal mucosal surfaces often being involved concomitantly. Superficial skin lesions may form crusts and have a verrucous appearance. The clinical appearance of bacillary angiomatosis can mimic that of cherry angiomas; pyogenic granulomas, particularly of the disseminated type; and lesions of Kaposi's sarcoma.

TABLE 31-15

Bacillary Angiomatosis

Clinical Features

Caused by gram-negative bacillus *Bartonella henselae*
Individuals with AIDS with rare exceptions
Solitary to hundreds of lesions
Any location, especially ocular, oral, GI mucosal surfaces
Reddish papules, nodules; skin-colored subcutaneous nodules
Ulcerated fungating lesions
Fever, malaise, anorexia
Hepatosplenomegaly

Histopathological Features

Resemblance to pyogenic granuloma
Often dome-shaped with epidermal collarettes
Vague lobular vascular configuration
Endothelial cells usually protuberant, i.e., have epithelioid features
Edema
Neutrophilic infiltrates with leukocytoclasis
Granular purplish material located interstitially corresponds to bacteria
Organisms stain with Warthin-Starry, Steiner, and Dieterle reactions
   but are gram- and acid-fast-negative

Differential Diagnosis

Lobular capillary hemangioma (pyogenic granuloma)
Angiolymphoid hyperplasia with eosinophilia
Kaposi's sarcoma
Angiosarcoma

Constitutional symptoms and signs may occur such as fever, malaise, anorexia, and hepatosplenomegaly. Visceral involvement should be investigated, and cases may be found to have underlying bacillary peliosis hepatis and peliosis splenis, conditions comprised of blood-filled cysts, rupture of which can be life threatening. It is important to recognize the manifestations of bacillary angiomatosis because the disease can be readily treated with antibiotics, such as oral erythromycin.

BA has been associated with a gram-negative bacillus, recently identified as *Bartonella* (formerly *Rochalimaea*) *henselae*, or, in one patient, *Bartonella quintana*.[55] The bacillus has been linked to domestic cats as the reservoir, and the cat flea, *Ctenocephalides felis*, as the potential vector of this newly recognized zoonotic infection.[56]

Histopathological Features   The vasculature appears lobulated at low power resembling that of pyogenic granuloma (Table 31-15).[54] The vessels appear rounded to somewhat branching in a very edematous background. Endothelial cells are variably protuberant and may seem epithelioid in appearance. Numerous neutrophils are seen throughout, with leukocytoclasis and sometimes forming microabscesses (Fig. 31-25). On close scrutiny, masses of finely granular purplish material are present in the interstitium. Older lesions fibrose, and the resemblance to Kaposi's sarcoma may be striking.

The finely granular masses are accumulations of bacilli. On silver impregnation stains (e.g., Warthin-Starry, Steiner, Dieterle) they appear as rod-shaped with rounded extremities (Fig. 31-26). Not apparent on H&E stains, the bacilli may sometimes be observed intracellularly. These bacilli are gram- and acid-fast-negative. The bacillus appears very similar to that of cat-scratch disease. Curiously, it also has a taxonomic relationship with *Bartonella bacilliformis*, the agent of verruga peruana, a disease with cutaneous lesions that clinically and histologically are virtually indistinguishable from BA and constitute the second stage of bartonellosis, a chronic endemic disease in some areas of Perú and adjacent regions of South America.

Differential Diagnosis   The clinicopathologic features allow distinction from vascular tumors such as lobular capillary hemangioma/pyogenic granuloma, angiolymphoid hyperplasia with eosinophilia (epithelioid hemangioma), Kaposi's sarcoma, and angiosarcoma. The most helpful features for the recognition of BA are the presence of neutrophils and the interstitial, finely granular aggregates. Silver stains and,

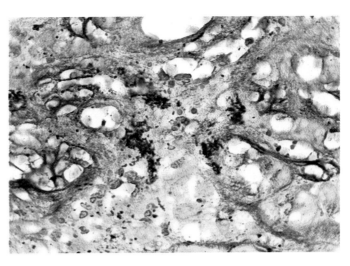

FIGURE 31-26 Bacillary angiomatosis. Interstitial debris stains positive (black) for bacteria (Steiner stain).

if needed, electron microscopy may be used to detect the bacilli and confirm the diagnosis. Although BA may show vague lobular aggregates of blood vessels, it lacks the well-organized lobular architecture that typifies pyogenic granulomas. In general, the latter findings are not observed in Kaposi's sarcoma. In particular, in contrast to Kaposi's sarcoma, bacillary angiomatosis lacks spindled cells, hyaline globules, and thin-walled vessels in "dissection" of dermal collagen. Moreover, the inflammatory cell infiltrate of Kaposi's sarcoma is predominantly lymphoplasmacytic.

Angiolymphoid Hyperplasia with Eosinophilia

Angiolymphoid hyperplasia with eosinophilia has many synonyms: *epithelioid hemangioma, subcutaneous lymphoid hyperplasia with eosinophilia, subcutaneous angiolymphoid hyperplasia with eosinophilia, atypical pyogenic granuloma, inflammatory angiomatous nodules with abnormal blood vessels, pseudopyogenic granuloma, papular angioplasia, atypical vascular proliferation with inflammation, intravenous atypical vascular proliferation, nodular angioblastic hyperplasia with eosinophilia and lymphofolliculosis,* and *histiocytoid hemangioma.* Angiolymphoid hyperplasia with eosinophilia (ALHE) is an entity that has evolved since the 1960s and has carried various names during that time.[57–62] Moreover, ALHE had been confused with Kimura's disease, a condition that differs clinicopathologically from ALHE and is now viewed as a separate entity.[59] Opinions regarding the pathogenesis of ALHE seem to favor a reactive vascular proliferation; however, origin as a primary vascular neoplasm or hemangioma must be considered.

Clinical Features   ALHE presents as single or multiple, pink to red-brown papules or plaques in the head and neck region of young to middle-aged adults, particularly women[57–62] (Table 31-16). The most common sites are the ear and forehead. Uncommonly, the trunk, extremities, and hands may be involved. Most lesions of ALHE are intradermal, but deeper extension into the subcutaneous tissue may occur, and occasionally the condition may arise as primary subcutaneous nodules. Peripheral blood eosinophilia is present in a minority of cases. Lesions of ALHE are usually asymptomatic, but on occasion there may be tenderness, pulsation, pruritus, or bleeding, either spontaneously or after minor trauma.

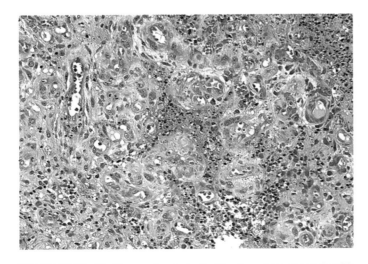

FIGURE 31-25 Bacillary angiomatosis. Proliferation of blood vessels with epithelioid endothelial cells. Note the interstitial neutrophils and basophilic debris.

TABLE 31-16

Angiolymphoid Hyperplasia with Eosinophilia

Clinical Features

Women more than men
Young to middle-aged adults
Head and neck region favored
Single or multiple, pink to red-brown papules or plaques
Peripheral blood eosinophilia, on occasion

Histopathological Features

Proliferation of blood vessels of variable diameter
Prominent endothelial cells
Enlarged, cuboidal or hobnail shape
Abundant eosinophilic to amphophilic cytoplasm and large vesicular
　　nuclei ("histiocytic" appearance)
Cytoplasmic vacuoles of variable size
Diffuse to nodular lymphocytic infiltrate
Lymphoid follicles
Variable numbers of eosinophils

Differential Diagnosis

Kimura's disease
Epithelioid hemangioendothelioma
Epithelioid angiosarcoma

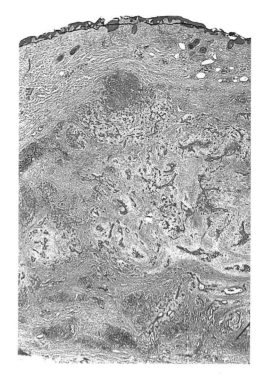

FIGURE 31-27 Angiolymphoid hyperplasia with eosinophilia. Low-power view of the vascular proliferation with peripheral rim of lymphocytes.

Histopathological Features ALHE shows blood vessel proliferation and inflammation[57-62] (Table 31-16) (Fig. 31-27). The vessels vary in diameter and are lined by prominent endothelial cells, a feature that is characteristic of ALHE and defines the entity (Fig. 31-28). These "histiocytic" endothelial cells led to the grouping of ALHE under the name *histiocytoid hemangioma*, a term used to encompass lesions of other organ systems that by light microscopy had cells with a similar appearance. However, the latter term (*histiocytoid hemangioma*) is eschewed by many, since such a category may encompass a diverse group of specific entities that may not necessarily be related. The endothelial cells are enlarged, cuboidal to "hobnail" in shape, with abundant eosinophilic to amphophilic cytoplasm and large vesicular nuclei (Fig. 31-28). Cytoplasmic vacuoles may be present and, when large, may distort the nucleus or coalesce into small lumina by merging with the vacuoles of other cells. There is an accompanying diffuse to nodular lymphocytic infiltrate, possibly with lymphoid follicles and germinal center formation. Variable numbers of eosinophils are present. There is zonation of the inflammatory infiltrate toward the periphery of the lesion. Occasional thrombi may be seen, and mitotic activity is generally inconspicuous to absent. Subcutaneous lesions, particularly those associated with arteriovenous malformations, tend to show prominent endothelial cell proliferation, sometimes forming solid intraluminal masses. Such solid proliferations of endothelial cells may obscure the true vascular nature of the lesion and occasionally lead to confusion in diagnosis.

Differential Diagnosis Clinicopathologic differences serve to differentiate ALHE from Kimura's disease. In particular, Kimura's disease lacks the characteristic endothelial cell of ALHE and is usually noted in young Asian males. A large subcutaneous mass occurs typically in the periauricular and submandibular regions. Commonly, there are associated manifestations such as lymphadenopathy, circulating eosinophilia, and increased serum levels of IgE. Distinctive histologic features of Kimura's disease include a florid lymphocytic infiltrate with prominent lymphoid follicles, germinal center vascularization, germinal center necrosis, sclerosis, and marked eosinophilia with or without eosinophil

abscess formation. There also are germinal center deposits of IgE and frequent involvement of skeletal muscle, salivary glands, and regional lymph nodes. Kimura's disease is considered to be the result of an immunologic reaction of allergic or autoimmune nature.

In comparison to ALHE, angiosarcoma generally has conspicuous cytologic atypia, frequent mitotic figures, piling up of cells, and lacks the inflammatory infiltrate of ALHE, although rare angiosarcomas can display substantial infiltrates. Solid areas of ALHE offer similarity in appearance to epithelioid angiosarcoma and even more so to epithelioid hemangioendothelioma. However, epithelioid angiosarcoma is generally a highly malignant appearing tumor that is more apt to be mistaken for poorly differentiated carcinoma than a lesion of ALHE. Epithelioid hemangioendothelioma (EH) is an angiocentric tumor that also may be

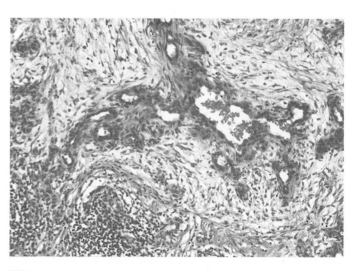

FIGURE 31-28 Angiolymphoid hyperplasia with eosinophilia. Multilayered epithelioid endothelial cells line the vascular structures.

mistaken for metastatic carcinoma. Vascular differentiation in EH is more primitive than that seen in ALHE and occurs primarily at the cellular level with the formation of vacuoles and intracellular lumina. The lesions are often desmoplastic, relatively noninflammatory, and frequently associated with a chondromyxoid matrix.

Microvenular Hemangioma

This hemangioma, also known as *microcapillary angioma*, with its characteristic histologic appearance of small dermal blood vessels was first described by Hunt and coworkers in 1991.[63] The clinicopathologic features of ten cases were presented, and 2 years later five additional cases were added to the literature by Aloi and colleagues.[64] Microvenular hemangioma is believed to be a type of acquired venous hemangioma. A very similar if not identical appearing angioma arising in young females under the hormonal influence of pregnancy or hormonal contraceptives has been referred to as *microcapillary angioma*.

Clinical Features   Microvenular hemangiomas (MVs) typically occur as solitary asymptomatic, small, enlarging, purple to red, plaques or nodules that favor the extremities of young to middle-aged adults of either sex (Table 31-17). In the original series, the patients (6 males, 4 females) ranged in age from 9 to 39 years (mean 28 years) and presented with lesions as large as 1 cm.[63] The later report showed similar demographics; however, the age range was extended to a 64-year-old woman who uniquely had two lesions, including the first described on the face.[64] Lesions in that series were slightly larger, between 1 and 2 cm. The duration of MV at presentation is usually brief, weeks to several months, but has been as long as 4 years. Clinically, MVs are generally viewed as a benign hemangioma, but the differential diagnosis has also included dermatofibroma and Kaposi's sarcoma.

Histopathological Features   The microvenular hemangioma is comprised of irregularly branching, small blood vessels, often with the appearance of collapsed venules[63,64] (Table 31-17) (Fig. 31-29). Lumina are generally inconspicuous, narrow to absent. Endothelial cells may, at times, be a little plump, but there is no cellular atypia. Some examples of MV have prominent epithelioid cells resembling those of epithelioid (histiocytoid) hemangioma. Glomeruloid aggregates of vessels can be seen in the deep dermis. These structures closely resemble those of lobular capillary hemangiomas and tufted hemangiomas.

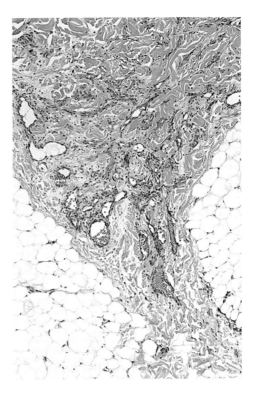

FIGURE 31-29   Microvenular hemangioma. Typical infiltrative growth pattern in lower dermis extending into the septum of the subcutaneous fat.

Examples of pyogenic granuloma merging with microvenular hemangioma have also been observed. There is a background of dermal desmoplasia with variably thickened dermal collagen. Inflammation and hemosiderin are generally scant or absent. Plasma cells and eosinophils are usually not observed. Immunohistochemically, the endothelial cells stain weakly for factor VIII–related antigen and strongly for Ulex europaeus lectin 1.

Differential Diagnosis   Microvenular hemangioma has a distinctive histologic appearance allowing little difficulty in diagnosis, although there may be some resemblance to stasis change, reactive angiogenesis in scars, early Kaposi's sarcoma, and the vascular proliferations in some lesions previously included under the name *sclerosing hemangioma*. The venular differentiation is also similar to that which may sometimes be seen in late stages of acquired tufted angioma and targetoid hemosiderotic hemangioma. Stasis change occurs in a clinical setting distinct from microvenular hemangioma, typically arising on the distal lower extremities of an individual with chronic venous insufficiency. Hemosiderin is abundant. Immature scars show irregularly arranged fibroblastic and vascular proliferations often associated with erythrocyte extravasation, hemosiderin deposition, and an inflammatory infiltrate that may contain a few plasma cells. This fibroblastic proliferation, red cell extravasation, and plasmacytic inflammation is lacking in microvenular hemangioma. Early Kaposi's sarcoma can be excluded by clinical setting along with the absence of angulated, irregular vascular spaces enveloping preexisting dermal blood vessels; plasma cells; hyaline (eosinophilic) globules; and, of course, any spindle cell population.

Targetoid Hemosiderotic Hemangioma

Also known as *hobnail hemangioma*, targetoid hemosiderotic hemangioma (THH) is a benign, possibly reactive, vascular lesion first described in 1988.[65] Additional cases have since been reported. THH is

---

TABLE 31-17

Microvenular Hemangioma

Clinical Features

Young to middle-age adults favored
Extremities most common site
Small, purple to red, plaques or nodules

Histopathological Features

Irregular branching, small blood vessels
Inconspicuous lumina
Variable degree of desmoplasia
Scant or absent inflammatory infiltrate

Differential Diagnosis

Stasis change
Scar
Early Kaposi's sarcoma
Sclerosing hemangioma/dermatofibroma

Targetoid Hemosiderotic Hemangioma

Clinical Features

Men more than women
Young adults favored
Diverse sites
Annular targetlike lesion: central violaceous papule surrounded by
    a pale rim and a more peripheral expanding ecchymotic ring

Histopathological Features

Early lesions:
    Widely dilated, irregular, thin-walled vascular lumina in the
        superficial dermis
    Endothelial cells flat to epithelioid
    Intraluminal papillary projections usually lined by a single layer of
        epithelioid endothelial cells
    Narrower, more angulated and inconspicuous vessels "dissecting"
        collagen bundles of the deeper reticular dermis
    Dermal edema, red blood cell extravasation, hemosiderin, little
        lymphocytic inflammation
Later lesions:
    Collapsed lumina
    Extravascular spindle cells
    Narrow, angulated, thin-walled vessels crisscross the dermis in
        "dissection" of collagen
    Variable hemosiderin deposition

Differential Diagnosis

Early Kaposi's sarcoma
Lymphangiomalike Kaposi's sarcoma
Benign lymphangioendothelioma

---

one of the histologic simulants of Kaposi's sarcoma, and knowledge of its clinicopathologic features is crucial to the avoidance of misdiagnosis. A role for trauma in the pathogenesis of THH has been suggested by some.

Clinical Features   THH typically presents as a solitary, annular, violaceous to purple papule 2 to 3 mm in diameter, with both a surrounding pale rim and a more peripheral ecchymotic ring giving a targetlike appearance (Table 31-18).[65] This ring expands peripherally and then eventually disappears. Late lesions may show only a purple-brown, slightly elevated papule. This event appears to be secondary to trauma or thrombosis and may not be a constant feature. This raises the question as to how many of the clinical (and histologic) features are primary and how many are secondary changes. The majority of patients to date have been men and young with an age range of 17 to 58 years. There is no apparent site preference.

One case of THH was reported as an acquired process developing in a congenital lesion of 17 years' duration, and another involved the trunk in the belt line, both cases suggesting a role for trauma in their development.

Histopathological Features   The histology of THH varies according to the duration or age of the individual lesion. The earliest finding is a proliferation of widely dilated and irregular, thin-walled vascular lumina in the superficial dermis (Table 31-18)[65] (Fig. 31-30). The endothelial cells are flat or conspicuously epithelioid. Intraluminal papillary projections lined by a single layer of epithelioid endothelial cells in "hobnail" fashion are often seen protruding into vascular lumina (Fig. 31-31).

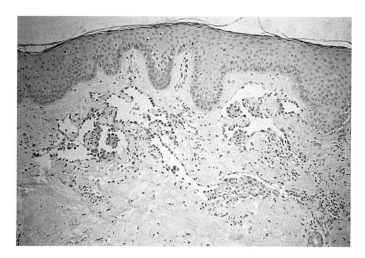

FIGURE 31-30   Targetoid hemosiderotic hemangioma. Superficial portion of lesion with irregular vascular lumina and prominent dissection of collagen bundles.

These plump endothelial cells may occasionally pileup and even obliterate vascular lumina. Intraluminal fibrin thrombi may be present.

Vessels deeper in the reticular dermis have an inconspicuous endothelial cell lining and become angulated and irregular, appearing to dissect collagen bundles. The vessels tend to be oriented around adnexal structures, such as eccrine coils. Other features of THH are dermal edema; variable, often intense red blood cell extravasation; hemosiderin deposition; and an inconspicuous to mild, predominantly lymphocytic, inflammatory infiltrate.

Overall on low-power magnification, THH gives a stratified appearance with ectatic vessels containing epithelioid endothelial cells at the top and angulated, inconspicuous vessels at the bottom. Mature lesions show most vascular lumina to be collapsed and increased cellularity of extravascular tissue. Spindle cells appear in close approximation to the vascular proliferation. Late lesions demonstrate collapsed, anastomosing, thin-walled vessels crisscrossing the dermis. Immunohistochemically, the endothelial cells of the targetoid hemosiderotic hemangioma stain weakly for factor VIII–related antigen and strongly with Ulex europaeus lectin 1.

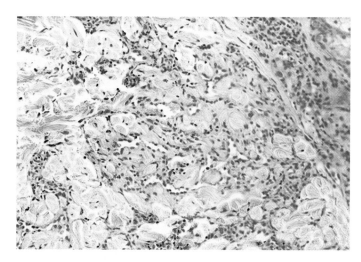

FIGURE 31-31   Targetoid hemosiderotic hemangioma. Deep portion of the process with angulated vessels lined by thin endothelial cells that dissect collagen.

Differential Diagnosis   Targetoid hemosiderotic hemangioma appears histologically as an atypical vascular lesion with similarity to Kaposi's sarcoma of the patchstage and lymphangiosarcomalike types and to benign lymphangioendothelioma. The clinical setting is helpful in differentiating these lesions because THH occurs as a solitary small lesion in healthy individuals. Outside of Africa, Kaposi's sarcoma is seen classically in the elderly or secondary to the acquired immunodeficiency syndrome. Lesions of Kaposi's sarcoma are typically multiple and of variable size. Benign lymphangioendothelioma is clinically distinct from THH and occurs as well-demarcated dermal plaques that are larger in size than THH and often reach considerable proportions.

THH shares histologic features with patches of KS. These similarities include angulated vascular lumina dissecting collagen bundles, erythrocyte extravasation, hemosiderin deposition, and, in late lesions, the presence of spindle cells. Differential features are present, however, and in particular the low-power appearance of THH shows stratification whereas Kaposi's sarcoma tends to be "bottom heavy." The papillary intraluminal projections and epithelioid endothelial cells of early lesions of THH are not features of KS. In contrast to patch-stage Kaposi's sarcoma, THH typically lacks plasma cells and is more apt to show significant erythrocyte extravasation and hemosiderin. A lymphoplasmacytic infiltrate is typical of early KS but is infrequent in THH, with plasma cells being identified focally in only one of the reported cases. Apoptotic endothelial cells may be seen in early KS but do not seem to be a feature of THH. Despite all these features, the overlap in features of THH and KS may be so great that clinicopathologic correlation is necessary to separate the lesions.

The lymphangiomalike variant of KS and lesions of benign lymphangioendothelioma can also be confused histologically with THH, particularly in regard to mature lesions of THH. In all these entities, relatively bland, empty, irregular blood vessels are found in dissection of dermal collagen. The clinical setting is important for the discrimination of these entities. Fortunately, patients with lymphangiomalike Kaposi's sarcoma have extensive, clinically typical KS. Histologically, benign lymphangioendothelioma lacks hemosiderin, extravasated erythrocytes, and plasma cells and clinically is quite different, being a much more extensive process than THH. In late lesions, THH needs to be differentiated from the vessel-rich variant of dermatofibroma, the sclerosing hemangioma.

Acro-Angiodermatitis

Also known as *stasis dermatitis*, *angiodermatitis*, or *pseudo-Kaposi's sarcoma*, acro-angiodermatitis (AA) is a reactive vasoproliferative condition first described in 1965 by Mali and colleagues.[66–69] Eighteen patients, with chronic venous insufficiency of the lower extremities, presented with violaceous plaques on the extensor surface of the foot and toes. In several patients, the diagnosis of Kaposi's sarcoma was a clinical consideration. Since this initial report, the characteristic constellation of reactive vascular proliferation, dermal fibrosis, and hemosiderin deposition has also been reported in the setting of arteriovenous malformations. The name, *acro-angiodermatitis* is a misnomer, as the spectrum of changes is reactive in nature and does not reflect an inflammatory dermatosis. This name, however, is preferable to the proposed alternative of *pseudo-Kaposi's sarcoma*.

Clinical Features   In a given population, the incidence of mild forms of stasis dermatitis parallels the incidence of chronic venous insufficiency (Table 31-19). In comparison to the incidence of chronic venous insufficiency, however, the florid clinical lesions described by Mali, and later by Strutton,[66] are relatively uncommon and are an exaggerated vasoproliferative response to venous stasis. Most affected patients are

TABLE 31-19

Acro-Angiodermatitis

Clinical Features

Chronic venous insufficiency
Venous stasis
Arteriovenous malformation/shunts
Middle age or older
Younger distribution with congenital or acquired AV causes
Scaly, violaceous papules, plaques, and nodules
Distal lower extremities, particularly extensor foot and toes
Accompanying stasis dermatitis
Extremity with AV malformation or hemodialysis shunt

Histopathological Features

Epidermal acanthosis and compact hyperkeratosis
Proliferation of small blood vessels with dilated, round lumina
Upper half of the dermis
Dermal edema and variable fibrosis
Extravasated erythrocytes and hemosiderin, especially perivascular
Inconspicuous mononuclear inflammatory infiltrate

Differential Diagnosis

Kaposi's sarcoma
Pyogenic granuloma, dermal type

middle-aged or older. In the original paper, males predominated, though the incidence of chronic venous insufficiency is higher in women.[62] Later reports, by a number of authors, have emphasized the occurrence of acro-angiodermatitis in younger patients with relative chronic venous insufficiency associated with arteriovenous malformations whether they be congenital or acquired. In particular, AA has been reported as an acquired, iatrogenic complication of arteriovenous shunts for hemodialysis. AA has been seen in venous stasis associated with paralytic feet, in the hypertrophied leg of a patient with the Klippel-Trenaunay syndrome, and in the setting of an above-the-knee amputation stump, attributed to chronic circulatory disturbance from a poorly fitting suction-type prosthesis.

The clinical lesions of acro-angiodermatitis are scaly, violaceous plaques, papules, and nodules. In chronic venous insufficiency of the lower extremities, the lesions are most numerous over the extensor surfaces of the toes and foot. They tend to spare areas of the foot where direct pressure, either extrinsic or intrinsic, is applied. Areas of sparing include points where adjacent digits contact each other or a shoe.[62] Lesions may also occur on the lateral aspect of the ankle and anterior lower leg.[67] Surrounding tissues are edematous and show changes of stasis dermatitis. Acro-angiodermatitis arising in the setting of arteriovenous malformation presents a similar clinical picture, limited to the extremity involved by the arteriovenous malformation. Because AA is a reactive, vasoproliferative response, it is not generally amenable to direct surgical approaches, and therapy to limit progression of lesions is directed at the underlying cause.

Histopathological Features   Reactive epidermal acanthosis and compact hyperkeratosis are frequent features of AA (Table 31-19). The most striking histologic changes involve the papillary and superficial to mid-reticular dermis. A proliferation of small blood vessels with dilated, round lumina are distributed throughout the dermis in a loose, vaguely lobular arrangement[66–69] (Fig. 31-32). The vessels tend to be relatively uniform in size and regular in contour. The endothelial cells are plump

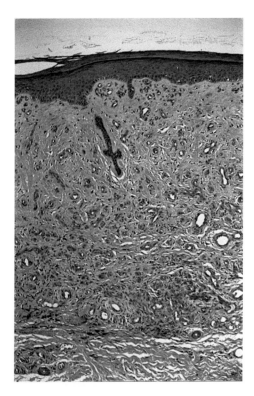

FIGURE 31-32   Acro-angiodermatitis. Subepidermal lobular vascular proliferation with deposition of hemosiderin.

and one cell layer in thickness. The cytologic features are bland. The neovascular proliferation is superimposed on a background of dermal edema and fibrosis. The contribution of each component varies from lesion to lesion and varies in individual lesions over time. The dermal edema may be quite pronounced, particularly in the papillary dermis. Fibrosis is more variable and ranges from inconspicuous, represented by a relatively sparse number of fibroblasts, to quite pronounced, with dense dermal fibrosis. Similar vascular proliferation is seen around sweat gland coils.

Extravasated erythrocytes are distributed in perivascular sites. The extent of erythrocyte extravasation is variable and often prominently associated with more superficial dermal vessels. Dermal deposition of hemosiderin may be quite exuberant and reflects chronic, ongoing erythrocyte extravasation and degradation. Hemosiderin deposition is most prominent in a perivascular pattern and may be extracellular or contained within dermal macrophages. An inconspicuous, mononuclear inflammatory infiltrate is an inconstant feature. Plasma cells are an infrequent component of the inflammatory infiltrate and never a prominent finding.

Differential Diagnosis   The clinical lesions of AA may closely resemble the lesions of classic Kaposi's sarcoma (KS). A clinical history of chronic venous insufficiency and a background of stasis changes should raise the consideration of AA. Certainly, the presence of a local AV malformation or fistula should prompt consideration of AA, but the possibility of an unsuspected AV malformation should not be overlooked when a diagnosis of AA or KS is entertained in a young individual. The microscopic features of AA are distinct from KS. The vessels of AA are arranged in a lobular pattern; have a round, regular contour; are centered in the papillary dermis; and show no tendency to localize around preexisting dermal structures. KS, in contrast, shows a haphazard arrangement of slitlike vascular spaces arranged around dermal structures. The

inflammatory infiltrate in KS is more pronounced than that of AA and contains more plasma cells.

The confusion of AA with lesions of KS occurs primarily when biopsies of either entity are interpreted in isolation from clinical data. Attention to clinical history, physical findings, and correlation of histologic findings should lead to the correct diagnosis. Chronic lesions of atrophie blanche (hyalinizing segmental vasculitis) may have similar vasoproliferative changes, usually associated with vascular fibrin deposits.

Also, the lobular pattern of vascular proliferation may be quite pronounced and may vaguely mimic the vascular proliferation of dermal pyogenic granuloma, a point emphasized by Le Boit in a paper that proposes the lobular proliferation of capillaries as the underlying process in a number of benign vascular tumors and reactive conditions.[68]

Intravascular Papillary Endothelial Hyperplasia

In 1923, Masson first described as vegetant intravascular hemangioendothelioma an unusual angiosarcomalike proliferation in organizing thrombi of hemorrhoidal veins.[70–73] However, the phenomenon received little attention until the last two decades, when the clinicopathologic features of intravascular papillary endothelial hyperplasia became better defined.

Clinical Features   Intravascular papillary endothelial hyperplasia (IPEH), also known as *Masson's tumor*, *intravascular angiomatosis*, or *vegetant intravascular hemangioendothelioma*, occurs in patients of all ages (Table 31-20).[70–73] The typical presentation is that of a slowly enlarging, often tender, blue to red, deep dermal to subcutaneous swelling or mass. IPEH occurs at diverse sites, the most frequent of which are the head and the extremities, particularly the fingers. The duration at presentation is often more than 1 year, and has been as long as 21 years. Multiple lesions appearing as violaceous papules and nodules on the lower extremities of an elderly woman have clinically mimicked Kaposi's sarcoma.

TABLE 31-20

Intravascular Papillary Endothelial Hyperplasia

Clinical Features

All ages
Diverse sites; head, extremities, fingers most common
Predilection for hemorrhoidal veins
Slowly enlarging swelling, often tender and blue to red
Dermal to subcutaneous location
Arises in skin in the absence of, or more commonly within, a
  preexisting vascular lesion

Histopathological Features

Intravascular papillary endothelial-lined structures with fibrous cores
Generally flattened endothelial cells
Underlying organizing, thrombotic matrix
Vascular lumina variably filled by the process
Mitotic figures absent or rare

Differential Diagnosis

Angiosarcoma
Glomeruloid hemangioma
Endovascular papillary angioendothelioma (Dabska tumor)

In native blood vessels, IPEH develops within arterial thromboemboli and venous thrombi, particularly those of hemorrhoids. In the skin, IPEH occurs as a pure form without any apparent prior lesion or, more commonly, as a focal change within a preexisting pyogenic granuloma or other hemangioma. IPEH has arisen within vascular malformations, hemangiomas of the blue rubber bleb nevus syndrome, and cervical cystic hygromas. IPEH has also been identified in unusual sites, such as the eyelid, oral mucosa, and tongue. Extravascular papillary endothelial hyperplasia has also been reported in an organizing hematoma of the thyroid gland. Surgical excision of IPEH is usually curative, although recurrence after excision has been reported.

Histopathological Features   IPEH shows conspicuous intravascular papillary structures that are formed by cores of fibrous tissue that are lined by endothelial cells that are generally flattened in appearance (Table 31-20) (Fig. 31-33). Endothelial cells at times, however, may be plump with mildly enlarged nuclei, and there may be some piling up. Mitotic figures are generally absent or rare. IPEH may virtually fill the lumina of some blood vessels. A characteristic feature in most cases is the presence of an underlying thrombotic matrix that appears to be undergoing the process of organization. The papillary projections result from the endothelialization of fragmented thrombotic material and the ingrowth of anastomosing capillaries. Immunohistochemically, IPEH shows a pattern of reactivity similar to that of organizing thrombi. Factor VIII–related antigen is only seen in advanced lesions.

Differential Diagnosis   The juxtaposition or fusion of adjacent papillae results in an irregular, vascular network reminiscent of the pattern seen in angiosarcoma. However, key histologic features in identifying IPEH are the thrombotic matrix, the intraluminal location, and the relative absence of both cytologic atypia and mitotic activity. Necrosis and solid cellular areas are absent. Glomeruloid hemangiomas differ from

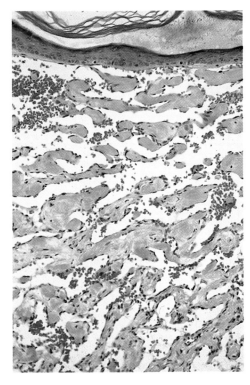

FIGURE 31-33 Intravascular papillary endothelial hyperplasia. Papillary fronds with thin endothelial cells and collagenous cores.

IPEH by showing conglomerates of blood-filled capillaries lined by endothelial cells that may display clear vacuoles and eosinophilic globules. In addition, IPEH has papillations with fibrous cores and is largely a process resulting from the organization of thrombotic matrix.

Angioendotheliomatosis

In 1959, Pfleger and Tappeiner described a rare vascular disorder that they subsequently named *angioendotheliomatosis proliferans systemisata*.[74,75] Over subsequent years, additional cases of angioendotheliomatosis were reported, and their disparate clinical courses illustrated that there were actually two distinct categories: reactive and malignant. Reactive angioendotheliomatosis is a benign process often associated with an underlying chronic infection, such as subacute bacterial endocarditis. Malignant angioendotheliomatosis is an intravascular malignant lymphoma that has also been termed *intravascular lymphomatosis* and *malignant intravascular lymphomatosis*.[76]

REACTIVE ANGIOENDOTHELIOMATOSIS

Also known as *angioendotheliomatosis proliferans systemisata*, *Tappeiner-Pfleger disease*, or *reactive forms of proliferating or systemic angioendotheliomatosis*, reactive angioendotheliomatosis (RAE) is extremely rare and includes the case described by Pfleger and Tappeiner, a patient reported by Gottron and Nikolowski 1 year earlier, and but a handful of others.[77–80] The earliest case was possibly reported by Merklen and Wolf in 1928 as "arterio-capillary endotheliitis." The etiology is unknown, but inflammatory or immunologic reactions and a pathogenesis involving a circulating angiogenic factor have been suggested. An endothelial proliferative response to bacterial antigens and to cryoproteins has been proposed.

Clinical Features   There is no age or sex predilection. Patients have varied from the first year of life to the eighth decade. Lesions of RAE are multiple and may occur as red-brown patches or plaques and purple-red nodules.[77–80] Sites of involvement have included the face, earlobes, trunk, and limbs. Necrosis and ulceration can occur. An associated infection may be present, the most common of which is subacute bacterial endocarditis but individual associations with pulmonary tuberculosis, Chagas' disease, and acute otitis media have been documented. Many cases have constitutional symptoms, such as fever, malaise, and weight loss.

Treatment is generally directed at the underlying disorder. Antibiotics, with or without systemic corticosteroids, are the most commonly employed therapy. Lesions of RAE generally resolve slowly over time, and no deaths from RAE have been reported.

Histopathological Features   Reactive angioendotheliomatosis shows dilated dermal and subcutaneous vessels that contain proliferations of small to enlarged endothelial cells that variably fill and often occlude vascular lumina (Fig. 31-34). Nuclei may appear vesicular. Fibrin thrombi may be present. Being endothelial in nature, the intraluminal cells of RAE react with endothelial markers. Most of the cells stain with factor VIII–related antigen and, to a lesser degree, with Ulex europaeus lectin 1.

Differential Diagnosis   The reactive form of angioendotheliomatosis must be distinguished from intravascular malignant lymphoma as discussed in the next section. The latter condition, malignant angioendotheliomatosis, displays cytologically malignant cells that mark as lymphoid cells by immunohistochemistry.

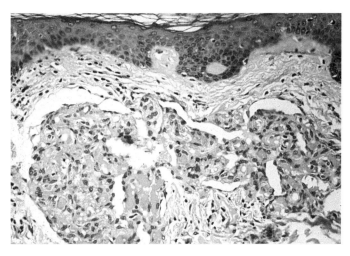

FIGURE 31-34 Reactive angioendotheliomatosis. Tufted proliferation of cells in intraluminal location.

Malignant Angioendotheliomatosis

Also known as *neoplastic angioendotheliosis, intravascular lymphomatosis, malignant intravascular lymphomatosis, angiotropic (intravascular) large-cell lymphoma,* or *cerebral angioendotheliomatosis,* malignant angioendotheliomatosis (MAE), in contrast to reactive angioendotheliomatosis, is an aggressive disease that generally is associated with progressive clinical manifestations leading to death.[76,81,82] The onset is insidious, and by the time MAE presents with neurologic and cutaneous manifestations, the course is rapidly fatal. This is not a vascular neoplasm but a lymphoma.

Clinical Features   Skin lesions present as tender, erythematous to purple, plaques and nodules over the trunk and extremities.[76,81,82] Typically, there are constitutional symptoms and signs of multiple-organ-system dysfunction. Cerebral involvement may result in a bizarre clinical picture of multifocal neurologic signs and progressive dementia, the etiology of which, particularly in the absence of cutaneous disease, may not become apparent until autopsy. Although there may be response to chemotherapy, the general prognosis of malignant angioendotheliomatosis is quite poor.

Histopathological Features   Malignant angioendotheliomatosis is similar to reactive angioendotheliomatosis in that dilated vascular lumina contain, or are occluded by, accumulations of cells and fibrin thrombi.[76,81,82] However, in contrast to the reactive form, cytologic atypia is prominent in malignant angioendotheliomatosis. Furthermore, mitotic figures are conspicuous, necrosis is more common, and extravascular tissue infiltration by a lymphomatous-appearing infiltrate can occur. Initial ultrastructural and histochemical studies erroneously supported the concept of an endothelial-derived neoplasm by alleging various features, such as Weibel-Palade bodies and factor VIII–related antigen expression. Additional studies, however, revealed the lymphomatous nature of most cases of malignant angioendotheliomatosis. Tumor cells react with lymphoid markers and fail to stain with endothelial cell markers. Prior reports of factor VIII–related antigen staining have not been corroborated or have been attributed to nonspecific staining, possibly secondary to the adsorption of platelet-derived factor VIII by tumor cells embedded in fibrin-platelet thrombi. Malignant angioendotheliomatosis may have either a T- or B-cell immunophenotype.

Differential Diagnosis   The presence of a cytologically malignant infiltrate of nonepithelioid, generally lymphoid-appearing cells filling

vascular lumina is distinct from the appearance of most other diseases, including that of metastatic carcinoma, and generally proclaims the diagnosis of malignant angioendotheliomatosis. Immunohistochemical staining for lymphoid markers is useful in confirming the diagnosis and in subclassifying the type of lymphoma.

Glomus Tumor

In 1924, Masson described the glomus tumor as a distinct neoplasm with morphologic similarities to the normal neuromyoarterial glomus, an arteriovenous shunt concerned with temperature regulation, located in the reticular dermis of the skin of the nail beds, the pads of the fingers and toes, the volar side of the hands and feet, the ears, and the center of the face.[83–89] This arteriovenous anastomosis consists of a vessel with a thick, cellular wall (Sucquet-Hoyer canal) connecting the two circulations prior to the ramification of the capillary bed. A neural network surrounds this thick-walled canal and peripherally there is a capsule of connective tissue.

Clinical Features   Glomus tumors can be classified into solitary and multiple types.[83–89] (Table 31-21) The typical solitary glomus tumor occurs in an adult as a small, blue-red nodule, less than 1 cm in diameter, in the deep dermis or subcutis of the extremities. The most common site is the subungual region of the finger where glomus tumors typically produce a triad of symptoms: pain, which may be paroxysmal; tenderness; and temperature sensitivity. Unusual sites of glomus tumors have included the stomach, rectum, cervix, vagina, mesentery, chest wall, bone, eyelid, and nose. An intravascular glomus tumor occurring within a vein of the forearm has been reported.

In contrast to solitary glomus tumors, multiple glomus tumors are uncommon, often present in childhood, are generally asymptomatic, arise in more proximal sites, only rarely occur subungually, and can be subdivided anatomically into whether they are regional or disseminated. Compared to the regional type, the disseminated form is often familial, with inheritance as an autosomal dominant trait. Congenital multiple plaquelike glomus tumors have been recently reported and are nonfamilial. In general, multiple glomus tumors are usually larger than solitary tumors and may reach several centimeters in size. Widespread glomangiomas presenting in infancy may mimic the blue rubber bleb nevus syndrome.

Glomangiosarcoma or malignant glomus tumor is exceedingly rare with just a few cases having been reported. These tumors typically have sarcoma accompanying a glomus tumor. The prognosis has been good without documented metastases, perhaps because early presentation secondary to pain has led to excision while the tumor is still small. However, because none of the cases have metastasized, some might question their designation as malignant. De novo glomangiosarcoma is exceedingly rare and must be distinguished from other round-cell sarcomas.

Histopathological Features   The histology of the glomus tumor is very distinctive.[83–89] (Table 31-21) The typical glomus cell is round or cuboidal with a round nucleus in amphophilic to eosinophilic cytoplasm and occurs in monotonous nests and sheets that are interrupted by many blood vessels, around which the glomus cells form collars (Figs. 31-35, 31-36). Depending upon the relative proportions of smooth muscle and blood vessels, glomus tumors have been subclassified as glomangioma and glomangiomyoma. Solitary glomus tumors are usually encapsulated, contain numerous small blood vessels, and are associated with ample nerve fibers.

Multiple glomus tumors generally appear as glomangiomas, tumors with large, irregularly shaped vascular spaces that may resemble those

TABLE 31-21

Glomus Tumor

Clinical Features

Solitary type
  Adults
  Nail beds, pads of fingers and toes, volar surfaces of hands and feet,
    ears, center of face
  Blue-red nodule
  < 1 cm
  Pain, often paroxysmal
  Tenderness
  Temperature sensitivity
Multiple type
  Childhood common
  Proximal ≫ distal sites
  Regional
  Disseminated, often familial
  Bluish nodules
  Often > 1 cm
Often asymptomatic

Histopathological Features

Solitary type
  Dermal or subcutaneous
  Well-circumscribed
  Encapsulated usually
  Nests and sheets of monotonous round or cuboidal cells
  Glomus cells cuff small vascular channels
  Round nucleus with amphophilic or eosinophilic cytoplasm
  Smooth muscle may be present (glomangiomyoma)
  Nerve fibers present
  Occasional myxoid stroma
Multiple type
  Large, irregularly shaped vascular (cavernous) channels
    (glomangioma)
  Usually fewer layers of glomus cells cuffing vessels
  Glomus cells may blend with smooth muscle (glomangiomyoma)
Immunohistochemistry
  Postive for vimentin, smooth-muscle actin, myosin, desmin
    (variable)
  Negative for factor VIII–related antigen, S-100 protein

Differential Diagnosis

Adnexal tumor
  Eccrine acrospiroma
  Chondroid syringoma (mixed tumor)
Mastocytoma
Melanocytic nevi (pseudoangiomatous)
Cavernous malformation
Hemangiopericytoma
Angioleiomyoma

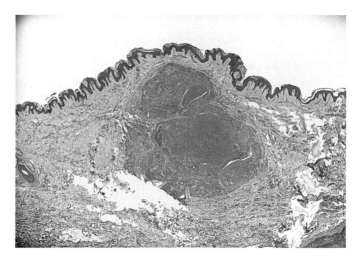

FIGURE 31-35   Glomus tumor. Solid variant.

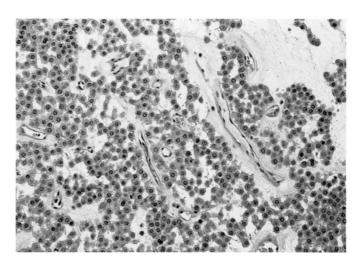

FIGURE 31-36   Glomus tumor. Solid variant. Note the similarities to an epithelial tumor. The tumor is composed of uniform cuboidal cells.

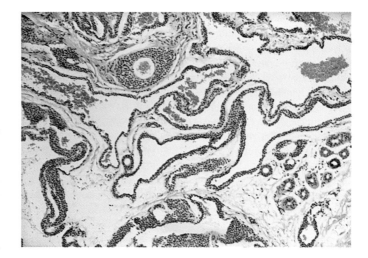

FIGURE 31-37   Glomus tumor (glomangioma). Cavernous vascular channels lined by several layers of glomus cells.

of a cavernous malformation (usually termed *hemangioma*) (Fig. 31-37). These spaces may be filled with blood or contain organized thrombi. Typically, only a few layers of glomus cells surround these large spaces, and some vessels may focally lack glomus cells. In contrast to the solitary painful tumors, nerve fibers about multiple glomus tumors are few. Glomangiomyomas are an uncommon variant of glomus tumor and show glomus cells blending with a population of smooth-muscle cells. These features are best seen at the periphery of large blood vessels. Solid forms are also seen with a remarkable epithelioid appearance of solid lobules of glomus cells with scant lumen formation.

Glomangiosarcomas are characterized by numerous mitoses, short spindle cells, disordered arrangement of cells, moderate pleomorphism, and single large nucleoli. Immunohistochemically, glomus tumors react positively for vimentin, smooth-muscle actin, and myosin, but are negative for factor VIII–related antigen, desmin (variable), and S-100. Ultrastructurally, the cells of glomus tumors show characteristics of modified smooth-muscle cells such as intracytoplasmic myofilaments with characteristic focal densities, numerous pinocytotic vesicles, and dense attachment plaques on cell membranes. These features suggest that glomus tumors are not derived from capillary pericytes as was once advocated but instead derive from smooth-muscle cells of the vascular part of the neuromyoarterial glomus.

Differential Diagnosis   The histology of glomus tumors is so characteristic that it is not readily confused with that of other tumors (Table 31-21). An exception might be the occasional glomangioma that exhibits only a subtle, multifocal population of glomus cells. However, careful scrutiny of such glomangiomas for the presence of glomus cells will avoid confusion with cavernous malformations (often termed *hemangioma*), including those hemangiomas that occur multiply in the setting of the blue rubber bleb nevus syndrome.

Hemangiopericytomas show a more spindled, irregular pattern of cells and particularly in the malignant forms are associated with hemorrhage, necrosis, and mitotic figures. Mastocytomas have their own monotonous proliferation of cells, but these unencapsulated tumors lack significant vascularity, and mast cells can be identified by metachromatic stains, if they are not readily recognized by light microscopy and experience. Glomus tumors appearing as cellular sheets of cells may evoke the epithelioid appearance of an adnexal tumor (eccrine acrospiroma or chondroid syringoma); however, the vascularity of glomus tumors combined with their lack of both ductal differentiation and epithelial mucin serve to differentiate these tumors. It should be noted that occasional glomus tumors may exhibit a strikingly myxoid stroma.

Pseudoangiomatous melanocytic nevi are usually not confused with glomus tumors, but, if there is doubt, the S-100 reactivity of nevi and not of glomus tumors will readily distinguish the two.

Finally, it should be noted that there is a normal anatomic structure, the glomus coccygeum, that is several millimeters in size and is located near the tip of the coccyx. It may be mistaken for a glomus tumor by those that are unaware of its existence.

Lymphangioma

Lymphangiomas are proliferations of variably dilated lymphatic vessels, usually present either at birth or within the first few years of life, and generally considered to be hamartomatous (malformations) in nature.[1–3,14,41,90,91] Various clinical types of lymphangioma have been reported: lymphangioma simplex (capillary lymphatic malformation), lymphangioma circumscriptum (localized and classic forms), cavernous lymphangioma (cavernous lymphatic malformation), and cystic hygroma, the latter entity perhaps being an extremely dilated form of cavernous hemangioma occurring on typical clinical sites. Many lymphangiomas have a deep component, and, in general, the features of the above types of lymphangioma form a continuum and may overlap, thus making the exact classification of individual cases difficult at times.

Clinical Features   *Lymphangioma simplex* appears in infancy as a solitary, rather well-defined, skin-colored dermal, mucosal, or subcutaneous lesion, often less than a few centimeters in size. The contour is usually smooth and slightly elevated.

Lymphangioma circumscriptum is the most common type of lymphangioma and clinically is characterized by cutaneous vesicles. Typically, the localized form is single and of small size. It may occur at any age and is the one form of lymphangioma that is most apt to arise beyond infancy. In contrast, the classic form of lymphangioma circumscriptum usually appears at birth or in early childhood, is generally of larger size, and is comprised of solitary or multiple patches. Common sites are the proximal extremities, limb girdle, neck, tongue, and buccal mucosa. The degree of involvement may at times be quite extensive. Both clinical forms of lymphangioma circumscriptum may include vesicles with a variably sanguinous or violaceous appearance due to presence of admixed red blood cells. Features similar to lymphangioma circumscriptum have developed as an acquired lesion in the setting of lymphedema subsequent to radical mastectomy and radiotherapy.

Cavernous lymphangioma (cavernous lymphatic malformation) is usually present at birth or by infancy. This large, ill-defined lesion may occur at many sites but favors the head, neck, mouth, and extremities. A particular subtype of cavernous lymphangioma, the cystic hygroma, has extensive, often deforming, cystic dilatations that generally occur on the neck but may involve the axilla, groin, popliteal fossa, mediastinum, and retroperitoneum.

Histopathological Features   Various lymphangiomas generally differ in the size of the lymphatic vessels.[1–3,14,41,90,91] Lymphangioma simplex is composed of small capillary-sized lymphatic vessels. Lymphangioma circumscriptum has dilated lymphatic channels occupying the superficial dermis. The overlying epidermis is often elevated and is variably thin to acanthotic. There may be papillomatosis and hyperkeratosis, particularly in the classic type of lymphangioma circumscriptum (Fig. 31-38). Also, in contrast to the localized type, this classic type has deeper extension of the lymphatic vessels into the lower dermis and subcutis. Cavernous lymphangiomas have widely dilated lymphatic channels occupying and expanding the dermis and subcutis (Fig. 31-39). The intervening stroma may be inapparent or variably fibrotic. Cystic hygromas show large unilocular or multilocular thin-walled cysts. Lymphangiomas generally show homogenous, lightly stained lymph fluid within their lymphatic spaces and may have a variable number of stromal lymphocytes. Red blood cells may at times be present within lymphatic lumina. A deeper cavernous lymphangioma may occasionally underlie the classic type of lymphangioma circumscriptum. Smooth-muscle bundles may be seen within the walls of some dilated lymphatic vessels in cavernous and cystic lymphangiomas.

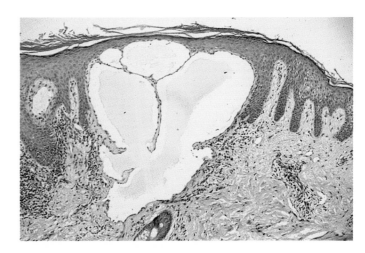

FIGURE 31-38 Lymphangioma circumscriptum. Large lymphatic lumen impinging upon the epidermis. Note the absence of red blood cells.

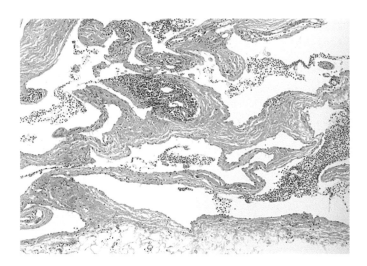

FIGURE 31-39 Cavernous lymphatic malformation. Widely dilated lymphatic channels are surrounded by fibrous tissue and lymphocytic infiltrates. The lumina contain proteinaceous material.

TABLE 31-22
Benign Lymphangioendothelioma

Clinical Features

Men and women equally affected
Childhood to elderly
Diverse sites
Well-demarcated dermal plaques, dull pink to violaceous
Variable size (3–30 cm)
Slow enlargement over time

Histopathological Features

Variable degree of dermal involvement, favoring the upper half
Thin-walled, irregular vascular channels "dissecting" collagen
Bland endothelial cells
Scant or absent mononuclear inflammatory infiltrate
Lack of plasma cells, extravasated erythrocytes, and hemosiderin

Differential Diagnosis

Low-grade angiosarcoma
Lymphangiomalike Kaposi's sarcoma
Lymphangioma circumscriptum

Differential Diagnosis The diagnosis of *lymphangioma* (or lymphatic malformation) may have to suffice when clinical correlation is lacking and when vessels of mixed size are present. Moreover, the presence of admixed erythrocytes within a particular lymphangioma may generate consideration of a hemangioma or mixed lesion (*hemolymphangioma* or *hemolymphatic malformation*). The papillary dermal component of lymphangioma circumscriptum bears similarity to that of an angiokeratoma, and the presence of intraluminal red blood cells, whether they be present de novo or secondary to trauma from a biopsy procedure, may contribute to misdiagnosis. Recognition of the deeper lymphatic component in the classic form of lymphangioma circumscriptum is useful in such situations. The diagnosis of cavernous and cystic lymphangiomas is seldom difficult, and the clinicopathologic features for the cystic hygroma, in particular, are quite unique.

Benign Lymphangioendothelioma

Also known as *angioendothelioma (lymphatic type)* or *acquired progressive lymphangioma*, benign lymphangioendothelioma is an entity that has undergone a nosological evolution over the three decades prior to Wilson Jones and colleagues' proposal of the name *benign lymphangioendothelioma* (BL) in 1990.[92,93] BL was previously described by Gold and Wilson Jones in the late 1960s under the name *angioendothelioma (lymphatic type)*. In the interim, a few cases were also reported as *acquired progressive lymphangioma*. BL is a rare entity that can offer diagnostic difficulty with low-grade angiosarcoma and the lymphangiomalike form of Kaposi's sarcoma.

Clinical Features The incidence of BL is relatively similar in males and females (Table 31-22). Patients range in age from 5 years to 69 years. The duration of clinical lesions before presentation has ranged from 3 months to 10 years. Sites of involvement are diverse and include thigh, forearm, chest, abdomen, and shoulder. Multiple sites of involvement, both synchronous and asynchronous, are documented. One case presented with a history of preceding trauma to the affected area.

Clinical lesions are well-demarcated dermal plaques that range in color from dull pink, to dusky, to violaceous. The lesional borders are usually clearly delineated from the surrounding, uninvolved skin.[92,93] Characteristically, the dermal plaques are painless and nontender. The plaques tend to slowly enlarge over time. In reported cases, the lesions

have ranged in size from 3 to 30 cm. Presentation as a subcutaneous nodule has been reported.

Excision of BL with attainment of clear margins is curative, and clinical recurrence after excision has not been reported. Regression of two asynchronous lesions after oral prednisolone therapy and spontaneous regression of a case of BL have been documented. The significance of lesional regression after steroid therapy is uncertain and requires further investigation. Most lesions tend to pursue a relatively static clinical course, slowly increasing in size over a period of years. There are no reports of malignant transformation.

Histopathological Features The epidermis is unremarkable. The lesions are dermal with a tendency to involve the midpapillary dermis and superficial to midreticular dermis (Table 31-22). Occasional lesions show full-thickness dermal involvement and may extend to involve superficial subcutaneous tissue.[92,93] The unifying histologic features, identified in all cases, are jagged, irregularly shaped vascular channels distributed between dermal collagen bundles (Fig. 31-40). The lumina of these thin-walled vascular spaces may be dilated or collapsed and inconspicuous. The vessels are intimately associated with the dermal collagen, appearing to dissect between the collagen bundles. The thin-walled vessels tend to be arranged in a horizontal array, although they may be quite haphazard in distribution. The endothelial lining is one cell layer in thickness. The cytologic features tend to be bland, although occasional plump or hyperchromatic endothelial cells are an acceptable finding. Pronounced cytologic atypia is not a feature of BL. A single case report describes occasional multinucleated endothelial cells. The largest series to date does not confirm this finding. Occasional, intraluminal papillary projections may be seen. Rarely, endothelial cells may detach from the vascular wall and appear to float freely within the vessel lumen. Mitotic activity is not a reported feature. The vascular spaces are typically empty but may contain a faintly eosinophilic, proteinaceous material. A scant, mononuclear, inflammatory infiltrate is a variable feature. Plasma cells, extravasated erythrocytes, spindle cell proliferation, and hemosiderin are not features typical of BL.

Immunohistochemical studies on a small number of cases have shown, in most cases, that endothelial cells of BL consistently react

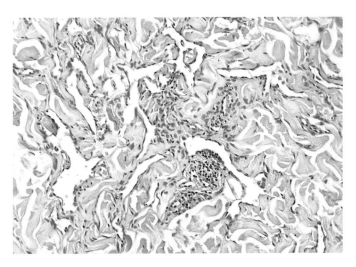

FIGURE 31-40   Benign lymphangioendothelioma. Thin-wall, infiltrative, staghorn-shaped vessels devoid of red blood cells.

with antibodies to Ulex europaeus 1. Staining with antibodies to factor VIII–related antigen is limited to normal intralesional and perilesional vessels. Tadaki and coworkers, in a single case, found no immunoreactivity to both Ulex europaeus 1 and factor VIII–related antigen. In any event, the pattern of immunoreactivity is not useful in distinguishing BL from other benign and malignant vascular proliferations. In a single case, electron microscopy failed to demonstrate Weibel-Palade bodies. The report did not comment on other electron microscopic features.

Differential Diagnosis   Benign lymphangioendothelioma is a histologic mimic of both low-grade or well-differentiated angiosarcoma and patch-stage Kaposi's sarcoma. The clinical setting for each of these entities is distinct, and an important caveat is that a diagnosis of BL should not be established on a small biopsy in the absence of clinical history. The earliest known case of BL was initially considered to be a low-grade angiosarcoma until its benign course and reevaluation led to a diagnosis of BL. Considering the relative histologic similarities of BL to AS, it seems likely that several early series of cutaneous angiosarcoma may have contained examples of BL, these constituting the rare cases of AS with an indolent course, good prognosis, and odd clinical presentation.

Cutaneous angiosarcomas, excluding the Stewart-Treves syndrome and postradiation angiosarcomas, are malignant tumors essentially confined to the head and neck of elderly individuals. If an adequate biopsy of AS is obtained, the degree of cytologic atypia far exceeds that acceptable for BL. In addition, extravasated erythrocytes, hemosiderin deposition, and an inflammatory tumor response are distinct from BL. Patch-stage lesions of Kaposi's sarcoma, in both the classic and epidemic forms, may be clinically subtle. In contrast to BL, however, they tend to be small and multiple and show clinical progression over a relatively short period. Histologic features of KS that are distinct from BL include the tendency for the neovascular channels of KS to localize around preexisting dermal structures and the presence of erythrocyte extravasation, hemosiderin deposition, and a dermal inflammatory infiltrate that nearly always includes plasma cells.

Lymphangioma circumscriptum has one or more patches of vesicles favoring the limb girdles; contains large, dilated lymphatic vessels raising the epidermis; and lacks the dissection of collagen pattern seen in BL. Giant-cell fibroblastoma may in some rare settings be confused with BL. The presence of the giant cells and the endothelial marker–negative pseudolumina should allow the correct diagnosis.

VASCULAR LESIONS WITH INDETERMINATE OR BORDERLINE STATUS

Epithelioid Hemangioendothelioma

Also known as *histiocytoid hemangioma, intravascular bronchioloalveolar tumor (IVBAT), sclerosing endothelial tumor, sclerosing angiogenic tumor, sclerosing interstitial vascular sarcoma,* or *sclerosing epithelioid angiosarcoma,* epithelioid hemangioendothelioma (EH) is a rare entity that has been reported as a biologically "borderline" neoplasm because of an occasional association with local recurrence or metastasis.[94–97] EHs in systemic organs have been known in the past as sclerosing endothelial tumor, sclerosing angiogenic tumor, sclerosing interstitial vascular sarcoma, sclerosing epithelioid angiosarcoma, and as a form of intravascular bronchioloalveolar tumor (IVBAT).

Clinical Features   EH is an angiocentric neoplasm that may be multifocal and has been described in soft tissue and in various organs such as lung, liver, and bone (Table 31-23).[94–97] EH presenting in the skin is rare and occurs in the upper and lower limbs of both sexes, favoring the third and fourth decades of life. Cutaneous EH is usually associated with involvement of underlying bone, although one case of EH limited to the skin of the palm has been reported. Cutaneous lesions of EH may be solitary or multiple. EH of soft tissue usually presents as a solitary, slightly painful mass. Cutaneous EH has varied from being asymptomatic dermal nodules to being associated with the severe burning pain, hyperesthesia, swelling, and hyperhidrosis of reflex sympathetic dystrophy.

The prognosis of EH is variable. Patients with EH of the lung and liver have a higher mortality than those with EH of soft tissue. Mortality

TABLE 31-23

Epithelioid Hemangioendothelioma

Clinical Features

Favors the third and fourth decades of life
Upper and lower extremities
Solitary or multiple skin lesions
Usually involves underlying bone
Occurs in other sites: soft tissue, lung, liver

Histopathological Features

Cutaneous tumors:
   Relatively inconspicuous vascularity
   Small vascular channels lined by cuboidal endothelial cells
Soft-tissue tumors: often angiocentric arising from medium to large veins
Hyaline to myxoid/myxochondroid stroma
Cords or solid nests of rounded or slightly spindled epithelioid cells
Intracytoplasmic vacuoles
Histologic separation
   Benign: cytologically bland, mitotic figures inapparent
   Malignant: cytologic atypia, more than 1 mitosis per 10 high-power
     fields, necrosis, focal spindling of cells

Differential Diagnosis

Metastatic carcinoma
Malignant melanoma
Epithelioid sarcoma
Epithelioid angiosarcoma
Angiolymphoid hyperplasia with eosinophilia

rates of 65, 35, and 13 percent, respectively, have been reported. Local recurrence and metastatic disease to regional lymph nodes or to lung may occur, yet less than one-half of the patients with metastases succumb to their disease. Histologically benign appearing forms of EH generally have a better prognosis than those that appear malignant, but histologically bland appearing lesions have occasionally been associated with metastasis and death.

Whether the relatively indolent tumors previously described as cutaneous epithelioid angiosarcoma belong to the spectrum of EH is unclear. Some of these patients experienced slow, protracted disease associated with numerous local recurrences and regional lymph node metastases.

Histopathological Features   EH displays "histiocytoid" or epithelioid-appearing endothelial cells that may be angiocentric and, in at least half of soft-tissue cases, arise from and expand the wall of a medium to large-size vein[94–97] (Table 31-23) (Fig. 31-41). A hyaline to myxoid or myxochondroid-appearing stroma is common. The endothelial cells appear as cords or solid nests of rounded or slightly spindled epithelioid cells. Small intracytoplasmic lumina appear as vacuoles, and on occasion these vacuoles are large and may distort the cell, mimicking the mucin-containing cells of an adenocarcinoma. Red blood cells may be present within the intracytoplasmic lumina. In contrast to the angiocentric pattern that may be seen with EH in soft tissue, the vascularity in cutaneous EH is relatively inconspicuous and, when present, generally consists of small vascular channels that may be lined by cuboidal endothelial cells.

"Benign"-appearing EH is cytologically bland without appreciable mitotic activity. In contrast, the features of "malignant"-appearing, clinically more aggressive cases of EH include significant cytologic atypia, more than one mitotic figure per 10 high-power fields, necrosis, and focal spindling of cells.

A reticulin stain will reveal a network of reticulin fibers outlining individual cells and groups of cells. Immunohistochemically, EH usually marks with both factor VIII–related antigen and Ulex europaeus lectin. The staining for factor VIII–related antigen is accentuated about intracytoplasmic lumina and varies in distribution and with the degree of tissue preservation. EH is considered to be negative for both epithelial membrane antigen and cytokeratin, although staining for keratin was observed in one case when frozen sections were utilized. By electron microscopy, EH shows features of endothelial cells such as Weibel-Palade bodies, pinocytotic vacuoles, and well-developed basal lamina. Abundant cytoplasmic intermediate filaments are present.

Differential Diagnosis   EH shares similarities to a variety of tumors that exhibit epithelioid histologic patterns. Among these are metastatic carcinoma, adenocarcinoma, malignant melanoma, angiolymphoid hyperplasia with eosinophilia (epithelioid hemangioma), epithelioid sarcoma, and epithelioid angiosarcoma. Carcinomas, malignant melanoma, and epithelioid angiosarcoma generally show significant cytologic atypia and mitotic activity that will distinguish them from most cases of EH. Mucin stains mark the vacuoles and signet-ring cells of adenocarcinoma but are negative in EH. Melanomas usually lack the intracytoplasmic vacuoles of EH and often show evidence of melanin pigment. ALHE may show intracytoplasmic vacuoles; however, ALHE characteristically exhibits well-developed vascularity lined by hobnail endothelial cells and has a prominent inflammatory infiltrate of lymphoid follicles and eosinophils. Epithelioid sarcoma perhaps has the closest similarity to EH, but epithelioid sarcoma will generally display a nodular arrangement of cells with central cores of necrotic debris and collagen. EH exhibiting a well-developed chondromyxoid matrix must be distinguished from chondrosarcoma and chordoma.

Immunohistochemistry is often important to the diagnosis of EH. A panel of antibodies should be used, and the pattern of reactivity will help in differentiating EH from its various mimickers. In particular, EH will show endothelial markers (factor VIII–related antigen, Ulex europaeus lectin) while being negative for the S-100 staining of malignant melanoma and the cytokeratin staining of both carcinomas and epithelioid sarcoma.

Kaposi's Sarcoma

This vascular neoplasm was first described by Kaposi in 1872 under the name of "idiopathic multiple pigmented sarcoma of the skin."[98–120] The skin is the most common site, but several other organ systems may be affected. Although KS has been endemic in Central Africa for some time, KS has been primarily known as a relatively rare tumor of the elderly until the advent of the acquired immunodeficiency syndrome (AIDS) and organ transplantation. With the increase in the number of cases of KS as well as the occurrence of the disorder in a younger population that is apt to have other, generally benign, vascular lesions, intimate knowledge of the disease spectrum of KS has become essential to correct diagnosis. This is particularly true for the diagnosis of early lesions of KS.

The isolation of herpesviruslike DNA sequences designated human herpesvirus 8 in KS from AIDS-related KS, African-endemic KS, and the Mediterranean form of KS, strongly suggests a role for this agent in the pathogenesis of KS.[121–123]

Clinical Features   The classic, chronic or "European," form of KS is an uncommon disease that generally affects individuals greater than 50 years of age and shows a strong predilection for men (Table 31-24).[98–101] There is an increased incidence of KS in Ashkenazic Jews and individuals of Mediterranean descent. KS typically begins on the distal lower extremities, either uni- or bilaterally. Over time, lesions may increase in number and arise more proximally. The upper extremities may become affected, and occasionally this may be the initial site of presentation. Characteristically, KS lesions evolve through stages as patches, plaques, and nodules, and clinical lesions of varying stages are often present in a single patient. Lesions may gradually coalesce, and nodules may eventually ulcerate. The clinical course of the classic form of KS is relatively indolent. Occasional lesions may regress while others progress. However, one should be aware that up to one-third of

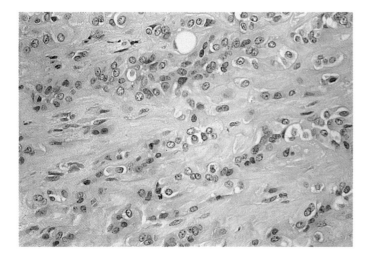

FIGURE 31-41 Epithelioid hemangioendothelioma. Cords of epithelioid cells in a fibrous stroma. Note the similarities to an infiltrative carcinoma.

Kaposi's Sarcoma

Clinical Features

Clinical forms of Kaposi's sarcoma
Classic (European)
    Predominantly men, older than 50 years old
    Ashkenazic Jews; Mediterranean descent
    Distal lower extremities
    Relatively indolent clinical course
African (endemic)
    Males, younger age distribution
    Nodular, florid, infiltrative, lymphadenopathic subgroups
AIDS-associated (epidemic)
    Homosexual men more than other risk groups
    Upper half of the body
    Early lesions, small, pink to light purple
    Disseminated disease
Immunosuppression
    Organ transplant recipients
    Disseminated disease

Histopathological Features

Patch stage
    Inconspicuous, irregular, angulated blood vessels
    Upper to entire reticular dermis
    Promontory sign
    Lymphocytic perivascular infiltrate, plasma cells
Plaque stage
    Vessels fill the dermis and involve the superficial subcutis
    Obvious spindle cells
    Slitlike spaces containing erythrocytes
    Extravasated erythrocytes, hemosiderin, apoptotic endothelial cells,
        hyaline globules
Nodular stage
    Extensive spindle cell infiltrate in fascicles and sheets
    Numerous slitlike spaces in sievelike pattern, containing
        erythrocytes
    Mitotic figures, variable numbers

Differential Diagnosis

Acro-angiodermatitis (pseudo-Kaposi's sarcoma)
Benign lympangioendothelioma
Targetoid hemosiderotic hemangioma
Immature scar
Bacillary angiomatosis
Angiosarcoma

---

patients with the classic form of KS subsequently develop a second primary neoplasm, often of hematopoietic origin.

In equatorial Africa, KS is a common neoplasm that accounts for 9% of malignant tumors in Ugandan males and up to 10% of registered cancers in other areas. Males again predominate, but this endemic African form of KS affects a younger population than the classic European variant, with the difference averaging a decade in most reports, and children are also affected. The disease can be subclassified into four clinical groups: nodular, florid, infiltrative, and lymphadenopathic. The nodular group presents with a limited number of circumscribed cutaneous nodules and pursues an indolent clinical course. The florid and infiltrative groups have more aggressive disease with extensive cutaneous lesions on one or more extremities, generally associated with involvement of

bone. The lymphadenopathic type occurs mainly in children in whom lymph node involvement is usually the sole manifestation, and in young adults who may have concomitant skin involvement.

AIDS-associated or epidemic KS occurs in a population of individuals with unique demographics. This new group of patients, at risk for an aggressive, often disseminated form of KS, is composed predominantly of homosexual men who comprise 95 percent of all cases. The remainder is comprised of intravenous drug users and other populations at risk for AIDS. All but very rare cases have serologic antibody titers to the human immunodeficiency virus type 1. However, cofactors in the pathogenesis of KS have been suspected, and indirect evidence for this is the drop in incidence of KS in the AIDS-affected homosexual population since the early 1980s. Upon initial medical presentation, lesions of KS are often small and few in number. They may be light purple or pink rather than deeply violaceous as with more established lesions of KS. The upper half of the body is frequently affected without the tendency of classic KS to first involve the distal lower extremities. Moreover, clinically normal skin of patients with well-developed AIDS show ultrastructural abnormalities similar to those of early KS, suggesting that they too are potential sites of involvement.

Another new group of patients at risk for the development of KS are patients receiving immunosuppressive agents, particularly organ transplant recipients. The incidence is low and after renal transplantation is estimated at 0.4 percent. As with classic KS, there is a propensity toward individuals of Jewish or Mediterranean descent. However, women are more frequently affected in this group than in the other clinical forms of KS. Cutaneous and visceral involvement occur, but no particular pattern of distribution has been emphasized. The clinical course is more aggressive than classic KS, with a significant percentage of patients perishing with disseminated disease. Lesions may regress with the reduction or withdrawal of immunosuppressive therapy.

Histopathological Features   The histology of cutaneous lesions associated with the various clinical forms of KS is essentially identical and will be described together according to their stage at presentation (Table 31-24). Although some authors feel there are subtle differences between classic and AIDS-associated KS, others have not confirmed this impression. The observed differences and diagnostic difficulty in AIDS-associated KS seem to relate to the subtle changes inherent in early lesions rather than differences unique to this form of KS.

For patch-stage KS, the earliest features are inconspicuous and on initial review may be mistaken as nondiagnostic or inflammatory. The alterations are mainly confined to the reticular dermis (involving the upper half or all of it). A variable, predominantly lymphocytic perivascular infiltrate is present and contains a variable number of plasma cells. Subtle vascular changes can be appreciated. The earliest of these is a proliferation of miniature or irregular, jagged blood vessels around normal or ectatic dermal blood vessels and about adnexal structures (Figs. 31-42, 31-43). The newly formed vessels may protrude into a vascular lumen or surround and partially isolate normal dermal structures; a feature referred to as the *promontory sign*. In some lesions, the vessels aggregate into clusters that resemble small hemangiomas. The endothelium may be inconspicuous or plump and a single layer in thickness and shows little atypia or mitotic activity. Irregular, branching, thin-walled bland vessels may be seen dissecting between collagen bundles. These neovascular channels tend to be contiguous with preexisting dermal blood vessels. In well-developed patch-stage lesions, KS involves the entire dermis.

A highly suggestive but subtle finding that may be seen only with careful examination of multiple levels of sections is the presence of small numbers of bland spindle cells in close association with the newly formed vessels. Other features that are relatively inconspicuous in patch-stage KS but may be seen are apoptotic endothelial cells, extravasated erythrocytes, hemosiderin, and hyaline globules. In con-

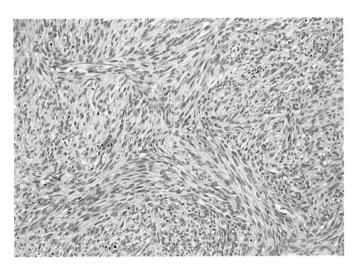

FIGURE 31-44   Kaposi's sarcoma, tumor stage. The compact spindle cell proliferation variant mimics other soft-tissue sarcomas.

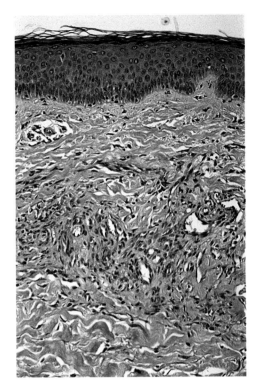

FIGURE 31-42   Kaposi's sarcoma, patch stage. This lesion exhibits irregular vascular channels and interstitial spindle-shaped cells.

trast to patch-stage KS, these features are best seen in well-developed plaques and nodules. Hyaline globules are small, faintly eosinophilic, PAS-positive, and diastase-resistant spheres that may be deposited extracellularly or may be seen intracellularly within macrophages. The globules most likely represent phagocytized red blood cells and their degenerative forms. They are a useful diagnostic criterion but are neither necessary nor sufficient for the diagnosis of KS. They may be seen in other neoplastic and inflammatory processes with abundant erythrocyte extravasation, such as angiosarcomas, pyogenic granulomas, and inflammatory granulation tissue.

Plaque-stage lesions of KS show further progression of the neoplastic process, filling the entire dermis and involving the superficial sub-

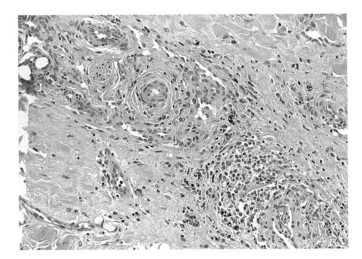

FIGURE 31-43   Kaposi's sarcoma, patch stage. Note the similarities with a banal chronic inflammatory process. The angulated thin-walled lumina are the clue for the diagnosis.

cutaneous tissue. The most characteristic feature of this stage is the presence of a significant spindle cell component. These relatively bland cells are dispersed between dermal collagen bundles and around preexisting dermal vessels. Between these spindle cells, irregular, cleft or slit-like spaces are formed, creating new, angulated vascular channels that contain small numbers of erythrocytes. Hemosiderin deposits and hyaline globules are more prominent than in patch-stage KS. The vasoproliferative changes of the patch stage persist at the periphery of plaques. The predominantly lymphocytic, perivascular inflammatory infiltrate persists along with its component of plasma cells.

Nodular lesions of KS show a further proliferation of spindle cells into intersecting fascicles and sheets (Fig. 31-44). Amidst these spindle cells are slitlike vascular spaces containing variable numbers of erythrocytes. The spindle cells show a degree of cytologic atypia that generally ranges from mild to moderate. Frank anaplasia of the spindle cell component is distinctly uncommon and is more frequently described in the endemic African form of KS. Apoptotic cells, hyaline globules, and hemosiderin deposition are all readily visible. Mitotic figures vary in number but may be frequent. The dermal lymphoplasmacytic inflammatory infiltrate persists, and at the periphery of the nodules ectatic blood vessels and lymphatics are generally noted.

Lymphangiomatous or lymphangiomalike lesions of KS have been reported as both a focal and predominant clinicopathologic pattern in otherwise typical Kaposi's sarcoma[119] (Fig. 31-45). The process usually involves the entire dermis and often extends into the superficial subcutaneous tissue. Angulated, irregular, narrow to ectatic, thin-walled vascular channels lined by a single layer of flattened, bland endothelium interconnect and dissect collagen bundles. The majority of the vascular spaces lack red blood cells. Features typical of KS such as a significant inflammatory infiltrate, extravasated erythrocytes, hemosiderin, and hyaline globules have not been reported. Occasional cases show sparse numbers of spindle cells in close association with the vascular elements, but these cells are never a prominent feature.

The histogenesis of KS is a subject open to some debate. Kaposi's sarcoma may be a lesion that arises from pluripotential stem cells variably differentiating toward blood-vessel endothelium. However, an alternative theory involves multicentric hyperplasia that combines lymphatic venular anastomoses with elements of both lymphatic and blood vessel endothelium.

Despite their erythematous clinical appearance, early lesions of KS typically have thin-walled vessels with a lymphaticlike histologic appearance. Enzyme histochemistry shows these vessels to have a staining profile of lymphatic endothelium. In contrast, ultrastructural exam-

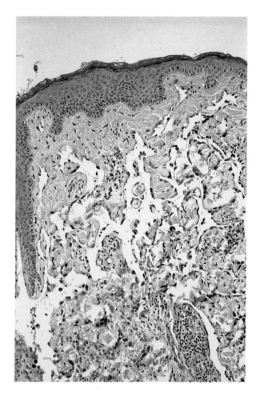

FIGURE 31-45   Kaposi's sarcoma, lymphangiomatous variant. There are highly irregular dilated vascular spaces that dissect collagen and surround other blood vessels.

inations of the endothelial cells in a minority of cases show Weibel-Palade bodies and, in general, display features of poorly differentiated blood vessels. Variable immunohistochemical results have been obtained, but endothelial cells of early KS are usually negative for factor VIII–related antigen and weakly positive for Ulex europaeus lectin 1. The spindle cells of nodular lesions of KS display only patchy reactivity for factor VIII–related antigen and show diminished reactivity for Ulex europaeus lectin 1. Moreover, it is doubtful that these two markers can reliably distinguish between blood vessel and lymphatic endothelium.

Differential Diagnosis   Difficulty in diagnosis usually occurs with early lesions of KS rather than the well-developed lesions of nodular-stage KS. Among the entities to be considered in the differential diagnosis of KS are acro-angiodermatitis, benign lymphangioendothelioma, targetoid hemosiderotic hemangioma (Table 31-25), early scar, bacillary angiomatosis, and angiosarcoma. More cellular lesions of KS must be differentiated from aneurysmal fibrous histiocytoma and from spindle cell hemangioendothelioma. The reader is referred to sections on the above topics for discussions of the differential features. In particular, histologic findings that are often important to the diagnosis of early Kaposi's sarcoma include: the promontory sign, plasma cells, and newly formed, thin-walled vessels that dissect dermal collagen. Important criteria of more evolved lesions include: spindle cells, slitlike spaces containing erythrocytes, hyaline globules, apoptotic cells, and hemosiderin deposition. It should be recognized, however, that there is a continuum of these features from patch to nodular stage.

Hemangiopericytoma

The hemangiopericytoma is a relatively rare soft-tissue neoplasm that is thought to derive from the pericyte.[124–128] The diagnosis is often difficult, since other soft-tissue tumors may be highly vascular and show hemangiopericytomalike patterns. Its occurrence in the skin proper is debatable.

Clinical Features   Hemangiopericytomas generally occur as deep-seated soft-tissue tumors in adults, with a median age of 45 years in one large series (Table 31-26). The most common sites are the lower extremities and the pelvic retroperitoneum, but the tumor has a wide distribution. Typically, the tumor arises as a painless mass that is often several centimeters in size by the time of clinical presentation. Hypoglycemia may be associated with large retroperitoneal lesions. Hemangiopericytomas are well-vascularized tumors, and excision is often complicated by hemorrhage.

Benign and malignant forms of hemangiopericytomas have been recognized. However, there are also intermediate or borderline cases of hemangiopericytoma that resist classification and make prognostication difficult. A median survival of 19 months was reported for malignant hemangiopericytomas. Malignant tumors frequently recur and metastasize.

Histopathological Features   Tumor cells are rounded or spindle-shaped and are present outside the numerous, admixed blood vessels (Table 31-26).[124–128] A reticulin stain will demonstrate that the endothelial cells of the vessels lie inside a delicate reticulin sheath and are thus separated from the peripheral population of tumor cells. The rich network of blood vessels has a varied morphology ranging from capillaries to large sinusoidallike spaces. The latter spaces often appear to divide in antlerlike or "staghorn" configurations (Fig. 31-46).

Malignant hemangiopericytomas are characterized by hemorrhage, necrosis, and increases in both cellularity and mitotic activity. The presence of 4 or more mitotic figures per 10 high-power fields has been associated with recurrence and metastasis, whereas benign hemangiopericytomas generally show fewer than 2 or 3 mitoses per 10 high-power fields.

Being derived from the pericyte, the hemangiopericytoma is generally negative for endothelial markers. Reactivity for Ulex europaeus 1 is absent, and factor VIII–related antigen is negative or only weakly positive. Conversely, the endothelial cells of the accompanying vasculature are richly stained by both markers. Hemangiopericytomas stain for vimentin and laminin but are negative for smooth-muscle actin and desmin. Ultrastructurally, basal lamina–like material is present and either partially or completely surrounds tumor cells. This feature, along with the presence of myogenic filaments and pinocytotic vessels, serves to support a diagnosis of hemangiopericytoma in a histologically compatible tumor.

Differential Diagnosis   Other soft-tissue tumors with a hemangiopericytomalike pattern must be considered before rendering a diagnosis of hemangiopericytoma. Among these tumors are solitary myofibromatosis, synovial sarcoma, extraskeletal mesenchymal chondrosarcoma, malignant schwannoma, and malignant fibrous histiocytoma. Immunohistochemical staining and ultrastructural examination are important adjuncts to diagnosis.

Monophasic forms of synovial sarcoma can cause particular confusion with hemangiopericytoma by light microscopy, but fortunately most synovial sarcomas show a biphasic pattern of glandlike areas and sarcomatous stroma. Immunohistochemical marking for cytokeratin is typical of synovial sarcomas but is absent in hemangiopericytomas. In particular, the diagnosis of synovial sarcoma should always be considered when a tumor is near a knee or other large joint, particularly in young adults. Extraskeletal mesenchymal chondrosarcoma has foci of well-differentiated cartilage and rarely bone. Areas of hypocellular, myxoid change are commonly seen in malignant schwannoma in contrast to the hemangiopericytoma. Malignant fibrous histiocytoma is more apt to show a storiform pattern than is hemangiopericytoma and may display pleomorphic or fascicular patterns. Moreover, the fascicular pattern of fibrosarcoma, synovial sarcoma, and malignant schwannoma is not a feature of hemangiopericytoma.

TABLE 31-25

Comparison of Histologic Features in Microvenular Hemangioma, Kaposi's Sarcoma (Patch Stage), Targetoid Hemosiderotic Hemangioma, and Lobular Capillary Hemangioma

	Major clinical features	Irregular anastomosing vascular spaces	Cytologic features of endothelial cells	Cellularity	Inflammation	Hemosiderin
Microvenular hemangioma	Single, small, purple to red lesions favoring the extremities of young to middle-aged adults	1+	Normal to plump	1–2+	0 to sparse lymphocytic	0–1+
Kaposi's sarcoma (patch stage)	Usually multiple, pink to purple, broad, flat lesions favoring the lower extremities of elderly men in the classic form; more disseminated in the AIDS-associated form	4+	Cells lining vessels normal; others spindle-shaped, hyperchromatic with variable atypia	0–1+	Sparse perivascular lymphocytes and plasma cells	0–3+
Targetoid hemosiderotic hemangioma	Single, small, annular, often targetlike lesions on the trunk and extremities of young to middle-aged adults	2–3+ with epithelioid fronds in early lesions	Normal to epithelioid	1–2+	0 to sparse lymphocytes (and variable but often intense red cell extravasation)	3–4+
Lobular capillary hemangioma	Single or multiple, rapidly growing lesions of the skin or mucosal surfaces of individuals of all ages	0–1+	Normal to rarely epithelioid	3–4+	0–4+ intense acute and chronic inflammation associated with ulcerated lesions	0–1+

TABLE 31-26

Hemangiopericytoma

Clinical Features

Adults
Asymptomatic, deep-seated soft-tissue mass
Most common sites: lower extremities and retroperitoneum
Hypoglycemia with large retroperitoneal tumors
Excision often complicated by hemorrhage

Histopathological Features

Rounded or spindled tumor cells
Numerous blood vessels of variable size
Sinusoidal spaces dividing in staghorn configuration
Histological separation
   Benign: less than 2 or 3 mitoses per 10 high-power fields
   Malignant: 4 or more mitoses per 10 high-power fields;
     hemorrhage, necrosis, increased cellularity

Differential Diagnosis

Synovial sarcoma
Extraskeletal mesenchymal chondrosarcoma
Malignant schwannoma
Malignant fibrous histiocytoma

Endovascular Papillary Angioendothelioma

Also known as *malignant endovascular papillary angioendotheliom* or *Dabska tumor*, this exceedingly rare vascular lesion was first reported by Dabska in 1969 as malignant endovascular papillary angioendothelioma of the skin in childhood.[129–131] However, the cumulative experience in the literature indicates that endovascular papillary angioendothelioma (EPA) has a generally good prognosis despite local invasion

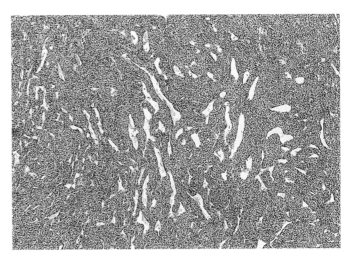

FIGURE 31-46 Hemangiopericytoma. Note characteristic antlerlike or staghorn pattern of vessels that is nonetheless shared by a number of other tumors.

and regional lymph node metastasis; it has become regarded as one of the "borderline" vascular tumors.

Clinical Features   Dabska reported 6 children, 4 months to 15 years of age, who presented with enlarging cutaneous lesions, 4 to 9 cm in diameter, occurring as either a diffuse swelling or an intradermal tumor on the head, neck, and extremities. Few additional cases have been reported.[129–131] Only one has occurred beyond childhood, a lesion on the left ear of a 54-year-old man. Two of Dabska's cases displayed regional lymphadenopathy, and another had tumor penetration through the frontal bone and into the cranial vault. Treatment consisted of wide excision supplemented in individual cases by radiotherapy or regional lymphadenectomy.

Local recurrence was observed only once but resolved with a second surgical procedure. Lymph node metastasis was seen in two children, one of which showed involvement of eight axillary lymph nodes. All the children were well without evidence of disease on follow-up examinations 4 to 16 years later. Acknowledging the favorable prognosis and the capacity of tumor for both local invasion and regional lymph node metastasis, Dabska viewed EPA as a variant of malignant angioendothelioma in childhood, possessing a limited degree of malignancy. It has been proposed that the lymph node inclusions might occur as a manifestation of regional endothelial proliferation rather than as evidence of metastatic disease.

Histopathological Features   The most characteristic feature of EPA is the presence of intraluminal papillary structures lined by endothelial cells showing pleomorphism, hyperchromatism, mitotic activity, and multilayered endothelium[129–131] (Fig. 31-47). Tumor cells appear to float free in the lumina either in clumps or as single cells. The central framework of the papillations can appear eosinophilic and hyalinized. Papillary formations resembling renal glomeruli may be seen. More cellular lesions reveal hemorrhage, cholesterol clefts, and areas of necrosis. Dabska reported a moderate degree of mitotic activity in EPA; however, later reports have described only rare mitoses and only mild cellular pleomorphism.

Vascular channels may show a cuboidal- to columnar-appearing endothelial lining, at times, with a hobnail appearance. Intravascular proliferations of endothelial cells may be arranged about hyaline globules,

a feature interpreted as the earliest form of fibrovascular stalk formation. The globules have the staining characteristics of basement membrane and ultrastructurally appear to be comprised of basal lamina–like material. A lymphocytic infiltrate may be prominent and may frequently intermingle with the endothelial cells. The latter association suggests that the endothelial cells of EPA show differentiation toward "high" endothelial cells of postcapillary venules.

Differential Diagnosis   Grossly, upon sectioning, and on low-power microscopic examination, EPA may have cystic spaces resembling a cavernous lymphangioma. The presence of the lymphocytic infiltrate supports this impression, but confusion in diagnosis is unlikely as soon as the proliferative endothelial nature of EPA is appreciated. In contrast to EPA, intravascular papillary endothelial hyperplasia (IPEH) has a generally flattened endothelial lining and an underlying thrombotic matrix. Both IPEH and angiosarcoma lack the hyaline globules and lymphocytic infiltrate of EPA. Angiosarcoma, an extremely rare tumor in childhood, also differs by showing conspicuous cytologic atypia and frequent mitotic figures. Compared with the flattened endothelium of glomeruloid hemangioma, EPA demonstrates intraluminal papillations lined by endothelium with variable but generally mild pleomorphism. The vascularity in EPA is more primitive, and cells within lumina may appear to float free as single cells or as clumps. The hemorrhage, cholesterol clefts, and necrosis of more cellular lesions of EPA are not features of glomeruloid hemangioma.

Retiform Hemangioendothelioma

Retiform hemangioendothelioma is a recently described vascular tumor that is considered a well-differentiated and low-grade form of angiosarcoma.[132] This tumor usually presents on the extremities of young adults. Although this tumor has a tendency for recurrence, metastatic spread appears to be very uncommon. Only one case with lymph node metastasis has been reported, and no deaths have occurred.

Histopathological Features   The tumor has a predominantly subcutaneous location and is composed of ill-defined arborizing thin-walled vessels lined by a monotonous population of small protuberant hobnail endothelial cells[132] (Fig. 31-48). The vascular architecture is reminis-

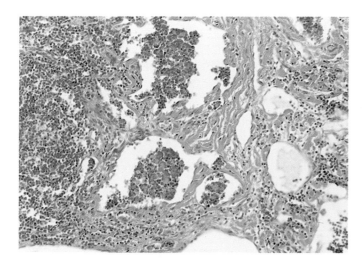

FIGURE 31-47 Endovascular papillary angioendothelioma (Dabska tumor). There are intraluminal papillary structures lined by multilayered endothelial cells that show atypia. The clumps of cells appear to float free in the lumina. (Courtesy of Dr. C.D.M. Fletcher.)

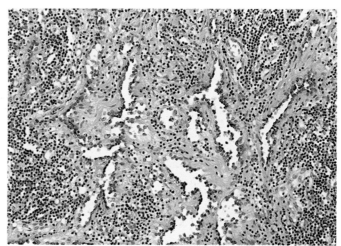

FIGURE 31-48 Retiform hemangioendothelioma. Branching and arborizing blood vessels are reminiscent of rete testis. (Courtesy of Dr. C.D.M. Fletcher.)

cent of rete testis. Frequently, the tumor is surrounded by a lymphocytic infiltrate, and in some cases lymphocytes are present within lumina of the neoplastic vessels. Solid areas of more epithelioid or spindled endothelial cells may be present.

Differential Diagnosis Retiform hemangioendothelioma and endovascular papillary angioendothelioma are considered together in the same section because they share clinical and histopathologic features; indeed, it has been recently proposed that these tumors represent the adult (retiform hemangioendothelioma) and pediatric (endovascular papillary angioendothelioma) counterparts of the same tumor. However, some histologic differences are recognized; papillary tufts, which are a striking feature in endovascular papillary endothelioma, are typically a focal finding when present in retiform hemangioendothelioma. In addition, the striking arborizing vascular channels that characterize retiform hemangioendothelioma are not usually present in endovascular papillary angioendothelioma. In contrast to endovascular papillary angioendothelioma and retiform hemangioendothelioma, targetoid hemosiderotic hemangioma (hobnail hemangioma) is well circumscribed; more superficial lesion and protuberant endothelial cells are only a focal histologic feature when present.

Kaposiform Hemangioendothelioma

Also known as *hemangioma with Kaposi's sarcoma–like features* or *Kaposi-like infantile hemangioendothelioma*, kaposiform hemangioendothelioma (KHE) is an exceedingly rare vascular tumor occurring almost exclusively in childhood and involving the soft tissue and skin.[133]

Clinical Features Most patients reported thus far have been under the age of 10 years with males and females equally affected.[133] The tumor most commonly presents as a soft-tissue mass, but the skin may be the initial site of involvement. The upper extremities have been most commonly involved, followed by the retroperitoneum and various other sites. Some tumors have developed in the context of a lymphangiomatosis or been associated with the Kasabach-Merritt phenomenon. Some lesions have exhibited locally aggressive behavior, but no patients have developed distant metastases. Because of the potential for locally aggressive disease, these tumors are considered to be borderline malignancies. Two patients have died from complications not directly related to the tumor.

Histopathological Features KHE when involving the skin and subcutis usually presents as a multinodular tumor composed of sheets of spindle cells often connected and surrounded by dense hyalinized fibrous tissue. The spindle cells comprising such nodules have elongated or crescent-shaped vascular spaces and exhibit minimal cytological atypia[133] (Fig. 31-49). Occasional rounded vascular lumina also may be observed. Among such spindle cell areas one may encounter fairly discrete aggregates of cytologically bland epithelioid endothelial cells (glomeruloid clusters). The latter cells often contain hemosiderin and hyaline globules. Well-formed vascular channels are often nested at the periphery of tumor nodules. In general, the mitotic rate is low (commonly fewer than 3 per 10 high-power fields). Inflammatory cell infiltrates containing lymphocytes and plasma cells are usually absent. The spindle cells comprising the tumor are positive for CD34 and generally negative for factor VIII–related antigen, Ulex europaeus lectin, and actin.

Differential Diagnosis The differential diagnosis includes Kaposi's sarcoma, capillary hemangioma, spindle cell hemangioendothelioma, and acquired tufted angioma. KHE generally affects younger individu-

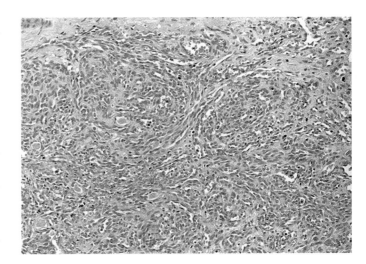

FIGURE 31-49 Kaposiform hemangioendothelioma. Note spindle cells and associated vascular channels that are elongated or have a crescent-shaped morphology, suggesting Kaposi's sarcoma. (Courtesy of Dr. H. Kozakewich.)

als, presents as a deep solitary mass, and shows no association with HIV or immunodeficiency to date. KHE does not show the diffusely infiltrative and multicentric pattern or the lymphoplasmacytic infiltrates noted in KS. In addition, KHE exhibits epithelioid cell aggregates, a feature not typically observed in KS. KHE differs from capillary hemangioma by demonstrating nodules of spindle cells with slitlike vascular channels resembling KS, frequent hemosiderin deposition, and the immunophenotype: factor VIII-, Ulex-, actin-, and CD34+. KHE does not contain the cavernous vascular spaces that typify spindle cell hemangioendothelioma. Tufted angioma is distinguished from KHE by discrete cellular nodules containing typical vascular channels and lacking fascides of spindle cells suggesting KS. In addition, there is intervening normal dermis between the tumor islands in tufted angioma.

MALIGNANT VASCULAR LESIONS

Angiosarcoma

Also known as *malignant hemangioendothelioma* or *lymphangiosarcoma*, angiosarcoma (AS) is a rare, malignant endothelial tumor that arises in skin, soft tissue, breast, bones, liver, and other viscera.[134–141] Cutaneous AS is the most common form of angiosarcoma. The prognosis for AS is poor. In one series of 72 patients with angiosarcoma of the face and scalp, one-half of the individuals died within 15 months of presentation.

Clinical Features In skin, AS most commonly arises in the scalp and face of the elderly, with men affected more frequently than women[134] (Table 31-27). AS may also occur in the setting of chronic lymphedema, often developing in a lymphedematous upper extremity as a late sequela of radical mastectomy as described by Stewart and Treves.[135] Other causes of lymphedema—idiopathic, filarial, traumatic, congenital hereditary lymphedema (Milroy's disease)[136] and morbid obesity—have also been implicated. Ionizing radiation has been linked to the development of AS with cases developing in the breast after radiation for breast cancer and in the abdominal region after irradiation of pelvic tumors.

AS generally appears as ill-defined, asymptomatic, red to violaceous patches, plaques, or nodules.[134,137–141] Satellite lesions are frequent. AS frequently presents with multifocal disease, and there is a tendency toward both local recurrence and distant metastasis. The clinical appearance of AS varies somewhat according to the degree of histologic dif-

TABLE 31-27

Angiosarcoma

Clinical Features

Clinical settings for cutaneous angiosarcoma:
    Scalp and face of the elderly—men more affected than women
    Postmastectomy (Stewart-Treves syndrome) and other causes of
      chronic lymphedema
    Postradiation therapy
Ill-defined, red to violaceous patches, plaques, and nodules
Extension well into adjacent, normal-appearing skin
Satellite lesions
Local recurrence and distant metastases

Histopathological Features

Angiomatous
    Individual or widely anastomosing vessels in dissection of collagen
      bundles
    Variably atypical endothelial cell lining, one or more layers
    Mixed inflammation, often with plasma cells
    Hemosiderin, variable extent
    Lymphangiomatous-appearing areas, minimal cytologic atypia
Spindled
    Bundles of spindled cells
    Cleftlike spaces containing erythrocytes
    Syncytium of cells with insignificant blood vessel formation
Undifferentiated/epithelioid
    Circumscribed nodules
    Sheets of epithelioid-appearing cells
    Intracytoplasmic lumen formation
    Cytologic atypia
    Prominent mitotic activity

Differential Diagnosis

Kaposi's sarcoma
Lymphangiomalike Kaposi's sarcoma
Hemangiopericytoma
Epithelioid angiosarcoma
    Poorly differentiated carcinoma
    Malignant melanoma
    Epithelioid hemangioendothelioma

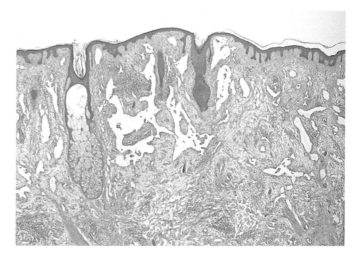

FIGURE 31-50   Angiosarcoma, well-differentiated type. Irregular thin-walled anastomosing vascular spaces dissect collagen throughout the dermis.

undifferentiated (Figs. 31-50 to 31-53). Individual tumors are composed of varying proportions of each pattern.

In angiomatous areas, vascular spaces that are distinctly individual or widely anastomosing are dispersed between dermal collagen bundles in a dissecting fashion (Fig. 31-50). The endothelium may be one to several cell layers in thickness and shows variable degrees of cytologic atypia. A mixed inflammatory response, often containing plasma cells, is usual. Hemosiderin deposition is variable. Some lymphedema-associated tumors have a lymphangiomatous appearance with irregular vascular channels devoid of erythrocytes dissecting dermal collagen bundles. The endothelium in these areas may be attenuated and show only subtle cytologic atypia. These foci are usually interspersed with more classic angiosarcomatous areas.

In spindle cell areas, spindled tumor cells are arranged in bundles that traverse the dermis in multiple directions, often enveloping adnexal structures. Cleftlike spaces and cracks containing erythrocytes are formed. The tumor may appear as a syncytium of cells without significant blood vessel formation.

"Undifferentiated" areas are usually encountered as circumscribed nodules within more characteristic areas of AS. Solid sheets of "epithelioid" tumor cells with abundant acidophilic cytoplasm and large, atyp-

ferentiation. Histologically more undifferentiated AS lesions may grow rapidly, with fungating and ulcerative appearances. Undifferentiated AS lesions may appear epithelioid and are high-grade neoplasms that generally affect deep, usually intramuscular, soft tissue and rapidly develop metastases. Cutaneous occurrence has been reported, although the few cases that have been described had a distinctly better prognosis than other undifferentiated AS. Such cutaneous tumors perhaps may fall into the spectrum of epithelioid hemangioendothelioma.

Retiform hemangioendothelioma has been described recently as a low-grade AS favoring the second to fourth decades of life and occurring most commonly on the upper and lower limbs (see above). The tumor has a good prognosis with frequent local recurrence but a low incidence of metastasis and no tumor-related deaths.

Histopathological Features   Cutaneous AS extensively infiltrates the dermis, with microscopic involvement extending well beyond the clinically apparent boundaries (Table 31-27).[134–141] The epidermis may be normal, atrophic, or ulcerated. Direct epidermal invasion or involvement of the papillary dermis usually does not occur. Three distinct patterns of proliferation have been described: angiomatous, spindled, and

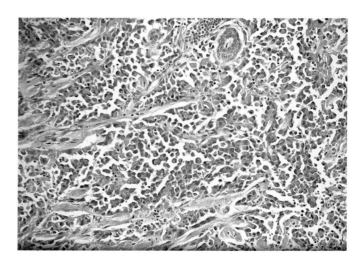

FIGURE 31-51   Angiosarcoma. Epithelioid endothelial cells in multilayered patterns fill vascular spaces and infiltrate the dermis.

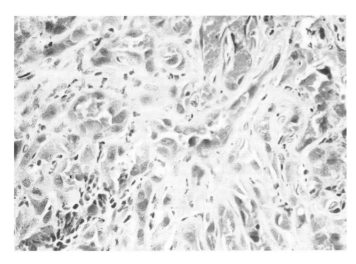

FIGURE 31-52 Angiosarcoma. Large atypical epithelioid endothelial cells protrude into vascular spaces.

ical nuclei expand the dermis (Figs. 31-51 to 31-53). Lumen formation is usually only evident at the intracytoplasmic level. Intralesional hemorrhage may be prominent.

Unusual variants of AS have been reported. An AS of the face contained many tumor cells with the appearance of granular cells. The newly described retiform hemangioendothelioma has a distinct retiform pattern of long arborizing vessels with a monomorphic hobnail endothelial lining. A lymphocytic infiltrate is usually present, and there are focal papillations similar to those of endovascular papillary angioendothelioma (Dabska's tumor).

Studies of AS have variably indicated blood vessel or lymphatic differentiation, and, therefore, the histogenesis of AS is controversial. Ultrastructurally, AS generally shows features of endothelial cells, and cases often suggest blood vessel differentiation. Immunohistochemical analysis has shown positivity for Ulex europaeus lectin 1, vimentin, laminin (a constituent of basal lamina), and other endothelial cell markers but often demonstrates only the variable presence or absence of factor VIII–related antigen. Furthermore, the immunohistochemical pattern can vary within tumors, suggesting mixed differentiation of both blood vascular and lymphatic endothelium. Further clarification of the histogenesis must await the development of additional endothelial markers.

Differential Diagnosis   Kaposi's sarcoma displays dissection of dermal collagen by newly formed vascular channels similar to that of angiomatous- and lymphangiomatous-appearing areas of AS. An important feature to be identified within AS is endothelial "layering" and cytologic atypia. In contrast, the endothelial lining of KS is usually inconspicuous and almost always one cell layer in thickness. Particular confusion, however, may still arise between the lymphangiomatous pattern of AS and the lymphangiomatous variant of KS. The clinical setting associated with each entity is very helpful as are areas of more typical AS identified in lymphedema-associated AS. In general, AS displays more intralesional variation than KS.

AS with a predominant spindle cell pattern may mimic plaques and nodules of Kaposi's sarcoma. Features of distinction include the identification of more angiomatous areas in AS and a degree of cytologic atypia exceeding that observed in even florid nodules of KS. The clinical context is also helpful, since AS is often confined to the head and neck of elderly individuals or unilaterally to a lymphedematous upper extremity. KS often does not involve such anatomic sites in older individuals.

In contrast to AS, hemangiopericytomas contain dilated sinusoidal spaces with a characteristic antlerlike or staghorn configuration lined by a single layer of flattened endothelial cells. A reticulin stain will further highlight differences between these two entities. In AS, the delicate reticulin sheath will be present peripheral to the inner lining of atypical endothelial cells, whereas in hemangiopericytoma the tumor cells will lie outside this reticulin sheath.

Epithelioid AS may be mistaken for poorly differentiated carcinoma or melanoma. Compounding the difficulty in distinction from carcinoma is the coexpression of cytokeratin and endothelial markers by epithelioid angiosarcoma.[139] This emphasizes the need for a broad panel of antibodies when such tumors are being evaluated.

Some squamous cell carcinomas have an intense acantholytic pattern, closely resembling the histology of well-differentiated AS. The demonstration of keratins and negative endothelial markers by immunoperoxidase stains is diagnostic.

REFERENCES

1. Hunt SJ, Santa Cruz DJ: Acquired benign and "borderline" vascular lesions. *Dermatol Clinic* 10:97–112, 1992.
2. Wassef M: Angiomes et malformations vasculaires cervico-céphaliques: Aspects histopatholigiques et classification. *Journal des Maladies Vasculaires (Paris)* 17:20–25, 1992.
3. Mulliken JB: A biologic classification of vascular birthmarks in, Boccalon H (ed): *Vascular Medicine.* Amsterdam, Elsevier Science Publishers, 1993, pp 603–614.
4. Takahashi K, Mulliken JB, Kozakewich HP, et al: Cellular markers that distinguish the phases of hemangioma during infancy and childhood. *J Clin Invest* 93(6):2357–2364, 1994.
5. Gold MH, Eramo L, Prendiville JS, et al: Hereditary benign telangiectasia. *Pediatr Dermatol* 6:194–197, 1989.
6. Perry WH: Clinical spectrum of hereditary hemorrhagic telangiectasia (Osler-Weber-Rendu disease). *Am J Med* 82:989, 1987.
7. Smith LL, Conerly SL: Ataxia-telangiectasia or Louis-Bar syndrome. *J Am Acad Dermatol* 12:681, 1985.
8. McGrae JD Jr, Winklemann RK: Generalized essential telangiectasia. *JAMA* 185:909, 1963.
9. Wilkin JK, Smith JG Jr, Cullison DA, et al: Unilateral dermatosomal superficial telangiectasia. *J Am Acad Dermatol* 8:468, 1983.
10. Picascia DD, Esterly NB: Cutis marmorata telangiectatica congenita: Report of 22 cases. *J Am Acad Dermatol* 20:1089, 1989.
11. Bean WB, Walsh JR: Venous lakes. *Arch Dermatol* 74:459, 1956.
12. Alcalay J, Sandbank M: The ultrastructure of cutaneous venous lakes. *Int J Dermatol* 26:645, 1987.
13. Epstein E, Novy FG Jr, Allington HV, et al: Capillary aneurysms of the skin. *Arch Dermatol* 91:335, 1965.
14. Bean WB: *Vascular Spiders and Related Lesions of the Skin.* CC Thomas, Springfield, IL, 1958.

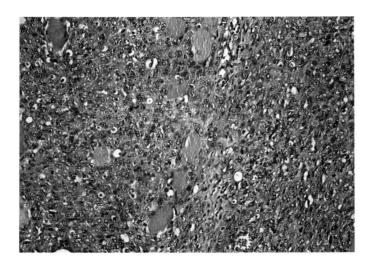

FIGURE 31-53 Angiosarcoma. High-grade, moderately differentiated neoplasm demonstrates sheets of tumor cells.

15. Wenzl JE, Burgert EO: The spider nevus in infancy and childhood. *Pediatrics* 33: 227–232, 1964.

16. Stevenson JR, Lincoln CS Jr: Angioma serpiginosum. *Arch Dermatol* 95:16–22, 1967.

17. Marriott PJ, Munro DD, Ryan T: Angioma serpiginosum-familial incidence. *Br J Dermatol* 93:701–706, 1975.

18. Suzuki Y, Nakamura N, Fukuoka K, et al: B-galactosidase deficiency in juvenile and adult patients: Report of six Japanese cases and review of literature. *Hum Genet* 36: 219–229, 1977.

19. Ishibashi A, Tsuboi R, Shinmei M: B-Galactosidase and neuraminidase deficiency associated with angiokeratoma corporis diffusum. *Arch Dermatol* 120:1344–1346, 1984.

20. Imperial R, Helwig EB: Angiokeratoma: A clinicopathologic study. *Arch Dermatol* 95: 166–175, 1967.

21. Rossi A, Bozzi M, Barra E: Verrucous hemangioma and angiokeratoma circumscriptum: Clinical and histologic differential characteristics. *J Dermatol Surg Oncol* 15: 88–91, 1989.

22. Enjolras O, Herbreteau D, Lemarchand F, et al: Hemangiomas and superficial vascular malformations: Classification. *J Mal Vasc* 17:2–19, 1992.

23. Jessen RT, Thompson S, Smith EB: Cobb syndrome. *Arch Dermatol* 113:1587,1977.

24. Uram M, Zubillaga C: Cutaneous manifestation of Sturge-Weber disease. *J Clin Neuropathol* 2:245–248, 1982.

25. Mullins JF, Naylor D, Redetsky J: The Klippel-Trenaunay-Weber syndrome. *Arch Dermatol* 85:120–124, 1982.

26. Viljoen D, Saxe N, Pearn J, Beighton P: The cutaneous manifestations of the Klippel-Trenaunay-Weber syndrome. *Clin Exp Dermatol* 12:12–17, 1987.

27. Rice JS, Fischer DS: Blue rubber-bleb nevus syndrome. *Arch Dermatol* 86:503, 1962.

28. Jorizzo JR, Ampara EG: MR imaging of blue rubber-bleb nevus syndrome. *J Comput Assist Tomogr* 10(4):686, 1986.

29. Bean WB: Dyschondroplasia and hemangiomata. *Arch Intern Med* 95:767, 1955.

30. Rao VK, Weiss SW: Angiomatosis of soft tissue: An analysis of the histologic features and clinical outcome in 51 cases. *Am J Surg Pathol* 16:764, 1992.

31. Imperial R, Helwig EB: Verrucous hemangioma: A clinicopathologic study of 21 cases. *Arch Dermatol* 96:247–253, 1967.

32. Klein JA, Barr RJ: Verrucous hemangioma. *Pediatr Dermatol* 2:191–193 1985.

33. Weiss SW, Enzinger FM: Spindle cell hemangioendothelioma: A low-grade angiosarcoma resembling a cavernous hemangioma and Kaposi's sarcoma. *Am J Surg Pathol* 10:521–530, 1986.

34. Scott GA, Rosai J: Spindle cell hemangioendothelioma: Report of seven additional cases of a recently described vascular neoplasm. *Am J Dermatopathol* 10:281–288, 1988.

35. Fletcher CD, Beham A, Schmid C: Spindle cell haemangioendothelioma: A clinicopathological and immunohistochemical study indicative of a non-neoplastic lesion. *Histopathology* 18:291–30, 1991.

36. Pellegrini AE, Drake RD, Qualman SJ: Spindle cell hemangioendothelioma: A neoplasm associated with Maffuci's syndrome. *J Cutan Pathol* 22:173–176, 1995.

37. Biberstein HH, Jessner M: A cirsoid aneurysm in the skin. *Dermatologica* 113:129, 1956.

38. Girard C, Graham JH, Johnson WC: Arteriovenous hemangioma (arteriovenous shunt): A clinicopathological and histochemical study. *J Cutan Pathol* 1:73, 1974.

39. Carapeto FJ, Garcia-Perez A, Winkelmann RK: Acral arteriovenous tumor. *Acta Derma Venerol* 57:155, 1977.

40. Connelly MG, Winkelmann RK: Acral arteriovenous tumor: A clinicopathologic review. *Am J Surg Pathol* 9:15–21, 1985.

41. Mulliken JB, Young AE: *Vascular Birthmarks: Hemangiomas and Malformations.* Philadelphia, Saunders, 1988, pp 63–76.

42. Kasabach HH, Merritt KK: Capillary hemangioma with extensive purpura: Report of a case. *Am J Dis Child* 59:1063, 1940.

43. Mills SE, Cooper PH, Fechner RE: Lobular capillary hemangioma: The underlying lesion of pyogenic granuloma: A study of 73 cases from the oral and nasal mucous membranes. *Am J Surg Pathol* 4:471–479, 1980.

44. Valentic JP, Barr RJ, Weinstein GD: Inflammatory neovascular nodules associated with oral isotretinoin treatment of severe acne. *Arch Dermatol* 119:871–872, 1983.

45. Cooper PH, McAllister HA, Helwig EB: Intravenous pyogenic granuloma: A study of 18 cases. *Am J Surg Pathol* 3:221–228, 1979.

46. Cooper PH, Mills SE: Subcutaneous granuloma pyogenicum: Lobular capillary hemangioma. *Arch Dermatol* 118:30–33, 1982.

47. Braunstein Wilson B, Greer KE, Cooper PH: Eruptive disseminated lobular capillary hemangioma (pyogenic granuloma). *J Am Acad Dermatol* 21:391–394, 1989.

48. Strohal R, Gillitzer R, Zonzits E, Stingl G: Localized vs generalized pyogenic granuloma: A clinicopathologic study. *Arch Dermatol* 127:856–861, 1991.

49. Padilla RS, Orkin M, Rosai J: Acquired "tufted" angioma (progressive capillary hemangioma): A distinctive clinicopathologic entity related to lobular capillary hemangioma. *Am J Dermatopathol* 9:292–300, 1987.

50. Wilson Jones E, Orkin M: Tufted angioma (angioblastoma): A benign progressive angioma, not to be confused with Kaposi's sarcoma or low-grade angiosarcoma. *J Am Acad Dermatol* 20:214–225, 1989.

51. Cho KH, Kim SH, Park KC, et al: Angioblastoma (Nakagawa)—is it the same as tufted angioma? *Clin Exp Dermatol* 16:110–113, 1991.

52. Ishikawa O, Nihei Y, Ishikawa H: The skin changes of POEMS syndrome. *Br J Dermatol* 117:523–526, 1987.

53. Chan JKC, Fletcher CDM, Hicklin GA, et al: Glomeruloid hemangioma: A distinctive cutaneous lesion of multicentric Castleman's disease associated with POEMS syndrome. *Am J Surg Pathol* 14:1036–1046, 1990.

54. Cockerell CJ, LeBoit PE: Bacillary angiomatosis: A newly characterized, pseudoneoplastic, infectious, cutaneous vascular disorder. *J Am Acad Dermatol* 22:501–512, 1990.

55. Koehler JE, Quinn FD, Berger TG, et al: Isolation of *Rochalimaea* species from the cutaneous and osseous lesions of bacillary angiomatosis. *N Engl J Med* 327:1625–1631, 1992.

56. Koehler JE, Glaser CA, Tappero JW: *Rochalimaea henselae* infection: A new zoonosis with the domestic cat as reservoir. *JAMA* 271:531–535, 1994.

57. Rosai J, Gold J, Landy R: The histiocytoid hemangiomas: A unifying concept embracing several previously described entities of skin, soft tissue, large vessels, bone, and heart. *Human Pathol* 10:707–730, 1979.

58. Rosai J: Angiolymphoid hyperplasia with eosinophilia of the skin: Its nosological position in the spectrum of histiocytoid hemangioma. *Am J Dermatopathol* 4:175–184, 1982.

59. Googe PB, Harris NL, Mihm MC Jr: Kimura's disease and angiolymphoid hyperplasia with eosinophilia: Two distinct histopathological entities. *J Cutan Pathol* 14:263–271, 1987.

60. Urabe A, Tsuneyoshi M, Enjoji M: Epithelioid hemangioma versus Kimura's disease: A study. *Am J Surg Pathol* 11:758–766, 1987.

61. Chan JK, Hui PK, Ng CS, et al: Epithelioid haemangioma (angiolymphoid hyperplasia with eosinophilia) and Kimura's disease in Chinese. *Histopathology* 15:557–574, 1989.

62. Olsen TG, Helwig EB: Angiolymphoid hyperplasia with eosinophilia: A clinicopathologic study of 116 patients. *J Am Acad Dermatol* 12:781–796, 1985.

63. Hunt SJ, Santa Cruz DJ, Barr RJ: Microvenular hemangioma. *J Cutan Pathol* 18: 235–240, 1991.

64. Aloi F, Tomasini C, Pippione M: Microvenular hemangioma. *Am J Dermatopathol* 15: 534–538, 1993.

65. Santa Cruz DJ, Aronberg J: Targetoid hemosiderotic hemangioma. *J Am Acad Dermatol* 19:550–558, 1988.

66. Strutton GF, Weedon D: Acro-angiodermatitis: A simulant of Kaposi's sarcoma. *Am J Dermatopathol* 9:85–89, 1987.

67. Kolde G, Worheide J, Baumgartner R, Brocker EB: Kaposi-like acro-angiodermatitis in an above-knee amputation stump. *Br J Dermatol* 120:575–580, 1989.

68. Le Boit PE: Lobular capillary proliferation: The underlying process in diverse benign cutaneous vascular neoplasms and reactive conditions. *Semin Dermatol* 8:298–310, 1989.

69. Marshall ME, Hatfield ST, Hatfield DR: Arteriovenous malformation simulating Kaposi's sarcoma (pseudo-Kaposi's sarcoma). *Arch Dermatol* 121:99–100, 1985.

70. Clearkin KP, Enzinger FM: Intravascular papillary endothelial hyperplasia. *Arch Pathol Lab Med* 100:441–444, 1976.

71. Kuo T-T, Sayers CP, Rosai J: Masson's "vegetant intravascular hemangioendothelioma": A lesion often mistaken for angiosarcoma. Study of seventeen cases located in the skin and soft tissues. *Cancer* 38:1227–1236, 1976.

72. Barr RJ, Graham JH, Sherwin LA: Intravascular papillary endothelial hyperplasia: A benign lesion mimicking angiosarcoma. *Arch Dermatol* 114:723–726, 1978.

73. Albrecht S, Kahn HJ: Immunohistochemistry of intravascular papillary endothelial hyperplasia. *J Cutan Pathol* 17:16–21, 1990.

74. Pfleger L, Tappeiner J: Zur Kenntnis der systemisierten Endotheliomatose der cutanen theliose? *Hautarzt* 10:359–363, 1959.

75. Tappeiner J, Pfleger L: Angioendotheliomatosis proliferans systematisata. *Hautarzt* 14:67–70, 1963.

76. Wick MR, Mills SE, Scheithauer BW, et al: Reassessment of malignant "angioendotheliomatosis": Evidence in favor of its reclassification as "intravascular lymphomatosis." *Am J Surg Pathol* 10:112–123, 1986.

77. Martin S, Pitcher D, Tschen J, et al: Reactive angioendotheliomatosis. *J Am Acad Dermatol* 2:117–123, 1980.

78. Eisert J: Skin manifestations of subacute bacterial endocarditis: Case report of subacute bacterial endocarditis mimicking Tappeiner's angioendotheliomatosis. *Cutis* 25:394–400, 1980.

79. Lazova R, Slater C, Scott G: Reactive angioendotheliomatosis: Case report and review of the literature. *Am J Dermatopathol* 18:63–69, 1996.

80. LeBoit PE, Solomon AR, Santa Cruz DJ, Wick MR: Angiomatosis with luminal cryoprotein deposition. *J Am Acad Dermatol* 27:969–973, 1992.

81. Sheibani K, Battifora H, Winberg CD, et al: Further evidence that "malignant angioendotheliomatosis" is an angiotropic large-cell lymphoma. *N Engl J Med* 314:943–948, 1986.

82. Bhawan J, Wolff SM, Ucci AA, et al: Malignant lymphoma and malignant angioendotheliomatosis: One disease. *Cancer* 55:570–576, 1985.

83. Carroll RE, Berman AT: Glomus tumors of the hand. *J Bone Joint Surg [Am]* 54A: 691–703, 1972.

84. Beham A, Fletcher CD: Intravascular glomus tumour; a previously undescribed phenomenon. *Virchows Arch A Pathol Anat Histopathol* 418:175–177, 1991.

85. Landthaler M, Braun-Falco O, Eckert F, et al: Congenital multiple plaquelike glomus tumors. *Arch Dermatol* 126:1203–1207, 1990.

86. Aiba M, Hirayama A, Kuramochi S: Glomangiosarcoma in a glomus tumor: An immunohistochemical and ultrastructural study. *Cancer* 61:1467–1471, 1988.

87. Gould EW, Manivel JC, Albores-Saavedra J, Monforte H: Locally infiltrative glomus tumors and glomangiosarcomas: A clinical, ultrastructural, and immunohistochemical study. *Cancer* 65:310–318, 1990.

88. Kaye VM, Dehner LP: Cutaneous glomus tumor: A comparative immunohistochemical study with pseudoangiomatous intradermal melanocytic nevi. *Am J Dermatopathol* 13:2–6, 1991.

89. Murray MR, Stout AP: The glomus tumor: Investigation of its distribution and behavior, and the identity of its "epithelioid" cell. *Am J Pathol* 18:183–203, 1942.

90. Whimster IW: The pathology of lymphangioma circumscriptum. *Br J Dermatol* 94:473–486, 1976.

91. Flanagan BP, Helwig EB: Cutaneous lymphangioma. *Arch Dermatol* 113:24–30, 1977.

92. Wilson Jones E, Winkelmann RK, Zachary CB, Reda AM: Benign lymphangioendothelioma. *J Am Acad Dermatol* 23:229–235, 1990.

93. Mehregan DR, Mehregan AH, Mehregan DA: Benign lymphangioendothelioma: Report of 2 cases. *J Cutan Pathol* 19:502–505, 1992.

94. Weiss SW, Enzinger FM: Epithelioid hemangioendothelioma: A vascular tumor often mistaken for a carcinoma. *Cancer* 50:970–981, 1982.

95. Weiss SW, Ishak KG, Dail DH, et al: Epithelioid hemangioendothelioma and related lesions. *Semin Diagn Pathol* 3:259–287, 1986.

96. Bollinger BK, Laskin WB, Knight CB: Epithelioid hemangioendothelioma with multiple site involvement: Literature review and observations. *Cancer* 73:610–615, 1994.

97. Marrogi AJ, Hunt SJ, Santa Cruz DJ: Cutaneous epithelioid angiosarcoma. *Am J Dermatopathol* 12:350–356, 1990.

98. Cox FH, Helwig EB: Kaposi's sarcoma. *Cancer* 12:289–298, 1959.

99. O'Brien PH, Brasfield RD: Kaposi's sarcoma. *Cancer* 19:1497–1502, 1966.

100. Rothman S: Remarks on sex, age, and racial distribution of Kaposi's sarcoma and on possible pathogenetic factors. *ActaUn Int Cancer* 18:326, 1962.

101. DiGiovanna JJ, Safai B: Kaposi's sarcoma: retrospective study of 90 cases with particular emphasis on the familial occurrence, ethnic background and prevalence of other diseases. *Am J Med* 71:779, 1981.

102. Safai B, Mike V, Giraldo G, et al: Association of Kaposi's sarcoma with second primary malignancies: Possible etiopathologic implications. *Cancer* 45:1472–1479, 1980.

103. O'Connell KM: Kaposi's sarcoma: Histopathological study of 159 cases from Malawi. *J Clin Pathol* 30:687–695, 1977.

104. Templeton AC: Kaposi's sarcoma. *Pathol Annu* 16:315–336, 1981.

105. Dorfman RF: Kaposi's sarcoma: With special reference to its manifestations in infants and children and to the concepts of Arthur Purdy Stout. *Am J Surg Pathol* 10:68S, 1986.

106. Friedman-Kien AE, Saltzman BR: Clinical manifestations of classical, endemic African, and epidemic AIDS-associated Kaposi's sarcoma. *J Am Acad Dermatol* 22:1237–50, 1990.

107. Garcia-Muret MP, Pujol RM, Puig L, et al: Disseminated Kaposi's sarcoma not associated with HIV infection in a bisexual man. *J Am Acad Dermatol* 23:1035–1038, 1990.

108. Harwood AR, Osaba D, Hofstader SL, et al: Kaposi's sarcoma in recipients of renal transplants. *Am J Med* 67:759–765, 1979.

109. Shmueli D, Shapira Z, Yussim A, et al: The incidence of Kaposi's sarcoma in renal transplant patients and its relation to immunosuppression. *Transplant Proc* 21:3209, 1989.

110. Chor PJ, Santa Cruz DJ: Kaposi's sarcoma. A clinicopathologic review and differential diagnosis. *J Cutan Pathol* 19:6–20, 1992.

111. Francis ND, Parkin JM, Weber J, Boylston AW: Kaposi's sarcoma in acquired immune deficiency syndrome (AIDS). *J Clin Pathol* 39:469–474, 1986.

112. Santucci M. Pimpinelli N, Moretti S, Gianotti B: Classic and immunodeficiency-associated Kaposi's sarcoma: Clinical, histologic, and immunologic correlations. *Arch Pathol Lab Med* 112:1214, 1988.

113. Niedt GW, Myskowski PL, Urmacher C, et al: Histology of early lesions of AIDS-associated Kaposi's sarcoma. *Mod Pathol* 3:64, 1990.

114. Ackerman AB: Subtle clues to diagnosis by conventional microscopy: The patch stage of Kaposi's sarcoma. *Am J Med* 1:165, 1979.

115. Blumenfeld W, Egbert BM, Sagebiel RW: Differential diagnosis of Kaposi's sarcoma. *Arch Pathol Lab Med* 109:123–127, 1985.

116. Gottlieb GJ, Ackerman AB: Kaposi's sarcoma: An extensively disseminated form in young homosexual men. *Hum Pathol* 13:882–892, 1982.

117. Kao GF, Johnson FB, Sulica VI: The nature of hyaline (eosinophilic) globules and vascular slits of Kaposi's sarcoma. *Am J Dermatopathol* 12:256, 1990.

118. Fukunaga M, Silverberg SG: Hyaline globules in Kaposi's sarcoma: A light microscopic and immunohistochemical study. *Lab Invest* 60:31A, 1989.

119. Gange RW, Wilson Jones E: Lymphangioma-like KS: A report of three cases. *Br J Dermatol* 100:327–334, 1979.

120. Holden CA: Histogenesis of Kaposi's sarcoma and angiosarcoma of the face and scalp. *J Invest Dermatol* 93:119S–124S, 1989.

121. Chang Y, Cesarman E, Pessin MS, et al: Identification of herpesvirus-like DNA sequences in AIDS-associated Kaposi's sarcoma. *Science* 266:1865–1869, 1994.

122. Dupin N, Grandadam M, Calvez V, et al: Herpesvirus-like DNA sequences in patients with Mediterranean Kaposi's sarcoma. *Lancet* 345:761–762, 1995.

123. Levy JA: A new human herpesvirus: KSHV or HHV8? [comment] *Lancet* 346:786, 1995.

124. Enzinger FM, Smith BH: Hemangiopericytoma: An analysis of 106 cases. *Hum Pathol* 7:61–82, 1976.

125. Hultberg BM, Daugaard S, Johansen HF, et al: Malignant haemangiopericytomas and haemangioendotheliosarcomas: An immunohistochemical study. *Histopathology* 12:405–414, 1988.

126. Schurch W, Skalli O, Lagace R, et al: Intermediate filament proteins and actin isoforms as markers for soft-tissue tumor differentiation and origin: III. Hemangiopericytomas and glomus tumors. *Am J Pathol* 136:771–786, 1990.

127. Porter PL, Bigler SA, McNutt M, Gown AM: The immunophenotype of hemangiopericytomas and glomus tumors, with special reference to muscle protein expression: An immunohistochemical study and review of the literature. *Mod Pathol* 4:46–52, 1991.

128. Nunnery EW, Kahn LB, Reddick RL, Lipper S: Hemangiopericytoma: A light microscopic and ultrastructural study. *Cancer* 47:906–914, 1981.

129. Dabska M: Malignant endovascular papillary angioendothelioma of the skin in childhood. *Cancer* 24:503–510, 1969.

130. Manivel JC, Wick MR, Swanson PE, et al: Endovascular papillary angioendothelioma of childhood: A vascular lesion possibly characterized by "high" endothelial cell differentiation. *Hum Pathol* 17:1240–1244, 1986.

131. Morgan J, Robinson MJ, Rosen LB, et al: Malignant endovascular papillary angioendothelioma (Dabska tumor): A case report and review of the literature. *Am J Dermatopathol* 11:64–68, 1989.

132. Calonje E, Fletcher CD, Wilson Jones E, Rosai J: Retiform hemangioendothelioma: A distinctive form of low-grade angiosarcoma delineated in a series of 15 cases. *Am J Surg Pathol* 18:115–125,1994.

133. Zukerberg LR, Nickoloff BJ, Weiss SW: Kaposiform hemangioendothelioma of infancy and childhood: An aggressive neoplasm associated with Kasabach-Merritt syndrome and lymphangiomatosis. *Am J Surg Pathol* 17(4):321–328, 1993.

134. Holden CA, Spittle MF, Jones EW: Angiosarcoma of the face and scalp, prognosis and treatment. *Cancer* 59:1046–1057, 1987.

135. Stewart FW, Treves N: Lymphangiosarcoma in postmastectomy lymphedema: A report of six cases in elephantiasis chirurgica. *Cancer* 1:64, 1948.

136. Offori TW, Platt CC, Stephens M, Hopkinson GB: Angiosarcoma in congenital hereditary lymphoedema (Milroy's disease)—diagnostic beacons and a review of the literature. *Clin Exp Dermatol* 18:174–177, 1993.

137. Mark RJ, Tran LM, Sercarz J, et al: Angiosarcoma of the head and neck: The UCLA experience 1955 through 1990. *Arch Otolaryngol Head Neck Surg* 119:973–978, 1993.

138. Girard C, Johnson WC, Graham JH: Cutaneous angiosarcoma. *Cancer* 26:868–883, 1970.

139. Fletcher CD, Beham A, Bekir S, et al: Epithelioid angiosarcoma of deep soft tissue: A distinctive tumor readily mistaken for an epithelial neoplasm. *Am J Surg Pathol* 15:915–924, 1991.

140. Rosai J, Sumner HW, Kostianovsky M, Perez-Mesa C: Angiosarcoma of the skin: A clinicopathologic and fine structural study. *Hum Pathol* 7:83–109, 1976.

141. McWilliam LJ, Harris M: Granular cell angiosarcoma of the skin: Histology, electron microscopy and immunohistochemistry of a newly recognized tumor. *Histopathology* 9:1205–1216, 1985.

TUMORS OF ADIPOSE TISSUE, MUSCLE, CARTILAGE, AND BONE

Andrew A. Renshaw / Christopher D. M. Fletcher

TUMORS OF ADIPOSE TISSUE

Tumors of adipose tissue are common in the skin and subcutaneous tissue (Table 32-1). Although most are lipomas, a variety of other lesions have been described with distinct clinical and pathologic features. Several of these have worrisome histologic findings that may lead to confusion with liposarcoma. Although liposarcomas are more common in deep soft tissues, liposarcomas of all types may occur superficially, albeit rarely. Recognition that atypical lipoma and well-differentiated liposarcoma are two terms for identical lesions has eliminated considerable confusion. The prognosis for these tumors depends not only on grade, but also site and age. Recently, characteristic cytogenetic features have been identified in some of these tumors.

Hamartomas

FOCAL DERMAL HYPOPLASIA

Clinical and Histopathological Features   Focal dermal hypoplasia is a rare congenital lesion that may be associated with anomalies of the skin, skeleton, eyes, and ears.[1,2] It is more common in women. The lesions may appear anywhere as yellow to red nodules in a reticular pattern. Histologically, the dermis is underdeveloped and replaced by mature adipose tissue. The surrounding dermal collagen fibers may be smaller than normal. Focal, total absence of skin may be present, suggesting clinical overlap with the congenital absence of the skin syndrome.

Differential Diagnosis   The differential diagnosis includes nevus lipomatous superficialis. This is also characterized by mature adipose tissue in the dermis, but occurs in adults, is not associated with other defects, and the surrounding collagen is normal.

NEVUS LIPOMATOUS SUPERFICIALIS

Clinical Features   Nevus lipomatous superficialis is a rare lesion of young adults most commonly presenting as unilateral lesions on the lower trunk or gluteal region.[3] These are skin colored papules that may coalesce into plaques with a cerebriform surface up to 10 cm in diameter.[4] Single and multiple lesions occur; multiple lesions occur in younger patients and often are grouped in a zonal distribution on the buttock. Solitary lesions overlap clinically and histologically with fibroepithelial polyps (skin tags). Only rare recurrences are reported.

TABLE 32-1

Tumors of Adipose Tissue

Mature Fat

+ Nothing = lipoma
+ Capillaries = angiolipoma
+ Spindle cells, collagen and myxoid change = spindle cell lipoma
+ Floret cells and often spindle cell areas = pleomorphic lipoma
+ Chondroblast-like cells and lipoblasts = chondroid lipoma
+ Smooth muscle = myolipoma
+ Brown fat = hibernoma

Immature Fat

+ Young age = lipoblastoma
+ Older age and lipoblasts = liposarcoma

Histopathological Features   Histologically, variable amounts of mature adipose tissue are present within the papillary dermis (Fig. 32-1). This often is clustered around blood vessels of the superficial dermal vascular plexus, which may be increased in number. The overlying epidermis may be normal, acanthotic, or hyperkeratotic.

Differential Diagnosis   When single, differentiation from a skin tag with herniation of adipose tissue may be impossible, but is of little clinical significance. Mature dermal melanocytic nevi can occasionally consist largely of "metaplastic" adipose tissue, obscuring the melanocytes. Distinction from focal dermal hypoplasia is discussed in the preceding text (above).

Benign Neoplasms

LIPOMA

Clinical Features   Lipomas are common, with an annual clinical incidence of at least approximately 0.1 percent of the population.[5] They comprise up to 5 percent of all benign tumors and 25 to 50 percent of all soft tissue tumors.[6] They are most common in the fifth and sixth decades.[6,7] They occur anywhere, but most are subcutaneous. The head and neck, arm, and upper thorax often are affected, whereas lesions of the lower leg and hand are distinctly uncommon.[5,8] Up to 7 percent are multiple; the latter are often more common in younger men.[5,6] Solitary

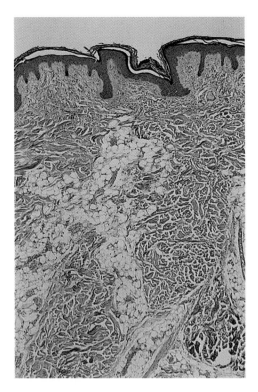

FIGURE 32-1   Nevus lipomatous superficialis. A polypoid lesion containing mature adipose tissue that extends into the papillary dermis.

lesions affect men and women equally. Most are less than 5 cm in diameter. Less than 1 percent recur; recurrence suggests incomplete excision or possibly atypical features.[7]

Histopathological Features   Lipomas are composed of lobules of mature adipose tissue enclosed in a thin fibrous capsule (Table 32-2). The adipocytes are uniform in size and appearance (Fig. 32-2). Fibrous tissue and scattered capillaries may also be present. Lesions with copious fibrous tissue are known as fibrolipoma. Occasional cases have metaplastic bone or cartilage. Degenerative changes, including foamy macrophages, lymphocytes, myxoid change, and calcification may be seen. Cytogenetically, lipomas are often associated with alterations of chromosomes 12q, 6p, and 13q.[9–11]

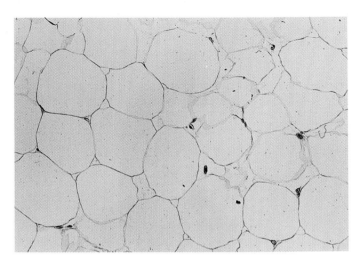

FIGURE 32-2   Lipoma. Uniformly sized adipocytes without atypia.

Differential Diagnosis   Adipose tissue hypertrophy is similar but lacks the circumscription of a lipoma or a capsule. However, some cases can not be distinguished histologically. Nodular-cystic fat necrosis is a rare lesion of uncertain origin that may be confused with lipoma. It occurs in adolescent boys and middle-aged women, may be related to trauma, and consists of infarcted adipose tissue with well-preserved cell outlines and no nuclei contained within a thin fibrovascular capsule.[12] The lack of nuclei distinguishes it from lipoma. Distinction from other benign adipose tissue tumors is discussed in the following pages. Liposarcoma is the most important lesion to exclude. Liposarcomas are discussed in the following text, but in general are defined by the presence of adipocytic atypia or lipoblasts, are often greater than 5 cm and commonly are located in the thigh.[5]

ANGIOLIPOMA

Clinical Features   Compared to lipomas, angiolipomas are one-fifth as common, occur at a younger age (17–24 years), are more commonly multiple, and often are painful (Table 32-3).[13] They occur most commonly in the forearm or on the trunk, but also in similar locations as lipomas. Grossly, they may be firmer than lipomas, usually measure less than 2 cm and are always subcutaneous. Angiolipomas are benign and cured by simple excision.

TABLE 32-2

Lipoma

Clinical Features

   Adults
   Upper body but overall wide distribution

Histopathological Features

   Mature adipose tissue
   Encapsulated

Differential Diagnosis

   Angiolipoma
   Lipomatosis
   Atypical lipoma/well differentiated liposarcoma

TABLE 32-3

Angiolipoma

Clinical Features

   Young adults
   Painful, often multiple
   Upper body

Histopathological Features

   Mature adipose tissue
   Capillaries (mainly peripheral)
   Fibrin thrombi

Differential Diagnosis

   Lipoma
   Hemangioma
   Kaposi's sarcoma
   Spindle-cell lipoma

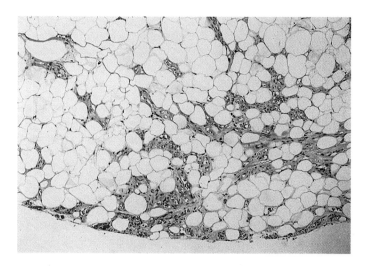

FIGURE 32-3 Angiolipoma. A mixture of mature adipocytes and capillaries that appear to be more concentrated around the periphery.

Histopathological Features   The lesion is encapsulated and composed of mature adipose tissue and a variably prominent capillary network that is often denser at the periphery (Table 32-3) (Fig. 32-3). The vessels may have a complex branching pattern and prominent pericytes. Fibrin microthrombi are present in almost all cases. Examples in which the vascular component comprises the bulk of the lesion are known as cellular angiolipomas.

Differential Diagnosis   In cases with few capillaries, distinction from lipoma may be difficult. The presence of fibrin thrombi may be helpful. Highly vascular lesions may be confused with hemangioma or even Kaposi's sarcoma.[14] In hemangiomas the capillaries radiate out from a central larger vessel, whereas in angiolipoma the capillaries are located peripherally and radiate inward. In contrast to angiolipoma, Kaposi's sarcoma has more poorly formed vascular spaces, solid aggregates of spindle cells, hyaline globules, and is poorly circumscribed. Spindle-cell lipomas with prominent vascularity may be similar, but present in older individuals, are solitary, and have organized arrays of spindle cells often associated with hyaline collagen bundles.[14] Fibrin thrombi are rare.

SPINDLE-CELL LIPOMA

Clinical Features   Spindle-cell lipoma occurs predominantly as a solitary subcutaneous mass in the shoulder and posterior neck of males between the ages of 45 and 70 (Table 32-4).[15] A significant minority of cases arise on the face. They comprise approximately 1.5 percent of adipocyte lesions and are 1/60th as common as lipoma but ten times as common as pleomorphic lipoma.[16] Local recurrence is rare.[16] Both spindle-cell and pleomorphic lipomas show karyotypic aberrations of 16q.[11]

Histopathological Features   Grossly the lesions are circumscribed, and average 4 cm (range 1–14 cm) (Table 32-4). Histologically, they are usually well-demarcated and composed of variable amounts of mature adipose tissue, uniform spindle cells in a mucinous matrix, and thick (ropey) bundles of refractile collagen (Fig. 32-4). Cases with virtually no fat occur. The spindle cells are small, with a single elongate nucleus and slender bipolar cytoplasmic processes. These cells stain positively for CD34 and often are oriented along bundles of collagen or form very short fascicles that are interspersed with the adipocytes. Mitoses are rare; pleomorphism and lipoblasts are not present. Most cases have

TABLE 32-4
Spindle-cell Lipoma

Clinical Features

    Adult males
    Subcutaneous location
    Shoulders, upper back, face

Histopathological Features

    Mature adipose tissue
    Bland spindle cells
    Ropey collagen
    Mucinous background
    Mast cells

Differential Diagnosis

    Pleomorphic lipoma
    Angiolipoma
    Neurofibroma/schwannoma
    Liposarcoma
    Hemangiopericytoma

numerous stromal mast cells. Cases with increased vascular areas and marked "pseudoangiomatous" degeneration have been described.[17,18] Exceptional cases may contain bone or cartilage.

Differential Diagnosis   The characteristic age, sex, and site are very helpful in making the diagnosis. Heavily vascular cases may be mistaken for angiolipoma (see the preceding text). Pleomorphic lipoma is distinguished by the presence of large bizarre cells, cells with multiple nuclei in a floret-like pattern, and occasional lipoblasts. Cases with a prominent spindle cell component may be confused with neurofibroma. However, in spindle-cell lipoma the nuclei are not as wavy, and the spindle cells are S100 negative (the adipocytes can be positive). Cases with a prominent mucinous background may be mistaken for myxoid liposarcoma. However, spindle-cell lipoma has very monotonous spindle-shaped cells, abundant thick collagen, lacks the characteristic "chicken wire" vascular pattern, and usually lacks lipoblasts. Cellular cases may be mistaken for well differentiated/sclerosing liposarcoma. Well-differentiated liposarcoma can contain thick bundles of collagen, but has a less uniform appearance, with large atypical cells clustered

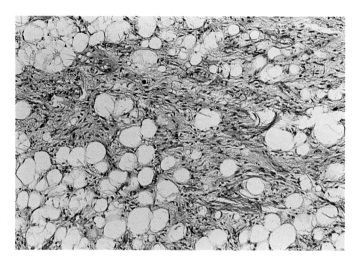

FIGURE 32-4 Spindle-cell lipoma. A mixture of mature adipocytes, ropey collagen and bland spindle cells in a myxoid matrix.

TABLE 32-5

Pleomorphic Lipoma

Clinical Features

Adult males
Subcutaneous tissue
Shoulders, upper back, face

Histopathological Features

Mature adipose tissue
Spindle-cell areas
Floret cells, bizarre cells, rare lipoblasts

Differential Diagnosis

Liposarcoma

---

around fibrous septa. Finally, very cellular lesions can resemble hemangiopericytoma. Hemangiopericytomas can contain mature adipose tissue.[19] However, the spindle cells of hemangiopericytoma more often are curved rather than straight, do not form discrete fascicles, and often are less associated with either ropey collagen or a mucoid background.

PLEOMORPHIC LIPOMA

Clinical Features Pleomorphic lipoma, like spindle-cell lipoma, occurs principally in the neck, upper back, and shoulders of men in the fifth to seventh decades (Table 32-5).[20,21] It is located in the subcutis almost exclusively. Twenty-five percent of cases have areas resembling spindle-cell lipoma, and essentially these lesions form a morphologic continuum. Both spindle-cell and pleomorphic lipomas show similar karyotypic aberrations of 16q.[11] Despite the worrisome cytologic features, pleomorphic lipomas are benign.

Histopathological Features Grossly the lesions are well circumscribed, range from 1 to 12 cm in diameter (average 4 cm), and resemble lipomas. Histologically they are not encapsulated, and characteristically have a mixture of variably sized fat cells with a varying number of pleomorphic enlarged cells (Fig. 32-5) (Table 32-5). These cells contain moderate amounts of eosinophilic cytoplasm, often are multinucleated,

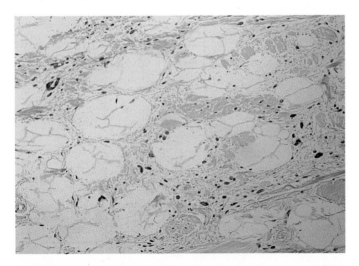

FIGURE 32-5 Pleomorphic lipoma. Atypical cells mixed with mature adipose tissue. The collagen and myxoid background are similar to that in spindle-cell lipoma.

and often have nuclei arranged in a circumferential pattern which has resulted in the term floret cell. The chromatin can be fine or smudgy and hyperchromatic. Rare lipoblasts, with cytoplasmic vacuoles indenting the nucleus, also can be found. Scarce mitoses may be present but necrosis is not observed.

Differential Diagnosis They may be distinguished in general from liposarcoma by their typical location, numerous floret cells greatly outnumbering any lipoblasts, and the absence of necrosis. In addition, in well differentiated/sclerosing liposarcoma the atypical cells and lipoblasts are concentrated along fibrous septa. Myxoid liposarcoma has a characteristic vasculature, numerous lipoblasts, and a uniform myxoid background. Collagen rarely is seen. Paradoxically, myxoid liposarcoma may be less atypical looking than pleomorphic lipoma. Pleomorphic liposarcoma has numerous lipoblasts and lacks floret cells. The atypical cells are so numerous that they form sheet like masses rather than being scattered between adipocytes.

CHONDROID LIPOMA

Clinical Features Chondroid lipoma is a recently described, rare, yet distinctive tumor.[22–24] It occurs more commonly in women over a wide age range and a variety of sites. The tumors are well circumscribed (1–11 cm) and located subcutaneously, within fascia, or intramuscularly. Whether these tumors show true chondroid differentiation is controversial but unlikely. To date, no recurrences or metastases have been reported.

Histopathological Features A mixture of mature adipose tissue interspersed with nests of round, vacuolated cells within a basophilic myxoid background is found. The vacuolated cells often have a prominent cytoplasmic border resembling chondrocytes. In some areas the vacuolated cells form cords superficially resembling myxoid chondrosarcoma. In addition, admixed with these cells are typical multivacuolated lipoblasts. Mitoses are rare. Numerous vessels with occasional fibrin thrombi also are present, as well as degenerative changes, including hemorrhage, sclerosis, and inflammation. PAS stains reveal intracellular glycogen; the lesions are reactive for S100, CD68, and vimentin.

Differential Diagnosis The lesion is unique. Chondroma lacks adipose tissue and has mature hyaline cartilage as well as multinucleated giant cells. Mixed tumors contain myoepithelial cells that may be univacuolated but rarely multivacuolated. Keratin and/or epithelial membrane antigen-positive epithelial cells should be present for the diagnosis.

Myxoid liposarcoma is distinguished by its characteristic vasculature, uniform myxoid background, and lack of vacuolated, chondroblast-like cells. Lesions without mature fat may be confused with extraskeletal myxoid chondrosarcoma, but the chondroblasts of extraskeletal myxoid chondrosarcoma are smaller, more uniform and round, and lack the extensive cytoplasmic vacuolization.

MYOLIPOMA

Clinical and Histopathological Features Myolipoma is an uncommon, recently recognized neoplasm occurring in adults but only infreqently arising in subcutaneous tissue.[25] No association with tuberous sclerosis has been found. Although deep lesions reached 25 cm in diameter, subcutaneous lesions were smaller, around 5 cm, and well circumscribed. The tumor is an intimate mixture (in varying proportions) of mature adipose tissue interspersed with well-differentiated smooth muscle, resembling a sieve. The muscle cells form only short irregular fascicles, in contrast to the long fascicles present in leiomyomas. The smooth muscle is reactive for both actin and desmin. No recurrences have been reported.

Differential Diagnosis The differential diagnosis includes spindle cell lipoma, liposarcoma, smooth muscle hamartoma, leiomyomas with fatty infiltration, and hemangiopericytoma with mature adipose tissue. The spindle cells of spindle-cell lipoma have scant cytoplasm, a mucoid background and are not immunoreactive for actin or desmin. Well-differentiated liposarcomas may have a smooth muscle component but also show adipocytic atypia and/or lipoblasts. Smooth muscle hamartoma may closely resemble this lesion, but usually is dermal and congenital. Leiomyomas with fatty infiltration have long regular fascicles, typically occur in the uterus, and rarely have such diffuse infiltration with fat. Hemangiopericytoma with adipose tissue does not form fascicles and is desmin negative.

ANGIOMYOLIPOMA

Angiomyolipomas are deep seated lesions that usually occur in the kidney but rarely may be located in other organs or in deep soft tissue. Approximately half are associated with tuberous sclerosis. The lesion is composed of mature adipose tissue, vascular channels of varying caliber, and an unusual eosinophilic spindle or round-cell component that is intimately associated with the vascular walls. Although this is often felt to represent smooth muscle, this component is immunoreactive for HMB45 as well as muscle markers. This lesion most likely is not related to superficial and subcutaneous lesions occasionally called angiomyolipomas, which probably represent angioleiomyomas with fatty metaplasia.

HIBERNOMA

Clinical Features Hibernomas are tumors of brown fat.[26] They arise usually in young to middle age adults (average age 36 years) and are commonly located between the scapulae or in the axilla (Table 32-6). They are most often subcutaneous, well-circumscribed, and measure up to 19 cm in diameter (mean 10 cm). Occasional examples are intramuscular. These tumors are benign.

Histopathological Features The tumor usually is lobulated. Three cell types are present.[27] Intermediate sized, polygonal cells with abundant granular, eosinophilic cytoplasm, and centrally placed nuclei often are most common (Table 32-6). Slightly larger cells with multiple cytoplasmic vacuoles that do not indent the centrally placed nucleus also are present. Occasionally the nuclei are eccentric. The third cell type resembles a mature adipocyte with a large solitary vacuole displacing the nucleus off to the side. A myxoid background may be present. The ultra-structural features differ from those of mature adipose tissue, and include pleomorphic mitochondria, basal lamina, and micropinocytotic vesicles.

Differential Diagnosis Diagnosis usually is straightforward. Focal areas of brown fat can be present in an otherwise typical mature lipoma. Hibernomas may be mistaken for liposarcomas, but the uniformity of the lesion, lack of mitoses, lack of atypia, and most important the lack of true lipoblasts (defined by their indented, hyperchromatic nuclei) argue against the diagnosis. Granular cell tumors and adult rhabdomyomas do not contain adipocytes.

MULTIPLE SYMMETRIC LIPOMATOSIS (MADELUNG'S DISEASE)

Multiple symmetric lipomatosis is characterized by unencapsulated masses of adipose tissue symmetrically located in the neck, shoulders, chest, abdomen, groin, or buttocks.[28,29] These lesions arise in subcutaneous tissue but spread deeply. Although generally asymptomatic, compression of airways and vital organs has been described. This condition is most common in adult males (20–52 years) and can be familial. Histologically the adipocytes are said to be smaller than normal and relatively uniform in size. Definitive diagnosis requires clinical correlation.

LIPOBLASTOMA/LIPOBLASTOMATOSIS

Clinical Features Lipoblastoma/lipoblastomatosis is rare and almost exclusively occurs in children less than 7 years old, predominantly in those less than 3.[30,31] Boys are more commonly affected (2:1). The lesions can be localized or diffuse and usually occur in the extremities. Localized forms are termed lipoblastoma and diffuse forms lipoblastomatosis. In subcutaneous sites, localized lobulated lesions less than 5 cm in diameter are most common. Although 15 to 20 percent of lesions recur (usually of the diffuse type), no metastases or deaths have been reported.

Histopathological Features Histologically the lesions mimic and may be almost identical to well-differentiated or myxoid liposarcomas (Table 32-7). At low power the tumor is distinctly lobulated or nested. At high power, numerous lipoblasts, a rich plexiform capillary network, and a myxoid matrix resemble myxoid liposarcoma. Lesions with mature adipocytes interspersed with lipoblasts and spindled or stellate

---

TABLE 32-6

Hibernoma

Clinical Features

  Young adults
  Upper back

Histopathological Features

  Granular cells
  Vacuolated cells
  Mature adipose tissue

Differential Diagnosis

  Lipoma
  Liposarcoma

TABLE 32-7

Lipoblastoma

Clinical Features

  Children
  Boys > girls
  Extremities usually
  Localized or diffuses

Histopathological Features

  Mature adipose tissue
  Often lobular growth pattern
  Lipoblasts
  Capillary network
  Spindle cells

Differential Diagnosis

  Liposarcoma

mesenchymal cells resemble well-differentiated liposarcoma. In general, however, nuclear atypia is absent in contrast to that in liposarcoma. Fibrous septa may be pronounced. Signet ring and multivacuolated lipoblasts both are present. In contrast to liposarcomas, rearrangements of chromosome 8 (der(8)) often are found cytogenetically.[32]

Differential Diagnosis   The primary differential diagnosis is with liposarcoma. Liposarcoma is rare in children, and the diagnosis must be made with caution. Liposarcomas in children occur at an older age, are more common in girls, are often located in the thigh, and usually involve deep soft tissues rather than subcutaneous sites.[33] Histologically, they lack lobulation, and have more nuclear atypia. Cytogenetic analysis may be of value in difficult cases.

Malignant Neoplasms

LIPOSARCOMA

Liposarcomas are most common in deep soft tissues, especially the thigh and retroperitoneum; however, they also occur, albeit relatively infrequently, in subcutaneous sites and rarely even in the dermis. There are several distinct types. Well-differentiated and myxoid liposarcomas are low-grade, pleomorphic, and round-cell liposarcomas are high grade. Taken together, most series show a male predominance and a mean age of 50 years (range 30–80).[34] However, myxoid and round-cell tumors tend to occur ten years earlier than well differentiated and pleomorphic tumors.

Well-Differentiated Liposarcoma, Sclerosing Liposarcoma, Atypical Lipoma

Well differentiated liposarcoma of deep soft tissues is a well-recognized entity. The same lesion occurs subcutaneously but has a markedly better prognosis, perhaps related to earlier detection and easier wide excision. Some authors prefer the term "atypical lipoma" to well differentiated liposarcoma since the clinical course is so indolent and these lesions have no potential to metastasize unless they become dedifferentiated.[35] However, the lesions are histologically identical, and the different terms are essentially synonyms.[36] Terminological preference depends heavily on liaison between surgeon and pathologist and in most instances we prefer to use both terms in the histology report. In this chapter we will use the term well-differentiated liposarcoma.

Clinical Features   Well-differentiated liposarcoma occurs in adults of either sex, mainly in the fourth to eighth decades (Table 32-8). Subcutaneous tumors are well-circumscribed, 2–20 cm in diameter (mean 10 cm), and have predilection for the upper and lower limb girdles. In subcutaneous lesions, recurrence is relatively infrequent. Metastases do not occur; however, dedifferentiation to a higher grade tumor (and hence an acquisition of metastatic potential) may rarely take place, although this is less common than in deep tumors.[37]

Histopathological Features   Histologically these lesions superficially resemble lipomas. However, the adipocytes vary in size, and fibrous septa (usually containing hyperchromatic spindle cells) often are present. The floret cells commonly seen in pleomorphic lipomas generally are not present; however, atypical stromal cells with enlarged hyperchromatic nuclei, atypical adipocytic nuclei, or vacuolated cytoplasm that indents a hyperchromatic nucleus (lipoblasts) are present (Fig. 32-6). Signet ring forms may also be observed but are hard to recognize reliably. When these atypical cells are identified among the adipocytes the term lipoma-like liposarcoma is used. When the atypical cells are associated with a predominant diffuse pattern of fine fibrosis and a relatively sparse adipocytic component the term sclerosing liposarcoma is used. Some tumors have areas with spindle cells and have been termed spindle-cell liposarcoma.[38] Cytogenetically, well-differentiated liposarcomas are associated with a ring or giant chromosome derived from the long arm of chromosome 12.[39]

Differential Diagnosis   The differential diagnosis includes lipoma, pleomorphic lipoma, spindle-cell lipoma, lipoblastoma, xanthomatous reactions, diffuse neurofibroma, and dermatofibrosarcoma protuberans (DFSP). The atypical cells distinguish this tumor from a lipoma. Pleomorphic lipomas have a rather well-defined clinical context (see the preceding text), and usually floret cells are noted rather than the smudgy atypical cells observed in well-differentiated liposarcoma. Spindle-cell lipomas have distinctive ropey (thick bundles of) collagen and lack lipoblasts. Lipoblastomas may be identical, but generally occur in children younger than 7 years of age, when the diagnosis of liposarcoma is rare indeed. Xanthomatous reactions have numerous foamy cells rather than cells with large fat vacuoles, are associated with inflammation, and lack atypia. Spindle-cell liposarcoma can be confused with either diffuse neurofibroma or dermatofibrosarcoma protuberans (DFSP). Recognition of the atypical adipocytes is most important for the correct diagnosis. In difficult cases, reactivity for neurofilament in neurofibroma and CD34 in DFSP may be helpful.

TABLE 32-8
Atypical Lipoma/Well-differentiated Liposarcoma

Clinical Features

    Adults
    Proximal extremities

Histopathological Features

    Mature adipose tissue, variably sized adipocytes
    Atypical cells
    Rare lipoblasts

Differential Diagnosis

    Lipoma

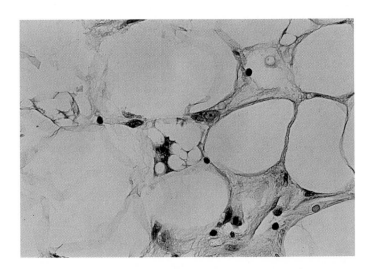

FIGURE 32-6 Well differentiated liposarcoma. Atypical Lipoma. Atypical cells are interspersed between adipocytes of various sizes. Note a lipoblast with multivacuolated cytoplasm indenting the nucleus.

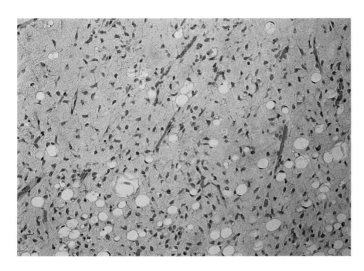

FIGURE 32-7   Myxoid liposarcoma. Lipoblasts, mainly of the signet ring type, and a prominent capillary network embedded in a myxoid matrix.

MYXOID LIPOSARCOMA

Clinical Features   The clinical presentation of myxoid liposarcoma is similar to that of well-differentiated liposarcoma, although it may occur at an earlier age and arises in the lower limb (particularly the thigh) in the vast majority of cases (see the preceding text). Like well-differentiated liposarcoma, pure myxoid liposarcoma is a low-grade tumor. Metastasis is rare from subcutaneous sites, but recurrences occur, as does transformation to a higher-grade lesion with a variably prominent round-cell component.

Histopathological Features   The tumor consists of a uniform myxoid matrix, a characteristic "chicken wire" like plexiform capillary network, numerous small relatively bland spindle cells, and a variable number of small lipoblasts, commonly of signet ring or bivacuolated type (Fig. 32-7) (Table 32-9). The most characteristic feature is the capillary network. The capillaries are evenly spaced, thin-walled, and slightly curved. Occasionally the myxoid matrix may form acellular pools creating a pseudovascular or alveolar appearance. This may be seen in other myxoid tumors. Cytogenetically, myxoid liposarcoma almost always has a t(12;16) (q13;p11) translocation that involves the transcription factor gene *CHOP*.[40]

TABLE 32-9

Myxoid Liposarcoma

Clinical Features

  Adults
  Proximal extremities

Histopathological Features

  Mature adipose tissue
  Myxoid background
  Lipoblasts, often signet ring-like lipoblasts
  Capillary network

Differential Diagnosis

  Myxofibrosarcoma
  Chordoma

TABLE 32-10

Round Cell Liposarcoma

Clinical Features

  Adults
  Proximal extremities

Histopathological Features

  Numerous undifferentiated cells
  Rare lipoblasts

Differential Diagnosis

  Undifferentiated sarcomas

Differential Diagnosis   Myxoid liposarcoma can be confused with soft tissue myxoma, superficial angiomyxoma, and myxofibrosarcoma (myxoid malignant fibrous histiocytoma). Myxomas are less cellular, lack the vascular network, and do not contain lipoblasts. Angiomyxomas lack lipoblasts and are characterized by numerous isolated vessels rather than a plexiform network of capillaries. Myxofibrosarcoma, similar to myxoid liposarcoma, is characterized by a prominent capillary network and spindle cells. However, the vessels are not as profuse and typically are slightly thicker and straighter than those in myxoid liposarcoma, and the spindle cells are more atypical in myxofibrosarcoma. In addition, lipoblasts are not present, and the lesion often has a distinctly multinodular growth pattern.

ROUND-CELL LIPOSARCOMA

Clinical and Histopathological Features   Round-cell liposarcomas can arise de novo but most often develop in a long-standing or recurrent low-grade myxoid liposarcomas (Table 32-10). Otherwise, the clinical presentation is similar to that of myxoid liposarcomas, although subcutaneous lesions are rare. Round-cell liposarcomas are characterized by a significant increase in cellularity (Fig. 32-8). The cells are smaller than adipocytes, and have enlarged hyperchromatic nuclei and prominent nucleoli. The cytoplasm may be scant or vacuolated. Despite the aggressive nature of the lesion (including eventual metastases in more than 50% of cases), mitoses usually are sparse.

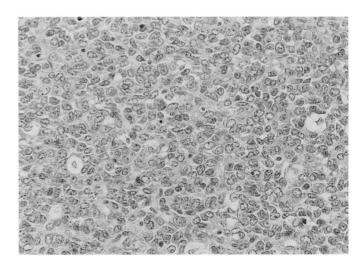

FIGURE 32-8   Round Cell Liposarcoma. Dense cellularity with rare, diagnostic, lipoblasts. The lesion merged elsewhere with more typical myxoid areas.

TABLE 32-11

Pleomorphic Liposarcoma

Clinical Features

   Adults
   Deep soft tissues

Histopathological Features

   Pleomorphic cells
   Spindle cells
   Lipoblasts

Differential Diagnosis

   Pleomorphic lipoma
   Myxofibrosarcoma
   Pleomorphic rhabdomyosarcoma
   Pleomorphic malignant fibrous histiocytoma

Differential Diagnosis   When seen as part of a low-grade liposarcoma, the diagnosis is straightforward. When a tumor is purely round-cell, the diagnosis may be very difficult and require a thorough search for lipoblasts. This type of liposarcoma also distinctively shows S100 positivity in the non-lipogenic cells in most cases.[41]

PLEOMORPHIC LIPOSARCOMA

Clinical and Histopathological Features   Pleomorphic liposarcomas are the least common type of liposarcoma, most often occur in the elderly, and subcutaneous examples are especially rare (Table 32-11). These tumors are among the most pleomorphic tumors of humans. They are cellular and can form fascicles, storiform patterns, or diffuse sheets. Cells with enlarged atypical nuclei are common (Fig. 32-9). Many of these have abundant eosinophilic cytoplasm, suggesting rhabdomyosarcomatous differentiation. However, by definition, some cells with sharply punched-out, lipid-containing cytoplasmic vacuoles and scalloping of the nucleus consistent with lipoblasts can be found.

Differential Diagnosis   The differential diagnosis includes mainly pleomorphic malignant fibrous histiocytoma (including atypical fibro-

xanthoma) and pleomorphic rhabdomyosarcoma. The identification of lipoblasts is key. Reactivity with S100 protein in liposarcoma may also be helpful.[41,42] In contrast to rhabdomyosarcoma, the tumor is negative for desmin and actin.

DEDIFFERENTIATED LIPOSARCOMA

Biphasic tumors characterized by the development of high-grade non-lipogenic sarcoma in the primary or recurrence of a well-differentiated liposarcoma have been termed dedifferentiated liposarcomas. They are more common de novo and in deep sites, but can arise in recurrences and subcutaneously. The dedifferentiated areas most often resemble pleomorphic malignant fibrous histiocytoma, myxofibrosarcoma, or rhabdomyosarcoma.[43] Although up to one-half will recur and at least 15 percent will metastasize, these dedifferentiated tumors may have a better prognosis than other "pleomorphic" sarcomas, perhaps reflecting their well-differentiated origins.

LIPOSARCOMA WITH MYOGENIC DIFFERENTIATION

Rarely, true liposarcomas can exhibit myogenic differentiation.[44–46] This is more common in deep-seated tumors, occurs in both well-differentiated and high-grade (including dedifferentiated) tumors, and can be present initially but is more common in recurrences. The muscle may be benign or malignant, and may show skeletal or smooth muscle differentiation, or both. Its presence does not appear to affect the prognosis.

MUSCLE

Smooth Muscle

Smooth muscle tumors occur mainly but not exclusively in adults (Table 32-12). Determining the prognosis of these lesions may be a difficult task for the pathologist. Prognosis is very dependent on site. Extremely bland lesions in some sites may still carry a risk for recurrence, although this may occur late.

CONGENITAL SMOOTH MUSCLE HAMARTOMA

Clinical and Histopathological Features   Smooth muscle hamartoma is a rare congenital lesion presenting in children up to 18 years old.[47,48] Clinically, they are most common on the torso, measure up to 10 cm in diameter, and may or may not occur in association with Becker's nevus (melanosis), an epidermal hamartoma exhibiting hyperpigmentation and hypertrichosis. Histologically, the lesion is composed of well-ordered non-cohesive fascicles of smooth muscle arranged in various directions within the dermis and subcutaneous tissue (Fig. 32-10). Adipocytes may also be present unusually high in the dermis. There may be an artifactual cleft between the lesion and the surrounding dermis.

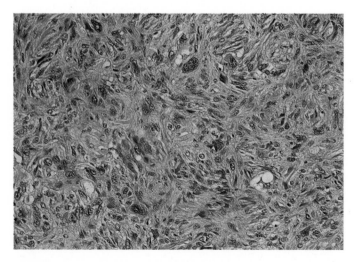

FIGURE 32-9   Pleomorphic Liposarcoma. Pleomorphic cells with rare diagnostic lipoblasts.

TABLE 32-12

Tumors of Smooth Muscle

Smooth Muscle

   + Nothing = leiomyoma
   + Vessels = angioleiomyoma
   + Mitoses, necrosis or atypia = leiomyosarcoma

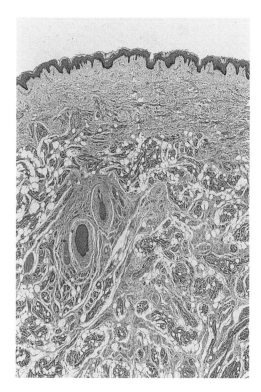

FIGURE 32-10 Congenital Smooth Muscle Hamartoma. Irregularly arranged smooth muscle bundles in the reticular dermis are interspersed with collagen, adipocytes, and adnexae.

Differential Diagnosis Diagnostically, the lesion may be associated with or distinct from Becker's nevus, which may have similar smooth muscle hyperplasia. However, Becker's nevus usually is not congenital, and the distinction is primarily clinical. Leiomyomas are also composed of smooth muscle, but the muscle bundles tend to form a single mass, whereas in hamartoma the bundles are discrete and surrounded by ordered collagen.

LEIOMYOMA

Clinical Features Smooth muscle tumors of the skin and subcutaneous tissues are uncommon and can be divided into pure leiomyomas and those arising in association with vascular structures, that is, angioleiomyomas.[49,50] Pure leiomyomas have no sex preference and generally arise in early adulthood (3rd to 4th decade). They can be separated into those that arise in the skin and nipple (dermal) and those associated with the external genitalia. Leiomyomas of the skin arise from the erector pilae muscles and tend to occur on the extensor surface of the extremities, and the trunk (Table 32-13). They are often multiple, painful, and less than 2 cm in diameter. Some cases are inherited as an autosomal dominant trait. Nipple lesions are similar and arise from areolar smooth muscle. Genital leiomyomas arise from dartos or vulvar smooth muscle. They are solitary, painless, well-circumscribed masses that may grow up to 15 cm in diameter and may be located in the subcutaneous tissue.

Separation of dermal and genital leiomyomas is most important for prognosis. Small, solitary dermal leiomyomas tend not to recur. Patients with multiple dermal leiomyomas often suffer recurrence (50%) and tend to develop subsequent lesions. Patients with genital leiomyomas tend usually to be disease free after 5 years of follow-up, but longer follow-up has shown the development of recurrences after periods as long as 15 years.[51]

TABLE 32-13

Pilar Leiomyoma

Clinical Features

　　Adults
　　Skin, nipples
　　Painful, often multiple

Histopathological Features

　　Ramifying fascicles
　　Spindle-shaped eosinophilic cells
　　Blunt-ended nuclei

Differential Diagnosis

　　Leiomyosarcoma
　　Dermatofibroma
　　DFSP
　　Neurofibroma
　　Dermatomyofibroma

Histopathological Features Histologically, dermal pilar leiomyomas are composed of numerous fascicles of smooth muscle and variable amounts of collagen arranged randomly throughout the dermis or subcutaneous tissue (Fig. 32-11). They are unencapsulated and infiltrative; involvement of hair follicles and adnexal glands is typical. The cells have abundant eosinophilic cytoplasm that may have a perinuclear vacuole; the nuclei are oval with blunt ends and evenly dispersed chromatin. Genital tumors are larger, usually better circumscribed, and centered in the subcutaneous tissues. They may have a pseudocapsule, focal calcifications, stromal myxoid change, and focal mitotic activity.[52] Any mitotic activity should raise the suspicion of malignancy. Epithelioid tumors have been described in the vulva.

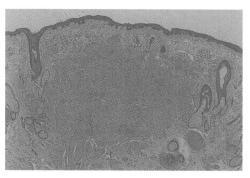

A

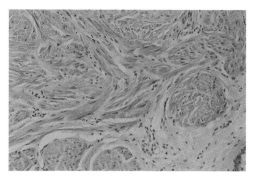

B

FIGURE 32-11 Pilar Leiomyoma. Ramifying bundles of eosinophilic spindle cells with elongate nuclei, abundant cytoplasm and no mitoses.

Differential Diagnosis   The differential diagnosis for these lesions includes dermatofibroma, dermatomyofibroma, dermatofibrosarcoma protuberans (DFSP), neurofibroma, fibromatosis, and leiomyosarcoma. Dermatofibroma is less fasicular, the cells tend to be rounder and more polymorphic, may surround collagen, and foamy macrophages may be present. DFSP has spindle cells but these tend to be wavy rather than straight, have pale rather than eosinophilic cytoplasm, form storiform patterns rather than fascicles, and are CD34-positive. Neurofibroma also has wavy nuclei, does not form fascicles, and is immunoreactive for S100 and neurofilament. Fibromatosis tends to have cells with more variable nuclei and paler cytoplasm and generally a less well-developed fasicular pattern. Low-grade leiomyosarcoma may be difficult to distinguish. Tumors larger than 2 cm that extend deep into the subcutis always should raise the suspicion of malignancy. The presence of mitotic activity, amounting to 1 or more per 10 hpf, or necrosis should also raise the possibility. In some cases definitive distinction may not be possible. In general, the diagnosis of leiomyoma should be reserved for small, superficial lesions without necrosis or mitoses or for cases in which multiple lesions are present. In occasional cases it may be appropriate to resort to the term "uncertain malignant potential."

ANGIOLEIOMYOMA (TABLE 32-14)

Clinical Features   Angioleiomyomas are solitary, often painful tumors of adults (average age 47 years) with a predilection for women (2:1); they occur mainly in the lower extremities, especially the lower leg and foot.[53] The lesion is benign and only rarely recurs.

Histopathological Features   Histologically, angioleiomyomas are well-circumscribed solid masses composed of coalesced vessels with prominent walls composed of smooth muscle and collagen (Fig. 32-12). They are commonly located in the subcutis. They have been divided in to three types, termed solid, cavernous, and venous.[53] Usually the vascular lumina are compressed, but occasionally they are large and dilated in the cavernous angioleiomyoma. The muscle of the vessel walls forms

TABLE 32-14

Angioleiomyoma

Clinical Features

    Adults, female predominance
    Lower extremity
    Painful, usually solitary

Histopathological Features

    Well-circumscribed, encapsulated
    Blood vessels
    Smooth muscle of vessel walls often in irregular concentric bundles
    Three types:
        solid
        cavernous
        venous
    Stromal hyalinization
    Myxoid change

Differential Diagnosis

    Leiomyoma
    Leiomyosarcoma
    Vascular anomaly
    Hemangioma

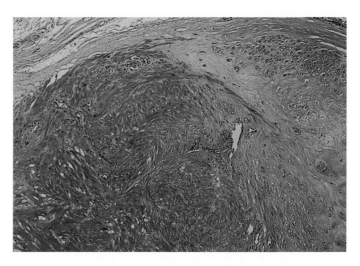

FIGURE 32-12   Angioleiomyoma. Smooth muscle cells arranged around compressed vascular spaces with focal areas of hyalinization.

irregular, often concentric bundles that merge with those of their neighbors. Stromal hyalinization or myxoid change is common. Rarely, mature adipose tissue is present. Small nerve fibers are detectable immunohistochemically.[54] Atypia, mitoses, and necrosis are rare.

Differential Diagnosis   The lesion should be distinguished from pilar leiomyoma and leiomyosarcoma. Leiomyoma is poorly circumscribed, lacks the vascular spaces, and the muscle does not emerge from vascular walls. Most leiomyosarcomas also lack the vascular spaces, although vascular leiomyosarcomas have been described.[55] Most important, leiomyosarcomas have cytologic atypia, mitoses, and necrosis. Cutaneous angiolipoleiomyomas (also reported as angiomyolipomas) are rare tumors composed of mature adipose tissue, smooth muscle, and vessels.[56] The relationship with renal angiomyolipomas is unclear but it seems most likely that this is a form of involutional metaplasia in an angioleiomyoma.

LEIOMYOSARCOMA

Clinical Features   Superficial (i.e., dermal and subcutaneous) leiomyosarcoma is most common between the ages of 40 and 80 years, although it has been described in teenagers.[57] These lesions are most common in the proximal extremities, especially the lower extremity and are generally less than 5 cm in maximum diameter.[58,59] Dermal tumors are felt to arise from erector pilae muscles, subcutaneous tumors from blood vessels. The prognosis is highly dependent on size and depth.[59] In general, tumors less than 5 cm in diameter have a much better prognosis. Up to 40 percent of dermal tumors recur but metastasis is extremely rare. In contrast, one-third of subcutaneous lesions metastasize and cause death.[58] In fact, most subcutaneous smooth muscle tumors of nonvascular type may have some malignant potential, given long enough follow-up (see the preceding text). For subcutaneous lesions, aneuploidy may be an additional unfavorable prognostic feature.[60] Neither epithelioid change, granular cell change, or myxoid change, all of which are occasional features, is prognostically important.

Histopathological Features   Histologically, leiomyosarcomas, particularly of the dermis, can closely resemble their benign counterparts with well-formed fascicles of spindle cells with abundant eosinophilic cytoplasm, and elongate blunt-ended nuclei (Table 32-15) (Fig. 32-13). The nuclei may be more vesicular and have nucleoli. The fascicles typically run at right angles to each other. Unlike leiomyomas, most tumors dis-

TABLE 32-15

Leiomyosarcoma

Clinical Features

Adults
Extremities
Dermal or subcutaneous

Histopathological Features

Smooth muscle
Mitoses
Atypia
Necrosis

Differential Diagnosis

Leiomyoma
Dermatofibroma
Fibromatosis
Myxofibrosarcoma
DFSP
Rhabdomyosarcoma
Granular cell tumor
Malignant melanoma
Neurothekeoma
Epithelioid sarcoma
Metastatic carcinoma
Metastatic leiomyosarcoma

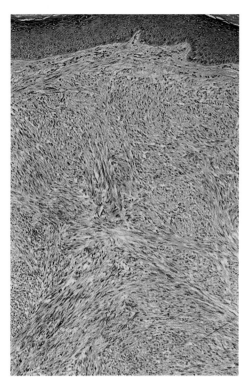

FIGURE 32-13 Leiomyosarcoma. Cellular spindle-cell lesion forming fascicles extending up to epidermis. Mitoses were present.

play some pleomorphism, mitotic activity, and/or necrosis; however, well-differentiated tumors may be difficult to differentiate from leiomyomas (see the preceding text). Some tumors are epithelioid, and composed of rounded cells that do not form fascicles and often have clear cytoplasm.[57] These are more common in the head and neck.[61] Others have abundant granular cytoplasm; still others have a myxoid background.[62,63] As with leiomyomas, dermal lesions often are highly infiltrative; by contrast, subcutaneous lesion appear more circumscribed and more commonly have degenerative changes such as hyalinization or myxoid change.

Immunohistochemically, these tumors typically are reactive for actin and often desmin, and some cases (<10%) express keratin.[57,64,65] Granular cell variants of leiomyosarcoma are negative for S100, but in addition to muscle markers, stain for NKIC3.[62]

Differential Diagnosis The distinction from leiomyoma can be difficult. In general, leiomyosarcomas occur in an older age group, and more commonly in the proximal extremity. Certainly, tumors that extend widely into the subcutis, are larger than 2 cm, have more than 1 mitosis per 10 hpf or necrosis at all should be diagnosed as benign with great trepidation. All of these features are more common in leiomyosarcomas (Table 32-16). In some cases absolute distinction may not be possible, and in these cases this uncertainty should be expressed in the report using such terms as "uncertain malignant potential." Distinction from dermatofibroma is based on greater fasicularity, more eosinophilic cytoplasm, lack of cytologic polymorphism, presence of foam and inflammatory cells, and the finding of

desmin reactivity. Fibromatoses have more poorly formed fascicles, paler cytoplasm, and generally are desmin negative. Distinction from myxofibrosarcoma (myxoid malignant fibrous histiocytoma) is based on fascicle formation, lack of mucin-containing vacuolated cells, and reactivity for actin and or desmin. Dermatofibrosarcoma protuberans has a storiform pattern rather than fascicles, more wavy nuclei, and reactivity for CD34. Embryonal rhabdomyosarcomas can have a spindle-cell appearance, especially in the paratesticular region, but such lesions are exceedingly rare in superficial soft tissue.[66,67] Detection of true rhabdomyoblasts with their abundant eosinophilic cytoplasm and eccentric nuclei can be helpful, as well as detection of sarcomeric structures by electron microscopy.

The granular, myxoid, and epithelioid variants can be confused with granular cell tumor, malignant melanoma, cellular neurothekeoma, epithelioid sarcoma, and metastatic carcinoma. Classic type granular cell tumors often are associated with pseudoepitheliomatous hyperplasia, do not form fascicles as frequently, are S100 positive and desmin and actin negative, and have characteristic ultrastructural features. S100 and or HMB45 reactivity in melanoma is typical and such lesions tend

TABLE 32-16

Features Useful in Distinguishing Cutaneous Leiomyoma from Leiomyosarcoma

	Leiomyoma	*Leiomyosarcoma*
Peak age	20–50	30–80
Site	Trunk, extensor extremities	Proximal lower extremities
Number	Often multiple	Solitary
Depth	More superficial	Usually extend more deeply
Size	Usually <2 cm	Often larger
Necrosis	Rare	Common
Mitoses	Rare (<1/10 hpf)	Often (>3/10 hpf)

TABLE 32-17

Tumors of Skeletal Muscle

Mature skeletal muscle = hamartoma
Immature strap-like skeletal muscle no necrosis or atypia = fetal rhabdomyoma
Large round eosinophilic cells with fibrillar cytoplasm = adult rhabdomyoma
Immature skeletal muscle with mitoses or atypia = rhabdomyosarcoma

---

also to have prominent nucleoli. Neurothekeoma has a distinctive lobular growth pattern, usually some myxoid alteration, and is actin negative. Epithelioid sarcoma tends to have a multinodular growth pattern and central areas of degenerate collagen or necrosis. Metastatic carcinoma should be suspected in cases with an appropriate clinical history and keratin reactivity.

Primary cutaneous leiomyosarcoma should be distinguished from metastatic leiomyosarcoma originating in deeper visceral tissues, which is one of the more common deep tissue sarcomas to metastasize to skin. Such metastases appear to be more common in the head and neck region, are typically dermal in location and tend to be better circumscribed and morphologically higher grade than their primary cutaneous counterparts. Clinical correlation is necessary.

Skeletal Muscle

Tumors showing skeletal muscle differentiation are most common in childhood (Table 32-17). Malignant tumors are far more common than benign tumors, and benign tumors may have immature features suggesting a malignant lesion.

RHABDOMYOMATOUS MESENCHYMAL HAMARTOMA

Rhabdomyomatous mesenchymal hamartoma is a rare congenital lesion predominantly affecting boys which may be associated with other developmental anomalies of the head and neck.[68,69] It usually presents as a small soft polyp in the head and neck region. Histologically, fascicles of mature striated myofibers are seen at all levels of the dermis, interdigitating with hair follicles and adnexal structures (Fig. 32-14).

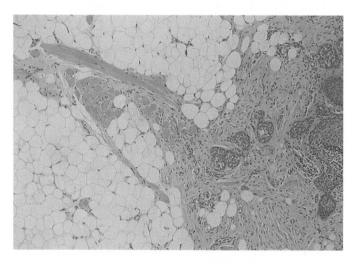

FIGURE 32-14 Rhabdomyomatous Mesenchymal Hamartoma. Irregular bundles of skeletal muscle underlie abnormal dermis.

TABLE 32-18

Rhabdomyoma

Clinical Features

  Boys <5 and men >60
  Head and neck commonest

Histopathological Features

  Immature skeletal muscle
  No mitoses or atypia

Differential Diagnosis

  Rhabdomyosarcoma
  Granular cell tumor

The fibers may form a central mass which rarely can ossify. Cross striations can be seen. Although both nevus lipomatosis superficialis and fibrous hamartoma of infancy have a variety of abnormally placed dermal tissues, they do not contain skeletal muscle. Benign Triton tumors contain muscle but are associated with nerves. Rhabdomyomas in childhood show relatively immature skeletal muscle differentiation rather than well-formed muscle fibers.

RHABDOMYOMA

Rhabdomyomas of cardiac origin are hamartomas and associated with tuberous sclerosis (Table 32-18). However, rhabdomyomas of skin and soft tissue are benign neoplasms and are not associated with any clinical syndromes. These rhabdomyomas can be divided into fetal and adult types.

Fetal Rhabdomyoma

Clinical and Histopathological Features Fetal rhabdomyomas typically occur as a solitary mass in the subcutaneous tissue of the head and neck region of boys less than 5 years of age.[70–72] Somewhat more mature but similar lesions occur in the genital areas of adult women.[73] They measure up to 12 cm in diameter, are well-circumscribed but not encapsulated. Histologically, bland, elongate spindle cells are present in a myxoid background. The cells show various stages of muscle differentiation, with poorly differentiated cells located centrally and more mature cells peripherally, but often the arrangement is haphazard (Fig. 32-15). Rudimentary fascicles may be present. Some cases may be quite cellular, and areas resembling adult rhabdomyoma with large ganglion-like cells may be present.[71,72] Mitoses, pleomorphism, and necrosis are absent. This lesion is benign.

Differential Diagnosis Atypical nuclei, hyperchromasia, and necrosis should raise the suspicion of rhabdomyosarcoma. Rhabdomyosarcomas have alternating hypercellular and hypocellular areas, are less circumscribed, do not "mature" peripherally, and may have a cambium layer if submucosal. Adult rhabdomyoma has a uniform population of large polygonal cells with abundant deeply eosinophilic cytoplasm (see the following). Rhabdomyomatous mesenchymal hamartoma is described in the preceding text.

Adult Rhabdomyoma

Clinical and Histopathological Features Adult rhabdomyomas also occur in the head and neck of males, with a predilection for the upper respiratory tract (Table 32-18).[71] The average age at presentation, however, is the sixth decade. Most are solitary but multiple lesions have

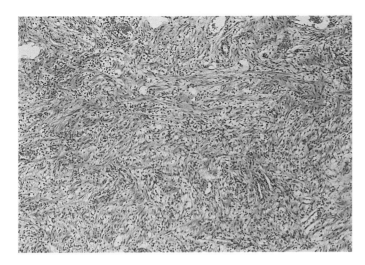

FIGURE 32-15   Fetal Rhabdomyoma. Spindle cells with elongated nuclei and cytoplasm. No mitoses were seen.

been reported.[74] They are well-circumscribed and composed of large polygonal or round cells with abundant eosinophilic cytoplasm, a large nucleus, and prominent nucleolus (Fig. 32-16). The nucleus may be eccentric or multiple. Occasional spider cells, with clear cytoplasm and thin strands of material extending from the nucleus to the cytoplasmic membrane are present. Cross striations, disorderly filamentous arrays, and crystalline material may be present in the cytoplasm. Mitoses are rare. Some cases have features of both adult and fetal types. Adult rhabdomyomas may recur, but aggressive behavior has not been seen.

Differential Diagnosis   Adult rhabdomyomas may be confused with granular cell tumors and pleomorphic rhabdomyosarcomas. Granular cell tumors are composed of slightly smaller cells with much smaller nuclei and nucleoli. The cytoplasm is generally paler and more granular. They are reactive for S100 and electron microscopy will show characteristic autophagocytic lyzosomes. Pleomorphic rhabdomyosarcomas typically occur in the extremities, are more infiltrative, and have far more cytologic atypia and mitoses.

TABLE 32-19
Rhabdomyosarcoma

Clinical Features

Mainly 0–20 years old
Males more than females
Head and neck, urogenital region, extremities

Histopathological Features

Small round blue cells, variable size
Eosinophilic cytoplasm
Strap or tadpole cells
Solid or alveolar pattern

Differential Diagnosis

Ewings/PNET
Lymphoma
Neuroblastoma
Granular cell tumor
Rhabdomyomas
Leiomyosarcoma

RHABDOMYOSARCOMA

Rhabdomyosarcomas most commonly arise in children, but are rarely primary in the skin. Three main subtypes have been described, embryonal, alveolar, and pleomorphic (Table 32-19).

Embryonal Rhabdomyosarcoma
Clinical Features   Embryonal rhabdomyosarcoma is the most common type of rhabdomyosarcoma. It occurs most frequently in the head and neck and urogenital regions of boys less than 8 years old.[75]

Histopathological Features   Histologically, noncohesive spindle- to round-shaped cells with a variable amount of cytoplasm are present in a myxoid background (Table 32-19) (Fig. 32-17). The cells have round to oval nuclei with open chromatin and inconspicuous nucleoli. Small amounts of eosinophilic cytoplasm may be present to one side of the cell or cytoplasm may be more profuse, giving rise to round, tadpole-, or strap-shaped rhabdomyoblasts. Mitoses and necrosis may be present.

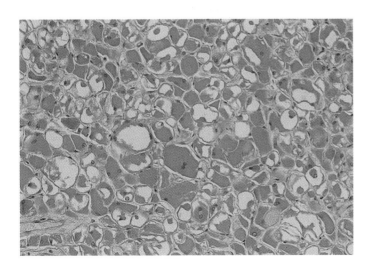

FIGURE 32-16   Adult Rhabdomyoma. Polygonal cells with abundant granular cytoplasm.

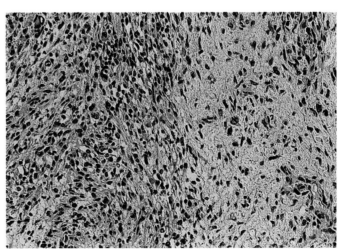

FIGURE 32-17   Embryonal Rhabdomyosarcoma. Small round to spindle-shaped cells with scant cytoplasm in a myxoid matrix.

When submucosal, the lesion may present as a polypoid mass protruding into the lumen and there may be a so-called cambium layer characterized by increased cellularity immediately beneath the epithelium. This subtype is termed botryoid. Another subtype, predominantly in the paratesticular region, has spindle cells in a fasicular or storiform pattern and is termed spindle cell.[66,67] Immunohistochemically, reactivity for muscle actin, desmin, and (in fewer cases) myoglobin or fast myosin is characteristic.[76] Ultrastructurally alternating thin and thick filaments with occasional Z bands can be demonstrated.

Differential Diagnosis   The differential diagnosis is long. Ewing's sarcoma/PNET does not have the eosinophilic cytoplasm, the eccentric nuclei, or desmin reactivity. Lymphoma does not have the eosinophilic cytoplasm and is positive for leukocyte common antigen. Neuroblastoma is distinguished by the neuropil background, less cytoplasm, and reactivity for neural markers. Granular cell tumors are more cohesive, with rounder cells and granular rather than fibrillary cytoplasm, have less prominent nucleoli and are reactive for S100. Rhabdomyomas are discussed in the preceding. The spindle cell subtype of rhabdomyosarcoma may be confused with a leiomyosarcoma or fibrosarcoma. Both lesions are uncommon in children. Leiomyosarcoma does not have cross striations by light microscopy or Z bands by electron microscopy. Fibrosarcoma has less eosinophilic cytoplasm and is desmin negative.

Alveolar Rhabdomyosarcoma

Clinical Features   Alveolar rhabdomyosarcomas are most common in adolescent boys and young men. The average age at presentation (12 years) is distinctly older than that of embryonal tumors (6 years) and less than that of the pleomorphic subtype (50 years).[77–79] Most tumors arise in the extremities, usually intramuscularly.

Histopathological Features   The initial descriptions emphasized the alveolar pattern, with cells lining up against thin fibrous septa to produce small spaces resembling lung tissue (Fig. 32-18). The cells may have a hobnail appearance, and are discohesive, with isolated cells lying free within these spaces. In contrast to embryonal rhabdomyosarcoma, the cells tend to be round rather than oval, with larger nuclei and sometimes with more abundant eosinophilic cytoplasm. Multinucleated cells

with the nuclei forming a peripheral wreath are a characteristic finding and some cases have strap cells as well.

Recently, greater emphasis has been placed on the nuclear rather than the architectural features.[79] Cases with a solid pattern without any evidence of alveolar septa but containing cells with larger, more pleomorphic nuclei, coarse chromatin, and prominent nucleoli were found to behave more like alveolar rather than embryonal rhabdomyosarcomas. A specific translocation, t(2;13)(q35;q14), has also been demonstrated in this type of rhabdomyosarcoma, and the breakpoint region has been cloned, allowing distinction from Ewing's sarcoma/PNET by cytogenetic analysis or RT-PCR.[80–82]

Differential Diagnosis   The alveolar pattern may suggest a vascular or epithelial neoplasm. Markers for CD31, CD34 and keratin are most helpful in these situations. As with embryonal rhabdomyosarcoma, in fact more so in view of the larger nuclear size, Ewing's sarcoma/PNET is also in the differential. The more prominent eosinophilic cytoplasm, the eccentric nuclei, and desmin staining are again helpful. Lymphoma is ruled out by reactivity with leukocyte common antigen.

Pleomorphic Rhabdomyosarcoma

Clinical and Histopathological Features   Pleomorphic rhabdomyosarcoma is most common in adults,[83] but comparable lesions occur also in children.[83,84] The limbs and limb girdles are the most common location. A sea of large polygonal cells with abundant eosinophilic cytoplasm forming irregular fascicles is typical (Fig. 32-19).

Differential Diagnosis   The differential diagnosis includes pleomorphic leiomyosarcoma. Ultrastructural demonstration of Z bands may be necessary for definitive separation. Distinction from pleomorphic malignant fibrous histiocytoma is based on immunoreactivity for actin and desmin, and ultrastructural demonstration of muscle differentiation.

PROGNOSIS

Rhabdomyosarcomas commonly spread to regional lymph nodes. Overall the 5-year survival for pediatric rhabdomyosarcoma is at least 55 percent.[85] The spindle cell, and botryoid subtype of embryonal rhab-

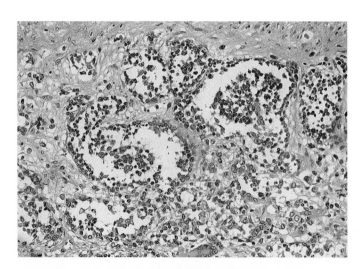

FIGURE 32-18   Alveolar Rhabdomyosarcoma. Round cells with scant cytoplasm forming structures reminiscent of pulmonary alveoli.

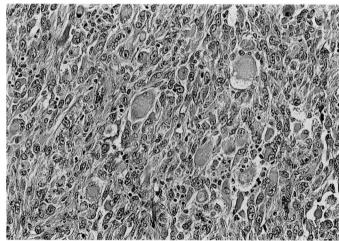

FIGURE 32-19   Pleomorphic Rhabdomyosarcoma. Spindle cells with abundant cytoplasm and large pleomorphic cells.

TABLE 32-20

Tumors of Cartilage

Mature cartilage = chondroma
Myxoid areas with cells in strands = myxoid chondrosarcoma

domyosarcoma do well.[66,67,86] Alveolar rhabdomyosarcoma has a worse prognosis than embryonal rhabdomyoarcoma.[79,87]

Pleomorphic tumors in adults and children do poorly.[83,84] Increasing age, stage, and deep location also are poor prognostic factors.[88]

CARTILAGE

Cartilage tumors in the skin and subcutaneous sites are infrequent (Table 32-20). The majority occur in the hands and feet and are benign, despite worrisome histologic features. In large cartilaginous masses occurring in superficial sites and showing significant cytologic atypia, the possibility of local spread or metastasis from a primary bone tumor always should be considered. Extraskeletal mesenchymal chondrosarcoma virtually never involves skin or subcutaneous tissue and is not discussed further here.

Extraskeletal Chondroma

Clinical and Histopathological Features   Extraskeletal chondromas are uncommon and present mainly in the hands and feet of adults in their fourth and fifth decades.[89–91] They are solitary, well-circumscribed, and usually less than 2 cm in greatest diameter, although large tumors have been reported occasionally. They are composed of variably cellular but generally mature hyaline cartilage that can calcify and even ossify (Fig. 32-20). Plump chondroblasts and giant cells are present. Myxoid areas and fibrosis may occur. In one series, all lesion had areas with marked nuclear pleomorphism, hyperchromasia, binucleation, and myxoid change. The lesion may appear more mature peripherally. Although these lesions may recur, multiple recurrences and metastases have not been reported.

Differential Diagnosis   The differential diagnosis includes osteochondroma, fibro-osseous pseudotumor, synovial chondromatosis, giant-cell tumor of tendon sheath, tumoral calcinosis, extraskeletal chondrosarcoma of myxoid or mesenchymal types, and mixed tumor (chondroid syringoma). Osteochondroma is connected to bone. Fibro-osseous pseudotumor is discussed in the following pages. Synovial chondromatosis is located within a joint or synovial tissue and usually comprises multiple nodules. Giant cell tumor of tendon sheath and tumoral calcinosis do not contain cartilage. Extraskeletal myxoid chondrosarcoma has more prominent myxoid areas, is less circumscribed, has cells in chains and nests rather than isolated in lacunae, is more cellular, and the cells are smaller. Generally mature cartilage is absent and tumor cells at the periphery appear undifferentiated. Mesenchymal chondrosarcoma can present in soft tissue, although rarely in the hands and feet. Diagnosis requires identification of the generally predominant small-cell undifferentiated component that rarely may be missing in small biopsies. Mixed tumors usually show a significant epithelial component that often contains ducts. Rarely mixed tumors contain a single-cell dispersion of epithelium indistinguishable from chondroma. However, the epithelial cells are positive for cytokeratin or epithelial membrane antigen.

Extraskeletal Myxoid Chondrosarcoma

Clinical Features   Extraskeletal myxoid chondrosarcoma is uncommon and occurs mainly in adults with a peak incidence in the fifth decade.[92,93] Men are more commonly affected (2:1). It favors the lower extremity and can present in subcutaneous tissue. Rare cases can present in children.[94] There is a 5-year survival of approximately 85 percent. However, the lesion is persistent, and long-term follow-up is not as favorable.[95]

Histopathological Features   Histologically the tumor is lobulated and consists of isolated, strands, ribbons, or small nests of cells in a myxoid or mucoid background (Fig. 32-21). The cells are oval, small, have scant amounts of eosinophilic cytoplasm, and round nuclei. Occasional cytoplasmic vacuoles can be found, but the extensive vacuolization, as in the physalliphorous cells of chordoma, is not seen. Lacunae formation rarely occurs. Some areas can be quite cellular, and focal areas of true

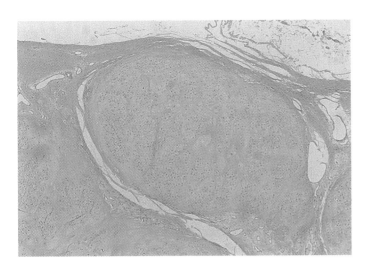

FIGURE 32-20   Extraskeletal Chondroma. Mature hyaline cartilage unattached to bone.

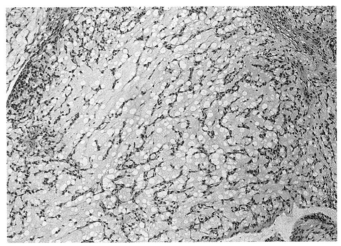

FIGURE 32-21   Extraskeletal Myxoid Chondrosarcoma. Lobulated myxoid neoplasm with small stellate cells with scant cytoplasm.

Hands and feet and fasciitis-like = fibro-osseous pseudotumor
Rapid onset and zonal = myositis ossificans
Lace-like osteoid and atypia = osteosarcoma

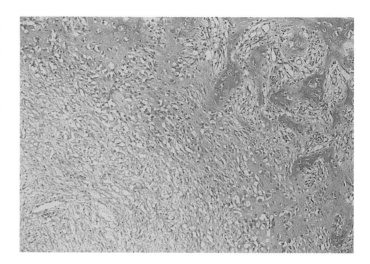

FIGURE 32-22   Fibro-osseous Pseudotumor. Irregular arrangement of bone, cartilage, and fibrous tissue that can be quite cellular.

cartilage and rarely metaplastic bone can be found. Some cases have cytoplasmic rhabdoid inclusions. Immunohistochemically the tumors may be reactive for S100 protein, but this is not a consistent finding.[96] Ultrastructural features of chondrocytes are seen, including rough endoplasmic reticulum, aggregates of microtubules, glycogen and lipid.[97] These tumors are characterized by a reciprocal t(9;22) translocation.[98]

Differential Diagnosis   The differential diagnosis includes myxoma, myxoid liposarcoma, myxofibrosarcoma (myxoid malignant fibrous histiocytoma), chordoma, chondroid syringoma, and cellular neurothekeoma. Myxoma is much less cellular. Myxoid liposarcoma has a characteristic vascular pattern and lipoblasts. Myxofibrosarcoma has a characteristic curvilinear vascular pattern and significantly more atypia. Chordoma contains physalliphorous cells and is keratin and epithelial membrane antigen positive. Chondroid syringoma has nests of cells, can display overt tubular differentiation, and typically is strongly positive for keratin and S100 protein. Ultrastructural examination reveals true epithelial and myoepithelial differentiation. Cellular neurothekeoma most commonly occurs in adolescents of young adults, involves the head and neck most commonly, is superficial (i.e., dermal), does not show chondroid differentiation, often has a distinct lobular pattern, shows neural differentiation, and usually is NKI/C3- and neuron-specific, enolase positive, and S100-negative.

BONE

Primary bone-forming lesions in skin and soft tissues are unusual; the most common lesion is myositis ossificans, a reactive lesion that histologically can mimic osteosarcoma (Table 32-21). Metaplastic bone formation in other lesions, such as pilomatrixoma or intradermal nevus, is probably more frequent.

Osteoma Cutis

Ossification in the skin commonly occurs with trauma or as a component of a variety of other neoplasms. Uncommonly ossification has been reported to follow acne vulgaris. Very rarely, ossification occurs in the absence of a demonstrable lesion and without a history of trauma. Such cases have been described as cutaneous osteoma or osteoma cutis.[99,100] They occur at any age and at any site. The bone appears mature in all cases and may be accompanied by marrow elements and inflammation. Cartilage and amorphous calcifications are rare. An underlying tumor should be excluded. Calcinosis cutis is differentiated by the presence of mature bone.

Fibro-osseous Pseudotumor

Clinical and Histopathological Features   Fibro-osseous pseudotumor (also called parosteal fasciitis and florid reactive periostitis) is a painful, reactive lesion occurring usually in the hands and less commonly the

feet of young adults (with a female predominance) and rarely in children.[101–103] A history of trauma usually is lacking and the lesion may be related to the periosteal surface of bone. It is a multinodular partially circumscribed mass less than 3 cm in diameter. Microscopically, spindle-cell areas, myxoid areas, irregular trabeculae of bone with osteoblastic rimming, areas of vascularity and giant cells, and occasionally cartilage can be seen (Fig. 32-22). Mitoses are common. The zonation of myositis ossificans is not seen. The combination of fibrous areas, myxoid areas, and increased vascularity often are similar to nodular fasciitis. The cellularity, mitoses, and osteoblastic activity may suggest a malignant neoplasm; however, the lesion is benign.

Differential Diagnosis   The differential diagnosis includes myositis ossificans, nodular fasciitis, osteochondroma, and osteogenic sarcoma. Anatomic location, a close association with bone and a lack of zonation distinguish it from myositis ossificans. Bone formation distinguishes it from nodular fasciitis. Osteochondroma has an orderly appearance with cartilage on the surface and underlying mature bone, often with marrow. Osteogenic sarcoma of the hand or foot is rare, and typically has more pleomorphism, with lace-like areas of osteoid, rather than the thicker seams of woven bone present in fibro-osseous pseudotumor.

Myositis Ossificans

Clinical Features   Myositis ossificans is a reactive lesion most commonly presenting in muscle but also arising in or extending into subcutaneous tissue of the extremities.[104–106] Cutaneous involvement is not a feature. It occurs mainly in young active men and may be related to trauma in up to 50 percent of cases. Rapid onset is characteristic. Grossly the lesion is well circumscribed, usually less than 6 cm, and often stone hard.

Histopathological Features   Histologically the lesion is zonal, with mature bone at the periphery and immature elements centrally (Fig. 32-23). The immature area has a loose myxoid to fibrous background with spindle cells that can become highly cellular and mitotically active. This can mimic nodular fasciitis or fibromatosis. Some cells are epithelioid, in particular in areas associated with bone. Osteoblasts are plump and can simulate malignant osteoblasts, but are not as atypical. The bone

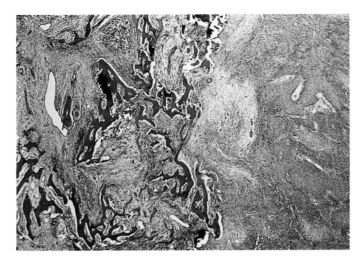

FIGURE 32-23 Myositis Ossificans. Zonation, the lesion forms more mature bone toward the periphery and is more cellular toward the center.

varies from mature to immature and usually is surrounded by abundant osteoblasts. Lace-like patterns of osteoid can rarely be seen, as well as areas of cartilage. In subcutaneous sites, the zonal phenomenon may not be as apparent. In these cases (sometimes known as fasciitis ossificans), the resemblance of the spindle-cell component to nodular fasciitis is critical for accurate diagnosis.

Differential Diagnosis   The principal differential diagnosis is osteosarcoma. The history of rapid onset is helpful, as well as the zonal pattern and resemblance to nodular fasciitis. Osteosarcoma generally has more atypia, atypical mitoses, and an infiltrative pattern. In difficult cases, rebiopsy at a later time may be useful. Nodular fasciitis lacks osteoid.

Extraskeletal Osteosarcoma

Clinical and Histopathological Features   Extraskeletal osteosarcoma is a rare neoplasm of adults (mean age 59 years) with a predilection for the extremities, especially the thigh.[107] Some cases are associated with prior radiation.[108] Although most are deep-seated lesions, cases con-

fined to the dermis and subcutaneous tissue have been described. All show at least focal areas of infiltration. By definition, the lesions contain osteoid intimately associated with atypical cells (Fig. 32-24). Areas of cartilage and areas resembling pleomorphic malignant fibrous histiocytoma are common. Rare cases of telangectatic osteosarcoma consisting of large dilated blood-filled spaces have been described.[109] Up to two-thirds recur, and at least two-thirds of patients develop metastases and die.

Differential Diagnosis   In contrast to osteosarcoma, myositis ossificans has a zoning phenomenon with more mature bone at the periphery and more immature areas centrally. Although osteosarcomas vary, in many the bone is central. The lack of markedly atypical cells in myositis ossificans also may be helpful. Distinction from fibro-osseous pseudotumor is discussed in the preceding text. Malignant fibrous histiocytoma and chondrosarcoma lack malignant osteoid.

REFERENCES

1. Goltz RW, Henderson RR, Hitch JM, Ott JE: Focal dermal hypoplasia syndrome. *Arch Dermatol* 101:1–11, 1970.
2. Hall EH, Terezhalmy GT: Focal dermal hypoplasia syndrome. *J Am Acad Dermatol* 9:443–451, 1983.
3. Wilson Jones E, Marks R, Pongsehirun D: Naevus superificialis lipomatosus. *Br J Dermatol* 93:121–133, 1975.
4. Fergin PE, MacDonald DM: Naevus superficialis lipomatosus. *Clin Exp Dermatol* 5:365–367, 1980.
5. Rydholm A, Berg NO: Size, site and clinical incidence of lipoma. *Acta Orthop Scand* 54:929–934, 1983.
6. Adair FE, Pack GT, Farrior JH: Lipomas. *Am J Cancer* 16:1104–1120, 1932.
7. Bick EM: Lipoma of the extremities. *Ann Surg* 104:139–143, 1936.
8. Truhan AP, Garden JM, Caro WA, Roenigk HH: Facial and scalp lipomas: Reports and study of prevalence. *J Dermatol Surg Oncol* 11:981–984, 1985.
9. Sreekantaiah C, Sandberg AA: Clustering of aberrations to specific chromosome regions in benign neoplasms. *Int J Cancer* 48:149–198, 1991.
10. Sreekantaiah C, Leong SPL, Karakousis CP, et al: Cytogenetic profile of 109 lipomas. *Cancer Res* 51:422–433, 1991.
11. Fletcher CDM, Akerman M, Dal Cin P, et al: Correlation between clinicopathological features and karyotype in lipomatous tumors. *Am J Pathol* 148:623–630, 1996.
12. Hurt MA, Santa Cruz DJ: Nodular-cystic fat necrosis. *J Am Acad Dermatol* 21: 493–498, 1989.
13. Howard WR, Helwig EB: Angiolipoma. *Arch Dermatol* 82:924–931, 1960.
14. Hunt SJ, Santa Cruz DJ, Barr RJ: Cellular angiolipoma. *Am J Surg Pathol* 14:75–81, 1990.
15. Enzinger FM, Harvey DA: Spindle cell lipoma. *Cancer* 36:1852–1859, 1975.
16. Fletcher CDM, Martin-Bates E: Spindle cell lipoma: A clinicopathological study with some original observations. *Histopathology* 11:803–817, 1987.
17. Warkel RL, Rehme CG, Thompson WH: Vascular spindle cell lipoma. *J Cutan Pathol* 9:113–118, 1982.
18. Hawley IC, Krausz T, Evans DJ, Fletcher CDM: Spindle cell lipoma: A pseudoangiomatous variant. *Histopathology* 24:565–569, 1994.
19. Nielsen GP, Dickersin GR, Provensal JM, Rosenberg AE: Lipomatous hemangiopericytoma. *Am J Surg Pathol* 19:748–756, 1995.
20. Shmookler BM, Enzinger FM: Pleomorphic lipoma: A benign tumor simulating liposarcoma. *Cancer* 47:126–133, 1981.
21. Azzopardi JG, Iocco J, Salm R: Pleomorphic lipoma: A tumour simulating liposarcoma. *Histopathology* 7:511–523, 1983.
22. Meis JM, Enzinger FM: Chondroid lipoma. A unique tumor simulating liposarcoma and myxoid chondrosarcoma. *Am J Surg Pathol* 17:1103–1112, 1993.
23. Kindblom LG, Meis-kindblom JM: Chondroid lipoma: An ultrastructural and immunohistochemical analysis with further observations regarding its differentiation. *Hum Pathol* 26:706–715, 1995.
24. Nielsen GP, O'Connell JX, Dickersin GR, Rosenberg AE: Chondroid lipoma: A tumor of white fat cells. *Am J Surg Pathol* 19:1272–1276, 1995.
25. Meis JM, Enzinger FM: Myolipoma of soft tissue. *Am J Surg Pathol* 15:121–125, 1991.
26. Novy FG, Wilson JW.: Hibernomas, brown fat tumors. *Arch Dermatol* 73:149–157, 1956.

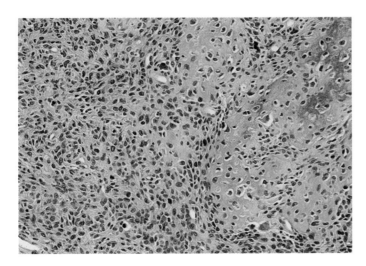

FIGURE 32-24 Extraskeletal Osteosarcoma. Atypical cells forming osteoid.

27. Gaffney EF, Hargreaves HK, Semple E, Vellios F: Hibernoma. *Hum Pathol* 14: 677–687, 1983.

28. Enzi G, Inelmen EM, Baritussio A, Dorigo P, Prosdocimi M, Mazzoleni F: Multiple symmetric lipomatosis. *J Clin Invest* 60:1221–1229, 1977.

29. Enzi G: Multiple symmetric lipomatosis: An updated clinical report. *Medicine* 63: 56–64, 1984.

30. Chung EB, Enzinger FM: Benign lipoblastomatosis. *Cancer* 32:482–492, 1973.

31. Mentzel T, Calonje E, Fletcher CDM: Lipoblastoma and lipoblastomatosis: A clinicopathologic study of 14 cases. *Histopathology* 23:527–533, 1993.

32. Fletcher JA, Kozakewich HP, Schoenberg ML, Morton CC: Cytogenetic findings in pediatric adipose tumors: Consistent rearrangement of chromosome 8 in lipoblastoma. *Genes Chrom Cancer* 6:24–29, 1993.

33. Shmookler BM, Enzinger FM: Liposarcoma occurring in children. *Cancer* 52:567–574, 1983.

34. Enzinger FM, Winslow DJ: Liposarcoma. A study of 103 cases. *Virchows Arch [Pathol Anat]* 335:367–388, 1962.

35. Evans HL, Soule EH, Winkelmann RK: Atypical lipoma, atypical intramuscular lipoma, and well differentiated retroperitoneal liposarcoma. *Cancer* 43:574–584, 1979.

36. Azumi N, Curtis J, Kempson RL, Hendrickson MR: Atypical and malignant neoplasms showing lipomatous differentiation. *Am J Surg Pathol* 11:161–183, 1987.

37. Weiss SW, Rao VK: Well-differentiated liposarcoma (atypical lipoma) of deep soft tissue of the extremities, retroperitoneum, and miscellaneous sites. *Am J Surg Pathol* 16:1051–1058, 1992.

38. Dei Tos AP, Mentzel T, Newman PL, Fletcher CDM: Spindle cell liposarcoma: A hitherto unrecognized variant of liposarcoma. *Am J Surg Pathol* 18:913–921, 1994.

39. Dal Cin P, Kools P, Sciot R, et al: Cytogenetic and fluorescence in situ hybridization investigation of ring chromosomes characterizing a specific pathologic subgroup of adipose tissue tumors. *Cancer Genet Cytogenet* 38:85–90, 1993.

40. Aman P, Ron D, Mandahl N, et al: Rearrangement of the transcription factor gene CHOP in myxoid liposarcoma with t(12;16)(q13;p11). *Genes Chrom Cancer* 5:278–285, 1992.

41. Dei Tos AP, Wadden C, Fletcher CDM: S-100 protein staining in liposarcoma: Its diagnostic utility in the high grade myxoid (round cell) variant. *Appl Immunohistochem* 4:95–101, 1996.

42. Hashimoto H, Daimaru Y, Enjoji M: S-100 protein distribution in liposarcoma. *Virchows Arch [Pathol Anat]* 405:1–10, 1984.

43. McCormick D, Mentzel T, Beham A, Fletcher CDM: Dedifferentiated liposarcoma. Clincopathologic analysis of 32 cases suggesting a better prognostic subgroup among pleomorphic sarcomas. *Am J Surg Pathol* 18:1213–1223, 1994.

44. Evans HL: Smooth muscle in atypical lipomatous tumors. *Am J Surg Pathol* 14: 714–718, 1990.

45. Tallini G, Erlandson RA, Brennan MF, Woodruff JM: Divergent myosarcomatous differentiation in retroperitoneal liposarcoma. *Am J Surg Pathol* 17:546–556, 1993.

46. Evans HL, Khurana KK, Kemp BL, Ayala AG: Heterologous elements in the dedifferentiated component of dedifferentiated liposarcoma. *Am J Surg Pathol* 18:1150–1157, 1994.

47. Berger TG, Levin MW: Congenital smooth muscle hamartoma. *J Am Acad Dermatol* 11:709–712, 1984.

48. Johnson MD, Jacobs AH: Congenital smooth muscle hamartoma. *Arch Dermatol* 125:820–822, 1989.

49. Stout AP: Solitary cutaneous and subcutaneous leiomyoma. *Am J Cancer* 29:435–469, 1937.

50. Fisher WC, Helwig EB: Leiomyoma of the skin. *Arch Dermatol* 88:78–88, 1963.

51. Newman PL, Fletcher CDM: Smooth muscle tumours of the external genitalia: Clinicopathologic analysis of a series. *Histopathology* 18:523–529, 1991.

52. Kilpatrick SE, Mentzel T, Fletcher CDM: Leiomyoma of deep soft tissue. *Am J Surg Pathol* 18:576–582, 1994.

53. Hachisuga T, Hashimoto H, Enjoji M: Angioleiomyoma. *Cancer* 54:126–130, 1984.

54. Fox SB, Heryet A, Khong TY: Angioleiomyomas: An immunohistochemical study. *Histopathology* 16:495–506, 1990.

55. Varela-Duran J, Oliva H, Rosai J: Vascular leiomyosarcoma. *Cancer* 44:1684–1691, 1979.

56. Fitzpatrick JE, Mellette R, Hwang RJ, Golitz LE, Zaim MT, Clemons D: Cutaneous angiolipoleiomyoma. *J Am Acad Dermatol* 23:1093–1098, 1990.

57. Swanson PE, Wick MR, Dehner LP: Leiomyosarcoma of somatic soft tissues in childhood. *Hum Pathol* 22:569–577, 1991.

58. Fields JP, Helwig EB: Leiomyosarcoma of the skin and subcutaneous tissue. *Cancer* 47:156–169, 1981.

59. Wile AG, Evans HL, Romsdahl MM: Leiomyosarcoma of soft tissue: A clinicopathologic study. *Cancer* 48:1022–1032, 1981.

60. Oliver GF, Reiman HM, Gonchoroff NJ, Muller SA, Umbert IJ: Cutaneous and subcutaneous leiomyosarcoma: A clinicopathological review of 14 cases with reference to antidesmin staining and nuclear DNA patterns studied by flow cytometry. *Br J Dermatol* 124:252–257, 1991.

61. Suster S: Epithelioid leiomyosarcoma of the skin and subcutaneous tissue. *Am J Surg Pathol* 18:232–240, 1994.

62. Mentzel T, Wadden C, Fletcher CDM: Granular cell change in smooth muscle tumours of skin and soft tissue. *Histopathology* 24:223–231, 1994.

63. Chen KTK, Hafez GR, Gilbert EF: Myxoid variant of epithelioid smooth muscle tumor. *Am J Clin Pathol* 74:350–353, 1980.

64. Lundgren L, Kindblom LG, Seidal T, Angervall L: Intermediate and fine cytofilaments in cutaneous and subcutaneous leiomyosarcomas. *APMIS* 99:820–828, 1991.

65. Brown DC, Theaker JM, Banks PM, Gatter KC, Mason DY: Cytokeratin expression in smooth muscle and smooth muscle tumours. *Histopathology* 11:477–486, 1987.

66. Cavazzana AO, Schmidt D, Ninfo V, et al: Spindle cell rhabdomyosarcoma. A prognostically favorable variant of rhabdomyosarcoma. *Am J Surg Pathol* 16:229–235, 1992.

67. Leuschner I, Newton WA, Schmidt D, et al: Spindle cell variants of embryonal rhabdomyosarcoma in the paratesticular region. A report of the Intergroup Rhabdomyosarcoma Study. *Am J Surg Pathol* 17:221–230, 1993.

68. Sahn EE, Garen PD, Pai GS, Levkoff AH, Hagerty RC, Maize JC: Multiple rhabdomyomatous mesenchymal hamartomas of skin. *Am J Dermatopathol* 12:485–491, 1990.

69. Farris PE, Manning S, Vuitch F: Rhabdomyomatous mesenchymal hamartoma. *Am J Dermatopathol* 16:73–75, 1994.

70. Dehner LP, Enzinger FM, Font RL: Fetal rhabdomyoma. *Cancer* 30:160–166, 1972.

71. Di Sant'Agnese PA, Knowles DM: Extracardiac rhabdomyomas: A clinicopathologic study and review of the literature. *Cancer* 46:780–789, 1980.

72. Kapadia SB, Meis JM, Frisman DM, Ellis GL, Heffner DK: Fetal rhabdomyomas of the head and neck. *Hum Pathol* 24:754–765, 1993.

73. Willis J, Abdul-Karim FW, di Sant-Agnese PA: Extracardiac rhabdomyomas. *Semin Diagn Pathol* 11:15–25, 1994.

74. Blaauwgeers MG, Troost D, Dingemans KP, Taat CW, Van den Tweel JG: Multifocal rhabdomyoma of the neck. *Am J Surg Pathol* 13:791–799, 1989.

75. Bale PM, Parsons RE, Stevens MM: Diagnosis and behavior of juvenile rhabdomyosarcoma. *Hum Pathol* 14:596–611, 1983.

76. Parham DM, Webber B, Holt H, Williams WK, Maurer H: Immunohistochemical study of childhood rhabdomyosarcomas and related neoplasms. *Cancer* 67:3072–3080, 1991.

77. Enterline HT, Horn RC: Alveolar rhabdomyosarcoma. A distinctive tumor type. *Am J Clin Pathol* 29:356–366, 1958.

78. Enzinger FM, Shiraki M: Alveolar rhabdomyosarcoma. An analysis of 110 cases. *Cancer* 24:18–31, 1969.

79. Tsokos M, Webber BL, Parham DM, et al: Rhabdomyosarcoma. A new classification scheme related to prognosis. *Arch Pathol Lab Med* 116:847–855, 1992.

80. Parham DM, Shapiro DN, Downing JR, Webber DL, Douglass EC: Solid alveolar rhabdomyosarcomas with the t(2;13). Report of two cases with diagnostic implications. *Am J Surg Pathol* 18:474–478, 1994.

81. Shapiro DN, Sublett JE, Li B, Downing JR, Naeve CW: Fusion of PAX3 to a member of the forkhead family of transcription factors in human alveolar rhabdomyosarcoma. *Cancer Res* 53:5108–5112, 1993.

82. Galili N, Davis RJ, Fredericks WJ, et al: Fusion of a fork head domain gene to PAX3 in solid tumour alveolar rhabdomyosarcoma. *Nat Genet* 5:230–235, 1993.

83. Gaffney EF, Dervan PA, Fletcher CDM: Pleomorphic rhabdomyosarcoma in adulthood. Analysis of 11 cases with definition of diagnostic criteria. *Am J Surg Pathol* 17:601–609, 1993.

84. Kodet R, Newton WA, Hamoudi AB, Asmar L, Jacobs DL, Maurer HM: Childhood rhabdomyosarcomas with anaplastic (pleomorphic) features. *Am J Surg Pathol* 17: 443–453, 1993.

85. Maurer HM, Beltangady M, Gehan EA, et al: The Intergroup Rhabdomyosarcoma Study Group-I. *Cancer* 61:209–220, 1988.

86. Newton WA, Gehan EA, Webber BL, et al: Classification of rhabdomyosarcomas and related sarcomas. *Cancer* 76:1073–1085, 1995.

87. Crist WM, Garnsey L, Beltangady MS, et al: Prognosis in children with rhabdomyosarcoma: A report of the Intergroup Rhabdomyosarcoma Studies I and II. *J Clin Oncol* 8:443–452, 1990.

88. La Quaglia MP, Heller G, Ghavimi F, et al: The effect of age at diagnosis on outcome in rhabdomyosarcoma. *Cancer* 73:109–117, 1994.

89. Dahlin DC, Salvador AH: Cartilaginous tumors of the soft tissues of the hands and feet. *Mayo Clin Proc* 49:721–726, 1974.

90. Chung EB, Enzinger FM: Chondroma of soft parts. *Cancer* 41:1414–1424, 1978.

91. Humphrey S, Pambakian H, McKee PH, Fletcher CDM: Soft tissue chondroma: A study of 15 tumours. *Histopathology* 10:147–159, 1986.

92. Enzinger FM, Shiraki M: Extraskeletal myxoid chondrosarcoma. *Hum Pathol* 3: 421–435, 1972.

93. Dardick I, Lagace R, Carlier MT, Jung RC: Chordoid sarcoma (extraskeletal myxoid chondrosarcoma). *Virchows Arch [Pathol Anat]* 399:61–78, 1983.

94. Hachitanda Y, Tsuneyoshi M, Daimaru Y, et al: Extraskeletal myxoid chondrosarcoma in young children. *Cancer* 61:2521–2526, 1988.

95. Saleh G, Evans HL, Ro JY, Ayala AG: Extraskeletal myxoid chondrosarcoma. *Cancer* 70:2827–2830, 1992.

96. Fletcher CDM, Powell G, McKee PH: Extraskeletal myxoid chondrosarcoma: A histochemical and immunohistochemical study. *Histopathology* 10:489–499, 1986.

97. DeBlois G, Wang S, Kay S: Microtubular aggregates within rough endoplasmic reticulum: An unusual ultrastructural feature of extraskeletal myxoid chondrosarcoma. *Hum Pathol* 17:469–475, 1986.

98. Sciot R, Dal Cin P, Fletcher C, et al: t(9;22)(q22-31;q11-12) is a consistent marker of extraskeletal myxoid chondrosarcoma: evaluation of three cases. *Mod Pathol* 8:765–768, 1995.

99. Roth SI, Stowell RE, Helwig EB: Cutaneous ossification. *Arch Pathol Lab Med* 76:44–54, 1963.

100. Peterson EC, Mandel SL: Primary osteomas of the skin. *Arch Dermatol* 87:626–632, 1963.

101. Dupree WB, Enzinger FM: Fibro-osseous pseudotumor of the digits. *Cancer* 58:2103–2109, 1986.

102. McCarthy EF, Ireland DCR, Sprague DL, Bonfiglio M: Parosteal (nodular) fasciitis of the hand. *J Bone Joint Surg* 58A:714–716, 1976.

103. Spjut HJ, Dorfman HD: Florid reactive periostitis of the tubular bones of the hands and feet. *Am J Surg Pathol* 5:423–433, 1981.

104. Johnson LC: Histogenesis of myositis ossificans. *Am J Pathol* 24:681–682, 1948.

105. Miller LF, O'Neill CJ: Myositis ossificans in paraplegics. *J Bone Joint Surg* 31A:283–294, 1949.

106. Ackerman LV: Extra-osseous localized non-neoplastic bone and cartilage formation (so-called myositis ossificans). *J Bone Joint Surg* 40A:279–298, 1958.

107. Chung EB, Enzinger FM: Extraskeletal osteosarcoma. *Cancer* 60:1132–1142, 1987.

108. Sordillo PP, Hadju SI, Magill GB, Golbey RB: Extraosseous osteogenic sarcoma. *Cancer* 51:727–734, 1983.

109. Mirra JM, Fain JS, Ward WG, Eckhardt JJ, Eilber F, Rosen G: Extraskeletal telangectatic osteosarcoma. *Cancer* 71:3014–3019, 1993.

CHAPTER 33

NEURAL AND NEUROENDOCRINE TUMORS

Zsolt B. Argenyi

During their histogenesis, cutaneous neural tumors either recapitulate or retain to a variable extent the architectural arrangement and cytologic components of the normal peripheral nerve. Therefore, familiarity with the normal histology of the peripheral nerve is essential for the correct characterization of neural tumors.[1] In short, the structural organization of the peripheral nerve follows a hierarchical arrangement of different compartments. The basic unit is the *nerve fiber*, which is composed of an axon (neurite) and the surrounding Schwann cells.[2] Axons are cytoplasmic extensions of neurons that are located in the central nervous system or in the sympathetic ganglionic chain. Axons become myelinated by multiple periaxonal rotation of the surrounding Schwann cells, thus creating a concentric layer of cytoplasmic membranes. Unmyelinated nerve fibers develop by invagination of the axons into the cytoplasm of the Schwann cells. In the next architectural compartment, several nerve fibers form nerve fascicles that are surrounded by a sheath, called a *perineurium*, whereas the space within the perineurium is referred to as *endoneurium*.[2] The perineurium is composed of a specialized cell type, the perineurial cell, which is in continuity with the pia-arachnoidal lining of the central nervous system. Besides the nerve fibers, the endoneurium also contains fibroblasts, capillaries, and mast cells. In the final organizational compartment, numerous nerve fascicles are grouped into nerve bundles that are held together by a protective sheath referred to as the *epineurium*.[2] The epineurium is made up of fibroblasts, collagen, and adipose tissue, but fine vascular structures also penetrate its wall. The sensory nerves are connected to various types of sensory corpuscles, e.g., pacinian, Meissnerian, Vater-Pacini, Krause, that are differentiated to specific sensory perceptions.

CLASSIFICATION

Cutaneous neural tumors represent either primary tumors of the peripheral nerves or ectopic-heterotopic tissues from the central nervous system or sympathetic ganglionic chain. Further classification is usually based on their assumed histogenetic differentiation. Table 33-1 contains one of the currently used classifications of cutaneous neural tumors.

PERIPHERAL NERVE SHEATH TUMORS

Neuromas

Synonyms: spontaneous neuroma, solitary circumscribed neuroma, palisaded encapsulated neuroma, true neuroma, amputation neuroma, traumatic neuroma, supernumerary digit

Neuromas represent hamartomatous proliferation of the nerve sheath components in which there is an approximate recapitulation of the normal structural arrangements of the peripheral nerve.[3,4] The constituent fibers have an axon-to-Schwann cell ratio close to the normal 1:1, which makes this group of tumors distinct from other nerve sheath neoplasms. From an etiologic standpoint, neuromas can be classified as spontaneous and traumatic types. The spontaneous type has two main forms: solitary, encapsulated type (solitary palisaded encapsulated neuroma) and multiple, nonencapsulated type.[3,4] Spontaneous neuromas are considered to be a form of primary hyperplasia of the nerve fibers without apparent antecedent tissue injury.[4]

Traumatic neuromas develop after sharp or blunt trauma of the peripheral nerve resulting in a partial or complete transection of the continuity of the nerve fibers.[1,3] After the transection of the nerve fibers, the distal end undergoes wallerian degeneration, whereas the fibers from the proximal end try to regenerate and reunite with the distal end. This attempt at regeneration often fails due to the severity of the damage and will result in an unorganized, irregular overgrowth of regrowing nerve fibers from the proximal end of the nerve. Traumatic neuromas developing after a complete transection of the nerves are called *amputation neuromas* and are reactive proliferations rather than true hamartomas or neoplasms.[1,3]

Clinical Features   Palisaded encapsulated neuroma develops in adults (mean age 45.5 years), with an approximately equal ratio of both genders. The majority of the lesions (close to 90 percent) manifest on the face, but they can occur anywhere on the body. The lesions are solitary, small (2 to 6 mm), skin-colored, firm or rubbery, dome-shaped, asymptomatic papules.[5,6] There is no increased association with neurofibromatosis or with the multiple endocrine neoplasia syndrome.

The multiple, nonencapsulated neuromas usually manifest as part of the *multiple mucosal neuroma syndrome*. In this syndrome, there are numerous soft, skin-colored or pink papules and nodules around the mucosal orifices, mainly around the lips, but they can be present in the oral cavity as well. This manifestation also can be part of the multiple endocrine neoplasia syndrome (type 2A), in which pheochromocytoma and medullary carcinoma of the thyroid commonly occur.[7]

Traumatic neuromas can occur at any age or gender but are obviously more prevalent in certain professions that make the individual prone to acute and chronic injuries. There is some predilection for these tumors on the extremities. They are usually solitary, skin-colored, often broad-based, firm papules and nodules at the sites of previous injury or trauma.[8] They can be asymptomatic, but older lesions often become sensitive and painful on pressure. Lancinating pain is considered characteristic for amputation neuromas.[8]

A special form of traumatic neuroma is the *supernumerary digit*, which occurs on the lateral-volar aspect of the hand in newborn and young infants. These lesions represent amputation neuromas at the site of the in utero separated extranumerary digit. Despite the term, they do not contain bone or cartilage of a true digit.[9]

Classification of Cutaneous Neural Tumors

Peripheral Nerve Sheath Tumors	Neural Heterotopias
Hamartomas	**Meningothelial**
Neuromas	Meningocele
Traumatic	Rudimentary meningocele
Spontaneous	Meningioma
Solitary, encapsulated	**Neuroglial**
Multiple, nonencapsulated	Nasal glioma
Variants	**Neuroblastic/ganglionic**
Neurofibromas	Metastatic neuroblastoma
Superficial	Primary primitive
Deep	Neuroectodermal tumor
Diffuse	Ganglioneuroma
Pigmented	**Miscellaneous**
Plexiform	Pigmented neuroectodermal
Variants	tumor of infancy
True nerve sheath neoplasms	
Schwannomas	
Common, solitary	
Ancient	
Cellular	
Plexiform	
Variants	
Nerve sheath myxoma	
Classic	
Cellular (neurothekeoma)	
Malignant peripheral nerve sheath tumor	
Miscellaneous	
Granular cell tumor	
Neuroendocrine carcinoma of the skin (Merkel cell carcinoma)	

Histopathological Features Palisaded, encapsulated neuroma is a well-circumscribed, round or oblong nodule located in the dermis, which on rare occasions has a polypoid configuration (Tables 33-2 and 33-3). The tumor is composed of tightly woven fascicles, which are often separated by clear clefts[5,6] (Fig. 33-1A). The cells in the fascicles are uniformly spindle-shaped with eosinophilic cytoplasm and ovoid or wavy nuclei. Mitotic figures are rare or absent. Occasionally, there is parallel arrangement of the nuclei, featuring a palisading pattern, although this is not a persistent feature (Fig. 33-1B). Classic Verocay bodies are not present. There is no appreciable fibrosis, chronic inflammation, or granulomatous reaction within the tumor.[10] A thin capsule-like structure separates the tumor from the surrounding dermis. However, this capsule is often incomplete near the epidermal aspect of the tumor. A connection with the adjacent nerves usually can be demonstrated on serially sectioned specimens. Variants of palisaded, encapsulated neuroma with a plexiform or multinodular growth pattern and highly vascular stroma have been reported.[11]

The morphologic features of spontaneous neuromas, in either solitary or multiple settings, are similar, with the exception of histologic encapsulation.

Traumatic or amputation neuromas are usually well-defined, nodular lesions located in the dermis or in the subcutis (Tables 33-2 and 33-4). The tumors are encased by a fibrous sheath, which is often incomplete at the distal end, where the regenerating fibers may infiltrate the adjacent stroma (Figs. 33-2A,B). The tumor nodules are composed of a chaotic tangle of regenerating nerve fascicles of various sizes and shapes separated by fibrous tissue, variable chronic inflammation, or less often, granulomatous reaction[3] (Fig. 33-1A, B). Mucinous changes are common in early lesions, especially in the regenerating perineurial spaces.[10] The regenerated individual fibers have a close to normal structural organization of typical Schwann cells, perineurial cells, and centrally located axons.

Immunohistochemically, the palisaded, encapsulated neuroma and traumatic neuroma share several features.[10] The constituent cells of the fascicles stain for S-100 protein. In traumatic neuroma, the perineurial cells in the surrounding sheaths are positive for epithelial membrane antigen. In palisaded, encapsulated neuroma, only the outer capsule reacts for this antigen, confirming a perineurial cell participation.[10] Silver impregnation and neural filament stains reveal that the fascicles are rich in axons in both lesions. In traumatic neuroma the axons follow the normal longitudinal arrangement in the proximal part of the tumor, but they become haphazardly and irregularly arranged toward the distal end.[6,10,12] Prominent myelinization is often present, as detected by antibodies to myelin basic protein and CD57 antigen.[12]

Differential Diagnosis Palisaded, encapsulated neuroma must be differentiated from other encapsulated spindle cell neoplasms such as solitary schwannoma and angioleiomyoma. Solitary schwannomas contain Antoni A and B type tissues with Verocay bodies and are devoid of axons by special stains. Angiomyolipomas are encapsulated, but the cytologic features are different. The cells have a more eosinophilic, finely fibrillary cytoplasm with blunt-ended nuclei that have a "bubbly" chromatin pattern. The tumor also lacks axons. Plexiform or multinodular variants of palisaded, encapsulated neuromas should be differentiated from plexiform variants of neurofibroma, schwannoma, and fibrohistiocytic tumors.

Traumatic neuroma can be differentiated easily from the other variants of neuromas based on the presence of scar, chronic inflammation, and a history of previous trauma. Painful plantar nodules, often referred to as *Morton's neuromas*, are no longer considered true neuromas but localized forms of interdigital neuritis with a complex etiology.

Neurofibromas

Synonyms: solitary neurofibroma, solitary nerve sheath tumor, plexiform nerve sheath tumor, multiple neurofibromatosis

Neurofibromas are hamartomatous proliferations of the various components of the neuromesenchyme, including Schwann cells, endoneurial fibroblasts, perineurial cells, and mast cells.[3,4] In this complex proliferation, however, the proportion of each cell type varies, providing the broad histologic manifestation of neurofibromas. Since axons do not duplicate, their relative proportion to the other cell components is less than the usual 1:1 axon-to-Schwann cell ratio of the normal nerve. The main histopathologic types of neurofibromas include (1) sporadic cutaneous type, (2) deep-seated encapsulated type, (3) diffuse type, (4) pigmented type, and (5) plexiform type, but other rare variants also exist.[1,3,4,13–16]

Clinical Features Sporadic neurofibromas are relatively common lesions in adults, and they affect both sexes equally (Table 33-5). They are soft or rubbery, dome-shaped or polypoid, skin-colored or tan papules or nodules. They may display a "button hole" sign on pinching. The are usually asymptomatic, but the pedunculated forms may become irritated.[7,14] A few lesions in a single patient, provided there are no other stigmata present, do not indicate neurofibromatosis; however, they still can be part of this syndrome. Contrary to this, the plexiform variant is considered pathognomonic for *neurofibromatosis*, particularly for type I manifestation.[1,3] The diffuse, deep-seated, and the pigmented variants are also more common in neurofibromatosis.[1]

TABLE 33-2

Histopathologic Diagnostic Features of Common Cutaneous Neural Neoplasms

Feature	Traumatic Neuroma	Palisaded, Encapsulated Neuroma	Solitary Superficial Neurofibroma	Solitary Schwannoma	Classic Nerve Sheath Myxoma	Cellular Neurothekeoma
Growth pattern	Well circumscribed at the proximal end, irregular at the distal end	Well circumscribed, nodular, rarely plexiform	Relatively well defined, but with infiltrative margins	Well circumscribed, nodular	Lobulated or plexiform	Fascicular or irregular sheaths and nests
Encapsulation	Partially by fibrous sheath	Yes, by perineurium	None	Yes, perineurium	Yes partially by perineurium	None
Architecture	Unorganized tangles of regenerating fascicles	Compactly arranged fascicles, separated by clefts	Variable matrix from the fine fibrillary to dense fibrotic	Antoni A type: hypercellular Antoni B type: hypocellular	Hypocellular, myxoid matrix	Solid proliferation of epithelioid or spindled cells
Cytologic features	Spindled cells with tapered, wavy nuclei	Spindled cells with tapered, wavy nuclei	Spindled cells with tapered, wavy nuclei, plump fibroblasts, mast cells	Spindled cells with tapered, wavy nuclei, mast cells	Stellate, spindled, and giant cells	Large epithelioid or spindled cells
Nuclear palisading and Verocay bodies	None	Variable palisading	Rarely	Yes	None	None
Nerve fibers	Irregularly arranged axons	Relatively well-organized axons	Rare, scattered axons	None or only at the origin	None	None
Other important features	Extensive fibrosis, rarely inflammation, macrophages	No fibrosis or inflammation	Fibrosis, myxoid, and vascular changes	Hemorrhage, thrombosis, hyalinization, cytologic atypia (ancient changes)	Mild cytologic atypia	Variable atypia, rare mitotic figures

TABLE 33-3

Palisaded and Encapsulated Neuroma

Clinical Features

Usually solitary
Predilection for the face of adults
Nondescript skin-colored papule or nodule suggesting a dermal nevus

Histopathological Features

Well-circumscribed nodule with incomplete encapsulation
Spindled cells arranged in short fascicles
Well-developed palisading of nuclei is usually not present

Differential Diagnosis

Schwannoma
Leiomyoma
Neurotized nevus
Other spindle-cell melanocytic tumors

TABLE 33-4

Traumatic Neuroma

Clinical Features

May occur at any site following trauma
Small skin-colored nodule or mass
Often painful

Histopathological Features

Circumscribed but unencapsulated
Mass composed of axons and Schwann cells admixed with fibrous tissue

Differential Diagnosis

Neurofibroma
Perineurioma

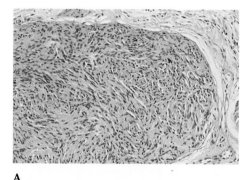

A

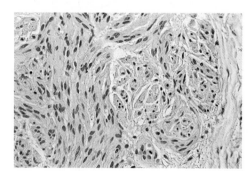

B

FIGURE 33-1 (*A*) Palisaded, encapsulated neuroma. Well-delineated, encapsulated dermal nodule (H&E stain; ×25). (*B*) The individual fascicles are compactly and relatively uniformly arranged and separated by narrow artificially produced clefts. Focal palisading of the nuclei is present (H&E stain; ×100).

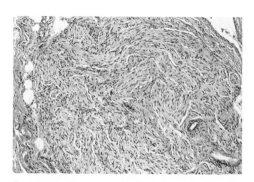

A

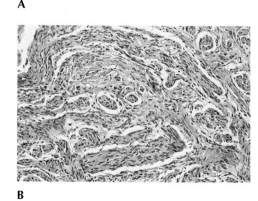

B

FIGURE 33-2 (*A*) Traumatic neuroma. The regenerating nerve fascicles have haphazard arrangement and are embedded in a markedly fibrotic stroma (H&E stain; ×25). (*B*) There is prominent variation in the size and shape of the fascicles, which are separated by scar tissue (H&E stain; ×50).

TABLE 33-5

Neurofibroma

Clinical Features

Skin-colored or tan polypoid papule or nodule
Soft or rubbery
May involve any cutaneous site
Plexiform pattern—pathognomonic of neurofibromatosis

Histopathological Features

Spindle cell proliferation, wavy nuclei with tapered ends
Often significant fibrosis
Occasional mucinous stroma
In general, not encapsulated
Mast cells are common
Plexiform variant is similar but with complex "wormlike" growth
   pattern

Differential Diagnosis

Neurotized nevus
Schwannoma
Trichodiscoma and related tumors
Dermatofibroma
Smooth-muscle neoplasms
Hypertrophic scar

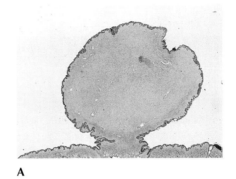

A

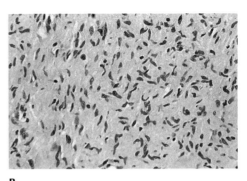

B

FIGURE 33-3 (*A*) Solitary, cutaneous neurofibroma. A well-defined but not encapsulated dermal nodule, which on occasion becomes pedunculated (H&E stain; ×5). (*B*) The slender spindle cells are haphazardly arranged in a fine fibrillary matrix (H&E stain; ×100).

The common solitary neurofibromas grow slowly and follow a benign course, whereas the deep-seated, diffuse, and plexiform variants may cause local infiltration and organ displacement. The plexiform type also has an increased probability of malignant transformation.[1] The typical presentation of plexiform neurofibroma is a baglike or twisted rope-like dermal or subcutaneous mass, often associated with redundant skin folds, hyperpigmentation, and hirsutism.[1,3,4] Beside plexiform neurofibroma, the other important clinical stigmata of *neurofibromatosis* include conjunctival Lisch nodules, café-au-lait spots, bilateral axillary freckling, numerous superficial and deeply located diffuse neurofibromas, and various soft tissue, bone, endocrine, and other types of neoplasms.[17] For a detailed description of the various types of neurofibromatoses, the reader is referred to the specific literature on this subject.[17]

Histopathological Features   The common solitary cutaneous neurofibromas are round, oblong, or polypoid nodules in the dermis. Although they are well-circumscribed, they are not encapsulated (Fig. 33-3*A*). The tumor is composed of proliferating delicate spindle cells with indistinct cytoplasmic membranes (Tables 33-2 and 33-5). The nuclei are wavy, with tapered ends and an evenly distributed chromatin pattern.[1,3,4] Mitotic figures should not be present. The cells are embedded in a finely fibrillary pale-pink collagenous stroma (Fig. 33-3*B*). The cellularity varies from densely cellular to a loosely arranged pattern. The stroma can be markedly fibrotic, edematous, myxomatous, and even vascular. The adnexa are surrounded but spared by the tumor. Mast cells are present in variable numbers throughout the lesion. Entrapped small nerve twigs, tactile bodylike structures, or pigmented dendritic cells may be observed. Although nuclear palisading can occur, Verocay bodies are not characteristic findings.[1,3]

When neurofibromas develop in the deeper and larger nerves, they initially remain encapsulated due to confinement by the perineurium. These types are sometimes referred to as *intraneural* neurofibromas.[4] In the deep-seated and diffuse types, the spindle cell proliferation is poorly defined and usually involves the subcutaneous fat. The tumor otherwise has similar features to the solitary type. The intraneural and diffuse (*extraneural*) types may be combined in the same lesion.[4]

Plexiform neurofibromas (Fig. 33-4) are composed of interconnecting bundles and fascicles of markedly expanded nerves that are usually surrounded by a fibrous encapsulation of the epineurium and adjacent connective tissue.[1,3,15] The superficial part, however, is usually not encapsulated, and the proliferating fascicles blend into the surrounding dermis. The individual fascicles display variable cellularity and often show edematous and mucinous changes. Cytologically, the cells are similar to the ones described in the solitary superficial form. Mild to moderate cytologic atypia is rare, and if associated with any mitotic activity, a malignant transformation should be considered seriously. In neurofibromatosis, plexiform neurofibroma and diffuse neurofibroma often coexist.[1]

Immunohistochemically, the cells in neurofibromas express variable antigens depending on the predominant cell types. These include S-100 protein, collagen type IV for Schwann cells, epithelial membrane antigen for perineurial cells, vimentin for fibroblasts and Schwann cells, and neural filaments and myelin basic protein for axons and myelin sheaths, respectively.[13]

Differential Diagnosis   The solitary superficial type of neurofibroma must be differentiated from other spindle cell neoplasms that are not encapsulated, such as dermatofibroma, hypertrophic scar, neurotized intradermal nevus, and traumatic neuroma. The diffuse deep-seated type and the pigmented variant may be confused with dermatofibrosarcoma protuberans and common blue nevus. The plexiform variant, which has the greatest clinical relevance due to its common association with von Recklinghausen's disease and the increased possibility of malignant transformation, should be separated from the plexiform schwannoma and the plexiform fibrohistiocytic tumor of infancy. All these can be differentiated relatively easily with the help of immunohistochemical markers.[18]

Schwannomas

Synonyms: neurilemoma, neurolemmoma, neurinoma, Schwann cell tumor, acoustic neuroma, perineurial fibroblastoma

Schwannomas are considered true nerve sheath neoplasms because they are composed almost entirely of proliferating Schwann cells. The Schwann cell proliferation takes place within the confines of the perineurium and displaces the remainder of the normal nerve fibers to the periphery of the tumor.[1,3] This histogenesis explains the three main features of schwannomas: the exclusive Schwann cell component, encapsulation, and the virtual lack of axons within the tumor. There are five main types of schwannomas: (1) the common solitary type,[19] which is almost invariably a benign neoplasm, (2) the ancient type, which represents a degenerated variant of the common type,[20,21] (3) the plexiform type, which displays cytologic features similar to the common type but which has a distinct growth pattern,[22,23] (4) the cellular type, which is a controversial entity originally conceptualized as a benign lesion in the deep soft tissues but which may represent a low-grade malignancy,[24,25] and (5) malignant schwannoma, one entity denoting a malignant transformation of a benign schwannoma.[26] Other less common variants, such as pigmented, glandular, epithelioid, also have been reported.[27,28]

Clinical Features   Common solitary schwannomas are tumors of adulthood; however, although rare, unusual congenital variants have been documented (Table 33-6). There is no significant predilection for either gender.[19] The lesions are usually solitary tumors, but rarely they can occur as multiple lesions, designated as *neurolemmomatosis*.[29] The tumors have a predilection for the flexor aspects of the extremities, followed by the head and neck areas and mediastinum, but even internal organs can be involved.

The average size of the tumors ranges between 1.5 and 3 cm, but extreme growth can occur, especially in body cavities. The usual appearance is that of a skin-colored or pink-yellow, deep dermal or subcutaneous well-defined nodule, which may be partially movable. Although the lesion in general is asymptomatic, it may be slightly painful or tender on palpation. Sensory or motor impairment can occur, but it is extremely rare.[1,19]

Cutaneous solitary schwannoma rarely can be part of neurofibromatosis type I, whereas the acoustic variant is more common in the type II manifestation of neurofibromatosis. The cutaneous tumors grow slowly following an almost invariably benign course, but they may encompass adjacent tissues and organs, necessitating their removal.

Histopathological Features   Common solitary schwannomas are ovoid or round tumors located in the deep dermis or subcutis (Tables 33-2 and 33-6). They are well-delineated by a thin, fibrous capsule. There are two main histologic patterns that are considered characteristic of schwannomas: the Antoni type A and type B tumors[1,3] (Fig. 33-5A). The *Antoni type A* pattern refers to a solid proliferation of Schwann cells forming compactly arranged fascicles and cords. The ovoid nuclei of the spindled Schwann cells often are arranged in a parallel fashion, referred to as *palisading*. When two rows of palisaded nuclei are separated by an acellular matrix, the resulting structures are designated as *Verocay bodies*[1,3] (Fig. 33-5B). Although nuclear palisading is nonspecific and can occur in other soft tissue tumors, it is quite common in schwannomas. Verocay bodies superficially resemble tactile bodies, but they do not have a sensory innervation. The cells constituting Antoni type A areas do not display significant cytologic atypia, and mitotic fig-

TABLE 33-6
Schwannoma

Clinical Features

Deep dermal or subcutaneous nodule
Up to 3 cm
May be painful
Predilection for flexor surface of extremities, and head and neck

Histopathological Features

Well-circumscribed, encapsulated, spindle cell proliferation
Alternating Antoni A and B areas
Palisaded nuclei
Cystic or myxoid degeneration is common
Thickened hyalinized vessel walls

Differential Diagnosis

Neuromas
Smooth-muscle neoplasms
Melanocytic neoplasms with spindle cell phenotype

ures are absent or extremely rare. *Antoni type B* tissue shows various degrees of cystic, edematous, or myxoid degeneration associated with vascular changes, thickened and hyalinized vessel walls, and fibrosis.[1,3] Thrombosis of the vessels, hemosiderin deposition, adjacent chronic inflammatory infiltrate, and increased numbers of mast cells are common. The degenerating cells often display variable nuclear atypia and pleomorphism, but mitotic figures are usually absent.

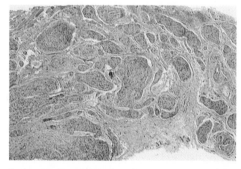

A

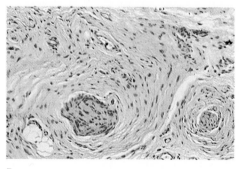

B

FIGURE 33-4   (*A*) Plexiform neurofibroma, superficial type. Interconnecting nerve fascicles of various size and shape infiltrating the dermis (H&E stain; ×2.5). (*B*) The spindle cells in a whorling pattern are embedded in variably fibromatous stroma (H&E stain; ×50).

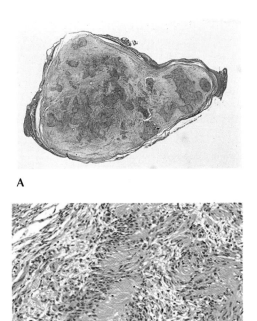

A

B

FIGURE 33-5 (*A*) Solitary schwannoma. The tumor is an encapsulated nodule consisting of hypercellular Antoni A, and hypocellular Antoni B types of tissues (H&E stain; ×5). (*B*) There is characteristic nuclear palisading and Verocay bodies with adjacent edematous stroma (H&E stain; ×66).

If the tumor is thoroughly sampled, its nerve origin can be recognized, as a rule, around the periphery of the lesion.[1,3]

Ancient schwannoma is composed almost entirely of Antoni type B tissue (Fig. 33-6). The degenerating cells may display prominent cytologic atypia, but no other features of malignancy are present.[20,21] Cellular schwannoma is usually a tumor of the mediastinum, retroperitoneum, and deep soft tissue. It is exceedingly rare in the skin. The tumor is a hypercellular mass of spindle-shaped cells, which form intertwining fascicles and cords (Fig. 33-7). Mild to moderate cytologic atypia and low mitotic rate (5 per 20 high-power fields) are characteristic. Atypical mitotic figures, necrosis, and invasion are absent.[24–26] Plexiform schwannoma is predominantly composed of Antoni type A tissue.[22,23] The proliferating cells form interconnecting fascicles and nodules extensively involving the dermis and subcutis (Fig. 33-8). The proliferation, however, remains mainly within the confines of the capsule. Mild to moderate cytologic atypia is common, but mitotic figures are rare or absent.[23] In contrast to the plexiform neurofibroma, this tumor is not considered pathognomonic of neurofibromatosis, and its malignant transformation is extremely rare.[23] Malignant schwannoma is a controversial entity because malignant transformation of a common solitary schwannoma is considered an extremely rare phenomenon.[1,26] The current prevailing view on malignant nerve sheath tumors is that they originate either de novo from a peripheral nerve or rarely from a preexisting neurofibroma.[1]

Immunohistochemically, schwannomas stain strongly for S-100 protein in the Antoni type A areas, whereas their capsule is positive for epithelial membrane antigen, supporting perineurial cell participation. Stains for axons either by silver impregnation or immunohistochemistry show lack of axons in the tumor itself, except where the nerve of origin is detected.[2]

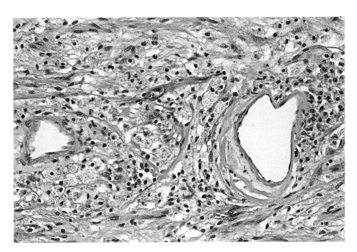

FIGURE 33-6 Ancient schwannoma. The lesion is composed of extensive areas of degenerative changes with stromal edema, vascular abnormalities, chronic inflammation, and foamy macrophages (H&E stain; ×100).

Differential Diagnosis Common solitary schwannoma must be differentiated from the encapsulated, palisaded neuroma and amputation neuroma, both of which contain abundant axons, as opposed to schwannoma. Angiomyomas are composed of spindle cells with more eosinophilic cytoplasm and characteristic nuclei. Since vascular and degenerative changes may mimic ancient schwannoma, immunohistochemical stains for smooth muscle–specific actin and desmin may be necessary to render a specific diagnosis. Plexiform schwannomas can be separated from plexiform neurofibromas by the complete absence of axons. The plexiform fibrohistiocytic tumor may represent a diagnostic problem, but it contains histiocytic cells and often multinucleated giant cells, and it does not stain for S-100 protein.[18]

Nerve Sheath Myxoma (Neurothekeoma)

Synonyms: pacinian neurofibroma, cutaneous lobular neuromyxoma, myxomatous perineurioma, bizarre cutaneous neurofibroma, myxoma of the nerve sheath, cellular neurothekeoma

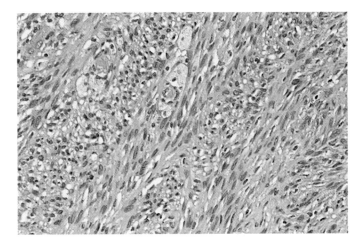

FIGURE 33-7 Cellular schwannoma. There is compact, fascicular proliferation of spindle cells with variable cytologic atypia and with rare mitotic figures (H&E stain; ×100).

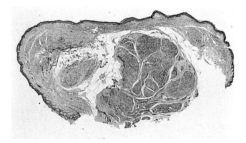

A

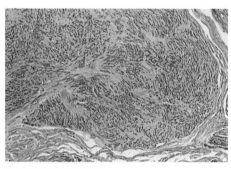

B

FIGURE 33-8   (*A*) Plexiform schwannoma. Interconnecting hypercellular nodules and fascicles infiltrating the dermis (H&E stain; ×2.5). (*B*) The individual fascicles are composed mainly of Antoni A type of tissue with common nuclear palisading and Verocay bodies (H&E stain; ×25).

head and neck areas.[32] Cellular neurothekeomas are firm, pink or red-brown papules and nodules that usually are less than 3 cm in diameter. Both variants are commonly asymptomatic, but on occasion they may become sensitive or tender. They are benign lesions, but they may recur if they are incompletely removed.

The term *nerve sheath myxoma* refers to a spectrum of neuromesenchymal tumors that are characterized by the proliferation of nerve sheath cells in a variably myxomatous stroma.[1,3] At one end of the spectrum, the tumors contain only sparse neuromesenchymal cells but in association with abundant myxomatous stroma. These tumors often are referred to as *classic nerve sheath myxomas*[30,31] because they were originally described under this term, or *mature nerve sheath myxomas*, because ultrastructurally and immunohistochemically they display characteristics of nerve sheath differentiation. At the other end of the spectrum are hypercellular tumors composed of immature cells in a scant or absent myxoid stroma. Such lesions display distinctly different features and deserve a different designation as *cellular neurothekeomas*.[32,33] Since these tumors often do not express the ultrastructural and immunohistochemical attributes of fully developed nerve sheath cells, they also are referred to as *immature nerve sheath myxomas*. They often demonstrate multiple lines of mesenchymal differentiation, i.e., fibrohistiocytic, myoid, and even chondroid features, in conjunction with primitive neural characteristics; not surprisingly, their histogenesis remains controversial.[31,32]

Clinical Features   Classic nerve sheath myxoma has been reported in middle-aged adults (average age 48.4 years),[32] occurring mainly on the head and upper extremities of female patients. However, these lesions can occur at any age, in either sex, and in any location (Table 33-7). The individual lesions are skin-colored or pink, soft to rubbery papules and nodules. Their clinical differential diagnoses include ganglions, myxoid cysts, dermal nevi, fibrolipomas, or adnexal neoplasms. Cellular neurothekeomas have been observed in younger adults (average age 24 years), with a female preponderance, at any body site but mainly in the

Histopathological Features   Classic nerve sheath myxoma usually is a well-delineated dermal tumor composed of interconnecting lobules and fascicles (Tables 33-2 and 33-7 and Fig. 33-9*A*). The fascicles contain abundant myxomatous stroma that is only sparsely cellular.[3,30] The component cells are variable: plump, spindle-shaped, slender, elongated with bipolar cytoplasmic extensions, or stellate (Fig. 33-9*B*). The nuclei are slightly hyperchromatic without prominent nucleoli. Mitotic figures are sparse or absent. Occasionally, multinucleated giant cells are present. The myxoid stroma is often separated by a partially preserved capsule or by condensation of the surrounding fibrous tissue. While adjacent nerve twigs often can be identified, direct connection with nerves usually is not readily discernible.

Immunohistochemically, the cells in the myxoid stroma react strongly to S-100 protein and collagen type IV and less intensely to neuron-specific enolase and Leu-7 (CD57) antigen.[30] When the capsule is preserved, a reaction to epithelial membrane antigen often is present. Neural filament stain for axons is usually negative. The myxomatous stroma is strongly positive for acidic mucopolysaccharides.[30]

Cellular neurothekeoma is an ill-defined, often infiltrative lesion occupying much of the dermis and even extending to the subcutis. The growth patterns are fascicular, plexiform, nodular, or nested, but a combination of these patterns also can occur[30–33] (Table 33-2 and Fig. 33-10*A*). The tumor is mainly composed of epithelioid cells with large ovoid nuclei, ample bright eosinophilic cytoplasm, and indistinct cytoplasmic membranes. The chromatin material often is concentrated around the nuclear membrane, and there is a prominent nucleolus (Fig. 33-10*B*). Spindle-shaped cells with plump or ovoid nuclei are also common, especially when the cells form nests or whorls.[34] Mitotic figures can be conspicuous, associated with various degrees of cytologic atypia.

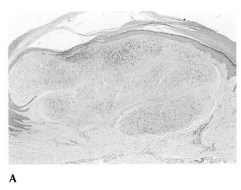

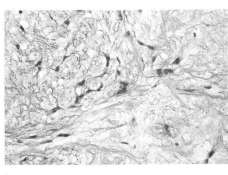

B

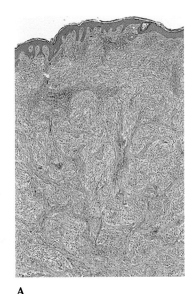

A

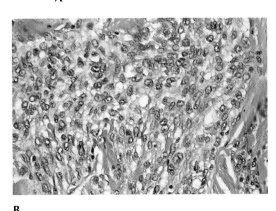

B

FIGURE 33-9 (*A*) Nerve sheath myxoma, classic type. Well-defined dermal nodules and fascicles with myxomatous stroma (H&E stain; ×10). (*B*) The mucinous stroma contains scattered spindle, polygonal, and stellatelike cells (H&E stain; ×100).

FIGURE 33-10 (*A*) Nerve sheath myxoma, cellular type, or cellular neurothekeoma. The tumor is composed of fascicles and nests infiltrating the dermis and subcutis without prominent myxomatous changes (H&E stain; ×10). (*B*) The tumor cells have eosinophilic cytoplasm, large, vacuolated nuclei, often with prominent nucleoli. Mitotic figures are scant (H&E stain; ×100).

Multinucleated cells also can be present. Myxoid material is usually scant or accumulated around the individual cell nests. Stromal changes, as in the classic variants, can occur, such as chronic inflammation, angioplasia, fibrosis, and hyalinization of collagen.[32] Occasionally, the overlying epidermis shows mild to moderate melanocytic hyperplasia. A direct association with nerve twigs is difficult to demonstrate.[30]

Immunohistochemically, cellular neurothekeomas show a variable and inconsistent reaction pattern. The cells do not, or only focally and weakly, react for S-100 protein.[30,33,34] The expression of Leu-7 (CD57), collagen type IV, and epithelial membrane antigen is similarly focal, weak, or absent. Sporadic positive reactions have been reported with NK1/C3, neuron-specific enolase, smooth muscle–specific actin, and CD34 antigens.[35] The tumor is consistently positive for vimentin only.

Differential Diagnosis Classic nerve sheath myxoma must be differentiated from the myxoid variant of neurofibroma, with axons demonstrable by special stains and usually some retained architecture of a neurofibroma. Focal cutaneous mucinosis and ganglion cysts may superficially resemble classic nerve sheath myxomas but do not display a plexiform or fascicular growth pattern, and their cells do not stain for S-100 protein.[30] Cellular neurothekeomas have a wider differential diagnosis, including epithelioid Spitz's nevus, deep-penetrating nevus, plexiform spindle cell nevus, and fascicular variants of cellular blue nevi. With the exception of the latter, these entities usually show epidermal melanocytic hyperplasia, often contain distinct pigmented cells, and all stain strongly for S-100 protein.[32,33] One must consider fibrohistiocytic lesions such as epithelioid cell histiocytoma and juvenile xanthogranuloma. However, careful study of histologic features and the adjunctive use of immunostaining should facilitate this discrimination.

Epithelioid variants of piloleiomyoma can be excluded based on their fine cytomorphologic features, their connection with existing pilar muscles, and the strong reaction with both smooth muscle–specific actin and desmin. In cases where the predominant cell type is spindle-shaped, plexiform fibrohistiocytic tumors must be excluded.

Granular Cell Tumor

Synonyms: granular cell nerve sheath tumor, granular cell myoblastoma, granular cell schwannoma, Abrikossoff's tumor

Granular cell tumor has a disputed histogenesis. A neural origin is postulated based on the observation that granular cells similar to those composed of these tumors are often observed within or adjacent to normal peripheral nerves.[36] The granular cells also express S-100 protein, Leu-7 (CD57) antigen, and myelin basic protein, as do normal peripheral nerves.[37] However, morphologically identical granular cells also have been described in various other nonneural neoplasms.[38]

TABLE 33-8

Granular Cell Tumor

Clinical Features

Adults, predilection for females
May occur at almost any site, predilection for tongue
Extremely rare malignant counterpart is often large, deep-seated, and
   unlikely to be encountered by dermatopathologist

Histopathological Features

Ill-defined infiltrative tumors
Large cells with abundant finely granular eosinophilic cytoplasm
Often associated with pseudoepitheliomatous hyperplasia, particularly
   in mucosal locations
Criteria for malignancy are not well established but include large size
   and mitotic activity

Differential Diagnosis

Xanthoma
Reticulohistiocytoma
Adult-type rhabdomyoma
Alveolar soft part sarcoma
Metastatic Leydig cell tumor and granular cell variant of renal cell
   carcinoma

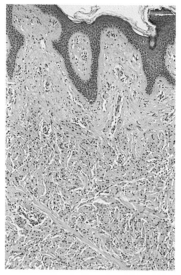

A

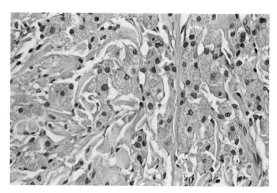

B

FIGURE 33-11 (*A*) Granular cell tumor. Indistinct, eosinophilic tumor cells forming nests and cords infiltrate the dermis and subcutis. The overlying epidermis is often acanthotic (H&E stain; ×25). (*B*) The tumor cells have polygonal shape, indistinct cytoplasmic membranes, and uniformly small, round nuclei. The cytoplasm has a characteristic fine granular appearance (H&E stain; ×100).

Clinical Features   Granular cell tumors usually present in adults with a 1:3 male-to-female ratio. In about 90 percent of the cases the tumor is solitary (Table 33-8). In the remaining 10 percent, multiple lesions are present, predominantly in blacks.[36] The most common site is the tongue, followed by the skin, various organs such as the gastrointestinal and upper respiratory tract, and skeletal muscle.[39]

In the skin, granular cell tumor presents as a skin-colored, firm, often verrucous or ulcerated nodule ranging in size from 0.5 to 3.0 cm.[36] The lesion is usually asymptomatic, but mild pruritus or tenderness may occur. Approximately 1 to 2 percent of granular cell tumors have a malignant course. The malignant variant is usually a rapidly growing nodule that frequently ulcerates.[40] Extensive local involvement and lymph node metastasis have been described.

Histopathological Features   Granular cell tumors form an ill-defined, often infiltrative mass in the dermis, frequently involving the subcutis (Table 33-8). The relatively large, polygonal cells are arranged in nests and cords, but infiltration as single cells or peculiar plexiform growth patterns also have been documented (Fig. 33-11*A*). The cells have an abundant, finely granular, faintly eosinophilic cytoplasm with small, round, centrally located nuclei[36] (Fig. 33-11*B*). Occasional tiny intracytoplasmic spherules with halos are present. Mitotic figures are rare or absent. The surrounding dermis is frequently fibrotic or hyalinized. Association with a peripheral nerve is extremely uncommon. The overlying epidermis often displays prominent pseudoepitheliomatous hyperplasia. Histopathologically, the malignant variant[40] may be indistinguishable from the benign lesion, whereas in other cases distinct cytologic atypia, increased mitotic activity, abnormal mitotic forms, and areas of necrosis are present. In the former case, only the clinical information about rapid growth, large size, and ulceration permits prediction of the malignant nature of the tumor.

The intracytoplasmic granules stain positively with the periodic acid–Schiff reaction, but they are diastase-resistant. Immunohistochemically, the cells are positive for S-100 protein, CD57 (Leu-7), peripheral nerve myelin proteins, neuron-specific enolase, and vimen-

tin.[37,41] Ultrastructurally, the intracytoplasmic granules are membrane-bound lysosomes and autophagosomes.[41]

Differential Diagnosis   Granular cell tumors often are associated with prominent pseudoepitheliomatous hyperplasia and may be misdiagnosed as squamous cell carcinoma. Cells of xanthomas contain fine cytoplasmic vacuoles rather than granules and are PAS-negative. Various other tumors, e.g., basal cell carcinoma, leiomyoma, leiomyosarcoma, and dermatofibroma, may contain granular cells.

Malignant Peripheral Nerve Sheath Tumor

Synonyms: malignant schwannoma, neurofibrosarcoma

Malignant peripheral nerve sheath tumor (MPNST) is usually a tumor of the deep soft tissues, head and neck areas, and retroperitoneum.[42] Approximately 50 percent of MPNSTs are associated with neurofibromatosis type I. Cutaneous involvement is the result of either direct extension from a deeply located tumor or malignant transforma-

TABLE 33-9

Malignant Peripheral Nerve Sheath Tumor

Clinical Features

Only rarely involves skin
Often associated with neurofibromatosis

Histopathological Features

Spindle cells with wavy nuclei
Cellular areas alternating with less cellular myxoid zones is
   characteristic
Increased cellularity adjacent to blood vessels
Only 50 percent of tumors are immunoreactive for S-100 protein
Tumors may show heterogeneous differentiation (i.e., rhabdomyo-
   blastic, cartilaginous, osseous)

Differential Diagnosis

Spindle cell melanoma, especially neurotropic melanoma
Monophasic synovial sarcoma
Fibrosarcoma

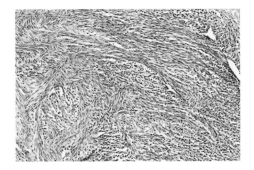

A

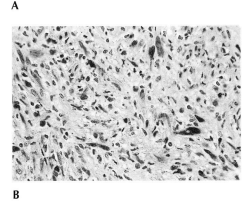

B

FIGURE 33-12   (*A*) Malignant peripheral nerve sheath tumor. The tumor is composed of intersecting and "sweeping" fascicles of spindle cells (H&E stain; ×25). (*B*) The tumor cells show marked cytologic pleomorphism, nuclear atypia, and increased mitotic figures (H&E stain; ×100).

tion of a preexisting neurofibroma, usually of the plexiform type. The probability of the latter occurrence has been estimated at about 4 percent.[43] The more generic term *malignant peripheral nerve sheath tumor* is favored over *malignant schwannoma* because cells other than Schwann cells can be present in the tumor. Furthermore, malignant transformation of benign schwannoma is exceedingly rare, and the term *malignant schwannoma* would incorrectly imply this histogenesis.

Clinical Features   MPNST is a tumor of adulthood; however, the cases that are associated with neurofibromatosis type I tend to occur in the younger age group. Whereas the sporadic form of MPNST is roughly equally common in both genders, it is more common in males when the tumor is associated with neurofibromatosis.[42] The tumor presents as a gradually growing, asymptomatic soft tissue mass, but pain, paresthesia, or weakness may occur at any stage of development. The sporadic type usually involves the main nerve trunks of extremities, whereas tumors associated with neurofibromatosis are more common on the trunk.[42,44] Sudden enlargement of a preexisting plexiform or solitary neurofibroma is always suspicious for malignant transformation. The overall clinical course is poor, especially in patients with associated neurofibromatosis; it is manifested by aggressive local recurrence, distant metastasis, and eventual death.[43]

Histopathological Features   The predominant histopathologic type of MPNST strongly resembles fibrosarcoma with spindle cells arranged in sweeping fascicles[42,43] (Table 33-9). This pattern is also referred to as *herring bone pattern* and often is composed of alternating hyper- and hypocellular areas (Fig. 33-12*A*). The constituent cells, however, differ from fibroblasts by their slender, wavy nuclei and indistinct cytoplasmic membranes. In addition, focal whorling, nuclear palisading, or tactile body–like structures may be present. Cytologic pleomorphism and nuclear atypia are variable (Fig. 33-12*B*). Mitotic activity greater than 1 per 20 high-power fields (HPFs) is considered a suspicious sign for malignancy.[42] Rare subtypes include elements of divergent differentiation, e.g., rhabdoid, cartilagenous, and osteoid (so-called Triton tumor), but glandular, epithelioid, and neuroblastic components also have been described.[42,43]

Immunohistochemically, only about 50 to 75 percent of MPNSTs stain for S-100 protein, which may be focal and weak.[42] In the remainder, the diagnosis can be quite difficult, especially if a direct connection with a peripheral nerve cannot be established. Other markers, including Leu-7 (CD57), myelin basic protein, and neuron-specific enolase and neural filaments,[42,43,45] are nonspecific but in the appropriate context can help to corroborate neural differentiation.

Differential Diagnosis   MPNST should be differentiated from fibrosarcoma, monophasic synovial sarcoma, leiomyosarcoma, and desmoplastic or neurotropic melanoma. Identification of the nerve of origin, cytologic features (especially the nuclear features), and the antigenic profile of these tumors should be helpful for making the definite diagnosis.

PRIMARY NEUROENDOCRINE CARCINOMA OF THE SKIN

Synonyms: Merkel cell carcinoma, trabecular carcinoma of the skin, primary small cell carcinoma of the skin, cutaneous APUDoma

Although the cells of primary neuroendocrine carcinoma of the skin (PNECS) and the normal Merkel cell, which is a specialized receptor cell of touch located in the basal layer of the epidermis, share several morphologic, immunohistochemical, and ultrastructural features, there is little evidence for a direct histogenetic relationship between the two.[46] Furthermore, other extracutaneous neuroendocrine tumors also display similar features; therefore, the conceptually more unifying term *primary neuroendocrine carcinoma of the skin* is preferred over *Merkel cell carcinoma.*[46]

Clinical Features   PNECS is most common in late adulthood, and it is slightly more prevalent in females. The tumor involves mainly the head

TABLE 33-10

Neuroendocrine (Merkel Cell) Carcinoma of Skin

Clinical Features

Predilection for head and neck of older adults
Solitary rapidly growing nodule

Histopathological Features

"Small, round, blue cell" tumor
Often nested or trabecular growth pattern
High mitotic rate and frequent single-cell necrosis, often zonal
   necrosis
Squamous differentiation not infrequently seen

Differential Diagnosis

Metastatic small cell carcinoma of lung and other sites
Lymphoma and leukemia
Small cell melanoma

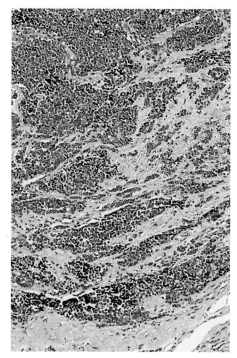

A

and neck areas, followed by the extremities and the buttocks (Table 33-10). The usual appearance is a pink-red or violaceous, firm, dome-shaped solitary nodule that grows rapidly.[46] Ulceration can occur. The biologic course is that of an aggressively growing, quickly metastasizing tumor with a usually fatal outcome.[46,47]

Histopathological Features   PNECS appears as a poorly defined dermal mass, frequently infiltrating the subcutaneous fat, fascia, and muscle. While it may show various growth patterns, a sheetlike growth is the most common, followed by the nested and trabecular types (Table 33-10) (Fig. 33-13A). Characteristically, the edge of the tumor shows a trabecular infiltrating pattern.[47] The tumor is composed of monotonously uniform, small, round to oval cells that are about two to three times larger than mature lymphocytes. The nuclei of these cells are ovoid with a finely dispersed chromatin material and distinct nuclear membranes. Nucleoli are usually not prominent (Fig. 33-13B). Mitotic figures are abundant. The cytoplasm is scant and faintly amphophilic. Extensive areas of necrosis, individual cell necrosis, and characteristic crush artifacts are common in PNECS.[46,47] Various peculiar types of differentiation have been described in PNECS, including rosettelike structures resembling Homer Wright rosettes of neuroblastoma, epidermotropic involvement with pagetoid spread, and eccrine and squamoid differentiation.[48,49] The adjacent stroma may show fibrosis, a lymphoplasmacytic infiltrate, and increased vascularity.

Immunohistochemically, PNECS demonstrates a characteristic perinuclear, globular-appearing reaction to low-molecular-weight cytokeratin, which corresponds to the ultrastructurally seen distribution of paranuclear whorls of intermediate filaments.[47,48,50] The cells also commonly express epithelial membrane antigens. In addition, there is a reaction with various neuroendocrine markers, including chromogranin, synaptophysin, somatostatin, calcitonin, vasoactive intestinal peptides, and others. These peptides are associated with the ultrastructurally demonstrable membrane-bound dense-core secretory granules.[47,48,50] The tumor also expresses neuron-specific enolase and occasionally neural filaments and cytokeratin 20, but reaction for S-100 protein is characteristically negative.[48,50,51]

Differential Diagnosis   There is a broad spectrum of small, round, blue cell tumors of various histogenesis that can be confused with PNECS. These include metastatic neuroendocrine carcinoma of the lung (small cell or oat cell carcinoma), poorly differentiated eccrine carcinoma, malignant lymphoma, metastatic neuroblastoma, primary peripheral

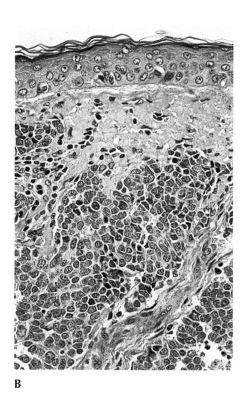

B

FIGURE 33-13 (*A*) Primary neuroendocrine carcinoma of the skin, Merkel cell carcinoma. The tumor forms irregular sheets and cords of hyperchromatic cells infiltrating the dermis (H&E stain; ×10). (*B*) The tumor cells have relatively uniform size, round to ovoid shape, with scant cytoplasm and fine "dusky" chromatin pattern (H&E stain; ×100).

TABLE 33-11

Immunohistochemical Differential Diagnostic Features of Small Round Cell Cutaneous Tumors

	S-100	CK	CEA	EMA	LCA	VIM	CHG	SYN-7	Leu-7	DES	AC	NSE	NF	CD99 (013)	CK20
PNECS (Merkel cell tumor)	−	+	−	+	−	−	+	+	−	−	−	+	+/−	NK	+
PNET (neuroblastoma)	−	−	−	−	−	+	+/−	+/−	+/−	−	−	+	+/−	+	−
Malignant lymphoma	−	−	−	−	+	+	−	−	−	−	−	−	−	+	−
Poorly differentiated eccrine carcinoma	+/−	+	+	+	−	−	−	−	−	−	−	−	−	NK	NK
Small cell melanoma	+	−	−	−	−	+	−	−	−	−	−	+	−	NK	−
Embryonal rhabdomyosarcoma	+/−	−	−	−	−	+	−	−	−	+	+	−	−	most −	−
Neuroblastoma	−	−	−	−	−	+	+/−	+/−	+/−	−	−	+	+	−	−
Small cell carcinoma	−	+	−	+	−	−	+	+	−	−	−	+	−	−	−

KEY: +, present; −, absent; +/−, variably present; NK, not known.
PNECS = primary neuroendocrine carcinoma of the skin; PNET = primitive neuroectodermal tumor; NF = neural filaments; AC = actin; S-100 = S-100 protein; CK = cytokeratin; CEA = carcinoembryonic antigen; EMA = epithelial membrane antigen; LCA = leukocyte common antigen; VIM = vimentin; CHG = chromogranin; SYN = synaptophysin; DES = desmin; NSE = neuron-specific enolase.

primitive neuroectodermal tumor, Ewing's sarcoma, malignant melanoma, and poorly differentiated squamous cell carcinoma.[46] These entities usually can be differentiated with the help of immunohistochemistry and electron microscopy, with the exception of metastatic small cell neuroendocrine carcinoma of any origin. However, the expression of neurofilament and cytokeratin 20 may help in the latter distinction and favor PNECS. The main immunohistochemical differential diagnostic features are summarized in Table 33-11.

NEURAL HETEROTOPIAS AND RELATED TUMORS

Cutaneous neural heterotopias are rare conditions, and they represent a broad spectrum of abnormalities of the cerebrospinal axis. Histogenetically, most of them are due to abnormal closure of the neural tube and its associated components, representing dysraphic conditions. A less common etiology of neural heterotopia is the result of abnormal migration and differentiation of neural crest cells despite a complete closure of the neural tube.[52] There are three major histopathologic manifestations of neural heterotopias in the skin: (1) meningeal, (2) neuroglial, and (3) neuroblastic/ganglionic abnormalities. Only the most common entities relevant to dermatopathologists are discussed here.

Heterotopic Meningeal Tissue

Cutaneous heterotopic meningeal tissues either represent herniations of the meningeal linings, as in the classic and rudimentary meningoceles as a result of congenital malformation, or they are autonomous proliferations of displaced meningothelial cells, defined as meningiomas.[53]

Clinical Features Rudimentary meningoceles are most common on the scalp along the cranial closure lines as skin-colored papules and nodules associated with alopecia or abnormal hair growth.[53–55]

Cutaneous meningiomas have three main forms of histogenesis, which also explains their clinical presentations.[56] In *type I*, the tumors are composed of arachnoid lining cells that are misplaced during embryogenesis. These lesions are usually congenital and are located on the scalp, forehead, and paravertebral regions. In *type II*, the tumors develop along the course of the cranial nerves and therefore are located mainly on the head, usually in adult patients. *Type III* lesions represent

cutaneous metastasis or direct extension of primary meningiomas of the arachnoid lining, and these carry the worst prognosis of the three types.[56]

Histopathological Features Rudimentary meningocele is an ill-defined mass of cavernous, pseudovascular spaces embedded in a markedly collagenous stroma. The spaces may be lined by elongated meningoendothelial cells characterized by eosinophilic cytoplasm, round or ovoid nuclei, and a fine chromatin pattern (Fig. 33-14). Similar cells dissect or wrap around collagen fibers, producing "collagen bodies."[55] No significant cytologic atypia or mitotic activity is present. Focal calcification and psammoma bodies may occur.[54,55]

Immunohistochemically, the meningoendothelial cells are positive for epithelial membrane antigen and vimentin.[54]

Differential Diagnosis Differential diagnosis includes cellular neurothekeoma, vascular neoplasms (particularly angiosarcoma), hemangiopericytoma, and giant cell fibroblastoma.

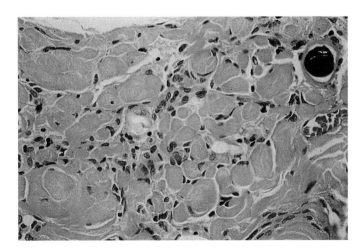

FIGURE 33-14   Rudimentary meningocele. The infiltrating meningoendothelial cells appear to dissect the dermal collagen creating "pseudovascular spaces." A psammoma body is present (H&E stain; ×100).

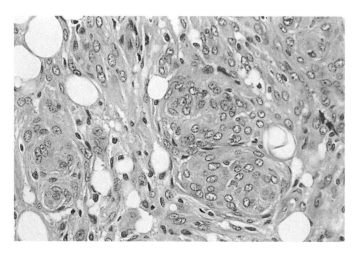

FIGURE 33-15 Primary cutaneous meningioma. The tumor has an infiltrative growth, and the epithelioid or spindle-shaped cells are often arranged in a whorl-like pattern (H&E stain; ×100).

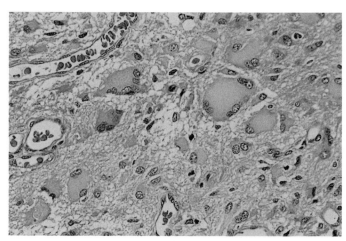

FIGURE 33-16 Nasal glioma. Gemistocytic astrocytes with abundant eosinophilic cytoplasm and multiple nuclei, and spindle-shaped fibrillary astrocytes are embedded in a foamy neuropil matrix (H&E stain; ×100).

CUTANEOUS MENINGIOMA

Histopathological Features Cutaneous meningioma is composed of a multinodular mass in the deep dermis or subcutis, often with an infiltrative growth pattern.[56–58] Depending on their histogenesis, the cells may show a variable degree of differentiation. In the most common form the spindle cells show a concentric, whorllike arrangement[56] (Fig. 33-15). The cells have oval nuclei with a vesicular chromatin pattern. Cytologic atypia can be predominant in type III lesions. Mitotic figures are rare in types I and II and variably increased in type III. Psammoma bodies often are present.[56,59]

Immunohistochemically, the constituent cells are positive for epithelial membrane antigen and vimentin, but other antigen expression, such as S-100 protein, neuron-specific enolase, and cytokeratins, also has been described in the various subtypes of meningioma.[51,59,60]

Differential Diagnosis Differential diagnosis includes metastatic squamous cell carcinoma, cutaneous adnexal neoplasms, hemangiopericytoma, cellular neurothekeoma, and cellular blue nevus. Their immunohistochemical profiles help to differentiate them from meningioma.

Heterotopic Neuroglial Tissue

There are three major forms of neuroglial tissue displacement from the central nervous system: (1) meningomyeloceles, (2) meningoencephaloceles, and (3) heterotopic brain tissue.[51,61] In the first two forms there is some degree of connection retained between the herniated brain tissue and the underlying structures, whereas in completely heterotopic brain tissue there is no apparent communication. The heterotopic brain tissue has a predilection for the perinasal areas; therefore, it is commonly designated as *nasal glioma*.[61] This is not a true neoplasm; therefore, the term is incorrect.

Clinical Features Nasal gliomas are firm, smooth-surfaced, skin-colored or pink, sometimes slightly vascularized nodules ranging in size between 1.0 and 5.0 cm. Approximately 60 percent of them are located extranasally on the bridge of the nose, whereas the remainder are located intranasally or in both locations.[61–63] Occasionally, there may

be some communication with the underlying central nervous system; therefore, thorough neuroradiologic imaging is mandatory before any cranial midline mass is biopsied to avoid cerebrospinal fluid leakage and possible consequent meningoencephalitis.[63]

Histopathological Features Nasal glioma forms an ill-defined, unencapsulated neuropillike mass in the dermis and subcutis. The adjacent stroma is usually markedly fibrotic and vascularized. On rare occasions, residual meningoendothelial cells may be present. The neuropillike tissue is composed of nests and strands of pale-staining, finely vacuolated or fibrillary glial tissue in which various types of astrocytes can be found.[53,62] Normal astrocytes have a round nucleus, a distinct nuclear membrane, and a prominent nucleolus, whereas fibrillary astrocytes are characterized by eosinophilic cytoplasmic processes. Gemistocytic astrocytes, with polygonal, eosinophilic cytoplasm and eccentric nuclei, as well as multinucleated giant cells, are also common (Fig. 33-16). Mature neurons with triangular cell bodies, large, open, eccentric nuclei, Nissle granules, and dendritic and axonal processes are present in variable numbers.[63,64] Occasionally, ductlike structures with ependymal cells, choroid plexus–like structures, and pigmented cells can be identified. No mitotic activity or destructive growth pattern has been described.[64]

Immunohistochemically, the glial tissue stains strongly for glial fibrillary acidic protein, the neurons react with neuron-specific enolase, and the axons label with antibodies to neural filaments.[52]

Differential Diagnosis Nasal glioma must be differentiated from ganglioneuroblastoma, dermoid cyst, and hemangioma. Ganglion cells can be differentiated from glial cells by their characteristic oval shape, large size, and eccentric nuclei with prominent nucleoli. Dermoid cysts contain tissues of all three germ layers, and hemangiomas are devoid of neuropillike tissue.

Heterotopic Neuroblastic Tissue and Their Tumors

Neuroblastic-ganglionic tumors are derived from the germinal neuroepithelium and/or from the neural crest. They represent a wide spectrum of clinicopathologic manifestations commonly referred to as *primitive neuroectodermal tumors.*[65,66] Primitive neuroectodermal tumors in the skin either represent *metastases* of neuroblastomas of the adrenals and/or the ganglionic chain or develop de novo from heterotopic neural crest cells.[65]

Clinical Features   Neuroblastoma is a common childhood neoplasm, and cutaneous metastasis is frequent. The metastases often manifest as multiple, blue or purple dermal papules or nodules resembling the "blueberry muffin" lesions of congenital rubella syndrome.[67] These nodules may blanch on stroking. Serum and urine catecholamine levels are typically elevated. The prognosis depends on the patient's age and the clinical stage. Spontaneous regression has been described in the stage IV-S type.[65,68]

Histopathological Features   Metastatic neuroblastoma is an ill-defined or infiltrative mass in the dermis and/or the subcutis. The mass is composed of atypical, small, dark cells with scant cytoplasm. The cells have larger nuclei than mature lymphocytes, with a coarse chromatin pattern. The cells form irregular nests, cords, or poorly cohesive sheets.[65] Rosette formation, by concentrically arranged tumor cells in double or multiple circles, is common. The center of the rosettes contains converging fine fibrillary material characteristic of Homer Wright–type rosettes (Fig. 33-17). Mitotic activity is high, and abnormal mitoses are abundant.[65,66] Extensive areas of necrosis and hemorrhage are common. As the tumor differentiates, the percentage of neuroblastomatous components decreases and the ganglioneuromatous elements proportionately increase, and eventually, the tumor may become a ganglioneuroma.[65]

Immunohistochemically, the cells variably react with the various neural and neuroendocrine markers, depending on their state of differentiation. These markers include neuron-specific enolase, S-100 protein, neurofilaments, synaptophysin, chromogranin, and CD99.[69]

Primary cutaneous primitive neuroectodermal tumors are exceedingly rare in the skin.[70–73] They usually manifest in adults as rapidly growing dermal and subcutaneous nodules. These highly aggressive neoplasms have an almost invariably fatal outcome. Histopathologically, they are composed of atypical, small, round blue cells similar to those of the classic neuroblastoma, but ganglionic or neuromatous differentiation is not characteristic. Primitive neuroectodermal tumor also shares the main immunohistochemical features with classic neuroblas-

toma.[70,71] However, mic-2 (O13) is commonly expressed by these tumors but not by neuroblastoma, facilitating distinction of the two tumors.

Differential Diagnosis   Both metastatic neuroblastoma and primary neuroectodermal tumor must be differentiated from other rosette-forming, small, round, blue cell tumors that may involve the skin.[46] These entities include primary neuroendocrine carcinoma of the skin (Merkel cell carcinoma), metastatic undifferentiated small cell carcinoma of the lung, extraskeletal Ewing's sarcoma, small cell malignant melanoma, rhabdomyosarcoma, poorly differentiated eccrine carcinoma, malignant lymphoma, and leukemic infiltrates. A summary of the cardinal differential diagnostic, immunohistochemical, and ultrastructural findings is provided in Table 33-11.

REFERENCES

1. Enzinger FM, Weiss SW: Benign tumors of peripheral nerves, in *Soft Tissue Tumors*, 3d ed. St. Louis, Mosby, 1995:821–888.
2. Ortiz-Hidalgo C, Weller RO: Peripheral nervous system, in Sternberg SS (ed): *Histology for Pathologists*, 1st ed. New York, Raven Press, 1992:169–193.
3. Harkin JC, Reed RJ: Tumors of the peripheral nervous system, in Armed Forces Institute of Pathology (ed): *Atlas of Tumor Pathology*, 2d series, fasc 3. Washington, Armed Forces Institute of Pathology, 1969:19–168.
4. Reed RJ, Harkin JC: Tumors of the peripheral nervous system, in Armed Forces Institute of Pathology (ed): *Atlas of Tumor Pathology*, 2d series, fasc 3, (supplement). Washington, Armed Forces Institute of Pathology, 1983:S1–S52.
5. Reed RJ, Fine RM, Meltzer HD: Palisaded, encapsulated neuromas of the skin. *Arch Dermatol* 106:865, 1972.
6. Dover JS, From L, Lewis A: Palisaded encapsulated neuromas: A clinicopathologic study. *Arch Dermatol* 125:386, 1989.
7. Gorlin RJ, Sedano HO, Vickers RA, et al: Multiple mucosal neuromas, pheochromocytoma and medullary carcinoma of the thyroid: A syndrome. *Cancer* 22:293, 1968.
8. Matthews GJ, Osterholm JL: Painful traumatic neuromas. *Surg Clin North Am* 51:1313, 1972.
9. Shapiro L, Juklin EA, Brownstein HM: Rudimentary polydactyly. *Arch Dermatol* 108:223, 1973.
10. Argenyi ZB, Santa Cruz D, Bromley C: Comparative light-microscopic and immunohistochemical study of traumatic and palisaded, encapsulated neuromas of the skin. *Am J Dermatopathol* 14:504, 1992.
11. Argenyi ZB, Cooper PH, Santa Cruz D: Plexiform and other unusual variants of palisaded encapsulated neuroma. *J Cutan Pathol* 20:34, 1993.
12. Argenyi ZB: Immunohistochemical characterization of palisaded encapsulated neuroma. *J Cutan Pathol* 17:329, 1990.
13. Megahed M: Histopathological variants of neurofibroma: A study of 114 lesions. *Am J Dermatopathol* 16:486, 1994.
14. Oshman RG, Phelps RG, Kantor I: A solitary neurofibroma on the finger. *Arch Dermatol* 124:1185, 1988.
15. Jurecka W: Plexiform neurofibroma of the skin. *Am J Dermatopathol* 10:209, 1988.
16. Mentzel T, Dei Tos AP, Fletcher CDM: Perineurioma (storiform perineurial fibroma): Clinicopathological analysis of four cases. *Histopathology* 25:261, 1994.
17. Riccardi VM: Von Recklinghausen neurofibromatosis (review). *N Engl J Med* 305:1617, 1981.
18. Argenyi ZB: Recent developments in cutaneous neural neoplasms. *J Cutan Pathol* 20:97, 1993.
19. Das Gupta TK, Brasfield RD, Strong EW, et al: Benign solitary schwannomas (neurilemomas). *Cancer* 24:355, 1969.
20. Dahl I, Hagmar B, Idvall I: Benign solitary neurilemmoma (schwannoma): A correlative cytological and histological study of 28 cases. *Acta Pathol Microbiol Immunol Scand [A]* 92:91, 1984.
21. Argenyi ZB, Balogh K, Abraham AA: Degenerative ("ancient") changes in benign cutaneous schwannoma: A light microscopic, histochemical and immunohistochemical study. *J Cutan Pathol* 20:148, 1993.
22. Woodruff JM, Marshall ML, Gowin TA, et al: Plexiform (multinodular) schwannoma: A tumor simulating the plexiform neurofibroma. *Am J Surg Pathol* 7:691, 1983.
23. Kao GF, Laskin WB, Olsen TG: Solitary cutaneous plexiform neurilemmoma (schwannoma): A clinicopathologic, immunohistochemical and ultrastructural study of 11 cases. *Mod Pathol* 2:20, 1986.
24. Woodruff JM, Godwin TA, Erlandson RA, et al: Cellular schwannoma: A variety of schwannoma sometimes mistaken for a malignant tumor. *Am J Surg Pathol* 5:733, 1981.

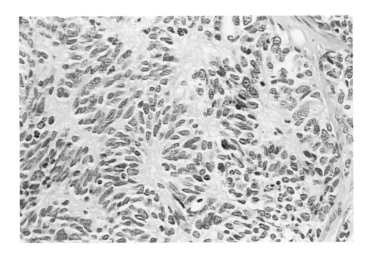

FIGURE 33-17   Cutaneous neuroblastoma. Poorly differentiated, small, round to ovoid, hyperchromatic cells form Homer Wright rosettes with characteristic central fibrillary material (H&E stain; ×100).

25. White W, Shiu MH, Rosenblum MK, et al: Cellular schwannoma: A clinicopathologic study of 57 patients and 58 tumors. *Cancer* 66:1266, 1990.

26. Woodruff JM, Selig AM, Crowley K, et al: Schwannoma (neurilemoma) with malignant transformation: A rare, distinctive peripheral nerve tumor. *Am J Surg Pathol* 18:882, 1994.

27. Carney JA: Psammomatous melanotic schwannoma: A distinctive, heritable tumor with special associations, including cardiac myxoma and the Cushing syndrome. *Am J Surg Pathol* 14:206, 1990.

28. Oda Y, Hashimoto H, Tsuneyoshi M, et al: Benign glandular peripheral nerve sheath tumor. *Pathol Res Pract* 190:466, 1994.

29. Shishiba T, Niimura M, Ohtsuka F, et al: Multiple cutaneous neurilemmomas as a skin manifestation of neurilemmomatosis. *J Am Acad Dermatol* 10:744, 1984.

30. Argenyi ZB, LeBoit PE, Santa Cruz D, et al: Nerve sheath myxoma (neurothekeoma) of the skin: Light microscopic and immunohistochemical reappraisal of the cellular variant. *J Cutan Pathol* 20:294, 1993.

31. Argenyi ZB, Kutzner H, Seaba MM: Ultrastructural spectrum of cutaneous nerve sheath myxoma/cellular neurothekeoma. *J Cutan Pathol* 22:137, 1995.

32. Barnhill RL, Mihm MC: Cellular neurothekeoma: A distinctive variant of neurothekeoma mimicking nevomelanocytic tumors. *Am J Surg Pathol* 14:113, 1990.

33. Barnhill RL, Dickersin GR, Nickeleit V, et al: Studies on cellular origin of neurothekeoma: Clinical, light microscopic, immunohistochemical, and ultrastructural observations. *J Am Acad Dermatol* 25:80, 1991.

34. Fletcher CDM, Chan JK-C, McKee PH: Dermal nerve sheath myxoma: A study of three cases. *Histopathology* 10:135, 1986.

35. Calonje E, Wilson-Jones E, Smith NP, et al: Cellular "neurothekeoma": An epithelioid variant of pilar leiomyoma? Morphological and immunohistochemical analysis of a series. *Histopathology* 20:397, 1992.

36. Apisarnthanarax P: Granular cell tumor: An analysis of 16 cases and review of the literature. *J Am Acad Dermatol* 5:171, 1981.

37. Regezi JA, Zarbo RJ, Courtney RM, et al: Immunoreactivity of granular cell lesions of skin, mucosa and jaw. *Cancer* 64:1455, 1989.

38. LeBoit PE, Barr RJ, Burall S, et al: Primitive polypoid granular-cell tumor and other cutaneous granular-cell neoplasms of apparent nonneural origin. *Am J Surg Pathol* 15:48, 1991.

39. Khansur T, Balducci L, Tavassoli M: Granular cell tumor: Clinical spectrum of the benign and malignant entity. *Cancer* 60:220, 1987.

40. Cadotte M: Malignant granular-cell myoblastoma. *Cancer* 33: 1417, 1974.

41. Buley ID, Gatter KC, Kelly PMA, et al: Granular cell tumours revisited: An immunohistological and ultrastructural study. *Histopathology* 12:263, 1988.

42. Brooks JJ: Malignant peripheral nerve sheath tumor (MPNST), in Antonioli DA, Carter D, Mills SE, Oberman HA (eds): *Diagnostic Surgical Pathology*, 2d ed. New York, Raven Press, 1994:147–229.

43. Enzinger FM, Weiss SW: Malignant tumors of peripheral nerves, in *Soft Tissue Tumors*, 3d ed. St. Louis, Mosby, 1995:889–928.

44. Herrera GA, deMoraes HP: Neurogenic sarcomas in patients with neurofibromatosis (von Recklinghausen's disease). *Virchows Arch Pathol Anat* 403:361, 1984.

45. George E, Swanson PE, Wick MR: Malignant peripheral nerve sheath tumors of the skin. *Am J Dermatopathol* 11:213, 1989.

46. Wick MR, Scheithauer BW: Primary neuroendocrine carcinoma of the skin, in Wick MR (ed): *Pathology of Unusual Malignant Cutaneous Tumors*. New York, Marcel Dekker, 1985:107.

47. Sibley RK, Dehner LP, Rosai J: Primary neuroendocrine (Merkel cell?) carcinoma of the skin: I. A clinicopathologic and ultrastructural study of 43 cases. *Am J Surg Pathol* 9:95, 1985.

48. Visscher D, Cooper PH, Zarbo RJ, et al: Cutaneous neuroendocrine (Merkel cell) carcinoma: An immunophenotypic, clinicopathologic, and flow cytometric study. *Mod Pathol* 2:331, 1989.

49. LeBoit PE, Crutcher WA, Shapiro PE: Pagetoid intraepidermal spread in Merkel cell (primary neuroendocrine) carcinoma of the skin. *Am J Surg Pathol* 16:584, 1992.

50. Layfield L, Ulich T, Liao S, et al: Neuroendrcrine carcinoma of the skin: An immunohistochemical study of tumor markers and neuroendocrine products. *J Cutan Pathol* 13:268, 1986.

51. Sibley RK, Dahl D: Primary neuroendocrine (Merkel cell?) carcinoma of the skin: II. An immunocytochemical study of 21 cases. *Am J Surg Pathol* 9:109, 1985.

52. Argenyi ZB: Cutaneous neural heterotopias and related tumors relevant for the dermatopathologist. *Semin Diagn Pathol* 13:60, 1996.

53. Berry AD III, Patterson W: Meningoceles, meningomyeloceles, and encephaloceles: A neuro-dermatopathologic study of 132 cases. *J Cutan Pathol* 18:164, 1991.

54. Marrogi AJ, Swanson PE, Kyriakos M, et al: Rudimentary meningocele of the skin: Clinicopathologic features and differential diagnosis. *J Cutan Pathol* 18:178, 1991.

55. Sibley DA, Cooper PH: Rudimentary meningocele: A variant of "primary cutaneous meningioma." *J Cutan Pathol* 16:72, 1989.

56. Lopez DA, Silvers DN, Helwig EB: Cutaneous meningiomas: A clinicopathologic study. *Cancer* 34:728, 1974.

57. Argenyi ZB, Thieberg MD, Hayes CM, Whitaker DC: Primary cutaneous meningioma associated with von Recklinghausen disease. *J Cutan Pathol* 21:549, 1994.

58. Nochomovitz LE, Jannotta F, Orenstein JM: Meningioma of the scalp: Light and electron microscopic observations. *Arch Pathol Lab Med* 109:92, 1985.

59. Gelli MC, Pasquinelli G, Martinelli G, et al: Cutaneous meningioma: Histochemical, immunohistochemical and ultrastructural investigation. *Histopathology* 23:576, 1993.

60. Theaker JM, Fleming KA: Meningioma of the scalp: A case report with immunohistological features. *J Cutan Pathol* 14:49, 1987.

61. Orkin M, Fisher I: Heterotopic brain tissue (heterotopic neural crest): Case report with review of related anomalies. *Arch Dermatol* 94:699, 1966.

62. Patterson K, Kapur S, Chandra RS: "Nasal gliomas" and related brain heterotopias: A pathologist's perspective. *Pediatr Pathol* 5:353, 1986.

63. Yeoh GPS, Bale PM, DeSilva M: Nasal cerebral heterotopia: The so-called nasal glioma or sequestered encephalocele and its variants. *Pediatr Pathol* 9:531–549, 1989.

64. Fletcher CDM, Carpenter G, McKee PH: Nasal glioma: A rarity. *Am J Dermatopathol* 8:341, 1986.

65. Joshi VV, Silverman JF: Pathology of neuroblastic tumors. *Semin Diagn Pathol* 11:107, 1994.

66. Dehner LP: Peripheral and central primitive neuroectodermal tumors: A nosologic concept seeking a consensus. *Arch Pathol Lab Med* 110:997, 1986.

67. Shown TE, Durfee MF: Blueberry muffin baby: Neonatal neuroblastoma with subcutaneous metastases. *J Urol* 104:193, 1970.

68. Evans AE, Chatten J, D'Angio GD, et al: A review of 17 IV-S neuroblastoma patients at the Children's Hospital of Philadelphia. *Cancer* 45:833, 1980.

69. Stevenson AJ, Chatten J, Bertoni F, et al: CD99 (p30/32^{MIC2}) neuroectodermal/Ewing's sarcoma antigen as an immunohistochemical marker: Review of more than 600 tumors and the literature experience. *Appl Immunohistochem* 2:231, 1994.

70. Argenyi ZB, Bergfeld WF, McMahon JT, et al: Primitive neuroectodermal tumor in the skin with features of neuroblastoma in an adult patient. *J Cutan Pathol* 13:420, 1986.

71. Nguyen AV, Argenyi ZB: Cutaneous neuroblastoma: Peripheral neuroblastoma. *Am J Dermatopathol* 15:7, 1993.

72. Tang CK, Hajdu SI: Neuroblastoma in adolescence and adulthood. *NY State J Med* 75:1434, 1975.

73. Aleshire DL, Glick AD, Cruz VE, et al: Neuroblastoma in adults: Pathologic findings and clinical outcome. *Arch Pathol Lab Med* 109:352, 1985.

LYMPHOID, LEUKEMIC, AND OTHER CELLULAR INFILTRATES

Cutaneous T-Cell Lymphomas (CTCL)

Guenter Burg / Werner Kempf / Andreas Haeffner / Beatrix Mueller / Reinhard Dummer

Cutaneous T-cell lymphomas (CTCL) represent the largest proportion (65%) of all primary cutaneous peripheral lymphomas (CL). They comprise lymphoproliferative disorders, which to some extent can be classified by an adaptation of the Kiel or other classifications for nodal lymphomas. The most common CTCL, mycosis fungoides (MF) and Sézary syndrome (SS), are monoclonal T-helper memory-cell lymphomas. However, CTCL include other disease entities showing biological and phenotypical differences from these prototypes. Immunophenotyping and polymerase chain reaction (PCR) of the T-cell receptor (TCR) genes and screening of the PCR products for sequence-specific mobility in acrylamide gels have increased the detection limit for clonal T-cells in the skin and help to define the relationship of CTCL to other lymphoproliferative disorders contributing to the early diagnosis of CTCL. The malignant clone of lymphoid cells in CTCL secretes a cytokine pattern of T-helper 2 cells (TH2), which might be responsible for the many systemic and laboratory changes found in CTCL patients.[1,2]

Classification

Many attempts have been made over the last decades to classify cutaneous lymphomas.[4-6] In general, classifications should be simple, reproducible, clinically relevant, and tranferable into other competing classification systems. Classifications of CTCL should be compatible with current classifications for nodal lymphomas.

For routine diagnostic purposes, morphology always has been and always will be in the future the "golden standard" for the classification of lymphoproliferative disorders, which have changed again and again over the years because of the development of new techniques for cell identification and our increasing understanding of lymphocyte ontogeny.

Rappaport's most useful classification into lymphocyte-rich, lymphocyte-poor, mixed cell, and histiocytic lymphomas—all forms nodular or diffuse—has been modified and replaced by others.[3,6,7] The most common classifications used today are the modified Kiel classification and the Working Formulation.[7-9] Recently, a Revised European American Lymphoma (R.E.A.L.)-classification has come under consideration.[10]

Extranodal tissues, including the skin, may provide unique environments for lymphomas; nevertheless we are dealing with the same pathogenetic processes as found in nodal lymphomas. Therefore, classifica-

tions of extranodal lymphomas should be adopted to the current classifications of nodal lymphomas, completing the basic concepts by specific organ-related requirements in order to reflect the biological uniqueness of extranodal lymphomas.

For cutaneous lymphomas, this basic concept is the Working Formulation or the updated Kiel classification, modified and supplemented as given in Table 34-1.[7,9]

Clinical Aspects

In contrast to cutaneous B-cell lymphomas (CBCL), in which the clinical presentation usually is relatively uniform, CTCL comprise a heterogeneous pattern of clinical features including patches of various sizes, plaques, tumors with or without ulceration, erythroderma, usually with some scaling, and many other variations.

Histomorphological and Cytomorphological Basis

STRUCTURAL DIFFERENCES BETWEEN SKIN AND LYMPH NODE

In contrast to lymph nodes, the skin is not a primary homing organ for lymphocytes. Nevertheless, comparable with the lymph node, it provides compartments, in which T-cells and B-cells home preferentially, respectively. This zonal structure is spherical in the lymph node, but flat in the skin (Fig. 34-1).

The different structural and cellular compositions provide a variety of functionally different compartments and microenvironments, respectively. The epidermis, the subepidermal papillary dermis, the periadnexal areas, and the subcutaneous tissue are typical microenvironments for T-cell infiltrates, containing dendritic reticulum cells, Langerhans cells, and postcapillary high endothelial venules, and correspond to the peri- and interfollicular regions of the secondary lymph-follicles. The mid and deep dermis and their perivascular spaces are compartments in which B-lymphocytes home preferentially.

COMPARTMENTS

The preferential involvement of the different compartments of the skin corresponds to the different nosologic subtypes of cutaneous lymphomas. The epidermis shows sponge-like disaggregation of keratinocytes by invading lymphocytes in pagetoid reticulosis. Epidermal

TABLE 34-1

Classification of Non-Hodgkin's Lymphomas According to Kiel and Working Classifications

Non-Hodgkin's Lymphomas

Kiel Classification	*Working Formulation*
T-cell Lymphomas	
Lymphomas of T-precursor cells T-lymphoblastic lymphoma/ leukemia*	ML, lymphoblastic
Lymphomas of peripheral T-cells T-chronic lymphocytic leukemia*	ML, small lymphocytic, consistent with CLL
Mycosis fungoides (MF)	Mycosis fungoides
Sézary syndrome	Sézary syndrome
Pagetoid reticulosis, circumscribed, disseminated ML, polymorphous	
Pleomorphic T-cell lymphoma, HTLV-1± small, medium, large	
Immunoblastic lymphoma, T-cell type (Ki-1+)	ML, large-cell, immunoblastic
B-cell Lymphomas	
B-chronic lymphocytic leukemia*	ML, small lymphocytic, consistent with CLL
Lymphoplasmacytoid immunocytoma	ML, small lymphocytic plasma-cytoid
Plasmacytoma	Extramedullary plasma-cytoma
Centroblastic/centrocytic lymphoma	ML, mixed small cleaved and large
Skin-associated lymphoid tissue (SALT) lymphoma(?)	
Centrocytic (mantle cell) lymphoma	ML, small cleaved
Immunoblastic lymphoma	ML, large cell, immuno-blastic
Burkitt's lymphoma	ML, small noncleaved, Burkitt

Rare and Distinct Forms of Lymphoproliferative and Related Disorders

Granulomatous slack skin/MF
Lymphoepithelioid lymphoma (Lennert)*
Midline granuloma*
Lymphomatoid papulosis
Systemic angioendotheliomatosis (angiotrophic lymphoma) (B > T)
Lymphomatoid granulomatosis (Liebow)*
Angiolymphoid hyperplasia with eosinophilia (Kimura)
Syringolymphoid hyperplasia with alopecia
Subcutaneous (lipotropic) T-cell lymphomas
Sinus histiocytosis with massive lymphadenopathy (Rosai-Dorfman)*
Peripheral T-cell lymphoma of the AILD-type**
T-cell rich large T-cell lymphoma
B-cell rich T-cell lymphoma
Large cell lymphoma of the multilobated cell type (B or T)
T-cell lymphoma expressing delta T-cell receptor

*Usually secondary involvement
**AILD = Angioimmunoblastic lymphadenopathy with dysproteinemia

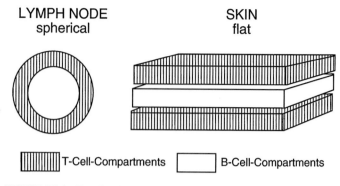

FIGURE 34-1   Functional structuring of T- and B-zones in lymph node and skin.

structures may be completely destroyed by the infiltrate in CD8+ CTCL.

Involvement of the epidermis and the papillary dermis typically is found in classical CTCL such as mycosis fungoides, in which single-cell epidermotropism is the most prominent feature, whereas intraepidermal (Pautrier's) microabscesses are much more frequently seen in the leukemic variant of CTCL, Sézary's syndrome.

Involvement of the junctional zone with edema and vacuolization in this area, but without significant epidermotropism, is a typical feature for large plaque parapsoriasis and early mycosis fungoides.

Localization of the infiltrate in the mid and deep dermis typically is found in cutaneous B-cell lymphomas (CBCL) or in high-grade malignant (large cell) lymphomas of both T- or B-cell phenotype, respectively.

The subcutaneous fat typically is involved in subcutaneous panniculitic T-cell lymphoma.[11,12] Tumor cells in the subcutaneous tissue usually are large blasts showing pleomorphic, anaplastic, or lobulated nuclei.

The periadnexal compartment around hair follicles, sebaceous glands, and sweat gland ducts provides microenvironmental conditions corresponding to the subepidermal papillary dermis. Diffuse superficial T-cell infiltrates arranged in a sleeve-like pattern along those structures may reach into the deep dermis.

Proliferations of lymphocytes may reside in the vascular lumina passively in intravascular lymphomatosis (former "angioendotheliomatosis proliferans systematisata").

The blood vessel walls and the perivascular spaces are the major sites of activity in lymphomatoid granulomatosis Liebow, in which angiodestructive lymphoid infiltrates accumulate in an angiocentric fashion.

GROWTH PATTERN

In nodal lymphomas, the description of nodular or diffuse growth patterns is used for the discrimination of lymphoma subtypes. In the skin, the terms nodular or diffuse reflect two different types of growth pattern that best can be compared with the three dimensions of a sphere or the two dimensions of a disc, respectively, and are completely different from their designations in nodal lymphomas. A small biopsy or punch biopsy from a nodular infiltrate exceeding the borders of the section owing to the smallness of the specimen, may simulate a diffuse infiltrate in the sense as used for the description of the lymph node and clearly could be detected as being nodular, if the biopsy would have been somehow larger or deeper.

In CTCL a diffuse cutaneous infiltrate involves the subepidermal grenz zone over a large area (Fig. 34-2) and is preferentially composed

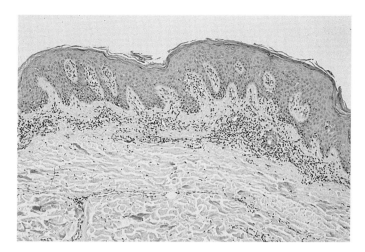

FIGURE 34-2   CTCL A diffuse infiltrate involving the subepidermal grenz zone (H&E magnification × 100).

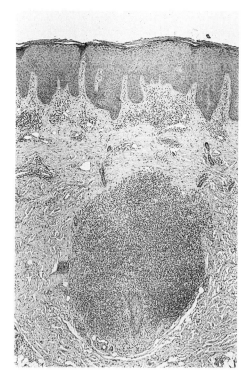

FIGURE 34-3   CTCL. Nodular cutaneous infiltrate primarily located within the dermis, growing centrifugally in three dimensions (H&E magnification × 25 [Z 3, 27]).

of T-lymphocytes and presents clinically as patches, flat plaques or virtually the entire cutaneous surface as in erythroderma. The typical growth pattern is horizontal in two dimensions, but vertical along adnexal structures. It is a typical feature of early stages and small-cellular types of CTCL.

Usually, a nodular cutaneous infiltrate is located primarily within the dermis and grows centrifugally in three dimensions (Fig. 34-3). This pattern is mostly found in CBCL or in primary or secondary high-grade malignant large cell lymphomas of both lineages, for example, mycosis fungoides transforming into high-grade malignant large cell lymphoma. Nodular growth patterns in the skin may be small, such as in lymphomatoid papulosis, or large without restriction to preferential T- and B-cell compartments.

There may be combinations of both growth patterns if, for example, tumorous lesions develop within patches or erythroderma.

PRINCIPAL CELL TYPES OF THE T-CELL SERIES AND ONTOGENY

Proliferating cells in malignant lymphomas partly retain morphological and functional properties that are found in normal cells of the lymphoid series along the differentiation pathway from the stem cell to the peripheral postthymic, well differentiated T-cell (Fig. 34-4). However, neoplastic cells may loose properties of normal cells or acquire other properties. Their origin may be obscured and render additional pheno- or genotyping mandatory in special cases, in which precise morphologic classification is not possible.

Small lymphocytes (Fig. 34-5A) correspond to the lymphocytes in the peripheral blood. In skin infiltrates, they appear as roundish nuclei with dark, homogeneously distributed chromatin; the small rim of cytoplasm usually cannot be seen by light microscopy.

The small cerebriform lymphocyte (Fig. 34-5B) is a variant of the well-differentiated peripheral T-cell, also referred to as Sézary-cell, Lutzner-cell, or mycosis fungoides cell, respectively. The characteristic hallmark is the increased nuclear folding and indentations, which can be roughly estimated in H&E paraffin sections, but are more precisely demonstrated in Giemsa-stained sections or semithin and ultrathin sections, and can be expressed as nuclear contour index or form factor, respectively.[13]

Pleomorphism of cells indicates that the nuclei are multishaped: Small, medium, and large variants exist (Fig. 34-6). The nuclei are irregularly shaped, folded, twisted, or serrated. The chromatin—somewhat in contrast to the small cerebriform cells—usually is dense. The cytoplasm is visible as a small rim in the small cell variants and abundant, sometimes with clear areas in the large pleomorphic variants. Pleomorphic cells are seen in small and large cell types of lymphomatoid papulosis, primary pleomorphic T-cell lymphoma and pleomorphic T-cell lymphoma evolving from mycosis fungoides or Sézary's syndrome. Small pleomorphic cells exhibit features of cerebriform cells in mycosis fungoides or Sézary's syndrome.

Multilobated cell types have mostly been described in large B-cell lymphomas, but also in T-cell lymphomas of the skin.[14] The neoplastic cells are characterized by medium sized to large mulberry- or cloverleaf-shaped multilobed nuclei.

Signet ring cell features with large cytoplasmic vacuoles or inclusions deforming the nucleus, so that it resembles a signet ring, also may occur in T-cell lymphomas that preferentially show primary skin involvement.[15]

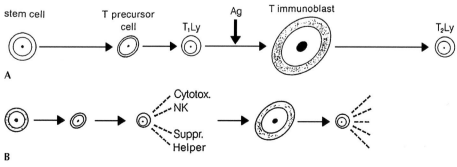

FIGURE 34-4   Ontogeny of T-cell differentiation.[7]

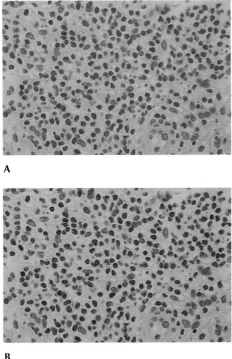

A

B

FIGURE 34-5 Cytomorphologic features in cutaneous T-cell lymphoma. *A.* Small, well-differentiated lymphocytes in chronic lymphocytic-leukemia, T-cell type (H&E magnification × 630). *B.* Typical cerebriform cells in mycosis fungoides (H&E magnification × 630).

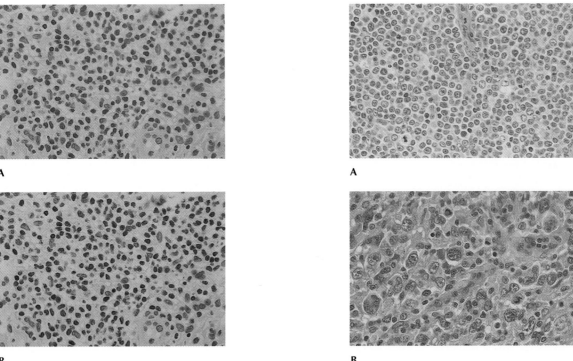

A

B

FIGURE 34-7 *A.* T-immunoblastic lymphoma (H&E magnification × 630). *B.* Anaplastic large cell lymphoma, showing densely packed atypical cells with large nuclei, abundant cytoplasm, and many mitoses (H&E magnification × 630).

T-lymphoblasts are characterized by gyrated nuclei with deep indentations leading to a convoluted aspect; the cytoplasm is moderate or abundant. These cells are characteristically found in prethymic lymphomas. The skin may be involved secondarily.

Originally, the term immunoblast was coined to describe precursors of plasma cells; however, cells of identical morphologic features may be precursors of peripheral T-lymphocytes (Fig. 34-7A) .The morphologic hallmark of both, T- and B-immunoblasts, is a large round or oval clear nucleus owing to coarse chromatin, and a prominent centrally located nucleolus. The cytoplasm usually is abundant, gray (Giemsa stain), or clear.

Large anaplastic lymphoid T-cells (Fig. 34-7B) morphologically do not correspond to any lymphoid cell in the normal or reactive lymph node. The tumor cells are large or giant with extreme irregularity of

nuclear shapes and sizes and are sometimes multinucleated. The chromatin is fine or coarse. The cytoplasm is abundant, gray or clear. The tumor cells grow cohesively, reminiscent of melanoma or carcinomas. In the past these cells have been misinterpreted as histiocytic or reticulum cells. The immunophenotype of large anaplastic cells characteristically is CD30+.

Special Features
In CTCL, there is a pronounced proliferation of postcapillary venules with high endothelial cells, typically seen in the T-region of secondary lymph follicles.

An edema predominantly in the upper dermis and the junctional area is a common feature of CTCL (Fig. 34-8), which later may be replaced by fibrosis.

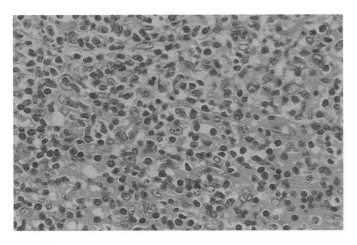

FIGURE 34-6 Large pleomorphic cells. Note the convolutions and indentations of nuclei (H&E magnification × 630).

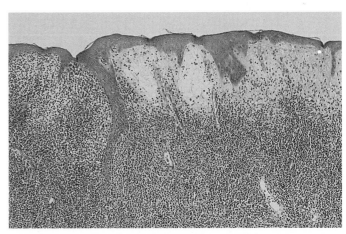

FIGURE 34-8 Mycosis fungoides, plaque-stage. Significant edema, simulating nonepidermotropic T-cell lymphoma (H&E magnification × 100).

Granulomatous features can be observed in some cases of mycosis fungoides and in granulomatous slack skin. The granulomatous component in the dermal infiltrate can vary from a few giant cells to large epitheloid granulomas (Fig. 34-9).

Neoplastic proliferations of lymphocytes mostly are accompanied by varying numbers of dendritic reticulum cells, macrophages, plasma cells, eosinophils, and reactive lymphocytes. Their presence partially may be owing to the TH2 cytokine pattern released by the tumor cells.

REPRODUCIBILITY OF MORPHOLOGIC CRITERIA IN LYMPHOPROLIFERATIVE SKIN INFILTRATES

Histopathologic diagnosis in CTCL has to be interpreted with caution owing to the lack of "golden standards" for histologic or cytologic evaluation. Significant interrater and intrarater variabilities have been reported, especially in the early stages of CTCL.[16-18]

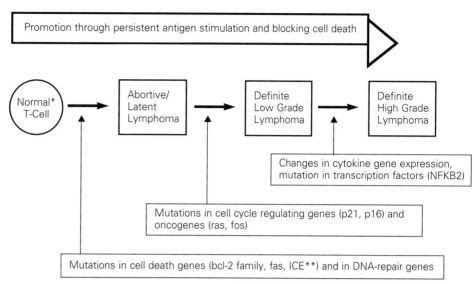

*Endogenous chromosomal instability may facilitate the susceptibility for exogenous mutagenic factors.
**ICE = Interleukin-1-beta converting enzyme

FIGURE 34-9   Pathogenetic model of multistage lymphoma genesis.

Special Techniques for the Diagnosis of Cutaneous T-cell Lymphomas

H&E stained sections always have been and will be the most reliable routine technique in the diagnosis and differentiation of CTCL. However, progress in lineage- and cell type identification by immunohistochemical phenotyping and molecular genotyping has led to a tremendous progress in the interpretation of histo- and cytomorphological findings.

IMMUNOPHENOTYPING

The most important T-cell associated antigens to be detected on T-lymphocytes are listed in Table 34-2. Antibodies working in formalin-fixed, paraffin-embedded sections (CD3, CD 43, CD30, MIB-1) are especially helpful when used in combination with B-cell associated antibodies. Other markers, such as CD4, CD8, CD5, CD 45RO, CD7, CD56, and CLA/HECA-452, have to be demonstrated in cryostat sections or in paraffin-embedded, formalin-fixed sections after antigen retrieval using microwave pretreatment or the immunomax technique.[19]

GENOTYPING

In the context of lymphoproliferative skin infiltrates, monoclonality should be regarded by definition as a sign of neoplastic proliferation. Clonal rearrangement of the T-cell receptor genes can be demonstrated by the Southern blot technique, if sufficient cells can be obtained from fresh or cryo-preserved material or by PCR-based amplification of DNA, if only a few tumor cells are present or if only formalin-fixed, paraffin-embedded material is available. The sensitivity of this procedure can be increased by denaturing (DGGE) or temperature gradient gel electrophoresis (TGGE).[20-22]

CYTOGENETIC TYPING

Genetic instability of T-cells (genotraumatic cells) may result in chromosomal aberrations, which can be detected by appropriate karyotyp-

ing.[23] Malignant T-cells of patients with CTCL often demonstrate multiple and complex chromosome aberrations with translocations of genes regulating cell proliferation or programmed cell-death (apoptosis).

Pathogenetic Aspects of Cutaneous T-cell Lymphomas

The hypothesis of an involvement of the human T-lymphotropic virus I (HTLV-I) in the pathogenesis of CTCL can no longer be supported, even if there are conflicting reports on this issue.[24-27] Other hypotheti-

TABLE 34-2

Monoclonal Antibodies Recommended for Immunophenotyping in T-cell Lymphoproliferative Skin Infiltrates

CD	Antibody	Specificity
CD2	Leu5, OKT11	T lymphocytes
CD3	Leu4, OKT3	Mature thymocytes, peripheral T lymphocytes
CD4	Leu3, OKT4	Helper/inducer T cells, some macrophages
CD5	Leu1, OKT1, Lyt2	T lymphocytes; less than 5 % of B lymphocytes
CD7	Leu9, WT1	T lymphocytes
CD8	Leu2, OKT8	Natural killer (NK) cells, suppressor/cytotoxic T cells
CD30	Ki-1, BerH2	Reed-Sternberg cells, Hodgkin cells, large cell anaplastic lymphoma, plasma cells
CD43	MT-1	T lymphocytes, monocytes, myeloid cells
CD45RO	UCHL-1	T lymphocytes, monocytes, myeloid cells
CD56	NCAM	Natural killer (NK) cells

cal models focus on antigen persistance, environmental factors, or the thymus bypass model.

There is increasing evidence that cancerogenesis is not a big bang-event, but a stepwise evolutionary process because of the accumulation of mutations in DNA repair genes, oncogenes, or tumor suppressor genes.[28] This concept of pathogenesis provides reasonable explanations for the broad spectrum of CTCL. We favor the following hypothesis (Fig. 34-9). Abnormal but not neoplastic lymphocytes showing chromosomal instability (genotraumatic lymphocytes) are driven into activation and reactive cell proliferation by an antigen, which may be viral or non-viral.[23,29] The risk of the occurrence of mutations in the susceptible "genotraumatic" cell clone increases with every new cell divisions, which usually is limited by controlling mechanisms leading to cell death in order to prevent cells with chromosomal aberrations from unlimited, neoplastic expansion. Such controlling mechanisms include programmed cell death (apoptosis), which can be blocked, for example, by overexpression of the *bcl-2* gene; and natural senescence of the cell leading to its natural death after 50 to 70 divisions, owing to cutting off repetitive base sequences at the end of each chromosomes (telomeres). Telomeres are responsible for the maintenance of structure and function of the chromosomes. The enzyme telomerase, commonly present in highly replicating cells such as keratinocytes or lymphocytes, shows a significant increase of activity in CTCL and may be responsible for the prevention of cell death caused by senescence in cells with unlimited proliferation and accumulation of mutations.[30] This results in the growth of a highly abnormal cell clone independent from external stimuli caused by autocrine or paracrine stimulation.

Common Clinicopathologic CTCL Entities Composed of Predominantly Small Cell Types

THE PARAPSORIASIS GROUP

About 100 years ago, Unna et al. described two cases of so-called parakeratosis variegata (Table 34-3).[31] Seven years later, Brocq introduced the term parapsoriasis because of the similarities of these conditions to psoriasis, seborrheic eczema, or lichen (paralichen).[32] He described three major subgroups, the common features of which are: (1) The long duration of the disease; (2) no reduction of general health; (3) the absence of pruritus; (4) superficial localization of the process involving the upper dermis and the epidermis leading to erythema and pityriasiform scaling; (5) resistance to topical treatment; and (6) histologically an infiltrate of round cells disposed about dilated blood vessels of the papillary dermis, edema in the papillary dermis, and foci of spongiosis and parakeratosis. Today another criterium can be added: (7) Lack of extracutaneous involvement.

Based mainly on clinical manifestations, Brocq differentiated the following subgroups.[32]

PARAPSORIASIS EN GOUTTES

Today, this form is referred to as pityriasis lichenoides chronica (synonymous with parapsoriasis guttata of Jadassohn and Juliusberg). Nosologically this disease has nothing to do with CTCL or any subtype of CTCL, for example, mycosis fungoides, as has been erroneously stated.[33,34]

PARAPSORIASIS LICHENOÏDE

Parapsoriasis lichenoïde consists of a network of "pseudo-" papular lesions with atrophy exhibiting a poikilodermic appearance.

TABLE 34-3

Primary Cutaneous T-Cell Lymphomas (CTCL)

Predominantly Small Cell Types
    Parapsoriasis group
        Small plaque parapsoriasis
        Large plaque parapsoriasis
    Mycosis fungoides
    Sézary syndrome
    Pagetoid reticulosis
Predominantly Large Cell Types
    Anaplastic large cell lymphoma
    Pleomorphic medium-sized and large T-cell lymphoma, HTLV +/−
    Immunoblastic lymphoma
    Lymphoblastic lymphoma
CTCL with Distinct Histological Features
    Lymphomatoid papulosis
    Granulomatous slack skin
    Subcutaneous panniculitis-like T-cell lymphoma
Adult T-cell Lymphoma/Leukemia
Rare and/or Provisional CTCL-Entities
    Cytotoxic/suppressor CD8+/CD4− T-cell lymphoma
    Gamma/delta-lymphoma
    CD56+ lymphoma
    Lineage crossover
    Juvenile granulomatous cutaneous T-cell lymphoma
    Syringolymphoid hyperplasia with alopecia
    Epstein-Barr virus (EBV)-associated CTCL

PARAPSORIASIS EN PLAQUES

This variant, formerly referred to by Brocq as "erythrodermies pityriasiques en plaques disséminées," is characterized by round or oval well-circumscribed macules (plaques), which are 2 to 6 cm in diameter. Today this variant is referred to as Brocq's disease; parapsoriasis, small patch (digitiform) type; digitate dermatosis; xanthoerythroderma perstans; chronic superficial dermatitis.

SMALL PLAQUE PARAPSORIASIS

Synonyms: Parapsoriasis en plaques disséminées (Brocq's disease); digitate dermatosis; xanthoerythroderma perstans; chronic superficial dermatitis

Clinical Features   Small plaque parapsoriasis (SPP) is characterized by oval or digitate patches, 2 to 6 cm in diameter, preferentially located on the lateral parts of the trunk, and showing a reddish or yellowish surface with "pseudoatrophic" wrinkling and slight pityriasiform scaling. The prognosis is exceptionally good. There have been no deaths reported thus far in patients with SPP. The disease can be controlled by topical therapy (glucocorticosteroids, phototherapy, PUVA). Since the disease may be confined to the skin, cure by early application of total body electron-beam therapy may be possible.

Histopathological Features   The histopathologic features of SPP are inconspicuous or spongiotic, as in the early stages of MF. The epidermis appears normal or shows slight acanthosis and spongiosis with patchy parakeratosis. Sparse perivascular lymphocytic infiltrates may be seen in the upper dermis, with or without minimal single-cell epidermotropism. Usually the latter cells are not atypical. In general, there is no edema in the upper dermis and no plasma cells or eosinophils are present (Fig. 34-10).

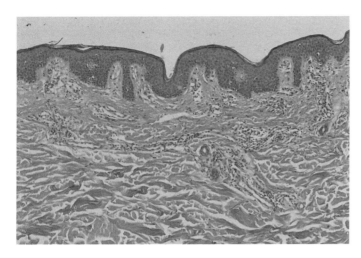

FIGURE 34-10 Parapsoriasis en plaque (small plaque parapsoriasis). Histologically, a sparse lymphocytic infiltrate is present in the upper dermis. Patchy parakeratosis, subepidermal edema. Unconspicuous single cells within the epidermis (H&E magnification × 200).

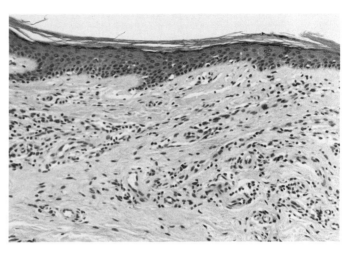

FIGURE 34-11 Large plaque parapsoriasis clinically presenting as poikiloderma. Atrophy of the epidermis. Relatively sparse lymphocytic infiltrate in the upper dermis with dilatation of blood vessels (H&E magnification × 100).

Immunology and Genetic Features   Phenotypically, the infiltrate in SPP is composed of CD4+ T-cells, intermingled with a few CD8+ cells and cannot be differentiated from eczematous reactions or from early stages of mycosis fungoides. Clonality is an inconstant finding in SPP and may be detected in a considerable number of cases.[35]

Differential Diagnosis   The major differential diagnoses include mild eczematous dermatitis, large plaque parapsoriasis, and the early stage of mycosis fungoides. The latter entities cannot be distinguished from SPP histologically without additional clinical information since the histopathological features are nonspecific. From a clinician's standpoint, it is important to distinguish these diseases because of their different prognosis and long-term management.

LARGE PLAQUE PARAPSORIASIS

Synonyms: Parapsoriasis en grandes plaques

Clinical Features   Usually a few large (> 10 cm in diameter) irregularly shaped, reddish, and fairly well demarcated lesions with pityriasiform scaling are localized to the trunk and/or extremities. The poikilodermatous variant of large-plaque parapsoriasis (LPP) often is located in light-protected areas such as the buttocks or female breasts and shows a characteristically reticular network of hyperpigmentation, depigmentation, atrophy, and telangiectasias. Therefore, it is also referred to as poikiloderma atrophicans vasculare. The prognosis generally is good. However, formation of infiltrative plaques and tumors may occur in later stages, indicating a close relationship to mycosis fungoides.

Histopathological Features   In the non-poikilodermatous form, the epidermis is normal or slightly acanthotic. Scattered lymphocytes are seen in the upper dermis with focal accumulation around papillary dermal vessels. Single-cell epidermotropism with arrangement of lymphocytes along the basal layer, if present, usually is very discreet. Typical Pautrier's microabscesses are lacking in the early patch lesions. However, some epidermotropism (with the lining up of lymphocytes in the basal layer) may occur or even intraepidermal microabscesses can be found on occasion in more developed lesions. In the poikilodermatous form, the epidermis is atrophic. In the upper dermis, there is a band-like lymphocytic infiltrate and dilatation of blood vessels (Fig. 34-11).

Immunology and Genetic Features   The lymphocytes express the T-helper memory phenotype CD 4+, CD 8–, CD 45RO+, and show positivity for *bcl-2*, indicating that accumulation of cells is caused by block of apoptosis rather than proliferation. Early CTCL lesions do not show the immunophenotypic aberrations seen in the advanced stages, but are indistinguishable from benign inflammatory cutaneous conditions.[36] T-cell receptor gene rearrangement studies may show clonality of the lymphocytic infiltrate in about 50 percent of cases.

Differential Diagnosis   There are no clear-cut histologic criteria to differentiate SPP, LPP, and early-stage mycosis fungoides. The situation is comparable with morphoea and progressive systemic scleroderma, which cannot be differentiated on histomorphological features. Nevertheless, the difference in clinical appearance and biological behavior makes it unacceptable to lump these diseases together.[33,37]

Atypical lymphocytes, sometimes showing a small halo around small- to medium-sized pleomorphic nuclei, lining up along the dermal-epidermal junction, Pautrier's microabscesses, edema in the upper dermis followed by fibrosis, favor the initial stages of mycosis fungoides; the latter features are regularly found in initial lesions of patients with MF or CTCL in advanced stages.

MYCOSIS FUNGOIDES

Mycosis fungoides is a peripheral non-Hodgkin's T-cell lymphoma, initially and preferentially presenting in the skin and showing distinct clinical and histological features in the plaque and tumor stage. It is the most common subtype of cutaneous lymphoma.

Clinical Features   Males are affected more often than females. The disease starts with irregular, well circumscribed, yellowish-red patches distributed all over the body and showing pityriasiform scaling (Table 34-4). Usually after several years the lesions may (or may not) progress to elevated plaques and tumors with or without ulceration. The sudden multifocal eruption of tumors without preceeding patches or plaques has been referred to as the d'emblée form of MF in former times. However, they are primary large-cell T-cell lymphomas, some of which are CD30 positive. Lymph nodes and internal organs may become involved in the later stages of the disease. Survival is usually less than 1 year with lymph node involvement. In the advanced stages, progression to a large

TABLE 34-4

Mycosis Fungoides

Clinical Features

Irregular patches with pityriasiform scaling
Evolution to plaques and nodular tumors in later stages
Disease progression over years in some patients with involvement
of lymph nodes and internal organs

Histopathological Features

Early stage
Perivascular lymphocytic infiltrate with small, well-differentiated
lymphocytes with round or cerebriform nuclei
Subepidermal edema and proliferation of postcapillary venules
Admixture of eosinophils and plasma cells
Plaque stage
Dense subepidermal infiltrate with significant epidermotropism of
single cells or cell clusters forming Pautrier's microabscesses
Tumor stage
Nodular dense infiltrate, blast transformation

Immunohistology

CD4+
CD45RO+
CD2+
CD3+
CD5+
CD7+ (in 30% of the lesions)
CD1−
CD8−
CD30−
Loss of T-cell antigens in tumor stage

Differential Diagnosis

Small and large plaque parapsoriasis
Sézary syndrome
Pagetoid reticulosis
Eczema

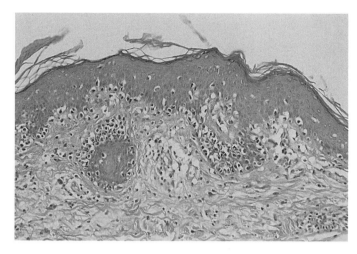

FIGURE 34-12   Mycosis fungoides. Lining up of atypical lymphoid cells along the basal epidermal layer in a patch lesion of a patient with advanced cutaneous T-cell lymphoma (H&E magnification × 160).

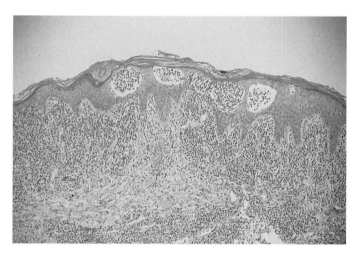

FIGURE 34-13   Plaque stage of mycosis fungoides showing dense epidermal infiltrate forming Pautrier's microabscesses (H&E magnification × 200).

T-cell lymphoma may be observed, which usually is associated with an aggressive clinical course.

Histopathological Features   In the early patch stage and in the plaque stage of MF, a T-cell pattern with a diffuse (disk-like) subepidermal and/or periadnexal infiltrate occurs. Epidermotropism is found to a variable degree, mostly as single cells or small clusters of cells, but rarely with typical intraepidermal Pautrier's microabscesses. Lymphocytes commonly line up along the dermal-epidermal junction (Fig. 34-12). In the early stages, the changes may not be disease-specific and thus are impossible to distinguish from eczematous or psoriasiform reactions.[18] However, early patch lesions in otherwise advanced-stage MF show typical features of epidermotropism of atypical cells.

In the plaque stage, there is a dense subepidermal infiltrate with significant epidermotropism of single cells or cell clusters forming Pautrier's microabscesses (Fig. 34-13).

In the tumor stage, the infiltrate is nodular, and in addition to the horizontal spread seen in the earlier stages, there is additional vertical growth, sometimes with loss of epidermotropism. The different stages are depicted in Fig. 34-14.

Cytomorphology shows predominantly small, well-differentiated lymphocytes with round or cerebriform nuclei. In the tumor stage, transformation to a blast stage may occur showing immunoblasts, lym-

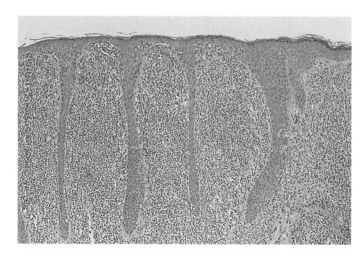

FIGURE 34-14   Tumor stage of mycosis fungoides showing a dense infiltrate involving all layers of the dermis, showing only slight epidermotropism (H&E magnification × 100).

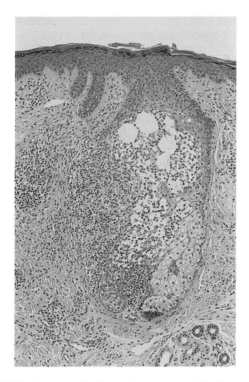

FIGURE 34-15   Cutaneous T-cell lymphoma showing follicular mucinosis due to infiltration of follicular epithelium by tumor cells with mucinous degeneration (H&E magnification × 100).

phoblasts, pleomorphic cells, or anaplastic cells, originating from the same clone.[38,39]

Distinctive features of MF include subepidermal edema, the proliferation of postcapillary venules, and an admixture of eosinophils, plasma cells, macrophages, and dermal dendritic cells.

Special Histologic Features   Small foci of sarcoidal granulomatous infiltrates with epithelioid cells and multinucleated giant cells sometimes are found within or beyond the predominant small cellular lympoid infiltrate.

Infiltration of follicular epithelium by tumor cells with mucinous degeneration is referred to as follicular mucinosis (Fig. 34-15).

Fibrosis is found in the papillary dermis following regression of the subepidermal infiltrate. Peritumoral fibrosis beyond the dermal infiltrate has been observed in 40 percent of MF cases.[40]

Eruptive epidermoid cysts and infiltration of eccrine structures also may be a special feature noted in MF patients.[41–43]

Other variants include verrucous or hyperkeratotic forms of MF, pustular, and acanthosis nigricans-like, hypo- and hyperpigmented, and purpura-like forms.[44]

Immunology and Genetic Features   The characteristic phenotype is CD1−, CD2+, CD3+, CD5+, CD4+, CD45RO+, CD8−, CD30−, and TCR+. Rare cases expressing a CD3+, CD4−, CD8+ mature T-cell phenotype, have been reported.[45] CD7 is expressed in one-third of the lesions. In the tumor stage, an aberrant phenotype with loss of T-cell antigens is a common finding. Expression of CD44v6 may be helpful as a prognostic marker for assessing metastatic potential and homing behavior of the tumor cells.[46]

TCR beta or gamma chain genes rearrange clonally in most cases including some large patch lesions. Two (or more) unrelated clones are seen in about 20 percent of cases as shown by cytogenetic analysis and RT-PCR analysis of TCR beta genes. Complex single cell abnormalities, resulting possibly from increased genetic instability, are another

characteristic feature. In cases with extracutaneous involvement, the same clone may be detected in either site.[47]

Differential Diagnosis   In the early stages of MF, differentiation from small plaque parapsoriasis on histological grounds alone usually is not possible. One must consider the clinical features and course of the disease. The nosologic relationship between large plaque parapsoriasis (LPP) and MF has not yet been completely resolved. Many cases of LPP never develop infiltrated plaques or tumors, and behave in a different manner from MF, which often leads to death within 5 years after diagnosis. Differentiation of plaque stage MF from Sézary syndrome is based on clinical and hematologic parameters. Pagetoid reticulosis shows a prominent intraepidermal dispersion of lymphoid cells. Tumorous non-MF forms of CTCL, including pleomorphic and anaplastic types of lymphoma, exhibit different cytologic features with large convoluted irregularly-shaped atypical nuclei, which may be difficult to distinguish from atypical cells in undifferentiated non-lymphoid tumors such as anaplastic melanoma.

SÉZARY SYNDROME

The Sézary syndrome (SS) is a leukemic, erythrodermic, low-grade malignant, peripheral T-cell lymphoma involving peripheral lymph nodes in most cases.

Clinical Features   Sézary syndrome is characterized by a pruritic erythroderma with edematous swelling of the skin, palmo-plantar hyperkeratosis, loss of hair, onychodystrophy, and swelling of peripheral lymph nodes. Involvement of the bone marrow is a rare event (Table 34-5).

The prognosis is worse than that of MF and depends on the number of circulating atypical CD4-positive cells. There may be tumorous infiltration in the advanced stages, resulting in leonine facies.

TABLE 34-5
Sézary Syndrome

Clinical Features

Pruritic erythroderma with edematous swelling of the skin
Palmo-plantar hyperkeratosis
Loss of hair and onychodystrophy
Enlargement of peripheral lymph nodes

Histopathological Features

Band-like infiltrate and edema in the upper dermis
Prominent epidermotropism with Pautrier abscesses
Small lymphocytes with convoluted/cerebriform nuclei

Immunohistology

CD2+
CD3+
CD5+
CD45RO+
CD8−
CD30−
Blood examination: >1000 Sézary cells/mm^3; CD4/CD8 ratio >10

Differential Diagnosis

Generalized atopic eczema
Drug reactions
Photosensitivity reactions

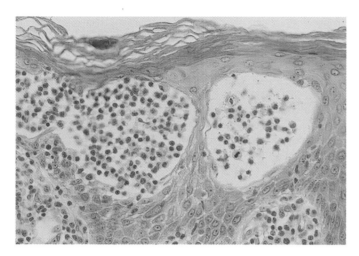

FIGURE 34-16   Intraepidermal Pautrier's microabscesses in Sézary-syndrome. Note large atypical cells indicating transformation into high-grade malignant lymphoma (H&E magnification × 400).

Histopathological Features   The histological features of MF and SS are similar, although there are some differences. For example, Pautrier abscesses are seen more frequently in SS (Fig. 34-16). There are differences also in the composition of the dermal infiltrate, which is less pleomorphic in SS and shows fewer eosinophils or plasma cells. The lymph nodes may show varying degree of involvement, ranging from scattered clusters of three to five atypical cells, which may be hard to detect, to complete effacement of the nodal structure by infiltrates of small atypical lymphocytes with a variable admixture of blast cells.

Immunology and Genetic Features   The lymphoid cells exhibit CD2+, CD3+, CD5+, CD45RO+, CD8−, and CD30−, which is similar to other low-grade CTCL, such as MF. In most cases, there is clonal rearrangement of TCR genes in the skin infiltrates, peripheral blood, and specifically involved lymph nodes.[47] The demonstration of the absence or presence of clonal rearrangement of TCR genes is still the most reliable technique for making the proper differentiation between nosologically and prognostically different erythrodermas. In the peripheral blood, demonstration of at least 1000 Sezary cells per mm^3 and the presence of an extended CD4+ T-cell population resulting in a significantly increased CD4/CD8 ratio (>10), are useful additional criteria in favor of SS.

Differential Diagnosis   Erythrodermas showing polyclonal lymphoid infiltrates may be seen in the red man syndrome, which includes generalized eczema in elderly patients, photosensitivity reactions, drug reactions, paraneoplastic syndromes, and other non-neoplastic erythrodermas.[49]

PAGETOID RETICULOSIS

In 1931 Ketron and Goodman described multiple lesions of the skin "apparently of epithelial origin" clinically resembling mycosis fungoides.[50] In 1939, Woringer and Kolopp reported a solitary plaque-like lesion on the arm of a 6-year-old boy.[51] The term pagetoid reticulosis was proposed by Braun-Falco et al. because of the clinical and the histological appearance.[52]

Only the localized form should be referred to as PR sensu strictu. This distinct nosologic entity can be regarded as an abortive, localized form of a peripheral CTCL of low-grade malignancy. Pagetoid reticulosis is nosologically closely related to MF in which the neoplastic cells are particularly dependent on the epidermal environment for growth. This extremely selective homing behavior, possibly in conjunction with

defense mechanisms of the host, limits the process and characterizes the abortive nature of this distinctive process.

Clinical Features   Pagetoid reticulosis presents as a solitary psoriasiform or bowenoid erythematous, scaling or crusting plaque, exhibiting centrifugal growth. In contrast to MF, PR never spreads to other sites of the body, to lymph nodes, peripheral blood, internal organs, or bone marrow.

Histopathological Features   The epidermis shows marked psoriasiform hyperplasia with para- and hyperkeratosis, including small abscess-like formations, containing serum, some neutrophils, and cellular debris. Sponge-like disaggregation of the epidermal cells by large atypical pagetoid cells that are singly disposed or arranged in clusters or nests, is a typical feature (Fig. 34-17). The pagetoid cells are devoid of intercellular bridges. The vacuolated, abundant cytoplasm stains faintly. The nuclei are large, sometimes convoluted, and hyperchromatic. Mitotic figures are rare.

At the edge of the lesion, the infiltrate is restricted to and appears to start within the basal layer of the epidermis. Single cells and small clusters of cells also are seen within the epithelia of adnexal structures. Toward the center of the lesion, the diffuse band-like infiltrate increasingly involves the upper dermis, showing small cerebriform lymphocytes.

Immunology and Genetic Features   Classical types of PR express the phenotype typical for MF: CD3+, CD4+, CD5+, and CD8−. There are reports on CD8+ cases or PR expressing a gamma/delta phenotype.[53,54] An immunological study using cell activation associated monoclonal antibodies has shown that the epidermotropic cells are activated T-cells.[55] Clonal T-cell receptor (TCR) gene rearrangement has been demonstrated in PR.[56]

Differential Diagnosis   Clinically the differential diagnosis includes solitary lesions of psoriasis, Bowen's disease, extramammary Paget's disease, or a localized eczematous reaction.

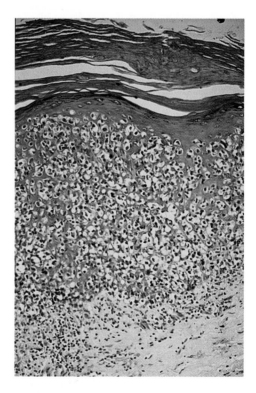

FIGURE 34-17   Sponge-like disaggregation of epidermal cells by atypical lymphoid cells in pagetoid reticulosis (H&E magnification × 200).

Predominantly Large Cell Types

The common hallmark of this group of non-MF/SS CTCL is the large size of the neoplastic lymphoid cell. On cytomorphological grounds, anaplastic large-cell lymphoma (ALCL)—usually expressing a CD30+ phenotype—and pleomorpic lymphoma can be differentiated as major subtypes of this group of CTCL.

The differentiation of various cytomorphologic subtypes of cutaneous large-cell lymphomas may have prognostic implications. Therefore, they can be referred to as showing predominantly anaplastic, pleomorphic, or immunoblastic cytomorphology. In terms of the immunophenotype, however, it is known that primary CD30-positive, localized CTCL have a favorable prognosis.

Clinical Features Predominantly large cell lymphomas usually present as tumors arising from normal appearing skin without pretumorous patch- or plaque-like stages and have been referred to as the d'emblée form of MF in the historical literature.[57] However, classical MF in the end stage of the disease may show transformation into large-cell lymphoma.[58,59]

ANAPLASTIC LARGE-CELL LYMPHOMA

Clinical Features Solitary or multiple nodules confined to one anatomic site usually are seen in anaplastic large-cell lymphoma (ALCL). The tumorous lesions occur on normal appearing skin without preceeding patches or plaques in most cases. There is little epidermal involvement or scaling, unless ulceration occurs in advanced tumor nodules.

Histopathological Features A nodular infiltrate extends through all levels of the dermis into the subcutis. Epidermotropism usually is present, but is not pronounced, showing a few single cells within the epidermis. The morphologic hallmark is the distinctive large, bizarre cells with large, round, irregularly shaped nuclei, abundant chromatin and one or more nucleoli. Cells may be multinucleated. The cytoplasm is abundant, clear, or eosinophilic. Tumor cells grow in dense cohesive sheets, reminiscent of melanoma or undifferentiated carcinoma (Fig. 34-7B). Clusters of small reactive lymphocytes are found within and around the tumorous proliferation. Eosinophils, plasma cells, and accessory cells, usually abundant in low-grade CTCL, often are lacking in ALCL.

Immunology and Related Features The large anaplastic cells typically show CD30 positivity. Moreover, T-cell-associated antigens (CD 43, CD45RO) are expressed with variable loss of pan-T-cell antigens (CD2, CD3, CD5). In contrast to nodal ALCL, primary cutaneous forms lack EMA and express the cutaneous lymphocyte antigen (CLA, HECA-452). Cytogenetic studies of primary cutaneous forms have not been reported thus far. Some cases of the systemic form have shown a t(2;5) translocation.

Differential Diagnosis The clinical differential diagnosis includes cutaneous B-cell lymphomas and non-lymphoid tumors. Distinction from other undifferentiated anaplastic large-cell tumors, especially melanoma, may be difficult, but usually can be made by appropriate immunohistochemical evaluation.

PLEOMORPHIC MEDIUM-SIZED AND LARGE T-CELL LYMPHOMA, HTLV+/−

Histopathological Features Pleomorphic cells are characterized by multishaped nuclei, which may be medium-sized or large. In addition small reactive lymphocytes, eosinophils and plasma cells may be pre-

sent. In the HTLV+ leukemic form (adult T-cell lymphoma/leukemia; ATL/L), significant epidermotropism with formation of intraepidermal microabscesses is observed.

Immunology and Related Features Tumor cells express T-cell-associated antigens (CD2, CD3, CD5), but usually lack CD7; most cases are CD4+, but rare cases of CD8+ have been reported. Usually there is a clonal rearrangement of TCR genes.

IMMUNOBLASTIC LYMPHOMA

Histopathological Features The tumorous infiltrate showing a nodular growth pattern, involves all layers of the dermis and often the subcutis. Usually, significant epidermotropism is lacking. The tumor cells are large immunoblasts showing a large round or oval nucleus with clear karyoplasma and a prominent, centrally located nucleolus. The cytoplasm is abundant and basophilic (Fig. 34-7A). In addition, many smaller and reactive cells are present.

Immunology and Related Features T-immunoblasts express major T-cell antigens, but also can lose their differentiation antigens in advanced stages. Molecular biology is the only way to reveal lineage fidelity in these cases.

LYMPHOBLASTIC LYMPHOMA

This is a prethymic precursor T-cell lymphoma with proliferation of large "convoluted" cells, which does not occur as a primary process in the skin.

CTCL with Distinct Histological Features

LYMPHOMATOID PAPULOSIS

Lymphomatoid papulosis (LyP) is a chronic lymphoproliferative disease with a benign course often persisting over decades, but malignant histologic appearance based on cytomorphology of atypical lymphocytes.

Clinical Features Lymphomatoid papulosis is a chronic, recurrent disease with papular, sometimes nodular or patchy, self-regressing eruptions, which heal with hyperpigmented scars after several weeks or months (Table 34-6). The number of lesions ranges from only a few to hundreds and are mainly located on the trunk, proximal parts of the limbs, and sometimes on the head. Females in the third and fourth decades are affected preferentially. Despite its malignant histologic appearance, the disease is benign and may persist up to 40 years.[60] A minority of cases (approximately 10%) progress to a malignant lymphoma. Molecular studies indicate a close nosologic relationship to Hodgkin's disease and anaplastic large cell lymphoma.[61]

There is increasing evidence that there is a spectrum of CD30-positive lymphoproliferative disorders, ranging from LyP to ALCL, with intermediate forms of the disease that are difficult to classify as clearly LyP or ALCL.

Histopathological Features Histologic features in LyP may vary considerably depending on the stage of the disease.[62] The predominant histological feature of a fully developed lesion, 2 to 3 weeks after initial presentation, is a nodular superficial and deep, sometimes wedge-shaped dermal infiltrate, which may invade the subcutaneous fat and shows variable epidermotropism (Fig. 34-18). Cytomorphologically, the infiltrate is composed of normal-appearing lymphocytes, with a

TABLE 34-6

Lymphomatoid Papulosis

Clinical Features

  Preferential localization: trunk, limbs, head
  Papular, nodular or patchy, self-regressing eruptions
  Healing with hyperpigmented scars
  Persistence over up to 40 years

Histopathological Features

  Nodular superficial and deep, sometimes wedge-shaped dermal
    infiltrate of normal appearing lymphocytes and medium-sized or
    large pleomorphic lymphoid cells with atypical mitoses
  Eosinophilic granulocytes and erythrocyte extravasation
  Neutrophils and necrosis with erosion in resolving lesions

Immunohistology

  CD30+
  CD3+
  CD4+
  CD5+
  CD8−
  CD15−
  EMA−
  PCNA, KI-67, MIB1+

Differential Diagnosis

  Pityriasis lichenoides varioliformis et acuta
  Leukocytoclastic vasculitis
  Lymphomatoid reactive infiltrates as from drugs

---

considerable number of medium-sized or large pleomorphic cells. Atypical mitoses (up to 70% of cases), eosinophilic granulocytes (46%), and erythrocyte extravasation (48%) are found frequently.[60] Resolving lesions (6–8 weeks old) show signs of necrosis with erosion and infiltration with neutrophils, resulting in scar formation. Special features, which can be seen at the same time in the same patient in different locations, include small-cell variants of LyP with predominantly small pleomorphic cells, arising from the same clone of neoplastic cells.

It has been proposed that LYP lesions, containing mainly large cells and small cells, be classified as type A and type B, respectively.

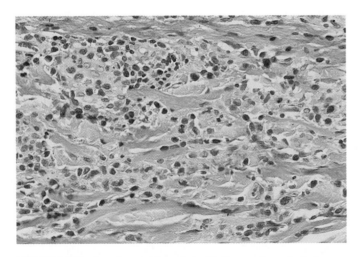

FIGURE 34-18 Lymphomatoid papulosis. Medium- to large-sized pleomorphic cells (H&E magnification × 630).

However, such a categorization may be of limited value since the proportion of large cells may differ from lesion to lesion in the same patient, and no significant prognostic implication has been demonstrated so far. There is no logical reason not to refer to these special features as predominantly large-cell (more than 50%), predominantly small-cell, or mixed.

Immunology and Related Features   The proliferating cells in LyP are activated helper T-cells and express the Hodgkin's disease-associated antigen Ki-1 (CD30).[63–66] They show the following marker profile: CD3+, CD4+, CD5+, CD8−, CD30+, CD15−, EMA−. The proliferating nuclear cell antigen (PCNA, Ki-67, MIB-1) is highly positive in most of the cases. Clonal rearrangement of T-cell receptor genes is found in most cases studied so far, giving evidence for one single clone in cases showing transformation into CTCL and Hodgkin's disease.[67,68]

Differential Diagnosis   Clinically, LyP resembles pityriasis lichenoides varioliformis et acuta (Mucha-Haberman) (PLEVA); however, the latter disorder shows more pronounced epidermal changes, an infiltrate extending into epidermis and a lack of CD30+, Ki67+ lymphoid cells in contrast to LyP. Nonetheless, a relationship between LyP and PLEVA cannot be dismissed altogether. Allergic vasculitis is distinguished by leukocytoclastic vasculitis with nuclear dust and damage to vessel walls.

GRANULOMATOUS SLACK SKIN

Clinical Features   The extremely rare condition known as granulomatous slack skin (GSS), originally was reported as "progressive, atrophying, chronic granulomatous dermohypodermitis," and was named for the striking clinical development of hanging bulky folds of lax skin in flexural areas.[69,70] The age of onset is between 15 and 50 years in most cases, but also may start in early childhood.[71,72]

Histopathological Features   The histopathological pattern in GSS shows a nodular or diffuse infiltrate throughout the dermis. It consists predominantly of small well-differentiated lymphocytes, as seen in mycosis fungoides. Significant epidermotropism as found in most low-grade malignant CTCL, usually is lacking in GSS. The histologic hallmark are huge multinucleated giant cells disseminated within the dermal infiltrate (Fig. 34-19). Differentiation from MF with granulomatous features may be difficult. However, in GSS, there is almost complete loss of elastic fibers in the papillary and reticular dermis. Fragments of the elastic fibers can be found as small inclusions in the cytoplasm of the giant cells.

Immunology and Related Features   The small lymphoid cells express a T-helper phenotype, being CD3+, CD4+, CD8−, CD30−. The giant cells are positive for lysozyme, S-100, CD, 68, and negative for MAC387 and vimentin.[71,72] Clonal TCR gene rearrangement have been demonstrated in most of the cases studied thus far.[72,73]

Differential Diagnosis   Cutis laxa usually shows slack skin folds without infiltration. The histologic features in GSS are very characteristic, showing giant cells distributed singly within the dermal lymphoid infiltrate, and usually without formation of epithelioid or sarcoid nodules as seen in granulomatous MF. Moreover, phagocytosis of elastic fibers is more prominent in GSS, resulting in the typical clinical feature of lax skin. Also there is slight single-cell epidermotropism in GSS; however, intraepidermal microabscesses are lacking.

Sarcoidosis shows solid nodules of epithelioid cells with only a few lymphocytes present. Granulomatous infiltrates, caused by infections (leprosy, deep fungi fungal infections, atypical mycobacteria), consist

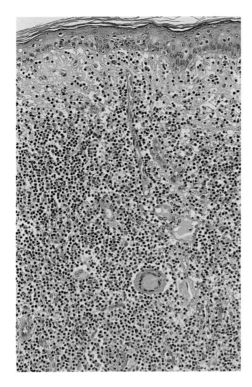

FIGURE 34-19 Granulomatous slack skin showing dense lymphoid infiltrate within the dermis with a prominent multinucleated giant cell (H&E magnification × 100).

of polymorphous infiltrates often including plasma cells, eosinophils, and other granulocytes. Elastorrhexis usually is lacking in the latter infections.

ANGIOCENTRIC, ANGIODESTRUCTIVE T-CELL LYMPHOMA

Clinical Features   Skin lesions showing erythroderma, infiltrating plaques or flat ulcerations, may precede pulmonary involvement by this form of lymphoma.

Histopathological Features   An angiocentric and angioinvasive infiltrate composed of an admixture of well-differentiated or cerebriform small lymphocytes and variable numbers of atypical lymphoid cells, immunoblasts, plasma cells, eosinophils, and histiocytes are seen (Fig. 34-20). The vascular occlusion, resulting from infiltration of blood vessel walls, usually is associated with ischemic necrosis with superficial ulceration.

Immunology and Related Features   The lymphoid cells express the T-cell markers CD2+, CD5+, CD4+, or CD8+ and often CD56+.[10] TCR and Ig genes are usually not rearranged.[10]

Differential Diagnosis   Granulomatous vasculitis showing histiocytes and lymphocytes arranged perivascularly with a variable admixture of granulocytes may be confused with the features in angiocentric lymphoma.

SUBCUTANEOUS PANNICULITIS-LIKE T-CELL LYMPHOMA

Clinical Features   Skin lesions simulate an erythema nodosum-type of panniculitis. The clinical course is either highly aggressive with systemic symptoms or non-aggressive. Hemophagocytic panniculitis ocurring in association with various systemic diseases such as connective tissue disease should be differentiated from subcutaneous T-cell lymphoma.[74]

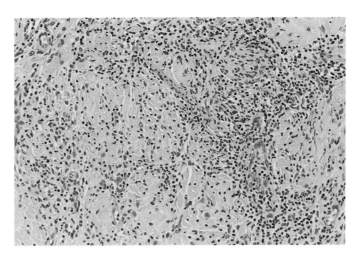

FIGURE 34-20 Angiocentric, angiodestructive T-cell lymphoma showing lymphoid infiltrates within the blood vessel walls (H&E magnification × 400).

Histopathological Features   The histopathologic hallmark of this type of CTCL is the subcutaneous localization and growth pattern of non-epidermotropic nodular infiltrates simulating panniculitis (Fig. 34-21).[11,12,75–77] Cytomorphologically, the tumor cells are small as in MF or large pleomorphic or anaplastic cells.[12]

Immunology and Related Features   Tumor cells show the T-cell-associated antigens CD2+, CD3+, CD5+, CD4+, CD8− or CD4−, CD8+, in rare cases expressing a gamma/delta phenotype and producing large amounts of gamma interferon.[12,78,79] Clonal rearrangement of the genes for the alpha/beta or gamma/delta chains of the T-cell receptor is found, in contrast to CD56+ NK-cell lymphomas which show a germline configuration.

Differential Diagnosis   Erythema nodosum and histiocytic cytophagic panniculitis may be confused with subcutaneous T-cell lymphoma.[74] Histiocytic cytophagic panniculitis is a reactive process associated with various systemic diseases and presents with a hemorrhagic diathesis owing to hemophagocytosis but no proliferation of lymphoid tumor cells (see Chapter 11). In erythema nodosum, granulomatous features (Miescher's nodules) may be observed, but are lacking in subcutaneous T-cell lymphoma.

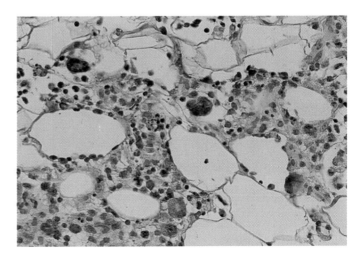

FIGURE 34-21 Subcutaneous panniculitic T-cell lymphoma with infiltration of small- to medium-sized pleomorphic cells (H&E magnification × 200).

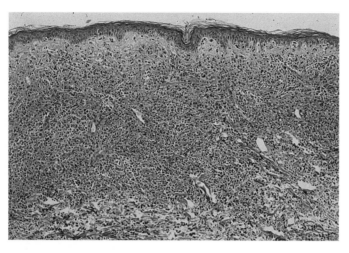

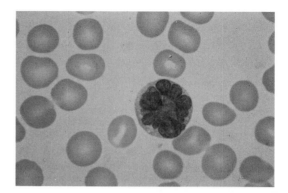

FIGURE 34-22B Adult T-cell leukemia associated with HTLV-1. Note lymphocyte with multilobated nucleus in peripheral blood.

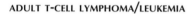

FIGURE 34-22A Adult T-cell lymphoma showing a diffuse infiltrate of medium- to large-sized pleomorphic cells with epidermotropism (H&E magnification × 200).

ADULT T-CELL LYMPHOMA/LEUKEMIA

The adult T-cell lymphoma/leukemia (ATL) is a lymphoproliferative disorder, etiologically associated with the human T-cell leukemia virus I (HTLV-I).

Clinical Features   An acute and a smoldering subtype can be differentiated. Skin involvement occurs in about 50 percent of the cases during the course of the disease, presenting as papules, nodules, or tumors, or as erythroderma. Typical laboratory findings are a leukemic blood picture sometimes in conjunction with anemia, hypoalbuminemia, hypergammaglobulinemia, and hypercalcemia.[80,81]

Histopathological Features   The skin lesions usually show a diffuse infiltrate of medium to large pleomorphic cells, with or without epidermotropism (Fig. 34-22A). The lymphoid cells often have multilobated nuclei (Fig. 34-22B).

Immunology and Related Features   There is a pronounced heterogeneity of the phenotype of neoplastic cells from patients with ATL. Usually, they show a helper/inducer T-cell phenotype (CD4+, CD8−); however, other phenotypic profiles may be seen in some of the cases (CD4−, CD8+ or CD4−, CD8−). In the endemic variants, integration of retroviral DNA into the host cell genome plays an important role in the etiopathogenesis of this distinct entity.

Differential Diagnosis   Differential diagnosis includes pleomorphic or anaplastic T-cell lymphomas.

Rare and/or Provisional Cutaneous T-cell Lymphomas

CYTOTOXIC/SUPPRESSOR CD8+/CD4− T-CELL LYMPHOMAS

These lymphomas show an aggressive course in most of the cases reported thus far.[45,82,83] There also have been reports of CD8-negative CTCL showing pagetoid or lymphoepithelioid features.[84,85]

GAMMA/DELTA+ LYMPHOMA

Cutaneous T-cell lymphomas of this type do not exhibit any specific clinical or histological features. Subcutaneous, pagetoid, erythrodermic,

and tumorous forms have been reported.[12,36,54,86,88] The clinical course is rapidly progressive in most cases, but also may be slowly progressive over many years.

CD56+ LYMPHOMA

Recently a unique primary cutaneous lymphoma has been described, presenting with bruise-like skin lesions, a CD4+, CD43+, CD2−, CD3−, CD8−, T-cell receptor negative phenotype of the medium- to large-sized lymphoid tumor cells, and an undetermined genotype (T-cell receptor beta and immunoglobulin heavy chain in germline configuration, no clonal T-cell receptor gamma population as detected by PCR-DGGE) and a rapid relapse after radiotherapy.[88]

LINEAGE CROSSOVER

Ten to twenty percent of central thymic-based lymphoblastic leukemias and lymphomas have immunoglobulin heavy (IgH) chain gene rearrangements in addition to a T-cell receptor (TCR) gene rearrangement (dual phenotype). In contrast to central T-cell leukemias and lymphomas, the mature (i.e., peripheral) T-cell malignancies rarely exhibit this phenomenon.[47] It is not clear whether this particular genomic feature could serve as a marker for a poorer prognosis in comparison to those lymphomas with only one clonal rearrangement.

JUVENILE GRANULOMATOUS CUTANEOUS T-CELL LYMPHOMA

Clinical Features   Patients with this type of lymphoma present with poikilodermatous patchy or nodular, localized or disseminated skin lesions, with onset in childhood or early adulthood (median age of six patients reported thus far, is 13 years, ranging from 4 to 23 years).[89] The course of the disease is slowly progressive. About 20 years after onset of the disease, two of six patients have developed nodal Hodgkin's disease (nodular sclerosis) and one patient developed an extracutaneous large-cell anaplastic Ki-1+ lymphoma; one patient died from cutaneous lymphoma and one patient was lost to follow-up 8 years after the onset of the disease at age 12.

Histopathological Features   Histology shows a patchy or nodular granulomatous infiltrate consisting of histiocytes, epithelioid cells and a few multinucleated giant cells with a variable admixture of small well-

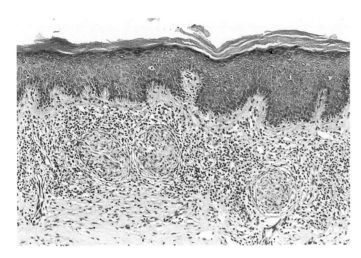

FIGURE 34-23   Juvenile granulomatous cutaneous T-cell lymphoma showing epithelioid granulomas in the upper dermis, surrounded by many lymphocytes (H&E magnification × 200).

differentiated lymphocytes (Fig. 34-23). Clonal rearrangement of TCR-genes has been reported.

Differential Diagnosis   This type of lymphoma may be easily confused with infectious granulomatous disorders and is associated with a high risk for the development of systemic lymphoma.

SYRINGOLYMPHOID HYPERPLASIA WITH ALOPECIA

This rare condition, like pagetoid reticulosis, is a localized CTCL presenting with a specific histomorphologic pattern that shows exclusive involvement of the sweat glands and ductal structures with small cerebriform lymphocytes around and between epithelial cells (Fig. 34-24). There also may be involvement of hair follicles leading to circumscribed alopecia without follicular mucinosis.[90]

EPSTEIN-BARR VIRUS (EBV)-ASSOCIATED CUTANEOUS T-CELL LYMPHOMAS

Recently, four patients with lymphoproliferative lesions of the skin characterized by recurrent necrotic, papulo-vesicles of the face have

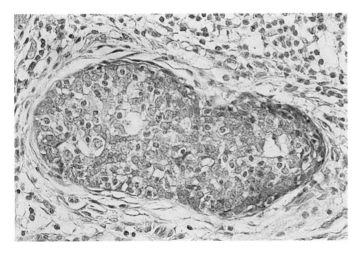

FIGURE 34-24   Syringolymphoid hyperplasia showing lymphocytes within and around sweat gland structures.

been reported.[92] Latent EBV infection was detected in the lymphoid cells from the skin lesions of all four patients. Histopathological alterations included epidermal necrosis, and a significant nodular lymphocytic infiltrate, expressing a memory helper T-cell phenotype, in the periadnexal and perivascular region. Three of the patients developed lymphoma several years after onset of the disease.

Cutaneous B-Cell Lymphoid Hyperplasia and Cutaneous B-Cell Lymphomas

Helmut Kerl / Lorenzo Cerroni

Cutaneous B-cell Lymphoid Hyperplasia

With the advent of new technics (immunophenotyping, molecular genetics) it has become clear that many lymphoid proliferations that were classified in the past as cutaneous B-cell lymphoid hyperplasia (pseudolymphoma) are in reality examples of low-grade malignant B-cell lymphomas with a favorable clinical behavior.

The term cutaneous B-cell lymphoid hyperplasia is still used, but it is not a specific diagnosis.[3,93,94] It is descriptive and refers to a heterogenous spectrum of diseases, that simulate malignant B-cell lymphomas clinically, histopathologically, or both.

Whenever possible, a diagnosis of cutaneous lymphoid hyperplasia should be avoided in favor of specific designations using the language of clinical dermatology.

The classical example of a cutaneous B-cell lymphoid hyperplasia (Table 34-7) is lymphadenosis benigna cutis (synonyms: lymphocytoma cutis and pseudolymphoma of Spiegler-Fendt)

TABLE 34-7

Cutaneous B-Cell Lymphoid Hyperplasia

Clinical Features

Solitary (or rarely multiple) nodules favoring the face (nose, earlobe), nipple, scrotum, and extremities
Both children and adults affected

Histopathological Features

Nodular, "top heavy," mixed-cell infiltrates
Small lymphocytes predominate, plasma cells, eosinophils, and histiocytes
Lymphoid follicles frequently present

Immunohistology

CD20+
CD79$_a$+
Polyclonal pattern (K +, L +)
Bcl-2−
MT2−
CD3+
CD4+

Differential Diagnosis

Cutaneous B-cell lymphoma
Lupus erythematosus

Clinical Features   Erythematous or red-brown to red-purple solitary nodules with a smooth surface are usually found. Agminated lesions in a region or disseminated papules may be observed rarely. Favored sites of involvement are the face (cheek, nose, earlobe), trunk (mammary area), scrotum, and extremities. Children and adults can be affected. The course of cutaneous B-cell lymphoid hyperplasia varies. The lesions may resolve with or without treatment.

Various stimuli can induce lesions of cutaneous B-cell lymphoid hyperplasia, among them insect bites (persistent nodules of scabies), drugs (antidepressant therapy), vaccinations, injections of antigens for hyposensitization, and tattoos. Often cases of cutaneous B-cell lymphoid hyperplasia are associated with infection by Borrelia burgdorferi (Borrelia-induced lymphocytoma). In many cases, however, a precise cause is not found.

Histopathological Features   Relatively symmetrical rather well-circumscribed nodular infiltrates, within the dermis and sometimes within the subcutaneous fat, can be observed. As a rule, the infiltrates are more dense in the upper part of the dermis than in the lower part. Germinal centers are frequently present (follicular type) (Fig. 34-25). Sometimes a non-follicular pattern without formation of germinal centers can be observed. An important diagnostic criterion is the mixed character of the infiltrate (Fig. 34-26). Although lymphocytes, especially small ones, nearly always are dominant, eosinophils, plasma cells, histiocytes, and giant cells often are found. The epidermis is not involved and usually is separated from the infiltrates of inflammatory cells by a thin zone composed of normal collagen bundles. Adnexal structures are spared.

These histopathological features frequently represent responses to infectious etiologies such as Borrelia burgdorferi. Drug-associated cutaneous lymphoid hyperplasia (antidepressants) usually reveal a mycosis fungoides-like pattern, but occasionally can also induce histopathological features similar to lymphadenosis benigna cutis.[95]

Immunology and Related Features   Immunohistological investigations reveal the presence B-cell compartments (CD20+) surrounded by T-

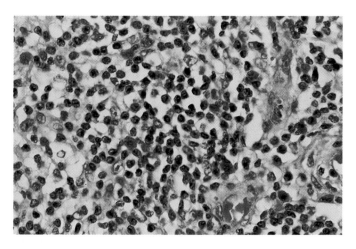

FIGURE 34-26   Cutaneous B-cell lymphoid hyperplasia. Mixed-cell infiltrate with small lymphocytes, lympho-plasmacytoid cells, eosinophils and histiocytes.

cell aggregations. The T-cells (CD45R[1], CD3+) may even predominate. Cases with germinal center formation (*Bcl-2*, CD45RA[MT2]-) are associated with a regular network of dendritic reticulum cells (CD21+). Analysis of Ig-light chain expression usually discloses a polyclonal proliferation of B-cells that express both kappa and lambda light chains.

Very few systematic molecular studies have been performed. Polyclonal Ig-gene rearrangements are usually observed.

Differential Diagnosis   The differentiation of cutaneous B-cell lymphoid hyperplasia from malignant cutaneous B-cell lymphomas sometimes is one of the most difficult problems in diagnostic dermatopathology (Table 34-8).[96,97] As a rule, but surely not always, cellular infiltrates in cutaneous B-cell lymphoid hyperplasia are relatively sym-

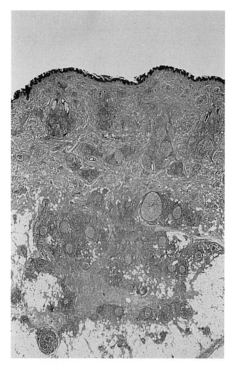

FIGURE 34-25   Cutaneous B-cell lymphoid hyperplasia (lymphadenosis benigna cutis). Nodular infiltrates with a follicular pattern.

TABLE 34-8

Histopathologic Criteria: B-cell Cutaneous Lymphoid Hyperplasia versus Malignant B-cell Lymphoma

Cutaneous B-cell hyperplasia	*Malignant B-cell lymphoma*
Symmetry	Asymmetry
Well-circumscribed	Less well-defined nodules
Nodular aggregates often	Diffuse or interstitial infiltrate often
Wedge-shaped pattern	Lack of wedge-shaped pattern
Involvement of upper part of the dermis usually greater than that of the lower dermis	Involvement of the lower part of the dermis equal to or greater than that of the upper dermis
Mixed-cell infiltrate: small lymphocytes, eosinophils, plasma cells, histiocytes	Monomorphous infiltrate of lymphocytes
	Atypical lymphocytes may predominate
Mitotic figures rare (only in germinal centers)	Mitotic figures frequent and everywhere
Adnexal structures spared	Adnexal structures often obliterated
No necrotic areas	Necrotic areas sometimes present
Vasculature prominent	Vasculature not prominent

metrical, rather well-circumscribed, and more dense in the upper part of the dermis than in the lower part of it (top heavy). Often the infiltrate in toto assumes the shape of a wedge pointing in the direction of the subcutaneous fat. In contrast, infiltrates in malignant B-cell neoplasms are more massive, asymmetrical, poorly circumscribed, and, frequently, are more or less equally distributed in the superficial and deep dermis, or more dense in the lower part of the dermis and subcutaneous fat (bottom heavy). There is a mixed character of the infiltrate in B-cell cutaneous lymphoid hyperplasia. In addition to lymphocytes, often there are eosinophils, plasma cells, histiocytes, and giant cells in contrast to the malignant counterpart in which the infiltrate is usually more monomorphous. Nuclear atypia and an increased number of mitotic figures are found more frequently in malignant lymphomas.

The histologic features of distinct lymphoid follicles with germinal centers, which have been misinterpreted in the past as characteristic criteria of a benign inflammatory process, are not reliable for the differential diagnosis lymphoma versus pseudolymphoma. Reactive follicles also may be present in lymphomas.

Other findings helpful in the differential diagnosis are the tendency of the cellular infiltrates in cutaneous lymphoid hyperplasia to spare the adnexa in contrast to lymphomas, where frequently the adnexal structures are involved by lymphomatous infiltrates, the prominent vascular pattern of thick-walled blood vessels lined by plump endothelial cells in cutaneous lymphoid hyperplasia and the absence of those features in lymphoma, and the presence of tingible bodies (lymphocytic nuclear debris engulfed by macrophages) in cutaneous lymphoid hyperplasia, but not in lymphomas.

Important for the diagnosis of a cutaneous lymphoid hyperplasia is the immunohistological demonstration of a polyclonal population of B-cells (either by staining of sIg-light chain restriction or by Ig-gene rearrangement analysis). However, there are clear exceptions to each of the above mentioned criteria. The diagnosis must then be based on a constellation of clinical and histological features including follow-up information.

Cutaneous B-cell Lymphomas

Cutaneous B-cell lymphomas (CBCL) are distinct clinical and morphological subtypes of extranodal lymphomas.[3,98,99] They can be defined as neoplasms of the immune system, characterized by a proliferation of B-lymphocytes that infiltrate the skin. The neoplastic cells frequently produce monoclonal immunoglobulins and the demonstration of light-chain restriction is an important diagnostic criterion.

Clinical Features Cutaneous B-cell lymphomas occur far more frequently than is generally believed.

The clinical manifestations are variable. The lesions may be single, regionally multiple, or generalized in distribution. Large, sometimes ulcerated tumors, nodules, or plaques of varying hues of red, blue, purple, and brown are very common. Erythematous macular-papular eruptions also can be observed. Subcutaneous masses are seen occasionally. In contrast to cutaneous T-cell lymphomas there is usually no scaling or erythroderma.

The lesions can be localized everywhere on the skin and may involve mucous membranes. Preferred locations are the head and neck, the back, and the lower extremities.

It is becoming clear that primary CBCL have an excellent prognosis and are potentially curable by therapy. The 5-year survival rate for primary CBCL is over 90 percent.

Histopathological and Cytomorphological Features Morphology remains the principal basis for defining CBCL. The optimal technical quality of the sections (fixation, embedding) is a precondition for a cor-

rect diagnosis. The specimen must be of sufficient size to reveal the critical information. Punch biopsies should be avoided.

The standard methods for the light microscopic diagnosis of CBCL include hematoxylin-eosin, Giemsa, and PAS-staining. The Giemsa stain is very useful for the recognition of a follicular pattern and it reveals precise cytologic details especially in large B-cell lymphomas. The PAS method helps in the identification of intracytoplasmic or intranuclear immunoglobulins in B-cells. The chloroacetate esterase reaction (Leder stain) is important for the exclusion of myeloproliferative disorders; it identifies normal and abnormal cells of the neutrophil series and mast cells.

As a rule CBCL present patchy infiltrates, a nodular growth pattern, or diffuse lymphoid aggregates. The infiltrates are predominantly perivascular and periadnexal and show a distribution at all levels of the dermis extending into the subcutaneous fat. The epidermis usually is not involved. A follicular pattern with germinal centers frequently is observed in CBCL. Superficial band-like infiltrates and epidermotropism—as in cutaneous T-cell lymphomas may be found rarely.

A major problem in the diagnosis of CBCL on morphological grounds is the admixture of other cell types. It may be difficult to distinguish the neoplastic clone from the reactive cells. This problem is especially evident in T-cell rich B-cell lymphomas.

In order to understand the different cytomorphologic appearances of the cells and their neoplastic counterparts it is necessary to mention the main pathways of the B-cell differentiation as illustrated in Fig. 34-27.[7]

In the bone marrow, stem cells give rise to B-precursor cells (pre-pre-B cells). They are the earliest detectable stage of B-cell differentiation: rearrangement of the immunoglobulin heavy chain gene has already begun, but immunoglobulins are not yet produced. Pre-B cells, in contrast, reveal intracytoplasmic mu heavy chain; they do not express surface Ig. Morphologically the B-precursor cells appear as lymphoblasts.

The next stage of antigen-independent B-cell differentiation is represented by the B1-lymphocytes, which express surface Ig; they correspond morphologically to small lymphocytes. On encountering antigenic stimulation, the B1-cells undergo blast transformation, proliferate, and differentiate into antigen-specific effector cells (B2-lymphocytes). Two pathways are possible: In one there is transformation into immunoblasts and then into lymphoplasmacytoid cells and plasma cells; in the other germinal centers that contain centroblasts and centrocytes are formed. The exact relationship between the immunoblast-plasma cell system and the germinal centers is not yet known.

Additional B-cell subtypes with characteristic morphological features are the marginal zone cells and the mantle cells of the inner follicle mantle. Marginal zone cells are closely related to monocytoid B-cells. The position of marginal zone cells in the B-cell differentiation pathway is not completely clear. They have the capacity to mature into plasma cells and appear to display specific homing patterns (extranodal marginal zone lymphoma, MALT-type lymphoma).

Principal Cell Types of the B-cell Series

LYMPHOBLASTS

Uniform appearing medium-sized cells with round, oval, or indented nuclei, fine chromatin, inconspicuous nucleoli, and scanty cytoplasm. These cells are found in precursor B-lymphoblastic lymphomas.

SMALL LYMPHOCYTES: B-TYPE

Small lymphocytes usually with a round nucleus, dense chromatin, and a small rim of cytoplasm. These cells correspond to those that are found in B-cell chronic lymphocytic leukemia.

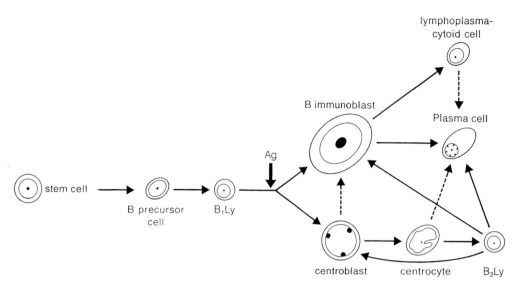

FIGURE 34-27   Scheme of B-cell development.[4]

LYMPHOPLASMACYTOID CELLS

Lymphoplasmacytoid cells are smaller than typical mature plasma cells. The nucleus resembles the nucleus of small lymphocytes and the cytoplasm is abundant and basophilic—as in plasma cells.

PLASMA CELLS

The typical mature plasma cells are also known as the Marschalko type plasma cells. They are characterized by a round, frequently eccentrically located, nucleus that exhibits the often-mentioned cartwheel or clock face pattern. The abundant cytoplasm is strongly basophilic and may show a paranuclear halo.

Lymphoplasmacytoid cells and plasma cells are found in immunocytomas and plasmacytomas.

GERMINAL CENTER CELLS

Two main types of lymphoid cells can be distinguished:

1. Centroblasts: Large cells with a narrow rim of cytoplasm and oval, vesicular nuclei containing one or more distinctive nucleoli, typically situated near the nuclear membrane.
2. Centrocytes: Smaller cells with irregular, sometimes cleaved nuclei, a fine chromatin pattern, and small nucleoli. The cytoplasm can be rarely identified.

The neoplastic counterparts of centroblasts and centrocytes are seen in follicle center lymphomas and in large B-cell lymphomas.

B-IMMUNOBLASTS

They have large round to oval vesicular nuclei with a particularly distinct nuclear membrane and very prominent centrally placed nucleoli. The cytoplasm is broad and basophilic. Large B-cell lymphomas of the immunoblastic type are composed of B-immunoblasts.

MARGINAL ZONE B LYMPHOCYTES

Small to medium-sized cells with moderately abundant pale cytoplasm. The nuclei are round or indented (centrocyte-like cells). Marginal zone

cells are found in marginal zone B-cell lymphomas. Besides B-lymphocytes, CBCL contain various other cell types. Macrophages (including T-zone histiocytes) are regularly distributed in any lymphoid infiltrate of the skin. Dendritic reticulum cells are an important component of germinal centers.

Immunohistological Features The application of monoclonal antibodies to routinely fixed paraffin-embedded material with the use of the microwave treatment technique for antigen retrieval enhances the staining quality and provides the basis for a reliable immunohistological analysis of CBCL.[100,101] Table 34-9 displays a selected panel of antibodies suitable for the diagnosis of B-cell lymphoid infiltrates.

The most useful B-cell markers are CD20 (L26) and CD79a (mb1), which detect nearly all lymphoid infiltrates of B-cell lineage (Fig. 34-28 A, B). Large cell lymphomas of B-cell type may reveal partial loss of one or more B-cell associated antigens.

Malignant B-cell populations usually show a clonal restriction to either kappa or lambda light chain, whereas benign infiltrates exhibit a polyclonal expression pattern of both light chains. Unfortunately, however, there are several cases of B-lymphoproliferative disorders, both benign and malignant, in which the cells do not express Ig or the Ig can not be detected.

In low-grade malignant lymphomas of B-cell lineage, aberrant expression of some T-cell associated markers can be observed. CD5 reacts with the cells of B-cell chronic lymphocytic leukemia and of mantle cell lymphoma. Another abnormal pattern of reactivity that may be indicative of a low-grade malignant B-cell lymphoma is the coexpression of CD20 (L26) and CD43 (MT1) ("normal" B-lymphocytes are CD43-negative).

Germinal centers can be detected by the use of CDw75 (LN1)-monoclonal antibody. LN1 positivity in interfollicular areas also can be found in malignant follicle center lymphomas.

TABLE 34-9

Immunohistology: Antibodies Useful for the Diagnosis of Cutaneous B-cell Lymphomas

Cluster/Antibody	Specificity
CD20/L26	B lymphocytes
CD79a/mb1	B lymphocytes
CDw75/LN1	B lymphocytes (germinal center cells)
Ig	B lymphocytes
CD5	T lymphocytes, B-CLL
CD10	Germinal center cells, common ALL antigen
CD23	B lymphocytes, monocytes
CD43/MT1	T lymphocytes, monocytes
CD45RA/MT2	T lymphocytes, B lymphocytes (mantle cell)
MIB-1	Proliferating cells
anti-DRC	Dendritic reticulum cells
anti-Bcl-2	*bcl-2* protein
KiM1p	Monocytoid B cells, monocytes

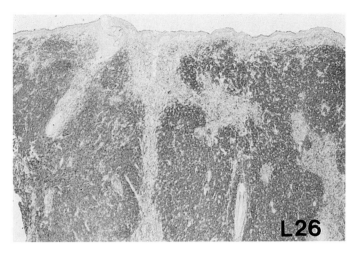

FIGURE 34-28 Cutaneous B-cell lymphoma. Immunohistology demonstrates CD20 (L26) reactivity of the neoplastic infiltrate.

Antibodies directed against the follicular dendritic reticulum cells demonstrate the network of dendritic reticulum cells in reactive and malignant germinal centers.

The assessment of proliferative activity with MIB-1 may be useful in identifying areas with the highest likelihood of containing tumor and to detect the transformation from a low-grade lymphoma to high-grade "blastic" disease.

CBCL almost always show a distinct T-cell population, which is usually numerically predominant.

Molecular Genetic Analysis   B-lymphoid malignancies can be studied using specific probes detecting rearrangements of the Ig heavy- or light-chain genes. However, a negative result does not exclude a diagnosis of malignant lymphoma.

Classification

Patients with involvement by cutaneous B-cell lymphomas can be divided into the following groups:

1. Primary cutaneous B-cell lymphomas: Cutaneous disease alone with no evidence of extracutaneous manifestations over a period of at least 6 months when complete staging has been performed.
2. Secondary cutaneous B-cell lymphomas: Extracutaneous disease and subsequent development of skin lesions.
3. Concurrent cutaneous B-cell lymphomas: Extracutaneous disease at the same time as the skin lesions diagnosed.

Clinico-pathologic correlation is extremely important in the accurate interpretation of CBCL. Adequate staging procedures should include laboratory investigation, chest X-ray, ultra-sound examination of lymph nodes and visceral organs, CT-scan, and bone marrow biopsy.

Primary cutaneous B-cell lymphomas (primary CBCL) comprise a broad spectrum of lymphomas with characteristic clinical, histopathologic, immunophenotypic, and molecular genetic findings. Thus, it is important that the various subtypes are appropriately classified as separate entities. It is also evident that lymphomas arising in lymphnodes and primary CBCL, which may show similar or comparable morphological features, are different with respect to clinical outcome. CBCL exhibit only rarely the typical cytogenetic and molecular alterations characteristic of node-based B-cell lymphomas. Modern classification systems (Kiel classification, Revised European American Classi-

fication), which are mainly used for nodal lymphomas,[7,10] therefore can not be applied satisfactorally for CBCL.[7,10]

In this chapter, we employ a modified scheme of the recently proposed *EORTC-Classification For Primary Cutaneous Lymphomas*, which is not only based on the currently available morphologic, immunologic and genetic technics, but also on well-defined clinical criteria (Table 34-10).

The most important subtypes of primary CBCL are follicle center lymphoma and immunocytoma.

Secondary cutaneous B-cell lymphomas can be observed in all types of B-cell lymphomas of lymphoid organs after dissemination and involvement of the skin. These lymphomas usually reveal the histopathological features, immunology, and genetic features and genotype of the original lymphoma. Prognosis usually is poor. Of special interest for dermatopathologists are specific skin infiltrates in B-cell chronic lymphocytic leukemia and B-lymphoblastic lymphoma.

FOLLICLE CENTER LYMPHOMA OF THE HEAD AND TRUNK

Synonyms: Centroblastic-centrocytic; follicular, small-cleaved, mixed or large-cell; reticulohistiocytoma of the dorsum (Crosti); large-cell lymphocytoma.

Follicle center lymphomas (Table 34-11) are defined as neoplasms of B-cells composed of germinal center cells, usually showing a follicular pattern with a mixture of centrocytes (cleaved follicle center cells) and centroblasts (large non-cleaved follicle center cells).[102–106]

Clinical Features   Patients present with solitary or grouped reddish papules, plaques or tumors that can be surrounded by erythematous patches. Preferential locations are the scalp and forehead or the back ("reticulohistiocytoma of the dorsum," according to Crosti).[105]

Primary cutaneous follicle center lymphoma represents probably the commonest subtype of primary CBCL.[102–106] Recurrences can be observed. Dissemination to extracutaneous sites is rare and follow-up data suggest that these patients have a favorable prognosis after adequate treatment.

Histopathological Features   These lymphomas are characterized by nodular or diffuse infiltrates within the whole dermis, often extending into the subcutaneous fat. Epidermotropism usually is not observed. A follicular pattern with germinal centers frequently is found (Figs. 34-29 and 34-30). The diffuse growth pattern does not exhibit follicular nodule formation. Sometimes, however, it may be difficult to recognize the follicular structures within the diffuse infiltrates.

The neoplastic follicles consist mainly of centrocytes and centroblasts; centrocytes predominate (Figs. 34-31A, B). The interfollicular areas and the diffuse component contain germinal center cells, small lymphocytes with a T-cell phenotype, some immunoblasts, and histiocytes.

Follicle Center Lymphoma of the Head and Trunk

Clinical Features

Preferential location: head and trunk
Solitary or regionally localized patches, papules, plaques, and
   tumors
Favorable prognosis

Histopathological Features

Nodular or diffuse infiltrates with follicular pattern
Mixture of germinal center cells: centrocytes and centroblasts

Immunohistology

SIg+
CD20+
CD79a+
DRC+
CD5−
CD43−
CD10 −/+

Differential Diagnosis

Cutaneous lymphoid hyperplasia
Marginal zone B-cell lymphoma
Immunocytoma

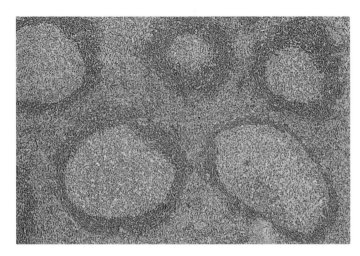

FIGURE 34-30   Primary cutaneous follicle center lymphoma. Note variation in the size of the neoplastic follicles.

The differences in *bcl-2* protein expression and incidence of t(14;18) translocations between nodal and cutaneous lymphomas suggest that different mechanisms may be involved in the pathogenesis of these neoplasms.

Differential Diagnosis   The major differential diagnosis in cases of cutaneous follicle center lymphomas is cutaneous lymphoid hyperplasia with follicular structures (lymphadenosis benigna cutis). Findings that enable the differentiation are summarized earlier in the chapter and Table 34-8.

In recent years, new interpretations have led to the revision of basic tenets about cutaneous lymphoproliferative diseases and many lesions that were considered to be cutaneous lymphoid hyperplasia have been

Immunology and Related Features   The tumor cells express surface Ig (monotypic, Fig. 34-32) and B-cell-associated antigens. They are CD5 and CD43 negative. CD45 RA (MT2), which is a useful marker in distinguishing follicle center lymphoma from benign follicular hyperplasia of the lymphnodes, reacts with less than 20 percent of primary cutaneous malignant follicular and is always negative in cutaneous pseudolymphomas. *bcl-2* Protein expression usually is negative. Within the follicular areas an organized network of follicular dendritic cells is present.

Clonal Ig rearrangement can be demonstrated in many cases. Interchromosomal (14;18) translocation, which has been shown to be very common in follicle center lymphomas of the lymphnodes, is extremely rare in primary CBCL and can be found in some secondary CBCL.[107]

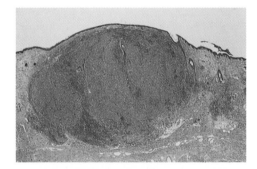

A

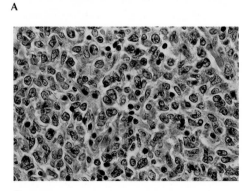

B

FIGURE 34-31   Primary cutaneous follicle center lymphoma. *A*. The follicular pattern is more difficult to recognize. *B*. Higher magnification shows a mixture of centrocytes and centroblasts.

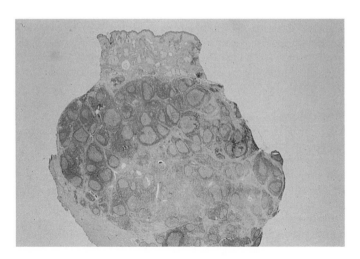

FIGURE 34-29   Primary cutaneous follicle center lymphoma extending into the subcutaneous fat.

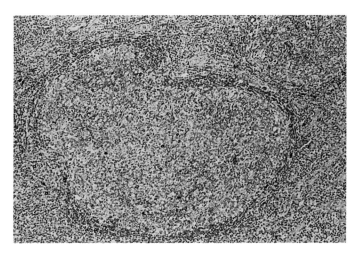

FIGURE 34-32 Primary cutaneous follicle center lymphoma stained for K-light chain. The follicles revealed K-light chain restriction. The mantle zone cells were polytypic.

reclassified as malignant lymphomas (e.g., follicle center lymphoma, marginal zone B-cell lymphoma).

The differential diagnosis also may include marginal zone B-cell lymphoma and immunocytoma, especially if follicles are present. Both are characterized by reactive polyclonal follicle centers. However, it may be difficult or impossible to differentiate the neoplastic cells (centrocyte-like cells) in marginal zone B-cell lymphoma from the centrocytes in follicular lymphoma.

IMMUNOCYTOMA

Synonyms: lymphoplasmacytoid; small lymphocytic; plasmacytoid lymphoma.

Immunocytoma (Table 34-12) is defined as a proliferation of small lymphocytes, lymphoplasmacytoid cells, and plasma cells showing monotypic intracytoplasmic immunoglobulins.

TABLE 34-12

Immunocytoma

Clinical Features

Preferential location: lower extremities
Solitary or localized skin tumors
Favorable prognosis
Borrelia burgdorferi may play a role in the pathogenesis

Histopathological Features

Nodular or diffuse infiltrates
Lymphoplasmacytoid cells, small lymphocytes, plasma cells
PAS + inclusions may be present
Sometimes reactive follicles

Immunohistology

Monotypic CIg+
CD20−
CD5−

Differential Diagnosis

Marginal zone B-cell lymphoma
Follicle center lymphoma
B-cell chronic lymphocytic leukemia
Cutaneous lymphoid hyperplasia

Clinical Features   Pink, bluish-red or reddish-brown plaques or dome-shaped solitary tumors are found especially on the lower extremities. Additional tumors can develop during the course of the disease. Generalized lesions in patients with primary skin manifestation are rarely found.

Primary cutaneous immunocytoma is different from nodal immunocytoma with respect to prognosis and responds excellently to therapy.[108,109]

There may be a link between immunocytoma and infectious diseases. Immunocytoma develops sometimes in patients with Borrelia burgdorferi infections, especially in areas affected by acrodermatitis chronica atrophicans.

Histopathological Features   The architectural pattern is characterized by dense nodular or diffuse infiltrates (Fig. 34-33A) with involvement of the dermis and subcutis. The epidermis is usually intact.

The predominating cell types are lymphoplasmacytoid cells and small lymphocytes (Fig. 34-33B). In addition mature plasma cells, which are frequently located in subepidermal aggregations or at the periphery of the infiltrate, a few immunoblasts, histiocytes, and eosinophils are found. PAS-positive intranuclear (Dutcher bodies) or intracytoplasmic inclusion bodies can be sometimes detected and represent a valuable diagnostic feature (Fig. 34-34). Reactive (polytypic) germinal centers rarely may be scattered within the infiltrate.

Immunology and Related Features   The tumor cells express monotypic cytoplasmic Ig. The lymphoplasmacytoid cells and the plasma cells show a negative staining with most B-cell associated markers (CD20) and also lack CD5. Variable numbers of T-lymphocytes are usually present.

Ig heavy and light chain genes are rearranged.

Differential Diagnosis   The distinction between immunocytoma and marginal zone B-cell lymphoma cannot always be made since both lymphoma types are probably closely related.

For the differentiation between immunocytoma and follicle center lymphoma, clinical features (localization) must be considered. Follicle center lymphoma reveals a follicular growth pattern with monotypic neoplastic germinal centers, a proliferation of centrocytes and centroblasts, and absence of cytoplasmic inclusions and cytoplasmic Ig.

B-cell chronic lymphocytic leukemia does not show PAS-positive globular intranuclear inclusions, CIg cannot be detected and CD5 (and CD23) staining is frequently positive.

Cutaneous lymphoid hyperplasia may be very difficult to distinguish from immunocytoma.

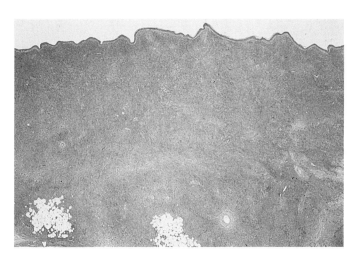

FIGURE 34-33 Primary cutaneous immunocytoma. Diffuse growth pattern.

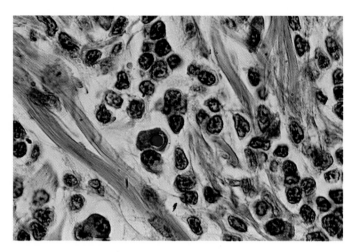

FIGURE 34-34 Primary cutaneous immunocytoma. Intranuclear globular PAS-positive inclusion (Dutcher body).

MARGINAL ZONE B-CELL LYMPHOMA

Synonyms: Monocytoid B-cell; extranodal low-grade B-cell lymphoma of MALT type; reticulohistiocytoma of the dorsum (Crosti)

Marginal zone B-cell lymphoma (MZL; Table 34-13) is a low-grade malignant lymphoma with morphologic evidence of differentiation into cells of the marginal zone that display tissue-specific homing patterns. Primary cutaneous MZL are closely related to immunocytomas, monocytoid B-cell lymphomas (nodal marginal zone B-cell lymphoma), and MALT-lymphomas.[7,110] The term SALT (skin associated lymphoid tissue)-lymphomas also has been used for these tumors.[111,112]

TABLE 34-13

Marginal Zone B-cell Lymphoma

Clinical Features

Preferential location: head, trunk, and extremities
Recurrent solitary or localized papules, plaques, and tumors
Excellent prognosis

Histopathological Features

Nodular or diffuse infiltrates
Small to medium-sized B cells with indented nuclei and abundant
    pale cytoplasm (centrocyte-like cells)
Plasma cells are frequent
Reactive lymphoid follicles may be present

Immunohistology

SIg+
CIg+ (50%)
CD20+
CD79a+
CD5−
CD10−
KiM1p+ (granular)
bcl 2+

Differential Diagnosis

Cutaneous lymphoid hyperplasia
Follicle center lymphoma
Mantle cell lymphoma
Immunocytoma

Clinical Features Recurrent localized red to reddish-brown papules, plaques, and tumors on the head, trunk and extremities are observed. The prognosis is excellent.

In a few cases an association with Borrelia burgdorferi can be established.[113]

Histopathological Features Patchy, nodular (Fig. 34-35A) or diffuse infiltrates, involving the dermis and subcutaneous fat, of small to medium-sized cells with indented nuclei, inconspicuous nucleoli and abundant pale cytoplasm (marginal zone cells, centrocyte-like cells, Figs. 34-35 B, C) can be observed. In addition plasma cells, lymphoplasmacytoid cells, small lymphocytes, and histiocytes are present.[114] Occasionally large blasts and eosinophils can be admixed. Reactive follicles may be seen and show a characteristic contrast with the pale staining perifollicular areas of marginal zone cell-populations. The epidermis is not involved.

Immunology and Related Features The centrocyte-like cells reveal a CD20+, CD79a+, CD5−, CD10−, and *bcl-2+* phenotype. In 50 percent of cases, a monoclonal distribution of Ig-light chains can be

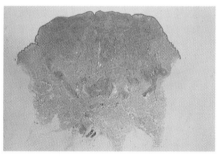

A

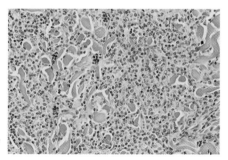

B

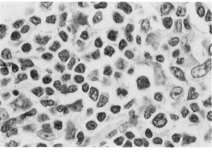

C

FIGURE 34-35 Primary cutaneous marginal zone B-cell lymphoma. *A.* Patchy and nodular infiltrates. Reactive follicles can be vaguely recognized. *B.* Marginal zone (centrocyte-like) cells with abundant pale cytoplasm. *C.* Marginal zone cells are a little larger than lymphocytes and show round to irregular nuclei. A few blast cells can be observed.

observed (especially in the plasma cells). Staining with the monocytoid B-cell related antibody Ki-M1p shows positive reactivity with a typical intracytoplasmic granular pattern.[7]

The genetic features are not well studied. Clonal Ig-heavy chain gene rearrangement has been observed in several cases.

Differential Diagnosis   Marginal zone B-cell lymphoma can be confused with cutaneous lymphoid hyperplasia, which is characterized by the polyclonality of B-cells.

Marginal zone B-cell lymphoma must be distinguished from follicle center lymphoma. As pointed out MZL may show follicles that are reactive and is characterized by an interfollicular proliferation of centrocyte-like cells, whereas in follicle center lymphoma, the neoplastic follicles with centrocytes and centroblasts reveal a monotypic light chain restriction.

Mantle cell lymphoma, which is not well-defined in the skin, is composed of relatively uniform small to medium-sized lymphocytes with an irregular nuclear contour.[115] Because of the cytological similarities it may be very difficult to differentiate this lymphoma from MZL. Neoplastic mantle cells express CD5 and *bcl-1* gene rearrangement can frequently be documented.

Immunocytoma is very similar to MZL suggesting that they may be related. In immunocytoma the cytological picture is more monotonous with proliferation of small lymphoid, lymphoplasmacytoid cells and plasma cells, which contain CIg. In MZL a characteristic cellular heterogeneity with predominance of centrocyte-like cells is observed and CIg is only expressed in about 50 percent of the tumor cells.

PLASMACYTOMA

Primary cutaneous plasmacytoma (Table 34-14) is defined as a monoclonal proliferation of plasma cells that develops in the skin in the absence of bone marrow involvement (extramedullary plasmacytoma).[116–118]

Clinical Features   The skin lesions are characterized by erythematous, reddish-brown or violaceous cutaneous/subcutaneous plaques or nod-

---

TABLE 34-14

Plasmacytoma

Clinical Features

Preferential location: head and trunk
Solitary or multiple nodules
The possibility of myeloma and paraproteinemia has to be excluded

Histopathologial Features

Nodular or diffuse aggregates of mature plasma cells
Atypical cells and multinucleate forms may be present

Immunohistology

CIg+
CD20−
CD79a+/−
LCA−

Differential Diagnosis

Reactive plasma cell proliferations
Inflammatory pseudotumor (plasma cell granuloma)
Immunocytoma

---

ules with predilection for the trunk and head. Solitary, clustered, or multiple tumors can occur, mostly in elderly male patients.

Primary cutaneous plasmacytoma is exceedingly rare. The prognosis is much more favorable than in patients with secondary skin involvement associated with multiple myeloma.

Histopathological Features   The tumor consists of dense nodules or sheets of plasma cells within the dermis and subcutis. The predominant cells represent mature or immature plasma cells with varying degrees of atypia (Fig. 34-36). Multinucleated plasma cells and mitoses also may be present, especially in secondary cutaneous plasmacytomas. Rarely Dutcher bodies and Russell bodies are found. Occasionally amyloid deposits or crystalloid intracytoplasmic inclusions within histiocytes can be demonstrated.[119]

Immunology and Related Features   The tumor cells contain CIg (usually of IgA-type) or express one light chain type. However, most B-cell-associated antigens and LCA are negative. It is important to mention that the immunohistochemical interpretation of plasmacytomas can lead to diagnostic errors because plasmacytomas sometimes show aberrant reactivities with HMB-45 and cytokeratins.

Molecular studies usually reveal rearrangement of IgH and light genes.

Differential Diagnosis   Plasmacytoma must be distinguished from reactive plasma cell proliferations, in which one can recognize a mixed-inflammatory cell infiltrate with polytypic plasma cells.

Distinction from cutaneous inflammatory pseudotumor (plasma cell granuloma) is possible by the detection of a polytypic lymphoplasmacellular and plasmacellular infiltrate.[120] In addition, cutaneous inflammatory pseudotumor is characterized by areas of hyalinized fibrosis that are not seen in plasmacytoma.

In contrast to immunocytoma, plasmacytoma does not contain lymphocytes.

LARGE B-CELL LYMPHOMA OF THE LEG

Synonyms: Centroblastic; B-immunoblastic; diffuse large cell, noncleaved lymphoma

This group consists of more aggressive malignant lymphomas that contain a predominant population of large B-cells.[3,98] Primary cutaneous large B-cell lymphomas develop frequently on the lower legs of elderly patients (Table 34-15).[121]

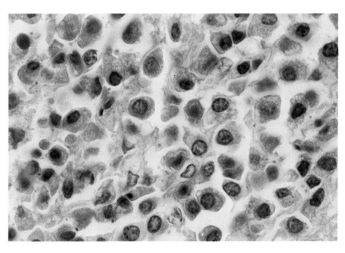

FIGURE 34-36   Cutaneous plasmacytoma consisting of Marschalkó type cells and atypical plasma cells.

TABLE 34-15

Large B-cell Lymphoma of the Leg

Clinical Features

Preferential location: lower leg
Solitary or multiple tumors
Older females predominate
In 50% of patients there is an aggressive course

Histopathological Features

Diffuse growth pattern
Large cells with features of immunoblasts and centroblasts
High mitotic rate; sometimes starry sky pattern

Immunohistology

SIg+
CIg+
CD20+
CD79a+
BCL-2+

Differential Diagnosis

Granulocytic sarcoma
Large cell anaplastic lymphoma
Histiocytic tumors
Metastases

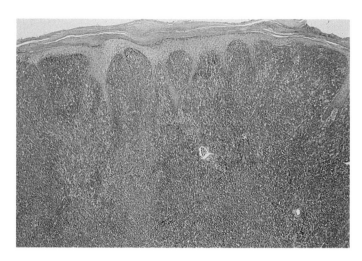

FIGURE 34-37   Primary cutaneous large B-cell lymphoma. Dense diffuse infiltrate with focal epidermotropism.

Granulocytic sarcoma, histiocytic neoplasms, metastases, or other non hematopoietic tumors can be excluded not only by morphology but also by applying a panel of monoclonal antibodies.

B-LYMPHOBLASTIC LYMPHOMA

Synonym: Precursor B-lymphoblastic leukemia/lymphoma

B-lymphoblastic lymphomas are neoplasms of precursor-B cells (pre-pre-B lymphoblasts, pre-B lymphoblasts and "mature" B lymphoblasts) (Table 34-16).

Clinical Features   Patients usually have acute lymphoblastic leukemia with bone marrow and peripheral blood involvement and secondary skin manifestations.

Sometimes a distinct entity of pre-B lymphoblastic lymphoma with primary cutaneous involvement is observed in young children. Especially on the head (scalp) and neck region solitary or multiple reddish-brown to bluish tumors can be observed.[122–125]

Patients with localized skin disease appear to have a relatively good prognosis.

Histopathological Features   Within the dermis and the subcutaneous fat dense diffuse monotonous infiltrates are found. Cytomorphologically the lymphoblasts are medium-sized cells with round, oval, or convoluted nuclei, fine chromatin, inconspicuous nucleoli, and scant cytoplasm. Mitoses are frequent, and a starry sky pattern may be seen (Fig. 34-38).

Immunology and Related Features   The cutaneous lymphoblastic lymphomas with the pre-B-cell phenotype express CD79a, CD19, TdT, CD10 (CALLA), CD34, and cytoplasmic μ heavy chains without surface immunoglobulin.

Systematic molecular studies have not been performed.

Differential Diagnosis   One must consider in the differential diagnosis myelomonocytic leukemia that shows a proliferation of immature granulocytic (Leder stain positive) and monocytic cells arranged in a figurate pattern.

Mantle cell lymphoma can be confused with lymphoblastic lymphoma. However the cytomorphology in mantle cell lymphoma with

Clinical Features   The clinical features are variable. Solitary or multiple reddish-brown or violaceous tumors localized on one (or sometimes both) lower legs are observed. Ulceration is common. The disease primarily affects older females (> 70 years of age). Relapses and extracutaneous involvement can occur. The prognosis is more unfavorable than that in the other primary CBL and the 5-year survival rate is approximately 50 percent.

Histopathological Features   There are dense diffuse infiltrates (Fig. 34-37) within the dermis and subcutis. Infiltration of the epidermis simulating a T-cell lymphoma rarely can be observed. Cytomorphologically the neoplastic cells resemble either immunoblasts (Fig. 34-37) or centroblasts. In several cases a subclassification between immunoblastic lymphoma or centroblastic lymphoma is not possible because a mixture of large cell types is found. Other lymphoid cells that can be observed are large cleaved cells, anaplastic large cells, multilobated cells, and centrocytoid centroblasts (morphology intermediate between a centrocyte and a centroblast). There are many mitotic figures. A starry sky pattern sometimes is present. Some cases reveal an extreme predominance of T-lymphocytes (T-cell rich B-cell lymphoma); it may be difficult to classify these lesions as large B-cell lymphomas.

Immunology and Related Features   Surface Ig and/or cytoplasmic Ig can be demonstrated. The neoplastic cells are CD20, CD79a (loss of antigen expression can be observed), and often *bcl-2* positive.

Detailed molecular studies have not yet been performed.

Differential Diagnosis   Large B-cell lymphomas must be distinguished from large-cell anaplastic lymphoma, which consists of CD30-positive large cells with irregularly shaped nuclei and giant cells resembling Reed-Sternberg cells.

TABLE 34-16

B-Lymphoblastic Lymphoma: Pre-B-cell Type

Clinical Features

Preferential location: head (scalp)
Solitary or multiple tumors
Sometimes primary cutaneous involvement, especially in young
  children

Histopathological Features

Dense diffuse monotonous infiltrates
Medium-sized lymphoblasts with scanty cytoplasm, round or con-
  voluted nuclei with fine chromatin and inconspicuous nucleoli
High mitotic rate

Immunohistology

CD79a+
CD19+
TdT+
CD10+
cMU+
CD34+

Differential Diagnosis

Myelo-monocytic leukemia
Mantle cell lymphoma
Merkel cell carcinoma
Metastatic neuroendocrine carcinoma

---

cleaved or irregularly shaped nuclei and the immunophenotype of the
neoplastic mantle cells (SIg+, CD5+, CD10−) are distinct from lymphoblastic lymphoma.

The differential diagnosis also may include Merkel cell tumor, which
is characterized by the co-expression of cytokeratin filaments (CK20),
neurofilaments, and metastatic neuroendocrine carcinoma, for example,
oat cell carcinoma developing in the lung.

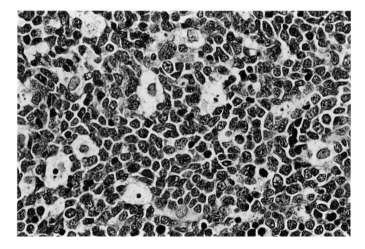

FIGURE 34-38 Primary cutaneous pre-B lymphoblastic lymphoma.
Monomorphous population of lymphoblasts. Prominent starry-sky pattern.

Cutaneous Hodgkin's Disease

Helmut Kerl / Lorenzo Cerroni

Hodgkin's disease is regarded as a distinct malignant lymphoma (Table
34-17) characterized by the presence of neoplastic Reed-Sternberg (RS)
cells in association with different patterns of reactive cells. The exact
nature of the RS-cells is still unknown but immunohistochemical and
molecular investigations are providing growing evidence that
Hodgkin's disease probably is a B-cell disorder (especially the lymphocyte predominance type of Hodgkin's disease).[126] A viral etiology is
possible since the Epstein-Barr virus genome has been detected frequently.

Clinical Features   Cutaneous involvement in patients with Hodgkin's
disease can be "non-specific" (zoster, prurigo, ichthyosis acquisita) or
the skin can be affected by specific infiltrates with Hodgkin and Reed-
Sternberg cells. Specific cutaneous manifestations are uncommon,
occurring in only about 1 percent of patients with systemic Hodgkin's
disease.[127,128]

The skin lesions usually are confined to the drainage area of affected
lymph nodes (retrograde lymphatic spread). In rare cases direct extension from underlying lymph nodes or hematogenous spread can be
observed. Primary cutaneous Hodgkin's disease also exists as demonstrated in the literature.[129]

Clinically, the lesions appear as localized erythematous papules and
plaques or reddish-brown to bluish, often ulcerated tumors. The trunk
seems to be the most common site of involvement, but all other sites of
the body may be affected.

Cutaneous Hodgkin's disease usually is manifested as advanced
(stage IV) disease and carries, a bad prognosis. In some patients, nodal

---

TABLE 34-17

Hodgkin's Disease

Clinical Features

Solitary or multiple papules, plaques, or tumors
Skin involvement most often results from retrograde lymphatic
  spread from involved lymph nodes
Unfavorable prognosis

Histopathological Features

Nodular or diffuse infiltrates
Hodgkin cells, Reed-Sternberg cells (in 50%)
Reactive component: lymphocytes, plasma cells, neutrophils,
  eosinophils, histiocytes
All four subgroups can be observed in the skin

Immunohistology

CD30+
CD15 +/−
CD45R−

Differential Diagnosis

Lymphomatoid papulosis
Anaplastic large cell lymphoma

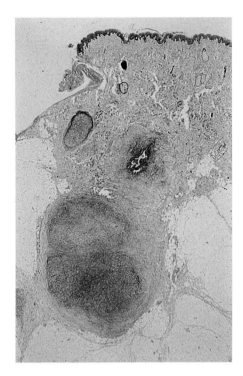

FIGURE 34-39   Cutaneous Hodgkin's disease, nodular sclerosis. Giemsa.

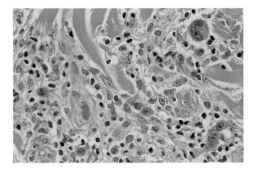

A

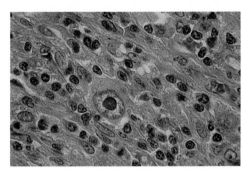

B

FIGURE 34-40   Cutaneous Hodgkin's disease. *A.* Reed-Sternberg cells set in a background of lymphocytes, histiocytes, and eosinophils. *B.* Hodgkin-cell.

Hodgkin's disease can be associated with second cutaneous lymphoproliferative diseases. Mycosis fungoides, lymphomatoid papulosis, anaplastic large-cell lymphoma, and granulomatous slack skin sometimes occur in the course of Hodgkin's disease or may eventuate in Hodgkin's disease.

Histopathological Features   All four subtypes of Hodgkin's disease can be observed in the skin (Fig. 34-39). Nodular sclerosis or mixed cellularity are recognized most frequently.[130] There are nodular or diffuse infiltrates within the dermis extending into the subcutaneous fat. Areas of fibrosis and/or sclerosis may be found. The epidermis is usually spared. Hodgkin cells are a constant finding, but typical RS-cells are present only in about 50 percent of the cases (Fig. 34-40A, B). The background of the infiltrate contains lymphocytes, histiocytes, plasma cells, eosinophils, and neutrophils.

It is well known that Hodgkin and Reed-Sternberg cells are not a unique feature of Hodgkin's disease. These cells have been found in a variety of conditions (lymphomatoid papulosis, anaplastic large cell lymphoma).

Immunology   Hodgkin and RS-cells reveal constant positivity for CD30 (BerH2), and negativity for CD45R (LCA); CD15 (LeuM1) is expressed frequently, but also may be negative.[130–132]

The accompanying infiltrate is composed mostly of T-lymphocytes.

Differential Diagnosis   Lymphomatoid papulosis resembles Hodgkin's disease morphologically. Clinically lymphomatoid papulosis differs by its benign course with generalized recurrent papular or papulonecrotic self-healing eruptions. Lymphomatoid papulosis shows histologically wedge-shaped epidermotropic infiltrates with large atypical (RS-like) cells. In contrast to Hodgkin's disease the phenotype of these cells is usually: CD30+, CD15−, and CD45R+ as well as expression of T-cell antigens in most cases.[132]

There may be a similarity of Hodgkin's disease to mycosis fungoides. Lymphocytes as solitary units and collections of cells within the

epidermis are not present in Hodgkin's disease. In advanced stages of mycosis fungoides associated with the development of tumors, progression to large-cell anaplastic lymphoma can be observed. In these lymphomas giant cells with features of RS-cells are seen.

In the differential diagnosis of cutaneous Hodgkin's disease, special attention should be given to exclude anaplastic large cell (CD30+) T-cell lymphoma. In Hodgkin's disease Hodgkin- and RS-cells are found in small numbers together with an appropriate polymorphous background of inflammatory cells. Anaplastic large-cell lymphoma is characterized by cohesive sheets of large blastic cells, occasionally with features of RS-cells. The large blastic cells are CD30+, CD15−, and frequently reveal an aberrant T-cell phenotype.

Cutaneous Extramedullary Hematopoiesis

Stefan   Hoedl   /   Helmut   Kerl

Synonyms: Myeloid metaplasia of the skin; neoplastic cutaneous myelofibrosis

Extramedullary hematopoiesis (Table 34-18) represents the occurrence of hematopoietic elements in organs other than the bone marrow.

Cutaneous extramedullary hematopoiesis (EMH) is a rare phenomenon and can be associated with a variety of pathologic conditions.[133–136] These comprise mainly myelofibrosis, myeloproliferative disorders, hemolytic anemias, and intrauterine infections.

The pathogenesis has not yet been elucidated. Whether this phenomenon may be an effect of compensatory demand due to progressive failure of the bone marrow, hematopoietic differentiation of pluripotent

TABLE 34-18

Cutaneous Extramedullary Hematopoiesis

Clinical Features

   Neonates
   Hemorrhagic purpuric eruptions of palms and soles
   Blueberry muffin spots
   Adults
   Papulo-nodular and plaque-like hemorrhagic-erythematous lesions
      especially on the trunk

Histopathological Features

   Diffuse or patchy perivascular/periadnexal infiltrates within the
      reticular dermis
   Erythroid, myeloid, and megakaryocytic cell series in various stages
      of maturation
   Myxoid stroma

Differential Diagnosis

   Myeloid and myelomonocytic leukemia

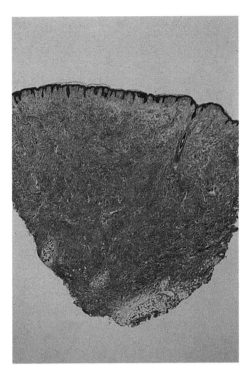

FIGURE 34-41   Cutaneous extramedullary hematopoiesis in a patient with primary myelofibrosis. Diffuse infiltrate within the dermis.

stem cells within the skin or metastatic colonization of the skin by atypical hematopoietic progenitor cells, remains to be determined.

Clinical Features   Hemorrhagic purpuric eruptions and the blueberry muffin syndrome can be observed in neonates.

Hemorrhagic purpuric eruptions are characterized by small reddish macules on palms and soles in neonates without a specific clinical disease. The eruptions are residual lesions of the physiologic dermal erythropoiesis during embryogenesis.

A rash of slightly elevated, purplish-red or dark blue papules and plaques appears in the postnatal period in the blueberry muffin syndrome. The underlying perinatal infections are summarized under the term TORCH (toxoplasma, other, rubella, cytomegalic inclusion virus, herpes). The lesions usually disappear spontaneously within a period of 4 to 6 weeks.

Cutaneous EMH in adults manifests as randomly scattered asymptomatic erythematous, brownish-red, or violaceous hemorrhagic papules, nodules, or small plaques. Most frequently the trunk (abdomen) of elderly males is involved. Cutaneous EMH in adults (neoplastic EMH) reflects a severe underlying disease of the hematopoietic system. Commonly primary myelofibrosis is the associated disorder, which may be diagnosed before or after the development of the skin lesions. Hepato-splenomegaly and enlarged lymph nodes are regular findings, and result from EMH in these organs.

EMH has also been described in benign tumors of the skin such as pilomatricoma (reactive EMH).

Histopathological Features   Patchy perivascular and periadnexal or diffuse infiltrates (Fig. 34-41) embedded in a loose myxoid stroma with abundant vessels are found mainly in the reticular dermis. The infiltrates may be composed of the erythroid, myeloid, and megakaryocytic series (trilinear extramedullary hematopoiesis) or of erythroid and myeloid (bilinear) or only myeloid cells. Higher power magnification reveals clusters of nucleated red blood cells with dark pyknotic spherical nuclei and bright red eosinophilic glassy refractile cytoplasm. Myeloid cells of various stages of maturation can be identified using the Leder stain. Megakaryocytes, which can be labeled with factor VIII-related antigen, are characterized by large atypical single or multiple nuclei and abundant eosinophilic cytoplasm.

Differential Diagnosis   In infants, the hemorrhagic eruptions of extramedullary hematopoiesis could be confused with true petechial hemorrhages in thrombocytopenia. Blueberry muffin lesions must be differentiated from metastases of congenital neuroblastoma (stage IVs).

The cellular composition may be represented only by myeloid cells. In these instances myeloid or myelo-monocytic leukemia, including congenital leukemia cutis, should be excluded. In contrast to cutaneous EMH, the infiltrates in myeloid and myelomonocytic leukemia are much denser. In addition immunophenotyping of the cells is helpful.

Cutaneous Leukemic Infiltrates

Stanislaw A. Buechner / W. P. Daniel Su

Leukemic infiltrates are defined as localized or disseminated infiltration of the skin by leukemic cells.[137–140] These infiltrates may be the initial clue to the presence of an underlying hematologic malignancy or may be present concomitantly with, and in some cases precede, the development of systemic leukemia.[141–143] Depending on the extent of infiltration, leukemic infiltrates can involve the epidermis, dermis, or subcutaneous fat and show variable cytomorphologic features that depend on cell differentiation and the origin of the neoplastic cells. The common histopathologic features shared by most leukemic infiltrates are a dense perivascular and periadnexal or a more diffuse infiltrate of atypical mononuclear cells, with frequent sparing of the subepidermal Grenz zone. The diagnosis of leukemic infiltrates is based on the recognition of the preponderant cell type and pattern of infiltration in the skin and on correlation with clinical and hematologic findings. However, the characterization of leukemic cells by cytomorphologic criteria alone is not always possible, and, in most instances, cytochemical and immuno-histochemical studies are necessary to identify accurately the origin of the leukemic cell infiltrate in the skin. Various nonspecific skin lesions may be associated with systemic leukemia in which there is no leukemic infiltration of the skin.[142–144] Dermatopathologists must approach leukemic infiltrates by being aware of the morphological diversity expressed by these neoplastic proliferations and of the difficulty in differentiating leukemic skin infiltrations from those of non-Hodgkin's lymphoma, nonhematopoietic neoplasms, and numerous nonspecific skin lesions.

Classification of Leukemias

In the French-American-British (FAB) classification, the leukemias have been classified into various clinicopathologic categories according to the presumed cell of origin and the morphological appearance of the bone marrow and blood leukemic cells.[145–147] The classification of leukemias in which leukemic skin infiltrates have been reported is shown in Table 34-19. Adult T-cell leukemia/lymphoma (ATLL) is a neoplasm of T cells associated with human T-cell leukemia virus type I (HTLV-I).[148,149] According to the FAB classification, chronic myelo-monocytic leukemia (CMMoL) is classified as a myelodysplastic syndrome.[150]

Incidence

The true incidence of leukemic skin infiltrates is difficult to determine accurately because specific skin lesions may have features that overlap those of various nonspecific manifestations that also may occur in this patient population. These lesions are rarely documented by histopathologic or immunohistochemical studies and, thus, do not allow for definitive diagnosis of specific skin lesions. Because of the uncertainties of case definition, the incidence reported varies from 1 to 50 percent, depending on the type of leukemia.[138,143] Specific skin lesions are more common in patients with acute nonlymphocytic leukemia, particularly in the monocytic and myelomonocytic subtypes. Skin involvement occurs in up to 30 percent of patients with acute monocytic leukemia (AMoL) or acute myelomonocytic leukemia (AMMoL).[137,138,143] Leukemic infiltrates have been reported to occur in 4 to 45 percent of patients with chronic lymphocytic leukemia (CLL).[143,151] Specific skin lesions are uncommon in acute lymphocytic leukemia (ALL) and are noted in about 1 percent of the patients. Specific skin lesions develop in approximately 10 percent of patients with acute myelocytic leukemia (AML).

TABLE 34-19

Classification of Leukemias

Myelogenous Leukemias	Lymphocytic Leukemias
Acute myelocytic leukemia (M3, AML)	Acute lymphocytic leukemia (ALL)
Acute myelomonocytic leukemia (M4, AMMoL)	Chronic lymphocytic leukemia (CLL)
Acute monocytic leukemia (M5, AMoL)	Adult T-cell leukemia/ lymphoma (ATLL)
Chronic myelocytic leukemia (CML)	Hairy cell leukemia (HCL)
Chronic myelomonocytic leukemia (CMMoL)	

MYELOCYTIC (GRANULOCYTIC) LEUKEMIA

Acute myelocytic leukemia (AML) accounts for about 50 percent of acute myeloid leukemias.[16] However, cutaneous leukemic infiltrates are uncommon during the course of AML. In a series of 877 patients with acute myeloid leukemia, only five patients with AML had leukemic skin infiltrates.[153]

Clinical Features   Clinically, the lesions are erythematous or violaceous, slightly elevated papules or nodules.[137,138,142,143] In some patients, papules may become confluent and give rise to plaque-like lesions. Hemorrhagic lesions may occur and nodules may ulcerate, especially if they enlarge progressively. The eruption may be widespread, but the most frequent areas of involvement are the trunk, extremities, neck, and face.[142] However, single large nodules or plaques do occur. Bullous hemorrhagic lesions and painful genital ulcers have been reported as an initial presentation of AML.[154,155] Leukemic gingivitis occurs in about 4 percent of patients.[156]

Specific skin lesions in chronic myelocytic leukemia (CML) are uncommon, with a reported incidence of 2 to 8 percent.[143,157] Juvenile CML, a rare malignancy in childhood, is characterized by a rapidly progressive course. Circinate erythematous annular plaques and nodules have been described in a few patients with juvenile CML.[159,160] Chloroma or granulocytic sarcoma is a rare manifestation of AML or CML that may concurrently present with the development of acute leukemia or may precede the disease by months to years.[160,162] Usually the lesions occur singly, but they occasionally are multiple. Individual lesions are erythematous, red-brown, or yellowish-green nodules or plaques.[163] The term chloroma was used originally because of the green color, which is owing to the presence of myeloperoxidase in the neoplastic tissue. However, many granulocytic sarcomas are colorless. Therefore, granulocytic sarcoma is the preferred term.

Histopathological Features   Biopsy specimens from specific skin lesions of AML or CML show a dense leukemic infiltrate in the upper and deep dermis that frequently extends to the subcutaneous tissue. It generally is separated from the epidermis by a narrow grenz zone, although the dermal-epidermal interface may be obliterated. The infiltrates usually have a diffuse distribution, but a preferential perivascular location may be seen (Fig. 34-42). In most cases, the infiltrate surrounds and infiltrates the dermal blood vessels, and leukemic cells may be found migrating through vessel walls. In some instances vascular injury and even frank vasculitis may be observed (leukemic vasculitis). The affected blood vessels may also contain intravascular clusters of atypical myeloid cells. Typically, the leukemic myeloid cells spread between the collagen bundles and permeate the lobules of subcutaneous tissue.[137,138,164] Most commonly, the leukemic infiltrate involves cutaneous appendages, with invasion of sebaceous glands, sweat glands, muscle fibers, and nerves (these structures tend to be destroyed by the tumor growth). Hemorrhage may be observed.

The infiltrate of AML is composed predominantly of large myeloblasts with round or oval vesicular nuclei and smaller cells with clefted nuclei. The cells stain positively with the chloroacetate esterase stain (Fig. 34-43). Immature atypical myeloid cells with bizarre nuclei frequently are present.[164] Mitotic figures are a consistent finding in the infiltrate of AML. Also, there may be admixtures of polymorphonuclear leukocytes, although the numbers are small. In CML, the infiltrate is more pleomorphic and dominated by granulocytes in various stages of differentiation, including atypical myelocytes, metamyelocytes, and neutrophils.[164] In granulocytic sarcoma, a diffuse, confluent infiltrate consisting of a mixture of immature myeloid cells ranging from large myeloblasts to myelocytes is present throughout the dermis and in the subcutaneous tissue.[160,162,163] The atypical hematopoietic cells may

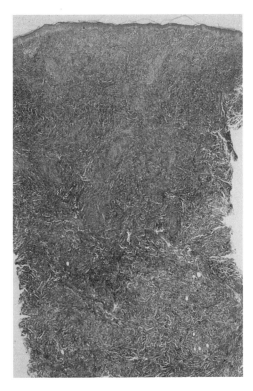

FIGURE 34-42   Acute myelocytic leukemia. Diffuse, dense infiltrate of leukemic cells (H&E magnification × 25).

show marked variation in size and nuclear configuration. Mature eosinophils admixed with eosinophilic myelocytes are observed regularly. Not uncommonly, an infiltrate of nonneoplastic inflammatory cells is seen in the leukemic infiltrate.

Histochemical and Immunohistochemical Findings   Staining for lysozyme and myeloperoxidase helps to identify mature and immature granulocytes in most cases of AML and CML.[163–165] Mature granulocytes are strongly positive for chloroacetate esterase and alpha-1-antitrypsin. CD43 (Leu-22) antibody, which is a marker for monocytes, T cells, and

granulocytes, is expressed strongly in most cases of AML and CML. In most cases of granulocytic sarcoma, the tumor cells show strong reactivity with antimyeloperoxidase and lysozyme.[163] Also, a variable proportion of leukemic cells stain with Leu-M1 (CD15), Leu-M5 (CD11c), and antineutrophil elastase (Fig. 34-44).

MONOCYTIC LEUKEMIA

Acute myelocytic leukemia accounts for between 2 and 10 percent of all cases of acute nonlymphocytic leukemia. Extramedullary disease is more common in AMoL than in other subtypes of leukemia; it is also associated with a worse prognosis. Patients with AMoL have the highest incidence of leukemic skin infiltrates, which are present in 10 to 30 percent of patients.[137,143,152]

Clinical Features   The specific skin lesions are violaceous to red-brown papules, nodules, and plaques.[137,138,142] Bullous lesions have been reported with AMoL.[166] The eruption occurs all over the body and may involve the face and scalp. Skin lesions may undergo rapid cycles of development and may resolve spontaneously. Leukemic gingival hyperplasia is the characteristic feature of AMoL, occurring in up to 60 percent of patients.[156] Ulceration, necrosis, and bleeding of the gums may occur. Rarely, leukemic skin infiltrates are observed before evidence of leukemic involvement is found in the bone marrow.[167] Congenital monocytic leukemia is a rare form. Among the 175 cases of congenital leukemia reported in the literature, 14 of the 41 patients with leukemic skin infiltrates had AMoL.[168] Skin lesions present as red-brown to purple papules and nodules and may have a "blueberry muffin" appearance.[69,70]

Histopathological Features   A dense perivascular or a more diffuse and confluent infiltrate is found predominantly in the dermis, but it often involves the lower part of the dermis and extends into the subcutis.[137,164,171] The epidermis usually is spared except for flattening of the rete ridge pattern. Prominent periadnexal aggregates of leukemic cells can be seen in addition to the diffuse infiltration. Infiltration and disruption of the cutaneous adnexa by leukemic infiltrates is present in some biopsy specimens. In most cases, thin rows of atypical cells migrating between collagen bundles, called an "Indian file" array, can be identified at the periphery of the infiltrate (Figs. 34-45 and 34-46). Cytologically, the infiltrate is composed of a monomorphous population of neoplastic cells of various sizes with large folded, or kidney-shaped, nuclei and a basophilic cytoplasmic seam.[164] Large atypical mononuclear cells with hyperchromatic, irregular nuclei frequently are present in the infiltrate (Fig. 34-47). Atypical mitotic figures usually are seen but may be few in number. A few granulocytes and extravasated erythrocytes are intermingled with the tumor cells.

Histochemical and Immunohistochemical Findings   The leukemic infiltrate in most cases of AMoL stains positively with antilysozyme.[153,165,171] Chloroacetate esterase usually is not present in AMoL, although a weak reactivity may be detected in a small proportion of patients. The tumor cells express leukocyte common antigen (CD45) and Leu-22 (CD43), whereas only weak staining is found with the antibody Leu-M1 (CD15) in part of the cells.[171] Although many available antibodies can be used on formalin-fixed and paraffin-embedded tissue, a panel of monoclonal antibodies used on frozen sections usually is required to identify a specific reaction pattern that is diagnostic for AML.[171] In staining frozen sections with markers for granulocytes and monocytes (Leu-M5 [CD11c], KiM7 [CD68], My7 [CD13], OKM14 [CD14], VIM 2 [CD65], and My9 [CD33]), positive reactions are found in approximately 85 percent of specimens (Fig. 34-44).[171]

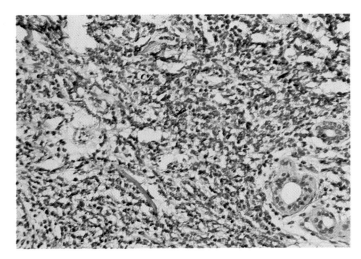

FIGURE 34-43   Acute myelocytic leukemia. Dense infiltrate of myelocytes demonstrated with chloroacetate esterase stain (H&E magnification × 250).

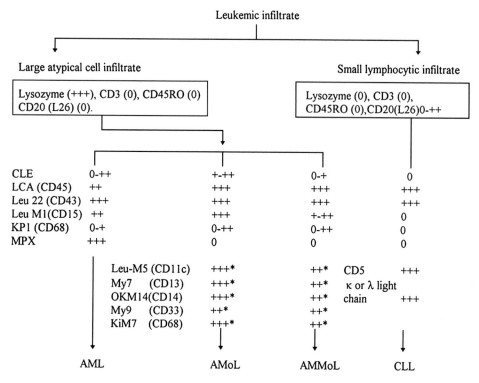

Leukemic infiltrate

Large atypical cell infiltrate

Lysozyme (+++), CD3 (0), CD45RO (0) CD20 (L26) (0).

Small lymphocytic infiltrate

Lysozyme (0), CD3 (0), CD45RO (0),CD20(L26)0-++

CLE	0-++	+-++	0-+	0
LCA (CD45)	++	+++	+++	+++
Leu 22 (CD43)	+++	+++	+++	+++
Leu M1(CD15)	++	+++	+-++	0
KP1 (CD68)	0-+	0-++	0-++	0
MPX	+++	0	0	0

Leu-M5 (CD11c)	+++*	++*
My7 (CD13)	+++*	++*
OKM14(CD14)	+++*	++*
My9 (CD33)	++*	++*
KiM7 (CD68)	+++*	++*

CD5   +++
κ or λ light chain   +++

AML   AMoL   AMMoL   CLL

FIGURE 34-44   Approach to leukemic infiltrates: immunohistochemical evaluation. AML, acute myelocytic leukemia; AMMoL, acute myelomonocytic leukemia; AMoL, acute monocytic leukemia; CLE, chloroacetate esterase; CLL, chronic lymphocytic leukemia; MPX, myeloperoxidase; 0, negative; +, fewer than 25 percent cells positive; ++, 25 to 50 percent cells positive; +++, more than 50 percent cells positive. *Staining on frozen sections.

MYELOMONOCYTIC LEUKEMIA

Myelomonocytic leukemia (AMMoL) represents 25 percent of all cases of acute non-lymphocytic leukemia.[172] In AMMoL, both granulocytic and monocytic precursors are present in varying proportions, and each cell line accounts for at least 20 percent of nucleated bone marrow cells. Leukemic mucocutaneous lesions are found in 13 to 27 percent of patients.[138,152,156] Specific skin lesions are very uncommon in CMMoL, and only a few cases have been reported.[173]

Clinical Features   Most patients have multiple, red or purple, asymptomatic papules, nodules, or plaques on the head, trunk, or extremities.[138,142] The gums are involved in approximately 18 percent of patients.[156] Specific infiltrations into scars of previous sites of catheter placement, trauma, burns, and herpes simplex may occur.[138,174] Rarely, the clinical features of the lesions may be atypical, and the initial appearance has been reported in some cases as a bullous, erythrodermic, or clinically benign-appearing cutaneous eruption.[175–177] A vesiculopapular rash mimicking chickenpox has been reported in AMMoL.[178] Less commonly, the leukemic skin infiltrates may be evident before leukemia is detected in the peripheral blood and bone marrow.[153,176]

Histopathological Features   There is a dense infiltrate of atypical mononuclear cells throughout the dermis and in the subcutaneous fat (Fig. 34-48). Overlying the infiltrate is a distinct grenz zone, separating it from the epidermis.[164,176,177] Occasionally, focal involvement of the epidermis may be seen.[179] The infiltrate consists of a mixture of pleomorphic monocytoid and myelogenous cells.[180] There are immature monocytes with irregularly shaped nuclei, mature monocytes, myeloblasts, myelocytes, and occasional eosinophils.[156,164] Mitotic fig-

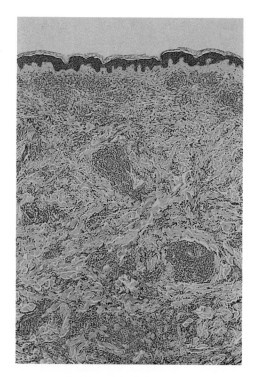

FIGURE 34-45   Acute monocytic leukemia. Diffuse leukemic infiltration of the whole dermis. Note the grenz zone and involvement of blood vessels and cutaneous appendages (H&E magnification × 12).

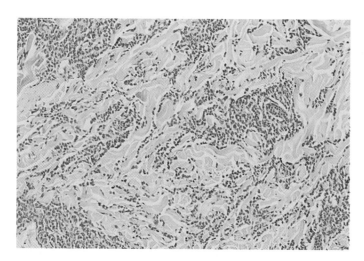

FIGURE 34-46   Acute monocytic leukemia. Leukemic cells infiltrate between the collagen bundles (H&E magnification × 32).

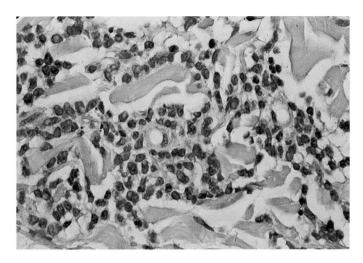

FIGURE 34-47   Acute monocytic leukemia. Large atypical mononuclear cells with hyperchromatic nuclei (H&E magnification × 320).

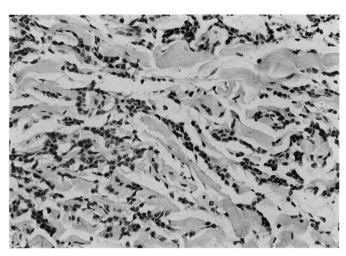

FIGURE 34-49   Acute myelomonocytic leukemia. Leukemic cells spread between collagen bundles (H&E magnification × 80).

ures may be seen. The tumor cells are arranged in strands and cords, spreading between collagen bundles (Fig. 34-49). In addition, infiltration and destruction of vessels and skin appendages is characteristic of AMMoL.

Histochemical and Immunohistochemical Findings   Most leukemic cells in the infiltrate stain strongly with antilysozyme. The neoplastic cells usually do not stain with chloroacetate esterase, although a weak reactivity may be found in some cells.[165] Immunophenotyping of the leukemic infiltrate shows that the major proportion of cells express macrophage-associated antigens (Leu 22 [CD43], Leu-M1 [CD15], KP1 [CD68], HAM56, and MAC387), although the number of reactive cells may vary greatly from patient to patient (Fig. 34-50).[153,165,179] In

addition, the expression of Leu-M5 (CD11c) and My7 (CD13), which are markers for monocytes and granulocytes, can be demonstrated in frozen sections (Fig. 34-44).[171]

Differential Diagnosis of Leukemic Myelogenous Infiltrates   The diagnosis of leukemic myelogenous skin infiltrates may be extremely difficult on routine histologic examination. Myelocytic, monocytic, and myelomonocytic leukemic infiltrates are compared in Table 34-20. The histologic differential diagnosis (Table 34-21) includes leukemic skin infiltrates of lymphocytic leukemia, non-Hodgkin's lymphoma, cutaneous lesions of Hodgkin's disease, malignant histiocytosis, Langerhan's cell histiocytosis, metastatic undifferentiated carcinomas, and various benign dermatoses such as granuloma faciale, erythema elevatum diutinum, mastocytosis, secondary syphilis, neutrophilic arthropod reactions, acute febrile neutrophilic dermatosis, Behçet's disease, and neutrophilic eccrine hidradenitis.[139,141,144,181] The histologic differentiation may be a problem, thus emphasizing the importance of clinicopathologic correlation in establishing a diagnosis. The presence of immature myeloid cells usually allows its differentiation from benign neutrophilic infiltrates. Erythema elevatum diutinum is ruled out by the presence of leukocytoclastic vasculitis. Neutrophils, pyknotic neu-

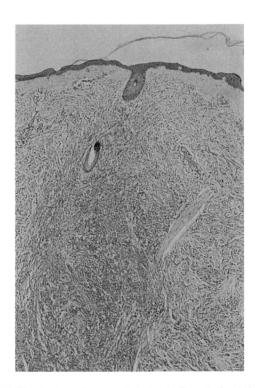

FIGURE 34-48   Acute myelomonocytic leukemia. Dense leukemic infiltrate in the dermis. Note infiltration and destruction of blood vessels and cutaneous adnexa (H&E magnification × 12).

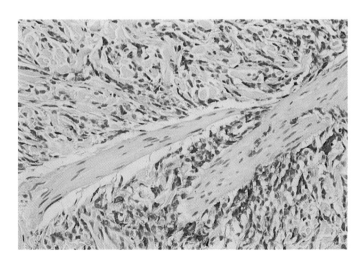

FIGURE 34-50   Acute myelomonocytic leukemia. Leukemic cells express Leu-M1 (CD15) antigen, which is present in monocytes and granulocytes. Note infiltration of the muscle bundles (Immunoperoxidase stain magnification × 80).

TABLE 34-20

Comparison of Myelocytic, Monocytic, and Myelomonocytic Leukemic Skin Infiltrates

	Myelocytic Leukemia	Monocytic Leukemia	Myelomonocytic Leukemia
Clinical Features			
Incidence	2–13%	10–30%	13–27%
Clinical description	Red papules and nodules; red-brown or yellowish-green nodules (chloroma); ulceration may occur	Violaceous papules and nodules	Red-purplish papules, nodules, or plaques Leukemic infiltration of scars may occur
Location	Widespread	Widespread	Widespread
Gingival involvement	Rarely (4%)	Common (>30%)	Common (18%)
Histopathological Features			
Level of leukemic involvement			
Epidermis	Usually no involvement	Usually no involvement	Usually absent, focal involvement may occur
Grenz zone	Usually present	Mostly present	Present
Upper and lower dermis	Usually involved	Involved, mainly the upper part	Involved
Subcutaneous tissue	Frequently involved	Usually involved	Mostly involved
Pattern of infiltrate	Usually diffuse, rarely nodular	Diffuse	Diffuse
Infiltration of adnexa	Mostly present	Prominent	Prominent
Cytomorphology of leukemic cells	Atypical myeloblasts with large irregularly shaped nuclei; atypical myelocytes, few neutrophils	Relatively uniform medium-sized and large monoblasts with folded or kidney-shaped nuclei; small monocytoid cells	Pleomorphic monoblasts with pale cytoplasm and irregular nuclei; myeloblasts, occasional eosinophils
Mitotic figures	Present	Rarely present	Occasionally present

trophil nuclei, and neutrophil fragments are hallmarks of acute neutrophilic dermatosis.[182]

Nonspecific cutaneous lesions usually are characterized by a mixed cellular infiltrate composed of mature granulocytes, macrophages, and lymphocytes. They may result from the pancytopenia and immunosuppression associated with leukemia or from adverse effects of treatment. Leukemic patients are prone to infections, which may be of viral, fungal, or bacterial origin for the skin lesions. The inflammatory infiltrate usually involves the superficial dermis and is composed mainly of lymphocytes and neutrophils. Special stains and tissue culture are helpful in confirming the diagnosis. Other frequently observed nonspecific lesions

TABLE 34-21

Differential Diagnosis of Leukemias

Cutaneous T-cell lymphomas	Lupus erythematosus
Cutaneous B-cell lymphomas	Lymphocytic infiltrate of Jessner
Hodgkin's disease	Lymphomatoid papulosis
Histiocytosis X	Actinic reticuloid
Malignant histiocytosis	Lymphocytoma cutis
Mastocytosis	Pityriasis lichenoides
Angioimmunoblastic lymphadenopathy	Pyoderma gangrenosum
	Sweet's syndrome
Lymphomatoid granulomatosis	Behçet's disease
Merkel cell carcinoma	Neutrophilic eccrine hidradenitis
Metastatic carcinomas	Erythema elevatum diutinum
Kaposi's sarcoma	Granuloma faciale
	Secondary syphilis
	Arthropod bite reactions

in leukemia include purpura and ecchymoses owing to thrombocytopenia. Numerous extravasated red cells are present in the dermis and subcutaneous fat. There is no evidence of vasculitis, but a mild perivascular infiltrate of mononuclear cells may be present. The histologic changes observed in drug eruptions include vacuolar alterations of the basal cell layer and a perivascular infiltrate composed predominantly of lymphocytes. However, in most instances, the histologic changes in drug eruptions are nonspecific. Unlike leukemic infiltrates, the infiltrate usually involves the epidermis. Eosinophils may be present in small numbers. Immunohistochemical studies of the nonspecific lesions show an infiltrate predominantly of T cells, which are positive for CD3, CD45, and CD45RO. CD20-positive B cells are scattered in the infiltrate. Lymphoid cells do not stain with lysozyme, myeloperoxidase, and chloroacetate esterase, which is an important feature that distinguishes these cells from myelogenous leukemic infiltrates.[165] Leukocyte common antigen (CD45) helps to exclude poorly differentiated carcinomas. Extensive staining with antilysozyme, antimyeloperoxidase, and chloroacetate esterase as well as expression of Leu-M1 (CD15) favors the diagnosis of AML.[153] A battery of special immunoperoxidase stains discussed above can be used on frozen sections to confirm the diagnosis of AML and AMMoL.[171] The differentiation of AML and AMMoL from malignant lymphoma and even poorly differentiated carcinoma may require the use of additional immunohistochemical techniques. The differential diagnosis of leukemic skin infiltrates is outlined in Table 34-20.

CHRONIC LYMPHOCYTIC LEUKEMIA

Chronic lymphocytic leukemia (CLL) is the most frequent form of leukemia in western countries, with an incidence of three to five new cases per 100,000 persons per year. Nearly all cases occur in persons older than 50 years, and the disease affects men twice as frequently as women. The clinical features of CLL are the result of the proliferation and accumulation of mature-appearing lymphocytes that, in most cases, represent a monoclonal B-cell population.[183]

Clinical Features   Specific skin lesions have been reported to occur in 8 percent of patients, although the reported incidence ranges from 4 to 45 percent.[143,151,184,185] The lesions are solitary—or more often, multiple—red or violaceous macules, papules, or nodules.[137,142,151] Large nodules may become necrotic and ulcerated. Nodules and tumors are most frequent, accounting for 23 to 50 percent of all lesions.[151,186] The development of nodules up to several centimeters in diameter has been described. The lesions tend to occur mainly on the face and scalp, but they have been reported on the trunk and extremities.[142] Specific skin involvement may also present as an exfoliative erythroderma.[185] However, the clinical lesions may have striking variations in their morphological features and distribution. Atypical manifestations may present as chronic paronychia, subungual nodules, plaques on the volar surface of the hands and fingers, finger clubbing with periosteal bone destruction, and papulovesicular eruptions.[54,151,187–189,191,192] Involvement of the mucous membranes is rare. Infiltrated plaques on the vulva and nodular lesions with or without ulceration of the oropharynx, tonsils, and palate may occur (Table 34-22).[145]

Histopathologic Features   The predominant feature of CLL is a dense superficial and deep dermal perivascular and periadnexal infiltrate that frequently involves the subcutaneous tissue (Fig. 34-51). Extensive involvement of the subcutaneous tissue usually is seen, particularly in large nodular lesions. There is a grenz zone of normal dermis between the uninvolved epidermis and the dermal infiltrate, although the infiltrate frequently extends close to the dermal-epidermal junction, with focal involvement of the epidermis.[164] However, prominent epidermotropism may be seen in T-cell CLL. Another frequent histologic finding is the involvement of dermal appendages, which is associated with occasional destruction of sweat glands and hair follicles. Less commonly, leukemic infiltrates may invade the walls of blood vessels. At higher magnification, the infiltrate is monomorphous and composed mainly of small- to medium-sized lymphocytes with a round nucleus

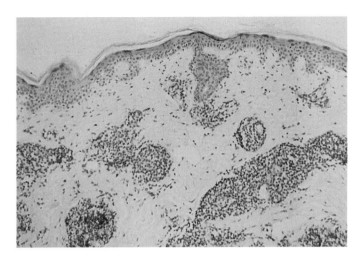

FIGURE 34-51   Chronic lymphocytic leukemia. Perivascular and periadnexal infiltrate in the reticular dermis (H&E magnification × 32).

and dense nuclear chromatin.[141,164] Large atypical lymphoid cells with irregular nuclei and prominent nucleoli occasionally are present. Rarely, a subepidermal bullous separation, accompanied by edema of the superficial dermis, may be present.[151,192]

Histochemical and Immunohistochemical Findings   The leukemic infiltrate in CLL is nonreactive with chloroacetate esterase staining and is consistently lysozyme-negative. The majority of the infiltrates do not stain with the T-cell markers CD45RO and CD3, whereas CD20 (L-26)—which preferentially stains mature normal B cells—is either negative or weakly positive in the abnormal B cells.[165] Characteristically, the neoplastic cells express CD5 antigen. The detection of a single idiotype or light chain on the cell surface in CLL is owing to the monoclonal proliferation of B cells. The immunoglobulin light chain restriction can be demonstrated with the use of markers for kappa and lambda light chains. Frozen sections may be required for optimal staining. The predominant SIg isotype in classic CLL is IgM or IgM and IgD.

HAIRY CELL LEUKEMIA

Hairy cell leukemia (HCL) is a rare lymphoproliferative malignancy of B-cell lineage that accounts for approximately 10 percent of chronic lymphocytic leukemias. A rare T-cell variant of HCL associated with HTLV exists.[194]

Clinical Features   Hairy cell leukemia is characterized by splenomegaly, pancytopenia, wasting, and weight loss. Lymphadenopathy is an inconsistent finding and may occur in 26 percent of patients.[195] Characteristic of HCL is the presence in the peripheral blood and bone marrow of uniform, mononuclear hairy cells with prominent cytoplasmic projections. Infections are the most common origin of cutaneous manifestations and account for 60 percent of cases.[196,197] Also, HCL is frequently associated with vasculitis.[196–198] Leukemic skin infiltrates are rarely observed in patients with HCL. They were seen in 48 (8%) of the 600 cases reported in the literature, but only eight cases were proved by skin biopsy.[199] In one series of 113 patients, only one had skin infiltration by leukemic cells.[196] The lesions usually are erythematous maculopapular eruptions.[199–201] Deep infiltrated nodules of HCL may be present.

TABLE 34-22

Leukemic Infiltrates of Chronic Lymphocytic Leukemia

Clinical Features

Peak incidence over 50 years of age
Males equal to females
Red or violaceous macules, papules, and nodules
Often ulcerated large nodule
Solitary and multiple
Exfoliative erythroderma
Located on face, scalp, trunk, and extremities
Rare involvement of mucous membranes

Histopathological Features

Dense monomorphous perivascular and periadnexal infiltrates
Predominantly in reticular dermis
Usually grenz zone
May involve subcutaneous tissue
Involvement of dermal appendages may occur
Small- to medium-sized lymphoid cells
Monoclonal B-cell proliferation
Expression of IgM and kappa or lambda light chains

Histopathological Features   The pathologic feature of cutaneous involvement is that of a dense, diffuse, or patchy infiltrate of uniform mononuclear cells. The epidermis and papillary dermis are spared, and on low-power microscopic examination, the infiltrate is seen predominantly in the upper dermis, mainly around vessels. The infiltrate also surrounds and invades the skin appendages. Less commonly, the infiltrate extends deeply throughout the entire dermis and into subcutaneous tissue. On high-power examination, the individual leukemic cells are small to medium in size and have an abundant, pale cytoplasm and hyperchromatic rounded or indented nuclei. Typically, the nuclei are separated from one another by clear cytoplasmic spaces. Cytoplasmic hairy projections cannot be seen in fixed tissue sections. There usually is a small number of neutrophils, eosinophils, and histiocytes. Mitoses are absent.[199,200]

Histochemical and Immunohistochemical Findings   Most infiltrating hairy cells stain strongly with tartrate-resistant acid phosphatase. The leukemic cells stain with the B-cell marker L26 (CD20) and express CD22 antigen.

ADULT T-CELL LEUKEMIA/LYMPHOMA

Adult T-cell leukemia/lymphoma (ATLL) is an aggressive lymphoproliferative disorder caused by the proliferation of CD4+ T cells infected with HTLV-I.[148,149,203,204] HTLV-I infection is endemic in the southwestern district of Japan, the Caribbean, South America, and central Africa.[149] The lifetime risk of developing ATLL among HTLV-I infected persons is 2.5 percent.[202]

Clinical Features   Adult T-cell leukemia/lymphoma occurs only in adults. The age at onset ranges from 24 to 85 years (average, 58 years).[202] The classification of ATLL is based on the clinical manifestations and laboratory findings and includes four types: the so-called acute, chronic, smoldering, and lymphoma types.[202,203] Acute ATLL is the most characteristic form of the disease and is characterized by a high-grade leukemia, generalized lymphadenopathy, hepatosplenomegaly, skin lesions, leukemic involvement of the bone marrow, and rapid clinical progression. Leukemic cells usually have large, highly convoluted nuclei, called "flower cells," and characteristically display the mature T-cell phenotype, CD4+, but lack CD7 and CD8 antigen expression.[202] A common feature is lytic bone lesions with an associated hypercalcemia. Patients with chronic ATLL usually present with skin lesions, but widespread systemic involvement is less common. In particular, smoldering ATLL presents with predominantly cutaneous manifestations and a protracted clinical course before giving rise to an acute, aggressive terminal phase. In addition to the clinical features, the diagnosis of ATLL is based on the presence of circulating antibodies against HTLV-I and monoclonal integration of the HTLV-I provirus in the tumor cell DNA.[202–205] In up to 77 percent of cases of ATLL, there is a cutaneous infiltration of malignant T cells. Cutaneous manifestations of ATLL can be quite variable and have been described as generalized erythroderma, maculopapular rash, nodules, plaques, and bullous lesions.[206–208]

Histopathological Features   There is a dense lymphoid infiltrate that is often concentrated around blood vessels and appendages. The infiltrate may diffusely involve the full thickness of the dermis and the subcutaneous fat. Exocytosis of atypical lymphoid cells into the epidermis, with or without intraepidermal clusters of cells forming the so-called Pautrier's microabscesses, is seen frequently. However, the nonepidermotropic pattern of infiltration may occur. The infiltrate consists of various small, medium-sized, or large lymphoid cells with markedly con-

voluted nuclei. Mitotic figures are common. Dermal edema may be prominent. Occasionally, eosinophils and a few plasma cells occur in the infiltrate. The perivascular infiltration is frequently associated with evidence of vasculitis, with destructive changes of blood vessels and extravasation of erythrocytes.[206–208]

Immunohistochemical Findings   Immunophenotyping with monoclonal antibodies shows that the predominant phenotype of the neoplastic cells in the skin of patients with ATLL is the helper T cell that expresses CD3, CD4, CD7, CD29, CD45RO, and HLA-DR but lacks CD45RA.[206,209]

Differential Diagnosis of Leukemic Lymphoid Infiltrates   Each of these leukemic lymphoid infiltrates may present difficulty in differential diagnosis, both with one another and with other disease processes characterized by an extensive lymphocytic infiltrate. The histologic differential diagnosis includes infiltrates of lupus erythematosus, pityriasis lichenoides, lymphomatoid papulosis, cutaneous lymphoid hyperplasia, actinic reticuloid, angioimmunoblastic lymphadenopathy, and cutaneous lymphomas (Table 34-21).[3] The presence of marked epidermotropism usually favors the diagnosis of cutaneous T-cell lymphoma over CLL. Lymphocytic infiltrate of the skin is characterized by a predominantly perivascular infiltrate composed of small lymphocytes. In addition, deposition of mucin may be seen in the reticular dermis. Pityriasis lichenoides is distinguished by the presence of epidermal necrosis, dyskeratosis, and exocytosis of lymphocytes. Lymphomatoid papulosis shows an infiltrate of large atypical cells with vesicular nuclei or atypical small lymphoid cells with cerebriform nuclei. Most cases of lymphomatoid papulosis consist of a proliferation of activated helper T cells expressing CD4, CD30, and other activation antigens. In contrast, the leukemic cells in HCL are morphologically uniform and usually stain with a B-cell marker.[196,200] At low-power magnification, leukemic infiltrates of CLL may be difficult to differentiate from cutaneous lymphoid hyperplasia, but the predominance of small mature lymphocytes, scattered large macrophages, and an admixture of plasma cells and eosinophils usually helps to exclude a malignant process. In addition, immunophenotyping of cutaneous lymphoid hyperplasia shows mixed infiltrates composed of a polyclonal B-cell population, T cells, and macrophages. Histologically, leukemic infiltrates of CLL can be confused with lymphoplasmacytic lymphoma. The presence of lymphoplasmacytoid cells and plasma cells with intracytoplasmic or intranuclear immunoglobulin inclusions (Dutcher bodies), which can be demonstrated with the periodic acid-Schiff stain, helps in the differential diagnosis.

The histopathologic differentiation of ATLL from other cutaneous T-cell lymphomas such as mycosis fungoides and Sézary syndrome may be difficult. Knowledge of the clinical features of ATLL and clinical shrewdness can usually solve these diagnostic dilemmas. The lack of damage to blood vessels and the deficiency of L-selectin (Leu-8)-positive cells help to distinguish cutaneous T-cell lymphoma from ATLL.[208,209] The demonstration of HTLV-I proviral integration in the clonal population of malignant T cells can help to differentiate ATLL from cutaneous T-cell lymphoma when the clinical presentation overlaps.[204]

REFERENCES

1. Dummer R, Kohl O, Gillessen J, Kagi M, Burg G: Peripheral blood mononuclear cells in patients with nonleukemic cutaneous T-cell lymphoma. Reduced proliferation and preferential secretion of a T helper-2-like cytokine pattern on stimulation. *Arch Dermatol* 129: 433-436, 1993.
2. Vowels BR, Cassin M, Vonderheid EC, Rook AH: Aberrant cytokine production by Sezary syndrome patients: Cytokine secretion pattern resembles murine Th2 cells. *J Invest Dermatol* 99:90–94, 1992.

3. Burg G, Braun-Falco O: *Cutaneous Lymphomas, Pseudolymphomas and Related Disorders.* New York: Springer, 1983.

4. Burg G, Dummer R, Kerl H: Classification of cutaneous lymphomas. *Dermatol Clin* 12:213–217, 1994.

5. Kerl H, Cerroni L, Burg G: The morphologic spectrum of T-cell lymphomas of the skin: a proposal for a new classification. *Semin Diagn Pathol* 8:55–61, 1991.

6. Rappaport H: *Tumors of the Hematopoietic System.* Washington, DC: Armed Forces Institute of Pathology, 1966.

7. Lennert K, Feller AC: *Histopathology of Non-Hodgkin's Lymphoma,* 2nd ed. Berlin: Springer, 1992.

8. Suchi T, Lennert K, Tu LY, Kikuchi M, et al: Histopathology and immunohistochemistry of peripheral T cell lymphomas: A proposal for their classification. *J Clin Pathol* 40:995–1015, 1987.

9. Working Formulation: The non-Hodgkin's lymphoma pathologic classification project. National Cancer Institute sponsored study of classification of non-Hodgkin's lymphoma. Summary and description of Working Formulation for clinical usage. *Cancer* 49:2112–2135, 1982.

10. Harris NL, Jaffe ES, Stein H, Banks PM, et al: A revised European-American classification of lymphoid neoplasms: A proposal from the International Lymphoma Study Group. *Blood* 84:1361–1392, 1994.

11. Gonzalez CL, Medeiros LJ, Braziel RM, Jaffe ES: T-cell lymphoma involving subcutaneous tissue. A clinicopathologic entity commonly associated with hemophagocytic syndrome. *Am J Surg Pathol* 15:17–27, 1991.

12. Burg G, Dummer R, Wilhelm M, et al: A subcutaneous delta positive T-cell lymphoma that produces interferon gamma. *N Engl J Med* 325:1078–1081, 1991.

13. McNutt NS, Crain WR: Quantitative electron microscopic comparison of lymphocyte nuclear contours in mycosis fungoides and in benign infiltrates in skin. *Cancer* 47:698–709, 1981.

14. Pinkus GS, Said JW, Hargraeves HK: Malignant lymphoma, T-cell type: A distinct morphological variant with large multilobated nuclei. Report of four cases. *Am J Clin Pathol* 72:540–550, 1979.

15. Vaillant L, Monegier DSC, Arbeille B, et al: Cutaneous T cell lymphoma of signet ring cell type: a specific clinico-pathologic entity. *Acta Derm Venereol* 73:255–258, 1993.

16. Burg G, Zwingers T, Staegemeir E, Santucci M: Interrater and intrarater variabilities in the evaluation of cutaneous lymphoproliferative T-cell infiltrates. EORTC-Cutaneous Lymphoma Project Group. *Dermatol Clin* 12:311–314, 1994.

17. Lefeber WP, Robinson JK, Clendenning WE, Dunn JL, Colton T: Attempts to enhance light microscopic diagnosis of cutaneous T-cell lymphoma (mycosis fungoides). *Arch Dermatol* 117:408–411, 1981.

18. Santucci M, Burg G, Feller AC: Interrater and intrarater reliability of histologic criteria in early cutaneous T-cell lymphoma. An EORTC Cutaneous Lymphoma Project Group study. *Dermatol Clin* 12:323–327, 1994.

19. Merz H, Malisius R, Mannweiler R, et al: Immunomax. A maximized immunohistochemical method for the retrieval and enhancement of hidden antigens. *Lab Invest* 73:149–156, 1995.

20. Volkenandt M, Wienecke R, Tiemann M: Detection of monoclonal lymphoid cell populations by polymerase chain reaction technology. *Dermatol Clin* 12:341–349, 1994.

21. Mielke V, Staib G, Boehncke WH, Duller B, Sterry W: Clonal disease in early cutaneous T-cell lymphoma. *Dermatol Clin* 12:351–360, 1994.

22. Wood GS, Haeffner A, Dummer R, Crooks CF: Molecular biology techniques for the diagnosis of cutaneous T-cell lymphoma. *Dermatol Clin* 12:231–241, 1994.

23. Kaltoft K, Hansen BH, Thestrup-Petersen K: Cytogenetic findings in cell lines from cutaneous T-cell lymphoma. *Dermatol Clin* 12:295–304, 1994.

24. Boni R, Davis-Daneshfar A, Burg G, Fuchs D, Wood GS: No detection of HTLV-I proviral DNA in lesional skin biopsies from Swiss and German patients with cutaneous T-cell lymphoma. *Br J Dermatol* 134:2 1996.

25. Lessin SR, Vowels BR, Rook AH: Retroviruses and cutaneous T-cell lymphoma. *Dermatol Clin* 12:243–253, 1994.

26. D'Ican M, Souteyrand P, Gasmi M, Desgranges C: Deleted HTLV retrovirus may be involved in the development of cutaneous T-cell lymphomas (letter). *J Invest Dermatol* 103:134, 1994.

27. Khan ZM, Sebenik M, Zucker-Franklin D: Localization of human T-Cell lymphotropic virus-1 tax proviral sequences in skin biopsies of patients with Mycosis fungoides by *in situ* polymerase chain reaction. *J Invest Dermatol* 106: 667–672, 1996.

28. Fearon ER, Vogelstein BA: A genetic model for colorectal tumorigenesis. *Cell* 61: 759–76, 1990.

29. Thestrup-Petersen K, Kaltoft K: Genotraumatic T cells and cutaneous T-cell lymphoma. A causal relationship? *Arch Dermatol Res* 287:97–101, 1994.

30. Taylor RS, Ramirez RD, Ogoshi M, Chaffins M, Piatyszek MA, Shay JW: Detection of Telomerase activity in malignant and nonmalignant skin conditions. *J Invest Dermatol* 759–765, 1996

31. Unna PG, Santi S, Pollitzer S: Ueber die Parakeratosen im allgemeinen und eine neue Form derselben (Parakeratosis variegata). *Monatsschr Prakt Dermatol* 10:404–412, 444–459, 1890.

32. Brocq L: Les parapsoriasis. *Ann Dermatol Syphilol* 3:433–468, 1902.

33. King ID, Ackerman AB: Guttate parapsoriasis/digitate dermatosis (small plaque parapsoriasis) is mycosis fungoides. *Am J Dermatopathol* 14:518–530, 1992.

34. Ackerman AB, White W: *Differential Diagnosis in Dermatopathology IV.* Philadelphia: Lea & Febiger, 1994.

35. Haeffner AC, Smoller BR, Zepter K, Wood GS: Differentiation and clonality of lesional lymphocytes in small plaque parapsoriasis. *Arch Dermatol* 131:321–324, 1995.

36. Ralfkiaer E, Wollf SA, Thomsen K, Geisler C, Vejlsgaard GL: T-cell receptor gamma delta-positive peripheral T-cell lymphomas presenting in the skin: a clinical, histological and immunophenotypic study. *Exp Dermatol* 1:31–36, 1992.

37. Burg G, Dummer R: Small plaque (digitate) parapsoriasis is an "abortive cutaneous T-cell lymphoma" and is not mycosis fungoides. *Arch Dermatol* 131:336–338, 1995.

38. Cerroni L, Rieger E, et al: Clinicopathologic and immunologic features associated with transformation of mycosis fungoides to large-cell lymphoma. *Am J Surg Pathol* 16: 543–552, 1992.

39. Schmoeckel C, Burg G, Braun-Falco O, Klingmüller G: Mycosis fongoide a forte malignité avec transformation cytologique. *Ann Dermatol Venereol* 108:231–241, 1981.

40. Geerts ML, Burg G, Schmoeckel C, Braun-Falco O: Alkaline phosphatase activity in non-Hodgkin's lymphomas and pseudolymphomas of the skin. *J Dermatol Surg Oncol* 10:306–312, 1984.

41. Aloi F, Tomasini C, Pippione M: Mycosis fungoides and eruptive epidermoid cysts: a unique response of follicular and eccrine structures. *Dermatology* 187:273–277, 1993.

42. Oliwiecki S, Ashworth J: Mycosis fungoides with a widespread follicular eruption, comedones and cysts. *Br J Dermatol* 127:54–56, 1992.

43. Radeff B, Merot Y, Saurat JH: Acquired epidermal cysts and mycosis fungoides. A possible pitfall in clinical staging. *Am J Dermatopathol* 10:424–429, 1988.

44. LeBoit PE: Variants of mycosis fungoides and related cutaneous T-cell lymphomas. *Semin Diagn Pathol* 8:73–81, 1991.

45. Agnarsson BA, Vonderheid EC, Kadin ME: CD8+ cutaneous T-cell lymphoma (letter). *Am J Dermatopathol* 13: 628–629, 1991.

46. Dommann SNW, Ziegler T, et al: CD 44v6 is a marker for systemic spread in cutaneous T-cell lymphomas. *J Cutan Pathol* 22:407–412, 1995.

47. Dommann SNW, Dommann-Scherrer CC, Dours-Zimmermann MT, Zimmermann DR, Kural-Serbes B, Burg G: Cutaneous pleomorphic T-cell lymphoma showing lineage cross-over of antigen receptor gene rearrangement. *Eur J Dermatol*, 6:96, 1996.

48. Imai S, Burg G, et al: Mycosis fungoides and Sezary's syndrome show distinct histomorpholoical features. *Dermatologica* 173:131–135, 1986.

49. Thestrup-Petersen K, Sogaard H, Zachariae H: The red man syndrome. Exfoliative dermatitis of unknown etiology: A description and follow up of 38 patients. *J Am Acad Dermatol* 18:1307–1312, 1988.

50. Ketron LW, Goodman MH: Multiple lesions of the skin apparently of epithelial origin resembling clinically mycosis fungoides. *Arch Dermatol* 24:758–777, 1931.

51. Woringer F, Kolopp P: Lésion érythématosquameuse polycyclique de l'avant-bras évoluant depuis 6 ans chez un garçonnet de 13 ans. *Ann Dermatol Syphilol* 10:945–958, 1939.

52. Braun-Falco O, Marghescu S, Wolff HH: Pagetoide Reticulose. *Hautarzt* 24:11–21, 1973.

53. Mackie RM, Turbitt ML: A case of pagetoid reticulosis bearing the T cytotoxic suppressor surface marker on the lymphoid infiltrate: Further evidence that pagetoid reticulosis is not a variant of mycosis fungoides. *Br J Dermatol* 110:89–94, 1984.

54. Berti E, Cerri A, Cavicchini S, Delia D, Soligo D, Alessi E, Caputo R: Primary cutaneous gamma/delta T-cell lymphoma presenting as disseminated pagetoid reticulosis. *J Invest Dermatol* 96:718–723, 1991.

55. Kaudewitz P, Burg G, Stein H, Klepzig K, Mason DY, Braun-Falco O: Monoclonal antibody patterns in lymphomatoid papulosis. *Dermatologic Clinics* 3:749–757, 1985.

56. Wood GS, Weiss LM, et al: T-cell antigen deficiencies and clonal rearrangements of T-cell receptor genes in pagetoid reticulosis (Woringer-Kolopp disease). *N Engl J Med* 318:164–167, 1988.

57. Vidal E, Brocq L: Etude sur le mycosis fungoide. *La France Médical* 2:946–1019, 1885.

58. Harrington CI, Slater DN: Mycosis fungoides with blast cell transformation. *Arch Dermatol* 114:611–612, 1978.

59. Braverman IM: Tranformation in cutaneous T-cell lymphoma. *J Invest Dermatol* 101:249–250, 1993.

60. Braun-Falco O, Nikolowski J, Burg G, Schmoeckel C: Lymphomatoide Papulose. Uebersicht und Beschreibung von 4 Patienten. *Hautarzt* 34:59–65, 1983.

61. Davis TH, Morton CC, Miller CR, Balk SP, Kadin ME: Hodgkin's disease, lymphomatoid papulosis, and cutaneous T-cell lymphoma derived from a common T-cell clone. *N Engl J Med* 326:1115–1122, 1992.

62. Burg G, Ziffer S, Ziffer UL: Light and electron microscopy in lymphomatoid papulosis, in Muller SA (ed). *Parapsoriasis.* Rochester: Mayo Foundation, 1990, pp. 78–81.

63. Burg G, Hoffmann FG, Nikolowski J, Schmoeckel C, Braun-Falco O, Stunkel K: Lymphomatoid papulosis: a cutaneous T-cell pseudolymphoma. *Acta Derm Venereol Stockh* 61:491–496, 1981.

64. Kadin M, Nasu K, Sako D, Said J, Vonderheid E: Lymphomatoid papulosis. A cutaneous proliferation of activated helper T cells expressing Hodgkin's disease-associated antigens. *Am J Pathol* 119:315–325, 1985.

65. Kaudewitz P, Burg G, Stein H, Klepzig K, Mason DY, Braun-Falco O: Monoclonal antibody patterns in lymphomatoid papulosis. *Dermatol Clin* 3:749–757, 1985.

66. Kaudewitz P, Stein H, Burg G, Mason DY, Braun-Falco O: Atypical cells in lymphomatoid papulosis express the Hodgkin cell-associated antigen Ki-1. *J Invest Dermatol* 86:350–354, 1986.

67. Weiss LM, Wood GS, Trela M, Warnke RA, Sklar J: Clonal T-cell populations in lymphomatoid papulosis. Evidence of a lymphoproliferative origin for a clinically benign disease. *N Engl J Med* 315:475–479, 1986.

68. Davis TH, Morton CC, Miller CR, Balk SP, Kadin ME: Hodgkin's disease, lymphomatoid papulosis, and cutaneous T-cell lymphoma derived from a common T-cell clone. *N Engl J Med* 326:1115–1122, 1992.

69. Convit J, Kerdel F, Goihman M., et al: Progressive, atrophing, chronic granulomatous dermohypodermitis. Autoimmune disease? *Arch Dermatol* 107:271, 1973.

70. Ackerman AB: *Histologic Diagnosis of Inflammatory Skin Diseases.* Philadelphia: Lea & Febiger, 1978.

71. LeBoit PE: Granulomatous slack skin. *Dermatol Clin* 12:375–389, 1994.

72. Camacho F, Burg G, Moreno JC, Campora RC, Villar JL: Granulomatous slack skin in childhood. *Ped Dermatol*, 14:204–208, 1997.

73. Puig S, Iranzo P, Palou J, et al: Lymphoproliferative nature of granulomatous slack skin. Clonal rearrangement of the T-cell receptor-gene. *Arch Dermatol* 128:562–563, 1992.

74. Winkelmann RK, Bowie EJW: Hemorrhagic diathesis associated with benign histiocytic, cytophagic panniculitis and systemic histiocytosis. *Arch Intern Med* 140:1460–1463, 1980.

75. Grange F, Avril MF, Duvillard P, Bosq J, Ollivaud L, Ortoli JC, Guillaume JC: Subcutaneous anaplastic Ki1+ large cell lymphoma with clinical aspect of panniculitis. *Ann Dermatol Venereol* 119 890–892, 1992.

76. Perniciaro C, Zalla MJ, White JJ, Menke DM: Subcutaneous T-cell lymphoma. Report of two additional cases and further observations. *Arch Dermatol* 129:1171–1176, 1993.

77. Mehregan DA, Su WP, Kurtin PJ: Subcutaneous T-cell lymphoma: a clinical, histopathologic, and immunohistochemical study of six cases. *J Cutan Pathol* 21:110–117, 1994.

78. Chan JKC, Tsang WYW, Lo ESF: Cutaneous angiocentric T-cell lymphoma and subcutaneous panniculitic T-cell lymphoma are distinct entities. *Mod Pathol* 9:109, 1996.

79. Wang CE, Su WPD, Kurtin PJ: Subcutaneous panniculitic T-cell lymphoma. *Int J Dermatol* 35:1–8, 1996.

80. Nagatani T, Miyazawa M, Matsuzaki T, Iemoto G, Ishii H, Kim ST, Baba N, Miyamoto H, Minato K, Motomura S, et. al: Adult T-cell leukemia/lymphoma (ATL): Clinical, histopathological, immunological and immunohistochemical characteristics. *Exp Dermatol* 1:248–252, 1992.

81. Arai E, Chow KC, Li CY, Tokunaga M, Katayama I: Differentiation between cutaneous form of adult T cell leukemia/lymphoma and cutaneous T cell lymphoma by in situ hybridization using a human T cell leukemia virus-1 DNA probe. *Am J Pathol* 144:15–20, 1994.

82. Urrutia S, Piris MA, Orradre JL, Martinez B, Cruz MA, Garcia AD: Cytotoxic/suppressor (CD8+, CD4−) cutaneous T-cell lymphoma with aggressive course. *Am J Dermatopathol* 12:603–606, 1990.

83. Marti RM, Estrach T, Palou J, Urbano IA, Gratacos J, Cervera R, Feliu E, Grau JM, Mascaro JM: Specific cutaneous lesions in a CD8+ peripheral T-cell lymphoma. *Int J Dermatol* 31:624–628, 1992.

84. Fujiwara Y, Abe Y, Kuyama M, Arata J, Yoshino T, Akagi T, Miyoshi K: CD8+ cutaneous T-cell lymphoma with pagetoid epidermotropism and angiocentric and angiodestructive infiltration. *Arch Dermatol* 126:801–804, 1990.

85. Kikuchi A, Naka W, Harada T, Nishikawa T: Primary CD8+ lymphoepithelioid lymphoma of the skin. *J Am Acad Dermatol* 29:419–422, 1993.

86. Avinoach I, Halevy S, Argov S, Sacks M: Gamma/delta T-cell lymphoma involving the subcutaneous tissue and associated with a hemophagocytic syndrome. *Am J Dermatopathol* 16:426–433, 1994.

87. Heald P, Buckley P, Gilliam A, Perez M, Knobler R, Kacinski B, Edelson R: Correlations of unique clinical, immunotypic, and histologic findings in cutaneous gamma/delta T-cell lymphoma. *J Am Acad Dermatol* 26:865–70, 1992.

88. Dummer R, Potoczna N, Haeffner AC, Zimmermann DR, Gilardi S, Burg G: A primary cutaneous non-T, non-B CD4+, CD56+ lymphoma. *Arch Dermatol* 132: 550–553, 1996.

89. Kempf W, Dummer R, Haeffner A, Mueller B, Dommann-Scherrer C, Zimmermann D, Panizzon R, Burg G: Juvenile granulomatous cutaneous T-cell lymphoma: a new entity in cutaneous lymphomas? (abstract). *Am J Dermatopathol* 1997 (in press).

90. Burg G, Schmockel C: Syringolymphoid hyperplasia with alopecia: A syringotropic cutaneous T-cell lymphoma? *Dermatology* 184:306–307, 1992.

91. Zelger B, Sepp N, Weyrer K, Grunewald K, Zelger B: Syringotropic cutaneous T-cell lymphoma. A variant of mycosis fungoides? *Br J Dermatol* 130:765–769, 1994.

92. Cho KH, Kim CW, et al: An Epstein-Barr virus-associated lymphoproliferative lesion of the skin presenting as recurrent nekrotic papulovesicles of the face. *Br J Dermatol* 134:791–796, 1996.

93. Caro WA, Helwig EB: Cutaneous lymphoid hyperplasia. *Cancer* 24:487, 1969.

94. Kerl H, Kresbach H: Lymphoretikuläre Hyperplasien und Neoplasien der Haut, in Schnyder UW (ed): Spezielle pathologische Anatomie. Berlin: Springer Verlag, 1979, p. 396.

95. Crowson AN, Magro CM: Antidepressant therapy. A possible cause of atypical cutaneous lymphoid hyperplasia. *Arch Dermatol* 131:925, 1995.

96. Rijlaarsdam JU, Meijer CJLM, Willemze R: Differentiation between lymphadenosis benigna cutis and primary cutaneous follicular center cell lymphomas: a comparative clinicopathologic study of 57 patients. *Cancer* 65:2301, 1990.

97. Kerl H, Ackerman AB: Inflammatory diseases that simulate lymphomas: Cutaneous pseudolymphomas, in Fitzpatrick TB, et al: *Dermatology in General Medicine.* New York: McGraw-Hill, 1993, p. 1315.

98. Kerl H, Kresbach H: Lymphoretikuläre Hyperplasien und Neoplasien der Haut, in Schnyder UW (ed): *Spezielle pathologische Anatomie.* Berlin: Springer Verlag, 1979, p. 351.

99. Willemze R, Rijlaarsdam JU, Beljaards RC, Meijer CJLM: Classification of primary cutaneous lymphomas. Historical overview and perspectives. *Dermatology* 189:8, 1994.

100. Cerroni L, Smolle J, Soyer HP, Martinez-Aparicio A, Kerl H. Immunophenotyping of cutaneous lymphoid infiltrates in frozen and paraffin-embedded tissue sections: A comparative study. *J Am Acad Dermatol* 22:405, 1990.

101. Wallace ML, Smoller BR. Immunohistochemistry in diagnostic dermatopathology. *J Am Acad Dermatol* 34:163, 1996.

102. Kerl H, Kresbach H. Germinal center cell-derived lymphomas of the skin. *J Derm Surg Oncol* 10:291, 1984.

103. Garcia CF, Weiss LM, Warnke RA, Wood GS: Cutaneous follicular lymphoma. *Am J Surg Pathol* 10:454, 1986.

104. Willemze R, Meijer CJLM, Sentis HJ, Scheffer E, van Vloten WA, Toonstra J, et al: Primary cutaneous large cell lymphomas of follicular center cell origin: A clinical follow-up study of 19 patients. *J Am Acad Dermatol* 16:518, 1987.

105. Berti E, Alessi E, Caputo R, Gianotti R, Delia D, Vezzoni P: Reticulohistiocytoma of the dorsum. *J Am Acad Dermatol* 19:259, 1988.

106. Pimpinelli N, Santucci M, Bosi A, Moretti S, Vallecchi C, Messori A, et al: Primary cutaneous follicular centre cell lymphoma: A lymphoproliferative disease with favourable prognosis. *Clin Exp Dermatol* 14:12, 1989.

107. Cerroni L, Volkenandt M, Rieger E, Soyer HP, Kerl H: bcl-2 Protein expression and correlation with the interchromosomal 14;18 translocation in cutaneous lymphomas and pseudolymphomas. *J Invest Dermatol* 102:231, 1994.

108. Rijlaarsdam JU, van der Putte SCJ, Berti E, Kerl H, Rieger E, Toonstra J, et al: Cutaneous immunocytomas: A clinicopathologic study of 26 cases. *Histopathology* 23:117, 1993.

109. LeBoit PE, McNutt NS, Reed JA, Jacobson M, Weiss LM. Primary cutaneous immunocytoma. A B-cell lymphoma that can easily be mistaken for cutaneous lymphoid hyperplasia. *Am J Surg Pathol* 18:969, 1994.

110. Isaacson PG, Norton AJ: *Extranodal Lymphomas.* Edinburgh: Churchill Livingstone, 1994.

111. Slater DN: MALT and SALT: The clue to cutaneous B-cell lymphoproliferative disease. *Br J Dermatol* 131:557, 1994.

112. Santucci M, Pimpinelli N, Arganini L: Primary cutaneous B-cell lymphoma: A unique type of low-grade lymphoma. Clinicopathologic and immunologic study of 83 cases. *Cancer* 67:2311, 1991.

113. Garbe C, Stein H, Dienemann D, Orfanos CE: Borrelia-burgdorferi-associated cutaneous B cell lymphoma: Clinical and immunohistologic characterization of four cases. *J Am Acad Dermatol* 24:584, 1991.

114. Cerroni L, Signoretti S, Kütting B, Annessi G, Metze D, Giannetti A, et al: Marginal zone B-cell lymphoma of the skin. *J Cut Pathol* 23:47, 1996.

115. Banks PM, Chan J, Cleary ML, Delsol G, De Wolf-Peeters C, Gatter K, et al: Mantle cell lymphoma. *Am J Surg Pathol* 16:637, 1992.

116. Torne R, Su WPD, Winkelmann RK, Smolle J, Kerl H: Clinicopathologic study of cutaneous plasmacytoma. *Int J Dermatol* 29:562, 1990.

117. Wong KF, Chan JKC, Li LPK, Yau TK, Lee AWM: Primary cutaneous plasmacytoma. Report of two cases and review of the literature. *Am J Dermatopathol* 16:392, 1994.

118. Tüting T, Bork K: Primary plasmacytoma of the skin. *J Am Acad Dermatol* 34:386, 1996.

119. Jenkins RE, Calonje E, Fawcett H, Greaves MW, Wilson-Jones E. Cutaneous crystalline deposits in myeloma. *Arch Dermatol* 130:484, 1994.

120. Hurt MA, Santa Cruz DJ: Cutaneous inflammatory pseudotumor. *Am J Surg Pathol* 14:764, 1990.

121. Vermeer MH, Geelen AMJ, van Haselen CW, van Voorst Vader PC, Geerts ML, van Vloten WA, et al: Primary cutaneous large B-cell lymphomas of the legs. *Arch Dermatol*, 132:1304–1308, 1996.

122. Grümayer ER, Ladenstein RL, Slavc I, Urban C, Radaszkiewicz T, Bettelheim P, et al: B-cell differentiation pattern of cutaneous lymphomas in infancy and childhood. *Cancer* 61:303, 1988.

123. Kamps WA, Poppema S: Pre-B-cell non-Hodgkin's lymphoma in childhood. *Am J Clin Pathol* 90:103, 1988.

124. Sander CA, Medeiros LJ, Abruzzo LV, Horak ID, Jaffe ES: Lymphoblastic lymphoma presenting in cutaneous sites: A clinicopathologic analysis of six cases. *J Am Acad Dermatol* 25:1023, 1991.

125. Knowles DM. Lymphoblastic lymphoma, in Knowles DM (ed): *Neoplastic Hematopathology.* Baltimore: Williams & Wilkins, 1992, p. 715.

126. Hummel M, Ziemann K, Lammert H, Pileri S, Sabattini E, Stein H: Hodgkin's disease with monoclonal and polyclonal populations of Reed-Sternberg cells. *N Engl J Med* 333:901, 1995.

127. Smith JL, Butler JJ: Skin involvement in Hodgkin's disease. *Cancer* 45:354, 1980.

128. White RM, Patterson JW: Cutaneous involvement in Hodgkin's disease. *Cancer* 55:1136, 1985.

129. Sioutos N, Kerl H, Murphy SB, Kadin ME: Primary cutaneous Hodgkin's disease: Unique clinical, morphologic, and immunophenotypic findings. *Am J Dermatopathol* 16:2, 1994.

130. Cerroni L, Beham-Schmid C, Kerl H. Cutaneous Hodgkin's disease: An immunohistochemical analysis. *J Cut Pathol* 22:229, 1995.

131. Moretti S, Pimpinelli N, Di Lollo S, Vallecchi C, Bosi A: In situ immunologic characterization of cutaneous involvement in Hodgkin's disease. *Cancer* 63:661, 1989.

132. Davis TH, Morton CC, Miller-Cassman R, Balk SP, Kadin ME: Hodgkin's disease, lymphomatoid papulosis, and cutaneous T-cell lymphoma derived from a common T-cell clone. *N Engl J Med* 326:1115, 1992.

133. Mizoguchi M, Kawa Y, Minami T, Nakayama H, Mizoguchi H: Cutaneous extramedullary hematopoiesis in myelofibrosis. *J Am Acad Dermatol* 22:351, 1990.

134. Schofield JK, Shun JL, Cerio R, Grice K: Cutaneous extramedullary hematopoiesis with a preponderance of atypical megakaryocytes in myelofibrosis. *J Am Acad Dermatol* 22:334, 1990.

135. Hoss DM, McNutt NS: Cutaneous myelofibrosis. *J Cut Pathol* 19:221, 1992.

136. Patel BM, Su WP, Perniciaro C, Gertz MA: Cutaneous extramedullary hematopoiesis. *J Am Acad Dermatol* 32:805, 1995.

137. Buechner SA, Su WPD: Leukemia cutis, in Arndt KA, Robinson JK, Leboit PE, et al (eds): *Cutaneous Medicine and Surgery.* Philadelphia: WB Saunders, 1996, pp. 1670–1673.

138. Su WPD: Clinical, histopathologic, and immunohistochemical correlations in leukemia cutis. *Semin Dermatol* 13: 223, 1994.

139. Dreizen S, McCredie KB, Keating MJ, et al: Leukemia-associated skin infiltrates. *Postgrad Med* 85:45, 1989.

140. Bluefarb SM: *Leukemia Cutis.* Springfield, IL: Charles C Thomas, 1960.

141. Longacre TA, Smoller BR: Leukemia cutis. Analysis of 50 biopsy-proven cases with an emphasis on occurrence in myelodysplastic syndromes. *Am J Clin Pathol* 100: 276, 1993.

142. Su WPD, Buechner SA, Li CY: Clinicopathologic correlations in leukemia cutis. *J Am Acad Dermatol* 11:121, 1984.

143. Ratnam KV, Khor CJ, Su WPD: Leukemia cutis. *Dermatol Clin* 12:419, 1994.

144. Piette WW: An approach to cutaneous changes caused by hematologic malignancies. *Dermatol Clin* 7:467, 1989.

145. Bennett JM, Catovsky D, Daniel MT, et al: Proposals for the classification of the acute leukaemias. French-American-British (FAB) cooperative group. *Br J Haematol* 33: 451, 1976.

146. Bennett JM, Catovsky D, Daniel MT, et al: Proposed revised criteria for the classification of acute myeloid leukemia. A report of the French-American-British Cooperative Group. *Ann Intern Med* 103:620, 1985.

147. Bennett JM, Catovsky D, Daniel MT, et al: Proposals for the classification of chronic (mature) B and T lymphoid leukaemias. French-American-British (FAB) Cooperative Group. *J Clin Pathol* 42:567, 1989.

148. Uchiyama T, Yodoi J, Sagawa K, et al: Adult T-cell leukemia: Clinical and hematologic features of 16 cases. *Blood* 50:481, 1977.

149. Davey FR, Hutchison RE: Pathology and immunology of adult T-cell leukemia/lymphoma. *Curr Opin Oncol* 3:13, 1991.

150. Bennett JM, Catovsky D, Daniel MT, et al: Proposals for the classification of the myelodysplastic syndromes. *Br J Haematol* 51:189, 1982.

151. Bonvalet D, Foldes C, Civatte J: Cutaneous manifestations in chronic lymphocytic leukemia. *J Dermatol Surg Oncol* 10:278, 1984.

152. Ricevuti G, Mazzone A, Rossini S, et al: Skin involvement in hemopathies: Specific cutaneous manifestations of acute nonlymphoid leukemias and non-Hodgkin lymphomas. *Dermatologica* 171:250, 1985.

153. Baer MR, Barcos M, Farrell H, et al: Acute myelogenous leukemia with leukemia cutis. Eighteen cases seen between 1969 and 1986. *Cancer* 63:2192, 1989.

154. Ochonisky S, Aractingi S, Dombret H, et al: Acute undifferentiated myeloblastic leukemia revealed by specific hemorrhagic bullous lesions (letter). *Arch Dermatol* 129:512, 1993.

155. Zax RH, Kulp-Shorten CL, Callen JP: Leukemia cutis presenting as a scrotal ulcer. *J Am Acad Dermatol* 21:410, 1989.

156. Dreizen S, McCredie KB, Keating MJ, et al: Malignant gingival and skin "infiltrates" in adult leukemia. *Oral Surg Oral Med Oral Pathol* 55:572, 1983.

157. Murphy WG, Fotheringham GH, Busuttil A, et al: Skin lesions in chronic granulocytic leukemia. Treatment of a patient with topical nitrogen mustard. *Cancer* 55:2630, 1985.

158. Buescher L, Anderson PC: Circinate plaques heralding juvenile chronic myelogenous leukemia. *Pediatr Dermatol* 7:122, 1990.

159. Heskel NS, White CR, Fryberger S, et al: Aleukemic leukemia cutis: Juvenile chronic granulocytic leukemia presenting with figurate cutaneous lesions. *J Am Acad Dermatol* 9:423, 1983.

160. Sun NC, Ellis R: Granulocytic sarcoma of the skin. *Arch Dermatol* 116:800, 1980.

161. McCarty KS Jr, Wortman J, Daly J, et al: Chloroma (granulocytic sarcoma) without evidence of leukemia: Facilitated light microscopic diagnosis. *Blood* 56:104, 1980.

162. Long JC, Mihm MC: Multiple granulocytic tumors of the skin: Report of six cases of myelogenous leukemia with initial manifestations in the skin. *Cancer* 39:2004, 1977.

163. Ritter JH, Goldstein NS, Argenyi Z, et al: Granulocytic sarcoma: An immunohistologic comparison with peripheral T-cell lymphoma in paraffin sections. *J Cutan Pathol* 21: 207, 1994.

164. Buechner SA, Li CY, Su WPD: Leukemia cutis. A histopathologic study of 42 cases. *Am J Dermatopathol* 7:109, 1985.

165. Ratnam KV, Su WPD, Ziesmer SC, et al: Value of immunohistochemistry in the diagnosis of leukemia cutis: Study of 54 cases using paraffin-section markers. *J Cutan Pathol* 19:193, 1992.

166. Grob JJ, Gabriel B, Horchowski N, et al: Bullous cutaneous localization with epidermotropism in monoblastic leukemia. [French]. *Ann Dermatol Venereol* 115:59, 1988.

167. Ohno S, Yokoo T, Ohta M, et al: Aleukemic leukemia cutis. *J Am Acad Dermatol* 22:374, 1990.

168. Resnik KS, Brod BB: Leukemia cutis in congenital leukemia. Analysis and review of the world literature with report of an additional case. *Arch Dermatol* 129:1301, 1993.

169. Gottesfeld E, Silverman RA, Coccia PF, et al: Transient blueberry muffin appearance of a newborn with congenital monoblastic leukemia. *J Am Acad Dermatol* 21:347, 1989.

170. Pujol RM, Lopez D, Badell I, et al: Congenital monoblastic leukemia and self-healing papulonodular cutaneous lesions [French]. *Ann Dermatol Venereol* 117:878, 1990.

171. Sepp N, Radaszkiewicz T, Meijer CJ, et al: Specific skin manifestations in acute leukemia with monocytic differentiation. A morphologic and immunohistochemical study of 11 cases. *Cancer* 71:124, 1993.

172. Lukens JN: Classification and differentiation of the acute leukemias, in Lee GR, Bithell TC, Foerster J, et al. (eds): *Wintrobe's Clinical Hematology,* vol 2, 9th ed. Philadelphia: Lea & Febiger, 1993, pp. 1873–1892.

173. O'Connell DM, Fagan WA, Skinner SM, et al: Cutaneous involvement in chronic myelomonocytic leukemia. *Int J Dermatol* 33:628, 1994.

174. Baden TJ, Gammon WR: Leukemia cutis in acute myelomonocytic leukemia. Preferential localization in a recent Hickman catheter scar. *Arch Dermatol* 123:88, 1987.

175. Horlick HP, Silvers DN, Knobler EH, et al: Acute myelomonocytic leukemia presenting as a benign-appearing cutaneous eruption. *Arch Dermatol* 126:653, 1990.

176. De Coninck A, De Hou MF, Peters O, et al: Aleukemic leukemia cutis. An unusual presentation of acute myelomonocytic leukemia. *Dermatologica* 172:272, 1986.

177. Eubanks SW, Patterson JW: Subacute myelomonocytic leukemia—an unusual skin manifestation. *J Am Acad Dermatol* 9:581, 1983.

178. Hoen B, Neidhardt AC, Aghassian C, et al: Acute myelomonocytic leukemia revealed by a chickenpox-like rash. *J Eur Acad Dermatol Venereol* 6:76, 1996.

179. Kaiserling E, Horny HP, Geerts ML, et al: Skin involvement in myelogenous leukemia: Morphologic and immunophenotypic heterogeneity of skin infiltrates. *Mod Pathol* 7:771, 1994.

180. Yam LT: Acute myelomonocytic leukemia: Coexistent cytochemical markers for monocytes and granulocytes in the leukemic cells. *So Med J* 72:670, 1979.

181. Wong TY, Suster S, Bouffard D, et al: Histologic spectrum of cutaneous involvement in patients with myelogenous leukemia including the neutrophilic dermatoses. *Int J Dermatol* 34:323, 1995.

182. Jordaan HF: Acute febrile neutrophilic dermatosis. A histopathological study of 37 patients and a review of the literature. *Am J Dermatopathol* 11:99, 1989.

183. Foerster J: Chronic lymphocytic leukemia, in Lee GR, Bithell TC, Foerster J, et al. (eds): *Wintrobe's Clinical Hematology,* vol 2, 9th ed. Philadelphia: Lea & Febiger, 1993, pp. 2034–2047.

184. Epstein E, MacEachern K: Dermatologic manifestations of lymphoblastoma-leukemia group. *Arch Intern Med* 60: 867, 1937.

185. Fayolle J, Coeur P, Bryon PA, et al: Cutaneous manifestations of chronic lymphoid leukemia. Apropos of 44 cases from a personal series of 430 cases of chronic lymphoid leukemia. [French]. *Ann Dermatol Syphiligr* (Paris) 100:5, 1973.

186. Beek CH: Skin manifestations associated with lymphatic-leucaemia. *Dermatologica* 96:350, 1948.

187. High DA, Luscombe HA, Kauh YC: Leukemia cutis masquerading as chronic paronychia. *Int J Dermatol* 24:595, 1985.

188. Simon CA, Su WPD, Li CY: Subungual leukemia cutis. *Int J Dermatol* 29:636, 1990.

189. Ausubel H, Levine ML, Shapiro L: Leukemia cutis manuum. *N Y State J Med* 70:2835, 1970.

190. Calvert RJ, Smith E: Metastatic acropachy in lymphatic leukemia. *Blood* 10:545, 1955.

191. Desvignes V, Bosq J, Guillaume JC, et al: Papulovesicular eruption of the face in chronic lymphoid leukemia [French]. *Ann Dermatol Venereol* 117:880, 1990.

192. Rosen LB, Frank BL, Rywlin AM: A characteristic vesiculobullous eruption in patients with chronic lymphocytic leukemia. *J Am Acad Dermatol* 15:943, 1986.

193. Batata A, Shen B: Immunophenotyping of subtypes of B-chronic (mature) lymphoid leukemia. A study of 242 cases. *Cancer* 70:2436, 1992.

194. Golomb HM, Catovsky D, Golde DW: Hairy cell leukemia: A clinical review based on 71 cases. *Ann Intern Med* 89:677, 1978.

195. Damasio EE, Spriano M, Repetto M, et al: Hairy cell leukemia: A retrospective study of 235 cases by the Italian Cooperative Group (ICGHCL) according to Jansen's clinical staging system. *Acta Haematol* 72:326, 1984.

196. Finan MC, Su WPD, Li CY: Cutaneous findings in hairy cell leukemia. *J Am Acad Dermatol* 11:788, 1984.

197. Carsuzaa F, Pierre C, Jaubert D, et al: Cutaneous findings in hairy cell leukemia: Review of 84 cases. *Nouv Rev Fr Hematol* 35:541, 1994.

198. Kurzrock R, Cohen PR: Mucocutaneous paraneoplastic manifestations of hematologic malignancies. *Am J Med* 99:207, 1995.

199. Arai E, Ikeda S, Itoh S, et al: Specific skin lesions as the presenting symptom of hairy cell leukemia. *Am J Clin Pathol* 90:459, 1988.

200. Lawrence DM, Sun NC, Mena R, et al: Cutaneous lesions in hairy-cell leukemia. Case report and review of the literature. *Arch Dermatol* 119:322, 1983.

201. Bilsland D, Shahriari S, Douglas WS, et al: Transient leukaemia cutis in hairy-cell leukaemia. *Clin Exp Dermatol* 16:207, 1991.

202. Yamaguchi K: Human T-lymphotropic virus type I in Japan. *Lancet* 343:213, 1994.

203. Hall WW: Human T cell lymphotropic virus type I and cutaneous T cell leukemia/lymphoma. *J Exp Med* 180:1581, 1994.

204. Arai E, Chow KC, Li CY, et al: Differentiation between cutaneous form of adult T cell leukemia/lymphoma and cutaneous T cell lymphoma by in situ hybridization using a human T cell leukemia virus-1 DNA probe. *Am J Pathol* 144:15, 1994.

205. Dosaka N, Tanaka T, Miyachi Y, et al: Examination of HTLV-I integration in the skin lesions of various types of adult T-cell leukemia (ATL): Independence of cutaneous-type ATL confirmed by Southern blot analysis. *J Invest Dermatol* 96:196, 1991.

206. Nagatani T, Miyazawa M, Matsuzaki T, et al: Adult T-cell leukemia/lymphoma (ATL)—clinical, histopathological, immunological and immunohistochemical characteristics. *Exp Dermatol* 1:248, 1992.

207. Chan HL, Su IJ, Kuo TT, et al: Cutaneous manifestations of adult T cell leukemia/lymphoma. Report of three different forms. *J Am Acad Dermatol* 13:213, 1985.

208. Maeda K, Takahashi M: Characterization of skin infiltrating cells in adult T-cell leukaemia/lymphoma (ATLL): Clinical, histological and immunohistochemical studies on eight cases. *Br J Dermatol* 121:603, 1989.

209. Nagatani T, Miyazawa M, Matsuzaki T, et al: Comparative study of cutaneous T-cell lymphoma and adult T-cell leukemia/lymphoma. *Semin Dermatol* 13:216, 1994.

CHAPTER 35

CUTANEOUS METASTASES

Randall J. Margolis

A metastasis is a neoplastic tumor no longer in continuity with and often not in close proximity to the primary malignant tumor.[1,2] In various studies, the frequency of cutaneous metastases ranges from 0.6 to 9 percent,[3–7] and in a recent study of 4020 patients with metastatic disease, 10.4 percent had cutaneous metastases.[8] Of those 420 patients with cutaneous metastases, the skin metastases were the first sign of extranodal disease in 7.6 percent of patients. In another study of 7316 cancer patients, 1 percent had cutaneous metastases at the time that their malignancy was diagnosed, and in 0.6 percent of these patients, the skin metastasis was the first sign of a malignancy.[9] Thus, although skin metastases are in general relatively uncommon, they may be the initial presentation of metastatic disease.

The greatest incidence of cutaneous metastases is in the fifth, sixth, and seventh decades, and the types of tumors that metastasize to the skin reflect the overall incidence of the primary tumors in the general population and their biologic behavior. From studies by Brownstein and Helwig,[3,4] the incidence of primary tumors in women and men with skin metastases are listed in Table 35-1. In women, the distribution was breast 69 percent, large intestine 9 percent, melanoma 5 percent, lung 4 percent, ovary 4 percent, sarcoma 2 percent, uterine cervix 2 percent, pancreas 2 percent, squamous cell carcinoma of the oral cavity 1 percent, and urinary bladder 1 percent. In men, the distribution was lung 24 percent, large intestine 19 percent, melanoma 13 percent, squamous cell carcinoma of the oral cavity 12 percent, kidney 6 percent, stomach

TABLE 35-2

Mechanisms of Metastases

Sequence of events:
1. Detachment from the primary tumor
2. Invasion and intravasation of tumor cells into a vessel
3. Passage through the blood or lymphatic circulatory system
4. Stasis within recipient tissue
5. Extravasation of cells from the circulation and invasion into the target tissue
6. Proliferation of tumor cells in the recipient site

6 percent, esophagus 3 percent, sarcoma 3 percent, pancreas 2 percent, salivary gland 2 percent, urinary bladder 2 percent, breast 2 percent, and prostate, thyroid, liver, and squamous cell carcinoma of the skin together 1 percent. Of note in this study of metastases seen in dermatologic consultation is the fact that the underlying malignancy was undiagnosed at the time of skin metastasis in 60 percent with lung cancer, 53 percent with renal cancer, and 40 percent with ovarian cancer. In men, skin metastases were the presenting sign in 37 percent, as opposed to only 6 percent in women, presumably because breast cancer can be diagnosed earlier in women than lung cancer in men. In a subsequent study by Lookingbill et al. regarding skin metastases in a population of patients with metastatic disease, the most frequent tumors to metastasize to the skin in women were breast (70.7 percent), melanoma (12 percent), ovary (3.3 percent), and unknown (3.0 percent).[8] In men they were melanoma (32.3 percent), lung (11.8 percent), colon and rectum (11.0 percent), oral cavity (8.7 percent), unknown (8.7 percent), larynx (5.5 percent), kidney (4.7 percent), and upper digestive tract (3.9 percent) (Table 35-1).

Although some tumors have contiguous spread or spread into incisional scars by direct extension, the pathway of regional or distant metastases is through lymphatic or blood vessels.[5] The mechanisms responsible for metastasis can be broken down into six conceptual steps[1,10–14] (Table 35-2).

CLINICAL AND MORPHOLOGICAL FEATURES

Cutaneous metastases can take a variety of forms and occur in a number of locations, although none of them are entirely specific either for the type of tumor or the site of the primary malignancy.

Metastatic tumors frequently are flesh-colored nodules or plaques; multiple lesions are more common than solitary lesions, and sometimes they have a zosteriform pattern.[15] Ulceration has been reported in 10 percent of breast carcinoma metastases, and 36 percent of melanoma

TABLE 35-1

Sites of Origin of Skin Metastases

Primary Site	Women (%)	Men (%)
Breast	69/70.7	2/2.4
Large intestine	9/1.3	19/11
Melanoma	5/12	13/32.3
Lung	4/2	24/11.8
Ovary	4/3.3	
Sarcoma	2/0	3/0
Uterine cervix	2/0.7	
Pancreas	2/0.3	2/0.8
Oral cavity	1/2.3	12/8.7
Bladder	1/1.3	2/2.4
Kidney	0/0	6/4.7
Stomach	0/0.7	6/0.8
Esophagus	0/0	3/2.4
Salivary gland	0/0	2/0
Prostate		1/0
Unknown primary site	0/3	0/8.7

SOURCES: Data from Brownstein and Helwig, 1972[4] and Lookingbill et al., 1993.[8]

TABLE 35-3

Types of Cutaneous Metastases from Breast Carcinomas

Clinical Type	Histopathological Features
Inflammatory: Erythematous patch that resembles cellulitis or figurate erythema	Dilatation and obstruction of lymphatics by tumor cells along with congestion of capillaries
En cuirasse (encasement in armor): Diffuse morphealike induration of the skin	Tumor cells in sheets and cords in association with dermal sclerosis
Telangiectatic carcinoma: Clustered, violaceous papulovesicles that may have associated hyperpigmentation	Both blood vessels and lymphatics filled with tumor cells
Nodular: Dermal nodules that may have ulceration and hyperpigmentation	Sheets and cords of tumor cells in the dermis
Alopecia neoplastica: Scarring alopecia with a smooth surface and some erythema	Tumor cell infiltration with dermal fibrosis and a loss of appendages
Paget's disease: Nipple or areola with persistent erythema, scaling, oozing, and crusting	The epidermis is permeated by cells lying singly and in groups; the cells are larger, rounder, and paler than the surrounding keratinocytes
Inframammary crease metastasis: Exophytic nodule or may resemble intertriginous dermatitis	Dermal infiltrate of tumor cells
Eyelid metastasis: Asymptomatic papules	Histiocytoid cells in 8 of 13 cases that resemble xanthoma, histiocytoma, or granular cell tumor

metastases are pigmented, according to Lookingbill et al.[8] Metastases from renal cell, thyroid follicular, and choriocarcinomas are frequently red-purple and hemorrhagic. Both renal cell and thyroid metastases, which often spread to bone, may produce a pulsating mass with a detectable bruit in the overlying skin.[5,8,16–19] Breast carcinoma is associated with eight types of cutaneous metastases if one includes Paget's disease, although none are unique to breast carcinoma[20] (Table 35-3). Inflammatory carcinoma is a red patch that resembles cellulitis or a figurate or gyrate erythema and results from the dilatation and obstruction of lymphatics by tumor cells and congestion of capillaries.[21,22] En cuirasse (encasement in armor) metastases have diffuse morphealike indurations of the skin resulting from dermal sclerosis in association with tumor cells.[23] Telangiectatic metastases are composed of clustered, violaceous papulovesicles that may have such prominent pigmentation that they resemble metastatic melanoma.[24,25] In the latter type of metastasis, both the blood vessels and lymphatics are filled with tumor, and the obstructed lymphatics are more superficial than those involved in inflammatory carcinoma.[26] Nodular metastatic lesions from the breast, in addition to being ulcerated, on occasion may also be pigmented and mimic pigmented basal cell carcinoma or malignant melanoma.[8,25,27]

Alopecia neoplastica is a form of scarring alopecia, as the name implies, secondary to a neoplastic process, such as metastatic breast carcinoma, and may be the initial presentation of the tumor.[28] It is characterized by alopecia, a smooth surface, and some red-pink erythema and needs to be distinguished from other forms of scarring alopecia[5] (see Chap. 10). In 1874, Paget first noted the association of breast carcinoma and "long persistent eczema" of the nipple and areola, now known as *Paget's disease of the breast*.[29] Extramammary Paget's disease involves the vulva, male genital area, perianal area, and rarely the axilla, external ear, and eyelid in association with underlying carcinomas.[30–33] Metastatic tumors of the inframammary crease may present as an exophytic nodule suggestive of a primary squamous or basal cell carcinoma or may resemble an intertriginous dermatitis.[34,35] The final variant is metastatic involvement of the eyelids. These are asymptomatic papules that in 8 of 13 reported cases have histiocytoid cells that resemble xanthoma, histiocytoma, or granular cell myoblastoma cells.[36]

Metastases are seen most often in the vicinity of the primary tumor.[8] Squamous cell carcinomas of the head and neck metastasize to actini-

cally damaged skin in the area and sometimes can be impossible to distinguish from primary cutaneous squamous cell carcinoma.[4] Breast and lung cancers frequently metastasize to the chest wall, and abdominal tumors, such as those arising in the gastrointestinal tract, ovary, or bladder, most often metastasize to the abdominal wall.[8] Umbilical metastases, called *Sister Joseph nodules*, come from intraabdominal malignancies that include tumors from the stomach, colon, pancreas, and bladder.[37–40] Lower abdominal and groin metastases originate from primary tumors in the cervix, urinary tract, prostate, and rectum.[3,4,41–45] Local metastases also may develop at the site of scars from previous surgical incisions, usually within a year of the procedure, or in unrelated surgical or traumatic scars.[5] Scar metastases at the excision site or as the first sign of metastatic disease have been seen with breast, ovarian, colorectal, liver, oral, laryngeal, lung, renal, and endometrial carcinomas.[5,8] In addition to occurring in scars, metastatic tumors may be seen in persistent fistulas after surgery.[46]

Distant cutaneous metastases have been reported in up to 39 percent of patients with metastases.[8] Melanoma, lung, and breast carcinoma most frequently metastasized to distant sites. Tumors associated with vascular invasion, which include melanoma, renal cell, thyroid follicular, and choriocarcinoma, are more frequently associated with distant metastases, and scalp metastases are disproportionately common in renal cell carcinoma.[3] Metastases to extremities are uncommon, usually occur late, are seen most often with melanoma and less often with breast, lung, kidney, and large intestine carcinomas.[3,8]

The time of onset of a cutaneous metastasis is variable and reflects the biologic behavior of the underlying malignancy. However, when a cutaneous metastasis does occur, it usually portends a poor prognosis.[5] Metastases to the skin can be delayed from 6 to 32 years with malignant melanoma, breast, renal cell, thyroid, colon, larynx, ovary, and bladder carcinomas.[5,16,47] Epithelioid cell sarcoma is a sarcoma that occurs on the extremities of young adults and is characterized by a long clinical course of local recurrences and distant metastases.[48,49]

Metastatic tumors can be classified broadly as adeno, squamous, undifferentiated, or miscellaneous carcinomas, although the site of origin is often unclear from the cutaneous metastasis.[5] Metastatic tumors also include sarcomas and cutaneous involvement by hematopoietic malignancies.

SITES OF ORIGIN OF METASTATIC TUMORS

Breast Carcinoma

In the most recent study available, cutaneous metastases from breast carcinoma account for 71 percent of the metastases in women and 2.4 percent of the metastases in men owing primarily to the difference in prevalence of this tumor in the two sexes.[8]

Clinical Features   Breast metastases frequently occur on the trunk, although they are seen less frequently on other parts of the body such as the upper extremities or scalp.[8] The cutaneous features include noninflammatory nodules along with presentations that are more closely associated with metastatic breast carcinoma[20] (Table 35-3). In addition to ductal carcinoma, other forms of breast carcinoma include lobular, tubular, cribriform, mucinous, and medullary carcinomas.[50,51]

Histopathological Features   Breast carcinoma metastatic to the skin may look like any type of primary invasive breast carcinoma. When the tumor is associated with other features, it gives rise to the various clinical patterns of cutaneous metastasis. In inflammatory carcinoma, tumor cells fill the lymphatics in the dermis and, in some cases, those found in the subcutaneous fat[5,52] (Fig. 35-1). Telangiectatic carcinoma has tumor cells in more superficially located lymphatics along with blood vessels congested with erythrocytes.[26] In nodular metastases, tumor cells predominate with some stromal fibrosis[24] (Fig. 35-2). In contrast to this, cancer en cuirasse has a predominantly fibrous stroma with a smaller portion of tumor cells (Fig. 35-3), and alopecia neoplastica has dermal fibrosis with a loss of hair follicles and an infiltrate of tumor cells.[5]

Invasive ductal carcinoma is the most common type of breast carcinoma. The epithelial cells have variable pleomorphism and infiltrate in sheets or cords of cells with or without glandular structures or signet-ring cells.[5,53] Infiltrating lobular carcinoma consists of small round to ovoid cells with scant cytoplasm, eccentric nuclei with little pleomorphism, and few mitoses. Intracytoplasmic lumina are most frequent in lobular carcinoma and are best seen with PAS–alcian blue stain or immunohistochemically with epithelial membrane antigen.[54] The Indian-file pattern of infiltration that is associated most often with this tumor consists of cords of cells in a single-file arrangement in a fibrotic stroma that was first described by Foote and Stewart; however, this pattern of infiltration does not appear to be associated exclusively with lobular carcinoma.[55,56] Other patterns include *alveolar*, with rounded

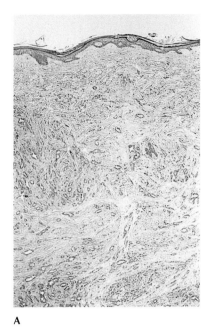

A

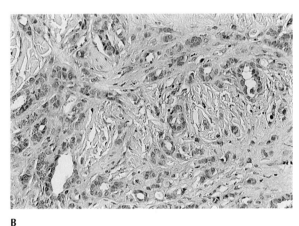

B

FIGURE 35-2   Nodular metastatic breast carcinoma. (*A*) Metastatic carcinoma with gland formation in association with a fibrotic stroma throughout the dermis. (*B*) Higher-power view of glandular tumor in a fibrotic stroma.

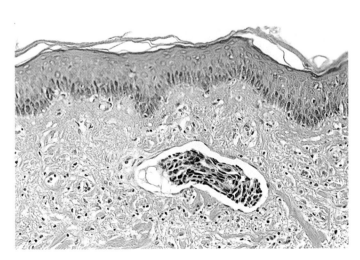

FIGURE 35-1   Inflammatory metastatic breast carcinoma. There is a dilated lymphatic vessel filled with a cluster of tumor cells.

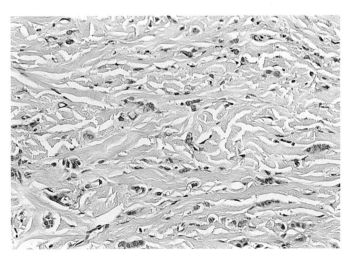

FIGURE 35-3   Cancer en cuirasse metastatic breast carcinoma. Small nests and strands of tumor cells in a so-called Indian-file pattern surrounded by dense, sclerotic collagen bundles.

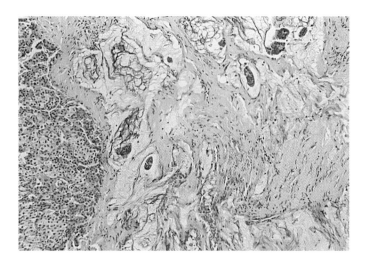

FIGURE 35-4 Colloid carcinoma of the breast in association with infiltrating ductal carcinoma, on the left. There is colloid carcinoma on the right with large spaces filled with extracellular mucin and small aggregates of tumor cells.

aggregates of 20 or more cells; *solid*, characterized by sheets of cells; *tubulolobular*, which has classic lobular infiltration along with microtubules with a single epithelial layer; and *mixed*.[57] Tubular carcinoma is made up of round to oval tubules lined by a single layer of cells larger than those seen in lobular carcinoma and frequently exhibiting apical snouts. There is little nuclear pleomorphism, mitoses are rare, and the tumor cells are embedded in a desmoplastic stroma. In tubular mixed carcinoma the glandular elements are seen in combination with more typical infiltrating ductal carcinoma.[51,58] Cribriform carcinoma resembles tubular carcinoma with tubules aggregated together in an irregular sievelike pattern.[59] Mucinous carcinoma, also referred to as *colloid* or *mucoid carcinoma*, consists of islands of uniform, small epithelial cells with hyperchromatic nuclei and a cribriform or papillary pattern in lakes of mucin[60] (Fig. 35-4). Medullary carcinoma has a poorly differentiated epithelial component with sheets of large, pleomorphic cells showing a high proportion of bizarre nuclei and many mitoses surrounded by a dense lymphoplasmacytic infiltrate.[61]

Differential Diagnosis   The various patterns of breast carcinoma each have their own list of conditions from which a cutaneous metastasis must be distinguished. A history of primary breast carcinoma is helpful, but care must be taken not to overlook another cutaneous primary or metastatic tumor.

Fibrotic nodules with diffuse infiltration of uniformly atypical sheets and cords of cells may suggest dermatofibroma, fibrosarcoma, desmoplastic melanoma, and Schwann cell tumors. When single-file rows or cords of deeply basophilic cells predominate, one may need to consider morphea-type basal cell carcinoma and malignant sweat gland tumors.[62] When there is gland formation with mucin, one should consider adenocarcinomas from gastrointestinal tract, lung, salivary gland, or lacrimal gland.[4,63] When there are islands of tumor cells in abundant mucin, one should consider mucinous carcinoma of eccrine glands or large intestine as the primary site.[64]

Special Stains and Immunohistochemistry   The mucin in tumor cells is PAS-positive and resistant to diastase and hyaluronidase but is sensitive to sialidase. It is positive for alcian blue at pH 2.5 but not pH 1 and 0.4, which is indicative of a nonsulfated mucin such as sialomucin, an epithelial mucin.[65] With immunoperoxidase studies, the cells are positive, as are many other epithelial cells, for epithelial membrane antigen and keratin. Using antibodies directed against gross cystic disease fluid protein-15 (GCDFP-15), the sensitivity, specificity, and positive predic-

tive value for metastatic breast carcinoma in the skin are 71, 91, and 94 percent, respectively. Antibodies against estrogen receptor protein (ERP) have a sensitivity, specificity, and positive predictive value of 73, 100, and 100 percent, respectively.[66] About 48 percent of breast carcinomas are positive for S-100 protein and 71 percent are positive for monoclonal carcinoembryonic antigen (CEA), and while this is not useful in distinguishing metastatic breast carcinoma from a primary sweat gland carcinoma, it is useful in excluding melanoma which is CEA-negative.[62,67–69]

Lung Carcinoma

Cutaneous metastases from lung carcinoma represent 12 to 24 percent of cutaneous metastases in men and 2 to 4 percent in women. Although only 1.5 percent of patients with lung cancer develop cutaneous metastases, such metastases occur in 52 to 60 percent of patients before the lung primary tumor is first recognized.[3,8,70] Chest, back, and abdomen are the most frequent sites of cutaneous metastasis, followed by the scalp and neck.[4]

Clinical Features   The usual presentation is a localized cluster of discrete, firm, nontender, flesh-colored nodules of recent onset and rapid growth to a certain size followed by a stationary period.[5] In addition, cutaneous metastases from the lung, in some cases, have a vascular appearance suggesting a hemangioma, pyogenic granuloma, or Kaposi's sarcoma.[5]

Histopathological Features   The types of carcinoma of the lung observed in the skin are adenocarcinoma (30 percent), squamous cell carcinoma (30 percent), and undifferentiated tumors, which include large cell undifferentiated and small (oat) cell carcinomas.[4,5] Much less commonly seen are bronchioalveolar, mucoepidermoid, carcinoid, and pulmonary sarcomas.[4,71,72]

Squamous cell carcinoma from the lung is usually moderately to poorly differentiated without evidence of epidermal origin. The tumor cells are dispersed in sheets and islands of epithelial cells with varying degrees of keratinization and intercellular bridges, and there are usually only a small number of whorls of squamous cells (pearls). The more atypical features of the keratinizing cells include large, bizarre cells, spindle cells, and clear cells with abundant mitotic figures, and, in the larger tumor foci, areas of central necrosis.[4]

Adenocarcinoma is usually moderately differentiated with small tubular and glandular structures that may have scattered, individual tumor cells with intracytoplasmic mucin. The tumor cells tend to have pleomorphic, hyperchromatic nuclei with numerous mitotic figures[4] (Fig. 35-5).

Large cell undifferentiated tumors consist of sheets of large, pleomorphic tumor cells with abundant cytoplasm, prominent nucleoli, and numerous mitoses. The giant cell variant has monster cells with bizarre nuclei and cells that frequently contain leukocytes. The clear cell variant is composed of sheets and islands of clear cells without other forms of differentiation.[73,74]

Small cell carcinoma is composed of islands, trabeculae, and rosettes of mildly pleomorphic cells that are somewhat larger than lymphocytes, with scant cytoplasm and hyperchromatic nuclei. There are frequent mitoses, and a crush artifact is a recognizable characteristic of these cells.[75]

Differential Diagnosis   Each of the variants of metastatic lung carcinoma needs to be distinguished from other tumors with a similar histopathologic pattern and correlated with the clinical history of the patient.

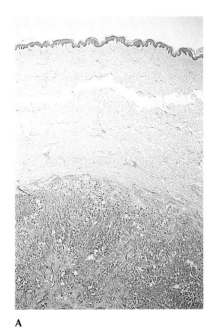

A

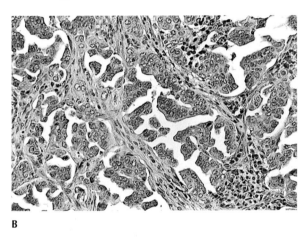

B

FIGURE 35-5   Metastatic adenocarcinoma from the lung. (*A*) Well-demarcated nodule of tumor in the reticular dermis with some glands. (*B*) Papillary adenocarcinoma.

Squamous Cell Carcinoma   A lung metastasis usually has no association with the overlying epidermis as is seen in a primary squamous cell carcinoma arising in the skin. Squamous cell carcinomas metastasizing to the skin usually arise from the oral cavity, lung, or esophagus and less often the uterine cervix, penis, or a distant skin site. Lesions from the oral cavity are often better differentiated than those from the lung, and appear in the region of the head and neck after the primary tumor has been recognized. A cutaneous metastasis from the esophagus may be the presenting lesion, and squamous cell carcinoma from the uterine cervix and penis occurred after the primary tumor was recognized.[5]

Adenocarcinoma   Most adenocarcinomas in the skin originate from the large intestine, lung, or breast. Those from the large intestine are often better differentiated than those from the lung. The former tumors show well-formed mucinous glandular epithelium or even large pools of mucin with a small amount of epithelium, as in mucinous carcinoma of the skin and a metastasis from the breast. Signet-ring cells that are char-

acteristic of adenocarcinoma of the stomach are seen only occasionally in metastases from the lung.[4,5]

Cutaneous metastatic lesions of undifferentiated type are usually from the breast or lung and less often from the stomach, liver, or urinary bladder.[5]

Large Cell Undifferentiated Tumor   This tumor, along with its giant cell, clear cell, and large cell neuroendocrine variants, needs to be differentiated from a sarcoma, such as rhabdomyosarcoma and malignant fibrous histiocytoma, a renal cell carcinoma, sebaceous carcinoma, a neuroendocrine tumor from some other site, and melanoma.[4,73]

Small (Oat) Cell Carcinoma   The differential diagnosis of this tumor includes skin adnexal carcinoma, metastatic melanoma, primary or metastatic neuroendocrine tumor (such as Merkel cell carcinoma in the skin or an oat cell carcinoma from another organ), malignant lymphoma, extraskeletal Ewing's sarcoma, and rhabdomyosarcoma.[76]

Special Stains and Immunohistochemistry   Squamous Cell Carcinoma   Like other squamous cell carcinomas, those from the lung are positive for cytokeratins and epithelial membrane antigen (EMA). Between 50 and 80 percent of squamous cell carcinomas from the lung are positive for carcinoembryonic antigen (CEA), while it is not seen in squamous cell carcinomas that arise in the skin.[69,77]

Adenocarcinoma   Lung primary tumors, like other adenocarcinomas, primarily from the breast and gastrointestinal tract, are PAS-positive and diastase-resistant and are positive for sialomucin. By immunoperoxidase, 70 to 100 percent are positive for CEA, like adenocarcinomas from other organs, although lung-derived adenocarcinomas are negative for gross cystic disease fluid protein-15 (GCDFP-15), as seen in breast carcinomas.[69,77,78]

Large Cell Undifferentiated Carcinoma   Large cell undifferentiated carcinomas from the lung are positive for cytokeratin and CEA, and negative for neuron-specific enolase (NSE), S-100 protein, and leukocyte common antigen (LCA).[73,77,79] They may be differentiated from a sarcoma such as rhabdomyosarcoma, which is positive for desmin; lymphoma, which is positive for leukocyte common antigen; and melanoma, which is positive for S-100 protein.[79–81] The clear cell variant of large cell undifferentiated carcinoma is positive for glycogen (PAS-positive, diastase-positive).[87] The latter tumor must be differentiated from a primary cutaneous clear cell sweat gland carcinoma, which is positive for both CEA and S-100 protein, and renal cell carcinoma, which is positive for glycogen and lipid, has numerous vessels with interstitial hemorrhage, and is negative for CEA and S-100 protein.[4,78,82] Sebaceous carcinoma, which is also in the differential diagnosis, is positive for lipids but not mucopolysaccharides, and the cells have a vacuolated cytoplasm.[4]

Small (Oat) Cell Carcinoma   Small (oat) cell carcinomas from the lung are positive for low-molecular-weight cytokeratins in a diffuse, perinuclear, granular pattern, and variably positive for neurofilaments, while Merkel cell carcinoma has paranuclear globular staining.[79,83] Small cell carcinomas from the lung are also positive for NSE and negative for S-100 protein, as are Merkel cell carcinomas, but 25 percent of small cell carcinomas that have neurosecretory granules by electron microscopy are positive for CEA, which is not seen in Merkel cell carcinomas.[77,83,84] For further differentiation of metastatic small cell carcinoma from the lung from other small cell tumors in the skin, see immunohistochemistry section in this chapter for neuroendocrine tumors and sarcomas.

Gastrointestinal Carcinoma

Carcinomas of the colon and rectum are the second most common primary tumors and the most frequent visceral tumors to metastasize to the skin in both men and women. The majority arise in the rectum and account for 11 to 19 percent of cutaneous metastases in men and 1.3 to 9 percent in women. Carcinoma of the large intestine is usually discovered before the cutaneous metastasis.[3,4,8] Cutaneous metastases from gallbladder and bile duct have been noted at the time that the initial tumor was recognized and as late as 40 years after the primary tumor was resected.[5,8] Cutaneous metastases from the stomach and pancreas usually occur prior to the discovery of the primary tumor.[3,8] The usual sites of metastases from gastrointestinal carcinomas are the abdominal wall, the perineum, and the umbilicus (Sister Joseph nodule).[3,4,8,37,85] In one series, 10 percent of metastases to the abdominal wall occurred in the umbilicus and 28 percent of those were of gastric origin.[85]

Clinical Features   Colon and rectal cutaneous metastases may present as flesh-colored sessile or pedunculated nodules, inflammatory carcinoma, grouped vascular nodules, or occasionally a perianal nodular and inflamed lesion suggestive of hidradenitis suppurativa.[9,45,86,87] Lookingbill et al.[8] found that in 11 of 18 patients with local metastases, most of these occurred in the abdominal incision site, and colorectal carcinoma also may metastasize to a colostomy site.[4,8] Gastric, pancreatic, and gallbladder carcinomas that metastasize to the skin usually present as nodules or sclerodermoid plaques.[5,8] In one case, a gastric carcinoma that metastasized to the scalp was associated with alopecia (alopecia neoplastica).[5]

Histopathological Features   Skin metastases from the large intestine are predominantly well-differentiated, mucin-secreting adenocarcinomas that in some cases may have a pattern of mucinous carcinoma. Less often they are poorly differentiated, and rarely they are so anaplastic that it is difficult to discern that they are of epithelial origin.[4]

Cutaneous metastases from the stomach are frequently anaplastic, infiltrating carcinomas in a loose or fibrotic stroma with varying numbers of signet-ring cells containing intracytoplasmic mucin.[4,5] Well-formed acini are observed only rarely, and only occasionally do gastric metastases present as a form of mucinous carcinoma.[4]

Differential Diagnosis   Cutaneous metastases from the gastrointestinal tract are most often adenocarcinomas, and those from the large intestine are the most well-differentiated mucin-secreting tumors.[4] A mucinous carcinoma from the gastrointestinal tract is often from the large intestine but may be indistinguishable from a metastasis from the lung or even a primary mucinous carcinoma of the skin. Rarely, such adenocarcinomas metastasize from a primary salivary gland, lacrimal gland, or esophageal or breast tumor.[63,88,89] Less well differentiated adenocarcinomas would be more likely to come from sites other than the large intestine in the gastrointestinal tract, such as stomach, pancreas, or gallbladder, as well as lung, breast, prostate, endometrium, ovaries, and endocervix.[4,5]

Gastric carcinomas are most often anaplastic with varying degrees of cellularity and numbers of signet-ring cells in a loose stroma. Although a cutaneous metastasis with this pattern, especially in a woman, is more likely to come from the breast, it is also observed in metastases from lung.[4,5]

Special Stains and Immunohistochemistry   Adenocarcinomas of the gastrointestinal tract contain sialomucin, which includes both neutral and nonsulfated acid mucopolysaccharides. It is PAS-positive and diastase-resistant, stains with alcian blue at pH 2.5 but not at pH 0.4, and is hyaluronidase-resistant.[64,90] By immunoperoxidase the cells are positive for cytokeratins and carcinoembryonic antigen (CEA) but not for GCDFP-15, ERP, prostate-specific antigen (PSA), or prostatic acid phosphatase (PAP).[78,91]

Oral Cavity Carcinomas

It has been shown that 8.7 percent of cutaneous metastases in men and 2.3 percent in women originate from the oral cavity.[8] They are almost all squamous cell carcinomas that present after the diagnosis of the primary tumor and are located in skin of the head and neck.[4,8]

Clinical Features   Cutaneous metastases derived from neoplasms of the oral cavity are frequently single or multiple nodules with or without ulceration, and in one series the cutaneous metastasis occurred at the site of surgery in 10 of 18 patients.[8]

Histopathological Features   Most of the metastases are moderately to well-differentiated squamous cell carcinomas in the deeper dermis and subcutaneous fat with no evidence of an epidermal origin, and the tumor cells sometimes involve perineural spaces and lymphatic vessels.[4]

Differential Diagnosis   Squamous cell carcinomas that metastasize to the skin usually originate in the oral cavity, esophagus, or lung, with the lung being the most common site of origin.[5] Less frequently, the primary tumor is in the uterine cervix, penis, or a distant cutaneous site.[5] In some cases, especially in ulcerated lesions, it may be impossible histologically to distinguish a metastasis from a primary squamous cell carcinoma.[4]

Special Stains and Immunohistochemistry   Special stains and immunohistochemical markers are not unique to metastatic tumors from the oral cavity.

Urinary Tract Tumors

It has been shown that 4.6 percent of cutaneous metastases originate from the kidney and 8.2 percent from the urinary bladder.[8] They are both seen more frequently in men than in women. While a cutaneous metastasis from renal cell carcinoma may be the first sign of the malignancy, metastases from the urinary bladder usually occur after recognition of the primary tumor.[5,8,92,93] In addition, a cutaneous metastasis from a renal cell carcinoma may occur 10 or more years after resection of the primary tumor.[5,47]

Clinical Features   Cutaneous metastases from renal cell and transitional cell tumors occur as either local metastases, often in surgical scars, or as distant metastases.[4,8] Metastases from renal cell carcinoma (hypernephroma) are seen more commonly on the head and neck, particularly the scalp, rather than in other areas of the body, and transitional cell carcinoma is seen most often on the trunk and extremities.[4,8,94]

Renal cell carcinoma metastases are solitary or widespread dermal nodules that are flesh colored or, more commonly, violaceous with a prominent vascularity as in Kaposi's sarcoma or pyogenic granuloma.[8,95,96] Transitional cell carcinoma metastases usually present as one or more flesh-colored dermal nodules[8,94] Less common types of metastases include warty papules and inflammatory plaques.[8,97,98]

Histopathological Features   Renal cell carcinoma is a type of clear cell adenocarcinoma. The metastatic nodules in the dermis are composed of large polyhedral cells with clear to finely granular cytoplasm and a central nucleus with little pleomorphism. The cells are arranged in sheets and cords with some gland formation and often a papillary component. The tumor cells are embedded in a delicate, highly vascular stroma with some extravasated erythrocytes and hemosiderin[4,99] (Fig. 35-6).

Transitional cell carcinoma that metastasizes to the skin consists of well-demarcated sheets and strands of large oval cells with small amounts of faintly basophilic to clear cytoplasm. There is some nuclear pleomorphism, and varying numbers of mitoses are seen. In addition, there may be some squamous differentiation and papillary formation with varying thicknesses of atypical epithelial cells covering a fine fibrovascular core. The metastatic tumor cells may be located in the dermis, either in between collagen bundles or in association with a desmoplastic stroma, in the subcutaneous fat, or in the lumina of vessels.[43,94]

Differential Diagnosis   Renal cell carcinoma must be differentiated from other clear cell carcinomas that on occasion metastasize to the skin (Table 35-4). These include primary tumors of the lung, liver, ovary, endometrium, cervix, and vagina.[99] Primary tumors of the skin that may resemble a renal cell carcinoma are clear cell hidradenoma (eccrine acrospiroma) and sebaceous tumors. In contrast to renal cell carcinoma, clear cell hidradenoma is usually multilobular and has prominent ductal structures but is not associated with prominent vascularity, hemorrhage, or hemosiderin deposition. Sebaceous tumors are not as vascular as renal tumors and have fine vacuolated cytoplasm.[4]

Transitional cell carcinomas from the urinary tract that metastasize to the skin are usually moderately to poorly differentiated and are difficult to differentiate form similar epithelial tumors from other sites or even a primary squamous cell carcinoma. Papillary metastases are more suggestive of a primary tumor in the urinary tract but need to be differentiated from transitional cell carcinomas from other sites such as the nasal pharynx.[43,94]

Special Stains and Immunohistochemistry   Renal cell carcinoma contains intracytoplasmic lipid and glycogen (PAS-positive and diastase-sensitive). In contrast, clear cell hidradenoma has no lipid, and sebaceous tumors exhibit lipid but little or no glycogen.[4] By immunoperoxidase, renal cell carcinoma is positive for cytokeratin and EMA. Although CEA and S-100 protein have been reported in some renal cell carcinomas, there was no immunoreactivity for either marker in the largest series of 70 cases. The latter finding is helpful in differentiating renal cell carcinoma from a primary clear cell hidradenoma and carcinoma or metastatic clear cell carcinoma from the lung or other organs, which is usually CEA-positive, and clear cell melanoma, which is S-100-positive.[62,82,100]

Genital Tract Tumors

In women, the most common genital tract tumors that metastasize to the skin are of ovarian (4 percent), endometrial (4 per-

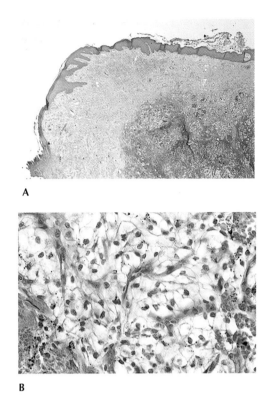

A

B

FIGURE 35-6   Metastatic clear cell adenocarcinoma from the kidney. (*A*) Well-demarcated nodule of tumor in the reticular dermis with clear cells and prominent extravasation of erythrocytes. (*B*) Sheets and cords of clear cells embedded in a delicate vascular stroma with some extravasated erythrocytes and hemosiderin deposition.

cent), and cervical (2 percent) origin.[8] Metastases from the latter tumors usually occur after recognition of the primary tumor, although a cutaneous metastasis from the ovary may be the initial manifestation of disease.[4] The trunk and pelvic areas are the primary sites of cutaneous metastases for each of these tumors, and ovarian metastases may involve the umbilicus.[4,8,37] Choriocarcinoma, which is usually a gestational tumor, frequently presents as a consequence of a metastasis, and

TABLE 35-4

Differentiation of Clear Cell Tumors

Tumor	Special Stains		Immunoperoxidase		
	Lipid	Glycogen	Cytokeratin	CEA	S-100 Protein
Renal cell carcinoma	+	+	+	−	−
Clear cell sweat gland tumors	−	+	+	+	+
Sebaceous tumors	+	−	+	−	−
Clear cell melanoma	−	−	−	−	+
Clear cell, large cell undifferentiated tumors of the lung	−	−	+	+	−

metastases to the skin are not uncommon.[17,101] In men, the primary tumor site is the prostate, which represents less than 1 percent of cutaneous metastases, and metastasis is seen most commonly in the pelvic area.[8,102]

Clinical Features   Cutaneous metastases from ovary, endometrium, and cervix are usually one or more skin-colored nodules that arise either in normal skin or in incisional scars.[8] Less often, ovarian metastases have erysipelaslike features.[103]

Prostate carcinomas in the skin usually consist of flesh-colored or violaceous nodules, and in some cases they resemble a pyoderma or have a zosteriform pattern that may result from growth along nerve sheaths.[22,104,105]

Histopathological Features   The histologic pattern of metastatic carcinoma of the ovary is usually that of a moderately to well-differentiated adenocarcinoma, often with a papillary configuration and psammoma bodies, which are small, laminated, calcified spherules[4,5] Endometrial carcinoma has the pattern of an adenocarcinoma with a solid and glandular pattern, and cutaneous metastases from the cervix are usually poorly differentiated squamous cell carcinomas.[93,106] Choriocarcinoma consists of cytotrophoblasts, which are large, cuboidal cells with vesicular nuclei and pale cytoplasm, and syncytiotrophoblasts, which are large cells with irregular nuclei and basophilic cytoplasm. Clusters of cytotrophoblasts are surrounded by sheets and cords of syncytiotrophoblasts in a plexiform pattern resembling chorionic villi.[17] Prostatic metastases to the skin are usually poorly differentiated adenocarcinomas with clusters and cords of cells with little gland formation that infiltrate dermal collagen bundles.[99,107] There may be pronounced epidermotropism.[108]

Differential Diagnosis   Metastatic adenocarcinoma from the ovary resembles papillary tumors from other sites such as colon, thyroid gland, stomach, and lung. Psammoma bodies may be observed in both ovarian carcinoma and papillary carcinoma of the thyroid gland.[99,109] Metastatic endometrial carcinoma usually does not have histologic features distinctive from adenocarcinomas from other organs, and metastatic cervical carcinoma cannot be discriminated from squamous cell carcinoma from other organs.[99] The differential diagnosis for choriocarcinoma includes sites of origin other than in the uterus. These include testes, ovaries, and mediastinum.[17]

Prostate carcinoma in the skin can have an infiltrative pattern, i.e., an Indian-file pattern, that is also observed in metastatic breast, stomach, pancreas, and oat cell carcinoma.[99] When epidermotropism is present, the differential diagnosis also includes metastatic tumors from the breast, colon, larynx, penis, and vagina, as well as melanoma.[108,110,111]

Special Stains and Immunohistochemistry   Ovarian adenocarcinomas are positive for CEA but negative for GCDFP-15, which is helpful in differentiating them from breast carcinoma.[78,112] The thyroid papillary carcinoma, which also has psammoma bodies, is positive for thyroglobulin.[113]

Choriocarcinoma is associated with high levels of circulating chorionic gonadotropin, which may be detected in the urine.[17]

Immunohistochemical staining of metastatic prostate carcinoma is positive for prostate-specific antigen and prostate acid phosphates.[107]

Neuroendocrine Tumors

Neuroblastoma, a tumor of adrenal origin, is the most common carcinoma seen at birth and is associated with cutaneous metastases in 32 percent of neonatal patients and 3 percent of patients of all ages.[114]

In older patients, carcinoid tumors occasionally metastasize to the skin, and this may be the first manifestation of the disease.[115,116] Bronchial carcinoids followed by those arising in the small intestines, including the appendix, are the most frequent primary tumors to metastasize to the skin.[115] Merkel cell carcinoma frequently recurs locally and metastasizes to distant sites, including skin.[117,118]

Thyroid carcinoma metastasizes to the skin in 1 percent of men and less often in women.[4] The 21 cases reported to date include follicular (6), papillary (5), giant cell (4), medullary (4), anaplastic (1), and follicular-papillary (1).[16] Papillary carcinoma relapses are sometimes delayed 20 to 30 years.[119]

Clinical Features   Neuroblastoma metastases are randomly scattered, firm, nontender, mobile, blue subcutaneous nodules that blanch for 30 to 60 min after being stroked.[120] Carcinoid tumors appear as single or multiple dermal or subcutaneous nodules that may be painful.[115,121,122] Metastases from Merkel cell carcinoma are usually firm, red-pink, nonulcerated nodules 0.4 to 0.8 cm in diameter.[123]

Thyroid carcinoma metastases may be flesh-colored or red-violet cutaneous nodules, often involving the scalp and abdomen; follicular carcinoma metastases may be pulsatile or have a bruit.[16,18,19]

Histopathological Features   Neuroblastoma exhibits clusters of small basophilic cells that have numerous mitoses and form rosettes in a fine, fibrillar, eosinophilic stroma.[120] Carcinoid tumor metastases in the dermis and subcutaneous fat are composed of islands, nests, and cords of uniform cells with round nuclei and clear or eosinophilic cytoplasm that occasionally contains eosinophilic granules.[116,121] Merkel cell carcinoma has anastomosing cords and bands and sheets and clusters of uniform, round basophilic cells with vesicular nuclei, scant cytoplasm, and numerous mitoses[83,124] (Fig. 35-7). Throughout the tumor there is cell necrosis and apoptosis, and there may be keratin pearls and foci of squamous differentiation. Sweat gland differentiation may be seen, and Merkel cell carcinoma has even been reported in association with a squamous cell, basal cell, and sweat gland carcinoma.[83]

Papillary carcinoma of the thyroid gland has an infiltrative pattern that consists of tubulopapillary structures with occasional psammoma bodies and dark, eosinophilic-staining colloid.[99,109] The "Orphan Annie" nuclei of papillary carcinoma of the thyroid are large, ovoid, ground glass–appearing, and grooved with small nucleoli.[125] Follicular thyroid carcinoma in the skin has trabeculae and follicles with intraluminal colloid.[126] Medullary carcinoma of the thyroid is composed of sheets of polygonal or plump spindle cells in a fibrovascular stroma that often contains lymphocytes and amyloid.[127]

Differential Diagnosis   Neuroblastoma and Merkel cell carcinoma must be differentiated from other small, round, blue cell tumors, which include small (oat) cell carcinoma, poorly differentiated sweat gland carcinoma, metastatic melanoma, malignant epithelioid schwannoma of superficial tissue (neurotropic/desmoplastic melanoma), extraskeletal Ewing's sarcoma, rhabdomyosarcoma, and malignant lymphoma.[76,128,129] The uniform small cells of a carcinoid tumor may look similar to those of a sweat gland carcinoma or a glomus tumor.[121]

The differential diagnosis for papillary tumors with metastases to the skin include papillary carcinomas of the thyroid and ovary, which may have psammoma bodies, as well as papillary carcinoma from the stomach and lungs.[99,109] Follicular carcinoma of the thyroid is unique because of the colloid in the follicles, and the anaplastic small cell variant of medullary carcinoma of the thyroid gland needs to be differentiated from other small cell carcinomas as well as a malignant lymphoma.[130]

Special Stains and Immunohistochemistry   Carcinoid tumors from the bronchus are of foregut origin (type 1), and they contain argyrophil

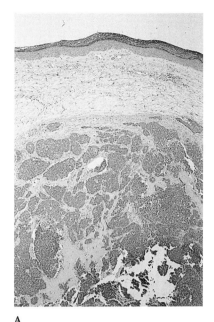

A

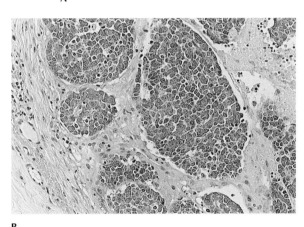

B

FIGURE 35-7   Metastatic Merkel cell carcinoma. (*A*) Well-demarcated nodule of tumor in the reticular dermis with sheets and cords of uniform basophilic cells. (*B*) Sheets and cords of uniform basophilic cells.

granules that can be impregnated with silver. Small intestine carcinoids are of midgut origin (type 2), and they contain argentaffin granules that stain with Fontana-Masson.[116]

By immunoperoxidase, the small, round basophilic cells in a neuroblastoma are positive for neuron-specific enolase (NSE) and neurofilaments, and the stromal spindle cells stain for S-100 protein, which suggests that they are cytodifferentiated cells like Schwann cells.[131] Carcinoid tumors are positive for NSE.[132] Merkel cell carcinomas have features of both neuroendocrine and epithelial differentiation. They have a distinct paranuclear or juxtanuclear globular staining pattern that resembles cytoplasmic inclusion bodies and perinuclear dots that are seen with antibodies to low-molecular-weight cytokeratins such as AE-1 and CAM-5.2 and neurofilaments.[79,83,133] They are also positive for epithelial membrane antigen, chromogranin, and NSE but negative for S-100 protein, carcinoembryonic antigen, and leukocyte common antigen.[83,129,133,134] Metastatic small cell carcinoma of the lung shows a diffuse perinuclear dotlike pattern with low-molecular-weight cytokeratins and a variable dotlike pattern with antibodies against neurofilaments.[79,83,133] In addition, although Merkel cell carcinoma is negative for CEA, approximately 50 percent of metastatic small cell carcinomas are reactive with CEA.[84]

Immunostaining is useful for the diagnosis of papillary and follicular thyroid carcinomas when they are reactive with thyroglobulin and medullary carcinoma with calcitonin.[113,135]

Sarcomas

Sarcomas metastasize to the skin in 3 percent of men and 2 percent of women with cutaneous metastases.[4] These include leiomyosarcoma, rhabdomyosarcoma, fibrosarcoma, chondrosarcoma, Ewing's sarcoma, osteogenic sarcoma, and undifferentiated sarcomas. Distant cutaneous metastases also may be seen from sarcomas that arise in the dermis, subcutaneous fat, or underlying soft tissue such as epithelioid cell sarcoma and malignant fibrous histiocytoma.[136,137] The metastases occur on the scalp, trunk, and extremities, and while they usually occur after recognition of the primary lesion, they also may be the first presentation of the tumor.[136,138]

Clinical Features   Metastatic sarcomas in the skin are firm, skin-colored or red-purple nodules that may be ulcerated and/or painful.[136,139]

Histopathological Features   Leiomyosarcoma is often a well-demarcated or infiltrating nodule in the dermis or subcutaneous fat with fascicles of spindle cells with eosinophilic cytoplasm and varying degrees of atypism[139] (Fig. 35-8). Rhabdomyosarcomas are usually poorly differentiated tumors that may have large, atypical cells with abundant eosinophilic cytoplasm and multinucleated giant cells or small, hyperchromatic cells with scant cytoplasm, in which case they are included in the differential diagnosis of small, round, blue cell tumors.[76,140] Only some of the tumors have elongated eosinophilic strap cells and recognizable rhabdomyoblasts with cross-striations in their cytoplasm.[141,142] Fibrosarcomas consists of fascicles of spindle cells often arranged in a herringbone pattern with few polygonal and giant cells.[143] Better-differentiated tumors have more spindle cells and collagen production, whereas poorly differentiated tumors have anaplastic cells and mitoses.[144,145] Malignant fibrous histiocytoma has several variants that include storiform-pleomorphic, xanthomatous, inflammatory, myxoid, angiomatoid, and giant cell types[146,147] (see Chap. 30). Chondrosarcomas are composed of undifferentiated round to spindle-shaped cells with malignant cartilage or chondroblasts in a myxoid matrix.[148,149] Osteogenic sarcoma is composed of varying admixtures of malignant osteoid and bone along with a spindle cell component that resembles fibrosarcoma or malignant fibrous histiocytoma.[150] Ewing's sarcoma is characterized by lobules of uniform small, round or oval cells with perilobular fibrosis.[151] Epithelioid sarcoma is composed of nodules of polygonal, epithelioid, and spindle cells with abundant eosinophilic cytoplasm and atypical nuclei that palisade around central areas of necrosis in association with a lymphocytic infiltrate at the periphery.[136]

Differential Diagnosis   The differentiation of various sarcomas from each other and from spindle cell or round cell tumors of epithelial origin has been made much easier by the advent of immunohistochemistry. However, there are light-microscopic findings that are of benefit in differentiating sarcomas from one another as well as from epithelial tumors.

The main tumor in the differential diagnosis of a metastatic fibrosarcoma in the skin is a primary dermatofibrosarcoma protuberans (DFSP). DFSP is located in the reticular dermis and has uniform spindle cells and a more pronounced storiform pattern as compared with fibrosarcoma.[152] It should be noted that DFSP may have myxoid areas and fibrosarcomatous changes in up to 25 percent of its total volume.[153,154] Nodular fasciitis is a benign lesion in the subcutaneous fat that arises from the fascia and, occasionally, from the septa of the subcutaneous

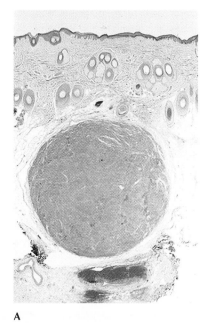

A

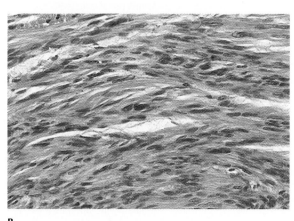

B

FIGURE 35-8 Metastatic leiomyosarcoma. (*A*) Well-demarcated nodule of tumor in the subcutaneous fat with brightly eosinophilic cells. (*B*) Interlacing fascicles of eosinophilic spindle cells with nuclear pleomorphism.

fat.[155] In contrast to fibrosarcoma, it has uniform fibroblasts and, in some cases, giant cells haphazardly arranged in a highly vascular myxoid stroma.[155,156] Atypical fibroxanthoma can be differentiated from malignant fibrous histiocytoma by its smaller size and more superficial location.[157] Well-differentiated metastatic leiomyosarcoma may have a similar infiltrative or well-demarcated pattern in the dermis or subcutaneous fat as that seen in primary leiomyosarcomas or even leiomyomas.[158] Metastatic leiomyosarcoma does not have a vascular origin as observed in subcutaneous leiomyosarcoma and angioleiomyoma and has more atypical smooth-muscle cells than are seen in leiomyoma. Anaplastic tumors with bizarre giant cells may resemble malignant fibrous histiocytoma.[159] Rhabdomyosarcomas composed of small, round blue cells need to be differentiated from other primary or metastatic tumors with similar cells. Pleomorphic rhabdomyosarcomas with a storiform pattern and bizarre multinucleated cells may resemble a malignant fibrous histiocytoma.[76,160] Ewing's sarcoma raises the differential diagnosis of small cell tumors. Epithelioid sarcoma must be distinguished from infectious and palisading granulomas.[161] It differs from malignant fibrous histiocytoma because of the absence of bizarre multinucleated cells and foam cells.

REFERENCES

1. Brodland DG, Zitelli JA: Mechanism of metastases. *J Am Acad Dermatol* 27:110, 1992.
2. Lambert WC, Schwartz RA: Metastasis (editorial). *J Am Acad Dermatol* 27:131–133, 1992.
3. Brownstein MH, Helwig EB: Patterns of cutaneous metastasis. *Arch Dermatol* 105:862–868, 1972.
4. Brownstein MH, Helwig EB: Metastatic tumors of skin. *Cancer* 29:1298–1307, 1972.
5. Brownstein MH, Helwig EB: Spread of tumors to the skin. *Arch Dermatol* 107:80–86, 1973.
6. Abrams HL, Spiro R, Goldstein N: Metastases in carcinoma: Analysis of 1000 autopsied cases. *Cancer* 3:74–85, 1950.
7. Spencer PS, Helm TN: Skin metastases in cancer patients. *Cutis* 30:119–121, 1987.
8. Lookingbill DP, Spangler N, Helm KF: Cutaneous metastases in patients with metastatic carcinoma: A retrospective study of 4020 patients. *J Am Acad Dermatol* 29:228–236, 1993.
9. Lookingbill DP, Spangler N, Sexton FM: Skin involvement as the presenting sign of internal carcinoma. *J Am Acad Dermatol* 22:19–26, 1990.
10. Zetter BR: The cellular basis of site-specific tumor metastasis. *N Engl J Med* 332:605–612, 1990.
11. Sobel ME: Metastasis suppressor genes. *J Natl Cancer Inst* 82:267–276, 1990.
12. Sporn MB, Todaro GJ: Autocrine secretion and malignant transformation of cells. *N Engl J Med* 303:878–880, 1980.
13. Sporn MB, Roberts AB: Peptide growth factors and inflammation, tissue repair, and cancer. *J Clin Invest* 78:329–332, 1986.
14. Folkman J, Greenspan HP: Influence of geometry on control of cell growth. *Biochim Biophys Acta* 417:211–236, 1975.
15. Matarasso SL, Rosen T: Zosterioform metastasis: Case presentation and review of the literature. *J Dermatol Surg Oncol* 14:774–778, 1988.
16. Vives R, Valcayo A, Menendez E, et al: Follicular thyroid carcinoma metastatic to the skin. *J Am Acad Dermatol* 27:276–277, 1992.
17. Cosnow I, Fretzin DF: Choriocarcinoma metastatic to skin. *Arch Dermatol* 109:551–553, 1974.
18. Auty RM: Dermal metastases from follicular carcinoma of the thyroid. *Arch Dermatol* 113:675–676, 1977.
19. Ginzberg E, Catz B, Nelson CL, et al: Hyperthyroidism secondary to metastatic functioning thyroid carcinoma. *Ann Intern Med* 58:684–690, 1963.
20. Schwartz RA: Cutaneous metastatic disease. *J Am Acad Dermatol* 33:161–182, 1995.
21. Cox SE, Cruz PD Jr: A spectrum of inflammatory metastasis to skin via lymphatics: Three cases of carcinoma erysipeloides. *J Am Acad Dermatol* 30:304–307, 1994.
22. Stahl D, Veien NK: Cutaneous metastases simulating other dermatoses. *Cutis* 26:282–284, 1980.
23. Hyde JN: Disseminated lenticular cancer of the skin: "Cancer en cuirasse." *Am J Med Sci* 103:235–245, 1892.
24. Parkes Weber F: Bilateral thoracic zosteroid spreading marginate telangiectasia—probably a variety of "carcinoma erysipelatodes" (C. Rasch)-associated with unilateral mammary carcinoma, and better termed "carcinoma telangiectaticum." *Br J Dermatol Syphilol* 418–423, 1933.
25. Newcomb WD: Unusual cutaneous metastases in carcinoma of the breast. *Lancet* 206:1056–1057, 1924.
26. Ingram JT: Carcinoma erysipelatodes and carcinoma telangiectaticum. *Arch Dermatol* 77:277–231, 1958.
27. Poiares-Baptista A, Abreu de Vasconcellos A: Cutaneous pigmented metastasis from breast carcinoma simulating malignant melanoma. *Int J Dermatol* 27:124–125, 1988.
28. Carson HJ, Pellettiere EV, Lack E: Alopecia neoplastica simulating alopecia areata and antedating the detection of primary breast carcinoma. *J Cutan Pathol* 21:67–70, 1994.
29. Paget J: On disease of the mammary areola preceding cancer of the mammary gland. *St Bartholomews Hosp Rep* 10:87–89, 1874.
30. Murrell TW, McMullan FH: Extramammary Paget's disease. *Arch Dermatol* 85:600–613, 1962.
31. Helwig EB, Graham JH: Anogenital (extramammary) Paget's disease: A clinical study. *Cancer* 16:387–403, 1963.
32. Fligiel Z, Kaneko M: Extramammary Paget's disease of the external ear canal in association with ceruminous gland carcinoma. *Cancer* 36:1072–1076, 1975.
33. Whorton CM, Patterson JB: Carcinoma of Moll's glands with extramammary Paget's disease of the eyelid. *Cancer* 8:1009–1015, 1955.
34. Waisman M: Carcinoma of the inframammary crease. *Arch Dermatol* 114:1520–1521, 1978.
35. Watson JR, Watson CG: Carcinoma of the mammary crease: A neglected clinical entity. *JAMA* 209:1718–1719, 1969.
36. Hood CI, Zimmerman LE: Metastatic mammary carcinoma in the eyelid with histiocytoid appearance. *Cancer* 31:793–800, 1973.
37. Powell FC, Cooper AJ, Massa MC, et al: Sister Mary Joseph's nodule: A clinical and histologic study. *J Am Acad Dermatol* 10:610–615, 1984.
38. Schwartz IS: Sister (Mary?) Joseph's nodule. *N Engl J Med* 316:1348–1349, 1987.
39. Miyashita M, Honjo M, Suzuki H, et al: A case of cutaneous metastases of gastric carcinoma showing peculiar clinical features. *J Dermatol (Tokyo)* 18:619–623, 1991.

40. Edoute Y, Ben-Haim SA, Malberger E: Umbilical metastasis from urinary bladder carcinoma. *J Am Acad Dermatol* 26:656–657, 1992.

41. Imachi M, Tsukamoto N, Kinoshita S, et al: Skin metastasis from carcinoma of the uterine cervix. *Gynecol Oncol* 48:349–354, 1993.

42. Williams JC, Heaney JA: Metastatic renal cell carcinoma presenting as a skin nodule: Case report and review of the literature. *J Urol* 152:2094–2095, 1994.

43. Schwartz RA, Fleishman JS: Transitional cell carcinoma of the urinary tract presenting with a cutaneous metastasis. *Arch Dermatol* 117:513–515, 1981.

44. Jones C, Rosen T: Multiple red nodules on lower abdomen. *Arch Dermatol* 128:1535–1538, 1992.

45. Nazzari G, Drago F, Malatto M, et al: Epidermoid anal canal carcinoma metastatic to the skin: A clinical mimic of prostate adenocarcinoma metastases. *J Dermatol Surg Oncol* 20:765–766, 1994.

46. Nishitani K, Nishitani H, Shimoda Y: Cutaneous invasion of mucinous adenocarcinoma of the appendix. *J Dermatol* 14:167–169, 1987.

47. Menter A, Boyd AS, McCaffree DM: Recurrent renal cell carcinoma presenting as skin nodules: Two case reports and review of the literature. *Cutis* 44:305–308, 1989.

48. Enzinger FM, Weiss WW: Malignant tumors of uncertain histiogenesis, in *Soft Tissue Tumors*, 2d ed. St Louis, Mosby, 1988:936–945.

49. Chase DR, Enzinger FM: Epithelioid sarcoma (diagnosis, prognostic indicators, and treatment). *Am J Surg Pathol* 9:241–263, 1985.

50. Dixon JM, Page DL, Anderson TJ, et al: Long term survivors after breast cancer. *Br J Surg* 72:445–448, 1985.

51. Ellis IO, Galea M, Broughton N, et al: Pathological prognostic factors in breast cancer: II. Histological type. Relationship with survival in a large study with long-term follow-up. *Histopathology* 20:479–489, 1992.

52. Sherry MM, Johnson DH, Page DL, et al: Inflammatory carcinoma of the breast. *Am J Med* 79:355–364, 1985.

53. Rosen PP: The pathological classification of human mammary carcinoma: Past, present and future. *Ann Clin Lab Sci* 9:144–156, 1979.

54. Quiencey C, Raitt N, Bell J, et al: Intracytoplasmic lumina: A useful diagnostic feature of adenocarcinoma. *Histopathology* 19:83–87, 1991.

55. Foote FW Jr, Stewart FW: A histologic classification of carcinoma in the breast. *Surgery* 19:74–99, 1946.

56. Wheeler JE, Enterline HT: Lobular carcinoma of the breast in situ and infiltrating. *Pathol Annu* 11:161–188, 1976.

57. Dixon JM, Anderson TJ, Page DL, et al: Infiltrating lobular carcinoma of the breast. *Histopathology* 6:149–161, 1982.

58. Parl FF, Richardson LD: The histologic and biologic spectrum of tubular carcinoma of the breast. *Hum Pathol* 14:648–698, 1983.

59. Page DL, Dixon JM, Anderson TJ, et al: Invasive cribriform carcinoma of the breast. *Histopathology* 7:525–536, 1983.

60. Clayton F: Pure mucinous carcinomas of the breast: Morphologic features and prognostic correlates. *Hum Pathol* 17:34–38, 1986.

61. Fisher ER, Kenny JP, Sass R, et al: Medullary cancer of the breast revisited. *Breast Cancer Res Treat* 16:212–229, 1990.

62. Swanson PE, Cherwitz DL, Newmann MP, et al: Eccrine sweat gland carcinoma: An histologic and immunohistochemical study of 32 cases. *J Cutan Pathol* 14:65–86, 1987.

63. Balin AK, Fine RM, Golitz LE: Mucinous carcinoma. *J Dermatol Surg Oncol* 14:521–512, 1988.

64. Mendoza S, Helwig EB: Mucinous (adenocystic) carcinoma of the skin. *Arch Dermatol* 103:68–78, 1971.

65. Baandrup U, Sogaard H: Mucinous (adenocystic) carcinoma of the skin. *Dermatologica* 164:338–342, 1982.

66. Ormsby AH, Snow JL, Daniel Su WP, et al: Diagnostic immunohistochemistry of cutaneous metastatic breast carcinoma: A statistical analysis of the utility of gross cystic disease fluid protein-15 and estrogen receptor protein. *J Am Acad Dermatol* 32:711–716, 1995.

67. Dwarakanath S, Lee AKC, DeLellis RA, et al: S-100 protein positive breast carcinoma: A potential pitfall in diagnostic immunohistochemistry. *Hum Pathol* 18:1144–1148, 1987.

68. Urabe A, Matsukuma A, Shimizi N, et al: Extramammary Paget's disease: Comparative histopathologic studies of intraductal carcinoma of the breast and apocrine adenocarcinoma. *J Cutan Pathol* 17:257–265, 1990.

69. Taylor CR: Lung, pancreas, colon and rectum, stomach, liver, in Taylor CR, Cote RJ (eds): *Immunomicroscopy: A Diagnostic Tool for the Surgical Pathologist*, 2d ed. Philadelphia, Saunders, 1994:302.

70. Ask-Upmark E: On location of malignant metastases with special regard to the behavior of primary malignant tumours of the lung. *Acta Pathol Microbiol Scand* 9:239–248, 1932.

71. Terashima T, Kanazawa M: Lung cancer with skin metastases. *Chest* 106:1448–1450, 1994.

72. Rudner EJ, Lentz C, Brown J: Bronchial carcinoid tumor with skin metastases. *Arch Dermatol* 92:73–75, 1965.

73. Gibbs AR, Whimster WF: Tumors of the lung and pleura, in Fletcher CDM (ed): *Diagnostic Histopathology of Tumors*. New York, Churchill-Livingstone, 1995:133.

74. Wang N, Seemayer TA, Ahmed MN, et al: Giant cell carcinoma of the lung. *Hum Pathol* 7:3–16, 1976.

75. Gibbs AR, Whimster WF: Tumors of the lung and pleura, in Fletcher CDM (ed): *Diagnostic Histopathology of Tumors*. New York, Churchill-Livingstone, 1995:130.

76. Jacinto CM, Grant-Kels JM, Knibbs DR, et al: Malignant primitive neuroectodermal tumor presenting as a scalp nodule. *Am J Dermatopathol* 13:63–70, 1991.

77. Said JW, Nash G, Tepper G, et al: Keratin proteins and carcinoembryonic antigen in lung carcinoma: An immunoperoxidase study of 54 cases, with ultrastructural correlations. *Hum Pathol* 14:70–76, 1983.

78. Wick MR, Lillemoe TJ, Copland GT, et al: Gross cystic disease fluid protein-15 as a marker for breast cancer: Immunohistochemical analysis of 690 human neoplasms and comparison with alpha-lactalbumin. *Hum Pathol* 20:281–287, 1989.

79. Battifora H, Silva EG: The use of antikeratin antibodies in the immunohistochemical distinction between neuroendocrine (Merkel cell) carcinoma of the skin, lymphoma, and oat cell carcinoma. *Cancer* 58:1040–1046, 1986.

80. Wick MR, Swanson PE: Soft tissue tumors, in Colvin RB, Bhan AK, McCluskey RT (eds): *Diagnostic Immunopathology*. New York, Raven Press, 1988:384–386.

81. Wick MR, Swanson PE: Soft tissue tumors, in Colvin RB, Bhan AK, McCluskey RT (eds): *Diagnostic Immunopathology*. New York, Raven Press, 1988:375–376.

82. Nadasdy T, Bane BL, Silva FG: Adult renal diseases, in Sternberg SS (ed): *Diagnostic Surgical Pathology*, 2d ed. New York, Raven Press, 1994: 1726.

83. Ratner D, Nelson BR, Brown MD, et al: Merkel cell carcinoma. *J Am Acad Dermatol* 29:143–156, 1993.

84. Wick MR, Swanson PE, Ritter JH, et al: The immunohistology of cutaneous neoplasia: A practical perspective. *J Cutan Pathol* 20:481–497, 1993.

85. Steck WD, Helwig EB: Tumors of the umbilicus. *Cancer* 18:907–915, 1965.

86. Weiner K: *Skin Manifestations of Internal Disorders (Dermadromes)*. St Louis, Mosby, 1947:565–569.

87. Graham BS, Wong SW: Cancer cellulitis. *South Med J* 77:277–278, 1984.

88. Smoller BR, Narurkar V: Mucoepidermoid carcinoma metastatic to the skin: An histologic mimic of a primary sweat gland carcinoma. *J Dermatol Surg Oncol* 18:365–368, 1992.

89. Nahass GT, Otrakji CJ, Gould E: Mucinous breast carcinoma: Single cutaneous metastasis. *J Dermatol Surg Oncol* 19:878–880, 1993.

90. Cawley EP, Hsu YT, Weary PE: The evaluation of neoplastic metastases of the skin. *Arch Dermatol* 90:262–265, 1964.

91. Bhan AK: Differentiation antigens and strategies in tumor diagnosis, in Colvin RB, Bhan AK, McCluskey RT (eds): *Diagnostic Immunopathology*. New York, Raven Press, 1988:200–201.

92. Cuckow P, Doyle D: Renal cell carcinoma presenting in the skin. *J R Soc Med* 84:497–498, 1991.

93. Brady LW, O'Neil EA, Farber SH: Unusual sites of metastases. *Semin Oncol* 4:59–64, 1977.

94. Hollander A, Grots IA: Oculocutaneous metastases from carcinoma of the urinary bladder: Case report and review of the literature. *Arch Dermatol* 97:678–684, 1968.

95. Rogrow L, Rotman M, Roussis K: Renal metastases simulating Kaposi sarcoma: Radionuclide scanning, an aid in diagnosis and treatment planning. *Arch Dermatol* 111:717–719, 1975.

96. Bates E, Knox JM, Wolf JE Jr: Metastatic renal cell carcinoma resembling a pyogenic granuloma. *Arch Dermatol* 114:1082–1083, 1978.

97. Langolis NEI, McClinton S, Miller ID: An unusual presentation of transitional cell carcinoma of the distal urethra. *Histopathology* 21:482–484, 1992.

98. Ando K-I, Goto Y, Kato K, et al: Zosteriform inflammatory metastatic carcinoma from transitional cell carcinoma of the renal pelvis. *J Am Acad Dermatol* 31:284–286, 1994.

99. McKee PH: Cutaneous metastases. *J Cutan Pathol* 12:239–250, 1985.

100. Penneys NS, Mehrdad N, Morales A: Carcinoembryonic antigen in benign sweat gland tumors. *Arch Dermatol* 118:225–227, 1982.

101. Elston CW: Gestational trophoblastic disease, in Fox H (ed): *Haines and Taylor's Obstetrical and Gynaecological Pathology*, 3d ed. Edinburgh, Churchill-Livingstone, 1987:1045–1078.

102. Tenjo S, Isomatsu M, Ueda K: Skin metastases from prostatic cancer. *Acta Dermatol (Kyoto)* 89:453–460, 1994.

103. Lever LR, Holt PJA: Carcinoma erysipeloides. *Br J Dermatol* 124:279–282, 1991.

104. Schellhammer PF, Milsten R, Bunts RC: Prostatic carcinoma with cutaneous metastases. *Br J Urol* 45:169–172, 1973.

105. Andrews GC: Carcinoma of the prostate with zosteriform cutaneous lesions. *Arch Dermatol* 104:301–303, 1971.

106. Damewood MD, Rosenchein NB, Grumbine FC, et al: Cutaneous metastasis of endometrial carcinoma. *Cancer* 46:1471–1475, 1980.

107. Steinkraus V, Lange T, Abeck D, et al: Cutaneous metastases from carcinoma of the prostate. *J Am Acad Dermatol* 31:665–666, 1994.

108. Segal R, Penneys NS, Nahass G: Metastatic prostatic carcinoma histologically mimicking malignant melanoma. *J Cutan Pathol* 21:280–282, 1994.

109. Elgart GW, Patterson JW, Taylor R: Cutaneous metastasis from papillary carcinoma of the thyroid gland. *J Am Acad Dermatol* 25:404–408, 1991.

110. Aguilar A, Schoendorff C, Lopez Rendondo MJ, et al: Epidermotropic metastases from internal carcinomas. *Am J Dermatopathol* 13:452–458, 1991.

111. Abernathy JL, Soyer HP, Kerl H, et al: Epidermotropic metastatic malignant melanoma simulating melanoma in situ: A report of 10 examples from two patients. *Am J Surg Pathol* 18:1140–1149, 1994.

112. Felix JC, Sherrod AE, Taylor CR: Gynecologic and testicular neoplasms, in Taylor CR, Cote RJ (eds): *Immunomicroscopy: A Diagnostic Tool for the Surgical Pathologist*, 2d ed. Philadelphia, Saunders, 1994:243.

113. Albores-Saavedra J, Nadji M, Civantos F, et al: Thyroglobulin in carcinoma of the thyroid: An immunohistochemical study. *Hum Pathol* 14:63–66, 1983.

114. Schneider KM, Becker JM, Krasna IH: Neonatal neuroblastoma. *Pediatrics* 36: 265–366, 1965.

115. Keane J, Fretzin DF, Jao W, et al: Bronchial carcinoid metastatic to the skin. *J Cutan Pathol* 7:43–49, 1980.

116. Brody HJ, Stallings WP, Fine RM, et al: Carcinoid in an umbilical nodule. *Arch Dermatol* 114:570–572, 1978.

117. Raaf JH, Urmacher C, Knapper WK, et al: Trabecular (Merkel cell) carcinoma of the skin. *Cancer* 57:178–182, 1986.

118. Wong SW, Dao AH, Glick AD: Trabecular carcinoma of the skin: A case report. *Hum Pathol* 12:838–840, 1981.

119. Tubiana M, Schlumberger M, Rougher P, et al: Long-term results and prognostic factors in patients with differentiated thyroid carcinoma. *Cancer* 55:794–804, 1985.

120. Lucky AW, McGuire J, Komp DM: Infantile neuroblastoma presenting with cutaneous blanching nodules. *J Am Acad Dermatol* 6:389–391, 1982.

121. Reingold IM, Escovitz WE: Metastatic cutaneous carcinoid. *Arch Dermatol* 82:971–975, 1960.

122. Archer CB, Rauch HJ, Allen MH, et al: Ultrastructural features of metastatic cutaneous carcinoid. *J Cutan Pathol* 11:485–490, 1984.

123. Wick MR, Goellner JR, Scheithauer BW, et al: Primary neuroendocrine carcinoma of the skin (Merkel cell tumors). *Am J Clin Pathol* 79:6–13, 1983.

124. Toker C: Trabecular carcinoma of the skin. *Arch Dermatol* 105:107–110, 1972.

125. Chan JKC: Papillary carcinoma of thyroid: Classical and variants. *Histol Histopathol* 5:241–257, 1990.

126. Caron PH, Moreau-Cabarrot A, Gorguet B, et al: Cutaneous metastasis from follicular carcinoma of the thyroid gland. *Thyroid* 3:235–237, 1993.

127. Ordonez NG, Samaan NA: Medullary carcinoma of the thyroid metastatic to the skin: Report of two cases. *J Cutan Pathol* 14:251–254, 1987.

128. Triche TJ, Askin FB: Neuroblastoma and the differential diagnosis of small-, round-, blue-cell tumors. *Hum Pathol* 14:569–595, 1983.

129. Wick MR, Kaye VN, Sibley RK, et al: Primary neuroendocrine carcinoma and small-cell malignant lymphoma of the skin. *J Cutan Pathol* 13:347–358, 1986.

130. Mendelsohn G, Baylin SB, Bigner SH, et al: Anaplastic variants of medullary thyroid carcinoma: A light microscopic and immunohistochemical study. *Am J Surg Pathol* 4:333–341, 1980.

131. Hachitanda Y, Tsuneyoshi M, Enjoji M: An ultrastructural and immunohistochemical evaluation of cytodifferentiation in neuroblastic tumors. *Mod Pathol* 2:13–19, 1989.

132. Gould VE, Lee I, Warren WH: Immunohistochemical evaluation of neuroendocrine cells and neoplasms of the lung. *Pathol Res Pract* 183:200–213, 1988.

133. Tope WD, Sangueza OP. Merkel cell carcinoma: Histopathology, immunohistochemistry, and cytogenetic analysis. *J Dermatol Surg Oncol* 20:648–652, 1994.

134. Drijkoningen M, De Wolf-Peeters C, Van Limbergen E, et al: Merkel cell tumor of the skin: An immunohistochemical study. *Hum Pathol* 17:301–307, 1986.

135. Chaiwun B, Cote RJ, Taylor CR: Diffuse neuroendocrine and endocrine systems, in Taylor CR, Cote RJ (eds): *Immunomicroscopy: A Diagnostic Tool for the Surgical Pathologist*, 2d ed. Philadelphia, Saunders, 1994:187–189.

136. Kusakabe H, Yonebayashi K, Sakatani S, et al: Metastatic epithelioid sarcoma with an N-ras oncogene mutation. *Am J Dermatopathol* 16:294–300, 1994.

137. Enion DS, Scott JL, Gouldesbrough: Cutaneous metastasis from a malignant fibrous histiocytoma to a limb skin graft donor site. *Br J Surg* 80:366, 1993.

138. Chen KTK: Scalp metastases as the initial presentation of malignant fibrous histiocytoma. *J Surg Oncol* 27:179–180, 1984.

139. Powell FC, Cooper AJ, Massa MC, et al: Leiomyosarcoma of the small intestine metastatic to the umbilicus. *Arch Dermatol* 120:402–403, 1984.

140. Ansai S, Takeda H, Koseki S, et al: A patient with rhabdomyosarcoma and clear cell sarcoma of the skin. *J Am Acad Dermatol* 31:871–876, 1994.

141. Agamanolis DP, Dasu S, Krill CE Jr: Tumors of skeletal muscle. *Hum Pathol* 17:778–795, 1986.

142. Wiss K, Solomon AR, Raimer SS: Rhabdomyosarcoma presenting as a cutaneous nodule. *Arch Dermatol* 124:1687–1690, 1988.

143. Pritchard DJ, Soule EH, Taylor WF, et al: Fibrosarcoma, a clinicopathologic and statistical study of 199 tumors of the soft tissue of the extremities and trunk. *Cancer* 33:888–897, 1974.

144. Chung EB, Enzinger FM: Infantile fibrosarcoma. *Cancer* 38:729–739, 1976.

145. Soule EH, Pritchard DJ: Fibrosarcoma in infants and children: A review of 110 cases. *Cancer* 40:1711–1721, 1977.

146. Kearney MM, Soule EH, Ivins JC: Malignant fibrous histiocytoma. *Cancer* 45: 167–178, 1980.

147. Kempson RL, Kyriakos M: Fibroxanthosarcoma of the soft tissues: A type of malignant fibrous histiocytoma. *Cancer* 29:961–976, 1972.

148. Enzinger FM, Shiraki M: Extraskeletal myxoid chondrosarcoma: An analysis of 34 cases. *Hum Pathol* 3:421–435, 1972.

149. Guccion JG, Font RL, Enzinger FM, et al: Extraskeletal mesenchymal chondrosarcoma. *Arch Pathol* 95:336–349, 1973.

150. Rao U, Cheng A, Didolkar MS: Extraosseous osteogenic sarcoma. *Cancer* 41: 1488–1499, 1978.

151. Patterson JW, Maygarden SJ: Extraskeletal Ewing's sarcoma with cutaneous involvement. *J Cutan Pathol* 13:46–58, 1986.

152. Taylor HB, Helwig EB: Dermatofibrosarcoma protuberans. *Cancer* 15:717–725, 1961.

153. Frierson HF, Cooper PH: Myxoid variant of dermatofibrosarcoma protuberans. *Am J Surg Pathol* 7:445–450, 1983.

154. Wrotnowski U, Cooper PH, Shmookler BM: Fibrosarcomatous change in dermatofibrosarcoma protuberans. *Am J Surg Pathol* 12:287–293, 1988.

155. Chung EB, Enzinger FM: Proliferative fasciitis. *Cancer* 36:1450–1458, 1975.

156. Price EB Jr, Siliphant WM, Shuman R: Nodular fasciitis, a clinicopathologic analysis of 65 cases. *Am J Clin Pathol* 35:122–136, 1961.

157. Enzinger EB: Atypical fibroxanthoma and malignant fibrous histiocytoma. *Am J Dermatopathol* 1:185, 1979.

158. Fields JP, Helwig EB: Leiomyosarcoma of the skin and subcutaneous tissue. *Cancer* 47:156–169, 1981.

159. Headington JT, Beals TF, Niederhuber JE: Primary leiomyosarcoma of skin: A report and critical appraisal. *J Cutan Pathol* 4:308–317, 1977.

160. Shin-ichi A, Takeda H, Koseki S, et al: A patient with rhabdomyosarcoma and clear cell sarcoma of the skin. *J Am Acad Dermatol* 31:871–876, 1994.

161. Enzinger FM: Epithelioid sarcoma: A sarcoma simulating a granuloma or a carcinoma. *Cancer* 26:1029–1041, 1970.

PART FIVE

DISORDERS OF NAILS AND THE ORAL MUCOSA

CHAPTER 36

DISORDERS OF THE NAIL APPARATUS

Aldo González-Serva

The pervasive misunderstanding of the nail unit as a skin equivalent rather than as an adnexal unit such as the hair follicle has complicated the evaluation and diagnosis of nail diseases.[1] After recognizing that the matrical and bed epithelia and stroma are not epidermis and dermis, a better appreciation of the microscopic findings in nail diseases has emerged.

The nail can be considered to resemble a flattened, cubist-like, hair follicle that is asymmetric (Fig. 36-1). The plate is laminar and enclosed by lip-shaped sides of unequal length. The plate-forming matrix is lateralized rather than enclosing the nail root (Fig. 36-2a). The intermediary epithelia surrounding the matrix, especially the bed epithelium, are its products as well, as are ultimately the resulting cuticular keratins that ensheath the plate (Fig. 36-2b).[2]

Regarding the dynamics of migration of the nail components, every layer of the nail unit moves forward alongside the plate in unison. Thus, the plate does not glide over the bed epithelium but is firmly attached to it in a parallel course. The bed ends at a predetermined site (the onychodermal band [Fig. 36-2c], which may be recognized clinically) and keratinizes fully in a zone known histologically as the solehorn. This keratinization may be described as onycholemmal keratinization.[3] On the opposite side, the true cuticle, which originates on the ventral side of the proximal nail fold, apposes the plate as it emerges, thus sealing the virtual space that otherwise would occur.

All the described onychal structures are encircled by cutaneous structures more akin to epidermis, which intersects with the emerging plate and epithelial and keratinous coverings. The rim of epidermoid keratin above the plate and the true cuticle is the rough eponychium, a nonessential and disposable semilunar spur that has erroneously been called "cuticle." Beneath the site of plate launching, beyond the solehorn, is the product of the bed epithelium—the hyponychial horn (or ventral cuticle). The latter structure lies above an intermediate epithelium, closer to epidermis, which is termed hyponychium. Keratins of onychal and epidermoid origin are blended in this hyponychial angle. This area of collision of nail and cutaneous epithelia, an half ostium of sorts, is a reservoir of information about past events in the matrix and bed. The nail plate is also a mirror of the same events. This realization supports the interpretation of nail diseases, from either scrapings or clippings of nail horn or plate, expressed earlier and still probably active at the time of the study. Thus fungi of the bed also will be at the subungual or hyponychial horn. Pigment associated with keratins will reflect a pigment-forming lesion of matrix or bed.

The melanocytic system of the nail consists of inconspicuous, non-pigmented cells in both matrix and bed, particularly in Caucasians.

When in the matrix, the melanocytes are more abundant in the distal matrix.

MICROSCOPIC SIGNS OF NAIL DISEASES

There are relatively limited histologic signs characterizing nail disease.[4] Some of the signs are noted in subungual horn and nail plate and may thus be diagnosed by noninvasive methods. Other signs are tissue-based and will need a biopsy for their detection. Excellent monographs of clinical and histologic features of nail diseases are now available.[5,6]

The choice of biopsy method should be influenced by the type of signs needed to secure specific diagnosis. Many diseases can be diagnosed or strongly suspected from scrapings and clippings of the nail. Plate dystrophy, subungual hyperkeratosis, and gross pigmentary deposits are the most important. However, knowing the source of the latter will require tissue examination. This more invasive approach will reveal epithelial changes such as epidermidalization or atypia. The presence of pigmented material or cells, atypical melanocytes, misplaced tissues, or neoplastic cells of other lineages, hemorrhage, and stromal changes—such as cellular infiltrates and myxoid degeneration—will require tissue for histologic examination as well.

More common signs of skin disease will be recognized in the perionychium, as essentially this is skin with the same type of patterns of disease as noted elsewhere.

RESOURCES FOR HISTOLOGIC DIAGNOSIS

The study of keratinous or tissue products of the nail with routine histology stained with Hematoxylin and Eosin is the mainstay of the diagnosis of nail diseases. Particularly helpful is the PAS stain, which habitually should accompany every study. For pigmentary disorders, iron and melanin stains are mandatory.

GROUP DIAGNOSIS OF NAIL DISEASES

The first issue to be addressed is whether the nail disorder is a plate dystrophy, a mass, or a pigmented lesion.

Most biopsies are obtained for the evaluation of nail dystrophy. This is the most difficult group of diseases to diagnose specifically; however, fortunately, most specimens fall into the triad of tinea, psoriasis and,

Anatomy of the Nail

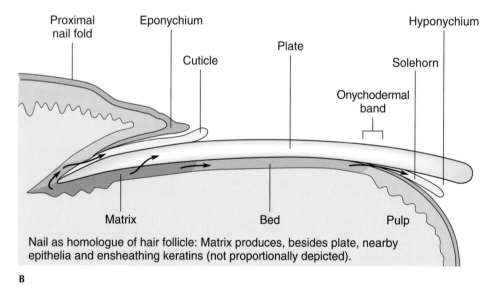

Eponychium
(false cuticle)

Cuticle

Hyponychium*
(space)

Solehorn*
(ventral cuticle)

Onychodermal
band

Lunula
(distal matrix)

Bed

*Under nail plate

A

Histology/Anatomy of the Nail

Proximal
nail fold

Eponychium

Cuticle

Plate

Hyponychium

Solehorn

Onychodermal
band

Matrix

Bed

Pulp

Nail as homologue of hair follicle: Matrix produces, besides plate, nearby
epithelia and ensheathing keratins (not proportionally depicted).

B

FIGURE 36-1 *A.* Clinical anatomy of the nail. The morphology of the plate is
the result of intimate accommodation of the nail structures to the subjacent bone.
The nail root rests over the proximal epiphysis of the distal phalanx whereas the
distal groove (at the site of onychodermal band and hyponychium) arches around
(and actually inserts, by specialized nail ligaments, on) the tuberositas unguium.
B. Diagram of nail structures.

much more rarely, lichen planus. Repeatable criteria for these diagnoses now are available.

DISEASES OF THE NAIL

This chapter emphasizes the disorders that are prone to be diagnosed histologically. Many others not discussed here can be diagnosed from other cutaneous or systemic signs. It is noteworthy to recognize that the nail unit is a domain of the skin, rather than a region, that expresses a wide spectrum of disorders, even if not diagnosable specifically by means of a biopsy.

Onychomycosis

Synonyms: Tinea unguium; dermatophytosis; nail ringworm

Fungal infections of the nail, the most frequent cause of nail disease, can be dermatomycetic (encompassing the cited synonyms), nondermatomycetic (such as mold infections), and yeast-related infections (mostly candidiasis).[7]

Clinical Features Regardless of etiologic agent, the fungal infections have been grouped as: distal/lateral subungual onychomycosis, superficial white or black onychomycosis, proximal subungual onychomycosis, and total dystrophic onychomycosis. Candidal onychomycosis stands apart. Isolation of the agent may be difficult, even if direct microscopy shows positive findings.

Histopathological Features The findings on direct microscopy may help to broadly identify organisms in nail plate or other nail tissue biopsies.[8] Besides the presence of the fungi, the nail tissues will undergo plate dystrophy and variable degrees of psoriasiform onychitis (Fig. 36-3a). The hyphae of dermatophytes are tubular, colorless, often refractile, and usually septate (Fig. 36-3b). In contrast, those of nondermatophytes will be thinner, more irregular and tortuous, and occasionally tan-brown. Conidia can also be seen with the latter infection. If this type of infection is suspected, fungal culture should be used for confirmation. Yeasts occur as pseudohyphae and spores.

In recent years, the biopsy of the plate alone, as clippings, has burgeoned as the method of choice for fast recognition leading to early treatment of onychomycosis.[9] The plate is variably penetrated by fungi in tunnels containing air but, more reliably, the subungual horn will invariably contain most organisms. PAS stain suffices in most cases for confirmation.

If a biopsy is done, the skin or epidermidalized bed epithelium show hyperkeratosis, both ortho- and parakeratotic, with Munro-like intracorneal microabscesses. Besides the presence of the fungi, the changes

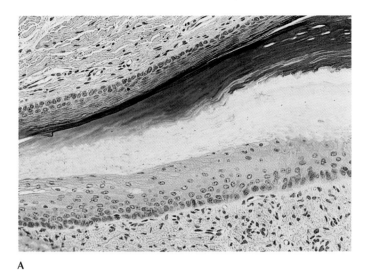

A

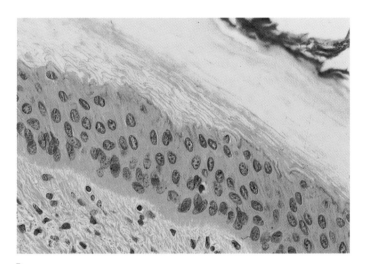

B

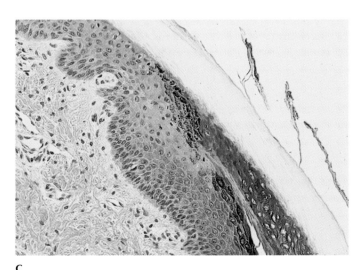

C

FIGURE 36-2 Histology of the nail (in newborn). *A*. The matrix epithelium is stratified and produces eosinophobic nail plate, mirrored by concurrent keratin of the ventral portion of the proximal nail fold (true cuticle). *B*. The bed epithelium is less stratified than the matrical one, with relatively monotonous upper and lower keratinocytes. *C*. The onychodermal band occurs wherein the bed epithelium clashes with the epidermis of the hyponychium. The entirety of the bed epithelium keratinizes and is extruded as the solehorn (ventral cuticle).

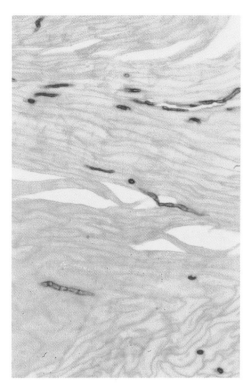

FIGURE 36-3 Tinea unguium. With PAS stain, septate hyphae are seen arranged parallel between sheets of the plate.

are similar to those of psoriasis. In superficial white onychomycosis, short and gnarled fungi are present in the superficial sheets of the plate. In contrast, fungi are present throughout the plate in proximal subungual onychomycosis and dystrophic onychomycosis. Candida also involve the whole thickness of the plate but pseudohyphae are distinct and accompanied by spores.

Differential Diagnosis The most important discrimination, prior to recognizing the fungal agents, is with psoriasis. After this relatively simple distinction is reached, one should realize that most fungal organisms identified in nails are not causing true infection. Commensal fungi can be seen in many biopsies. Even secondarily colonizing fungi may be observed in nonmycotic disorders such as psoriasis and lichen planus, among others.

Psoriasis

Synonyms: Pustular psoriasis; acrodermatitis continua of Hallopeau

Clinical Features Involvement of the nail is commonly seen, in up to 50 percent of patients, with psoriasis and is even more prevalent in patients with psoriatic arthropathy.[10,11] The abnormalities are zonal and related to the involved portion of the nail apparatus. Pits, transverse grooves, and other surface irregularities in the plate are related to damage to the matrix. An affected bed may exhibit discolorations, onycholysis, and splinter hemorrhages. If the bed and hyponychium are involved, subungual hyperkeratosis will be prominent.

Histopathological Features The histopathological alterations depend on the site of the disease, which may involve any part of the nail (Fig. 36-4). However, the basic pattern is that of psoriasiform onychitis with spongiform pustulation. In the proximal nail fold, the process is similar to psoriasis elsewhere in the skin. Matrical involvement results in pits,

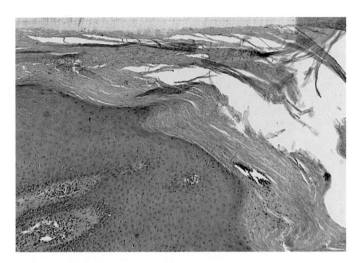

FIGURE 36-4   Psoriasis. The receding hyponychium, now occupying the space of former nail bed (onycholysis), is epidermidalized and hyperkeratotic. Besides keratinocytic pallor and agranulosis of the epithelium and papillomatosis of the bed stroma, there is a microabscess within the horn. No fungi are demonstrated with special stains.

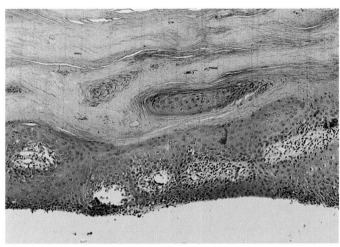

FIGURE 36-5   Lichen planus. Epidermidalized nail bed epithelium, appearing under dystrophic plate, is associated with lichenoid lymphocytic infiltrate.

which are dislodged psoriatic scale-like islands of variable width and length, according to the breadth and lapse of injury to the proximal matrix. If these parakeratotic islands with neutrophils originate in papules of the middle and distal matrix, punctate leukonychia will follow. The matrical damage will result in an overall thick, crumbly plate. When matrix and bed are affected, the spongiform pustulation will be the basis for the salmon patch and onycholysis. Involvement in the bed will produce epidermalization of its epithelium with resulting subungual hyperkeratosis. If the longitudinally oriented ectatic vessels of the bed exude erythrocytes, splinter hemorrhages will ensue.

Differential Diagnosis   The main differential diagnosis is onychomycosis. The microscopic changes may be identical, although psoriasis is usually more parakeratotic. The mainstay of the discrimination is the finding of fungi in onychomycosis.

   Another distinction is with eczematous onychitis, given that psoriasis in the nail may show eczematoid features. Other psoriasiform disorders, such as Reiter's syndrome and parakeratosis pustulosa, are either indistinguishable or very hard to separate from psoriasis.

Lichen Planus

Clinical Features   Onychal lichen planus may occur in 1 to 10 percent of patients with lichen planus elsewhere, but may be rarely confined to the nails, particularly in children.[12] The disorder varies in intensity, extension, or number of nails or portions of nails involved. Besides the common presentation, a hypertrophic variant is recognized. Onychomycosis can supervene in lichen planus of the nail.

Histopathological Features   The most devastating clinical features result from involvement of the matrix (Fig. 36-5).[13] According to severity of damage, only dystrophic plates may develop or, in many cases, complete destruction of the matrix will eventuate in loss of plate with scarring and adhesion of proximal nail fold to the nail mesenchyme (pterygium) (Fig. 36-5). If damage is limited, the impairment of the matrix will produce thinner and/or shorter plates. When the process is intermittent in the matrix, pits and irregularities are noticeable (20-nail dystrophy). Microscopic findings may not be sufficient for an unequivocal diagnosis as the disease evolves into a relatively nonspecific end

stage. The most diagnostic pattern is one similar to that of lichen planus in skin, namely, lichenoid onychitis with a band-like lymphocytic infiltrate near vacuolated basal keratinocytes. There is also hyperkeratosis with hypergranulosis. Plasma cells may be present.[14] If burnt-out, the nail field will become atrophic and epidermidalized, often permanently, and difficult to discriminate from that resulting from external trauma.

Differential Diagnosis   If the highly characteristic features of lichen planus are identified, few other differential diagnoses are practical. The main problem is with healed lichen planus in which the residual changes will be less than pathognomonic and practically indistinguishable from lichen simplex chronicus of the nail following external rubbing or other mechanical trauma. If onychomycosis supervenes, care should be taken not to miss lichen planus that may be obscured by infection.

Paronychia

This is infectious onychitis of the nail folds. Acute paronychia is bacterial, secondary to Staphylococcus aureus. Chronic paronychia is a disorder often associated with Candida albicans infection.

Clinical Features   The features of acute paronychia are those of acute pyogenic infection, namely, an abscess or cellulitis. Pseudomonas may be an offender.[15] Chronic paronchia will combine proliferative elements of fibrosing granulation tissue with foci of suppuration.

Histopathological Features   In acute paronchia, a collection of purulent material is present near a disrupted lateral or proximal fold (Fig. 36-6). A hangnail may be a preceding event. Interstitial neutrophilic exudate may be seen as well.

   Chronic paronchia has minimal or variable epidermal hyperplasia with spongiosis and scale-crust. The dermal infiltrate is composed of lymphocytes, histiocytes, and numerous plasma cells. Dilated vessels in an edematous stroma are prominent. If Candida organisms are present, they will be located in the cornified layer and will be neither invasive nor associated with granulomas.

Differential Diagnosis   Each paronychia has to be distinguished on the basis of etiology. Chronic paronychia can conceivably be bacterial, as candidal paronychia can be acute. Some tumors, including amelanotic melanoma, may mimic paronychia. Rarely, fixed drug eruption may resemble paronychia clinically.[16]

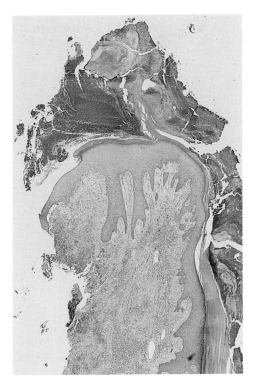

FIGURE 36-6   Acute paronychia. The proximal nail fold, protuberant and crusted (not unlike a hangnail), contains mixed inflammatory cell infiltrate (mostly suppurative), along with fibrosing granulation tissue reaction.

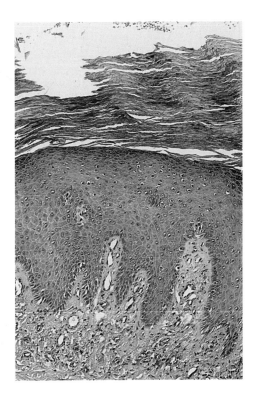

FIGURE 36-7   Traumatic onychitis (lichen simplex chronicus onychalis). The lichenified bed epithelium, now with mature squamous metaplasia (epidermidalization), is orthokeratotic. The bed stroma (never referred to as dermis) is fibrotic, reflecting a subjacent scar.

Traumatic Onychitis

Clinical Features   The results of trauma in the nail field include: hemorrhage, lichenification, and scar. The nail hemorrhage may be of splinter type or, more overt and of an acute nature, intralaminar hemorrhage (within the plate) and subungual hematoma. The trauma also can be enhanced by an abnormal protuberance of bone or cartilage under the nail plate as in the case of a subungual corn (heloma durum) above an exostosis or osteochondroma.

Other complications of external trauma are nail dystrophy, misplacement of the matrix and anomalous growth of new plate, and even, longitudinal melanonychia.[17-19]

Histopathological Features   Hemorrhage can be recognized histologically by extravasation of erythrocytes in the matrical-bed stroma and beneath or within the plate. Hematein, rather than hemosiderin (negative for iron stain), is identified. Benzidine stain may be used to detect disintegrated red blood cells and their products.[20]

Lichenification is a common final pathway to many disorders of the nail unit (Figs. 36-7 and 36-8). Be it derived from associated external trauma or, possibly, from self-perpetuating damage by abnormal epidermoid horn of various inflammatory disorders lodged between the plate and epithelia, the process is the same and may be erroneously taken for the primary disorder. The macerated lichenification of heloma durum, with clavus-like hyperkeratosis, is the equivalent of picker's nodule.

Scar results from mechanical damage tearing tissues. A protruding scar in the matrix will result in a split nail plate. If present in the bed or in the proximal nail fold, a scar will also induce dystrophic change in the plate.

Differential Diagnosis   Nail hemorrhage is the common differential diagnosis for pigmented lesions. A nail plate biopsy will usually discriminate between blood and melanin. The former may be freshly extravasated erythrocytes or hemolyzed products and pigments in or under the nail plate. Melanin, in contrast, can be easily discerned in the plate as opaque brown granules that are argyrophilic. Hemorrhages from other etiology, such as subacute bacterial endocarditis, cholesterol embolism and antiphospholipid syndrome, should be kept in mind.[21,22]

Lichenification, when secondary to protracted trauma, is usually accompanied by evidence of mechanical trauma, that is, hemorrhage and/or fibrosis.

A scar has to be distinguished from sclerosing conditions of the lamina propria of the nail, such as that following lichen planus.

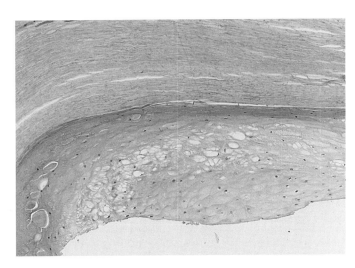

FIGURE 36-8   Traumatic onychitis (above exostosis). The macerated bed epithelium, also epidermidalized and hyperkeratotic, shows hydropic swelling and degeneration of keratinocytes. Subungual hyperkeratosis also indicates compression trauma of nail structures against the hard nail plate (and shoe).

Verruca

Clinical Features This human papilloma virus-induced lesion can be either periungual or subungual. If under the plate, the latter can be minimally affected. Trauma may contribute to persistence and refractoriness to treatment.

Histopathological Features The ungual wart is similar to the verruca vulgaris of skin. There is prominent digitated epithelial hyperplasia with koilocytotic (clear cell) changes of the upper strata and hyperkeratosis. The cytopathic changes are less pronounced than in palmo-plantar verruca. The lesion may become inflamed following trauma.

Differential Diagnosis Besides the common wart, there is an authochtonous variety of verruca known as the onycholemmal horn.[23] This lesion develops at the proximal and lateral folds and shows onycholemmal differentiation, namely, a proliferation of large polygonal keratinocytes without a granular layer, resembling that of trichilemmal and onycholemmal cysts.

A much rarer entity which may be warty is mucinous syringometaplasia of the distal bed.[24] This process is characterized by a focal invagination lined by squamous epithelium. There are eccrine coils and ducts with mucinous cells. The ducts drain into the epidermoid invagination.

Finally, the verrucous lesions of incontinentia pigmenti and epidermal nevus must be distinguished from viral warts. Another condition to be excluded when a "wart" is clinically noted is Bowen's disease.[25]

Cysts

The cysts in the nail are a broad group of lesions that differ in histogenesis and clinical expression. They may be minuscule and subclinical like the subungual epidermoid inclusions ("epidermal buds") or similar to epidermal buds but with nail dystrophy.

Others are indistinguishable from so-called epidermal inclusion cysts of the skin and are known as implantation epidermoid cysts (keratin cyst, squamous epithelial cyst, traumatic cyst).

Clinical Features Cysts of sufficient size will produce a subungual mass. Some of them will involve subjacent bone. A history of trauma is almost always elicited, except in the incidentally found subungual epidermoid inclusions.

Histopathological Features The implantation epidermoid cyst is unilocular, lined by thin epidermoid epithelium and filled with orthokeratin.

The subungual epidermoid inclusions are protrusions of the bed epithelium into the uppermost bed stroma. Although often asymptomatic, many of them may be associated with marked hyperplasia of the bed epithelium. This disorder will result in subungual hyperkeratosis, onycholysis and, rarely, a shortened dystrophic nail plate.

Finally, some cysts may contain epithelium that resembles that of the bed (and trichilemmal cysts) and are hence called onycholemmal cysts (Fig. 36-9).

Differential Diagnosis Some malignant neoplasms may be partly or largely cystic, such as the malignant proliferating onycholemmal cyst.[26]

Onychomatricoma

This newly described tumor is also known as filamentous tufted tumor in the matrix of a funnel-shaped nail.[23]

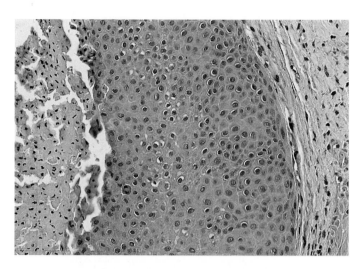

FIGURE 36-9 Onycholemmal cyst. In subungual location, a cyst resembling trichilemmal (pilar) cyst is identified. The content is parakeratotic, not separated from the epithelium by a granular layer.

Clinical Features This neoplasm produces a markedly overcurved plate (in transverse fashion) with excessive longitudinal ridging and a yellow longitudinal band.

When the plate is avulsed, the exophytic tumor in the matrix is digitated and filiform, being encased in a curved plate that offers a mirror-like funnel to the exuberant proliferation.

Histopathological Features Microscopically, the neoplasm is matrical, of lobular pattern, formed by basaloid keratinocytes. At the base of the lobules are narrow columns of densely arranged elongated cells with dark nuclei (similar to those in the matrical keratogenous zone). If these columns become dislodged, invaginations resembling hair follicle infundibula replace the formerly solid cores in the endophytic columns of cells.

Differential Diagnosis Unlike onychomatricoma, a *verruca* is epidermoid rather than basaloid and matrical. It also shows prominent keratinization and thick epithelium. The *invaginated fibrokeratoma with matrix differentiation* is mainly composed of a broad-based stromal fibrous nodule.[27]

Fibroma

This is a complex group of hamartomas and benign neoplasms that overlap and are sometimes difficult to distinguish unequivocally.

Clinical Features The periungual fibromas and fibrokeratomas are sessile or filiform masses that occur in digital skin or around the nail field, as well as in nail tissues where they arise in the proximal or distal nail fold or under the plate. The true fibroma, in contrast, is nodular and deep, always endophytic, even though it may be protuberant. However, it does not exhibit hyperkeratosis nor epidermal collarettes as observed in fibrokeratomas and periungual fibromas.

Histopathological Features The *periungual fibroma* is essentially an angiofibroma. The accompanying epidermal hyperplasia is ancillary. On the other hand, the *fibrokeratoma* is a fibrotic proliferation, with numerous fibroblasts, lined by prominent epidermal hyperplasia with hyperkeratosis. This lesion can be very large and invaginated.[27,28] Collagenous, cellular (fibroblastic) and edematous patterns have been described.[29] The *true fibroma* is composed of dense and hyaline colla-gen bundles, both aligned irregularly and interspersed among few fibroblasts. Elastic fibers are often few in number or absent. It is a deep and poorly circumscribed nodule located in reticular dermis or nail stroma.

Differential Diagnosis   The most important differential diagnosis of each fibroma of this taxonomically confusing group is with the other entities in this group, given the subtle variations that distinguish each one. It is noteworthy that periungual warts may resolve as relatively persistent angiofibromatous papules. A fibrokeratoma differs from a supernumerary digit in that the latter contains nerve trunks in its core, mainly near the base of the lesion. Infantile digital fibromatosis is richly spindle-celled, with frequent paranuclear inclusion bodies in up to 2 percent of fibroblasts.

Digital Myxoid Pseudocyst

Synonyms and Pathogenesis: Synovial cyst; dorsal finger cyst; cuta-neous myxoid or mucoid cyst

Clinical Features   This common disorder occurs in the proximal nail fold or under the proximal matrix. Attachment, through a stalk, to the distal interphalangeal joint has been proposed and occasionally found. This is not, however, sufficient evidence to claim herniation of syn-ovium as the source of the cavity of the pseudocyst. It may just reflect the ganglion-like degeneration of nail stroma, a surrogate of teno-syn-ovial tissue, or of nearby real teno-synovial structures.

Histopathological Features   The lesion is a pseudocyst without a gen-uine epithelial or even synovial lining. Some alignment and compres-sion of marginal fibroblasts may give the impression of pseudosynovial lining but the changes are not those of pseudosynovial metaplasia else-where. An ill-defined wall of fibro-connective tissue surrounds the lesion. The cavity is filled with mucoid material. The area initially is tra-versed by cobweb-like loose myxomatous tissue with few fibroblasts prior to cavitation. If the tense mucin-filled cavity erodes upward, the epidermis or the nail epithelia may rupture and evacuation of mucin may occur. Resealing of the defect and ongoing myxoid degeneration of soft tissues will be responsible for recurrence of the lesion, unless fully treated.[30]

Differential Diagnosis   A resolving abscess from chronic paronychia may enter into the differential diagnosis. If the mucin is drained, the resulting changes may suggest a scar. When epithelial necrosis occurs above a myxoid cyst, the traumatic changes may resemble those over-lying exostosis or ostechondroma. A true myxoma is never cavitated and contains numerous and prominent stellate fibroblasts.

Osteo-Cartilaginous Tumors

Synonyms and Pathogenesis: This group of entities is related because of common clinical signs and histologic features. It includes exostosis, osteochondroma, enchondroma, osteoid osteoma and solitary bone cyst. The first two constitute the bulk of the presentations.

Clinical Features   The classical triad for exostosis (pain, nail defor-mity and radiographic abnormalities) may apply to the rest of these enti-ties. A history of trauma is often noted.

Exostosis is an exophytic lesion, either single or multiple (as in the multiple exostosis syndrome).[31,32] Osteochondroma, enchondroma, osteoid osteoma and solitary bone cyst are intraosseous disorders.[33] The former may be multiple (as in Ollier's dyschondroplasia and in Maffucci's syndrome, in which there are also multiple vascular malfor-mations in soft tissue).

Histopathological Features   The exostosis is a protuberant prolifera-tion of mature bone surmounted by a fibrocartilaginous cap. An osteo-chondroma, not clearly distinguished from exostosis, is also a sessile or polypoid tumor of mature bone capped by mature cartilage. The enchondroma is a nodule of hyaline cartilage with haphazardly disposed chondrocytes that are often pleomorphic. The osteoid osteoma contains a nidus of disarrayed thick bone trabecules.[34] The very rare subungual bone cyst is cavitated reparative fibrotic tissue with giant cells.

Differential Diagnosis   First of all, exostosis and osteochondroma must be distinguished but that is difficult histologically. Enchondroma must be differentiated cytologically from chondrosarcoma (the latter is a distinct yet rare complication of osteochondroma and enchondroma). Osteoid osteoma is identical histologically to benign osteoblastoma.[2] If protuberant, any of the ossified and, therefore, calcified tumors may be mimicked by occasional subungual calcifications of the nail bed or nearby soft tissues and by circumscribed calcinosis cutis.

Glomus Tumor

This rare tumor is mostly observed in the hand, particularly in the sub-ungual area.

Clinical Features   The glomus tumor is a small (less than 1 cm), bluish red, and intensely painful lesion.[35] Some tumors may produce slight plate deformity with ridging and fissuring. A history of trauma is fre-quent. After surgical excision, recurrence is relatively high (10–20% of cases). Some cases may be associated with neurofibromatosis.[36]

Histopathological Features   This well circumscribed and encapsulated solid tumor is biphasic and highly organoid. Besides afferent arterioles and efferent venules, there are numerous vessels enmeshing small and round cuboidal cells. The cells are uniform and contain dark nuclei and comparatively pale cytoplasm. Many nerves are also present.

Differential Diagnosis   Other vascular tumors may resemble the glo-mus tumor on cursory examination. Among them, angioleiomyoma may have a complex net of vessels as well, but eosinophilic spindle-shaped smooth muscle bundles define the latter.

Squamous Cell Carcinoma

Clinical Features   Squamous cell carcinoma in situ (Bowen's disease) may be polydactilous, usually involving the hands more often than the feet. Rarely, pigmented bands are noted.[37,38] Squamous cell carcinoma, as other tumors of the nail unit, may give rise to a painful mass or swelling that may mimic traumatic and primarily inflammatory dis-orders.

Histopathological Features   Squamous cell carcinoma in situ is simi-lar to that noted in skin, namely, a keratinizing proliferation of atypical keratinocytes throughout the epithelium of the periungual epidermis, bed or matrix. It may be pigmented.[39]

Squamous cell carcinoma consists, as in other sites, of a bulky and invasive proliferation of atypical keratinocytes with anaplasia and dyskeratosis.[40,41] The invasion of nearby stroma is jagged and irregular, more infiltrative than pushing.

Verrucous carcinoma (epithelioma cuniculatum) is an exo-endophytic neoplasm with deep burrows and fistulas, strikingly well-differentiated and deeply invasive, with expansive and pushing rather than classically infiltrating margins. Bone invasion is frequently noted.[42]

Differential Diagnosis　Squamous cell carcinoma in situ has to be distinguished from verrucae displaying atypia or of the nearby in situ component of an invasive squamous cell carcinoma.[25]

Squamous cell carcinoma presents few problems in recognition. The distinction from keratoacanthoma probably remains the most important one.

Verrucous carcinoma must be distinguished from keratoacanthoma, verrucae, pseudoepitheliomatous hyperplasia, and conventional squamous cell carcinoma.

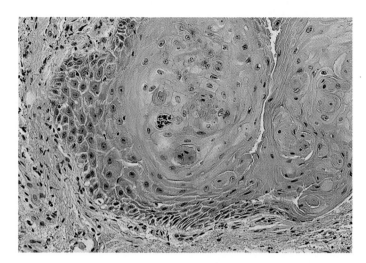

FIGURE 36-10　Keratoacanthoma. A cluster of glassy keratinocytes, one among many is identified. Prominent dyskeratosis and a small neutrophilic abscess are noted toward the center of the cluster.

Keratoacanthoma

Clinical Features　This entity may be subungual or periungual, either as solitary or multiple painful lesions.[43] It should be emphasized that the subungual keratoacanthoma (KA) does not behave like or even morphologically resemble cutaneous KA. It is of longer duration (more than 1 year), rapidly erodes bone and often does not regress.

Histopathological Features　Subungual KA has a narrow, more vertically oriented profile than common KA but otherwise is composed of deeply infiltrating aggregates of large pale (glassy) keratinocytes with keratohyalin granules and prominent dyskeratosis (Fig. 36-10).[44,45] The structure is centered around a keratin-plugged crater delimited by prominent lips. Compared to conventional KA, it is less inflamed (with fewer neutrophils and eosinophils), does not show fibrosis at the base, and readily infiltrates the subjacent bone.

Differential Diagnosis　Given the peculiar features of subungual KA, its distinction from squamous cell carcinoma can be difficult. Despite a similar sex distribution (male > female) as squamous cell carcinoma, KA often presents as a mass, occurs in a younger population, is rarer, grows faster, and is of shorter duration than squamous cell carcinoma. It also may be multiple, may erode bone (which may be reconstituted), and is rarely associated with a history of trauma.

Histologically, the well-differentiated appearance of large keratinocytes, arranged in large aggregates with central dyskeratosis, and at the base of a crater, favors KA. The unusually progressive course of KA raises the differential diagnosis of endophytic—rather than more easily recognized exophytic—verrucous carcinoma. In the opinion of the author, some KAs which do not regress but rather destroy structures inexorably are in fact verrucous carcinomas.

Typical Melanocytic Proliferations (Benign Melanocytic Hyperplasia), Including Ephelis, Simple Lentigo, and Melanocytic Nevi

These entities are very frequent causes of longitudinal melanonychia. The latter feature results from melanin granules in the growing plate derived from the segment of matrix involved by the melanocytic activation or proliferation.

Clinical Features　Longitudinal melanonychia is a brown-black band that indicates a melanin-producing lesion of the matrix. The same type of lesion in the bed, a non–plate-forming portion of the nail, results in a pigmented spot that is discrete and immobile. All the cited entities may produce a band that is narrow, sharply circumscribed and homogeneous.

Histopathological Features　Melanocytic hyperplasia, which may be the equivalent of an ephelis (freckle), shows either hyperpigmentation with or without slightly increased numbers of melanocytes. It is essentially a well demarcated pigmented macule in the matrix.

A simple lentigo exhibits an increased number of melanocytes singly disposed in a variably hyperplastic epithelium.

A rare melanocytic nevus, either acquired or congenital, contains nests of melanocytes in variably hyperpigmented rete ridges.[46–48]

Differential Diagnosis　The longitudinal melanonychia derived from neoplastic disorders (lentigo and nevus) has to be distinguished from the same phenomenon secondary to the freckle-like lesions with hyperactive melanocytes. The latter lesions may be related to ethnicity (Africans and Asians), may be spontaneous or congenital, follow trauma (such as friction or radiation), or be associated with the Laugier-Hunziker-Baran syndrome.[49,50]

These benign causes of longitudinal melanonychia have, in turn, to be distinguished from early melanoma, also characterized by a pigmented band. However, this band usually is wider, darker and/or variegated, and less well circumscribed than a benign pigmented band. It reflects a larger, more irregular and heterogeneous neoplasm of the matrix (see the following).

Atypical Melanocytic Proliferation, Including Melanoma In Situ

These lesions encompass atypical melanocytic proliferation or the early stage of melanoma in situ.[51] It has also been addressed as recurrent or persistent melanocytosis with histologic features that simulate melanoma.

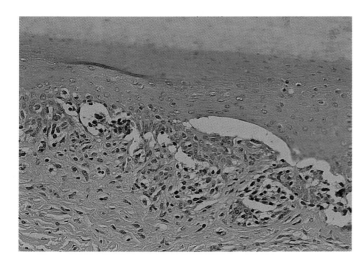

FIGURE 36-11   Melanoma, microinvasive. In the matrical epithelium, mostly basally located, are small yet hyperchromatic melanocytes that are irregularly arranged as single cells and in variably confluent nests. Few melanocytes are subtly present in the bed stroma.

Clinical Features   This early phase of acral melanoma may present as longitudinal melanonychia and, occasionally, as Hutchinson's sign (spread of pigmentation in the nail folds).[52,53]

Histopathological Features   On biopsy of the nail plate, the melanin granules are distributed broadly and, more important, throughout the whole thickness of the plate. This is a reflection of the usually wide and lengthy extension of the primary lesion. A problem in its recognition is the relatively uniform melanocytes near the junction of the matrix (practically always the source of melanoma in situ). However, the process may be cellular, and nuclear pleomorphism and other signs of malignancy may be obvious (prominent nucleoli, increased or abnormal mitoses, longitudinally branching dendritic melanocytes). If nests are formed, they are usually small, only slightly pleomorphic, and almost always nevoid. The latter characteristics account for the relative reluctance of pathologists to accept such a subtle proliferation as malignant. Regardless of terminology applied to such a lesion, complete removal of the lesion is mandatory.[54]

Hutchinson's sign may be seen histologically as the continuation of the same matrical and/or bed-extended proliferation of melanocytes in the epidermoid epithelia of epo- and hyponychium or the epidermis of the nail folds.

Differential Diagnosis   The differential diagnosis includes the entities discussed above, ephelis, lentigo, nevus, and invasive melanoma. As mentioned above the diagnosis of these various lesions is based on frequency, disposition, and degree of atypia of melanoctyes (see Chapter 27).

Melanoma (Also see Chapter 27)

Clinical Features   Although early melanomas may present with a longitudinal melanotic streak, more advanced tumors may give rise to a fully pigmented flat or tumorous mass in the nail field and periungual tissues.[55] The pigmented band usually has the same characteristics as melanoma in situ. More advanced melanomas may be amelanotic and be accompanied by destruction of the plate and ulceration. Melanotic whitlow (Hutchinson's sign) is very frequently found at this stage.[56]

Histopathological Features   As discussed in Chapter 27, the criteria for diagnosis include variable degrees of the following: a lesion of sufficient breadth, asymmetry, poor circumscription, increased numbers of atypical basilar melanocytes reaching confluence (Fig. 36-11), aggregates of atypical melanocytes that are irregularly sized and shaped, and pagetoid spread.[57]

Differential Diagnosis   The main pitfall is the misdiagnosis of melanoma as a simple lentigo, nevus or an atypical intraepithelial melanocytic proliferation (see Chapter 27 for further discussion).

REFERENCES

 1. González-Serva A: Structure and Function [Chapter 2], in Scher RK DRI (ed): *Nails: Therapy, Diagnosis, Surgery*. Philadelphia: W.B. Saunders, 1990, 11–30.
 2. González-Serva A: The nail bed: A conceptual revision. (Abstract). *J Cut Pathol* 14(6):357, 1987.
 3. González-Serva A: Onycholemmal keratinization: Ensheathing and fastening of the nail plate (Abstract): *J Invest Dermatol* 98(4):582, 1992.
 4. Jerasutus S: Histology and Histopathology (Chapter 2), in Scher RK DRI (ed): *Nails, Therapy, Diagnosis, Surgery*. Philadelphia: W.B. Saunders, 52–75, 1990.
 5. Baran R, Dawber RPR (eds): *Diseases of the Nails and Their Management*, 2nd ed. Oxford, London: Blackwell Scientific, 1994.
 6. Zaias N: *The Nails in Health and Disease*. Norwalk, CT: Appleton & Lange, 1990.
 7. Arenas R: [Onychomycosis. Clinico-epidemiological mycological and therapeutic aspects] Las onicomicosis. Aspectos clinico-epidemiologicos, micologicos y terapeuticos. *Gac Med Mex* 126(2):84–89, 1990.
 8. Pierard GE, Arrese JE, Pierre S, et al: [Microscopic diagnosis of onychomycoses]. *Ann Dermatol Venereol* 121(1):25–29, 1994.
 9. Suarez SM, Silvers DN, Scher RK, Pearlstein HH, Auerbach R: Histologic evaluation of nail clippings for diagnosing onychomycosis [see comments]. *Arch Dermatol* 127(10): 1517–1519, 1991.
10. Farber EM, Nall L: Nail psoriasis. *Cutis* 50(3):174–178, 1992.
11. Lavaroni G, Kokelj F, Pauluzzi P, Trevisan G: The nails in psoriatic arthritis. *Acta Derm Venereol Suppl* (Stockh) 186:113, 1994.
12. Peluso AM, Tosti A, Piraccini BM, Cameli N: Lichen planus limited to the nails in childhood: Case report and literature review. *Pediatr Dermatol* 10(1):36–39, 1993.
13. Tosti A, Peluso AM, Fanti PA, Piraccini BM: Nail lichen planus: Clinical and pathologic study of twenty-four patients. *J Am Acad Dermatol* 28(5 Pt 1):724–730, 1993.
14. Roustan G, Hospital M, Villegas C, Sanchez Yus E, Robledo A: Lichen planus with predominant plasma cell infiltrate. *Am J Dermatopathol* 16(3):311–314, 1994.
15. Molina DN, Colon M, Bermudez RH, Ramirez Ronda CH: Unusual presentation of Pseudomonas aeruginosa infections: A review. *Bol Asoc Med PR* 83(4):160–163, 1991.
16. Baran R, Perrin C: Fixed-drug eruption presenting as an acute paronychia. *Br J Dermatol* 125(6):592–595, 1991.
17. Price MA, Bruce S, Waidhofer W, Weaver SM: Beau's lines and pyogenic granulomas following hand trauma. *Cutis* 54(4):246–249, 1994.
18. Kato N: Vertically growing ectopic nail. *J Cutan Pathol* 19(5):445–447, 1992.
19. Baran R: Nail biting and picking as a possible cause of longitudinal melanonychia. A study of 6 cases. *Dermatologica* 181(2):126–128, 1990.
20. Hafner J, Haenseler E, Ossent P, Burg G, Panizzon RG: Benzidine stain for the histochemical detection of hemoglobin in splinter hemorrhage (subungual hematoma) and black heel. *Am J Dermatopathol* 17(4)362–367, 1995.
21. Turakhia AK, Khan MA: Splinter hemorrhages as a possible clinical manifestation of cholesterol crystal embolization. *J Rheumatol* 17(8):1083–1086, 1990.
22. Frances C, Piette JC, Saada V, et al: Multiple subungual splinter hemorrhage in the antiphospholipid syndrome: A report of five cases and review of the literature. *Lupus* 3(2):123–128, 1994.
23. Haneke E, Franken J: Onychomatricoma. *Dermatol Surg* 21(11):984–987, 1995.
24. Scully C, Assad A: Mucinous syringometaplasia. *J Am Acad Dermatol* 11:503–508, 1984.
25. Kaiser JF, Proctor Shipman L: Squamous cell carcinoma in situ (Bowen's disease) mimicking subungual verruca vulgaris. *J Fam Pract* 39(4):384–387, 1994.
26. Alessi E, Zorzi F, Gianotti R, Parafioriti A: Malignant proliferating onycholemmal cyst. *J Cutan Pathol* 21(2):183–188, 1994.
27. Perrin C, Baran R: Invaginated fibrokeratoma with matrix differentiation: A new histological variant of acquired fibrokeratoma. *Br J Dermatol* 130(5):654–657, 1994.
28. Hashiro M, Fujio Y, Tanaka M, Yamatodani Y: Giant acquired fibrokeratoma of the nail bed. *Dermatology* 190(2):169–171, 1995.
29. Kint A, Baran R, DeKeyser H: Acquired digital fibrokeratoma. *J Am Acad Dermatol* 12:816–821, 1985.

30. Miller PK, Roenigk RK, Amadio PC: Focal mucinosis (myxoid cyst). Surgical therapy [see comments]. *J Dermatol Surg Oncol* 18(8):716–719, 1992.

31. Kato H, Nakagawa K, Tsuji T, Hamada T: Subungual exostoses—clinicopathological and ultrastructural studies of three cases. *Clin Exp Dermatol* 15(6):429–432, 1990.

32. Jetmalani SN, Rich P, White CR Jr: Painful solitary subungual nodule. Subungual exostosis (SE). *Arch Dermatol* 128(6):849, 852, 1992.

33. Schulze KE, Hebert AA: Diagnostic features, differential diagnosis, and treatment of subungual osteochondroma. *Pediatr Dermatol* 11(1):39–41, 1994.

34. Brown RE, Russell JB, Zook EG: Osteoid osteoma of the distal phalanx of the finger: A diagnostic challenge. *Plast Reconstr Surg* 90(6):1016–1021, 1992.

35. Belanger SM, Weaver TD: Subungual glomus tumor of the hallux. *Cutis* 52(1):50–52, 1993.

36. Sawada S, Honda M, Kamide R, Niimura M: Three cases of subungual glomus tumors with von Recklinghausen neurofibromatosis. *J Am Acad Dermatol* 32(2 Pt 1):277–278, 1995.

37. Goodman G, Mason GTOB: Polydactylous Bowen's disease of the nail bed. *Australas J Dermatol* 36(3):164–165, 1995.

38. Baran R, Eichmann A: Longitudinal melanonychia associated with Bowen's disease: Two new cases [letter]. *Dermatology* 186(2):159–160, 1993.

39. Sau P, McMarlin SL, Sperling LC, Katz R: Bowen's disease of the nail bed and periungual area. A clinicopathologic analysis of seven cases. *Arch Dermatol* 130(2):204–209, 1994.

40. Guitart J, Bergfeld WF, Tuthill RJ, Tubbs RR, Zienowicz R, Fleegler EJ: Squamous cell carcinoma of the nail bed: A clinicopathological study of 12 cases. *Br J Dermatol* 123(2):215–222, 1990.

41. Patel DU, Rolfes R: Squamous cell carcinoma of the nail bed. *J Am Podiatr Med Assoc* 85(10):547–549, 1995.

42. Tosti A, Morelli R, Fanti PA, Morselli PG, Catrani S, Landi G: Carcinoma cuniculatum of the nail apparatus: Report of three cases. *Dermatology* 186(3):217–221, 1993.

43. Evole Buselli M, Botella Estrada R, Hernandez Marti M, Fortea Baixauli JM, Aliaga Boniche A: [Subungual keratoacanthoma] Queratoacantoma subungueal. *Med Cutan Ibero Lat Am* 18(2):145–147, 1990.

44. Allen CA, Stephens M, Steel WM: Subungual keratoacanthoma. *Histopathology* 25(2):181–183, 1994.

45. Oliwiecki S, Peachey RD, Bradfield JW, Ellis J, Lovell CR: Subungual keratoacanthoma—a report of four cases and review of the literature. *Clin Exp Dermatol* 19(3):230–235, 1994.

46. Brantley SK, Das SK: Junctional nevus of the nailbed germinal matrix. *J Hand Surg Am* 16(1):152–156, 1991.

47. Shukla VK, Hughes LE: How common are benign subungual naevi? *Eur J Surg Oncol* 18(3):249–250, 1992.

48. Tosti A, Baran R, Morelli R, Fanti PA, Peserico A: Progressive fading of longitudinal melanonychia due to a nail matrix melanocytic nevus in a child [letter]. *Arch Dermatol* 130(8):1076, 1994.

49. Wong DE, Brodkin RH, Rickert RR, McFalls SG: Congenital melanonychia. *Int J Dermatol* 30(4):278–280, 1991.

50. Haneke E: [Laugier-Hunziker-Baran syndrome] Laugier-Hunziker-Baran-Syndrom. *Hautarzt* 42(8):512–515, 1991.

51. Cho KH, Kim BS, Chang SH, Lee YS, Kim KJ: Pigmented nail with atypical melanocytic hyperplasia. *Clin Exp Dermatol* 16(6):451–454, 191.

52. Ishihara Y, Matsumoto K, Kawachi S, Saida T: Detection of early lesions of "ungual" malignant melanoma. *Int J Dermatol* 32(1): 44–47, 1993.

53. Kechijian P: Subungual melanoma in situ presenting as longitudinal melanonychia in a patient with familial dysplastic nevi. *J Am Acad Dermatol* 24(2 Pt 1):283, 1991.

54. Molina D, Sanchez JL: Pigmented longitudinal bands of the nail. A clinicopathologic study. *Am J Dermatopathol* 17(6):539–541, 1995.

55. Dawber RP, Colver GB: The spectrum of malignant melanoma of the nail apparatus. *Semin Dermatol* 10(1):82–87, 1991.

56. Baran R, Kechijian P: Hutchinson's sign: A reappraisal. *J Am Acad Dermatol* 34(1):87–90, 1996.

57. Blessing K, Kernohan NM, Park KG: Subungual malignant melanoma: Clinicopathological features of 100 cases. *Histopathology* 19(5):425–429, 1991.

DISORDERS OF ORAL MUCOSA

Sook Bin Woo

Oral and maxillofacial pathology is the specialty of dentistry and pathology that concerns itself with the study, diagnosis, and management of all developmental, inflammatory, infectious, neoplastic, and metabolic diseases relating to the teeth, the maxilla and mandible, the major and minor salivary glands, and the oral mucosa. Systemic diseases as well as drug interventions often manifest in the oral cavity and comprise an important category of oral disease. Overlap with other pathology disciplines occurs not uncommonly when lesions occur on the lips, perioral skin, sinonasal tract, and the oropharynx.

This chapter focusses on the more common oral mucosal diseases encountered in a pathology practice. As in the practice of dermatopathology, the importance of a thorough understanding of the clinical aspects and dynamic evolution of each entity cannot be overemphasized.

DEVELOPMENTAL CONDITIONS

Fordyce Granules

Synonyms: Ectopic sebaceous glands

Fordyce granules are intraoral sebaceous glands that are present in approximately 80 percent of the population.[1] Because of this high prevalence, they are viewed as a normal anatomic variation of oral mucosa. They are more commonly noted in adults rather than children probably because they become prominent after puberty because of hormonal influences.

Clinical Features   They occur as yellow-to-white papules measuring 1 to 3 mm in diameter and present symmetrically on the buccal mucosa, upper and lower labial mucosa, lip vermillion, and the retromolar areas, although rarely they may also be seen on the tongue, gingiva, and palate.

Histopathological Features   They consist of normal sebaceous glands that may communicate with the surface epithelium via a duct. Occasionally, there may be hyperplasia of the sebaceous acini, retention of secretions with pseudocyst formation, and even adenomatous change.[2–4] In one report, a hair follicle and hair shaft were present.[5] There is no risk for malignant transformation.

Differential Diagnosis   Most Fordyce granules are diagnosed on clinical findings alone and there is usually no need for a biopsy. If biopsied, it is unlikely that the presence of well-organized sebaceous units would be mistaken for a pathologic process other than Fordyce granules. Some salivary gland neoplasms (usually those found in the major glands) may

exhibit focal sebaceous differentiation within an obviously neoplastic process.

Cannon's White Sponge Nevus

Synonyms: Leukoedema exfoliativum mucosae oris; congenital leukokeratosis mucosa oris; naevus spongiosus albus mucosae

White sponge nevus is an uncommon, autosomal dominant, mucosal condition with a high degree of penetrance and variable expressivity, affecting primarily the oral mucosa, although genital, anal, laryngeal, and esophageal mucosal involvement also have been documented.[6–8] There are no concomitant skin lesions, although ocular coloboma have been described in one report.[9]

Clinical Features   Onset is in early childhood. The buccal mucosa is thickened and white with soft and spongy folds and creases, and an overall boggy appearance. Involvement is usually bilateral and the labial mucosa, alveolar ridge mucosa, floor of the mouth, and tongue may show similar changes. It is asymptomatic and may undergo periods of exacerbation and remission. Tetracycline and penicillin have been reported to improve lesions.[10,11]

Histopathological Features   There is parakeratosis, epithelial hyperplasia with cytoplasmic clearing of the spinous cells, and eosinophilic para- and peri-nuclear condensations, the last being most readily observed in the vacuolated cells, particularly on cytologic smears.[12] These condensations are characteristic for white sponge nevus (Fig. 37-1). Dyskeratosis may or may not be a feature. Some spinous cells may exhibit nuclear degeneration and be anucleate. Bacterial colonization may be a result of chronic trauma. The lamina propria is usually devoid of inflammation. Rarely, epidermolytic changes are noted.[13]

Ultrastructurally, the cells show segregation of organelles with some areas being completely devoid of organelles. There is abnormal aggregation of tonofilaments into dense clumps, corresponding to the para- and peri-nuclear condensations and the superficial cells contain Odland bodies (membrane coating granules) but without transfer of granules into the intercellular space.[12,14] White sponge nevus may be a result of abnormal keratinization and faulty desquamation.

Recent investigations revealed a mutation in differentiation specific keratins K4 and/or K13, in a domain critical for keratin filament stability.[15,16]

Differential Diagnosis   White sponge nevus may be differentiated from pachyonychia congenita, dyskeratosis congenita, and Darier's disease by the lack of concomitant skin lesions. Leukoedema does not

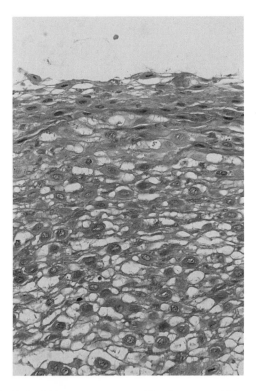

FIGURE 37-1 White sponge nevus. Keratinocytes exhibit perinuclear eosinophilic condensations.

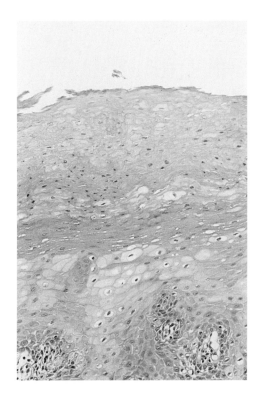

FIGURE 37-2 Leukoedema. Ballooned cells, compact cells, and superficial degenerated and anucleate cells.

show the perinuclear eosinophilic condensations and clinically, the lesions of leukoedema disappear when the mucosa is stretched. The histology of chronic cheek chewing is discussed in the following section. In some cases of white sponge nevus, there may be a component of chronic cheek chewing present histologically since the lesions protrude and may be inadvertently traumatized.

Leukoedema

Leukoedema is a fairly common mucosal condition reported to be present in 4 to 90 percent of the general population.[17] This wide variation in prevalence figures is likely a reflection of the variation in criteria used for diagnosis, differences in examination conditions, and differences in population groups and oral habits. The prevalence of leukoedema may appear to be higher in African Americans, because the pigmented nature of their mucosa allows this white lesion to be more visible.

Some consider this condition to be a variation of the norm because it is so widespread. However, its occurrence has been associated with the use of tobacco products, chewing of coca leaves and smoking of cannabis, and many believe that leukoedema occurs as a result of local insult to the mucosa since in some cases, cessation of smoking results in resolution of the lesions.[18–21]

Clinical Features   Both children and adults may present with this lesion. The buccal mucosa and sometimes the labial mucosa has a pale milky white or grey, opalescent appearance with crinkly folds and wrinkles. When the mucosa is stretched, the white crinkly appearance disappears or diminishes. The mucosa is not as white or thickened as noted in white sponge nevus.

Histopathological Features   The mucosa may or may not be thinly parakeratinized. There is acanthosis with the formation of broad rete

ridges. The mid-level spinous cells are swollen and vacuolated (so-called "intracellular edema"). Towards the surface, they flatten out and become eosinophilic. Another layer of vacuolated and ballooned cells are present beyond the flattened cells (Fig. 37-2).[22]

Ultrastructurally, the swollen cells of the mid-epithelium consists of cytoplasmic vacuolations with the cellular organelles displaced against the cytoplasmic and nuclear membranes. The vacuolations contain clumped glycogen-like material, and abnormal mitochondria are noted. The superficial ballooned cells contain membrane-bound spaces that contain remnants of organelles, keratohyalin-like granules, and clumped chromatin.[22] These features have been interpreted as reversible degenerative changes in the mid-epithelium and irreversible degenerative changes in the superficial cells, possibly owing to an overlying irritant.

Differential Diagnosis   Para- and perinuclear eosinophilic condensation and dyskeratosis is seen in white sponge nevus but not leukoedema. The three layers of vacuolated cells, flattened cells and superficially ballooned cells are typical for leukoedema. Parakeratosis and associated bacterial colonization may be present in areas that are chronically traumatized. Indeed, biopsies of the linea alba may be identical to leukoedema supporting superficial mucosal injury as an etiologic factor.

INFECTIOUS CONDITIONS

Median Rhomboid Glossitis

Synonym: Central papillary atrophy of the tongue

Median rhomboid glossitis represents at least in part, a form of erythematous candidiasis that involves the tongue dorsum. It had been thought to be a developmental anomaly caused by failure of the two lateral tongue processes to overgrow the tuberculum impar in the area anterior to the foramen cecum.[23] Perhaps it is the anomalous mucosa that predisposes to the development of candidiasis.

Clinical Features This condition is rare in children (which would be unusual if this was a primarily developmental entity). The prevalence rate is 0.1 to 1.0 percent of adults.[23] The lesion presents as a slightly painful, oval to rhomboidal, discrete, erythematous, depapillated, often nodular area in the midline posterior dorsum of the tongue anterior to the circumvallate papillae.[24] Treatment with antifungals may reduce symptoms and erythema but will rarely result in complete resolution (which would be unusual if this is purely candidiasis).

Histopathological Features There is atrophy of the tongue papillae with parakeratosis, and the presence of spongiotic pustules associated with candidal hyphae, in most but not all cases. There usually is a psoriasiform epithelial hyperplasia with confluent rete ridges, papillary edema, and a variable chronic inflammatory infiltrate in the connective tissue.[24] Some biopsies, if deep and taken from the midline, may contain the median raphe of the tongue. This appears as a homogenously hyalinized, hypocellular, and avascular band beneath the mucosa, into which the muscle fibers of the tongue decussate.

Differential Diagnosis Benign migratory glossitis also consists of a psoriasiform mucositis, but will not contain evidence of candidal infection.

Hairy Leukoplakia

Synonyms: Viral leukoplakia

First described in HIV-infected individuals, hairy leukoplakia is an EBV infection of the mucosa that also occurs in non-HIV infected immunocompromised individuals, particularly organ transplant recipients, and rarely in immunocompetent individuals.[25–27] In HIV infection, hairy leukoplakia is predictive of AIDS, which generally develops within 2 years of the diagnosis of hairy leukoplakia.[28] Some investigators question EBV as the etiologic agent in oral hairy leukoplakia.[29,30]

Clinical Features The lateral border of the tongue is the most frequently involved site, sometimes with extension onto the dorsum. The buccal and labial mucosae are the next most common sites. Hairy leukoplakia occurs as a painless white plaque that has a corrugated, shaggy ("hairy") surface with parallel furrows running at right angles to the lateral tongue border. When on the dorsum or the buccal mucosa, the furrowed nature is less noticeable and it may appear as a homogenous dense white plaque.

Histopathological Features There is parakeratosis with surface corrugations, as well as epithelial hyperplasia. Candidal hyphae are often present in the keratin layer but importantly, are usually unassociated with spongiotic pustules. Clusters of pale-staining somewhat vacuolated cells in the superficial one-third may show either condensation of chromatin against the nuclear membrane, or prominent, dense nuclear inclusions (Fig. 37-3).[31] Eosinophilic keratinized cells may insinuate between these clusters of vacuolated cells. There is no evidence of dysplasia, and inflammation in the lamina propria is insignificant. Epstein-Barr virus may be demonstrated by immunohistochemical stains, in situ hybridization or polymerase chain reaction in the majority of cases. Human papilloma virus occurs concurrently in 15 to 60 percent of cases, although its presence at all has been disputed.[32–34]

Differential Diagnosis Prominent dense nuclear inclusions and chromatin condensation, and not just vacuolation of the cells, are character-

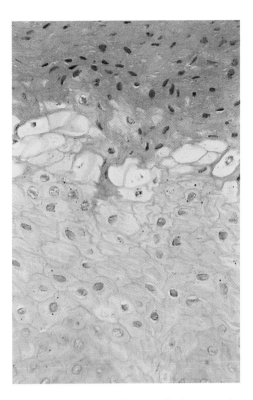

FIGURE 37-3 Hairy leukoplakia. Ballooned cells showing nuclear condensations and eosinophilic dense nuclear inclusions.

istic of hairy leukoplakia. Vacuolated cells are reminiscent of those seen in leukoedema or white sponge nevus. However, their distribution in hairy leukoplakia is patchy and may require a careful search. Chronic bite injuries may also give rise to leukoedematous changes and a superficial shaggy or "hairy" appearance to the keratin. Candidal colonization is a secondary phenomenon and a primary diagnosis of candidiasis should not be made.

Focal Epithelial Hyperplasia

Synonyms: Heck's disease; multifocal papilloma virus epithelial hyperplasia

Focal epithelial hyperplasia is a squamo-papular mucosal disorder caused by HPV-13 and -32.[35,36] It has been reported frequently in the Inuits and in the American Indian population. Africans, Cape Malays, Caucasians, and Arabs also have been shown to be affected. The prevalence rate varies from 7 to 13 percent of susceptible populations. Up to 25 percent of patients may have another member of the household similarly affected and in general most afflicted individuals come from a low socioeconomic class, suggesting horizontal transmission.[37,36]

Clinical Features Although most often noted in children, adults may also be affected. The disorder presents as multiple mucosal-colored or pale pink, papules with smooth or papillary surfaces. Individual papules may coalesce to form larger plaques. The labial mucosa, buccal mucosa and tongue are frequently involved. The lesions regress after a few months or years.[37,36]

Histopathological Features There is an exophytic squamous epithelial proliferation with or without papillomatosis. Hyperparakeratosis, if present, is mild. Rete ridges are usually broad and may be confluent at the base of the lesion. Koilocytes are noted superficially as in other

HPV-associated lesions. The so-called "mitosoid" figures represent nuclear degeneration and karyorhexis.[38,36]

Differential Diagnosis   Condyloma acuminatum and oral florid papillomatosis are important differential diagnoses. Condylomas have an obviously papillary surface, and acanthosis is much more pronounced than in focal epithelial hyperplasia. They may also contain HPV-13 and -32.[38] Oral florid papillomatosis tends to involve the pharyngeal tissues as well. The clinical presentation is more helpful than histologic features in differentiating between these lesions.

INFLAMMATORY CONDITIONS

Recurrent Aphthous Ulcer

Synonym: Canker sore; aphthous stomatitis

Recurrent aphthous ulcers of the minor variety is a recurrent ulcerative condition of the mouth that afflicts approximately 20 percent of the population. Predisposing local and systemic conditions include trauma, hypersensitivity to food, hematinic deficiencies, inflammatory bowel disease, immunoglobulin deficiencies, Behcet's disease, neutropenia and some collagen vascular disorders; and major aphthous ulcers are seen in HIV infection. One variant of minor aphthous ulcers occurs in early childhood as part of the FAPA (fever, adenitis, pharyngitis, aphthae) syndrome.[39] Although aphthous ulcers are likely associated with mild immune dysregulation, no clear evidence exists yet for autoimmunity as its etiopathogenesis.[40]

Clinical Features   The minor form occurs in teenagers and adults. They are evanescent, painful discrete ulcers, single or multiple, less than 1 cm in diameter with an erythematous border, that occur on the nonkeratinized mucosa and heal within 1 to 2 weeks. Common sites are the buccal and labial mucosa, ventral/lateral tongue and soft palate. The herpetiform type occurs in crops of many small ulcers, whereas the major type (Sutton's disease, periadenitis mucosae necrotica recurrens) measure greater than 1 cm and take weeks if not months to heal, often with scarring.[41]

Histopathological Features   The ulcer base contains granulation tissue with acute and chronic inflammatory cells and an overlying fibrin clot that contains many neutrophils unless the patient is neutropenic. The adjacent epithelium may exhibit reactive atypia. Underlying skeletal fibers, if penetrated by inflammatory cells, exhibit myositis. Vasculitis and thrombi formation are usually secondary phenomena.[42]

Differential Diagnosis   If there is significant stromal eosinophilia associated with myositis and proliferation of large, mononuclear histiocyte-like cells, a diagnosis of traumatic ulcerative granuloma should be made (see the following section). The presence of true vasculitis may be seen in the oral ulcers of Behcet's disease. A search for HSV and CMV should be made in biopsies from HIV seropostive individuals since such viral infections often present as aphthous-like ulcers clinically.

Traumatic Ulcerative Granuloma

Synonym: Traumatic ulcerative granuloma with tissue eosinophilia; traumatic eosinophilic granuloma/ulcer of the tongue; granuloma eosinophilium diutinum; Riga-Fede disease

This is a not uncommon condition that is most likely of traumatic origin since a clinically and histologically identical lesion has been experimentally reproduced in rat tongues after crush injury.[43] However, a history of trauma may be present in less than half the cases. The term Riga

Fede disease refers to sublingual ulcers in infants and young children caused by the trauma of rubbing the tongue against erupting teeth. It is also seen in patients with familial dysautonomia who are indifferent to pain and who are unaware of injuring themselves.[44]

Clinical Features   Males are affected more than females in a 5:1 to 2:1 ratio and it tends to occur in infants during eruption of the primary dentition, and in adults (Riga-Fede's disease).[45,46] Although most traumatic ulcers of the oral mucosa heal within a 2-week period, traumatic ulcerative granuloma may persist for more than 1 month raising the suspicion for a carcinoma, the reason for biopsies in the older population. The tongue is affected in 50 to 75 percent of cases with the lip and buccal mucosa as the next most frequent sites.

Traumatic ulcerative granuloma may present as an indurated ulcer or as a rapidly enlarging ulcerated mass. It heals uneventfully after biopsy or on its own although it may take several months, depending on the size of the lesion.

Histopathological Features   Beneath the ulcerated epithelium is a mass of granulation tissue that may be exuberant and exophytic. There is a polymorphous inflammatory infiltrate that extends deep into the tissues often into the muscle and salivary gland, and a large number of large mononuclear histiocyte-like cells with pale vesicular nuclei and eosinophils are constant findings (Fig. 37-4). In almost all cases, bundles of degenerating muscle fibers are also identified. Mast cells and Langerhans cells may be abundant.[45,47]

Differential Diagnosis   The atypical histicytic granuloma contains sheets of large mononuclear cells, often with cellular pleomorphism and mitoses, resembling a lymphoma.[48] However, the lesion is polyclonal and self-limiting. Another consideration is Langerhans cell histiocytosis. The cells in traumatic ulcerative granuloma lack the convoluted nuclei typical for that entity and the lesions regress with no treatment.

Benign Migratory Glossitis

Synonyms: Geographic tongue; erythema migrans; erythema areata migrans; erythema circinata

The evanescent nature of this fairly common inflammatory tongue condition has resulted in its prevalence rate being reported as between 1 and 14 percent of the population.[49] Patients with generalized pustular

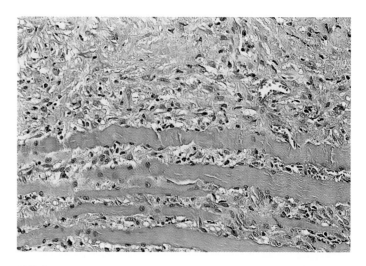

FIGURE 37-4   Traumatic ulcerative granuloma. A mononuclear cell infiltrate with eosinophils insinuate between skeletal muscle fibers.

psoriasis and Reiter's syndrome may exhibit lesions of migratory glossitis in 17 to 70 percent of cases.[50,51] An atopic diathesis has been suggested as a contributory factor in its development.[52]

Clinical Features   This condition affects adults in a male:female ratio of 1:2.[53] The tongue presents with irregular, map-like areas of depapillation and atrophy that is erythematous, often but not invariably outlined by a slightly raised, yellow-white serpiginous or circinate border. When located on mucosa other than the tongue, the term erythema migrans is used. Other common sites are the buccal and labial mucosa, gingiva, and palate.[54] The lesions wax and wane and there may be pain, burning, and sensitivity to acidic and spicy foods.

Histopathological Features   There is atrophy of the filiform papillae on the tongue dorsum with or without hyperkeratosis. Spongiotic pustules and sometimes microabscesses unassociated with candidal hyphae are present superficially (Fig. 37-5). The epithelium is acanthotic with leukocyte exocytosis and often confluence of the retes at the bases. There is papillary edema, thinning of the suprapapillary plate, vascular ectasia, and a variable lymphoplasmacytic infiltrate, all features of a psoriasiform mucositis.[49]

Differential Diagnosis   Stains for fungi should be performed routinely because candidiasis characteristically produces a psoriasiform mucositis. Areas adjacent to ulcers may also have similar histologic findings, although these are localized to the edge of the ulcer.

Cheilitis Glandularis

This is an unusual condition of the lip (usually lower), of unknown etiology, although there is some association with actinic cheilitis, atopic

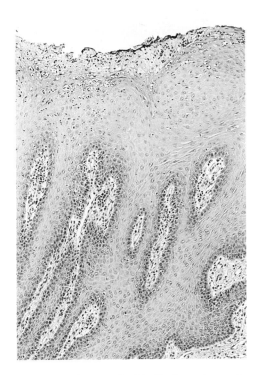

FIGURE 37-5   Benign migratory glossitis. Parakeratosis, atrophy of filiform papillae and spongiotic pustules characterize migratory glossitis.

diatheses, and factitial injury.[55] This bears no relationship to cheilitis granulomatosa, although lip swelling is present in both.

Clinical Features   This is a disorder of adults. Three clinical forms are recognized: simple, superficial suppururative (Baelz's disease) and deep suppurative (cheilitis glandularis apostematosa). In all cases, the lip is enlarged and often everted with areas of nodularity. In the simple type, crusting may occur with associated beads of mucus on the lip surface. Pain is more prominent in the suppurative type and ductal orifices may exude purulent material. Cases of squamous cell carcinoma arising from this condition may be a reflection of increased exposure to the sun because of lip eversion, as well as exposure to tobacco products rather than cheilitis glandularis representing a premalignant process.[56]

Histopathological Features   The glands contain a chronic interstitial inflammatory infiltrate with acinar atrophy, sialodochitis, and often, a purulent exudate within dilated and metaplastic ducts (Fig. 37-6).[57,58] In the simple type, the findings are less severe and suppuration is usually absent. In many cases, actinic cheilits may be concurrently present. The finding of hyperplasia of the mucous glands has been disputed.[55]

Differential Diagnosis   Distal obstruction of the salivary glands especially by sialoliths may cause similar histologic changes of a chronic sclerosing sialadenitis. In such cases, the sialoliths are identified in the ducts, usually of the upper lip.

Orofacial Granulomatosis

Synonyms: Cheilitis granulomatosis; Miescher's disease; Melkersson-Rosenthal syndrome

Some investigators use this term to refer only to granulomatous inflammation not associated with other systemic conditions such as Crohn's disease or sarcoidosis, whereas others use it to designate a condition characterized by orofacial swelling that histologically consists of noninfectious granulomatous inflammation regardless of whether there is a known systemic eiotlogy. Oral manifestations of the aforenamed systemic conditions may predate systemic findings.

Orofacial granulomatosis has been attributed to an abnormal immune response to a variety of antigens including microorganisms, food, and food additives. There may be a genetic predisposition and many patients have been reported to be atopic.[59]

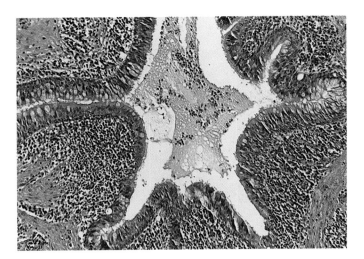

FIGURE 37-6   Cheilitis glandularis. Dilated excretory duct with luminal suppuration and periductal acute and chronic inflammation.

Clinical Features There is only a slight female predilection (1.1:1).[60,61] The most common clinical presentation is painless, persistent swelling of the upper and/or lower lips, sometimes with vesicles occurring symmetrically or unilaterally. If only the lips are involved, the clinical diagnosis of cheilitis granulomatosa is made. If the patient presents with the triad of cheilitis granulomatosa, fissured tongue, and facial nerve palsy, the diagnosis of Melkersson-Rosenthal syndrome applies. Some consider cheilitis granulomatosa alone (Miescher's disease) as the oligosymptomatic form of Melkersson-Rosenthal syndrome. In addition, patients may present with gingival swelling (up to 30%), erythema, and erosions, not unlike what may be seen in oral Crohn's disease.[60–62]

Histopathological Features Within the lamina propria are noncaseating granulomas often containing multinucleated giant cells (Fig. 37-7). These granulomas are usually present in small numbers and may be poorly formed so that multiple sections may be needed before they can be definitively identified. The surrounding tissues may be edematous and contain scattered chronic inflammatory cells, often in a peri- and paravascular location.[60,61] Dilated lymphatics may be present superficially. If salivary glands are present, granulomas should be sought within the gland parenchyma. Stains for organisms are negative and the granulomas should contain no identifiable foreign material. Since the condition may wax and wane, the appearance of granulomas may not be demonstrable in all patients.[63]

Differential Diagnosis The granulomas of orofacial granulomatosis are indistinguishable from those of Crohn's disease and the patient should be evaluated for gastrointestinal signs and symptoms. Granulomas of sarcoidosis usually contain asteroid bodies and tend to be well formed. Wegener's granulomatosis presents with "strawberry gingivitis." The histologic changes consist of pseudoepitheliomatous hyperplasia, vasculitis, abscesses, and a mixed inflammatory infiltrate in addition to granulomas. Ascher's syndrome consists of double lip, blepharochalasis, and nontoxic thyroid enlargement, but the biopsy does not contain granulomas.

Pyostomatitis Vegetans

This is a rare pustular and vegetating mucosal disorder that is associated with inflammatory bowel disease in 50 to 70 percent of cases, and is thought to represent the mucosal counterpart of pyodermatitis vegetans.[64–66] There is also an association with liver disease. Although originally thought to represent a form of pemphigus vegetans or vulgaris, pyostomatitis vegetans is now thought to be distinct from pemphigus.

Clinical Features Multiple painful small yellowish-white papules, ulcers and pustules are noted on the mucosa, sometimes with a linear, serpentine or "snail track"-like configuration, and sometimes in clusters and crops. The surrounding mucosa may be markedly erythematous and friable with nodular excrescences and vegetative plaques. Generally, the bowel symptoms precede the oral lesions by about 1 year, although oral lesions may predate them.[64] Skin lesions are present in approximately 50 percent of cases.[64,65]

Histopathological Features There is epithelial hyperplasia with marked spongiosis, and the formation of suprabasilar clefts. Intra-epithelial abscesses composed of neutrophils and eosinophils are characteristic and often there are similar abscesses in the edematous connective tissue papillae (Fig. 37-8). A polymorphic inflammatory infiltrate is present in the lamina propria. Direct immunofluorescence studies may reveal weak patchy positive staining for IgA and C3.[64,65] It has been suggested that such immunoreactivity may be a secondary phenomenon owing to chronic tissue destruction.

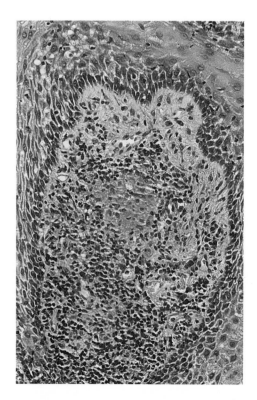

FIGURE 37-7 Orofacial granulomatosis. Non-necrotizing granulomatous inflammation in the lamina propria.

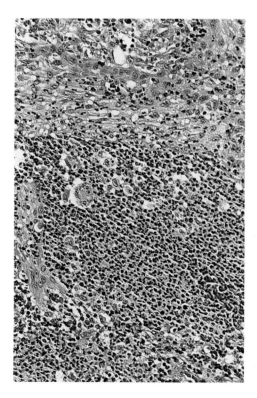

FIGURE 37-8 Pyostomatitis vegetans. Eosinophilic abscesses are present.

Differential Diagnosis   Pemphigus vegetans rarely involves the oral mucosa without obvious skin involvement although histologically, they may be indistinguishable. Direct immunofluorescence studies usually are strongly positive in pemphigus lesions and weak in pyostomatitis vegetans. The epithelial hyperplasia may be so florid that the differential diagnosis of acantholytic squamous cell carcinoma may be suggested. The latter would show cytologic atypia and pleomorphism beyond the range encountered in reactive lesions and direct immunofluorescence studies are negative.

Necrotizing Sialometaplasia

Necrotizing sialometaplasia is an uncommon inflammatory condition characterized by ulceration of the mucosa overlying infarcted salivary glands. It is believed to result from ischemia to the gland. Such vascular compromise has been variably attributed to local trauma, epinephrine from local anesthetics, Raynaud's phenomenon and adjacent tumors impinging on the blood supply.[67] Nevertheless, many cases occur idiopathically. It may be confused with a malignant process because of rapid onset, the clinical appearance, and histopathology.

Clinical Features   There is a slight 2:1 male predilection and it tends to occur in middle age. The mucosa of the posterior hard palate and associated glands is affected in 70 to 80 percent of cases, with two-thirds of cases occurring unilaterally. Necrotizing sialometaplasia may also occur in the labial mucosa, retromolar pad, tongue, major salivary glands, and upper respiratory tract.[67,68]

The lesion usually begins as an ulcer that may or may not be painful, often with preceding swelling. After a few weeks, a sizable mass of necrotic tissue may exfoliate and rapid healing ensues. The average length of time that the ulcer is present is 5 weeks.

Histopathological Features   The salivary glands exhibit preservation of its usual lobular architecture and this is a very important feature present in all lesions provided an adequate biopsy is obtained. In early lesions, coagulative necrosis of the acini predominates, whereas in more advanced lesions, squamous metaplasia of the ducts and pseudoepitheliomatous hyperplasia of the overlying mucosa may be pronounced. There may be extensive mucous pooling and extravasation around acini even in early lesions with accompanying acute and chronic inflammation.[67,69] The islands of squamous epithelium usually are cytologically bland with occasional evidence of reactive atypia. Small vessels in the area often exhibit thrombosis and occlusion.

Differential Diagnosis   The preservation of the normal lobular architecture of the glands is the single most important histologic parameter that helps to distinguish necrotizing sialometaplasia from mucoepidermoid carcinoma and squamous cell carcinoma. In addition, in mucoepidermoid carcinoma, there is proliferation of mucous cells, admixed with squamous cells in a disorganized fashion, forming islands of tumor cells that vary in shape and size. Infiltration of the adjacent structures usually is evident. Squamous cell carcinoma will exhibit significant cytologic atypia and pleomorphism with infiltration of the adjacent tissues.

Morsicatio Buccarum

Synonym: Morsicatio mucosae oris; pathominia mucosae oris

The term "morsicatio buccarum" should be reserved for its primary, less common and more extensive form that is a result of a chronic mucosal chewing or biting habit. Histologic changes caused by bite trauma may occur as an incidental finding in a localized fashion associ-

ated with another lesion such as a fibroma, that has been inadvertently traumatized because of its exophytic nature.

Clinical Features   A cheek and lip chewing habit is more often encountered in the teenage years (1 to 2%) with an even sex distribution. Patients may be unaware of the habit. The most common locations are the buccal and labial mucosa. The mucosa appears greyish white with an irregular shaggy surface, focal erosions, erythema and sometimes ulcerations.[70,71] It is often possible to peel off some of the white strands of macerated surface mucosa.

Histopathological Features   There is marked hyperparakeratosis and the surface of the keratin is shaggy and irregular with fissures and clefts rimmed by many bacterial colonies (Fig. 37-9).[72] It is common to see changes of leukoedema superficially and previous reports of leukoedema have noted the presence of bacteria.[73] It is likely that in cases of leukoedema, the thickening of the epithelium caused the mucosa to be chronically traumatized. Conversely, local chronic irritation such as a chewing habit may cause changes of leukoedema.

Differential Diagnosis   It is common to see leukoedematous changes in the hyperplastic epithelium, although morsicatio buccorum is clinically distinct from leukoedema. Unlike hairy leukoplakia, there is no clumping of the chromatin against the nuclear membrane and no concomitant candidiasis.

Oral Lichen Planus

This is a common condition of the mucosa with a prevalence rate of 1 to 2 percent. Although many cases are idiopathic, a lichenoid mucosal reaction (similar clinically and histologically) may be seen in mucosal drug eruptions, and in contact stomatitides associated with dental

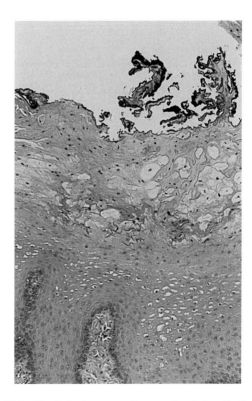

FIGURE 37-9   Morsicatio buccarum. Hyperparakeratosis with fissures and papillary projections rimmed by bacterial colonies.

restorations. The use of cinnamon-containing dentrifices and chewing gum may result in the occurrence of oral lichenoid reactions, although more commonly, they present as painful, erythematous areas with only faint peripheral lichenoid striations. Drugs that have been implicated include antihypertensive agents, nonsteroidal antiinflammatory drugs, and antirheumatologic agents.[74] Discoid lupus erythematosus and chronic oral graft-versus-host disease may result in oral lesions that are clinically and histologically similar to oral lichen planus. There appears to be an association of lichen planus with chronic liver disease and in particular hepatitis C.[75,76]

The rate of malignant transformation of lichen planus has been reported to be between 0.4 and 6.0 percent.[77] Some investigators believe that oral lichen planus has an innate premalignant potential. Others believe that the preexisting lichen planus lesions are actually premalignant epithelial dysplasias that have lichenoid features, that subsequently undergo carcinomatous change.[78] Supporting this latter theory is the finding that many of the reported cases of malignant transformation have a history of tobacco use.

Oral lichen planus results from a complex interplay between cellular and molecular signals that begin with alteration of keratinocyte antigens by an endogenous or exogenous agent. T lymphocytes, Langerhans cells, mast cells, and endothelial cells together with their cytokines and adhesion molecules are all involved in the induction and effector phases that lead to progression and chronicity.[79]

Clinical Features   Females are affected twice as often as males and most are adult or middle-aged. Concurrent skin lesions are present in 4 to 44 percent of cases.[74] Six clinical types have been identified, and they can be grouped into reticular, papular/plaque, and atrophic/ulcerative/bullous. The bullous type is rare since most bullae in the mouth rupture within a short period of their appearance, appearing ulcerated or atrophic. The first two groups of lesions generally are asymptomatic, whereas the last group tends to be painful. Many patients have combinations of these types and generally, reticular white areas suggestive of Wickham's striae are present at the periphery. Lesions wax and wane and patients report they are worse during stressful times.

Any part of the mucosa may show oral lichen planus, with the favored sites being buccal mucosa, labial mucosa, tongue, and gingiva. Some patients have the atrophic/erosive/bullous form of lichen planus on the gingiva that clinical presents as "desquamative gingivitis" (see the following).

Histopathological Features   There is para or orthokeratosis. The epithelium is attenuated or eroded in the atrophic/erosive type, often with small ulcerations, and somewhat hyperplastic in the reticular and plaque type. There is leukocyte exocytosis, an increase in the number of Langerhans cells and variable apoptosis. Sawtooth rete ridges may be seen. The basal cells are degenerated and the basement membrane is thickened. A bandlike lymphohistiocytic infiltrate hugs the connective tissue–epithelium interface. Some cases exhibit subepithelial bullae formation or complete desquamation of the epithelium. Melanophages and incontinent melanin may be present in the lamina propria in dark-skinned individuals. Plasma cells are prominent if there is overlying ulceration and possibly, if associated with a contact stomatitis. Eosinophils are not usually encountered.

In some cases, nodular peri and paravascular lymphocytic aggregates may be a prominent feature, sometimes with lymphoid follicles within the lymphoid band (Fig. 37-10). Some, but not all of such cases are associated with hypersensitivity reactions to cinnamon.[80]

Differential Diagnosis   In cicatricial pemphigoid, the basal cells are intact and the lymphocytic band is usually not as dense. Lupus erythe-

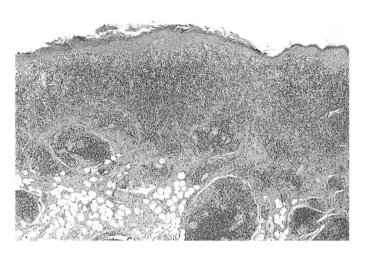

FIGURE 37-10   Lichen planus. Lichenoid mucositis with nodular peri- and paravascular lymphocytic infiltrate.

matosus shows hydropic degeneration of the basal cells, alternating epithelial atrophy and hyperplasia or rete ridges and perivascular lymphocytic infiltrates. Both these entities can be confirmed with direct immunofluorescence studies. The epithelial changes are less marked and the lymphocytic infiltrate sparse in oral chronic graft-versus-host disease because of systemic immunosuppression. Importantly, lichenoid dysplasias represent epithelial dysplasia that incites a lichenoid tissue reaction.

An entity that clinically and histologically resembles erosive lichen planus called chronic ulcerative stomatitis exhibits speckled nuclear anti-IgG deposits on direct immunofluorescence, against a putative stratified epithelium-specific antinuclear antibody.[81]

Desquamative Gingivitis

This is a clinical term used to describe a distinctive form of gingivitis that may represent one of several pathologic entities, the histology of which have been described in other sections.

Clinical Features   There is a 4:1 female predilection, with patients being adults or middle-aged. The gingiva is painful, and diffusely erythematous with areas of vesiculation, erosion, and desquamation, often covered by a white membrane that may represent a fibrin clot or the roof of a collapsed bulla. A positive Nikolsky sign may be present. Half the patients will present with only gingival involvement, whereas others may show involvement of other oral, mucosal, and skin sites.[82,83]

Histopathological Features   In approximately half the cases, direct immunofluorescence studies are consistent with cicatricial pemphigoid, whereas one-fourth each are consistent with lichen planus or are nonspecific.[83] Less commonly, desquamative gingivitis may be a manifestation of pemphigus vulgaris, linear IgA disease, or epidermolysis bullosa acquisitia.

Plasma Cell Gingivitis

This condition was first described in the early 1970s and its etiology was putatively ascribed to a component of chewing gum.[84] Sporadic cases continue to be reported, of unknown etiology.

Clinical Features   The gingiva (usually anterior maxilla) is markedly erythematous, edematous, and painful. Ulceration is unusual.[85] In the chewing gum-associated cases, there was concomitant cheilitis and glossitis.[84] In some idiopathic cases, there is accompanying supraglottic and laryngeal involvment with accompanying hoarseness and/or sore throat.[86]

Histopathological Features   The epithelium is markedly hyperplastic with spongiosis and sometimes, superficial microcyst and pustule formation. Dyskeratotic cells may be present. The lamina propria contains sheets of plasma cells that do not display atypia and are polyclonal with immunohistochemical studies. Dilated capillaries and scattered lymphocytes are noted in areas where the plasma cell infiltrate is less dense. Eosinophils are not a feature.[85]

Differential Diagnosis   Monoclonality of the plasma cell infiltrate must be ruled out since the differential diagnosis includes extramedullary plasmacytoma histologically. An intense plasmacytic infiltrate in the gingival tissues and periodontium is not uncommon in severe chronic periodontal disease but would not clinically resemble the entity plasma cell gingivitis.

ORAL NODULES AND EPULIDES

Mucocele

Synonym: Mucous cyst

This is a common condition of the lower labial mucosa and floor of mouth caused by mucous extravasation and pooling in the interstitium as a result of traumatic disruption of the integrity of the excretory salivary duct. Sometimes a distal obstruction causes retention of mucous within the cystically dilated duct. In either event, the term mucocele may be applied although the latter may also be referred to as a "salivary duct cyst." Floor of mouth lesions are sometimes termed ranulas.

Clinical Features   The mucocele occurs as a dome-shaped, sessile, bluish, translucent, usually painless swelling on the lower labial mucosa, floor of mouth, and any other site that has underlying salivary glands. There may be a history of the cyst filling up and draining periodically.

Histopathological Features   A pool of mucinous material containing muciphages and often neutrophils is present in the interstitium, sometimes abutting the epithelium. It is surrounded by condensed granulation tissue containing muciphages and variable numbers of chronic inflammatory cells (Fig. 37-11). It is therefore, not a true cyst. A portion of the salivary duct, often exhibiting squamous metaplasia may be present at the periphery and the associated minor salivary glands exhibit varying degrees of chronic inflammation, ductal ectasia, acinar atrophy, and interstitial fibrosis. In late stages, only a nodule of granulation tissue with occasional muciphages remain. A small number of mucoceles sometimes called "salivary duct cysts," consist of cystically dilated excretory ducts filled with mucous usually exhibiting squamous metaplasia of the lining epithelium.

Differential Diagnosis   The partially organized mucocele may be mistaken for a minor salivary gland tumor. The presence of muciphages with granulation tissue and chronic inflammatory cells and the absence of proliferation of ductal or epidermoid cells differentiate a mucocele from neoplastic processes. Salivary gland tumors are exceedingly rare on the lower labial mucosa.

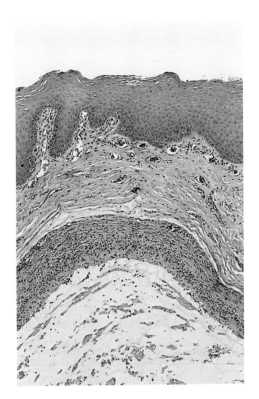

FIGURE 37-11   Mucocele. Cyst-like cavity surrounded by granulation tissue.

Fibromas

Synonym: Fibrous hyperplasia; fibroepithelial polyp, bite fibroma, irritation fibroma

This is a very common condition of the oral mucosa and occurs at sites that are commonly traumatized. It is not a true neoplastic process but rather a reactive proliferation of fibrous tissue.

Clinical Features   Fibromas usually present on the buccal or lower labial mucosa, and lateral border of the tongue, all common sites of bite trauma. The nodule usually is dome-shaped, sessile or pedunculated, soft, mucosal-colored, and may show areas of ulceration and/or whiteness.

A variant of the fibroma called the giant cell fibroma tends to be located on the gingiva and tongue and often has a papillary surface clinically.[87,88]

Histopathological Features   There is a proliferation of fibrous tissue, usually with low cellularity, and scattered blood vessels. The overlying epithelium may be attenuated or hyperplastic, and there is usually hyperkeratosis (Fig. 37-12). Focal areas of myxoid degeneration and mucinous change may be encountered and occasionally, scattered lymphocytes are noted. Although some fibromas may contain a few lipocytes, others contain significant amounts of fat. If so, a diagnosis of fibrolipoma is appropriate.

The giant cell fibroma has a papillary surface configuration and usually exhibits epithelial hyperplasia in the form of spiky rete ridges. Just beneath the epithelium are numerous plump stellate-shaped and often bi- or multi-nucleated giant fibroblasts (Fig. 37-13).[87,88] Occasionally, the nuclei may have a wreath-like configuration. Ultrastructurally, the giant fibroblasts have been noted to contain microfilaments, dense bodies, and junctional complexes, thus resembling myofibroblasts.

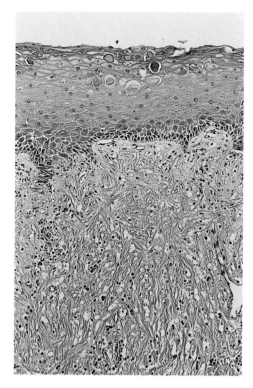

FIGURE 37-12   Fibroma with flattened epithelium and surface "plasma pooling."

Epulis Fissuratum

Synonym: Inflammatory fibrous hyperplasia; denture-associated epulis

The benign overgrowth of fibrous tissue that characterizes this condition is caused by an ill-fitting denture sliding on and traumatizing the soft tissues at the edges of the denture flange.

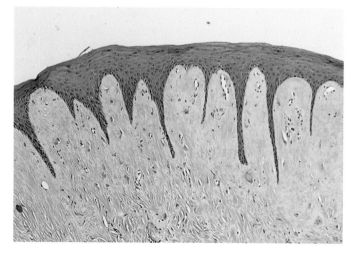

FIGURE 37-13   Giant cell fibroma with stellate-shaped and binucleated fibroblasts with epithelial hyperplasia.

Clinical Features   There is a female predilection for this condition that for obvious reasons occurs in older individuals. There are papulous and ridged folds of soft tissue, usually in the buccal maxillary and mandibular sulci, often with a prominent central fissure into which the denture flange fits. The surface may have papillary, ulcerated, or erythematous areas.

Histopathological Features   The overlying epithelium is often hyperplastic and pseudoepitheliomatous hyperplasia is not unusual. There may be parakeratosis, focal ulcerations, and areas of candidal infection. The bulk of the tissue consists of hyperplasia of fibrous tissue, sometimes with many ectatic vessels. A lymphocytic infiltrate is invariably present, and sometimes, lymphoid nodules and osseous and cartilagenous metaplasia also may be noted. Salivary glands, if present, may demonstrate chronic sialadenitis.

Differential Diagnosis   Pseudoepitheliomatous hyperplasia may be mistaken for squamous cell carcinoma in this elderly population but there is lack of atypia, true invasion, or mitotic activity. Cartilagenous metaplasia is a well-recognized phenomenon in these lesions and should not be overdiagnosed.

Inflammatory Papillary Hyperplasia of the Palate

Synonym: Denture hyperplasia

This condition is caused by wearing an ill-fitting maxillary denture and/or wearing a denture continuously, even when asleep at night.[89]

Clinical Features   The palatal mucosa under the denture is covered by soft, pebbly, fibrous nodules that coalesce, resulting in a cobblestone appearance.

Histopathological Features   This is essentially similar to the histopathology of epulis fissuratum except that the fibrous hyperplasia has a papillary configuration.

Differential Diagnosis   See section on epulis fissuratum.

Gingival Nodules

The term "epulis" refers to any growth on the gingiva or alveolar mucosa. The six gingival nodules that are reactive in nature are fibrous hyperplasia or fibroma, pyogenic granuloma (not uncommon during pregnancy, at which time they may be referred to as granuloma gravidarum), peripheral ossifying fibroma, peripheral giant cell granuloma, drug-induced gingival hyperplasia, and the parulis (Figs. 37-14 through 37-16).[90–93]

The first five entities are reactive and thought to arise as a reparative process in response to chronic irritation from deposits of dental calculus, poorly adapted dental restorations, orthodontic braces, and other local factors. They occur on the marginal gingiva and at least a portion of the lesion rests against the teeth. Histopathologically, it is not unusual to see combinations of pyogenic granuloma, peripheral ossifying fibroma, and peripheral giant cell fibroma within one lesion.

The parulis usually occurs on attached or nonattached gingiva at a distance from the teeth. Its presence almost always indicates an underlying intrabony odontogenic infection.

All present as nodules varying in size from a few mm to 1 to 2 cm. They may be mucosa-colored when small. Larger ones are usually erythematous and/or ulcerated. Drug-induced hyperplasias affect the gingiva diffusely over time.

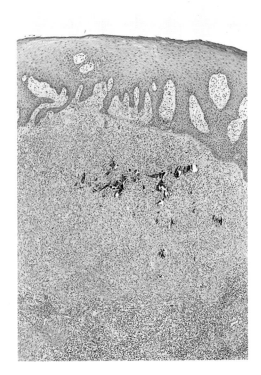

FIGURE 37-14   Peripheral ossifying fibroma. Cellular fibrous tissue with deposition of osteoid and calcifications.

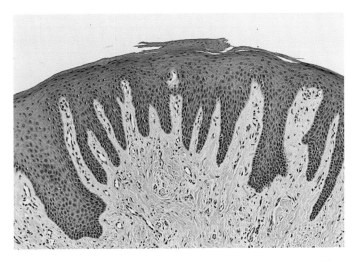

FIGURE 37-16   Dilantin-induced gingival hyperplasia. Elongated rete ridges and fibrous tissue proliferation.

Table 37-1 summarizes the clinical and histologic findings, as well as the differential diagnoses of these lesions.

PIGMENTED LESIONS

Amalgam Tattoo

Amalgam used in dental restorations may be inadvertently implanted into the mucosa via tears in the mucosa during placement of a restoration, may fall from an extracted tooth into its socket, or may be present

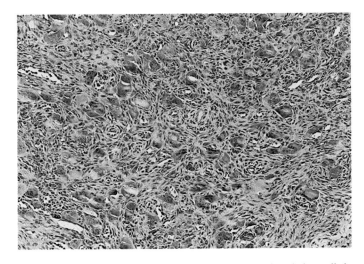

FIGURE 37-15   Peripheral giant-cell granuloma. Multinucleated giant cells in a vascular stroma.

at the site of a retrograde root canal filling. It is the most common cause of exogenous pigmentation in the oral cavity.

Clinical Features   The most common locations for amalgam tattoos are the gingiva adjacent to the restoration, and the buccal mucosa.[94] The tattoo is macular and appears black, or slate grey and may have discrete or ill-defined borders. If of sufficient size, the particles may show up as a radiodensity on dental radiographs.

Histopathological Features   Dark brown to black, coarse and/or fine granules are present in the lamina propria and sometimes within the cytoplasm of macrophages. The silver content of amalgam stains the reticulin fibers within the stroma and in the basement membrane of blood vessels and the epithelium, and nerve twigs (Fig. 37-17). There may or may not be a foreign body reaction around the particles.[94]

Differential Diagnosis   Graphite tattoos are often seen in the palatal mucosa of children who fall with pencils held between the teeth. Although clinically similar to amalgam tattoos, the particles tend to be coarse and do not stain the reticulin fibers. Tattoos performed for cosmetic reasons in some Middle Eastern and African cultures usually involve extensive areas of the anterior gingiva and are not metallic in nature. In cases where the diagnosis is not immediately apparent, energy dispersive X-ray microanalysis of the content of the particles may be helpful.[95]

Oral Melanotic Macule

This is a common condition of the oral mucosa caused by increased deposition of melanin and occasionally, very mild melanocytic hyperplasia. It is probably reactive in nature but is unlikely to have sun damage as its primary etiology.

Clinical Features   This occurs mainly in adults with a male:female ratio of 1:2. Approximately one-third of cases occur on the vermilion of the lower lip (labial melanotic macule); other sites include the gingiva, buccal mucosa, and palate. They are discrete, usually solitary, evenly tan-brown or black macules that are less than 1 cm in diameter.

Histopathological Features   There is absent or mild hyperkeratosis, and usually insignificant or mild epithelial hyperplasia. There is an

TABLE 37-1

Gingival Nodules

Entity	Clinical Features	Histopathological Features	Differential Diagnosis
Pyogenic granuloma	Often seen during pregnancy; may regress postpartum	Proliferation of endothelial cells and capillaries	Capillary hemangiomas are similar histologically
Peripheral ossifying fibroma	Marginal gingiva	Cellular fibroblast-like proliferation with deposition of osteoid, woven bone or cementum-like droplets	A bony spicule is composed of lamellar bone with periosteum and no spindle cell proliferation
Peripheral giant cell granuloma	May rest in a cup-shaped depression in the bone; 10% recurrence rate; unlike intra-osseous counterpart, no association with hyper-parathyroidism	Proliferation of multinucleated giant cells of osteoclast-type, mononuclear cells in stroma, siderophages, dilated capillaries; "Grenz" zone may be present	Central giant cell granuloma eroding through bone; lack of foreign material and epithe-lioid histiocytes excludes other granulomatous processes
Drug-induced fibrous hyperplasia	Usually involves gingiva diffusely and rare in edentulous areas; dilantin, cyclosporine and Ca^{2+} channel blockers are common etiologic agents	Proliferation of fibrous tissue and some granulation tissue with variable inflammation. In dilantin hyperplasia, elongated "test tube" ridges may be present	Gingival fibromatoses is similar histologically but tends to be hereditary and presents at an early age
Parulis	Usually not on marginal gingiva; indicates tooth has pulpal or periodontal infection	Edematous granulation tissue, acute and chronic inflam-mation and microab-scesses, may see neutrophil "tract"	Lack of mucin and muciphages as well as location excludes mucocele

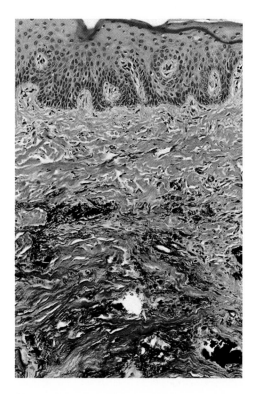

FIGURE 37-17 Amalgam tattoo. The silver in dental amalgam stains the base-ment membrane of blood vessels and epithelium.

increase in the amount of melanin in the basal cells, especially at the tips of the rete ridges. Melanocytic hyperplasia, if present, is usually very mild with no atypia and no nesting.[96–98] Melanin is present in the lam-ina propria and there are variable numbers of melanophages, incontinent melanin, and scattered lymphocytes.

Differential Diagnosis   Unlike ephelides, oral melanotic macules are not related to sun exposure and therefore the color varies little through-out the year. Unlike lentigo and melanoacanthosis, they show minimal melanocytic hyperplasia and insignificant epithelial hyperplasia. Lentigo maligna and superficial spreading melanoma are characterized by a proliferation of atypical melanocytes. The melanotic macule may be indistinguishable from oral pigmentation associated with Peutz-Jegher's, Albright's, and Addison's diseases.

Oral Melanoacanthosis

Synonym: Oral melanoacanthoma

Oral melanoacanthosis is a reactive hypermelanosis of the oral mucosa that has a characteristic clinical presentation. The original reports refer to it as "oral melanoacanthoma," and it shares some histo-logic similarities with skin melanoacanthoma. However, unlike skin melanoacanthomas, oral melanoacanthosis occurs in young adult African-American females, and are self-remitting.[99,100]

Clinical Features   This is a condition that is most commonly encoun-tered in young African-American adults with a 1:3 male to female ratio. Typically, the lesion presents as a solitary dark brown macule that may have a slightly roughened surface, usually on the buccal or labial

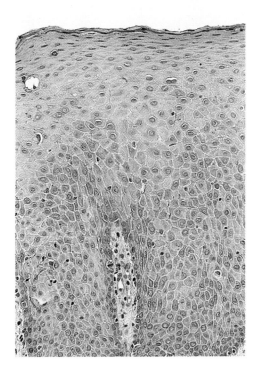

FIGURE 37-18   Oral melanoacanthosis. Dendritic melanocytes occupy the entire epithelium.

mucosa, that spreads laterally and may grow several centimeters within a few weeks. It does not ulcerate and is not indurated.[100] They regress spontaneously or after removal of offending physical stimuli, and may recur.[99]

Histopathological Features   There is acanthosis and increased deposition of melanin in the basal cells. There is hyperplasia of benign pigment-laden dendritic melanocytes throughout the thickness of the epithelium (Fig. 37-18). Rarely, there may be spongiosis. A lymphocytic infiltrate is present in the lamina propria with scattered melanophages, eosinophils, and vascular ectasia.[97,99,100]

Differential Diagnosis   Oral melanotic macules do not exhibit the marked acanthosis and dendritic melanocytic hyperplasia seen in melanoacanthosis. The benign appearance of the melanocytes differentiates this entity from dysplastic nevomelanocytic lesions and melanoma.

TOBACCO-ASSOCIATED ORAL MUCOSAL CONDITIONS

Tobacco used in different forms gives rise to clinically distinct lesions. The clinical features, histopathology, and differential diagnoses of nicotinic stomatitis, smokeless tobacco keratoses, submucous fibrosis, and leukoplakia are compared in Table 37-2 and (Figs. 37-19 and 37-20).[101–107] Submucous fibrosis is seen primarily in people who chew betel quid, such as in subcontinental Indians and South East Asian populations.[108–112] Leukoplakia has a strong association with tobacco use and because of its prevalence and malignant potential, will be discussed separately in the following section.

Leukoplakia

Synonyms: Leukokeratosis

The World Health Organization (WHO) defines oral leukoplakia, the most common pre-malignant mucosal lesion, as "any white patch that does not rub off and does not conform to a known oral white lesion." The prevalence of leukoplakia in the general population ranges from 2 to 4 percent, and leukoplakia occurs in up to 14 percent in smokers.[113,114] More than 70 percent of patients who have leukoplakia use tobacco products.[115]

Clinical Findings   Leukoplakia is twice as common in adult males as females. Several different clinical forms are recognized: homogenous, speckled (erythroleukoplakia), verrucous, and nodular. Very often, a plaque will exhibit combinations of these forms. Early leukoplakic plaques tend to be greyish white and established lesions tend to be densely opaque with verrucous and/or nodular areas. Although any oral site may present with leukoplakia, the two most common sites are the buccal mucosa and gingiva.[113,115]

There is a form of extensive leukoplakia that tends to occur in elderly women, called proliferative verrucous leukoplakia, of which only half the cases are associated with tobacco use.[116] These extensive lesions develop over 10 or 20 years from homogenous leukoplakias: 57 percent develop squamous cell carcinoma and 30 percent verrucous carcinoma on long-term follow-up.

Histopathological Features   The criteria for the diagnosis of oral epithelial dysplasia may be divided into architectural changes such as endophytic growth and bud- or tear drop- shaped rete ridges (Fig. 37-21). Cytologic features include maturation disarray, basal cell hyperplasia, increased nuclear:cytoplasmic ratio, pleomorphism, and increased mitotic activity.[117] Some use the term "squamous intraepithelial neoplasia" (SIN) to designate such dysplasias.[118]

Papillomatosis per se is not a sign of dysplasia but dysplasia is often seen in biopsies from patients with proliferative verrucous leukoplakia. Papillomatosis is a constant feature of the entity "verrucous hyperplasia" that may be the precursor lesion to verrucous carcinoma or papillary squamous cell carcinoma.[119]

A band-like lymphocytic infiltrate typifies lichenoid dysplasia. Some believe these represent malignant transformation of oral lichen planus, whereas others believe that the lichenoid infiltrate is an immunologically mediated reaction to the epithelial dysplasia.[120]

Lesions on the floor of mouth, ventral tongue, and soft palate have a higher association with dysplasia or carcinoma at the time of first biopsy than other sites.[117,121] When leukoplakias are followed, malignant transformation occurs in up to 24 percent of all cases with long term follow-up and in 36 percent of patients with preexisting epithelial dysplasia.[115]

Differential Diagnosis   Inflammatory epithelial atypia may be seen in association with candidiasis, the latter sometimes being mistaken for leukoplakia. A lichenoid lymphocytic reaction to epithelial dysplasia should not mistakenly be underdiagnosed as lichen planus.

Erythroplakia

Synonym: Erythroplasia

Erythroplakia (similar to erythroplasia of Queyrat) is a clinical red plaque that cannot be attributed to any other specific oral condition.

TABLE 37-2

Tobacco-Associated Mucosal Diseases

Entity	Offending Agent	Clinical Findings	Histopathological Features	Differential Diagnosis
Nicotinic stomatitis	Heat from smoking (esp. pipe smoking; reverse smoking)	Whitened palatal mucosa; white papules with central red puncta; regresses when patient stops smoking	Hyperkeratosis and acanthosis; excretory (extralobular) salivary ducts exhibit squamous metaplasia, periductal lymphocytic infiltrate; usually no dysplasia	Necrotizing sialometaplasia exhibits more extensive metaplastic change in intralobular ducts; focal injury to palate
Smokeless tobacco keratosis	Snuff or chewing tobacco; severity proportional to length of exposure and brand of tobacco	Filmy grey white opalescence at area of contact; may become leathery; reversible on stopping habit	Hyperpara or orthokeratosis with spires of parakeratin ("chevrons"); acanthosis, leukoedematous changes, mild chronic inflammation; perivascular PAS+ cuff; dysplasia in <1% of cases; HPV in 20%	Leukoedema does not exhibit "chevron" formation
Submucous fibrosis	Chewing betel quid (composed of tobacco, betel leaf, areca nut, slaked lime, condiments); areca nut stimulates collagen synthesis and inhibits collagen degradation	Usually in women; progressive limitation of mouth opening, burning sensation, palpable fibrous bands in mucosa with rigidity and pallor; does not regress with cessation of habit	Epithelial atrophy, dense collagenization of lamina propria with hyalinization and loss of vascularity in late stages; dysplasia in percent of cases; malignant transformation in 3–8% of cases	Systemic sclerosis will demonstrate + serologic markers for autoimmune disease; lichen sclerosis et atrophicus contains a lichenoid lymphocytic band
Leukoplakia	Mainly cigarette smoking	White plaque(s); may be thin or thick homogeneous or speckled with red areas, smooth or verrucous, nodular +/or papillary	Hyperpara or orthokeratosis, acanthosis, sometimes papillomatosis; dysplasia in situ or invasive carcinoma in 10–20% of cases; malignant transformation on followup in small percent of cases	

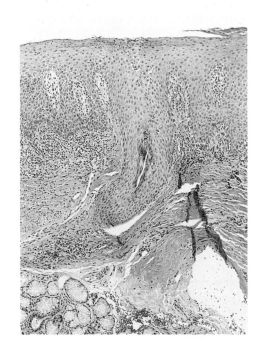

FIGURE 37-19 Nicotinic stomatitis. Squamous metaplasia of the ducts with sialodochitis.

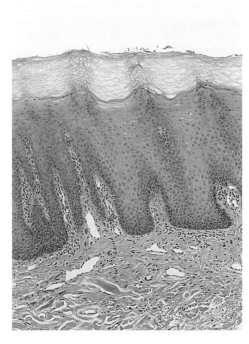

FIGURE 37-20 Smokeless tobacco keratosis. Coagulation and degeneration of superficial cells with "chevron" formation.

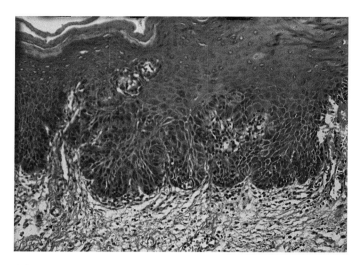

FIGURE 37-21 Moderate epithelial dysplasia typified by budding of rete ridges and maturation disarray involving less than 2/3 of epithelium.

Clinical Features   This is an uncommon condition of older men characterized by a discrete erythematous plaque that has a velvety surface. It is more often seen adjacent to, or admixed within a leukoplakia (erythroleukoplakia).

Histopathological Features   Up to 90 percent of cases exhibit epithelial dysplasia, carcinoma-in-situ or squamous cell carcinoma at the time of biopsy.

Differential Diagnosis   Nonspecific inflammation of the oral mucosa, atrophic candidiasis, and erosive lichen planus may resemble erythroplakia clinically. Epithelial changes beyond what one would expect for a reactive atypia are seen in erythroplakia.

Oral Epithelial Malignancies

Squamous cell carcinomas comprise more than 90 percent of all intraoral malignancies and constitute 3 percent of all malignancies diagnosed in the United States. Many of them occur in a pre-existing leukoplakia or erythroplakia.

Tobacco is the single most important risk factor for the occurrence of intraoral carcinoma. Alcohol may act synergistically with tobacco in the occurrence of leukoplakia but its use alone is not associated with a higher prevalence of these lesions. Iron deficiency anemia such as Plummer Vinson syndrome predisposes to oral cancer, as does a history of syphilis (probably because of treatment with arsenicals). HPV-16 and -18 have been identified in oral squamous cell carcinomas, verrucous carcinomas, and in normal healthy mucosa.[122] The role of candida as an etiopathogenetic agent is controversial.[123]

Clinical Features   The prevalence increases with increasing age. It may present as an ulcer that is painless, indurated, and shows no tendency to heal. It may be associated with a change in the nature of a pre-existing leukoplakia that becomes focally nodular, verrucous, or erythematous. It may appear as a rapidly-growing, fungating mass.

The most common sites are tongue (usually posterior), floor of mouth, soft palate, and gingiva/alveolar mucosa.

Histopathological Features   Squamous cell carcinomas of the oral cavity when excised in toto may be well, moderately, or poorly differentiated. There is variable pleomorphism and stromal invasion must be

present. Sometimes, involvement of salivary excretory ducts may give rise to ductal carcinomas-in-situ at a distance from the surface. There is some evidence to suggest that like melanomas, the thickness of the tumor may have some prognostic significance, with increasing thickness correlating with increased risk of metastasis and reduced survival.[124,125]

Differential Diagnoses   It is sometimes difficult to differentiate between papillary well-differentiated squamous cell and verrucous carcinomas, a carcinoma strongly associated with smokeless tobacco use. In the latter, there is minimal cytologic atypia, with prominent endophytic frond-like epithelial proliferations and keratin clefts. Keratin pearl formation, especially in the depths of the tumor occurs rarely, if at all, and there should be no evidence of individual cell invasion of the stroma.[126,127]

Other less well-recognized variations of squamous cell carcinomas include the spindle-cell carcinoma, adenosquamous carcinoma, adenoid squamous carcinoma, and basaloid squamous cell carcinoma.

Half of all spindle-cell carcinomas occur on the lower lip, with the tongue as the second most common site. They show reactivity for both vimentin and keratin even within the spindle cells, which are uniformly S-100 negative. A banal squamous cell carcinoma often is present within the tumor and the overlying epithelium is dysplastic.[128,129]

Adenosquamous carcinoma consists of a combination of a surface squamous cell carcinoma together with an underlying adenocarcinoma of the salivary ducts that often, but not invariably stains for mucin intracytoplasmically.[130] Some consider these to be variants of a mucoepidermoid carcinoma.

The majority of adenoid squamous cell carcinomas (also known as pseudoglandular and acantholytic squamous cell carcinoma) arise on the lower lip vermilion. The tumor forms duct-like structures within islands of tumor cells as a result of acantholysis.[131] Unlike adenosquamous carcinoma, these are not true ducts.

Basaloid squamous cell carcinoma arise primarily in the base of tongue and pharynx and consists of islands of basaloid cells usually with prominent necrosis and stromal hyalinization, associated with overlying squamous epithelial dysplasia. In addition to being keratin positive, the tumor cells also are often EMA, CEA, S-100 and NSE positive.[132,133]

REFERENCES

1. Halperin V, et al: Occurrence of fordyce glands, benign migratory glossitis, median rhomboid glossitis, and fissured tongue in 2,478 dental students. *Oral Surg* 6: 1072–1077, 1953.
2. Koutlas I, Yaholnitsky B: Oral sebaceous retention phenomenon. *J Periodontol* 65: 186–188, 1994.
3. Lipani C, Woytash J, Greene G: Sebaceous adenoma of the oral cavity. *J Oral Maxillofac Surg* 41:56–60, 1983.
4. Ferguson J, Geary C, MacAlister A: Sebaceous cell adenoma. Rare intra-oral occurrence of a tumor which is frequent marker of Torre's syndrome. *Pathology* 19:204–208, 1987.
5. Baughman R, Heidrich P: The oral hair: an extremely rare phenomenon. *Oral Surg Oral Med Oral Pathol* 49:530–531, 1980.
6. Jorgensen R, Levin S: White sponge nevus. *Arch Dermatol* 117:73–76, 1981.
7. Nichols G, et al: White sponge nevus. *Obstet Gynecol* 76:545–548, 1990.
8. Krajewska I, Moore L, Brown J: White sponge nevus presenting in the esophagus: Case report and literature review. *Pathology* 24:112–115, 1992.
9. Wright S, Levy I: White sponge naevus and ocular coloboma. *Arch Dis Child* 66:514–516, 1991.
10. Alinovi A, Benoldi D, Pezzarossa E: White sponge nevus: Successful treatment with penicillin. *Acta Derm Venereol (Stockh)* 63:83–85, 1983.
11. Lim J, Ng S: Oral tetracycline rinse improves symptoms of white sponge nevus. *J Am Acad Dermatol* 26:1003–1005, 1992.
12. Morris R, et al: White sponge nevus. Diagnosis by light microscopic and ultrastructural cytology. *Acta Cytol* 32:357–361, 1988.
13. Aloi F, Molinero A: White sponge nevus with epidermolytic changes. *Dermatologica* 177:323–326, 1988.

14. Frithiof L, Banoczy J: White sponge nevus (leukoedema exfoliativum mucosae oris): Ultrastructural observations. *Oral Surg* 41:607–622, 1976.

15. Rugg E, et al: A mutation in the mucosal keratin K4 is associated with oral white sponge nevus. *Nat Genet* 11:450–452, 1995.

16. Richard G, et al: Keratin 13 point mutation underlies the hereditary mucosal epithelial disorder white sponge nevus. *Nat Genet* 11:453–455, 1995.

17. Martin J: Leukoedema: a review of the literature. *J Nat Med Assoc* 84:938–940, 1992.

18. Hamner J, et al: An epidemiologic and histopathologic study of leukoedema among 50,915 rural Indian villagers. *Oral Surg Oral Med Oral Pathol* 32:58–65, 1971.

19. Axell T: Leukoedema: An epidemiologic study with special reference to the influence of tobacco habits. *Commun Dent Oral Epidemiol* 9:142–146.

20. Darling M, Arendorf T: Effects of cannabis smoking on oral soft tissues. *Commun Dent Oral Epidemiol* 21:78–81, 1993.

21. Gupta P, et al: Effect of cessation of tobacco use on the incidence of oral mucosal lesions in a 10-yr follow-up study of 12,212 users. *Oral Dis* 1:54–58, 1995.

22. Van-Wyk C, Ambrosio S: Leukoedema: ultrastructural and histochemical observations. *J Oral Pathol* 12:319–329, 1983.

23. Baughman R: Median rhomboid glossitis: A developmental anomaly? *Oral Surg* 31:56–65, 1971.

24. Wright B: Median rhomboid glossitis: Not a misnomer. *Oral Surg* 46:806–814, 1978.

25. Greenspan D, Greenspan J: Significance of oral hairy leukoplakia. *Oral Surg Oral Med Oral Pathol* 73:151–154, 1992.

26. Schiodt M, Norgaard T, Greenspan J: Oral hairy leukoplakia in an HIV-negative woman with Behcet's syndrome. *Oral Surg Oral Med Oral Pathol Oral Radiol Endodont* 79:53–56, 1995.

27. Eisenberg E, Krutchkoff D: Incidental oral hairy leukoplakia in immunocompetent persons. *Oral Surg Oral Med Oral Pathol* 74:322–323, 1992.

28. Greenspan D, et al: Risk factors for rapid progression from hairy leukoplakia to AIDS: A rested case control study. *J Acq Immunodefic Syn* 4:652–658, 1991.

29. Brehmer-Andersson E, et al: Oral hairy leukoplakia: Pathogenetic aspects and significance of the lesion. *Acta Derm Venereol (Stockh)* 74:81–89, 1994.

30. Mabruk MJ: Detection of Epstein-Barr virus DNA in tongue tissues from AIDS autopsies without clinical evidence of oral hairy leukoplakia. *J Oral Pathol* 24:109–112, 1995.

31. Sciubba J, Brandsma J, Schwartz M: Hairy leukoplakia. An AID-associated opportunistic infection. *Oral Surg Oral Med Oral Pathol* 67:404–410, 1989.

32. Eversole L, Stone C, Beckman A: Detection of EBV and HPV DNA sequences in oral "hairy" leukoplakia by in situ hybridization. *J Med Virol* 26:217–277, 1988.

33. Ficarra G, et al: Epstein-Barr virus and human papillomavirus detection in oral hairy leukoplakia and normal oral mucosa or HIV-infected patients. *Int Conf AIDS* 7:254(abst#MB 2290), 1991.

34. Fernandez J, et al: Oral hairy leukoplakia: A histopathologic study of 32 cases. *Am J Dermatopathol* 12:571–578, 1990.

35. Beaudenon S, et al: A new type of human papillomavirus associated with oral focal epithelial hyperplasia. *J Invest Dermatol* 88:130–135, 1987.

36. Carlos R, Sedano H: Multifocal papilloma virus epithelial hyperplasia. *Oral Surg Oral Med Oral Pathol* 77:631–635, 1994.

37. Harris A, Van-Wyk C: Heck's disease (focal epithelial hyperplasia): A longitudinal study. *Commun Dent Oral Epidemiol* 21:82–85, 1993.

38. Garlick J, Taichman L: Human papillomavirus infection of the oral mucosa. *Am J Dermatopathol* 13:386–395, 1991.

39. Scully C, Porter S: Recurrent aphthous stomatitis: current concepts of etiology, pathogenesis and management. *J Oral Pathol Med* 18:21–27, 1989.

40. Porter S, Scully C: Aphthous stomatitis: An overview of aetiopathogenesis and management. *Clin Exp Dermatol* 16:235–243, 1991.

41. Bagan J, et al: Recurrent aphthous stomatitis. A study of the clinical characteristics in 93 cases. *J Oral Pathol Med* 20:395–397, 1991.

42. Savage N, Seymour G, Kruger B: T-lymphocyte subset changes in recurrent aphthous stomatitis. *Oral Surg Oral Med Oral Pathol* 60:175–181, 1985.

43. Bhaskar S, Lilly G: Traumatic granuloma of the tongue (human and experimental). *Oral Surg* 18:206–218, 1964.

44. Eichenfield L, Honig P, Nelson L: Traumatic granuloma of the tongue (Riga-Fede disease): association with familial dysautonomia. *J Pediatr* 116:742–744, 1990.

45. Elzay R: Traumatic ulcerative granuloma with stromal eosinophilia (Riga-Fede's disease and traumatic eosinophilic granuloma). *Oral Surg* 55:497–506, 1983.

46. Sklavounou A, Laskaris G: Eosinophilic ulcer of the oral mucosa. *Oral Surg* 58:431–436, 1984.

47. El-Mofty S, Wick M, Miller A: Eosinophilic ulcer of the oral mucosa. *Oral Surg Oral Med Oral Pathol* 75:716–722, 1993.

48. Eversole L, et al: Atypical histiocytic granuloma. *Cancer* 55:1722–1729, 1985.

49. Marks R, Radden B: Geographic tongue: A clinico-pathological review. *Austr J Dermatol* 22:75–79, 1981.

50. Pogrel M, Cram D: Intraoral findings in patients with psoriasis with a special reference to ectopic geographic tongue (erythema circinata). *Oral Surg Oral Med Oral Pathol* 66:184–194, 1988.

51. Zelickson B, Muller S: Generalized pustular psoriasis. *Arch Dermatol* 127:1339–1345, 1991.

52. Marks R, Czarny D: Geographic tongue: Sensitivity to the environment. *Oral Surg* 58:156–159, 1984.

53. Brooks J, Balciunas B: Geographic stomatitis: Review of the literature and report of five cases. *J Am Dent Assoc* 115:421–424, 1987.

54. Espelid M, et al: Geographic stomatitis: Report of 6 cases. *J Oral Pathol* 20:425–428, 1991.

55. Swerlick R, Cooper P: Cheilitis glandularis: A re-evaluation. *J Am Acad Dermatol* 10:466–472, 1984.

56. Michalowski R: Cheilitis glandularis, heterotopic salivary glands and squamous cell carcinoma of the lip. *Br J Dermatol* 74:445–449, 1962.

57. Winchester L, et al: Cheilitis glandularis: A case affecting the upper lip. *Oral Surg Oral Med Oral Pathol* 62:654–656, 1962.

58. Lederman D: Suppurative stomatitis glandularis. *Oral Surg Oral Med Oral Pathol* 78:319–322, 1994.

59. Oliver A, et al: Monosodium glutamate-related orofacial granulomatosis. *Oral Surg Oral Med Oral Pathol* 71:560–564, 1991.

60. Worsaae N, Christensen K, Schiodt M: Melkersson-Rosenthal syndrome and cheilitis granulomatosa. *Oral Surg Oral Med Oral Pathol* 54:404–413, 1982.

61. Allen C, et al: Cheilitis granulomatosa: Report of six cases and review of the literature. *J Am Acad Dermatol* 23:444–450, 1990.

62. Plauth M, Jenss H, Meyle J: Oral manifestations of Crohn's disease. *J Clin Gastroenterol* 13:29–37, 1991.

63. Zimmer W, et al: Orofacial manifestations of Melkersson-Rosenthal syndrome. *Oral Surg Oral Med Oral Pathol* 74:610–619, 1992.

64. Thornhill M, Zakrzewska J, Gilkes J: Pyostomatitis vegetans: Report of three cases and review of the literature. *J Oral Pathol Med* 21:128–133, 1992.

65. Storwick G, et al: Pyodermatitis-pyostomatitis vegetans: A specific marker for inflammatory bowel disease. *J Am Acad Dermatol* 31:336–341, 1994.

66. Healy C, et al: Pyostomatitis vegetans and associated systemic disease. A review and two case reports. *Oral Surg Oral Med Oral Pathol* 78:323–328, 1994.

67. Brannon R, Fowler C, Hartman K: Necrotizing sialometaplasia. *Oral Surg Oral Med Oral Pathol* 72:317–325, 1991.

68. Wenig B: Necrotizing sialometaplasia of the larynx. A report of two cases and a review of the literature. *Am J Clin Pathol* 103:609–613, 1995.

69. Abrams A, Melrose R, Howell F: Necrotizing sialometaplasia. *Cancer* 32:130–135, 1973.

70. Sewerin I: A clinical and epidemiologic study of morsicatio buccarum/labiorum. *Scand J Dent Res* 79:73–80, 1970.

71. Van-Wyk C, Staz J, Farman A: The chewing lesion of the cheeks and lips: Its features and prevalence among a selected group of adolescents. *J Dent* 5:193–199, 1977.

72. Glass L, Maize J: Morsicatio buccarum et labiorum (excessive cheek and lip biting). *Am J Dermatopathol* 13:271–274, 1991.

73. Hjorting-Hansen E, Holst E: Morsicatio mucosae oris and suctio mucosae oris. *Scand J Dent Res* 78:492–499, 1970.

74. Scully C, El-Kom E: Lichen planus: Review and update on pathogenesis. *J Oral Pathol* 14:431–458, 1985.

75. Bagan J, et al: Oral lichen planus and chronic liver disease: A clinical and morphometric study of the oral lesions in relation to transaminase elevation. *Oral Surg Oral Med Oral Pathol* 78:337–342, 1994.

76. Cribier B, et al: Lichen planus and hepatitis C virus infection: An epidemiologic study. *J Am Acad Dermatol* 31:1070–1072, 1994.

77. Barnard N, et al: Oral cancer development in patients with oral lichen planus. *J Oral Pathol Med* 22:421–424, 1993.

78. Eisenberg E, Krutchkoff D: Lichenoid lesions of oral mucosa. *Oral Surg Oral Med Oral Pathol* 73:699–704, 1992.

79. Walsh L, et al: Immunopathogenesis of oral lichen planus. *J Oral Pathol Med* 19:389–396, 1990.

80. Miller R, Gould A, Bernstein M: Cinnamon-induced stomatitis venenata. *Oral Surg Oral Med Oral Pathol* 73:708–716, 1992.

81. Beutner E, et al: Ten cases of chronic ulcerative stomatitis with stratified epithelium-specific antinuclear antibody. *J Am Acad Dermatol* 24:781–782, 1991.

82. Rogers III R, Sheridan P, Nightingale S: Desquamative gingivitis: Clinical, histopathologic, immunopathologic and therapeutic observations. *J Am Acad Dermatol* 729:729–735, 1982.

83. Nisengard R, Rogers III R: The treatment of desquamative gingival lesions. *J Periodont* 58:167–172, 1987.

84. Kerr D, McClatchey K, Regezi J: Idiopathic gingivostomatitis. *Oral Surg* 32:402–423, 1971.

85. Sollecito T, Greenberg M: Plasma cell gingivitis. *Oral Surg Oral Med Oral Pathol* 73:690–693, 1992.

86. Timms M, Sloan P: Association of supraglottic and gingival idiopathic plasmacytosis. *Oral Surg Oral Med Oral Pathol* 71:451–453, 1991.

87. Houston G: The giant cell fibroma: A review of 464 cases. *Oral Surg Oral Med Oral Pathol* 53:582–587, 1982.

88. Savage N, Monsour P: Oral fibrous hyperplasias and the giant cell fibroma. *Aust Dent* 30:582–587, 1985.

89. Bhaskar SJB III, Cutright D: Inflammatory papillary hyperplasia of the oral mucosa: Report of 341 cases. *J Am Dent Assoc* 81:949–952, 1970.

90. Zain R, Fei YJ: Fibrous lesions of the gingiva: A histopathologic analysis of 204 cases. *Oral Surg Oral Med Oral Pathol* 70:466–470, 1990.

91. Katsikeris N, Kakarantza-Angelopoulou E, Angelopoulos A: Peripheral giant cell granuloma. Clinicopathologic study of 224 new cases and review of 956 reported cases. *Int J Oral Maxillo Surg* 17:94–99, 1988.

92. Bonetti F, et al: Peripheral giant cell granuloma: Evidence for osteoclastic differentiation. *Oral Surg Oral Med Oral Pathol* 70:471–475, 1990.

93. Dongari A, McDonnell H, Langlais R: Drug-induced gingival overgrowth. *Oral Surg Oral Med Oral Pathol* 76:543–548, 1993.

94. Buchner A, Hansen L: Amalgam pigmentation (amalgam tattoo) of the oral mucosa. A clinicopathologic study of 268 cases. *Oral Surg Oral Med Oral Pathol* 49:139–147, 1980.

95. Hartman L, Natiella J, Meenaghan M: The use of elemental microanalysis in verification of the composition of presumptive amalgam tattoo. *J Oral Maxillo Surg* 44:628–633, 1986.

96. Buchner A, Hansen L: Melanotic macule of the oral mucosa. A clinicopathologic study of 105 cases. *Oral Surg Oral Med Oral Pathol* 48:244–249, 1979.

97. Sexton F. and J. Maize, *Melanotic macules and melanoacanthomas of the lip. Am J Dermatopathol* 9:438–444, 1987.

98. Ho K, et al: Labial melanotic macule: A clinical, histopathologic, and ultrastructural study. *J Am Acad Dermatol* 28:33–39, 1993.

99. Tomich C, Zunt S: Melanoacanthosis (melanoacanthoma) of the oral mucosa. *J Dermatol Surg Oncol* 16:231–236, 1990.

100. Goode R, et al: Oral melanoacanthoma. Review of the literature and report of ten cases. *Oral Surg Oral Med Oral Pathol* 56:622–628, 1983.

101. Schwartz D: Stomatitis nicotina of the palate. *Oral Surg* 20:306–315, 1965.

102. Reddy C, et al: Changes in the ducts of the glands of the hard palate in reverse smokers. *Cancer* 30:231–238, 1972.

103. Archard HO, Tarpley TM Jr: Clinicopathologic and histochemical characterization of submucosal deposits in snuff dipper's keratosis. *J Oral Pathol* 1:3–11, 1972.

104. Axell T, Mornstad H, Sundstrom B: The relation of the clinical picture to the histopathology of snuff dipper's lesions in a Swedish population. *J Oral Pathol* 5:229–236, 1976.

105. Greer G, Schroeder K, L. Crosby L: Morphologic and immunohistochemical evidence of human papillomavirus capsid antigen in smokeless tobacco keratoses from juveniles and adults. *J Oral Maxillo Surg* 46:919–929, 1988.

106. Bouquot J, Glover E, Schroeder K: Leukoplakia and smokeless tobacco keratosis are two separate precancers. Second International Congress on Oral Cancer, New Delhi, India, 1991:6 (abstr).

107. Sciubba J: Oral leukoplakia. *Crit Rev Oral Biol Med* 6:147–160, 1995.

108. Canniff JP, Harvey W, Harris M: Oral submucous fibrosis: Its pathogenesis and management. *Br Dent J* 160:429–434, 1986.

109. Harvey W, et al: Stimulation of human buccal fibroblasts in vitro by betel nut alkaloids. *Arch Oral Biol* 31:45–49, 1986.

110. Pillai R, Balaram P, Reddiar K: Pathogenesis of submucous fibrosis. *Cancer* 69:2011–2020, 1992.

111. Maher R, et al: Role of areca nut in the causation of oral submucous fibrosis: A case-control study in Pakistan. *J Oral Pathol Med* 23:65–69, 1994.

s112. Rajendran R: Oral submucous fibrosis: Etiology, pathogenesis, and future research. *Bull WHO* 72:985–996, 1994.

113. Bouquot J, Gorlin R: Leukoplakia, lichen planus, and other oral keratoses in 23,616 white Americans over the age of 35 years. *Oral Surg Oral Med Oral Pathol* 61:373–381, 1986.

114. Salonen L, Axell T, Hellden L: Occurrence of oral mucosal lesions, the influence of tobacco habits and an estimate of treatment time in an adult Swedish population. *J Oral Pathol Med* 19:170–176, 1990.

115. Silverman S, Gorsky M, Lozada F: Oral leukoplakia and malignant transformation. *Cancer* 53:563–568, 1984.

116. Hansen LS, Olson JA, Silverman S Jr: Proliferative verrucous leukoplakia. *Oral Surg Oral Med Oral Pathol* 60:285–298, 1985.

117. Lumerman H, Freedman P, Kerpel S: Oral epithelial dysplasia and the development of invasive squamous cell carcinoma. *Oral Surg Oral Med Oral Pathol Oral Radiol Endodont* 79:321–329, 1995.

118. Crissman J, Zarbo R: Dysplasia, in situ carcinoma and progression to invasive squamous cell carcinoma of the upper aerodigestive tract. *Am J Surg Pathol* 13(suppl):5–16, 1989.

119. Shear M, Pindborg J: Verrucous hyperplasia of the oral mucosa. *Cancer* 46:1855–1862, 1980.

120. Eisenberg E: Lichen planus and oral cancer: Is there a connection between the two? *J Am Dent Assoc* 123:104–108, 1992.

121. Waldron C, Shafer W: Leukoplakia revisited: A clinicopathologic study of 3265 oral leukoplakias. *Cancer* 36:1386–1392, 1975.

122. Scully C: Viruses and oral squamous carcinoma. *Eur J Cancer B Oral Oncol* 28B:57–59, 1992.

123. O'Grady J, Reade P: Candida albicans as a promoter of oral mucosal neoplasia. *Carcinogenesis* 13:783–786, 1992.

124. Spiro R, et al: Predictive value of tumor thickness in squamous cell carcinoma confined to the tongue and floor of the mouth. *Am J Surg* 52:345–350, 1986.

125. Mohit-Tabatabai M, et al: Regulation of thickness of floor of mouth stage I and II cancers to regional metastasis. *Am J Surg* 152:351–353, 1986.

126. Medina J, Dichtel W, Luna M: Verucous-squamous carcinomas of the oral cavity: A clinicopathologic study of 104 cases. *Arch Otolaryngol* 110:437–440, 1984.

127. Kamath V: Oral verrucous carcinoma: An analysis of 37 cases. *J Craniomaxillo Surg* 17:309–314, 1989.

128. Ellis G, Corio R: Spindle cell carcinoma of the oral cavity. *Oral Surg Oral Med Oral Pathol* 50:523–534, 1980.

129. Ellis G, et al: Spindle-cell carcinoma of the aerodigestive tract. *Am J Surg Pathol* 11:335–342, 1987.

130. Ellis G, et al: Adenosquamous carcinoma, in Ellis GL, Auclair PL, Gnepp DR (eds): *Surgical Pathology of the Salivary Glands*. Philadelphia: W.B. Saunders, 1991, 455–459.

131. Jones A, Freedman P, Kerpel S: Oral adenoid squamous cell carcinoma: A report of three cases and review of the literature. *J Oral Maxillo Surg* 51:676–681, 1993.

132. Banks E, et al: Basaloid squamous cell carcinoma of the head and neck. *Am J Surg Pathol* 16:939–946, 1992.

133. Raslan W, et al: Basaloid squamous cell carcinoma of the head and neck: A clinicopathologic and flow cytometric study of 10 new cases with review of the English literature. *Am J Otolaryngol* 15:204–211, 1994.

K.S. Stenn / J.A. Carlson / Bernard Ng /
A. Del Rosario / K.J. Busam / G.S. Wood

NORMAL SKIN HISTOLOGY

K.S. Stenn / J.A. Carlson / Bernard Ng / A. Del Rosario

General

This chapter is written with the intention of presenting the essence of skin histology and biology for the use of the practicing dermatopathologist. General references for further study are appended.

Phylogeny

All organisms are separated from the environment by a wall (i.e., a plasma membrane for unicellular organisms or an integument for higher organisms). For the invertebrates integument is made of a single-layered epithelium embellished by an acellular matrix like chitin, mucin, and so on. For vertebrates integument is multicellular, allowing for ease of renewal and formation of multicellular appendages (i.e., scales, feathers, and hair).

Overall Structure of Skin

FUNCTION

In biology, structure reflects function. If one considers the function of skin, its structure can only be viewed as a truly amazing evolutionary achievement. Skin serves to protect from and communicate with the environment. It must prevent water loss or gain, prevent ingress of parasites or noxious chemicals, protect against electromagnetic radiation, and support temperature regulation. It must serve to express the needs and intentions of one individual to another.

STRUCTURE

Mammalian skin consists of three layers: (1) the outer multilayered epithelium, the epidermis, which serves as the environmental barrier, (2) the underlying connective tissue–rich dermis, moors the epidermis and gives strength to the whole organ, and (3) the deepest layer, the subcutis, is an adipose tissue serving as a thermal insulator, a cushion, and an energy store.

HETEROGENEITY

A fundamental theme in skin histology and function is the regional variation of skin structure from site to site (Figs. App-1 to App-3). This is reflected at all levels of skin biology involving clinical, histologic, and biochemical aspects: character of skin surface, density of hair or sweat glands and their placement, thickness of epidermis or subcutis, expression of specific keratins or lipids. Accepting bilateral symmetry, no two centimeters of skin are identical.

DEVELOPMENT OF SKIN

General

In general, skin ontogeny follows the phylogeny of integument. Skin morphogenesis occurs in two stages: an embryonic period (months 1 and 2) and a fetal period (month 3 to term). Initially, the epidermis is single-layered but with time acquires multiple layers. The dermis is initially a poorly defined, cell-numerous, highly hydrated, proteoglycan-rich layer joining the primitive epidermis to a fascial plane. Later, it becomes more collagenous and less hydrated. The epidermis and its appendages mature earlier than the dermis.

Epidermal Development

The epidermal layer is composed initially of simple epithelium. At 2 months it is made of a deep basal and a periderm layer. The periderm consists of a layer of flat epithelial cells, with intercellular desmosomes and a surface containing microvilli. Periderm is thought to play a role in fluid transport. During the end of the third fetal month an intermediate cell layer forms between the basal and periderm layers. At this time the basal layer expresses the keratin cytoskeleton proteins: K5/K14 are expressed in the basal cells, K1/K10 in the intermediate cells, and K8/K19 in the periderm. By the end of the sixth fetal month the periderm sheds and the epidermis acquires an aqueous barrier. During the final 3 months, development of the epidermis becomes complete and the adnexa become functional. At this time the epidermal-dermal junction shows rete ridge and dermal papilla formations. In adolescence, the eccrine and pilosebaceous (hair, sebaceous, and apocrine) structures enlarge in select regions. With age, the epidermis thins and the epidermal-dermal junction flattens.

Dermal Development

The dermis of the embryo consists of mesenchymal cells rich in proteoglycans containing a high water content. In the fetal stage the dermis matures with increasing collagen and decreasing glycosaminoglycans.

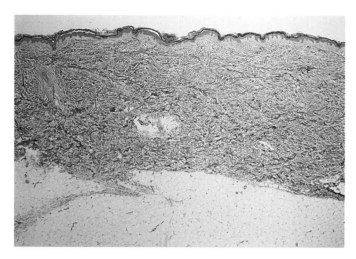

FIGURE APP-1   Skin of calf. Note thickness of dermis and sparse number of skin appendages.

Mature elastin is not found until 6 months postnatum. With age the dermis becomes thin, collagen becomes increasingly cross-linked, and adnexa drop-out.

EPIDERMIS

General

Epidermal cells proliferate in the basal layer; on differentiation basal cells progress outward to form the spinous, granular, and cornified layers (Fig. App-4). Proliferation and differentiation are exquisitely controlled so that there is an equilibrium between growth and desquamation.

Basal Layer

Most epidermal cell growth arises from the basal layer; however, cells making up the basal layer are not homogenous: There are actively proliferating cells and cells that divide very slowly. At the base of the rete ridges the cells are small, pigmented, and have a smooth basal membrane; these cells proliferate slowly, whereas the suprabasal cells in this

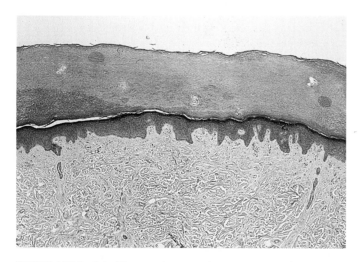

FIGURE APP-2   Sole. The stratum corneum is compacted, orthokeratotic, and much thicker than the epidermis.

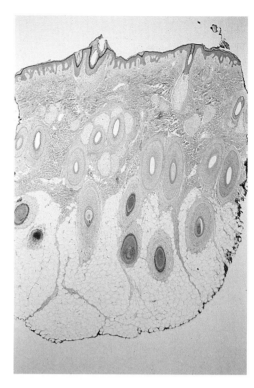

FIGURE APP-3   Scalp. The most striking finding is the presence of numerous terminal anagen follicles.

area show active DNA synthesis. In contrast, basal cells above the dermal papillae are larger cells, columnar in shape, pigmented, and have serrated inferior margins; these cells proliferate slowly and appear to play a sustentacular role. In general, one daughter cell of each cell division leaves the basal layer to differentiate. The total epidermal turnover time is about 26 to 42 days.

Suprabasal Layers and Keratinocyte Differentiation

LAYERS

Once a cell leaves the basal layer it begins to differentiate, acquiring more cell contacts and a developed cytoskeleton. In its progression from basal to cornified layers, keratinocytes differentiate to acquire characteristics of the recognized histologic strata: basal, spinous, granular, and cornified.

CYTOSKELETON

A critical element of keratinocyte function is its highly organized cytoskeleton. Although supported by actin filaments, the cytoskeleton is composed of keratin intermediate filaments. Keratin is composed of a family of 20 fibrous proteins that are grouped into two classes, acidic and basic, type I and type II, respectively. Keratin filaments consist of a pair of keratins, one representative from each class. Unique keratin pairs are found in unique epidermal sites, for example, K5 and K14 in the basal layer, K1 and K10 in the suprabasal layer, K6, K16, and K17 in palmar/plantar skin, K4 and K13 in suprabasal mucous membranes. It is the integrity of this keratin cytoskeleton that gives the epidermis its strength. Mutations in any one of these keratins lead to a pathologic state, for example, *epidermolysis bullosa simplex* (K5 or K14), *epidermolytic hyperkeratosis* (K1 or K10), *white sponge nevus* (K4 or K13).

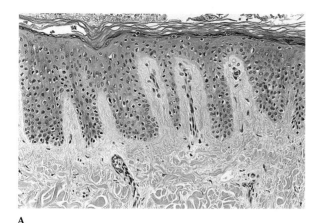

A

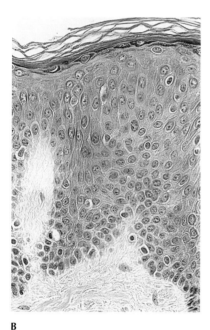

B

FIGURE APP-4 (A) Normal epidermis showing basal layer, granular layer, and basket-weave stratum corneum. (B) Higher magnification showing individual melanocytes in basal layer and maturation of epidermis.

CORNIFIED ENVELOPE

As the keratinocytes move upward, their structure is augmented by producing an envelope of highly cross-linked proteins just below the plasma membrane. This envelope is made of unique proteins including involucrin, pancornulins, keratolinin, and loricrin, all of which serve as substrates for a keratinocyte transglutaminase that cross-links these protein elements together (by means of epsilon-amino [gamma glutamyl] lysine bonds), entrapping keratins in the process, to make the highly resistant cornified structure.

Keratohyalin

As keratinocytes move outward they mature by accumulating an increasingly dense cytoskeleton. The keratin filament association is assisted by intermediate filament–associated proteins (IFAPs). One such protein, the nonmembrane-bound basophilic protein profilaggrin, accumulates in the granular layer as the keratohyalin granules. In the supragranular layer this very large (600 kDa) highly phosphorylated polymer becomes dephosphorylated and abruptly breaks down to its

filaggrin monomer units. This 50-kDa protein has the property to aggregate keratin filaments. Abnormalities in this molecule and its processing are implicated in the pathogenesis of *ichthyosis vulgaris*.

Desmosomes and Other Cell Junctions

For epidermal integrity keratinocytes of the epidermis must be tightly bonded to each other and to the basement membrane zone. There are four types of junctions in the epidermis: two intercellular junctions, desmosomes and intercellular adherens junctions; and two cell-to-substratum junctions, hemidesmosome and focal contacts. Desmosomes are highly specialized points of contact made of symmetric structures with a widened intercellular space bisected by a midline plate. A pair of submembranous electron-dense mats, called plaques, reinforce the membrane and serve as sites for filament association. Although desmosomes are symmetric, hemidesmosomes are asymmetric, serving to attach basal cell to the basal lamina.

Adherens junctions and focal contacts resemble immature desmosomes and hemidesmosomes, respectively, each having diffuse cytoplasmic mats and associated filaments. The building blocks of these junctions are: molecules that span the membrane and make the intercellular/stromal connection, and molecules that interface the membrane to the cytoskeleton. The transmembrane components of the cell-stromal junctions are members of the integrin superfamily. For example, the transmembrane integrin of the hemidesmosome is $\alpha6\beta4$; this integrin is mutated in the patient with *junction epidermolysis bullosa*. A second transmembrane adhesion protein in the hemidesmosome is bullous pemphigoid antigen, BPA-2, which is altered in *bullous pemphigoid, herpes gestationis,* and *cicatricial pemphigoid.* The transmembrane components of the intercellular junctions are members of the cadherin family, such as desmogleins and desmocollins. When the integrity of these proteins is disturbed, a blistering disease results, for example, antibodies to desmoglein-1 result in *pemphigus foliaceus,* and antibodies to desmoglein-3 result in *pemphigus vulgaris.* Although actin microfilaments insert into and provide the important structure in the adherens junctions from cell to cell or from cell to basal lamina, the keratin filaments insert into the desmosome and make up the important structure for desmosomes and hemidesmosomes. Molecules interfacing the transmembrane molecules to the cytoskeleton include plakoglobin and desmoplakin in desmosomes and bullous pemphigoid antigen, BPA-1, in the hemidesmosome; this protein is disturbed in *bullous pemphigoid.*

Permeability Barrier and the Membrane-Coating Granules

An isolated epidermal preparation exposed to an aqueous dye will show that the dye penetrates the epidermis from below to a point in the outer granular layer and from above to the same layer. This aqueous barrier is constituted in the outer epidermis by the secretion from the differentiating keratinocytes of lipid-rich lamellar bodies (Odland bodies, membrane-coating granules) (Fig. App-5). These vesicles fuse with the plasma membrane of granular layer keratinocytes and release their constituents into the intercellular space. Since the lamellar body is rich in highly hydrophobic glycolipids and sterols, the intercellular space becomes highly hydrophobic. The outer epidermis is conceived as being structured as brick and mortar: The cells make up the protein-rich bricks, and the intercellular space makes up the lipid-rich mortar.

Desquamation

Once keratinocytes differentiate fully and form the highly resistant and impermeable epidermis, the cells are called on to desquamate. This

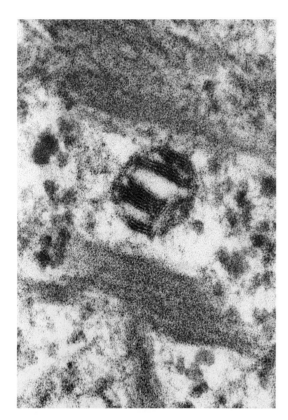

FIGURE APP-5 Keratinosome (membrane-coating granules/Odland body) in intercellular space of epidermal spinous layer.

process is highly controlled and involves an active process that is poorly understood. It is clear that the epidermis sheds as individual cells and that the dyshesion process can be delayed under pathologic states. Although the mechanism of desquamation is not known, we recognize that the lamellar body is not only lipid-rich but also enzyme-rich. Interestingly, the patient with deficiency in steroid sulfatase also suffers from *recessive X-linked ichthyosis*.

DERMAL-EPIDERMAL JUNCTION

The interface between the epidermis and the dermis is the epidermal-dermal junction, or the basement membrane zone (BMZ). This region must serve to moor the epidermis to the dermis, give support to the basal cells, and serve as a barrier to cells and molecules localized in either compartment. The BMZ consists of (1) the basal cell plasma membrane; (2) a lucent layer, as seen by electron microscopy, the lamina lucida; and (3) a dense layer, as seen by electron microscopy, the lamina densa, or basal lamina (Fig. App-6). The basal cells interface the BMZ with hemidesmosomes. Coursing through the lamina lucida from the basal cell to the lamina densa are minute filaments containing the protein laminin-5 (kalinin/epiligrin/nicein). When this protein is disrupted, *junctional epidermolysis bullosa* and *cicatricial pemphigoid* result. The lamina densa is rich in type IV collagen, entactin, and heparin sulfate proteoglycan. Analogous to the glomerular basement membrane, heparin sulfate may play a role in regulating molecular traffic between these tissues. Mooring the lamina densa to the dermis are anchoring fibrils, made of type VII collagen, which extend to anchoring plaques in the upper dermis. Mutation of type VII collagen is found in the patient with *dystrophic epidermolysis bullosa*.

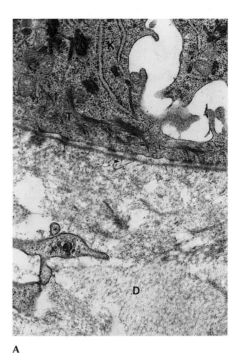

A

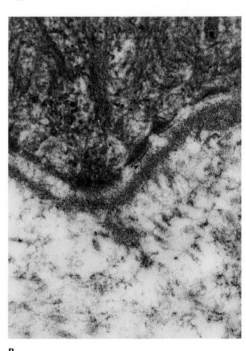

B

FIGURE APP-6 Basement membrane zone (BMZ): (*A*) note the hemidesmosomes with prominent overlying tonofilaments and underlying lamina lucida then lamina densa (K-keratinocyte; D-dermis; T-tonofilaments; arrow-anchoring fibrils); (*B*) higher power electron micrograph of the BMZ showing anchoring filaments (arrowed) extending from hemidesmosome to lamina densa.

IMMUNE FUNCTION OF SKIN

General

The skin serves as the first front for an immune response, another important defense function. It affects this function by means of a population of dendritic antigen processing cells by means of cytokines produced by the epidermis, and by means of lymphocytes that reside in the dermis.

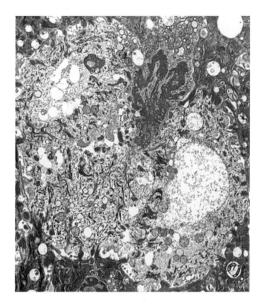

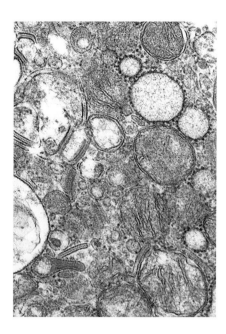

FIGURE APP-7 Langerhans' cells with characteristic Birbeck granules (*right*).

Langerhans' Cells

Langerhans' cells represent one member of the family of immunostimulatory dendritic cells of the immune system. They were discovered as a population of cells located in the suprabasal epidermis that have a dendritic structure and stain with gold salts. By electron microscopy this cell demonstrates unique features. (1) It contains a characteristic organelle, the Birbeck granule, which shows a racket shape. The granule is thought to be cell-membrane-derived and to play a role in antigen processing. (2) Its nucleus is lobulated and frequently convoluted. (3) It has clear cytoplasm lacking keratin filaments, desmosomes, and melanosomes (Fig. App-7). In H&E sections, Langerhans' cells appear as clear cells with reniform nuclei lying in intraspinous lacunae. As Langerhans' cells are thought to leave the epidermis in their antigen processing function, it is not surprising to find these cells in the dermis and lymph nodes. Many surface markers have been identified on these cells, including CD45; MHC class I antigens of the HLA-A, -B, and -C loci; class II alloantigen encoded by HLA-D; and S-100 protein. Langerhans' cells play a role in delayed type hypersensitivity reactions and skin allograft rejection. Reduction in their ability to present antigen is thought to play a role in the early stages of epidermal tumors, such as *squamous cell carcinoma*.

Cytokines

It has been recognized in the last decade that the epidermal keratinocyte is capable of active secretion. Cytokines released by these cells may influence cell growth, the inflammatory response, and the immune response. For example, keratinocytes secrete interleukins (e.g., IL-1α, IL-1β, IL-4, IL-6, IL-8, etc.), colony-stimulating factors (e.g., GM-CSF, G-CSF, M-CSF), interferons (IFN-α, IFN-β), growth factors (TGF-α, TGF-β, PDGF, NGF, EGF, FGF), and TNFα.

Dermal Dendrocytes

In the dermis is a population of cells related to the Langerhans' cell, which also have antigen presenting properties (Fig. App-8). These cells have prominent dendritic membrane processes and are highly motile. They are bone marrow–derived, express high levels of MHC class II molecules and factor XIIIa antigen, but do not express T-cell, B-cell, NK-cell markers. Although they stain for CD34, they lack Birbeck granules.

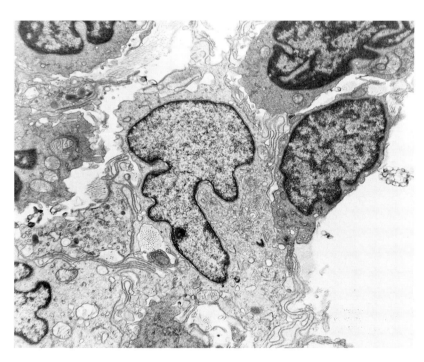

FIGURE APP-8 Dermal dendrocyte. Note dendritic processes, numerous Birbeck granules in cytoplasm, and lobulated nucleus. (Courtesy G. R. Dickersin.)

PIGMENTATION

General

Skin color results predominantly from the presence of melanins in epidermal and hair shaft cells, but carotenoids in the epidermis, oxyhemoglobin in dermal capillaries, and deoxyhemoglobin in dermal venules also contribute. Cutaneous melanization is essential to protection from electromagnetic radiation.

Melanin

Melanins are high-molecular-weight, chemically inert, polymerized oxidation products of tyrosine. Eumelanins range in color from brown to black; pheomelanins are reddish-brown and differ from eumelanins by their solubility in dilute alkali and high sulfur content. Melanins result from the action of the aerobic copper-containing oxidase, tyrosinase, on the substrates tyrosine and dihydroxyphenylalanine. Oxidation of the latter leads to the formation of dopaquinone, which cyclizes and polymerizes to form melanin. The melanins absorb strongly throughout the ultraviolet and visible range of electromagnetic radiation.

Melanocytes

Melanins are synthesized and packaged within neural crest–derived cells, melanocytes. These cells migrate from the neural crest during the eighth week of fetal life, to rest within the basal layer of the epidermis. The number of melanocytes per unit area of skin is constant for any individual within a given animal species; so the melanocyte density in heavily pigmented humans essentially equals that of lightly pigmented individuals. The significant differences between different individuals lie in the amount of melanin produced by the melanocyte, how it is packaged, and how it is transferred.

Melanin is packaged and transferred from the melanocyte in melanosomes, lysosomelike, laminated bodies derived within the Golgi. Synthesized within the endoplasmic reticulum, tyrosinase is later transferred to the immature melanosome. The extent of melanosome melanization is described by four stages: stage I, the melanosome is a spherical membranous vesicle; stage II, the organelle is oval and shows numerous filaments with a distinctive periodicity; stage III, the internal structure becomes obscured by melanin deposits; stage IV, the organelle becomes melanin-packed without discernible internal structure (Fig. App-9).

By means of abundant dendritic projections the basal layer melanocyte distributes melanosomes to a family of keratinocytes, referred to as the epidermal melanin unit. Approximately 36 keratinocytes are supplied by one melanocyte. In H&E sections melanocytes in skin are seen as cells sitting below the basal layer with elongated oval nuclei surrounded by a clear space in a ratio of about one melanocyte to four basal keratinocytes. Most of the dendrites contact basally situated keratinocytes, though a few stretch into the suprabasal layers. Passage of melanosome to keratinocytes involves the movement of melanosomes into the dendritic tips and active phagocytosis of the tips by the receiving keratinocyte. In lightly pigmented individuals melanosomes within the dendrites are clumped and less mature (very few stage III or IV melanosomes), whereas in heavily pigmented individuals melanosomes are individually placed and mostly stage IV. By a poorly understood mechanism, melanosomes are distributed to the generative population of basal cells and sit in a supranuclear position—optimally serving to protect against genomic damage by radiation.

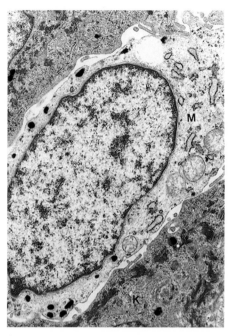

A

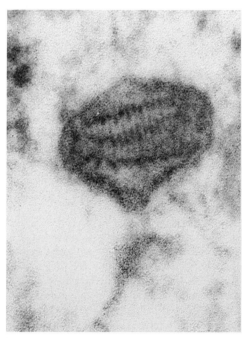

B

FIGURE APP-9 Melanocyte: (*A*) note scattered compound membrane-bound melanosomes in surrounding keratinocytes (M-melanocyte; K-keratinocyte); (*B*) melanosome showing elliptical configuration and striated internal structure.

DERMIS

Stroma

The strength of the skin is owing to the structure of the dermis, which is made of connective tissue packed in a highly organized fashion to give maximal stretchability and strength. The dermis consists of two compartments: The first, made of loosely packed, fine fibrillar stroma is called papillary dermis when it interfaces the epidermal BMZ, and adventitial dermis when it surrounds vessels, nerves, and adnexa. The second, lying deep to the papillary dermis contains coarse collagen bundles and is called reticular dermis. The major connective tissue molecules composing the dermis are collagens, elastin complex, and proteoglycans. Collagen constitutes 75 percent of the dry weight of skin. The predominant interstitial collagens of the dermis, type I and type III, are both present in the papillary and reticular dermis. In general, type III collagen bundles are smaller than type I. The dermis is 80 to 90 percent type I collagen and 8 to 12 percent type III collagen. Several minor collagens also are found: collagen type V, another interstitial collagen, is found in the papillary and adventitial areas, and collagen type VI is found throughout the reticular dermis.

Elastic fibers are thought to bring the skin back to normal configuration after it is stretched. Elastic fibers have an amorphous and fibrillar component. Several proteins have been associated with the fibril, but the best characterized is the molecule fibrillin. Mutations of fibrillin are found in patients with Marfan syndrome. The amorphous component that is referred to as elastin is made of tropoelastin monomers. The polymer constitutes a protein rich in hydrophobic amino acids with unique intermolecular cross-links referred to as isodesmosine and desmosine, cross-links formed between four lysyl residues on the tropoelastin molecule. Elastin microfibrils found in the papillary dermis are referred to as oxytalan fibers; these fibers extend down from the BMZ to the junction between the papillary and reticular dermis. Here the oxytalan fibers interact with a horizontal elastin network called elaunin. Elaunin is predominantly microfibrillar but also contains some amorphous elastin. The elaunin fibers connect to the mature elastin complex, which extends throughout the reticular dermis. Mature elastin is predominantly amorphous with embedded microfibrillar components.

Buried in the fibrous stroma of the dermis is a ground substance made of proteoglycans (PG) and glycosaminoglycans (GAG). The proteoglycans are large molecules with a protein core and GAG side chains. Hyaluronic acid, a protein-free GAG, associates with the core proteins. The major PG/GAGs found in the dermis are chondroitin sulfate–dermatan sulfate in the dermis and chondroitin-6-sulfate in the BMZ. A small dermatan sulfate molecule, decorin, binds to type I collagen by its core protein, where it may influence fibrillogenesis. Since the PG/GAG can bind up to 1000 times their own volume of water, these molecules play a major role in dermal hydration, dermal volume, and compressibility. Generally, PG/GAGs are not easily detected by H&E staining except when present in large amounts, as in lupus erythematosus or a focal (papular) mucinosis.

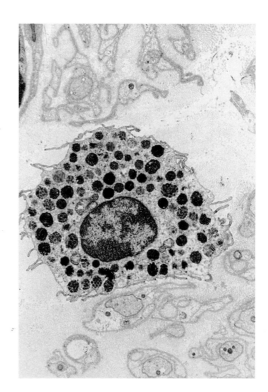

FIGURE APP-10 Mast cell with its distinctive scroll containing secretory granules (courtesy of Simone Petrocine).

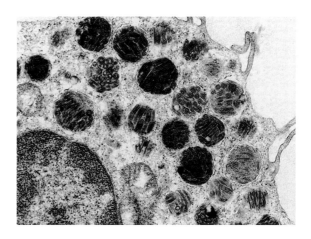

Cells of the Dermis

The major cells of the dermis are fibroblasts, macrophages, and mast cells (Fig. App-10). Although such cells are most common in the papillary and adventitial dermis, they also are found between fibrous bundles in the reticular dermis. Small collections of lymphocytes are also seen about vessels. Although morphologically similar, the fibroblasts of the dermis have been found to be heterogeneous; for example, fibroblasts of the papillary dermis differ from those in the reticular dermis in growth and biosynthetic properties. A population of dendritic cells are present in the dermis that manifest immunologic properties (see the preceding).

Blood Vessels

The primary function of cutaneous blood flow is thermoregulatory. There are two major horizontal dermal plexuses, a deep one at the level of the dermal-subcutis junction and a superficial one at the

papillary–reticular dermis junction (Fig. App-11). Capillary loops branch off the arterial vessels of the superficial plexus and project into the dermal papilla. The capillary loops have arterial characteristics within the confines of the dermal papilla and join the venous channels of the superficial plexus. The differential character of the capillary wall into arterial and venous portions is important since it is the venous limb of the capillary that is most sensitive to histamine and thus is the site of inflammatory cell and exudate release. Throughout the dermis, direct vertical vascular channels link the plexuses and feed the adnexa. The venules in the deep plexus contain valves in contrast to the venules of the superficial plexus. The caliber of vessel walls, particularly dermal vessels, generally is greater in the lower limbs. Dermal blood flow is controlled by arteriovenous anastomoses, which are composed of modified arterial, intermediate, and venous segments. In fully developed anastomoses (Sucquet-Hoyer canals) found in acral skin, the intermediate portion is tortuous and shows a fully developed glomus body. In

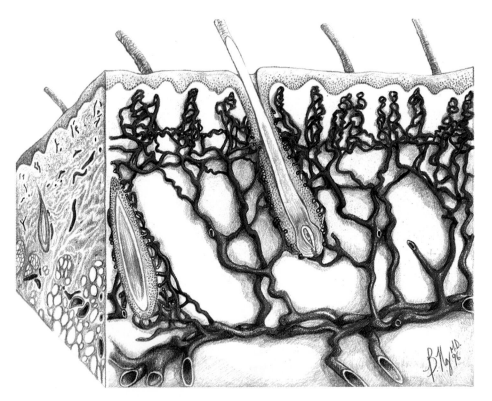

FIGURE APP-11   Illustration of vascular plexuses; superficial plexus, deep vascular plexus, and adventitial (adnexal) plexus.

these areas 60 percent of dermal blood flow courses through these shunts. Blood flow is regulated at these points by a tissue reaction in response to a stimulus (e.g., cold) mediated by sympathetic nerve or circulating pressor agents.

Lymphatics

Serving as a passage for clearing protein, fluid, and cells from the skin, are the lymphatic vessels that essentially follow the distribution pattern of the blood vessels in skin.

Normally, cutaneous lymphatics are difficult to see except in obstructive conditions such as lymphedema or vascular metastases. Lymphatics in the uppermost dermis are endothelium-lined, thin-walled, and blind-ending channels. They are distinguished from the blood vessels of the superficial plexus by their thin walls, prominent endothelial cell nuclei, and elastin-free valves (Fig. App-12). In the lower limbs larger lymphatic vessels (trunks) with muscular walls can be distinguished from arteries by the absence of an internal elastic lamina.

Nerves

Extending as myelinated radicles of the musculocutaneous branches, nerves of the skin form in the skin a deep and superficial plexus (Fig. App-13). Epineural connective tissue surrounds small branches while perineural and endoneural sheaths surround fiber bundles; Schwann cells surround individual fibers. Dermal nerves have both somatic sensory and sympathetic autonomic fibers that distribute together. Sympathetic nerves branch to innervate sweat glands, smooth muscle of vessel walls, and the arrector pili muscle. Sensory fibers, which may have free or specialized endings, are variably distributed. Cutaneous receptors include free nerve endings (e.g., hair follicle and Merkel

cell–associated), and those with encapsulate endings (e.g., Meissner's, pacinian, and Ruffini). Free terminals are the most important of the cutaneous receptors found in the dermis at all levels, but are particularly numerous in the papillary dermis just beneath the BMZ. Free nerve endings in acral skin provide more precise localization and project singly into the dermal papillae without overlapping distribution. Pencillate fibers are the major component of the subepidermal neural network in hairy skin. The three corpuscular receptors have a capsule and an inner core with both neural and nonneural elements. Meissner's corpuscles have an asymmetric lamellated core, are found within the uppermost dermal papilla, and are oriented perpendicular to the surface. Pacinian corpuscles, oval to round nerve endings located in the deep dermis/subcutis of many body parts, contain concentric lamellae separated by spaces containing proteinaceous fluid.

Free nerve endings also associate with Merkel cells. Merkel cells rest immediately above the basal layer of the epidermis in all skin types and are present at a density of 30 to 60 cell/mm^2. Although the cell is thought to derive from the primitive epidermis, the Merkel cell manifests a mix of epithelial and neural characteristics. Although the cell contacts adjacent keratinocytes by normal desmosomes, it also contains characteristic neurosecretory granules that are placed in the cytoplasm adjacent to the associated nerve axon. When the Merkel cell associates with an axon, it is thought to play a mechanosensory role; when it is located independent of an axon, it is thought to play a paracrine role. This cell contains a cytoskeleton made of the following keratins: K8, K18, K19, K20. It is notable that K20 is a specific marker for Merkel cells in the skin. This cell is thought to play a secretory role because it contains within it vasoactive intestinal peptide, neuron-specific enolase, substance P, and dynorphin, among others.

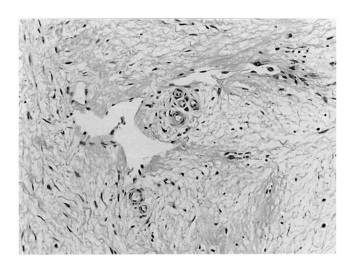

FIGURE APP-12   Lymphatic spaces not normally evident are dilated here by chronic lymphedema. Note the lack of walls, prominent endothelial cells, and presence of valves.

DERMAL APPENDAGES

Hair

The hair follicle arises as an invagination of the primitive epidermis. In most areas the follicle forms an angle with the epidermis. On the side of the follicle giving rise to the obtuse angle (with respect to the epidermis) the follicle shows specific differentiations: at the midportion, a smooth muscle (arrector pili), above this the sebaceous duct and gland, and above this point, in certain regions, an apocrine gland. In fact, then, the hair follicle is more than hair, it is really a pilosebaceous organ or apparatus.

Illustrative of the marked heterogeneity of skin is the hair follicle. Probably no two follicles are identical, accepting bilateral symmetry. Follicles and their shaft product differ in size, color, curl, androgen sensitivity, and so on. With maturation two follicle types are recognized: vellus and terminal (Fig. App-14). The terminal follicle is large and grows into the subcutis; the shaft it produces also is large, coarse, and pigmented. The vellus follicle is small and superficial; it produces a short, fine, unpigmented shaft. In select body regions androgen-sensitive follicles are induced to switch from a vellus to a terminal morphology by androgen exposure with the onset of adolescence. Hair is present on all surfaces of the body except the palms and soles, ventral aspects of fingers and toes, inner aspect of prepuce and glans penis, and the inner parts of the vulva.

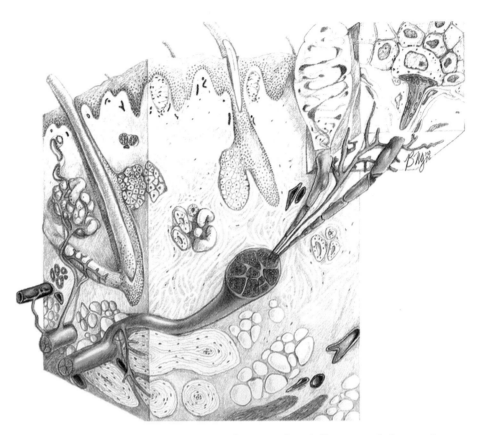

FIGURE APP-13 Illustration of cutaneous innervations: unmyelinated efferent sympathetic nerves that supply arterioles, eccrine glands, apocrine glands, and hair errector muscles, and mostly myelinated somatic sensory nerves that supply specialized end-organs (e.g., Meisner corpuscles and Pacini corpuscles), Merkel cells, and free dermal nerve endings. Not illustrated here are free nerve endings to hair follicles.

The pilosebaceous organ is divided into three regions: (1) an infundibular region that extends from the epidermis to the sebaceous duct, (2) an isthmus, or middle, region from the sebaceous duct to the insertion of the muscle, and (3) an inferior region that extends from the muscle to the follicle bulb.

The inferior follicle is that region that shows the greatest changes over the cycle. During the growth, or anagen, phase the inferior portion of a terminal follicle extends into the subcutis (Fig. App-15). After a variable period of time, depending on the site of the follicle (e.g., scalp follicles have a growth period of 2 to 6 years, whereas eyelashes have a growth period of 4 months), the follicle receives a signal that causes it to stop growing. In the regressive phase, called catagen (Fig. App-16A), the lower follicle atrophies by apoptosis, a process of individual cell controlled death, and then enters a nongrowing rest phase, telogen (Fig. App-16B). In telogen the follicle consists only of the permanent portions, namely, the infundibulum and the isthmus. At the end of telogen the hair shaft sheds. In the scalp, 80 to 85 percent of hair follicles are in the anagen phase, 1 to 2 percent in catagen phase, and 10 to 20 percent are in telogen phase. About 100 hairs are shed per day.

The hair shaft is synthesized within the inferior portion of the follicle. The lowest portion of the follicle is termed the bulb or matrix (Fig. App-15B). From this portion the layers of the follicle and the cells making up the shaft are formed. To produce a shaft, the cells of the bulb exhibit a rate of growth equal to that of the cells in bone marrow and intestinal epithelium. By mechanisms that we do not yet understand, follicle growth depends on influences arising from the mesenchyme of the follicular papilla and the surrounding connective tissue sheath. In the absence of the papilla, follicle growth ceases.

The papilla also is thought to initiate follicle growth from the telogen phase. That cells with stem cell characteristics are found in the bulge region of the follicle (a region underlying the insertion of the muscle), it is thought that stimuli from the papilla induce the telogen follicle stem cells to proliferate and give rise to a population of cells that will generate the next hair shaft.

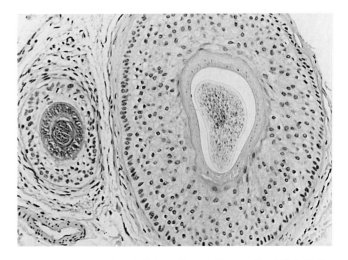

FIGURE APP-14 Terminal follicle (*right*) and adjacent vellus follicle (*left*) cut in cross section.

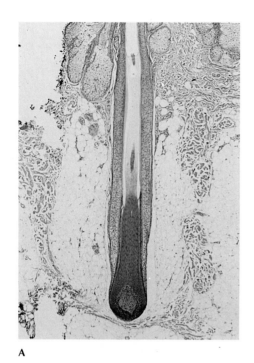

A

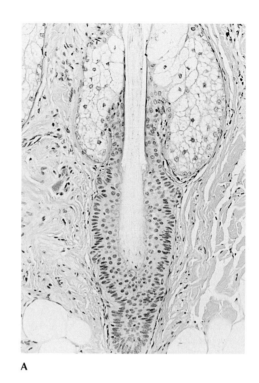

A

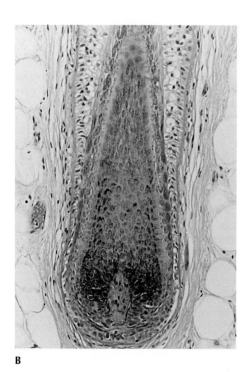

B

FIGURE APP-15 Follicular bulb: (*A*) low-power view of terminal anagen follicle; (*B*) divisions of hair bulb from the follicular papilla, melanocytes and matrical cells, hair shaft formation, inner root sheath, to outer root sheath.

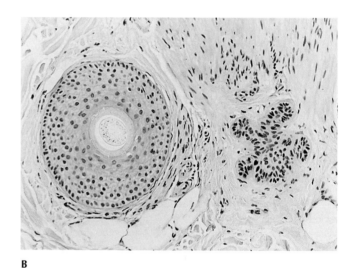

B

FIGURE APP-16 Cross sections of the hair cycle: (*A*) terminal follicle in catagen phase of hair cycle; (*B*) telogen follicle (*right*) adjacent to an anagen follicle (*left*).

The follicle actually consists of a series of concentric cylinders that form in the bulb and move progressively upward. The outermost cylinder comprises the outer root sheath (ORS); it serves to separate the whole organ from the dermis. The ORS does not move outward. Inside of the ORS is the inner root sheath (IRS). It consists of an outermost layer, Henle's layer, which is the first of the lower follicle layers to keratinize, and an inner cylinder, Huxley's layer, which also keratinizes

early but contains, in addition, trichohyalin granules. (These structures show a homology to the intermediate filament–associated proteins and the keratohyalin granules of the epidermis.) The IRS molds the shaft and moves with it on its voyage to the skin surface. The innermost cylinder of the follicle is the hair shaft itself. It is moored to the IRS by means of its cuticle that interdigitates with the cuticle of the IRS. Cells of the shaft cortex are tightly cohesive and contain a highly developed cytoskeleton composed of unique hard keratins (class I Hal-4, and class II Hb1-4) and intermediate filament–associated proteins (sulfur-rich, and tyrosine-glycine-rich components). Some hair shafts contain a medulla located in the centermost shaft; the medulla is made of vacuolated cells that also contain prominent trichohyalin granules. Shaft cortex cells are pigmented by melanocytes, which reside within the bulb at

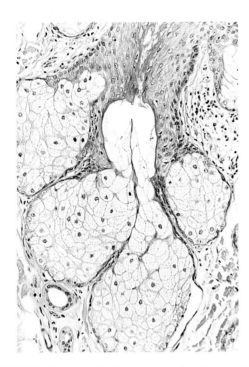

FIGURE APP-17   Sebaceous gland emptying into the sebaceous duct.

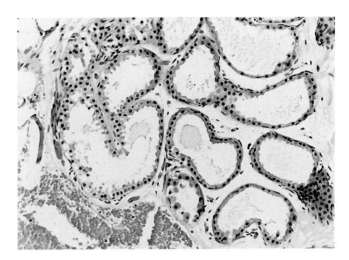

FIGURE APP-18   Apocrine gland secretory coils are typically dilated and contain cells with conspicuous cytoplasm showing decapitation secretion.

the papilla interface. The follicular melanocytes distribute melanosomes to the upward moving keratinocytes (trichocytes) as they mature.

Sebaceous Gland

The sebaceous gland arises as an outgrowth of the pilosebaceous apparatus. Except for acral skin this gland is found in follicles of all regions. The secretory epithelium grows from the periphery of the lobule where basaloid cells divide, move toward the duct, differentiate by accumulating foamy cytoplasmic lipid vacuoles, losing cytoplasmic organelles, and finally erupting (holocrine secretion) in the sebaceous duct and emptying into the pilary canal or directly onto the skin surface at certain sites (nipples, areolae, eyelids, and labia minora) (Fig. App-17). Sebum contains glycerides and free fatty acids, wax esters, and squalene. Sebaceous secretions are stimulated by androgen hormones, which enhance sebaceous cell growth and differentiation. Sebum serves not only as an emollient for the hair and skin surface but also to process the separation of the hair shaft from the surrounding IRS. Shaft-sheath separation occurs within the hair follicle at the level of the sebaceous duct.

Apocrine Gland

Although it is commonly thought to be restricted to very specific regions (e.g., axilla, mammary line, inguinal region, etc.), the apocrine gland actually can be found irregularly wherever hair is found. This tubular gland has a single-layered secretory portion that consists of one cell type (Fig. App-18). Apocrine secretion is stimulated by local or systemic adrenergic stimuli. The secretions are stored by the secretory epithelium and are released in a pulsatile fashion (not continuous as they are for eccrine secretions). One might find in a microscopic field contiguous contracted and dilated secretory portions of the gland. Although apical cleavage of the apocrine cap is characteristic (so-called apocrine secretion), these glands also manifest merocrine and holocrine secretory events.

In contrast to the double-layered eccrine duct, the apocrine duct often is triple layered. The luminal layer surface has microvilli, and the luminal cytoplasm is rich in keratin filaments giving a hyaline appearance to the inner duct by light microscopy.

Apocrine secretion is described as viscid and milky pale. It is protein-rich and lipid-poor. These secretions are thought to be odorless on production but then acquire the typical axillary odor by bacterial action.

Eccrine Gland

Also a tabular structure, the eccrine gland develops directly as a downgrowth of the primitive epidermis. It consists of five parts: a secretory segment, a coiled duct, a straight duct, intraepidermal coil, and eccrine pore. The secretory coil is surrounded by a basal lamina that entraps a discontinuous layer of myoepithelial cells (Fig. App-19A). The gland is made of clear serous cells and a lesser number of dark, granule-containing mucous cells. Serous cells are peripheral in the segment and mucous cells are luminal. Both cells are secretory and their main function is to produce sweat for the control of excessive heat. Although the cells are tightly coherent at the luminal surface, the lateral walls are plicated, allowing for channel formations between cells. The general principle of eccrine secretion begins with a cholinergic stimulus that depolarizes the lateral infolded serous cell membranes, allowing sodium flow into the cell followed by interstitial fluids. As the sodium ion osmotic gradient draws fluid into the serous cell and saturates it, sodium is transported into the gland lumen. The initial secretory product is isotonic. The coiled duct distal to the secretory portion is made of two cell layers: luminal cells that bear microvilli and basal cells. In the coiled duct, sodium is taken up from the isotonic sweat and the final sweat becomes hypotonic. The straight duct consists of two cylindrical layers of cells connected by desmosomes; the luminal cytoplasm is keratin filament–rich. Finally, the acrosyringium enters the epidermis within a rete ridge (Fig. App-19B). Within the epidermis the eccrine ductal cells remain distinct from the epidermal cells. Eccrine glands are found in highest density in the palms, soles, forehead, and axillae.

Apoeccrine Sweat Glands

In adults, axillary glands having the morphology of both apocrine and eccrine epithelium have been identified. This unique gland's secretory

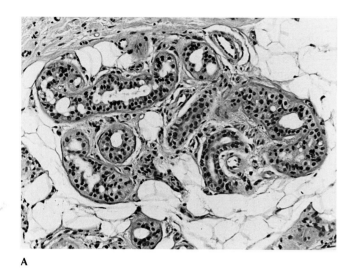

A

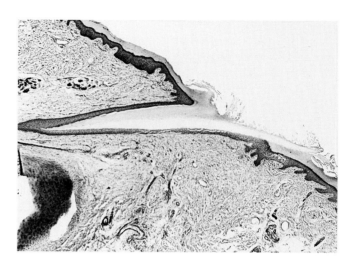

FIGURE APP-20 Nail: nail matrix continuous with the nail plate which overlies the nail bed; the proximal nail fold overlies the nail plate.

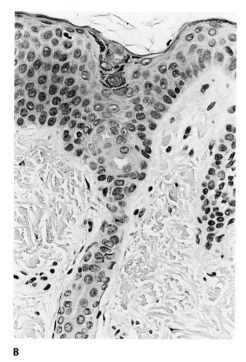

B

FIGURE APP-19 Eccrine gland: (*A*) eccrine secretory coil within subcutis; (*B*) acrosyringium and dermal duct.

activity and proximal duct are similar to the eccrine gland, but its secretory component is indistinguishable from an apocrine gland. These ducts open directly onto the skin surface.

Nail

The nail serves as a protective covering for the tip of the digit. It too is a derivative of the primitive epidermis. The nail matrix is an epithelial invagination along the proximal margin of the nail apparatus, which gives rise to the nail plate (Fig. App-20). As the germinative portion of the nail, the matrix consists of a stratified squamous epithelium of basal cells that sit on connective tissue just above the periosteum of the distal digit. With nail plate differentiation, the cells leave the basal region and push outward. These cells fill with keratin filaments in the absence of keratohyalin, they make and discharge membrane-coating granules, and

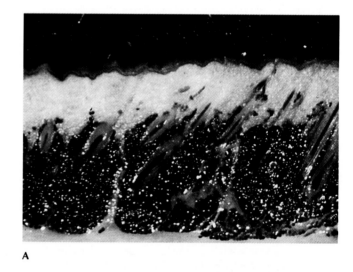

A

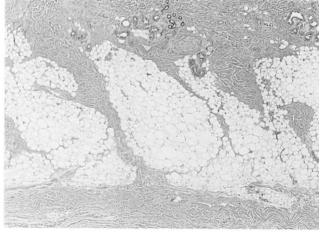

B

FIGURE APP-21 Subcutis: (*A*) Osmium stains adipocytes black highlighting the architecture of the subcutis (osmium stain, no magnification). (Courtesy of Richard Sagebiel, MD.) (*B*) The subcutis of the lower leg showing adipose tissue lobules surrounded by fibrous septa that vary in thickness.

they form cornified envelopes. The nail plate moves distally entirely by growth pressure arising from the matrix. The nail bed epithelium plays a passive roll in this movement. Nails grow about 0.1 mm per day on average, with growth faster in the summer than winter, and fingernails faster than toenails.

The nail plate is embedded by upfoldings of the surrounding skin that form the lateral and proximal nail folds. The keratin layer of the proximal fold adheres to the nail plate surface as the cuticle. The plate moves over the nail bed, which consists of a thin epidermis lacking a granular layer. The nail bed epidermis has an undulating rete pattern that runs parallel to the direction of the nail plate growth and gives subtle ribbing to the plate. Capillaries feeding the nail bed course along the rete parallel to the direction of growth. The hyponychium extends from the nail bed to the distal groove. This layer keratinizes like the epidermis with granular and desquamating layers.

SUBCUTIS

Below the fibrous and structurally strong dermis and resting on a fascial plane is the subcutis, a layer of adipose tissue organized into lobules separated by loose fibrous connective tissue septa (Fig. App-21). Within the septa are blood vessels, lymphatics, and nerves. The nature of the subcutis varies from site to site; for example, it is thin in acral skin, thick over abdominal skin, and manifests fibrous dermal projections in arm skin.

LABORATORY METHODS

Klaus J. Busam

The mainstay of dermatopathology is the examination of skin biopsies following fixation in formalin, embedding in paraffin, and staining with hematoxylin-eosin (H&E). This technique has been quite durable in the history of histopathology because it offers many advantages: It is relatively quick, inexpensive, suitable for most practical needs, and relatively easy to master. However, it cannot answer all the questions that a case may pose at the diagnostic level. Therefore, pathologists have always searched for additional methods to analyze their histologic material.

SPECIAL STAINS

There is an extensive battery of "special" stains listed in texts discussing histologic techniques.[1,2] Few of them are of practical value for the diagnostic dermatopathologist. A synopsis of some of the stains that appear relevant for a modern dermatopathology laboratory are listed in Table App-1.

Stains for Microorganisms

Perhaps the most important of all the special stains in the practice of dermatopathology are stains that help to identify microorganisms. This includes the modifications of the Gram stain, such as by Brown and Hopp, for most bacterial organisms; the methenamine silver stain or Periodic acid–Schiff (PAS) stain for fungi and parasites; and the Ziehl-Neelson or Fite stain for acid-fast bacilli. Silver stains, such as according to Dieterle, Warthin-Starry, or Steiner, are commonly used to identify spirochetes (syphilis, Lyme disease) or the organisms in cat-scratch disease and bacillary angiomatosis (*Rochalimaea*). Leishmania is best identified by a Giemsa stain.

Periodic Acid–Schiff (PAS) Stain

This stain demonstrates mucosubstances, basement membrane material, fibrinoid material, and glycogen in a specific fashion when combined with diastase digestion. The staining reaction yields a pink to red color. An intensely bright red homogeneous material within vessels suggests cryoglobulins. The PAS stain is also useful in highlighting most types of fungi and parasites.

Giemsa Stain

This technique is very useful for the demonstration of lymphoreticular cells, including mast cells. It is also used to highlight microorganisms such as leishmania.

Mucicarmine Stain

This technique has been recommended for epithelial mucins (i.e., adenocarcinoma), and to stain the capsule of cryptococcus. A positive reaction yields a reddish color.

Toluidine Blue

This stain is used to document metachromasia. Most acid mucosubstances will show metachromasia at higher pH value. Toluidine blue is used most often to identify mast cells.

Stain for Hemosiderin

In the Prussian blue reaction, hydrochloric acid splits off the protein bond to the iron, allowing the potassium ferrocyanide to combine specifically with the ferric iron to form ferric ferrocyanide. The reaction leaves a blue color.

Stains for Melanin

In the Fontana-Masson method, an ammoniacal silver solution is used without a reducing bath. Only substances capable of reducing directly silver salts (i.e., argentaffin material) such as melanin are demonstrated as grayish-black pigment. This stain is not entirely specific for melanin. Some metabolic products of minocin, for example, also stain with this method.

Von Kossa Stain for Calcium

In this technique, silver is substituted for calcium in calcium salts; this silver is then reduced to yield a black metallic color.

Trichrome Stains

In this stain, phosphotungstic or phosphomolybolic acid is used in combination with several anionic dyes. This stain primarily is used in the evaluation of extracellular material, in particular collagen such as in fibromatoses or connective tissue nevi. Its practical application also includes peculiar phenomena such as the identification of small globular structures in infantile digital fibromatosis.

Reticulin Stain

This method highlights reticulin fibers. It has traditionally been used to distinguish carcinoma (groups of cells surrounded by fibers) from sarcoma (single cells surrounded by fibers).

Elastic Fiber Stain

In the Verhoeff-van Gieson stain, elastic fibers are outlined with a strong black color. Its main application is in the demonstration of arterial injury and in connective tissue nevi.

Amyloid Stains

A number of stains are available to demonstrate amyloid material. Most laboratories use the Congo red stain. This stain needs to be combined with polariscopic examination, which yields an apple-green birefringent appearance. However, one needs to be cautious in interpreting this stain, because excess dye retained in the tissue may give a false-positive signal.

ENZYME HISTOCHEMISTRY

Because of the complexity of the techniques involved in enzyme histochemistry, the need for fresh material, and the relative nonspecificity of most of the reactions, this technique has only very limited applications nowadays. In dermatopathology, the methods most commonly used are chloracetate esterase, also known as Leder stain, for the identification of mast cells or hematopoietic cells of the myeloid lineage, and the dopa reaction to identify cells of the melanocytic lineage.[2]

IMMUNOHISTOCHEMISTRY

Technical Aspects

Several methods are applicable to the evaluation of skin biopsies. The most commonly used technique is an immune complex method with an enzyme antibody conjugate.[3] This conjugate is typically an enzyme, such as horseradish peroxidase or alkaline phosphatase. Enhancing techniques using biotin and avidin frequently are used.

A number of steps have been suggested to increase the sensitivity of these procedures. The aim is to expose the epitope that may otherwise be masked. Such "unmasking" techniques include digestion of the tissue with proteolytic enzymes or heat-treatment, such as with microwaves.

In addition to labeling an antibody with an enzyme, there are also a number of fluorescent probes available. Immunofluorescence can be performed either directly (DIF) with a probe, such as fluorescein isothiocyanate (FITC) label, or indirectly (IF). For direct immunofluorescence, a skin biopsy is submitted in saline (Table App-2) or, if immediate processing cannot be performed, in Michelle's medium. On arrival of the specimen in the laboratory, frozen sections are prepared, and these are labeled in a one-step method with fluorescence probe–tagged antibodies that are directed against human immunoglobulins, serum proteins, or complement factors. A signal then is obtained by visualizing antibody binding by excitation of the fluorescent label by ultraviolet light using a fluorescence microscope.[4]

Indirect immunofluorescence (IF) differs from direct immunofluorescence in that it does not probe the patient's skin directly, but rather analyzes the presence of circulating antibodies against cutaneous antigens in the patient's serum. For this method, the patient's serum is obtained and then allowed to incubate with substrate tissue. Subsequently, the target tissue is labeled with fluorescent-tagged antibodies as described for direct immunofluorescence. If the patient's serum contained circulating antibodies to antigens present in the target tissue, a positive

signal would be obtained. With indirect immunofluorescence, semiquantitative analysis can be performed by determining titers of antibodies.[5]

Saline-split skin preparations are an addition to the methodology of indirect immunofluorescence (Table App-3) and they are used mainly in the distinction between bullous pemphigoid and epidermolysis bullosa acquisita.[7] This technique requires that biopsies of normal skin must be obtained from human volunteers. They are subsequently incubated with $1M$ sodium chloride at $4°C$ for 72 h, and then the epidermis is separated from the dermis manually. The cleavage occurs between the lamina lucida and the remainder of the epidermal basement membrane, which allows localization of the bullous pemphigoid antigen to the roof of the artificially induced blister, whereas the epidermolysis bullosa acquisita antigen is located in its base. Although a properly done saline-split skin procedure is very valuable methodology, it is tedious, which explains why it is routinely used only in a few laboratories.

Applications in Nonneoplastic Diseases

BULLOUS DISEASES

Immunofluorescent studies play an important role in the evaluation of primary bullous disorders, because some of these disorders show a fairly specific reaction pattern (Tables App-4 to App-6).

Intraepidermal Blisters

This includes mainly variants of pemphigus. Immunohistologically, one typically observes a mosaiclike intercellular labeling of the acantholytic epidermis by DIF, in virtually all forms of pemphigus (Fig. App-22).

TABLE APP-1

Common Special Stains in Dermatopathology

Stain	Application	Results
H&E	Routine	Nuclei: blue; cytoplasm; red Collagen, muscles, nerves: red
PAS/diastase	Fungi, parasites	Wall of organisms: red
	Glycogen (e.g., in trichilemmoma)	Glycogen: red on PAS; clear after diastase digestion
	Basement membrane thickening (e.g., LE)	Basement membrane: pink/red
	Cryoglobulinemia	Cryoprecipitates: bright red
Mucicarmine	Adenocarcinomas	Mucin: red
	Cryptococcus	Capsule: red
Toluidine Blue	Mast cells	Metachromatically purple
Giemsa	Mast cells	Metachromatically purple
	Leishmania	Blue
Masson's trichrome	Fibrosis	Collagen: green; nuclei, muscle: dark red
	Infantile digital fibromatosis	Hyaline globules: red
Van Gieson	Arterial injury	Elastic fibers: black
Von Kossa	Calcium	Black
Congo red	Amyloid	Green under polarized light
Fontana	Melanin	Black
Prussian blue	Hemosiderin/iron	Black
Gram stain	Bacteria	Depending on method used (Gram-positive: usually blue; Gram-negative: usually red)
Methenamine-silver	Fungi, parasites	Black
Dieterle/Steiner/ Warthin-Starry	Spirochetes, *Rochalimaea*	Black
AFB/Fite	Acid-fast bacilli	Red

TABLE APP-2

TABLE APP-2

Optimal Sites for Skin Biopsy for Direct Immunofluorescence

Optimal Site(s) for Skin Biopsy

Disease	Lesional	Perilesional	Distant Normal
Pemphigus		X	
Bullous pemphigoid		X	
Cicatricial pemphigoid		X	
Epidermolysis bullosa acquisita (EBA)		X	
Herpes gestationis		X	
Dermatitis herpetiformis		X	
Linear IgA dermatosis		X	
Bullous lupus erythematosus		X	
Leukocytoclastic vasculitis			X
Porphyria cutanea tarda		X	
Erythema multiforme	X		
Lichen planus	X		

SOURCE: J.D. Fine: *Bullous Diseases*. Igaku-Shoin. New York, 1993.

IgG, in particular IgG1, is the most common immunoreactant. Other immunoglobulins are rarely deposited. Deposition of C3 occurs, but is infrequently seen.[6]

In pemphigus erythematosus, linear deposits of IgG, IgM, IgA, and/or C3 may be detectable at the epidermal basement membrane zone in addition to the intercellular labeling typical of the other variants of pemphigus.[7]

Subepidermal Blisters

Immunofluorescence plays a critical role in the distinction between a number of subepidermal bullous disorders.[8–11] This disease group includes bullous pemphigoid (BP), herpes gestationis (HG), dermatitis herpetiformis (DH), bullous disease of childhood, linear IgA dermatosis, bullous lupus erythematosus, and epidermolysis bullosa acquisita. In all of these diseases, a blister is formed by cleavage of the skin at the basement membrane zone, either in the lamina lucida or lamina densa.

Bullous pemphigoid, herpes gestationis, and epidermolysis bullosa acquisita all demonstrate linear continuous staining of the basement membrane zone by direct immunofluorescence for IgG and for C3 (Fig. App-23). The distinction of these three entities from each other depends mainly on the clinical findings. If epidermolysis bullosa cannot reliably be separated from bullous pemphigoid on clinical grounds alone, indirect immunofluorescence on saline split-skin preparations would be helpful (see the preceding). It has also been suggested that if this technique is not available, one might also attempt to localize the site of immune complex deposition by staining the tissue sections for type IV collagen. This type of collagen is a major component of the lamina densa. It will remain in the base of the blister in bullous pemphigoid–herpes gestationis, but resides in the roof of the bulla in epidermolysis bullosa acquisita.

Linear IgA dermatosis and chronic bullous dermatosis of childhood share the same immunofluorescence pattern: Linear deposits of IgA along the basement membrane zone. In dermatitis herpetiformis, on the other hand, IgA deposits are found in a patchy granular distribution in the dermal papillae (Fig. App-24). Complement C3 also is frequently deposited in each of these disorders. Occasionally, one may also find deposition of IgG or IgM.

In bullous lupus erythematosus, usually a number of immunoglobulins and complements are deposited along the basement membrane in the blister base, essentially showing the same patterns as in other lesions of lupus erythematosus.[11]

TABLE APP-3

Indirect Immunofluorescence in Selected Cutaneous Diseases Using the Split-Skin Preparation

Site of Antibasement Membrane Autoantibody Binding to Sodium Chloride–Separated Normal Human Skin Dermoepidermal Junction

Epidermal Portion Only	Epidermis and Dermis	Dermal Portion Only
Bullous pemphigoid (most commonly)	Bullous pemphigoid (rare)	EBA*
Cicatricial pemphigoid (some)		Bullous eruption of systemic lupus erythematosus
Chronic bullous dermatosis of childhood (IgA-class autoantibody)		Cicatricial pemphigoid (some)

*Use of 1.0*M* NaCl-split human skin as the tissue substrate increases the likelihood of detecting autoantibodies to at least an 85 percent positivity rate.
SOURCE: J.D. Fine: *Bullous Diseases*. Igaku-Shoin. New York, 1993.

CONNECTIVE TISSUE DISEASE

Immunofluorescence also may be helpful in the evaluation of connective tissue disease, in particular, for the diagnosis of lupus erythematosus. Immunoglobulins (IgG, IgM, IgA, IgE) and complements (C1q, C3, C4, C5) are commonly found along the basement membrane of lesional skin in discoid lupus erythematosus (DLE) (Fig. App-25).[12,13] The pattern of deposition typically is granular. In systemic lupus erythematosus (SLE), such granular deposits of immunoglobulins and complement is not only seen in lesional skin, but also in clinically normal appearing skin. The phenomenon that normal appearing skin may show deposition of immunoglobulins and complements has been used diagnostically in the so-called "lupus band test."[14] This test may help in the distinction between SLE and DLE. Although in DLE, a lupus band test should be negative, a positive test is found in approximately 60 percent of patients with SLE. A positive test in sun-protected normal skin in a patient with SLE has been suggested also to be of prognostic value, implying a worse prognosis. In patients with SLE, immunoglobulins and complements are not only found along the basement membrane zone, but also around the vessels and diffusely between collagen bundles.

Positive immunofluorescence findings also are seen commonly in a number of other examples of connective tissue disease, such as in mixed connective tissue disease, scleroderma, or dermatomyositis. In most cases, the immunofluorescence pattern is fairly nonspecific and usually adds little useful information.

VASCULITIS

Positive immunofluorescence findings are commonly seen in many cutaneous vasculitides.[14] Many times it is difficult to decide whether the deposition of immunoglobulins and complements in damaged vessels is primary or secondary. The diagnostically most useful application of immunofluorescence studies in vasculitides is

Direct Immunofluorescence Findings in Specific Bullous Diseases

Localization of Immune Deposits	Pattern of Deposition	Immunoreactant(s) Present	Disease(s)
Intraepidermal	Epidermal cell surface	IgG, complement	Pemphigus family
		IgA	Intraepidermal IgA dermatosis
Dermoepidermal junction	Linear, homogeneous	IgG, complement	Bullous pemphigoid
			Herpes gestationis
			Cicatricial pemphigoid
			EBA
		Multiple Igs, complement, and/or fibrin	Cicatricial pemphigoid
			EBA
			Lupus erythematosus
		IgA	Linear IgA dermatosis (adult)
			Chronic bullous dermatosis of childhood
	Linear, nonhomogeneous (shaggy, smudged, fibrillar, and/or granular)	Multiple Igs, complement, and/or fibrin	Lupus erythematosus
	Granular, focal	IgA	Dermatitis herpetiformis
Other upper dermis	Cytoid bodies	Multiple Igs, complement, and/or fibrin	Lichen planus
	Interstitial perivascular (smudged, broad) and/or dermoepidermal junction	Multiple Igs, complement, and/or fibrin	Porphyria cutanea tarda
Intravascular	Granular	IgM, complement, and/or fibrin	Vasculitis
			Erythema multiforme

SOURCE: J.D. Fine: *Bullous Diseases*. Igaku-Shoin, New York, 1993.

in the evaluation of Henoch-Schoenlein purpura.[15] In this clinical setting, the demonstration of IgA deposits by immunofluorescence is paramount for establishing the diagnosis (Fig. App-26).

them have been applied to formalin-fixed and paraffin-embedded tissue. The detection system usually relies on enzyme-conjugated antibodies (peroxidase or phosphatase) and not on immunofluorescence. One of the more frequently employed antibodies in this context are antibodies

LICHENOID DERMATITIS

Positive immunofluorescence findings may also be seen in lichen planus–lichen planopilaris and some drug-induced dermatitides. Positive staining often is observed in so-called "colloid" bodies, which frequently represent immunoglobulin-encrusted keratinocytic material. Staining may be seen for IgM, IgG, IgA, C3, or fibrin. Drug-induced dermatitides can show a very broad spectrum of immunofluorescence patterns and lack specificity.[16]

IMMUNOHISTOLOGY OF INFECTIOUS DISEASES

Direct antibodies have been developed for the detection of infectious agents. Most of

Indirect Immunofluorescence Patterns Observed in Selected Autoimmune Bullous Diseases

Indirect Immunofluorescence Pattern and Autoantibody Class	Representative Diseases and Frequency
Epidermal cell surface intercellular—IgG class	Pemphigus vulgaris (in majority of cases)
Dermoepidermal junction–specific—IgG class	Bullous pemphigoid (in >80% of cases) Cicatricial pemphigoid (in <10% of cases) EBA (in >40% of cases)
Dermoepidermal junction–specific—IgA class	Chronic bullous dermatosis of childhood (in majority of cases)

SOURCE: J.D. Fine: *Bullous Diseases*. Igaku-Shoin. New York, 1993.

TABLE APP-6

Staining Patterns of Specific Antibodies to Inherited EB Skin via the Immunofluorescence Antigenic Mapping Technique

Specific Basement Membrane Antibodies and Site of Binding within Induced or Spontaneous Blisters in Inherited EB

Type of Inherited EB	Anti-bullous pemphigoid antigen; anti α6β4 integrin	Anti-laminin	Anti-type IV collagen; Anti-LDA-1
EB simplex	Dermal base	Dermal base	Dermal base
Junctional EB	Epidermal roof	Dermal base	Dermal base
Dystrophic EB	Epidermal roof	Epidermal roof	Epidermal roof

SOURCE: J.D. Fine: *Bullous Diseases*. Igaku-Shoin. New York, 1993.

to herpes simplex virus type I or II. A number of antibodies to other viral or bacterial organisms are available.

Applications in Neoplastic Skin Diseases (Table App-7)

CUTANEOUS LYMPHOID INFILTRATES

Immunohistology plays an invaluable role in the characterization of lymphoid cells.[17,18] A list of commonly used markers in the evaluation of lymphoid infiltrates is provided in Table App-7. The application of these markers is guided by the differential diagnosis formulated based on the cytology and distribution of the infiltrate in routine H&E-stained sections. A thorough investigation of the cell phenotype requires the availability of fresh tissue for cryostat sections (Table App-8).

Epidermotropic Infiltrates

This includes cutaneous T-cell infiltrates, in particular, mycosis fungoides, atypical T-cell reactions, such as lymphomatoid papulosis, lymphomatous drug reactions, lymphomatous lichenoid, or spongiotic dermatitides and actinic reticuloid. It has been said that the phenotype of the T-cell infiltrate in mycosis fungoides is different from other

processes, such as actinic reticuloid. Mycosis fungoides, for example, typically has a predominant population of CD4+ cells expressing other T-cell markers as well (CD2, CD3, CD5) and often some decrease in CD7.[19,20] On the other hand, actinic reticuloid and some lymphomatoid dermatitides tend to retain pan T-cell markers and contain a larger proportion of CD8 cells.[22] It is important not to put too much weight on these findings, however, since mycosis fungoides may have an uncharacteristic phenotype, and reactive lesions may mimic the immunophenotype of mycosis fungoides. CD30 is a useful antibody if lymphomatoid papulosis is suspected, since the condition typically contains T lymphocytes expressing this activation marker.[20]

Deep Lymphoid Infiltrates

Bulky deep dermal lymphoid infiltrates generally suggest a B-cell phenotype. These infiltrates are readily identified as reactive if immunohistochemical studies demonstrate a mixture of B cells and T cells and the B cells lack light chain restriction. If frozen tissue is available, the demonstration of light chain restriction is perhaps the most useful test in diagnostic immunohistology of lymphoid infiltrates because it proves presence of a clonal neoplastic B-cell population.[24] Unfortunately, light chain immunostains are very difficult to perform technically and many times they are difficult to interpret. If a deep T-cell infiltrate is present, CD30 may again be a useful marker if lymphomatoid papulosis or CD30+ lymphoma is suspected.

NONLYMPHOID HEMATOPOIETIC INFILTRATES

Immunohistochemical studies also are important in the evaluation of hematopoietic infiltrates other than lymphoid cells. This includes Langerhans' cell proliferation and leukemias.[26,27] Langerhans' cells still are best recognized immunohistochemically by CD1a, which unfortunately requires fresh tissue as substrate. Paraffin sections of Langerhans' cell histiocytoses stain fairly reliably for S-100 protein, HLA-DR, and CD43.

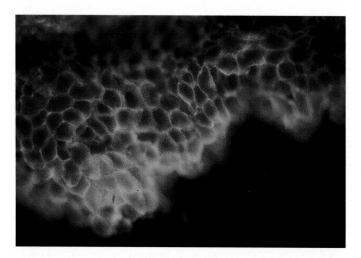

FIGURE APP-22 Immunofluorescence of pemphigus. Note intercellular immunofluorescence pattern within epidermis.

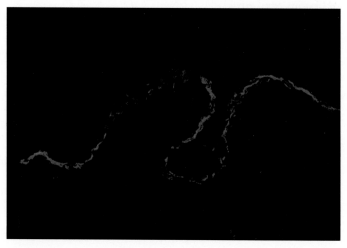

FIGURE APP-23 Immunofluorescence of bullous pemphigoid. There is linear deposition of immunoreactants in basement membrane zone.

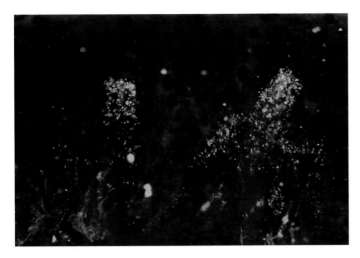

FIGURE APP-24 Immunofluorescence of dermatitis herpetiformis. Note striking granular deposition of IgA in dermal papillae. (Courtesy of Grant J. Anhalt.)

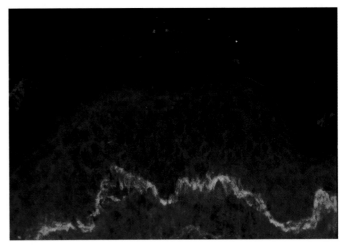

FIGURE APP-25 Immunofluorescence of lupus erythematosus. Note thick linear band of immunoreactants along dermal-epidermal junction.

FIGURE APP-26 Immunofluorescence of Henoch-Schoenlein purpura. Immunoreactants are deposited in vessels in dermas.

Most leukemic infiltrates of the skin are myeloid. Markers useful in the recognition of myeloid leukemia include myeloperoxidase, chloracetate esterase, Leu-M1 (CD15) and KP-1 (CD68).

EPITHELIOID NEOPLASMS

Cytokeratins and epithelial membrane antigen (EMA) remain the most important markers of epithelial differentiation.[28,29] Their application usually is needed for the evaluation of undifferentiated primary tumors or metastases. They need to be used in conjunction with the most likely mimics, such as melanoma or lymphoma (Table App-9). Certain markers, such as thyroglobulin, GCDFG, calcitonin, or prostate-specific antigen, may be helpful to identify possible primary sites.

MELANOCYTIC NEOPLASMS

A number of markers are available that aid in the identification of a lesion as melanocytic in origin.[26,27] This is most often needed in the evaluation of poorly differentiated (generally amelanotic) primary or metastatic tumors that suggest melanoma. Primary tumors that may mimic melanoma include spindle cell squamous cell carcinoma, atypi-

---

TABLE APP-7

Lymphoid Markers

B-cell markers

CD 10 (CALLA): Marks precursor B cells and granulocytes. Present in follicular center cell lymphomas (FCC), precursor B cell ALL; absent in maltomas

CD19: Pan B-cell marker

CD20 (L26): Pan B-cell marker; best B-cell marker on paraffin sections

CD22: Pan B-cell marker

CD45RA: Pan B-cell marker

Light chains: Demonstration of monotypic plasma cells (cryostat or paraffin sections)

T-cell markers

CD1a (T6): Thymocytes and Langerhans' cells

CD2: Pan T-cell marker

CD3: Pan T-cell marker

CD4: T cell and macrophages; T helper cells

CD5: T cell and subsets of B cells

CD7: Precursor T, T subsets, and natural killer cells. One of the first markers lost in CTCL

CD8: T subsets, NK cells, T suppressor cells

CD43 (Leu-22): T cells, macrophages, and granulocytes (e.g., chloromas)

TdT: Immature B cells and T cells

UCHL-1: Best Pan T-cell marker in paraffin sections

CALLA–Common acute lymphoblastic leukemia antigen
ALL–Acute lymphoblastic leukemia antigen

---

cal fibroxanthoma, leiomyosarcoma, malignant peripheral nerve sheath tumor, and neuroendocrine carcinoma. Whenever a lesion is suspected to be melanocytic it is important to apply a panel of antibodies, including antibodies positive for those lesions that enter into the differential diagnosis.

Although a large number of melanocytic markers have been developed, only two are widely used: S-100 protein and HMB-45. Neuron-specific enolase may on occasion also be useful. S-100 protein is by far the most sensitive marker for melanocytes, but it is not specific. It is also expressed in Schwann cells, astrocytes, Langerhans' cells, chondrocytes, and several other cell types. HMB-45 stains melanocytes in

Lymphoma Panels

Fixed tissue: suspected T-cell lymphoma
  UCHL-1:   to confirm T-cell phenotype
  CD30 (Ki-1):   in LYP or large-cell lymphoma
  L26:   to evaluate for presence of B cells suspected in B-cell lymphoma
  L26:   to confirm B-cell phenotype
  UCHL-1:   to evaluate for presence of T cells
  Light chains: demonstration of monotypic cells
Frozen tissue: suspected T-cell lymphoma
  CD2, CD4, CD8, CD7, CD43, CD1a, CD30
  Suspected B-cell lymphoma
  CD2, CD20, CD22, lambda, kappa

Poorly Differentiated Tumors

	Cytokeratins	S-100	HMB-45	LCA
Carcinoma	+	−	−	−
Melanoma	−	+	+	−
Lymphoma	−	−	−	+

Soft Tissue Tumors

	S-100	AE1/AE3	HHF-35	SM-ACT	Desmin	CD34	Other
Neural origin							
Schwannoma	+	−	−	−	−	−	−
Neurofibroma	+/−	−	−	−	−	−	−
Perineurioma	−	−	−	−	−	−	EMA+
MPNST		+/−	+/−	+/−	+/−	−	−
Muscle origin							
Smooth muscle	−	−	+/−	+	−	−	
Skeletal muscle	−	−	+/−	−	+	−	
Glomus tumor	−	−	+/−	+	−	−	
Fibrous origin							
DFSP	−	−	+/−	+/−	−	+	
FH	−	−	+/−	+/−	−	+/−	
Fibroma	−	−	−	−	−	−	
SFT	−	−	+/−	+/−	−	+	

AE1/AE3 = cytokeratin; HHF-35 = smooth muscle specific actin; SM-ACT = smooth muscle actin; EMA = epithelial membrane antigen; MPNST = malignant peripheral nerve sheath tumor; DFSP = dermatofibrosarcoma protuberans; FH = fibrous histiocytoma; SFT = solitary fibrous tumor.

several nevi, notably the blue nevi, Spitz nevi, and the intraepidermal components of atypical (dysplastic) nevi and some ordinary nevi, as well as many melanoma cells. It is not entirely specific for melanocytes. Positive staining for this marker has been observed in a variety of non-melanocytic lesions, including angiomyolipoma, some breast cancers, and gliosarcomas. It should be noted that the vast majority of desmoplastic melanomas are negative for HMB-45. Almost of all of them, however, stain for S-100 protein.

SOFT TISSUE NEOPLASMS

Immunohistology is essential in the evaluation of poorly differentiated soft tissue neoplasms. The main role is to confirm suspected histogenesis or differentiation. A list of markers relevant in the workup of sarcomas is provided in Table App-10.

SMALL-CELL NEOPLASMS

Many different neoplasms can assume a small cell phenotype. This includes metastatic small-cell carcinoma, cutaneous neuroendocrine (Merkel cell) carcinomas, small-cell sweat gland carcinoma, sarcomas such as ES/PNET, neuroblastoma, or alveolar rhabdomyosarcoma, small-cell lymphomas, and small-cell melanomas. Immunophenotypic studies are paramount in the differential diagnosis of small-cell neoplasms (Table App-11).

CYTOGENETICS

The main application of solid tumor cytogenetics in dermatopathology is in the evaluation of sarcomas, since a surprising number of sarcomas have characteristic karyotypic abnormalities and gene rearrangements.[31] A list of diagnostically useful cytogenetic alterations in cutaneous sarcomas is provided in Table App-12. If fresh tissue is available, conventional karyotypes may be obtained. The development of fluorescent in situ hybridization allows cytogenetic analysis also on archival material.

ELECTRON MICROSCOPY

The main applications of electron microscopy to diagnostic dermatopathology is in the field of congenital bullous disorders, certain storage diseases, and tumor pathology. Ultrastructural studies are the gold standard for the localization of the cleavage site in the disease group of epidermolysis bullosa congenita. Electron microscopy is very helpful in identifying intracellularly stored or deposited material, such as intralysosomal electron-dense lamellar bodies in Fabre's disease, or characteristic fibrils in amyloid.

In the differential diagnosis of neoplastic disorders, ultrastructural studies play a role in the identification of Birbeck granules in Langerhans' cell proliferations. They may also reveal useful information in a number of other neoplasms, such as melanosomes in melanoma, desmosomes and

Small-Cell Neoplasms

	LCA	PAS	013	Des	CK	CK20	NSE	NF	S-100
Small-cell CA	−	−	−	−	+	−	+/−	−	−
Merkel-cell CA	−	−	−	−	+	+	+/−	−	−
Small-cell sweat gland CA	−	−	−	−	+	−	?	?	+
Ewing's/PNET	−	+	+	−	+/−	−	+/−	+/−	−
Alveolar rhabdomyosarcoma	−	+/−	−	+	−	−	+/−	−	−
Neuroblastoma	−	−	−	−	−	−	+	+	−
Lymphoma	+	−	−	−	−	−	−	−	−
Melanoma	−	−	−	−	−	−	+/−	−	+

LCA = leukocyte common antigen; PAS = periodic acid–Schiff stain; 013 = CD99; DES = desmin; CK = cytokeratin; CK20 = cytokeratin 20; NSE = neuron specific enolase; NF = neurofilament; S-100 = S-100 protein.

tonofilaments in epithelial tumors, myofibrils in myogenic tumors, electron-dense core granules in neuroendocrine neoplasms, perinuclear bundles of intermediate filaments in epithelioid sarcoma, Weibel-Palade bodies in angiosarcoma, or rhomboid crystals in alveolar soft part sarcoma.

POLARISCOPIC EXAMINATION

Polariscopic examination is useful in evaluating certain foreign material such as suture material, wood splinters, beryllium, zirconium, or silica. It is also helpful to highlight some endogenous deposits, such as uric acid crystals in gout or oxalate crystals.

It should be used routinely in the evaluation of granulomatous tissue reactions. It is an ancillary technique in the Congo red stain to evaluate for amyloid.

Cytogenetics of Cutaneous Neoplasms

Tumor	Karyotypic Abnormality	Genes
Melanoma	Heterogenous abnormality, various deletions (e.g., 1, 6, 9)	?
DFSP	Ring chromosome (17, 22), trisomy 5	?
Alveolar rhabdomyosarcoma	t(2;13)(p36;q14)	PAX3-FKHR
	t(1;13)(p36;q14)	PAX7-FKHR
Embryonal rhabdomyosarcoma	+2q, +8, +20, del 1	?
ES/PNET	t(11;22)(q24;q12)	FLI-1-EWS
Clear cell sarcoma	t(11;22)(q13;q12)	ATF-1-EWS
Neuroblastoma	del (1p)	?
MPNST	+1	?
Lipoma (ordinary)	Rearrangements of 12q, 14-15, 6p, 13q	HMGC-1
Spindle cell lipoma	Rearrangements of 16q, 13q	?
Giant cell tumor of tendon sheath	+7, +5	?

DFSP = dermatofibrosarcoma protuberans; ES/PNET = Ewing's sarcoma/primitive neuroectodermal tumor; MPNST = malignant peripheral nerve sheath tumor.

MOLECULAR BIOLOGIC TECHNIQUES FOR THE DIAGNOSIS OF CUTANEOUS LYMPHOMAS

Gary S. Wood

This section focuses on the principal molecular biologic methods that have been developed to study cutaneous lymphoid infiltrates. It is presented as a review divided into six parts: (1) antigen receptor genes, (2) Southern blot analysis, (3) gene amplification techniques, (4) major findings, (5) clinical applications, and (6) conclusions.

ANTIGEN RECEPTOR GENES

Immunoglobulin (Ig) molecules are the antigen-specific receptor of B cells.[31] Each Ig molecule is a protein heterodimer consisting of two heavy chains and two light chains linked by disulfide bridges. Each B cell and its clonal progeny express Ig molecules containing only one of two possible types of Ig light chains (kappa or lambda). This is known as Ig light chain restriction. T-cell receptors (TCRs) are glycoproteins, composed of two possible combinations of heterodimers usually linked by disulfide bridges, in association with the CD3 complex.[31] Four different protein chains of the human TCR are involved in antigen binding: α, β, γ, and δ. The TCR is expressed on the cell surface of lymphocytes as an $\alpha\beta$ or $\gamma\delta$ heterodimer and is responsible for antigen recognition. Each Ig and TCR protein chain consists of three to four distinct regions encoded by gene segments called variable (V), diversity (D), joining (J), and constant (C). Whereas V, J, and C segments are found in each gene, D segments are only present in the TCRβ and δ genes. The V, D, and J genes are involved in forming the variable region of the Ig and TCR proteins. This region includes the antigen recognition site. The C region is responsible for other functions, such as signal transduction, oligomerization, secretion, passage across physiologic barriers, and interaction with other immune molecules like complement and Fc receptors.

During maturation of T cells and B cells from hematopoietic progenitor cells into functionally active lymphocytes, antigen receptor genes are assembled from one segment each of the V, D, J, and C gene sets through a series of DNA recombination events, collectively referred to as gene rearrangement, followed by posttranscriptional splicing and translation. The VDJ joining is mediated by specific enzymes collectively referred to as recombinases, and is orchestrated by recombinase activation gene-1 (RAG-1) and RAG-2. These two genes are coexpressed at substantial levels only in primary lymphoid tissue and in cell lines that resemble precursor lymphocytes. The result is the creation of one intact, continuous V-, (D) J-, coding sequence at an antigen receptor gene locus. This is subsequently joined to a C-region coding segment by posttranscriptional splicing of mRNA. The diversity of Igs and TCRs is owing to the many possible combinations among the different gene segments. In addition, the rearrangement itself creates diversity by small deletions or insertions of nucleotides at the V-D, D-J, and V-J

junctions. The random nucleotide insertions are known as N regions. Consequently, the amino acid sequences at the junctions of V, D, and J segments demonstrate extreme hypervariability.

During thymic development, T lymphocytes are generated by several molecular events and by positive and negative selection. The present model of thymic T-cell development suggests that hematopoietic stem cells enter the thymus through the cortex with their TCR genes in the germline (unrearranged) configuration. In addition to the acquisition of T-cell differentiation antigens on their surface, many T lymphocytes undergo rearrangement of the TCRγ and δ chain genes. Some of these T cells then express the TCR$\gamma\delta$ protein heterodimer throughout their lives. Others undergo subsequent rearrangement of their TCRα and TCRβ genes, and replace their TCR$\gamma\delta$ heterodimer with a TCR$\alpha\beta$ heterodimer. TCRδ gene rearrangements are frequently deleted during TCRα gene rearrangement because the δ gene is embedded within the α gene. Although its expression is suppressed, the rearranged TCRγ chain remains intact within the genome.

During their development, B cells also undergo a hierarchy of antigen receptor gene rearrangements. The heavy chain (IgH) genes are rearranged first. If a productive rearrangement occurs, then the kappa light chain genes are rearranged. If these genes are abortive, then the lambda light chain genes are rearranged. Because kappa rearrangements are successful more often than not, there is usually a 2:1 ratio of B cells expressing kappa versus lambda light chains. As with T cells, if a B cell fails to rearrange its Ig genes successfully, then it is deleted via apoptosis.

As B cells mature, they progress through a series of phenotypic and genetic alterations involving Ig genes.[32] When a naive B cell migrates to the lymph node from the marrow, it is IgM^+IgD^+ and has functional IgH gene rearrangements; however, the V_H region within the rearranged Ig gene retains its germline sequence and has not yet undergone any of the V_H somatic point mutations involved in the antigen selection phase of B-cell differentiation that results in a better fit between antibody and antigen. Once the naive B cell is exposed to its corresponding antigen, it enters the germinal center where it loses IgD expression and undergoes successive rounds of V_H somatic point mutation and proliferation. Once this process is completed, the B cell enters the postgerminal center memory B-cell phase in which it has stable V_H point mutations and is either IgM^+ or has switched to another Ig heavy chain isotype. These phenotypic and genetic alterations will allow us to determine the differentiation (or point of maturational arrest) exhibited by B-cell lymphoma tumor clones. In addition, the distribution of point mutations within antigen-relevant (e.g., complementarily determining) versus antigen-irrelevant (e.g., framework) regions of the V_H gene allows us to determine the degree to which these B-cell clones have been antigen-selected.

864

Molecular Biologic Techniques for the Detection of Cutaneous T-Cell Lymphoma

Method	Sensitivity	Time	Comments
Southern blot analysis	10^{-2}	1 to 2 weeks	Not optimal for small specimens or sparse CTCL infiltrates
Non–tumor-specific PCR clonality assays	10^{-3}–10^{-4}	A few days	Reasonable compromise among sensitivity, specificity, simplicity, and rapidity of assays
Tumor-specific PCR clonality assays	10^{-5}–10^{-6}	Initially 1 to several weeks to obtain tumor-specific oligonucleotides; thereafter, a few days to analyze new specimens	Requires diagnostic index specimen from which tumor-specific primers and/or probes are made; best suited for detailed case studies

SOUTHERN BLOT ANALYSIS

In this and the following sections, the most common molecular biologic assays for assessing B-cell and T-cell clonality are described. Key features of these assays are summarized in Table App-13.

Southern blot analysis is an assay that detects rearrangement of Ig and TCR genes from their germline configuration.[31,33] As generally performed, however, it offers no information about clone-specific nucleotide sequence or the particular V, D, J, and C segments involved in the rearrangement. The sensitivity limit of this method is about 5 percent, that is, the percentage of clonal DNA in the DNA sample has to be at least 5 percent. In nonlymphatic tissues, such as skin in which a considerable amount of DNA is contributed by various cell types, this limitation can be particularly problematic.

Figure App-27 summarizes the most important steps involved in this procedure and Fig. App-28 illustrates representative results. Key factors in Southern blot analysis include restriction enzymes, hybridization probes, and the stringency of hybridization and wash conditions. Restriction enzymes are bacteria-derived endonucleases that cleave double-stranded DNA at or near a specific nucleotide sequence recognized by that enzyme. At present, more than 100 different restriction enzymes are available. The incubation of genomic DNA with one of these enzymes results in DNA restriction fragments of many lengths. These fragments are separated according to their length using agarose gel electrophoresis. Separated DNA fragments are transferred by vacuum or capillary action onto a nylon membrane. The membrane is incubated with a DNA fragment (probe) that is known to hybridize with (be complementary to) the sequence of interest. Radiolabeled IgH and TCR-β probes are the ones used most commonly to investigate the clonality of Ig and TCR gene rearrangements in lymphoproliferative disorders. Autoradiography is used to detect the band(s) where the radiolabeled probe has hybridized and to compare these bands to known germline and positive control bands. The number of bands varies depending on the restriction enzyme used. The positions of these bands reflect the difference in size of the rearranged DNA fragment(s) compared with the fragment(s) characteristically produced from DNA in the unrearranged or germline configuration of the relevant gene. There is no combination of a single restriction enzyme with a single probe that detects all corresponding gene rearrangements. Thus, more than one restriction enzyme digest is usually studied by Southern blot analysis.

During recent years, a tremendous amount of information concerning the clonality of cutaneous lymphoproliferative disorders has been derived by Southern blot analysis of immunoglobulin and TCR gene rearrangements. The skin diseases that have been shown to contain

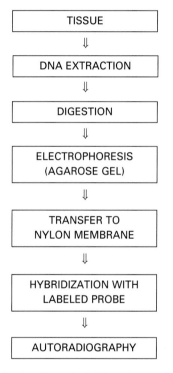

FIGURE APP-27 Southern blot analysis. The major steps involved in Southern blot analysis of TCR and Ig gene rearrangements in genomic DNA extracted from lesional tissues are summarized.

dominant monoclonal or oligoclonal lymphoid cells by means of this technique are listed in Table App-14.

POLYMERASE CHAIN REACTION (PCR)-BASED ASSAYS

PCR is a procedure in which small regions of DNA can be amplified geometrically in vitro by means of a thermostable DNA polymerase purified from the bacterium *Thermophilus acquaticus* (so-called *Taq* polymerase).[31,33,34] Short fragments of single-stranded DNA known as oligonucleotide primers are used in repeated cycles of heating and cooling. This allows denaturation of the double-stranded template DNA into single-stranded DNA, annealing of the primers to complementary sequences on the single-stranded template DNA, and synthesis of new copies of the template DNA by primer extension.

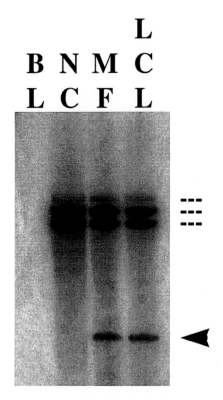

FIGURE APP-28 Detection of clonal TCRβ gene rearrangements by Southern blot analysis. Shown is an autoradiogram of genomic DNA digested with *Bgl* II restriction endonuclease and probed with a radiolabeled Jβ1/Jβ2 DNA probe. Germline bands are marked with dashes and clonally rearranged bands are marked with an arrow. BL; blank lane; NC, negative control; MF, mycosis fungoides; LCL, CD30+ large cell lymphoma from the same patient showing an identical clonal band. This was confirmed by nucleotide sequencing.

TCR-Based PCR Clonality Assays

As a result of genetic events occurring during their thymic development, many T lymphocytes expressing the αβ heterodimer also contain clonal TCRγ rearrangements.[34,35] Therefore, molecular approaches for the analysis of clonality may focus on either TCRβ or TCRγ rearrangements. In the TCRβ gene, only the V and C genes contain consensus sequences that are highly conserved and thus the most suitable as tem-

TABLE APP-14

Cutaneous Lymphoproliferative Disorders: T-Cell and B-Cell Clonality as Determined by Southern Blot Analysis

Disorder	Dominant Clonality[a]
Mycosis fungoides/Sézary syndrome	T cell[b]
Other cutaneous lymphomas	T cell
Regressing atypical histiocytosis	T cell
Granulomatous slack skin	T cell
Lymphomatoid papulosis	T cell > none
Pityriasis lichenoides and varioliformis acuta	T cell
Angioimmunoblastic lymphadenopathy	T cell > none
Malignant histiocytosis	T cell > B cell
Cutaneous B-cell lymphomas	B cell
Cutaneous lymphoid hyperplasia	None > B cell > T cell

[a]Usually dominant clonality is monoclonal but in some cases it can be biclonal or oligoclonal.
[b]Some early patch/thin plaque lesions lack dominant clonality by Southern blot analysis owing to the limited sensitivity of this assay.

plates for PCR consensus primers capable of detecting the vast majority of TCRβ gene rearrangements. Because these V and C regions are separated by large introns within the rearranged gene, genomic DNA cannot be used for PCR amplification of the TCRβ rearrangement. Instead, the target sequence must be transcribed from TCRβ mRNA into TCRβ cDNA. These extra steps are a relative disadvantage of methods involving TCRβ amplification because handling RNA is much more complicated than handling DNA owing to its fast degradation by ubiquitous RNase. Attempts to circumvent this problem by using Vβ and Jβ consensus primers have been less than fully successful because of the sequence diversity of these regions. In contrast, conserved regions in the Vγ and Jγ gene segments are close together (400 to 700 base pairs) in the rearranged TCRγ gene. This allows the use of genomic DNA for PCR amplification of TCRγ gene rearrangements. Furthermore, the relatively high degree of homology among various Vγ segments and among Jγ segments means that only a small number of different consensus primers are required to amplify most TCRγ gene rearrangements. Therefore, several PCR-based T-cell clonality assays focus on the rearranged TCRγ gene.

After amplification using Vγ and Jγ primers, the TCRγ PCR products must be screened for dominant clonal TCR gene rearrangements. At least three methods have been used to accomplish this. These include DGGE, TGGE, and cRNA electrophoresis.[34,35] Figure App-29 shows the key steps of TCRγ PCR in combination with DGGE. Representative results are illustrated in Fig. App-30. DGGE involves the electrophoresis of PCR products in a polyacrylamide gel that contains an increasing gradient of chemical denaturants, specifically formamide and urea. This type of electrophoresis separates the PCR products according to their nucleotide sequence as well as their size. The gradient in the gel causes local denaturation of domains within double-stranded DNA fragments and the resultant formation of melted, single-stranded DNA domains at various points along the gradient in the gel. This alteration reduces the mobility of the DNA fragment in the gel, causing all fragments of identical sequence to accumulate at the same position in the gel. Polyclonal PCR products appear as a diffuse smear, whereas bands are seen in the case of a dominant clone constituting at least 0.1 to 1 percent of the total specimen DNA. The sensitivity threshold depends on the background content of polyclonal T cells in the specimen. TGGE is similar in principle to DGGE, except that a gradient of temperature rather than chemical denaturants provides the conditions for the sequence-dependent melting of PCR products. A third approach to the separation of TCRγ products begins with their transcription into cRNA. The cRNA frag-

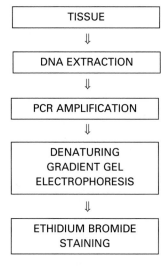

FIGURE APP-29 PCR/DGGE. The major steps involved in the amplification and separation of TCRγ gene rearrangements in genomic DNA extracted from lesional tissues are summarized.

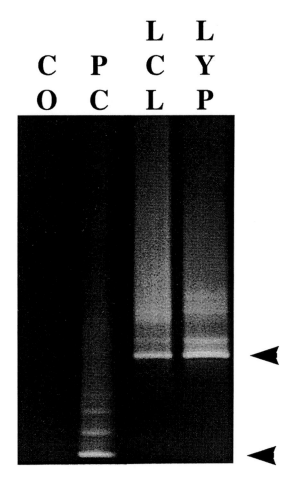

FIGURE APP-30   PCR/DGGE. Detection of clonal TCRγ gene rearrangements by PCR combined with DGGE. Shown is a photograph of an ethidium bromide–stained gel after DGGE of TCRγ PCR products that were amplified using consensus primers for Vγ 1–8 and Jγ 1–2. CO, carry over negative control; PC, positive control; LCL, CD30+ large cell lymphoma; LYP, lymphomatoid papulosis from the same patient showing a matching clonal band (upper arrow) indicating an identical nucleotide sequence. The lower arrow shows the position of the clonal band in the PC lane.

ments then are separated by electrophoresis in a polyacrylamide gel. Because single-stranded cRNA displays multiple conformational polymorphisms depending on its sequence, a dominant clone constituting at least 0.01 to 0.1 percent of total specimen cells can be detected by the presence of discrete bands. These bands represent the cRNA conformational polymorphisms of dominant TCRγ gene rearrangements.

In addition to these TCRγ gene-based methods, non–tumor-specific PCR assays have been developed for the detection of clonal TCRβ rearrangements. One of these methods involves reverse transcription of TCRβ mRNA into cDNA followed by multiple separate PCRs, each specific for TCRβ gene rearrangements involving one or two of the 24 known Vβ families. PCR products are then electrophoresed in a special agarose gel. The presence of a sharp band indicates a dominant clonal TCRβ gene rearrangement. The sensitivity of this method ranges from 0.01 to 10 percent of total cDNA, depending on whether the clone is diluted by nonlymphoid or polyclonal T-cell cDNA, respectively.

Ig-Based PCR Clonality Assays

PCR assays involving IgH gene rearrangements have been used to assess the clonality of B-cell lymphoproliferative disorders.[36] Strategies range from a single V_H/J_H consensus primer set, to nested consensus primers, to a single consensus J_H primer combined with a set of V_H con-

sensus primers, each specific for a different V_H family or subfamily (V_H1, 2, 3, 4a, 4b, 5, and 6). PCR products then are electrophoresed through gels designed to produce a discrete band when a dominant clonal IgH rearrangement is present and diffuse smears when it is not. As with TCR-based PCR assays, these Ig-based PCR methods are more sensitive than genomic Southern blot analysis of Ig gene rearrangements.

Tumor-Specific PCR Clonality Assays

These techniques depend on the strategy of isolating and sequencing the monoclonal antigen receptor gene rearrangement from a diagnostic specimen and then using this tumor-specific dominant sequence to generate tumor-specific probes or PCR primers.[34] These tools can be applied to detect tumor involvement in additional nondiagnostic tissue samples from the same patient; however, they are not useful for studying other patients because they are specific for only one unique tumor clone. These tumor-specific assays use several different technical approaches that target various antigen receptor genes. A recently developed PCR-RNase protection assay (PCR-RPA) has the advantage that, although it is clone-specific, it requires neither analysis of nucleotide sequences nor synthesis of tumor-clone specific DNA primers or probes. It involves analysis of TCRγ gene rearrangements and has a sensitivity of 0.001 percent or 1 of 10^5 cells.

PCR Assays Other than Clonality

In addition to their use for detecting dominant clonality, genomic Southern blot and PCR assays can be used to study other tumor cell characteristics such as whether they contain the t(14;18) translocation (common among follicular B-cell lymphomas), the t(2;5) translocation (common among lymph node–based CD30+ anaplastic large cell lymphomas), or HTLV-1 retrovirus (a defining feature of adult T-cell leukemia/lymphoma).[33]

MOLECULAR BIOLOGIC FINDINGS

Molecular biologic studies combined with immunophenotypic analyses have significantly advanced our understanding of cutaneous lymphoproliferative disorders in recent years. CTCL has been shown to be a neoplasm of mature CD4+ memory T cells belonging to the skin-associated lymphoid tissue (SALT), which includes those lymphocytes and antigen-presenting cells that traffic between the skin and peripheral lymph nodes.[33–35,37] Using PCR-based methods, the monoclonality of early CTCL as well as advanced CTCL has been established. In fact, PCR techniques have allowed the recognition that some cases of chronic, nonspecific dermatitis harbor occult T-cell clones. These cases are referred to as "clonal dermatitis."[35] Some of these patients have progressed to overt CTCL, indicating that at least some cases of clonal dermatitis represent a precursor to CTCL. Molecular staging studies have shown that small numbers of CTCL cells can be found throughout the body in samples of morphologically normal lymph node, marrow, and blood even in early-stage IA disease.[38] This suggests that tumor cells can traffic throughout the SALT system at low levels and that CTCL is a neoplasm of a T-cell circuit rather than a particular tissue. Studies of diseases associated with CTCL, such as large cell lymphoma, lymphomatoid papulosis, and Hodgkin's disease, have shown that these diseases share a common clonal origin when they arise in the same patient.[39] Taken together, these findings allow us to conceptualize of CTCL and associated diseases as an array of lymphoproliferative disorders sharing a common monoclonal ancestry beginning with a single mature SALT T cell that undergoes one or more genetic alterations resulting in clonal dermatitis, then progression to overt CTCL, followed by additional somatic mutations responsible for creating subclones of the original tumor which manifest themselves clinically as advanced-stage CTCL and other CTCL-associated diseases.

Similarly, CBCL has been shown to be a monoclonal B-cell neoplasm of the skin that in some cases is preceded by cutaneous lymphoid hyperplasia (CLH)—a clinicopathologically benign lymphoid infiltrate usually containing immunophenotypically polyclonal B cells.[39–42] Molecular biologic studies have shown that some CLH cases harbor occult dominant B-cell clones and may progress to overt CBCL containing the same dominant clone. In aggregate, these studies suggest that CLH, clonal CLH, and CBCL exist as clinicopathologically defined points along a continuum of cutaneous B-cell lymphoproliferative disease.

CLINICAL APPLICATIONS

Diagnosis

The detection of dominant clonal lymphoid populations has been used to confirm a suspected diagnosis of lymphoma in patients whose clinicopathologic features were suggestive, but not diagnostic. The rationale for this approach is based on two observations. First, well-developed lymphoma lesions are clearly monoclonal tumors. Second, with rare exception, dominant lymphoid clones have not been reported in unequivocally inflammatory infiltrates or in normal tissues.[31,33,35,43] For example, the molecular biologic demonstration of dominant T-cell clonality has been used to establish or confirm a diagnosis of CTCL in patients with patch-type MF, large plaque parapsoriasis, idiopathic erythroderma, and follicular mucinosis.[13] In some instances, Southern blot analysis has been sufficient, whereas in other cases PCR-based techniques have been required to detect the dominant T-cell clone. This has been especially true for very small specimens or for those in which the neoplastic T-cell clone was diluted excessively by normal cell constituents, reactive T cells, or a combination of both cell types.

Although it is generally true that TCR gene rearrangements are indicative of T-cell lymphomas and Ig gene rearrangements are indicative of B-cell lymphomas, some lymphomas may exhibit both.[31,33] Therefore, it is helpful to supplement gene rearrangement studies with immunophenotypic data in order to achieve the clearest possible interpretation of lineage and clonality during immunodiagnostic workup of an unknown case. In addition, it is important to emphasize that the demonstration of a monoclonal lymphoid population, per se, cannot be equated with the diagnosis of lymphoma. Clinicopathologic correlation is essential. There are several clinically benign lymphoproliferative disorders that are known to contain dominant T-cell or B-cell clones in a variable proportion of cases. These include lymphomatoid papulosis, pityriasis lichenoides, and cutaneous lymphoid hyperplasia.[42]

Staging

Because molecular biologic analysis of Ig and TCR gene rearrangements is significantly more sensitive than light microscopy for the detection of tumor cells, molecular biologic methods have increased the sensitivity of lymphoma staging. For example, among eight lymph nodes diagnosed as showing only reactive, dermatopathic changes by light microscopy, six were positive for CTCL by Southern blot analysis.[34] Southern blot analysis has also proven superior to light microscopy in detecting involvement of the peripheral blood in CTCL.[34] PCR-based techniques have further enhanced this sensitivity and have detected sites of involvement missed by Southern blot analysis. PCR techniques have detected CTCL involvement in microscopically uninvolved extracutaneous tissues, and even in clinically normal-appearing skin containing only very sparse, nonspecific lymphoid infiltrates histopathologically.[37,43,44] The impressive sensitivity of molecular biologic analysis for detecting dominant Ig and TCR gene rearrangements (about 10^{-2} for Southern blot analysis and 10^{-3} to 10^{-6} for various PCR techniques) raises important questions regarding clinical relevance. For example, although we know that histopathologically detectable lymph node involvement is a poor prognostic sign in CTCL, we do not yet know the clinical relevance of histopathologically occult involvement detected solely by molecular biologic means.[42] Yet, it is known that remissions of long duration can be induced in many but not all patients with clinical stage I CTCL. In addition, some studies have suggested that aggressive therapy initiated early in the course of disease might improve survival and chances for cure. Prospective molecular biologic staging of early CTCL might help define subgroups of patients most likely to benefit from various therapeutic regimens or those with the best prognosis regardless of therapy.

Disease Monitoring

In addition to their use in the initial diagnosis and staging of cutaneous lymphoma patients, molecular biologic techniques have also been used to monitor the response of the disease to treatment. For example, it has been shown that the skin can serve as a reservoir of clinically occult residual disease in CTCL.[43]

CONCLUSIONS

It is apparent that, in addition to their value in the early diagnosis and staging of cutaneous lymphomas, molecular biologic assays are valuable in monitoring the response to therapy, detecting early relapse, and improving understanding of the compartmentalization and trafficking of tumor cells. In order to reap the full clinical benefit from this new information, however, it will be important to perform prospective long-term studies designed to determine the clinical significance of molecular biologic data. In addition, the complexity of cutaneous lymphoproliferative disorders dictates that molecular biologic clonality data should never be interpreted in a vacuum. In skin disease, dominant clonality does not always imply clinical malignancy. The proper diagnosis of CTCL and other cutaneous lymphoproliferative diseases requires the thoughtful integration of molecular biologic data with the clinicopathologic and immunophenotypic findings.

GENERAL REFERENCES AND RECOMMENDED FURTHER READING

Fitzpatrick TB, Eisen AZ, Wolff K, et al: *Dermatology in General Medicine*, 4th ed. New York: McGraw-Hill, 1993, pp. 87–473.

Goldsmith LA: *Physiology, Biochemistry and Molecular Biology of the Skin*, 2nd ed. New York: Oxford University Press, 1991, pp. 1–1529.

Leigh IM, Lane EB, Watt FM: *The Keratinocyte Handbook*. Cambridge: University Press, 1994, p. 566

REFERENCES

1. Bancroft JD, Cook HC: *Manual of Histological Techniques and Their Diagnostic Application.* Edinburgh: Churchill Livingston, 1994.

2. Johnson WC: Histochemistry of the skin, in Spicer S (ed): *Histochemistry in Pathologic Diagnosis.* New York: Marcel Dekker, 1984, 665–694.

3. Rosai J: Special techniques in surgical pathology, in Rosai J (ed): *Ackerman's Surgical Pathology*, 8th ed. St Louis: Mosby, 1996, 29–62.

4. Rodriguez HA, McGavran MH: A modified dopa reaction for the diagnosis and investigation of pigment cells. *Am J Pathol* 52:219–227, 1969.

5. Beutner EH, Chorzelski TP, Kumar V: *Immunopathology of the Skin*, 3rd ed. New York: Wiley, 1987.

6. Ceballos P, Jimenez-Acosta F, Penneys NS: Immunohistochemical techniques in non-neoplastic conditions. *Sem Dermatol* 8:276–282, 1989.

7. Gammon WR, Fine JD, Forbers M, Briggaman RA: Immunofluorescence on split skin for the detection and differentiation of basement membrane zone autoantibodies. *J Am Acad Dermatol* 27:79–87, 1992.

8. Beutner EH, Jordan RE, Chorzelski TP: The immunopathology of pemphigus and pemphigoid. *J Invest Dermatol* 51:63–80, 1968.

9. Farmer ER: Subepidermal bullous diseases. *J Cutan Pathol* 12:316–321, 1985.

10. Helm KF, Peters MS: Immunodermatology update: The immunologically-mediated vesiculobullous diseases. *Mayo Clin Proc* 66:187–202, 1991.

11. Gately LE III, Nesbitt LT Jr: Update on immunofluorescent testing in bullous diseases and lupus erythematosus. *Dermatol Clin* 12:133–142, 1994.

12. Mutasim DF, Pelc NJ, Supapannachart N: Established methods in the investigation of bullous disease. *Dermatol Clin* 11:399–418, 1993.

13. Pardo RJ, Pennesy NS: Location of basement membrane type IV collagen beneath subepidermal bullous diseases. *J Cutan Pathol* 17:336–341, 1990.

14. Braverman IM, Yen A: Demonstration of immune complexes in spontaneous and histamine-induced lesions and in normal skin of patients with leukocytoclastic vasculitis. *J Invest Dermatol* 64:105–112, 1975.

15. Faile-Kuyper Eh Dela, Kater L, Koviker CJ, et al: IgA-deposits in cutaneous blood vessel walls and mesangium in Henoch-Schoenlein syndrome. *Lancet* 1:892–893, 1973.

16. Knowles DM, Chadburn A, Inghirami G: Immunophenotypic markers useful in the diagnosis and classification of hematopoietic neoplasms, in Knowles DM (ed): *Neoplastic Hematopathology*. Baltimore: Williams & Wilkins, 1992.

17. Burke J: Malignant lymphomas of the skin: Their differentiation from lymphoid and non-lymphoid cutaneous infiltrates that simulate lymphoma. *Sem Diagn Pathol* 2:169–182, 1985.

18. Perksin SL, Kjeldsberg CR: Immunophenotyping of lymphomas and leukemias in paraffin-embedded tissues. *Am J Clin Pathol* 99:362–373, 1993.

19. Kaplan EH, Leslie WT: Cutaneous T-cell lymphomas. *Curr Opin Oncol* 5:812–818, 1993.

20. Filippa DA, Ladanyi M, Wollner N, et al: CD30 (Ki-1) positive malignant lymphomas: Clinical, immunophenotypic, histologic, and genetic characteristics and differences with Hodgkin's disease. *Blood* 87:2905–2917, 1996.

21. Emile JF, Wechsler J, Brousse N, et al: Langerhans' cell histiocytosis: Definitive diagnosis with the use of monoclonal antibody 010 on routinely paraffin-embedded samples. *Am J Surg Pathol* 19:636–641, 1995.

22. Ratnam KV, Khor CJL, Su WPD: Leukemia cutis. *Dematol Clin* 12:419–431, 1994.

23. Battifora H: Diagnostic uses of antibodies to keratins. *Prog Surg Pathol* 8:1–15, 1988.

24. Thomas P, Battifora H: Keratins vs. epithelial membrane antigen in tumor diagnosis: An immunohistochemical comparison of five monoclonal antibodies. *Hum Pathol* 18:728–734, 1987.

25. Wick MR, Swanson PE, Ritter JH, et al: The immunohistology of cutaneous neoplasia: A practical perspective. *J Cutan Pathol* 20:481–497, 1993.

26. Busam KJ, Barnhill RL: Biopsies, tissue processing and special studies, in Barnhill RL (ed): *Pathology of Melanocytic Nevi and Malignant Melanoma*. Boston: Butterworth-Heineman, 1996, 13–20.

27. Ruiter D, Broecker E-B: Immunohistochemistry in the evaluation of melanocytic tumors. *J Clin Pathol* 38:7–15, 1985.

28. Miettinen M: Immunohistochemistry of soft tissue tumors: Possibilities and limitations in surgical pathology. *Annu Pathol* 5:1–36, 1990.

29. Ladanyi M: The emerging molecular genetics of sarcoma translocations. *Diagn Mol Pathol* 4:162–173, 1995.

30. Sklar J: Antigen receptor genes, in Knowles DM (ed): *Neoplastic Hematopathology*, 1st ed. Baltimore: Williams & Wilkins, 1992, 215–244.

31. Tamaru J, Hummel M, Marafioti T, et al: Burkitt's lymphomas express V_H genes with a moderate number of antigen-selected somatic mutations. *Am J Pathol* 147:1398–1407, 1995.

32. Medeiros LJ, Bagg A, Cossman J: Application of molecular genetics to the diagnosis of hematopoietic neoplasms, in Knowles DM (ed): *Neoplastic Hematopathology*, 1st ed. Baltimore: Williams & Wilkins, 1992, 263–298.

33. Wood GS: Cutaneous lymphoproliferative disorders: Strategies for molecular biological analysis and their major findings. *Springer Semin Immunopathol* 13:387–399, 1992.

34. Wood GS, Tung RM, Haeffner AC, et al: Detection of clonal T-cell receptor γ gene rearrangements in early mycosis fungoides/Sezary syndrome by polymerase chain reaction and denaturing gradient gel electrophoresis (PCR/DGGE). *J Invest Dermatol* 103:34–41, 1994.

35. Ramasamy I, Brisco M, Morley A: Improved PCR method for detecting monoclonal immunoglobulin heavy chain rearrangement in B cell neoplasms. *J Clin Pathol* 45:770–775, 1992.

36. Veelken H, Sklar JL, Wood GS: Detection of low-level tumor cell trafficking to allergic contact dermatitis induced by mechlorethamine in patients with mycosis fungoides. *J Invest Dermatol* 106:685–688, 1996.

37. Veelken H, Wood GS, Sklar J: Molecular staging of cutaneous T cell lymphoma: Evidence for systemic involvement in early disease. *J Invest Dermatol* 104:889–894, 1995.

38. Wood GS, Crooks CF, Uluer AZ: Lymphomatoid papulosis and associated cutaneous lymphoproliferative disorders exhibit a common clonal origin. *J Invest Dermatol* 105:51–55, 1995.

39. Wood GS, Ngan B-Y, Tung R, et al: Clonal rearrangement of immunoglobulin genes and progression to B-cell lymphoma in cutaneous lymphoid hyperplasia. *Am J Pathol* 135:13–19, 1989.

40. Rijlaarsdam U, Bakels V, van Oostveen JW, et al: Demonstration of clonal immunoglobulin gene rearrangements in cutaneous B-cell lymphomas and pseudo-B-cell lymphomas: Differential diagnostic and pathogenetic aspects. *J Invest Dermatol* 99:749–754, 1992.

41. Hammer E, Sangueza O, Suwanjindar P, et al: Immunophenotypic and genotypic analysis in cutaneous lymphoid hyperplasia. *J Am Acad Dermatol* 28:426–433, 1993.

42. Wood GS: The benign and malignant cutaneous lymphoproliferative disorders including mycosis fungoides, in Knowles DM (ed): *Neoplastic Hematopathology*, 1st ed. Baltimore: Williams & Wilkins, 1992, 917–952.

43. Lessin SR, Benoit BM, Jaworsky C, et al: Skin as a reservoir of minimal residual disease in cutaneous T cell lymphoma after complete clinical response to biological response modifier therapy. *J Invest Dermatol* 100:507, 1993.

44. Volkenandt M, Soyer HP, Kerl H, et al: Development of a highly specific and sensitive molecular probe for detection of cutaneous lymphoma. *J Invest Dermatol* 97:137, 1991.

INDEX

Page numbers followed by f or t indicate illustrations or tables.

871

ISBN 0-07-005726-5

90000>